Postgraduate Textbook of
Clinical Orthopaedics

Postgraduate Textbook of
Clinical Orthopaedics

EDITED BY

NIGEL H. HARRIS MA FRCS
Honorary Consultant Orthopaedic Surgeon
St Mary's Hospital
London
Orthopaedic Surgeon to
The Football Association and
Arsenal Football Club
London

AND

ROLFE BIRCH MChir FRCS
Orthopaedic Surgeon
The Royal National Orthopaedic Hospital Trust
London and Stanmore

FOREWORD BY

CHRISTOPHER L. COLTON
MBBS FRCS FRCS(Ed)

SECOND EDITION

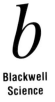

Blackwell
Science

© 1995 by
Blackwell Science Ltd
Editorial Offices:
Osney Mead, Oxford OX2 0EL
25 John Street, London WC1N 2BL
23 Ainslie Place, Edinburgh EH3 6AJ
238 Main Street, Cambridge
  Massachusetts 02142, USA
54 University Street, Carlton
  Victoria 3053, Australia

Other Editorial Offices:
Arnette Blackwell SA
  1, rue de Lille, 75007 Paris
  France

Blackwell Wissenschafts-Verlag GmbH
  Kurfürstendamm 57
  10707 Berlin, Germany

  Feldgasse 13, A-1238 Wien
  Austria

First published 1983
by John Wright and Sons Ltd, Bristol
Second edition 1995

Set by Setrite Typesetters Ltd, Hong Kong
Printed and bound in Great Britain
at the University Press, Cambridge

DISTRIBUTORS

Marston Book Services Ltd
PO Box 87
Oxford OX2 0DT
(*Orders*: Tel: 01865 791155
       Fax: 01865 791927
       Telex: 837515)

North America
Blackwell Science, Inc.
238 Main Street
Cambridge, MA 02142
(*Orders*: Tel: 800 215-1000
            617 876-7000
       Fax: 617 492-5263)

Australia
Blackwell Science Pty Ltd
54 University Street
Carlton, Victoria 3053
(*Orders*: Tel: 03 347-0300
       Fax: 03 349-3016)

A catalogue record for this title
is available from the British Library

ISBN 0-632-02902-1

Library of Congress
Cataloging-in-Publication Data

Postgraduate textbook of clinical orthopaedics
  edited by Nigel H. Harris, Rolfe Birch;
  foreword by Christopher L. Colton—2nd edn.
       p.   cm.
  Includes bibliographical references
  and index.
  ISBN 0-632-02902-1
  1. Orthopedics. I. Harris, Nigel H.
  II. Birch, Rolfe.
  [DNLM: 1. Orthopedics. WE 168 P8571995]
RD731.P58 1995
617.3—dc20
DNLM/DLC
for Library of Congress

Contents

List of Contributors

P. J. Abernethy FRCS
Consultant Orthopaedic Surgeon, Princess Margaret Rose
Orthopaedic Hospital, Edinburgh

P. M. Aichroth MS FRCS
Consultant Orthopaedic Surgeon, Chelsea and Westminster
Hospital; Wellington Knee Surgery Unit, The Wellington
Hospital, London

A. Al-Kutoubi MD FRCR DMRD
Consultant Radiologist, Department of Diagnostic Radiology,
St Mary's Hospital, London

A. A. Amis PhD CEng MIMechE
Reader in Orthopaedic Biomechanics, Biomechanics Section,
Department of Mechanical Engineering, Imperial College of
Science, Technology and Medicine, London

B. G. Andrews FRCS
Consultant Orthopaedic Surgeon, Queen Mary's University
Hospital, London

B. M. Ansell CBE MD FRCS FRCP
Consultant Rheumatologist, Windsor Hospital Group, Windsor

M. Bell MBBS BSc FRCS
Consultant Orthopaedic Surgeon, Royal Hallamshire Hospital,
Sheffield

R. Birch MChir FRCS
Orthopaedic Surgeon, The Royal National Orthopaedic Hospital
Trust, Stanmore, Middlesex

G. Bonney MS FRCS
Honorary Consultant Orthopaedic Surgeon, St Mary's Hospital,
London

C. J. K. Bulstrode MCh FRCS(Orth)
Clinical Reader in Orthopaedic Surgery, Nuffield Orthopaedic
Centre, Oxford

A. Cassoni MRCP FRCR
Senior Lecturer, Department of Oncology, University College
London Medical School, London

M. Catto MD FRCPath
Formerly Reader in Orthopaedic Pathology, University of
Glasgow at Western Infirmary, Glasgow

S. S. Coleman MD
Professor of Orthopaedic Surgery, The University of Utah School
of Medicine, Division of Orthopaedic Surgery, Salt Lake City,
USA

S. M. Craig MD
Associate Attending, Lenox Hill Hospital, New York, USA

R. A. Dickson MA ChM FRCS DSc
Professor of Orthopaedic Surgery, Department of Orthopaedic
Surgery, St James's University Hospital, Leeds

J. C. Drennan MD
Professor of Orthopaedics, University of New Mexico, School of
Medicine; Medical Director, Carrie Tingley Hospital,
Albuquerque, New Mexico

A. Fairney MD FRCP FRCPath
Senior Lecturer and Consultant in Chemical Pathology, St Mary's
Hospital Medical School; Head of Department, Diagnostic
Chemical Pathology, St Mary's Hospital Trust, London

H. Firth MA BMBCh MRCP DCH
Senior Registrar, Department of Medical Genetics, Churchill
Hospital, Oxford

J. A. Fixsen MChir FRCS
Consultant Orthopaedic Surgeon, Great Ormond Street Hospital
for Children NHS Trust, London

H. L. Frankel OBE MB FRCP
Consultant in Spinal Injuries, National Spinal Injuries Centre,
Stoke Mandeville Hospital NHS Trust, Aylesbury, Bucks

N. H. Harris MA FRCS
Honorary Consultant Orthopaedic Surgeon, St Mary's Hospital,
London; Orthopaedic Surgeon to the Football Association and
Arsenal Football Club

P. J. L. Holt FRCP
Reader in Rheumatology and Consultant Physician, Department
of Rheumatology, University of Manchester, Manchester

F. T. Horan MSc FRCS
Medical Director, Princess Royal Hospital, Haywards Heath,
West Sussex

D. M. Hunt FRCS
Consultant Orthopaedic Surgeon, Department of Orthopaedics,
St Mary's Hospital, London

S. M. Huson MB MRCP
Consultant Clinical Geneticist, Department of Medical Genetics,
Churchill Hospital, Oxford

J. N. Insall MD
Professor of Orthopaedic Surgery, Cornell University Medical
College, New York, USA

J. R. Johnson FRCS
Consultant Orthopaedic Surgeon, St Mary's Hospital, London;
The Royal National Orthopaedic Hospital, Stanmore, Middlesex

I. G. Kelly MD BSc MB FRCS
Consultant Orthopaedic Surgeon, Orthopaedic Department,
Glasgow Royal Infirmary, Glasgow

H. B. S. Kemp MS FRCS
Honorary Consultant Orthopaedic Surgeon, Institute of
Orthopaedics and Royal National Orthopaedic Hospital Trust,
London

B. E. Kendall FRCP FRCR
Consultant Neuroradiologist, Lysholm Radiological Department,
National Hospital for Neurology and Neurosurgery, London

R. E. King MD
Director of Orthopaedic Residency Training Program, Georgia,
Baptist–Scottish Rite Hospitals, Atlanta, Georgia, USA; Clinical
Professor of Orthopaedic Surgery, Emory University, Atlanta,
Georgia, and Tulana University, New Orleans, Louisiana, USA

A. K. Kour MMed (Surg) FRCS (Glas)
Senior Lecturer, Department of Orthopaedic Surgery, National
University of Singapore, Singapore

V. P. Kumar FRCS (Ed) FRCS (Glas)
Associate Professor, Department of Orthopaedic Surgery,
National University of Singapore, Singapore

R. S. M. Ling OBE MA BM (Oxon) Hon FRCS (Ed) FRCS
Honorary Consultant Orthopaedic Surgeon, Princess Elizabeth
Orthopaedic Hospital, Exeter

R. H. Luff Bsc MBBS FRCS
Consultant in Rehabilitation Medicine, King's College Hospital
(Dulwich), East Dulwich, London

M. S. McMahon MD
Department of Orthopaedic Surgery, Lenox Hill Hospital,
New York, USA

P. Maquet
Consultant Orthopaedic Surgeon, Liège, Doct. h. c. Univ. Paris
XII, 25 Thier Bosset, Aywaille, Belgium

L. J. Micheli MD
Associate Clinical Professor of Orthopaedic Surgery, Harvard
Medical School; Director, Division of Sports Medicine, The
Children's Hospital, Boston, Massachusetts, USA

H. Phillips Bsc Hons MB FRCS
Consultant Orthopaedic Surgeon, The Orthopaedic Department,
Norfolk and Norwich Hospital, Norwich, Norfolk

R. W. H. Pho FRCS
Professor in Orthopaedic Surgery, Department of Orthopaedic
Surgery, National University of Singapore, Singapore

R. G. S. Platts MA MD
Honorary Consultant to the Department of Orthotics, The Royal
National Orthopaedic Hospital, Stanmore, Middlesex

D. F. Powell MD
Director, State of Georgia Juvenile Amputee Clinic, Atlanta,
Georgia, USA

J. A. S. Pringle FRCS
Senior Lecturer/Honorary Consultant Pathologist, Institute of
Orthopaedics and Royal National Orthopaedic Hospital Trust,
London

G. Ravichandran FRCS
Consultant in Spinal Injuries, Spinal Injuries Unit, Northern
General Hospital NHS Trust, Sheffield

T. S. Renshaw MD
Professor of Orthopaedic Surgery, Yale University School of
Medicine, New Haven, Connecticut, USA

M. Saleh MB ChB MSc (Bioeng) FRCS (Lond) FRCS (Ed)
Senior Orthopaedic Lecturer/Honorary Consultant, Northern
General Hospital NHS Trust, Sheffield

K. Satku MMed (Surg) FRCS (Ed)
Senior Lecturer, Department of Orthopaedic Surgery, National
University of Singapore, Singapore

W. N. Scott MD
Orthopaedic Surgeon, Institute for Orthopaedics and Sports
Medicine, New York, USA

G. R. Scuderi MD
Co-Director, Institute for Orthopaedics and Sports Medicine,
Beth Israll Medical Center — North Division, New York, USA

M. H. Seifert MB FRCP
Consultant Physician and Honorary Senior Lecturer in Medicine,
Department of Rheumatology, St Mary's Hospital, London

R. M. Smith MA MD FRCS
Senior Lecturer and Consultant Orthopaedic Surgeon, Academic
Unit of Orthopaedic Surgery, St James's University Hospital,
Leeds

S. Sooriakumaran MBBS LRCP MRCS FRCS (Eng) FRCS
(Ed) FRCS (Glas)
Consultant in Rehabilitation Medicine, Queen Mary's University
Hospital, London

R. L. Souhami MD FRCP
Head of Department, Department of Oncology, University
College London Medical School, London

W. A. Souter FRCSE
Consultant Orthopaedic Surgeon, Princess Margaret Rose
Orthopaedic Hospital, Edinburgh

J. M. Stevens DRACR FRCR
Consultant Radiologist, St Mary's Hospital, London

D. J. Stoker FRCP FRCR FRCS
Consulting Radiologist, The Institute of Orthopaedics, Royal
National Orthopaedic Hospital, London

M. Swann FRCS
Consultant Orthopaedic Surgeon, Windsor Hospital Group,
Windsor

A. B. Swanson MD FACS
Director of Orthopaedic and Hand Surgery, Blodgett Professional
Building, Grand Rapids, Michigan, USA

G. de Groot Swanson MD
Orthopedic Surgeon, Blodgett Professional Building, Grand
Rapids, Michigan, USA

A. J. Timperley FRCS (Ed)
Consultant Orthopaedic Surgeon, North Devon District Hospital,
Barnstable

J. K. Tucker
Consultant Orthopaedic Surgeon, The Orthopaedic Department,
Norfolk and Norwich Hospital, Norwich, Norfolk

T. G. Wadsworth MCh Orth LL M FRCS FRCSE FACS
Honorary Consultant Orthopaedic and Hand Surgeon, The Royal
Hospitals Trust (St Bartholomew's, The London and The London
Chest Hospitals)

Preface to the Second Edition

It is 12 years since publication of the first edition — longer than was planned. However, the extended gestation period has the advantage that account can be taken of the momentous changes in some aspects of orthopaedic practice. We nevertheless apologize to those contributors who have had to revise their manuscripts.

The book has been extensively revised and new chapters added to reflect the changes in orthopaedic practice during the last 10 years or so.

It follows that the knowledge and experience required by an editor has increased significantly. It is for this reason that the senior editor (NHH) is delighted and honoured to welcome Rolfe Birch as joint editor.

In the paediatric section the importance of genetics is reflected by a chapter devoted to this subject.

The general and special topic sections contain much new material, including femoral and tibial osteotomy, cementless hip replacement, more detail about arthroscopy, magnetic resonance imaging and computed tomography investigations, microsurgical techniques and amputations.

It is only a minority of orthopaedic surgeons who engage in cervical spine operations. We think it appropriate therefore that this difficult subject should be reviewed in some detail. We are particularly pleased to include George Bonney's learned account which is based on extensive practical experience.

In view of the steady increase in claims for medical negligence, particularly in orthopaedics, we included a chapter on this aspect of orthopaedics about which we should all be aware.

We hope the book serves a useful addition to the trainee surgeon's library, and not only for the purpose of passing examinations. We think the more experienced surgeon will find it useful for reference.

We have good reason to be grateful to John Harrison who gave valuable advice at the very early stages of preparation, and without whose help this edition would have foundered.

We especially wish to thank Christopher Colton for finding the time to read the manuscripts and write a foreword.

We gratefully acknowledge the hard work of Mary-Clare Swatman and Emmie Williamson who have diligently and with great expertise processed the manuscripts through production.

We admire the skilful artwork of David Gardner and thank him for his efforts.

Finally, it is a pleasure to record our sincere thanks to Blackwell Science for their co-operation and infinite patience during the long period of the book's preparation.

N. H. H.

Preface to the First Edition

The art and science of orthopaedics have changed remarkably in the past ten years; the success of joint replacement, improvement of implant materials and new investigative techniques are only three examples. It is indeed a most exciting and rewarding time to train for a career in orthopaedics.

The aim of this book is to provide an authoritative account of the common and not so common orthopaedic conditions specifically for the young surgeon during his training. Now more than ever he has to cover a wide field of knowledge and absorb all the many recent advances. It is hoped that this book will enable him to do so without too often having recourse to numerous monographs. However, it is appreciated that additional reading is essential and to this end extensive references have been provided. The material should be of value to the established orthopaedic surgeon who needs to refer to subjects that are not part of his regular experience. Those who are working for higher surgical diplomas will find certain sections of the book useful for reference.

Acute trauma and operative detail have been excluded as a matter of policy; inevitably this has meant that some difficult decisions have had to be made. I decided that it was entirely reasonable to include a discussion on the clinical aspects and management of peripheral nerve and tendon injuries, for example, which so often present problems long after the acute injury has occurred.

There are several books on operative orthopaedic surgery and it therefore seemed inappropriate to include details of technique. Nevertheless, all contributors have given guidance on the indications for operation and, where appropriate, discussed the relative merits of the different procedures, in some instances including a certain amount of operative detail.

Orthopaedic surgery will only continue to make significant advances in the future if we invest wisely, and to this end I can think of no better way of doing so than by ensuring that our trainee surgeons have the benefit of the knowledge and experience of their seniors. I hope that this book will form a part of such an investment, and I am indebted to the contributors who have given up their valuable time for this purpose.

I am pleased to acknowledge the valuable assistance that I have had from Robert MacKenney and David Hunt, who have diligently read many of the scripts and offered valuable criticism. During discussion, in the early stages, of the book's content and other general matters, I received valuable advice from Sir Henry Osmond-Clarke, John Sharrard and Graham Apley; I am most grateful to them for their help and encouragement. A considerable amount of typing has been done under sometimes difficult circumstances; in this respect I am most appreciative of all the hard work done by Sheila Fletcher and Julia Bucknall. I particularly wish to express my gratitude to the late Frank Price, who was responsible for all the artist's drawings; his service to medical textbooks will be sadly missed. Finally, it gives me great pleasure to acknowledge the unfailing courtesy and co-operation that I have received from John Wright & Sons Ltd. In particular I must mention Roy Baker and his secretary Dagmar Lee for the considerable assistance they have given me at all times. Jane Walker has been untiring in her efforts to correct the scripts; she has discovered errors which I most certainly would have missed had it been left to me, and has made valuable suggestions for improvement of the text. Without the help and kindness of all these people this book could not have been produced.

N. H. H.

Foreword

In 1983, I was prudent enough to purchase my personal copy of Nigel Harris's *Postgraduate Textbook of Clinical Orthopaedics*, which he so kindly autographed for me.

This book has been a constant reference work for me ever since. It has proven invaluable, not only in clinical practice, but also as a reliable authority and bibliographic source for medico-legal work. For this reason I was fascinated to read the new chapter devoted to medico-legal matters, one which Nigel Harris is eminently qualified to write. Any orthopaedic surgeon who accepts instructions in this field will skip this at his or her peril.

Ours is an expanding and evolving specialty and, notwithstanding the encyclopaedic care with which that first book was prepared, the time is ripe for a revised and augmented edition. I was delighted to hear last year that such a revision was imminent and then honoured to be asked to write its foreword.

The foreword of the inaugural edition was contributed by Dr Frank Stinchfield of New York who so rightly pointed out that each practising orthopaedic surgeon should have a personal copy. This advice applies today with an even greater imperative (if that were possible) to this new work.

A foreword should not be a book review and I shall refrain from commenting upon the format and content in detail. As the title states, this book is aimed at the postgraduate. Such a reader may well use it both for primary study and for revision. In the UK, as in many countries of the world, health care is consuming ever-increasing slices of the national financial cake and there is a global drive to rationalize, structure and render more cost-effective surgical training and evaluation. Training periods are shortening and study is becoming more intense over a widening field. This produces the need for single, up-to-date and authoritative works. This book fulfils this role admirably and constitutes, by its comprehensive coverage of its subject, at the same time a syllabus for learning and a ready source of knowledge. I would expand Dr Stinchfield's advice and additionally urge every orthopaedic surgical trainee to acquire a personal copy.

For the practising orthopaedic specialist, this book will be equally invaluable as a reliable source of reference and for revision. It will be with growing confidence that such surgeons will come to appreciate the research that has gone into its preparation. The editors have chosen a team of authors, each outstanding in the subject addressed, who have given to the surgical world its prime orthopaedic textbook. This book sets the standard against which future similar works are to be judged. I congratulate Nigel Harris for his inspiration and continued dedication, and he and his co-editor, Rolfe Birch, for their monumental achievement.

Professor Christopher Colton
1995

Section I
Paediatric Orthopaedics

Chapter 1
Genetic Aspects of Orthopaedics

H. Firth & S.M. Huson

INTRODUCTION

The advent of recombinant DNA technology (Pembrey, 1987; Weatherall, 1991) has led to a resurgence of interest in genetic disease in the last decade. Molecular biologists now have the tools available to clone and sequence the entire human genome. The genes responsible for the major single gene disorders that present in orthopaedic practice, e.g. neurofibromatosis type 1, Marfan's syndrome and osteogenesis imperfecta, have all been isolated.

The technology is now being applied to more common diseases with polygenic inheritance, e.g. diabetes, ischaemic heart disease and various forms of arthritis. The first clinical application of developments in DNA technology for single gene disorders is usually in pre-natal and pre-symptomatic diagnosis. In the long term there is hope that by understanding disease pathogenesis, preventive treatment will follow.

Not all developments in medical genetics have been confined to the field of molecular biology. The laboratory researcher depends on DNA samples from patients with well-characterized disease. In the process of collecting such samples, many clinical researchers have looked again at the natural history of the particular disease to provide improved information about natural history for genetic counselling and by which potential treatment can be assessed. The field of congenital malformation syndromes and dysmorphology is also rapidly developing, in terms of both our ability to diagnose rare syndromes (Winter and Baraitser, 1991) and to look at the biological mechanisms that underlie the development of congenital malformations.

As a result of extensive media coverage of the developments in genetic research and the formation of lay groups for many genetic diseases (Contact a Family Directory of Specific Conditions and Rare Syndromes), patients and their families are also better informed. This in turn puts pressure on health professionals to keep updated about the research developments that may affect patients in their care. This chapter attempts to summarize the impact of the new developments in genetics for patients with genetic disease who are seen in the orthopaedic clinic. The clinical management of the majority of the conditions discussed here from the genetic viewpoint is described elsewhere in the book. The coverage of the chapter is not exhaustive but it is hoped that it will point the way to useful reference sources. Good general clinical genetic texts are available (Harper, 1988; Emery and Rimoin, 1990; Gelehrter and Collins, 1990).

For many patients with genetic disease involving the musculoskeletal system, a multidisciplinary approach with combined paediatric, genetic and orthopaedic input turns out to be the best. Each specialist, however, needs to be able to identify the patient who will benefit from the expertise of their colleagues. The importance of this cannot be over-emphasized and is succinctly summarized by Michael Goldberg in the foreword to his excellent book, *The Dysmorphic Child*: *An Orthopaedic Perspective*:

There was a time once when life for the orthopaedic surgeon was simpler. A physical finding was considered a diagnosis. A club foot was a club foot and polydactyly meant that the extra finger would soon be off. Associated problems were often not known or not recognised. If the orthopaedic deformity turned out to be merely the tip of the iceberg, the surprises were treated as they came along.

But no longer. The geneticist's and paediatrician's interest in congenital malformations of the musculo-skeletal system has blossomed. These practitioners have become the leaders of multi-disciplinary clinics that previously were the bailiwick of orthopaedic surgeons. Is the

3

orthopaedist destined to become the surgeon—technician of the future—charged only with the mechanical correction of deformity and allowing the challenge of diagnosis to fall entirely to others? Perhaps so, but like it or not, the non-orthopaedic aspects of the child's disease may easily ruin one's surgical results, making at least a cursory interest in diagnosis essential.

There is an important corollary: many children who carry as a diagnosis the names of some well known syndromes have musculo-skeletal deformity as a constant feature. When the orthopaedic disease is just one component of the child's multiple birth defects, it is often not recognised and is occasionally overlooked entirely.

PRINCIPLES OF MEDICAL GENETICS

Prevalence of genetic disease

Population-based studies have shown that at least 5.3% of live-born individuals can be expected to develop diseases with an important genetic component by the age of 25 years (Baird *et al.*, 1988). This total is composed of multifactorial disorders (4.64%), chromosome anomalies (0.18%), single gene disorders (0.36%) and other disorders (0.12%) where the precise mechanism was not identified. If all congenital anomalies are included as part of the genetic load, then at least 7.9% of the population have a genetic disorder by the age of 25 years. These figures exclude important genetic disorders with late onset, e.g. Huntington's disease and the family cancer syndromes. Genetic disease and congenital malformation are an important cause of morbidity and mortality, particularly in children; they account for up to 30% of paediatric hospital admissions, and they are an important cause of death under the age of 15 years.

Genes and chromosomes

Each nucleated cell of the body contains a complete set of the individual's genetic material. The smallest unit of inheritance is the gene, and it is estimated that the human genome contains 50 000−100 000 genes. There are two copies of each gene. The genes are packaged on chromosomes, and the human cell contains 46 chromosomes arranged in 23 pairs; one of the pair, and therefore one copy of every gene, comes from each parent. Both sexes have pairs 1−22, and the 23rd pair is the sex chromosomes; women have two X chromosomes and men an X and a Y chromosome.

The genetic disease that develops is very dependent on the 'genetic level' at which problems arise. For example, children with chromosome disorders usually have intellectual handicap in association with multiple congenital anomalies; in comparison, those with a single gene disorder may show quite specific effects on just one body system. The different kinds of disorders that are at least in part genetically determined are summarized in Table 1.1.

Chromosomal disorders

The correct chromosome complement in humans was identified in 1956 and the first chromosome disorders defined in 1959. The first disorders recognized were those with an abnormal number of chromosomes, e.g. Down's syndrome with an extra chromosome 21. Each chromosome can be identified by light microscopy (Fig. 1.1). During metaphase the two chromatids of each chromosome are joined at the centromere. The short arm of the chromosome is designated p (petit) and the long arm q. Chromosomes were first studied using solid staining techniques with which only fairly obvious chromosome rearrangements could be identified. With the introduction of chromosome banding in the 1970s, the characteristic black and white patterns specific to each chromosome became obvious (Fig. 1.1) and over the years more and more subtle deletions, duplications and translocations have been identified (Kingston, 1989).

The incidences of abnormalities of the autosomes (numbers 1−22) and the sex chromosomes are about the same. Abnormalities of the sex chromosomes usually have a relatively mild phenotypic effect. Those involving autosomes cause disorders with multiple congenital malformations, almost invariably in association with intellectual handicap. It is beyond the scope of this book to describe specific chromosome syndromes in detail. The majority of children with major chromosome anomalies will have been diagnosed in the neonatal period and present to the orthopaedic surgeon for assessment of treatment for particular malformations. Some older children, however, may have been discharged from regular paediatric follow-up and only attend the ortho-

Table 1.1 Diseases with a genetic aetiology

Chromosomal disorders, e.g. Down's syndrome
Single gene disorders (5710 now catalogued by McKusick)
Congenital malformations and other common diseases
  (e.g. diabetes mellitus) exhibiting polygenic inheritance
Disorders of mitochondrial DNA
Disorders due to somatic cell mutation, e.g. cancer

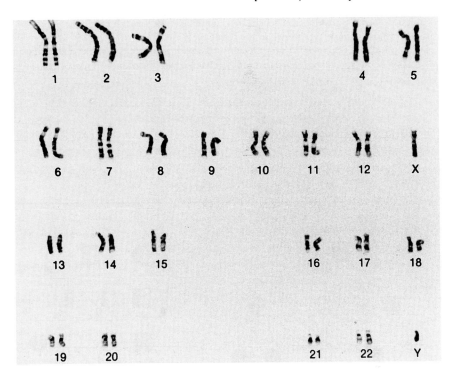

Fig. 1.1 A normal human male karyotype (with permission of Greenwood Medical Centre).

paedic clinic. If the cause of their problems has not been identified and no chromosome study has been done for several years, it can be worth considering repeating the investigation because of the improved standard of analysis now available.

Mendelian inheritance

> Those characteristics that are transmitted entire, or almost unchanged by hybridisation, and therefore constitute the characters of the hybrid, are termed dominant, and those that become latent in the process, recessive.
>
> *Gregor Mendel* (1865)

Mendelian diseases are defined as those that are the result of a single mutant gene and are inherited in simple patterns similar to or identical with those described by Mendel for certain discrete characters in garden peas. Mendelian diseases are referred to as *autosomal* if they are caused by a gene on the autosomes and *X-linked* if on the X chromosome. There are no major disorders caused by genes on the Y chromosome.

The two copies of each gene may be identical or different. The alternative forms of a gene at a given genetic locus are referred to as *alleles*. When those alleles at a locus are identical the individual is said to be *homozygous* or a *homozygote*. If the alleles are different, the individual is referred to as *heterozygous* or a *hetero-*

zygote. The word *genotype* is used to refer to an individual's genetic composition and *phenotype* to the observed effects on the individual of a given genotype. The end phenotype is the result of the interaction of a given genotype with environmental factors. Following Mendel, *dominant* conditions are those that are expressed in the heterozygote, i.e. they have one abnormal or *mutant* allele and one normal or *wild-type* allele. Recessive conditions are those where the individual needs to be homozygote for a mutant allele for there to be a phenotypic effect.

McKusick (1992) has maintained a catalogue of mendelian loci in man since the mid-1960s, which is now in its tenth edition. The increase in recognized mendelian traits since the first edition has been enormous, and there are now over 4000 recognized human mendelian traits (Table 1.2).

The mode of inheritance of most genetic diseases has been deduced from family trees or pedigrees. The standard symbols used in drawing a pedigree are shown in Fig. 1.2 alongside pedigrees showing typical autosomal dominant, autosomal recessive and X-linked recessive patterns of inheritance. The person who brings the family to medical attention is called the proband or index case (also sometimes the propositus or proposita) and is indicated by an arrow. Different generations within a pedigree are indicated by Roman numerals and an individual within a given generation by an Arabic numeral.

Table 1.2 Increase in number of genetic loci identified in McKusick's catalogue. Numbers in parentheses refer to loci not fully identified or isolated (those without an asterisk in the catalogue)

	Mendelian inheritance in man		
Phenotype	1966 (first edition)	1978 (fifth edition)	1992 (tenth edition)
Autosomal dominant	269 (+568)	736 (+753)	2470 (+1241)
Autosomal recessive	237 (+294)	521 (+596)	647 (+984)
X-linked	68 (+51)	107 (+98)	190 (+178)
Total	574 (+913)	1364 (+1447)	3307 (+2403)
Grand total	1487	2811	5710

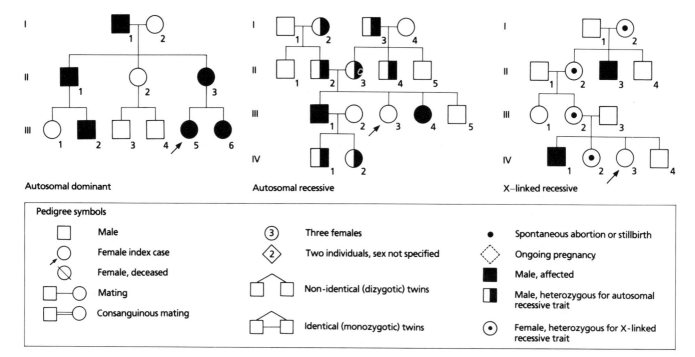

Fig. 1.2 Pedigrees showing different types of mendelian inheritance and standard pedigree symbols.

Autosomal dominant disorders

These include many of the serious and more common genetic diseases of adult life, e.g. familial hypercholesteraemia, Huntington's disease and polyposis coli, which affect both men and women. An affected person is heterozygous for the abnormal allele of the gene and has a 1 in 2 chance of passing the abnormality to any children, whether male or female. The segregation of a dominant gene is shown in Fig. 1.3. An autosomal dominant pedigree is usually recognized by the fact that both sexes are equally affected, there are affected individuals in every generation, and there is male-to-male transmission. Dominant inheritance seems straight-

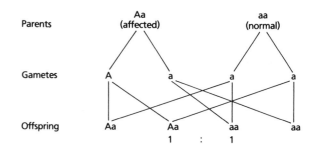

Fig. 1.3 Segregation of a dominant gene. a = mutant allele, A = normal allele.

forward at first glance. There are, however, some features of dominant inheritance that can make genetic counselling complicated. These are:

1 Variable age of onset—many dominant disorders show no phenotypic effect in childhood. For example, in Huntington's disease the mean age of symptom onset is approximately 40 years. Individuals at risk of the condition therefore do not know whether they have inherited the disease at the crucial time in their lives when they are planning families and careers. This situation is changing for some disorders now, with the availability of pre-symptomatic diagnosis using DNA markers, and this is discussed in a later section (see p. 14). In genetic counselling for diseases like Huntington's disease, an age of onset curve is used to calculate the residual risk a person has of carrying the gene, given the present age and the fact that no signs of the disease have appeared.

2 Variable expressivity—the nature and severity of the phenotype of a mutant gene are a reflection of its expressivity. Variable expression is a common feature of dominant conditions. For example, in neurofibromatosis type 1 a parent with only café au lait spots and a few dermal neurofibromas may have a child with severe scoliosis or pseudoarthrosis. Some doctors feel it is unnecessary to alarm families who are experiencing few problems from a particular disorder about all the different complications that could occur in their children. Experience in genetic counselling clinics suggests that this is the wrong approach. If a person is not given adequate information and then has a severely affected child, the feeling of guilt is exacerbated. With today's level of media coverage about genetic disease, the parents may learn about the disease in detail from a newspaper article or the television; they then feel cheated by their doctor with a consequent loss of faith in the doctor–patient relationship.

3 Variable penetrance—penetrance of a gene refers to whether all individuals who carry the mutant gene show a phenotypic effect. On a pedigree, non-penetrance manifests itself by apparently 'skipped' generations, i.e. an affected grandparent has an affected grandchild through a phenotypically normal but obligate gene carrier. The significance of reduced penetrance in the clinical setting is that phenotypically normal individuals cannot be fully reassured that their child will not inherit the disorder. In clinical practice care must be taken not to confuse a person only very mildly affected due to variable expression, where the risk to children would be 1 in 2, with a gene carrier phenotypically normal due to reduced penetrance, where the risk to children would be less.

4 'True' dominant conditions—homozygosity for dominant genes is uncommon, unless two people with the same disorder marry. Social factors mean that this is more likely to happen for certain conditions, e.g. those leading to short stature, such as achondroplasia. 'True' dominance is used to describe dominant genes when the heterozygous and homozygous genotypes give the same phenotype, e.g. Huntington's disease. In other diseases, the homozygous state is much more severe, e.g. in homozygous achondroplasia where the phenotype is one of a lethal skeletal dysplasia.

5 Mutation—although for some disorders the pedigree will go back many generations, in others it is common to see affected children with normal parents. This is usually due to new gene mutation: in other words a mis-copy in the gene occurs when either the ovum or the sperm is formed. If a disorder significantly affects an individual's ability to reproduce, either because it causes death at a young age or interferes with the ability to form relationships or physically reproduce, then it is more likely that new mutations will occur. For example, the majority of cases of achondroplasia arise by new mutation. For some loci, increased paternal age at the time of conception may increase the risk of new mutation.

As is the case for reduced penetrance, new mutation must not be confused with variable expression, and therefore detailed examination of the parents of an apparently isolated case is essential. Even so, the risk of recurrence might be slightly raised due to a phenomenon known as *gonadal mosaicism*. This means that one of the parents is phenotypically normal but has a gonadal clone of cells containing the abnormal gene. Tuberous sclerosis is a dominant disorder where gonadal mosaicism is observed, and the parents of an apparently isolated case have a recurrence risk of about 5%. On the other hand, in neurofibromatosis type 1 pure gonadal mosaicism seems to be a rare event, if it occurs at all. Several families have been reported, however, in which a parent with apparently segmental neurofibromatosis (the features of neurofibromatosis type 1 limited to one segment of the body) has produced children with full-blown neurofibromatosis type 1. These cases are presumed to represent *gonosomal mosaics*; in other words, they have abnormal clones of cells both in their somatic tissue and the germ line.

Autosomal recessive inheritance

The segregation pattern of an autosomal recessive disorder is shown in Fig. 1.4. Individuals who are heterozygous for a recessive gene show no major phenotypic effect, though there may be minor changes in the gene product that can be used as a basis for carrier tests,

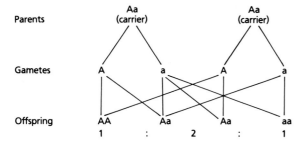

Fig. 1.4 Segregation of a recessive gene. a = mutant allele, A = normal allele.

e.g. reduced enzyme levels. The disease phenotype is only expressed in individuals who are homozygous, and expression of the disease is more uniform than in dominant disorders. In addition, the phenotypic effect of many recessive disorders is apparent from early childhood, if not from infancy. Many have a more severe overall prognosis than the dominantly inherited diseases.

Within a family, there is usually no history of the disorder, the affected child being born to healthy parents. Although the abnormal gene itself may have passed through many generations of the family in the heterozygote state (Fig. 1.2), the affected children usually only appear in one generation. This is because, unless two relatives marry, the chance is low of two carriers for most recessive conditions marrying. Once an affected child is born the risk of having another affected child is 1 in 4. Siblings of affected individuals often present for genetic counselling. They have a two-thirds risk (Fig. 1.4) of being a carrier, but unless they marry another carrier, there will be no risk of them having affected offspring. For example, in cystic fibrosis with a carrier frequency of about 1 in 25 in the British population, the risk to offspring will be two-thirds (the risk of the partner with the affected sibling being a carrier) multiplied by 1 in 25 (the spouse's population risk) multiplied by 1 in 4 (the risk of having an affected child if they were both carriers), i.e. 1 in 150.

All humans carry a few recessive genes. In certain populations particular recessive genes are more common. For example, in Northern Europe cystic fibrosis occurs with a birth incidence of 1 in 2000 and there is a carrier frequency of 1 in 25; Tay—Sachs disease is common in Ashkenazi Jews, sickle cell disease in black populations and other haemoglobinopathies in certain Mediterranean countries and parts of Asia.

The only situation in which affected children will definitely appear in the next generation in a recessive disorder is when two affected individuals marry. In this situation all the children will be affected. In practice,

this situation seldom arises because of the severe phenotypic effect of many recessive disorders. It occasionally occurs in the deaf community, when two individuals with the same kind of severe congenital sensorineural deafness marry.

X-linked inheritance

Males and females each inherit one of their mother's X chromosomes. A baby will be female if it inherits an X chromosome from its father and male if it inherits a Y chromosome (Fig. 1.5). There are both recessive and dominant X-linked conditions.

X-LINKED RECESSIVE

An X-linked recessive pedigree is characterized by affected males in different generations. The disease is transmitted through healthy female carriers; heterozygous females occasionally show mild disease features.

A female carrier will transmit the disease gene to half of her daughters and half of her sons (Fig. 1.5a). All the daughters of an affected male will be carriers and all the sons healthy. Most X-linked diseases cannot be transmitted by healthy males. As many X-linked diseases are severe or lethal during childhood, cases do arise by new mutation. Great caution must be exercised, however, in

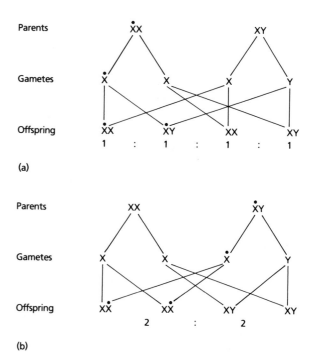

Fig. 1.5 Segregation of an X-linked gene. (a) Heterozygous mother (chromosome carrying gene marked with dot). (b) Heterozygous father.

concluding that apparently isolated cases arise through a new mutation. If there have only been females in the previous generations, then the disease will not have been expressed in the males and the female relatives could still be carriers. Genetic counselling and carrier testing in women in X-linked pedigrees is a complex process and probably best left to a clinical geneticist. Many genetic departments have genetic registers for X-linked recessive disorders where the female relatives of an affected male, e.g. with Duchenne muscular dystrophy, are contacted to undergo carrier testing at an appropriate age.

X-LINKED DOMINANT

In X-linked dominant diseases both males and heterozygous females are affected. As the disorders can only be transmitted by affected males or females, there will be an excess of affected females. In some disorders the condition is lethal in the male. In this case there will be fewer males than expected in the families, all of them will be healthy, and there will be an excess of females half of whom will be affected. X-linked vitamin D-resistant rickets is an example of a X-linked dominant disorder.

Polygenic or multifactorial inheritance

The genetic component of disease is variable; some disorders are entirely environmental in causation and others are wholly genetic. There is a large group of disorders, which have an appreciable genetic contribution, that do not follow mendelian inheritance nor are they associated with chromosome abnormalities. The terms *multifactorial* or *polygenic* inheritance have been used to describe the aetiology of these disorders. Normal traits inherited in this way include height and intelligence; common diseases include ischaemic heart disease and diabetes mellitus. Another group of conditions that shows multifactorial inheritance includes many of the common birth defects, e.g. neural tube defect and club foot.

The factor that distinguishes these disorders from those showing mendelian inheritance is that more than one genetic locus contributes to the phenotype. Multifactorial conditions result from the additive effect of a number of genetic loci and a number of external factors, e.g. environment. The risk of development of a particular disorder in a given population shows a normal distribution; most people have an intermediate risk, with a few at either end with a very high or very low risk of inheriting the disorder (Fig. 1.6) (Carter, 1969, 1970).

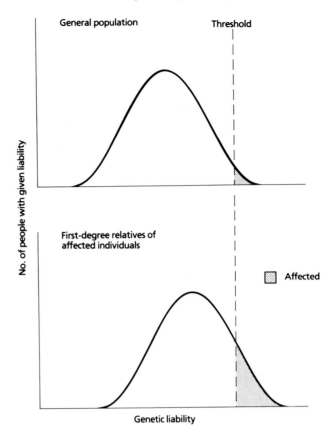

Fig. 1.6 Threshold model of multifactorial inheritance.

At a pathogenetic level, it is presumed that a particular genotype predisposes an individual to respond to external influences to produce the problem, while other genotypes protect against its development. A particular threshold of genetic liability must be reached before the problem can develop. In families with one or more affected individuals the liability curve is shifted to the right and therefore more individuals are above the threshold of liability and are affected (Fig. 1.6). Even individuals with a high genetic liability may not be affected if they are exposed to a favourable environment. The degree to which liability is determined by genetic vs. environmental factors is referred to as *heritability*. The heritability of particular disorders has been established by studying the disease incidence in the general population and in relatives of affected subjects. The concept of heritability is easily appreciated by looking at data from studies of identical and non-identical twins. In disorders with a high degree of heritability, the concordance in identical twins will approach 100%. As the degree of heritability decreases, so also will the degree of concordance.

In the clinical setting, empirical risk data are available for most diseases or malformations showing polygenic inheritance. Empirical risk data are derived from family studies of affected individuals. One rider must be added, which is that before using such data it is important to establish that the studies were done in a population similar to the one in which the counselling is taking place. Certain populations have an increased genetic disposition to some disorders over others. A number of general rules are predicted by the multifactorial model:

1 The risk is greatest among first-degree relatives. It is rare to find a significantly increased risk beyond second-degree relatives, and even then the risk is small. Dominance and recessiveness do not apply; the risks to siblings and children are the same.

2 Risk increases with the number of affected relatives. In mendelian inheritance the risk is the same for any pregnancy. In multifactorial inheritance, multiple affected individuals suggest an increased genetic liability and therefore increase the recurrence risks.

3 Differential risks to relatives of an affected proband increase as the prevalence of the disease or malformation in the general population decreases. For a common disorder, the genetic threshold in the general population is presumed to be lower anyway, so there is a smaller difference between the genetic liability of the population at large and that of the affected individual.

4 The risk increases with the severity of malformation or disease, as it is assumed that the more severe the defect, the greater the genetic liability.

5 When the sex incidence of the disorder is unequal in the general population, the risk is higher for relatives of patients of the rarer sex. This is because they must have had a greater genetic liability for the problem to have developed in them. For example, congenital dislocation of the hip is sixfold more common in girls than in boys, and the recurrence risk for offspring and siblings of affected boys is higher than for affected girls.

Cytoplasmic inheritance

The ovum, unlike the sperm, contains cytoplasm as well as a nucleus. The phenotype of certain disorders is probably influenced or wholly determined by cytoplasmic elements, including biochemical factors and mitochondrial DNA, and these are always maternally derived. The congenital form of myotonic dystrophy is an example of a disease probably accounted for by (as yet unidentified) cytoplasmic factors.

Mutations in mitochondrial DNA (Poulton, 1992) are now recognized to be responsible for a number of specific disease phenotypes, which when inherited are exclusively maternally transmitted, e.g. Leber's optic atrophy.

Diseases caused by somatic mutation

In all the disorders discussed above the genetic tendency is inherited. It is now clear that genetic change in the somatic (non-germ-line) cells of the body are the cause of cancer. Cell division and differentiation are controlled by a number of genes, both within particular cell types and in related cell populations. Malignant transformation of a given cell population is associated with a series of acquired mutations in the genes involved in the regulatory process. For some cancers these somatic changes occur more easily because of an inherited gene predisposing to their occurrence. Such cancer susceptibility genes segregate within the family in an autosomal dominant mode of inheritance and predispose to the development of the particular cancers and related benign tumours at a relatively young age (Hodgson and Maher, 1993). Examples of this are the rare family cancer syndromes, which include familial retinoblastoma, von Hippel−Lindau disease and polyposis coli. In addition, for some common cancers, particularly breast, ovary and colon, there are single genes that predispose to their development in some families.

Somatic mutation of disease genes in early embryonic life can give rise to phenotypic expression being limited to a particular segment of the body. The best recognized group of disorders is those showing segmental distribution of the genetic cutaneous disorders where the limited phenotypic effect is obvious. For example, in segmental neurofibromatosis, café au lait spots and neurofibromas are limited to specific dermatomes (Fig. 1.7).

Other genetic phenomena influencing phenotype

Although in the above descriptions the principles of mendelian and multifactorial inheritance seem straightforward in the clinical setting, exceptions to any set of rules are often observed. In recent years the importance of two phenomena that contribute to some of these exceptions has become apparent.

GENOMIC IMPRINTING

This refers to the differential expression of genetic material, at either chromosomal or allelic level, depending on whether the genetic material has come from the male or female parent (Hall, 1990). An example of this in man is found in two syndromes that cause intellectual handicap, but with quite different associated features. In Prader−Willi syndrome, children are born with profound hypotonia and have difficulty feeding in infancy.

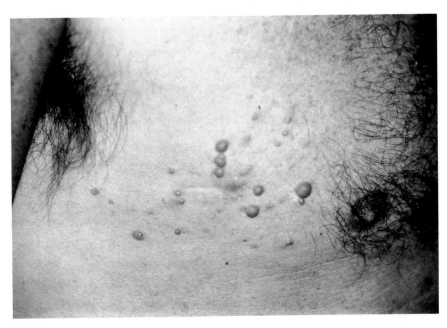

Fig. 1.7 Segmental neurofibromatosis. Dermal neurofibromas are limited to a segment of the upper right chest.

As they grow older the feeding difficulties are superseded by hyperphagia; the older child with Prader–Willi syndrome is obese and there is a characteristic facial appearance. In Angelman's syndrome, the intellectual handicap is associated with profound limitation of speech, ataxia and epilepsy. Both syndromes are associated with deletion of the same part of chromosome 15, but in Prader–Willi syndrome, it is the paternal chromosome 15 in which the deletion has occurred and in Angelman's syndrome the maternal chromosome 15. The phenotypes also arise if children do not inherit one chromosome 15 from each parent, but acquire both their copies from one parent. Two copies of maternal chromosome 15 (or *maternal disomy*) leads to Prader–Willi syndrome and two of paternal chromosome 15 (*paternal disomy*) to Angelman's syndrome.

In the clinical setting, imprinting is therefore being explored as a possible reason for the wide variation seen in some disorders. With an imprinting effect, pedigrees would show that severely affected children are only born to affected parents of a particular sex.

ANTICIPATION

This describes the increasing severity of a genetic disorder in successive generations (Harper *et al.*, 1992). Although clinical observers first reported this observation in association with diseases such as myotonic dystrophy and Huntington's disease several decades ago, other authors (principally geneticists!) have argued that it was secondary to ascertainment bias. In the last decade, however, one clinical study (Howeler *et al.*, 1989) showed clear evidence that it was a real observation in myotonic dystrophy. This was closely followed by the identification of a molecular basis for anticipation with the cloning of the genes responsible for myotonic dystrophy, fragile X syndrome and Huntington's disease (Suthers *et al.*, 1992; Huntington's Disease Collaborative Research Group, 1993). In each condition the mutation is a trinucleotide repeat sequence, and the number of repeats increases in successive generations, roughly correlating with disease severity.

Molecular genetics

During the past decade, advances in the field of molecular genetics, commonly known as recombinant DNA technology or genetic engineering, have revolutionized the pre-symptomatic and pre-natal diagnosis of the major single gene disorders. DNA diagnosis is only the first practical application of this research. In the long term it is hoped that through understanding disease pathogenesis, satisfactory treatments will be developed. Before DNA testing, there were no pre-natal or pre-symptomatic tests available for many single gene disorders, and many couples when given a recurrence risk of 1 in 4 or more simply opted to have no further children. The other development that has made pre-natal diagnosis easier is the use of chorionic villus sampling to obtain fetal material, which can be done at about 10 weeks of pregnancy, much earlier than amniocentesis; the techniques of pre-natal diagnosis are discussed in a later section. The impact of DNA testing for four common conditions is summarized in Table 1.3.

A detailed description of the techniques used to isolate and clone genes and of molecular analysis of genetic disease is beyond the scope of this chapter. A few major aspects will be covered briefly, not expecting readers to fully understand all the technical aspects of the procedures but rather that they become familiar with names used to describe the different procedures. This should prove to be helpful both in the clinical setting and because of the huge number of scientific papers involving molecular genetic analysis now being published. The interested reader will find user-friendly detailed descriptions in Weatherall (1991), Davies and Read (1988) and Strachan (1992).

ISOLATING DNA

The starting point for any form of molecular analysis is a DNA sample. DNA can be isolated by a series of simple steps from any cell type that has a nucleus, including white blood cells, amniotic cells, chorionic tissue, or skin. Sufficient DNA for multiple diagnostic procedures can be obtained from 10 ml of blood. Once the DNA has been extracted the sample can be stored for many years. It is important that when patients are dying from a genetic disease, it is considered whether it might be helpful for a sample of their DNA to be stored. Analysis of the sample would not help the patient, but it may be of use for counselling relatives about their own

risks of the disease in the future. For example, in cystic fibrosis the tests are much more accurate if the gene mutation in the affected individual in the family is known.

CUTTING AND SORTING THE DNA INTO MANAGEABLE SIZES

This is done by a group of bacterial enzymes that can cut double-stranded DNA where they recognize particular base sequences; these enzymes are called *restriction endonucleases*. The restriction enzymes are named after the bacterium from which they are isolated, e.g. Eco (*Escherishia coli*), Hinf (*Haemophilus influenzae*). In human DNA the presence/absence of some of the enzyme cutting sites is variable and inherited as a mendelian trait, and this is the basis for a group of genetic markers called *restriction fragment length polymorphisms* (RFLPs). Once the DNA has been cut using the restriction enzyme, the pieces can be sorted by size using gel electrophoresis. The DNA can be stored permanently in the sorted form by *Southern blotting*. In this technique, the DNA from the gel is transferred onto a permanent filter by passing a salt solution through the gel and filter into a stack of paper towels (Fig. 1.8).

DNA PROBES

These are used to identify the DNA of interest on the filter of genomic DNA. The probe used may either

Table 1.3 Advances in pre-natal and/or pre-symptomatic diagnosis for some common genetic diseases through DNA testing

Disease	'Pre-DNA'	'Post-DNA'
Duchenne muscular dystrophy	Pre-natal: no direct test Carrier females offered fetal sexing on amniocentesis or chorionic villus sampling with termination of males Pre-symptomatic: carrier tests using creatinine kinase and pedigree information; many women left with intermediate carrier risk	Pre-natal and pre-symptomatic: direct mutation studies of dystrophin gene give 100% accurate testing. If mutation not identified, gene marker studies used which are usually ≥95% accurate
Cystic fibrosis	Pre-natal: amniotic fluid alkaline phosphatase at around 17–18 weeks, approximately 95% accurate Pre-symptomatic: no carrier test available	Pre-natal: direct mutation or genetic marker studies on material obtained at chorionic villus sampling Pre-symptomatic: carrier tests using direct mutation or genetic marker analysis
Myotonic dystrophy	Pre-natal: no tests available Pre-symptomatic: clinical examination, electromyography and slit-lamp examination. Problems with variable age of onset	Pre-natal and pre-symptomatic: direct mutation testing. This has shown previous pre-symptomatic diagnosis to be unsatisfactory; in particular the polychromatic lens crystals are not specific for myotonic dystrophy

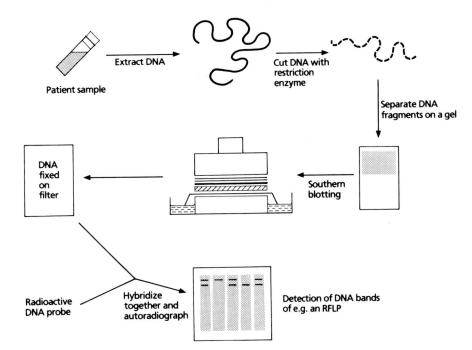

Fig. 1.8 Detection of human DNA variation using radioactive DNA probe and Southern blotting.

consist of the DNA of all or part of a disease gene or be a segment of 'anonymous DNA' that is known to identify a DNA polymorphism. The DNA on the filter is single-stranded and, therefore, when mixed with the DNA probe, the probe binds to its complementary sequence. As the probe is labelled (usually with a radioactive label), subsequent autoradiography of the filter shows the DNA sequences recognized by the probe. In direct gene analysis, the mutation may have resulted in an affected individual having a band on the autoradiograph of different molecular size or if the gene is deleted, no band at all. In RFLP analysis, the probe is used to light up the different alleles of the polymorphism in the individuals being studied.

POLYMERASE CHAIN REACTION

The methods of Southern blotting and probe hybridization described above are fairly time consuming. For many diagnostic DNA tests, the polymerase chain reaction (PCR) is now preferred because of its relative speed and the fact that only small amounts of DNA are needed. Using PCR it is possible to selectively amplify defined DNA target sequences present within a heterogeneous collection of DNA sequences, e.g. the total DNA sample from the given individual. The sequence amplified can either be part of a disease gene in direct mutation testing or the area around a DNA polymorphism. It is this technique that has made pre-implantation

genetic diagnosis testing possible, when the DNA from one or two cells of the early embryo is studied (Handyside *et al.*, 1992).

DNA POLYMORPHISMS

Study of the human genome has been revolutionized by the ability to detect the large number of sites in it that show variation between individuals. This has provided a new series of DNA polymorphisms or markers. As these are inherited in a mendelian fashion, they can be used in genetic linkage studies to track a nearby disease gene through a family. There are several different kinds of DNA polymorphism. RFLPs are polymorphisms created by the presence/absence of a restriction site. This gives rise to different sizes of DNA fragments, which can be detected by a DNA probe or PCR. The limitation of RFLP analysis is that there are usually only two alleles, thus limiting the informativeness of the marker. More powerful markers, with multiple alleles, are those based on variation in length of a given piece of DNA due to repeat sequences of variable number. For example, interspersed throughout the genome are microsatellite DNA families which consist of small arrays of tandem repeats of base pair sequence (usually of one to four base pairs). The number of repeats vary within the population, but are usually stably inherited within a given family.

MAPPING AND CLONING DISEASE GENES

Before the development of DNA technology, the chromosomal location of very few disease genes was known. Even on the X chromosome, although the X-linked pattern of inheritance for a given disease localized the gene to the X chromosome, the exact location of the gene on the X chromosome was usually unknown. When the new technology developed, the first group of disorders for which the genes were isolated and localized was those in which the protein or enzyme involved was already known, e.g. the haemoglobin disorders. As the RNA in human reticulocytes is almost entirely globin mRNA, it was possible to make purified mRNA for single globin chains and from these make complementary DNA probes. With these it was possible to isolate the globin genes from libraries of human DNA, characterize their fine structure and then compare normal structure with that of DNA from patients with haemoglobin disorders. Once a DNA gene probe is available, it can be localized to a particular position on a chromosome by standard mapping methods, e.g. *in situ hybridization* or using a *somatic cell hybrid panel*.

For diseases of which the pathogenesis is not understood, DNA technology offers ways to map and isolate genes without needing to know the gene product. This approach has become known as 'reverse genetics', as the traditional approach of working from protein back to gene has been reversed and the gene is first identified and then the protein product predicted from the base pair sequence. The first step is to map the gene to a position on a particular chromosome. For an autosomal disease, this can be compared with searching for a needle in a haystack! There may, however, be clues to the chromosomal localization, such as:

1 Chromosome rearrangements through the disease gene—when patients with single gene disorders are also found to have chromosome rearrangements, it must be considered whether the chromosome rearrangement is responsible for the disease having developed. It was such a rearrangement that gave the clue to the localization of the Duchenne muscular dystrophy gene. A series of girls was found with classical Duchenne muscular dystrophy who all had an X chromosome translocation through exactly the same area of the X chromosome. It was presumed that the translocation was through the Duchenne muscular dystrophy gene and that this was why the girls had developed the disease. This speculation turned out to be correct and led to the successful cloning of the disease gene.

2 Man/mouse homology—large areas of the mouse genome are found to have been preserved in evolution through to man. Therefore, if a mouse model is known for a particular disease and the mouse gene lies in an area showing homology with the human genome, that area of the human genome is a good starting point.

3 Candidate genes—although there may be no formal proof that a particular protein is the gene product, there will be some proteins for which the genes have already been isolated that are likely candidate genes. For example, when studying the skeletal dysplasias, the collagen genes were a good starting point for analysis, and indeed, it turned out to be mutation in collagen genes that caused a number of these diseases, including oesteogenesis imperfecta.

If there are no clues to the disease localization, family linkage studies are undertaken. DNA samples are collected from a number of families with the disorder under study, and the segregation of DNA markers from all over the genome is studied in the family panel. The aim is to find a DNA marker linked to the disease gene, which is recognized by the fact that the same marker allele will be inherited by all affected individuals. As DNA markers are now scattered throughout the human genome, it is simply a matter of methodically working through each chromosome to identify the disease localization. Once the chromosomal localization of the gene is known, further molecular techniques are available to isolate the disease gene by what is referred to as *positional cloning*.

DNA DIAGNOSIS OF GENETIC DISEASE

Once closely linked genetic markers have been identified for a given disease, they can be used for DNA diagnosis. Their only limitation is that their accuracy depends on the distance of the marker from the disease gene. The further away the marker, the more likely it is to be separated from the disease by recombination at meiosis and to give a wrong result. For clinical use, markers tend only to be applied when they are at least 95% accurate. The situation is improved if markers on either side of the disease gene are available as this makes the prediction even more accurate. The limitation of using genetic markers is that blood samples from several family members are needed (Fig. 1.9), usually including two or more people affected by the disease. Samples from unaffected spouses are also often needed, so that it can be seen which markers the children inherited from the affected parent and which from the unaffected. In Fig. 1.9 a family with neurofibromatosis type 1 is seeking advice. In this family the grandfather (I-1) has the disease, which he passed to his daughter (II-1), who would now like to know if her newborn baby (III-1) is affected. A DNA marker with two alleles, 1 and 2, has been used. In the informative

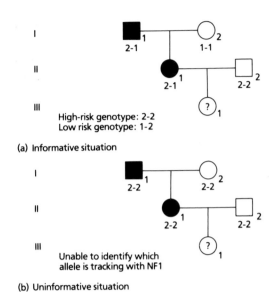

High-risk genotype: 2-2
Low risk genotype: 1-2

(a) Informative situation

Unable to identify which
allele is tracking with NF1

(b) Uninformative situation

Fig. 1.9 Pre-symptomatic diagnosis of neurofibromatosis type 1 using a DNA marker. (a) Informative situation. (b) Uninformative situation. Reproduced with permission from Huson and Hughes, 1993.

situation (Fig. 1.9a) the 2 allele tracks with neurofibromatosis type 1. If the child has a 2−2 genotype she is at high risk of disease, but if she has a 1−2 genotype she is at low risk, as the 1 allele is inherited from her unaffected maternal grandmother and the 2 allele from her father. The problem with DNA markers is that if everyone in the family has the same marker typing or certain key affected individuals are homozygous for the marker, the situation is uninformative; this is illustrated in Fig. 1.9b. The gene-tracking approach is also limited for some diseases in which cases arise by new mutation. In neurofibromatosis type 1 50% of cases arise by new mutation, and this severely limits the use of gene markers for molecular genetic diagnosis.

Once the gene itself has been cloned, the DNA diagnostic method used depends on the mechanism of mutation. In a few diseases it has been shown that all affected individuals have the same kind of mutation, and if this is the case then direct DNA testing for the mutation itself is possible, e.g. myotonic dystrophy, Huntington's disease. For other genes, however, the mutations have been difficult to identify and are different in each family. Looking for many different mutations is very time consuming and often not practical at a service level, particularly when large genes are involved. For example, in neurofibromatosis type 1, mutations have been identified in only approximately 10% of the patients studied. In this situation reliance still has to be placed on genetic marker studies for pre-natal and pre-

symptomatic diagnosis. Once the gene is cloned, however, markers from within the gene itself are usually available, and these are more accurate than linked markers.

PRACTICE OF CLINICAL GENETICS

Genetic counselling

In the UK, each health region now has a regional genetic service providing genetic counselling and laboratory analysis for families with genetic disease. The clinical genetic service comprises clinical geneticists, who before training in clinical genetics have usually had professional training in general medicine, obstetrics, or paediatrics. Some families with particularly distressing disease need much more contact than out-patient clinics alone, and this kind of support is usually given by specialist genetic nurses or genetic counsellors working alongside the clinical geneticist. Genetic clinic consultations are usually longer than the average out-patient appointment and may last for 1 h or more. Many clinical geneticists write letters summarizing the consultation not only to the referring physician but also to the family.

The process of genetic counselling is well summarized in the following definition, which was adopted by the American Society of Human Genetics in 1975 (Ad Hoc Committee on Genetic Counselling, 1975):

Genetic counselling is a communication process which deals with the human problems associated with the occurrence, or the risk of occurrence, of a genetic disorder in a family. This process involves an attempt by one or more appropriately trained persons to help the individual or family to:

1 comprehend the medical facts, including the diagnosis, probable course of the disorder, and the available management;

2 appreciate the way heredity contributes to the disorder, and the risk of recurrence in specified relatives;

3 understand the alternatives for dealing with the risk of recurrence;

4 choose the course of action which seems to them appropriate in view of their risk, their family goals, and their ethical and religious standards, and to act in accordance with that decision; and

5 to make the best possible adjustment to the disorder in an affected family member and/or to the risk of recurrence of that disorder.

For particular groups of disorders, combined clinics between clinical geneticists and other disciplines can be helpful. A good example in the orthopaedic field is in skeletal dysplasias, where management is usually best provided by an orthopaedic surgeon but a clinical geneticist can provide diagnostic assistance and genetic counselling to the families at the same clinic. For example, in Oxford a specialist neurofibromatosis/scoliosis clinic is run with a clinical genetics team and an orthopaedic surgeon specializing in scoliosis in attendance. This enables the families with neurofibromatosis to have both a general disease check-up from the clinical geneticist and their scoliosis reviewed at one appointment.

Referral to the clinical geneticist

An accurate diagnosis is critical to the process of genetic counselling. For this reason, clinical geneticists have often developed expertise in recognizing the underlying syndromal diagnosis in children with multiple congenital anomalies. Many genetic centres have a consultant geneticist with a particular interest in 'dysmorphology'. Children with multiple congenital anomalies and no unifying diagnosis represent one group of patients who may benefit from a genetic assessment. Families with major single gene disorders are another. Many parents who have had a child with a major isolated malformation, e.g. spina bifida, also seek genetic advice. Much less commonly, parents are so distressed by an isolated less severe malformation, e.g. a unilateral extra/missing digit, that the extra time available in the genetic consultation can be helpful in helping them to accept the problem.

Clinical geneticists see many families in whom the underlying genetic diagnosis has been missed or the broader implications of a diagnosis not discussed because the specialist was concentrating solely on the presenting problem, e.g. scoliosis in neurofibromatosis type 1 and Marfan's syndrome, Achilles tendon tightening in myotonic dystrophy. Another easy mistake is to assume that the presenting patient is the only affected individual in a family without examining the parents. In some conditions, e.g. the dominant arthrogryposes and the conditions with split hand/split foot deformity, the variation in expression can be marked and people may not realize that they have minor disease manifestations.

In the subsequent sections of this chapter, a limited number of genetic orthopaedic conditions is reviewed in more detail, though the coverage is far from exhaustive and mainly presents a geneticist's perspective. It is recommended that interested readers with unanswered questions should consult Goldberg (1987), who gives an excellent overview of the differential diagnosis and other disease features of the different genetic musculoskeletal

problems (excluding skeletal dysplasias). Much of Goldberg's emphasis is on trying to break the habit of accepting a physical sign as a diagnosis. Syndactyly, polydactyly, congenital amputations and club hands are all examples of malformations that are often associated with syndromes. The presence of the abnormalities should prompt the surgeon to ask:

1 Are there concealed malformations elsewhere?
2 Might problems with other organ systems develop in the future?
3 Is it genetically determined?
4 How will a syndromic diagnosis alter management?

The aim is not that orthopaedic surgeons become able to diagnose all genetic syndromes (clinical geneticists would be redundant!), but that they can recognize which patients may benefit from referral to a clinical geneticist. Helpful points to consider in assessing these patients are:

1 A pregnancy history and maternal illnesses, e.g. maternal myasthenia gravis can cause arthrogryposis in the offspring.
2 A family history—have other people in the family got this problem?
3 Examine the 'whole' patient, not just the region of interest.
4 Look closely at the parents if a dominant disorder is suspected.
5 Bilateral deformities are more likely to be 'genetic', but the degree of severity can be very variable.

PRE-NATAL DIAGNOSIS

The pre-natal diagnosis of orthopaedic disorders occurs in two settings: first, and more commonly, the unexpected detection of a skeletal anomaly by routine obstetric ultrasonography, and secondly, the planned employment of fetal ultrasonography, chorionic villus sampling, or amniocentesis to investigate a pregnancy at high genetic risk. Table 1.4 gives an indication of the variety of orthopaedic disorders that can be detected by ultrasonography, together with the approximate gestational age at which they can first be adequately visualized with current scanning techniques.

If a skeletal malformation is detected by obstetric ultrasonography, the nature of the problem and its likely prognosis will need to be discussed with the parents. For example, in the case of a mild unilateral talipes equinovarus the implications for the pregnancy are likely to be relatively minor. Management might include a detailed ultrasonographic scan to exclude oligohydramnios and associated anomalies, a careful family history, and a discussion of the likely management

Table 1.4 Some structural congenital anomalies identified by mid-trimester ultrasonography

Anomaly	Approximate gestation (weeks) at which anomaly can be first identified by ultrasonography
Axial skeleton	
Anencephaly	14
Spina bifida	18–22
Hemivertebrae	20–22
Sacral agenesis	18
Appendicular skeleton	
Transverse limb reduction defects	14
Longitudinal limb reduction defects	18
Polydactyly	20
Syndactyly	22
Positional deformities	
Talipes equinovarus	18
Severe skeletal dysplasias	18–20

of the newborn baby. Alternatively, and fortunately more rarely, a serious condition such as a lethal skeletal dysplasia is detected. More problematic is the detection of a major but non-lethal structural anomaly, e.g. a proximal transverse limb-reduction defect. Depending on the gestational age at which such a defect is recognized, the parents may be faced with deciding whether or not to continue the pregnancy. In such a situation they will be guided both by medical advice regarding the likely prognosis and treatment of the skeletal deformity and by their own moral and religious beliefs.

Gauging the likely outcome of the pregnancy when a structural anomaly, e.g. radial aplasia, is detected in a low-risk situation is often difficult because the differential diagnosis is very wide (including trisomy 18, Fanconi's syndrome, thrombocytopenia-absent radius (TAR) syndrome). It is usually somewhat easier in a high-risk situation where a specific diagnosis is being checked, e.g. Holt–Oram syndrome with variable limb defects and congenital heart disease, and the family are fully aware of the implications of the diagnosis from their personal experience or that of a close relative. When decision-making revolves around the likely prognosis and treatment, the parents may be referred by their obstetrician or geneticist to an orthopaedic specialist for further information.

Five different approaches are available for a pre-natal diagnosis of orthopaedic disorders:

1 Delineation of structural anomalies by ultrasonography, e.g. polydactyly.
2 Real-time analysis of fetal movements and range of joint mobility, e.g. arthrogryposis.
3 Analysis of DNA obtained from cells in chorionic villi or amniotic fluid, e.g. osteogenesis imperfecta.
4 Analysis of biochemical end products in samples of chorionic villi or amniotic fluid, e.g. mucopolysaccharidoses.
5 Biochemical study of products of the fetoplacental unit found in maternal blood, e.g. α-fetoprotein in neural tube defects.

These approaches may each be employed independently, but as they are largely complementary, they are often used in combination.

Techniques employed in pre-natal diagnosis

ULTRASONOGRAPHY

Ultrasonography has been used increasingly in obstetric practice since the early 1970s. While initially used predominantly for dating purposes, based on measurement of the fetal biparietal diameter, and to identify single or multiple gestations, the increasing resolution of detail by improved scanning equipment now enables a detailed structural examination of the fetus at 18–20 weeks of gestation, often referred to as an 'anomaly scan'. Many women are now offered such a scan as part of routine obstetric care.

In the normal fetus the skeleton is readily visualized by transabdominal ultrasonography (Fig. 1.10). The bones become visible sonographically at approximately the time ossification begins. Ossification of the clavicle and mandible begins at 8 weeks of gestation, and all of the appendicular long bones, phalanges, ileum and scapula have begun to ossify by the end of the first trimester. The metacarpals and metatarsals ossify between 12 and 16 weeks. The pubis, talus and calcaneous ossify during the fifth and sixth months of pregnancy, but ossification of the remaining tarsals and all of the carpal bones does not begin until after birth (Mahoney, 1990).

The long bones may all be measured ultrasonographically. Such measurements are clearly highly dependent on gestation. Tables of normal data giving mean values and standard deviations for fetal limb bone length in the second and third trimester are available. Such charts may be used to demonstrate the progressive relative shortening of the long bones which occurs in many of the skeletal dysplasias. Where pre-natal diagnosis is based largely on fetal limb measurements, a first trimester dating ultrasonographic scan (based on measure-

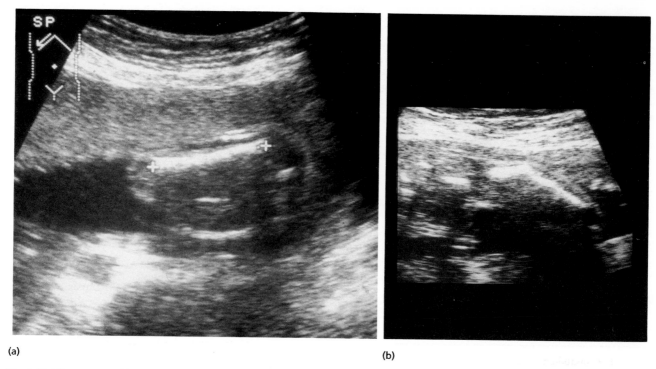

(a)   (b)

Fig. 1.10 Ultrasonographic scans at 23 weeks of gestation. (a) Normal femur. (b) Femur showing marked proximal angulation in a fetus with osteogenesis imperfecta type 3.

ment of crown–rump length) is highly desirable, as ensuing measurements can then be accurately plotted using this information and subsequent visits for serial ultrasonographic scans in the second trimester can be planned.

Transvaginal ultrasonography affords better resolution of detail in the first trimester than transabdominal scanning. Some lethal forms of skeletal dysplasia can be diagnosed at the end of the first trimester, but such scanning is not in routine use. While transvaginal ultrasonographic scanning promises much in the earlier diagnosis of structural congenital anomalies, limitations are clearly imposed by the smaller size of the structures to be visualized and the tolerance of the measurements, together with the gestation at which ossification occurs.

Ultrasonography has so far been discussed as a means of obtaining fetal measurements, but it may also be used to display the position of the fetal limbs, which is abnormal in conditions such as talipes equinovarus, and to demonstrate the range of movement of fetal joints, abnormal in conditions such as arthrogryposis.

When counselling parents of children born with skeletal deformities, the question is often asked why, if a scan was performed, the problem was not detected antenatally. Clearly gestation is a major factor (Table 1.4), but the level of scanning is also important (Royal College of Physicians, 1989). If primary level scanning is used

the main information obtained, e.g. measurement of biparietal diameter, is only sufficient to date the pregnancy; large structural defects, e.g. an absent forearm, may be easily missed and minor problems, e.g. polydactyly, would be most unlikely to be detected. For most planned pre-natal diagnosis, tertiary level scanning is appropriate. For low-risk obstetric patients the relatively simple manoeuvre of measuring fetal femur length will enable the pre-natal identification of many fetal skeletal anomalies, particularly the severe skeletal dysplasias.

CHORIONIC VILLUS SAMPLING

This technique is used to obtain cells from the chorionic plate (developing placenta) in the first trimester of pregnancy. The cells can be analysed directly or the sample cultured to increase the yield. The chorionic villi are a rich source of DNA, which can be extracted for molecular genetic analysis. Alternatively, the sample may be subjected to cytogenetic or biochemical study.

Chorionic villus sampling is a relatively new technique, becoming established in obstetric practice during the 1980s. Sampling is usually performed at approximately 10 weeks of gestation under ultrasound guidance. Either a percutaneous transabdominal route using a 20-gauge spinal needle can be used to obtain a sample of chorionic villi, or a flexible catheter can be introduced

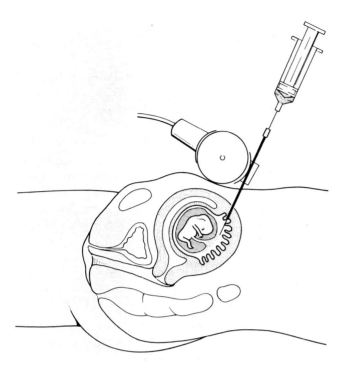

Fig. 1.11 Transabdominal chorionic villus sampling.

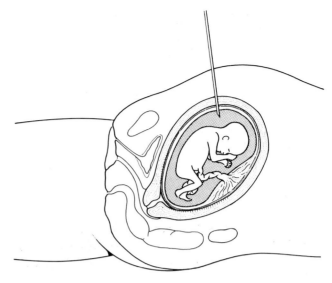

Fig. 1.12 Amniocentesis.

transcervically to reach the chorionic plate (Fig. 1.11).

The added miscarriage rate attributable to chorionic villus sampling has been the subject of several large randomized trials (Canadian Collaborative CVS–Amniocentesis Clinical Trial Group, 1989; MRC Working Party on the Evaluation of Chorionic Villus Sampling, 1991) and is of the order of 2–3%. When chorionic villus sampling is carried out before 10 weeks of gestation, there is probably a very small risk of the procedure causing limb and other defects in the fetus (Rodeck, 1993).

AMNIOCENTESIS

This technique is used to obtain samples of amniotic fluid at approximately 16 weeks of gestation. A 22-gauge spinal needle is introduced via a percutaneous transabdominal route into the amniotic fluid space and 10–20 ml of fluid withdrawn (Fig. 1.12). The added miscarriage rate attributable to the procedure is of the order of 1% (Tabor *et al.*, 1986). Initial concerns about an increased risk of postural malformation (congenital dislocation of the hip and club foot) following amniocentesis have been disproved in a case-controlled study (Wald *et al.*, 1983).

RADIOGRAPHY

In almost all circumstances high-resolution ultrason-

ography has superseded pre-natal radiography in the analysis of skeletal malformations.

GENETIC ASPECTS OF SOME COMMON CONGENITAL MALFORMATIONS SEEN IN ORTHOPAEDIC PRACTICE

This section considers the genetic aspects of congenital dislocation of the hip, club foot, spina bifida, idiopathic scoliosis and arthrogryposis. With the exception of arthrogryposis, all of these conditions exhibit polygenic or multifactorial inheritance.

The theoretical aspects of polygenic inheritance are discussed in the previous section. For practical purposes the recurrence risk in these conditions is based on empirical risks derived from surveys of affected individuals and their relatives. The risks are significantly increased for first-degree relatives (parents, siblings, children) and are of the order of 3–10%, but become small (1–3%) when second-degree relatives are considered (grandchildren, nephews, nieces) and fall close to the population risk for third-degree (first cousins) and more distant relatives.

Congenital dislocation of the hip

In congenital dislocation of the hip, the femoral head is displaced outside the acetabulum before birth. Congenital subluxation defines the situation when the femoral head remains in articular contact with the outer margin of the acetabulum. The term acetabular dysplasia refers to shallowness of the acetabulum, which invariably accompanies late-diagnosis congenital dislocation of the hip, but may occur without displacement of the femoral head. Genetic counselling is seldom requested for this condition, as its effects are largely remediable.

Environmental factors, e.g. breech presentation, firstborn, multiple pregnancy, oligohydramnios and winter season of birth, are undoubtedly important, but familial clustering and a higher concordance rate for monozygotic than dizygotic twins suggest an important genetic element (Table 1.5).

The most important single genetic determinant in congenital hip dislocation is, without doubt, fetal sex. Congenital dislocation occurs approximately sixfold more often in girls than in boys. The reason for this is not understood, but it may be mediated by the production of hormones, e.g. oestrone, by the female fetus. An important consequence of this observation is that the recurrence risks are skewed depending on the sex of the individual at risk (Table 1.5). Other important genetic factors include the depth of the acetabulum and joint laxity.

In a survey of acetabular dysplasia it was found that apparently normal parents of patients with congenital dislocation had a shallower acetabulum than the control group (Wynne-Davies, 1970). The normal distribution of acetabular depth in both controls and parents of children with congenital dislocation suggests that the configuration of the acetabulum is governed by a multiple gene system. The observation that the more severe the degree of dysplasia in the parents of a child with the condition, the higher the incidence of congenital dislo-

cation in the siblings of the child (Wynne-Davies, 1970) provides further support for this hypothesis. Several studies have noted an increased incidence of generalized joint laxity in infants with congenital dislocation of the hip. Joint laxity appears to act independently from acetabular configuration in predisposing a fetus to congenital dislocation of the hip (Czeizel et al., 1975).

The principal value of recognizing the genetic contribution in congenital dislocation of the hip is that appropriate neonatal screening procedures, e.g. clinical examination by an experienced orthopaedic surgeon or paediatrician and neonatal ultrasonography of the acetabular cavity, can be offered to subsequent siblings and offspring of affected individuals.

Club foot

Many primary causes of club foot, particularly neurological conditions, must first be excluded. Idiopathic congenital club foot comprises three distinct entities: talipes equinovarus, talipes calcaneovalgus and talipes metatarsus varus. All three forms are inherited in a multifactorial but independent manner; for example, in a survey of relatives of 340 patients with talipes equinovarus, 2.9% had talipes equinovarus, while talipes calcaneovalgus and talipes metatarsus varus were very uncommon (Wynne-Davies, 1964).

TALIPES EQUINOVARUS

Environmental factors, e.g. oligohydramnios, are

Table 1.5 Congenital dislocation of the hip: genetic aspects

		Concordance	
		Monozygotic	Dizygotic
Twin studies			
Idelberger	1951	10/29	3/109
Kambara and Sasakawa	1954	15/21*	3/6†
Wynne-Davies	1970	1/2	1/3
Czeizel et al.	1975	3/6	0/11

		Recurrence risk (%)		
Individual affected	Individual at risk	Overall	Male	Female
One sibling	Siblings	6	1	11
One parent	Children	12	6	17
One parent plus one child	Children	36		
Second-degree relative	Nephews, nieces	<1		

* Twins classified as monochorionic.
† Twins classified as biovular.

important. The male sex is more susceptible, with a male:female ratio of 2:1. The recurrence risk for siblings is approximately 3% (Wynne-Davies, 1964), though this is skewed by the uneven sex distribution such that the risk for siblings of a male patient is lower (2%) than for a female patient (5%).

TALIPES CALCANEOVALGUS

This anomaly occurs nearly twice as commonly in girls, giving a male:female ratio of 0.6:1. The overall recurrence risk for siblings is 4.5% (Wynne-Davies, 1964).

TALIPES METATARSUS VARUS

Environmental factors include overcrowding in multiple pregnancies and lying prone post-natally. Girls are affected slightly more often than boys. The overall recurrence risk for siblings is 4.5% (Wynne-Davies, 1964).

Spina bifida and anencephaly

The incidence of live-born children with neural tube defects (spina bifida and anencephaly) has declined dramatically in the UK in recent years. This is partly due to a natural decline in the incidence, probably attributable to improvement in the nutritional status of pregnant women and partly to the widespread introduction of antenatal screening procedures.

Both spina bifida and anencephaly arise very early in embryogenesis, by the end of the fourth week from conception, with failure of complete closure of the neural tube (Langman, 1975). The recurrence risks for neural tube defects are summarized in Table 1.6. In general, the recurrence risk is equally distributed for spina bifida and anencephaly, regardless of which condition the index case had.

Considerable confusion arises over the term spina bifida occulta. In 'true' spina bifida occulta the spinal cord remains within the spinal canal and there is no external sac, but there is a significant spinal defect, usually

Table 1.6 Anencephaly and spina bifida: recurrence risks

Individual affected	Risk (%)
One sibling	3
Two siblings	6
One second-degree relative (uncle/aunt or half-sibling)	1–2
One third-degree relative	<1
One parent	3

lumbosacral and often marked by a pigmented or hairy patch of skin or a midline dimple. Occasionally, subtle neurological signs can be elicited in the legs or there is a history of bladder dysfunction. In 'radiological' spina bifida occulta failure of midline fusion of the neural arch is discovered incidently in one or two vertebrae in the lumbosacral region on a radiograph taken for backache or some unrelated symptom. There are no accompanying dermatological or neurological signs. It is crucial to distinguish these two varieties, because 'true' spina bifida occulta carries the same recurrence risk as anencephaly or spina bifida, while individuals with 'radiological' spina bifida occulta are not thought to be at increased risk for neural tube defects.

Antenatal screening for neural tube defects is now offered to most pregnant women in the UK. The screening programme is based on the level of α-fetoprotein present in maternal blood at a given gestation, usually 16 weeks. The level of α-fetoprotein is increased in a number of situations, e.g. multiple pregnancy or where the fetus is more advanced in gestation than thought, and also in neural tube defects and defects of closure of the anterior abdominal wall. Using a cut-off value of 2.3 times the median value of α-fetoprotein for a given gestation, more than 95% of open neural tube defects will be detected, and of those mothers with a 'positive' screen, approximately 10% will be carrying a fetus with a neural tube defect. Pregnant women with a positive screen are offered detailed ultrasonographic examination of the fetal head and spine and sometimes an amniocentesis for estimation of the amniotic fluid levels of α-fetoprotein and cholinesterase. These further investigations should enable pre-natal diagnosis of affected fetuses and provide reassurance to those mothers with a false-positive screening result. Some indication of the likely prognosis for an affected pregnancy can be given by the level and extent of the lesion as determined ultrasonographically.

Women with a high risk of an affected pregnancy by virtue of their previous pregnancy history or a family history either in their own or their partner's family should be offered peri-conceptual vitamin supplementation with folic acid. A recently published randomized controlled trial demonstrated that peri-conceptual supplementation with folic acid, 4 mg/day, resulted in a dramatic decrease in recurrence risk to approximately 1% (MRC Vitamin Study Group, 1991). As supplementation needs to be started before conception, it is most important that women at increased risk are identified and the topic discussed before they attempt to become pregnant. Folic acid is continued until the end of the first trimester.

Idiopathic scoliosis

This may be either infantile or adolescent. The two varieties are distinguished not only by age of onset, but also by the sex ratio (infantile scoliosis is more common in males, adolescent scoliosis has a male:female ratio of 0.075:1) and by the direction of the curve (predominantly left-sided for infantile scoliosis and right-sided in adolescent scoliosis).

Environmental factors predominate in the aetiology of infantile scoliosis, which is almost invariably associated with plagiocephaly. They include breech presentation, prematurity, post-natal immobility and an excess of births during the winter months. The recurrence risk for first-degree relatives (siblings and children) of individuals with infantile scoliosis is approximately 2.6% (Wynne-Davies, 1968).

Female sex is a major genetic factor in the aetiology of adolescent idiopathic scoliosis. Twin studies show a concordance in monozygotic twin pairs that is nearly twice that in dizygotic pairs. The recurrence risk for first-degree relatives of an individual with a curve of 20° or greater, determined radiologically, was 11.1%, 2.4% for second-degree relatives and 1.4% for third-degree relatives (Riseborough and Wynne-Davies, 1973). Using a lower threshold for diagnosis of the index case gives reduced recurrence risks as would be predicted if inheritance follows a polygenic mode. Thus, using a 10° curve determined radiologically as the criterion for diagnosis gives recurrence risks of 6.8%, 1.6% and 1.0%, respectively, for first-, second- and third-degree relatives (Cowell *et al.*, 1972).

Arthrogryposis

This is a generic term covering a group of conditions of diverse aetiologies characterized by multiple congenital contractures. Any process that restricts fetal movement may lead to the development of congenital contractures. Congenital myopathies and neuropathies, abnormal fetal connective tissue and limitation of space within the uterus, as in a multiple pregnancy or bifid uterus, may result in limitation of fetal movement and the consequent development of contractures. It is also important to remember two maternal diseases that can cause arthrogryposis: myasthenia gravis and myotonic dystrophy.

Approximately one-third of patients have amyoplasia, also called 'classic' arthrogryposis or arthrogryposis multiplex congenita. The differential diagnosis for the remainder is very extensive, including more than 100 conditions (Hall, 1990). Hall distinguishes three categories of congenital contracture based on clinical findings: (i) primarily musculoskeletal involvement; (ii) musculoskeletal involvement plus other system malformations or anomalies; and (iii) musculoskeletal involvement plus central nervous system dysfunction and/or mental retardation. Initial subdivision into these categories is helpful before seeking a specific diagnosis within each category.

Achieving a specific diagnosis is important, as the recurrence risk varies from virtually zero in the case of amyoplasia, which is a sporadic disorder, to 50% for some varieties of distal arthrogryposis, which are dominantly inherited. For children with arthrogryposis and central nervous involvement, the recurrence risk averages 10–15%, suggesting that a high proportion of these cases is caused by single gene disorders with an autosomal recessive pattern of inheritance. Where no specific diagnosis can be reached, the recurrence risk to unaffected parents of an affected child, or of the affected individual with arthrogryposis for their own children, is in the range 3–5% (Hall, 1990). This empirical risk reflects the relative proportion of sporadic, single gene and polygenic disorders in the residual group of undiagnosed conditions causing arthrogryposis.

Pre-natal diagnosis is possible for some forms of arthrogryposis using real-time obstetric ultrasonography to evaluate fetal movements and range of joint mobility (Bendon *et al.*, 1987). Studies at 16, 20, 24 and 32 weeks of gestation are recommended. If a couple are at risk for an affected pregnancy, pre-natal diagnosis should be offered to them. Even in a situation where no recurrence is anticipated, e.g. in amyoplasia, visualization of normal fetal movement on an ultrasonographic scan may provide much-valued reassurance to the parents.

SOME SINGLE GENE DISORDERS WITH MUSCULOSKELETAL AND OTHER SYSTEM INVOLVEMENT

The clinical presentation and management of the major single gene disorders that present to the orthopaedic surgeon are discussed from an orthopaedic perspective elsewhere in the book. Most of the conditions described in the chapters on neuromuscular diseases (Chapter 3) and skeletal dysplasias (Chapter 2) are single gene disorders. For many of these conditions the orthopaedic management will be the mainstay of treatment. Other than for advice on the genetics of the condition and availability of pre-natal tests where appropriate, the clinical geneticist is seldom involved in the ongoing management of the patient.

There are, however, some autosomal dominant disorders with multisystem involvement in which the musculoskeletal problem may be only one of several presentations of the disorder. The danger for patients with this group of disease is that each time a problem occurs, the respective specialist may offer excellent care for that problem but forget to advise ongoing monitoring of the disease as a whole. It is often the role of the clinical geneticist to help to coordinate the care of such patients between the different specialties and provide ongoing monitoring for development of disease complications with the general practitioner. The authors have seen affected parents for genetic counselling in whom the diagnosis has only been made after the birth of an affected child with the same condition. Alternatively, the parent may have had expert treatment for a particular complication of the genetic disease in childhood and may even have been told the name of the disease but no one remembered to mention that it was genetic! This section does not cover all disorders that fall into this category exhaustively, but concentrates on a limited number of examples either because they are particularly common, e.g. neurofibromatosis, or because they can be used to demonstrate particular genetic principles. The section on neurofibromatosis is more extensive than the others because of its relative frequency and the authors' particular interest in the condition.

Neurofibromatosis

It is now recognized that there are several distinct types of neurofibromatosis, the recognition of which is important as the management and genetic counselling for each is different. In older textbooks patients with all forms of the disease tended to be described collectively as having 'von Recklinghausen's disease'.

NEUROFIBROMATOSIS TYPE 1

The most common form of neurofibromatosis, type 1, was formerly called peripheral or von Recklinghausen's neurofibromatosis. It is one of the most common autosomal dominant disorders with a birth incidence of about 1 in 2500 of the population (Huson *et al.*, 1988; Huson and Hughes, 1993). Approximately half the cases seen will have no family history and represent new gene mutations.

The major defining features of neurofibromatosis type 1, which are present in virtually all patients eventually, are *café au lait spots*, *dermal neurofibromas* and *Lisch nodules*. Café au lait spots are flat brown patches on the skin. They are asymptomatic and have no predilection for malignant change. In the general population 10% of

people have one or two spots, but in neurofibromatosis type 1 six or more are present. They are usually present from the first year or two of life and are therefore the first disease feature that can be checked for in children. As the child grows the other pigmentary feature that may develop is freckling in the axilla, groin, around the base of the neck and in the submammary area in girls.

As patients with neurofibromatosis type 1 reach their teens, the majority begin to develop dermal neurofibromas, which are benign tumours developing at the very ends of the peripheral nerves. They appear as small purplish lumps on the skin that can be very soft on palpation (Fig. 1.13). Some patients occasionally complain that they itch. The number of dermal neurofibromas that develop during a patient's life is extremely variable; some people have very few even in late adult life, while occasional patients are covered from head to foot. There is no treatment that can prevent these lesions developing and management at the present time simply involves removing those lesions that cause the patient problems from a cosmetic viewpoint or because they have grown larger than usual.

Lisch nodules are melanocytic hamartomas of the iris. They never cause symptoms, but are a useful sign to confirm the diagnosis in children with no family history. They cannot usually be seen with the naked eye and require slit-lamp examination, when they appear as raised, round lesions that are smooth and usually brown in colour.

In addition to these major defining features, there are two minor disease features — *macrocephaly* and *short stature*. Among the patients in the Welsh population study (Huson *et al.*, 1988), 45% had head circumferences at or above the 97th centile; 32% of patients were at or below the 3rd centile for height. The height measurements were compared with unaffected siblings in the families and showed that affected males were 8 cm and females 7.62 cm below expected height, purely because of having neurofibromatosis type 1.

Complications of neurofibromatosis type 1

These are listed in Table 1.7 and can affect any of the major systems of the body. The problem for the patient and the patient's family is that their recurrence cannot be predicted, even within families. In the past many patients with neurofibromatosis type 1 did not even realize that problems that arose were related to their disease — the author has seen many patients who had excellent treatment for scoliosis complicating neurofibromatosis without realizing that the two problems were related. Those patients who are unlucky enough to

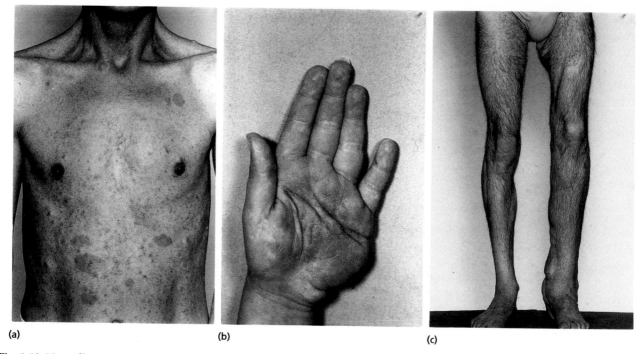

(a)　　　　　　　　　　(b)　　　　　　　　　　(c)

Fig. 1.13 Neurofibromatosis type 1. (a) Café au lait spots and dermal neurofibromatosis in an adult male. (b) Diffuse plexiform neurofibroma of right palm of child. (c) Diffuse plexiform neurofibroma of left leg. The patient had had epiphyseal plating at the knee in his teens to prevent further disproportion.

develop one or more complications may find themselves visiting several different specialist clinics and their care not being coordinated. For this reason it is now recommended that patients with neurofibromatosis type 1 have annual follow-up visits to one particular clinic offering a general health check for disease complications. In childhood this is usually offered by the paediatrician, for adults the general practitioner may well adopt the role of overall monitoring of the disease and referring to specialist colleagues if the patient develops disease complications. No single complication of the disease occurs often enough to warrant regular screening investigations, such as cranial neuro-imaging. The disease complications that can present to the orthopaedic surgeon are discussed briefly below. The orthopaedic management of the major ones (scoliosis and pseudoarthrosis) are discussed in other chapters (Chapters 4 and 8.2).

Scoliosis. In the South Wales population study of neurofibromatosis type 1, 5% of the patients had scoliosis that required surgery and a further 6% had minor curves that the patient had either not been aware of or had been treated conservatively. In a large series of patients with scoliosis, Winter *et al.* (1979) found that 1% had neurofibromatosis type 1. The classic description is of two main varieties of curve, the dystrophic and the idiopathic, the latter having a much better prognosis. Crawford estimated that there is a 7:1 ratio of idiopathic to dystrophic curve in the population with neurofibromatosis type 1 (Crawford, 1989; Fairbank, 1993).

Pseudoarthrosis of the long bones. Pseudoarthrosis appearing in any long bone in infancy often turns out to be associated with neurofibromatosis type 1. The most common sites are the tibia and/or fibula, though pseudoarthrosis has been observed in other long bones, particularly the radius and ulna. In the South Wales population study (Table 1.7) 2% of the patients had pseudoarthrosis of the tibia with or without the fibula, which had resulted in non-union and eventual below-knee amputation, and another 1% of patients had less severe forms. In series of patients with tibial pseudoarthrosis presenting to orthopaedic clinics, between 50% and 90% of cases are reported to have neurofibromatosis type 1 (Fairbank, 1993).

Other skeletal abnormalities. Although scoliosis and pseudoarthrosis are the symptomatic complications that present to the orthopaedic surgeon, other skeletal abnormalities are seen in neurofibromatosis type 1 and the surgeon should be aware of them. These include *vertebral scalloping,* which is often seen on spinal radiographs of adult patients with neurofibromatosis type 1 but seldom

Table 1.7 Prevalence of complications of neurofibromatosis type 1 in a population-based study in South Wales (Huson *et al.*, 1988; Huson and Hughes, 1993)

Complication	Prevalence (%)
Plexiform neurofibromas	
All lesions	30
Large lesions of head and neck	3
Limb/trunk lesions with significant skin/bone hypertrophy	5.6
Education	
Special school education	2.9
Remedial class education	23.5
Normal education, specific learning difficulties	5.9
Scoliosis	
Requiring surgery	4.4
Less severe	5.2
Pseudoarthrosis of tibia and fibula	
Resulting in non-union and eventual below-knee amputation	2.2
Less severe forms	1.5
Lamboidal suture defect	0.75
Malignancy secondary to neurofibromatosis type 1 (peripheral nerve tumours, pelvic rhabdomyosarcoma)	2.9
Symptomatic CNS tumours (including optic glioma)	1.5–2.2
Spinal neurofibromas	1.5
Acoustic neuroma	0
Epilepsy	
No known cause	4.4
Secondary to disease complications	2.2
Others	
Hypsarrhythmia	1.5
Aqueduct stenosis	1.5
Meningoangiomatosis*	0.75
Gastrointestinal neurofibromas	2.2
Renal artery stenosis	1.5
Phaeochromocytoma	0.75
Duodenal carcinoid	1.5
Delayed puberty (no underlying cause)†	1.5
Congenital glaucoma	0.75
Juvenile xanthogranuloma	0.75

Complications (which would have been symptomatic) *not* seen in study population but definitely associated with neurofibromatosis type 1

Thoracic meningocoele	Presumed frequency ≤1%
Sphenoid wing dysplasia	
Atypical forms of childhood leukaemia	
Cerebrovascular disease	

* Diagnosis of neurofibromatosis type 1 not certain, may have had type 2 disease.
† Possibly not increased incidence above general population.

causes symptoms. *Thoracic meningocoeles* have been reported to occur, but are a rare complication. They are sometimes found incidentally when a patient with neurofibromatosis type 1 undergoes chest radiography for other reasons, or they may be symptomic, presenting as a large soft-tissue or cystic mass protruding from the mediastinum. They may be accompanied by structural defects in the pedicle, enlargement of the intervertebral foramina and vertebral body anomalies. In a review of 70 cases of thoracic meningocoele, of which 85% had neurofibromatosis type 1, Miles *et al.* (1969) reported severe paraplegia in only six and minor neurological impairment in seven, though nearly one-quarter had significant pain.

The skull is another area of the body that can have skeletal defects which may or may not be associated with symptoms. Patients may have *sphenoid wing dysplasia*, often associated with a facial plexiform neurofibroma which will present with obvious swelling around the orbit. In the absence of a plexiform neurofibroma, the sphenoid wing dysplasia usually presents as a pulsatile enophthalmos. The author has seen several patients with this defect who have not been aware of it. Another skull defect of which the patient rarely complains are *lamboidal suture defects*—these are usually found on skull radiographs done for other reasons; clinically a defect in the skull is found as the lamboidal suture is palpated.

Occasionally, cyst-like lytic lesions of the bones are seen and may cause diagnostic confusion with McCune–Albright syndrome. The latter is characterized by one or more areas of café au lait pigmentation in association with polyostotic fibrous dysplasia and sexual precocity. The café au lait pigmentation in McCune–Albright syndrome tends to cover larger areas of the body than the spots in neurofibromatosis type 1. The borders tend to be more jagged, and were compared to the 'coast of Maine' by Albright. The smooth borders in neurofibromatosis type 1 have been compared to the 'coast of California'. Although these distinctions are generally true, the café au lait spots in neurofibromatosis type 1 can have jagged edges, and therefore the border shape of the pigmentation cannot be relied on as a distinguishing feature.

Plexiform neurofibromas. These are quite distinct from dermal neurofibromas, particularly in that the largest lesions are usually present from the first 1–2 years of life. In the Welsh population study (Huson *et al.*, 1988), 27% of patients had plexiform neurofibromas; of these 1% had large lesions of the head and neck and 6% particularly large lesions on the trunk or limbs associated with significant hypertrophy of the underlying bone or overlying skin.

Clinically, two types of plexiform neurofibromas can be recognized. The majority of lesions are *diffuse plexiform neurofibromas*—these present as large subcutaneous swellings with ill-defined margins ranging from a few centimetres in diameter to those involving a whole area of the body. Their consistency is usually soft,

though occasionally hypertrophied nerves can be palpated within the mass. The skin overlying the lesion is often abnormal due to a combination of hypertrophy, café au lait pigmentation, or hypertrichosis. When these lesions involve the limbs and are particularly large, they can be associated with overgrowth of the underlying bone and present to the orthopaedic surgeon because of limb length discrepancy.

Much rarer are the *nodular plexiform neurofibromas*. In these lesions, the abnormality is confined to the nerves of a particular area, where there are multiple neurofibromatous lesions on the major nerves. For example, patients may present complaining of persistent pain in the buttock region and on imaging multiple neurofibromas are seen in the major nerves of that area.

Peripheral nerve neurofibromas. The dermal neurofibromas, which are actually cutaneous lesions, seldom cause symptoms. This is in contrast to neurofibromas that develop within the major peripheral nerves. No study has looked at exactly how many patients develop these lesions, but it may be in the region of 5–10%. They usually cause symptoms and patients present with acute paraesthesiae because the lesions are painful to touch. Surgical removal by someone with experience in peripheral nerve surgery is imperative.

Preparation of the patient with neurofibromatosis type 1 for operation. When patients are prepared for an operation, it is important to consider other disease complications that could affect the operation. Of particular importance would be an undiagnosed phaechromocytoma, so symptoms of such lesions should be sought and the blood pressure carefully checked. Similarly, in assessing patients with neurofibromatosis type 1 and scoliosis, it is important to check whether they have spinal neurofibromas that may complicate an operation (Fairbank, 1993).

NEUROFIBROMATOSIS TYPE 2

The major disease feature in neurofibromatosis type 2 is bilateral acoustic neuromas. These occur in nearly all patients, but are often associated with tumours elsewhere in the nervous system, particularly cranial meningiomas and spinal schwannomas or meningiomas. In a significant proportion of patients there are some overlapping cutaneous features in common with neurofibromatosis type 1. They may have one or two café au lait spots, though to have six is extremely unusual, and one or two cutaneous or peripheral nerve tumours. This often leads to confusion as to which type of neurofibromatosis is present. The peripheral nerve tumours in type 2 disease are usually schwannomas rather than neurofibromas. It is important that orthopaedic surgeons with an interest in peripheral nerve surgery are aware of this distinction. When young patients present with multiple peripheral nerve schwannomas, serious consideration should be given to whether or not this is an initial presentation of neurofibromatosis type 2. In a recent UK study of the disease (Evans *et al.*, 1992), a small but significant group of patients had presented with peripheral nerve tumours before becoming symptomatic from their acoustic neuromas, and the significance of the peripheral nerve tumours in association with a family history of deafness had been ignored. The other peripheral sign of the disease which has only recently been appreciated is that approximately two-thirds of patients have posterior lens opacities, though symptomatic cataract is unusual.

The importance of identifying neurofibromatosis type 2 is that the acoustic neuromas in the disease tend to become symptomatic at a relatively late stage. As they are by then large, surgery is extremely difficult. Once the disease is suspected in an individual, or someone is at 50% risk of inheriting it from one of their parents, it is essential that regular disease monitoring is initiated, including brain-stem evoked responses and cranial neuro-imaging (Evans *et al.*, 1992).

OTHER FORMS OF NEUROFIBROMATOSIS

The other best recognized form of neurofibromatosis is segmental neurofibromatosis (Fig. 1.7). In this form of the disease, the features are limited to one segment of the body surface, which may be either unilateral or bilateral. The importance of recognizing such patients is that they would not be expected to be at risk of the generalized complications of the disease. Also, as it is assumed their mutation has arisen at a somatic level, only a few patients will be expected to have germ cell involvement and therefore the risk of their having children with neurofibromatosis type 1 is not the usual 50% and may only be 1–2%, though the exact risk is difficult to estimate.

Riccardi (1992) has suggested that there may be as many as four other types of neurofibromatosis, in addition to the ones reviewed above. The authors' own feeling is that these are not sufficiently defined at the present time and that if they exist at all they are extremely rare. For the practising clinician, the take-home message is that if patients do not immediately fall into the clinical spectrum of neurofibromatosis type 1 or 2 or segmental neurofibromatosis, then it may be worth a clinician with a particular interest in neurofibromatosis assessing them

to see exactly what kind of neurofibromatosis is present. The importance of doing this is because of the genetic and management implications. For disorders similar to type 2 disease, detailed follow-up with careful monitoring for development of acoustic neuromas is essential, whereas in disorders similar to type 1 disease a general physical examination is all that is recommended.

In recent years there have been major advances in the molecular genetics of neurofibromatosis types 1 and 2. The gene for type 1 is on chromosome 17 and for type 2 on chromosome 22, molecular confirmation of the fact that they are quite distinct disorders. The genes for both disorders have now been cloned, and work is beginning on unravelling disease pathogenesis. DNA markers are now available for pre-symptomatic and pre-natal diagnosis of both types of neurofibromatosis (Huson and Hughes, 1993).

Marfan's syndrome

This is an autosomal dominant condition with an incidence of approximately 1 in 10 000 of the population; 25–30% of cases have no family history and represent new gene mutations. Cardinal disease features are skeletal changes ('the marfonoid habitus') in association with lens dislocation and cardiovascular disease in the form of aortic dilation with or without dissection. The disease phenotype is extremely variable, however, and assessment of first-degree relatives of affected individuals should not simply rely on clinical examination but include ophthalmological and cardiac assessments (Godfrey, 1993). Affected individuals can have cardiovascular and/or eye involvement without major skeletal changes.

The major orthopaedic problem in Marfan's syndrome is scoliosis. Other problems include protrusio acetabulae and painful feet, presumably related to the long, narrow, foot shape seen in the syndrome (Goldberg, 1987) (Fig. 1.14). Orthopaedic management of the condition is not reviewed here, other than to point out that when a patient is identified by an orthopaedic surgeon it is important to refer on for assessment and long-term follow-up by someone with an interest in the condition. In the past many people with Marfan's syndrome have died at a young age because of aortic dissection. If the degree of aortic dilatation is monitored and a prophylactic operation undertaken when it reaches a critical degree, the fatal complication of aortic dissection can be avoided. To provide coordinated care for patients with Marfan's syndrome and to avoid them having to attend many different specialty clinics, many centres now run Marfan's syndrome clinics where combined cardio-

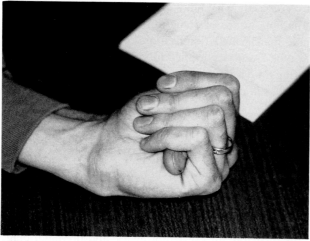

(a)

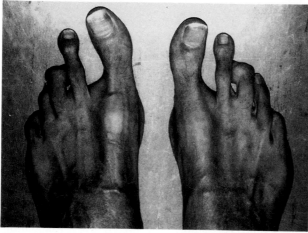

(b)

Fig. 1.14 Marfan's syndrome. (a) Steinberg thumb sign. The long digits, narrow hand and hyperextensible joints allow the thumb to extend beyond the ulnar surface of the hand when held as shown. (b) Long toes, some with flexion contractures.

logical, ophthalmological and genetic opinion is available on the same day.

DIFFERENTIAL DIAGNOSIS AND DIAGNOSTIC CRITERIA

One of the major problems in assessing patients with possible Marfan's syndrome is distinguishing those with the actual disease from members of families where the body habitus is part of familial variation and not part of a disease as such. The major clinical features of Marfan's syndrome are listed in Table 1.8 and the differential diagnosis of the condition in Table 1.9. At present, assessment is based purely on clinical examination, including a detailed cardiovascular and ophthalmo-

logical assessment. The diagnostic criteria are shown in Table 1.8 (Beighton *et al.*, 1988).

There has recently been major progress in our understanding of the pathogenesis of Marfan's syndrome (Godfrey, 1993). Mutations in the fibrillin gene on chromosome 16 have been found to be the cause of Marfan's syndrome. It is hoped that this research will soon lead to a diagnostic test for the condition. Direct mutation analysis, however, may not be the answer, as the mutations in the gene are proving hard to identify and vary between different families.

Myotonic dystrophy

The clinical features of myotonic dystrophy are described in detail and illustrated in Chapter 3 (Fig. 3.4, p. 58). As it is both relatively common as a genetic disease and is a multisystem disorder, it is included in this section to highlight some of the genetic aspects of the condition and some disease features that make regular follow-up of affected individuals advisable.

Myotonic dystrophy is one of the more common forms of muscular dystrophy with a birth incidence of 1 in 7000. It is inherited as an autosomal dominant condition, but disease expression is extremely variable as summarized in Table 1.10 (Harper, 1989). The disease demonstrates the phenomenon of anticipation, with affected individuals in successive generations showing a more severe phenotype. This has recently been shown to be due to the nature of the gene mutation (Suthers *et al.*, 1992) which involves a triplet repeat of DNA within the gene that increases in size in successive generations. The myotonic dystrophy gene is on chromosome 19 and encodes for a protein kinase that has been named myotonin.

MANAGEMENT OF PATIENTS WITH MYOTONIC DYSTROPHY

Once the diagnosis of myotonic dystrophy has been made it is important that patients are aware of the multisystem nature of their disease. The most important points are:
1 The patient knows that the anaesthetist must be warned about the disease because of the anaesthetic complications.
2 Patients are offered annual review with electrocardiography to monitor for the development of cardiac conduction abnormalities.
3 Patients are aware of the association of the disease with cataracts, so that if visual deterioration occurs, they can seek appropriate ophthalmological assessment.

Table 1.8 Clinical features and diagnostic criteria of Marfan's syndrome. Clinical features are listed in approximate order of decreasing specifity. Major disease manifestations are marked by an asterisk

---

Skeletal
  Anterior chest deformity, particularly asymmetrical pectus excavatum/carinatum
  Dolichostenomelia not due to scoliosis
  Arachnodactyly
  Scoliosis
  Thoracic lordosis or reduced thoracic kyphosis
  Tall stature, compared to unaffected 1° relatives
  High, narrow arched palate and dental crowding
  Protrusio acetabulae
  Congenital flexion contractures
  Joint hypermobility

Ocular
  Ectopia lentis*
  Flat cornea
  Enlarged globe
  Retinal detachment
  Myopia

Cardiovascular
  Dilatation of ascending aorta*
  Aortic dissection*
  Aortic regurgitation
  Mitral regurgitation due to mitral valve prolapse

Pulmonary
  Spontaneous pneumothorax
  Apical bleb

Skin and integument
  Striae distensae
  Inguinal and other hernias (umbilical, diaphragmatic, incisional)

Central nervous system
  Dural ecstasia—lumbosacral meningocoele, dilated cisterna magna*
  Learning disability (verbal performance discrepancy)
  Hyperactivity ± attention deficit disorder

Diagnostic criteria
In the absence of an unequivocally affected first-degree relative: involvement of the skeleton and at least two other systems with one major manifestation. N.B. Homocystinuria must be excluded
In the presence of at least one unequivocally affected first-degree relative: involvement of at least two systems, one major manifestation preferred but depends on family's phenotype

---

4 Patients are aware of the wide variation within families and the risk to women with the disease (even if mildly affected) of having children with the severe congenital form.

Genetic counselling

Once a patient with myotonic dystrophy has been diagnosed, it is important that any first-degree relatives are offered assessment. This is a condition where the doctor cannot rely on affected individuals complaining of symptoms because of the wide variation of the disease. The assessment of at-risk individuals used to consist of clinical and slit-lamp examination plus electromyography; however, if these were normal in young adulthood because of the late onset of the disease in some people, there was still a small but significant risk of carrying the gene. Fortunately, with the cloning of the gene, all individuals with the disease have been found to have the same mutation which is easily tested for in the laboratory. Direct DNA testing has therefore superseded the older methods of assessment. Indeed, DNA testing

Table 1.9 A limited differential diagnosis of the marfanoid habitus (Godfrey, 1993; Goldberg, 1987)

Syndromes with overlapping features
Congenital contractural arachnodactyly
Stickler's syndrome
Achard–Thiers syndrome
(skeletal changes limited to hands and feet with arachnodactyly
   and joint laxity)

Syndromes with similar body habitus
Klinefelter's syndrome (47,XXY)
Mosaic trisomy 8 (may also have joint contractures)
Nemaline myopathy
Multiple endocrine neoplasia type 3
   (marfanoid habitus, mucosal neuromas, phaeochromocytomas
   and medullary carcinoma of thyroid)
Megaduodenum–megacystis syndrome
   (marfanoid habitus, intestinal pseudo-obstruction)
Goodman camptodactyly syndrome B
Syndrome of nerve deafness, eye anomalies and marfanoid habitus
Diaphyseal dysplasia (Camurati–Engelmann syndrome)

Table 1.10 Range of clinical features in myotonic dystrophy

Congenital myotonic dystrophy
Seen in children of affected mothers; pregnancy history may include polyhydramnios and reduced fetal movements. Children have neonatal hypotonia with or without joint contractures and facial weakness. Developmental delay and mental retardation become obvious in first year of life

Classical adult presentation
Onset of symptoms (usually initially grip myotonia) late teens or early twenties. Characteristic pattern of wasting and weakness of certain voluntary muscle group ensues. Multisystem involvement (see Chapter 3)

Mild adult presentation
Usually ascertained via affected children. May show polychromatic lens crystals or pre-senile cataracts only. Occasionally myotonia but no muscle weakness

has shown that one of the signs that used to be relied on, polychromatic lens crystals, is not as specific for myotonic dystrophy as first thought. A small percentage of individuals who had been labelled as affected on the basis of this sign alone have now been shown not to carry the myotonic dystrophy gene.

Unfortunately, one of the more common presentations of the disease in a family is via the birth of a congenitally affected child. In the Oxford Health Region, with a population of approximately 2.6 million, one or two babies are born each year with this condition who are the first people to be diagnosed in their families. Sometimes their mothers have previously sought medical advice about symptoms from grip myotonia and been told that it was nothing to worry about. Once a woman has symptomatic myotonic dystrophy, even if it is very mild, when she has children there is a 1 in 2 risk of them inheriting the (dominant inheritance) gene, and an approximately 20% risk of having a child with the congenitally affected form of the disease. There is evidence that the more severe the disease in the mother the greater her risk of having a congenitally affected child (Koch *et al.*, 1991). When a woman has had one affected child with the congenital myotonic dystrophy phenotype her subsequent children, who inherit the gene, will be similarly affected. Fortunately with the detection of the gene mutation, 100% accurate pre-natal diagnosis can now be offered to women at risk of having children with congenital myotonic dystrophy. It is not known why some women are predisposed to have children with this form of the disease; initial research looking at size variation of the gene mutation suggests that this is not the sole answer and there may be another, possibly cytoplasmic, factor involved in the development of congenital myotonic dystrophy.

Ehlers–Danlos syndrome

This is much rarer than the other disorders reviewed in this section. A minimum incidence of 1 in 150 000 was estimated in one survey in the south of England (Beighton, 1970a). It is included in the chapter to draw attention to the concept of *heterogeneity* of genetic conditions—heterogeneity refers to the fact that different mutations can cause a similar phenotype. *Allelic heterogeneity* refers to different mutations at the same locus, whereas *locus heterogeneity* refers to mutations at different loci. Within Ehlers–Danlos syndrome, subtypes showing all three kinds of mendelian inheritance are recognized. As in neurofibromatosis, the other important point arising from subclassification is that the various disease types are associated with quite different morbidity and mortality. The subtypes of Ehlers–Danlos are summarized in Table 1.11.

The cardinal features of Ehlers–Danlos syndrome (Beighton *et al.*, 1986; Beighton, 1993) are:
1 Skin abnormality—the skin is hyperextensible (Fig. 1.15) and has a soft, velvety, doughy texture. The skin is fragile, there is easy bruising and scar formation is poor. Minimal trauma can cause a gaping wound and healing results in wide, shiny scars as if it had occurred by secondary intention. The scars are most apparent over the knees, shins, elbows, forehead and chin, and have been likened to cigarette paper or papyrus. Repeated trauma and the tendency for wound dehiscence

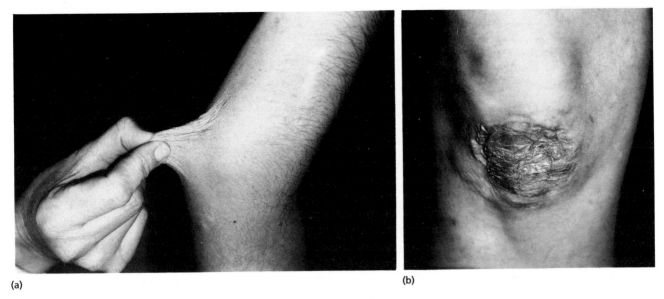

(a) (b)

Fig. 1.15 Ehlers−Danlos syndrome. (a) Hyperextensible skin. (b) Abnormal scarring.

result in a collection of purplish connective tissue nodules often developing over the elbows and knees; these are known as molluscoid pseudotumours.

2 Joint hypermobility — some infants with Ehlers− Danlos syndrome have such marked hyperextensibility that they are mistakenly labelled as being 'floppy infants'. The rheumatological and orthopaedic implications of Ehlers−Danlos syndrome have been the subject of several reviews (Beighton and Horan, 1969; Beighton, 1970b; Beighton, 1972; Goldberg, 1987). Effusions and pain can follow exercise, and presentation to the paediatric rheumatologist is not uncommon. The hyperextensibility improves with age, but in individuals with very hypermobile joints the gait may always be abnormal and is broad based, often with short, hesitant steps. About 20% of adults continue to have instability and chronic effusions of the knees, ankles, elbows and thumbs. Dislocation occurs in about 25% of patients, can involve any joint, and be acute, chronic, or repetitive.

3 Connective tissue fragility — the connective tissue of all parts of the body is affected, and the basic defect is thought to concern the organization of collagen bundles into an intermeshing network. Genetically determined abnormalities in collagen structure or processing have been recognized in some forms of Ehlers−Danlos syndrome (Beighton, 1993).

The degree of connective tissue involvement varies in the different types (Table 1.11). Arterial involvement is a particular feature of Ehlers−Danlos types I and IV.

Here sheer force from normal activity can result in spontaneous arterial rupture. During childhood and adolescence multiple aneurysms may develop in the arteries of the major extremities, viscera and brain, particularly in the popliteal, femoral and axillary arteries. Caution must be exercised in assessment of the aneurysm because of the danger of increasing the problem through trauma at catheterization, and non-invasive methods of evaluation are preferred if this is possible. In some patients the veins dilate and become varicose, but their fragility prevents effective surgical stripping.

The supporting structure of the colon, bladder and uterus is weakened and diverticula may develop. Sudden rupture of a hollow viscus is well recognized, e.g. intestine or uterus. Spontaneous pneumothorax is also a feature, as is mitral valve prolapse. Hernias are also common, but repair is difficult and they often recur.

Although the subclassification of Ehlers−Danlos syndrome shown in Table 1.11 is helpful, as with many other conditions some patients cannot neatly be categorized. The message for the orthopaedic surgeon (Goldberg, 1987) is that in assessing a patient with hypermobile joints, examination of the skin and a family history may provide clues as to whether the underlying diagnosis is Ehlers−Danlos syndrome. The importance of recognizing the condition is that surgical management may be altered because of the problems with scarring and connective tissue fragility.

Table 1.11 Subclassification of Ehlers−Danlos syndrome

Cardinal features
Hyperextensible skin
Dystrophic scarring
Easy bruising
Joint hypermobility
Connective tissue fragility

Classification

Type	Name, clinical features and basic defect (if known)	Mode of inheritance
I	Gravis. Cardinal manifestations in severe degree	Autosomal dominant
II	Mitis. Cardinal manifestations in mild degree	Autosomal dominant
III	Hypermobile type. Marked articular hypermobility, moderate dermal hyperextensibility, minimal scarring	Autosomal dominant
IV	Vascular. Variable stigmata. Severe bruising, hyperpigmentation and/or scarring. Thin skin with prominent veins. Vascular rupture. Colonic perforation. Characteristic facial appearance. All forms have defect of type III collagen	
	IV-A Acrogeric type	Autosomal dominant
	IV-B Acrogeric type	Autosomal recessive
	IV-C Ecchymotic type	Autosomal dominant
V	X-linked type. Cardinal manifestations in moderate degree	X-linked
VI	Ocular−scoliotic type. Cardinal manifestations in severe degree, plus eye involvement (microcornea, scleral perforation, retinal detachment) and scoliosis	
	IV-A Decreased lysyl hydroxylase activity	Autosomal recessive
VII	Arthrochalasis multiplex congenita. Cardinal manifestations with marked articular hypermobility, short stature and micrognathia	
	VII-A Structural defect of pro-α_1-(1) collagen	Autosomal dominant
	VII-B Structural defect of pro-α_2-(1) collagen	Autosomal dominant
	VII-C Procollagen *N*-proteinase deficiency	Autosomal recessive
VIII	Periodontitis type. Cardinal manifestations in moderate degree. Aggressive periodontitis, gingival recession, early tooth loss	Autosomal dominant
IX	Vacant	
X	Fibronectin abnormality. Cardinal manifestations but skin texture normal. Petechiae. Striae distensae. Platelet aggregation defect corrected by fibronectin	Autosomal recessive

ACKNOWLEDGEMENTS

The authors are grateful to Mark Selinger for providing Figs 1.11 and 1.12 and Lyn Chitty and David Griffen for Fig. 1.10.

REFERENCES

Ad Hoc Committee on Genetic Counselling (1975) *Am. J. Hum. Genet.* **27**, 240−242.
Baird P.A., Anderson T.W., Newcombe H.B. and Lowry R.B.

(1988) Genetic disorders in children and young adults: a population study. *Am. J. Hum. Genet.* **42**, 677–693.

Beighton P. (1970a) *The Ehlers–Danlos Syndrome.* London, William Heinemann Medical Books.

Beighton P. (1970b) Ehlers–Danlos syndrome. *Ann. Rheum. Dis.* **29**, 332–333.

Beighton P. (1972) Articular manifestations of the Ehlers–Danlos syndrome. *Semin. Arthritis Rheum.* **1**, 246–261.

Beighton P. (1993) The Ehlers–Danlos syndrome. In Beighton P. (ed) *McKusick's Heritable Disorders of Connective Tissue*, 5th edn. St Louis, Mosby–Year Book Inc., pp. 189–251.

Beighton P. and Horan F. (1969) Orthopaedic aspects of the Ehlers–Danlos syndrome. *J. Bone Joint Surg.* **51B**, 444–453.

Beighton P., de Paepe A., Danks D. *et al.* (1988) International nosology of heritable disorders of connective tissue, Berlin 1986. *Am. J. Med. Genet.* **29**, 581–594.

Bendon R., Digman P. and Siddiqui T. (1987) Prenatal diagnosis of arthrogryposis multiplex congenita. *J. Pediatr.* **111**, 942–946.

Canadian Collaborative CVS–Amniocentesis Clinical Trial Group. (1989) Multicentre randomised clinical trial of chorion villus sampling and amniocentesis. *Lancet* **i**, 1–6.

Carter C.O. (1969) Genetics of common disorders. *Br. Med. Bull.* **25**, 52–57.

Carter C.O. (1970) Multifactorial genetic disease. *Hosp. Pract.* **5**, 45–59.

Contact a Family Directory of Specific Conditions and Rare Syndromes (1991). London, Contact a Family.

Cowell H.R., Hall S.N. and MacEwen G.D. (1972) Genetic aspects of idiopathic scoliosis. *Clin. Orthop.* **86**, 123–131.

Crawford A. (1989) Pitfalls of spinal deformities associated with neurofibromatosis in children. *Clin. Orthop.* **245**, 29–42.

Czeizel A., Tusuady G., Vaczo G. and Vizkelety T. (1975) The mechanism of genetic predisposition in congenital dislocation of the hip. *J. Med. Genet.* **12**, 125–130.

Davies K.E. and Read A.P. (1988) *Molecular Basis of Inherited Disease.* Oxford, IRL Press.

Emery A.E.H. and Rimoin D.L. (eds). (1990) *Principles and Practice of Medical Genetics*, 2nd edn. Edinburgh, Churchill Livingstone.

Evans D.G.R., Huson S.M., Neary W., Newton V., Blair V., Donnai D. and Harris R. (1992) A clinical study of type 2 neurofibromatosis. *Q. J. Med.* **304**, 603–618.

Fairbank J. (1993) Neuromuscular and skeletal manifestations of neurofibromatosis. In Huson S.M. and Hughes R.A.C. (eds) *The Neurofibromatoses: a Clinical and Pathogenetic Overview.* London, Chapman and Hall, pp. 275–304.

Gelehrter T.D. and Collins F.S. (1990) *Principles of Medical Genetics.* Baltimore, Williams and Wilkins.

Godfrey M. (1993) The Marfan syndrome. In Beighton P. (ed) *McKusick's Heritable Disorders of Connective Tissue*, 5th edn. St Louis, Mosby–Year Book Inc., pp. 51–135.

Goldberg M.J. (1987) *The Dysmorphic Child. An Orthopaedic Perspective.* New York, Raven Press.

Hall J.G. (1990) Genomic imprinting: review and relevance to human diseases. *Am. J. Hum. Genet.* **46**, 857–873.

Hall J.G. (1990) Arthrogryposis (multiple congenital contracture). In Emery A.E.H. and Rimoin D.L. (eds) *Principles and Practice of Medical Genetics*, 2nd edn. Edinburgh, Churchill Livingstone.

Handyside A.H., Lesko J.G., Tarin J.J., Winston R.M.L. and Hughes M.R. (1992) Birth of a normal girl after in vitro fertilization and preimplantation diagnostic testing for cystic fibrosis. *N. Engl. J. Med.* **327**, 905–909.

Harper P.S. (1993) *Practical Genetic Counselling*, 4th edn. London, Butterworth and Co.

Harper P.S. (1989) *Myotonic Dystrophy*, 2nd edn. London, W.B. Saunders Co.

Harper P.S., Harley H.G., Reardon W. and Shaw D.J. (1992) Anticipation in myotonic dystrophy: new light on an old problem. *Am. J. Hum. Genet.* **51**, 10–16.

Hodgson S.V. and Maher E.R. (1993) *A Practical Guide to Human Cancer Genetics.* Cambridge, Cambridge University Press.

Howeler C.J., Busch H.F.M., Geraedts J.P.M., Niermeyer M.F. and Staal A. (1989) Anticipation in myotonic dystrophy: fact or fiction. *Brain* **112**, 770–797.

Huntington's Disease Collaborative Research Group. (1993) A novel gene containing a trinucleotide repeat that is expanded and unstable on Huntington's disease chromosomes. *Cell* **72**, 1–20.

Huson S.M. and Hughes R.A.C. (1993) *The Neurofibromatoses: a Clinical and Pathogenetic Overview.* London, Chapman and Hall.

Huson S.M., Harper P.S. and Compston D.A.S. (1988) Von Recklinghausen neurofibromatosis: a clinical and population study in South East Wales. *Brain* **111**, 1355–1381.

Idelberger K. (1951) *Die erbpathologic der sogenannten angeborenen.* H'uftverrenkung, M'unchen und Berlin Urban & Schwarzenberg.

Kambara H. and Sasakawa Y. (1954) On twins with congenital dislocation of the hip. *J. Bone Joint Surg.* **36A**, 186–187.

Kingston H.M. (1989) *ABC of Clinical Genetics.* London, British Medical Association.

Koch M.C., Grimm T., Harley H.G. and Harper P.S. (1991) Genetic risks for children of women with myotonic dystrophy. *Am. J. Hum. Genet.* **48**, 1084–1091.

Langman J. (1975) *Medical Embryology*, 3rd edn. Baltimore, Williams and Wilkins.

McKusick V.A. (1992) *Mendelian Inheritance in Man*, 10th edn. Baltimore, Johns Hopkins University Press.

Mahoney B.S. (1990) The extremities. In Nyberg D.A., Mahoney B.S. and Pretorius D.H. (eds) *Diagnostic Ultrasound of Fetal Anomalies: Text and Atlas.* St Louis, Mosby–Year Book Inc., pp. 493–562.

Miles J., Pennybacker J. and Sheldon P. (1969) Intrathoracic meningocele: its development and association with neurofibromatosis. *J. Neurol. Neurosurg. Psychiatry* **32**, 99–100.

MRC Vitamin Study Group. (1991) Prevention of neural tube defects: results of the Medical Research Council Vitamin Study. *Lancet* **238**, 131–137.

MRC Working Party on the Evaluation of Chorionic Villus Sampling. (1991) Medical Research Council European Trial of chorionic villus sampling. *Lancet* **i**, 1491–1499.

Pembrey M. (1987) Impact of molecular biology on clinical genetics. *BMJ* **925**, 711–713.

Poulton J. (1992) Mitochondrial DNA and genetic disease. *Bioessays* **14**, 763–768.

Riccardi V.M. (1992) *Neurofibromatosis: Phenotype, Natural History and Pathogenesis*, 2nd edn. Baltimore, Johns Hopkins University Press.

Riseborough E.J. and Wynne-Davies R. (1973) A genetic survey of idiopathic scoliosis in Boston, Massachusetts. *J. Bone Joint Surg.* **55A**, 974–982.

Rodeck C. (1993) Fetal development after chorionic villus sampling. *Lancet* **i**, 468–469.

Royal College of Physicians. (1989) *Prenatal Diagnosis and Genetic Screening. Community and Service Implications. A Report of the Royal College of Physicians.*

Strachan T. (1992) *The Human Genome.* Oxford, BIOS Scientific Publishers.

Suthers G.K., Huson S.M. and Davies K.E. (1992) Instability versus predictability: the molecular diagnosis of myotonic dystrophy. *J. Med. Genet.* **29**, 761–765.

Tabor A., Madsen M., Obel F. *et al.* (1986) Randomised controlled trial of genetic amniocentesis in 4606 Low-risk women. *Lancet* **i**, 1287–1293.

Wald N.J., Teizian E., Vickeis P.A. and Weatherall J.A.C. (1983) Congenital talipes and hip malformation in relation to amniocentesis: a case control study. *Lancet* **ii**, 246–249.

Weatherall D.J. *The New Genetics and Clinical Practice*, 3rd edn. Oxford, Oxford University Press.

Winter R.M. and Baraitser M. (1991) *Multiple Congenital Anomalies. A Diagnostic Compendium.* London, Chapman and Hall.

Winter R.B., More J.H., Bradford D.S., Lonstein J.E., Pedras C.V. and Weber A.H. (1979) Spine deformity in neurofibromatosis. *J. Bone Joint Surg.* **61A**, 677–694.

Wynne-Davies R. (1964) Family studies and the cause of congenital club foot, talipes equinovarus, calcaneovalgus and metarsus varus. *J. Bone Joint Surg.* **46B**, 445–463.

Wynne-Davies R. (1968) Familial (idiopathic) scoliosis, a family survey. *J. Bone Joint Surg.* **50B**, 24–30.

Wynne-Davies R. (1970) A family study of neonatal and late-diagnosis congenital dislocation of the hip. *J. Med. Genet.* **7**, 315–333.

Chapter 2
Skeletal Dysplasias

F.T. Horan

INTRODUCTION

Syndromes that are characterized by generalized or localized faults in skeletal growth are known as skeletal dysplasias. They are rare, and many show established patterns of heredity. The term *dysplasia* implies a generalized abnormality in growth or development, whereas *dysostosis* denotes maldevelopment of a single bone or body segment. Both types of disorder may be described under the heading of skeletal dysplasias.

Many skeletal dysplasias have a characteristic individual appearance and are easily recognized. Because of their rarity, however, their features may not be widely known. The first attempt at classification and delineation of these disorders was made by Sir Thomas Fairbank, who built up a unique collection of radiographs and clinical descriptions of affected patients during the first half of this century. He published his observations in a classic monograph *An Atlas of General Affections of the Skeleton*, and this book became the basis for all subsequent investigation.

Wider recognition of these syndromes has resulted in the formation of specialist units devoted to their study and management. Consequently, the problems that may be associated with such disorders are now more widely appreciated, and proper advice can be given concerning prognosis and patterns of transmission.

The last decade has seen the application of molecular genetic studies to this group of disorders, and the underlying genetic defect has been identified in some. As reviewed in Chapter 1, this is a rapidly advancing field. No attempt has been made here to report on advances in molecular genetics, as it was felt they may well be out of date by the time of publication. Readers will find the most up-to-date overviews of these disorders in McKusick's *Mendelian Inheritance in Man* and in his *Heritable Disorders of Connective Tissue* (1992; 1993). For families under their care requiring specific genetic advice, physicians can consult their local clinical genetic service.

CLASSIFICATION

Because the nature of the underlying defect is usually uncertain, classification of skeletal dysplasias is difficult. It seems certain that the basic abnormality is at a biochemical level, resulting in modification of the formation and structure of bone. This is plainly true in such disorders as the mucopolysaccharidoses or Gaucher's disease, where there are obvious deposits of partly degraded metabolites in bone substance. In some forms of osteogenesis imperfecta the basic abnormality in the structure of the collagen is now known, but the reason for its deficiency is uncertain. In disorders showing sclerosis and hyperostosis, there is a deficiency in the control of deposition and breakdown of calcium salts in the bone substrate, but many of these syndromes also demonstrate abnormalities in modelling. Whether the latter are secondary to the deficiencies in control of calcium deposition or are due to a separate mechanism with imbalance in the normal cycle of bone growth and breakdown is not known. In other disorders the growth plate itself is abnormal. The entire structure may be involved, but disturbance in growth may be confined to either the epiphysis or the metaphysis.

In 1964 Rubin published his *Dynamic Classification of Bone Dysplasias*. He based his method on assessment of the major anatomical site of the abnormality, namely whether it lay in the epiphysis, the growth plate, the metaphysis or the diaphysis. Subsequent classifications have been broadly based on that of Rubin. In 1969 a meeting was convened in Paris by the European Society of Paediatric Radiology to discuss the nomenclature and classification of the constitutional skeletal disorders. Increased interest in the description of these syndromes had resulted in a proliferation of eponyms and misleading terminology. This meeting produced the International Nomenclature of Constitutional Disorders of Bone, which was published in 1970. The broad principles of Rubin's classification were used, but the emphasis was on agreement in nomenclature rather than accurate classification. Further revisions of nomenclature have taken place at similar meetings since. The simple classification used in this chapter is loosely based on the Paris nomenclature and is used only as an aid to general categorization and description (Table 2.1). It does not imply any certain understanding of the underlying abnormalities.

Description of syndromes

Many syndromes involving degrees of dysplasia of a bone have been described, and most of these are very rare. Detailed accounts of these abnormalities can be found in the books listed in the bibliography at the end of this chapter.

Dwarfism

This describes a pathological diminution of height below the lower end of the normal range for the population. There can be no absolute definition of dwarfism, as the height of an individual is principally determined by race or ethnic grouping, and shortness of stature can only be decided by comparison within a peer group.

Dwarfism is classified as being proportionate, with equal involvement of all bony segments, or disproportionate. The latter group is divided into short-limb and short-trunk forms.

Table 2.1 A simple classification of skeletal dysplasias

Disorders around the growth plate
  Predominantly epiphyseal involvement
  Predominantly metaphyseal involvement
  With major vertebrae involvement
Changes in bone density
  Increased
  Decreased
Craniotubular disorders
Craniofacial abnormalities
Vertebral anomalies
Storage disorders
Abnormalities of cartilage and fibrous tissue
Miscellaneous disorders

DISORDERS AROUND THE GROWTH PLATE

These interfere with longitudinal bone growth and may result in some degree of short stature or, when severe, dwarfism. They are broadly divisible into three groups:
1 Those that involve principally the epiphyseal side of the growth plate with failure to produce a normal ossific nucleus.
2 Those that show metaphyseal abnormality with derangement of the normal process of endochondral bone formation which takes place at the metaphyseal side of the growth plate.
3 In the first two groups involvement of the vertebrae is either absent or relatively minor. The third group comprises the conditions which show a major disorder of vertebral growth in association with abnormality of the epiphyses or metaphyses, or sometimes both. Marked shortness of stature or dwarfism is found.

Predominantly epiphyseal involvement

MULTIPLE EPIPHYSEAL DYSPLASIA (Fig. 2.1)

This is a relatively common skeletal dysplasia and is a heterogeneous condition, comprising a number of disorders ranging from the mild (Ribbing) to the severe (Fairbank) type. There is irregularity of epiphyseal growth, usually affecting joints symmetrically. The epiphyses of the major joints are most commonly affected, and the condition may present with problems of walking in childhood. The digits are stubby in some forms, and a minor degree of vertebral involvement may

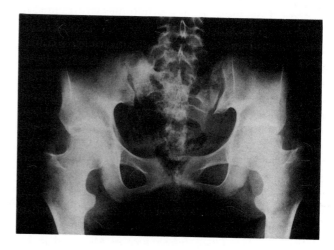

Fig. 2.1 Multiple epiphyseal dysplasia. Note abnormality of both femoral capital epiphyses.

occur. Many forms of multiple epiphyseal dysplasia, however, give surprisingly little trouble, and the diagnosis may not be made until symptoms arise from the premature onset of degenerative changes in weight-bearing joints in adults.

In childhood radiographs show retarded development of the epiphyses of the long bones with late appearance of the ossific nucleus, which may become flattened and irregular. The capital femoral epiphyses are usually involved. This may lead to a mistaken diagnosis of Perthes' disease, and a skeletal survey should be undertaken before the latter disorder is ever diagnosed as occurring in both hips. Familial dysplasia of the upper femoral epiphyses has been described and is inherited as an autosomal dominant trait.

In the adult the appearance of the joints may be surprisingly normal, but early osteoarthritic changes of the weight-bearing joints are commonly encountered and, when severe, will require operative treatment. Multiple epiphyseal dysplasia is usually inherited as an autosomal dominant trait.

CHONDRODYSPLASIA PUNCTATA (STIPPLED EPIPHYSES)

Stippling of the epiphyses may occur in a number of conditions including multiple epiphyseal dysplasia, spondyloepiphyseal dysplasia, hypothyroidism and fetal warfarin syndrome, but the term *stippled epiphyses* has also been used as an alternative name for chondrodysplasia punctata.

This latter condition has two principal forms. In the more common Conradi−Hunnerman type, the severely affected children may be stillborn, but the majority survive to enjoy a normal life span. Infants have a flat face with a depressed nasal bridge and atrophic skin changes. Congenital cataracts may be present. Asymmetric limb shortening, joint contracture and scoliosis may occur. Epiphyseal stippling may be visible in radiographs of the long bones, vertebrae and pelvis up to the age of 4 years, after which the epiphyses may remain irregular and resemble epiphyseal dysplasia. The condition is usually inherited as an autosomal dominant trait.

In the severe rhizomelic form, most infants are still-born or die in the first year of life. Marked proximal limb shortening is present in addition to the features described above. The punctate stippling of the epiphyses is obvious, particularly in relation to the vertebrae. The pattern of inheritance is autosomal recessive.

Predominantly metaphyseal involvement

ACHONDROPLASIA (Figs 2.2 and 2.3)

This is the most common form of dwarfism and is apparent at birth. There is some spinal involvement but the metaphyseal abnormalities predominate. The limbs are disproportionately short with the proximal segment

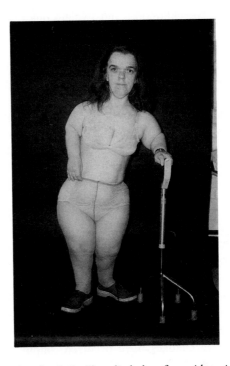

Fig. 2.2 Achondroplasia. Short-limb dwarfism with typical facies and trident hands. A tripod is used to walk because of limb weakness secondary to lumbar canal stenosis.

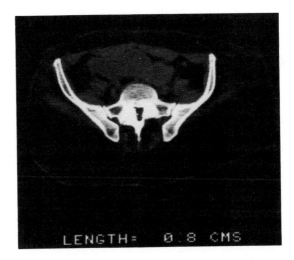

Fig. 2.3 Achondroplasia. Computed tomographic scan of the lumbosacral region of an adult showing gross narrowing of the spinal canal.

particularly affected. The forehead is prominent, the nasal bridge depressed and the fingers short and stubby with a 'trident' appearance. The children walk late, and have a characteristic appearance with a prominent abdomen, lumbar lordosis and hip flexion contractures. An upper lumbar kyphosis may be present in infancy, but often disappears after walking has commenced. If it persists it increases the danger of the development of cord compression in later life. Genu varum usually appears in late childhood, and a valgus deformity of the ankle may occur.

The radiographic appearances are characteristic. The calvarium is relatively large and the base of the skull underdeveloped. The limb bones are short and wide with irregular metaphyses, but the epiphyses are normal. The pelvis shows squared iliac wings and a small greater sciatic notch. The pedicles of the lumbar spine are short, and the interpedicular distance decreases from the upper to the lower lumbar spine with consequent narrowing of the spinal canal. The posterior border of the vertebrae may be scalloped.

The most important problems of management concern the back and legs. A narrow spinal canal may produce signs of cord compression. The symptoms tend to be progressive with numbness and paraesthesiae in the legs often a presenting feature. Wide decompression of the canal may be necessary to prevent gradual disablement.

The varus deformity of the knees should be corrected by osteotomy to restore vertical alignment before degenerative changes have occurred. Impingement of the lateral malleolus of an over-long fibula may occur with a valgus ankle producing local pain.

Achondroplasia can be inherited as an autosomal dominant trait, but most cases result from new mutations.

HYPOCHONDROPLASIA

The clinical and radiographic appearances of this condition suggest a mild form of achondroplasia, but the two conditions are quite distinct genetically. In hypochondroplasia the cranium, facies and fingers are normal and stature is less stunted. Spinal changes are usually present, but to a much lesser degree than in achondroplasia. Radiographs of the pelvis may show a horizontally placed sacrum and short femoral necks. Such changes may be mild, however, and the clinical stigmata minimal. The condition may remain undiagnosed. It is inherited as an autosomal dominant trait.

METAPHYSEAL CHONDRODYSPLASIA

The metaphyseal chondrodysplasias are a composite group of disorders in which the principal deformity lies in the metaphyses of the long bones. The most common of this group is the Schmid type in which moderate short stature, bow legs and bilateral coxa vara may be apparent in early childhood and persist into maturity. The lumbar spine is usually lordotic. Radiographs show cupping and splaying of the metaphyses of the long bones with an appearance resembling healing rickets. Abnormality of the metaphysis of the neck of the femur may produce coxa vara, which may necessitate valgus osteotomy. Corrective osteotomy about the knees may also be required. The condition is inherited as an autosomal dominant trait.

Other forms of metaphyseal chondrodysplasia include the Jansen type, originally described in 1934, and the McKusick type (cartilage–hair hypoplasia).

FAMILIAL HYPOPHOSPHATAEMIA (VITAMIN D-RESISTANT RICKETS) (see Chapter 14)

This is a metabolic disorder that is inherited as an autosomal dominant trait and may present in childhood with abnormalities of the legs. It may be confused with a metaphyseal chondrodysplasia. Deformity of the legs becomes apparent after walking has started, and bow legs, knock knees or a windswept appearance may develop. The skeletal deformities vary from minimal to severe and are progressive throughout childhood, stabilizing by the third decade. Radiographs taken in an active phase show irregular, wide metaphyses with normal epiphyses. The skeleton is porotic and pseudofractures may be present. Treatment is by massive doses of vitamin D, but requires supervision by a specialist metabolic unit. The deformities should be corrected by operation, but will recur unless the biochemical abnormality is controlled.

Major vertebral involvement

SPONDYLOEPIPHYSEAL DYSPLASIA

In this group of disorders, changes are principally in the vertebral bodies and the epiphyses of the long bones, particularly the femur, but mild metaphyseal involvement may be present. Two forms are generally recognized: the *congenita*, in which abnormalities are apparent at birth, and the *tarda*, in which the features are much less severe and are seen later in childhood.

Spondyloepiphyseal dysplasia congenita is characterized by short-trunk dwarfism, with a barrel chest and pectus carinatum associated with marked lumbar lordosis. The hands and feet are normal, but genu valgum or varum may occur. Club foot, cleft palate and myopia have also been described. In the adult the weight-bearing joints, e.g. the hips, may show early degenerative changes.

Radiographs show that the epiphyses appear late, particularly in the hip, which may also show coxa vara. The vertebral bodies are flat and in infancy appear pear-shaped on the lateral view. The odontoid process may be hypoplastic. In the limbs the proximal epiphyses are most affected. The hands are likely to be normal, but there may be irregularity in the carpus.

The odontoid hypoplasia may lead to atlantoaxial instability with cord compression, and operative stabilization may be required. Malalignment of the hips and knees should be treated with corrective osteotomy. Most cases encountered are sporadic, but autosomal dominant inheritance has been established in some patients.

In spondyloepiphyseal dysplasia tarda the appearances are variable, and there may be no obvious clinical change in those most mildly affected. Relative shortness of the trunk may be appreciated by mid-childhood, and investigation of low back pain may draw attention to the underlying condition. Adults may present with osteoarthritic changes of the hips and knees.

Radiographic examination will show generalized platyspondyly with a humped appearance of the posterosuperior portion of the vertebral body on the lateral view. Mild dysplastic changes are present in the proximal major joints. X-linked recessive, autosomal dominant and autosomal recessive inheritance patterns have been reported, illustrating the heterogeneity of the condition.

PSEUDO-ACHONDROPLASIA (Fig. 2.4)

A variable degree of short-limbed dwarfism is present, which may be very severe, but the normal craniofacial appearance prevents confusion with achondroplasia. There is always some degree of spinal abnormality and genu valgum or varum may occur. The radiographic changes are present in infancy and progress through childhood. The vertebral deformities may vary. An oval shape of the body may be seen in early childhood, with later platyspondyly. Odontoid hypoplasia may be present. The shape may become more normal towards puberty. The pelvis appears hyperplastic, with flattened acetabulae, and the epiphyses and metaphyses of the long bones are abnormal. The tubular bones are short and broad.

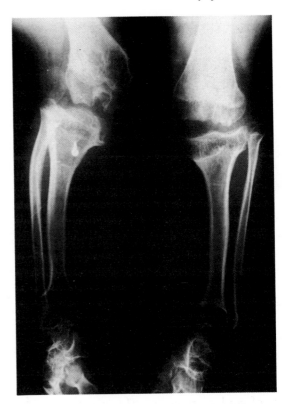

Fig. 2.4 Pseudo-achondroplasia. Short, broad, tubular bones with marked epiphyseal irregularity and broadening of the metaphyses. Reproduced by permission of Professor P. Beighton, Cape Town, South Africa.

The condition is heterogeneous, and both dominant and recessive forms have been reported.

Deformities in the hips and knees may require corrective osteotomy, and later degenerative changes in the major joints may warrant replacement arthroplasty.

DIASTROPHIC DYSPLASIA (Fig. 2.5)

The features of this very rare form of short-limb dwarfism are present at birth, with short limbs, stiff equinus feet and proximally set 'hitchhiker' thumbs. The palate may be cleft, and a cystic swelling may be seen on the pinna. Joint contractures and stiffness present problems by late childhood. Scoliosis is often severe and may cause cord compression. Rigid deformed feet may impair mobility. Intelligence is normal.

Radiographic examination shows abnormality of the epiphyses of the long bones and flaring of the metaphyses. Both the metacarpal and metatarsal bones are wide and shortened, particularly that of the thumb. The iliac wings are flared. The capital femoral epiphyses appear late, and the femoral heads are flat and irregular with short, broad, varus necks. The acetabulae are

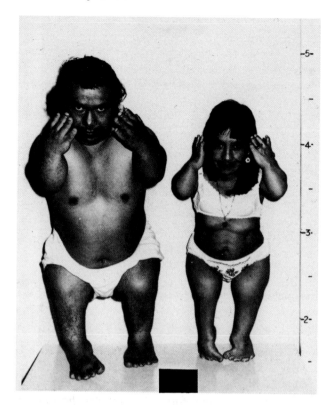

Fig. 2.5 Diastrophic dysplasia in a brother and sister. Reproduced by permission of Professor P. Beighton, Cape Town, South Africa.

widened. Although the spine may be normal at birth, a severe progressive kyphoscoliosis develops in infancy.

The rigid equinus feet present a problem in management. Late operation has proved valueless, and early correction of the feet with release of contractures of the hip and knee is thought to give the best results. The severe kyphoscoliosis may be best treated by early fusion, as progression does not occur after late childhood.

The condition is inherited as an autosomal recessive trait.

MORE UNCOMMON SYNDROMES

Metatropic dysplasia presents at birth with short limbs and a trunk of normal length, but in late infancy a rapidly progressive kyphoscoliosis results in short-trunk dwarfism.

The spondylometaphyseal dysplasias are a heterogeneous group of disorders which present with disproportionate short stature and variable skeletal changes. The principal radiographic findings are platyspondyly and metaphyseal irregularity, with the epiphyses being abnormal in some forms.

Kniest dysplasia is a rare form of dwarfism that resembles metatropic dysplasia and is apparent at birth or in early infancy.

CHANGES IN BONE DENSITY

Increased bone density

OSTEOPETROSIS (Figs 2.6 and 2.7)

The term osteopetrosis has been loosely used to describe a number of conditions in which radiographs show a generalized increase in bone density. The name should strictly be applied to the specific abnormality described in this section. Osteopetrosis is a heterogeneous condition, but two distinct forms are recognized — an adult tarda or benign autosomal dominant type and an infantile malignant autosomal recessive variety — though intermediate forms may be encountered. The autosomal recessive type is very rare. Stillbirth is common and surviving infants show anaemia, hepatosplenomegaly, cranial nerve palsy and delayed dentition; they die in early childhood from overwhelming infection or haemorrhage.

The tarda form may not give rise to clinical symptoms, but can present with evidence of cranial nerve compression, particularly facial palsy and deafness, or with

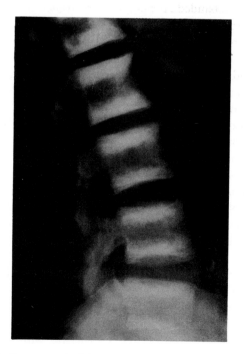

Fig. 2.6 Osteopetrosis. Sclerosis of the vertebral end-plates gives a 'banded' appearance. Reproduced by permission of Professor P. Beighton, Cape Town, South Africa.

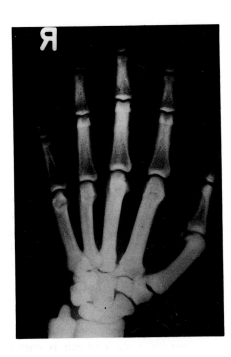

Fig. 2.7 Osteopetrosis. Radiograph of the hand of an adult with the tarda form. Reproduced by permission of Professor P. Beighton, Cape Town, South Africa.

pathological fractures. Tooth extraction may be difficult and lead to osteomyelitis of the jaw.

Radiographs of the skull show a thick calvarium with basal sclerosis. In the spine, vertebral end-plate sclerosis may give a banded appearance, the 'rugger jersey' spine. The cortices of the long bones are widened and dense, but there is little disturbance of modelling. In infancy and childhood the long bones may show central diaphyseal and metaphyseal thickening, giving an 'endobone' or 'bone within a bone' appearance. The infantile form is usually fatal. Bone marrow transplants have given promising results, however, and apparent permanent remission has been obtained in a number of children. The appearances of the radiographs in these cases have been converted from the classic appearances of the condition to a seemingly normal film.

Pathological fractures may occur in the tarda form, but they have been successfully treated by traction, immobilization in a cast and internal fixation. Operation may prove difficult because of the hardness of the bone, but there have been reports of some patients in whom the bone has been more like chalk than marble. Facial palsy and deafness may require decompression of the appropriate cranial nerve.

PYCNODYSOSTOSIS

In this rare disorder shortness of stature is associated with generalized bone density. The face is small and triangular and the mandible is underdeveloped, with an obtuse angle. The hands are short and square with stubby fingers. Dentition is abnormal.

Radiographs show generalized sclerosis, but with little abnormality of modelling. The skull has a large calvarium with wide suture lines, persistent fontanelles, wormian bones and a hypoplastic facial skeleton. The terminal phalanges are short and irregular. Madelung's deformity may be present.

Clinically, affected persons may have surprisingly little disability. Transverse fractures may occur in the long bones and usually heal without problems by the standard methods of treatment. The condition is inherited as an autosomal recessive trait.

Decreased bone density

OSTEOGENESIS IMPERFECTA (Fig. 2.8)

Bone fragility is the principal feature of this relatively common disorder, which is remarkable for its heterogeneity with considerable variation in the degree of severity in the different forms. Several classifications of the disorder have been produced, and the variability of the patterns of inheritance indicates that there are a number of closely related conditions grouped under the heading of osteogenesis imperfecta. Research into the condition has indicated that the basic abnormality is a genetic defect in collagen structure, which varies from type to type. The generalized nature of the disorder is

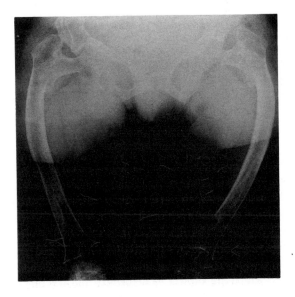

Fig. 2.8 Osteogenesis imperfecta. Gross femoral bowing. Reproduced by permission of Professor P. Beighton, Cape Town, South Africa.

indicated by associated features, e.g. poor scar formation, joint laxity, a bruising tendency and abnormal dentition. It is still useful, however, to consider the clinical features of osteogenesis imperfecta under the classification into 'congenita' and 'tarda' forms.

Many babies with the congenita type are stillborn or die early from intracranial haemorrhage. At birth the head is large with a soft calvarium and wide fontanelles, and disproportionate shortening of the limbs may be evident. Radiographs of the skull show poor ossification of the calvarium, with wide sutures and numerous wormian bones. There may be multiple fractures of the ribs and the long bones. The vertebrae are normal at birth, but if the infant survives they become flattened or biconcave and spinal deformities may appear. The limb bones may be either short and wide, the 'thick bone' type, or slender with narrow cortices, the 'thin bone' type. The genetics of the congenita form are uncertain; some children have an autosomal recessive condition, but other cases may be the consequence of new mutations in the dominant gene.

The tarda form usually presents with fractures in early childhood due to bone fragility. Subsequently, fractures may occur frequently or in some cases occasionally, until the tendency diminishes in early adulthood. Fracture healing is rapid with the occasional patient producing hyperplastic callus which can be mistaken for osteomyelitis or osteosarcoma. Malignant change has been reported in hyperplastic callus. The other features are variable. The sclerae are characteristically blue, but the shade varies with age and race and in several varieties the sclerae are white. The features of a generalized collagen disorder noted above may occur, and otosclerosis produces deafness in about 20% of adults. Radiographs demonstrate a generalized porosity of the skeleton. The long bones are gracile and deformed with evidence of healed fractures. The calvarium shows poor ossification with a bitemporal bulge and wormian bones. The vertebral bodies are flat and biconcave. Some patients are encountered who are mildly affected, however, and are only diagnosed because of investigation into affected relatives, an isolated fracture or when examined because of other problems.

Inheritance in the tarda form is usually autosomal dominant, but in a few patients an autosomal recessive pattern has been described.

Treatment of the bone fragility depends on the degree of skeletal deformity encountered. The major long bones, which are subject to deformity and fracture, are best stabilized by intramedullary rods (Figs 2.9 and 2.10). Stabilization of spinal deformities is extremely difficult.

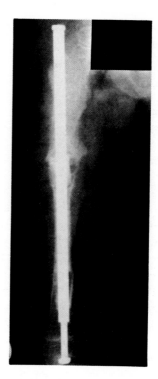

Fig. 2.9 Osteogenesis imperfecta. Radiograph of the left femur of a child 10 weeks after insertion of a Bailey–Dubow telescoping rod. Reproduced by permission of Dr R.B. Gledhill, Phoenix, Arizona, USA.

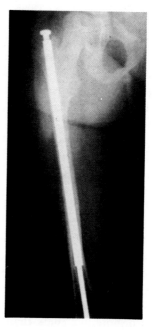

Fig. 2.10 Osteogenesis imperfecta. The same femur as shown in Fig. 2.9 2 years later. Reproduced by permission of Dr R.B. Gledhill, Phoenix, Arizona, USA.

Craniotubular disorders

The principal characteristics of this group are an increase

in bone density and abnormality of skeletal modelling in the skull and long bones.

CRANIOMETAPHYSEAL DYSPLASIA

Gradual enlargement of the skull and the mandible distorts the appearance of the face and jaw, but the condition does not worsen in the adult. Paranasal bossing may be seen in infancy, but tends to regress in adolescence. Many patients develop facial palsy and deafness due to cranial nerve compression, and this is the usual mode of presentation. Pathological fractures do not occur. The radiographic changes appear in childhood. The skull shows progressive sclerosis and thickening, which is most marked at the base. The mandible, clavicles and ribs are wide and undermodelled. The metaphyses of the long bones are broad, and this undermodelling is most marked in the lower femur, which may be club shaped. The condition may be very mild and is inherited as an autosomal dominant trait, though a severe autosomal recessive form has been described.

METAPHYSEAL DYSPLASIA (PYLE'S SYNDROME)

Clinical abnormality is usually restricted to a valgus deformity at the knee. Radiographs show flaring of the metaphyses of the tubular bones, but changes are most marked at the knee where the lower end of the femur presents an 'Erlenmeyer flask' appearance. Pyle's syndrome is inherited as an autosomal recessive trait, and the apparently normal heterozygote carrier may be recognized by the presence of undermodelling of the lower end of the femur on radiographic examination.

DIAPHYSEAL DYSPLASIA (CAMURATI–ENGELMANN SYNDROME)

This rare condition presents in childhood with pain and weakness of the legs, which show a reduction in soft tissue bulk. Symptoms vary in severity and usually resolve in late adolescence. Radiographs of the long bones show cortical widening and sclerosis of the metaphyses and diaphyses, principally in the tibia and femur. Thickening of the calvarium is occasionally encountered. Diaphyseal dysplasia is inherited as an autosomal dominant condition.

OTHER CRANIOTUBULAR DISORDERS

Rare syndromes which show abnormalities of density and modelling of the skeleton include endosteal hyperostosis, when the presenting symptom is deafness and radiographs show sclerosis of the cranium and long bones, and sclerosteosis. This latter abnormality is transmitted as an autosomal recessive condition and most reported cases have been from South Africa. Severe progressive hyperostosis and overgrowth of the skeleton produce facial distortion and gigantism. Compression of the appropriate cranial nerve may give deafness and facial palsy. A raised intracranial pressure may require emergency craniotomy.

CRANIOFACIAL ABNORMALITIES

Many disorders of the craniofacial skeleton occur as isolated examples, but there is a group of syndromes in which maldevelopment is found principally in the facial skeleton, and which demonstrates recognizable patterns of inheritance. Craniostenosis, resulting from premature closure of the sutures of the skull, may be present and the resulting shape of the head will depend on the sutures involved. The growth and development of the brain may be affected secondarily. Craniofacial dysostosis (Crouzon's syndrome) shows craniostenosis, mid-facial hypoplasia, hypertelorism, proptosis and nasal beaking, producing a frog-like facies. There are no other skeletal or visceral abnormalities.

A group of syndromes exhibits craniofacial abnormalities with severe syndactyly. The degree and distribution of syndactyly and skull abnormality vary considerably. Acrocephalosyndactyly type 1, the classic Apert's syndrome, is characterized by a high, broad forehead, a flat occiput and mid-facial hypoplasia. The hands and feet show bone and soft tissue syndactyly of the second and fourth digits, with variable involvement of the first and fifth, forming the 'sock foot' and 'mitten hand' deformities. The incidence of intellectual impairment and infant mortality is high. Acrocephalosyndactyly type 2, Carpenter's syndrome, is distinguished by the additional presence of extra digits and structural cardiac malformation.

Procedures for cranio-orbital reconstruction have been developed which can greatly improve the appearance in these abnormalities, and when carried out early may lessen the possibility of mental impairment. Reconstruction of the hands is preferably undertaken in early childhood before schooling begins.

VERTEBRAL ANOMALIES

Although abnormalities of development of the vertebrae are present in a number of bone dysplasias, there are two groups in which local spinal anomalies are the principal feature.

Klippel–Feil syndrome (Fig. 2.11) (see also Chapter 7) occurs as a distinct entity and as a major component of the cervico-oculoacoustic (Wildervanck's) syndrome and the oculoauriculovertebral (Goldenhar's) syndrome in which deafness is the major complication. The posterior hairline is low, and the neck is short with a limited range of movement. Radiographs show fusion of two or more cervical vertebrae, and hemivertebrae may be present. Localized fusions may be seen in the thoracic spine and ribs. Sprengel's deformity is present in about one-third of the patients and dorsal or lumbar kyphosis or a scoliosis may occur. Abnormalities of the renal tract may be present. Although most patients are asymptomatic, neck pain and symptoms due to compression of the cervical nerve root or spinal cord may require treatment.

The spondylocostal dysostoses are a heterogeneous group of disorders in which the trunk is short due to thoracic asymmetry and spinal deformity. Thoracic vertebrae and ribs show variable degrees of fusion and failure of segmentation.

Sprengel's deformity—congenital elevation of the scapula—may occur as an isolated entity, but is commonly seen in association with anomalies of the vertebrae and ribs. The high, small scapula is associated with an omovertebral bone in about one-third of cases, and the associated muscles may be absent or hypoplastic. The degree of cosmetic and functional deformity is related to the height of the scapula, and most patients do not require treatment. Operative correction may be undertaken when indicated.

STORAGE DISORDERS

The absence or an insufficient quantity of a specific enzyme may result in the accumulation of partly degraded material within the cell. These storage disorders are classified according to the type of substance that collects in the cell. The mucopolysaccharidoses as a group produce characteristic skeletal changes, as does Gaucher's disease of the mucolipidoses.

Abnormal quantities of such mucopolysaccharides as dermatin, keratin and heparin sulphate accumulate in the urine in the mucopolysaccharidoses, and their identification has assisted in the delineation of individual syndromes. Such categorization has been carried further by histochemical studies of cultured fibroblasts, which have allowed identification of specific enzyme defects, and genetic studies are well advanced to identify the individual genes responsible.

Clinically, the mucopolysaccharidoses are distinguished by varying degrees of facial coarsening, short stature, corneal clouding, hepatosplenomegaly, skeletal dysplasia and intellectual impairment. The radiographic features of the mucopolysaccharidoses are basically similar, with a large skull and thick calvarium, a 'J'-shaped pituitary fossa and wide, oar-shaped ribs. The immature vertebrae are ovoid with anterior beaking, but become flattened as they develop. The pelvis shows flaring of the iliac wings with dysplastic acetabulae, and tubular bones are short and undermodelled with irregular epiphyses. There is generalized osteoporosis. Hurler's syndrome (mucopolysaccharidosis 1-H) and Hunter's syndrome (mucopolysaccharidosis II) are the most common such disorders encountered and will be described here.

Mucopolysaccharidosis I-H (Hurler's syndrome)

Infants appear normal until towards the end of their first year, when the gradual onset of persistent rhinorrhoea, stiff joints, thoracolumbar kyphosis, chest deformity and facial coarsening becomes apparent. By the age of 2 years the characteristic facies and enlarged tongue, hepatosplenomegaly, corneal clouding, joint stiffness and cardiac anomalies are established. Death occurs from respiratory or cardiac failure, usually before the age of 10 years.

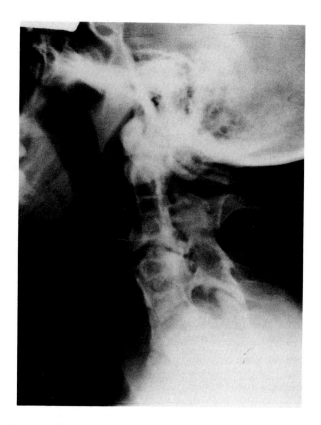

Fig. 2.11 Klippel–Feil syndrome.

The radiographic appearances are as described above with a thoracolumbar gibbus, valgus femoral necks and dysplastic hip joints. The digits are short and stubby. The syndrome is inherited as an autosomal recessive trait.

Mucopolysaccharidosis II (Hunter's syndrome)

This disorder is inherited as an X-linked recessive trait and is therefore seen only in males. Mild and severe forms are recognized clinically.

Children with the severe form resemble those with Hurler's syndrome, but are less affected. Corneal clouding and mental impairment are not so marked, but deafness is common. Death usually occurs before adolescence. In the mild form the disease progresses more slowly. There is shortness of stature with moderate facial coarsening, flexion contracture of the fingers and hepatosplenomegaly. There may be no mental impairment and survival into adulthood is usual. The radiographic changes in mucopolysaccharidosis II are characteristic of the mucopolysaccharidoses, but are less severe.

Gaucher's disease (Fig. 2.12)

The infantile and juvenile forms of this disease are lethal due to the accumulation of cerebrosides within the central nervous system. The non-neuropathic form usually presents in early adulthood with splenomegaly or dyshaemopoiesis, though persistent, dull bone pain, due to bone destruction and the accumulation of Gaucher's cells, may be the first symptom. Pseudo-osteomyelitis may be difficult to differentiate from true pyogenic osteomyelitis. Aseptic necrosis of the head of the humerus and of the femur is common. Considerable disability may result, requiring replacement arthroplasty.

The radiographic appearances show deposits of Gaucher's cells, which give a foamy appearance with areas of bone absorption, widening of the marrow cavity and cortical thinning. An 'Erlenmeyer flask' deformity of the lower end of the femur may be present, and avascular necrosis noted at the sites mentioned above.

Gaucher's disease is inherited as an autosomal recessive trait.

ABNORMALITIES OF CARTILAGE AND FIBROUS TISSUE

Diaphyseal aclasia (multiple exostoses)

Variable numbers of exostoses arise from the growth

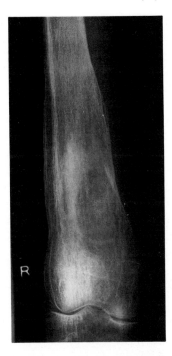

Fig. 2.12 Gaucher's disease. The lower femur shows an 'Erlenmeyer flask' deformity with areas of bone absorption. Reproduced by permission of Professor P. Beighton, Cape Town, South Africa.

plate of the long bones, occasionally from the scapulae and pelvis and very occasionally from the skull or vertebrae. The lesions are bony but capped with cartilage. They usually cause little harm, but at some sites, particularly the neck of the femur, they may interfere with local growth and produce deformity. Problems may arise from pressure on adjacent soft tissue structures, as the outgrowths continue to enlarge until skeletal maturity is achieved. Between 5 and 10% of affected patients may develop chondrosarcoma, particularly in relation to exostoses in the scapula or pelvis. Suspicious lesions may be monitored by bone scans. Radiographs show that a typical lesion protrudes from the epiphysis or adjacent metaphysis and points away from the growth plate. Metaphyseal expansion and irregularity may produce local deformity, particularly at the wrist, ankle and upper femur. Diaphyseal aclasia is inherited as an autosomal dominant trait.

Enchondromatosis (Ollier's disease) (Fig. 2.13)

Aggregations of unossified cartilage in the metaphyses of the long bones produce sites of localized swelling, which may be confined to a single bone, one limb, or be widespread. The hands, the lower ends of the radius and ulna and the knees are affected most commonly.

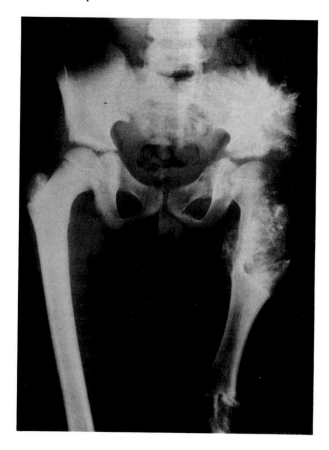

Fig. 2.13 Enchondromatosis affecting left side of the pelvis and left leg. Reproduced by permission of Professor P. Beighton, Cape Town, South Africa.

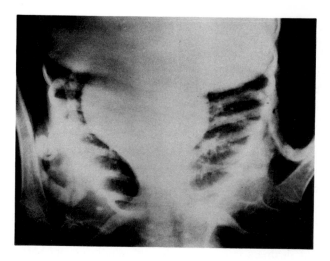

Fig. 2.14 Fibrodysplasia ossificans progressiva. Plaques of bone have formed across the chest and linking the scapula to the upper arm. Reproduced by permission of Professor P. Beighton, Cape Town, South Africa.

Expansion of the phalanges may produce marked swelling of the fingers, which can inhibit function. Fractures occur through the weakened bone and disparity of limb length may arise when an affected part fails to grow normally. The presence of enchondromas around the knee may give rise to valgus or varus deformity.

When associated with multiple haemangiomas, enchondromatosis comprises Maffuci's syndrome. Malignant change is rare in Ollier's disease, but an incidence of about 20% has been reported for the lesions in Maffuci's syndrome.

No hereditary pattern has been established for enchondromatosis.

Fibrous dysplasia ossificans progressiva (Fig. 2.14)

In this rare disorder inflammatory swellings develop, usually over the upper back, neck and shoulders. The lesions subside after several weeks, but eventually calcify and bony plaques may be laid down in the fascial planes, intermuscular septa and tendon attachments. The disease may present at any time between infancy and adulthood, but the first symptoms commonly appear in late childhood. A short hallux and sometimes a short thumb may be apparent at birth. The degree of disability may be profound or relatively mild.

Treatment with steroids has met with some success in the acute phase of the disorder. Operative removal of the plaques of bone may be helpful in attempting to improve the mobility of the severely crippled, but the bone tends to reform. The use of diphosphonates may help to suppress this.

The disorder is transmitted as an autosomal dominant trait.

MISCELLANEOUS DISORDERS

Within this group lie several abnormalities that do not fall into any convenient category for classification. The more common of these disorders will be briefly discussed.

Osteopoikilosis

Numerous small sclerotic foci, principally at the ends of long bones, but also seen in the pelvis, can be demonstrated on radiographs. There are usually no clinical manifestations, but about 15% of patients show patches of multiple, sessile nodules on the skin which are called dermatofibrosis lenticularis disseminata. Osteopoikilosis is inherited as an autosomal dominant trait.

Melorheostosis

The radiographic appearance of this rare, non-genetic condition is striking (Fig. 2.15). There is an irregular hyperostosis of the cortices of affected long bones which appears to 'flow' down the limb from one bone to the next. The flat bones may show sclerotic patches. Clinically, the skin over the affected bone is sometimes thickened and painful, and the associated joints may be stiff. In children, joint contractures may present a major clinical problem and are extremely resistant to treatment.

Osteopathia striata

The diagnosis of osteopathia striata is made on radiographic examination only (Fig. 2.16), as there are no special clinical features. The films show linear hyperostotic streaks in the metaphyses of the long bones and the ilia. An autosomal dominant pattern of inheritance is well established. Osteopathia striata may occur in association with cranial sclerosis. This is an autosomal dominant condition which may present with deafness due to cranial nerve compression. Osteopathia striata is also seen in association with a number of other bone dysplasias.

Craniocleidal dysplasia

In the newborn the sutures are palpably broad and the

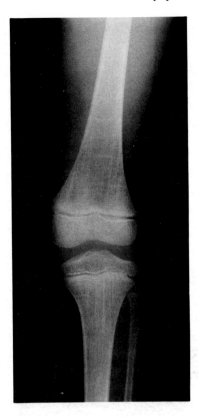

Fig. 2.16 Osteopathia striata. Reproduced by permission of Professor P. Beighton, Cape Town, South Africa.

calvarium ossifies slowly. Closure of the fontanelles and sutures is delayed and wormian bones persist. As the child develops the chest appears narrow and the shoulders hypermobile due to the absence or underdevelopment of the clavicles. Dysplasia of the neck of the femur may result in coxa vara. The vertebrae show delayed maturation and the pelvic bones may be hyperplastic at maturity. Caesarian section may be required in the event of pregnancy. The syndrome has an autosomal dominant pattern of inheritance.

Larsen's syndrome

Infants present as 'floppy babies' with generalized joint laxity, which may be associated with dislocation of the hips, knees and head of the radius. Talipes equinovarus may be present. The face has a flattened appearance due to mid-facial hypoplasia. The stature is short. Radiographic examination confirms the joint dislocations and may demonstrate spinal anomalies. The calcaneum has an additional ossification centre which may appear in late infancy. The place of operation in the management of the joint dislocations is uncertain, and a thorough trial of conservative care should be undertaken before surgery is contemplated.

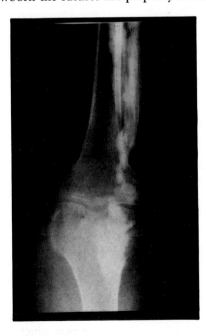

Fig. 2.15 Melorheostosis. Reproduced by permission of Professor P. Beighton, Cape Town, South Africa.

Chondroectodermal dysplasia (Ellis–van Creveld syndrome)

In this rare form of disproportionate dwarfism, the middle and distal portions of the limbs are particularly underdeveloped. Post-axial polydactyly may be present, the nails are sparse and the hair fine. Structural cardiac defects are common. The disorder has been encountered principally in the Amish religious sect in Pennsylvania, USA, and is inherited as an autosomal recessive condition.

Hereditary osteo-onychodysplasia (nail–patella syndrome)

The principal characteristics of this syndrome are the absence or hypoplasia of the nails and patellae. The associated skeletal features may include iliac horns, dislocation of the radial heads and hypoplasia of the scapula. Few problems are encountered apart from dislocation of the patellae or retropatellar discomfort on exercise. Patients are otherwise normal, but about one-third are said to develop renal problems in later life.

The nail-patella syndrome is inherited as an autosomal dominant trait.

Madelung's deformity

This deformity of the wrist shows volar subluxation of the carpus of the radius, dorsal subluxation of the distal end of the ulna and shortening and bowing of the radius. The abnormality may occur after damage to the lower epiphysis of the radius, as a primary anomaly that is unilateral and non-genetic, and as a component of dyschondrosteosis when bilateral. Dyschondrosteosis is a mild form of mesomelic dwarfism.

SUMMARY

This account of the skeletal dysplasias is, of necessity, brief. The rarity of the syndromes is such that the orthopaedic surgeon in average practice will encounter few in his lifetime. Some familiarity with the conditions is necessary, however, so that when encountered the proper advice and management can be instituted. For the most part such conditions are best handled in units specially devoted to the study of clinical genetics. In such centres the more profoundly affected patients are able to obtain sound advice and counselling. They are able to meet others who may be similarly afflicted, and the growth of self-help associations for the more common syndromes is an indication of the need that such patients have for sympathetic help and support.

REFERENCES

McKusick V.A. (1992) *Mendelian Inheritance in Man*, 10th edn. Baltimore, Johns Hopkins Press.
McKusick V.A. (1993) *Heritable Disorders of Connective Tissue*, 5th edn. St. Louis, C.V. Mosby.

FURTHER READING

Bailey J.A. II (1973) *Disproportionate Short Stature*. Philadelphia, W.B. Saunders.
Beighton P. (1978) *Inherited Disorders of the Skeleton*. Edinburgh, Churchill Livingstone.
Beighton P. and Cremin B.J. (1980) *Sclerosing Bone Dysplasias*. Berlin and New York, Springer-Verlag.
Bergsma D. (ed) (1979) *Birth Defects Compendium*, 2nd edn. New York, Alan R. Liss (The National Foundation–March of Dimes).
Carter C.O. and Fairbank T.J. (1974) *The Genetics of Locomotor Disorders*. London, Oxford University Press.
Cremin B.J. and Beighton P. (1978) *Bone Dysplasias of Infancy*. Berlin and New York, Springer-Verlag.
Goldberg M.J. (1987) *The Dysmorphic Child*. New York, Raven Press.
Gorlin R.J., Pindborg J.P. and Cohen M.M. Jr. (1990) *Syndromes of the Head and Neck*, 3rd edn. New York, McGraw-Hill.
Horan F.T. and Beighton P. (1982) *Orthopaedic Problems in Inherited Skeletal Disorders*. Berlin and New York, Springer-Verlag.
Kaufman H.J. (ed) (1973) Intrinsic diseases of bones. *Prog. Pediatr. Radiol.* **4**.
Maroteaux P. (1979) *Bone Disease of Children*. Philadelphia, J.B. Lippincott.
Smith D.W. (1982) *Recognizable Patterns of Human Malformations*, 3rd edn. Philadelphia, W.B. Saunders.
Smith R., Francis M.J.O. and Houghton G.R. (1983) *The Brittle Bone Syndrome*. London, Butterworth.
Spranger J.W., Langer L.O. and Wiedermann H.R. (1974) *Bone Dysplasias*. Stuttgart, Fischer.
Warkany J. (1971) *Congenital Malformations*. Chicago, Year Book Medical Publishers.
Wynne-Davies R. and Fairbank T.J. (1976) *Fairbank's Atlas of General Affections of the Skeleton*, 2nd edn. Edinburgh, Churchill Livingstone.
Wynne-Davies R., Hall C.M. and Apley A.G. (1985) *Atlas of Skeletal Dysplasias*. Edinburgh, Churchill Livingstone.

Chapter 3
Neuromuscular Diseases

T.S. Renshaw & J.C. Drennan

INTRODUCTION

Acquiring a broad knowledge of the neuromuscular diseases is an important, but not an easy, task for the orthopaedic surgeon (Table 3.1). Many diseases have common features and as research progresses, conditions that were formerly grouped together as a single entity are now being differentiated and their study becomes more and more complex. Progress in understanding the pathophysiology has exceeded progress in successfully treating many diseases. Whereas many conditions are still considered to be incurable, this does not mean that they are untreatable and much can be done to improve individual quality of life, even with the more rapidly fatal of the neuromuscular diseases.

Assessment of a patient with any neuromuscular disorder begins with the patient's history and the genetic history of the family, and includes a careful physical examination and other studies, e.g. serum levels of muscle enzymes, electrophysiological studies, sophisticated analysis of tissue obtained by muscle or nerve biopsy and specialized radiographic studies.

The history should include the onset of the weakness, the developmental history and motor milestones. It should be noted whether weakness is constant or intermittent and whether it is improving, static, or worsening. A functional assessment of the activities of daily living must be recorded, as well as the patient's ambulatory status and endurance. Environmental factors, e.g. the use of alcohol, drugs, or exposure to toxins, should be noted. A history of endocrinological abnormalities including dysfunction in the thyroid, parathyroid, or adrenal glands or diabetes mellitus is important. Finally, a thorough family history is essential and, if indicated, parents, siblings and other relatives of the patient should be examined.

Physical examination must include ambulatory status, sitting or standing balance and posture, patterns of weakness, and the physiological state of muscle groups including tone and excursion, as well as quantifying their strength. Also important are assessments of joint stability, the presence or absence of contractures, the configuration of the spine, and a complete neurological examination.

Once a diagnosis has been established, prompt genetic counselling and education of the patient and the family regarding the natural history of the disorder and the overall planned management are essential.

MUSCULAR DYSTROPHIES

The muscular dystrophies are a group of genetically transmitted diseases, most of which are progressive and associated with muscle wasting and weakness. They are identified by eponyms, by descriptions of anatomical involvement, by biochemical abnormalities, by microscopic abnormalities and by pathological muscle behaviour.

Duchenne muscular dystrophy

This is the most common of the muscular dystrophies and is also known as pseudohypertrophic muscular dystrophy of childhood. Genetic transmission is X-linked recessive, with approximately one-third of new cases arising as spontaneous mutations. This condition, therefore, theoretically occurs only in males, though females may be afflicted through carrier expressivity (the Lyon hypothesis), in Turner's syndrome (45,X chromosome pattern), or as the offspring of a carrier female and an afflicted male (exceptionally unlikely). The incidence in live male births is approximately 1 in 5000. In this disease a defect at the Xp21 locus is responsible for a paucity or absence of dystrophin, which is a protein normally present in the muscle cell membrane in the region of the triadic junctions; its

Table 3.1 Summary of clinical features of conditions discussed in this chapter

Duchenne muscular dystrophy
X-linked recessive (Xp21); males only
Progressive muscle degeneration
Calf pseudohypertrophy (fibrosis)
Most live 20–25 years
Equinovarus foot deformities in 99%
Progressive scoliosis in 90%

Becker muscular dystrophy
Similar clinically, but milder than Duchenne type
More protracted course

Emery–Dreifuss muscular dystrophy
X-linked recessive (Xq28); males only
Late childhood onset, very slowly progressive
Elbow flexion contractures, stiff neck, talipes equinus
Atrial cardiac conduction defects

Limb girdle muscular dystrophy
Autosomal recessive, usually adolescent onset
Hip and shoulder (biceps, deltoid) weakness, then distal spread
No cardiac involvement, scoliosis rare

Facioscapulohumeral muscular dystrophy
Autosomal dominant with variable onset and expressivity
Weak facial and scapular fixator muscles
Deltoid and rotator cuff muscles usually remain good
Late spread of weakness to hips and tibialis anterior muscles
Life expectancy often normal

Scapuloperoneal muscular dystrophy
Variable inheritance patterns
Weakness of shoulder, tibialis anterior and peroneal muscle
  groups
Very slow progression, normal longevity

Congenital muscular dystrophy
Autosomal recessive or isolated finding
Profound neonatal hypotonia and often respiratory problems
Variable prognosis, some early death, some stabilize or improve
Spine, hip, foot problems common

Differential diagnosis of floppy infant
Cerebral palsy; congenital myopathy; cervical spinal cord lesion;
  Down's syndrome; Prader–Willi syndrome; hypoxia;
  septicaemia; spinal muscular atrophy; congenital muscular
  dystrophy; benign congenital hypotonia; metabolic diseases

Myotonia congenita (Thomsen's disease)
Autosomal dominant or recessive
Myotonia after rest and cold, relieved by exercise
Generalized muscle hypertrophy common
Many improve over time; medical problems not usually severe

Myotonic dystrophy (Steinert's disease)
Autosomal dominant (defect on the long arm of chromosome 19)
Variable severity, facial muscle wasting, foot deformities, scoliosis
  common
Often other system problems

Earlier onset, means more severe involvement and increased
  mental retardation

Congenital myopathies
Autosomal dominant or sporadic
Static or very slowly progressive clinical course
Similar clinical findings in all types
Weak in proximal muscles
Often floppy
Scoliosis, hip dysplasia, foot deformities common

Inflammatory myopathies
Acquired autoimmune diseases
Systemic illness, weakness, myalgia
Contractures, skin lesions, exacerbations and remissions
Limb girdle muscles first involved

Fibrodysplasia (or myositis) ossificans progressiva
Onset in first decade
Fascial planes, ligaments, tendons ossify (not muscles)
Neck and back involved first, then limbs
Short first ray of hands and feet
Ends in severe ankylosis and respiratory death
Muscle biopsy unwise, leads to more ossification

Arthrochalasis multiplex congenita
Often autosomal dominant; no skin changes
Hypermobility of joints; often hypotonia
No weakness, normal neurologically
Hip dysplasia common, also patellofemoral instability

Arthrogryposis multiplex congenita
Cause unknown, not genetic; not progressive
Most have deficient anterior horn cells
Contractures worse distally
Club foot common; also knee, hand, elbow contractures
Hip dysplasia and scoliosis possible

Congenital absence of muscles
Well compensated, seldom needs treatment
Pectorals, then trapezius most common
Usually unilateral
Absent quadriceps may be reconstructible

Cerebral palsy
Non-progressive, caused by brain lesion
Spastic most common; mixed, athetoid, ataxic, hypotonic less
  common
Common patterns are diplegia, hemiplegia, quadriplegia
Operations usually very beneficial

Hereditary spinocerebellar ataxia
Also known as Friedreich's ataxia
Usually autosomal dominant, but occasionally recessive
Progressive degenerative central and peripheral nervous system
  disease
Weakness, ataxia, nystagmus, dysarthria, difficult hand fine
  motor control
Pes cavovarus, scoliosis, wheelchair by third decade

Table 3.1 *Continued*

Spinal muscular atrophy
Autosomal recessive, fifth chromosome defect
Progressive anterior horn cell and motor nerve fibre disease; fasciculations
Proximal greater than distal weakness; scoliosis very common
Spectrum of severity

Acute anterior poliomyelitis
Poliomyelitis virus; effective vaccine
Viral infection of anterior horn cells and brain-stem motor nuclei with range from temporary weakness to permanent paralysis
Lower limbs more commonly involved
Acute phase may last 3–4 months, recovery may continue for up to 2 years

Myelomeningocoele
Saccular posterior herniation of neural tissue and meninges; usually lumbar, thoracolumbar, or sacral
Hydrocephalus and Chiari–Arnold syndrome often associated
Lower limb paralysis, deformities, sensory loss and scoliosis are common

Amyotrophic lateral sclerosis
Unknown inheritance pattern
Motor neurone degeneration
Usually adult onset, death within 3 years
Relentless progression to involve all muscles

Acute idiopathic post-infectious polyneuropathy
Guillain–Barré syndrome
More than 50% of cases follow a viral infection by 2–4 weeks
Symmetrical ascending motor paralysis
Can ascend to bulbar paralysis
Many cases have severe muscle pain
Maximum paresis in 1–4 weeks, then recovery over 3–6 months
10% mortality; 20% permanent sequelae

Hereditary motor and sensory neuropathies
Some autosomal dominant, some recessive; usually progressive
Most have intrinsic hand and foot atrophy and ankle dorsiflexor and evertor weakness
Variable degrees of involvement within families

Congenital indifference to pain
Many types, some genetic
Self-mutilation and biting, occult fractures
Neuropathic arthropathy later

Myasthenia gravis
Unknown inheritance; autoimmune disease
Involves females more often than males; three types in children
Excessive weakness after activity or stress
Bulbar, ocular, shoulder girdle involvement early, then generalized
Variable clinical course, remissions and relapses

absence ultimately results in cell death. Much research is now being directed at genetic manipulations to induce dystrophin synthesis.

Pregnancy and delivery are usually normal, as are the initial developmental milestones of head control and the ability to sit upright. Walking may occur at the normal time, though 50% of cases have delayed independent walking.

Weakness is symmetrical, with earliest and most severe involvement of the muscles first formed in the embryo, those of the pelvic and shoulder girdles. Spurious 'improvement' in some patients may be noted during the period of 4–7 years of age and is explained by the processes of normal growth and development and increase in motor ability outstripping progression of the disease. As skeletal muscle usually requires 30–40% loss of mass before clinical weakness is detectable, the apparent 'normal' functioning of children with this disease during the first few years of life is understood. Eventually, all skeletal muscles are involved, the posterior tibial, facial and extraocular muscles remaining intact longest. The early gait is a wide-based waddle with increased lumbar lordosis (Fig. 3.1). Progressive contracture of the triceps surae group produces a toe-walking gait and the ability to run is never attained. Shoulder weakness is apparent with a positive Meryon sign, a 'slipping through' when attempts are made to pick a child up by lifting under the axillae (Fig. 3.2). The child has trouble climbing stairs and eventually Gowers' sign, the necessity to use the arms to assist in rising from the floor, becomes apparent (Gowers, 1879).

The ability to maintain independent ambulation deteriorates, and most affected children stop walking by the age of 9–12 years. Once confined to a wheelchair, the development and progression of flexion contractures, particularly of the major joints, and progressive equino-varus foot deformities occur. The onset of progressive scoliosis, initially flexible, but later becoming fixed, is seen in more than 90% of patients after ambulation is lost. With further progressive weakness, patients become confined to bed, the last remaining functional muscles being the diaphragm, the muscles of swallowing, facial muscles, extraocular muscles, and intrinsic muscles of the hands and feet. Death is usually precipitated by respiratory failure or pneumonia, though cardiac failure, resulting from involvement of the heart muscle, may be the terminal event.

Physical findings in Duchenne muscular dystrophy show weakness of the proximal muscles of greater magnitude than that found in the distal muscles and lower extremity weakness that is often slightly greater than weakness in the upper limbs. The gluteal muscles

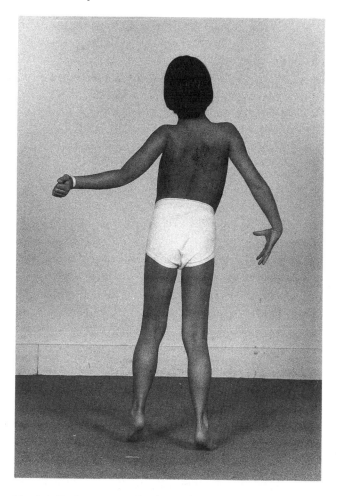

Fig. 3.1 Duchenne muscular dystrophy. Note the characteristic toe-walking, wide-based gait and hyperlordosis of the spine seen in mid-childhood.

are usually involved first, followed by the quadriceps and then the foot dorsiflexors. The gastrocnemius and soleus muscles also become weak and have a firm, rubbery consistency on palpation. This is the result of pseudohypertrophy, in which fat and fibrotic tissue replace muscle (Fig. 3.3). Neurologically, sensation is intact. Stretch reflexes are absent in the upper extremities and the quadriceps early, but the triceps surae maintains its activity for a longer period. The Babinski reflex remains negative. Sphincter function remains intact and dysphagia does not occur. Intelligence testing in these patients shows generally lower function than in normal controls, though normal or above normal intelligence may occur.

In most cases, the diagnosis is made from the family history and the clinical findings, particularly the pattern of muscle weakness and the pseudohypertrophy of the triceps surae group. Laboratory data are confirmatory,

the most striking finding being the extremely marked elevation of creatine phosphokinase early in the course of the disease, with values usually several hundred times greater than normal. These levels gradually fall during the course of the disease as muscle mass is replaced by fibrous tissue. Approximately three-quarters of the patients show electrocardiographic changes because of cardiomyopathy. Electromyographic studies characteristically show small polyphasic potentials with increased recruitment of motor neurones with effort. Fibrillation potentials are also often seen in advanced stages of the disease. Muscle biopsy findings include increased fibrosis, small groups of basophilic-staining fibres and groups of undifferentiated type II fibres.

TREATMENT

Included in the management of Duchenne muscular dystrophy are genetic counselling, identification of the carrier state, and a specific, individualized treatment programme for each patient. Although treatment is palliative, advances in multispecialty management, including physiotherapy, orthotics, pulmonary therapy, and orthopaedic surgery, have prolonged function and probably survival in recent years. Early in the disease, treatment is aimed at preventing joint contractures by a passive range of motion exercises. Some advocate night splints to delay equinovarus deformity of the foot and ankle, but often these fail or are not well tolerated. Active power building exercises to the weaker muscles are probably of no benefit.

When it is apparent that the child's ability to walk is in jeopardy, surgery and orthotic support are most worthwhile. The goals at this stage are to keep the patient as mobile and independent as possible so that the benefits of ambulation can help to delay the appearance of contractures and general physiological deterioration. This is the proper time for surgical intervention. Equinovarus deformities of the feet and ankles and sometimes hip flexion contractures prohibit a stable base of support and interfere with walking. If operation is delayed until walking ceases, the wheelchair-bound patient will never walk again. It has been shown that the appropriately timed release of contractures and the use of lightweight orthoses can prolong standing or walking by 2–5 years (Siegel, 1986). In the foot, the major deforming forces are the triceps surae and posterior tibial muscles. Percutaneous tenotomy alone is sufficient for the triceps surae and in some cases also for the posterior tibial muscle. Many, however, recommend transfer of the posterior tibial muscle through the interosseous membrane to the dorsum of the foot.

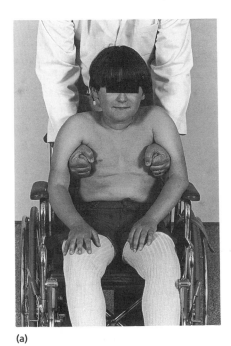 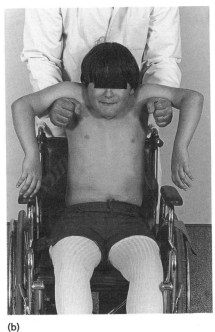 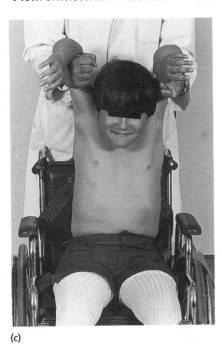

(a) (b) (c)

Fig. 3.2 (a−c) Meryon sign: a 'slipping-through' as an attempt is made to lift a patient with profound shoulder muscle weakness.

Although non-phasic, this transfer acts as an eversion, dorsiflexion tenodesis, removes a major deforming force, and may be superior to tenotomy for preventing recurrent equinovarus. When performed just before the termination of independent walking, the child tolerates the procedure quite well and is able to stand and walk in postoperative casts within 1−2 days. Advanced equinovarus with fixed bony deformity may require percutaneous medullostomy of the talus and calcaneus as advocated by Siegel (1986).

The hip flexors and tensor fascia latae are the other major contracted muscles at this stage, and subcutaneous release through a very limited incision is indicated if the flexion contracture of the hip exceeds 30° in an ambulatory patient or becomes painful in late stages of the disease in a non-ambulatory individual. Release of such contractures may allow a patient with end-stage Duchenne dystrophy to sleep on the back and may facilitate the use of lower extremity orthoses for transferring in and out of the wheelchair. Knee flexion contractures seldom become significant (greater than 20°) until a child has long since lost the ability to stand, even with orthotic control. If they become painful late in the disease process, hamstring tenotomies and serial splints may be helpful.

Any operation in this disease must not cause excessive pain and must be followed by immediate mobilization of the patient, as postoperative bedrest rapidly accelerates weakness and atrophy; a loss in strength of 1−3%/day is not uncommon. The patient should be standing in plaster casts or braces within 24 h of operation. Physiotherapy is resumed on the day of operation, and when soft tissues have healed, lower limb orthoses are applied. These are essential to provide support and prevent recurrent deformity in all postoperative patients. This must be understood by the patient and the parents before any operation. The most commonly used orthosis features a quadrilateral ischial seat, spring-loaded, drop-lock knee hinges and solid ankle joints.

Scoliosis develops in over 90% of patients with Duchenne muscular dystrophy, its onset occurring after independent ambulation has been lost. Probably more than 90% of those with scoliosis have continued progression of the spinal deformity and will ultimately require stabilizing spinal surgery. Because the risk is so high, mild spinal deformities must be aggressively followed and operations performed when appropriate. The natural history of untreated progressive scoliosis in Duchenne muscular dystrophy is substantial interference with sitting balance, respiratory function (a thoracic curve decreases pulmonary function by 4% for every 10° of curvature) and generalized physical discomfort. Spinal orthoses serve only to slow, but not to prevent, progression of scoliosis, and therefore are contraindicated in Duchenne muscular dystrophy, serving only to 'buy false time' while pulmonary function deteriorates.

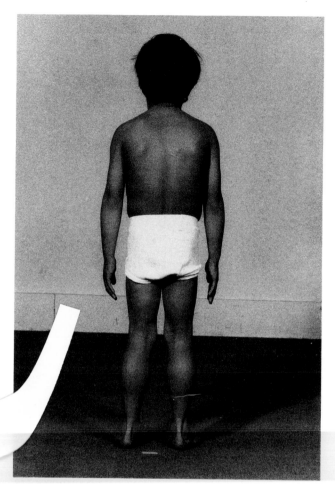

Fig. 3.3 Pseudo-hypertrophy of the triceps surae group in a boy with Duchenne muscular dystrophy.

As long as forced vital capacity and forced expiratory volume remain above 25% of predicted, it is rare for a patient to require prolonged ventilatory support in the postoperative period. Function less than 20% of predicted may prohibit operation, the likelihood of permanent postoperative ventilatory dependency being too high. Therefore, any curve that reaches 40° should be surgically stabilized, unless the pulmonary function is less than 20% of predicted. Similarly, if pulmonary function deteriorates to close to 30% of predicted, then any curve over 10–15° should be surgically stabilized. The procedure of choice is a one-stage posterior spinal fusion using segmental instrumentation, either sublaminar wires or multiple hooks, with fixation from the second thoracic level to L5 or the pelvis, depending on the absence or presence of fixed pelvic obliquity. Abundant homograft bank bone is essential to ensure the development of a solid fusion mass.

An aggressive attitude towards the treatment of Duchenne muscular dystrophy is most beneficial for the patient. Even as the disease reaches its terminal stage, occupational therapy and devices to improve the activities of daily living can prolong the child's ability to help care for himself. Ethical questions, such as whether or not to institute ventilatory support, are best decided by the patient and the family before the terminal stage.

Becker muscular dystrophy

A disease similar to Duchenne muscular dystrophy, but milder in form, was described in 1955 by Becker and Kiener. This is an X-linked recessive condition with the same genetic defect at the Xp21 locus as that of Duchenne muscular dystrophy. It occurs in a ratio of about one case to nine of the severe Duchenne type. Usually onset is noted between 5 years and the third decade of life. The overall clinical course is much slower, and it may be asymmetrical but begins with similar proximal weakness of hip and shoulder musculature, the tendency towards toe walking, and the characteristic calf muscle pseudohypertrophy. Independent ambulation may continue into or beyond the third decade and patellar subluxation, secondary to quadriceps weakness, is sometimes seen. Triceps strength is prolonged and assists in rising from a seated position. The gait is waddling with abductor insufficiency and hyperlordosis. Equinocavovarus foot deformity is common. Scoliosis may develop in ambulatory patients. Mental retardation is rare in Becker dystrophy.

Laboratory findings include marked elevation of the creatine phosphokinase and similar, but milder, electrocardiographic changes occurring later than with Duchenne muscular dystrophy. Muscle biopsy shows foci of atrophy similar to denervation, as well as findings of degeneration and regeneration.

Treatment for Becker muscular dystrophy is similar to that for Duchenne muscular dystrophy, with the overall goals being prolonged ambulation, prevention of contractures and control of scoliosis.

Benign autosomal muscular dystrophy

Another form of pseudohypertrophic muscular dystrophy occurs in females as well as males and appears to be autosomal recessive in inheritance type. It runs a much more benign course than the Duchenne type. According to Kloepfer and Emery (1969), this disease is about one-sixth as common as Duchenne muscular dystropy.

Emery–Dreifuss muscular dystrophy

This genetic condition is an X-linked, recessively transmitted disease (Emery and Dreifuss, 1966). The defect is at the gene locus Xq28. Its onset is typically during or after late childhood and is characterized by difficulty in running, stiffness of the neck and spine in extension, elbow flexion contractures and triceps surae contractures with talipes equinus. Cardiac arrhythmias, particularly atrial conduction defects, are common and often are detected only by monitoring. Mild, very slowly progressive muscle weakness is the rule in this syndrome, particularly involving the biceps, triceps, triceps surae and anterior tibial muscles. Creatine phosphokinase is moderately elevated. Muscle biopsy demonstrates focal atrophy and dystrophic changes.

Treatment of Emery–Dreifuss muscular dystrophy consists of correcting the equinus deformity of the ankle and preventing or correcting elbow flexion contractures by using alternating night splints or dropout casts. Because of the occurrence of cardiac conduction defects, a pacemaker may be indicated.

Limb girdle muscular dystrophy

This disease is transmitted by autosomal recessive inheritance and is characterized by a progressive, sometimes asymmetrical, weakness of the musculature of the shoulders and hips. When shoulder weakness is noted first, the prognosis is usually better. The onset is most commonly in the adolescent or young adult years, but it can occur in early childhood. Life expectancy is somewhat reduced but variable, as diaphragmatic involvement may occur and lead to alveolar hypoventilation.

The most common distribution pattern is a slowly progressive weakness from proximal to distal, particularly in the lower extremities, though marked atrophy of shoulder girdle musculature with concomitant weakness of the paraspinal muscles is seen in adults. Periods of apparent arrest of progression are not unusual. Gait is characterized by proximal weakness and waddling, secondary to abductor insufficiency. Running and stair climbing are impaired, and hyperlordosis compensates for weakness of hip extensor muscles. There is often a positive Gowers' sign. In the later stages, joint contractures are common, but these are usually not as severe as with other muscle diseases. Spinal deformities are also much less common, though paraspinal muscle weakness often leads to low back pain. Marked involvement of the biceps and deltoid muscles is common in limb girdle dystrophy, whereas the brachioradialis and extensor digitorum brevis muscles remain strong. This is an important clinical feature distinguishing this condition from fascioscapulohumeral dystrophy. Patients with limb girdle dystrophy have normal intelligence and no cardiomyopathy.

Creatine phosphokinase levels may be normal, but usually are moderately elevated, and muscle biopsy gives results consistent with myopathy. Electromyographic studies show small polyphasic potentials with occasional high-frequency discharges, also consistent with myopathy.

Treatment principles in limb girdle dystrophy are to maintain joint motion and muscle strength and to utilize a cane, crutches, or a walker before wheelchair dependency during the later stages of the disease. In those patients with intractable low back pain, surgical treatment has been disappointing, and conservative methods should be employed.

Fascioscapulohumeral dystrophy

This disease, also know as Landouzy–Dejerine dystrophy, is inherited by the autosomal dominant pattern, affecting both sexes equally. Expressivity is extremely variable, not only between but also within families. The disease can be manifest as a severe infantile form, noted within the first few years of life, which is often a rapidly progressive disease. The child drools excessively and does not smile. By the end of the first decade, severe scoliosis may have developed and the ability to walk has been lost. On the other hand, the disease may not be noted until the second decade of life or beyond.

Clinical weakness is noted in the facial muscles with a weak transverse smile and difficulty squeezing the eyelids, whistling, or wrinkling the forehead. The upper arm and shoulder muscles are involved, particularly the muscles of scapular fixation, and high-riding scapulae are common. Winged scapulae are noted on arm abduction. In contrast to limb girdle muscular dystrophy, the brachioradialis and deltoid muscles and muscles of the rotator cuff appear less involved than the other shoulder muscles, particularly the rhomboid and the pectoral muscles. Progression is usually slow, spreading distally to involve the hips and later the tibialis anterior muscles, producing foot drop usually 10–15 years after the onset of the disease. Hyperlordosis is the consequence of hip extensor muscle weakness. In the upper extremities, wrist and finger extensors are eventually involved, but the extensor digitorum brevis is usually spared and may appear hypertrophied. In slowly progressive cases, life expectancy may be normal and the disease may appear to be quiescent for periods of time.

The diagnosis of this condition is based on the clinical

presentation of the patient and the family history. Muscle enzyme levels are either normal or slightly to moderately elevated, and electromyographic and muscle biopsy studies show characteristic myopathic changes.

Treatment for fascioscapulohumeral dystrophy attempts to maintain muscle power and range of motion as long as possible. Surgical stabilization of the spine may be indicated with progressive scoliosis. Scapulothoracic fusion may benefit a minority of patients with early-onset disease that substantially interferes with upper extremity function, e.g. over-head dressing, or activities related to employment. Stabilizing the scapula to the chest wall allows the deltoid improved mechanical advantage in abducting the humerus.

Scapuloperoneal dystrophy

In this condition, muscle weakness is confined mostly to the shoulder, tibialis anterior and peroneal muscle groups. No single inheritance pattern has been established. About 50% of patients show associated facial muscle weakness and, therefore, this may be a variant of fascioscapulohumeral dystrophy. Clinically, progression is slow, ambulation is usually maintained, and life expectancy is normal.

Scapulohumeral dystrophy

This is a very uncommon condition, with shoulder girdle weakness that is slowly progressive. There is no facial muscle involvement. Late pelvic girdle and lower extremity involvement may occur. Loss of ambulation is not characteristically seen.

Hereditary distal myopathy

This myopathy is an autosomal dominant disease, usually beginning after the fourth decade, though occasional cases have been reported as early as infancy. Initial involvement appears to affect the intrinsic muscles of the hands and the tibialis anterior and gastrocnemius groups. In the majority of cases, progression is extremely slow.

Congenital muscular dystrophy

Infants with congenital muscular dystrophy have profound hypotonia at birth, with facial involvement and difficulty with sucking and swallowing. Respiratory infections and aspiration are common. The disease is more commonly an isolated finding, but some cases are inherited by an autosomal recessive pattern. The clinical course is variable, with some patients seemingly stabil-

izing in mid-childhood or improving, whereas others follow a rapid downhill course with early demise caused by respiratory insufficiency. Manifestations include multiple contractures and trunk weakness with paralytic kyphosis or lordosis, sometimes associated with the early development of scoliosis. Hip subluxation or dislocation is also common. Intellectual function is usually normal, but mental retardation may occur. Cardiomyopathy is not usually present.

Muscle enzyme levels may be normal or moderately elevated, and electromyography shows myopathic changes. Muscle biopsies reveal dystrophic changes with extensive fibrosis.

Early treatment includes a range of motion exercises and orthotics to prevent contractures and provide trunk and extremity support. Because of the compromised respiratory muscles, a soft thoracolumbosacralorthosis (TLSO) is often all that is needed to allow sitting. Equinovarus foot and ankle deformities are common and respond to percutaneous tenotomies or lengthenings and ankle/foot orthoses.

The floppy infant

The floppy infant presents as a differential diagnosis of muscular hypotonia, which is particularly evident in the axial and proximal appendicular muscle groups. The infant often demonstrates inability to extend the neck and spine against gravity and does not assume some of the normal infant postures. Decreased resistance to a passive range of motion occurs at the proximal joints. When propped in the sitting position, poor head control, inappropriate for chronological age, is usually seen. Unfortunately, the diagnosis may be extremely difficult or impossible to make in very early infancy, but prompt further investigation is mandatory because the prognosis, depending on the diagnosis, may govern the intensity of the initial treatment.

The differential diagnosis of the floppy infant includes cerebral palsy, Prader–Willi syndrome, perinatal hypoxia secondary to such conditions as aspiration pneumonia or infant respiratory distress syndrome, Down's syndrome, metabolic diseases, septicaemia, severe systemic illness, congenital myopathies, paralytic conditions including quadriplegia secondary to birth trauma, benign congenital hypotonia, spinal muscular atrophy and congenital muscular dystrophy.

Ocular myopathies

Involvement of the extraocular muscles may be the presenting sign of other types of neuromuscular disease.

Progressive ocular myopathy, also known as ocular dystrophy, is a slowly progressive muscle disease, which begins with ptosis and then extraocular muscle weakness. This is usually an autosomal dominant condition, with sporadic cases being more common in women and rare cases of autosomal recessive pattern also described. Gradually, facial muscles become involved and later, weakness in the limbs is seen. This condition usually begins in the third decade of life. The muscle enzyme levels are normal, electromyographic patterns are myopathic, and ragged red fibres have been described on muscle biopsy. Patients with progressive ocular myopathy also have an abnormal sensitivity to curare, with profound weakness occurring in response to very small doses of this drug.

Another form of ocular myopathy is oculopharyngeal dystrophy, also an autosomal dominant condition, which usually begins in the third decade of life. This condition is characterized by asymmetrical ocular muscle weakness and dysphagia, caused by weakness of the muscles of swallowing. In the later stages, weakness of the proximal limb musculature is also seen. The diagnosis is based on clinical findings, mild-to-moderate elevation of creatine phosphokinase levels, myopathic findings on electromyography, and occasionally electrocardiographic abnormalities. Abnormalities of oesophageal motility are also detectable.

A third type of ocular myopathy is oculocranial somatic neuromuscular disease with ragged red fibres. This is a progressive disease arising during the first two decades of life, consisting of extraocular muscle weakness, ptosis, and often retinitis pigmentosa and optic atrophy. Generalized muscle fatigue occurs during exercise. Abnormalities may occur in virtually any organ system of the body, and include mental retardation, deafness, cardiomyopathy and heart block, limb spasticity, ataxic gait and pharyngeal weakness. Structural abnormalities of mitochondria have been identified in this disease.

Drug-induced myopathies

The aetiology of these conditions is evident from the history in most cases. One of the two most common drug-induced myopathies is that caused by chronic or excessive steroid administration, which presents initially with proximal muscle weakness and becomes more generalized with time if the underlying cause is not rectified. The other common myopathy is induced by excessive consumption of alcohol on either an acute or chronic basis.

The acute form follows excessive ingestion and is characterized by substantial pain, tenderness, weakness, and sometimes swelling in the larger muscles of the limbs. Creatine phosphokinase level is markedly elevated, and biopsy will show necrotizing myopathy with excessive lipid and glycogen in fibres. Muscle necrosis may result in myoglobinuria and renal failure. The chronic form is a proximal appendicular muscle weakness and is slowly progressive unless the underlying cause is rectified.

Other agents that have been implicated in progressive muscle weakness include antineoplastic agents and drugs such as quinine or chloroquine, which are sometimes used to treat muscle cramps or spasms. Excessive intake of diazacholesterol can cause myotonia, clofibrate may produce peripheral muscle cramps, and the chronic ingestion of licorice, diuretics and laxatives may produce proximal muscle weakness secondary to hypokalaemia. Excessive exogenous thyroid supplements can also produce generalized weakness, as can drug-induced hypocalcaemia.

MYOTONIC SYNDROMES

Myotonia is defined as the inability to rapidly relax skeletal muscle fibres after voluntary or induced contraction. It is associated with repetitive discharges of the muscle cell membrane, appearing on an electromyogram as repetitive trains of action potentials that increase and decrease in amplitude and frequency, the so-called 'dive-bomber effect'. Because of the membrane involvement, blockade of the neuromuscular junction with curare or interruption of the motor nerve supply will not diminish myotonia induced by percussion of the muscle belly. Myotonia may be seen as a side-effect of the drug clofibrate and has been associated with thyroid dysfunction, acid maltase deficiency, Schwartz–Jampel syndrome, hypokalaemic conditions and carcinoma of the lung. It is usually exacerbated by cold, fatigue, or stress, but may not be found in the advanced stages of the disease when muscle mass has been lost.

Myotonia congenita

This condition, also known as Thomsen's disease, has two varieties. The first is an autosomal dominant trait described by Thomsen (1876) in his own family and detectable at birth. Usually all voluntary muscles are affected, but the condition may be very mild. It is a non-progressive disease.

A second variety, more common than the first and thought to be an autosomal recessive trait, nevertheless occurs more commonly in males. Its onset is most often noted about the age of 5–6 years, and the myotonia is more severe than in the first type. There is generalized muscle stiffness after resting, which is aggravated by cold and relieved by exercise or use. With decreasing myotonia, strength increases. Generalized muscle hypertrophy is common but not always present, and strength is normal or near normal, though there may be some distal atrophy or weakness. This condition sometimes improves over time.

The clinical diagnosis of these conditions is not difficult. Electromyographic studies show increased excitability and rhythmic myotonic discharges without evidence of dystrophic potentials. Enzyme studies show normal or slightly elevated levels, and muscle biopsy shows generalized hypertrophy with absence of type 2B fibres. Contractures and other fixed deformities requiring surgical treatment do not occur in these conditions, and although no medication affects the course of the disease, therapeutic trials of phenytoin, quinidine, or procainamide may occasionally be indicated. The beneficial effects of these medications are relatively short, usually disappearing within 2–3 months. For this reason, medical treatment is most useful during times of undue stress or exposure to cold.

Myotonic dystrophy

This disease is also known as Steinert's disease or dystrophia myotonica (Steinert 1909). It is an autosomal dominant condition with a defective gene on the long arm of chromosome 19. It is usually first noticed in adolescence, but may be seen much earlier. These patients have a classic facial appearance with wasting of the muscles in the temporal and other facial areas, drooping of the lower lip, lid lag, general sagging of the face and wasting, particularly in the sternomastoid muscles (Fig. 3.4).

In its most severe manifestation the condition is inherited from the mother, and the infant is severely hypotonic at birth. There may be sucking and breathing difficulties which gradually improve. Severe talipes equinovarus is common and mental retardation is usually severe. Motor milestones are delayed and there has been little intrauterine movement. The infant does not show the electromyographic findings of myotonia, and muscle biopsy at this stage shows delayed maturation, appearing as fetal muscle. The severely affected child may require early respiratory support, aggressive treatment of contractures and talipes equinovarus, and ultimately speech therapy for severe dysarthria.

With later onset, there can be great variation of affliction within the same family. Patients usually first notice weakness in the hands and feet with stiffness and difficulty in releasing a grasp. Weakness of ankle dorsiflexion and knee extension is also seen relatively early and the overall weakness progresses from distal to proximal. Weakness is a greater problem for patients than myotonia. Exceptions to this are dysarthria, secondary to myotonia of the tongue, and dysphagia, caused by pharyngeal myotonia. The myotonia tends to

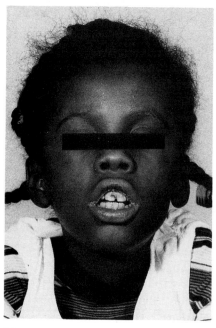

(a)

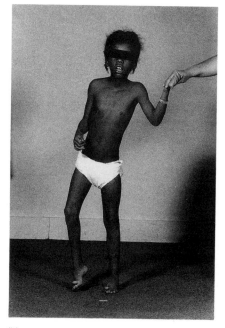

(b)

Fig. 3.4 Girl with myotonic dystrophy (Steinert's disease) demonstrating (a) facial muscle weakness and (b) weakness of knee extension and foot dorsiflexion. She required surgical correction of the rigid equinovarus foot deformities.

decrease as weakness progresses. Scoliosis may develop and usually responds to orthotic treatment. As a general rule, the earlier the onset, the more severe the mental retardation and the more rapid is the course of the disease. The disease may be genetically enhanced, with each succeeding generation demonstrating symptoms earlier and with more severe involvement.

Associated findings may include cataracts and endocrinological abnormalities, e.g. testicular atrophy, infertility, menstrual irregularity and thyroid dysfunction. Cardiac conduction abnormalities are seen in over half of the patients. In addition, these patients may be extremely susceptible to drugs, e.g. morphine or barbiturates, that depress the respiratory centres. Some patients have abnormal carbohydrate metabolism with a diabetic-type glucose tolerance curve. Facial characteristics include temporalis temple wasting, lid lag, frontal balding and hyperostosis of the frontal cranium with enlargement of the sinuses.

Electromyographic findings are classic and diagnostic, and muscle enzyme levels are slightly elevated. Muscle biopsy shows type 1 fibre atrophy and occasional internal nuclei, ring fibres and sarcoplasmic masses.

Treatment includes physical therapy, orthotics for distal lower extremity weakness or scoliosis, and occasionally operative stabilization of the foot to prolong walking ability. The hypersensitivity of these patients for certain depressant drugs must be kept in mind.

Paramyotonia congenita

This rare autosomal dominant disease was first described by Eulenberg in 1886. It is commonly detected shortly after birth and unlike other varieties of myotonia, exercise may make the condition worse instead of better. It affects the facial muscles, forearms and hands more than other areas. The myotonia may occur only following exposure to cold, and some patients may experience episodes of flaccid weakness similar to periodic paralysis.

Other types of myotonia

Other forms of myotonia include myotonia acquisita and Schwartz–Jampel syndrome. The former condition is characterized by myotonia precipitated by stress or sudden trauma. Exposure to certain chemicals or drugs may also precipitate myotonia. Schwartz–Jampel syndrome, also known as chondrodystrophic myotonia, includes myotonia, short stature, skeletal dysplasia, blepharal spasm and facial abnormalities. Intelligence is normal in this condition, and inheritance is likely to be of the autosomal recessive pattern.

CONGENITAL MYOPATHIES

Congenital myopathies can present with comparable clinical findings and generally carry a similar prognosis. These autosomal dominant abnormalities are classified by histochemical and electron microscopic evaluation of skeletal muscle. The patient may present in infancy as a hypotonic or 'floppy' baby or in early childhood, with delayed motor milestones. Weakness is predominantly found in the pelvic and shoulder girdles and is either static or very slowly progressive. Enzyme studies are usually normal.

Central core disease

This non-progressive congenital myopathy demonstrates a wide clinical spectrum of muscle involvement (Shy and McGee, 1956). Scoliosis, congenital dislocated hip and talipes equinovarus may require surgical correction, whereas a report of malignant hyperthermia may require medical management. Histochemical visualization using the NADH-tetrasodium reductase reaction demonstrates that the central portion of the muscle fibre is void of oxidative enzymes and phosphorylase. Electron microscopy demonstrates an almost complete absence of mitochondria and sarcoplasmic reticulum in this area.

Nemaline myopathy

This mild, non-progressive myopathy presents in early childhood and is characterized by elongated facies and high-arched palate (Shy *et al.*, 1963). Skeletal changes are similar to those of arachnodactyly and include pectus carinatum, scoliosis, and pes cavus (Fig. 3.5). Diminished pulmonary function tests suggest the need for controlled ventilation with inhalation anaesthetic agents coupled with avoidance of muscle relaxants. One-third of the cases are sporadic and the course may be fatal with severe involvement of pharyngeal and respiratory muscles. Gomeri trichrome stain demonstrates rod bodies in contrast to the blue-green colour of the muscle fibres.

Myotubular myopathy

These patients exhibit a generalized infantile weakness which includes axial musculature. Involvement of the extraocular and facial muscles results in the typical facies, which include ptosis, squint and a doleful expression. Muscle biopsy demonstrates a striking resemblance between the striated muscle and the myotubes of fetal life (Spiro *et al.*, 1966). Although the

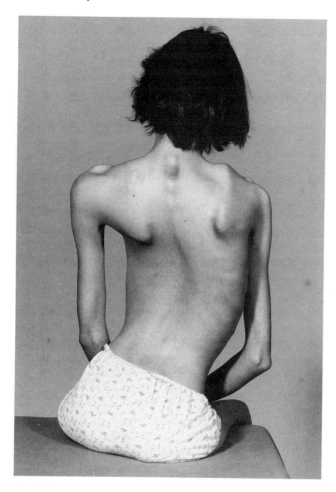

Fig. 3.5 Nemaline myopathy. Note atrophy in the shoulder and upper extremity muscles and scoliosis.

condition may be related to the arrest of development of the muscle, the fibre size remains normal. Histochemically, the central portion of the fibre is devoid of activity with ATPase reaction stain.

Congenital fibre-type disproportion

These patients present in infancy with generalized hypotonia and may have significant contractures including torticollis at birth. Congenital dislocated hip commonly occurs and over half will develop scoliosis because of paresis of the axial musculature. The weakness is greatest in infancy, when the infant is susceptible to life-threatening respiratory infection, and subsequently either stabilizes or slowly improves. In this myopathy, type 1 fibres are smaller and more numerous than type 2 on ATPase stain preparation (Brooke, 1973; Brooke and Engel, 1969). Additionally, some fibres contain internal nuclei and occasional rods.

INFLAMMATORY MYOPATHIES

Inflammatory reactions that primarily affect muscles include acquired illnesses, e.g. polymyositis or dermatomyositis, and genetic conditions, e.g. fibrodysplasia ossificans progressiva.

Polymyositis

This condition is an acquired, diffuse, inflammatory disease of muscle, usually beginning in early or midchildhood and is more commonly seen in females. More common in children, it is sometimes associated with skin manifestations and termed dermatomyositis.

The disease usually begins with a skin rash, fever and other systemic symptoms and ultimately results in diffuse muscle weakness and hyporeflexia. The muscles of the shoulder, pelvic girdles and the trunk are usually the most severely involved. The course of this disease may be acute and rapid or chronic, the acute form being more likely to both show skin changes and affect mucosal surfaces. Joint contractures are the rule with the chronic disease while pain, muscle stiffness and tenderness to palpation are seen in both forms. Exacerbations and remissions are characteristic of this condition.

Creatine phosphokinase levels are markedly elevated in polymyositis and electromyography shows spontaneous fibrillation potentials at rest. Muscle biopsies demonstrate chronic inflammatory cell infiltration, fibrosis, myonecrosis and some areas of regenerative changes. The biopsies should be done on a partially involved muscle.

Treatment of the acute stage includes rest and moist heat for symptomatic control, as well as the use of adrenocorticosteroids, with immunosuppressive agents and antineoplastic drugs being reserved for patients failing to respond to the steroids. Treatment of the chronic stage includes physiotherapy to maintain the range of motion and muscle strength, orthotics for prevention of contractures and occasionally operation for resistant joint deformities.

Dermatomyositis

The onset of this condition is most common in childhood, but it can occur at any age with another peak of incidence in the fifth and sixth decades. Dermatomyositis also appears to be slightly more common in females. It usually begins with systemic symptoms, e.g. irritability, malaise and fever. Sometimes there is an antecedent illness or a stressful event. Most cases demonstrate a heliotropic or violaceous rash, particularly over the eyes and malar regions in a classic butterfly distribution. Erythema may also be noted over the extensor surfaces of joints and may be precipitated by the photosensitivity of these patients. The skin lesions may appear before or after the development of weakness and other muscle symptoms.

Initially, the muscles may appear swollen, particularly in the limb girdle musculature, but the muscles may become tender, brawny and indurated as the disease progresses and joint contractures may develop. While pain may be present as a deep aching sensation with associated tenderness to palpation, at least one-third of the patients have no symptoms of muscle pain.

The course of this disease is variable. A patient may have an acute onset with a fulminating course or may have complete recovery with no medical treatment whatsoever. Other cases may show remissions and relapses with complete or incomplete recovery between these episodes. Still other cases show an indolent, chronic course. In most cases, the limb girdle muscles are affected first and then gradually more distal muscles become involved. There is a predilection for muscles of the anterior neck, and although facial muscle involvement and bulbar symptoms are rare, dysphagia is common late in the course of this condition and patients may ultimately require supplemental feeding. Severe forms of dermatomyositis that are not steroid responsive may develop calcifications, which are localized to the subcutaneous tissue and may form suppurative ulcers requiring excision of the thickened calcified tissue (Bowyer *et al.*, 1983).

This condition shows marked elevation of the levels of creatine phosphokinase and other muscle enzymes, and while an elevated erythrocyte sedimentation rate is a nonspecific finding, it can be a useful guide for following the course of the disease. Electromyographic findings are similar to those in polymyositis with short, low polyphasic potentials seen at rest. Muscle biopsies are similar to those for polymyositis, except that in dermatomyositis perifascicular atrophy is more prominent.

It is essential to note that there is a definite relationship between adult-onset dermatomyositis, and less often polymyositis, and the concomitant existence of neoplasia, which is estimated to occur in 10–20% of cases of dermatomyositis. Therefore, a search for carcinoma or other malignancy must be undertaken in any adult patient who has either of these conditions.

Treatment of dermatomyositis is similar to that for polymyositis, including physiotherapy and orthotic control during the acute phase and occasionally surgery for the release of chronic contractures. Drug treatment consists of steroids and may also include the use of other immunosuppressants and antineoplastic agents.

Fibrodysplasia ossificans progressiva

This is a rare, progressive, familial disease. It begins in the first decade of life, usually being noted within the first 3 years. The initial findings are small, painful swellings which regress and leave indurated lumps. Subsequently, calcification and ossification occur in fascial planes, tendons, ligaments and aponeuroses. The resultant extensive bone masses impede the action of muscles and may eventually result in ankylosis of joints (Connor and Evans, 1982). The neck and back areas are most commonly involved, followed by the face, shoulder and pelvic girdle areas, which results in loss of motion generally by the time the child is 10 years old. The muscles of the eyes, larynx, perineum, diaphragm, tongue and heart are spared. Nevertheless, slow progressive ankylosis is the usual rule and death, generally due to respiratory sufficiency, occurs in adult life in a patient who is often completely immobile by that time.

Patients with fibrodysplasia ossificans progressiva always have phalangeal abnormalities with a short first ray of the hands and feet. Syndactyly, polydactyly, external ear deformities, deafness, spina bifida, hallux valgus and mental retardation may also be noted. The diagnosis is made from the clinical picture, as no biochemical abnormalities have yet been identified. Muscle biopsy is most unwise in these patients, as trauma to muscle is almost always followed by more extensive ossification in the local fascial planes and interstitial tissues, though not in the muscle tissue itself.

No treatment has proved universally effective, and efforts at surgical excision have proved disappointing and generally result in a more extensive bone formation.

OTHER MUSCLE CONDITIONS

Arthrochalasis multiplex congenita

This is often a familial condition, which may be inherited as an autosomal dominant trait. It is characterized by hypermobility of joints and muscle hypotonia, but no weakness and no diminution of tendon reflexes. Intelligence is normal. The absence of any skin changes may differentiate it from the various forms of Ehlers–Danlos syndrome. Patients with arthrochalasis multiplex congenita present early in childhood with marked laxity and hypermobility of most joints, often leading to subluxation and frank dislocation, particularly of the hips and the patellofemoral joints (Fig. 3.6). Scoliosis may also develop. Although these children lead a relatively normal life, the treatment of bilateral hip dislocation can be exceedingly difficult, often requiring repeated operative procedures, particularly redirectional and realignment osteotomies and capsular plications.

Arthrogryposis multiplex congenita

Arthrogryposis (curved joint) is a motor pathway disorder, most often with decreased anterior horn cells in the spinal cord, which results in myofibrosis, joint capsular thickening, loss of motion and fusiform limbs. To the orthopaedic surgeon, arthrogryposis multiplex congenita is a specific diagnosis. To the neurologist, paediatrician, or geneticist, it usually simply means stiffness of joints. The classic 'orthopaedic' arthrogryposis, a static condition with decreased anterior horn cells in the spinal cord, is found in about 90% of cases. A much less common type, myopathic arthrogryposis, may be a variant of congenital muscular dystrophy. In these latter cases, the clinical presentation is similar to that of the

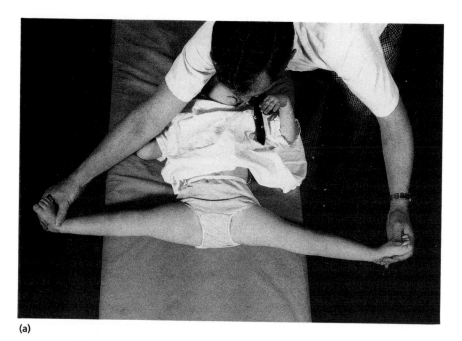

(a)

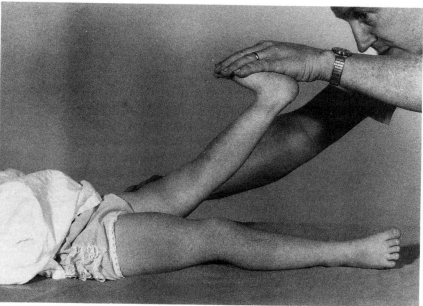

(b)

Fig. 3.6 Hypermobility of (a) the hips (b) the knees and ankles in a girl with arthrochalasis multiplex congenita. Extensive surgical treatment was required for bilateral congenital hip dysplasia.

anterior horn cell type, but the central and peripheral nervous systems are normal. A third variant, distal arthrogryposis, involves only the hands and feet.

In the most common type of arthrogryposis, the clinical findings are fusiform joints without creases, limited free motion to a sudden block, and more severe involvement distally (Fig. 3.7). Muscle mass is decreased and once the infantile fat distribution disappears, most patients have decreased subcutaneous fat stores. The condition occurs in approximately 1 in 3300 live births, a positive family history is rare, and other systems are not usually involved, though there is a 15% incidence of inguinal hernia associated with arthrogryposis. Intelligence is normal and sensation is intact. Approximately 60% of patients have quadrimelic involvement, 30% have lower extremities only involved, and 10% have either upper extremity involvement or distal arthrogryposis. Three-quarters of patients will gain the ability to walk.

In early infancy, an aggressive physical therapy programme to increase the range of motion of the knees and elbows is important. Other joints do not respond well. Splinting and orthotics may be necessary to maintain the gains. The aim of treatment for the foot is a plantigrade, braceable foot by the age of 2 years. Club foot occurs in 85% and is usually severe. Early manipulation will help maintain skin vascularity, but definitive treatment requires operation, either posteromedial release in the first year of life or talectomy after 12–18 months of age. Ankle–foot orthotics will be necessary to skeletal maturity or beyond, and triple arthrodesis may be required after the age of 10 years. Recurrent deformity during adulthood can be managed by supramalleolar osteotomy. Convex pes valgus develops in 10% of cases and will probably require surgical correction after the age of 6 months.

Knee contractures occur in 90% of patients, flexion being much more common than extension. Knee flexion deformity in the infant may be improved by a physiotherapy programme and/or serial dropout splinting, aiming to reduce flexion contractures to 20° or less. Following the infant physiotherapy programme, the arc of knee motion, but not its magnitude, may be changed by soft tissue release, osteotomy, or using slowly distractive external fixator devices. Knee extension deformity seldom needs treatment unless there is hyperextension, a condition often associated with congenital dysplasia or dislocation of the hip. Knee hyperextension may respond to physiotherapy and splinting, but may require quadricepsplasty and anterior capsulotomy if the child is older than 6 months.

The hip is involved in two-thirds of patients with arthrogryposis, approximately 20% having congenital dislocation, half of these being bilateral. When there is associated knee hyperextension, the knees should be treated first. Unilateral hip dislocation should be treated by open reduction, often combined with femoral shortening and derotational osteotomy. In cases of bilateral high-riding hip dislocation and severe involvement, it is wise not to attempt to treat the hips.

Considering the upper extremity in arthrogryposis, the aim is to maintain sufficient function for the activities

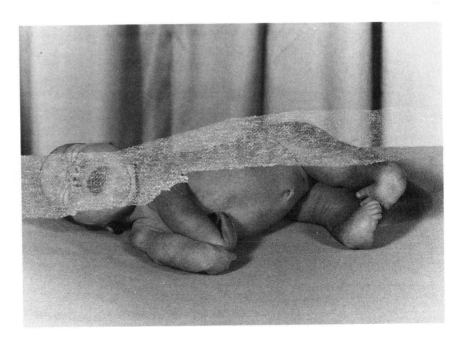

Fig. 3.7 Infant with arthrogryposis multiplex congenita showing the severe joint deformities present at birth in this condition.

of daily living, and not cosmesis. The entire upper extremity should be considered as a unit, and several years should be allowed to pass before assessing function. The patient must be able to reach the mouth with one hand and the perineum with the other. In addition, both hands should come together in the midline for manipulating objects. One elbow must be capable of full, stable extension to help the patient rise from a chair or use crutches. With the exception of severe thumb-in-palm deformity, treatment of the hand should not be undertaken, as this is almost certain to result in loss of function. A range of motion exercises and splinting for the hand and wrist have not been of benefit. Elbow flexion contractures may respond to physiotherapy in infancy, keeping in mind that one hand must be able to reach the head. The opposite elbow may require release to provide extension. Elbow extension contractures are more common than flexion contractures. Again, it is important to leave one straight. The other may require operation after the age of 6 years in the form of tricepsplasty, posterior capsulotomy, tendon transfers and then splinting or orthotic control. Internal rotation contracture of the shoulder is common and usually requires no treatment. A range of motion exercises for the shoulder have not been helpful. With severe involvement, proximal derotational osteotomy of the humerus before elbow correction may be of benefit.

Parents of patients with arthrogryposis should understand that multiple operative procedures are likely to be needed in severe cases, and also that it is impossible to achieve perfect muscle balance. Therefore, prolonged splinting or orthotic control may be necessary during the growth years. In general, it is desirable to correct lower limb deformities before walking age, whereas operations to improve the function of the upper limbs are best left until the child is 5−6 years old so that functional capacity can be more appropriately assessed and compliance with post-operative rehabilitation programmes will be more likely. Scoliosis occurs in about 20−30% of patients with arthrogryposis. Orthotic treatment can be successful in some curves of 25−40° in growing children. For larger curves, spinal stabilization by instrumentation and surgical fusion has been successful.

Congenital absence of muscles

This group of anomalies seldom requires specific orthopaedic treatment, but nevertheless has implications for function and is also important because there are often other associated anomalies. The pectoral muscles, followed by the trapezius, are the most commonly deficient groups. These anomalies are usually unilateral and are often quite well compensated by other muscle groups. In Poland's syndrome, absence of the sternal head of the pectoralis muscle is usually associated with syndactyly and other limb anomalies, as well as cardiac abnormalities. Congenital absence of abdominal muscles may be associated with respiratory insufficiency and also with defects of other internal organs and hip dysplasia. Absence of the quadriceps group of muscles may require reconstruction by tendon transfer.

Duplicated or accessory muscles, though sometimes mistaken for soft tissue tumours, are usually of no clinical significance.

Congenital muscle contractures

Contracture of musculotendinous units noted at, or shortly after, birth may be truly idiopathic or may be the result of blunt trauma with subsequent haemorrhage, oedema and then fibrosis in the muscle. Most commonly involved is the sternocleidomastoid muscle, causing congenital muscular torticollis. This condition may also be a myopathy. In most cases passive stretching exercises are curative, while others ultimately require surgical resection or lengthening of the involved units. A less common site for congenital contracture is the quadriceps region, the patient presenting with an extension contracture of the knee or even recurvatum or dislocation at birth. Dislocation of the patellofemoral joint is also quite common in this condition.

A similar clinical picture can be seen following multiple intramuscular injections into the quadriceps muscle during infancy. In these cases, the pathology is scarring and fibrosis of the muscle, most often seen in the vastus lateralis and vastus intermedius regions. In such cases, treatment is almost always operative, requiring a comprehensive exposure and appropriate musculotendinous elongation. Other contractures produced by repeated injection are noted to occur in the deltoid and gluteal musculature and may also require surgical release.

NEUROLOGICAL DISEASES

Brain and spinal cord

CEREBRAL PALSY

This is a disorder of movement and posturing caused by a static brain lesion, whose manifestations can change with growth and development. It occurs in 1−5 in 1000 live births and is caused by brain damage during the period of early brain growth. Common pre-natal causes include infection, exposure to toxins, e.g. drugs or alcohol, and congenital malformations of the brain. Peri-natal causes are most commonly prematurity, which usually leads to the diplegic pattern of involvement, anoxia, which may produce total involvement and quadriplegia, and trauma, which can produce variable patterns of involvement. Post-natal infection, trauma and vascular accidents can produce the brain lesion. A maternal history of infertility or fetal wastage is also associated with a higher incidence of cerebral palsy.

Patterns of motor involvement are classified both physiologically and anatomically. Physiological types are: (i) spastic (the most common), which shows increased muscle tone, slow movement and commonly contractures; (ii) athetoid, characterized by writhing movements with contractures being less common; (iii) mixed, which is usually a combination of spastic and athetotic involvement; (iv) ataxic, associated with cerebellar signs; and (v) hypotonic, usually a stage through which the infant with spastic cerebral palsy passes. Anatomical types include: (i) quadriplegia, with involvement of all four extremities; (ii) diplegia, with the lower extremities more severely involved than the upper extremities; (iii) hemiplegia, with unilateral involvement more severe in the upper extremity; and (iv) double hemiplegia. Less common types are monoplegia, triplegia and paraplegia involving only the lower extremities.

Several other defects are often associated with cerebral palsy. The most common is mental retardation, occurring in about two-thirds of all patients and seen most often in those with quadriplegia and least often in the athetoid and hemiplegic types. Seizures have been noted in 30–50% of patients, the hemiplegic type being at greatest risk. Other problems include learning disorders, emotional and personality derangements, visual defects, e.g. strabismus, visual field abnormalities and refractive errors, hearing impairment and disorders of speech.

In patients with the athetoid or mixed types of cerebral palsy, operation should be considered with caution and trepidation. Muscle releases and tendon lengthenings and transfers are unpredictable in these groups and may result in a more disabling deformity than existed before operation; they are more predictable in the spastic group. In general, it is advisable to perform operations after 5 years of age, when the patient is old enough to cooperate with the physician and physiotherapist. Procedures to prevent hip subluxation or dislocation, however, should not be deferred. It is vital in any procedure to consider the effects of altering any one musculotendinous unit or joint on the remainder of the limb, the pelvis and the spine. Employing preoperative gait analysis is of great benefit to improve surgical planning. If multiple corrections are needed, it is best to perform these under one anaesthetic, in order to minimize hospitalization and recovery time.

Spastic quadriplegia

Priorities, in order of importance, for the person with cerebral palsy are: communication; activities of daily living; mobility in the environment; and walking. Only 20% of patients with spastic quadriplegia will walk. The objectives in managing a patient with spastic quadriplegia are to maintain a straight spine and level pelvis; located, mobile, painless hips; mobile knees for sitting and bracing for transfer; plantigrade feet; appropriate adaptive equipment, including wheelchairs; and recognition and management of malnutrition, gastro-oesophageal reflux, seizures and other problems.

The prevalence of scoliosis in cerebral palsy parallels the neurological deficit and is most common in patients with spasticity and quadriplegia, occurring in up to 65% of patients in these groups. The use of an orthosis may improve sitting balance and slow curve progression in order to 'buy time' for beneficial spinal growth in immature patients, but only about 15% of progressive curves respond to spinal orthotic treatment, the remainder continuing to progress and requiring surgery. Custom-made seating devices are appropriate for patients in whom surgery is contraindicated and for those with residual deformity following spinal fusion. Spinal fusion should be considered for curves greater than 40° at any age, as scoliosis in cerebral palsy usually shows continued progression throughout adult life.

Hip subluxation and/or dislocation most commonly occurs in patients with the quadriplegic pattern. Flexors and adductor muscles overpower their antagonists and when combined with femoral anteversion and valgus, as well as pelvic obliquity and retained neonatal reflexes, hip instability may result. Because pain may occur in up to 50% of patients with hip dislocations, efforts at keeping the hips located are worthwhile. For the young child with a hip at risk for subluxation or dislocation, soft tissue releases and splinting are in order. An established subluxation may require varus derotational osteotomy, as well as soft tissue releases and sometimes pelvic osteotomy. A hip that has been dislocated for less than 1 year and has a reasonably good acetabulum may be appropriate for open reduction with femoral shortening, varization and derotation, and the addition of an appropriate pelvic osteotomy. A painful, established dislocation may be best treated by proximal femoral resection at the subtrochanteric level and covering of the bone end with a muscular cuff. Older patients with osteoarthritic hips respond well to total hip replacement arthroplasty or arthrodesis.

Spastic diplegia

Most patients with spastic diplegia will be able to walk. Many types of treatment are available. The role of neurodevelopmental therapy is currently being widely advocated in many centres, yet it remains very difficult to determine whether or not such therapy improves or accelerates the patient's own processes of maturation and development of the nervous system. Most physicians agree that after the age of 7–8 years, such therapy is of very limited use. Physiotherapy has little or no proven value in improving tone or diminishing the functional impairments of cerebral palsy, but it is of great value in postoperative rehabilitation and in minimizing progressive contractures. Manipulation and splinting are appropriate for mild foot and ankle equinus deformities or knee, elbow, or hand flexion contractures, but will fail painfully in patients with significant spasticity. Selective dorsal rhizotomy, a relatively recent treatment, can produce significant tone reduction while maintaining some voluntary control and intact sensation. It appears best suited for a patient with severe spasticity but good underlying strength who is capable of ambulation.

The use of drugs, e.g. diazepam, for postoperative spasms has been of benefit in cerebral palsy, but other drugs have not been successful in attempts to alter tone and improve function. The most commonly used and important group of drugs in cerebral palsy is the anticonvulsants. Gait analysis has been of substantial benefit in defining and documenting gait pathology, both before and after operation. It appears more accurate and objective than static examination and human observation and helps to avoid the staging of operative procedures.

Treatment of specific problems in spastic diplegia follows.

Hallux valgus is common, and whereas tendon transfers and osteotomies may be successful, they often fail. Metatarsophalangeal arthrodesis of the first ray in 10° of dorsiflexion is nearly always successful.

Pure *equinus deformity* of the foot and ankle responds to surgical elongation of the triceps surae by one of several methods. A post-operative ankle/foot orthosis is usually necessary to improve gait. *Equinovarus deformity* of the foot and ankle is best treated by Achilles tendon lengthening and either posterior tibial tendon lengthening or split posterior tibial tendon transfer. With *fixed hindfoot varus deformity*, a lateral closing wedge calcaneal osteotomy is of benefit. A post-operative ankle/foot orthosis is necessary. With *equinovalgus deformity*, Achilles tendon lengthening may be combined with peroneus brevis lengthening for mild cases, but more commonly, with significant valgus, requires subtalar arthrodesis (Fig. 3.8) and post-operative orthotic support.

A common problem is increased *external tibial torsion*, causing progressive valgus of the foot and loss of the foot lever arm length that is necessary for augmenting knee extension. This is corrected by supra-malleolar derotational osteotomy.

Knee flexion contractures are often associated with hip flexion contractures and a crouched gait. Treatment by medial hamstring lengthening, in conjunction with appropriate correction of hip flexion contractures, is successful. In cases with associated co-spasticity of the rectus femoris muscle throughout the gait cycle, distal transfer of the rectus femoris tendon, either medially to the sartorius muscle or laterally to the iliotibial band, will preserve knee flexion in swing phase and prevent changing a crouched gait to a stiff-legged, knee extension gait.

Hip flexion contractures are addressed by release or recession of the iliopsoas musculature. If the patient is ambulatory, intramuscular tenotomy of the psoas tendon at the pelvic brim saves strength and effectively reduces hip flexion contracture.

In-toeing in spastic diplegia is most often caused by excessive femoral anteversion. This is treated by proximal femoral derotation osteotomy, above the level of the lesser trochanter, and associated medial hamstring lengthening to compensate for the increased hamstring

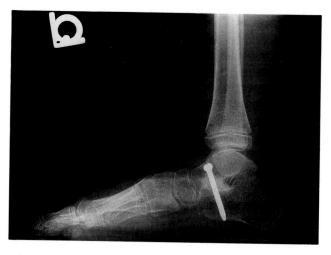

Fig. 3.8 Radiograph showing solid subtalar arthrodesis achieved by screw fixation and autologous bone grafting.

tightness produced by external rotation of the distal component of the osteotomy.

Post-operative management for surgical patients with spastic diplegia includes a short leg splint for a period of 2—3 weeks after Achilles tendon lengthening, followed by the application of an ankle/foot orthosis. After hamstring lengthening, simple knee splints are adequate, and traction and prone lying prevent recurrence during the first few days after hip releases. The use of diazepam for 4—5 days will help to reduce post-operative muscle spasms. A passive range of motion exercises should begin at 4—5 days after operation, gait training can be resumed at 1 week, and resistance exercises begun at 3 weeks after operation. In summary, the gait in spastic diplegia can often be improved by careful preoperative gait analysis, surgery performed at the age of 5—8 years (or sooner if needed), simultaneous correction of all deformities to avoid staging and then rapid rehabilitation.

Spastic hemiplegia

This presents a continuum of severity which has been classified into four types (Winters *et al.*, 1987). Operative results are very predictable in spastic hemiplegia. In type I, the tibialis anterior muscle is weak but the triceps surae group is not tight. The patient walks with a 'foot-drop' gait. This is best treated by an appropriate ankle/foot orthosis. In type II hemiplegia there is weakness of the tibialis anterior muscle and associated spasticity in the triceps surae group and tibialis posterior muscle. This produces an equinovarus foot, often associated with knee hyperextension in the late stance phase of gait. Treatment includes Achilles tendon lengthening, posterior tibialis tendon lengthening or split transfer, and an appropriate ankle/foot orthosis. In type III hemiplegia, the features of type II are present with, in addition, usually quadriceps and hamstring co-spasticity with a stiff-legged gait. Appropriate treatment includes lengthening of the Achilles, tibialis posterior and hamstring tendons and, usually, distal rectus femoris tendon transfer. A post-operative ankle/foot orthosis is used. Type IV hemiplegia has the features of type III with the addition of hip flexor and adductor spasticity. Treatment is the same as for type III involvement with the addition of iliopsoas lengthening and adductor release. Again, an ankle/foot orthosis is necessary after operation.

The upper extremity

Upper limb deformities are most commonly treated in the spastic hemiplegic patient. Orthotic treatment is poorly tolerated and seldom beneficial, but operation has an established role. To gain a perspective on the role of operative treatment, it must be remembered that these patients have sensory derangements, particularly proprioceptive and stereognostic deficiencies, which are permanent and will profoundly affect function, regardless of the operative result. Once a child has reached school age and has developed patterns of hand use, however, appropriate operations can improve the function of a 'helper' hand and certainly improve cosmesis. The most commonly performed procedures are those designed to correct or improve deformities of elbow flexion, wrist flexion and pronation, finger flexion and thumb-in-palm. Night splinting may be useful to prevent hand contractures. Other than for postoperative rehabilitation, physiotherapy has no proven value.

Overall, operations are indicated in the upper limb in fewer than 5% of patients with cerebral palsy. Pre-operative electromyographic studies are valuable; if a muscle is continuously spastic, then tendon lengthenings and release of contractures are appropriate; if it is phasic and has voluntary control, tendon transfers may be successful.

HEREDITARY SPINOCEREBELLAR ATAXIA

This disease, also known as Friedreich's ataxia, is a progressive condition that is usually an autosomal dominant trait, but occasionally is of autosomal recessive inheritance pattern. It is a degenerative disease of the central and peripheral nervous systems and is characterized by weakness, ataxic gait, nystagmus, dysarthria and difficulty with fine motor control of the hands. Symptoms are most often first noted between midchildhood and early adolescence. Cardiac abnormalities, including cardiomyopathy, dysrhythmias and coronary artery disease, are found in 90% of patients. Deficient position and vibration sense, loss of deep tendon reflexes and positive long tract signs occur, and progressive dementia develops. Nerve conduction studies show slight decreases in motor conduction velocities and often a marked decreased in sensory action potentials. Electrocardiographic changes may reflect myocardial fibrosis, and muscle biopsies often show the changes of denervation atrophy. Musculoskeletal problems include progressive pes cavovarus in the majority of patients, and approximately 80% will develop scoliosis (Fig. 3.9). This spinal deformity may respond well to orthotic treatment, but is usually progressive. Surgical stabilization has been effective.

The course of the disease is one of steady progression with remissions or plateaux being relatively uncommon

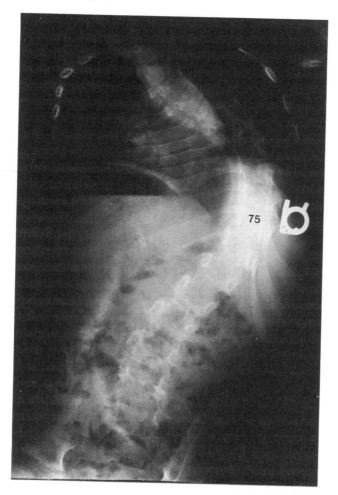

Fig. 3.9 Severe scoliosis in a patient with hereditary spinocerebellar ataxia.

occurrences. By the third decade most patients have lost their ability to walk, and death, usually brought on by progressive bulbar involvement, often occurs around the age of 40 years.

Orthopaedic treatment of this condition consists of maintenance of joint motion, minimizing contractures by preventive splinting, and operation to correct foot deformity or arrest progressive scoliosis if the prognosis is appropriate. The use of orthotics to improve balance for walking has been unsuccessful and usually rejected by the patient. Many patients who have lost the ability to walk and then developed severe equinovarus foot deformities, prefer adaptive footwear to triple arthrodesis.

SPINAL MUSCULAR ATROPHY

This is a progressive degenerative disease of the lower motor neurone cell body and the peripheral motor nerve fibres. Weakness is symmetrical, more profound proximally than distally, and usually involves the lower extremities to a greater extent than the upper ones. It is inherited as an autosomal recessive condition and may be manifested in various forms, ranging from the severe progressive form beginning pre-natally and causing death within the first year of life to a very mild form with onset in late childhood or adolescence and a very slow rate of progression. Motor neurones of cranial nerve nuclei are often involved. Sensation is unaffected. The cause is a defect in the fifth chromosome.

Approximately 50% of patients are classified as having type I spinal muscular atrophy, also known as acute Werdnig–Hoffman disease. These patients show decreased pre-natal activity as reported by their mothers and lack of spontaneous movement at birth or in the first few weeks of life, with marked generalized muscle weakness, hypotonia and atrophy. Deep tendon reflexes are absent. Fasciculations are seen in skeletal muscle groups, and the tongue and cranial nerve involvement results in a paralytic type of facies, weakness of the cry, and extremely difficult swallowing and feeding. Breathing is primarily diaphragmatic with retraction of intercostal spaces producing paradoxical respiration. Fixed deformities may develop with early hip adduction contracture, knee flexion contracture and external rotation contracture of the shoulder. This disease is rapidly progressive with death often occurring before the age of 1 year, the most common cause being respiratory failure. An occasional patient survives into early or mid-childhood. Electromyography shows degeneration, and muscle biopsy reveals clusters of type 1 fibres and large group atrophy. Treatment is supportive, using seating devices to provide upright trunk and head support.

Type II spinal muscular atrophy is known as chronic Werdnig–Hoffman disease. Onset is most often noted during the later part of infancy or shortly after the first birthday. Although the earliest motor milestones, e.g. head control, develop normally, sitting is delayed and these patients only very occasionally achieve the ability to walk with or without external support. In this type of the disease, the lower extremities appear to be more severely involved than the upper ones, and the proximal musculature appears weaker than the distal (Fig. 3.10). Deep tendon reflexes are absent, but the respiratory muscles and the cranial nerves are less involved. Approximately 50% of this group show fasciculations of the tongue. Most patients have hand tremors, but facial muscles are usually spared. Intelligence is normal. Although this is a progressive disease, in many cases progression can be extremely slow and orthopaedic

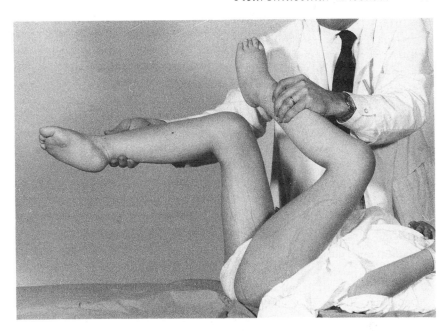

Fig. 3.10 Severe contractures of the hips, knees and feet in a patient with type II spinal muscular atrophy. More intensive care could have minimized these deformities.

management may offer a significant improvement in quality of life. All patients with type II disease develop scoliosis, which may require early orthotic treatment, though this often fails; operative stabilization is then required. Cardiomyopathy is rare, and the prognosis usually depends on respiratory involvement. Creatine phosphokinase levels may be normal or slightly increased.

Type III spinal muscular atrophy, also known as Kugelberg–Welander disease, is usually detected after walking begins. These patients show an abductor insufficiency gait, Gowers' sign and difficulty with running or climbing stairs. Fasciculations of the tongue are less common in this type. Deep tendon reflexes may be normal or slightly diminished, but ankle jerks are usually absent. As with type II disease, the proximal and lower extremity musculature appear to be more significantly involved, while wrist extensors and intrinsic muscles of the hand demonstrate the least involvement. Creatine phosphokinase level may be moderately increased. Some of these patients may have myocardial involvement with conduction abnormalities. The prognosis for this type of spinal muscular atrophy is excellent for long-term survival, the disease often being very slowly progressive. Nevertheless, most patients require a wheelchair by mid-adult life. Treatment is similar to that described for patients with type II spinal muscular atrophy. It should be noted that scoliosis is nearly a constant finding in types I, II and III spinal muscular atrophy.

Type IV spinal muscular atrophy is the mildest type and usually presents during the first two decades. These patients show minimal proximal and lower extremity muscular involvement. They do not lose their ability to walk. Life expectancy is normal and disability is mild.

ACUTE ANTERIOR POLIOMYELITIS

This acquired condition is caused by one of three types of poliomyelitis virus. Dissemination of the infection via the haematogenous route occurs from proliferative sites in the lymph nodes of the alimentary tract. Symptoms at this stage are usually confined to gastrointestinal discomfort, pharyngitis and low-grade fever. Only a small percentage of these patients have central nervous system invasion, but then often with disastrous results.

The central nervous system infection has a predilection for destruction of large motor cells, particularly in the anterior horn of the spinal cord and in the brain-stem motor nuclei. Involvement ranges from temporary interruption of function to total destruction of the cells themselves. The ensuing loss of muscle strength is variable and depends on the degree of involvement of motor neurones to specific muscles or on a more diffuse pattern which at the extreme may result in total paralysis of virtually the entire body including the lower bulbar musculature.

The distribution of paralytic involvement may not be related to anatomical nerve root distribution. Statistically, the lower cervical and mid-lumbar cord segments show the greatest incidence of involvement. Proximal muscles are more commonly involved and commonly develop paresis, whereas more distal muscles are more likely to be paralysed. The lower limbs, with a predilection for hip abductors, the quadriceps and medial hamstrings, are affected twice as often as the upper limbs where weakness of the pectoral muscles, deltoid and triceps is most often seen. Distally in the leg, the tibialis anterior and posterior muscles and long flexor and extensor muscles of the toes are most commonly involved. Progressive destruction of neurones may occur rapidly or may continue for a period of 3–4 months before the acute infection subsides.

Most of the clinical recovery of muscle power occurs during the first month following the acute stage of the disease, but recovery can continue for up to 2 years. During the acute phase, there is a strong tendency for rapid development of fibrotic contractures in fascia, muscle sheaths and tendons, particularly in the fascia lata and hamstring tendons, pectoral fascia and flexors of the elbow. These contractures often occur independently of the pattern of muscle involvement.

Diagnosis during the acute phase is based on the clinical picture with generalized symptoms and often signs of meningismus. The onset of muscle weakness may be seen as early as the first or second day. Spinal fluid examination often shows a slight elevation of the protein level and a mild-to-moderate lymphocytosis.

Although there is no specific treatment directed against the virus itself, this disease serves as a classic model for preventive medicine. The large epidemics recorded during the 19th and the first half of the 20th century no longer occur in countries where vaccination programmes and modern plumbing have been instituted. Treatment in the acute phase consists of general supportive measures, sedation, maintenance of appropriate nutrition and analgesics. Of paramount importance is comprehensive physiotherapy to prevent flexion contractures by maintaining a passive range of motion of all joints and relieving painful myospasm. Hot packs may be helpful during the exercise periods. It is also critically important to watch for signs of bulbar paralysis, particularly with respiratory muscle involvement, which may necessitate tracheostomy and mechanical ventilation.

After the acute stage, which may last up to 2 months, the patient enters the convalescent stage in which further active rehabilitation and mobilization are beneficial. Continued recovery may be expected for up to 2 years, though any muscle that is significantly weakened or paralysed after the first 6 months is unlikely to show any meaningful future improvement in strength. Serial documentation of muscle power is essential during the convalescent stage and overall treatment is directed at the prevention and correction of contractures. In addition to continuing the range of motion and power-maintaining exercises, orthotic devices may help in preventing deformity, improving function, or protecting

a weakened part. Fixed soft tissue contractures may require surgical elongation or division, particularly at the hip where significant iliotibial band involvement can influence deformities at the knee, hip and lumber spine. Hamstring lengthening may be required at the knee. At the ankle, stretching of the Achilles tendon and at the foot, release of the plantar fascia and intrinsic musculature, may also be indicated. The value of osteotomies and arthrodeses is well established for the reconstruction of the sequelae of poliomyelitis. Particularly at the end of the first year of treatment, therapeutic efforts are usually best directed at operative reconstructive procedures and orthotic utilization, as the maximum benefit of physiotherapy usually has been reached before this time.

Although the specific management of permanent paralysis during the chronic stage (beyond 2 years from onset) is beyond the scope of this chapter and has been well reviewed in many classic orthopaedic textbooks, it is appropriate to re-emphasize the principles of tendon transfer, an operative approach that can be of great benefit in static paralytic conditions. The tendon is mobilized with its muscle, nerve and blood supply intact and reinserted into bone to substitute for an ineffective musculotendinous unit. Recent advances in microvascular and microneurological surgery have allowed transfer of muscle and tendon units from one limb to another, re-establishing vascular and neurological continuity with remarkable success in some instances.

The primary indication for tendon transfer may be to improve function, to enhance joint stability or to improve muscle balance. Technical prerequisites for successful tendon transfer include:

1 Absence of joint contractures.
2 Sufficient power (not less than MRC grade 4) and cross-sectional area in the transferred muscle to perform its expected function.
3 Adequate excursion of the musculotendinous unit without scarring or adhesions.
4 A straight line of pull of the resultant transfer.
5 A phasic muscle, if possible, should be transferred, as non-phasic muscles usually function as tenodeses.
6 The transfer should cross one joint only, or at least as few as possible.
7 The musculotendinous transfer should be asked to perform one function only.
8 Whenever possible the tendon should be routed in the subcutaneous tissues.
9 The unit should be attached under appropriate tension.

POST-POLIO SYNDROME

Post-polio syndrome has recently emerged as a specific clinical entity (Bradley *et al.*, 1987). The diagnosis is essentially one of exclusion and is based on criteria that include: (i) the confirmed history of paralytic polio; (ii) partial to fairly complete neurological and functional recovery; (iii) a period of neurological and functional stability of at least 15 years duration; (iv) the onset of two or more of the following health problems since achieving a period of stability: unaccustomed fatigue; muscle and/or joint pain; new weakness in muscles previously affected and/or unaffected; functional loss; cold intolerance; and new atrophy; and (v) no other medical diagnosis to explain these health problems. The median age of onset of acute polio for these patients was 7 years. Those with onset over 10 years of age are more prone to develop post-polio syndrome, because older children are more likely to have severe poliomyelitis. Two-thirds of patients with post-polio syndrome are female with the onset generally 30 years after the acute episode of paralytic poliomyelitis.

Fatigue may be noted in previously affected muscles, particularly those used during ambulation or employment of a cane. These patients should be managed conservatively by reducing their activity level, changing the time and duration of exercises, and perhaps introducing a cane or a wheelchair on a part-time basis. Non-steroidal anti-inflammatory agents have been effective.

MYELOMENINGOCOELE

This condition is perhaps the most complex and demanding congenital anomaly of the central nervous system in which survival does occur. Before the advent of antibiotics, most patients died in early infancy. Now, with intensive efforts by teams of specialists, including neurosurgeons, orthopaedic surgeons, urologists and paediatricians, prolonged survival is possible even in severely affected individuals.

The incidence of this disorder has been reported to be 1–4 in 1000 births, with a subsequent increase to 1 in 20 if one child in a family has the condition and 1 in 10 if two siblings have been born with central nervous system malformation. Currently, the aetiology of myelomeningocoele is considered multifactorial, with the inheritance pattern probably modified by unknown teratogenic agents and environmental factors. The specific pathogenesis is also unknown, with two hypotheses attracting the most support. The first implicates the failure of closure of the neural tube, while the second proposes rupture of an initially closed neural tube.

The term 'myelomeningocoele' specifically refers to a saccular herniation of neural tissue and meningeal elements. This occurs most often in the lumbar, thoracolumbar and sacral regions, followed by the cervical area. While the vast majority occurs posteriorly, anterior myelomeningocoele has also been reported. The condition of myelomeningocoele is easily differentiated from both meningocoele, which contains only a sac of meningeal tissues without neural elements, and rachischisis, where there is no actual herniation but simply open exposure of a dysplastic spinal cord. Myelomeningocoele is commonly associated with cerebellar and brain-stem anomalies, and caudal herniation of these structures through the foramen magnum can occur, which is thought to be caused by pressure gradients between intracranial and spinal canal components.

Many other anomalies are often found in association with a myelomeningocoele. These may severely compromise the patient's chance of survival and have led physicians to develop selective criteria to determine which severely involved newborns should receive neonatal neurosurgical treatment. Lorber (1971, 1974) identified an exceptionally poor prognosis for patients with paralysis above the level of L3, a significant rigid congenital lumbar kyphosis, a grossly enlarged head secondary to hydrocephalus and the presence of other major congenital anomalies. Recent advances in pre-natal diagnosis, including amniotic fluid α-fetoprotein and acetylcholinesterase determinations, ultrasonography, fetography and fetoscopy, have made pre-natal screening and diagnosis possible with extremely high confidence levels.

Although the diagnosis is obvious at birth, assessment of the neonate with myelomeningocoele must include a general paediatric examination with emphasis on the cardiac, genitourinary, gastrointestinal and pulmonary systems. Further study should include evaluation of the presence or absence of hydrocephalus and increased intracranial pressure; evaluation of both the motor and sensory neurological levels; neurological reflexes; evaluation of the entire spine as well as the spinal lesion itself; and finally, orthopaedic evaluation of hip, knee and foot deformities which occur because of the muscle imbalance across the joints. Lack of proper antagonists produces active muscle shortening and subsequent joint contracture. Structural bony deformity develops because of the muscle imbalance, which may be enhanced by the intra-uterine position.

Initial treatment of this complex condition begins with closure of the spinal lesion by an experienced team within the first 24 h in order to prevent infection and preserve neurological function. When congenital lumbar kyphosis is present, resection of the osteochondral lumbar laminar bar will significantly aid in skin closure, and this limited procedure is recommended because these neonatal patients are at considerable risk for more extensive procedures (Drennan, 1976). Hydrocephalus occurs in more than 50% of these patients and may require ventriculoperitoneal shunting. Later assessment and management of the urinary tract are essential. Programmes of intermittent catheterization are now widely accepted and are of significant benefit in protecting the urinary function of these patients.

Operations, which include soft tissue releases and tendon transfers, should be performed after 8 months of age and after the spinal lesion, hydrocephalus and renal status are stabilized. Minimizing post-operative immobilization will help to reduce osteoporosis and subsequent fractures, which are common after prolonged immobilization in patients with myelomeningocoele. Preventive orthoses are useful in maintaining correction and improving lower extremity function.

The chief aims of treatment of the hips are mobility and symmetry. Hip dysplasia and subsequent dislocation are common in patients with mid-lumbar level lesions and are the result of weakness of hip abductors and extensors with muscle imbalance. Early abduction splinting is recommended. Posterior transfer of the adductor origin to the ischium, coupled with transfer of the external oblique muscle to the greater trochanter, may be necessary. When prevention of progressive hip dysplasia has been ignored or has failed more extensive measures, e.g. femoral osteotomy, open reduction and pelvic reconstructive surgery, may be indicated.

The knee must be free of deformity when walking is a consideration. Before fixed contractures develop, splints and orthoses may be effective. Operation is recommended to permit proper orthotic utilization when a fixed flexion deformity exceeds 20°. Operative approaches may include hamstring release or transfer, joint capsulotomy, or in the young adolescent, supracondylar femoral osteotomy. Hyperextension is seldom a clinical problem and quadriceps lengthening procedures are most commonly done in paralysed, nonambulatory patients who require knee flexion for better wheelchair positioning.

Virtually every possible foot and ankle deformity has been described in myelomeningocoele. This is the most common orthopaedic problem and generally requires operation. Proper alignment of the osseous structures, coupled with muscle balancing procedures, are needed to prevent recurrence. Long-term orthotic utilization is necessary.

Over 50% of patients with myelomeningocoele will have a deformity of the spine, the most common being paralytic scoliosis. It is important to remember, however, that 20% also have congenital scoliosis with structural anomalies of the vertebrae. Progressive congenital scoliosis cannot be treated by orthotic means and demands fusion of the involved segments as soon as progression is proved. Progression of paralytic scoliosis is the rule, and in the skeletally immature patient, may be temporarily treated by orthotic means. The Milwaukee brace, total contact jacket and the thoracic suspension orthosis have all been successful. Curves greater than 40° and those not controlled by bracing should be stabilized by surgical fusion with internal fixation. Small curves may be treated by posterior fusion alone, but larger curves or those with markedly deficient posterior elements will also require anterior fusion (McMaster, 1987). Segmental instrumentation, as advocated by Allen and Ferguson (1979), has been very successful in many centres.

Either a tethered spinal cord or hydromyelia can be associated with scoliosis in myelomeningocoele. Release of tethering or ventricular shunting may result in the arrest of scoliotic progression in some cases (Lindseth, 1976). In some cases of scoliosis and fixed pelvic obliquity, correction of the spinal deformity or hip joint contracture will not produce a level pelvis. Lindseth (1978) has devised a bilateral pelvic osteotomy to correct up to 3 cm of fixed pelvic obliquity.

The problem of persistent or developing kyphosis presents a difficult challenge, fraught with complications. Most surgeons favour excision of the cephalad limb of the kyphosis and perform circumferential fusion with posterior instrumentation (Lindseth and Slezer, 1979; Hedemann and Gillespie, 1987).

AMYOTROPHIC LATERAL SCLEROSIS

This condition is also known as motor neurone disease and is characterized by degeneration of motor neurones throughout the nervous system. The inheritance pattern is unknown, but some cases appear to be an autosomal dominant trait; 5% of patients have a positive family history of the disease. Although the onset can occur at any age, this is not a condition often seen in children, the usual onset occurring between the ages of 50 and 60 years. A variable distribution of muscle wasting, weakness and fasciculation, more likely to be distal than proximal, is usually the first sign. In the majority of cases, the disease progresses rapidly to involve almost all muscles in the body, including the bulbar muscles. Because of this, signs of both upper and lower motor neurone disease are present. Approximately 25% of patients have a slower progression of the disease. The usual course, however, is rapid deterioration with loss of ambulatory ability within 1−2 years and death secondary to respiratory failure usually within 3 years of the onset of symptoms.

Diagnosis is made from the clinical picture of the disease, aided by certain laboratory findings. Electromyography shows fasciculations, giant polyphasic potentials and widespread fibrillations. There may be evidence of delayed motor conduction velocities. Muscle enzyme levels are elevated in approximately 50% of patients and muscle biopsy shows areas of denervation.

Treatment of this condition is directed towards prolonging the patient's independence in the activities of daily living. A portable suction device is often useful in helping the patient to handle the pooled secretions in the posterior pharynx. The use of quinine or diazepam may help to dispel the often troublesome night-time leg cramps that occur, and late in the disease, portable oxygen may promote a restful night's sleep by alleviating the hypoxia caused by respiratory insufficiency. At the present time, there are no therapeutically effective drugs for treating this disease.

Peripheral nerve disorders and other types of neurological disease

ACUTE IDIOPATHIC POST-INFECTIOUS POLYNEUROPATHY

This disease, also called Guillain−Barré syndrome, is characterized by symmetrical segmental motor paresis of the extremities and sometimes of the trunk. More than half the patients report a viral infection or influenza vaccine inoculation 2−4 weeks before the onset of the clinical syndrome. The initial clinical presentation may vary in the rate of progression of the disease, which begins distally in the lower extremities and spreads in a proximal and craniad pattern such that in the most severe cases, the bulbar and respiratory muscles can be affected. Many patients have severe pain, particularly in the back and limbs which may mimic poliomyelitis. The syndrome progresses for 1−2 weeks with maximum paresis developing in 1−4 weeks. Sensory involvement is usually slight.

Recovery may take 3−6 months and, paradoxically, often the more rapid the onset, the better the prognosis. Patients with the most severe level of involvement have the worst prognosis. The subacute and chronic cases with their continuing activity result in a worsening prognosis. The mortality is estimated to be 10% with nearly 20% of the patients being left with permanent musculoskeletal sequelae.

Based on the clinical picture, the diagnosis may be confirmed by cerebrospinal fluid examination which shows a normal cell count with an increase in protein levels. These levels reach their peak at approximately 2−3 weeks after onset. An electromyogram in this condition shows delay in both sensory and motor nerve conduction velocities.

General support remains the most important treatment, including the possible need for tracheotomy for respiratory insufficiency. Orthopaedic treatment is directed at foot deformities, which develop because of muscle imbalance and may require tendon transfers or corrective bony procedures before orthotic control can be accomplished. Occasionally, in a chronic case, paralytic scoliosis develops which requires a spinal fusion (Berman and Tom, 1976). Current authors (Patten, 1986) recommend the use of plasma exchange, particularly in those patients with tetraplegia who require ventilation. Corticosteroids and cytotoxic immunosuppressive therapy also have been utilized.

HEREDITARY MOTOR AND SENSORY NEUROPATHIES

Intrinsic atrophy and weakness are prominent features of this group of peripheral neuropathies (Dyck and Lambert, 1968). Patients demonstrate slow progression of weakness with minor sensory abnormalities, generally have a positive family history and may demonstrate considerable variation in the degree of involvement within a given family.

Type I

This is the most common form and consists of the hypertrophic form of Charcot−Marie−Tooth disease, including hereditary areflexic dystaxia (Roussy−Lévy syndrome). This autosomal dominant disease presents most commonly during the second decade of life with a mild cavus or clawing of the toes (Fig. 3.11). Eventually, an equinocavovarus deformity gradually develops, and the patient experiences difficulty in running and progressive localization of weight-bearing to the lateral metatarsal heads. Upper extremity involvement begins later in the second decade, with progressive difficulty in fine motor activities due to atrophy of the intrinsic muscles. Peripheral motor nerve conduction velocities are reduced to less than one-half the expected value because of the repeated episodes of demyelination and remyelinization of the peripheral nerve.

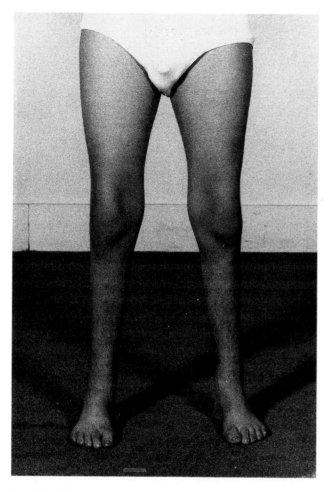

Fig. 3.11 Muscle wasting from the distal thigh to the intrinsic muscles of the feet in a patient with peroneal muscular atrophy (Charcot–Marie–Tooth disease).

Type II

This form represents the neuronal form of Charcot–Marie–Tooth disease and is inherited as an autosomal dominant disease. Onset occurs late in the second or third decade of life with more profound distal extremity weakness than in type I. The flail foot develops a calcaneal cavus deformity and the characteristic stork-leg appearance is seen because of focal atrophy of the distal one-third of the quadriceps and hamstrings. Upper extremity involvement is less pronounced. Conduction velocities are slightly reduced or normal.

Type III

This represents the hypertrophic neuropathy of infancy (Déjérine–Sottas disease) and is an autosomal recessive trait. Cavus foot deformity and palpably enlarged peripheral nerves may be noted in infancy, and delayed lower extremity motor milestones are common. Sensory functions are diminished in a stocking–glove type of distribution. Pes cavus and drop-foot deformities are common and require active management. Spinal deformity develops in most patients and ambulation is lost during the third or fourth decade of life. Patients with type III disease demonstrate markedly slow motor nerve conduction times and an elevation in cerebrospinal fluid protein.

Type IV

Refsum's disease is a rare condition transmitted as an autosomal recessive trait with onset in childhood or puberty. The disease can be differentiated from Friedreich's ataxia because it is characterized by remissions and relapses. Anosmia, progressive deafness, and night blindness are common initial findings. Orthopaedic problems include scoliosis, pes equinus and pes cavus. Elevation of serum phytanic acid levels is pathognomonic of this disease. Cerebrospinal fluid protein levels are markedly elevated, and motor nerve conduction velocities are slow.

Management

Foot deformity is the most common skeletal problem requiring orthopaedic management in these patients with progressive neurological loss. Young patients benefit from soft tissue operations, e.g. combined plantar–intrinsic release and a staged posterior tibial transfer to the second or third cuneiform bone. Triple arthrodesis is not recommended because the long-term results are generally unsatisfactory as the patient develops ankle instability and painful degenerative arthritis (Wetmore, 1989). Fixed bony deformity is more appropriately managed by a combination of calcaneal and metatarsal osteotomies. A posterior displacement calcaneal osteotomy is effective in correcting the calcaneocavus deformity of type II neuropathy. Post-operative ankle/foot orthotics should be employed following either soft tissue or bony procedures. Claw-toe deformities can be managed by a Jones procedure.

CONGENITAL INDIFFERENCE TO PAIN

Several different conditions have as a common feature either relative or absolute congenital indifference to pain. They must be differentiated for prognostic and therapeutic reasons. The most common presenting sign occurs after the deciduous teeth have appeared and consists of biting of the fingers, toes, lips, or tongue. It is also noted that the child does not cry or react to burns or injuries. Fractures and acute surgical abdominal conditions may be undetected, with a resultant risk of increased morbidity or mortality. When fractures occur, the diagnosis is usually delayed and malunion or non-union may develop. Excessive callus formation about such fractures is characteristic in these children, who may be mistaken for the 'battered child syndrome'.

Changes of neuropathic arthropathy (Charcot's disease) are often seen in major weight-bearing joints, particularly the ankle or knee. These include repeated haemarthrosis, synovial hypertrophy and secondary joint instability due to ligamentous laxity. Orthotic control of such joints may be difficult because of the imperception of pain and occasionally arthrodesis is required. Even then, an initially successfully fused joint may show eventual breakdown and pseudoarthrosis.

The major principle of treatment of such children is to attempt to convince the child to avoid trauma and also to educate the parents to look frequently for signs of injury or infection.

The classic condition in this group was described as congenital insensitivity to pain (Dearborn, 1932). In this condition, the threshold for perception of painful stimuli is normal, but these stimuli are not considered noxious by the patient. The senses of touch and temperature are usually intact, but anhidrosis and mental retardation are often associated. The entire body is involved, but other sensory functions are all normal. There is no known genetic transmission for this condition.

A different condition, *congenital sensory neuropathy*, is an autosomal recessive condition which does not progress. All sensory functions are affected, distally more than proximally. There is usually self-mutilation of the fingers with progressive loss of their length. Nerve conduction studies show grossly abnormal sensory velocities and skin biopsies reveal loss of myelinated nerve fibres. Mental retardation, retinitis pigmentosa, anhidrosis and loss of hearing are often associated findings.

Another condition, *Lesch–Nyhan syndrome*, presents with mental retardation, choreoathetosis and self-mutilation. This is an X-linked recessive condition which is caused not by insensitivity to pain, but rather by uncontrolled aggression against the self or others. A specific defect, the absence of hypoxanthine–guanine phosphoribosyltransferase, has been identified in Lesch–Nyhan syndrome, which leads to excessive levels of uric acid in the serum. Spasticity in the hip flexor and adductor muscles is sometimes seen in this syndrome.

Familial dysautonomia, also known as Riley–Day syndrome, is an autosomal recessive trait found in people of Jewish descent. It is characterized by insensitivity to pain, feeding difficulties, hyposalivation, loss of the corneal reflex, absence of fungiform papillae of the tongue, postural hypotension, emotional lability, poor coordination and hyporeflexia. Difficulties with temperature regulation are also seen. The indifference to pain can be incomplete and may increase with ageing. Other associated problems include gastro-oesophageal reflux, vomiting and aspiration pneumonia. Peripheral nerve biopsies show absence of unmyelinated nerve fibres in peripheral and autonomic nerves. A rigid progressive scoliosis, which is difficult to treat orthotically because of the decreased sensation, is a common feature of this condition.

Familial sensory neuropathy with anhidrosis is an autosomal recessive condition characterized by mostly intact sensation, but loss of temperature perception, anhidrosis and mental retardation.

Hereditary sensory radicular neuropathy is an autosomal dominant disease with degenerative changes seen in the dorsal root ganglion. This condition is often first noted in late childhood and is usually confined to the distal lower extremities for a long period of time. Sweating is normal. All sensory functions are usually affected, with deep tendon reflexes also absent. Late in its course, involvement of the upper extremities often occurs.

MYASTHENIA GRAVIS

This is characterized by an abnormally excessive fatiguability in voluntary muscles after activity or stress. In almost all cases, the bulbar, extraocular and shoulder girdle muscles are involved. The disease is more common in females, with a peak incidence of onset in the second decade. When males are involved, the peak age is the fifth to sixth decade. A positive family history for myasthenia gravis is found for 5% of patients, but the exact inheritance pattern is unknown. This is an auto-immune disease in which antibodies to the acetylcholine receptor sites block the neuromuscular junctions. Weakness is greatest late in the day, but strength tends to return with rest.

In children, three types of myasthenia gravis are seen. First, a transient neonatal myasthenia gravis occurs in approximately 15% of the offspring of mothers with the disease. This is secondary to transplacental passive transfer of the antibody to the acetylcholine receptor. Although this condition may be severe and life-threatening during the first 2 weeks of life, complete recovery is the rule and usually occurs within the first 3 months, probably because the maternal antibody is by then inactivated by the infant. The second childhood type is persistent neonatal myasthenia gravis. This is seldom seen under the age of 1 year and presents with ptosis, extraocular motor weakness, dysphagia, respiratory distress and generalized weakness. The mother does not have myasthenia gravis and this condition may be of autosomal recessive inheritance. It is a progressive condition. The third type is juvenile myasthenia gravis, which develops after the age of 10 years. This also presents with ptosis and extraocular weakness, as well as extremity weakness, more notably proximally than distally and more prominent in the upper than the lower extremities. There is a high titre of anti-acetylcholine receptor antibodies. This is also a progressive condition and is more common in females.

In adults, the clinical course is variable, but usually shows relapses and remissions. In one-quarter to one-third of patients the condition is non-progressive and does not require treatment. The remainder show either rapid or slow progression, and in general the worse the initial weakness, the worse is the prognosis. The most common cause of death in advanced myasthenia gravis is respiratory failure.

The diagnosis of myasthenia gravis is based on the clinical picture and a positive edrophonium chloride test. Within 1 min after injection of this drug, the patient experiences marked improvement in motor strength. In contrast to a normal subject the cholinergic side-effects, e.g. excessive perspiration, salivation and lacrimation, are absent. The circulating antibody to the acetylcholine receptor has been identified in the blood of about 90% of patients with myasthenia gravis. The thymus gland is probably the site of antibody production, and in this respect it is interesting to note that 70% of patients with myasthenia gravis have thymic hyperplasia and 10% have thymomas. Muscle biopsies demonstrate atrophy of type 2 fibres, which may be generalized or focal. Electromyographic studies show progressive diminution in the amplitude of evoked potentials, particularly at low frequencies. This is the electrical counterpart of fatigue on repeated muscle contraction.

Treatment of myasthenia gravis is primarily pharmacological, though in the advanced stages orthotic devices and aids for the activities of daily living may be extremely useful. The most common drugs used to treat this condition are anticholinesterase medications, adjusted empirically to obtain the maximal effect (Levinson 1987). Thymectomy has a role, either to excise a proven thymoma or in patients with hyperplasia who do not respond to medication, particularly in those over 50 years of age. The use of corticosteroids may be of benefit to older patients uncontrolled by other medication. Antineoplastic agents are reserved for patients unresponsive to corticosteroids or thymectomy. In severe myasthenic crisis, plasmapheresis may be required.

REFERENCES

Allen B.L. and Ferguson R.L. (1979) The operative treatment of myelomeningocele spinal deformity. *Orthop. Clin. North Am.* 10, 845–861.

Becker P.E. and Kiener F. (1955) Eine neue x-chromosomale Muskeldystrophie. *Arch. Psychiatr. Z. Neurol.* 193, 427–488.

Berman A.T. and Tom L. (1976) The Guillain–Barré syndrome in children. Orthopedic management and patterns of recovery. *Clin. Orthop.* 116, 61–65.

Bowyer S.L., Blane C.E., Sullivan D.B. *et al.* (1983) Childhood dermatomyositis: factors predicting functional outcome and development of dystrophic calcification. *J. Pediatr.* 103, 882–888.

Bradley W.C., Tandan R. and Robison S.H. (1987) Clinical subtypes, DNA repair efficiency and therapeutic trials in the post-polio syndrome. *Birth Defects* 23, 343–360.

Brooke M.H. (1973) A neuromuscular disease characterized by fibre types disproportion. In Kakulas B. (ed) *Proceedings of the Second International Congress on Muscle Disease*. Perth, Australia, November 1971. Amsterdam, Excerpta Medica.

Brooke M.H. and Engel W.K. (1969) The histographic analysis of human muscle biopsies with regard to fibre types: four children's biopsies. *Neurology* 19, 591–605.

Connor J.M. and Evans D.A. (1982) Fibrodysplasia ossificans progressiva. The clinical features and natural history of 34 patients. *J. Bone Joint Surg.* 64B, 76–83.

Dearborn G. van M. (1932) A case of congenital general pure analgesia. *J. Nerv. Ment. Dis.* 75, 612–614.

Drennan J.C. (1976) Management of neonatal myelomeningocele. In *Instructional Course Lectures*. The American Academy of Orthopedic Surgeons. St. Louis, C.V. Mosby, vol. 25, pp. 65–70.

Dyck P.J. and Lambert E.H. (1968) Lower motor and primary sensory neuron diseases with peroneal muscular atrophy. Part I. Neurologic, genetic, and electrophysiologic findings in hereditary polyneuropathies. Part II. Neurologic, genetic, and electrophysiologic findings in various neuronal degenerations. *Arch. Neurol.* 18, 603–619.

Emery A.E. and Dreifuss F.E. (1966) Unusual type of benign X-linked muscular dystrophy. *J. Neurol. Neurosurg. Psychiatry* 29, 338–342.

Eulenberg A. (1886) Über eine familiäre, durch 6 Generationen verfolgbare Form kongenitaler Paramyotonic. *A. Neurol.* 5, 265.

Gowers W.R. (1879) *Pseudohypertrophic Muscular Paralysis*. London, J. and A. Churchill Ltd.

Hedemann J.S. and Gillespie R. (1987) Management of myelomeningocele kyphosis in the older child by kyphectomy and segmental spinal instrumentation. *Spine* 12, 37–41.

Kloepfer H.W. and Emery A.E.H. (1969) Genetic aspects of neuromuscular disease. In Walton J.N. (ed) *Disorders of Voluntary Muscle*, 2nd edn. London, J. and A. Churchill, p. 683.

Levinson A.I., Zweiman B. and Lisak R.P. (1987) Immunopathogenesis and treatment of myasthenia gravis. *J. Clin. Immunol.* 7, 187–197.

Lindseth R.E. (1976) Treatment of the lower extremity in children paralyzed by myelomeningocele. In *Instructional Course*

Lectures. The American Academy of Orthopedic Surgeons. St. Louis, C.V. Mosby, vol. 25, p. 76–82.

Lindseth R.E. (1978) Posterior iliac osteotomy for fixed pelvic obliquity. *J. Bone Joint Surg.* **60A**, 17–72.

Lindseth R.E. and Slezer L. (1979) Vertebral excision for kyphosis in children with myelomeningocele. *J. Bone Joint Surg.* **61A**, 699.

Lorber J. (1971) Results of treatment of myelomeningocele. An analysis of 524 unselected cases with special reference to possible selection for treatment. *Dev. Med. Child Neurol.* **13**, 279–303.

Lorber J. (1974) Selective treatment of myelomeningocele: to treat or not to treat? *Pediatrics* **53**, 307.

McMaster M.J. (1987) Anterior and posterior instrumentation and fusion of thoracolumbar scoliosis due to myelomeningocele. *J. Bone Joint Surg.* **69B**, 20.

Patten E. (1986) Therapeutic plasmapheresis and plasma exchange. *Crit. Rev. Clin. Lab. Sci.* **23**, 147–175.

Shy G.M. and McGee K.R. (1956) A new congenital nonprogressive myopathy. *Brain* **79**, 610–621.

Shy G.M., Engel W.K., Somers J.E. *et al.* (1963) Nemaline myopathy: a new congenital myopathy. *Brain* **86**, 793–810.

Siegel I.M. (1986) *Muscle and Its Diseases*. Chicago, Year Book Medical Publishers.

Spiro A.J., Shy G.M. and Gonatas N.K. (1966) Myotubular myopathy. *Arch. Neurol.* **14**, 1–14.

Steinert H. (1909) Myopathologische Beitrage: I. Über des klinische und anatomische Bild des Muskelschwunds der Myotoniker. *Dtsch. Z. Nervenheilk.* **37**, 58.

Stern W.G. (1923) Arthrogryposis multiplex congenita. *JAMA* **81**, 1507–1510.

Thomsen J. (1876) Tonische Krampfe in willkurlich beweglichen Muskeln in Folge von erebter psychischer Disposition. *Arch. Psychiatr. Nervenkr.* **6**, 706.

Wetmore R.S. and Drennan J.C. (1989) Long term results of triple arthrodesis in Charcot–Marie–Tooth disease. *J. Bone Joint Surg.* **71A**, 417–422.

Winters T.F. Jr., Gage J.R. and Hicks R. (1987) Gait patterns in spastic hemiplegia in children and young adults. *J. Bone Joint Surg.* **69A**, 437–441.

FURTHER READING

Alberts M.J. and Roses A.D. (1989) Myotonic muscular dystrophy. *Neurol. Clin.* **7**, 1–8.

Alexander M.A. and Steg N.L. (1989) Myelomeningocele: comprehensive treatment. *Arch. Phys. Med. Rehabil.* **70**, 637–641.

Anderson B.J. and Brown T.C. (1989) Congenital myotonic dystrophy in children — a review of ten years' experience. *Anaesth. Intensive Care* **17**, 320–324.

Bakker E., Bonten E.J., den Dunnen J.T. *et al.* (1989) Carrier detection and prenatal diagnosis of Duchenne/Becker muscular dystrophy (D/BMD) by DNA-analysis. *Prog. Clin. Biol. Res.* **306**, 51–67.

Beals R.K. (1966) Spastic paraplegia and diplegia: an evaluation of non-surgical and surgical factors influencing the prognosis for ambulation. *J. Bone Joint Surg.* **48A**, 827.

Beals R.K. and Crawford A. (1976) Congenital absence of pectoral muscles. A review of twenty-five patients. *Clin. Orthop.* **119**, 166–171.

Binder H. and Eng G.D. (1989) Rehabilitation management of children with spastic diplegic cerebral palsy. *Arch. Phys. Med. Rehabil.* **70**, 482–489.

Bird T.D. (1989) Hereditary motor–sensory neuropathies. Charcot–Marie–Tooth syndrome. *Neurol. Clin.* **7**, 9–23.

Bleck E.E. (1975) Locomotor prognosis in cerebral palsy. *Dev. Med. Child Neurol.* **17**, 18–25.

Bodensteiner J. (1988) Congenital myopathies. *Neurol. Clin.* **6**, 499–518.

Bray G.M., Kaarso M. and Ross R.T. (1965) Ocular myopathy with dysphagia. *Neurology* **15**, 678–684.

Brooke M.H. (1977) *A Clinician's View of Neuromuscular Diseases*. Baltimore, Williams and Wilkins.

Bunch T.W. (1988) The therapy of polymyositis. *Mt. Sinai J. Med.* **55**, 483–486.

Caro I. (1989) Dermatomyositis as a systemic disease. *Med. Clin. North Am.* **73**, 1181–1192.

Close J.R. and Todd F.N. (1959) The phasic activity of the muscles of the lower extremity and the effect of tendon transfer. *J. Bone Joint Surg.* **41A**, 189–208.

Copeland S.A. and Howard R.C. (1978) Thoracoscapular fusion for facioscapulohumeral dystrophy. *J. Bone Joint Surg.* **60B**, 547–551.

Crandall R.C., Birkebak R.C. and Winter R.B. (1989) The role of hip location and dislocation in the functional status of the myelodyspolastic patient. A review of 100 patients. *Orthopedics* **12**, 675–684.

Dimon J.H., Funk F.J. Jr. and Wells R.E. (1965) Congenital indifference to pain with associated orthopedic abnormalities. *South. Med. J.* **58**, 524–529.

Drachman D.B. and Kuncl R.W. (1989) Amyotrophic lateral sclerosis: an unconventional autoimmune disease? *Ann. Neurol.* **26**, 269–274.

Drachman D.B., de Silva S., Ramsay D. *et al.* (1987) Humoral pathogenesis of myasthenia gravis. *Ann. N.Y. Acad. Sci.* **505**, 90–105.

Drachman D.B., McIntosh K.R., De Silva S. *et al.* (1988) Strategies for the treatment of myasthenia gravis. *Ann. N.Y. Acad. Sci.* **540**, 176–186.

Drennan J.D. (1978) Neuromuscular disorders. In Lovell W.W. and Winter R.B. (eds) *Pediatric Orthopaedics*, Vol. I. Philadelphia, Lippincott, pp. 239–318.

Drummond D.S., Rogala E., Templeton J. *et al.* (1974) Proximal hamstring release for knee flexion and crouched posture in cerebral palsy. *J. Bone Joint Surg.* **56A**, 1598–1602.

Dubowitz V. (1989) The Duchenne dystrophy story: from phenotype to gene and potential treatment. *J. Child Neurol.* **4**, 240–250.

Dwyer A.F. (1973) Experience of anterior correction of scoliosis. *Clin. Orthop.* **93**, 191–206.

Dwyer F.C. (1959) Osteotomy of the calcaneum forpes cavus. *J. Bone Joint Surg.* **41B**, 80–86.

Emery A.E. (1987) X-linked muscular dystrophy with early contractures and cardiomyopathy (Emery–Dreifuss type). *Clin. Genet.* **32**, 360–367.

Fenichel G.M. (1988) Congenital muscular dystrophies. *Neurol. Clin.* **6**, 519–528.

Fenichel G.M. (1989) Myasthenia gravis. *Pediatr. Ann.* **18**, 432–438.

Gage J.R. (1990) Surgical treatment of knee dysfunction in cerebral palsy. *Clin. Orthop.* **253**, 45–54.

Gamble J.F., Rinsky L.A. and Bleck E.E. (1990) Established hip dislocations in children with cerebral palsy. *Clin. Orthop.* **253**, 90–99.

Gardner W.J. (1960) Myelomeningocele, the result of rupture of the embryonic neural tube. *Cleve. Clin. Q.* **27**, 88–100.

Gardner W.J. (1968) Rupture of the neural tube? *Clin. Neurosurg.* **15**, 57–79.

Gardner-Medwin D. (1979) Controversies about Duchenne muscular dystrophy. (2) Bracing for ambulation. *Dev. Med. Child Neurol.* **21**, 659–662.

Genkins G., Kornfeld P., Papatestas A.E. *et al.* (1987) Clinical experience in more than 11 000 patients with myasthenia gravis. *Ann. N.Y. Acad. Sci.* **505**, 500–513.

Goldner J.L. (1974) Upper extremity tendon transfer in cerebral palsy. *Orthop. Clin. North Am.* **5**, 389–411.

Goldner J.L. (1988) Surgical reconstruction of the upper extremity in cerebral palsy. *Hand Clin.* **4**, 223–265.

Green N.E. (1987) The orthopaedic management of the ankle, foot, and knee in patients with cerebral palsy. In *Instructional Course Lectures*. The American Academy of Orthopedic Surgeons. St. Louis, C.V. Mosby, vol. 36, pp. 253–265.

Green W.T. and Banks H.H. (1962) Flexor carpi ulnaris transplant and its use in cerebral palsy. *J. Bone Joint Surg.* **44A**, 1343–1352.

Grob D., Arsura E.L., Brunner N.G. *et al.* (1987) The course of myasthenia gravis and therapies affecting outcome. *Ann. N.Y. Acad. Sci.* **505**, 472–499.

Guillain G., Barré J.A. and Strohl A. (1916) Sur un syndrome de radiculo-nevrité avec hyperalbummose du liquide cephalorachidien sans réaction cellulaire. Remarques sur les caractères cliniques et graphiques des réflexes tendineux. *Bull. Mem. Soc. Med. Hop. Paris* **40**, 1462.

Guthkelch A.N. (1986) Aspects of the surgical management of myelomeningocele: a review. *Dev. Med. Child Neurol.* **28**, 525–532.

Hall J.G. (1989) Arthrogryposis. *Am. Fam. Physician* **39**, 113–119.

Hass J. and Hass R. (1958) Arthrochalasis multiplex congenita. Congenital flaccidity of the joints. *J. Bone Joint Surg.* **40A**, 663–674.

Hensinger R.N. and MacEwen G.D. (1976) Spinal deformity associated with heritable neurological conditions: spinal muscular atrophy, Friedreich's ataxia, familial dysautonomia, and Charcot–Marie–Tooth disease. *J. Bone Joint Surg.* **58A**, 13–24.

Herron L.D., Westin G.W. and Dawson E.G. (1978) Scoliosis in arthrogryposis multiplex congenita. *J. Bone Joint Surg.* **60A**, 293–299.

Hoffer M.M., Feiwell E., Perry R. *et al.* (1973) Functional ambulation in patients with myelomeningocele. *J. Bone Joint Surg.* **55A**, 137–148.

Jones E.T. and Knapp D.R. (1987) Assessment and management of the lower extremity in cerebral palsy. *Orthop. Clin. North Am.* **18**, 725–738.

Jozefowicz R.F. and Griggs R.C. (1988) Myotonic dystrophy. *Neurol. Clin.* **6**, 455–472.

Kallen B. (1968) Early embryogenesis of the central nervous system with special reference to closure defects. *Dev. Med. Child Neurol.* **16**(Suppl.), 11.

Ketenjian A.Y. (1978) Scapulocostal stabilization for scapular winging in facioscapulohumeral muscular dystrophy. *J. Bone Joint Surg.* **60A**, 476–480.

Kilbrick S. (1954) Myasthenia gravis in the newborn. *Pediatrics* **14**, 365–386.

Koman L.A., Gelberman R.H., Toby E.B. *et al.* (1990) Cerebral palsy. Management of the upper extremity. *Clin. Orthop.* **253**, 62–74.

Kugelberg E. and Welander L. (1956) Heredofamilial juvenile muscular atrophy simulating muscular dystrophy. *Arch. Neurol.* **75**, 500.

Levinson A.I., Zweiman B. and Lisak R.P. (1987) Immuno-pathogenesis and treatment of myasthenia gravis. *J. Clin. Immunol.* **7**, 187–197.

Levitt R.L., Canale S.T., Cooke A.J. *et al.* (1973) The role of foot surgery in progressive neuromuscular disorders in children. *J. Bone Joint Surg.* **55A**, 1396–1410.

Little W.J. (1861) On the influence of abnormal parturition, difficult labours, premature birth and asphyzia neonatorum on the mental and physical condition of the child especially in relation to deformities. *Lancet* **ii**, 378.

McKibbin B. (1971) Conservative management of paralytic dislocations of the hip in myelomeningocele. *J. Bone Joint Surg.* **53B**, 758.

McKibbin B. (1973) The use of splintage in the management of paralytic dislocation of the hip in spina bifida cystica. *J. Bone Joint Surg.* **55B**, 163–172.

Macri J.N., Weiss R.R., Tillitt R. *et al.* (1976) Prenatal diagnosis of neural tube defects. *JAMA* **235**, 1251–1254.

Makin M. (1953) The surgical treatment of Friedreich's ataxia. *J. Bone Joint Surg.* **35A**, 425–436.

Menelaus M.B. (1976) The hip in myelomeningocele. Management directed towards a minimum number of operations and a minimum period of immobilization. *J. Bone Joint Surg.* **58B**, 448–452.

Menelaus M.B. (1976) Talectomy for equinovarus deformity in arthrogryposis and spina bifida. *J. Bone Joint Surg.* **53B**, 468–473.

Miller G. (1989) Myopathies of infancy and childhood. *Pediatr. Ann.* **19**, 439–453.

Moosa A. (1974) The feeding difficulty in infantile myotonic dystrophy. *Dev. Med. Child Neurol.* **16**, 824–825.

Mustard W.T. (1959) A follow-up study of iliopsoas transfer for hip instability. *J. Bone Joint Surg.* **41B**, 289–298.

Neville B.G. (1988) Selective dorsal rhizotomy for spastic cerebral palsy. *Dev. Med. Child Neurol.* **30**, 395–398.

Oppenheim W.L. (1990) Selective posterior rhizotomy for spastic cerebral palsy. A review. *Clin. Orthop.* **253**, 20–29.

Parsons D.W. and Seddon H.J. (1968) The results of operations for disorders of the hip caused by poliomyelitis. *J. Bone Joint Surg.* **50B**, 266–273.

Phelps W.M. (1957) Long-term results of orthopedic surgery in cerebral palsy. *J. Bone Joint Surg.* **39A**, 53–59.

Pinsky L. and DiGeorge A.M. (1966) Congenital familial sensory neuropathy with anhidrosis. *J. Pediatr.* **68**, 1.

Plotz P.H., Dalakas M., Leff R.L. *et al.* (1989) Current concepts in the idiopathic inflammatory myopathies: polymyositis, dermatomyositis, and related disorders. *Ann. Intern. Med.* **111**, 143–157.

Ramsey P.I. and Hensinger R.N. (1975) Congenital dislocation of the hip associated with central core disease. *J. Bone Joint Surg.* **57A**, 648–651.

Rang M. and Wright J. (1989) What have 30 years of medical progress done for cerebral palsy? *Clin. Orthop.* **247**, 55–60.

Refsum S., Salomonsen L. and Skatvedt M. (1944) Heredopathia atactica polyneuritiformis in children. *J. Pediatr.* **35**, 335–343.

Rinsky L.A. (1990) Surgery of spinal deformity in cerebral palsy. Twelve years in the evolution of scoliosis management. *Clin.*

Orthop. **253**, 100—109.

Roussy G. and Lévy G. (1934) A propos de la dystasie aréflexique héréditaire: contribution à l'étude de la genèse des maladies familiales et de leur parenté entre elles. *Rev. Neurol.* **2**, 763—773.

Russman B.S. and Gage J.R. (1989) Cerebral palsy. *Curr. Probl. Pediatr.* **19**, 65—111.

Ryerson E.W. (1923) Arthrodesing operations on the feet. *J. Bone Joint Surg.* **5**, 453.

Samilson R.L. and Bechard R. (1973) Scoliosis in cerebral palsy: incidence, distribution of curve patterns, natural history and thoughts on etiology. In Ahstrom J.P. (ed) *Current Practice in Orthopedic Surgery.* St. Louis, C.V. Mosby, vol. 5, pp. 183—205.

Schneider M. and Balon K. (1977) Deformity of the foot following anterior transfer of the posterior tibial tendon and lengthening of the Achilles tendon for spastic equinovarus. *Clin. Orthop.* **125**, 113—117.

Scrutton D. (1989) The early management of hips in cerebral palsy. *Dev. Med. Child Neurol.* **32**, 108—116.

Sharrard W.J.W. (1955) The distribution of permanent paralysis in the lower limb in poliomyelitis. A clinical and pathological study. *J. Bone Joint Surg.* **37B**, 540—558.

Sharrard W.J.W., Zachary R.B. and Lorber J. (1967) Survival and paralysis in open myelomeningocele with special reference to the time of repair of the spinal lesion. *Dev. Med. Child Neurol.* **13**(Suppl), 35.

Siegel I.M., Miller J.E. and Ray R.D. (1968) Subcutaneous lower limb tenotomy in the treatment of pseudohypertrophic muscular dystrophy. Description of technique and presentation of twenty-one cases. *J. Bone Joint Surg.* **50A**, 1437—1443.

Smith R., Russell R.G.G. and Woods C.G. (1976) Myositis ossificans progressiva. Clinical features of eight patients and their response to treatment. *J. Bone Joint Surg.* **58B**, 48—57.

Spencer G.E. Jr. (1967) Orthopedic care of progressive muscular dystrophy. *J. Bone Joint Surg.* **49A**, 1201—1204.

Spencer G.E. Jr. and Vignos P.J. Jr. (1962) Surgical management of spinal deformities in spina bifida. *J. Bone Joint Surg.* **44A**, 234—242.

Sriram K., Bobechko W.P. and Hall J.E. (1972) Surgical management of spinal deformities in spina bifida. *J. Bone Joint Surg.* **54B**, 666—676.

Strongwater S.L. (1988) Overview and clinical manifestations of inflammatory myositis: polymyositis and dermatomyositis. *Mt. Sinai J. Med.* **55**, 435—446.

Thrush D.C., Morris C.J. and Salmon M.V. (1972) Paramyotonia congenita: a clinical histochemical and pathological study. *Brain* **95**, 537—552.

Tirosh E. and Rabino S. (1989) Physiotherapy for children with cerebral palsy. Evidence for its efficacy. *Am. J. Dis. Child.* **143**, 552—555.

Tooth H.H. (1886) *The Peroneal Type of Progressive Muscular Atrophy.* London, Lewis.

Tuffanelli D.L. and Lavoie P.E. (1988) Prognosis and therapy of polymyositis/dermatomyositis. *Clin. Dermatol.* **6**, 93—104.

Victor M., Hayes R. and Adams R.D. (1962) Oculopharyngeal muscular dystrophy: a familial disease of late life characterized by dysphagia and progressive ptosis of the eye. *N. Engl. J. Med.* **267**, 1267—1272.

Vignos P.J., Spencer G.E. and Archibald K.C. (1963) Management of progressive muscular dystrophy of childhood. *JAMA* **184**, 89—96.

Ward W.T., Wenger D.R. and Roach J.W. (1989) Surgical correction of myelomeningocele scoliosis: a critical appraisal of various spinal instrumentation systems. *J. Pediatr. Orthop.* **9**, 262—268.

Werdnig G. (1891) Zwei fruhinfantile hereditare Falle von progressiver Muskelatrophie unter dem Bilde der Dystrophie, aber auf neurotischer Grundlage. *Arch. Psychiatr. Nervenkr.* **22**, 437.

Wessel H.B. (1989) Spinal muscular atrophy. *Pediatr. Ann.* **19**, 421—427.

Wilson P.D. (1920) Posterior capsulotomy in certain flexion contractures of the knee. *J. Bone Joint Surg.* **11**, 40—58.

Witkowski J.A. (1989) Dystrophin-related muscular dystrophies. *J. Child Neurol.* **4**, 251—271.

Wright T. and Nicholson J. (1973) Physiotherapy for the spastic child: an evaluation. *Dev. Med. Child Neurol.* **15**, 146—163.

Yount C.C. (1926) The role of the tensor fasciae femoris in certain deformities of the lower extremities. *J. Bone Joint Surg.* **8**, 171—193.

Zellweger H., McCormick W.F. and Mergner W. (1967) Severe congenital muscular dystrophy. *Am. J. Dis. Child.* **114**, 591.

Zweiman B. (1989) Theoretical mechanisms by which immunoglobulin therapy might benefit myasthenia gravis. *Clin. Immunol. Immunopathol.* **53**, 83—91.

Chapter 4
The Spine

R.M. Smith & L.J. Micheli

INTRODUCTION

Disorders of the spine in general, and the paediatric spine in particular, produce more controversy and variability of approach than most other areas of orthopaedic practice. The principal problem is scoliosis, where much of the literature is unclear and the lack of prospective controlled trials before the widespread acceptance of highly interventional forms of management is alarming.

Problems begin when an attempt is made to define the normal range of spinal structure and function in order to diagnose a pathological deformity or dysfunction (Steindler, 1955). After diagnosis, it is important to consider the natural history of the disorder together with its short-term or long-term impact on the patient's function, which may be very difficult to determine (Risser and Ferguson, 1936; Nachemson, 1968; Nilsonne and Lundgren, 1968). The orthopaedic literature has devoted much attention to the cataloguing of spinal deformities and the description of operative techniques, but has seldom addressed the subsequent effect of these deformities or interventions on the spinal function of the patient (Risser and Norquist, 1958; Blount and Millencamp, 1977; Curtis *et al.*, 1979; Moskowitz *et al.*, 1980; Cochran *et al.*, 1983).

In recent years, however, much has been learned or re-learned with regard to the essential basic science of scoliosis, though a healthy scepticism is necessary when faced with many of the 'advances' (Nachemson, 1987). It is now clear that when the essential nature of the deformity and its biomechanics are properly understood, these provide a rational basis from which the assessment and management of the most complex spinal deformities follow in a logical fashion along principles no different from the other skeletal deformities of childhood.

ANATOMY AND FUNCTION

The human spine is a segmental column of connected bony and ligamentous elements, extending from the base of the skull to the pelvis. Components at each level are similar, bony vertebrae articulating with each other through the intravertebral discs, posterior facet joints and ligaments. The specific anatomy of the facet articulations, ligamentous constraints and musculotendinous attachments change progressively along the spine, resulting in the flexibility of the cervical spine, stability of the dorsal spine, and 'flexible' stability of the lumbar spine (Steindler, 1955).

The spine serves as the central mechanical axis of the torso, transmitting the weight of the upper head and body. It provides for major muscle attachment and contributes considerably to the mechanical efficiency of locomotion (Smith, 1987) and of the function of the upper limbs (Davis *et al.*, 1965). The costovertebral joints provide attachment for the ribs, and therefore the spine contributes to protection of the vital thoracic organs and to the mechanics of respiration. This is of particular importance to an orthopaedic surgeon, as severe spinal deformities can result in lethal deterioration of pulmonary function. Finally, the spine is not simply a bony strut, but harbours the spinal cord and cauda equina. Considerations of neural damage either by disease, deformity, or iatrogenic means are of critical importance.

The normal contour of the spine consists of a series of linked curves in the sagittal plane (Fig. 4.1). While the usual contour of the cervical spine is a slight forward angulation, or lordosis, it is flexible enough to assume any posture. The dorsal or thoracic spine is normally kyphotic, a posture that gives it major biomechanical advantages. It is now clear that the sagittal plane alignment is of major importance in spinal stability and the pathogenesis of the deformities of scoliosis (Leatherman and Dickson, 1988). In North America, it is considered that 40° of kyphosis, as measured by the Cobb technique, is normal, while 0–40° is defined as hypokyphosis and more than 40° as hyperkyphosis. The term 'thoracic

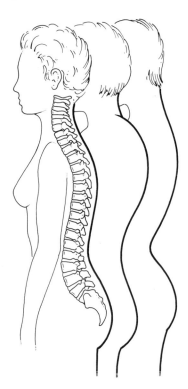

Fig. 4.1 The normal contour of the spine consists of a series of linked curves in the sagittal plane, with cervical lordosis, thoracic kyphosis and lumbar lordosis.

lordosis' refers to a true forward angulation, or lordosis, of the thoracic spine (Scoliosis Research Society, 1981). The term hypokyphosis should not be confused with lordosis as seen in every case of idiopathic scoliosis.

The 'normal' degree of lordosis of the lumbar spine has not yet been determined. While 40° of lordosis, analogous to the normal 40° of kyphosis of the thoracic spine, is often cited as the upper limit of normal, clinical observation suggests that it may be more useful to measure the lumbar spine alone, from the top of the vertebral body of L1 to the bottom of L5, and then to measure the lumbosacral lordosis across L5 to S1 separately. This is of importance in severe spondylolisthesis and post-fusion loss of the lumbar lordosis, a relatively new but difficult problem.

CLINICAL PICTURE

The paediatric patient with a spinal problem may present with a number of typical complaints. Essentially these are: spinal deformity; back pain; a neurological deficit; a functional problem with spinal stability, walking or sitting; or problems with a distal limb. Each major symptom may present in isolation or in combination

to a variety of physicians, and the identification of the spinal origin of the problem may be easy or quite obscure.

Spinal deformity accounts for a large proportion of the patients. They may present after noticing the deformity themselves, or more often after a family member or school teacher has noted the deformity. In the USA school screening programmes refer many patients. The most common presentation is the adolescent girl with a right-sided rib hump due to late-onset idiopathic scoliosis. A lack of appreciation that the rib hump is what the patient is complaining of is one of the most important problems in scoliosis management. Most patients with spinal deformity have a small inconsequential deformity, which is their only complaint and requires no treatment.

Back pain is a much more important symptom in a child than in an adult and is always assumed to be caused by a specific pathological process until proved otherwise. Spinal injuries, infections, inflammatory conditions and tumours are important to consider. Scoliosis in particular is not a painful condition, and like other back pain presentations demands careful investigation, often with computed tomography (CT), magnetic resonance imaging (MRI), or bone scanning.

The presence of a neurological deficit is of great importance, particularly if changing in degree. This can present as any combination of motor, sensory, or functional deficit and the development of a deformity, commonly a pes cavus or clawing of the toes, is particularly sinister. These are particularly associated with congenital deformities, when lesions such as dorsal hemivertebrae or diastematomyelia may be responsible. Neurological deficit may also present with changes in urological function signifying cord tethering, an important feature seen in myelodysplasia patients. Patients with major pre-existing neurological impairment must be assessed in the light of this and its effect on their general functional ability, specifically with regard to walking ability or sitting stability.

On occasion patients with abnormalities of leg length, gait, or specific problems with hip or knee present with a spinal anomaly, most often lumbar scoliosis, and need appropriate assessment.

PATIENT ASSESSMENT

As a number of serious and progressive childhood diseases may initially present with a spinal curve, a complete evaluation with clinical attention to both history and physical examination is essential in investigating the child with spinal deformity.

History

A careful history is the basis of the general assessment, and attention to the manner of onset, mode of presentation and time course can be helpful in making the correct diagnosis. The neonatal history and developmental milestones should be determined, as well as any major illnesses, injuries, or hospitalizations. The age at onset of the condition, rate of progression of symptoms or deformity, associated symptoms including presence of pain, weakness, shortness of breath, or other neurological symptoms, are important.

Determination of the state of maturation and relative growth is essential. In girls, menarche or the adolescent growth spurt signify a major reduction in scoliosis curve progression potential and are therefore very important. Additionally, a family history of spinal disorders or neuromuscular disorders should be determined, as well as any other attempt at evaluation or treatment of the spinal disorder in the past.

Physical examination

A complete physical examination, with particular attention to the spinal and neuromuscular systems, should be carried out (Hoppenfield, 1976); this involves undressing the patient to allow adequate exposure. It is essential to seek associated signs, e.g. the skin stigmata of spinal dysraphism (Fig. 4.2) or neurofibromatosis, when café au lait spots or nodules may be seen. In a child suspected of having congenital scoliosis, particular attention should be devoted to the cardiac and genitourinary evaluation, because of the high incidence of associated anomalies in these systems (MacEwen *et al.*, 1972).

Careful attention should be devoted to evaluation of the conformation of the hands and feet. Congenital anomalies of the digits are also commonly seen in association with congenital scoliosis (Winter *et al.*, 1968), and cavovarus feet, particularly if unilateral or if associated with anisomelia, increase the suspicion of spinal dysraphism or diastematomyelia (Fig. 4.3). Pectus excavatum or carinatum is often associated with spinal deformities, and there may be a representation of the rotational deformity seen by inequalities of breast prominence.

The child should be put at ease and initially examined standing erect with the hands at the sides and feet together. From behind, any asymmetry can be seen noting the shoulder height, trunk balance and loin symmetry. A rapid assessment of leg lengths can be made from the level of the iliac crests and the general trunk balance assessed in both the sagittal and coronal planes (Fig. 4.4). While observed from behind the child should then be asked to bend forward as if to touch the toes. This is the 'forward bend test'; it is very important and used as the primary assessment to screen and follow the progress of scoliosis (Ashworth and Ersil, 1981), as it increases the rotational prominence associated with scoliosis and throws it into profile so that it is easy to see (Figs 4.5, 4.6). Both thoracic rib humps and hollows and loin asymmetry stand out in this position. The hump corresponds to the side of the curve convexity, with a right thoracic rib hump and a left loin hump usually reflecting a right thoracic, left lumbar curve pattern (White, 1971). Kyphosis is best seen when this position is observed from the side (Fig. 4.7).

In addition to surface topography and spinal alignment, spinal mobility is assessed with attention to flexion and extension, lateral flexion and rotation. The relative stiffness or mobility of any spinal deformity will be seen together with the potential for correction. In paralytic

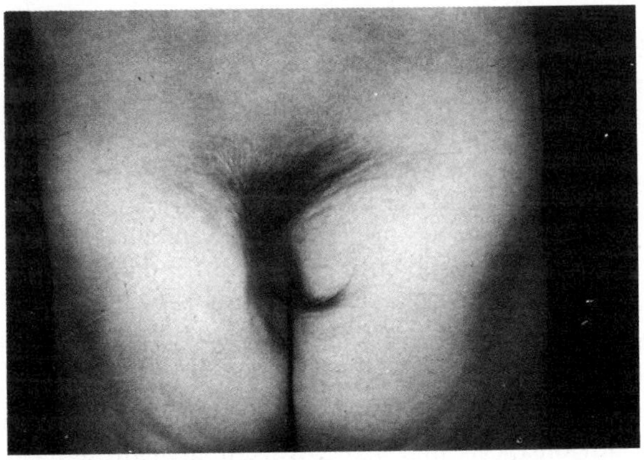

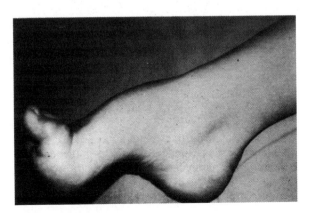

Fig. 4.2 Hairy patch over the lumbar spine in a child with diastematomyelia and congenital scoliosis.

Fig. 4.3 Pes cavus in a child with diastematomyelia.

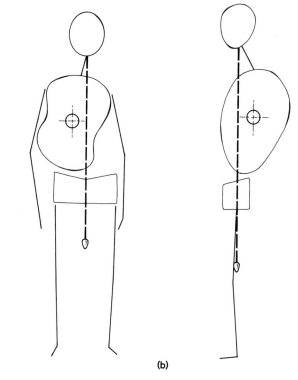

(a)   (b)

Fig. 4.4 Spinal deformity can result in decompensation of the torso in either (a) coronal or (b) sagittal planes.

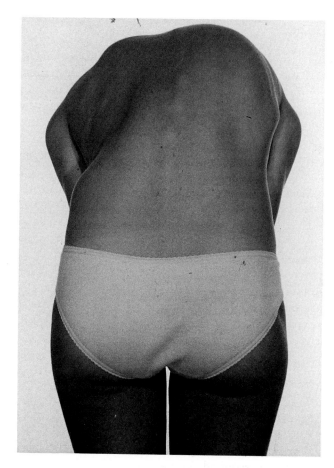

Fig. 4.5 The forward bend test to show the rib hump in a case of late-onset idiopathic scoliosis.

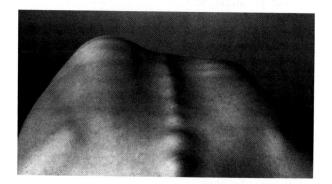

Fig. 4.6 Observing the child bending forward from above facilitates the determination of an associated rib hump.

scoliosis, elimination of gravity by lifting the patient under the arms will help assess curve mobility. In a child with tight lumbodorsal fascia and hamstrings, the lumbar spine will be obviously 'tight', and forward bending may be limited. In addition, much of the bending may be observed in the lower thoracic spine and thoracolumbar junction, and the lumbar spine exhibits relatively little motion. This pattern can be seen in children with lumbar disease, acute discitis, or spondylolysis. In those with dorsal round-backing or Scheuermann's kyphosis the local deformity will be obvious.

The child is then examined on a couch; watching the child climb (if possible) onto the couch allows a general assessment of mobility and general functional abilities, which is particularly important when a severe chronic disability is present. It is then preferable to examine the patient face down to look for focal spinal tenderness or a palpable step and then assess the hip rotation in extension and ankle reflexes before asking the child to roll over to complete the assessment of the lower extremity. In a neurologically impaired patient, sitting stability should be assessed by asking the patient to sit holding the hands in the air to see if balance can be maintained and also if it can be recovered after a gentle push. Finally, it is useful to watch the patient walk, when a characteristic gait abnormality may be seen. A child or adolescent with a herniated disc or spasm due to spondylolisthesis may have little or no pain and only moderate back stiffness, but may demonstrate a striking asymmetry of gait.

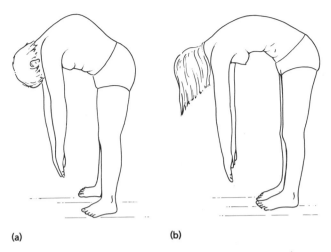

Fig. 4.7 Forward bending helps to accentuate dorsal round-backing, which is best seen from the side. (a) Tight lumbodorsal fascia or hamstrings. (b) Symmetric bending of the dorsal spine and flattening of the lumbar spine.

Imaging

The recent advances in imaging techniques have particular applications in spinal conditions. Plain anteroposterior and lateral radiographs provide much of the basic information required for most spinal conditions. The curves of a scoliotic deformity are obvious; specific lesions are also seen, e.g. congenital bony anomalies, fractures or stress lesions such as spondylolistheses, bone or soft tissue loss or swelling with inflammatory or infective processes, or the rare spinal tumour. Oblique views, particularly of the lumbar spine, are useful in spondylolisthesis and plain uniplanar tomography has a similar role in identifying particular lesions. Bone scanning is also useful to identify areas of increased bone activity including stress lesions or pseudoarthroses, infective of inflammatory lesions or tumours (Gilday *et al.*, 1975). Bone scanning is the best method to identify an osteoid osteoma, which takes up isotope avidly and shows very obviously.

In order to assess the spinal anatomy in more detail, both CT with sagittal and three-dimensional reconstructions and MRI are very useful and are now used instead of myelography or more invasive techniques in most situations (Sheldon *et al.*, 1977). These two scanning methods provide complementary methods of tissue assessment, MRI being particularly useful in looking at soft tissues and neurological structures within the spinal canal (Berns *et al.*, 1989). Obscure cord abnormalities are now easy to see, but in the presence of scoliosis even these advanced techniques are difficult to interpret as the spine twists in and out of the plane of the sections. It is essential that the images are assessed with the help of a radiologist familiar with the three-dimensional nature of scoliosis, with the questions being asked and with the problems faced by the surgeon. Good communication is essential. Occasionally standard or CT myelography will prove to be the best imaging technique.

As most spinal deformities require regular assessment over time, there is now increased awareness of the potential dangers of exposure to X-rays, and it becomes imperative to obtain the maximal amount of information from a minimal number of radiographs (DeSmet and Asher, 1981). The 'scoliosis series', which is used in many hospitals as a routine examination for a child with suspected scoliosis, usually consists of standing and supine anteroposterior views of the spine, as well as standing lateral and anteroposterior bending views which are taken either supine or upright. In most cases, this degree of exposure is totally unnecessary, and recent studies have shown that posteroanterior views of the spine decrease the exposure of the breasts and ovaries to less than one-third without significantly affecting the accuracy of curve measurement.

Similarly, the bending views of the spine provide little more information on the relative flexibility of the spine than careful physical examination with lateral bending and should not be part of a screening examination for scoliosis. These views may be necessary in the event of operative intervention as an aid in assessing the placement of instrumentation, but are not indicated for screening or initial diagnosis. The standing lateral radiograph is also useful particularly in the presence of pathological kyphosis.

The standing posteroanterior view of the dorsolumbar spine is the only examination required to assess the scoliotic patient adequately. If possible, this should be done on a full-length cassette and with proper bracketing, so that the patient is exposed from the neck to the top of the iliac crest only and with appropriate screening. Finally, a radiograph taken of the left hand and wrist is of particular use in order to assess bone age (Greulich and Pyle, 1959; Tanner *et al.*, 1975). This provides an assessment of the amount of growth remaining and therefore the potential for continued progression of the deformity.

SCOLIOSIS

The word 'scoliosis' is derived from the Greek *skolios*, which means bent. In clinical practice, scoliosis is a deformity characterized by lateral curvature of the spine away from the medial sagittal plane of the body (Fig. 4.8). It can be caused by a wide variety of different insults, including abnormalities of vertebral development, growth and local neurological function. In classifying scoliosis, it is first divided for clarity into structural and non-structural scoliosis (Goldstein and Waugh, 1973).

Non-structural scoliosis is a lateral curvature of the spine in which there is no vertebral rotation. These curves are usually mild, and the spine shows normal mobility. It tends to be seen with postural abnormalities, e.g. leg length inequalities, and in the presence of the muscular spasm associated with leg length inequality, a prolapsed intervertebral disc, local inflammatory disease, or spinal tumour. It is characteristic of non-structural scoliosis that if the underlying cause is dealt with the scoliosis resolves.

Structural scoliosis is characterized by the presence of vertebral rotation with underlying structural change of the vertebrae themselves and loss of normal spine flexibility (Riseborough and Herndon, 1975). Beyond this simple division, scoliotic deformities are usually classified by aetiology, as shown in Table 4.1 (Goldstein, 1969).

Idiopathic scoliosis

The most common form of scoliosis is known as idiopathic scoliosis. This deformity is the key to the

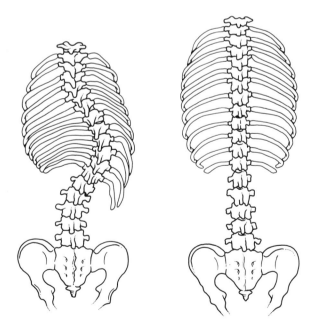

Fig. 4.8 Scoliosis is a lateral displacement of the spine in the coronal plane.

Table 4.1 Aetiological classification of scoliosis (Goldstein, 1969)

Idiopathic (no other aetiological condition present)
Infantile (onset 0–3 years)
  Resolving
  Progressive
Juvenile (onset 4–9 years)
Adolescent (onset from 9 years onward)

Congenital
Deformity due to abnormal bone development
  Congenital scoliosis
    Failure of formation
      Complete unilateral (hemivertebra)
      Partial unilateral (wedge vertebrae)
    Failure of segmentation
      Partial or unilateral (bar)
      Complete or bilateral (fusion)
    Mixed
  Congenital kyphosis
    Failure of formation
    Failure of segmentation
    Mixed
  Congenital lordosis
Deformity due to abnormal spinal cord development
  Myelodysplasia scoliosis
  Myelodysplasia kyphosis
  Myelodysplasia lordosis
Deformity due to mixed causes (spinal dysraphism)
  Meningomyelocoele
  Meningocoele
  Diastematomyelia

Neuromuscular
Neuropathic
  Lower motor neurone disease, e.g. poliomyelitis
  Upper motor neurone disease, e.g. cerebral palsy
  Others, e.g. syringomyelia
Myopathic
  Progressive, e.g. muscular dystrophy
  Static, e.g. cerebral palsy
  Others, e.g. Friedreich's ataxia
  Unilateral myelia

Associated with neurofibromatosis

Mesenchymal disorders
Congenital, e.g. Marfan's syndrome or Morquio's syndrome
Acquired, e.g. rheumatoid arthritis
Others, e.g. juvenile apophysitis

Trauma
Vertebral, e.g. fracture, irradiation, or surgery
Extravertebral, e.g. burns or thoracoplasty

Secondary to irritative phenomena (transient spinal curvatures)
Associated with nerve root irritation, osteoid osteoma, or spinal
  cord tumours

Others
Includes metabolic, nutritional, and endocrine problems

understanding and treatment of spinal deformity in general and forms the basis of the work load of a spinal deformity surgeon. The understanding of this complex deformity has increased considerably over the last few years, particularly with regard to its essential three-dimensional nature (Deacon *et al.*, 1984a; Dickson *et al.*, 1984; Dickson and Archer, 1986). The established deformity involves major changes in spinal alignment in all three planes of the body, always consisting of scoliosis (lateral curvature), lordosis and rotation. The commonly used description 'kyphoscoliosis' is incorrect when applied to the idiopathic deformity; the kyphosis is an illusion caused by vertebral rotation and the presence of a rib hump.

The presence of underlying lordosis at the curve apex was well known to 19th century physicians (Dods, 1824; Adams, 1865). After the discovery of X-rays before the turn of the century, simple pathoanatomical descriptions were replaced by radiographic analysis, and the vertebral abnormalities of congenital scoliosis and bony destruction of tuberculosis were rapidly identified. Study of the idiopathic curve was really only confused, however, as the dominant radiographic feature is the lateral curvature and the rotation, though evident, is not easy to define and completely obscures the sagittal plane lordosis. This is probably the principal reason for the poor general understanding of the basic anatomy of idiopathic scoliosis and of the widespread use of the term kyphoscoliosis, which is quite inaccurate. Accurate accounts of the scoliotic deformity have appeared only sporadically, but Roaf (1966) noted the underlying deformity while Deane and Duthie (1973) and Deacon *et al.* (1984b) consistently identified the apical lordosis and confirmed that the apical vertebrae themselves were lordotic.

Idiopathic scoliosis is usually divided into three types: infantile (onset between birth and 3 years of age); juvenile (onset between the ages of 3 and about 10 years); and adolescent idiopathic scoliosis (onset associated with puberty). In the UK, this classification has largely been abandoned in favour of a description of early-onset scoliosis, which starts during the first few years of childhood, and late-onset scoliosis, equivalent to the adolescent idiopathic condition. The early-onset or infantile idiopathic form of deformity is usually considered to occur with some frequency in the UK, but is seldom encountered in the USA (McMaster and McNicol, 1979). The late-onset deformity constitutes the great majority of spinal deformities seen in Western practice.

EPIDEMIOLOGY AND NATURAL HISTORY

Over the last 20 years, a considerable amount of information has been assembled on the prevalence of scoliosis in the community. In many states of the USA there are mandatory school screening programmes for spinal deformity, and accordingly, many minor degrees of body, trunk and back asymmetry are referred to clinics for assessment. A careful assessment of all these curves, particularly in overview, has shown that many are simply anomalies of trunk asymmetry and there is often no rotation in association with a slight spinal curvature. A non-structural curve associated with a pelvic tilt due to a minor leg length inequality is responsible for 40% of the screened abnormalities. As the curve size increases, however, the proportion of patients with a significant spinal scoliosis markedly increases. The community prevalence of scoliosis with curves between 5° and 10° is about 7%, while for curves over 20° it is about 0.2% (1 in 500). As curve size increases, not only does the proportion of spinal scoliosis increase, but so does the proportion of girls, which reaches more than 4:1 for curves over 15°.

One of the most important features of idiopathic scoliosis is its potential for progression with growth. Clinical treatment would be much simpler if this was universal, consistent and predictable, but unfortunately it is not. In a screened population referred because of a trunk inclination of 5° or more, 70% have a static non-progressive deformity, in 10–20% the curve will regress, and in only 10–20% will it progress 5° or more. Even fewer will have curve progression to a degree that is clinically important. The population eventually identified by significant curve progression are predominantly girls with right thoracic curves. The large number of children with minor anomalies of body topography identified by screening procedures have what is called 'schooliosis' rather than scoliosis and have little significant deformity. Difficulties with understanding the natural history, doubts about the effectiveness of conservative treatment, the economic consequences and the clinical overload caused by the large number of inconsequential anomalies referred to spinal clinics have led to the current UK policy of not screening for scoliosis.

IMAGING

Much of the confusion with regard to idiopathic scoliosis has arisen because of the difficulty of assessing radiographs of the severe deformity, as discussed above. Essentially, vertebral rotation produces a series of oblique projections of the curve on both the posteroanterior (Fig. 4.9) and the lateral radiographs of the patient; this conceals the true size and anatomy of the apical deformity. In order to demonstrate the true size of the deformity, a posteroanterior radiograph must be taken perpendicular to the coronal plane of the apical vertebra and not to the patient (Fig. 4.10). This is described as the 'plan d'éléction' of Stagnara (DuPeloux *et al.*, 1965). A further radiograph taken at 90° to the 'plan d'éléction' produces a true, derotated, lateral view of the curve apex and will demonstrate the apical lordosis (Fig. 4.11). Figure 4.12 shows a reproduction of an 1824 woodcut (Shaw, 1824); this is the posterior aspect of a spine with marked scoliosis. It beautifully illustrates the anatomy of a typical idiopathic curve, the rotation is such that almost a lateral view of the curve apex is seen, and the lordosis is obvious.

Despite the imaging problems caused by curve rotation, the gold standard for measurement of scoliosis is the Cobb angle. This measures the angles subtended between the end vertebrae of the curve and gives a simple figure in degrees. It is extremely important to note the limitations of this measurement; this angle is measured on a two-dimensional projection of a rotated three-dimensional deformity, which becomes increasingly more inaccurate as the curve rotates. Major changes in the curve can occur out of the plane of measurement, and major measurement errors are common.

In response to this difficulty and in order to reduce the amount of radiation to which patients are exposed, various other methods for measuring body topography have been raised. The scoliometer (Bunnell, 1984) is perhaps the most widely used and the most simple; it is a level that can be laid on the rotational prominence to give a figure for the inclination of the deformity. Other techniques include the Moire fringe technique, in which a fine mesh is projected onto the patient's back and then photographed to produce a contour-like effect (Fig. 4.13). More recently, Turner-Smith (1982) has produced

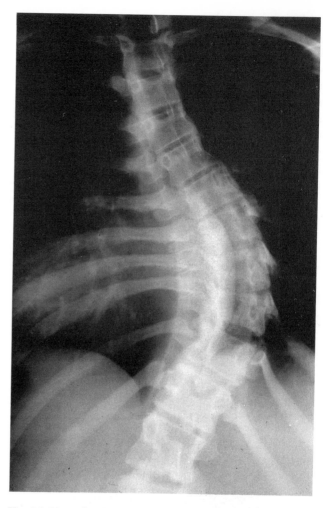

Fig. 4.9 Typical right thoracic structural scoliosis.

the integrated shape-imaging system, in which a beam of light is projected down the patient's back, detected by a TV camera, and analysed by computer. This produces a series of outlines of the surface shape of the patient's back and a computed measurement of the underlying

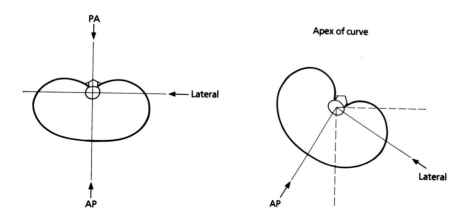

Fig. 4.10 The effect of vertebral rotation on the projection of the radiographic view of scoliosis.

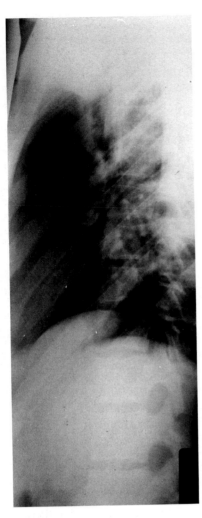

Fig. 4.11 Apical lordosis seen on a derotated lateral radiograph.

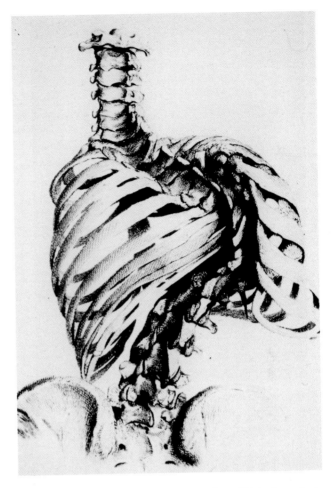

Fig. 4.12 Reproduction of an illustration from 1824 of a scoliotic specimen showing marked rotation with an obvious apical lordosis. (From Shaw, 1824.)

spinal deformity (Harris *et al.*, 1984). In recent years, many other workers have demonstrated computer graphic systems that produce a full three-dimensional image of spinal deformities. These have not yet reached clinical practice, however, but will become a common method of assessing spinal deformity.

PATHOGENESIS

Idiopathic scoliosis has for many years been the diagnosis of exclusion after all other possible causes of spinal deformity have been eliminated. Most aetiological hypotheses assume it to be a subclinical form of one or other recognizable cause of scoliosis. Evidence suggesting neuromuscular, metabolic, dietary, or congenital vertebral growth anomalies in these apparently normal children has been presented. While there is no doubt that there is a genetic tendency for children to become scoliotic (Wynne-Davies, 1968; Cowell *et al.*, 1972;

Rogola *et al.*, 1978; Carr, 1990), no consistent deficit in any other system has been found.

Although several workers (Zuk, 1962; LeFebvre *et al.*, 1971) have identified increased electrical activity in muscles on the convex side of the deformity, it is now felt that this is secondary to the presence of the curvature. Investigations of connective tissue function in scoliosis have not shown clear-cut anomalies (Stearns *et al.*, 1955; Ponseti, 1968; Ponseti *et al.*, 1972; Francis *et al.*, 1977). The most important contribution to the study of scoliosis in recent years has been the renewed interest in the underlying presence of lordosis as a biomechanical initiator of the deformity (Somerville, 1952; Deacon *et al.*, 1984a,b). The difficulty in identifying apical lordosis has been discussed, but it has been suggested this apical lordosis itself is the primary lesion favouring rotation and subsequent lateral curvature with growth. Although this analysis is not new (Heuer, 1927; Somerville, 1952; Wittebol, 1956; Roaf, 1966), it has

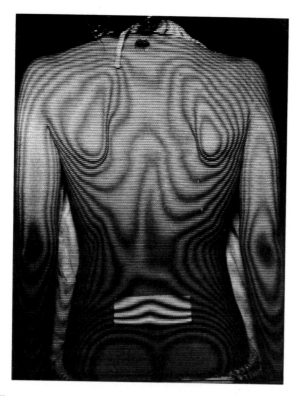

Fig. 4.13 Moire fringe photograph showing asymmetry of the back in a child with scoliosis.

recently received enthusiastic support and considerable evidence in its favour has been presented (Deacon *et al.*, 1984a,b; Dickson *et al.*, 1984; Dickson and Archer, 1986; Smith and Dickson, 1987; Smith *et al.*, 1991b).

Lordosis in the thoracic region lies in front of the normal axis of vertebral rotation, which with the shape of the vertebral bodies and the alignment of the facet joints in the thoracic region exposes this segment to rotation when the spine is flexed forward and the anterior column is placed under compression. Normal thoracic kyphosis is rotationally stable under compression and does not rotate into scoliosis. The rotational instability of lordosis has been demonstrated biomechanically (Somerville, 1952; Roaf, 1966) and experimentally (Smith and Dickson, 1987), and has been shown to produce all of the typical structural vertebral features of idiopathic scoliosis (Dickson and Archer, 1986; Smith *et al.*, 1991b). The changes of vertebral shape in the transverse and coronal plane are effects secondary to the rotation of the lordosis (Smith *et al.*, 1991b).

The lordosis theory is attractive in that it offers explanations of all the major features of idiopathic scoliosis, the deformity being a purely mechanical buckling of an extreme spinal shape in the sagittal plane, which may even be part of the normal spectrum of sagittal plane spinal alignment. No systemic abnormality is suggested, and the relationship between curve progression and the period of rapid vertebral growth is easily explained. The prevalence of right thoracic scoliosis is explained by the normal asymmetry of the spine to the right in the mid-thoracic region (Sabatier, 1777) and is probably due to the presence of the descending aorta on the left side at that level. The increased prevalence of the deformity in girls may be due to the normal flattening of thoracic kyphosis in children at about the age of 11–12 years (Willner, 1981), which corresponds to the earlier growth spurt in girls placing them at risk from vertebral buckling with growth. All curves of the spine need to be balanced in other regions and in all three planes to allow the pelvis to sit square and the head to face forward. Scheuermann's kyphosis is often associated with an area of scoliosis, but it has been demonstrated (Deacon *et al.*, 1985) that this area of scoliosis is seen adjacent to the kyphosis, where compensatory lordosis buckles the spine to the side to produce the slight curvature. The association of kyphosis and lordosis balances overall, and prevents the progression of these deformities to any major degree.

There is no doubt that lordosis is the essential feature in the development of idiopathic scoliosis, and evidence is mounting that it may be the primary cause of the deformity. Much of this evidence, however, is confused by the presence of secondary bony changes in the established deformity, which often obscures the initial pathogenetic lesion. Several longitudinal studies are now investigating the natural history and development of typical scoliotic deformities from straight spines, which perhaps develop lordosis first in the sagittal plane.

Increased awareness of the three-dimensional nature of spinal deformity is the major event that has taken place in the basic science of spinal deformity during the last 10 years, and an appreciation of this concept is essential before embarking on treatment. It is interesting to note that the more modern forms of treatment, including wiring to a pre-bent (kyphotic) Harrington rod and the Cotrel–Dubousset or TSRH (Texas Scottish Rite Hospital) spinal instrumentation systems, all pay particular attention to the three-dimensional aspects of the deformity.

Consequences of scoliosis

There are three principal consequences of severe idiopathic scoliosis, which are: the personal and social stigma of severe deformity; an increased morbidity and mortality from cardiopulmonary compromise; and long-term back pain.

DEFORMITY

There is no doubt that severe spinal deformity produces a serious cosmetic disfigurement and a risk of significant problems with social life, reported low marriage rates, high divorce rates, and psychiatric illness to the extent of suicide (Bengtsson *et al.*, 1974). How much this is relevant, however, to the child with a 30° thoracic curve and a small rib hump at the end of growth is highly questionable. The common surgical case with 40° or more of thoracic curve usually has a noticeable rib hump, but this is not marked compared with the very severe deformity of 90° with a major disfigurement where a sharp 'razor-back' rib deformity can be seen. Trunk imbalance contributes significantly towards cosmetic deformity and may be a more obvious problem than rotational prominence, particularly with a single curve. Despite their alarming radiological appearance, most double curves compensate for each other and may not produce a major cosmetic problem.

CARDIOPULMONARY FUNCTION

A less common but much more serious problem is the association of scoliosis with cardiopulmonary compromise, as described by Hippocrates (400 BC):

> And in those cases where the gibbosity is above the diaphragm, the ribs do not expand properly in width, but forward and the chest become sharp pointed and not broad, and they become affected with difficulty with breathing and hoarseness; for the cavities which inspire and expire the breath do not attain their proper capacity.

There is no doubt that major spinal deformities can be associated with reduction of pulmonary function (Nilsonne and Lundgren, 1968; Nachemson, 1968) due to a general reduction in lung capacity and an increase in stiffness of the whole respiratory unit (Smith *et al.*, 1991a). Those with the most seriously reduced pulmonary function are at risk of early death from opportunistic chest infection (Reid, 1965). Significant pulmonary deficit is extremely rare, however, and is found almost exclusively in patients with severe early-onset deformities and those with associated neurological deficits (Dickson, 1985; Muirhead and Conner, 1985; Branthwaite, 1986; Smith *et al.*, 1991a). Reduction in respiratory function is often given as an argument for treatment in children with late-onset scoliosis. When these children are examined in a scoliosis clinic, it is often quite clear that they have no respiratory deficit and are involved in energetic athletic pursuits typical of other children of their age. A recent review of dancers at the New York Ballet showed that 26% of them had scoliosis measuring between 10 and 30° (Warner *et al.*, 1986); clearly, their deformities were not affecting their athletic abilities and not causing any significant morbidity. These late-onset cases do not develop significant pulmonary compromise and should have their treatment planned accordingly. Only children who have a significant deformity of the thoracic spine and the chest wall during the very early years of life have any long-term problems with respiratory function due to the deformity alone. This occurs with severe, early-onset idiopathic scoliosis or congenital deformities, and although these are the most difficult cases, it is essential to attempt to prevent the progression of this form of the deformity.

SCOLIOSIS AND BACK PAIN

Idiopathic scoliosis is not a painful condition; if pain is a presenting feature detailed investigation of the cause of the scoliosis is essential. The question of later back pain due to the presence of a scoliosis has been addressed by several authors. Nachemson (1968) in particular has proposed that there is little difference in back pain between patients with and without spinal deformities. Other evidence suggests that although the incidence of pain may not be increased, it is often more persistent and difficult to treat (Jackson *et al.*, 1983), particularly in those patients with major deformities in the thoracolumbar and lumbar spine. As it is still unclear whether patients with scoliosis have more back pain than the general population, this factor should not be considered when planning treatment. Recently, Edgar and Mehta (1988) have suggested that previous treatment by spinal fusion reduces the severity of late low back pain.

Late-onset idiopathic scoliosis

The typical late-onset deformity presents in the early teens, usually after a family member or school teacher has noticed an asymmetry, sometimes in the loin, or a rib hump perhaps after a screening examination. These features of the rotational component of scoliosis are most obviously seen in the forward bend test (see Fig. 4.5). A full history-taking and examination should be conducted as described above, and radiographs should be obtained to assess the deformity and exclude the presence of a congenital vertebral anomaly.

MANAGEMENT

Having confirmed the diagnosis, most curves are then measured by the Cobb method and conventional

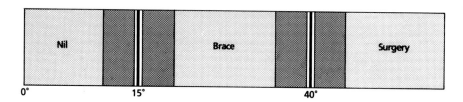

Fig. 4.14 Conventional treatment plan for idiopathic scoliosis of increasing severity of curvature.

treatment is prescribed according to the magnitude of the curvature (Fig. 4.14). Deficiencies of the Cobb angle method of measurement have led to its abandonment in some centres, and some surgeons base their treatment purely on the body topography of the patient and on the cosmetic acceptability or unacceptability of deformity (Leatherman and Dickson, 1988).

Patients with a Cobb angle of 15−20° are treated by observation. Although this is necessary, the vast majority does not progress and the mild deformity remains acceptable. It is important to follow these children with non-radiographic means to reduce X-ray exposure, using the Bunnell scoliometer, Moire fringe technique, or integrated shape-imaging system according to local practice. In many clinics, children are taught exercises to strengthen the abdomen and postural muscles of the spine, but no evidence has ever been presented to show that these are of any real benefit. Larger curves in the region of 20−30° are commonly treated by conservative means, and when greater than 40° operative treatment is considered.

Non-operative treatment

When a curve greater than 20° has shown its tendency to progress by a sustained increase in the Cobb angle of 5° or more, it is usually considered for conservative treatment. This takes the form of bracing, using an external thoracolumbosacral orthosis. For a few years electrospinal stimulation (the Scoliotron) was prescribed, but it has now been accepted that this form of treatment does not alter the natural history of the condition (Goldberg et al., 1988).

The standard method of attempting to influence the progression of small curves is still spinal bracing. The efficacy of bracing in preventing further progression is now also highly controversial, however, and although studies have been presented apparently confirming that braces diminish progression (Blount and Millencamp, 1977; Edmondson and Morris, 1977; Carr et al., 1978; Emans et al., 1986), other data suggest that such aggressive conservative treatment does not influence the natural history (Dickson, 1985; Kehl and Morrissy, 1988; Focarile et al., 1991; Goldberg, personal communi-

cation). Bracing for idiopathic scoliosis is a hotly debated topic; its death knell is finally beginning to sound and the results of current studies will be very important.

Bracing remains the mainstay of conservative treatment, principally in North America, where the standard brace is the Milwaukee brace (Fig. 4.15) which is really a cervicothoracolumbosacral orthosis. It has a plastic pelvic mould from which uprights are attached carrying thoracic pads and a cervical band. Initially this brace was used as a distraction device, but this produced major problems with the patient's teeth and now the chin strap is really only used as a postural reminder, with most of the correction being applied through pads attached to the uprights (Blount and Moe, 1973). Most physicians feel that continuous bracing use is needed for success, and it is usually prescribed for 23 h each day with a short period of time out for bathing and exercise to maintain some spinal flexibility. Other centres favour an underarm orthosis, of which the best known is the Boston brace (Fig. 4.16). This is a low-profile orthosis,

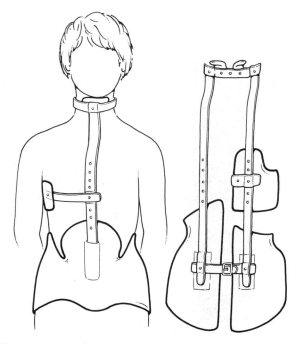

Fig. 4.15 Milwaukee brace with a pelvic ring opening posteriorly and three upright struts connected by a neck ring above.

which comes in prefabricated shapes to which pads and liners can be applied. The advantages of low braces include increased cosmesis with better acceptance of the orthosis and function within the brace. They are said to be as effective as the Milwaukee brace (Stanish *et al.*, 1975; Micheli *et al.*, 1980), but this may only represent the overall failure of all bracing systems (Focarile *et al.*, 1991).

Several different mechanisms have been proposed to explain brace function (Scoliosis Research Society, 1979). The early theory of mechanical straightening by distraction and lateral compression is clearly incorrect, and distraction is no longer part of the force applied. The Boston brace applies forces behind and below each apical segment in order to realign and derotate. There is no real evidence that braces work like a biofeed-back device, stimulating postural alignment reflexes in the scoliotic child. Leatherman and Dickson (1988) suggested that the temporary improvement seen during brace wearing is due to restriction of forward flexion, which reduces the compression force on the anterior column and therefore the buckling moment. As rotation and lordosis are the primary problems, it is clear that the brace cannot work in this plane to pull the lordosis back into a rotationally stable kyphotic alignment.

Overall, the Cobb angle and spinal balance can be improved while the brace is worn, but the rotation remains unchanged (Goldberg, personal communication). Conservative treatment is usually continued until spinal maturity, assessed by closure of the iliac apophyses (Risser sign) and the bone age. There is some controversy, however, regarding the relationship of these to spinal maturity. After the brace is removed, there is a consistent increase in the Cobb angle, so that after 1 year or more of follow-up, 70–80% of patients have a similar deformity to the pre-brace situation, 10% have a lesser deformity and 10–20% are worse. A proportion of these will have progressed to the extent that an operation is required. Overall, these data are ominously similar to those obtained from the standard natural history studies.

Bracing is not without cost and is not acceptable as a form of treatment to many adolescent girls. Houghton *et al.* (1987) showed very poor compliance even in a relatively well-motivated population. Having observed patients with scoliosis in the UK and USA, it is clear that there is a definite difference in treatment expectations, demands and acceptance of bracing on either side of the Atlantic, which makes direct comparisons of these aspects of treatment difficult.

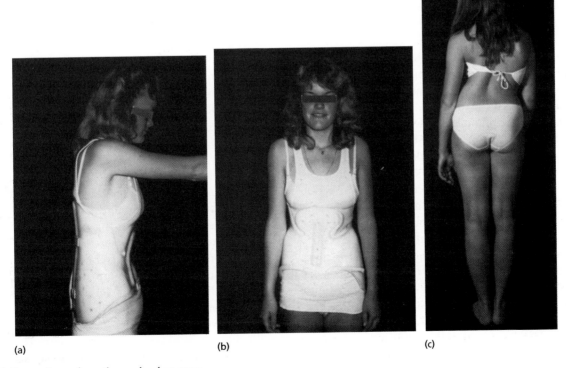

(a) (b) (c)

Fig. 4.16 Boston brace for a thoracolumbar curve.

Operative treatment

Operative treatment of idiopathic scoliosis has advanced considerably in recent years with major developments in the design and application of spinal instrumentation systems. The basis of treatment, spinal fusion, is now usually combined with instrumentation for stability and correction of the deformity. It is most commonly achieved after a posterior subperiosteal approach to the spine, but in some situations an anterior approach to fusion is employed.

Posterior surgery.   Surgical fusion of the spine for scoliosis was developed in the early part of the 20th century by Hibbs (1924) and initially involved a considerable amount of bed-rest and correction with turnbuckle casts; pseudoarthrosis was common. The operation is still performed for some deformities associated with congenital scoliosis. Intra-operative attention to detail is essential, with excision and grafting of each facet joint and meticulous cleaning and decortication of each vertebra out to the transverse processes. Bone graft is added to increase the fusion mass; this is usually harvested from one posterior iliac crest, but fusion rates using processed allograft bone are equally as good and this is often essential in the absence of adequate bone stock.

The incidence of pseudoarthrosis after an attempted fusion was considerably reduced by the implantation of metal stabilizing devices (Moe and Valuska, 1966). Harrington developed his instrumentation between 1949 and 1954, initially operating without fusion, but then modifying his instrumentation and adding a fusion to counteract the high incidence of metal fatigue and implant failure in his early patients (Harrington, 1960; Harrington, 1962). This proved a remarkable advance and significantly reduced the incidence of pseudoarthrosis.

The basis of Harrington instrumentation is distraction between hooks placed into the posterior elements of the neutral vertebrae at either end of the scoliosis. A variety of hooks is available for different sites. A sharp hook is inserted into the facet joint over the most superior neutral vertebra after the inferior margin of the inferior facet of the vertebra above has been cut square. Care must be taken to correctly site this hook to avoid it cutting out at an early stage. Some surgeons prefer a bifid hook to help prevent this (Houghton, personal communication). The blunt lower hook is inserted into the spinal canal at the level of the lower neutral vertebra; it normally has a round hole but a square hole can be used to obtain some rotational control of the rod. Special deeper hooks are available to fit round the lumbar lamina or sacral ala. After distraction the whole

system is held in place by locking the vanes of the upper part of the rod against the upper hook. Harrington also designed a compression system using hooks, nuts and a threaded flexible rod which can be used on the curve convexity and placed on the transverse processes or onto the lamina themselves (Fig. 4.17).

In parallel with other systems of internal fixation in orthopaedic surgery, recent developments have produced many different devices, most of which provide much more control of individual spinal segments and much more stability of fixation. In many situations, these newer techniques obviate the need for post-operative casts or braces (Dubousset *et al.*, 1986). The Cotrel–Dobousset system is now widely favoured in the USA. Multiple hooks are used along the instrumented segment, allowing separate areas of spinal distraction and compression on a single rod. The rod is pre-bent to a slight curve accommodating the partly corrected scoliosis and then rotated as a whole carrying the vertebrae with it. This produces a sustained derotation effect of 25–30% (Cundy *et al.*, 1990; Hall and Webb, 1990). A cross-linked second rod adds considerable stability, such that a post-operative spinal support is not needed (Fig. 4.18). Segmental spinal fixation can also be achieved using rods and sublaminar wires, first used by Luque (Luque and Cordoso, 1977; Luque, 1980), or using a rectangle and sublaminar wires (Hartshill rectangle). This form of segmental spinal instrumentation with sublaminar wiring systems is used principally in patients with neurological scoliosis, as many surgeons are concerned about the potential problems due to the passage of sublaminar wires and their long-term presence in the spinal canal in idiopathic cases. With modifications, however (principally attempting to wire back the spine into true kyphosis by pre-bending the rod to the corrected spinal shape), this technique has produced the maximum curve correction and derotation effect yet achieved in idiopathic scoliosis (Dickson and Archer, 1987).

Anterior surgery.   The anterior approach to the thoracolumbar spine via a thoracotomy or thoracoabdominal retroperitoneal approach allows resection of the intervertebral discs or parts of the vertebral bodies themselves, anterior fusion and instrumentation (Figs 4.19, 4.20). Considerable mobility of the scoliotic segment can be produced, allowing more correction over a shorter segment than by posterior surgery. This is logical as anterior procedures produce a considerable improvement in vertebral mobility by removal of the discs, allowing the overlong anterior column to shorten with correction and the lordosis to be corrected towards kyphosis. This also diminishes the risks from operation

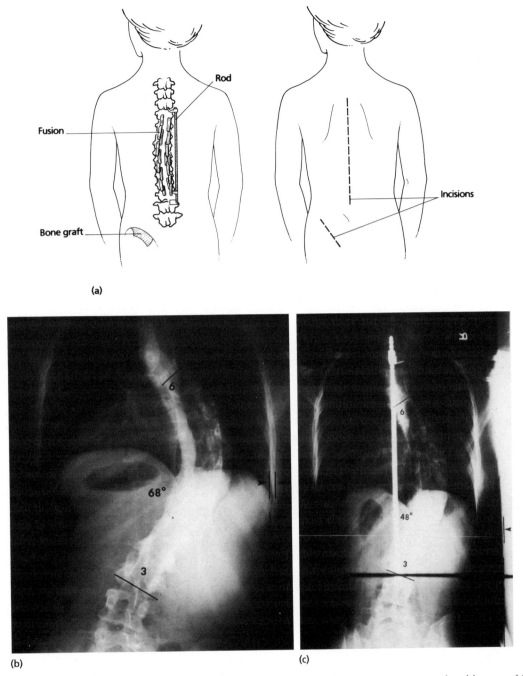

Fig. 4.17 (a) Posterior spinal fusion with decortication of posterior elements, insertion of a Harrington rod and bone grafting. (b) Decompensated, previously fused curve of 68°. (c) Curve corrected to 48° following instrumentation and re-fusion.

by allowing shortening rather than lengthening of the spinal column with correction.

Anterior surgery was initially championed by Hodgson for tuberculosis of the spine (Hodgson and Stock, 1956; Fang *et al.*, 1964; Hodgson, 1965). Hodgson initially favoured an anterior opening wedge osteotomy for angular spinal deformities, a technique that is now considered too risky to the neurological

structures within the spinal canal and has been abandoned in favour of closing wedge techniques. This was popularized by several surgeons in the USA, including Leatherman (1969) and Hall (1972).

Anterior instrumentation allows significant correction of the deformity at the time of the anterior fusion. The Dwyer system is a series of vertebral body screws attached via a cable on the curve convexity which is

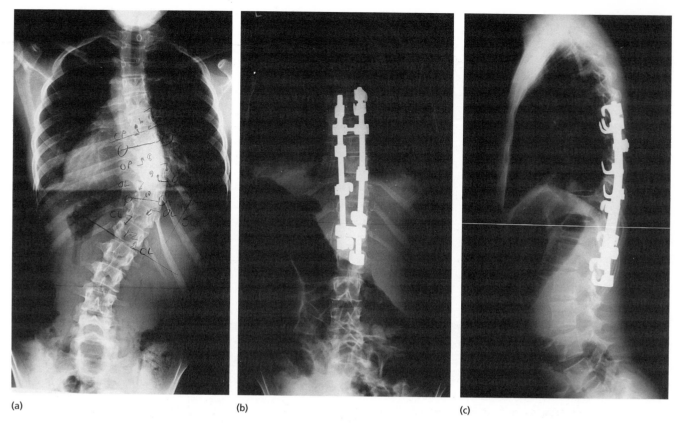

(a)   (b)   (c)

Fig. 4.18 Idiopathic scoliosis treated by the Cotrel–Dubousset system. (a) Pre-operative plane. (b) Post-operative correction in the anteroposterior plane. (c) Post-operative correction in the lateral plane.

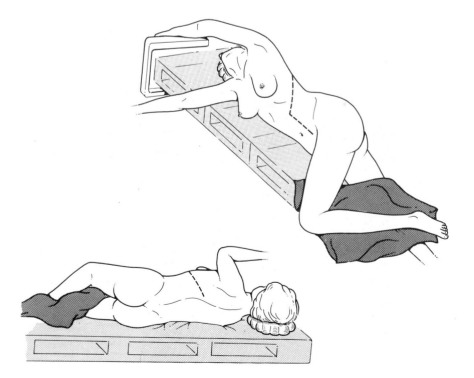

Fig. 4.19 Anterior exposure of the spine is attained by a transthoracic, retroperitoneal approach.

tightened to obtain correction (Dwyer, 1973; Dwyer and Schafer, 1974). It is mainly used as anterior instrumentation in the lordoscoliosis of myelodysplasia and other neuromuscular conditions, but is also occasionally indicated for idiopathic cases (Fig. 4.20). Modifications of anterior instrumentation have led to the development of the Zielke (Zielke and Berthet, 1978) and subsequent (Webb–Morley) anterior instrumentation systems. The Zielke system consists of much improved instrumentation for the insertion of the apparatus and better designed screws, which are tightened together via a flexible threaded rod and nuts. This produces fewer instrumentation problems and has expanded the indications significantly (Griss *et al.*, 1984).

Surgical philosophy.   In general, the results of surgical treatment have progressively improved over the years with less chance of pseudoarthrosis, less instrumentation failure and apparently better correction of the deformity. When the three-dimensional nature of idiopathic scoliosis is considered, however, the correction of the deformity obtained is generally disappointing, particularly with respect to the rotational prominence with which the patient presented. In addition, correction is only obtained with fusion of a long segment of the spine which carries its own associated problems.

The original Harrington distraction instrumentation can correct 50% of the coronal plane curvature of idiopathic scoliosis. It does not address the rotational prominence, however, and provides very little correction of this. What the patient does gain is partial correction of the Cobb angle and a fusion which to some degree prevents progression and stops forward flexion of the involved segment, thereby reducing rotation with flexion. As a late-onset deformity presents near the end of growth, however, when the progression potential is limited and there is no risk of either respiratory embarrassment or neurological compromise, it is principally a problem of disfigurement.

Clearly, surgical treatment should be directed at improving the presenting cosmetic complaint. What the patient wants treated is the problem that presented: a rib hump and the worry of it progressing (Leatherman

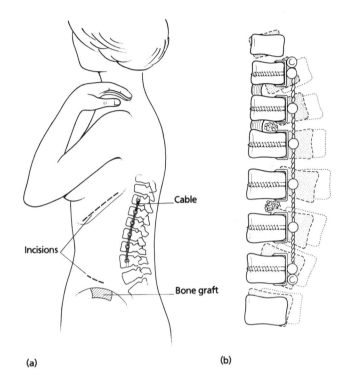

(a)   (b)

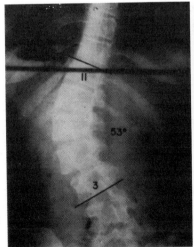
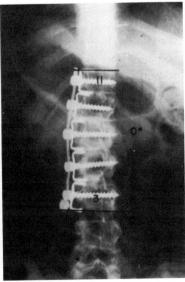

(c)

Fig. 4.20 (a,b) Dwyer instrumentation is performed anteriorly between adjacent vertebral bodies, with removal and fusion of intervening disc spaces, and acts as a tension band on the convex side of the curve. (c) Dramatic mechanical correction can often be attained.

and Dickson, 1988). The addition of a small Harrington compression system on the curve convexity, opposite a simple distraction system, may help a little, but significant derotation and correction of the rib hump can only be obtained with a segmental instrumentation system, either the Harrington rod with Luque wires as used by Dickson (Dickson and Archer, 1987; Leatherman and Dickson, 1988), or by the Cotrel–Dubousset (CD) or TSRH instrumentation (Cundy *et al.*, 1990; Hall and Webb, 1990) which allows some correction of the sagittal plane element of the deformity and as a secondary effect achieves some derotation. The surgeon's aim should be to lift and derotate the vertebral lamina on the curve concavity to bring the lordosis back into kyphosis and hence reduce the rib hump. Cotrel–Dubousset instrumentation (Cotrel *et al.*, 1988) obtains this derotation by turning the rod and provides sustained derotation of about 25% of the initial deformity, with significant improvement of the rib hump. Even better derotation can be obtained using a square-ended Harrington rod pre-bent into a kyphotic shape, to which the vertebrae are drawn and derotated with sublaminar wires. The latter procedure has been shown to produce a sustained correction of about 60% of both the Cobb angle and vertebral rotation with a significant improvement in the rib hump and the appearance of the patient.

As the curve size increases, the changes in vertebral shape make the curve too stiff for adequate correction to be obtained by a posterior procedure alone. In order to gain an adequate correction in the larger curves (over 70–80°), it is necessary to shorten the anterior column with a preliminary anterior stage. An anterior dissectomy provides anterior shortening and curve mobility which aid correction and an increased margin of safety from neurological damage by reducing the chance of a cord traction injury. It also provides for an anterior fusion for late stability. In less mature cases excision of the anterior growth plates removes the driving force behind further progression of rotation.

Complications. While there is no doubt that modern instrumentation systems and surgical techniques are significant advances, the risks carried by this sort of surgery must also be considered. These include the general risks of major surgery, problems related to the fusion itself and the risk of neurological damage.

After fusion, there is no doubt that curve progression is halted in the vast majority of cases of late-onset scoliosis, but in cases where there is still spinal growth rotational progression often continues unabated. This is known as the 'crank shaft' phenomenon. The problem is worse in younger patients and with larger curves and it

is one of the major difficulties in treating early-onset deformity. After posterior fusion only, anterior growth continues; with any incompletely corrected rotated lordosis, this growth can only be directed to produce further progression of rotation, in effect creating experimental scoliosis in a child with a posterior tether (Smith and Dickson, 1987). The addition of an anterior growth arrest has been shown necessary to halt this phenomenon (Grivas *et al.*, 1990; Shufflebarger, 1991).

In recent years it has become quite clear that long, and especially low (below L3) (Aaro and Ohlund, 1983; Cochran *et al.*, 1983), spinal fusions severely restrict spinal mobility, and with the original posterior Harrington distraction rod lumbar kyphosis or flat-back is produced (Kostuik *et al.*, 1988; Fabry *et al.*, 1989). Surgeons specializing in scoliosis are now seeing a considerable number of patients returning 10–15 years after their initial, long, Harrington fusion with a flat lumbar profile and serious pain and fatigue in the low back and thighs due to the abnormal alignment of the lumbar spine. This is known as flat-back syndrome and is proving very difficult to treat. The surgical salvage procedure is usually a posterior closing wedge osteotomy of the lower lumbar spine with compression instrumentation in order to recreate lumbar lordosis (Kostuik *et al.*, 1988; LaGrone, 1988).

Failure of fusion with pseudoarthrosis may be asymptomatic, but often presents with instrumentation failure. Symptomatic patients are best investigated with a bone scan, though conventional tomography aligned in the correct plane may be useful. Revision with refusion and reinstrumentation (Floman *et al.*, 1982) may be necessary.

The most feared complication of scoliosis treatment is neurological damage. A recent survey of members of the British Scoliosis Society suggests a prevalence of neurological lesions in the region of 4% (Dove, 1986). This includes, however, several minor transient and minimal deficits as well as the occasional rare major deficit or even paraplegia. The risk of a significant deficit is probably in the region of 1–1.5%. It has been suggested that the use of sublaminar wires may carry a higher risk of neurological lesions and an incidence as high as 17% (Wilbur *et al.*, 1984) has been reported, though it must be said that this figure is excessive. MacEwen *et al.* (MacEwen *et al.*, 1975) reported a survey of the Scoliosis Research Society that revealed a neurological complication rate of less than 1%. Risk factors, particularly a tethered spinal cord suggested by a spinal bifida occulta, any congenital spinal lesion, or skin stigmata of spinal dysraphism demand preliminary investigation of the patient with CT myelography or MRI. The risk of neurological damage is reduced by preliminary use of an anterior column shortening procedure (Leatherman and Dickson, 1988).

In order to immediately identify a neurological change and attempt to avoid a permanent neurological complication, patients are monitored during the operation with various forms of electrical spinal cord monitoring systems (Machida *et al.*, 1985). In the UK, Jones and Edgar (Jones *et al.*, 1981; Jones *et al.*, 1983) have considerable experience in this technique and have reported three minor cord problems in 138 operated cases. Most surgeons also use the 'wake-up test' (Hall *et al.*, 1978), in which the patient is partly woken after the correction has been obtained to confirm that they are able to move their feet. A loss of the monitoring readings, an increase in their latency, or a failure to pass a wake-up test is a reason to remove the instrumentation in order to remove the tension on the cord. In fortunate cases, this results in resolution of the neurological deficit. Investigations are continuing to determine the degree of change that can be accepted on a spinal cord monitor and also to design systems to monitor the motor side of the cord.

Surgical exposure of the spine with fusion and instrumentation is a major procedure that is often associated with heavy blood loss. The current international fear about the transmission of viral agents by blood transfusion has led to particular concerns among spinal surgeons. Several techniques, including controlled hypotensive anaesthesia, autodonation of the patient's blood for several weeks before the procedure and autotransfusion of blood spilled during the operation using a cell-saving machine are widely applied.

It must be emphasized that although there are significant advantages of spinal fusion for scoliosis, there are also serious risks. Modern instrumentation considerably improves the cosmetic results of surgical treatment and measures have been taken to make operations safer and the complications fewer than before. Many now consider, however, that idiopathic late-onset deformity is a problem of disfigurement and that before operative treatment the risks and rewards of any procedure should be carefully considered with both patient and family.

Specific curve patterns

The principles of treatment have been outlined above, but management of each individual curve type depends on its site and size together with the patient's progression potential and the current level of cosmetic unacceptability. The types of curve seen in idiopathic scoliosis are shown in Fig. 4.21. In late-onset cases the principal indication for surgery is cosmesis (Dickson and Archer, 1987; Leatherman and Dickson, 1988). For flexible deformities, with a Cobb angle up to 60−70°, posterior surgical instrumentation is usually satisfactory provided that a system designed to derotate the spine is used. Examples of typical instrumentation systems are shown in Figs 4.18, 4.20, 4.22. Patients with single curves often have a significant cosmetic defect and may be out of balance more than those with double curves, who may show minimal cosmetic disfigurement, despite an alarming radiographic appearance, as both the rotation and lateral curvature are balanced producing a relatively stable alignment.

Posterior fusion of thoracolumbar curves often requires a low fusion in the lumbar spine, which seriously reduces the remaining mobile vertebral segments. These curves are best dealt with from in front, where a relatively short segment can be fused and better spinal mobility maintained.

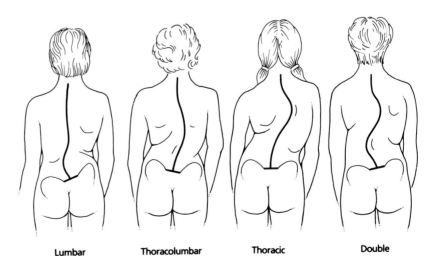

Fig. 4.21 The different curve patterns of idiopathic scoliosis.

Lumbar   Thoracolumbar   Thoracic   Double

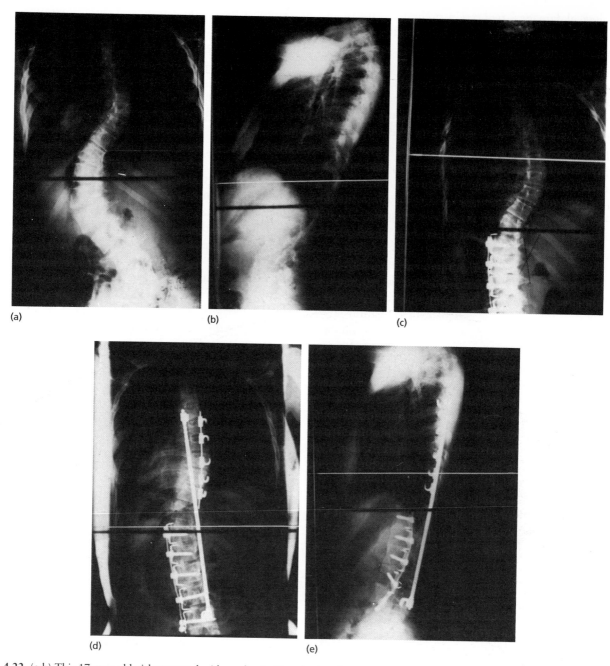

(a)   (b)   (c)

(d)   (e)

Fig. 4.22 (a,b) This 17-year-old girl presented with mechanical low back pain on activity. Standing radiographs revealed a right thoracic curve of 50° and a left thoracolumbar curve with 3 out of 4 rotation of 80°, with decompensation posteriorly and to the left. Two operations were required for correction, with (c) first-stage anterior Dwyer instrumentation to correct the decompensation, and (d,e) second-stage Harrington distraction and compression instrumentation to stabilize both curves.

Late cosmetic surgery

In some cases, rotation can still progress after instrumentation, and occasionally patients present dissatisfied with the rotational correction. A considerable amount of work on body topography and spinal deformity has

been performed and the results of late costoplasties for residual rib hump deformities discussed in detail (Broome *et al.*, 1990). Costoplasty is sometimes combined with the initial surgical procedure if there is still a residual rib hump after instrumentation (Dickson and Archer, 1987).

Early-onset idiopathic scoliosis

This is the new name for infantile idiopathic scoliosis. In contrast to the late-onset deformity, the early age of development of this condition and its high progression potential can produce severe deformities (Fig. 4.23) at a time when lung growth is incomplete (Branthwaite, 1986; Smith *et al.*, 1991a), so that in addition to a severe deformity it can produce severe cardiopulmonary compromise with its associated morbidity and mortality. Affected children can fail to thrive due to respiratory failure (Smith *et al.*, 1991a). The early-onset deformity appears to occur in low-birth-weight, hypotonic babies (Mehta, 1984). Boys are affected slightly more commonly than girls, and although thoracic curves are most common the other curve patterns are seen.

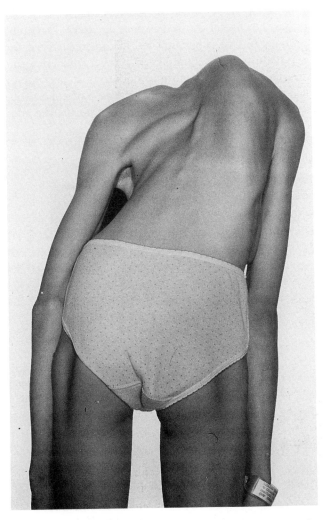

Fig. 4.23 Forward bend test to show the severe rib hump in early-onset idiopathic scoliosis. There is a potential for severe deformity and significant cardiopulmonary compromise.

Most importantly, it has been shown that two clinical forms of the early-onset deformity exist: one in which the curve resolves with growth, accounts for 95% of cases, but a small proportion has severe progression potential (Mehta, 1984). Mehta's rib–vertebrae angle difference (Mehta, 1972) was described to try to differentiate at an early stage which curve had the serious progression potential; it probably represents the degree of vertebral rotation at the curve apex. Cases in whom the rib–vertebrae angle difference is over 20° and increasing tend to show severe progression and require treatment, and those in whom it is under 20° and reducing resolve with growth.

MANAGEMENT

The mainstay of treatment of progressive early-onset deformity in a young child, often 2–3 years old, is the application of serial extension, derotation and flexion casts. The success of cast treatment probably reflects the malleability of the skeleton at this early age, and the curve can often be influenced favourably, particularly in experienced hands.

Unfortunately, occasional cases still progress and produce very severe, rotated lordoscolioses with a foreshortened trunk and a high risk of respiratory compromise. Several operative options are available, none of which is entirely satisfactory. For many years posterior fusion alone was in favour (Winter, 1977; McMaster and McNicol, 1979); unfortunately, posterior fusion in a very young child causes the serious problem of the crankshaft phenomenon as discussed above, and this procedure should now be abandoned. Clearly, in order to treat early-onset idiopathic scoliosis operatively, a procedure that overcomes the altered biomechanics and directs growth favourably is necessary; it should correct the sagittal plane curvature and balance anterior and posterior spinal growth. Various attempts at this have been made, including the insertion of subcutaneous Harrington rods which are periodically distracted to increase posterior spinal growth (Harrington, 1960), though this does not have a reputation of success.

The addition of segmental fixation with wires, or in the younger child with tapes, to pre-bent rods has been applied in the hope that the spine will grow along the rods and the wires slip with growth. These are called trolley procedures. Unfortunately, they are often not successful (Hall, personal communication), as the posterior exposure of the young spine can often lead to a spontaneous fusion and a crankshaft effect can occur. An attempt has been made to combine a trolley procedure with an anterior vertebral epiphysiodesis in order to reduce anterior growth and balance the spinal curvatures, and has produced promising preliminary results (Grivas *et al.*, 1990). In parallel, Shufflebarger (1991) has shown that the crankshaft phenomenon does not occur when an anterior apical fusion is added to the posterior procedure.

As curves increase, it becomes necessary, particularly in juveniles, to gain more correction at the bony level, especially with the rigid deformity. Posterior instrumentation must then be combined with anterior disc excision, to allow for shortening of the anterior column and production of an anterior fusion. As curve size increases further and rigidity supervenes, the only corrective procedure is a two-stage wedge vertebrectomy of the curve apex as advocated by Leatherman and Dickson (1979). This procedure is a major closing wedge vertebrectomy performed in two stages with visualization of the dural sac during closure of the wedge.

The aim of operative treatment of early-onset scoliosis is to improve the patient's appearance, halt curve progression with preservation of the maximum growth potential and preserve cardiopulmonary function. Unfortunately, no procedure to date has been shown to improve cardiopulmonary function; there is usually a reduction in pulmonary function after surgery as the deformed chest can actually be rendered stiffer in the immediately after operation and in the short term (Baydur *et al.*, 1990; Smith *et al.*, 1991a). A period of elective ventilation is common after surgery as the patient recovers from respiratory dependence.

The risks of major spinal surgery for these children should not be taken lightly and need to be considered with the parents and sometimes the patients themselves throughout the treatment programme. This form of operative approach to spinal deformities should only be considered by surgeons who have a special interest and experience in spinal deformities and who have the facilities to deal with the serious potential complications.

Congenital scoliosis

This is a deformity of the spine associated with a primary malformation of the vertebral elements. Although secondary changes in vertebral shape may occur, the primary lesion is often due to failure of segmentation or of formation of the spinal column, and as such is often associated with anomalies of the spinal nerves and spinal cord. Certain forms of bony malformation have a reputation for producing a rapidly progressive spinal deformity at an early age, which can be associated with major problems with rib and chest development and cardiopulmonary compromise as in early-onset scoliosis

(McMaster and Ohtsuka, 1982; McMaster and David, 1986).

When first assessing a congenital spinal lesion, it is important to define the underlying anatomy of the anomaly. Sometimes it is not easy to see the anomaly on plain radiographs. Associated anomalies of the ribs, which may be fused or missing (Fig. 4.24), are suggestive. The simple diagnosis of a jumbled or scrambled spine should not be accepted, and an attempt should be made to analyse the anomaly so that an assessment of the progression potential can be made, though this is not always possible (Fig. 4.25).

The primary bony deformities can be divided into failures of formation, as in wedged or hemivertebrae, and failures of segmentation, as in a block vertebra or unilateral vertebral bars extending over several segments. Although the pattern of vertebral deformity is a good guide to the progression potential of the curve, it is variable and the deformity should be regularly reassessed so that the clinical course becomes apparent. Particular combinations of congenital lesions are recognized for their deforming potential. As with other spinal deformities, the amount of deformity increases at the time of the growth spurts and therefore causes particular problems in the neonatal period and again during the adolescent growth spurt.

Spinal deformity is always initiated during the phase

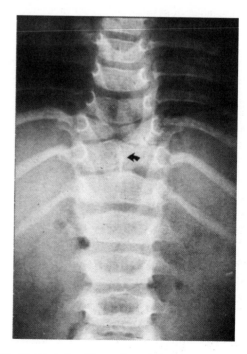

Fig. 4.24 Congenital malformation of the spine with diastematomyelia. Note the widened intrapedicular distance and bony spicule.

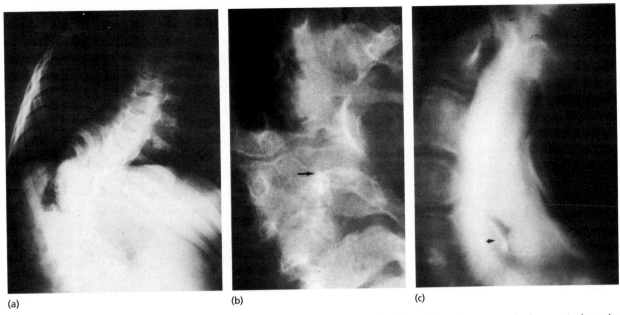

(a)   (b)   (c)

Fig. 4.25 (a) Child with severe congenital scoliosis with many bony anomalies. (b) Plain radiographs suggested a bony spicule at the thoracolumbar junction. (c) Myelography confirmed the presence of diastematomyelia.

of spinal development, and like other congenital lesions can be associated with anomalies in other organs. In addition to the rib fusions mentioned above, there is a higher prevalence of genital, urinary and cardiac anomalies (MacEwen *et al.*, 1972); 20% of patients have urinary anomalies and routine intravenous pyelography or ultrasonography is recommended in all cases of congenital scoliosis. Skin and soft tissue anomalies are often seen, and hairy patches, dimples, haemangiomas or lipomas in the lumbosacral region are particularly important as they may be associated with areas of underlying spinal diastrophism (Figs 4.25, 4.26, 4.27). Associated neurological deficits that occur with congenital scoliosis need to be considered carefully. The child who presents with a cavovarus foot (McMaster and Ohtsuka, 1982), particularly one developing in the juvenile period, has a neuromuscular problem affecting that foot until proved otherwise. The typical lesions to be found are those associated with a tethered spinal cord, including the many degrees of spina bifida, and diastematomyelia (Figs 4.25, 4.26).

Diastematomyelia is a lesion in which the spinal cord is bifid around a bony or fibrous bar which joins the centre of the back of the vertebral body with the inner surface of the underlying lamina (Fig. 4.27). It is suggested that with differential growth of the bony and neural elements, the spinal cord is put under tension by

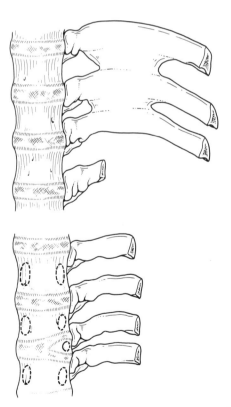

Fig. 4.26 Fused ribs in association with congenital malformation of the spine.

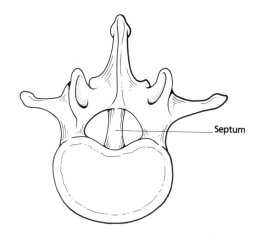

Septum

Fig. 4.27 Relationship of diastematomyelia to the neural canal.

this bar, causing progressive neurological damage, though this is probably an oversimplified explanation. Major problems can follow correction of a spinal deformity when the cord is tethered by diastematomyelia (Winter *et al.*, 1974). The radiological features are shown in Fig. 4.25. The bar is often not seen and the important sign is increased interpedicular distance. Identification of diastematomyelia or suspicion of a spinal cord tether requires detailed investigation with CT myelography or MRI and referral for neurosurgical advice. Even in the absence of a specific lesion, all cases of congenital scoliosis should be considered to have a potential for spinal cord tethering, and the presence of an underlying lesion of the cord must be excluded before treatment. The risk of spinal cord injury during instrumentation is considerably higher than during instrumentation for idiopathic curves, and it is even more important not to lengthen the spinal column during correction.

Simple lesions of vertebral formation or segmentation produce a simple coronal plane growth imbalance of the spine. Congenital spinal deformities, however, can also produce changes in the sagittal plane, leading to the same biomechanical instability to rotation as in idiopathic scoliosis. It is not uncommon to see a congenital lesion in the cervicothoracic region produce sharp kyphosis of this area; the thoracic spine develops compensatory lordosis which then buckles to the side to produce a typical pattern of idiopathic deformity. It is important to identify the underlying congenital lesion because of the reasons outlined above, but only recently has attention been drawn to the sagittal plane deformity of congenital lesions. It is clearly as important as in idiopathic scoliosis (Deacon *et al.*, 1990).

The individual lesions of congenital scoliosis have now been classified with regard to their individual pro-

gression potential (Winter *et al.*, 1968; MacEwen *et al.*, 1972; Winter, 1977). A block vertebra, in which there is symmetrical loss of growth over two or three vertebrae, has usually little potential to produce a progressive deformity. A simple wedged vertebra on one side of the spine tends to produce a slight kink in the spine at that level, but seldom produces a deformity that increases significantly with growth. An individual hemivertebra very occasionally causes problems at the lumbosacral or cervicothoracic region through interference with local spinal balance. If a hemivertebra is found in association with increasing deformity, then it is conventionally treated by posterior fusion (Winter and Moe, 1982). Some surgeons prefer convex epiphysiodesis in order to balance spinal growth with time (McMaster, 1990) or even excision of the hemivertebra (Hall, personal communication). An unsegmented bar has more progression potential than a hemivertebra, and the worst combination is the presence of an unsegmented bar on one side of the spine and a hemivertebra on the other.

MANAGEMENT

In order to assess the need for intervention, the individual features of the deformity must be considered. These include the particular nature and anatomy of the underlying vertebral anomaly, the degree of deformity present at the time of assessment, and of course the age of the patient. A young patient with an already severe deformity associated with an unsegmented bar and a contralateral hemivertebra needs an operation, while a single hemivertebra in the thoracic region of a 7–8-year-old child with little obvious deformity and no clinical functional deficit only needs watching while growth is completed. The presence of an associated neurological lesion is, of course, important, as is consideration of the potential for cardiopulmonary compromise.

Operative treatment

Several elective possibilities are available. While most surgeons agree that posterior spinal fusion is an easy and applicable technique, it is usually used with a simple convex stabilization, e.g. tapes, in infants (Hall, personal communication). Correction of these rigid curves requires great care to be exercised because the associated potential for neurological tethering increases the risk of a neurological lesion. Spinal instrumentation is usually used to stabilize and maintain a degree of correction. When there is severe deformity, an anterior procedure to allow some correction and shortening of the column is essential. In more severe and rigid deformities, the recommended technique is an anteroposterior, staged, closing wedged osteotomy as described above (p. 95). It is even more important in congenital scoliosis that this wedge should be a closing wedge, as the danger of neurological compromise is higher.

One particular congenital problem that warrants special mention is congenital scoliosis located at the cervicothoracic junction. These curves usually consist of combinations of paired hemivertebrae and may be associated with Klippel–Feil syndrome of the cervical spine (see p. 120). Such curves may show little evidence of progression or change until adolescence, at which point progression may result in an unsightly lateral tilting of the head. They can be most safely managed by *in situ* posterior spinal fusion, but sometimes require postoperative immobilization with a halo jacket in order to correct some of the head tilt which may have already developed.

Fortunately, most congenital curves do not produce severe clinical deformity. It is important to emphasize that treatment of spinal deformity should be treatment of the patient's actual deformity and not of the radiographs, because the radiographs can be fascinating. A combination of congenital defects that produces a kink in the spine first to one side and then to the other may produce little visible deformity and can eventually produce a relatively straight column and a balanced torso overall, and not require operative treatment. As with complex surgery for idiopathic scoliosis, the complex congenital cases that require operative treatment must only be treated by those with a wide experience of the techniques.

Scoliosis associated with spina bifida

In addition to the lesions of segmentation described above, developmental problems with formation of the posterior arch produce the typical lesions of spina bifida with meningomyelocoele and myelodysplasia. These patients have a serious neurological deficit in addition to their spinal anomaly, both of which can contribute to the development of scoliosis. In addition to their lower limb problems, patients may develop a spinal deformity which may affect walking or sitting balance and progress with growth. Failure of closure of the neural tube can produce a spectrum of lesions ranging from the commonly found spina bifida occulta, which is only important when associated with a tethered spinal cord, to the full lesion of spina bifida aperta with severe neurological loss.

The major spinal deformities of myelodysplasia fall into one of two characteristic patterns. The first is collapsing lordoscoliosis with a long C-shaped deformity and marked pelvic obliquity in association with subluxation or even dislocation of the hip on the high side and a pressure sore on the low side (Fig. 4.28). This may impair sitting stability so that these patients have to use their arms to hold themselves up. The loss of sitting stability is the principal indication for surgical treatment. Posterior spinal fusion and instrumentation is very difficult due to lack of healthy posterior soft tissue cover and poor formation of the posterior elements. A preliminary anterior procedure with extensive discectomies throughout the lumbar spine for anterior fusion, followed by instrumentation with the Dwyer, Zielke, or one of the newer systems, is essential (Floman *et al.*, 1981b). The posterior stage is very challenging due to the deficiency of the posterior elements, soft tissues and skin. The use of trans-pedicular screws, sublaminar wiring systems and the Galveston technique instrumentation to the pelvis can often provide fixation and stability of the spinal correction.

The second spinal deformity seen with myelodysplasia is severe kyphosis in the lumbar region. There is a short sharp kyphosis, usually present at birth and often progressing rapidly to severe deformity. These children usually have no distal cord function (Hall and Poitras, 1977) (Fig. 4.29). The aetiology of this deformity is

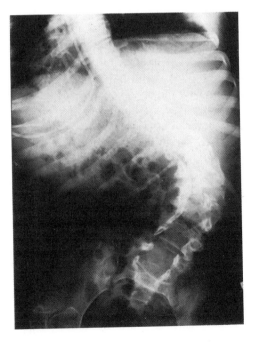

Fig. 4.28 Child with myelodysplasia and progressive thoracolumbar scoliosis. Note dysraphism from D12 to the sacrum.

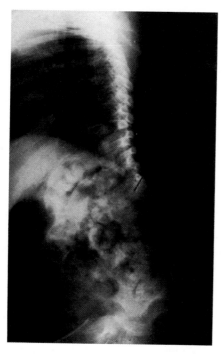

Fig. 4.29 Severe gibbus deformity in a 3-year-old child with myelodysplasia.

quite simple; where the posterior elements fail to meet there is no functioning posterior support, and any functioning tissue is in front of the spine and produces a marked anterior tether. Even the aorta can bowstring across the acute kyphosis, and tissue as anterior as the rectus abdominis forms a major component of the tether. These patients often suffer ulceration over the kyphus and seating problems. Operative treatment of these lesions is complex, requiring neurosurgical and plastic skills to deal with the neural contents of the spinal canal and the poor posterior skin cover. A kyphectomy with combined anterior and posterior approaches may be required with sacrifice of the spinal cord remnant if functionless (Hall and Poitras, 1977; McMaster, 1988).

Neuromuscular scoliosis

A number of different conditions affecting the neuromuscular system (Chapter 3) can be associated with spinal deformity. Anterior poliomyelitis, cerebral palsy, the spinocerebellar degenerative diseases, the muscular dystrophies, the spinal muscle atrophies (including both Werdnig–Hoffman disease and Kugelburg–Welander disease) and relatively rare conditions, e.g. syringomyelia, can all be associated with spinal deformity (Balmer and MacEwen, 1970; Siegal, 1973; Blount and Millencamp, 1977). Given the very different ways in which these conditions affect the neuromuscular system, it must be expected that the incidence, age of onset, curve pattern, rate of progression and the associated spinal deformities will vary. Despite this, certain generalities can be applied to these conditions.

Every child with a neuromuscular condition can develop spinal deformity and should be watched carefully for the onset and progression of spinal deformity. Once a curve has developed, it is likely to progress rapidly. Overall, two types of curve develop, the first being essentially a simple, unsupported flop to the side seen in children who are basically wheelchair-bound. The curve is correctable by traction or suspension and may, while flexible, be supported by bracing or appropriate seating while the child is in the wheelchair. These curves are long, C-shaped curves and represent collapsing kyphosis. With time vertebral growth accommodates to the curve, stiffness develops and correctability is lost.

The second form displays an idiopathic pattern of deformity and typical, rotated, lordoscoliosis occurs. Muscular imbalance and intrinsic unbalanced biomechanics combine to make these curves progress inexorably, soon becoming stiff and unmanageable. External support by bracing is difficult, and is poorly tolerated because of the heavy burden of disability and high incidence of skin breakdown, particularly in children with movement disorders or sensory deficits. The presence of the neurological disease increases the risk of pulmonary insufficiency from associated muscle weakness, e.g. Duchenne dystrophy, and bracing can contribute to this by effectively constricting the already compromised chest.

While spinal fusion is often required in these deformities, careful patient selection is essential. The reason for operation in each case must be clear in the minds of the surgeon, patient and family, and the possible risks and rewards fully assessed. Associated deformities, such as pelvic obliquity or hip contractures, and most importantly the patient's functional ability and problems, must be taken into account in managing these deformities. The best indications for operation include:
1 Loss of sitting stability due to spinal deformity.
2 The development of any curve in Duchenne dystrophy is an indication for fusion to help maintain respiratory function. This is done as soon as the patient becomes wheelchair-bound.
3 On very rare occasions, in order to improve quality of life by improving trunk posture for nursing purposes.
4 In the mildly affected child with good function, the same indications for treatment as discussed above for idiopathic scoliosis apply.

The loss of walking ability is not a direct indication for spinal fusion, as the spine is seldom the cause; fusion robs the patient of useful spinal mobility and often ends walking completely.

In many cases, extensive fusion of the spine may be required across the cervicothoracic or lumbosacral junction, with an increased possibility of pseudo-arthrosis. Combined anterior and posterior fusions and instrumentation are often required to attain adequate correction, stabilization and fusion and to resist the deforming force in many of these curves (McNeice *et al.*, 1980; Floman *et al.*, 1981b; Leatherman and Dickson, 1988).

The Luque system (Galveston technique) is particularly useful for paralytic curves (Fig. 4.30). An additional advantage of this technique is that sufficient internal stabilization can be provided by the instrumentation alone, so that additional post-operative external stabilization with a cast or brace may not be required (Allen and Ferguson, 1981). This is often combined with Dwyer, Zielke, or newer anterior instrumentation and fusion.

Other causes of spinal deformity

As has been noted earlier in this chapter, spinal deformity may be associated with a great variety of diseases.

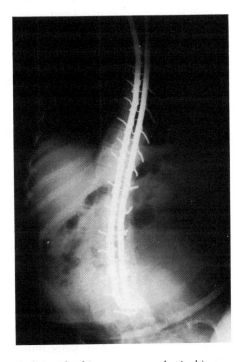

Fig. 4.30 Radiograph of Luque segmental spinal instrumentation for severe neuromuscular scoliosis.

Neurofibromatosis may result in severe deformities of the spine, including those short sharp curves associated with areas of dystrophic vertebrae which may be rapidly progressive (Chaglassion *et al.*, 1976). This deformity often requires both anterior and posterior fusion, as there may be severely dysplastic vertebrae at the curve apex with poor bone stock for fusion; these operations are only for the spinal expert (Winter *et al.*, 1979). Associated neural compression can occur in these deformities and must be carefully ruled out.

Osteogenesis imperfecta can also be associated with rapidly progressive scoliosis. Once a progressive curve is detected, early fusion should be considered. Instrumentation can be used, despite the poor quality of bone, with adjunctive acrylic fixation of proximal and distal hooks (Dawson *et al.*, 1973).

Radiation injury of the spine, such as that occurring after radiation for Wilms' tumour, can also result in short, sharp, scoliotic deformities, usually at the thoracolumbar junction (Riseborough, 1977).

Finally, tumours or infections of the spine may present with reactive scoliosis. A particularly deceptive lesion is osteoid osteoma, which can remain undetected while attention is directed to the associated reactive scoliosis. The underlying lesion can be identified by loss of a pedicle on a plain radiograph, and it stands out easily on a bone scan (Floman *et al.*, 1981a).

KYPHOSIS

Kyphosis, or posterior angulation of the spine, is the opposite deformity from idiopathic scoliosis; it is rotationally stable and represents brittle rather than plastic failure of the column (Dickson and Archer, 1986). There is, of course, normal thoracic kyphosis, the normal range of which probably has an upper limit of 40–50°.

Co-existent kyphosis and scoliosis occur when an area of the spine adjacent to the kyphosis develops compensatory lordosis and then rotates to the side (Deacon *et al.*, 1985); the kyphosis itself does not rotate. As with scoliosis, it is useful to consider the potential problems the patient will face, including deformity, pain and the development of a neurological deficit due to the angulation of the spinal canal over the kyphus, which can increase with growth.

Assessment

In addition to routine history-taking and examination, a simple plain radiograph is the principal method of assessment. The kyphotic deformity does not rotate, so the Cobb technique is a relatively accurate method of determining the degree of deformity. The measurement is taken as the angle subtended from the top of the uppermost vertebra of the curve to the bottom of the lower vertebral body (Fig. 4.31). The principal inaccuracy is finding the top of the upper vertebra and measuring to the edge of a rib by mistake. If an unusual situation or a case with neurological problems presents, additional imaging with CT or MRI may be required.

Aetiology

Kyphotic deformities are usually classified by aetiology as congenital or acquired. There has to be a loss of length in the anterior column or increase in the posterior column.

CONGENITAL KYPHOSIS

As in congenital scoliosis, deformation of spinal elements in congenital kyphosis may be due to either a failure of formation (usually of the anterior portion of the vertebral body) or a failure of segmentation (again of the anterior vertebral body), with subsequent overgrowth of the posterior elements and resultant kyphosis (Tsou, 1977) (Fig. 4.32). It is very important to determine whether kyphosis is congenital in origin, as a management of this deformity can be hazardous and the possibility of neurological compromise as a result of progression of the deformity with growth or with attempted correction is great.

If correction of rigid congenital kyphosis is attempted using distraction techniques, e.g. skeletal traction or Harrington distraction rods, the spinal cord or nerve

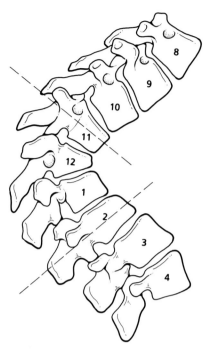

Fig. 4.31 The Cobb technique is used to measure the degree of kyphotic deformity. The angle subtended by the intersection of the top of the most angled vertebra above and the bottom of the most angled vertebra below is determined.

roots can be compressed against the anterior knuckle of bone with paralysis or paraparesis resulting (Fig. 4.33). If neural compromise has occurred as a result of growth alone, anterior decompression in the spine with removal of the apical vertebra may be required in addition to fusion. In common with congenital scoliosis, different patterns of bony anomaly exist; those with marked growth imbalance are at particular risk of progression

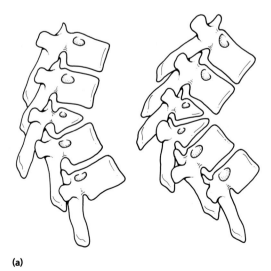

(a)

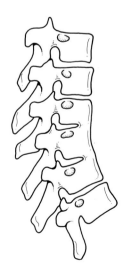

(b)

Fig. 4.32 Congenital anomalies of the spine (a) with failure of formation or (b) with failure of segmentation of the vertebral bodies can progress to severe kyphosis and neurological compromise.

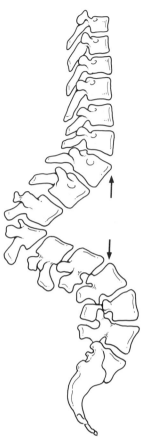

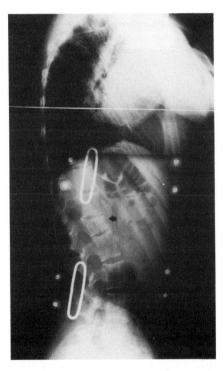

Fig. 4.34 Localized kyphus at the thoracolumbar junction following an old compression fracture.

Fig. 4.33 Distraction of the spine across a rigid kyphotic deformity risks neurological compromise.

and possibly of neurological compromise. Prophylactic posterior fusion may be necessary, as a dorsal hemivertebra that extrudes backwards into the spinal canal is a deformity that commonly puts the neural structures at risk.

ACQUIRED KYPHOSIS

Kyphotic deformities may develop in children as a result of acquired diseases. Spinal trauma, producing anterior column compression and localized short gibbus of the spine, is a typical example (Fig. 4.34). In children this can be complicated by subsequent growth and an increasing kyphosis occasionally develop (Whitesides, 1977). These lesions commonly occur at the thoracolumbar junction, with associated hyperlordosis of the lumbar spine below and subsequent low back pain, in addition to posterior decompensation of the spine.

Unfortunately, post-traumatic kyphosis is a common and serious problem after extensive laminectomy, e.g. for spinal tumours. These decompressions are best per-

formed as a combined approach by orthopaedic and neurosurgeons, allowing intra-operative posterior stabilization. This form of kyphosis is often a problem at the cervicothoracic or thoracolumbar junctions, and subsequent management can be difficult; it is much better prevented. If not fused initially, any child who undergoes an extensive laminectomy should be regularly observed for this condition.

Spinal tuberculosis (Pott's disease)

Historically in the West and currently worldwide tuberculosis is certainly one of the most important causes of acquired kyphosis in children. Hodgson *et al.* (1960) demonstrated the efficacy of anterior decompression and fusion as an aid in eradicating the disease and in preventing further deformity. In some cases, chronic neurological deterioration was avoided using these anterior spinal techniques.

Even in cases where the infectious process has been eradicated, however, as with effective chemotherapy, sufficient destruction of growth plates and bony elements anteriorly may have occurred that progressive deformity and late neurological compromise may result, even into young adulthood.

SCHEUERMANN'S KYPHOSIS AND POSTURAL
ROUNDBACK

The spectrum of idiopathic kyphotic deformities ranges
from just outside normal to postural round-back
and Scheuermann's kyphosis. Opinion varies as to
whether these represent degrees of severity of the same
entity, or whether they represent two distinct entities
(Scheuermann, 1936; Bradford, 1977). The adolescent
growth spurt appears to figure prominently in both. As
it is now clear that idiopathic scoliosis is a deformity due
to lordosis, it is interesting to consider the conditions at
the other end of the spectrum of spinal shape in the
sagittal plane. It has been suggested (Leatherman and
Dickson, 1988) that this spectrum runs from idiopathic
scoliosis (lordosis) to Scheuermann's disease (kyphosis),
with the normal range in between. Lordosis is biomechanically unstable in rotation and therefore produces
scoliosis with growth, while kyphosis is stable and
remains as a midline deformity. This is an attractive
theory and explains the whole spectrum of idiopathic
spinal deformities on simple biomechanical grounds.

With established kyphosis, the lumbodorsal fascia
and hamstrings are tight, and there is accentuated lumbar
lordosis and increased dorsal kyphosis, though many
dispute which comes first. If the dorsal kyphosis is
relatively mild, correctable when the child lies flat and
not associated with wedging of vertebral bodies, it is
called postural round-back. If, however, structural
changes have occurred in the spine and the deformity
is not reversible, it is then established Scheuermann's
kyphosis. Sorenson (1964) described the diagnostic
criteria for Scheuermann's kyphosis; at least three consecutive vertebrae must be involved, each must have at
least 5° of wedging and there are end-plate changes
(Fig. 4.35).

The most common form of Scheuermann's kyphosis is
seen in the mid thoracic region (type I), but there is also
a form (known as apprentice's spine or type II) that
occurs at the thoracolumbar junction. In the latter form
particularly, pain is a common feature, while in type I
cosmetic considerations are important. Although
Scheuermann's kyphosis is often described as epiphysitis,
suggesting an inflammatory process at the vertebral end-
plates, inflammatory changes have not been identified
at biopsy. This condition has also been classed as
an osteochondritis, along with Legg–Calvé–Perthes
disease, Osgood–Schlatter disease, osteochondritis
dissecans and others, but there is increasing evidence
that this classification is inadequate. Perhaps it is only
one extreme of the spinal shape spectrum with secondary
changes in bone growth, as Dickson suggests.

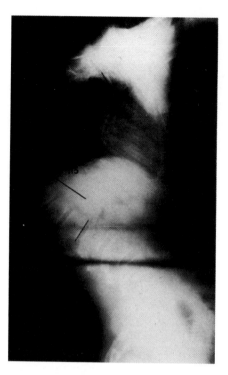

Fig. 4.35 Scheuermann's kyphosis of severe degree (115°) with
anterior vertebral wedging.

An alternative is the microtrauma theory, which
suggests that in the adolescent growth spurt tight lumbar
lordosis develops, normal excursion of the lumbar spine
in forward bending is limited, and bending occurs higher
in the spine—in the thoracic spine—or at the thoracolumbar junction. This results in excessive compression of the vertebral bodies anteriorly at these levels,
with subsequent injury and deformation.

Clinical management

Patients with adolescent-onset kyphosis may present
because of clinical deformity or because of backache.
Back pain may be located in the upper back, but is often
seen at the thoracolumbar junction. Initial physical
evaluation should determine the relative stiffness of the
kyphus, the presence of associated lumbar lordosis, any
decreased flexibility of the muscles and fascia about the
back and pelvis, and associated deformities. Any scoliosis
is often mild and in the associated lordotic segment,
which is protected from significant rotation by the
adjacent rotationally stable kyphotic segment (Deacon
et al., 1985). In addition, a careful neurological evaluation, particularly in the lower extremities, is indicated.
As noted above, the incidence and risk of neurological
compromise in association with kyphotic deformities is
high, particularly with the congenital type.

Radiographic evaluation should include both antero-posterior and lateral spine views. The degree of kyphus is determined using the Cobb technique (Fig. 4.31), and structural changes at the apex of the curve are noted as well as the stage of skeletal maturity. Radiographs should be carefully assessed to ensure that there are no congenital deformities or destructive deformities at the kyphotic apex.

CONSERVATIVE TREATMENT

As kyphosis remains in one plane, biomechanically it is easy to brace by simply pushing the spine into extension. This is the basis of the standard treatment, which can be applied by bracing or casting techniques often combined with extension exercises. The brace can be a Milwaukee-type brace with a free posterior compression pad (Fig. 4.36), along with a dorsal hyperextension and antilordotic exercise programme, but in some patients a low-profile brace can be used (Fig. 4.37). Obliterating the lumbar lordosis also helps by causing compensatory thoracic extension. Brace treatment tends to achieve correction at the more flexible parts of the spine with less effect on the wedged segment (Smith *et al.*, 1991b). While bracing is usual in the USA, serial plaster hyperextension casts are used extensively in Europe. They are effective but are less well accepted than braces.

SURGICAL TREATMENT

In cases of severe kyphotic deformities, usually those greater than 70° with a marked stiff kyphotic segment, operative correction may be considered. The indication for surgery in idiopathic kyphosis depends on the patients, acceptance of the deformity and the presence or absence of pain or neurological symptoms. Posterior fusion alone with heavy Harrington compression instrumentation can satisfactorily realign the spine if preoperative extension radiographs show that the deformity can be reduced to kyphosis of 50° or less (Bradford, 1975; Taylor *et al.*, 1979; Otsuka *et al.*, 1990). In more severe deformities, correction of the rigid apex requires a first-stage anterior release with discectomy and fusion before posterior instrumentation and fusion (Herndon *et al.*, 1981) (Fig. 4.38). In Europe some surgeons combine anterior fusion with kyphosis distraction instrumentation and strut grafting. Bradford (1986) has demonstrated the efficacy of the two-stage approach for correction of this deformity, but has cautioned about the potential for complications associated with this intervention.

In congenital kyphosis, early recognition of a progressive deformity may allow satisfactory treatment by posterior fusion alone. If kyphosis of greater than 60° has already occurred, anterior release and fusion may be

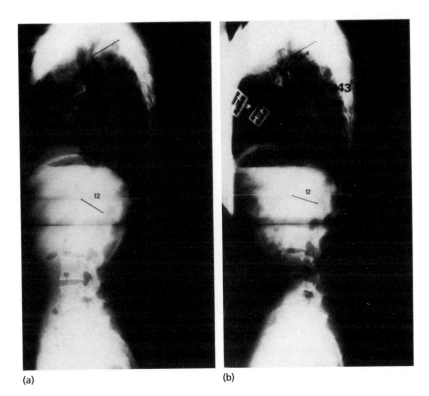

Fig. 4.36 (a) Scheuermann's kyphosis of 55°. (b) Deformity corrected to 43° in a Milwaukee-type brace.

(a)　　　　(b)

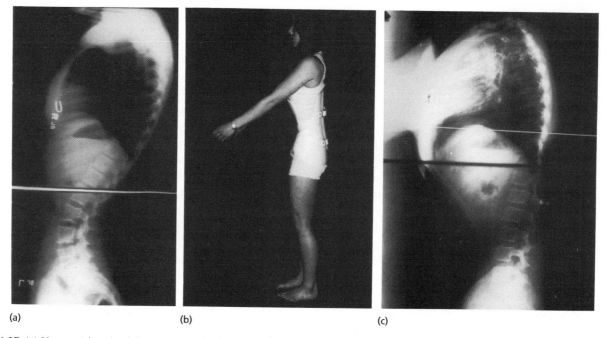

(a)   (b)   (c)

Fig. 4.37 (a) Young girl with adolescent round-back, increased lumbar lordosis and posterior decompensation of the spine. (b) In a low-profile Boston brace. (c) Lateral radiograph showing spine straightening in the brace.

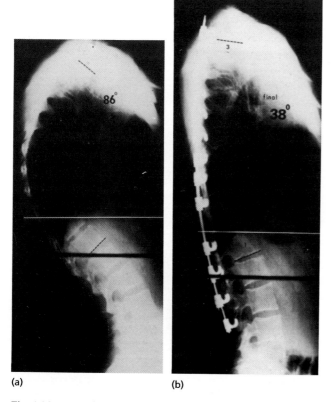

(a)   (b)

Fig. 4.38 (a) Kyphosis of 86° in a 15-year-old boy with back pain. (b) Correction of this deformity to 38° with anterior release and posterior fusion with Harrington compression instrumentation.

required, particularly in type II or incomplete segmentation kyphosis. In the type I lesion, where serious deformity has already occurred, discectomies and *in situ* spinal fusions alone may be appropriate (Winter, 1977). If neurological compromise has occurred, however, anterior cord decompression with strut grafting and fusion may be required.

SPONDYLOLYSIS AND SPONDYLOLISTHESIS (see also Chapter 22)

Spondylolisthesis is the slipping forward of one vertebral body on the body lying caudal to it. It is far more common at the lumbosacral level than at other spine levels until about the age of 50 years, when degenerative forms appear and predominate, often at the L4–L5 levels or higher in the lumbar spine. Spondylolisthesis was first described in 1782 by a Belgian obstetrician, Herbineaux, because of the mechanical problems presented by severe spondylolisthesis during childbirth.

Robert (1854) described the discontinuity in the pars interarticularis region of the neural arch (spondylolysis) that is found in most cases of spondylolisthesis in younger people. Neugebauer noted in 1888 that spondylolisthesis can occur either by discontinuity or by elongation of the pars.

Classification

Most modern authors (Newman, 1963; Wiltse *et al.*, 1974) accept the classification of spondylolisthesis into five types, namely dysplastic (or congenital), isthmic (spondylolytic), traumatic, degenerative and pathological (Fig. 4.39).

Dysplastic or *congenital spondylolisthesis* is associated with hypoplastic instability of the lumbosacral facet joints and spina bifida of L5 and S1. High degrees of slippage occur, usually together with elongation and/or occasionally fracture of the pars interarticularis. This type of spondylolisthesis is twice as common in females as in males.

Isthmic (spondylolytic) spondylolisthesis has a bilateral discontinuity in the pars interarticularis as its primary lesion (Wiltse *et al.*, 1975). The isthmic type is the most common form of spondylolisthesis before the age of 50 years. Isthmic spondylolysis is felt to be a fatigue fracture, with both hereditary and environmental predispositions to the lesion. For example, Caucasian men have about a 6% incidence of spondylolysis, but Caucasian women and North American blacks have a less than 3% incidence (Roche and Rowe, 1951). Some Inuit tribes, in contrast, have a 50% incidence of pars defects (Stewart, 1953). Wiltse (1962) noted a 26% incidence of spondylolysis in the first-order relatives of patients with spondylolisthesis, and considered inheritance to be most consistent with a single recessive gene with incomplete penetrance.

The environmental element in the development of spondylolysis is interesting, because this lesion has never been seen at birth. It only occurs in man, the only mammal with lumbar lordosis and an upright posture. The acquired nature of spondylolysis is highlighted by the example of female gymnasts who have an incidence of pars defects at least three to four times greater than that of their non-gymnastic peers (Jackson *et al.*, 1976). Although spondylolysis usually has a hereditary basis or is associated with chronic stresses, the pars fracture is occasionally secondary to an acute injury, usually severe lordotic stress to the lower lumbar spine.

Traumatic spondylolisthesis is rare, with bilateral acute fractures through the neural arch outside the pars interarticularis, always secondary to severe trauma and usually involving acute neurological deficits. In contrast

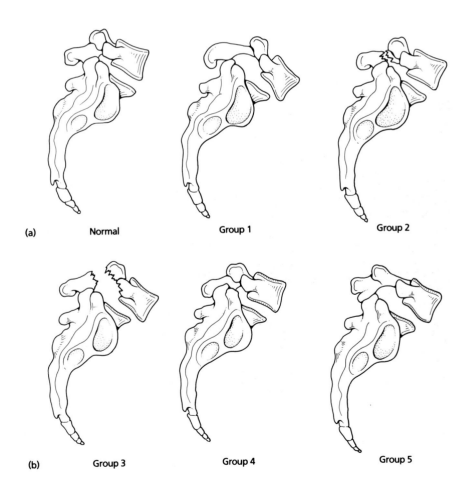

(a)   **Normal**   **Group 1**   **Group 2**

(b)   **Group 3**   **Group 4**   **Group 5**

Fig. 4.39 Types of spondylolisthesis. (a) Normal; Group 1, dysplastic (congenital lumbosacral subluxation); Group 2, isthmic (spondylolytic). (b) Group 3, traumatic; Group 4, degenerative; Group 5, pathological (attenuated pedicles).

to other types, acute spondylolytic lesions usually heal if held in good position.

Degenerative spondylolisthesis is unknown before middle age. It is found only with degenerative arthritis of the lumbar facets and will not be further discussed here.

Pathological spondylolisthesis is another rare type, which has intrinsic mechanical insufficiency of the bone tissue in the neural arch as its primary lesion. Osteogenesis imperfecta and osteoporosis are two representative conditions associated with pathological spondylolisthesis. This type of spondylolisthesis involves repeated pars microfractures, often leading to elongation deformation of the neural arch and forward slip.

Clinical presentation

Spondylolisthesis has two basic clinical presentations in childhood and adolescence. Symptomatic patients with mild degrees of isthmic spondylolisthesis predominantly have low back pain, sometimes with leg pain but seldom with overt neurological deficit. Clinical deformity in these patients, with only slight radiographic slip, is usually minimal (Fig. 4.40a,b) and indeed many patients, even those with forward slip of L5 on S1 of up to 50%, may be symptom free. The aetiology of the back pain in mild-to-moderate spondylolytic spondylolisthesis is not clear, though it is felt by many to be related more to the bony instability than to any slight nerve root compression.

The classic presentation of severe spondylolisthesis with a high degree of slip is that of leg, buttock and back pain with hamstring spasm. Initially, small degrees of slip take the L5 vertebrae forward on S1, but as the slip continues L5 tilts off the front of the sacrum and relative lumbosacral kyphosis occurs. The varied pain syndromes in severe spondylolisthesis are often secondary to combinations of foraminal compression of the L5 nerve roots and anterior compression of the cauda equina by the posterosuperior corner of the sacrum against the posterior elements of L4. Hamstring spasm is very common, but is not easily explained. Perhaps it is a reflex attempt to pull against the sacrum angling forward. The physical appearance of the child with a severe slip is characteristic, with lumbosacral kyphosis tucking the buttocks in. A foreshortened trunk (Fig. 4.41) is often evident, with a palpable lumbosacral step, and the patient walks with an ugly gait with flexed hips and knees. Kyphosis of L5 on S1 remains the primary deformity to be considered in understanding and treating the axial malalignment.

Scoliosis can occur with severe spondylolisthesis and is usually lumbosacral 'sciatic' scoliosis secondary to the asymmetric muscle spasm associated with nerve root irritation. Neurological signs are variably present. Sphincter dysfunction can occur, even though associated disc protrusions are very rare with spondylolisthesis in adolescence and childhood. Progression of slip can be rapid or slow, usually being most rapid during the adolescent growth spurt.

Diagnosis

With the marked deformity described above the diag-

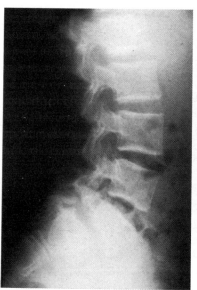

(a)

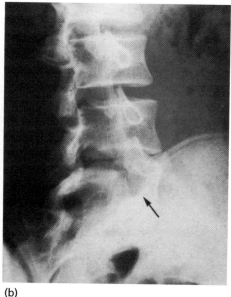

(b)

Fig. 4.40 Diagnosis of spondylolisthesis/ spondylolysis by radiography. (a) Standing lateral radiograph showing mild spondylolisthesis. (b) Spondylolysis demonstrated on an oblique radiograph.

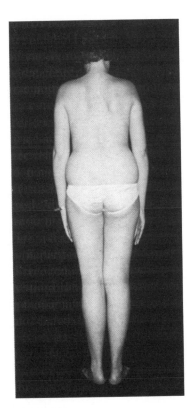

Fig. 4.41 Classic appearance of severe spondylolisthesis. Note the shortened trunk and heart-shaped upper contour of the buttocks from posterior rotation of the sacrum and pelvis.

nosis of severe spondylolisthesis is obvious. Radiological examination is necessary to confirm the problem, which is best seen on a standing lateral film of the lumbosacral spine (Fig. 4.40a). Oblique radiographs or tomography may sometimes be required to demonstrate spondylolysis (Fig. 4.40b), which is shown by the appearance of a break or a collar across the 'Scottie dog's' neck, the illusion created by the projection of the posterior vertebral elements on the oblique view.

Meyerding's classification of the percentage of slip is widely used and is as follows: grade I spondylolisthesis, 0–25%; grade II, 25–50%; grade III, 50–75%; and grade IV, more than 75% (Fig. 4.42a) (Meyerding, 1932). Boxall *et al.* (1979) introduced other measurements in addition to the simple degree of slip. The most useful is the slip angle (Fig. 4.42b), which represents the degree of forward tilting of the L5 body on the sacrum and correlates well with both clinical deformity and rate of progression.

Treatment

ISOLATED SPONDYLOLYSIS

Asymptomatic patients with spondylolysis without slip require no treatment at any age. While spondylolysis without spondylolisthesis has traditionally been considered unlikely to cause symptoms in skeletally immature patients, young athletes may present with low back pain and spondylolysis, with or without a history of acute onset of pain or injury. A physical examination in this situation may be non-diagnostic, or it may reveal only a lower lumbar tenderness or pain on hyperextension of the lumbar spine. Spondylolysis may be unilateral and may be visible only on oblique radiographs (Fig. 4.40b), or by tomography or CT when the gantry angle has to be reversed in order to line up with the pars defect. Sometimes the only finding on a plain radiograph is a sclerotic pedicle on the unfractured side, which represents a confusing compensatory hypertrophic reaction (Sherman *et al.*, 1977). Both the sclerotic pedicle and the pars defect will show increased uptake on radionuclide bone scanning. Increased activity of the pars defect is a feature carrying a good prognosis for healing and resolution of symptoms with bracing. If a unilateral or bilateral symptomatic pars defect shows no increased uptake on radionuclide scanning, healing may be less likely, but resolution of symptoms with bracing is still quite possible (Steiner and Micheli, 1985).

An individual who remains symptomatic with painful spondylolysis unresponsive to conservative treatment is a candidate for operation. This may include simple *in situ* posterolateral fusion to the sacrum in the case of L5 lesions, or *in situ* fusion of the pars defect with transverse process to spinal process wiring (Micheli, 1985).

It must also be remembered that many adolescents and children with simple spondylolysis have no symptoms, and other causes of back pain must be ruled out before embarking on treatment directed at the pars lesion. The differential diagnosis of back pain in young people includes neoplasm or infection of bone (Wenger *et al.*, 1978), neural elements (Tachkjan and Matson, 1965), or retroperitoneum, as well as disc prolapse.

The preferred spinal orthosis in the treatment of symptomatic spondylolysis and of progressive spondylolisthesis, with or without symptoms, is an anterior opening polypropylene antilordotic brace with prefabricated components in variable degrees of lumbar flexion (Fig. 4.43). It is individually fitted and used only in conjunction with an aggressive physiotherapy programme to maintain abdominal muscle tone and hip

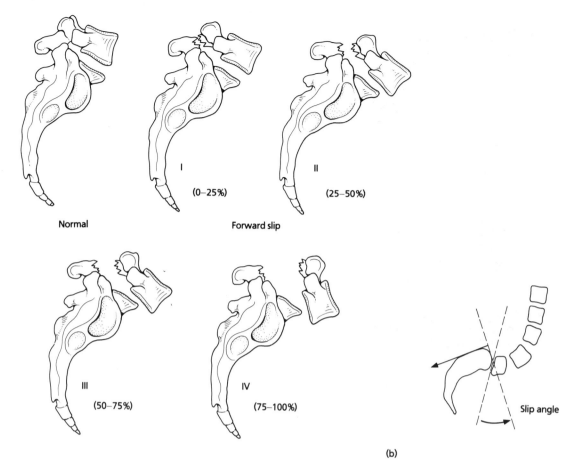

(a)

(b)

Fig. 4.42 Measurement of spondylolisthesis. (a) Meyerding grade (percentage of forward slip). (b) Slip angle.

flexor and hamstring flexibility. The brace acts on the lumbar lordosis above the unstable lumbosacral segment to reduce the shearing forces across the lumbosacral junction. Some centres use hyperextension pantaloon spica casts to reduce severe spondylolisthesis, which act primarily on the kyphotic sacrum by levering through the maximally extended hip joints.

DYSPLASTIC AND ISTHMIC SPONDYLOLISTHESIS

Asymptomatic spondylolisthesis in childhood and adolescence may simply be observed until slip reaches 25%. At this point, institution of antilordotic bracing and physiotherapy to maintain abdominal muscle tone should be considered, particularly if L5 is beginning to tilt and is trapezoidal in shape; such trapezoidal shape of L5 and rounding off of the anterior edge of S1 predispose to rapid forward slip. If anterior slip reaches one-third of the length of S1, bracing, physiotherapy and activity restriction are considered as a minimum of treatment, even in the absence of symptoms. Such

asymptomatic children should be followed with a standing lateral lumbosacral radiograph no less often than every 4–6 months. If further slip occurs in asymptomatic children but is no more than grade II, bilateral intertransverse fusion can be carried out, usually from L4 to the sacral alae, packing cancellous bone graft in the facet joints as well as the lateral gutters (Hensinger *et al.*, 1976). The patient is mobilized in a plastic orthosis during the second post-operative week.

SYMPTOMATIC PATIENTS

The child or adolescent with back or leg pain in spondylolisthesis is unlikely to have another source for his pain, in contrast to the adult with spondylolisthesis. Attention should be directed towards this lesion in such symptomatic young people, and management quickly moves beyond abdominal strengthening exercises and activity restriction to antilordotic bracing if symptoms do not improve greatly in a few weeks. If neither the symptoms nor the progressive spondylolisthesis are controlled by opening plastic orthosis must be worn until the fusion is radiographically sound (usually after 4−6 months).

If the spondylolisthesis is 50% or more, particularly if the tilt angle is 30° or more (Boxall *et al.*, 1979), the intertransverse fusion has to go to at least L4. The spondylolisthesis can be partially reduced and stabilized by employing Harrington distraction rods (Fig. 4.44) or more recently a wired-in Luque box. The treatment of severe spondylolisthesis is quite varied, with many surgeons preferring to fuse *in situ*, no matter how severe the deformity (Hensinger *et al.*, 1976), usually keeping patients with high-grade slip supine in a pantaloon spica cast for 3 months before allowing ambulation in a brace. Other centres, following Ascani's and Scaglietti's technique (Scaglietti *et al.*, 1976), apply hyperextension body casts pre-operatively for 3−4 months to reduce the deformity before carrying out posterior fusion with internal fixation of the upper lumbar spine to the sacrum. Other surgeons again (Bradford, 1979; DeWald *et al.*, 1981) employ both posterior and anterior fusions for grade III or grade IV spondylolisthesis, both to facilitate more complete reduction and to ensure high rates of fusion. Even with these two-stage fusions, most authors recommend 3 months of recumbency. Recent experience with segmental fixation using pedicle screws and fusion holds promise for both stabilization and, in some cases, reduction of the slip (Dick and Schnebel, 1988).

Brief mention must be made of the Gill procedure (Gill *et al.*, 1955) — the removal of the loose posterior elements of L5 (rattle fragment) in isthmic spondylolisthesis — if only to condemn its isolated use in children. While this form of limited posterior decompression may occasionally be useful in symptomatic adults, the Gill procedure will only hasten slip in an immature patient unless simultaneous arthrodesis is performed.

TRAUMATIC SPONDYLOLISTHESIS

Minimally displaced traumatic spondylolisthesis will usually heal with spinal immobilization. Severe degrees of displacement will usually require open reduction and internal fixation, particularly if a partial neurological deficit is present. The internal fixation technique, and indeed the open reduction technique, must be tailored to the individual needs of the particular anatomical situation.

SCOLIOSIS ASSOCIATED WITH SPONDYLOLISTHESIS

If spasm occurs, lumbar scoliosis can develop secondary to spondylolisthesis. It is a typical non-structural

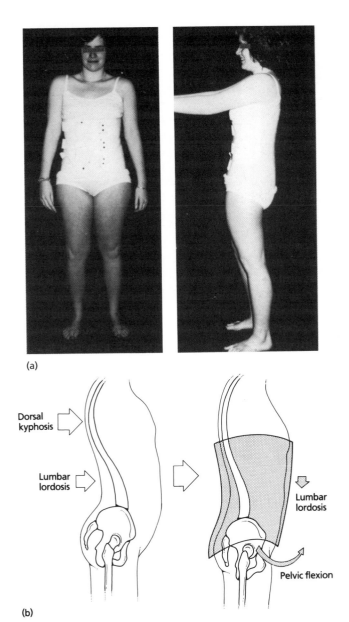

(a)

(b)

Dorsal kyphosis

Lumbar lordosis

Lumbar lordosis

Pelvic flexion

Fig. 4.43 Bracing for spondylolysis and spondylolisthesis. (a) Anterior opening polypropylene antilordotic brace. (b) Forces exerted by the brace on the lumbosacral junction.

bracing and the exercise programme, then surgical stabilization is required. For patients with grade I spondylolisthesis with no tilting of L5, the authors suggest a one-level lumbosacral intertransverse fusion. If the slip is a grade II type and the tilt angle is up to 30°, bilateral intertransverse fusion from L4 to the sacrum is preferred as the L5 transverse process is too far forward and the fusion mass would lie too horizontal and at a major biomechanical disadvantage. Immobilization is required when the operative discomfort settles, and an anterior

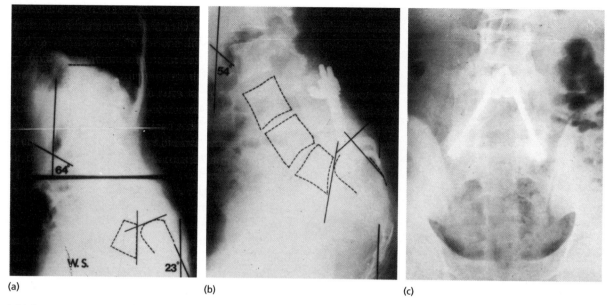

Fig. 4.44 Instrumentation and fusion in the treatment of severe spondylolisthesis. (a) Pre-operative lateral radiograph. (b) Post-operative lateral and (c) anteroposterior radiographs showing partial reduction with Harrington rods and solid L3–S1 arthrodesis.

scoliosis and will resolve when solid lumbosacral arthrodesis is achieved. If lumbosacral scoliosis associated with spondylolisthesis has some structural elements (and shift of the trunk without adequate compensation above by another small scoliotic curve), meticulous postoperative body casting techniques may be needed to restore balance (Goldstein *et al.*, 1976). If structural scoliosis that seems totally independent of the spondylolisthesis is present, it should be treated as an independent problem. This is true even if surgical stabilization of the scoliosis down to or near the spondylolisthesis is necessary, as such arthrodesis seems not to affect the natural history of the spondylolisthesis itself.

DISCITIS (see also Chapter 15, p. 420)

Discitis is a non-specific term for a spectrum of inflammatory conditions involving the intervertebral disc and the adjacent vertebral end-plates in skeletally immature individuals. It usually occurs in the lower thoracic or lumbar spine (Menelaus, 1964; Smith and Taylor, 1967; Wenger *et al.*, 1978). The classic presentation is a child with back pain and stiffness, fever, increased erythrocyte sedimentation rate and radiographic narrowing of an intervertebral disc space at a level consistent with the symptoms. Traditionally, a bacterial aetiology has been favoured, but trauma, apophysitis (e.g. Scheuermann's kyphosis), or idiopathic disc space calcification may be the cause of symptoms in some of these patients.

Anatomy and pathology

The intervertebral disc in skeletally immature patients has numerous vascular connections to the bone vertebral end-plates (Somogyi, 1964), which in turn have been shown to be readily accessible to bacteria or septic emboli from the general circulation (Wiley and Trueta, 1959). This makes direct haematogenous spread of bacteria to the intervertebral disc a plausible aetiology for disc space infection in children. In adults older than 30 years, however, intradiscal vascular channels are rare (Coventry *et al.*, 1945), and disc space infection may be secondary to late invasion from a paravertebral abscess or advanced vertebral osteomyelitis. This may account for the much poorer prognosis and resistant nature of adult disc space infection compared with symptomatic disc space narrowing noted in childhood, even when groups with similar organisms cultured from the involved discs are compared.

Clinical presentation

A child with discitis usually has several days of malaise and pyrexia, often preceded by an upper respiratory tract infection. Most children will have some element of back pain, postural abnormality (loss of lumbar lordosis, loss of thoracic kyphosis) and back stiffness. Two other distinct presentations have been noted by Wenger *et al.* (1978) in their review of 41 patients in Toronto. In one, abdominal pain is the primary complaint, usually being an ache of gradual onset radiating from the upper abdominal quadrants towards the pubic symphysis. Although these patients have no localizing signs in the abdomen, extensive diagnostic studies of the abdomen and contents are often made before intra-abdominal pathology can be ruled out. This means that abnormalities of the spine in this group are usually noted only late, often several weeks after presentation (the mean duration of symptoms before diagnosis was more than 6 weeks in the Toronto series). A third distinct presentation found in young children (mean age about 2 years) is characterized by difficulty in walking or standing, sometimes to the point of refusing to do either. Localizing findings are often not noted on an initial examination, but once the diagnosis of discitis is reached, localized spinal tenderness and spasm are usually noted. Spinal cord tumour may be an early diagnostic consideration in this group (Tachkjan and Matson, 1965).

Diagnosis

When a child presents in any of the above ways, a full blood count, erythrocyte sedimentation rate, urinalysis, blood cultures, and anteroposterior and lateral plain radiographs of the entire spine should be obtained as a minimum. If the radiographs reveal disc space narrowing, particularly if associated with any peridiscal erosion of the vertebral end-plates, a radionuclide scan,

e.g. with technetium diphosphonate, is probably not necessary to make the diagnosis (Fig. 4.45). If radiographs are normal, technetium bone scanning is indicated.

Use of technetium bone scanning in the diagnosis of discitis is a recent great advance (Gilday *et al.*, 1975; Treves *et al.*, 1976) (Fig. 4.46). If a scan is positive, it usually obviates the need for other studies, such as abdominal contrast studies or myelography. False-positive and false-negative rates associated with radionuclide scanning in the diagnosis of discitis are not available, but judicious comparison of the scan with radiographs should eliminate most confusion of discitis with fractures, Scheuermann's kyphosis and other conditions.

The syndrome of *idiopathic disc calcification* (Asadi, 1959; Melnick and Silverman, 1963) can be diagnosed if fluffy calcific densities appear in the nucleus pulposus at the symptomatic level 1–2 weeks following the onset of symptoms in the cervical or thoracic spine. This usually occurs in a clinical background virtually indistinguishable from that of discitis. Symptoms usually last 3–4 weeks, but may be intermittent for 1 year or more. The calcification may disappear in a few months or may be permanent.

False-negatives have not been reported with the use of bone scanning to diagnose discitis, though a plain radiograph can certainly still fail to show definite disc space

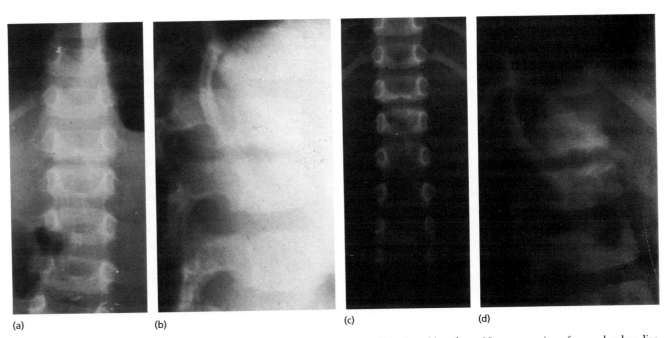

(a)   (b)   (c)   (d)

Fig. 4.45 Disc space narrowing in discitis. (a,b) 4-year-old male with sore, stiff back and low fever. Note narrowing of upper lumbar disc space. Symptoms resolved after 6 weeks in a body cast. (c,d) Radiographs 1 year later show restoration of disc space height.

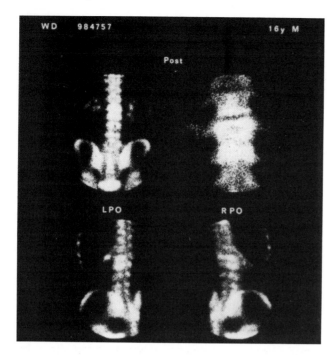

WD   984757   16y M

Post

LPO   RPO

Fig. 4.46 Positive technetium scan shaving discitis in a 16-year-old with back pain and malaise. Plain radiographs were normal. The scan shows greatly increased uptake around the disc space, strongly suggestive of discitis.

narrowing at a time in the disease process when the radionuclide uptake is intense.

The use of disc space or vertebral body aspiration in the diagnosis of discitis and related conditions should be reserved for patients with persistent symptoms despite adequate treatment or if tuberculosis, other fungal infection, or neoplasia is strongly suspected. When performed in discitis, aspiration and cultures have been positive in about 40–50% of cases and almost always for *Staphylococcus aureus* (Speigel *et al.*, 1972).

Treatment

Resting the spine is the most important element in the treatment of discitis, whether the disorder is thought to be primary vertebral osteomyelitis, primary pyogenic discitis, or an idiopathic aseptic inflammatory lesion of the disc. Some favour simple bed-rest until signs and symptoms resolve; others add a body jacket to make the resting of the spine more complete. Still other physicians add antibiotics, particularly if the patient has toxaemia on presentation or if symptoms do not resolve within a few days of resting the spine. Wenger *et al.* (1978) suggest intravenous antibiotics until the patient can walk and move comfortably, usually 2–3 days after beginning treatment, with an additional arbitrary 3

weeks of oral therapy; they suggest either a cephalosporin or any penicillinase-resistant synthetic penicillin as satisfactory.

The authors' preference in treatment is to put all children to bed initially, and to immobilize them in a light body jacket in a neutral position for about 4 weeks if symptoms do not disappear within 1 week of starting bed-rest. Antibiotics are given only if patients present in toxic fashion, if blood cultures are positive, or if there is no response to the body jacket.

Sequelae

The authors have had no experience of the formation of frank paravertebral abscess in association with discitis, though it has been reported in the literature. Spontaneous interbody fusion as a complication of discitis has been reported, but is rare. Gradual restitution of the disc space to its pre-morbid height with remodelling of the eroded vertebral end-plates is the usual course.

Wenger *et al.* (1978) reported two patients in the Toronto series who required posterior spine fusions to control symptoms of back pain that persisted, despite their usual course of treatment with antibiotics and immobilization.

THE CERVICAL SPINE (see also Chapter 21)

Klippel–Feil syndrome

In 1912 Klippel and Feil described a patient with a low posterior hair-line, shortening of the neck and marked restriction of neck motion, who was found at autopsy to have complete fusion of the cervical spine. Klippel–Feil syndrome currently refers to all patients with any element of cervical fusion, only a minority of whom will have the three clinical findings originally described. Of greatest functional significance is the relation of the extent of cervical fusion to the stability of the C1–C2 articulation. Extensive mid- and lower cervical fusion can lead to compensatory hypermobility in the upper cervical spine that is potentially dangerous or even lethal. Recent investigations, particularly by Hensinger *et al.* (1976), have shown important abnormalities associated with Klippel–Feil syndrome (Table 4.2).

ASSOCIATED CONDITIONS

The scoliosis associated with Klippel–Feil syndrome (60%) is often congenital in nature, but is not necessarily so. High thoracic scoliosis associated with Klippel–Feil syndrome may indeed cause more problems than the

Table 4.2 Extraspinal abnormalities associated with Klippel—Feil syndrome

Abnormality	Incidence (%)
Renal anomalies	35
Sprengel's deformity	30
Deafness	30
Synkinesia	20
Facial asymmetry/neck web/torticollis	20
Congenital heart disease	14

syndrome itself. For example, decompensated progressive high thoracic scoliosis in association with a stiff cervical spine may not only be associated with very severe clinical deformity (Fig. 4.47), but may also interfere with binocular vision. In addition, there can be severe restriction of rib cage movement associated with congenital thoracic curves. It is obvious that scoliosis associated with Klippel—Feil syndrome needs careful, continued, observation and often vigorous treatment throughout the growing years and beyond.

Renal abnormalities are found in 35% of patients with Klippel—Feil syndrome (Hensinger *et al.*, 1976), with most of them being asymptomatic at least during childhood, sometimes until irreparable damage has been done to the genitourinary system. Intravenous pyelography is recommended as a routine procedure for all children with Klippel—Feil syndrome. The most common

anomaly in the renal system is unilateral absence of a kidney.

Hearing impairments of various kinds, up to and including deafness, are reported in over 30% of patients with Klippel—Feil syndrome (Palant and Carter, 1972). No single, characteristic, audiological anomaly is found. All patients should undergo early audiometric testing to permit early speech and language training where it is appropriate.

Synkinesia, or mirror motions, is found in about 20% of patients. Its aetiology is unclear, though it is suspected to be connected with incomplete decussation of the phyramidal tracts through the cervical region (Gunderson and Solitaire, 1968). This condition appears to improve somewhat as the patient matures, though two-handed activities that require reciprocal movements with the two hands may always be difficult for these patients.

Congenital heart disease is noted in more than 10% of patients with Klippel—Feil syndrome (Morrison and Scott, 1968), with ventricular septal defect being the most common lesion.

ORTHOPAEDIC PROBLEMS

Hypermobility in the unfused cervical joints leads to most of the orthopaedic problems in the cervical region for patients with Klippel—Feil syndrome. Specifically, there are three high-risk patterns of movement in the cervical spine which can be closely correlated with late

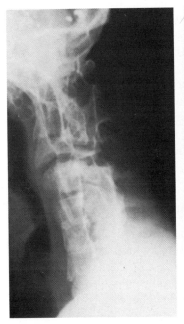 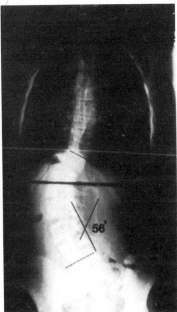

Fig. 4.47 Scoliosis associated with Klippel—Feil syndrome in a 13-year-old girl with multiple cervical spine segmentation defects and severe progressive thoracolumbar scoliosis. There were no apparent anomalies in the scoliotic spinal segments.

instability or degenerative osteoarthritis (Fielding *et al.*, 1978):

1 Pattern 1 consists of fusion of C2 and C3 with occipitalization of the atlas (McRae, 1954). This leads to greatly accentuated flexion and extension at the C1—C2 level, and hypermobility of the odontoid is very common with advancing age.

2 Pattern 2 consists of complete or nearly complete cervical fusion with an abnormal occipitocervical junction. This pattern again concentrates enormous forces about an abnormal odontoid or hypoplastic ring of C1. The long cervical fusion does not influence prognosis so much if the C1—C2 articulation is totally normal.

3 High-risk pattern 3 consists of any pattern where there is a single, open interspace between two, long, fused segments. This clear example of force concentration can be seen on radiographs at the level at which the cervical spine seems to hinge.

TREATMENT OF ORTHOPAEDIC PROBLEMS RELATED TO KLIPPEL—FEIL SYNDROME

The treatment of scoliosis has been dealt with briefly in a previous section (see p. 102). Treatment of secondary instability is of major concern. Patients at risk from abnormal cervical motion are advised to avoid contact sports. It is difficult to generalize about the indication, for surgical stabilization at the cost of further decreasing a patient's already severely limited range of cervical motion. The utmost caution should be given to the treatment of symptoms suggesting nerve root or cord compression. Combined evaluations by neurologists, neurosurgeons and orthopaedic surgeons are essential in dealing with cervical spines that contain so many more abnormal components than are found in the normal spine.

Treatment of the cosmetic deformities associated with Klippel—Feil syndrome has been in general unrewarding, though the use of scapular mobilization procedures, such as the Woodward procedure (Woodward, 1961) in treating Sprengel's deformity, has occasionally been valuable.

Congenital anomalies of the odontoid

The odontoid originates from the first cervical sclerotome as the original centrum of C1. It becomes separated from C1 and later fuses with the rest of the axis. At birth, the tip of the odontoid is typically unossified and is represented by a V-shaped cleft. At about the age of 3 years, a small ossification centre appears within the

V-shaped cleft. This is known as the ossiculum terminale, and it fuses with the remainder of the odontoid by the age of 12 years (Rothman and Simeone, 1975). The physis at the base of the dens is present at birth and until fusion, usually by the age of 6 years, it lies well below the level of the superior articular facets of the axis. It should never, therefore, be confused with fractures of the odontoid, which almost always lie well above this level.

Congenital or acquired abnormalities of the odontoid are of clinical significance in proportion to the amount of instability of C1 on C2 with which they are associated. Gross instability of C1 on C2 can lead to sudden death. Congenital abnormalities of the odontoid range from complete absence to hypoplasia of the os odontoideum, which represents a potential or actual separation of the odontoid process from the body of C2. Such os odontoideum can have either a congenital or developmental basis, with case reports in the literature clearly demonstrating the development of os odontoideum where a radiographically normal odonto process had been present earlier (Fielding and Griffin, 1974).

EVALUATION OF ODONTOID ANOMALIES

Open-mouth, anteroposterior and lateral radiography of the upper cervical spine are essential in initial evaluation of odontoid anatomy. Tomography is often necessary because of the density of structures overlying the areas of interest. Flexion and extension lateral radiographs of the upper cervical spine are also very important, with attention directed to the amount of anteroposterior displacement of C1 on C2 during flexion and extension. Fielding *et al.* (1978) note that if measurements are taken from a line projected superiorly from the anterior border of the body of the axis to the posterior border of the anterior arch of the atlas, any measurement of displacement greater than 4 mm is considered pathological. In addition, Fielding's 'rule of thirds' is useful in evaluating the space available for the cord, as normally in the upper cervical spine one-third of the available space is taken up by the odontoid, a second third of the space is taken up by the cord, and the remaining third is normally soft tissue.

SPECIFIC ABNORMALITIES

Aplasia is an extremely rare abnormality recognizable any time after birth from the open-mouth radiograph and characterized by absence of the basilar portion of the odontoid. Hypoplasia is similarly recognizable in the open-mouth view as a shortened peg of odontoid projecting minimally, if at all, above the lateral facets. Os odontoideum is recognized radiographically as a centrally radiolucent oval ossicle with sclerotic borders usually located where the normal odontoid tip would be found. Tomography may be necessary to detect os odontoideum, which may be virtually impossible to differentiate from a non-union following an odontoid fracture in early childhood. Odontoid non-unions generally have irregular margins, though not necessarily so (Fig. 4.48).

Clinical findings associated with the various aforementioned odontoid dysplasias are secondary to instability of C1 on C2. These symptoms can, therefore, range from none to those associated with severe myelopathy. Fatigue, specific weakness and a variety of upper motor neurone signs and symptoms are relatively commonly found (Schiller and Nieda, 1957; Rowland *et al.*, 1958).

Treatment of C1—C2 instability associated with odontoid dysplasia

The basic treatment for C1—C2 instability is stabilization of C1 on C2. Once the diagnosis is made in children, it is usually more conservative to proceed with surgical stabilization than to expect a child to curtail his activity. The posterior approach is standard for a C1—C2 fusion, using the technique of Gallie. If there is abnormality at the articulation between the skull and C1, then the fusion may have to be extended to the skull (Fig. 4.49).

Occipitocervical synostosis

This involves varying degrees of congenital union between the base of the skull and C1. Tomography is often necessary to clarify abnormalities in this region, which commonly involve fusion of at least the anterior arch of the atlas into the occiput. Atlantoaxial instability is found in at least one-half of the patients with occipitocervical synostosis. A common non-bony anomaly of this region involves posterior encroachment on the upper cervical cord by a constricting band of dura. Both this finding, and the finding of herniation of the cerebellar tonsils, can be demonstrated by myelography.

Most patients have a clinical appearance similar to that of Klippel—Feil syndrome, with associated extra-cervical conditions similar in range to those associated with Klippel—Feil syndrome.

Treatment of occipitocervical synostosis and the commonly found instability lying just inferior to it is hazardous. The distorted anatomy makes attempts at reduction before C1—C2 fusion attractive in some ways, but still hazardous.

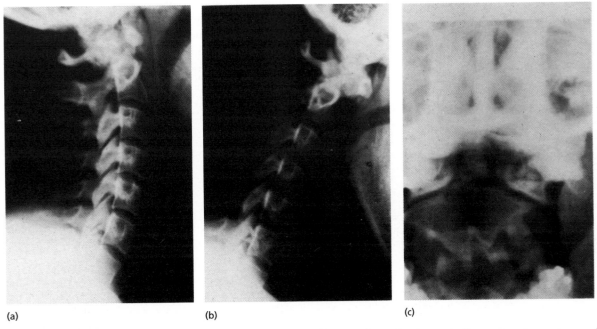

(a) (b) (c)

Fig. 4.48 Os odontoideum in a 16-year-old girl with neck ache and stiffness, and occasional arm tingling and weakness, 1 year after an automobile accident. She originally was thought to have cervical sprain. Abnormal mobility of C1 and C2 was confirmed with voluntary flexion—extension views. (a) Neutral. (b) Flexion. (c) Anteroposterior view.

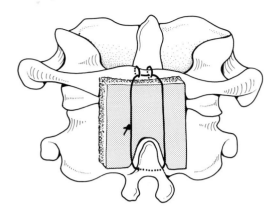

Fig. 4.49 Gallie fusion for C1–C2 instability. A carefully shaped block of corticocancellous iliac bone graft is wired snugly to the lightly decorticated posterior elements of C1 and C2 with no. 20 wire as illustrated. Post-operative immobilization depends on the cervical bone stock and patient cooperation. A Kirschner wire may be driven across the C2 spinous process to provide further fixation for the wire.

Congenital muscular torticollis

This is a commonly observed condition during the first 2 months of life, due to sternocleidomastoid muscle contracture with tilting of the head toward the involved side and rotation of the chin toward the contralateral shoulder (Jones, 1968) (Fig. 4.50). A small knot of tissue is often palpable in the involved sternocleidomastoid muscle in the first 2–3 weeks of life (Coventry and Harris, 1959). This has been suggested by some to represent a residual of birth trauma. If the condition is allowed to persist or is progressive, asymmetry of the face and skull can ensue due to the infant's lying consistently with his head turned one way as he sleeps.

AETIOLOGY

Most observers agree that fibrosis of the sternocleidomastoid muscle body is a part of this condition (Coventry and Harris, 1959; Jones, 1968). There is no complete agreement as to whether it is due to idiopathic occlusion of venous outflow from the muscle (Brooks, 1922). In 75% of cases, the lesion occurs on the right side, and 20% of children with congenital muscular torticollis have some element of congenital hip dysplasia (Hummer and MacEwen, 1972). Very occasionally, apparent congenital muscular torticollis can be due to bony abnormality within the cervical spine, making radiography of the cervical spine wise in a persistent case.

TREATMENT

Stretching exercises are appropriate treatment for the young infant with congenital muscular torticollis and can be expected to produce complete resolution within a few months in about 90% of cases (Coventry and Harris, 1959). The exercises consist of gentle stretching of the head to position the ear opposite the contracted muscle to the opposite shoulder and touching the chin to the ipsilateral shoulder. In addition, the child should be placed in his crib so that he will always tend to turn towards his toys so as to stretch out his deformity.

Operation is only occasionally necessary in congenital muscular torticollis and should usually be delayed for at least 2 years after birth to make certain that persistent stretching will not produce correction. As long as open release of the contracted muscle is carried out before the child is of school age, good resolution of any facial

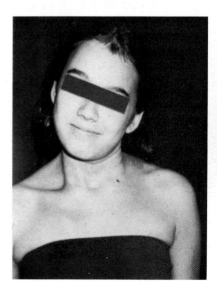

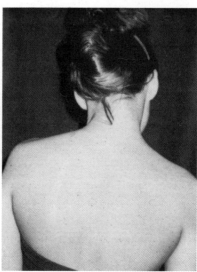

Fig. 4.50 Congenital muscular torticollis. Classical presentation, with the head turned away from but tilted towards the side of the tight sternocleidomastoid muscle.

asymmetry can be expected (Coventry and Harris, 1959).

Distal release is all that is usually required, provided that both heads of the sternocleidomastoid muscle are sectioned and the deep fascia is also completely divided (Staheli, 1971). The distal skin incision occasionally leads to the formation of an unattractive scar. Only very occasionally is a proximal incision at the mastoid process necessary. Post-operatively, the child should undergo passive stretching exercises similar to those before surgery.

Torticollis due to bony anomalies

Childhood torticollis can be caused by a number of bony anomalies, all of which are much less common than the congenital muscular variety (Table 4.3). Basically, bony torticollis is due to congenital or acquired anomalies of the craniocervical junction, and most of the congenital causes have been mentioned in the previous section. Of the acquired anomalies, by far the most common is atlantoaxial rotary subluxation (Fielding and Hawkins, 1977), which seems to involve a ligamentous laxity of the C1–C2 facet joints, usually following an upper respiratory tract infection. It may also occur spontaneously following trauma and may occasionally occur when the patient is turning his neck through an apparently normal range of movement. In

Table 4.3 Differential diagnosis of torticollis

Congenital
Congenital muscular torticollis
Occipitocervical bony anomalies
Webbing of neck skin

Acquired
Neurogenic (tumours, cranial nerve palsies, etc.)
Inflammatory (pyogenic, rheumatic, tuberculous)
Traumatic (overt or hidden)
Idiopathic

such a situation the patient is suddenly unable to return his head to a neutral position.

The radiographic features of atlantoaxial rotary subluxation or 'fixation' are definite when demonstrated, but are often difficult to demonstrate because of malalignment of the head, often due to discomfort of the patient. Cineradiography is an excellent technique in demonstrating movement of C1 and C2 together (fixation of C1 on C2) during attempts at rotation. Tomography may also elucidate the abnormal rotation or the atlantoaxial articulation (Fig. 4.51).

The classic clinical appearance of atlantoaxial rotary fixation is the so-called 'cock robin' position, with the head tilted to one side and rotated to the opposite side with slight cervical flexion. In acute cases, the child will

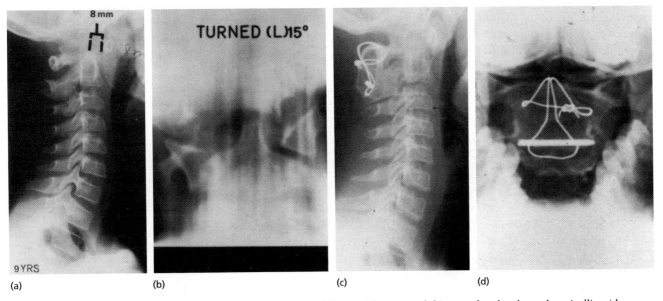

(a)   (b)   (c)   (d)

Fig. 4.51 Atlantoaxial rotary subluxation (fixation) in a 10-year-old boy with a 6-month history of neck ache and torticollis with no history of trauma. (a) An 8 mm interval between the odontoid and the arch of C1 confirmed anterior subluxation. (b) A rotary component of the subluxation was confirmed by tomography, with the right side of C1 displaced anteriorly and distally on C2. (c,d) Nearly complete elimination of the deformity and complete relief of symptoms following C1–C2 fusion by a modified Gallie technique.

not allow his head to be moved at all, nor will he move it spontaneously. An important point differentiating atlantoaxial rotary displacement from muscular torticollis is that in the former condition it is the long sternocleidomastoid muscle that is in spasm as it 'tries' to correct the subluxation. Symptoms in this condition usually consist of neck stiffness and discomfort on any attempted movement from the 'cock robin' position. Neurological signs and symptoms are rare but may occur with severe displacement. Long-standing fixation can lead to facial asymmetry and visual difficulty.

Treatment of atlantoaxial rotary fixation in very acute cases often consists only of a collar, analgesics and perhaps muscle relaxants. In cases of more than 24–36 h duration, head halter traction is useful. If there is an element of anterior displacement of the atlas on the axis, Fielding (1964) suggests that after reduction is achieved, immobilization in a firm collar should be continued for at least 6 weeks. He suggests that there is some potential for permanent atlantoaxial instability and that careful follow-up is necessary.

Very occasionally, patients with severe rotary fixation may require halo traction and, in very occasional cases with very resistant deformity and symptoms, a C1–C2 fusion may be necessary (Fielding and Hawkins, 1977).

Basilar impression

This consists of an indentation of the floor of the skull about the foramen magnum. In this rare situation, the tip of the odontoid is located more cephalad than normal, and the cervical spine appears to 'indent' the base of the skull. This may lead to encroachment of the upper cervical spine on the brain stem with a resulting variety of neurological symptoms resembling those of posterior fossa or spinal cord tumours, syringomyelia, etc.

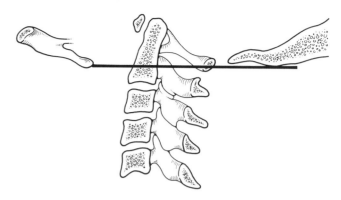

Fig. 4.52 Evaluation for basilar impression by lateral craniometry. McGregor's line is drawn from the upper surface of the posterior edge of the hard palate to the most caudal point of the occipital curve of the skull. Basilar impression is present if the tip of the odontoid is more than 4–5 mm above McGregor's line.

Chamberlain (1939) classically described basilar impression:

> The changes shown by the roentgenogram give the impression of softening of the base of the skull and molding through the force of gravity. It is as though the weight of the head has caused the ears to approach the shoulders while the cervical spine, refusing to be shortened, has pushed the floor of the posterior fossa upward into the brain space.

Such basilar impression may occur as a primary developmental anomaly (often associated with a spectrum of other cranial and vertebral defects) or as a secondary phenomenon from actual softening of the base of the skull, as in rickets or Paget's disease.

The details of the radiographic assessment of basilar impression are well represented by McGregor (1948) and McRae (1954). McGregor's line is the most useful radiographic screening test for basilar impression, because it is easily constructed at all ages, as: 'a line

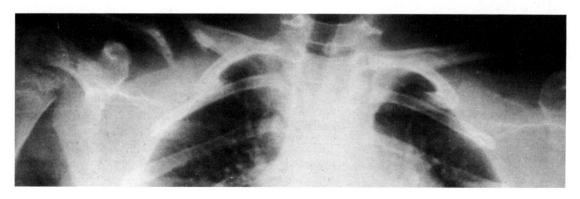

Fig. 4.53 Pseudarthrosis of the right clavicle in an 8-year-old boy with a history of fall on the shoulder 1 year previously. A mid-clavicular lump with local pain and tenderness was noted following the fall.

drawn from the upper surface of the posterior edge of the hard palate to the most caudal point of the occipital curve in the true lateral roentgenogram' (Fig. 4.52). McGregor defined 4–5 mm as the upper limit of the mean distance (range, 2–6 mm). Should McGregor's measurement be suggestive, tomography can be employed to obtain the more accurate but difficult measurements of McRae (1954), Chamberlain (1939), or Fischgold and Metzger (1952). McRae noted that if the tip of the odontoid is below the foramen magnum, then symptoms are unlikely to occur.

Basilar impression may be severe and yet asymptomatic. A search for other possible causes or associated symptoms should be carried out before treatment directed at the basilar impression is instituted. Posterior cord impingement may require laminectomies of C1 and C2, and tight posterior dural bands may also require division (DeBarros *et al.*, 1968). Anterior cord impingement by the odontoid may require occipitocervical reduction and arthrodesis. Anterior excision of an impinging, irreducible odontoid is rare, but may demand consideration of anterolateral excision of the odontoid (Whitesides and Pendleton, 1975).

CLAVICLE

The clavicle seldom presents a significant orthopaedic problem in childhood. Although often fractured, the clavicle routinely heals in children whether displaced or not and whether immobilized or not. Instances of apparent non-union of the clavicle following injury are almost always previously unrecognized cases of congenital pseudarthrosis.

Congenital pseudarthrosis of the clavicle (Alldred, 1963)

This rare condition usually represents deficiency or absence of the central portion of the bone, always affecting the right clavicle when it occurs and almost never associated with other bony anomalies. The lateral half may be absent unilaterally or bilaterally. Total absence is quite uncommon, except in cleidocrania dysostosis.

In congenital pseudarthrosis, a painless lump is noted in infancy near the mid-clavicle with painless mobility of the superficial sternal fragment on the deeper acromial fragment. The deformity increases with age. Onlay bone grafting is recommended in early childhood to prevent progression of deformity and symptoms or instability. Intramedullary internal fixation at the time of grafting is preferred (Fig. 4.53).

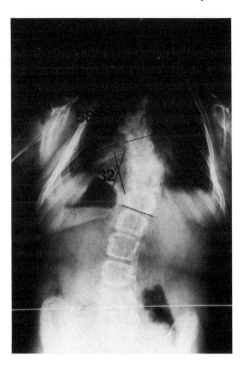

Fig. 4.54 Cleidocranial dysostosis in a 14-year-old girl with associated thoracic scoliosis. Note the tapering thorax and absence of the clavicles.

Cleidocranial dysostosis (Fitzwilliams, 1910)

In cleidocranial dysostosis, bilateral total or subtotal absence of the clavicle is associated with a characteristic cranial deformity, with broadening of the skull and delayed ossification of the cranium. The shoulders slope severely due to absence of the clavicles. An affected child is usually asymptomatic and no treatment is necessary (Fig. 4.54).

REFERENCES

Aaro S. and Ohlund G. (1983) The effect of Harrington instrumentation on the sagittal configuration and mobility of the spine in scoliosis. *Spine* 8, 570–575.

Adams W. (1865) *Lectures on the Pathology and Treatment of Lateral and Other Curvature of the Spine* (2nd edn. 1882). London, Churchill.

Alldred A.J. (1963) Congenital pseudoarthrosis of the clavicle. *J. Bone Joint Surg.* 45B, 312–319.

Allen B.L. Jr. and Ferguson R.L. (1981) The place for segmental spinal instrumentation in the treatment of spine deformity. Scoliosis Research Society Meeting, Montreal, Canada, 1981.

Asadi A. (1959) Calcification of intervertebral discs in children. *Am. J. Dis. Child.* 97, 282.

Ashworth M.A. and Ersil A.K. (1981) The measurement of rib hump inclination — a potential aid in scoliosis screening. *Orthop. Trans.* 5, 33–34.

Balmer G.A. and MacEwen G.D. (1970) The incidence and treatment of scoliosis in cerebral palsy. *J. Bone Joint Surg.* **52B**, 134–141.

Baydur A., Swank S.M., Stiles C.M. *et al.* (1990) Respiratory mechanics in anesthetized young patients with kyphoscoliosis. Immediate and delayed effects of corrective spinal surgery. *Chest* 97, 1157–1164.

Bengtsson G., Fallstrom K., Jansson B. *et al.* (1974) A psychological and psychiatric investigation of the adjustment of female scoliosis patients. *Acta. Psychiatr. Scand.* **50**, 50–59.

Berns D.H., Blaser S.I. and Modic M.T. (1989) Magnetic resonance imaging of the spine. *Clin. Orthop.* **244**, 78–100.

Blount W.P. and Moe J.H. (1973) *The Milwaukee Brace.* Baltimore, Williams and Wilkins.

Boxall D., Bradford D., Winter R. *et al.* (1979) Management of severe spondylolisthesis in children and adolescents. *J. Bone Joint Surg.* **61A**, 479–495.

Bradford D.J. (1977) Juvenile kyphosis. *Clin. Orthop.* **128**, 45–55.

Bradford D.J. (1979) Treatment of severe spondylolisthesis. *Spine* **4**, 423–429.

Bradford D.S. (1986) Instrumentation of the lumbar spine. An overview. *Clin. Orthop.* **203**, 209–218.

Bradford D.S., Moe J.H., Montairo F.J. and Winter R.B. (1975) Scheuermann's kyphosis – results of surgical treatment by posterior spine arthrodesis in twenty-two patients. *J. Bone Joint Surg.* **57A**, 439–448.

Branthwaite M.A. (1986) Cardiorespiratory consequences of unfused idiopathic scoliosis. *Br. J. Dis. Chest* **80**, 360–369.

Brooks B. (1922) Pathologic changes in muscles as a result of disturbances of circulation. *Arch. Surg.* **5**, 188–216.

Broome G., Simpson A.H.R.W. and Houghton G.R. (1990) The modified Schollner costoplasty. *J. Bone Joint Surg.* **72B**, 894–900.

Bunnell W.P. (1984) An objective criterion for scoliosis sreening. *J. Bone Joint Surg.* **66A**, 1381–1387.

Carr A.J. (1991) Annual Meeting of the British Scoliosis Society, Southampton. Family Stature in Adolescent Idiopathic Scoliosis. *J. Bone Joint Surg.* Supp I, 30.

Carr W.A., Moe J.H., Winter R.B. *et al.* (1978) Long-term follow-up of patients treated with Milwaukee brace. *Orthop. Trans.* **2**, 279–280.

Chaglassion J.H., Riseborough E.J. and Hall J.E. (1976) Neurofibromatosis scoliosis – natural history and results of treatment in thirty-seven cases. *J. Bone Joint Surg.* **58A**, 695–702.

Chamberlain W.E. (1939) Basilar impression (platybasia): a bizarre developmental anomaly of the occipital bone and the upper cervical spine with striking and misleading neurologic manifestations. *Yale J. Biol. Med.* **11**, 487–496.

Cochran T., Irstam L. and Nachemson A. (1983) Long-term anatomic and functional changes in patients with adolescent idiopathic scoliosis treated by Harrington rod fusion. *Spine* **8**, 576–584.

Cotrel Y., Dubousset J. and Guillaumat M. (1988) New universal instrumentation in spinal surgery. *Clin. Orthop.* **227**, 10–23.

Coventry M.D. and Harris L.B. (1959) Congenital muscular torticollis in infancy. *J. Bone Joint Surg.* **41A**, 815–822.

Coventry M.D., Ghormley R.K. and Kerndhan J.W. (1945) The intervertebral disc: its microscopic anatomy and pathology. *J. Bone Joint Surg.* **27B**, 233–247.

Cowell H.R., Hall J.N. and MacEwen G.D. (1972) Genetic aspects of idiopathic scoliosis. *Clin. Orthop.* **86**, 121–131.

Cundy P.J., Paterson D.C., Hillier T.M. *et al.* (1990) Cotrel–Dubousset instrumentation and vertebral rotation in adolescent idiopathic scoliosis. *J. Bone Joint Surg.* **72B**, 670–674.

Curtis R.S., Dickson J.H., Harrington P.R. *et al.* (1979) Results of Harrington instrumentation in the treatment for severe scoliosis. *Clin. Orthop.* **144**, 128–134.

Davis P.R., Troup J.D. and Burnard J.H. (1965) Movements of the thorax and lumbar spine when lifting: a chronocyclophotographic study. *J. Anat.* **99**, 13–26.

Dawson E., Moe J.H. and Pedras C.V. (1973) Spinal deformity in neurofibromatosis – natural history, classification and treatment. *J. Bone Joint Surg.* **55A**, 1321–22.

Deacon P., Archer I.A. and Dickson R.A. (1984a) The anatomy and biomechanics of spinal deformity. *J. Bone Joint Surg.* **66B** 289.

Deacon P., Flood B.M. and Dickson R.A. (1984b) Idiopathic scoliosis in three dimensions: a radiographic and morphometric analysis. *J. Bone Joint Surg.* **66B**, 509–512.

Deacon P., Berkin C.R. and Dickson R.A. (1985) Combined idiopathic kyphosis and scoliosis: an analysis of the lateral spine curvatures associated with Scheuermann's disease. *J. Bone Joint Surg.* **67B**, 189–192.

Deacon P., Newman R.J. and Dickson R.A. (1991) Congenital spine deformities: the influence of biomechanical factors on the development and progression of the deformity. Annual Meeting of the British Scoliosis Society. Southampton. *J. Bone Joint Surg.* Supp I, 33.

Deane G. and Duthi R.B. (1973) A new projectional look at articulated scoliotic spines. *Acta. Orthop. Scand.* **44**, 351–365.

DeBarros M.D., Farias W., Ataide L. *et al.* (1968) Basilar impression and Arnold–Chiari malformation: a study of 66 cases. *J. Neurol. Neurosurg. Psychiatry* **31**, 596–605.

DeSmet A.A., Asher M.A. and Fritz S.L. (1981) A method for minimizing radiation exposure from scoliosis radiographs. *Orthop. Trans.* **5**, 33.

DeWald R.I., Fault M.S., Taddario R.F. *et al.* (1981) Severe lumbosacral spondylolisthesis in adolescents and children. *J. Bone Joint Surg.* **63A**, 619–626.

Dick W.T. and Schnebel B. (1988) Severe spondylolisthesis. Reduction and internal fixation. *Clin. Orthop.* **232**, 70–79.

Dickson R.A. (1985) Conservative treatment for idiopathic scoliosis. *J. Bone Joint Surg.* **67B**, 176–181.

Dickson R.A. and Archer I.A. (1986) Biomechanics of spinal deformity. *J. Bone Joint Surg.* **68B**, 682.

Dickson R.A. and Archer I.A. (1987) The surgical treatment of late-onset idiopathic thoracic scoliosis: the Leeds procedure. *J. Bone Joint Surg.* **69B**, 709–714.

Dickson R.A., Lawton J.O., Archer I.A. *et al.* (1984) The pathogenesis of idiopathic scoliosis: biplanar spinal asymmetry. *J. Bone Joint Surg.* **66B**, 8–15.

Dods A. (1824) *Pathological Observations on the Rotated or Contorted Spine, Commonly Called Lateral Curvature Derived from Practice.* London, T. Cadell in the Strand; Edinburgh, Blackwood.

Dove J. (1986) Segmental spinal instrumentation: British Scoliosis Society Morbidity Report. *J. Bone Joint Surg.* **68B**, 680.

Dubousset J., Graf H., Miladi L *et al.* (1986) Spinal thoracic and derotation with CD instrumentation. *Orthop. Trans.* **10**, 36.

DuPeloux J., Fauchet R., Faucon B. *et al.* (1965) Le plan d'élection pour l'éxamen radiologique des kyphoscolioses. *Rev. Cir. Orthop.* **51**, 517–524.

Dwyer A.F. (1973) Experience of anterior correction of scoliosis.

Clin. Orthop. **93**, 191–214.

Dwyer A.F. and Schafer M.F. (1974) Anterior approach to scoliosis. Results of treatment in fifty-one cases. *J. Bone Joint Surg.* **56B**, 218–224.

Edgar M.A. and Mehta M.H. (1988) Long-term follow-up of fused and unfused idiopathic scoliosis. *J. Bone Joint Surg.* **70B**, 712–716.

Edmondson A.S. and Morris J.T. (1977) Follow-up study of Milwaukee brace treatment in patients with idiopathic scoliosis. *Clin. Orthop.* **126**, 58–62.

Emans J.B., Kaelin A., Bancel P. *et al.* (1986) The Boston bracing system for idiopathic scoliosis. *Spine* **11**, 792–801.

Fabry G., Van Melkebeek J. and Bockx E. (1989) Back pain after Harrington rod instrumentation for idiopathic scoliosis. *Spine* **14**, 620–624.

Fang H.S.Y., Ong G.B. and Hodgson A.R. (1964) Anterior spinal fusion—the operative approaches. *Clin. Orthop.* **35**, 16–33.

Fielding J.W. (1964) Normal and selected abnormal motion of the cervical spine from the second cervical vertebra to the seventh cervical vertebra based on cineroentgenography. *J. Bone Joint Surg.* **46A**, 1779–1781.

Fielding J.W. and Griffin P.P. (1974) Os odontoideum: an acquired lesion. *J. Bone Joint Surg.* **56A**, 187–190.

Fielding J.W. and Hawkins R.J. (1977) Atlanto-axial rotatory fixation. *J. Bone Joint Surg.* **59A**, 37–44.

Fielding J.W., Hensinger R.N. and Hawkins R.J. (1978) The cervical spine. In Lovell W.W. and Winter R.B. (eds) *Pediatric Orthopaedics*. Philadelphia, J.B. Lippincott, pp. 545–548.

Fischgold H. and Metzger J. (1952) Etude radiotomographique de l'impression basilaire. *Rev. Rhum. Mal. Osteoartic.* **19**, 261–264.

Fitzwilliams D.C.L. (1910) Hereditary cranio-cleido dysostosis. *Lancet* **ii**, 466.

Floman Y., Kenan S., Sabata S. *et al.* (1981a) Osteoblastoma and osteoid osteoma of the axial skeleton. Scoliosis Research Society Annual Meeting. Montreal, September 1981.

Floman Y., Penny J.N., Micheli L.J. *et al.* (1981b) Combined anterior and posterior spinal fusion in seventy-three spinally deformed patients: indications, results and complications. *Orthop. Trans.* **5**, 24.

Floman Y., Penny J.N., Micheli L.J. *et al.* (1982) Osteotomy of the fusion mass in scoliosis. *J. Bone Joint Surg.* **64A**, 1307–1316.

Focarile F.A., Bonaldi A., Giarolo M-A. *et al.* (1991) Effectiveness of nonsurgical treatment for idiopathic scoliosis. Overview of available evidence. *Spine* **16**, 395–401.

Francis M.J.O., Smith R. and Sanderson M.C. (1977) Collagen abnormalities in idiopathic adolescent scoliosis. *Calcif. Tissue Res.* **22** (Suppl.), 381–384.

Gilday D.L., Paul D.J. and Paterson J. (1975) Diagnosis of osteomyelitis in children by combined blood pool and bone imaging. *Radiology* **117**, 331–340.

Gill G.G., Manning J.G. and White H.L. (1955) Surgical treatment of spondylolisthesis without spine fusion. *J. Bone Joint Surg.* **37A**, 493.

Goldberg C., Dowling F.E., Fogarty E.E. *et al.* (1988) Electrospinal stimulation in children with adolescent and juvenile scoliosis. *Spine* **13**, 482–484.

Goldstein L.A. (1969) Terminology committee report. In *Proceedings of the 4th Annual Meeting of the Scoliosis Research Society*. Los Angeles, California.

Goldstein L.A. and Waugh T.R. (1973) Classification and terminology of scoliosis. *Clin. Orthop.* **93**, 10–22.

Goldstein L.A., Haake P.W., DeVanny J.R. *et al.* (1976) Guidelines for the management of lumbosacral spondylolisthesis associated with scoliosis. *Clin. Orthop.* **117**, 135–148.

Greulich W.W. and Pyle S.I. (1959) *Radiographic Atlas of Skeletal Development of the Hand and Wrist*, 2nd edn. Stanford, Stanford University Press; London, Oxford University Press.

Griss P., Harms J. and Zielke K. (1984) In Dickson R.A. and Bradford D.S. (eds) *Management of Spinal Deformities*. London, Butterworth, pp. 193–236.

Grivas T.B., Webb J.K. and Burwell R.G. (1990) The effects of epiphysiodesis and rodding for early onset idiopathic scoliosis. Annual Meeting of the British Scoliosis Society, Southampton. *J. Bone Joint Surg.* Supp I, 32.

Gunderson C.W. and Solitaire G.B. (1968) Mirror movements in patients with Klippel–Feil syndrome: neuropathologic observations. *Arch. Neurol.* **18**, 675–679.

Hall D.J. and Webb J.K. (1991) Harlow Wood experience with Cotrel Dubousset instrumentation. Annual Meeting of the British Scoliosis Society, Southampton Posterior instrumentation and fusion for idiopathic scoliosis. A comparison of five techniques. *J. Bone Joint Surg.* Supp I, 32.

Hall J.E. (1972) The anterior approach to spinal deformities. *Orthop. Clin. North Am.* **3**, 81–98.

Hall J.E. and Poitras B. (1977) The management of kyphosis in patients with myelomeningocele. *Clin. Orthop.* **128**, 33–40.

Hall J.E., Levine C.R. and Sudhir K.G. (1978) Intraoperative awakening to monitor spinal cord function during Harrington instrumentation and spine fusion. Description of procedure and report of three cases. *J. Bone Joint Surg.* **60A**, 533–536.

Harrington P.R. (1960) Surgical instrumentation for management of scoliosis. *J. Bone Joint Surg.* **42A**, 1448.

Harrington P.R. (1962) Treatment of scoliosis. Correction and internal fixation by spine instrumentation. *J. Bone Joint Surg.* **44A**, 591–610.

Harris J.D., Jefferson R.S. and Turner Smith A.R. (1984) Measurement of back shape using ISIS scanning. In *Proceedings of the 3rd International Symposium on Surface Topography and Spinal Deformity*. Oxford, 1984.

Hensinger R.N., Lang J.R. and MacEwen G.D. (1976) Surgical management of spondylolisthesis in children and adolescents. *Spine* **1**, 207–217.

Herbineaux G. (1782) *Traité sur des Accouchements Laborieux, et sur les Polypes de la Matrice*. Brussels, J.L. DeBowbers.

Herndon W.A., Emans J.B., Micheli L.J. *et al.* (1981) Combined anterior and posterior fusion for Scheuermann's kyphosis. *Spine* **6**, 125–130.

Heuer F. (1927) *Zur Theorie der Skoliose. Hessisches Artzteblatt No. 18 and FF*. Quoted by Wittebol (1956).

Hibbs R.A. (1924) A report on 59 cases of scoliosis treated by fusion operation. *J. Bone Joint Surg.* **6**, 3–37.

Hippocrates on the Articulations (400 BC) In *The Genuine Works of Hippocrates*, vol. 2. Translated by Adams F. London, Sydenham Society (1848).

Hodgson A.R. (1965) Correction of fixed spinal curves. *J. Bone Joint Surg.* **47A**, 1221–1227.

Hodgson A.R. and Stock F.E. (1956) Anterior spine fusion. *Br. J. Surg.* **44**, 266–275.

Hodgson A.R., Stock F.E., Fang H.J. *et al.* (1960) Anterior spine fusion—the operative approach and pathological findings in 412 patients with Pott's disease of the spine. *Br. J. Surg.* **48**, 172–178.

Hoppenfield S. (1976) *Physical Examination of the Spine and*

Extremities. New York, Appleton-Century-Crofts.

Houghton G.R., McInerney A. and Tew T. (1987) Monitoring true brace compliance. *Orthop. Trans.* **2**, 105.

Hummer D.D. Jr. and MacEwen G.D. (1972) The coexistence of torticollis and congenital dysplasia of the hip. *J. Bone Joint Surg.* **54A**, 1255–1256.

Jackson D.W., Wiltse L.L. and Cirincione R.J. (1976) Spondylolysis in the female gymnast. *Clin. Orthop.* **117**, 68–73.

Jackson R.P., Simmons E.H. and Stripinis D. (1983) Incidence and severity of back pain in adult idiopathic scoliosis. *Spine* **8**, 749–756.

Jones P.G. (1968) *Torticollis in Infancy and Childhood.* Springfield, Illinois, C.C. Thomas.

Jones S.J., Edgar M.A., Ransford A.O. *et al.* (1981) Spinal cord monitoring during scoliosis surgery. *J. Bone Joint Surg.* **63B**, 631–632.

Jones S.J., Edgar M.A., Ransford A.O. *et al.* (1983) A system for the electrophysiological monitoring of the spinal cord during operations for scoliosis. *J. Bone Joint Surg.* **65B**, 134–139.

Kehl D.K. and Morrissy R.T. (1988) Brace treatment in adolescent idiopathic scoliosis. An update on concepts and technique. *Clin Orthop.* **229**, 34–43.

Klippel M. and Feil A. (1912) Anomalie de la colonne vertebrale par absence des vertebres cervicales: cage thoracique remontant jusqu'à la base du crâne. *Bull. Soc. Anat. Paris* **87**, 185–188.

Kostuik J.P., Maurais G.R., Richardson W.J. *et al.* (1988) Combined single stage anterior and posterior osteotomy for correction of iatrogenic lumbar kyphosis. *Spine* **13**, 257–266.

LaGrone M.O. (1988) Loss of lumbar lordosis. A complication of spinal fusion for scoliosis. *Orthop. Clin. North Am.* **19**, 383–393.

Leatherman K.D. (1969) Resection of vertebral bodies. *J. Bone Joint Surg.* **51A**, 206.

Leatherman K.D. and Dickson R.A. (1979) Two stage corrective surgery for congenital deformities of the spine. *J. Bone Joint Surg.* **61B**, 326–328.

Leatherman K.D. and Dickson R.A. (1988) *The Management of Spinal Deformities.* London, Wright.

LeFebvre J., Triboulet-Chassevant A. and Missirliu J.F. (1971) Electromyographic changes in idiopathic scoliosis. *Arch. Phys. Med.* **42**, 710–711.

Luque E.R. (1980) Segmental spinal instrumentation: a method of rigid internal fixation of the spine to induce arthrodesis. *Orthop. Trans.* **4**, 391.

Luque E.R. and Cordoso A. (1977) Treatment of scoliosis without arthrodesis or external support. Preliminary report. *Orthop. Trans.* **1**, 37–38.

MacEwen G.D., Bunnell W.P. and Sriram K. (1975) Acute neurological complications in the treatment of scoliosis. A report of the Scoliosis Research Society. *J. Bone Joint Surg.* **57A**, 404–408.

MacEwen G.D., Winter R.B. and Hardy J.H. (1972) Evaluation of kidney anomalies in congenital scoliosis. *J. Bone Joint Surg.* **54A**, 1451–1454.

McGregor M. (1948) The significance of certain measurements of the skull in the diagnosis of basilar impression. *Br. J. Radiol.* **21**, 171–181.

McMaster M.J. (1988) The long-term results of kyphectomy and spinal stabilization in children with myelomeningocele. *Spine* **13**, 417–424.

McMaster M.J. (1990) Congenital scoliosis. British Scoliosis Society Instructional Course, Southampton.

McMaster M.J. and David C.V. (1986) Hemivertebrae as a cause of scoliosis: a study of 104 patients. *J. Bone Joint Surg.* **68B**, 588–595.

McMaster M.J. and McNicol M.F. (1979) The management of progressive infantile idiopathic scoliosis. *J. Bone Joint Surg.* **61B**, 36–42.

McMaster M.J. and Ohtsuka K. (1982) The natural history of congenital scoliosis: a study of 251 patients. *J. Bone Joint Surg.* **64A**, 1128–1147.

McNeice G., Raso J., Gillespie R. *et al.* (1980) Rod design criteria for instrumentation without fusion. *Orthop. Trans.* **4**, 37.

McRae D.L. (1954) Bony abnormalities in the region of the foramen magnum: correlation of the anatomic and neurologic findings. *Acta Radiol.* **40**, 335–354.

Machida M., Weinstein S.L., Yamada T. *et al.* (1985) Spinal cord monitoring. Electrophysiological measures of sensory and motor function during spinal surgery. *Spine* **10**, 407–413.

Mehta M.H. (1972) The rib vertebra angle in the early diagnosis between resolving and progressive infantile scoliosis. *J. Bone Joint Surg.* **54B**, 230–243.

Mehta M.H. (1984) Infantile idiopathic scoliosis. In Dickson R.A. and Bradford D.S. (eds) *Management of Spinal Deformities.* London, Butterworth, pp. 101–120.

Melnick J.C. and Silverman F.N. (1963) Intervertebral disc calcification in childhood. *Radiology* **80**, 339–408.

Mellencamp D.D., Blount W.P. and Anderson A.J. (1977) Milwaukee brace treatment of idiopathic scoliosis. Late results. *Clin. Orthop.* **126**, 47–57.

Menelaus M.B. (1964) Discitis: an inflammation affecting the intervertebral discs in children. *J. Bone Joint Surg.* **46B**, 16–23.

Meyerding H.W. (1932) Spondylolisthesis. *Surg. Gynecol. Obstet.* **54**, 371–377.

Micheli L.J. (1985) Sports following spinal surgery in the ÿung athlete. *Clin. Orthop.* **188**, 152–157.

Micheli L.J., Hall J.E. and Miller M.E. (1980) Use of a modified Boston brace for back injuries in athletes. *Am. J. Sports Med.* **8**, 351–356.

Moe J.H. and Valuska J.W. (1966) Evaluation of treatment of scoliosis by Harrington instrumentation. *J. Bone Joint Surg.* **48A**, 1656–1657.

Morrison S.G. and Scott L.P. (1968) Congenital brevicollis (Klippel–Feil syndrome) and cardiovascular anomalies. *Am. J. Dis. Child.* **115**, 614–620.

Moskowitz A., Moe J.H., Winter R.B. *et al.* (1980) Long-term follow-up of scoliosis fusion. *J. Bone Joint Surg.* **62A**, 364–376.

Muirhead A. and Conner A.N. (1985) The assessment of lung function in children with scoliosis. *J. Bone Joint Surg.* **67B**, 699–702.

Nachemson A. (1968) A long-term follow-up study of non-treated scoliosis. *Acta. Orthop. Scand.* **39**, 466–476.

Nachemson A. (1987) *All that Glitters is not Gold.* Guest Lecture, Annual Meeting of the British Scoliosis Society, Leeds.

Neugebauer F.L. (1888) A new contribution to the history and etiology of spondylolisthesis. Translated from the German report and reprinted in *Clin. Orthop.* (1976) **117**, 4–22.

Newman P.H. (1963) The etiology of spondylolisthesis. *J. Bone Joint Surg.* **45B**, 39–59.

Nilsonne U. and Lundgren K.D. (1968) Long-term prognosis in idiopathic scoliosis. *Acta Orthop. Scand.* **39**, 456–465.

Otsuka N.Y., Hall J.E. and Mah J.Y. (1990) Posterior fusion for Scheuermann's kyphosis. *Clin. Orthop.* **251**, 134–139.

Palant D.L. and Carter B.L. (1972) Klippel—Feil syndrome and diseases. *Am. J. Dis. Child.* **123**, 218—221.

Ponseti I.V. (1968) The pathogenesis of adolescent scoliosis. In Zorab P.A. (ed) *Proceedings of the 2nd Symposium on Scoliosis: Causation*. Edinburgh, E. and J. Livingstone, pp. 60—63.

Ponseti I.V., Pedrini V. and Dohrman S.H. (1972) Biochemical analysis of intervertebral discs in idiopathic scoliosis. *J. Bone Joint Surg.* **54A**, 1793.

Reid L. (1965) Autopsy study of the lungs in kyphoscoliosis. In Zorab P.A. (ed) *Proceedings of a Symposium on Scoliosis: Action for the Crippled Child Monograph*, 1965, pp. 71—77.

Riseborough E.J. (1977) Irradiation induced kyphosis. *Clin. Orthop.* **128**, 101—106.

Riseborough E.J. and Herndon J.H. (1975) *Scoliosis and Other Deformities of the Axial Skeleton*. Boston, Little, Brown and Co.

Risser J.C. and Ferguson A.B. (1936) Scoliosis: its prognosis. *J. Bone Joint Surg.* **18**, 667—670.

Risser J.C. and Norquist D.M. (1958) A follow-up study of the treatment of scoliosis. *J. Bone Joint Surg.* **40A**, 555—569.

Roaf R. (1966) The basic anatomy of scoliosis. *J. Bone Joint Surg.* **48B**, 786—792.

Robert J. (1854) *Monatssch. Geburtskd. Frauenkr.* **5**, 81.

Roche M.B. and Rowe G.G. (1951) The incidence of separate neural arch and coincident bone variation. *Anat. Rec.* **109**, 223.

Rogola E.J., Frummond D.S. and Crurr J. (1978) Scoliosis: incidence and natural history — a prospective epidemiological study. *J. Bone Joint Surg.* **60A**, 173—176.

Rothman R.H. and Simeone F.A. (1975) *The Spine*. Philadelphia, W.B. Saunders, p. 58.

Rowland L.P., Shapiro J.H. and Jacobsen H.G. (1958) Neurological syndromes associated with congenital absence of the odontoid process. *Arch. Neurol. Psychiatry* **80**, 286—291.

Sabatier (1777) Traite complete d'anatomie. Paris (Quoted by Farkas, 1941).

Scaglietti O., Frontino G. and Bartolozzi P. (1976) Technique of anatomical reduction of lumbar spondylolisthesis and its surgical stabilization. *Clin. Orthop.* **117**, 164.

Scheuermann H.W. (1936) Kyphosis juvenilis. *Fortschr. Geb. Rontgenstr.* **53**, 1—16.

Schiller F. and Nieda I. (1957) Malformations of the odontoid process. Reports of a case and clinical survey. *Calif. Med.* **86**, 397—398.

Scoliosis Research Society (1979) *Spinal Orthotics Workshop Report*. Seattle, Washington, Scoliosis Research Society.

Scoliosis Research Society (1981) *Terminology Committee Report*. Seattle, Washington, Scoliosis Research Society.

Shaw J. (1824) *Engravings Illustrative of a Work on the Nature and Treatment of the Distortions of which the Spine and the Bones of the Chest are Subject*. London, Hurst, Rees, Orme, Brown and Green.

Sheldon J.J., Serlands T. and Leborgne T. (1977) Computerized tomography of the lower lumbar vertebral column. *Radiology* **124**, 113—118.

Sherman F.C., Wilkinson R.H. and Hall J.E. (1977) Reactive sclerosis of a pedicle and spondylolysis in the lumbar spine. *J. Bone Joint Surg.* **59A**, 49—54.

Shufflebarger H.L. (1991) Prevention of the crankshaft phenomenon. Annual Meeting of the American Academy of Orthopaedic Surgeons. Anaheim, California.

Siegal I.M. (1973) Scoliosis in muscular dystrophy. *Clin. Orthop.* **93**, 235—238.

Smith R.F. and Taylor T.L.F. (1967) Inflammatory lesions of intervertebral discs in children. *J. Bone Joint Surg.* **49A**, 1508—1520.

Smith R.M. (1987) Experimental spinal deformity. MD Thesis, The University of Leeds.

Smith R.M. and Dickson R.A. (1987) Experimental structural scoliosis. *J. Bone Joint Surg.* **69B**, 576—581.

Smith R.M., Hamlin G.W. and Dickson R.A. (1991a) Respiratory deficiency in experimental idiopathic scoliosis. *Spine* **16**, 94—99.

Smith R.M., Pool R., Butt W.P. *et al.* (1991b) The transverse plane deformity of structural scoliosis. *Spine*, **16**, 1126—1129.

Somerville E.W. (1952) Rotational lordosis: the development of the single curve. *J. Bone Joint Surg.* **34B**, 421—427.

Somogyi G. (1964) Blood supply of the fetal spine. *Acta Morphol. Acad. Sci. Hung.* **12**, 261—274.

Sorensen K.H. (1964) *Scheuermann's Juvenile Kyphosis: Clinical Appearances, Radiography, Aetiology and Prognosis*. Copenhagen, Munksgaard.

Speigel P.G., Kengla K.W., Isaacson A.S. *et al.* (1972) Intervertebral disc space inflammation in children. *J. Bone Joint Surg.* **54A**, 284—296.

Staheli L.T. (1971) Muscular torticollis: late results of operative treatment. *Surgery* **69**, 469—473.

Stanish W., Hall J.E., Miller W. *et al.* (1975) The Boston scoliosis orthosis. *Orthot. Prosthet.* **29**, 7—11.

Stearns G., Chen J-Y., McKinley J.B. *et al.* (1955) Metabolic studies of children with idiopathic scoliosis. *J. Bone Joint Surg.* **37A**, 1028—1034.

Steindler A. (1955) *Kinesiology of the Human body*. Springfield, Illinois, Charles C. Thomas.

Steiner M.E. and Micheli L.J. (1985) Treatment of symptomatic spondylolysis and spondylolisthesis with the modified Boston brace. *Spine* **10**, 937—943.

Stewart T.D. (1953) The age incidence of neural arch defects in Alaskan natives, considered from the standpoint of etiology. *J. Bone Joint Surg.* **35A**, 937—950.

Tachkjan M.O. and Matson D.D. (1965) Orthopaedic aspects of intraspinal tumors in infants and children. *J. Bone Joint Surg.* **47A**, 223—248.

Tanner J.M., Whitehouse R.H., Marshall W.A. *et al.* (1975) *Assessment of Skeletal Maturity and Prediction of Adult Height (TW2 method)*. London, Academic Press.

Taylor T.C., Wenger D.R., Stephen J. *et al.* (1979) Surgical management of thoracic kyphosis in adolescents. *J. Bone Joint Surg. [Am.]* **61**, 496—503.

Treves S., Khettry J., Broker E.H. *et al.* (1976) Osteomyelitis: early scintigraphic detection in children. *Pediatrics* **57**, 173—186.

Tsou P.M. (1977) Embryology of congenital kyphosis. *Clin. Orthop.* **128**, 18—25.

Turner-Smith A.R. (1982) A television scanning technique for topographic body measurements. SPIE Conference: Biostereometrics '82. San Diego, California, 1982.

Warner M., Brooks Gunn J. and Hamilton W.G. (1986) Scoliosis and fractures in young ballet dancers. *N. Engl. J. Med.* **314**, 1348—1353.

Wenger D., Bobechko W.P. and Gilday D.L. (1978) The spectrum of intervertebral disc space infection in children. *J. Bone Joint Surg.* **60A**, 100—108.

White A.A. III. (1971) Kinematics of the normal spine as related to scoliosis. *J. Biomech.* **4**, 405—411.

Whitesides T.E. (1977) Traumatic kyphosis of the thoracolumbar spine. *Clin. Orthop.* **128**, 78–92.

Whitesides T.E. Jr. and Pendleton E.B. (1975) Lateral approach to the upper cervical spine for treatment of upper cervical and occipito-cervical disorders. *J. Bone Joint Surg.* **57A**, 1025.

Wilbur R.G., Thompson G.H., Shaffer J.W. *et al.* (1984) Postoperative neurological deficits in segmental spinal instrumentation. A study using spinal cord monitoring. *J. Bone Joint Surg.* **66A**, 1178–1187.

Wiley A.M. and Trueta J. (1959) The vascular anatomy of the spine and its relationship to pyogenic vertebral osteomyelitis. *J. Bone Joint Surg.* **41B**, 796–809.

Willner S. (1981) Spinal pantograph—a non-invasive technique for describing kyphosis and lordosis in the thoraco-lumbar spine. *Acta Orthop. Scand.* **52**, 525–529.

Wiltse L.L. (1962) The etiology of spondylolisthesis. *J. Bone Joint Surg.* **44A**, 539–560.

Wiltse L.L., Newman P.H. and McNab I. (1974) Classification of spondylolysis and spondylolisthesis. *Clin. Orthop.* **117**, 23.

Wiltse L.L., Widell E.H. Jr and Jackson D.W. (1975) Fatigue fractures: the basic lesion in isthmic spondylolisthesis. *J. Bone Joint Surg.* **57A**, 17–22.

Winter R.B. (1977) Congenital scoliosis. *Clin. Orthop.* **128**, 26–32.

Winter R.B. and Moe J.H. (1982) The results of spinal arthrodesis for congenital spinal deformity in patients younger than 5 years old. *J. Bone Joint Surg.* **64A**, 419–432.

Winter R.B., Moe J.H. and Eiles V.E. (1968) Congenital scoliosis, a study of 130 patients. *J. Bone Joint Surg.* **50A**, 1–15.

Winter R.B., Haven J.J., Moe J.H. *et al.* (1974) Diastematomyelia and congenital spine deformities. *J. Bone Joint Surg.* **56A**, 27–39.

Winter R.B., Moe J.H., Bradford D.S. *et al.* (1979) Spine deformity in neurofibromatosis. A review of one hundred and two patients. *J. Bone Joint Surg.* **61A**, 677–694.

Wittebol P. (1956) Idiopathic scoliosis (an experimental investigation). *Arch. Chir. Neerl.* **8**, 269–279.

Woodward J.W. (1961) Congenital elevation of the scapula. Correction by release and transplantation of muscle origins. *J. Bone Joint Surg.* **43A**, 219–228.

Wynne-Davies R. (1968) Familial (idiopathic) scoliosis—a family survey. *J. Bone Joint Surg.* **50B**, 24–30.

Zielke K. and Berthet A. (1978) VDS—Ventrale Derotation Spondylodese—vorlaeufiger Bericht ueber 58 falle. *Beitr. Orthop. Traumatol.* **25**, 85–103.

Zuk T. (1962) The role of spinal and abdominal muscles in the pathogenesis of scoliosis. *J. Bone Joint Surg.* **44B**, 102–105.

Chapter 5
The Limping Child

D.M. Hunt

INTRODUCTION

The cause of limp in childhood is not just a question asked in examinations, but is a problem often faced in the out-patient or emergency department and by general practitioners. It causes anxiety because the reason for the limp can be obscure, and indeed there may not even be an identifiable cause. Surprisingly, little has been written about a structured approach to the clinical assessment of limp.

In this chapter, the cause of limp will be classified, a system of clinical assessment will be outlined, more sophisticated techniques will be mentioned and the commoner causes of limp described in more detail.

ASSESSMENT OF LIMP

A logical approach to the cause of a limp in a child is directed towards the site of the pathology resulting in the limp. It may be in the foot or toes, the ankle, tibia, knee, femur, or hip. It can also be in the spine or central nervous system, or it may not be in the musculoskeletal system at all. It may arise from the abdomen, e.g. in appendicitis, or from inflamed lymph glands in the abdomen or groin.

A careful history may indicate the site of pain, remembering the possibilities for referred pain. The history will come from the mother, and it is wise to accept that she is right even if no limp is demonstrable. Examination of each of the possible sites or systems will be laborious, particularly in a distressed child, but with patience, the site of maximal tenderness will be revealed. Subsequent blood investigations—full blood count, erythrocyte sedimentation rate and C-reactive protein combined with the appropriate radiographs, bone scans, or ultrasonography—will reveal the cause.

Frustratingly, often all investigations will be negative. Positive reassurance of the parents is a matter of clinical judgement.

Formal gait analysis is not a routine clinical investigation. The clinical approach to the assessment of limp will indicate the type of limp. Gait analysis is of interest in the assessment of gait in conditions such as cerebral palsy, though simple video filming can be as useful at a practical level.

Classification of limp

It is possible to classify a limp in a child under a number of broad headings, before a definitive diagnosis is revealed.

ANTALGESIC LIMP

This limp is due to pain. The site of the pain can be identified by a combination of the history from the child and the parents, and by clinical examination for tenderness or reluctance to move a joint.

SHORT LEG LIMP

Clinical examination will indicate leg length inequality due either to fixed deformity or actual discrepancy in the lengths of the bones of either leg.

PARALYTIC LIMP

This can only be diagnosed in the presence of a clinically demonstrable neurological abnormality. Mild cerebral palsy can be a difficult diagnosis in a very young child, even when walking. A neurogenic cause of limp must be considered when no other abnormality can be found.

STIFF LEG

A painless, stiff joint can occasionally be the cause of a limp in childhood.

TRENDELENBERG LIMP

This is due to abnormal function of the hip abductors. It may be associated with paralytic limp. It is usually specific for congenital dislocation of the hip in childhood, though other causes — usually associated with pain — can also give a Trendelenberg-positive gait, such as slipped upper femoral epiphysis.

Age

The final factor in an appraisal of limp in a child is the importance of age. Certain causes can be discounted on the grounds of age. Other causes occur typically at certain ages.

Following full clinical examination of a limping child, and classification of the limp, it is possible to consider the causes of the limp in each case (Table 5.1).

COMMON CAUSES OF LIMP

The conditions usually associated with limp in childhood are: (i) congenital dislocation of the hip; (ii) Perthes' disease; and (iii) slipped upper femoral epiphysis. None of these is the most common cause of a limp, which is without doubt irritable hip syndrome. It is these conditions that will be considered in more detail in this chapter.

Irritable hip syndrome

Irritable hip or transient synovitis is the most common cause of a painful hip in childhood, usually between 5 and 10 years of age. It occurs in 1 in 1000 children (Adams, 1963) and is probably as common in boys as in girls. There is commonly a history of preceding upper respiratory tract viral infection in approximately 50% of cases, but no specific viral antibodies have been identified (Blockey and Porter, 1968; Dunkerton, 1990). There is no evidence that it is a precursor of Perthes' disease, and only 1.5% of patients with established Perthes' disease have a history of a previous episode of hip irritability (Spock, 1959).

The child presents with a painful leg, inability to bear weight, and thus a limp. All movements are restricted, but particularly abduction in flexion. The radiograph is typically normal, the effusion being too small to show on plain radiography. It may, however, be seen on an ultrasound scan (Fig. 5.1) and this is now the investigation of choice in the early stages (Bickerstaff *et al.*, 1990). If the symptoms settle quickly, and the ultrasound scan showed an effusion, radiography is unnecessary.

Table 5.1 Possible causes for each type of limp

Antalgesic gait
Irritable hip syndrome
Stress fracture
Acute infection
   Septic arthritis or osteomyelitis
Tuberculosis
Perthes' disease
Slipped upper femoral epiphysis
Acute arthritis
Hypermobility syndrome
Juvenile chronic arthritis
Congenital pseudarthrosis of tibia
Osteoid osteoma and other bone tumours

Short leg
Congenital short femur
Coxa vara
Growth arrest
Hemiatrophy and hemihypertrophy

Paralytic
Cerebral palsy
Spina bifida
Progressive neuropathy
Poliomyelitis
Post-infective neuropathy
   Guillain–Barré syndrome
Transverse myelitis
Diastematomyelia
Spondylolisthesis
Spinal cord tumours
Hysteria

Stiff leg
Limp associated with talipes equinovarus
   or vertical talus
Post-traumatic or post-infective joint
   stiffness

Trendelenberg gait
Congenital dislocation of the hip
Poliomyelitis
Coxa vara
Perthes' disease
Post-infective destruction of the hip
Slipped upper femoral epiphysis

Only if the symptoms do not settle or irritability recurs should radiography be performed.

C-reactive protein concentration and erythrocyte sedimentation rate may be mildly elevated, and there may be a slight fever.

The symptoms settle in a few days with bed-rest, paracetamol and skin traction to the affected limb. Only if it does not are radiography and aspiration of the joint undertaken.

Even when the symptoms have settled, the hip moves

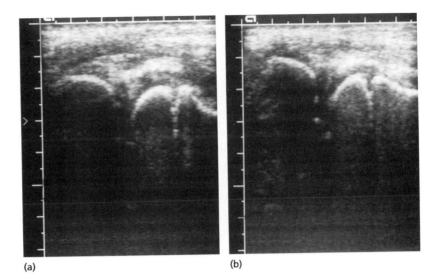

Fig. 5.1 (a) Ultrasonographic scan of hip effusion. (b) Ultrasonographic scan of a normal hip.

(a)   (b)

normally and the erythrocyte sedimentation rate and temperature are normal, the child may persist with a limp for some weeks. In the absence of any abnormality, reassurance is all that is required, but follow-up radiography will be necessary.

Congenital dislocation of the hip

It is uncommon, but still seen too often, that congenital dislocation of the hip is not diagnosed before a child begins to walk. Neonatal screening programmes have established the incidence of hip instability at birth: in the first 3 days, instability can be detected in up to 10 in 1000 births (Fredensborg, 1976); after 3 days, approximately 80% of unstable hips spontaneously stabilize, giving the true incidence of 1.5 in 1000 (Von Rosen, 1962). Screening has not eliminated late presentation of dislocated hips, however, which has an incidence of about 0.1 in 1000 births. These are the hips that present as limps in children just starting to walk.

AETIOLOGY

The common aetiological factors are well known. Congenital dislocation of the hip is six times more common in girls. It is more likely in the first born; it occurs in 20% of children born by breech presentation or by Caesarian section. The incidence is 5% if there is a positive family history, but where a parent and the first-born child are affected, subsequent children have a 36% chance of being affected (Wynne-Davis, 1973). Congenital dislocation of the hip is also more common in the presence of other deformities, e.g. plagiocephaly, infantile scoliosis with abduction and adduction con-

tractures of the hips (skew baby syndrome) (Fig. 5.2) or talipes equinovarus.

CLASSIFICATION AND PATHOLOGY

It is not sufficient to consider congenital dislocation of the hip as a single condition. The failure of screening programmes to eliminate the late diagnosis suggests that the possibility exists of a hip that is normal at birth and later progresses to dislocation. Indeed, the term congenital dislocation of the hip should be replaced by congenital and developmental hip instability or dysplasia (DDH). The condition then, includes the following groups: (i) ligamentous clicks; (ii) neonatal instability; (iii) true congenital dislocation; (iv) irreducible dislocation; and (v) late dislocation. This classification is purely clinical but is still a useful working classification. It is now possible to classify hips by the ultrasonographic appearance (Graf and Schulen, 1986). Ultrasonography

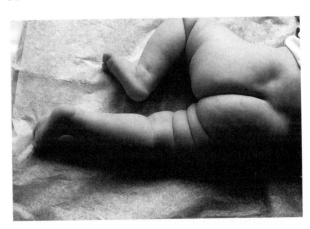

Fig. 5.2 Abduction/adduction of the hips in skew baby syndrome.

has identified hips that, although clinically normal, may progress to dislocation, and it demonstrates hips that although easily dislocatable, will relocate and stabilize without treatment.

Ligamentous clicks

The importance of the ligamentous click has long been a subject for debate. This is the hip in which, during routine clinical examination, a small, palpable click is elicited. It is quite different from the solid 'clunk' felt when the dislocated hip is relocated in Ortolani's manoeuvre. Indeed, these two words, which are often used together and so cause confusion, should be dropped. Less than 2% of ligamentous clicks are significant (Allan *et al.*, 1985). They have nothing to do with dislocated hips, and the word should not be used to describe a hip that is dislocatable. Ligamentous clicks can be found in 10% of newborn babies and indicate transient joint laxity only. When present, they are an indication for ultrasonographic examination only.

Neonatal instability

This describes the newborn child in whom the hip is located normally, but on examination the hip is dislocatable. These hips stabilize spontaneously in the first few days. They are the hips identified by Barlow's modification of Ortolani's manoeuvre, when a normally located hip can be dislocated out of the back of the normal acetabulum. As expected, the ultrasonographic examination will be normal.

True congenital dislocation

This is the group in which screening is essential, because these are the hips requiring treatment. The acetabulum is deficient, and the hip lies dislocated. It will not spontaneously relocate and stabilize. On examination, Ortolani's sign is positive, but the hip will redislocate unless splinted. The ultrasonographic examination is abnormal.

Irreducible dislocation

This group differs from the above in that Ortolani's sign will not be positive, because the head of the femur cannot be relocated without excessive force, and damage can be done. There is limited abduction of the affected hip, and the adductors are contracted, suggesting a neuromuscular element in the pathology of this condition. Because there is no 'clunk' of relocation on

examination, and there may not even be a click, these hips are easily missed on clinical screening examination. The importance of looking for asymmetry of abduction in the newborn cannot be overemphasized. Ultrasonographic examination will demonstrate the dislocation with an abnormal acetabulum. Simple splinting will not be appropriate. These children will require a period of traction, possibly an adductor tenotomy, and then splinting or even open reduction.

Late dislocation

Ultrasonographic examination can identify the hip that is dysplastic and at risk of progressing to true late dislocation. This may be associated with a ligamentous click at birth. The possibility puts a strong case for routine ultrasonographic screening of hips at birth.

SCREENING

Ortolani's manoeuvre and Barlow's modification of it have been mentioned. Until Ortolani described this test in 1937, it was widely believed that it was not possible to diagnose a dislocated hip until the child started walking.

Screening programmes have been practised for many years, mainly carried out by paediatricians, community medical officers or general practitioners, but also by orthopaedic surgeons and now radiologists. It is important that a consistent and thorough programme is established in each health district. For example, it is usual now for a child to be examined clinically within 24 h of birth, at 6 weeks, and checked again between 6 and 9 months, with a final check at 18 months.

Examination

Ortolani described examining both hips simultaneously (Ortolani, 1937). Part of Barlow's modification was to examine each hip individually, using the other hand to hold the opposite femur, and thus the pelvis, steady (Barlow, 1966). It is essential to any screening programme that all examiners test the hips in the same way.

The child is laid supine on a firm surface, with the legs together. The hips and knees are then fully flexed (Fig. 5.3a–c). The tibia is held in the web space between the index finger and thumb, with the thumb on the front of the femur, and the middle finger over the greater trochanter. Pressure is applied vertically along the shaft of the femur into the examining couch, pushing the head of the femur up out of the back of the acetabulum, so dislocating the hip. It is possible to feel the head slip

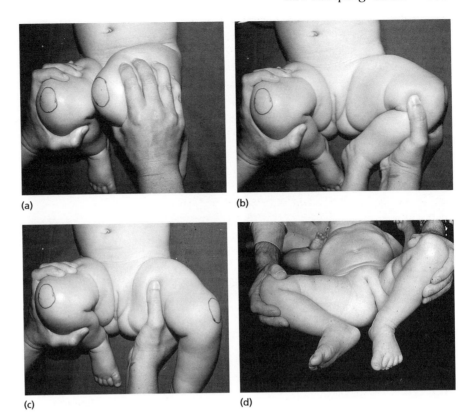

Fig. 5.3 Examination of the hips.

(a)   (b)   (c)   (d)

up over the posterior rim of the acetabulum. This is Barlow's test. Now both hips are abducted simultaneously as Ortolani described, still with the middle finger on the greater trochanter. This finger lifts the trochanter and the head of femur forward, as the hip is abducted. If the hip is dislocated, the first thing that will be noted is that abduction is limited on that side. If the hip has been dislocated throughout and is irreducible, limitation of abduction is all that will be noted. This is a vital sign, and itself is an indication for ultrasonographic examination. If a hip is reducible, it will relocate with a deep 'clunk' and the movement of the head rolling into the acetabulum will be felt, as distinct from a click, where no movement is felt. This is Ortolani's sign.

It is important to repeat the test, one hip at a time. The hips and knees are again flexed, and a posterior force applied through both hips. Holding one hip to stabilize the pelvis, Ortolani's manoeuvre is carried out on the other hip. Finally, with the leg in full abduction, the leg is released and the head of the femur held between finger and thumb, and rocked backwards and forwards.

Occasionally, a hip that may have been considered normal up until now can be rolled in and out of the acetabulum posteriorly by this manoeuvre. The same procedure is then applied to the other hip. It is important

to remember that other signs, e.g. asymmetry of skin creases, are unreliable in the newborn, and only become significant after the age of 6 months.

In the older child, the only sign may be limitation of abduction with or without asymmetry of skin creases (Fig. 5.3d). When the child is walking there will be a Trendelenberg positive gait.

ULTRASONOGRAPHIC EXAMINATION

The failure of screening programmes to eliminate late diagnosis of congenital dislocation of the hip has sustained interest in alternative diagnostic techniques. With real-time ultrasonography, it is possible to provide high-resolution images of the developing femoral head and acetabulum, and to provide dynamic images of the hip while it is being examined clinically, thus combining the advantages of ultrasonography and clinical examination (Clarke *et al.*, 1985; Bellmore *et al.*, 1989). The newborn hip can then be classified ultrasonographically into four grades, from normal (grade I) through to grade IV, which is the irreducible, dislocatable hip (Figs 5.4 and 5.5) (Graf and Schulen, 1986). The advent of ultrasonography, however, has not finally eliminated the late diagnosis of congenital dislocations, the reasons for which are still not clear. There is also the problem of

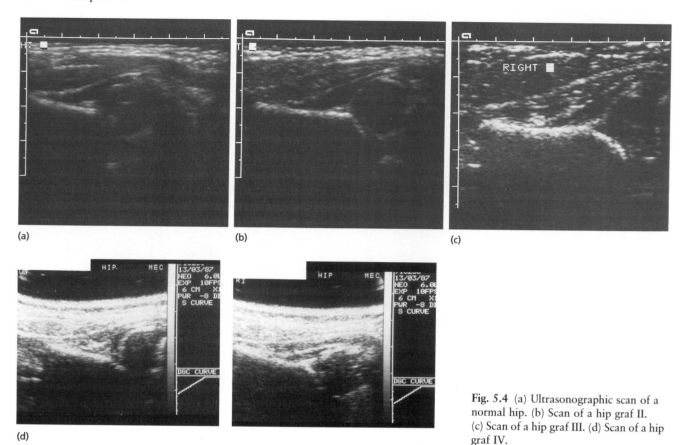

(a)   (b)   (c)

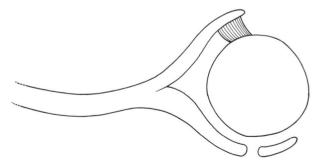

(d)

Fig. 5.4 (a) Ultrasonographic scan of a normal hip. (b) Scan of a hip graf II. (c) Scan of a hip graf III. (d) Scan of a hip graf IV.

whether the critical (type IIc) hip, which is normal on clinical examination, should be treated by splinting, as is practised in Europe. The small but significant risk of inducing avascular necrosis of the femoral head by splinting may mitigate against the theoretical advantage of preventing progression of these hips to dislocation. The answer to this is not yet established.

TREATMENT

When to start treatment for the true congenital dislocation is still debated. It does not matter. Sometime in

the first month is all that is important. It seems that if the majority of dislocatable hips will stabilize spontaneously in the first few weeks, then it is unnecessary to treat all dislocatable hips immediately. The ultrasonographic examination is very helpful; when a hip is abnormal on ultrasonography and clinical examination, treatment should not be delayed.

Treatment in the newborn involves splinting of the hip in flexion of more than 90° and some abduction. It must be stressed that abduction should not be forced, as too much abduction obstructs the blood supply to the growing femoral head, causing avascular necrosis. The risk of this with any form of splintage may be as high as 10% (Kalamachi and Macfarlane, 1982).

The type of splint is not important — it is the preference and established routine of the surgeon. The author's own choice is the Pavlik harness, which is effective, flexible and most readily accepted by parents (Fig. 5.6).

It is essential to establish that the hip is relocated in the harness. This can now be demonstrated ultrasonographically (Fig. 5.7) thus making radiography unnecessary; however, if there is some doubt, a radiograph in the harness should be obtained. The harness remains in place for 3 months, when it is removed and a further ultrasonographic scan and radiograph are obtained

Fig. 5.5 Diagramatic representation of an ultrasonographic scan of the hips.

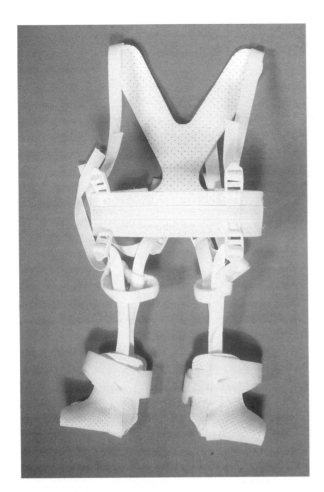

Fig. 5.6 Pavlik harness.

about 1 week later to show location of the hip and adequate development of the acetabulum. If there is deficiency of the acetabulum, splinting can be continued up to 6 months, either with the Pavlik harness if the child is small, or with a Denis Browne splint (Fig. 5.8).

Failure of treatment

In addition to the risk of avascular necrosis, splinting the newborn hip will fail to reduce or to hold reduced in approximately 10% of cases (Ramsay *et al.*, 1976).

Late diagnosis

Congenital dislocation of the hip after the newborn period is subdivided into four groups: (i) 3–9 months; (ii) 9–18 months; (iii) 18 months to 3 years; and (iv) over 3 years.

3–9 months. This group also includes those hips that

the Pavlik harness has either failed to reduce or has not held in reduction. The problem is to reduce and hold the hip reduced, without damaging the blood supply to the growing femoral head. This period is the danger period when the ossifying femoral head is most susceptible. (Lloyd Roberts and Swann, 1966).

If the dislocation is first diagnosed under 6 months of age and the hip is reducible, a trial of splinting in a Pavlik harness or Denis Browne splint can be undertaken. If the hip is not reducible, a trial of reduction by admission to hospital and traction on gallows (Fig. 5.9) or an abduction frame should be performed. Abduction should not be more than 60° at this age. If the hip relocates easily, splinting in a plaster hip spica is applied for 6 weeks, at which time arthrography is performed. If an in-turned limbus, preventing full reduction, is demonstrated (Fig. 5.10), limited exposure of the hip with open reduction and excision of the limbus only is justified in this age group. The limited anteromedial approach described by Ludloff can be used (Ludloff, 1913; Mau *et al.*, 1971). Although access to the limbus is more difficult by this approach, this is outweighed by the advantage of access to the adductors, psoas and transverse ligament of the acetabulum. If care is taken of the medial circumflex vessels, the risk of damage to the blood supply to the femoral head is minimal.

Concentric relocation of the head of the femur will result in excellent development of the acetabulum (Harris *et al.*, 1975), and no bony procedure is required. The more usual outcome of established dislocation in this age group is that the hip fails to reduce with traction. The decision then lies between open reduction or abandoning treatment until after 9 months of age, when traction into full abduction of 90° can be undertaken with less fear of avascular necrosis. The incidence of avascular necrosis is 19% in infants treated by this method under 6 months of age (Palmer, 1963).

9–18 months. In this age group, closed reduction with traction will result in a satisfactory reduction of the dislocation in 60% of cases (Wilkinson, 1985). The full programme of gallows traction consists of increasing abduction out to 90° with an adductor tenotomy if the adductors are tight and give discomfort during the process of abduction. Cross-traction can also be used for the last 4–5 days. The whole programme should take approximately 3 weeks. A trial of reduction is undertaken if the radiograph at the end of abduction shows apparent relocation. After 6 weeks in a plaster hip spica with the hips flexed more than 90° and abducted no more than 60° (Fig. 5.11), arthrography is performed. If the hip is not concentrically reduced or an in-turned

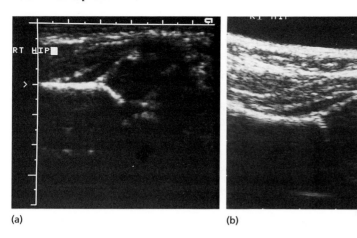

(a)   (b)

Fig. 5.7 Ultrasonographic scans of hips in a harness. (a) Normal hip. (b) Abnormal hip.

limbus is present, formal open reduction through an anterolateral approach is carried out.

The acetabulum is cleared of the limbus, ligamentum teres and transverse ligament, and the head then reduced. At the same time a Salter innominate osteotomy is performed to reconstruct the acetabulum (Fig. 5.12) (Barrett *et al.*, 1986). After a further 6 weeks in a spica, an upper femoral osteotomy is occasionally required to realign the leg while maintaining reduction. If so, a further 6 weeks in a plaster hip spica is prescribed, followed by 3 months in a Denis Browne splint. If osteotomy is not required, the Denis Browne splint is applied at this stage.

This treatment protocol will result in good or excellent

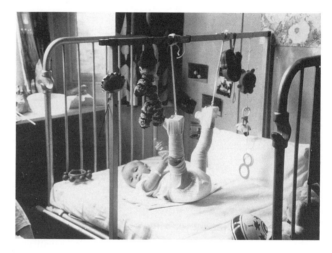

Fig. 5.9 Gallows traction.

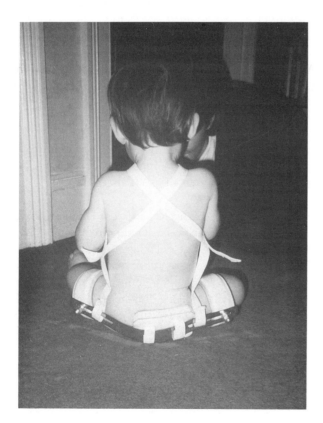

Fig. 5.8 Denis Browne splint.

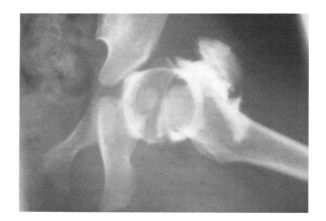

Fig. 5.10 Arthrogram, inturned limbus.

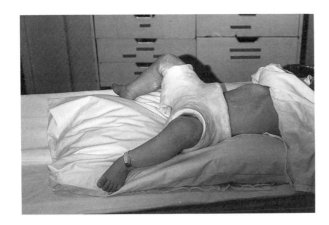

Fig. 5.11 Hip spica.

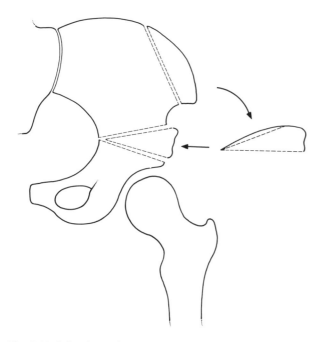

Fig. 5.12 Salter innominate osteotomy.

results in 75% of cases, with an incidence of avascular necrosis of about 5% (Salter and Dubor, 1974; Barrett *et al.*, 1986).

18 months to 3 years. After the age of 18 months, conservative treatment with traction is unlikely to succeed. Some surgeons favour a period of traction to stretch the soft tissues and thus prevent avascular necrosis and subsequent redislocation. It is also reasonable to progress straight to open reduction. This may be carried out exactly as for the younger age group, but reduction may be difficult at operation; the instability may be so great that femoral shortening and removal of a segment of femur from just below the lesser trochanter

is required. This can be combined with a derotation osteotomy of the femur (Fig. 5.13). An acetabular reconstruction can be done at the same time or delayed by 6 weeks to allow the child to recover from the first procedure. If femoral shortening is not required, the open reduction is combined with an innominate osteotomy.

Over 3 years. The only difference between this and the previous group is that femoral shortening is almost always required. Again, innominate osteotomy should be delayed, though good results have been reported following full open reduction, femoral shortening and innominate osteotomy at one operation (Dmitriou, 1989).

The question always asked in this group what is the upper age limit? Arbitrarily the age of 6 years is given as the upper limit, after which it is better not to treat. There is, however, the option of Colonna pericapsular acetabuloplasty, whereby the lax, stretched capsule is tightened over the head of the femur, encouraging the development of a false acetabulum (Colonna, 1966; Pozo *et al.*, 1987).

In older children who have been treated, persistent acetabular dysplasia can occur and give rise to pain and aching in early adolescence. Acetabular reconstruction is indicated to prevent progression to full osteoarthritis. The shelf procedure described by Wainwright (1976) is a straightforward and reliable technique (Fig. 5.14). Alternatively Chiari displacement osteotomy can be used, though it carries a significant risk of complications (Chiari, 1974; Benson and Evans, 1976; Matsuno, 1992).

RESULTS OF TREATMENT

How effective is treatment for congenital dislocation of the hip? Does the Pavlik harness always work? What

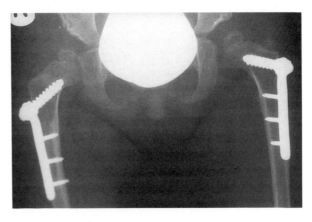

Fig. 5.13 Femoral osteotomies.

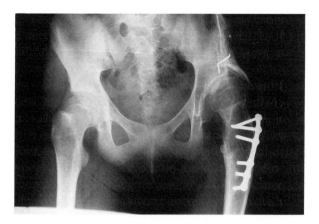

Fig. 5.14 Shelf procedure for acetabular dysplasia.

Table 5.2 Grading of avascular necrosis in treated congenital dislocation of the hip. After Salter (1969)

Grade	Classification	Radiographic changes
I	Temporary	Delayed less than 1 year Fragmentation Rapid recovery No deformity
II	Partial	Delayed more than 1 year Fragmentation Density of part of head Slow recovery Residual coxa magna
III	Total	Delayed more than 1 year Small nucleus Broadening of neck Increased density Residual coxa magna, coxa plana, coxa vara

sort of hip results from closed or open reduction for late diagnosed congenital dislocation of the hip? These questions are not easy to answer, but are the essence of the management of congenital dislocation of the hip. It is possible to produce a hip that is worse than one that has never been treated. It must never be forgotten that a congenitally dislocated hip has a good range of movement and is pain-free until degenerative changes set in. Failed treatment can produce a hip that is stiff and painful.

The results of treatment of congenital dislocation of the hip are assessed by measurements of the acetabulum and femoral heads on radiographs. These measurements are the acetabular index (Klieberman and Lieberman, 1936), the centre–edge angle (Wiberg, 1939) and avascular necrosis (Salter *et al.*, 1969) (Table 5.2). These measurements are shown in Figs 5.15–5.17.

Pavlik harness

The Pavlik harness will result in normal hips in 80% of dislocated hips diagnosed at birth. In the 20% failures, the harness either fails to hold or achieve reduction, results in a dysplastic hip, or produces avascular necrosis, an iatrogenic tragedy. The overall rate of avascular necrosis is 2.38% (Grill *et al.*, 1988). These results are comparable with those of other forms of splint and only serve to stress the importance of using any form of splint correctly and with care.

Closed reduction

Under the age of 2 years, closed reduction by traction and subsequent splinting can produce good results in 80% of cases, though the older the child, the less likely this method is to succeed (Morel, 1975). Even if the

procedure is successful, these children may require pelvic osteotomy to provide adequate acetabular cover.

Over the age of 2 years, traction can only produce good results in 40% of cases (Schoenecker and Strecker, 1984). Avascular necrosis occurs in over 50% of those treated by traction. Traction is not recommended for children over 2 years old. Open reduction with femoral shortening can produce good results in 85% of cases in this age group.

Open reduction

A number of workers prefer open reduction to traction even in very young children, claiming an incidence of

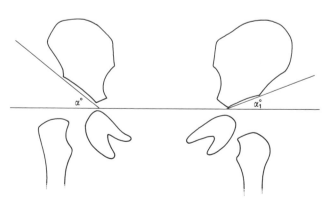

Fig. 5.15 Acetabular index: α°.

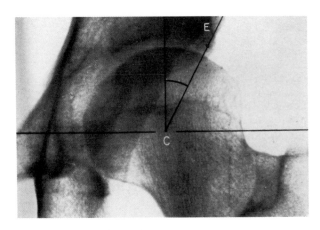

Fig. 5.16 Centre—edge angle.

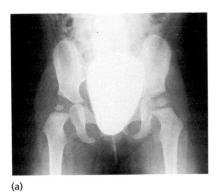

(a)

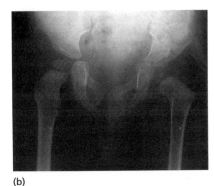

(b)

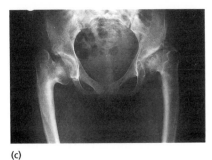

(c)

Fig. 5.17 Avascular necrosis.

avascular necrosis less than 5% and good results for acetabular development (Weinstein, 1987).

Closed or open reduction before the age of 2 years and open reduction with or without femoral shortening after the age of 2 years will result in excellent or good hips in 80% of cases. The 20% fair or poor results will comprise acetabular dysplasias, redislocations and 5—10% avascular necrosis. When a redislocation occurs after open reduction, only 33% will obtain an acceptable result with subsequent surgical treatment (McClusky *et al.*, 1988).

Summary

The aim of treatment either by closed or open means is not only stable reduction. There must be adequate reduction within the acetabulum without soft tissue imposition. This is obvious in open reduction, but in closed reduction the absence of soft tissue imposition can only be demonstrated by arthrography. Failure to identify and remove soft tissue will give a poor result (Renshaw, 1981). Adequate reduction before the age of 3 years results in good acetabular development (Harris *et al.*, 1975). Improvement in the acetabulum can occur up to 8 years after reduction (Lindstrom *et al.*, 1979).

The major studies referred to above all show that the age at which reduction is obtained is more important than the method of reduction and splinting. They all identify three groups according to the age at reduction and relate this to the end result (Table 5.3).

In the 20% who do not achieve a good result from primary treatment and have persistent acetabular dysplasia or worse, there is the risk of early degenerative arthritis. Wiberg (1939) showed that the centre—edge angle predicts the age of onset of osteoarthritis (Table 5.4); however, these measurements did not take into account whether Shenton's line was broken and whether there was lateral subluxation of the hip. It has since been shown that if Shenton's line is broken and there is lateral subluxation, significant arthritis occurs by the age of 42 years (Cooperman *et al.*, 1983).

Table 5.3 Results of treatment of DDH

Group	Age (years)	Centre—edge angle	Acetabular index	Result
I	<1 yr	24°	<20°	Good
II	1—2 yrs	22°	20—25°	Satisfactory
III	>2 yrs	20°	>25°	Fair

On the other hand, the centre—edge angle and acetabular index correlate poorly with the age of onset of osteoarthritis in the absence of lateral subluxation; some patients with a very low centre—edge angle do not develop significant arthritis until the sixth decade. There is a trend, however, which suggests that arthritis will develop earlier, the smaller the centre—edge angle (Table 5.4).

Table 5.4 Osteoarthritis in DDH

Centre—edge angle	Mean age of onset of osteoarthritis (years)
<5°	34
5—10°	46
10—15°	55
15—20°	65+

Perthes' disease

This is the classic cause of limp in a child aged about 5 years. It is, in fact, far less common than irritable hip syndrome in this age group, but the importance of establishing the diagnosis gives this condition appropriate prominence.

It is remarkable that in the same year—1910—only 15 years after the discovery of X-rays, three people independently published papers on this condition, which they called variously pseudo-coxalgia, osteochondritis deformans juvenilis and coxa plana. These were Calve (1910) from Berc in France, Legg (1910) from Boston and Perthes (1910), who was in fact the last to publish. Waldenstrom (1909) had described the condition 1 year earlier, but failed to achieve eponymous status, presumably because he wrongly attributed it to a variant of tuberculosis.

INCIDENCE

The incidence of Perthes' disease is variable. For example, it is much higher in the USA, where it is 1 in 1200 children (Molloy and MacMahon, 1967) than in the UK, where it is 1 in 12 500. Even within the UK there is a large variation, with 1 in 6000 in Merseyside and 1 in 11 500 in Wessex (Barker *et al.*, 1980). It is also extremely rare in black children, at less than 1 in 200 000 (Herring, 1989).

The condition occurs four times more commonly in boys, 10% of cases have bilateral disease, and the peak age to be affected is 4 years, with a range from 1 to 14 years.

AETIOLOGY

Avascular necrosis of part of the femoral head is the pathological process in Perthes' disease, but why the growing femoral head is so vulnerable remains obscure. Experimentally, raising the pressure of the fluid in the hip capsule can occlude venous drainage and produce a lesion in small dogs simulating Perthes' disease (Kemp, 1969).

It has been shown that a double infarct is required to produce the pathological changes of Perthes' disease, a single infarct being insufficient to do so (Inoue *et al.*, 1976). Venographic studies have demonstrated vascular abnormalities in the femoral neck, with abnormal filling of the femoral diaphysis and venous blockage of the neck (Green and Griffin, 1987), which indicates that venous occlusion rather than arterial obstruction is the cause of Perthes' disease. Perthes' disease is not, however, associated with the transient synovitis that might be expected if tamponade and venous occlusion were the whole story (Landin *et al.*, 1987).

There is no evidence for genetic inheritance of Perthes' disease, but it is more likely in low birth-weight children born towards the end of a family of older parents, particularly if born by breech presentation (Wynne-Davies, 1980). Children with Perthes' disease also show delay in skeletal development, particularly in the distal parts of the limbs, and failure of growth hormone levels to increase with age (Burnwell *et al.*, 1986).

NATURAL HISTORY

Legg (1927) said that after 10 years of follow-up, most patients with Perthes' disease would have pain, but few would be incapacitated. It has since been a widely held view that 20 years after Perthes' disease, patients will have some pain, but lead normal lives. Ratliff (1956) reported a 17-year follow-up showing that 25% of patients had deformed heads and severe pain. This series was followed for a further 20 years (Ratliff, 1967, 1977). Surprisingly, the number of poor outcomes did not increase over the 40 years. In other words, if the outcome for a particular patient is likely to be poor, this will be apparent in 10—20 years.

These findings tended to suggest that the outcome of Perthes' disease is determined at the time of onset of the disease and will not be affected by treatment. Evans and Lloyd Roberts (1958) indicated that treatment did not have much affect on the outcome, because either with or without treatment 30% did well, 30% had fair results and 30% did badly. On reviewing this work, however, Catterall (1971) formed the view that there were two types of the disease: one with less than half of the head showing radiographic involvement, which had a good prognosis particularly in younger children, and the second type with more than half the head involved, which had a poor prognosis, particularly if the child was more than 6 years old at the onset of the disease. It was the attempt to classify the unclear area in between these two groups that resulted in Catterall's classification. Nevertheless, the point was still made that overall there was no difference between the treated and the untreated groups (Table 5.5).

Subsequent studies (Brotherton and McKibbin, 1977; McAndrew and Weinstein, 1984) confirmed that treatment has little overall effect on the outcome, and almost all cases have osteoarthritis by the age of 65 years and 40% will have had total hip replacement, whereas few (6%) have by 35 years of age.

In an attempt to define that group, variously reported as between 6% and 20% of all cases, in whom early disabling osteoarthritis occurs, Catterall analysed the radiographs of almost 400 cases and produced his classification into four groups (Fig. 5.18). In addition, Catterall introduced the concept of the 'head at risk', which is a combination of clinical and radiological signs (Table 5.6). Gage (1933) described the radiological sign in which the lateral part of the femoral epiphysis and metaphysis are defective, as though a small 'bite' has been taken out (Fig. 5.19). Catterall was then able to show that in groups II, III and IV, particularly if 'at risk' signs were present, the number of good results fell and the number of poor results increased, but that with prospective treatment by femoral osteotomy based on this classification, the number of good results can be improved (Table 5.7). Most importantly, the number of poor results is reduced by treatment. This means that fewer patients will be severely incapacitated by the age of 35 years, suggesting that treatment in selected cases is worthwhile. Similarly, Petrie and Bitenc (1971) showed that treatment by abduction plaster casts reduced the number of poor results as did prolonged bed-rest and abduction (Brotherton & McKibbin, 1977) (Table 5.8).

Stulberg et al. (1981) proposed an alternative classification based on the radiographic appearance at the end of healing of the femoral head, and indicated that in the severe group (type 5) symptomatic osteoarthritis would be present after 40 years.

Treatment can therefore affect the outcome of the disease. The problem still remains of identifying which cases will benefit from treatment, for in addition to the radiographic changes, the age at onset of the disease has prognostic importance. Evans (1958) indicated that for those with onset under 6 years the prognosis was good. Onset after 6 years increased the number of poor results, and good results were not seen when the age of onset was after 8 years.

INDICATIONS FOR TREATMENT

The Catterall classification is difficult to apply in practice, and it relies on good-quality radiographs. Salter and Thompson (1984) simplified it to a two-part classification based on the extent of the subchondral fracture seen on an early lateral radiograph of the hip (Fig. 5.20):
1 Group A: child younger than 6 years; subchondral fracture involves less than half the head; no 'at risk' signs.

Table 5.5 Outcomes of patients with Perthes' disease with or without treatment (data from Catterall, 1971)

	Outcome (% of patients)		
	Good	Fair	Poor
Untreated	58	23	17
Treated	58	25	15

Table 5.6 Catterall's 'head at risk'

Clinical signs	Radiological sign
Older child	Gage's sign (Fig. 5.19)
Heavy child	Lateral calcification
Progressive loss of movement	Diffuse metaphyseal reaction
Adduction contracture	Lateral subluxation of head

Table 5.7 Outcomes of femoral osteotomy in patients at risk in Perthes' disease

	Outcome (% of patients)		
	Good	Fair	Poor
All cases	57	19	24
Group II, III and IV at risk	31	28	41
All cases untreated	57	19	24
Groups II–IV treated	67	25	8

Table 5.8 Outcomes of bed-rest and abduction in at-risk patients with Perthes' disease

	Outcome (% of patients)		
	Good	Fair	Poor
Brotherton and McKibbin, 1977	49	38	15
Petrie and Bitenc, 1971	60	30	9

2 Group B: child older than 6 years; subchondral fracture involves more than half the head; 'at risk' signs present.

Fractures involving less than half the head constitute group A; fractures involving more than half the head constitute group B and correspond to Catterall groups

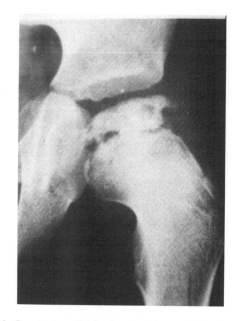

Fig. 5.19 Gage's sign. (Reproduced with permission from Catterall, 1971.)

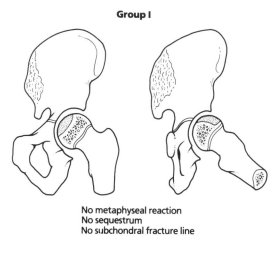

Group I

No metaphyseal reaction
No sequestrum
No subchondral fracture line

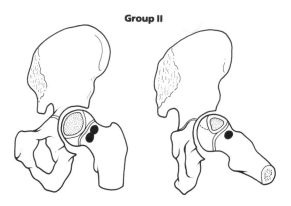

Group II

Sequestrum present—junction clear
Metaphyseal reaction—antero/lateral
Subchondral fracture line—anterior half

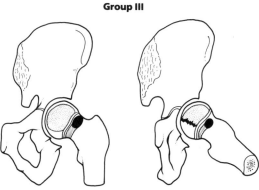

Group III

Sequestrum—large—junction—junction sclerotic
Metaphyseal reaction—diffuse antero/lateral area
Subchondral fracture line—posterior half

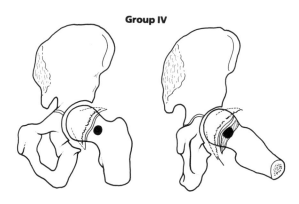

Group IV

Whole head involvement
Metaphyseal reaction—central or diffuse
Posterior remodelling

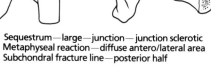

Fig. 5.18 Catterall classification of Perthes' disease. (Reproduced with permission from Catterall A., 1982, Legg-Calvé-Perthes' Disease. London, Churchill Livingstone.)

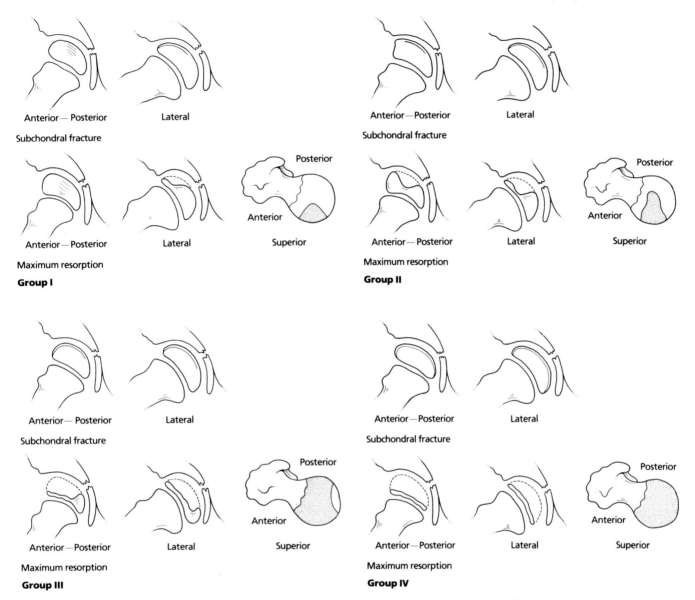

Anterior — Posterior   Lateral

Subchondral fracture

Anterior — Posterior   Lateral   Posterior / Anterior / Superior

Maximum resorption

Group I

Anterior — Posterior   Lateral

Subchondral fracture

Anterior — Posterior   Lateral   Posterior / Anterior / Superior

Maximum resorption

Group II

Anterior — Posterior   Lateral

Subchondral fracture

Anterior — Posterior   Lateral   Posterior / Anterior / Superior

Maximum resorption

Group III

Anterior — Posterior   Lateral

Subchondral fracture

Anterior — Posterior   Lateral   Posterior / Anterior / Superior

Maximum resorption

Group IV

Fig. 5.20 Salter–Thompson classification. (Reproduced with permission from Salter and Thompson, 1984.)

III and IV. If the 'at risk' signs and the age of the child are taken into account, these two broad groups can be identified simply. Provided that the child fits into one of the groups, the prognosis and place of treatment is clear, i.e. group B needs treatment.

Where there is a mixture of these parameters, e.g. a child older than 6 years with only minimal involvement, treatment is indicated only on the clinical signs, e.g. in a heavy, older child with limited abduction. This child will clearly need some form of treatment.

Finally, the stage of the disease at the time of diagnosis is an indicator of the need for treatment. If this is not clear on a radiograph, it can be established by arthro-graphy. Perthes' disease can be divided into three stages of active disease. Stage I is the earliest, before the femoral head has collapsed. Stage II: treatment will not be successful, but may prevent further deformity. Stage III is when healing has occurred. Treatment in some form may help remodelling of the femoral head.

TREATMENT

Two themes run through the history of the treatment of Perthes' disease. The first is that treatment is based on the three principles of containment of the femoral head within the acetabulum, weight relief and early mobilization. The second is that treatment in any form reduces the number of poor results rather than increasing the number of good results. Thus, treatment must be directed only towards those children whose prognosis is poor, and of course, treatment must do no harm.

Legg treated his cases by bed-rest, traction and hip spicas. Subsequently, the ischial-bearing weight-relieving caliper was used until it was shown that this does not alter pressure across the joint.

The principle of containment was probably introduced by A.O. Parker in Cardiff, and was used by both Rowley Bristow and Platt; however, it was first reported by Eyrebrook in 1936. The method was that of prolonged recumbency (up to 2 years) and wide abduction splinting followed by mobilization in abduction broomstick plasters (Fig. 5.21), which were maintained for up to another 2 years. While this method produced no poor results (Brotherton and McKibbin, 1977), it was noted to have severe psychological effects on the children. Even more absurd was the introduction of the Snyder sling following a report of a single case treated by a weight-bearing sling (Snyder, 1947), with a good result. The sling was then widely used around the world for many years. A modification was produced by Harrison *et al.* (1969) (Fig. 5.22), but the next advance was the introduction of mobile abduction plasters by Petrie and Bitenc (1971); these patients were allowed to bear weight. Again, few poor results were reported so the myth of weight relief was dispelled. Treatment was further simplified by the introduction of the Atlanta Scottish Rite brace (Fig. 5.23), which has been reported to have an equally good effect on reducing the number of poor results from 50% in controls to 24% (Purvis *et al.*, 1980).

A more logical and accurate method of containment is to place the head in the position of containment as

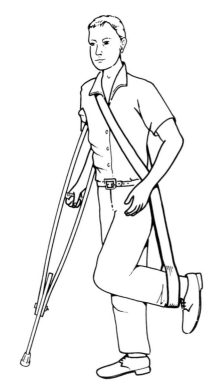

Fig. 5.22 Snyder sling.

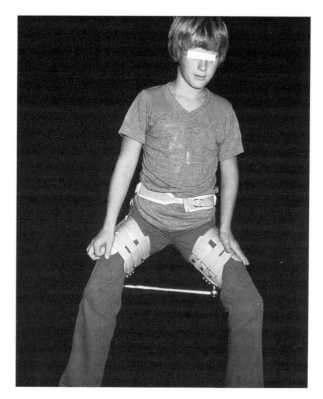

Fig. 5.23 Atlanta Scottish Rite brace.

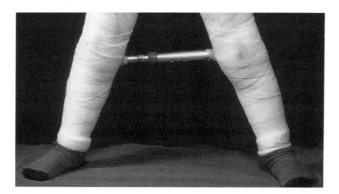

Fig. 5.21 Broomstick plasters.

demonstrated by arthrography, and to hold it there by acetabular (innominate) osteotomy (Salter, 1973) or by femoral osteotomy (Lloyd-Roberts *et al.*, 1976) (Fig. 5.24). Although this represents a major intervention, it avoids the need for prolonged recumbency and splinting. Patients do, however, have a short leg limp for some time after femoral osteotomy and stiffness of the hip after an innominate osteotomy. The results of femoral osteotomy are poor when undertaken late in the disease process, when healing is established and when the child is older than 8 years. In such cases, when the head is severely involved, shelf acetabuloplasty is a better option (Van der Heyden and Van Tongerloo, 1980) (Fig. 5.25).

Treatment can now be summarized as follows:
1 Symptomatic treatment for hip instability (bed-rest, traction, analgesia) for the young patient under 6 years, regardless of the degree of involvement.
2 For the child aged 6–8 years, bed-rest, traction, analgesia and progressive abduction in broomstick or Petrie casts, which can be continued, or containment achieved surgically, as defined by arthrography, either by femoral or innominate osteotomy, if the disease is diagnosed early.
3 Over 8 years old, weight relief and abduction plasters, or shelf acetabuloplasty.

This can be summarized on the algorithm in Fig. 5.26.

RESULTS OF TREATMENT

The complexity of the classification of Perthes' disease, the timing of onset of the disease, the age of the child at onset, and the relatively small number of patients in each group has meant that even now, no statistically

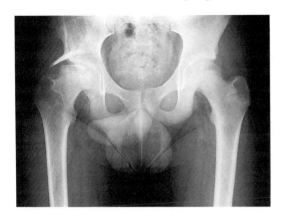

Fig. 5.25 Shelf operation.

significant difference has ever been shown between any of the different types of treatment, or even between treatment and no treatment. Furthermore, there has never been a comparison with a completely untreated group (Herring, 1989). This has led the Perthes' Study Group to comment:

It is difficult to draw firm conclusions about the relative merits of the three ambulatory treatment methods (crutches, abduction splints and femoral

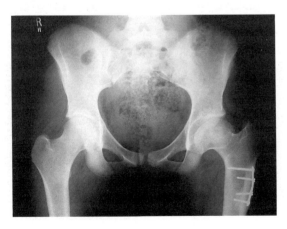

Fig. 5.24 Femoral osteotomy.

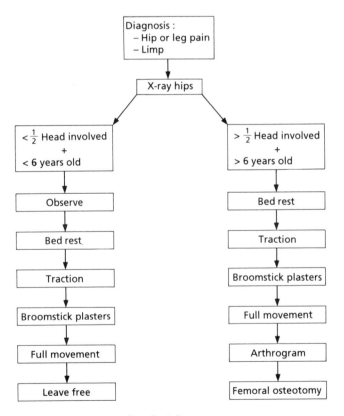

Fig. 5.26 Treatment of Perthes' disease.

osteotomy) because of the differences in prognosis of the patients in the treatment groups (Stulberg *et al.*, 1983). In other words, there is little to chose between any of the methods of treatment at present available.

Slipped upper femoral epiphysis

In the older child above the age of 11 years, the important cause of limp is slipped upper femoral epiphysis. It is still a diagnosis that is too often missed. Indeed, there is on average a 3-month delay from the onset of symptoms to making the diagnosis.

INCIDENCE

Developmental slipping of the proximal femoral epiphysis occurs between the ages of 11 and 16 years, with a peak at 13 years of age. It is then associated with the adolescent growth spurt. It is three times more common in boys, and when it does occur in girls it is almost always before menarche. It occurs in approximately 4 in 100 000 population, but is twice as common in the black population. It is thought to be bilateral in 20% of cases, but in as many as 40% there may be some abnormality of the unaffected hip (Bloomberg *et al.*, 1978). The left hip is most commonly affected, though the reason for this is obscure (Colton, 1987).

AETIOLOGY

Slipped epiphysis occurs in skeletally and sexually immature children, occurring on average 18 months before the proximal femoral epiphysis fuses. In girls menarche is delayed, and the slip almost always occurs before the onset of menstruation. The slip occurs during the growth spurt.

The actual cause of slipping of the epiphysis is obscure. The most attractive theory is that there is an imbalance between sex hormones and growth hormone; growth hormone weakens the physis, whereas sex hormones strengthen it. Thus, the child deficient in sex hormones who is growing rapidly is more likely to sustain a slipped epiphysis. This has never been proved, and in fact only 25% of children with a slip are of the classic obese, hypogonadal type. Slipped epiphysis is, however, associated with hypothyroidism and conditions affecting the pituitary, e.g. craniopharyngioma or fracture of the base of the skull. It is of note that patients with hormone deficiencies start to slip when treatment with growth hormone, thyroxine, or sex hormones is started.

Trauma is the precipitating episode in most cases, either minor repetitive trauma or a more significant injury giving an immediate slip, but not so great as to cause a fracture or fracture separation of the epiphysis.

PATHOLOGY

The slip always occurs posteriorly about an axis in the centre of the intertrochanteric region (Griffiths, 1975). A decreased extent of anteversion of the femoral neck is associated with slipping (Gelberman *et al.*, 1986). The soft tissue attached to the femoral head remains intact, and new bone is laid down on the back of the femoral neck producing the typical appearance of the chronic slip (Fig. 5.27). The soft tissue can rupture anteriorly, giving an acute on chronic slip. Histologically, the anterior synovium is initially oedematous and vascular, but is later replaced by a thin, fibrous layer (Howorth, 1966). The growth plate is thickened, and there is distortion of the normal columnar arrangement of the collagen fibres crossing the physis. In summary, the combination of a thickened physis during the growth spurt with deficiency of its collagen matrix, possibly abnormally rotated or angulated, which is subjected to an excessive load, predisposes to slipping of the proximal femoral epiphysis.

CLINICAL SIGNS

Slipped upper femoral epiphysis is the diagnosis that has replaced tuberculosis as the major cause of a young adolescent presenting with pain in the knee. Sometimes patients will persevere in insisting that the pain is in the knee, which must be why the diagnosis is still missed and accounts for the 3-month average delay between the onset of symptoms and diagnosis. Most patients, however, also have pain in the affected hip and they complain

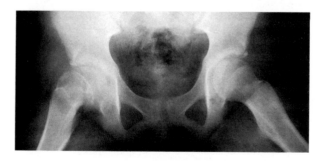

Fig. 5.27 Bilateral slipped upper femoral epiphyses. The head of the femur on the left has also started to slip.

of stiffness. All patients walk with a limp, and the affected leg is externally rotated. Movement may be quite good unless the slip is very acute, when there will be significant muscle spasm. In these circumstances, but usually not otherwise, there will be some local tenderness. Flexion is minimally reduced, with the leg tending to fall more into external rotation on flexion. Internal rotation in flexion is limited due to the relatively retroverted femoral neck impinging on the anterior acetabulum. It is also limited in extension, but not so much. This difference is more marked in the acute condition, when the synovium on the front of the femoral neck is inflamed. Abduction and adduction are similarly limited. There may be 1−2 cm of shortening of the leg.

The importance of examining the hip in a child presenting with knee pain and intermittent limp cannot be overemphasized, and radiographs of the hips should be obtained.

INVESTIGATIONS

The diagnosis rests on radiological examination. However, 11% of cases cannot be diagnosed on the anteroposterior projection, and therefore a lateral view is essential (Bloomberg *et al.*, 1978).

The most consistent sign on the anteroposterior view is blurring of the metaphysis, but in addition, the epiphyseal height is reduced, the growth plate is widened in early cases and Shenton's line may be broken with some extension of the inferior metaphysis below the acetabulum. Trethowan's line should be looked for, but is only positive when a substantial slip has occurred (Fig. 5.28). For more accurate diagnosis and for the effective planning of treatment, the standard Billing's view should be taken in every case (Billing, 1954). This is a standard lateral view of the proximal femur taken as an anteroposterior view of the pelvis with the hip flexed, abducted and externally rotated. This allows the angles subtended by the femoral head on the neck and shaft to be measured. These are normally 90°, and the mean of the two measured angles is taken and subtracted from 90°, giving an angle of slip.

TREATMENT

For the purposes of planning treatment, slipped upper femoral epiphysis is divided into two groups: acute and acute-on-chronic or chronic. Within these groups, management is determined by the degree of slip, which can be classified as three grades. Grade I is a slip of up to one-third of the physis or 30° on the Billing's view.

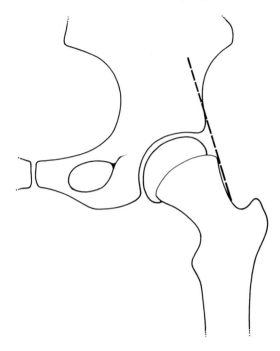

Fig. 5.28 Trethowan's line.

Grade II is an intermediate group of up to 50% slip or 30−50° on the Billing view. Grade III is the difficult, severe group of more than 50% or 50° slip.

Acute slip

Less than 30° slip. Several series over a long time have established that in this group, fixation of the femoral head *in situ* by whatever method results in a very satisfactory hip in over 85% of cases, with significant degenerative change only 20 years or more later (Wilson, 1936; Boyer *et al.*, 1981). This serves to condemn the practice of manipulation, which only results in any improvement in position in less than 40%, and of these 40% more than two-thirds will develop avascular necrosis (Griffiths, 1975).

Traction alone should also be avoided. It is unlikely to improve the position of the femoral head, and if it does, it carries the same risk as manipulation of subsequent avascular necrosis. Since the introduction of the cannulated screw systems, a single, cannulated screw is the author's preferred method of fixation of the femoral head, avoiding the increased risks associated with multiple pin fixation (Fig. 5.29).

30−50° slip. In this group, the risks associated with manipulative reduction are even greater, and the temp-

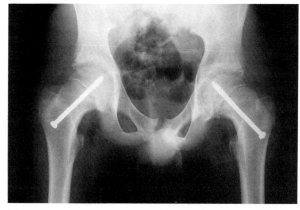

(a)

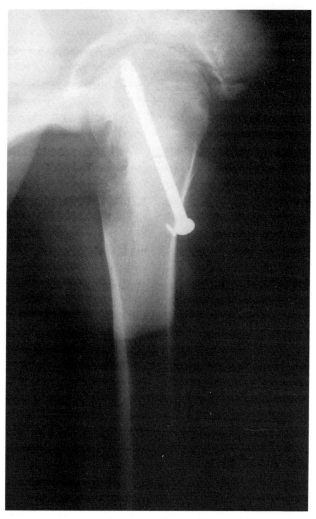

(b)

Fig. 5.29 Single cannulated screw fixation. (a) Anteroposterior view. (b) Lateral view.

tation must be resisted. The treatment of choice then rests between fixation *in situ* and the technique described by Heyman and Herndon (1954), in which an anterior approach to the hip is made, and the knob of bone that is the protruding anterior part of the neck of the femur excised to prevent abutment and subsequent limitation of internal rotation. The epiphysis is then fused by laying a graft across the plate anteriorly. This technique has been shown to be at least as good as multiple pin fixation, and given the technical difficulties of pin insertion with the more severe slips, it is a good option (Weiner *et al.*, 1984). On the other hand, multiple pin fixation can result in excellent remodelling in over 50% of cases with no late symptoms at 15 years (O'Brien and Fahey, 1977). This can be predicted if the tri-radiate cartilage is open at presentation, which is usually the case (Jones *et al.*, 1990). Given the greater simplicity of fixation *in situ* with a single cannulated screw, the author's choice is fixation *in situ* in this group.

More than 50° slip.   There is no doubt that this rare group does exist. Pinning *in situ* can be done, and should be, if in doubt, though it is difficult. Excision of the anterior neck and bone graft epiphysiodesis is also difficult and has the worrying problem that over half the neck is removed.

It is in this group, together with the severe acute-on-chronic or chronic group, that open reduction and fixation of the upper femoral epiphysis can be undertaken by the Dunn or Fish techniques (see below).

Acute-on-chronic or chronic slip

Less than 30° slip.   Treatment in this group is as for acute slip.

30–50° slip.   Treatment is also as for acute slip, with fixation *in situ* being the treatment of choice. Only in the chronic group, who may present after the tri-radiate cartilage is closed, does excision of the anterior femoral neck and bone graft epiphysiodesis have a place.

More than 50° slip.   In this group there is a considerable new bone formation on the posterior aspect of the femoral neck, and it can be hard to identify the original neck. Even though extensive remodelling can occur, there is persistent loss of internal rotation and early onset of osteoarthritis. The options are either open reduction and fixation of the femoral head, or a form of subtrochanteric osteotomy, readjusting the line of weight-bearing without opening the hip joint and jeopardizing the blood supply to the femoral head.

The principle of open reduction and internal fixation, described by Dunn in (1964), is to reduce the femoral epiphysis by shortening the neck, excising the new bone formed on the back of the neck while preserving the delicate soft tissue hinge, which contains the blood supply to the epiphysis, at the back of the femoral neck. Dunn described removal of the greater trochanter and a lateral approach to the hip, giving excellent exposure. There is a significant risk of avascular necrosis of the femoral head with this technique: 1 case in 40 in chronic slips and 5 in 24 in acute-on-chronic in his series (Dunn and Angel, 1978).

Fish modified the surgical exposure to undertake the same procedure from an anterolateral approach, reporting only one case of avascular necrosis in 42 cases (Fish, 1984).

Although these procedures require skill and patience, they do give the opportunity for anatomical reduction as well as fixing the epiphysis to prevent further slip and to promote early fusion. These are not provided by an extracapsular trochanteric osteotomy.

The techniques of choice for extracapsular osteotomy are either Griffiths' trochanteric, subcervical osteotomy or Southwick's subtrochanteric osteotomy (Southwick, 1967; Griffiths, 1975). The main difference between these two techniques is that the Griffith procedure is done at the pertrochanteric level, the Southwick at the level of the lesser trochanter. They are technically demanding and require precise pre-operative planning.

They have the disadvantage that it is difficult to pin the slipping epiphysis at the same time. It is then necessary to pin the slip *in situ*, which is difficult, and later undertake the osteotomy. Long-term follow-up of these procedures is surprisingly not available; however, it does seem that failure to fully correct the geometry of the proximal femur predisposes to early osteoarthritis in about 40% of cases after 20 years, which is not very different from the results of pinning *in situ* alone (Ireland and Newman, 1978).

PREFERRED TREATMENT

The choice and the technique of treatment still remains controversial, and a personal philosophy has to be followed. Pinning *in situ*, preferably using a single cannulated screw for all slips up to 50%, cannot be faulted. For an acute-on-chronic 50% slip when the epiphyseal plate is open, the Heyman and Herndon open fusion is preferable. For severe slips, pinning *in situ* with a later subtrochanteric osteotomy must be the best advice for the surgeon who only treats these cases occasionally. For the surgeon who is likely to be referred cases by his colleagues, open reduction by the Dunn or Fish technique will produce the best results.

COMPLICATIONS

The complications of slipped epiphysis are the complications of failed diagnosis or complications of treatment. Failed diagnosis results in a severely deformed hip and a painful, shortened, externally rotated leg, with early-onset osteoarthritis. The complications of treatment are either those directly associated with insertion of pins, or the later consequences of surgical treatment, namely chondrolysis and avascular necrosis.

The insertion of pins is not a benign procedure. Perforation of the joint and damage to the acetabular cartilage or to the blood supply by perforation of the back of the femoral head can occur. Pins can break or back out, resulting in further slip. Infection following insertion of pins is not unknown, and fracture of the femur through a pin site can occur. For these reasons, the practice of prophylactic pinning of the unaffected hip should now be discouraged. One case of chondrolysis of a normal hip as a direct result of prophylactic pinning is enough to persuade most surgeons to discontinue this practice. If a patient can be relied on to attend follow-up, it is sufficient to wait for the first sign of symptoms in the opposite leg before resorting to pinning the femoral head. Needless to say, the onset of symptoms, even without radiographic changes, is enough to justify pinning. For all these reasons, the insertion of multiple pins is being discontinued in favour of a single cannulated screw.

Chondrolysis

This is acute necrosis of the articular cartilage of the hip. The cause is unknown, but it is more likely to occur in black children, so it cannot entirely be attributed to operative technique. It may be an autoimmune phenomenon, and raised levels of IgM and IgG have been recorded. Chondrolysis can occur after any form of treatment. Overall, it occurs in 24% of cases of slipped femoral epiphysis, and in as many as 50% if the pin penetrates the joint. The incidence is even higher after subtrochanteric osteotomy. After open reduction and fixation of the Dunn or Fish type, the incidence of chondrolysis is reported as only 10–15%.

Chondrolysis produces a stiff, painful joint with reduction of the joint space on a radiograph. A form of fibrous ankylosis occurs. Gradually the movement returns, but the pain may worsen. Finally, after at least 2 years, the joint space may increase as seen on a radiograph, and there may be surprising recovery of the range of movement. Treatment, apart from anti-inflammatory agents and gentle mobilization, should be avoided. The only real option is arthrodesis, and then only when one side is affected. If the child is large and overweight, arthrodesis is difficult and disabling.

Avascular necrosis

This occurs occasionally in cases treated by rest alone, but it is more usually the result of treatment. In particular it is caused by manipulation of the hip, when 50% of cases will be affected overall, otherwise the incidence is about the same as for chondrolysis, with some necrosis occurring in about 30% of cases. It occurs after pinning or open reduction more than after subtrochanteric osteotomy alone.

REFERENCES

Adams J.A. (1963) Transient synovitis of the hip joint in children. *J. Bone Joint Surg.* **45B**, 471.

Allan D.B., Gray R.H., Scott T.D., Tonkin M., Hughes J.R. and Evans G.A. (1985) The relationship of ligamentous clicks arising from the newborn hip and congenital dislocation. *J. Bone Joint Surg.* **67B**, 491.

Barker D.J.P., Dixon E. and Taylor J.F. (1978) Perthes' disease of the hip in three regions of England. *J. Bone Joint Surg.* **60B**, 478.

Barlow T.G. (1966) Congenital dislocation of the hip in the newborn. Early diagnosis and treatment of congenital dislocation of the hip in the newborn. *Proc. R. Soc. Med.* **59**, 1103.

Barrett W.P., Staheli L.T. and Chew D.E. (1986) The effectiveness of the Salter innominate osteotomy in the treatment of congenital dislocation of the hip. *J. Bone Joint Surg.* **68A**, 79–87.

Bellmore M.C., Lam A.H. and Wayn B. (1989) The infant hip: real time assessment of hip stability. *J. Bone Joint Surg.* **71B**, 882.

Benson M.K.D. and Evans D.C.J. (1976) The pelvic osteotomy of Chiari: an anatomical study of the hazards and misleading radiographic appearances. *J. Bone Joint Surg.* **58B**, 164.

Bickerstaff D.R., Neal L.M., Booth A.J., Brennan P.O. and Bell M.J. (1990) Ultrasound examination of the irritable hip. *J. Bone Joint Surg.* **72B**, 549–553.

Billing L. (1954) Roentgen examination of the proximal femur end in children and adolescents. *Acta Radiol. Scand. Suppl. (Stockh.)* 110.

Blockey N.J. and Porter B.B. (1968) Transient synovitis of the hip: a virological investigation. *BMJ* **4**, 557.

Bloomberg T.J., Nuttall J. and Stoker D.J. (1978) Radiology in early slipped capital femoral epiphysis. *Clin. Radiol.* **29**, 657–667.

Boyer D.W., Mickelson M.R. and Ponsetti I.V. (1981) Slipped capital femoral epiphysis. *J. Bone Joint Surg.* **63A**, 85–95.

Bradley J., Wetherill M. and Benson M.K.D. (1987) Splintage for congenital dislocation of the hip. *J. Bone Joint Surg.* **69B**, 257–263.

Brotherton B.J. and McKibbin B. (1977) Perthes' disease treated by prolonged recumbency and femoral head containment. *J. Bone Joint Surg.* **59B**, 8.

Burwell R.G., Vernon C.L., Dangerfield P.H. *et al.* (1986) Raised somatomedin activity in the serum of young boys with Perthes' disease, revealed by bio-assay: a disease of growth transition? *Clin. Orthop.* **209**, 129.

Calve L. (1910) Sur une forme particulaire de pseudo-coxalgia gréffée sur des déformations caracteristiques de l'extrémétie superieure du femur. *Rev. Chir.* **30**, 54.

Catterall A. (1971) The natural history of Perthes' disease. *J. Bone Joint Surg.* **35B**, 37–53.

Chiari K. (1974) Medial displacement osteotomy of the pelvis. *Clin. Orthop. Rel. Res.* **98**, 55.

Clarke N.M.P., Theodore Hakke H., McHugh P., Myung Lee, Borns P.F. and Macewen G.D. (1985) Real time ultrasound in the diagnosis of congenital dislocation and dysplasia of the hip. *J. Bone Joint Surg.* **71B**, 882.

Colonna P.C. (1966) Capsular arthroplasty for congenital dislocation of the hip. Indictions for technique. *J. Bone Joint Surg.* **47**, 437.

Colton C.L. (1987) In: *Recent Advances in Orthopaedics.* Edinburgh, Churchill Livingstone.

Cooperman D.R., Wallenstein R. and Stulberg S.T. (1983) Acetabular dysplasia in the adult. *Clin. Orthop.* **175**, 79.

Dimitriou J. (1989) Surgical treatment of congenital dislocation of the hip in children over the age of three years with a one stage procedure — long term results. *Combined meeting of the Hellenic Association of Orthopaedics and Trauma and British Orthopaedic Association.*

Dunn D.M. (1964) The treatment of adolescent slipping of the upper femoral epiphysis. *J. Bone Joint Surg.* **46B**, 621–629.

Dunn D.M. and Angel J.C. (1978) Replacement of the femoral head by open operation in the severe adolescent slipping of the upper femoral epiphysis. *J. Bone Joint Surg.* **60B**, 394–403.

Evans D.L. (1958) Legg–Calvé–Perthes' disease. A study of late results. *J. Bone Joint Surg.* **40B**, 168–181.

Evans D.L. and Lloyd Roberts G.C. (1958) Treatment in Legg–Calvé–Perthes' disease. A comparison of in-patient and out-patient methods. *J. Bone Joint Surg.* **40B**, 182.

Eyrebrook A.L. (1936) Osteochondritis deformans coxae juvenilis in Perthes' disease. The results of treatment by traction in recumbency. *Br. J. Surg.* **24**, 166–182.

Fish J.B. (1984) Cuneiform osteotomy of the femoral neck in the treatment of slipped capital femoral epiphysis. *J. Bone Joint Surg.* **66A**, 1153–1168.

Fredensborg N. (1976) The results of early treatment of typical congenital dislocation of the hip in Malmo. *J. Bone Joint Surg.* **58B**, 272.

Gage H.C. (1933) A possible sign of Perthes' disease. *Br. J. Radiol.* **6**, 295.

Gelberman R.H., Cohen M.S., Shaw B.A., Kasser J.R., Griffin P.P. and Wilkinson R.H. (1986) The association of femoral retroversion with slipped capital femoral epiphysis. *J. Bone Joint Surg.* **68A**, 1000–1007.

Graf R. and Schulen P. (1986) Sonographie in der Orthopaedie. In *Braun Gunter Schwerk. Ultradiagnostik 4. Erg. Lfg. 7.* Ecomed Verlag.

Green N.E. and Griffin P.P. (1987) Intra-osseous venous pressure in Legg–Perthes' disease. *J. Bone Joint Surg.* **64A**, 666.

Griffiths M.G. (1975) Acute slipping of the capital femoral epiphysis. *J. Bone Joint Surg.* **57B**, 113.

Grill F., Bensahel H., Candell J., Dungel P., Matasovic T. and

Vizkelty T. (1988) The Pavlik harness in the treatment of the congenitally dislocating hip: a report on a multicentre study of the European Paediatric Orthopaedic Society. *J. Paediatr. Orthop.* **8**, 1.

Harris N.H., Lloyd-Roberts G.C. and Gallien R. (1975) Acetabular development in congenital dislocation of the hip. *J. Bone Joint Surg.* **57B**, 46.

Harrison M.H.M., Turner M.H. and Nicholson F.J. (1969) Coxa plana. Results of a new form of splinting. *J. Bone Joint Surg.* **51A**, 1057–1069.

Herring J.A. (1989) Legg–Calvé–Perthes' disease. A review of current knowledge. *American Academy of Orthopedic Surgeons. Institutional Course Lectures* **38**, 309–315.

Heyman C.H. and Herndon C.H. (1954) Epiphysiodesis for early slipping of the upper femoral epiphysis. *J. Bone Joint Surg.* **36A**, 539–555.

Howorth B. (1966) Pathology. Slipping of the capital femoral epiphysis. *Clin. Orthop. Rel. Res.* **48**, 33–48.

Inoue A., Freeman M.A., Vernon-Roberts B. *et al.* (1976) The pathogenesis of Perthes' disease. *J. Bone Joint Surg.* **58B**, 453.

Ireland J. and Newman P.H. (1978) Triplane osteotomy for severe slipped upper femoral epiphysis. *J. Bone Joint Surg.* **60B**, 390–393.

Jones J.R., Paterson D.C., Hillier T.M. and Foster B.K. (1990) Slipped capital femoral epiphysis: an assessment or remodelling after pinning. *J. Bone Joint Surg.* **72B**, 1093–1094, 1100.

Kalamachi A. and MacFarlane R. (1982) The Pavlik harness. Results in patients over three months of age. *J. Pediatr. Orthop.* **2**, 3.

Kemp H.B.S. (1969) Experimental Perthes' disease. *J. Bone Joint Surg.* **51B**, 178.

Klieberman S. and Lieberman H.S. (1936) The acetabular index in infants in relation to congenital dislocation of the hip. *Arch. Surg.* **32**, 1049.

Landin L.A., Danklsson L.G. and Wattsgard C. (1987) Transient synovitis of the hip. *J. Bone Joint Surg.* **69**, 328.

Legg A.T. (1910) An obscure affection of the hip joint. *Boston Med. Surg. J.* **162**, 202.

Legg A.T. (1927) The end results of coxa plana. *J. Bone Joint Surg.* **9**, 26.

Lindstrom J.R., Ponsetti I.V. and Wenger D.R. (1979) Acetabular development after reduction in congenital dislocation of the hip. *J. Bone Joint Surg.* **61A**, 112.

Lloyd-Roberts G.C. and Swann M. (1966) Pitfalls in the management of congenital dislocation of the hip. *J. Bone Joint Surg.* **48B**, 666.

Lloyd-Roberts G.C., Catterall A. and Salomen P.B. (1976) A controlled study of the indications for and the results of femoral osteotomy in Perthes' disease. *J. Bone Joint Surg.* **58B**, 31–36.

Ludloff K. (1913) The open reduction of congenital dislocation of the hip by an anterior incision. *Am. J. Orthop. Surg.* **10**, 438.

MacAndrew M.P. and Weinstein S.L. (1984) A long term follow-up of Legg–Perthes' disease. *J. Bone Joint Surg.* **66A**, 860–869.

McClusky W.P., Bassett G.S., More-Garcia G. and MacEwen G.D. Failed open reduction for congenital hip dislocation. 55th Annual Meeting of the American Academy of Orthopedic Surgeons, 1988.

Matsuno T., Ichioka Y. and Kaneda K. (1992) Modified Chiari pelvic osteotomy. A long term follow-up study. *J. Bone Joint Surg.* **74A**, 470–478.

Mau H., Doz D.R., Dorr W.M., Henkel L. and Lutsche J. (1971) Open reduction of congenital dislocation of the hip by Ludloff's method. *J. Bone Joint Surg.* **53A**, 1281.

Morel G. (1975) The treatment of congenital dislocation and subluxation of the hip in the older child. *Acta Orthop. Scand.* **46**, 364.

O'Brien E.T. and Fahey J.J. (1977) Remodelling of the femoral neck after *in situ* pinning for slipped capital femoral epiphysis. *J. Bone Joint Surg.* **59A**, 62–68.

Ortolani M. (1937) Un segno polonoto e sua importanza per la diagnosi precoce di pre-lussazione congenita dell'anca. *Paediatria* **45**, 129.

Palmer K. (1963) Examination of the newborn hip for congenital dislocation of the hip. *Dev. Med. & Child Neurol.* **5**, 45.

Perthes G.C. (1910) Uber arthritis deformans juveniles. *Dtsch. Z. Chir.* **107**, 11.

Petrie J.G. and Bitenc I. (1971) The abduction, weight-bearing treatment in Legg–Perthes' disease. *J. Bone Joint Surg.* **53B**, 54–62.

Pozo, J.L., Cannon S.R. and Catterall A. (1987) The Colonna Hey-Groves arthroplasty in the late treatment of congenital dislocation of the hip. *J. Bone Joint Surg.* **69B**, 220–228.

Purvis J.M., Dimon J.H. III and Meehan P.L. (1980) Preliminary experience with the Scottish Rite abduction orthosis for Legg–Perthes' disease. *Clin. Orthop.* **150**, 49–53.

Ramsey P.L., Lasser S. and MacEwan G.D. (1976) Congenital dislocation of the hip. The use of the Pavlik harness in the child in the first six months of life. *J. Bone Joint Surg.* **58A**, 1000.

Ratliffe A.H.C. (1956) Pseudocoxalgia: a study of the late results in the adult. *J. Bone Joint Surg.* **38B**, 498.

Ratliffe A.H.C. (1967) Perthes' disease. A study of 34 hips observed for 30 years. *J. Bone Joint Surg.* **49B**, 102.

Ratliffe A.H.C. (1977) Perthes' disease. A study of 16 patients followed up for 40 years. *J. Bone Joint Surg.* **59B**, 248.

Renshaw R.S. (1981) Inadequate reduction of congenital dislocation of the hip. *J. Bone Joint Surg.* **63A**, 1114–1121.

Salter R.B. (1973) Legg–Perthes' disease—treatment by innominate osteotomy. *American Academy of Orthopaedic Surgeons: Instructional Course Lectures* **22**, 309–316.

Salter R.B. and Dubor J-P. (1974) The first 15 years experience with innominate osteotomy in the treatment of congenital dislocation and subluxation of the hip. *Clin. Orthop.* **98**, 72–103.

Salter R.B. and Thompson G.H. (1984) Legg–Calvé–Perthes' disease: the prognostic significance of the sub-chondral fracture and a two group classification of the femoral head involvement. *J. Bone Joint Surg.* **66A**, 479–489.

Salter R.B., Kostuik J. and Dallas R. (1969) Avascular necrosis as a complication of treatment for congenital dislocation of the hip in young children. *Can. J. Surg.* **12**, 44–61.

Schoenecker P.L. and Strecker W.B. (1984) Congenital dislocation of the hip in children. Comparison of the effects of femoral shortening and of skeletal traction in treatment. *J. Bone Joint Surg.* **66A**, 21–27.

Snyder C.F. (1947) A sling for use in Perthes' disease. *J. Bone Joint Surg.* **29**, 524–526.

Southwick W.O. (1967) Osteotomy through the lesser trochanter for slipped capital femoral epiphysis. *J. Bone Joint Surg.* **49A**, 807–835.

Stulberg S.D., Cooperman D.R. and Wallensten R. (1981) The natural history of Legg–Calvé–Perthes' disease. *J. Bone Joint Surg.* **63**, 1095–1108.

Van der Heyden A.M. and Van Tongerloo R.B. (1980) Shelf operation in Perthes' disease. *J. Bone Joint Surg.* **63B**, 282–283.

Von Rosen S. (1962) Diagnosis and treatment of congenital dislocation of the hip in the newborn. *J. Bone Joint Surg.* **44B**, 284.

Wainwright D. (1976) The shelf operation for hip dysplasia in adolescence. *J. Bone Joint Surg.* **58B**, 159.

Waldenstrom H. (1909) Der obere tuberkulose collumherd. *Z. Orthop. Chir.* **24**, 487.

Weiner D.S., Weiner S., Melbu A. and Hoyt W.A. (1984) A 30 year experience with bone graft epiphysiodesis in the treatment of slipped capital femoral epiphysis. *J. Pediatr. Orthop.* **4**, 145–152.

Weinstein S.L. (1987) Anteromedial approach to reduction of congenital hip dysplasia. *Strategies Orthop. Surg.* **225**, 62.

Wiberg G. (1939) Studies on dysplastic acetabula and congenital subluxation of the hip joint. *Acta Chir. Scand. Suppl.* **58**, 1939.

Wilkinson J.A. (1985) *Congenital Displacement of the Hip Joint.* New York, Springer Verlag.

Wilson P.D. (1936) Conclusions regarding treatment of slipped upper femoral epiphysis. *Surg. Clin. North Am.* **16**, 733–752.

Wynne-Davis R. (1973) *Heritable Disorders in Orthopaedic Practice.* Oxford, Blackwell Scientific Publications.

Wynne-Davies R. (1980) Some aetiological factors in Perthe's disease. *Clin. Orthop.* **150**, 12.

Chapter 6
Disorders of the Knee in Children

P.M. Aichroth

INTRODUCTION

The knee is a hinge joint with a large, irregular and complex synovial cavity. It is a modified hinge, for some rotation is allowed with the two major bones articulating as a roller in a trough. Their incongruous surfaces produce point loading, and movement is a combination of rolling, gliding and rotation. The main extensor tendon expands the anterior aspect of the joint, and in this tendon is the largest of the sesamoid bones, the patella, which articulates with the anterior femoral condyle and in flexion tucks into the intercondylar notch. There are capsular condensations which produce the medial collateral and posterior oblique ligaments. The lateral collateral ligament should be considered extracapsular. The cruciate ligaments lie within the joint cavity and invaginate the synovium. The rather flat tibial plateaux are rendered concave to receive the femoral convexities by means of semilunar fibrocartilaginous rims—the menisci. The only exception to this is the discoid lateral meniscus, and this structure should be considered as a congenital malformation and not as an embryonic remnant.

The first sign of the limb bud in the embryo is at the end of the fourth week. The mesenchyme then condenses axially and is converted initially into the cartilaginous skeleton and later into bone. The joint cavity forms at the third month as a mass of undifferentiated mesenchyme, which becomes looser and then forms a cavity, the cellular lining of which becomes synovium. Mesenchyme may persist in this cavitated area to form the articular menisci.

OSSIFICATION AROUND THE KNEE

The femur ossifies at the centre of the future shaft at the end of the second month of intrauterine life. The ossific centre of the femoral condyles is usually present at birth.

It appears in boys between the eighth month and birth, but in girls may appear as early as the seventh month of intrauterine life. The lower femoral epiphysis remains unfused until the age of 17 years in girls and until 18 or even 19 years in boys, when the epiphyseal line ossifies. The tibia is similarly ossified from centres in the shaft, the upper 'growing end' and the lower epiphysis. The upper tibial epiphysis develops an ossific centre at the eighth month of intrauterine life in girls and just before or after birth in boys. This proximal epiphysis may fuse as late as 19 or even 20 years in boys and 2—3 years earlier in girls. The upper tibial epiphysis includes the upper half of the tibial tubercle, and there is usually an additional ossific centre here, appearing at the age of 12—13 years (Fig. 6.1)

Patellar development

The patella is preformed in cartilage and is usually seen by the third month of intrauterine life. It is cartilaginous at birth, and a bony centre appears at the third year in girls and the fourth or even fifth year in boys. Sometimes the ossific centre may be bipartite or multipartite and may be confused with a fractured patella by the unwary. Ossification is completed about the age of puberty.

Irregularity of ossification of the femoral condylar epiphysis

Throughout childhood the edge of the ossific nucleus of the lower femur is irregular. At the distal epiphysis boundary the advancing front of ossification may produce multiple areas that resemble small loose bodies. This has given rise to confusion with osteochondritis dissecans and has been implicated in the aetiology of this condition. Smillie (1960) feels that some cases of osteochondritis dissecans in the juvenile are actually ossification abnormalities. There is, however, a very

157

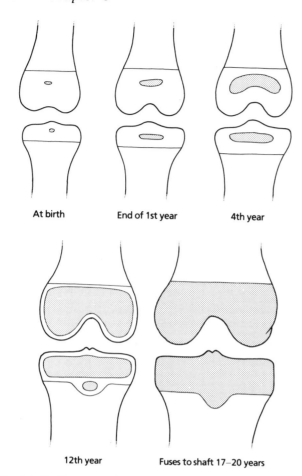

At birth   End of 1st year   4th year

12th year   Fuses to shaft 17–20 years

Fig. 6.1 Ossification at the knee.

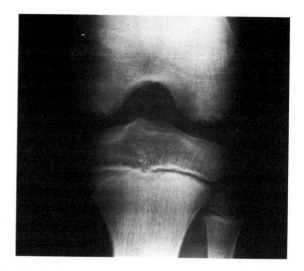

Fig. 6.2 Ossification defects — femoral condyles.

definite difference in the radiological appearance of the two conditions. In the ossification irregularity producing an ossicle effect, the proximal edge of the fragment does not fit into a crater (Fig. 6.2). In the child with osteochondritis dissecans, the bony fragment fits exactly the crater in the epiphyseal bone (Fig. 6.3). The articular cartilage in this latter situation is fractured and can be readily observed arthroscopically. Several patients with knee symptoms and ossification irregularity, as seen in Fig. 6.4, have been examined arthroscopically by the author and no lesion has been seen. A definite 'fragment-in-crater' must therefore be identified radiologically before osteochondritis dissecans is suspected in a child of this age.

SPECIAL FEATURES OF THE IMMATURE KNEE

The child's knee is lax, particularly in young girls. Although this state predisposes to easier patellar subluxation or dislocation, it does protect against significant ligament tears. Certainly, major knee disruptions do occur in the child's knee, but fractures of the femur above or the tibia below are more common in the child whose teenage or adult counterpart would sustain a major ligament injury. Laxity of the ligaments allows a greater range of physiological varus, valgus and recurvatum at the knee, and this must be borne in mind when examining joint stability. Comparison with the other side is always necessary.

Ligament laxity certainly has its advantages in the child, for ligament and capsular strains are much less common. General joint laxity allows easy observation of the synovial cavity by arthroscopy in a child, for the bones may be readily separated by traction and by

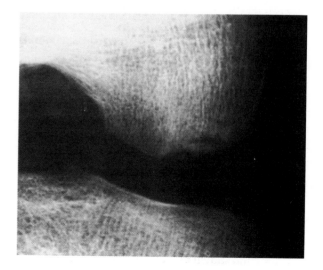

Fig. 6.3 Osteochondritis dissecans in an infant.

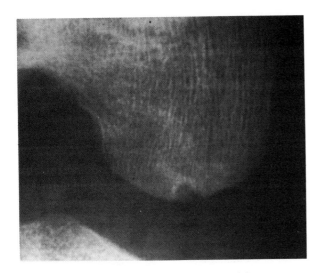

Fig. 6.4 Small ossification defect — femoral condyle.

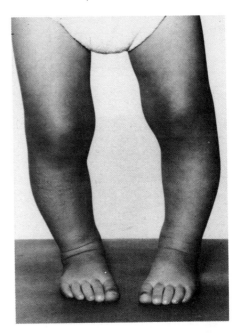

Fig. 6.5 Physiological genu varum in the toddler.

valgus and varus forces. In a child with congenital and sometimes familial joint laxity, recurrent dislocation of the patella may be present as well as congenital dislocation of the hip.

Physiological varus and valgus of the knee during development

During the first year of life the knee tends to lie in varus. The patella may be difficult to feel in the chubby infantile knee, but when the legs are positioned in neutral with the patellae facing exactly anterior, this curvature is present in most infants and is marked in some. During the toddler stage until the age of 3 or 4 years, this position is again often seen (Fig. 6.5). The traditional thought that this was due to a bunched nappy pad between the legs cannot apply, for any restriction to hip adduction must only affect the hip and not the knee position nor growth. The varus appearance of the knees at this stage may appear worse due to some associated internal rotation of the lower limbs with increased anteversion of the femoral neck. This is a very common condition, which often worries the mother of her first child and accounts for a substantial percentage of referrals to a paediatric orthopaedic clinic. Careful explanation of this condition to the mother is important at this initial stage, otherwise repeated visits to the clinic may be demanded by the parents during the next few years while the knee is straightening and the anteversion is derotating. Full correction of the internal rotation deformity does not always occur (see Chapter 10, p. 259).

In the child shown in Fig. 6.6, not only did the parents refuse to accept that the legs were normal while they were in the varus stage and repeatedly returned to the clinic for 'bow legs', but later, when the child's knees were in physiological valgus, they were just as adamant about this deformity. The child's knees passed from varus at the age of 2 years to valgus at the age of 5 years (Fig. 6.7) and, of course, developed into beautiful straight legs eventually. It is important to stress the normality of

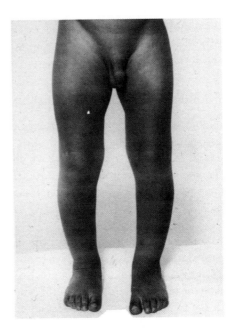

Fig. 6.6 Physiological genu varum.

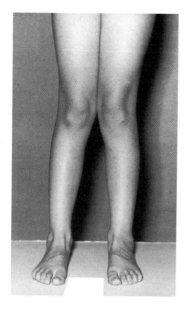

Fig. 6.7 Physiological genu valgum.

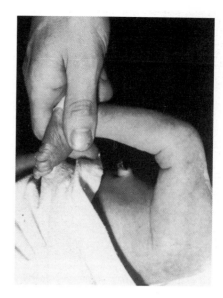

Fig. 6.8 Congenital dislocation of the knee.

this state not only to the parents but also to their general practitioner. The problem of deciding when the normal varus or valgus becomes pathological is very difficult; it may be a question of degree of angulation, and this will be discussed later in the chapter (p. 163). There may also be widespread joint abnormalities, e.g. epiphyseal dysplasias or the metaphyseal dysplasia of Blount's disease.

CONGENITAL ABNORMALITIES

Congenital abnormalities of this joint are rare. A discoid meniscus is the most commonly seen and is described later under meniscal abnormalities.

Congenital dislocation of the knee

This is seldom seen, either in one knee or bilaterally. It may be associated with congenital dislocation of the hip and is present in Larsen's syndrome, in which there are multiple congenital dislocations of joints together with a specific facies. The deformity is more common in females with a female:male ratio of 2:1 or 3:1 (Wynne-Davies, 1973).

The child is born with the knee in gross recurvatum with the angulation as much as, or even more than 90°. The tibia is not only hyperextended, but is also anteriorly displaced on the femoral condyle (Fig. 6.8). The posterior aspects of the femoral condyles are seen and felt in the popliteal fossa. It is impossible to bring this hyper-extended knee down to even the neutral position, and

this differentiates the full dislocation from the much more benign condition—congenital genu recurvatum. There never appears to be an associated vascular problem in the lower limb, though the popliteal fossa structures are tight in hyperextension. In all seven patients treated by this author there was a synovial cavity present, and this was confirmed by arthrography after treatment had begun. Laurence (1967) made a full and detailed assessment of patients seen in London during the preceding years. He concluded that the presence or absence of a synovial cavity decided the prognosis. Most babies in whom the hyperextended knee was such that a synovial cavity was present responded to conservative care. Those in whom no such cavity was found usually required operative exploration with lengthening of the quadriceps apparatus. Curtis and Fisher (1969), however, did not find arthrography helpful and stated that artrograms were technically difficult to produce in the hyperextended knee.

NON-OPERATIVE TREATMENT

Conservative care with traction and manipulation is usually effective and often produces full correction. Skin traction tapes are carefully applied and regularly inspected to make sure that no undue pressure arises. Traction is then applied with a gallows-type arrangement (Fig. 6.9), and the physiotherapist and the mother are instructed to regularly manipulate the hyperextended knee. In most cases the knee will gradually reduce to the neutral position and then start to flex.

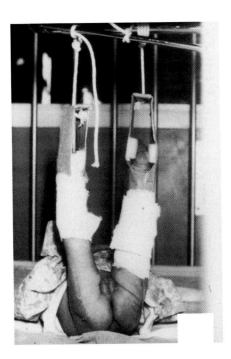

Fig. 6.9 Traction to reduce gross hyperextension in congenital dislocation of the knee.

In view of the importance of the presence or absence of the synovial cavity, it has always been the author's practice to undertake arthrography at this stage. Every child so investigated, however, has been the possessor of a definite synovial cavity, and this investigation may be of academic interest only. A traction and manipulation regimen may have to continue for several weeks before a flexion range is achieved, but in the majority of cases a full range of flexion will eventually be attained. Once flexion is achieved, serial plasters and regular physiotherapy manipulations continue and the child may attend as an out-patient. As the child later matures, the knee treated in this way appears to be perfectly normal in the majority, but residual hyperextension may be noted in some.

OPERATIVE TREATMENT

Continued hyperextension of the knee with an inadequate range of flexion so that 90° is unachievable will necessitate knee exploration and quadriceps lengthening. It is difficult to know when this is best undertaken, but it should be left until the movement range is static and, preferably, the child is walking. The quadriceps tendon and aponeurosis are lengthened by a V–Y plasty technique. The knee should then fully flex and any restricting bands are divided. The joint is left in approximately 45° of flexion in a plaster cast for the next 4 weeks before

mobilization. If the knee is left too flexed, at 90°, then a severe extension lag may persist following the period of immobilization.

Congenital genu recurvatum

This is a similar problem to congenital dislocation of the knee. The tibia may undergo subluxation on the femur, but does not dislocate (Fig. 6.10). A flexion range is always present, though initially inadequate, and regular stretching and manipulation are required. A full flexion range should be achieved by conservative means.

Congenital short quadriceps muscle

This is another rare condition, with progressive fibrosis of one or more components of the quadriceps musculature (Hnevkovsky, 1961). It may be associated with congenital heart defects, in which case the contracture may be acquired due to ischaemia of the quadriceps muscle following cardiac catheterization, for it has been seen in the same leg as the femoral arterial introduction of a catheter. Operative correction appears to be necessary, with elongation of the quadriceps muscle.

Congenital dislocation of the patella

Congenital lateral dislocation of the patella is rare and is difficult to diagnose in a small baby. It is the cause of a fixed, flexed, contracture of the knee at birth, and

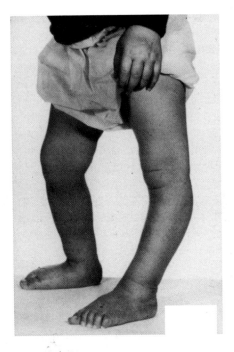

Fig. 6.10 Congenital genu recurvatum.

secondary deformities may develop in untreated cases (Green and Waugh, 1968). The knee should be treated by operation when the infant is large enough to make patellar reposition possible. Quadriceps lengthening is usually necessary in a fashion similar to that described previously if it proves impossible to reposition the patella without full flexion of the joint.

Patellar ossification abnormalities

Bipartite or multipartite patellae are seen very regularly. The junior doctor may decide that such an abnormal radiological appearance indicates a patellar fracture, but may be baffled by the minor injury that preceded the consultation. Almost all patellae with ossification defects of this type are normal in shape, size and articulation and are asymptomatic. In some teenagers, however, the patella is expanded and irregular, particularly on the lateral side, and in these individuals pain develops. The pain may be intermittent during activity and is due to abnormal articulation between the lateral expansion of the patella and the lateral femoral condyle. Eventually, degenerative changes localized to this site may develop. Continued symptoms from the abnormal patellar lump and articulation may necessitate removal of the separate ossicle through the epiphyseal–cartilage junction.

Other patellar abnormalities are rare and usually cause no symptoms. The child whose knee is illustrated in Fig. 6.11 had a patella magna with a large knee cap malarticulating with the femur, producing pain and gross patellar crepitus.

ACQUIRED ABNORMALITY

There are multiple causes of knee joint deformity, and these may be divided into the following categories:

1 Growth disturbances: unexplained growth of the epiphyseal growth plates may produce a varus or valgus deformity.
2 Metabolic: in rickets there is an abnormality of growth due to imperfect calcification and bone formation at the growth plate.
3 Epiphyseal growth abnormality: epiphyseal dysplasia multiplex congenita and spondyloepiphyseal dysplasias will produce curvatures at the knee.
4 Conditions that damage the epiphysis: septic arthritis and some rare tumours may damage the epiphyseal and the articular cartilage, producing gross deformity.
5 Damage to the epiphyseal growth plate: some fractures and fracture–dislocations at the physis will be responsible for deformity at the knee.
6 Paralytic and soft tissue contractures: spina bifida and spastic conditions will produce muscle imbalance leading to flexion contractures. Old poliomyelitis may lead to genu recurvatum.
7 Metaphyseal abnormality: Blount's disease may affect the growth plate, producing genu varum.

During growth, genu valgum may be considered physiological unless it reaches 10–11 cm of inter-malleolar separation and persists or increases until the age of 11 or 12 years. The cosmetic aspect is then usually unacceptable, and there is some evidence that continued deformity into adulthood does produce mechanical stresses that lead to osteoarthritis. It is difficult to be certain, however, of the degree of varus or valgus that produces future pathology. The knee in many Arab races is in a natural position of varus, and in some cases may reach a very substantial degree of angulation. Osteoarthritis of the knee in this group of patients is common.

Treatment of valgus or varus deformities may be undertaken by selective epiphyseal stapling in the

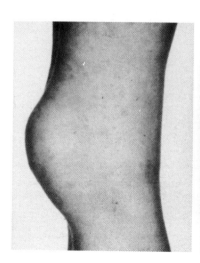
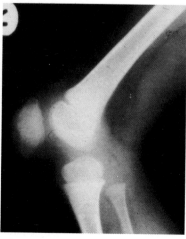

Fig. 6.11 Patella magna.

immature knee, though osteotomy around the knee may be necessary in the older child.

Medial or lateral epiphyseal stapling

It is usually necessary to temporarily stop the growth of one side of both the lower femoral and upper tibial growth plates. In a valgus deformity the medial sides of the growth plates are stapled in the child at an early enough age to allow sufficient growth potential of the lateral part of the epiphysis. Stapling the lateral side is necessary in a varus deformity. A longitudinal incision is used to explore the lower femur and upper tibia, and the exact position of the growth plate is identified by subperiosteal dissection and is confirmed radiologically using an image intensifier. At least three staples are positioned symmetrically over one side of the tibia and femur, accurately straddling the physis (Fig. 6.12). As a general rule, medial stapling is undertaken when the valgus reaches 10 cm of intermalleolar separation at a bone age of 10−11 years in girls and 12−13 years in boys.

Rickets

Deformity in rickets, of whatever type, is due to bending as a result of microfractures and epiphyseal displacement. The knees are most commonly affected, and genu varum results. Correction of the metabolic defect with vitamin D or calciferol administration produces reversal

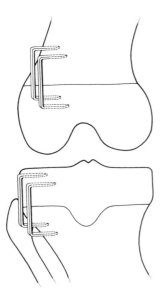

Fig. 6.12 Staples inserted laterally to prevent lateral growth at the knee in genu varum.

of these changes, and with growth the deformity decreases. Rickety deformity may be severe, however, and joint alignment may never completely recover at the end of skeletal growth. An osteotomy may therefore be required, and this is most satisfactorily performed at the supracondylar region of the lower femur.

SUPRACONDYLAR OSTEOTOMY OF THE FEMUR

An osteotomy−osteoclasis technique is ideal in children. Through a vertical lower femoral incision, the condylar and supracondylar regions are exposed and the epiphyseal growth plate is identified. It is always wise to confirm this radiologically with an image intensifier. An osteotomy is then performed with the power saw penetrating the femur to the medial cortex, but not actually dividing it. A second saw cut at an appropriate angle is then made to excise a wedge calculated to be of a size correct for the angular deformity adjustment. In a growing child it is preferable to leave the wedge open and to put back into the gap the nibbled cancellous bone from the excised wedge. The wound is then closed with drainage and an external cast applied with the knee still in the deformed position. This is maintained for 2−3 weeks, during which time the osteotomy becomes sticky with early union. After this interval, the knee is now bent under anaesthetic into its correct position and a new cast is applied with the knee straight. The advantage of this osteotomy−osteoclasis technique is the absence of unwanted displacement of the osteotomy site, which may occur with a complete osteotomy. Internal fixation devices are also avoided. In older, more mature children, however, an internal fixation device of a blade plate-type may be required to maintain the osteotomy position.

Epiphyseal dysplasias

The valgus deformity present in dysplasia epiphysealis multiplex congenita may be severe, and even after correction may recur in a vigorous manner. In this situation a double osteotomy of both the supracondylar region of the femur and the upper tibial zone just beneath the growth plate may be required. The tibial and femoral epiphyses are both deformed and may regrow in an angulated fashion, necessitating a further operative correction.

Deformity following septic arthritis

Epiphyseal destruction in septic arthritis may be severe, and a valgus or varus deformity will result with shortening. An opening wedge osteotomy is advocated for this, and not only corrects the deformity but also provides some lengthening of the bone.

OPENING WEDGE OSTEOTOMY

Through a vertical supracondylar incision, the growth plate is identified as before. A supracondylar osteotomy is performed leaving the cortex on the convex side of the deformity intact. The bone cut is then prised open on the concave side and a corticocancellous graft from the iliac crest is shaped and inserted. A blade plate is used to maintain the position and is secured with screws to prevent the grafted wedge from closing. Complete weight relief is demanded for a long period of 3 months to allow the graft to unite and revascularize without fear of collapse. Formal leg lengthening using the Wagner apparatus was necessary in the child shown in Fig. 6.13, as the shortening was still 8 cm.

Epiphyseal plate damage due to fracture

Salter and Harris (1963) have outlined the types of fractures that affect the growth plate (Fig. 6.14), and premature fusion of one area of the plate will lead to deformity. Excision of this area of bone and the insertion of a fat graft allows the chondrocytes of the growth

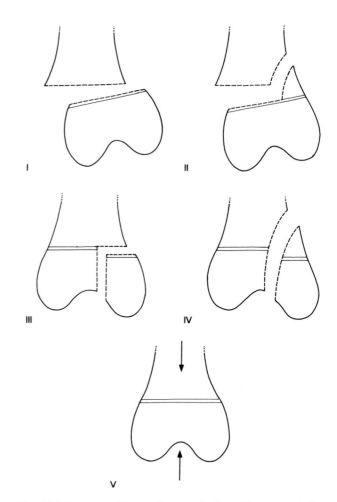

Fig. 6.14 Fractures affecting the growth plate. The prognosis for growth is good in types I, II and III, but may be poor in types IV and V. (From Salter and Harris, 1963, with permission.)

plate to grow across and to allow regrowth in a more balanced fashion (Langenskiöld, 1975).

EXCISION OF FUSED EPIPHYSEAL GROWTH PLATE AND FAT TRANSPLANT

Langenskiöld (1975) has described a technique whereby a fused portion of the plate is identified radiographically. The fused bone may be then identified through an osteotomy or through a drilled tunnel, and the affected bone is drilled and nibbled away, leaving a cavity which is filled with a fat graft. It may be necessary to combine this procedure with a corrective osteotomy (Fig. 6.15).

Blount's disease

Tibia vara, or Blount's disease, is a developmental abnormality producing marked genu varum as a result

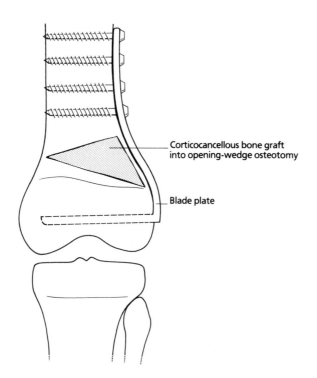

Fig. 6.13 An opening wedge osteotomy of the supracondylar region with insertion of an iliac crest graft.

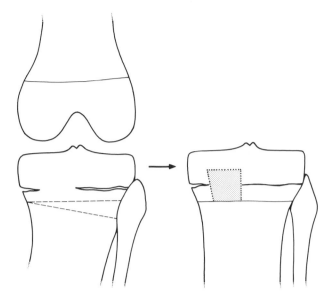

Fig. 6.15 A varus deformity produced by medial epiphyseal fusion following a type IV fracture. The fused area is approached through a tibial osteotomy and excised. The space is filled with a fat graft.

of a growth disturbance of the medial side of the upper tibial growth plate. The angulation is, in fact, below the knee at the upper tibial metaphysis which itself is disturbed in shape (Fig. 6.16). There is a high incidence of this deformity in West Africans, West Indians and American Blacks. These children are noted to walk earlier than their Caucasian counterparts and they also have more lax ligaments and joints. Golding and McNeil-Smith (1963) conclude that this type of tibia vara is caused by a failure of growth of the posteromedial part of the upper tibial epiphysis. There is an infantile type of

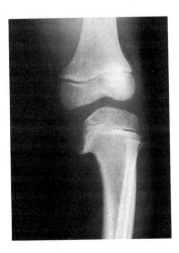

Fig. 6.16 Blount's disease.

the disease and a later adolescent variety developing between the ages of 8 and 13 years, with 90% of children being affected unilaterally. Spontaneous correction seldom occurs, and Langenskiöld and Riska (1964) strongly suggest that operative correction should be undertaken before the age of 8 years. A combination of tibial osteotomy, epiphyseodesis and lengthening may be required in severe cases.

SEPTIC ARTHRITIS

The general features of septic arthritis are outlined in Chapter 15, p. 411. Septic arthritis of the knee is now seldom seen in the UK, for this is a joint which seems fairly resistant to infection. Nevertheless, an ill child may present with a high fever and an immobile lower limb, with a swollen, tender and slightly flexed knee joint. Any movement of the limb in general is painful and any attempt to even approach the knee is resisted by the child, who is greatly apprehensive of any local attention to this area.

The usual route of infection is by haematogenous spread, though direct inoculation of organisms into the synovial cavity may occur when the child kneels on a nail or spike. *Staphylococcus aureus* is still the most common organism, but *Haemophilus influenzae* and the pneumococci and meningococci are detected frequently. *Escherichia coli*, salmonellae and *Brucella* organisms are seldom found. Clinical diagnosis is usually relatively easy with the features described above. Investigations include a high white cell count and polymorphonuclear leucocytosis, a high erythrocyte sedimentation rate and a positive blood culture in some cases. A radiograph usually shows an effusion, and at a much later stage erosions and joint destruction will become obvious.

The major differential diagnosis is between primary septic arthritis and lower femoral osteomyelitis, where the most distal part of the metaphysis is within the synovial area of the suprapatellar pouch. Septic arthritis is characterized by more swelling with a tight effusion, and even a minimal amount of joint movement produces acute agony. The effusion that accompanies lower femoral osteomyelitis is smaller, and the tenderness is localized to the lower femur with the joint being a little more mobile. A radiograph will give no help in the early stage, but an isotope bone scan will usually localize the increased blood flow to the metaphyseal region of the femur in osteomyelitis and to a much more diffuse region of the whole knee area in septic arthritis.

Treatment

Antibiotics are administered, preferably intravenously, as soon as the blood culture sample has been taken. A combination is necessary, and this should include a synthetic penicillin of the cloxacillin type, e.g. flucloxacillin, or alternatively fusidic acid to deal with penicillin-resistant staphylococci. Ampicillin, a cephalosporin, or another antibiotic active against *H. influenzae* and other Gram-negative organisms should be given. The antibiotics must be reviewed as soon as results are available from the first cultures from either the blood or synovial sample.

Aspiration of the joint must be undertaken under a general anaesthetic as soon as the child can be prepared. Decompression at the earliest stage is vital to preserve the articular cartilage from enzymic attack with bacteriological infection within the synovial cavity. The synovial sample will reveal either frank pus or a very cloudy synovial fluid which should be Gram-stained as well as cultured and sent for assessment of sensitivities. Once bacteriological infection is confirmed, the joint must be fully decompressed and irrigated, either by open operation or preferably by arthroscopic irrigation. The latter technique is ideal, allowing synovial crevasses, recesses and pockets to be washed out. Once this technique has been used the operator will realize how much more efficient this method is compared with even wide open inspection. Redivac drains must then be inserted, and this is again very easy to perform through the arthroscope. Irrigation and drainage may be undertaken using two Redivac tubes, and an antibiotic or an antibacterial−antifungal irrigation fluid is used. The joint should be splinted until more comfortable and all signs of infection have resolved. Slow return to weight-bearing then occurs and the antibiotics should be administered for several weeks, certainly well beyond the time when the erythrocyte sedimentation rate returns to normal.

Only by early and vigorous treatment along these lines is destructive arthropathy avoided. Chronic granulomatous infection with tuberculosis is occasionally seen, and diagnosis and treatment follow the same principles. The destructive effect is decreased by synovectomy and in some cases prolonged splinting and non-weight-bearing are important. If joint surface destruction is very severe, a knee fusion will be necessary when the child is large enough, and caliper control may be necessary in the interim period.

THE IRRITABLE KNEE

A swollen, painful knee may be due to a major infection as described above or, more commonly, to traumatic or transient synovitis. Traumatic synovitis occurs with a direct blow to the knee and is common in the normal active child. Direct injury causes an outpouring of synovial fluid from the traumatized synovial epithelium. In severe direct injuries haemarthroses may occur from synovial damage, but osteochondral fractures, cruciate ligament or capsular tears must be suspected if frank blood is aspirated from a very swollen, painful joint.

There are many other causes of transient synovitis similar to those seen more commonly in the hip joint. The child may have an infection, such as rubella or mumps, producing synovitis that develops before the overt stage of the disease. Monarticular synovitis may also develop without obvious cause, but often a history of recent infection of the upper respiratory tract or the gastrointestinal tract is given. In some children monarticular synovitis may be the first sign of a specific arthropathy (juvenile chronic arthritis). In others there may be an internal mechanical derangement or patellar abnormality. The effusion may persist, the child will tend to limp, and the quadriceps musculature will waste.

Full investigation to exclude all the specific diagnoses outlined above must be undertaken vigorously and appropriate treatment instituted. There still remains, however, a group of children in whom a definite diagnosis cannot be made, and although some of these will turn out to have a pauci-articular type of rheumatoid arthritis, many continue with a persistent, slowly resolving synovitis or even recurrent synovitis. It is presumed that these are due to a viral infection, though this is never proved. Arthroscopy and synovial biopsy through the arthroscope are indicated whenever the synovitis persists. Discoid meniscus is often missed clinically but detected arthroscopically, and with the use of this instrument other pathologies may become evident.

It is important to rest the child's knee in the acute irritable stage, but when chronic non-specific synovitis persists, normal activities and even quadriceps building exercises from a physiotherapist may be necessary to prevent muscle wasting. Further immobility may actually lead to more synovial effusion. There is a group of children, particularly young teenage girls, in whom traumatic or simple synovitis persists by producing an immobilization syndrome, sometimes voluntarily. Those children with emotional problems may then become 'knee cripples', and their treatment depends on a combination of sympathetic but firm physiotherapy and psychotherapy.

MECHANICAL DERANGEMENTS

Table 6.1 lists the various abnormalities seen in 130 consecutive patients with a painful swollen knee who were reviewed at the 'problem knee clinics' set up at the Westminster Children's Hospital and the Hospital for Sick Children, Great Ormond Street, London, UK. The most common derangements were found to be unstable patella and osteochondritis dissecans. The other internal derangements included the meniscus abnormalities, but of these a discoid lateral meniscus abnormality was the most common.

Symptoms

Although knee pain in the child is certainly a feature of knee pathology, it may be caused by abnormalities in other areas, e.g. hip abnormalities, particularly transient hip synovitis. Perthes' disease and slipped capital femoral epiphysis often produce pain that the child describes as being in the knee region. Thigh pain is rare in knee pathology, but the knee symptoms may radiate inferiorly, particularly when the lateral compartment is involved. Swelling in the knee is obvious, particularly so when the muscles are wasted above. A feeling of 'giving way' is usually described by the child who has instability due to patellar subluxation or due to movement of a loose body. A child complaining of locking must be carefully interrogated, for surgical locking, where there is a mechanical block to extension, is always indicative of a true internal derangement with a cartilage tear or loose body. A feeling of 'catching' as felt in osteochondritis dissecans or chondromalacia patellae is sometimes interpreted as locking. Stiffness of the joint may also be a parental synonym for locking. A loose body may be recognized by a child, and may be the source of some classroom amusement, as it acts like a 'joint mouse'

popping in and out of various parts of the joint. Clicking of the joint may be described accurately and the classic loud snap of the discoid meniscus may be demonstrated by the child to the surgeon or to the amused party audience, for it is commonly painless and often very loud.

Examination

This is performed along the same lines as for the adult. A greater deal of ligament and joint laxity, however, must be allowed for in the normal paediatric knee. The patella and its instability must be carefully assessed, for this derangement is so common. The popliteal fossa must be carefully examined for a Baker's cyst, which may be found in this site.

Special investigations

RADIOGRAPHIC EXAMINATION

Routine anteroposterior and lateral views must usually be supplemented by an intercondylar view (tunnel view), if osteochondritis dissecans in the classic site is to be detected. The routine patellar view is a skyline projection, but this may be supplemented by other views, as described by Ficat and Hungerford (1977).

ARTHROGRAPHY

This has a place in the diagnosis of internal derangements and is also important in assessing the synovial cavity and its various abnormalities. A discoid meniscus or a torn meniscus may be diagnosed by arthrography, but as a general anaesthetic usually has to be given for this investigation in the young child, it is often thought preferable to view the joint through an arthroscope. The accuracy of arthrography in general radiological departments is in the region of 70%, and this figure may rise in very specialized units to 95% (Freiberger and Kaye, 1979).

MAGNETIC RESONANCE IMAGING (Fig. 6.17)

Magnetic resonance imaging is now playing an important role in the diagnosis of various internal derangements. It is important in the assessment of menisci and ligaments, and being totally non-invasive it is taking over the diagnostic role that arthrography used to play. The accuracy is now very high, but the same problems of diagnosis in a child's knee are present in magnetic resonance imaging as in arthrography, for the child

Table 6.1 Abnormalities seen in the knees of 130 children (up to age 14 years)

	Number of cases
Dislocating patella	50
Osteochondritis dissecans	38
Irritable knee	16
Meniscus	
Tears	3
Discoid	9
Cysts	3
Proven chondromalacia patellae	4
Others	7

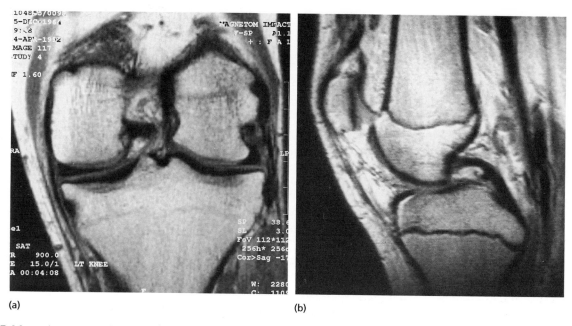

(a)   (b)

Fig. 6.17 Magnetic resonance imaging of the knee. (a) Anteroposterior view; (b) lateral view, showing normal menisci and posterior cruciate ligament.

must remain very still for a relatively long time. As these scanning machines improve, they will be of increasing importance in the diagnosis of knee disorders.

ARTHROSCOPY

This is currently the most important and definitive of the diagnostic tools used in a child's knee. Before the introduction of the arthroscope, the clinical accuracy of diagnosis of internal derangements, even in easier adults, remained in the region of 70% and in children very much lower (Bedford *et al.*, 1979; Zaman and Leonard,

1981). The improved diagnostic accuracy when using the arthroscope is remarkable and in experienced hands approaches 100% (Jackson and Dandy, 1976). The technique in children is exactly as for adults. The child's lax joint makes inspection even easier than in most adult knees, and derangements of the menisci and femoral condyles may be seen without problem (Fig. 6.18).

Arthroscopic surgical procedures

Operative arthroscopy is now important in the treatment of many children's knee problems. Meniscal tears may

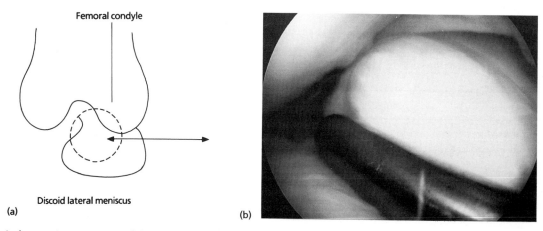

Femoral condyle

Discoid lateral meniscus

(a)   (b)

Fig. 6.18 Arthroscopic appearance of the discoid lateral meniscus.

be removed and peripheral meniscal injuries resutured. A discoid meniscus may be trimmed and osteochondritis dissecans fragments internally fixed or removed. Fine microsurgical scissors, knives, punches and rongeurs are used, and powered burrs and meniscotomes are important in these arthroscopic procedures.

It must be stressed again that internal derangements of the child's knee may be difficult to diagnose, and there is no indication for open arthrotomy purely to explore the joint. The arthroscope opens up much more of the joint cavity to inspection than exploratory arthrotomy.

Meniscal lesions

Tears of the meniscus may occur in a young child's knee, but the lesion is rare. A medial bucket-handle tear is sometimes seen in the first decade, but increasingly so as the child enters the teenage years. The symptoms and signs are exactly as outlined in adults, but often a youngster 'plays on' with severe symptoms and even a locked knee. A meniscus tag with surrounding cystic change occurs in children with the same features as in adults. The diagnosis is made on the symptoms and signs, sometimes with help from the arthrogram. The importance of the arthroscope in the child must be stressed, and the arthroscope and endoscopic instruments are used for removal of the bucket-handle portion, loose bodies and meniscal tags by the experienced arthroscopist.

Discoid lateral meniscus

In a review of 52 patients between the ages of 4 and 18 years, the clinical diagnosis of discoid lateral meniscus was found to be difficult. The history was often vague and unhelpful, and only 38% of the knees demonstrated a severe and loud clunk on examination, which is usually thought to be characteristic of this disorder. Lateral pain was more commonly detected, but joint-line tenderness was an unreliable sign. Arthroscopy was an essential investigation in view of the inaccuracy of clinical diagnosis. Difficulty may be encountered when using the lateral approach and particularly when attempting to move the arthroscope from the medial to the lateral compartment. It is important to use a medial approach on these occasions. Osteochondritis dissecans of the lateral femoral condyle was an associated abnormality found in 11% of the knees.

The discoid meniscus may tear and completely lock the knee. Alternatively, the lateral disc may remain intact throughout life, never detected until autopsy. If

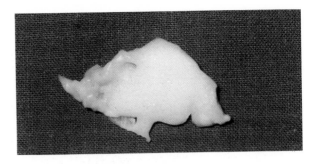

Fig. 6.19 Discoid meniscus excised.

the discoid meniscus is torn but peripherally stable, it may be trimmed arthroscopically. If the posterior attachment is deficient a total meniscectomy will be required (Fig. 6.19). The symptoms are often minor, and if at arthroscopy the disc is untorn and stable the child should be treated conservatively.

Osgood–Schlatter disease

Avulsion of a minor flake from the bone at the tibial tubercle occurs in this condition, which particularly affects vigorous young teenagers. Boys are more commonly affected, but athletic schoolgirls do not escape. The child complains of pain, tenderness and swelling at the insertion of the patellar tendon into the tibial tubercle. Exercise, particularly kicking and jumping, aggravates the symptoms, which are most marked during and after activity. A direct blow or fall onto the swollen tubercle produces excessive pain. On clinical examination, the joint itself is normal but the tubercle is prominent and selectively tender. There may be a bursa at the tendon insertion and this produces a fluctuant mass which adds to the prominence of the tubercle (Fig. 6.20).

The radiographic appearance is that of an avulsion flake from the tibial tubercle, combined with reparative callus at this site (Fig. 6.21). As the disease continues the bony mass may enlarge and become quite ugly. There has been much discussion over the years as to the aetiology of this condition, with osteochondrosis being commonly implicated. There seems little doubt, however, that the problem is one of an avulsion flake fracture.

TREATMENT

In most children the symptoms settle spontaneously. For a period of time during the acute symptoms, avoidance of the heaviest sports activities should be recommended, but it seems excessive to immobilize the knee joint

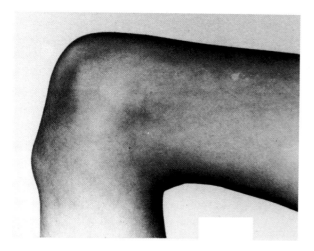

Fig. 6.20 Osgood–Schlatter disease.

further. If the symptoms persist for more than 18 months–2 years, exploration may be advocated.

Removing the avulsed fragment from within the tendon, removing the associated bursa and drilling the bone–tendon junction have all been advocated. The same results may have occurred if the child, the parents and the surgeons waited for natural resolution of the pain. The prominence of the tibial tubercle, however, usually persists.

Larsen–Johansson syndrome

A similar avulsion flake with associated pain and tenderness may occur at the superior insertion of the patellar tendon into the lower pole of the patella. The symptoms are similar to those of Osgood–Schlatter disease, with pain during and after exercise, and the disease particularly affects high jumpers. There is selective tenderness at this site. The radiographic appearance is shown in Fig. 6.22. Rest and controlled physical activity are all that are required in most cases, but in some children with chronic local pain, exploration and curettage of the bone fragments appear to be curative.

Osteochondritis dissecans

This is a condition of the knee in which a segment of articular cartilage and subchondral bone separates, either completely or partially, from the joint surface. The femoral condyle is usually involved, a patellar lesion is sometimes seen, and very occasionally the upper tibial plateau may be affected. The separated segment presents articular hyaline cartilage with normal chondrocytes alive and producing matrix, but the bony fragment is avascular. The fragment may heal and restore the joint surface, it may remain attached to the crater and hinge in this site, producing an internal derangement, or it may shed from the joint surface to form a loose body. The loose body may then increase in size as the articular

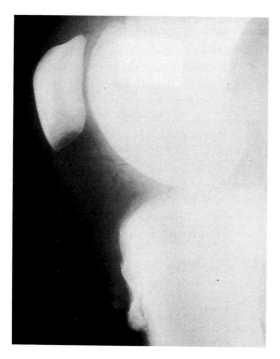

Fig. 6.21 Osgood–Schlatter disease. Avulsion fragments are seen in the patellar tendon.

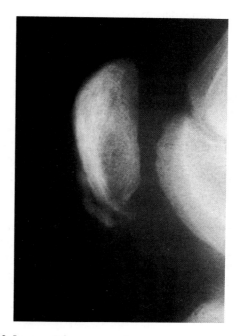

Fig. 6.22 Larsen–Johansson syndrome.

hyaline cartilage proliferates and surrounds the bony nidus (Fig. 6.23).

CLINICAL FEATURES

In a view of 150 patients with osteochondritis dissecans, unilateral lesions were found in 74% and bilateral lesions in 26%. The sex incidence was predominantly male in the ratio of about 2:1, with 68% of males affected and 32% of females. A history of injury of a substantial nature was present in 46% of the patients who presented with osteochondritis dissecans; the age range of onset is depicted in Fig. 6.24. The sites of lesions affecting the femoral condyle are shown in Fig. 6.25.

There were many associated internal derangements of the menisci and ligaments in patients with osteochondritis dissecans. Anterior lesions of the lateral femoral condyle were commonly associated with patellar dislocation and, as mentioned above, a lateral femoral condyle lesion on the weight-bearing surface has been described with a discoid meniscus. Most young people with osteochondritis dissecans give a history of substantial sporting activity, and Table 6.2 illustrates the breakdown of the athletic ability of 134 patients with osteochondritis dissecans.

AETIOLOGY

König (1887–1888) was the first to name the disease 'osteochondritis dissecans', and since that time there has been a substantial debate as to whether the lesion is due to trauma. Paget (1870) described cases in which knee injuries produced loose bodies, but his opponents felt

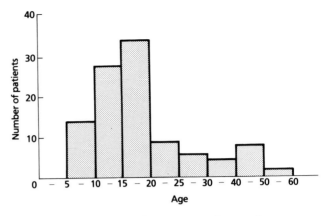

Fig. 6.24 Osteochondritis dissecans: age of onset of symptoms (range, 6–53 years; mean age, 18 years).

that avascular necrosis was the prime cause. Smillie (1960) feels that there are many different aetiological factors, all of which contribute to various types of osteochondritis dissecans.

Clinical factors

From the review described it was found that trauma occurred in one-half of patients seen with osteochondritis dissecans. Athletic ability and regular sporting activity, with the multiple stresses and strains that these entail, were factors common to the majority of cases, and many patients were extremely good athletes. Many other patients had associated mechanical derangements of the menisci, the ligaments and patellar instability. Kennedy *et al.* (1966) demonstrated that osteochondral fractures of most parts of the weight-bearing surfaces of the femoral condyles could be produced in cadavers with strong axial compression and rotary forces.

An experiment was set up in animals to follow the natural course of experimental osteochondral fractures

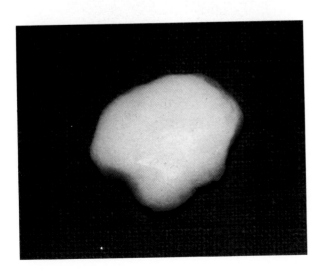

Fig. 6.23 Loose body from the knee joint.

Table 6.2 Sporting ability of 134 patients with osteochondritis dissecans.

	Percentage
Excellent (international or county standard)	10
Good (league or school first team)	45
Moderate (regular participation)	20
Poor (nil)	25

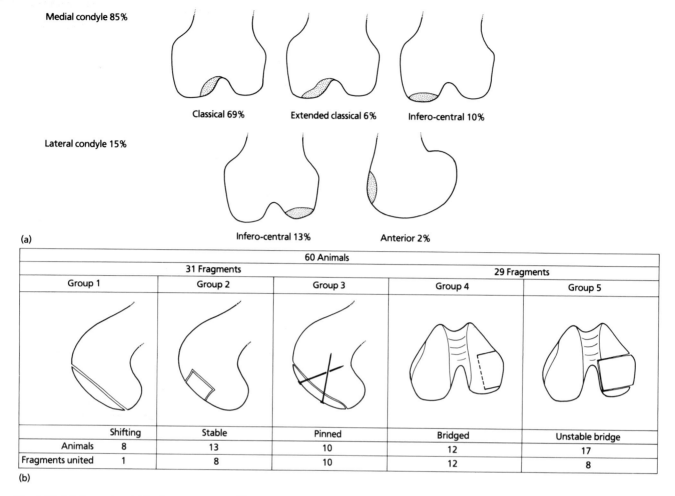

(a)

60 Animals				
31 Fragments			29 Fragments	
Group 1	Group 2	Group 3	Group 4	Group 5

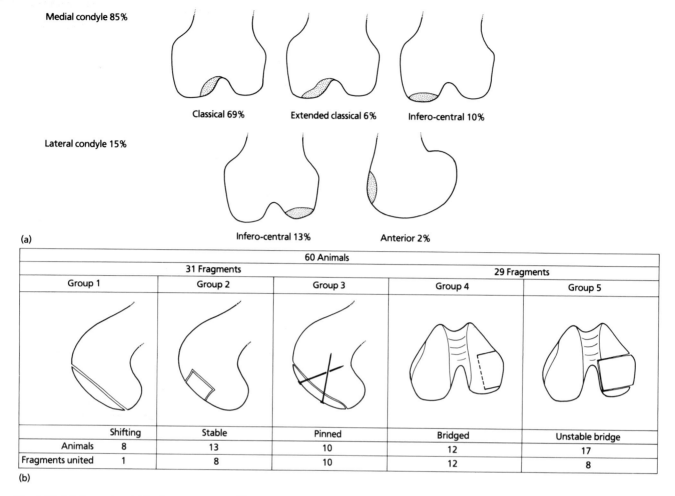

	Shifting	Stable	Pinned	Bridged	Unstable bridge
Animals	8	13	10	12	17
Fragments united	1	8	10	12	8

(b)

Fig. 6.25 (a) Osteochondritis dissecans: sites of lesions. (b) Experimental osteochondral fractures: union rate.

of various types, and an attempt was made to relate these findings to osteochondritis dissecans with the help of a cadaver demonstration. Various cuts through the hyaline articular surface and the subchondral bone were made. It was found that those fragments cut in such a way that shift occurred on weight-bearing did not unite, and the non-united osteochondral fracture closely resembled osteochondritis in humans. Those fragments that were cut in such a way that they were stable in their crater or were stabilized by internal fixation rapidly united, leaving a stable articular surface. Dye was then placed on the medial patellar facet of cadavers and the knee joint was re-articulated. The medial femoral condyle was stained in increasing flexion of the joint, and it was noted that this area of the medial femoral condyle was the classic site of osteochondritis dissecans (Fig. 6.26). Falls onto the patella in flexion may cause injury at this site. It was concluded that osteochondritis dissecans is a non-united osteochondral or subchondral fracture (Aichroth, 1971a,b).

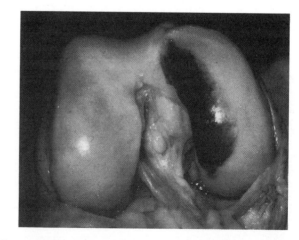

Fig. 6.26 The classic site of osteochondritis dissecans — medial femoral condyle.

DIAGNOSIS

The diagnosis is made from the clinical presentation combined with a history of the joint giving way, locking, or producing a loose body. Radiographs are usually characteristic, but full views must be obtained and in particular tunnel and skyline views. An arthrogram offers little help in the diagnosis.

NATURAL HISTORY AND MANAGEMENT

The natural history of the lesion is that the fragment *in situ* will heal in many cases, particularly in children. If it does not heal, movement of the fragment in the crater produces a feeling of repeated 'giving way'. The fragment may hinge and produce a major internal derangement with locking. The fragment may fully loosen to produce a loose body with the characteristic symptoms and signs of pain, swelling and repeated locking, as the fragment jams between the joint surfaces. While the fragment is loosening or hinging, the crater may fill up with some fibrocartilaginous material, and at a much later stage when the loose body has separated for many years, it may be very difficult to find the crater from which the fragment came because the fibrocartilaginous resurfacing may be extremely good.

If the fragment remains *in situ*, and if the patient is young, the lesion may heal. It is important to review the patient both clinically and radiologically at intervals, and in view of the aetiological factors mentioned, it is reasonable to decrease the heaviest sporting activities. It is unlikely in the fanatical teenage athlete that total absence of sports will be possible. It is recommended that these children alter their sporting activities to decrease pressure on the knee, but it is not recommended that the children are immobilized nor put into plaster casts. The evils of immobility and quadriceps wasting outweigh the advantages of such treatment.

In osteochondritis dissecans arthroscopy is the only definite way of assessing stability (Fig. 6.27).

HEALING OF OSTEOCHONDRITIS DISSECANS

The author's group has recently assessed 21 children up to the age of 14 years with osteochondritis dissecans in an effort to determine which of them heal and which are less likely to do so (Crawfurd *et al.*, 1990). They all had stable osteochondral lesions *in situ*, and 13 healed quite spontaneously while eight did not. Those who did not heal went on to form loose bodies or hinge fragments, and those who healed were shown to be united either radiologically or by 'second-look' arthroscopy. Those

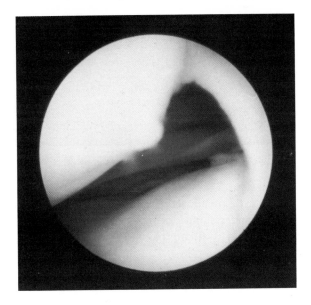

Fig. 6.27 Stable osteochondritis dissecans: arthroscopic appearance.

lesions that healed were surprisingly on the weight-bearing surfaces, and those that tended not to heal were in the classic site on the inter-condylar region of the medial femoral condyle.

TREATMENT

If the fragment remains stable and *in situ* but symptomatic, drilling the fragment has some advantages. It certainly may heal faster and revascularization is possibly stimulated by this procedure. Nevertheless, the healing rate is probably only 50% and the technique cannot be completely relied on. Drilling may be undertaken arthroscopically, with bone wires inserted through one or two sites on the articular hyaline cartilage drilling through the fragment. Alternatively, drilling may be from the condylar side entering the fragment but not perforating the hyaline cartilage. Image intensification radiological control is required for this type of fragment drilling. The relief of pain is often remarkable after drilling (Bradley and Dandy, 1989).

Compression screw fixation is the ideal method of internally fixing an unstable fragment. Over the years many internal fixation devices have been used, from Smillie's pins to Herbert compression screws. This technique has advantages in many situations, though bone grafting in addition may be required. The problem, however, is that even with this technique fixation and union are not always secured (Fig. 6.28). A fragment that is loose will be covered on the condylar surface with fibrocartilaginous material, and similarly the crater may

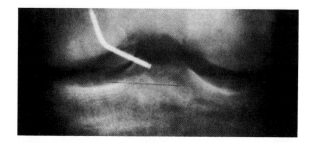

Fig. 6.28 A loosened pinned fragment and bent pin.

be lined with pseudoarthrosis material. The fibrocartilaginous material must be removed from both surfaces before fixation is attempted, and even then the results are variable.

Internal fixation can only be undertaken in certain situations, and the remainder of the fragments should be excised and the crater prepared by drilling and curettage to allow the outgrowth of fibrocartilage. Cartilaginous resurfacing over this crater may be quite remarkable in speed and thickness, and by 9 months resurfacing is usually very substantial when inspected at second-look arthroscopy.

MANAGEMENT PLAN FOR OSTEOCHONDRITIS DISSECANS

1 A lesion in the child may often heal, and so a young person with an osteochondral defect should be treated conservatively and followed both clinically and radiologically. The fragment may be seen to heal progressively, but if stability is in any doubt arthroscopy should be undertaken.
2 If at arthroscopy the fragment is *in situ* and the symptoms have been substantial, drilling the lesion may be helpful. Drilling, however, should not be considered curative in all cases.
3 The unstable fragment may sometimes be internally fixed with a compression screw. If it is a large fragment and lends itself to internal fixation because it fits back perfectly, curettage of the crater and internal fixation is often successful. Bone grafting may sometimes be required in the crater at the time of internal fixation of the fragment.
4 If the fragment is unsuitable for internal fixation, removal of fragment, curettage of the crater and drilling of the subchondral bone layer will promote fibrocartilaginous resurfacing.
5 Radiological and clinical reviews will be required. If a large fragment has been excised or the stability of the fragment is in any doubt, then a second-look arthroscopy will be necessary.

Dislocation of the patella

Almost all patellar dislocations are over the lateral femoral condyle. A few are interarticular, with the patella standing on its side in the intercondylar region, and very occasionally the patella may dislocate medially. Congenital patellar dislocation does occur (Green and Waugh, 1968) and may be the cause of an unexplained congenital flexion contracture of the knee.

Patellar dislocation appears to be due to different causes in adults than in children. In children the dislocation occurs recurrently or persistently (Fig. 6.29) due to some structural abnormality in the majority, whereas in adults the dislocation usually follows a traumatic incident. Structural abnormalities of the knee are much less common in adults. In children the patella may dislocate on one occasion or it may become recurrent. Habitual dislocation occurs when the knee cap dislocates at every flexion and extension range, and a persistent dislocation occurs when the patella is constantly over the lateral femoral condyle. Girls are much more commonly affected than boys.

In a recent review of 46 patients with 59 knee joints with patellar dislocations, nine were affected bilaterally; 11 of these patients had persistent dislocations and 25 had recurrent patellar dislocations. The associated abnormalities found in this group of patients are listed in Tables 6.3 and 6.4. Two further associated abnormalities were not specifically looked for in this series: increased femoral neck anteversion leading to excessive internal rotation at the hip (and usually associated with

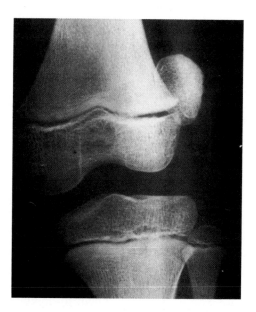

Fig. 6.29 Persistent dislocation of the patella.

Table 6.3 Abnormalities associated with persistent patellar dislocation in 11 patients

	Number of patients
Nail−patella syndrome (bilateral)	3
Vastus lateralis contracture*	3
Gross congenital ligament laxity	2
Significant trauma	1

* The cause of this was thought to be neonatal thigh injections.

Table 6.4 Abnormalities associated with recurrent patellar dislocation in 35 patients

	Number of patients
Congenital lax ligaments	11
Valgus knees	4
Congenital dislocation of the hip	3
Spastic hemiparesis	2
Marfan's syndrome	1
Ehlers−Danlos syndrome	1
Turner's syndrome	1
Peroneal muscular atrophy	1

a generalized increase in joint laxity) and structural deficiency of the lateral femoral condyle.

SYMPTOMS

The children or their parents complain of frequent falls, the knee giving way and sometimes a description of the knee cap being 'out of place'. It is interesting to note that in this group of young people pain is minimal, whereas in adults the painful symptoms are the most predominant. In persistent dislocations symptoms are often absent or minimal, and the joint 'giving way' is the most common presentation. In older children the symptoms alter somewhat, and pain becomes the more prominent feature, in adolescents, symptoms of a loose body may develop when an osteochondral fracture of the patella or the femoral condyle occurs.

CLINICAL SIGNS

Persistent or recurrent dislocation of the patella may be observed. A lateral kick of the patella is often noted when the flexed knee is slowly extended. Subluxation or dislocation occurs on passive lateral movement of the patella, and there is always a positive 'apprehension sign', when the patella is moved laterally and the patient becomes apprehensive, tenses his quadriceps musculature, looks worried and prevents the examiner from

further subluxing the knee cap. Tenderness over the medial retinaculum is commonly present, and this may be due to a medial internal derangement. There is often associated generalized ligament laxity in these children, and this is often quite marked.

RADIOLOGICAL SIGNS

1 Tangential osteochondral fractures (Fig. 6.30): in the skyline view a small fragment of bone may be avulsed from the medial patellar border and lies in the capsule. It is the telltale sign of recurrent patellar dislocation, but it has been found that this tangential fracture is much less common in children than adults.
2 Patella alta (Fig. 6.31): there are many methods for assessing a high patella and Blackburne's description (1977) is recommended (Fig. 6.31). Approximately 50% of patients with a recurrent dislocation of the patella show a patella alta.

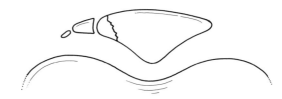

Fig. 6.30 Tangential osteochondral fracture of the medial patellar facet in patellar dislocation.

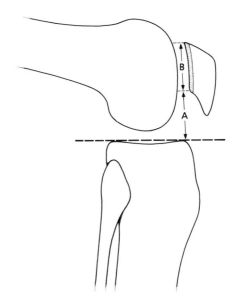

Fig. 6.31 Patella alta. In the normal knee the measurement A = B. In patella alta, A is larger than B. (B is the length of the articular surface of the patella.)

3 Osteochondral fractures of the lateral femoral condyle: from time to time osteochondritis dissecans or a fresh osteochondral fracture occurs on the anterior aspect of the lateral femoral condyle at the site where the patella crashes over this bony prominence.

4 Hughston's patellar views (Fig. 6.32): tangential views of many types have been used to show patellar tilt. There may be some confusion if the knee is swollen with an effusion, as this may in itself produce a tilted patella.

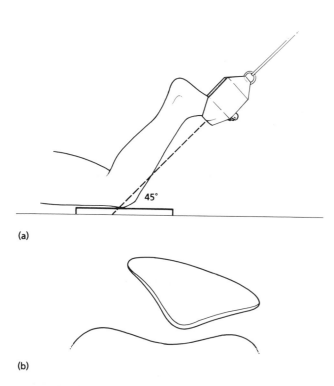

(a)

(b)

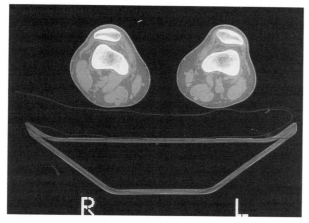

(c)

Fig. 6.32 (a) Radiological technique for obtaining skyline view of patella. (b) Skyline projection shows patella tilt. (c) Computed tomographic scan of both knees with patellar subluxation syndrome. Both patellae are laterally placed and the femoral sulcus is almost absent.

TREATMENT

In a congenital dislocation, a flexion contracture persists and this should be treated operatively. Persistent dislocation may produce minimal discomfort, but knee stability is poor and again operative treatment is indicated. Infrequent dislocations may be treated conservatively, but frequent dislocations in children should be treated by operative correction. It is always worth trying a course of quadriceps strengthening exercises, even if operative treatment is likely to be necessary; in a few less severe cases operation may be avoided.

Operative treatment

Over the past 100 years a large number of bony and soft tissue operations have been described. The Hauser tibial tubercle transposition is contraindicated in children because it may cause premature closure of the tibial growth plate, resulting in genu recurvatum. Patellectomy is also contraindicated, because the extensor apparatus may continue to dislocate after removal of the bone. Soft tissue operations are legion, and lateral release, Campbell's operation to pull the patella medially with a strip of patellar expansion, semitendinosus transfer and Goldthwaite's operation to transpose half the patellar tendon have all been advocated. The author has found that lateral release alone is usually insufficient, but a combination of long lateral release and repositioning of the patella by means of a Goldthwaite/Roux-type half-patellar tendon transfer produces the required result. The half-patellar tendon is transposed beneath an osteoperiosteal flap for good stability (Fig. 6.33), and the operation has been successful in both persistent and recurrent dislocations in childhood.

SUMMARY

Lateral patellar dislocations in children may be recurrent, habitual, or persistent. In children there are very often abnormalities of knee joint structure, and joint and ligament laxity constitutes the most important predisposing condition. A combined release and repositioning soft tissue operation appears to be the most successful procedure.

BURSAE AROUND THE KNEE

Every tendon at and around the knee has a potential related bursa (Fig. 6.34). The more common cystic swellings in this region are described below.

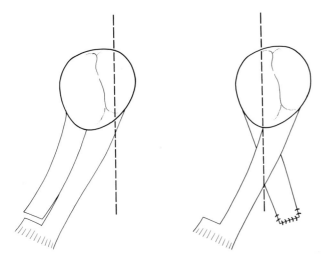

Fig. 6.33 Half-patellar tendon transfer after long lateral release.

Baker's cyst

Morrant Baker in the last century described a cystic mass in the popliteal fossa of children. The cyst is a constantly swollen bursa related to the semimembranosus tendon, and although it arises from this medial hamstring, it usually presents as a central popliteal fossa mass. It is fluctuant and transilluminant, and it can reach moderately large proportions but seldom produces symptoms apart from the presence of a lump noted by the parent when the child's knee is fully extended. The

majority of Baker's cysts appear spontaneously, often persisting for 1–2 years before resolution. Exploration and excision are advisable if the cyst rapidly increases in size or if there is any doubt whatsoever concerning the diagnosis. The differential diagnoses include enlarged popliteal lymph nodes, tumours attached to the popliteal nerve, soft tissue sarcomas and a popliteal aneurysm. A cyst that is definitely fluctuant and transilluminant, however, is most likely to be a semimembranosus bursa of Baker and should be left alone.

The adult knee sometimes presents with a similar semimembranosus bursa, but more commonly there is a mass of synovium or a knee joint synovial pouch, which swells in the popliteal fossa due to an associated knee effusion, synovitis, or other pathology affecting the joint as a whole. The posterior synovial pouch may become large and may interfere with venous return from the leg. A posterior synovial cyst may also burst and leak synovial fluid into the popliteal fossa and into the calf musculature, producing a synovial 'pseudocyst'. Pain and swelling of the lesion may be mistaken for a sudden deep vein thrombosis, and many patients have been hospitalized and anticoagulated with this mistaken diagnosis.

Pre-patellar bursa (housemaid's knee)

The normal bursal sac separating the anterior patella from skin and scanty subcutaneous tissue may become swollen due to the constant irritation of kneeling or a direct blow on the prominence of the patella. A fluctuant mass develops over the patella, which may rapidly become inflamed and is often secondarily infected. The portal of entry of bacteria may be a graze or laceration near the knee, infected eczema, or athlete's foot more distally. Treatment of the inflamed bursa depends on the prevention of further mechanical irritation, rest and anti-inflammatory medication. In the cellulitis (infective) stage, antibiotics will be effective, but pus rapidly forms and the large abscess that results will require incision and drainage.

Infrapatellar bursa (vicar's knee)

The bursal sac that is present superficial to the patellar tendon may be also inflamed by prolonged 'kneeling in prayer' position. The high jumper's lesion is a strain of the upper attachment of the patellar tendon to the bone of the inferior pole of the patella, and this patellar tendonitis may be associated with an infrapatellar bursa. The treatment follows that outlined above.

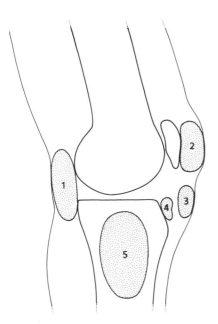

Fig. 6.34 Bursae around the knee. (1) Baker's cyst. (2) Pre-patellar bursa. (3) Intrapatellar bursa. (4) Tibial tubercle. (5) Subsartorial bursa.

Tibial tubercle bursa

The bursal sac becomes inflamed in association with Osgood–Schlatter disease deep to the inferior attachment of the patellar tendon at the tibial tubercle. If Osgood–Schlatter disease is treated operatively, it is important to look for this bursa and to remove it.

Subsartorial bursa (pes anserinus bursa)

This occurs over the medial upper tibia, well below the joint line where it should not be confused with a meniscal cyst. The lump may become large and painful and may interfere with joint function. It is a swelling of the normal bursal sac related to the insertion of sartorius, gracilis and semitendinosus muscle into the upper medial tibia. Its excision is usually necessary, as it produces increasing symptoms.

Biceps femoris bursa

A less common bursa may be found related to the biceps tendon insertion into the fibular head. It may also be related to the tendon at a higher point in the lateral popliteal fossa. The bursa may be confused with a ganglion arising from the superior tibiofibular joint and both abnormalities usually require excision.

REFERENCES

Aichroth P.M. (1971a) Osteochondritis dissecans of the knee: a clinical survey. *J. Bone Joint Surg.* **53B**, 440–447.

Aichroth P.M. (1971b) Osteochondral fractures and their relationship to osteochondritis dissecans of the knee: an experimental study in animals. *J. Bone Joint Surg.* **53B**, 448–454.

Bedford A., Aichroth P.M. and Hutton P. (1979) Arthroscopy — the first hundred are the worst. *J. R. Soc. Med.* **72**, 6–12.

Blackburne J.S. and Peel T.E. (1977) A new method of measuring patellar height. *J. Bone Joint Surg.* **59B**, 241–242.

Bradley J. and Dandy D.J. (1989) Results of drilling osteochondritis dissecans before skeletal maturity. *J. Bone Joint Surg.* **71B**, 642–644.

Crawfurd E.J.P., Emery R.J.H. and Aichroth P.M. (1990) Stable osteochondritis dissecans — does the lesion unite? *J. Bone Joint Surg.* **72B**, 320.

Curtis B.H. and Fisher R.L. (1969) Congenital hyperextension with anterior subluxation of the knee: surgical treatment and long-term observations. *J. Bone Joint Surg.* **51A**, 255–269.

Ficat R.P. and Hungerford D.S. (1977) *Disorders of the Patello-Femoral Joint.* Paris, Masson.

Freiberger R.H. and Kaye J.J. (1979) *Arthrography.* New York, Appleton-Century-Crofts.

Golding J.S.R. and McNeil-Smith J.D.G. (1963) Observations on the aetiology of tibia vara. *J. Bone Joint Surg.* **45B**, 320–325.

Green J.P. and Waugh W. (1968) Congenital lateral dislocation of the patella. *J. Bone Joint Surg.* **50B**, 285–289.

Hnekovsky O. (1961) Progressive fibrosis of the vastus intermedius muscle in children: a cause of limited knee flexion and elevation of the patella. *J. Bone Joint Surg.* **43B**, 318–325.

Jackson R.W. and Dandy D.J. (1976) *Arthroscopy of the Knee.* New York, Grune and Stratton.

Kennedy J.C., Grainger R.W. and McGraw R.W. (1966) Osteochondral fractures of the femoral condyles. *J. Bone Joint Surg.* **48B**, 436–440.

König F. (1887–1888) Uber freie Körper in den Gelenken. *Dtsch. Z. Chir.* **27**, 90–109.

Langenskiöld A. (1975) An operation for partial closure of an epiphyseal plate in children and its experimental basis. *J. Bone Joint Surg.* **57B**, 325–330.

Langenskiöld A. and Riska E.B. (1964) Tibia vara (osteochondrosis deformans tibiae): a survey of seventy-one cases. *J. Bone Joint Surg.* **46A**, 1405–1420.

Laurence M. (1967) Genu recurvatum congenitum. *J. Bone Joint Surg.* **49B**, 121–134.

Paget J. (1870) On the production of some of the loose bodies in joints. *St. Bartholomew's Hosp. Rep.* **6**, 1–4.

Salter R.B. and Harris W.R. (1963) Injuries involving the epiphyseal plate. *J. Bone Joint Surg.* **45A**, 587–622.

Smillie I.S. (1960) *Osteochondritis Dissecans.* Edinburgh, E. and S. Livingstone.

Twyman R.S., Desai K. and Aichroth P.M. (1991) Long-term follow-up of osteochondritis dissecans of the knee in children. *J. Bone Joint Surg. [Br.]* **73B**, 461–464.

Wynne-Davies R. (1973) *Hereditable Disorders in Orthopaedic Practice.* Oxford, Blackwell.

Zaman M. and Leonard M.A. (1981) Meniscectomy in children: results in 59 knees. *Injury* **12**, 425–428.

Chapter 7
The Foot

J.A. Fixsen

INTRODUCTION

Anxiety about foot deformities and foot problems is a very common reason for referral to a paediatric orthopaedic clinic. The most common complaints are in-toeing and flat feet.

IN-TOEING

It is important to remember that this condition may well be due to a more proximal condition in the legs, e.g. medial tibial torsion, persistent femoral anteversion, or a generalized problem such as cerebral palsy (see Chapters 3 and 10). This underlines the importance in all children's foot problems of examining the whole child and not just looking at the foot and lower leg.

Metatarsus varus or adductus

This condition is also known as hookfoot or skewfoot. It is the most common foot condition causing in-toeing. It is usually noticed in the first 3 months of life or when the child starts to stand and walk. The parents become anxious, either about the in-toe appearance or because they feel the child is tripping up over its own feet. This is particularly common when the child starts to walk, as at this age all children are liable to frequent falls.

On examination, the child is normal except for the varus deformity of the forefoot (Fig. 7.1a). Most important, the heel is in neutral or valgus and not in varus. This distinguishes the condition immediately from congenital talipes equinovarus, with which it is often confused (Fig. 7.1b). Unless the condition is associated with a neurological problem, e.g. meningomyelocoele or spinal dysraphism, there is no wasting of the calf muscles. This again distinguishes it from congenital talipes equinovarus. The forefoot is in varus with a concave medial border to the foot and a convex lateral

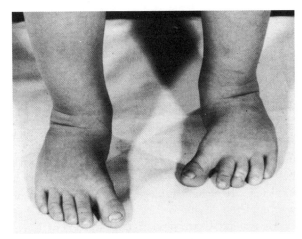

(a)

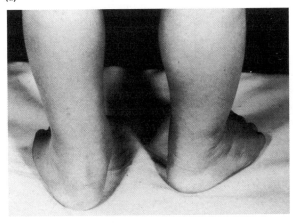

(b)

Fig. 7.1 Bilateral metatarsus varus. Note (a) the marked forefoot varus with hallux varus, the concavity of the medial border of the foot and the convexity of the lateral border of the foot, and (b) the valgus of the hindfoot.

border. The maximum prominence is over the base of the fifth metatarsal. When the child tries to stand the varus deformity is often increased with a high medial arch and supination of the foot due to action of the

179

invertors of the foot. Clinically, the forefoot is nearly always passively correctable, at least to the neutral position, and the foot is supple. Radiographs confirm the varus deformity of the metatarsals and the valgus position of the bones of the hindfoot (Fig. 7.2).

There are two definitive papers on the natural history of this common disorder. Ponseti and Becker (1966) stated that only 11% of feet suffering from this condition needed any treatment at all. The deformity may appear to deteriorate during the second year of life and then improve spontaneously to a normal or near normal foot with a mild valgus heel. If correction is necessary, this should be by serial plasters usually applied at the age of 6 months for a period of 8–12 weeks, changing the plasters every 2–3 weeks. They pointed out that Denis Browne hobble boots or splints (Fig. 7.3) do not control this deformity adequately. The plasters have to be applied carefully with the hindfoot supinated before the forefoot is corrected, otherwise the plaster will tend to increase the valgus deformity of the heel. They recommend plasters only for those feet that are rigid, severely deformed and not correctable passively. Only two out of 379 patients required operative correction. Rushforth (1978) confirmed these findings. In his series, where no treatment was given, 86% of feet corrected completely; 10% had mild persistent deformity which was completely asymptomatic; 4% had deformed stiff feet. He was unable to predict, until the age of 3 years, which feet would fail to correct spontaneously. It is an

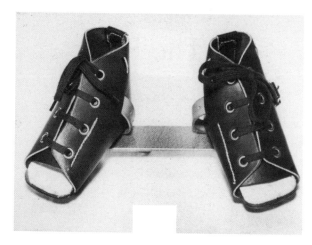

Fig. 7.3 Denis Browne hobble boots with bar. Note the heel-retaining strap which is most important for keeping the heel well down in the boot.

interesting general observation that this condition is seldom, if ever, seen in an adult. It is tempting to suggest that metatarsus primus varus with adolescent hallux valgus (Fig. 7.4) is the end-result of this condition, but few if any patients with this condition give a history of metatarsus varus or in-toeing in childhood. Bleck (1983) advised a more radical early approach to conservative treatment. He accepted that the pressures of 'the public attitude to deformity' among his treatment population

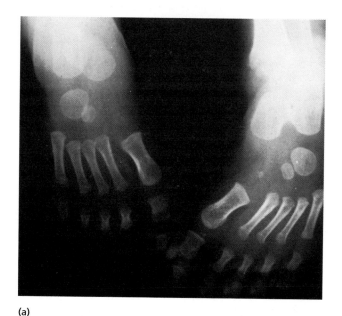

(a)

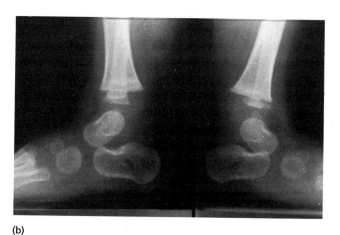

(b)

Fig. 7.2 Radiographs of a left metatarsus varus for comparison with a right normal foot. (a) Anteroposterior view. Note the normal appearance of the hindfoot on the affected side. (b) Lateral view. Again note the normal hindfoot.

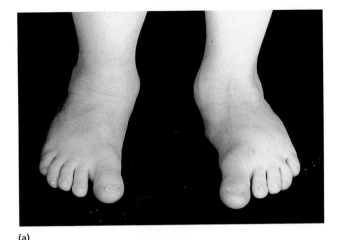

(a)

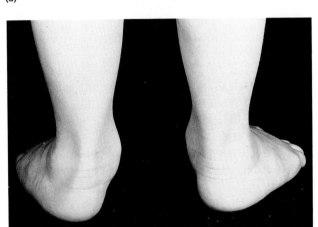

(b)

Fig. 7.5 (a) Persistent true metatarsus varus, the so-called S-shaped or serpentine foot. Note (b) the valgus heels (these patients may have a ball-and-socket ankle joint).

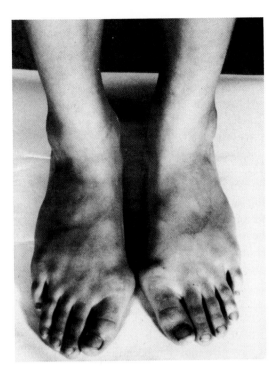

Fig. 7.4 Adolescent hallux valgus associated with metatarsus primus varus. Note the characteristic broadening of the forefoot and a tendency to develop a bunionette over the fifth metatarsal.

did not allow him to wait for spontaneous resolution, though he could not predict with certainty at the time of treatment which feet would definitely not correct with time.

Metatarsus varus seems to be becoming more common. It has been suggested that the present practice of nursing babies prone encourages the condition to persist. This practice is valuable in other ways, however, and as the condition appears to be benign, this should not be used as an argument against the prone lying position in early infancy. In 1921, Bankart pointed out that this condition was a separate entity and not a forme fruste of club-foot as was often stated at that time. He suggested an abnormality of the tibialis anterior as the causative factor. More recently, Browne and Paton (1979) described an anomalous insertion of the tibialis posterior tendon in 14 feet. Selection for operation was based on a fixed adduction deformity of the forefoot, which was 30° or more and not improving with passive manipulations by the parents and the physiotherapist. At operation, the insertion of the tibialis posterior tendon was found to be by a small slip only to the navicular bone. The main bulk of the tendon bypassed the navicular bone, being inserted further forward and laterally. Traction on the tendon reproduced the deformity. Cor-

rection was obtained by transferring the tibialis posterior tendon into the navicular bone and a medial capsulotomy of the naviculocuneiform joint followed by a plaster cast for 6 weeks. The authors comment on the difficulty in selecting patients who require operative treatment in a condition with such a high spontaneous correction rate.

A rare variety of metatarsus varus was described by Lloyd-Roberts and Clark (1973) as the S-shaped or serpentine foot (Fig. 7.5). In this condition, the deformity is rigid and resists conservative treatment. The valgus of the heel is particularly difficult to treat, and this may be due to a ball-and-socket abnormality of the ankle joint. Lloyd-Roberts and Clark considered this condition as a separate entity that is rare and often familial. Kite (1967) described 12 serpentine feet in 2818 patients with forefoot deformities and noted the strong hereditary influence in these cases. Lloyd-Roberts and Clark (1973) advised treating the rigid forefoot, but did not feel that the hindfoot and ankle deformities justified ankle arthrodesis.

In those few patients who fail to respond to conservative treatment, the forefoot can be corrected surgically, either by the tarsometatarsal release operation described by Heyman *et al.* (1958) or by multiple metatarsal osteotomies. Tarsometatarsal release is an extensive procedure in which all the tarsometatarsal joints are mobilized. Heyman *et al.* (1958) described the results in only nine operations for metatarsus varus. The other patients in their series were suffering from talipes equinovarus. Most patients were operated on over the age of 3 years and under the age of 7 years. They reported good or excellent results in all nine patients. Postoperatively, 3–4 months in plaster are required. The procedure can realign the foot adequately, but may result in some stiffness and thickening in the mid-foot. Multiple metatarsal osteotomies are seldom performed. There is a risk of vascular damage, as in the Lisfranc fracture dislocation of the mid-foot. Recently, Stark *et al.* (1987) reported a 41% overall failure rate of this operation and a 50% incidence of a painful dorsal prominence at the site of the surgical scar in a review of operations performed over a period of 18 years. Berman and Gartland (1971) reported good results in children over the age of 6 years. They emphasized the need for care in avoiding damage to the anterior tibial artery and to the deep branch of the peroneal nerve in the foot. Pin fixation was used to stabilize the first and fifth metatarsals, and the foot was immobilized in plaster for 6 weeks.

The orthopaedic surgeon faced with this common condition with such a high spontaneous recovery rate can happily advise a 'wait and see' policy for at least the first 3 years of life. If the foot appears very rigid in the early stages, then serial plasters will probably be effective. If, at the age of 3 years, there is still a significant varus deformity that is rigid and uncorrectable, then exploration and release of the tibialis posterior, if it is anomalous, are worthwhile. If this abnormality is not present, then release of the abductor hallucis and capsulotomy of the first metatarsocuneiform joint may correct the foot. If the foot is still not correctable, then a tarsometatarsal release up to the age of 6 years will correct the foot. Finally, over the age of 6 years multiple metatarsal osteotomies can be considered.

FLAT FEET

There is no accurate definition of this common condition. Clinically, if the medial longitudinal arch of the foot touches the ground on weight-bearing or is nearer the ground than the observer feels it should be, then the foot is considered to be flat. More accurate methods using weight-bearing mats and weight-recording foot plates are available. It is important to understand the normal development of the foot and the medial longitudinal arch. At birth, the most common position of the foot is in calcaneovalgus and no arch is present. When the child first starts to stand, it usually does so on a wide base with the feet externally rotated and everted (Fig. 7.6). There is a large pad of fat on the medial side of the foot which almost invariably looks flat at this time. As walking and balance become established during the second and third years, the feet tend to come together and the medial arch appears. In late walkers, because the foot is larger, the flattening of the medial arch is much more obvious and often causes great concern. Unless the natural history of the development of the medial arch is understood, a large number of children may be treated unnecessarily with modifications to their shoes, e.g. arch supports or wedges, which are quite unnecessary.

Feet may also look flat because of the position of the legs. Common normal variants such as genu valgum, which is present to some degree in 80% of children at the age of 3–4 years, will inevitably make the foot look flat (Fig. 7.7). Similarly, internal rotation of the leg from the hip due to persistent femoral anteversion will produce a flat-footed in-toe gait (Fig. 7.8). Morley (1957), in a most useful survey of flat feet and knock knees in normal children in North London, showed that at 18 months 97% of children have flat feet. By the age of 10 years, only 4% of children still have flat feet. Some of these children had been treated with shoe modifications

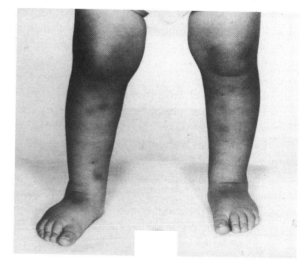

Fig. 7.6 Normal child, aged 18 months, showing the normal planovalgus foot at this age before the medial arch develops.

during this period with no evidence of any beneficial effect.

Flat foot remains a therapeutic dilemma. In some populations, up to 35% have flat feet with no apparent ill effects. There is often a strong familial and racial tendency to this condition. In this country, according to Morley (1957), there is a 90–95% spontaneous recovery rate with no treatment. The problem remains of how to select those patients who need treatment and avoid unnecessary treatment in a large proportion of the population?

The majority of flat feet are mobile, pain-free and show no evidence of neurological abnormality. Such feet are usually completely asymptomatic. They are often familial. Treatment is only necessary when shoe wear is excessive and occasionally to allay acute parental anxiety. In such cases, measures such as insoles, heel cups, or wedging, can help to prevent deformity of the shoe. Some authors, e.g. Rose (1962), claim that this sort of treatment can alter the shape of the foot. Against a 90–95% spontaneous recovery rate, however, it is very difficult to prove that this type of treatment really does alter the basic shape of the foot. The most useful clinical test for this mobile type of foot is either to ask the patient to stand on tiptoe or to passively dorsiflex the big toe (Jack's (1953) toe-raising test) and see whether the medial arch is restored. For many years

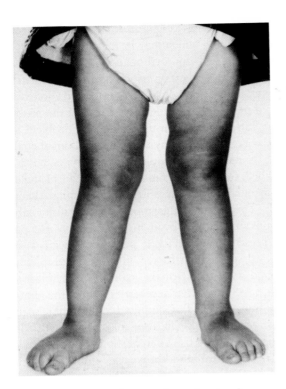

Fig. 7.7 Child with normal genu valgum showing the apparent flat foot that this produces.

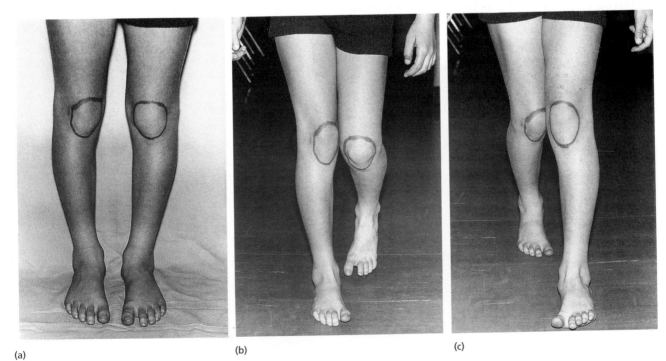

(a) (b) (c)

Fig. 7.8 (a–c) Child with the typical stance and appearance of persistent femoral anteversion. Note the internal rotation of the legs from the hip, giving rise to mild squinting patellas, apparent lateral bowing of the tibias and in-toeing at the feet.

exercises have been prescribed for flat feet. Electromyographic studies by Basmajian and Stecko (1963), however, showed that under normal relaxed standing conditions muscle function is not important in maintaining the arch of the foot. The medial longitudinal arch is dependent on the configuration of the bones, joints, joint capsules and ligaments. Therefore, there seems little point in performing specific foot exercises for short periods each day as they are unlikely to have any effect on the shape of the foot.

Rose *et al.* (1986) published the results of a 25-year study designed to distinguish normal anatomical variants from pathological conditions. They concluded that the test for flat foot should relate to function and be dynamic rather than static. They showed that children progressively developed a medial arch with time, so that the broad feet of pre-school children became normal with time irrespective of whether they had any treatment or not. They confirmed that Jack's great toe extension test, in which the medial arch rises and there is lateral tibial rotation when the big toe is dorsiflexed, is the most useful test for dynamic function of the medial arch. Wenger *et al.* (1989) in a very important prospective study showed that a flexible flat foot in a young child improves with growth. Treatment with corrective shoes or inserts or specially designed insoles does not alter the natural history of the condition in any way.

There is a small but important group of patients with flat feet in whom the feet are stiff or excessively mobile, painful, or show muscular weakness or spasticity. These feet need careful investigation for the underlying cause of the deformity, which may be local but is commonly a more generalized non-orthopaedic problem. Although treatment with wedges or insoles may be helpful in these patients, it must not obscure the need to discover and treat, if possible, the underlying cause of the problem.

The stiff flat foot is usually due to a problem in the subtalar region. This may be a localized tarsal coalition which is partial or complete. Many types have been described: the most common are talocalcaneal and calcaneonavicular bars. These are often familial (Leonard, 1974). They are often asymptomatic until the subtalar region is stressed, e.g. by an inversion strain. The patient then presents with marked peroneal spasm, so-called 'peroneal spastic' flat foot. Oblique radiographs of the foot and axial views of the subtalar joint (Harris and Beath, 1948) are often necessary to show the abnormal bar of bone (Fig. 7.9). Computed tomographic scanning is also very helpful. The foot may also be stiff due to spasticity resulting from cerebral palsy or a more localized neurological condition, e.g. spinal dysraphism, which should always be looked for.

The painful flat foot is commonly associated with stiffness and muscle spasm. Pain may be due to trauma, infection, juvenile chronic arthritis which often presents in the ankle or subtalar joint, localized osteochondritis, e.g. Köhler's disease, and tumours, e.g. an osteoid osteoma in the calcaneum or talus. Weakness and hypermobility of the foot may be seen in children with conditions such as generalized joint laxity, muscular

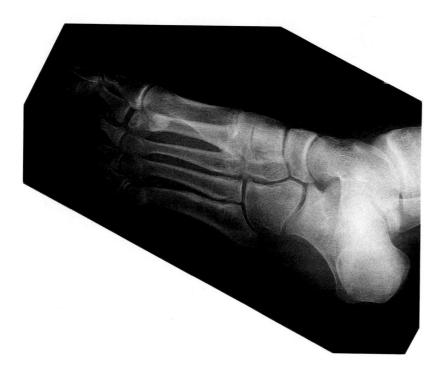

Fig. 7.9 Oblique radiograph of a patient with peroneal spastic flat foot showing an incomplete calcaneonavicular bar.

dystrophy, Marfan's syndrome, osteogenesis imperfecta, spinal muscular atrophy, or Down's syndrome.

In all these patients the first step is to make as accurate a diagnosis as possible. Once this has been done and appropriate measures taken for the causative condition, then the local flat foot problem can be dealt with. These children usually need support for the foot in the form of footwear modifications or insoles. Sometimes a below-knee calliper is necessary. If conservative measures fail, subtalar arthrodesis as described by Grice (1952) or even a triple arthrodesis at maturity can be considered.

CONGENITAL TALIPES EQUINOVARUS (CLUB-FOOT)

This is one of the oldest and best known of all orthopaedic conditions. Hippocrates described it and wrote about its treatment. In this condition both the forefoot and the hindfoot are in equinus and varus (Fig. 7.10). It is important to recognize that the condition affects the leg as well as the foot. There is always wasting of the calf muscles, and the foot on the affected side is always shorter than on the normal side (Fig. 7.11). One of the

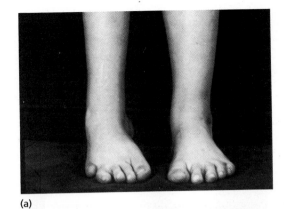

(a)

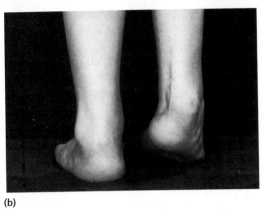

(b)

Fig. 7.11 Patient, aged $3\frac{1}{2}$ years, with a relapsed right congenital talipes equinovarus. Note (a) the equinus and varus of the heel and the varus and supination of the forefoot and (b) the scar of the previous posteromedial release operation.

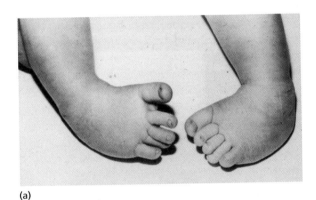

(a)

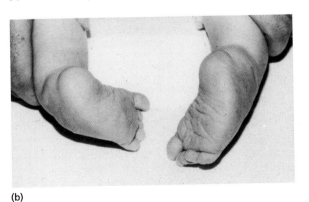

(b)

Fig. 7.10 Patient with bilateral congenital talipes equinovarus. Note that both the forefoot (a) and the hindfoot (b) are in equinus and varus.

greatest problems in this condition is describing its severity. There is a spectrum of the disorder ranging from mild positional deformity, which corrects easily in the first or second week of life, through to completely rigid deformity as seen in conditions such as arthrogryposis or lumbar agenesis (Fig. 7.12). The degree of rigidity is very difficult to measure or record in any objective manner. The condition must be distinguished from metatarsus varus, in which the forefoot is in varus but the hindfoot is in neutral or valgus.

The incidence of the condition in the UK is about 1−2 in 1000 live births. There is a strong family history in that if the condition runs in the family, the chances of having a child with talipes equinovarus are increased 20−30 times (Wynne-Davies, 1964). Unlike congenital dislocation of the hip, it is not associated with any particular position *in utero* or with birth rank. It is two to three times more common in males than in females.

It is most important when faced with a child with a club-foot to examine the whole child carefully to ascertain whether the condition is primary, idiopathic

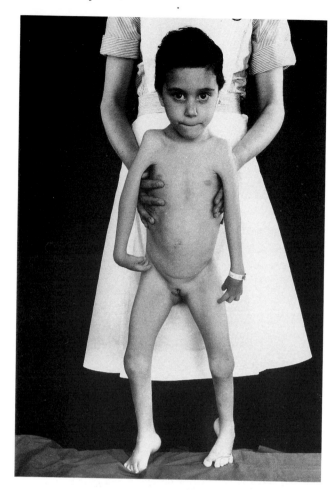

Fig. 7.12 Typical patient with arthrogryposis congenita multiplex affecting all four limbs. Note the severe talipes equinovarus, the marked wasting of the shoulder girdle, tubular limbs and contractures of the wrists and hands.

and unassociated with any other abnormality, or secondary to a wide variety of other congenital problems. The conditions that should be looked for are the following:

1 Neurological conditions, such as myelomeningocoele, spina bifida occulta, in which there may be a tell-tale patch of hair, naevus, skin dimple, or lipoma over the spine (Fig. 7.13), and lumbar agenesis. Careful palpation of the spine in the newborn is often an easier way than radiography for determining whether there is a significant spinal anomaly.

2 Local abnormalities such as constriction rings or tibial dysplasia may cause very severe equinovarus deformities (Fig. 7.14).

3 Generalized abnormalities such as arthrogryposis congenita multiplex cause very severe rigid deformities in many joints including the feet, which are common in severe equinovarus.

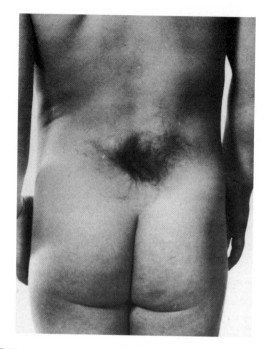

Fig. 7.13 Patient with spinal dysraphism affecting the lower lumbar spine. Note the prominent hairy patch over the site of the lesion.

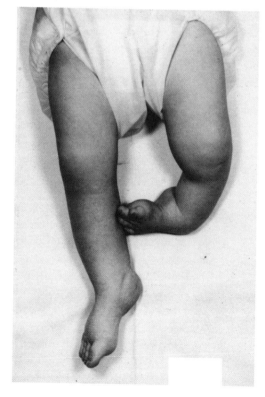

Fig. 7.14 Congenital absence of the tibia. Note the marked shortening of the lower leg and severe equinovarus position of the left foot.

4 Talipes equinovarus may be associated with other congenital abnormalities, such as tracheo-oesophageal fistula, anorectal atresia and congenital heart defects.

Finally, a number of chromosome abnormalities such as trisomy 13 and 18 and types of dwarfism such as diastrophic dwarfism may be associated with club-feet. It must also be remembered that an equinovarus deformity can be acquired following poliomyelitis, cerebral palsy, or trauma to the lateral popliteal nerve and the soft tissues of the posteromedial side of the leg, as in burns.

The cause of idiopathic talipes equinovarus is unknown, though a great deal has been written about this subject. Sir Denis Browne (1955) was an enthusiastic advocate of intrauterine moulding, but it seems doubtful that this could explain the familial tendency and the marked anatomical changes that have been found in the feet of early fetuses. Isaacs *et al.* (1977) put forward some convincing electron microscopic studies supporting a neurological cause for this condition. Certainly, the wasting of the muscles and the similarity in appearance of the severe club-foot seen in myelomeningocoele, lumbar agenesis and arthrogryposis make this an attractive hypothesis.

For many years, several authors have written about the anatomical findings; an important study was published by Ippolito and Ponseti in 1980. They studied in detail five fetal feet between the ages of 16 and 19 weeks. Great care was taken to ensure that these were idiopathic club-feet and not secondary to other abnormalities. They found extensive changes even at this early age. The tarsal bones were misshapen and smaller than normal, and there was a decrease in the size and number of fibres in the distal one-third of the muscles of the posterior and medial aspect of the leg, with an increase in the fibrous tissues in these muscles, tendon sheaths and fasciae. The ligaments on the posterior and medial aspects of the ankle joint were pulled into the joint by severe plantar flexion and varus of the talus, with thickening of the distal Achilles tendon and the posterior capsule of the ankle. On the basis of these findings, Ippolito and Ponseti (1980) postulated a retracting fibrosis as the primary aetiological factor in club-feet. This important paper not only emphasizes how extensive are the changes in club-foot at an early stage of fetal development, but also could explain the persisting problems with recurrent deformity after apparently excellent corrective treatment. Again, it underlines the difficulty in describing objectively and accurately the severity of this complex deformity.

Treatment

An immense amount has been written about the treatment of this deformity. Despite many treatment regimens, however, the overall results are not impressive. In most large series approximately 50% of cases respond to conservative treatment and the remaining 50% require operative treatment which often has to be repeated, due either to failure to obtain full correction at the time of previous treatment or to recurrence following apparently full and adequate correction. Treatment should start as soon as possible after birth. Hippocrates recommended manipulations and bandaging, and most surgeons still advise repeated gentle manipulation and splinting, either with strapping (Fig. 7.15) or plasters or a splint, such as the Denis Browne splint. Even in the most severe and rigid feet this type of conservative treatment is worth trying.

There have been few comparative studies of these three methods. Fripp and Shaw (1967) published a comparison between repeated daily stretching and strapping, serial plasters and the Denis Browne splint. Their results were heavily in favour of the stretching and strapping, but only 20 patients were treated with plasters. The Denis Browne splint did not work well, even in the hands of its originator. Basically, the principle of

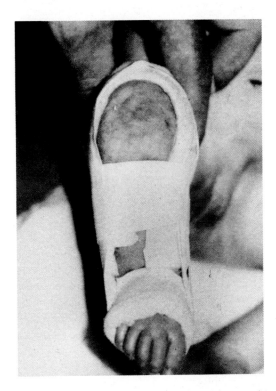

Fig. 7.15 Congenital talipes equinovarus treated by stretching and strapping method.

repeated gentle manipulation to stretch the foot into the correct position seems to be widely accepted. How to hold the correction once it is obtained following manipulation depends on the preference of the surgeon and the local conditions. Strapping allows daily manipulations but needs careful supervision and may be difficult to cope with in hot countries due to skin problems. Plasters need to be expertly applied and are usually changed weekly, and so the number of manipulations is markedly reduced compared with the strapping method. Finally, the Denis Browne splint can be used as a simple static splint to maintain correction but does not work as a dynamic self-manipulator as its originator suggested.

The vital point in conservative treatment is to know when full correction has been obtained and when spurious correction is being produced by too forceful manipulation against an unyielding deformity. Clini-

cally, the foot must dorsiflex and evert above neutral. The heel must be in calcaneus and the head of the talus, which is initially laterally displaced, must be replaced in its proper position relative to the calcaneum and the forefoot. Anteroposterior and lateral radiographs of the foot taken in a standard way can be helpful (Davis and Hatt, 1955) (Fig. 7.16). The lateral radiograph of the foot should be taken with the tibia as near as possible at a right angle to the foot. This will then show the talocalcaneal angle and whether the fibula is in its normal position or has been displaced backwards by forcing the foot upwards without fully correcting the external rotation of the talus. It will also reveal a spurious forefoot correction or rocker-bottomed foot, where the forefoot has been forced into dorsiflexion but the hindfoot equinus is not corrected (Fig. 7.17). The anteroposterior view will show whether the angle

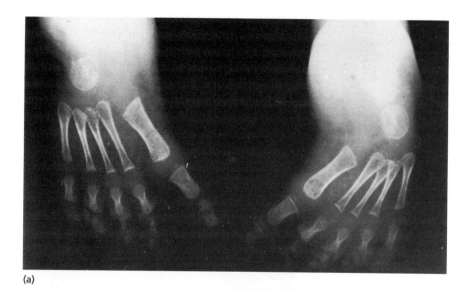

(a)

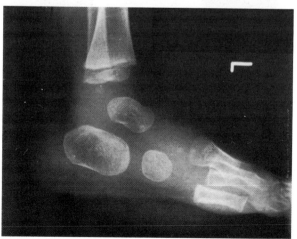

(b)

Fig. 7.16 (a) Anteroposterior radiograph showing congenital talipes equinovarus on the left and a normal foot on the right. Note the marked varus of the forefoot and the fact that the talus and the oscalcis on the left point laterally instead of the normal position as shown by the foot on the right. (b) Lateral radiograph of an uncorrected talipes equinovarus. Note that both the talus and the os calcis are still in equinus.

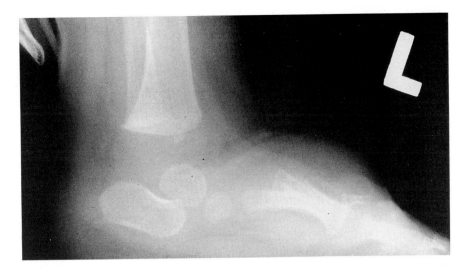

Fig. 7.17 Lateral radiograph of a foot following treatment for congenital talipes equinovarus showing spurious correction giving rise to a typical rocker-bottomed foot, i.e. the os calcis and talus are still in equinus, though the forefoot has been pushed up producing a midfoot breech.

between the talus and calcaneum has been restored to normal and whether the forefoot has been reduced on the hindfoot by realigning the first metatarsal with the talus. The anatomy and clinical features of uncorrected club-foot are well summarized by Swann *et al.* (1969). Scott *et al.* (1984) made some important observations on the anatomy of dorsiflexion in club-foot and the nature of the tethers that prevent adequate correction of the foot.

Once it is clear that conservative treatment is failing to adequately correct the foot, an operation should be considered. Until recently, operation at approximately 3 months of age was recommended. Long-term follow-up of such early surgery by Ghali *et al.* (1983), Green and Lloyd-Roberts (1985) and Hutchins *et al.* (1985), however, has been unable to show any correlation on statistical grounds between the time of operation and the quality of end-results. As a result many surgeons now advise leaving the foot if conservative treatment fails until the age of 9–12 months before considering surgery, particularly if this is of an extensive nature. The type of surgery varies widely. At the conservative end of the spectrum Laaveg and Ponseti (1980) advise percutaneous lengthening of the Achilles tendon and continued plaster casts. At the opposite extreme Clark (1968) and Turco (1971) advise radical posterior and medial release. The problem again is the tremendous variation in severity of this disorder, and whether a primary idiopathic club-foot or one of the many difficult cases associated with other abnormalities is being considered. Harrold and Walker (1983) published perhaps the only paper in which an attempt has been made to classify by a simple clinical method the severity of the deformity when first seen by the surgeon and relate this to the end-result of treatment. Even in the mildest postural type of club-foot

approximately 10% came to operation, and in their so-called severe type, i.e. any foot which had more than 20° of residual equinus and varus when the surgeon tried to correct it when it was first seen, 90% required operative treatment.

The work by Ippolito and Ponseti (1980) shows that the deformity is present early in fetal life and the abnormalities are very considerable. If conservative treatment fails to achieve full correction in 3–4 months, then surgery is indicated. Surgery should obtain full correction, but should avoid excessive dissection which can lead to over-correction, stiffness, fibrosis and recurrent deformity. This is particularly important if Ippolito and Ponseti's theory of a retracting fibrosis is correct. Usually, conservative treatment is successful in realigning the forefoot on the hindfoot in equinus, except in the very rigid cases. The problem is then the hindfoot equinus, which can be corrected by a posterior release (Attenborough, 1966). This involves Z-lengthening of the Achilles tendon, posterior capsulotomy of the ankle and subtalar joints, division or elongation of the tibialis posterior and flexor digitorum communis muscles, and elongation of the flexor hallucis longus muscle. If the abductor hallucis and plantar ligaments are tight, they should be released from the medial and plantar surface of the calcaneum. This will usually completely correct the heel and the forefoot on the hindfoot. This type of posterior surgery releasing tendinous tethers rather than fixed joint deformity can probably be undertaken early as part of continued conservative treatment provided adequate splinting is maintained until the child starts to walk. If, however, there is a more extensive fixed joint deformity, the more extensive operation described by Turco (1979) and the peritalar operation involving both medial, lateral and posterior aspects of the hindfoot described by Simons (1985) have to be considered. Turco (1979) did not recommend his operation under the age of 1 year, and Simons advised that the foot should be at least 8 cm in length before considering his extensive operation. Stiffening the foot should be avoided if possible, as shown by Laaveg and Ponseti (1980) in a carefully selected series of idiopathic club-feet followed up for 10–27 years, in which mobility of the foot was more important to the final functional result than perfect anatomical alignment.

The next crucial point to consider is relapse or recurrence. In the majority of reported series at least 50% of feet relapse and need some further treatment following the primary treatment. Most surgeons recommend splinting after initial correction has been obtained. The author prefers the Denis Browne hobble splint (see Fig. 7.3, p. 180) which is worn all the time except for 1 h in the morning and afternoon until the child is trying to stand. It is then left off when the child is active but applied at night and when the child is resting. Once the child is walking the splint is only worn at night. The author prefers the children to continue wearing a night splint until the age of 3–4 years if possible, but not if it is causing serious problems with sleeping. The hobble boots may be changed for an equinus night boot (Fig. 7.18) once the lower leg is long enough for this splint to be effective. The long-term studies by Green and Lloyd-Roberts (1985) and Hutchins *et al.* (1985) were unable to show any statistical correlation between those patients who had received long-term postoperative splinting and those who had not had any form of long-term splinting. As a result the place of splinting other than before the child walks and for short periods after coming out of plaster remains doubtful in the prevention of further deformity in club-feet.

The foot is watched at regular intervals. The most common early problem is failure to establish dorsiflexion and eversion. If this is not established within 6 months of the initial correction, or the child persists in supinating the foot on dorsiflexion, then a tibialis anterior tendon transfer to the lateral side of the foot should be considered. Laaveg and Ponseti (1980) used this transfer to the third cuneiform only. Imhauser (personal communication) in Cologne has had very impressive results applying this transfer in almost every case to obtain powerful eversion. Once eversion is obtained he is prepared to transfer the tendon back again if the foot is going into too much pronation.

Despite strenuous efforts recurrence of equinus and varus does occur. The lateral radiograph is most valuable in assessing this situation. Repeat posterior or posteromedial release is then necessary. This can be a difficult

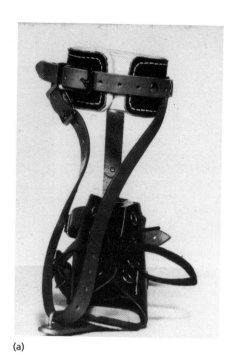

(a)

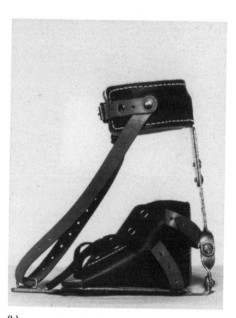

(b)

Fig. 7.18 (a,b) Equinus night boot.

operation and is never successful unless full correction can be obtained at the time of operation. Inevitably, it is liable to give rise to increasing stiffness in the foot. The other major type of relapse is the mid-foot breach or bean-shaped foot (Fig. 7.19). Here the calcaneum is corrected but the talus is still displaced laterally. This gives rise to the so-called 'flat-topped' talus in the lateral radiograph and the fibula is displaced posteriorly. In the anteroposterior radiograph the talonavicular alignment

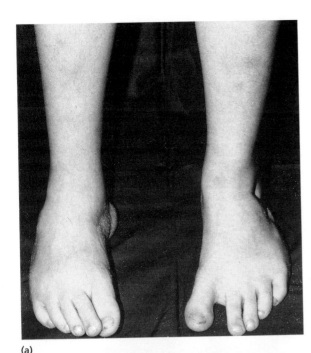

(a)

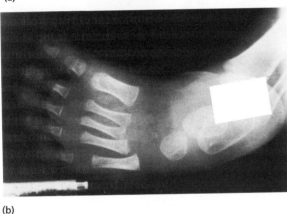

(b)

Fig. 7.19 (a) Relapsed clubbed feet, worse on the right than the left, giving rise to so-called 'mid-foot breech' or 'bean-shaped foot'. (b) Anteroposterior radiograph of a bean-shaped foot.

has not been corrected. The navicular with the forefoot is still displaced medially on the talus. This deformity responds well to the Dillwyn Evans (1961) operation. In this procedure the vital steps are: first, to correct any residual hindfoot equinus; second, to fully mobilize the navicular from its medially displaced position on the talus through a medial incision; finally, to remove a calcaneocuboid wedge to swing the forefoot round on the hindfoot in a manner reminiscent of the dome-shaped or Brackett osteotomy of a long bone. This can give excellent results, but should probably not be performed under the age of 4 years. Certain points must be watched; the procedure can increase the cavus and pronation of the forefoot and should not be done in

patients with an already pronated forefoot. Some of the deformity may be at the tarsometatarsal joints (Lowe and Hannon, 1973) and not at the talonavicular, calcaneocuboid level. If this is not recognized overcorrection may occur at the talonavicular, calcaneocuboid level, which produces an S-shaped or serpentine foot. Finally, removal of too large a calcaneocuboid wedge can produce a very flat, stiff, everted foot.

If the forefoot deformity is at the tarsometatarsal level, as in metatarsus varus, the tarsometatarsal release of Heyman *et al.* (1958) may be used under the age of 6 years. Over the age of 6 years metatarsal osteotomies are indicated. If there is a very severe mid-foot breach with the fibula severely displaced backwards, it is logical to correct this by a medial rotation osteotomy of the tibia (Lloyd-Roberts *et al.*, 1974), followed by a lateral wedge tarsectomy. This will produce a reasonably shaped but short and stiff foot. Finally, at maturity triple arthrodesis is still the classical operation for correcting rigid bony deformity. This can produce a reasonable foot to go in a shoe, but it is stiff with significant functional impairment. As such it represents the failure of earlier treatment.

The other operation that can be used in the totally rigid incorrectable foot is talectomy (Fig. 7.20). This has been of great value in arthrogryposis, lumbar agenesis and occasionally in meningomyelocoele (Menelaus, 1971). This can give a plantigrade foot, though it corrects the hindfoot deformity better than the forefoot deformity. The whole of the talus must be removed. The calcaneum is temporarily stabilized on the tibia by a Kirschner wire, which is retained for 6–8 weeks. A portion of the Achilles tendon should be excised to prevent it causing recurrent equinus. If part of the cartilaginous talus is not removed it will grow and cause troublesome recurrence.

Congenital talipes equinovarus in all its varied forms remains an unsolved problem. Orthopaedic surgeons will continue to struggle with its treatment and argue about this fascinating condition until its aetiology is better understood and more accurate and objective methods of assessment are available.

CONGENITAL VERTICAL TALUS (CONGENITAL CONVEX PES VALGUS)

This is a very rare disorder. It occurred in only 1 of 131 patients attending a special clinic for congenital foot deformities of the newborn (Osmond-Clark, 1956). It can occur as an isolated abnormality or in association with other disorders, e.g. meningomyelocoele, arthro-

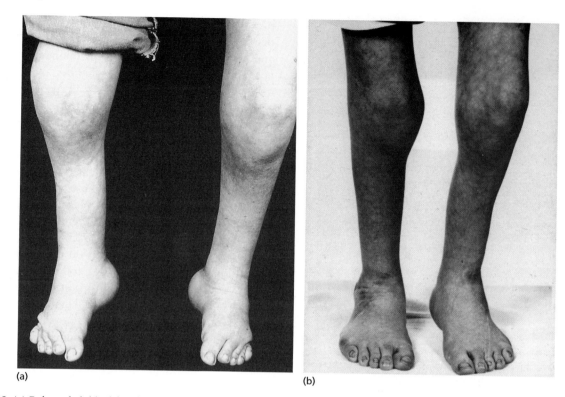

Fig. 7.20 (a) Relapsed clubbed feet following posterior release in arthrogryposis. (b) The same patient post-talectomy. Note that the left heel is off the ground but this is due to fixed flexion at the left knee and not to fixed equinus of the left foot.

gryposis, trisomy 18 and Freeman−Sheldon syndrome (craniocarpotarsal dystrophy).

The condition must be distinguished from severe calcaneovalgus foot, severe idiopathic flat foot, the valgus everted foot of cerebral palsy and the rocker-bottomed foot produced by spurious overcorrection of a congenital talipes equinovarus (Lloyd-Roberts and Spence, 1958). The salient features are that the hindfoot is in rigid equinus and the forefoot is in rigid calcaneus and eversion (Fig. 7.21). A lateral radiograph in neutral will confirm the hindfoot equinus (Fig. 7.22) and a lateral radiograph in full plantar flexion (Eyre-Brook, 1967) will confirm that the forefoot is not reduced on the hindfoot in full plantar flexion. Unless these criteria

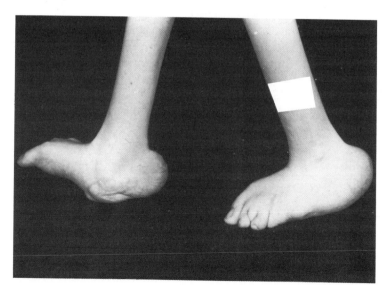

Fig. 7.21 Bilateral congenital vertical talus. Note the rocker-bottom shape of the foot, the rounded heel, the hindfoot still in equinus and the forefoot in calcaneus and valgus.

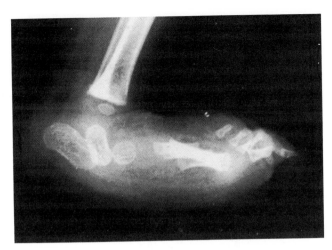

Fig. 7.22 Lateral radiograph of a congenital vertical talus. Note the hindfoot equinus, the vertical talus and the forefoot in calcaneus.

are fulfilled the condition cannot be considered a true congenital vertical talus. The crux of the deformity is a dorsal dislocation of the navicular on the head of the talus. The navicular bone does not ossify until the age of 3 years, but its position can be deduced from the position of the ossified first metatarsal in children under this age. In older patients the vertically placed talus shows a characteristic hourglass deformity, and the anterior portion of the calcaneum becomes narrowed and beak shaped.

Silk and Wainwright (1967) recommended repeated plastering in full plantar flexion to correct the forefoot on the hindfoot. This was followed by elongation of the Achilles tendon and posterior capsulotomy of the ankle joint to correct the hindfoot. The great majority of surgeons writing about this condition, however, have had no success with conservative treatment and a variety of operations has been described. They all involve open reduction of the dorsally dislocated navicular on the talus, with correction of the hindfoot and stabilization of the talonavicular joint in its correct position. Osmond-Clark (1956) used a peroneus brevis transfer to the neck of the talus; Harrold (1967) advocated Kirschner wire fixation; Eyre-Brook (1967) excised a wedge of the navicular bone which was inserted beneath the neck of the talus; Stone (1963) advised removal of the navicular bone and transfer of the tibialis anterior to the neck of the talus. Duckworth and Smith (1974), in reviewing the treatment of this condition in association with meningomyelocoele, which probably represents a separate type of the deformity, advised transfer of the tibialis anterior to the neck of the talus and the peroneus brevis to the tibialis posterior.

Any one surgeon's experience of this condition is likely to be small because of its rarity. In general, as long as both the hindfoot equinus and the forefoot calcaneus and eversion are fully corrected and the talonavicular dislocation satisfactorily reduced and stabilized by a posterior, medial and lateral approach to the foot deformity, then with or without the removal of the navicular bone a satisfactory plantigrade, but usually rather stiff foot, is obtained (Colton, 1973) (Fig. 7.23).

CONGENITAL TALIPES CALCANEOVALGUS

This is the opposite deformity to talipes equinovarus. The heel is in calcaneus and the forefoot dorsiflexed and everted (Fig. 7.24). This is the most common position of the foot in the newborn infant. When examining the newborn it is normal to be able to dorsiflex the foot so that the dorsum of the foot touches the front of the tibia. However, there should be a normal range of plantar flexion. The calcaneovalgus foot will usually only come down to about the neutral position or even less. This position of the foot is particularly common in children born by the breech presentation or with marked intra-uterine moulding. It is, therefore, often seen in first-born

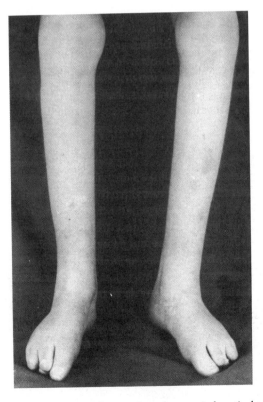

Fig. 7.23 Bilateral surgical correction of congenital vertical talus.

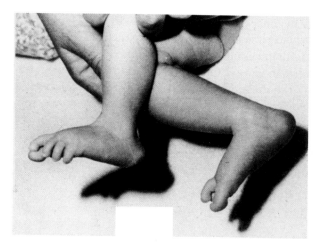

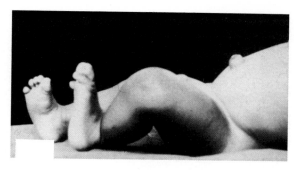

Fig. 7.25 Left tibia recurvatum. Note the marked calcaneovalgus of the left foot and the right metatarsus varus.

Fig. 7.24 Bilateral calcaneovalgus feet. Note that compared with congenital vertical talus the heels are in calcaneus and not equinus.

children and following pregnancies in which there has been oligohydramnios.

It is important to look for other problems in the child with a calcaneovalgus foot. In the leg there may be hyperextension of the knee (genu recurvatum) or very occasionally posterior bowing of the tibia itself (tibia recurvatum) (Fig. 7.25). It can be associated with congenital dislocation of the hip in 5% of patients (Wynne-Davies, 1973). Limitation of abduction of the hip associated with this condition should be looked for, as it may indicate a hip dysplasia or be part of the so-called 'moulded baby' syndrome (Lloyd-Roberts and Pilcher, 1965), which includes plagiocephaly, torticollis, idiopathic infantile scoliosis, pelvic obliquity and a calcaneus foot (Fig. 7.26). In the spine all forms of spinal dysraphism should be considered.

Usually congenital talipes calcaneovalgus responds rapidly to gentle maternal stretching. Some authors (Giannestras, 1973), however, recommend the use of plasters and splints, but in the author's experience this

is only necessary in severe and resistant cases. If the condition persists beyond 3–4 months of age, the presence of some generalized condition, usually a neurological problem, should be carefully sought. It should be distinguished from congenital vertical talus in which the deformity is rigid and the hindfoot fixed in equinus while the forefoot is in calcaneus. In older children the treatment is the same as for flat feet unless the condition is associated with neuromuscular problems, e.g. meningomyelocoele or cerebral palsy, where tendon transfer or division are sometimes necessary. Persistent severe calcaneovalgus may require treatment with shoe modifications, below-knee calipers or even subtalar arthrodesis (Grice, 1952).

PES CAVUS OR HIGH-ARCHED FOOT

The forefoot is in equinus, or plantaris as it is sometimes called, in relation to the hindfoot. As a result, when standing the medial, and to a lesser extent the lateral, longitudinal arch of the foot is raised and the heel is in calcaneus and commonly also varus (Fig. 7.27). The toes are commonly clawed. The weight is taken on the heads of the metatarsals and the heel with little or no weight

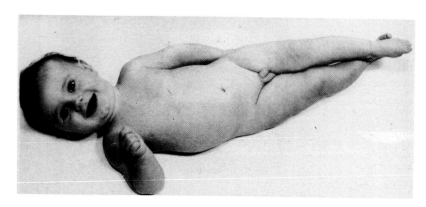

Fig. 7.26 So-called 'moulded baby' syndrome with plagiocephaly (not seen well in this photograph), a tendency to lie in a curve convex to the right, adduction of the left hip and the pelvis tilted up on the left.

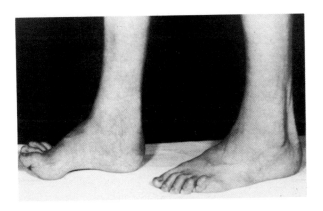

Fig. 7.27 Right pes cavus. Note the high arch and clawing of the toes.

being taken on the lateral border of the foot as in the normal foot.

The patient usually presents with a shoe wear problem or with problems from clawing of the toes. Pain over the metatarsal heads is rare in children, but common in adolescents and adults. Alternatively, the patient may present with a clumsy gait, a history of frequent falls and inversion strains due to an underlying neurological problem.

Brewerton *et al.* (1963), in a survey of so-called 'idiopathic' pes cavus, showed that in two of three cases a neurological abnormality could be found if carefully looked for. The lesion may be local in the foot, in the peripheral nerve, the spinal cord, or at a cortical level. The most common neurological condition in the series of Brewerton *et al.* was peroneal muscular atrophy. Other conditions that should be considered are anterior poliomyelitis, spinal dysraphism, meningomyelocoele, cord tumour, muscular dystrophies, Friedreich's ataxia and cerebral palsy. A family history is common, even when no definite neurological abnormality can be demonstrated. It is, therefore, necessary to enquire about the condition in other members of the family and if possible to examine them. It is important to establish any underlying cause of the deformity as this will have a considerable bearing on the course and prognosis of the deformity, particularly if the underlying problem is a progressive and disabling one, such as muscular dystrophy or Friedreich's ataxia. Expert neurological advice should be sought and investigations such as electromyography, nerve conduction studies, nerve biopsy, muscle biopsy and myelography may be indicated.

Pes cavus is seldom seen in very young children. However, there is one type that is called true congenital pes cavus, or pes arcuatus, which is sometimes seen. It is often not noticed at birth, but comes to light when the child first starts to wear shoes and the high arch causes problems. The toes are not usually clawed, and there is no evidence of an underlying neurological abnormality in these patients.

Coleman (1983), in his excellent book on complex foot deformities in children, pointed out that there are basically two types of pes cavus. Calcaneocavus is characteristic of the paralytic neurological diseases, e.g. poliomyelitis and spinal muscular atrophy, and there is marked forefoot cavus and hindfoot calcaneus. These feet may go into either varus or valgus depending on the imbalance due to the muscular weakness. The second type of pes cavus is the cavovarus foot typical of peroneal muscular atrophy and the peripheral neuropathies, which are now better classified as hereditary motor and sensory neuropathies (Harding and Thomas, 1980). In this type of foot the main characteristic is marked forefoot pronation of the first, second and sometimes third metatarsal, which in the presence of a mobile subtalar joint induces varus of the heel and inversion of the whole foot. The block test described by Coleman (1983) is most useful in demonstrating this type of cavovarus foot, and the logical operative treatment is medial release of the forefoot cavus and varus, combined if necessary with osteotomy of the first and second metatarsals to elevate the pronated forefoot and thereby correct the cavovarus foot without having to resort to bone and joint excising operations, e.g. wedge tarsectomy. It is important that orthopaedic surgeons distinguish clinically and radiologically between these two types of cavus foot, and the block test is very useful in deciding on the right type of surgical treatment for these feet.

Orthopaedic treatment consists initially of conservative measures, namely advice about shoe wear and relieving pressure on the metatarsal heads with a metatarsal pad or insole. If necessary special surgical shoes can be prescribed. In some cases during the growing period the height of the longitudinal arches can be reduced by the Steindler strip operation (Steindler, 1920), in which the plantar ligaments and intrinsic muscles are released from the calcaneus. If the block test is positive, a more radical medial release as described by Coleman (1983) can be used to elevate the pronated forefoot and correct the cavovarus.

Clawing of the toes can be corrected before the deformities become fixed by the Girdlestone flexor to extensor tendon transfer (Taylor, 1951). The clawing or so-called Z-deformity of the big toe can be corrected by a Robert Jones tendon transfer of the extensor hallucis longus to the neck of the first metatarsal with tenodesis or arthrodesis of the interphalangeal joint of the big toe.

In conditions such as peroneal muscular atrophy, where there is weakness of dorsiflexion and eversion, tibialis posterior tendon transfer to the lateral border of the foot can be very useful, even though the condition is slowly progressive. If there is fixed varus of the heel a lateral wedge calcaneal osteotomy, as described by Dwyer (1963), is an excellent procedure. At maturity, if there is a fixed cavus deformity of sufficient severity, a mid-tarsal osteotomy, either removing a dorsal wedge or the tarsal V-osteotomy described by Japas (1968), will correct the deformity. If there is significant equinus and varus as well as cavus then a triple arthrodesis is usually necessary.

Finally, if there is severe calcaneocavus as seen in the paralytic type of foot, Elmslie's two-stage arthrodesis (Cholmeley, 1953) can be considered. In this procedure, at the first stage the plantar fascia is stripped and a dorsally based wedge excised in the mid-tarsal region to correct the forefoot on the calcaneus hindfoot. After 6 weeks in plaster, at the second stage a posteriorly based wedge is excised from the subtalar joint to correct the calcaneus heel and produce a plantigrade foot. Elmslie used half the Achilles tendon, which he stapled to the back of the tibia as a tenodesis, but it is doubtful if this really contributed to the success of the procedure. Transfer of the flexor hallucis longus, flexor digitorum longus and peronei into the Achilles tendon can also be added where there is marked weakness of the soleus and gastrocnemius muscles, as in poliomyelitis. This is a very radical procedure, and the posterior displacement osteotomy of the os calcis described by Mitchell (1977) can be very useful and avoids the extensive bone and joint excision required by the Elmslie procedure.

CALCANEAL APOPHYSITIS (SEVER'S DISEASE)

This condition was originally thought to be a form of osteochondritis of the calcaneal apophysis (Sever, 1912) (Fig. 7.28). However, the appearance of increased density and fragmentation in the calcaneal apophysis has now been shown to be a normal radiological finding.

The child, usually between the ages of 7 and 13 years, presents with an intermittent limp and pain over the insertion of the Achilles tendon on the calcaneum. The pain typically comes on during or after exercise. It is worst when barefoot or wearing shoes with no heels, e.g. plimsolls. The condition is now believed to be a chronic strain of the insertion of the Achilles tendon, similar to the very common strain of the insertion of the patellar ligament on the tibial tubercle (Osgood–Schlatter disease). On examination the pain is accurately localized

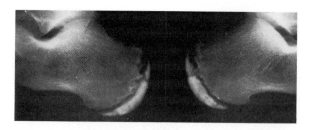

Fig. 7.28 Left Sever's disease. Note that the right os calcis apophysis looks exactly the same as the left but in fact is causing no symptoms.

to the insertion of the Achilles tendon. It is not above the heel over the tendon itself, as in Achilles tendon tendonitis which is seen in older patients.

The condition often remits spontaneously. Some reduction of activity may be necessary and the wearing of a slightly raised heel or a felt or sorbothane shock-absorbing pad under the heel will also relieve the strain on the tendon. Finally, if symptoms are severe and persistent, a short period of enforced rest in a below-knee plaster may be necessary. In the differential diagnosis, osteomyelitis of the calcaneum and an osteoid osteoma should be considered, particularly in persistent cases, as both can be difficult to diagnose.

KÖHLER'S DISEASE (OSTEOCHONDRITIS OF THE TARSAL NAVICULAR)

This condition was described by Köhler in 1908. The child, commonly between the ages of 3 and 6 years, presents with pain over the medial side of the mid-tarsus. Sometimes there is tenderness and swelling over the tarsal navicular and limping after exercise. In some patients the local signs are so marked that a diagnosis of osteomyelitis or even neoplasm has been considered and the bone biopsied. The biopsy shows avascular necrosis of the bone similar to Perthes' disease of the hip joint. Radiography shows increased density, flattening and fragmentation of the ossific nucleus of the navicular bone (Fig. 7.29). Waugh (1958) made a careful study of the condition and showed that it recovers spontaneously. Cox (1958) was unable to demonstrate any long-term sequelae of this disorder.

Most cases settle satisfactorily with no special treatment, but if necessary a short period in a below-knee plaster may be indicated. The condition must be differentiated from a strain of the insertion of the tibialis posterior tendon onto the tubercle of the navicular. In some patients there is a large accessory navicular

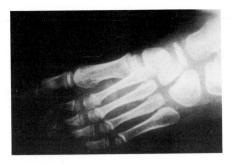

Fig. 7.29 Oblique radiograph of left Köhler's disease. Note the flattening and fragmentation of the navicular bone.

bone which causes pain and problems with shoe wear (Fig. 7.30). In adolescent girls this is sometimes sufficiently troublesome to justify excision of the prominence. Care must be taken not to damage the insertion of the tibialis posterior and to remove sufficient bone when excising the bony prominence.

FREIBERG'S DISEASE OR INFRACTION (KÖHLER'S SECOND DISEASE)

Freiberg (1914) described a condition of the second metatarsal head in which it appeared crushed, as if an infraction had occurred (Fig. 7.31). The aetiology is uncertain. Smillie (1955) and Braddock (1959) suggested that the cause was traumatic. The condition occurs in adolescence and is more common in girls. It can occur in other metatarsal heads and causes pain, local swelling and stiffness of the affected metatarsophalangeal joint.

In the acute stage a below-knee walking plaster may be necessary. For chronic symptoms a metatarsal insole or pad can be used. Sometimes in adult life excision of the damaged metatarsal head may be necessary.

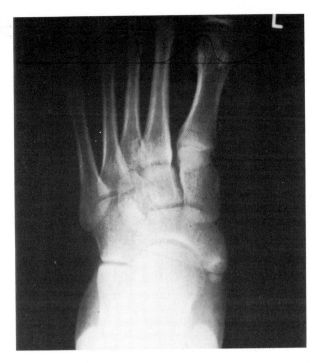

Fig. 7.30 Radiograph showing an accessory navicular bone.

PAIN IN THE HEEL

A number of conditions can cause pain in the heel in children. Calcaneal apophysitis has already been described (p. 196).

Trauma

Trauma to the heel following a fall is common. Often the heel is simply bruised, but fractures of the calcaneum can be easily overlooked unless axial views (Rang, 1974) or computed tomographic scans are taken. In the

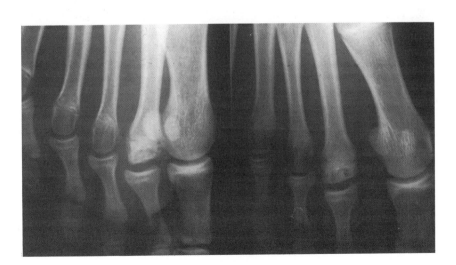

Fig. 7.31 Radiograph of the left foot showing Freiberg's osteochondritis of the second metatarsal head.

young child a foreign body such as a needle or piece of glass may be an unexpected finding on the radiograph.

Infection

Osteomyelitis in the calcaneum may be of the acute (Antoniou and Conner, 1974) or subacute (Harris and Kirlakdy-Willis, 1965) type (see Chapter 15). It is easily mistaken for calcaneal apophysitis until an abscess cavity appears on the radiograph (Fig. 7.32).

Infection in the talus is usually subacute or chronic (Antoniou and Conner, 1974) and is commonly mis-diagnosed as a simple sprain or ligamentous injury in the early stages before radiographic changes appear. Disease of the talus seems to be more common in children under the age of 4 years and should be con-sidered in a child with localized tenderness over the talus and a raised erythrocyte sedimentation rate. Acute infec-tion usually responds to antibiotics, but curettage may be necessary if there is evidence of abscess formation.

Juvenile chronic arthritis

This diagnosis must be considered in a patient with persistent pain and swelling of more than 3 months' duration in the ankle or subtalar region (Fig. 7.33). The knee and ankle are the most common joints affected in the pauciarticular group, and the knees, wrists and ankles in the polyarticular group (Arden and Ansell, 1978). In the spondylitic HLA B27 positive subgroup, calcaneal spurs and erosions of the calcaneum in relation

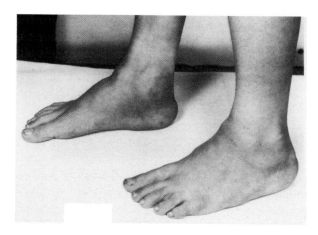

Fig. 7.33 Patient, aged 3 years, with juvenile chronic arthritis affecting the ankle and subtalar joints. Note the marked swelling apparent around the ankle and subtalar joints.

to the insertion of the Achilles tendon are some of the most characteristic early radiographic findings. Early referral to a rheumatologist is advised if this diagnosis is suspected.

NEUROPATHIC FRACTURES

In children with diminished sensation, particularly due to conditions such as spinal dysraphism or peripheral sensory neuropathy, fractures may be relatively pain free. The child presents with marked swelling and red-ness and all the signs of an apparent infection of the foot. However, the typical radiographic appearance of a

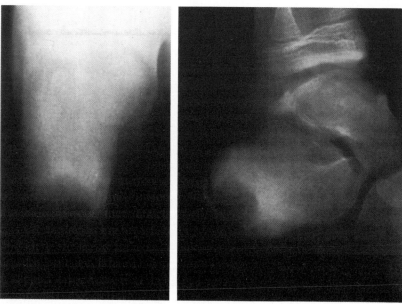

(a)   (b)

Fig. 7.32 (a) Lateral and (b) axial views of the hindfoot showing a large chronic osteomyelitic cavity in the os calcis.

neuropathic fracture with abundant callus can be seen. It is very easy to suspect either bone infection or a tumour in these circumstances (Fig. 7.34).

CURLY AND OVERRIDING TOES

Flexion and medial rotation deformities of the lateral three toes are extremely common (Fig. 7.35). Parents often bring their children to the clinic for advice during the first year of life. The condition is nearly always symptom free, but parents are worried about future problems with walking and footwear. There is often a strong family history. On examination the toe or toes are flexed and medially rotated, but nearly always passively fully correctable.

In the past conservative treatment by 'over and under' strapping was strongly advocated (Trethowan, 1925). However, Sweetnam (1958) in a review of the value of such treatment showed that there was no evidence that strapping or splinting had any long-term effect on the condition. Such treatment was often abandoned by the parents after a trial as being both tedious and ineffective. The majority of cases either improve spontaneously or remain static causing few or no symptoms. In the occasional rare case of a persistent fixed deformity causing troublesome symptoms, flexor to extensor

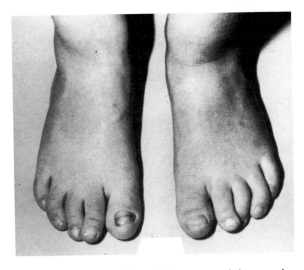

Fig. 7.35 Child with curly lateral three toes and the second toe overlapping the third toe.

tendon transfer can be performed. Simple flexor tendon tenotomy is an attractive alternative. Good results have been reported by Menelaus and Ross (1984) from this day-case procedure. Arthrodesis of the interphalangeal joints can be carried out at maturity if necessary.

Overlapping or dorsal displacement of the second toe is very common (Fig. 7.36). Minor syndactyly with the third toe and hypoplasia of the second toe are also commonly seen. Provided the toe can be passively reduced between the first and third toes and there is no fixed deformity, no treatment is necessary. Usually when weight-bearing commences the toes spread apart and the dorsal displacement is reduced. Major degrees of syndactyly occasionally warrant plastic surgery. Very occasionally a fixed deformity may require surgical correction.

Overriding or overlapping of the fifth toe is also common, but represents a definite fixed congenital deformity which does not correct with time (Fig. 7.37). The toe is usually hypoplastic. It is medially deviated and lies above and overlapping the fourth toe. Conservative measures of strapping and splinting will not correct this deformity. Some patients manage perfectly satisfactorily with the uncorrected deformity and no symptoms. However, those who have troubles with footwear and pressure over the deformed toe require operative correction. Butler's operation, described by Cockin (1968), and VY-plasty (Wilson, 1953) can both give good results but must be performed carefully with attention to detail, otherwise the deformity recurs to the dissatisfaction of both the patient and the surgeon. In such cases amputation remains the only satisfactory solution to the problem.

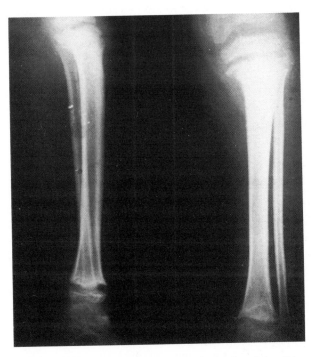

Fig. 7.34 Anteroposterior and lateral radiographs of the tibia showing neuropathic epiphyseal slips at both upper and lower ends in a child with meningomyelocoele and loss of pain sensation.

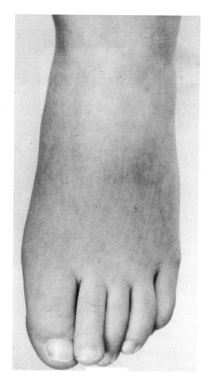

Fig. 7.36 Overlapping second toe.

HALLUX VALGUS AND HALLUX RIGIDUS

Hallux valgus

Hallux valgus occurs in children and adolescents as well as in adults (see Fig. 7.4, p. 181). In the past poorly fitting footwear was blamed for the development of this deformity. However, the condition seen in children is commonly inherited and a strong family history can usually be elicited. It is normally associated with a varus

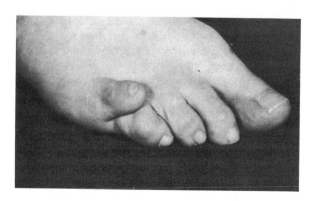

Fig. 7.37 Overriding fifth toe.

deformity of the first metatarsal (metatarsus primus varus). There has been considerable debate in the past as to which is the primary deformity. Probably both conditions develop simultaneously (Hardy and Clapham, 1951). It is often associated with valgus everted or pronated feet, particularly in children with cerebral palsy.

Symptoms are rare in childhood but increase, particularly in girls, when fashionable shoes start to be worn in adolescence. On account of the strong family history the child is often first examined when symptom-free because the parents are worried because he or, much more commonly, she may develop a severe deformity and symptoms in adult life like the older members of the family. Splints, insoles and exercises have no effect on the deformity (Cholmeley, 1958). Specialized surgical shoes are not usually necessary in children unless the deformity is associated with other disabilities, e.g. cerebral palsy or spina bifida. Operative correction should not be considered, if possible, before the age of 12 or 13 years.

The radiological classification described by Piggott (1960) is most useful in differentiating which feet are likely to progress and develop increasing problems with age. Piggott showed that the normal valgus inclination of the first metatarsophalangeal joint is 0–20°. From 20–25° if the joint was still congruous the toe was considered to be 'deviated'. In this situation the deformity may or may not progress with age and should simply be watched. If, however, the deformity was over 25° and the joint was already subluxing then progression and increasing symptoms would almost certainly occur. Operative correction was indicated in these patients. In children and adolescents operative treatment is seldom indicated, particularly in the former. The subject is further discussed in Chapter 26.

Hallux rigidus

Hallux rigidus is rare in children. The child presents with pain over the big toe on walking and often cannot run. The condition is more common in girls than in boys, unlike the adult form which is much more common in men.

On examination there is local tenderness over the first metatarsophalangeal joint and marked limitation and discomfort on dorsiflexion of the big toe. Often there is a history of injury to the toe, such as stubbing the toe or the toe being squashed by a heavy object. Changes compatible with osteochondritis dissecans are commonly seen on the radiograph if looked for carefully (Goodfellow, 1966). Taken together with the common history of injury or repeated minor trauma, these may well represent an osteochondral fracture.

Treatment with a metatarsal bar or rocker may allow the condition to settle satisfactorily. A short period in a below-knee plaster may be necessary. If conservative treatment fails, an operation will have to be considered. In adolescence, dorsal wedge osteotomy of the proximal phalanx (Bonney and McNab, 1952) gives good results. This operation should only be done if there is still 30° of plantar flexion at the first metatarsophalangeal joint and radiographic changes are minimal. Arthrodesis or a Keller's procedure should only be considered after growth is finished.

STRESS FRACTURES

The typical 'march' fracture of the second and third metatarsals is seldom seen in children. However, in uncorrected talipes equinovarus of whatever cause, stress fractures of the fourth or fifth metatarsal can occur because excessive weight is taken on the outer border of the foot. The child presents with pain, limp and deterioration in walking and the position of the foot. There is local tenderness over the shaft of the fourth or fifth metatarsal. Radiographs will often show the fracture or at least periosteal new bone at the site of the fracture.

TUMOURS

Tumours in the foot in children are rare. They can arise from any tissue in the foot, and usually present with persistent pain and swelling. A definitive diagnosis is made by biopsy. Osteoid osteomas can be particularly difficult to diagnose, and a bone scan is very useful in establishing this diagnosis.

REFERENCES

Antoniou D. and Conner A.N. (1974) Osteomyelitis of the calcaneus and talus. *J. Bone Joint Surg.* **56A**, 338–345.

Arden G.P. and Ansell B.M. (1978) *Surgical Management of Juvenile Chronic Polyarthritis.* London, Academic Press, New York, Grune and Stratton.

Attenborough C.G. (1966) Severe congenital talipes equinovarus. *J. Bone Joint Surg.* **48B**, 31–39.

Bankart A.S.B. (1921) Metatarsus varus. *BMJ* **2**, 685.

Basmajian J.V. and Stecko G. (1963) The role of the muscles in arch support of the foot. *J. Bone Joint Surg.* **48B**, 660–665.

Berman A. and Gartland J.J. (1971) Metatarsal osteotomy for the correction of adduction of the fore-part of the foot in children. *J. Bone Joint Surg. Am.* **53A**, 498–505.

Bleck E.E. (1983) Metatarsus adductus. Classification and relationship to outcomes of treatment. *J. Pediatr. Orthop.* **3**, 2–9.

Bonney G. and McNab I. (1952) Hallux valgus and hallux rigidus—critical survey of operative results. *J. Bone Joint Surg.* **34B**, 366–386.

Braddock G.T.F. (1959) Experimental epiphysial injury and Freiberg's disease. *J. Bone Joint Surg.* **41**, 154.

Brewerton D.A., Sandifer P.H. and Sweetnam D.R. (1963) The aetiology of pes cavus. *BMJ* **2**, 659–661.

Browne D. (1955) Congenital deformities of mechanical origin. *Arch. Dis. Child.* **30**, 37.

Browne R.S. and Paton D.F. (1979) Anomalous insertion of the tibialis posterior tendon in congenital metatarsus varus. *J. Bone Joint Surg.* **61B**, 74–76.

Cholmeley J.A. (1953) Elmslie's operation for the calcaneus foot. *J. Bone Joint Surg.* **35B**, 46–49.

Cholmeley J.A. (1958) Hallux valgus in adolescence. *Proc. R. Soc. Med.* **51**, 903–906.

Clark J.M.P. (1968) Early detection and management of the unreduced club foot. *Proc. R. Soc. Med.* **61**, 779–782.

Cockin J. (1968) Butler's operation for an over riding fifth toe. *J. Bone Joint Surg.* **50B**, 78–81.

Coleman S.S. (1983) *Complex Foot Deformities in Children.* Philadelphia, Lea and Febiger.

Colton C.L. (1973) The surgical management of congenital vertical talus. *J. Bone Joint Surg.* **55B**, 566–574.

Cox M.J. (1958) Köhler's disease. *Postgrad. Med. J.* **34**, 588–591.

Davis L.A. and Hatt W.S. (1955) Congenital abnormalities of the foot. *Radiology* **64**, 818–825.

Duckworth T. and Smith T.W.D. (1974) The treatment of paralytic convex pes valgus. *J. Bone Joint Surg.* **56B**, 305–313.

Dwyer F.C. (1963) Osteotomy of the calcaneum for pes cavus. *J. Bone Joint Surg.* **45B**, 67–75.

Evans D. (1961) Relapsed club foot. *J. Bone Joint Surg.* **43B**, 722–733.

Eyre-Brook A.L. (1967) Congenital vertical talus. *J. Bone Joint Surg.* **49B**, 618–627.

Freiberg A.H. (1914) Infraction of the second metatarsal bone. *Surg. Gynecol. Obstet.* **19**, 191.

Fripp A.T. and Shaw N.E. (1967) *Club Foot.* Edinburgh and London, Earl and Livingstone.

Ghali N.N., Smith R.B., Clayden A.D. and Silk F.F. (1983) Results of pantalar reduction in the management of congenital talipes equinovarus. *J. Bone Joint Surg.* **65B**, 1–7.

Giannestras M.J. (1973) *Foot Disorders. Medical and Surgical Management*, 2nd edn. London, Henry Kimpton.

Goodfellow J. (1966) Aetiology of hallux rigidus. *Proc. R. Soc. Med.* **59**, 821–824.

Green A.D.L. and Lloyd-Roberts G.C. (1985) Results of early posterior release in resistant club foot. A long term review. *J. Bone Joint Surg.* **67B**, 588–593.

Grice D.S. (1952) An extra-articular arthrodesis of the subastragular joint for correction of paralytic flat feet in children. *J. Bone Joint Surg.* **34A**, 927–940.

Harding A.E. and Thomas P.K. (1980) The clinical features of hereditary motor and sensory neuropathy types I and II. *Brain* **103**, 259–280.

Hardy R.H. and Clapham J.C.R. (1951) Observations on hallux valgus. *J. Bone Joint Surg.* **33B**, 376–391.

Harris R.I. and Beath T. (1948) Aetiology of peroneal spastic flat foot. *J. Bone Joint Surg.* **30B**, 624–634.

Harris N.H. and Kirkaldy-Willis W.H. (1965) Primary subacute pyogenic osteomyelitis. *J. Bone Joint Surg.* **47B**, 526.

Harrold A.J. (1967) Congenital vertical talus in infancy. *J. Bone Joint Surg.* **49B**, 634–643.

Harrold A.J. and Walker C.J. (1983) Treatment and prognosis in congenital club foot. *J. Bone Joint Surg.* **65B**, 8–11.

Heyman C.H., Herndon C.H. and Strong J.M. (1958) Mobilization of the tarso-metatarsal joints for the correction of resistant adduction of the fore-part of the foot in congenital club foot or congenital metatarsus varus. *J. Bone Joint Surg.* **40A**, 299–310.

Hutchins P.M., Foster B.K., Paterson B.T. and Cole E.A. (1985) Long term results of early surgical release in club foot. *J. Bone Joint Surg.* **67B**, 791–799.

Ippolito E. and Ponseti I.V. (1980) Congenital club foot in the human foetus. *J. Bone Joint Surg.* **62A**, 8–22.

Isaacs H., Handelsman J.E., Badenhost M. *et al.* (1977) The muscles in club foot. A histological, histoclinical and electron microscopic study. *J. Bone Joint Surg.* **59B**, 465–472.

Jack E.A. (1953) Naviculo-cuneiform fusion in the treatment of flat foot. *J. Bone Joint Surg.* **35B**, 75–82.

Japas L.M. (1968) Surgical treatment of pes cavus by tarsal 'V' osteotomy. *J. Bone Joint Surg.* **50A**, 927–944.

Kite J.H. (1967) Congenital metatarsus varus. *J. Bone Joint Surg.* **49A**, 388.

Köhler A. (1908) Über eine häufige bisher anscheinend und bekannte Erkrankung einzelner kindlicher Knochen. München. *Munch. Med. Wochenschr.* **55**, 1923.

Laaveg S.J. and Ponseti I.V. (1980) Long term results of treatment of congenital club foot. *J. Bone Joint Surg.* **62A**, 23–81.

Leonard M.A. (1974) The inheritance of tarsal coalition and its relationship to spastic flat foot. *J. Bone Joint Surg.* **56B**, 520–526.

Lloyd-Roberts G.C. and Clark R.C. (1973) Ball and socket ankle joint in metatarsus adductus varus. *J. Bone Joint Surg.* **55B**, 193–196.

Lloyd-Roberts G.C. and Pilcher M.F. (1965) Structural idiopathic scoliosis in infancy. *J. Bone Joint Surg.* **47B**, 520–523.

Lloyd-Roberts G.C. and Spence A.J. (1958) Congenital vertical talus. *J. Bone Joint Surg.* **40B**, 33–41.

Lloyd-Roberts G.C., Swann M. and Catterall A. (1974) Medial rotation osteotomy for severe residual deformity in club foot. *J. Bone Joint Surg.* **56B**, 37–43.

Lowe L.W. and Hannon M.A. (1973) Residual adduction of the forefoot in treated congenital club foot. *J. Bone Joint Surg.* **55B**, 809–813.

Menelaus M.B. (1971) Talectomy for equinovarus deformity in arthrogryposis and spina bifida. *J. Bone Joint Surg.* **53B**, 468–473.

Menelaus M.B. and Ross E.R.S. (1984) Open flexor tenotomy for hammer toes and curly toes in childhood. *J. Bone Joint Surg.* **66B**, 770–771.

Mitchell G.P. (1977) Posterior displacement osteotomy of the calcaneus. *J. Bone Joint Surg.* **59B**, 233–235.

Morley A.J.M. (1957) Knock-knee in children. *B.M.J.* **2**, 976–979.

Osmond-Clark H. (1956) Congenital vertical talus. *J. Bone Joint Surg.* **38B**, 334–341.

Piggott H. (1960) Natural history of hallux valgus in adolescence and early adult life. *J. Bone Joint Surg.* **42B**, 749–760.

Ponseti I.V. and Becker J.R. (1966) Congenital metatarsus adductus. *J. Bone Joint Surg.* **48A**, 702–711.

Rang M. (1974) *Children's Fractures*. Philadelphia and Toronto, J.B. Lippincott.

Robertson D.E. (1967) Primary acute and subacute localized osteomyelitis and osteochondritis in children. *Can. J. Surg.* **10**, 408–413.

Rose G.K. (1962) Correction of the pronated foot. *J. Bone Joint Surg.* **44B**, 642–647.

Rose G.K., Welton C.A. and Marshall T. (1986) The diagnosis of flat foot in the child. *J. Bone Joint Surg.* **67B**, 71–78.

Rushforth G.F. (1978) The natural history of hooked forefoot. *J. Bone Joint Surg.* **60B**, 530–532.

Scott W.A., Hosking S.W. and Catterall A. (1984) Club foot. *J. Bone Joint Surg.* **66B**, 71–76.

Sever J.W. (1912) Apophysitis of the oscalcis. *N. Y. Med. J.* **95**, 1025.

Silk F.F. and Wainwright D. (1967) The recognition and treatment of congenital flat foot in infancy. *J. Bone Joint Surg.* **49B**, 628–633.

Simons G.W. (1985) Complete subtalar release in club feet part 1 and 2. *J. Bone Joint Surg.* **67A**, 1044–1055, 1056–1065.

Smillie I.S. (1955) Freiberg's infraction (Köhler's second disease). *J. Bone Joint Surg.* **37**, 580.

Steindler A. (1920) Stripping of the os calcis. *J. Orthop. Surg.* **2**, 8.

Stark K.G., Johansen J.E. and Winter R.B. (1987) The Heyman Herndon tarso-metatarsal capsulotomy for metatarsus adductus. Results in 48 feet. *J. Pediatr Orthop.* **7**, 305–310.

Stone K.H. (1963) Congenital vertical talus. A new operation. *Proc. R. Soc. Med.* **56**, 12.

Swann M., Lloyd-Roberts G.C. and Catterall A. (1969) The anatomy of the uncorrected club foot. *J. Bone Joint Surg.* **51B**, 263–269.

Sweetnam D.R. (1958) Congenital curly toes, an investigation into the value of treatment. *Lancet* **ii**, 398–400.

Taylor R.G. (1951) The treatment of claw toes by multiple transfers of flexor into extensor tendons. *J. Bone Joint Surg.* **35B**, 539–542.

Trethowan W.H. (1925) The treatment of hammer toe. *Lancet* **i**, 1257–1258.

Turco V.J. (1971) Surgical correction of the resistant club foot. *J. Bone Joint Surg.* **53A**, 477–497.

Turco V.J. (1979) Resistant congenital club foot—one stage postero-medial release with internal fixation. *J. Bone Joint Surg.* **61A**, 805–814.

Waugh W. (1958) The ossification and vascularisation of the tarsal navicular and their relation to Köhler's disease. *J. Bone Joint Surg.* **40B**, 765–777.

Wenger D.R., Maudlin D., Speck G., Morgan D. and Lieber R.L. (1989) Corrective shoes and inserts as treatment for flexible flat foot in infants and children. *J. Bone Joint Surg.* **71A**, 800–810.

Wilson N.N. (1953) VY correction for varus deformity of the fifth toe. *Br. J. Surg.* **41**, 133–135.

Wynne-Davies R. (1964) Family studies and the cause of congenital club foot. *J. Bone Joint Surg.* **46B**, 445–463.

Wynne-Davies R. (1973) *Inheritable Disorders in Orthopaedic Practice*. Oxford, Blackwell Scientific Publications.

Chapter 8
Other Developmental Abnormalities

Chapter 8.1
The Upper Limb

J.A. Fixsen

INTRODUCTION

The effects of congenital abnormalities are cosmetic and functional. In the upper limb appearance can seldom be improved and the surgeon should concentrate on function. Reconstructive procedures demand a good deal of cooperation from the patient, and most children under 5 years old cannot cope. Any operation that requires post-operative rehabilitation should be postponed until after that age. Of course a child's intellectual and emotional development depends on his ability to perceive and to manipulate. Operative procedures that do not require post-operative rehabilitation should be undertaken as soon as possible for this reason. Beware the apparently functionless appendage in a neonate. Pressure to remove it (from the child's parents) is often great, but unless it is just a tag it should be preserved for it may become useful later.

CONGENITAL ELEVATION OF THE SHOULDER (SPRENGEL'S SHOULDER)

The arm bud appears in the third week of intrauterine life at the level of the fifth cervical to the first thoracic vertebra. The scapula develops within the arm bud in the fifth week of intrauterine life. Over the next 3 months it descends to its normal position level with the second to the seventh thoracic vertebrae. Failure of this descent gives rise to congenital elevation of the scapula, so-called Sprengel's deformity (1891). The condition is occasionally familial, in which case the inheritance is dominant. It is often associated with other congenital abnormalities in the neighbouring tissues.

Clinically, the scapula lies at a higher level than normal and it is smaller than normal. The superior angle is rotated upwards and forwards (Fig. 8.1.1). It may be joined to the cervical spine by a fibrous or bony omovertebral bar. This bar arises from the superior angle or

the medial third of the upper border of the scapula and attaches to the spinous process, the lamina or the transverse process of the cervical vertebrae in the region from the fourth to the seventh cervical vertebrae. The attachment to the scapula may be by bone, cartilage, fibrous tissue, or even a true joint. The surrounding shoulder girdle musculature is commonly defective. In particular the trapezius muscle may be weak or even absent. The rhomboids and levator scapulae may be hypoplastic. The serratus anterior muscle can be weak and the pectorals, latissimus dorsi and sternocleidomastoid muscles may also be affected.

Associated abnormalities are common: ribs may be fused or absent; cervical ribs may be present. There may be associated brevicollis (Klippel–Feil syndrome).

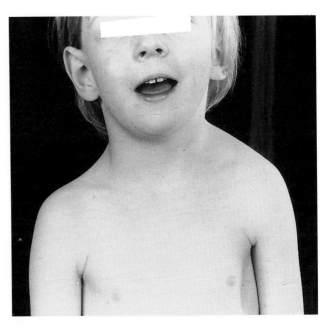

Fig. 8.1.1 Congenital elevation of the left shoulder (Sprengel's shoulder).

Vertebral anomalies, e.g. scoliosis, hemivertebrae and spina bifida occulta, can occur in the cervical and upper thoracic spine. In the arm the humerus may be short. The clavicle may be hypoplastic and sometimes it fails to articulate with the acromion. In a number of cases thenar hypoplasia has been recorded.

In unilateral cases the asymmetry of the shoulders usually becomes obvious soon after birth, though it may not be recognized until after the child starts to stand. In bilateral cases the neck appears abnormally short and the shoulders hunched. Both sexes are equally affected, but the condition is more common on the left side than the right. The neck looks fatter and shorter on the affected side. Abduction and external rotation of the arm are limited on the affected side; this limitation is due to loss of scapulothoracic rather than scapulo-humeral movement. This gives rise to some functional impairment in the arm as well as the cosmetic deformity.

An anteroposterior radiograph showing both shoulders is helpful in confirming the diagnosis (Fig. 8.1.2). Further radiographs of the chest and cervical spine are import-ant to show up the commonly associated rib and spinal anomalies. Oblique and lateral views of the scapula may demonstrate an omovertebral bar.

Treatment

Exercise may be helpful to encourage full use of the arm and shoulder, but it will not restore scapulothoracic movement to normal. Various operative procedures have been described to try and pull the scapula down to its normal position. Green (1957) described the procedure in which the muscles connecting the scapula to the trunk are divided at their scapular insertion. The omovertebral bar, if it is present, is removed. The supraspinous portion of the scapula is excised extraperiosteally. The scapula is displaced distally and held in position for 3 weeks by a traction wire to an external plaster spica. Woodward (1961) described a procedure in which instead of dividing the scapular muscles at their insertion on the scapula, they were divided from the spinous processes to allow depression of the scapula. These and other similar procedures involve extensive dissection, and they can produce large and often ugly scars. There is a small but definite incidence of damage to the brachial plexus if the scapula is pulled down too forcefully. Cosmetically the simplest operation is to excise the prominent angle of the scapula extraperiosteally and the omovertebral bar if it is present.

Campbell and Wilkinson (1979) described a vertical osteotomy of the scapula 2 cm from its medial border. This is combined with excision of the omovertebral bar, the superior angle of the scapula and any fibrous tether-ing bands. The lateral portion of the scapula is then displaced caudally improving both the range of abduction at the shoulder and the cosmetic appearance. Even this operation, which is less extensive than those of Green (1957) and Woodward (1961), was associated with one minor brachial plexus palsy, which fortunately re-covered, and slight winging of the scapula in another patient in a small series of 11 patients. In all these operations, particular care should be taken with the skin

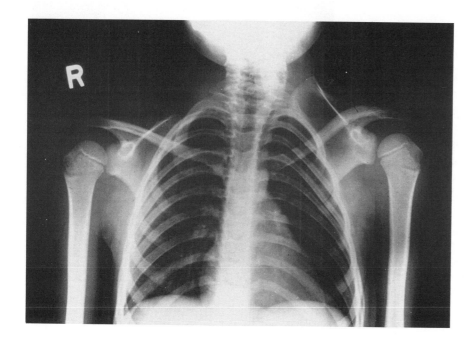

Fig. 8.1.2 Anteroposterior radiograph of a left Sprengel's shoulder. Note the elevation of the superior angle of the scapula and the rib anomalies.

to avoid hypertropic scarring, which is very common in this region.

CONGENITAL PSEUDARTHROSIS OF THE CLAVICLE

This is a rare condition. The child usually presents at or soon after birth with a painless swelling over the middle third of the clavicle (Fig. 8.1.3). Radiographs show established pseudarthrosis with the bulbous lateral end of the sternal half of the clavicle overlying the tapering medial end of the acromial half (Fig. 8.1.4). The lesion is nearly always on the right side. Congenital pseudarthrosis must be distinguished from a birth fracture of the clavicle, in which there is usually a history of traumatic delivery and early callus formation is seen on the radiograph. The other condition to be considered is cleidocranial dysostosis, in which both clavicles are

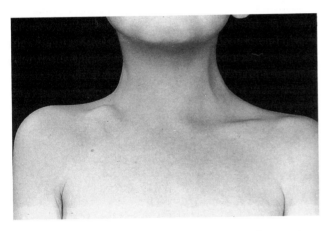

Fig. 8.1.3 Pseudarthrosis of the right clavicle. Note the prominent lump over the mid-clavicle.

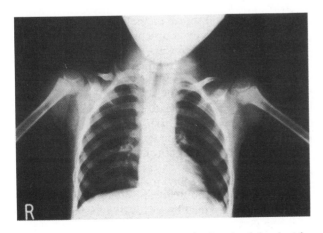

Fig. 8.1.4 Radiograph of a right pseudarthrosis of the clavicle.

deficient or absent and there are associated bony abnormalities in the skull, pelvis and facial bones.

It is now accepted that the clavicle develops in cartilage and not in membrane, as was previously thought. There is argument, however, as to whether there are one or two ossification centres. Alldred (1963) suggested that pseudarthrosis of the clavicle arose from failure of the two centres of ossification (Fawcett, 1913) to fuse. Lloyd-Roberts *et al.* (1975) made some interesting observations. They related the predominant right-sidedness of the lesion to the anatomical finding that the right subclavian artery normally lies higher than the left. They pointed out that one of the very few left-sided cases of pseudarthrosis (Gibson and Carroll, 1970) also had dextrocardia and an abnormally high left subclavian artery. Furthermore, they noted that a significantly large proportion of their patients had abnormally elevated first ribs or cervical ribs. They therefore proposed that pressure from the subclavian artery, accentuated by an abnormally high first rib or a cervical rib, produces the pseudarthrosis. They also observed that bilateral cases have a strong family history or are associated with cleidocranial dysostosis, in which abnormal elevation of the upper ribs on both sides is characteristic.

The pseudarthrosis does not unite spontaneously. Function is good but the prominent lump is unsightly. The condition responds well to excision of the pseudarthrosis and bone grafting, using either a block of iliac bone or rib to bridge the gap and internal fixation usually with a threaded pin. It is suggested that this operation is best done between the ages of 2 and 4 years (Alldred, 1963). Over the age of 8 years fusion is less certain. The alternative to bone grafting is simply to excise the prominent lateral end of the sternal half of the clavicle.

CONGENITAL CORACOCLAVICULAR BAR

Shoulder pain and stiffness may lead to the discovery of a bar of bone between the coracoid process and the clavicle. The bar may be incomplete; it lies within the substance of the conoid and trapezoid coracoclavicular ligaments. The pain is probably due to impingement of the anterior edge of the supraspinatus muscle on the bony bar. The stiffness is due to tethering of the scapula.

Symptoms can be lessened by removal of the bar. This is most easily achieved via an anterior parasagittal incision. Enough of the bar should be removed to ensure full coracoclavicular movement and decompression of the supraspinatus. The coracoclavicular ligament complex should not be removed completely; this leads to accelerated degeneration of the acromioclavicular joint.

HUMERUS VARUS

Some babies are found to have limited abduction of one shoulder, and radiography reveals a varus deformity of the humeral head. The aetiology of this disorder is not known, but malunion of a fracture seems likely. The limitation of movement is not usually severe, and no treatment is indicated. Where movement is less than 90°, however, corrective osteotomy helps. The operation should be delayed until the child is over 5 years old. The upper humerus is approached through a skin cleavage incision anteriorly. The anterior edge of the deltoid muscle is pushed laterally and the long head of the biceps medially. The humerus is divided below the surgical neck and a laterally based wedge is excised from the distal fragment. The osteotomy is fixed with a four-hole plate, guarding the proximal humeral growth plate (Fig. 8.1.5). The arm should be protected with a triangular sling until union is established (Lucas and Gill, 1947).

CONGENITAL RETROVERSION OF THE HUMERAL HEAD

Recurrent instability of the shoulder in a child may be due to congenital retroversion of the humeral head. This condition is often bilateral. The child complains of catching and locking of the shoulder. Examination reveals recurrent posterior dislocation; the humeral head jumps out posteriorly in internal rotation and flexion. Reduction is usually easily achieved by the child. Symptoms may be lessened by rotation osteotomy of the

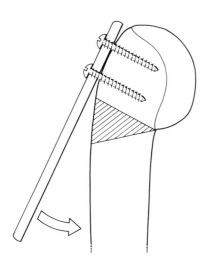

Fig. 8.1.5 Correction of humerus varus.

humerus, reducing the humeral head retroversion by about 30°. The operation is most easily performed through the anterior approach employed for humerus varus. The humerus is divided below the surgical neck, the lower fragment rotated internally about 30° and the osteotomy fixed with a four-hole plate.

ABDUCTION CONTRACTURE OF THE DELTOID MUSCLE

Children with an inability to fully adduct the arm are seen on occasion. The arm stands out from the side like a scarecrow's. Attempts to adduct the arm simply depress the scapula. A taut band of fibrous tissue is palpable in the substance of the acromial part of the deltoid muscle. The aetiology is obscure, but some cases are thought to be due to fibrosis following injection into the deltoid muscle (Grove and Goldner, 1974). Some may be due to congenital abnormalities of the muscle, for this condition may be seen in a bilaterally symmetrical form, sometimes in association with similar contractures in the abductors of the hips.

Whatever the cause, the condition is amenable to operative excision of the fibrous band. The operation should be done as soon as the contracture interferes with function, for delay may lead to irreversible contracture of the shoulder. Through a skin cleavage-line incision the fibrous band in the muscle is excised. The defect should be closed with a few absorbable sutures and the shoulder protected for about 10 days with a sling.

CONGENITAL DISLOCATION OF THE SHOULDER

Stiffness of the shoulder in an infant may be due to dislocation. It is diagnosed when the child fails to move the arm. The condition is usually associated with a difficult delivery. There may be a complicating fracture of the clavicle or the humerus, or even a brachial plexus palsy. Diagnosis rests on the interpretation of the radiograph, and this is not straightforward. The small size of the ossific nuclei near the shoulder may make all but the most severely displaced dislocations difficult to identify. If there is any doubt the other (normally mobile) shoulder should be radiographed in the same projection.

Uncomplicated dislocations in the neonate may be reduced by very gentle manipulation, under anaesthetic if necessary. Should this fail, or should complications make manipulation impossible, then an open reduction should be done.

Through an anterior cleavage-line incision the

shoulder is approached between the deltoid and pectoralis major muscles. The subscapularis muscle is divided taking care to anchor the medial stump with a marking suture. The capsule is opened and the dislocated joint exposed. The glenoid cavity is cleared of adherent capsule and the dislocation reduced. The subscapularis muscle is repaired after assessing the stability of the reduction. It may not be possible to suture the muscle end-to-end after a posterior dislocation, in which case the medial stump should be sutured to the tough perichondrium over the humeral head. Conversely, the subscapularis muscle may be very slack after reduction of an anterior dislocation, in which case the muscle should be sutured with overlapping to accommodate the slackness. The limb is immobilized with a sling and a thoracic bandage for about 10 days and then gentle active mobilization is allowed.

Associated fractures heal rapidly and remodelling neutralizes most deformity. Brachial plexus palsies need no urgent treatment and are dealt with later, depending on their severity.

CONGENITAL SYNOSTOSIS OF THE CERVICAL VERTEBRAE/BREVICOLLIS (KLIPPEL–FEIL SYNDROME)

In 1912 Klippel and Feil described this syndrome and the classical triad of short neck, low posterior hairline and limitation of neck movement (Figs 8.1.6, 8.1.7 and 8.1.8). By no means all patients show all the features of this triad (Gray *et al.*, 1964). Perhaps the most common finding is limitation of movement, particularly lateral movement of the neck.

The anomaly is due to a failure of normal segmentation of the mesodermal somites of the neck during the third to eighth week of fetal life. It is not surprising, therefore, that it is commonly associated with Sprengel's shoulder, which develops at the same time. Scoliosis occurs in 60% of cases and the bony anomalies often involve the upper thoracic spine and ribs. Associated non-bony defects are important. Hensinger *et al.* (1974) pointed out the importance of screening these patients for genitourinary anomaly, hearing loss, neurological problems and cardiopulmonary defects. The management of these disorders is often more important than the orthopaedic problem. The genetics of the condition have not been fully worked out, but some families show a dominant inheritance (Wynne-Davies, 1973).

Clinically, the patient will usually show limitation of neck movements, particularly laterally. In severely affected cases the head seems to rise directly from the shoulders and the posterior hairline is on a level with the

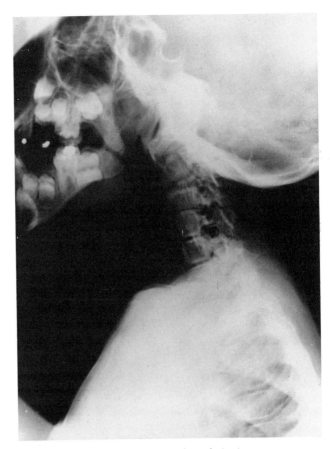

Fig. 8.1.6 Klippel–Feil syndrome (lateral view).

shoulders. Facial asymmetry and torticollis either due to the bony anomaly or a tight sternocleidomastoid muscle are common. Webbing of the neck from the mastoid to the acromion process also occurs. Scoliosis and kyphosis must be looked for. Assessment of the urinary tract, cardiopulmonary function, hearing and nervous systems should also be considered. Accurate radiological diagnosis is often difficult due to the neck being obscured by the shoulders, mandible and occiput. Lateral tomography in flexion and extension and computed tomography may be necessary to fully elucidate the extent of the spinal fusion. Apart from fusion of vertebral bodies, hemivertebrae, flattening and widening of the vertebral bodies, hypoplasia of the discs and cervical spina bifida are often present. It should be remembered that these anomalies often extend into the upper thoracic spine and are associated with scoliosis or kyphosis. When evaluating the spinal deformity radiographs of the whole spine should be taken and not just of the obviously affected area, otherwise defects below this area will be missed.

There is little that can be offered in the way of treatment for the neck deformity. Physiotherapy is unlikely

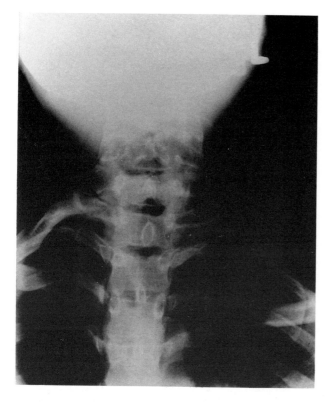

Fig. 8.1.7 Klippel—Feil syndrome (anteroposterior view).

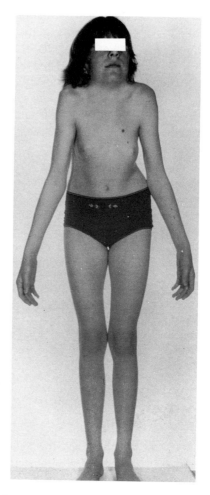

Fig. 8.1.8 Severe Klippel—Feil syndrome. Note elevation of both shoulders and the 'no neck' appearance.

to increase the range of movement significantly. If there is a definite tight sternocleidomastoid muscle it may be worthwhile releasing this, but full correction is often prevented by the bony anomaly. Similarly, if the webbing is severe plastic surgery can reduce this. If there is an associated Sprengel's shoulder, treatment of this deformity will help cosmetically, but is unlikely to improve the range of movement at the neck. It is doubtful whether cervicalization of the upper thoracic segment by bilateral resection of the first four ribs (Bonola, 1956) is justifiable, in view of the magnitude of the surgery and the possible complications to the brachial plexus, for what is a cosmetic deformity. The associated scoliosis often requires bracing and surgery. Traction, particularly use of the halopelvic apparatus, should be approached with caution as the cervical spine in this condition is more susceptible to neurological and vascular damage. Genitourinary problems can be severe and Klippel and Feil's original patient died of renal failure. Stark and Borton (1973), in their review of hearing loss in this condition, stressed the importance of this problem and its deleterious effect on the development of speech and language. Finally, the interesting condition of synkinesia or 'mirror motion' (Bauman, 1932) should be noted. In this condition the patient makes involuntary paired movements of the hands, i.e. the patient is unable to move one hand without making a reciprocal movement in the opposite hand. This is said to be due to inadequate or incomplete decussation of the pyramidal tracts and a dysraphic cervical cord.

STERNOCLEIDOMASTOID TORTICOLLIS
(see also p. 209)

Torticollis means 'twisted neck' or 'wry neck'. In childhood it may present at or shortly after birth as a transient postural torticollis which corrects spontaneously or with a minimum of physiotherapy (Hulbert, 1950). It may be associated with a sternocleidomastoid tumour, which is commonly noticed in the first 4 weeks of life or, finally, it may present as a contracture of the sternocleidomastoid muscle — muscular torticollis — at any age from 3—6 months up to adolescence.

There has been considerable discussion about the

cause of this condition. Pathologically, a sternocleidomastoid tumour consists of dense fibrous tissue with no evidence of haemorrhage or haemosiderin in the muscle. In muscular torticollis the sternocleidomastoid muscle shows marked fibrosis with the contracture commonly affecting the clavicular head of the muscle.

There is a high incidence of torticollis in breech presentations, forceps deliveries and in first-born children (MacDonald, 1969). The condition is also much more common on the right side. It is often associated with ipsilateral mandibular asymmetry, facial asymmetry, plagiocephaly, postural scoliosis and congenital hip and foot deformities. Dunn (1973), in a study of over 20 000 newborn infants, confirmed these findings and postulated an intrauterine postural deformity due to persistent acute lateral flexion with rotation of the neck in intrauterine life, causing venous occlusion and ischaemia of the muscle. This supports previous work by Brooks (1922) and Middleton (1930).

The patient presents with the head tilted to the affected side and the chin rotated towards the opposite side (Fig. 8.1.9). Rotation towards the affected side and lateral flexion away from it are limited but not painful. In the newborn it is important to look for other signs of moulding deformity, namely plagiocephaly, facial asymmetry, postural scoliosis, limitation of abduction at the hip and foot deformities. A sternocleidomastoid tumour may be palpable in the first 3 months of life but

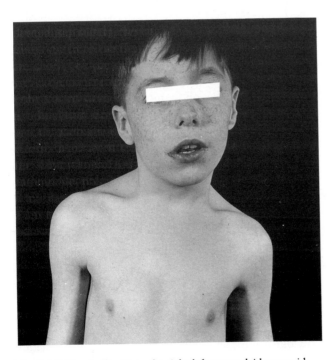

Fig. 8.1.9 Torticollis. Note the tight left sternocleidomastoid muscle causing elevation of the right shoulder.

then resolves. In older patients the sternocleidomastoid muscle on the affected side is visible and palpable as a tight cord. Facial asymmetry and postural scoliosis are commonly present. In fact, the patient may be referred as a problem of scoliosis and not torticollis at all.

There are several important conditions to consider in the differential diagnosis. A radiograph of the cervical and upper thoracic spine is mandatory in these patients. Skeletal anomalies, e.g. hemivertebrae or brevicollis (Klippel−Feil syndrome), must be excluded. Trauma causing subluxation or dislocation of the cervical spine must be considered. Inflammatory conditions of the spine, e.g. tuberculosis, and of the cervical soft tissues, e.g. cervical adenitis, should be excluded. Hyperaemia following soft tissue inflammation may cause hypermobility of the upper cervical vertebrae giving rise to torticollis and a subluxation of the vertebrae, which can be very worrying. It is important when interpreting radiographs of the cervical spine in young children to be aware of the range of normal variations (Cattell and Filtzer, 1965). Ophthalmic disorders, spinal tumours and occasionally psychiatric causes can also give rise to torticollis.

Treatment

Transient postural torticollis of the newborn usually corrects spontaneously. Torticollis in conjunction with a sternocleidomastoid tumour will usually respond to passive stretching which is taught to the parents by the physiotherapist. In muscular torticollis in older children, a trial of passive stretching may be worthwhile but often an operation is necessary.

Subcutaneous tenotomy of the lower end of the contracted sternocleidomastoid muscle has been practised since Roman times (Hulbert, 1950). However, most surgeons prefer open division in view of the risk of damage to the vital structures that lie beneath the muscle during a closed operation. Division of the muscle can be performed at its lower or upper end or occasionally, in very severe cases in older patients, at both ends. It is seldom necessary to excise the contracted portion of the muscle or the sternocleidomastoid tumour. Most surgeons prefer to divide the muscle at its lower end through a skin-crease incision just above the clavicle. It is important to see the whole of the lower end of the muscle and to release the contracture, completely dividing not only the muscle but also any other tight fascial bands, which can be demonstrated by rotating and laterally flexing the neck away from the affected side during the operation. Care must be taken not to damage the important structures, e.g. the carotid vessels and jugular veins, that lie in close proximity to the muscle. The skin incision should be sutured with care to avoid an unsightly scar. Division of the muscle at its upper end is technically more difficult. There is also the risk of damage to the spinal accessory nerve. The scar is, however, hidden behind the ear.

Post-operatively, intensive physiotherapy is necessary to re-educate the patient to hold his head straight and to prevent the muscle rejoining in its shortened position. A collar is often helpful. The enthusiastic cooperation of the patient is important. Occasionally it may be necessary to use a plaster or brace to hold the head in the over-corrected position for some weeks if physiotherapy is failing to maintain correction or the necessary patient cooperation is not forthcoming. Recurrence of the deformity is seldom seen if it has been adequately corrected at the first operation and the correction has been maintained by post-operative physiotherapy. Once the deformity has been corrected the facial asymmetry can correct up until the age of 18–20 years, when growth in the facial bones ceases. It is important, however, to warn patients that it takes a long time for the facial asymmetry to disappear and the older the patient the less likely it will disappear completely.

CONGENITAL ANKYLOSIS OF THE ELBOW

This is a very rare anomaly. It may occur in isolation, in which case it is usually bilateral. It may also occur in association with other anomalies, e.g. absence of the ulna or radius and fusion or absence of bones in the wrist and hand, in which case it is usually unilateral (Fig. 8.1.10). The lower end of the humerus is fused to the radius or ulna or both. Congenital ankylosis of other joints may be present. Attempts to construct a mobile elbow joint are disappointing. Osteotomy may be worthwhile to place the forearm and hand in a more functional position.

CONGENITAL DISLOCATION OF THE RADIAL HEAD

This is one of the more common congenital anomalies of the upper limb (Wynne-Davies, 1973) (Fig. 8.1.11). It may occur as an isolated lesion or in association with other abnormalities. The dislocation may be anterior, posterior, or lateral. It must be distinguished from an old, unreduced traumatic dislocation. In about 40% of cases it is bilateral. The isolated defect is commonly inherited as an autosomal dominant trait (Wynne-Davies, 1973). It may be associated with a wide variety

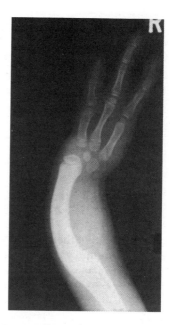

Fig. 8.1.10 Radiograph of humeroulnar synostosis (ankylosis of the elbow). Note that this is associated with a severe form of radial club hand with only three fingers and a small remnant of the proximal end of the radius present on the radiograph.

of syndromes, including acrocephalopolysyndactyly (Carpenter's syndrome), acrocephalosyndactyly (Apert's syndrome), chondroectodermal dysplasia (Ellis–Van Creveld syndrome), craniocarpotarsal dystrophy (Freeman–Sheldon syndrome), de Lange's syndrome Russell–Silver syndrome, Nievergelt's syndrome, onycho-osteodystrophy (nail–patella syndrome), arthrogryposis, Klinefelter's syndrome and joint laxity syndromes, e.g. Ehlers–Danlos syndrome.

The condition seldom causes symptoms in a child, but limitation of full flexion in anterior dislocation and full extension in posterior dislocation may be present. McFarland (1936) pointed out that congenital dislocation could be distinguished from traumatic dislocation by the radiographic appearance. In congenital dislocation the head of the radius is rounded, the capitulum is deficient and the posterior border of the proximal ulna bowed forwards. In congenital posterior dislocation the head of the radius is thinned and attenuated, and the normal convexity of the ulna exaggerated. Almquist *et al.* (1969) confirmed these findings. However, Lloyd-Roberts and Bucknill (1977) suggested that the same appearances could be produced in some isolated unilateral anterior dislocations by old unrecognized trauma, possibly due to non-accidental injury.

In old traumatic lesions Lloyd-Roberts and Bucknill (1977) advocate replacement of the radial head and reconstruction of the annular ligament using a strip of

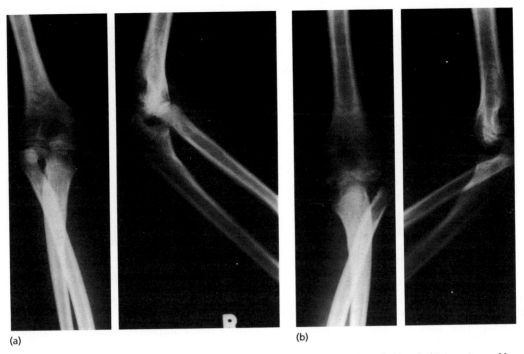

(a) (b)

Fig. 8.1.11 (a) Anteroposterior and lateral views of a patient with anterior dislocation of the radial head. (b) Anterior and lateral views of a patient with posterior dislocation of the radial head.

the triceps tendon. In true congenital cases, however, such reconstruction has seldom proved satisfactory. Excision of the radial head is not recommended while the child is still growing. If the radial head produces symptoms in adolescence or adult life, however, then excision can be useful.

RADIOULNAR SYNOSTOSIS

This deformity may be unilateral or bilateral; sometimes it is associated with a dislocated radial head on the opposite side. There are three main types of deformity — severe, intermediate and mild. In the most severe or 'headless' form the upper end of the radius is absent and the radial shaft fused to the ulna (Figs 8.1.12 and 8.1.13). In the intermediate type the upper third of the radius and ulna is fused. The radial head is present but deformed and often in subluxation or dislocated. In the mild form the radial head is malformed. The radius and ulna are not joined by bone but by an abnormal interosseous ligament. Some cases show a dominant inheritance, and the condition can be associated with other syndromes such as acrocephalosyndactyly (Apert's syndrome), arthrogryposis and Klinefelter's syndrome.

If the forearm is fixed in a fairly neutral position, the condition is often not noticed until the child goes to school. This is because the patient can compensate for

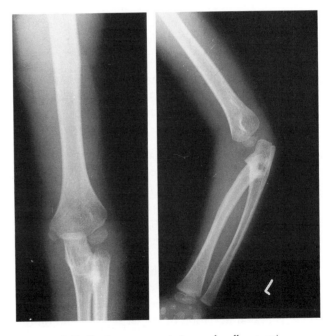

Fig. 8.1.12 Radioulnar synostosis (severe headless type) (anteroposterior and lateral views).

the loss of supination and pronation in the forearm by rotating the arm from the shoulder. If the arm is fixed in full pronation then the deformity is more obvious and disabling. Operative attempts to separate the synostosis

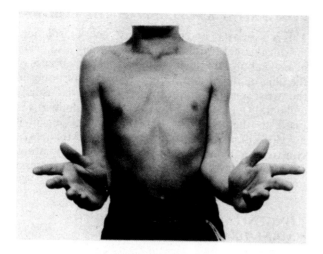

Fig. 8.1.13 Patient with radioulnar synostosis trying to supinate.

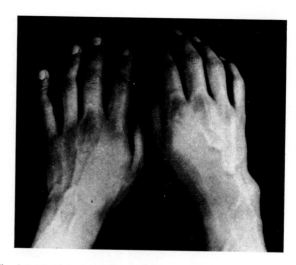

Fig. 8.1.14 Right Madelung's deformity. Note the radial deviation of the hand and the prominence of the lower end of the ulna on the right side.

are very disappointing. Kelikian and Doumanian (1957) described a swivel that they used initially for post-traumatic cases. They suggested that this could be used in congenital cases. Tachdjian (1972) reported disappointing experience with this procedure in congenital cases, however, due to the associated soft tissue abnormalities. For patients with the arm in extreme pronation corrective osteotomy to bring the forearm to a more neutral position may be worthwhile.

MADELUNG'S DEFORMITY (CONGENITAL SUBLUXATION OF THE INFERIOR RADIOULNAR JOINT)

In this deformity, described by Madelung in 1879, there is defective growth and premature fusion of the lower radial epiphysis in its anteromedial quadrant. As a result the distal end of the radius is tilted abnormally antero-medially. The distal end of the ulna becomes excessively long and undergoes posterior subluxation. The lunate bone comes to lie deeply between the lower end of the radius and ulna.

The clinical appearance is characteristic (Fig. 8.1.14). The distal end of the ulna is unduly prominent posteriorly. The radius is shortened and anteriorly bowed. There is lateral deviation of the wrist and hand on the forearm. The condition is more common in females. The patient commonly complains of the unsightly appearance, weakness and sometimes aching pain in the wrist. There is limitation of dorsiflexion and increased palmar flexion at the wrist. Supination is usually full, but pronation often limited.

Radiographs show the lower end of the ulna is enlarged and distorted. The ulnar epiphysis is abnor-

mally dense and the epiphyseal plate sloping. The growth plate of the radius slopes steeply medially and is fused at its ulnar end. The proximal row of the carpus is distorted into a 'V' with the lunate bone at the apex of the 'V' lying between the radius and ulna. In the lateral view the distal end of the ulna is in posterior subluxation and the normal anterior tilt of the radial epiphysis is increased (Fig. 8.1.15).

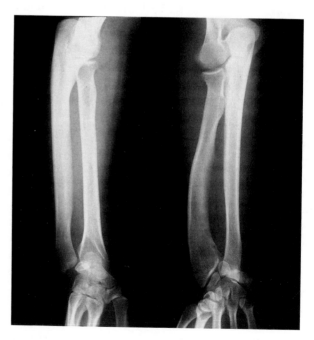

Fig. 8.1.15 Anteroposterior and lateral views of a Right Madelung's deformity. Note the subluxation of the lower end of the ulna and the increased angulation of the lower end of the radius in the anteroposterior view.

Madelung's deformity may be caused by a variety of conditions. It may be idiopathic or associated with skeletal dysplasias, e.g. osteochondromatosis (Ollier's disease) and multiple hereditary exostosis. It is sometimes seen in gonadal dysgenesis (Turner's syndrome). It may follow trauma to the medial part of the lower radial epiphysis. Autosomal dominant inheritance has been reported, but no large genetic surveys are available.

Treatment

In many patients no treatment is necessary. Conservative treatment has little to offer, though a wrist support may sometimes be helpful. The distal end of the ulna is unsightly and can be resected. A more complete correction of the deformity can be attempted by a step-cut shortening osteotomy of the distal ulna combined with an open-wedge osteotomy of the distal radius. This type of operation is best done at maturity when the epiphyses have fused. Henry and Thorburn (1967) reported good results from wrist fusion in two patients with persistent pain.

RADIAL CLUB-HAND (PARAXIAL RADIAL HEMIMELIA, CONGENITAL ABSENCE OF THE RADIUS)

Radial club-hand, or paraxial radial hemimelia, is one of the more common upper limb skeletal defects. Birch-Jensen (1949) reported an incidence of 1 in 30 000 births. A considerable number of cases followed ingestion of the drug thalidomide during pregnancy. There is no family history in the vast majority of patients, but a few familial instances have been reported. The condition may occur as an isolated defect. It is commonly bilateral. It must be remembered that it can be associated with a very wide variety of other congenital anomalies, in particular cardiac defects in Holt–Oram or heart–hand syndrome, which is of dominant inheritance, and blood dyscrasias, e.g. Fanconi's anaemia, where there is a pancytopenia and thrombocytopenia with absent radii (TAR) syndrome.

On examination, the radius may be completely absent or in milder cases only the distal end is deficient (Figs 8.1.16 and 8.1.17). The ulna is usually short and bowed laterally. The hand is radially deviated up to 90–100° on the forearm. The thumb and fingers may be normal, but usually the thumb is absent or significantly hypoplastic. The index and middle fingers can also be involved. The radial side of the carpus is nearly always affected. The scaphoid bone and trapezium are usually absent.

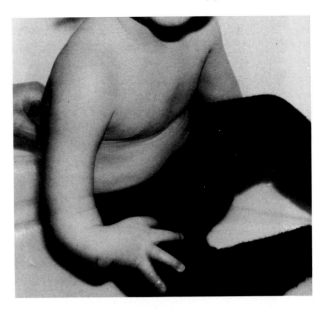

Fig. 8.1.16 Patient with a right radial club-hand. Note the absence of the thumb and the prominence of the lower end of the ulna, which is markedly short.

It is important to realize that the soft tissues on the radial side of the forearm and hand are also affected. Absence or deficiency of the muscles arising from the common extensor origin and the radius is common. In particular, the index profundus tendon may be absent, which will seriously influence any attempt to pollicize the index finger. The joints of the fingers on the radial side may show marked stiffness or even ankylosis, similar to that seen in arthrogryposis. Finally, the elbow is often stiff and sometimes ankylosed. As a result the radial deviation of the hand may actually prove to be beneficial in allowing the more normal ulnar fingers to reach the mouth.

Treatment

There is considerable debate about the management of this deformity. Lloyd-Roberts (1971) advocated a very conservative approach and pointed out the excellent function shown by many patients who had had no corrective surgery or splinting. He emphasized the importance of not sacrificing function for cosmesis. Particular care should be taken in patients with persistent stiffness or ankylosis of the elbow and where absence of the thumb, stiffness and hypoplasia of the index and middle fingers leave the ulnar two fingers as the dominant functional side of the hand. This approach inevitably means accepting a considerable cosmetic deformity. Lamb (1977) also stressed the paramount

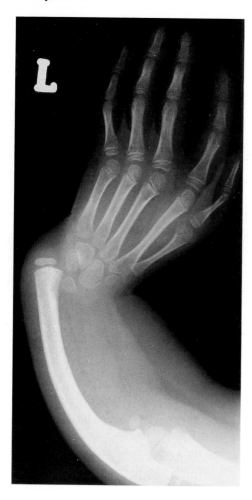

Fig. 8.1.17 Radiograph of a radial club-hand. The thumb is present but the hand is markedly radially deviated and there is only a minute remnant of the proximal end of the radius. The ulna is short and bowed.

importance of accurate functional assessment of the hand and arm. Special attention should be paid to hand function both in the deviated position and when splinted as straight as possible. Basing his comments on extensive experience Lamb advised splinting from birth, which is continued at night only once the child starts to use his hands. If there is limitation of elbow flexion in the absence of bony ankylosis, this is mobilized as far as possible. At the age of 3–4 years centralization of the hand on the ulna is undertaken. The lower end of the ulna is implanted in a slot in the carpus, the depth of which equals the diameter of the ulna, as recommended by MacCon (1974), to ensure stability. A Kirschner wire is used for internal fixation and external splinting is maintained at night for at least 6 months. Following centralization and a further period of careful functional assessment and observation, pollicization of the radial

digit for absence or gross hypoplasia of the thumb can be considered if there is active flexion in the terminal joint of this digit.

Flatt (1977) recommends splinting from birth by serial plasters followed by a plastic gutter splint. Once maximum correction has been achieved by splinting, any remaining soft tissue contracture is released surgically, usually before the age of 2 years. An important point to remember in any operation on the radial side of the forearm and hand in this condition is that the median nerve commonly lies immediately beneath the deep fascia and may easily be damaged by the unwary. For patients with gross displacement and where soft tissue release cannot provide adequate correction of the deformity, Flatt recommends operative centralization of the hand on the ulna at about 1 year of age. Detailed descriptions of this important procedure are given by both Lamb (1977) and Flatt (1977). Flatt quoted a 65% incidence of absence of the thumb in radial aplasia and a further 10% incidence of gross hypoplasia of the thumb. In these patients the index finger tends to undergo spontaneous or autopollicization. He felt that it is logical to complete this process by formally constructing a thumb from the index finger. He warned that this can often be surgically difficult and that the correct indications for pollicization in these patients are difficult to define. Clearly this is not a field for the surgeon who only treats the occasional patient. Treatment needs very careful thought and planning. The operation itself can be technically taxing even for those accustomed to operating on the hand in small children. If pollicization is to be performed, early centralization by the age of 12–18 months is advised by many hand surgeons.

Both Lamb and Flatt felt that the cosmetic benefits of centralization and, where necessary, pollicization offer very considerable advantages over the conservative approach, provided function can be retained and, if possible, improved by these procedures.

CONGENITAL ABSENCE OF THE ULNA (ULNAR DYSMELIA, PARAXIAL ULNAR HEMIMELIA)

This condition is much more uncommon than radial club-hand (Figs 8.1.18 and 8.1.19). There is a spectrum of the disorder ranging from simple hypoplasia to complete absence of the ulna. Ogden *et al.* (1976) divide the condition into three main types according to the radiological appearance at or shortly after birth (see below). They point out that there may be multiple highly variable associated deformities of the elbow, wrist and hand. The elbow may be ankylosed in flexion or extension. If there

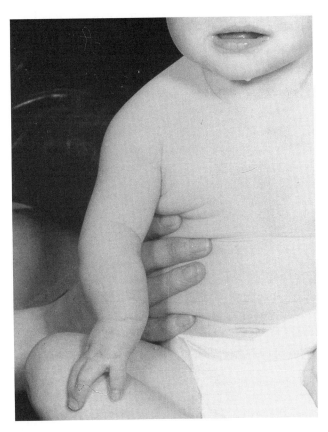

Fig. 8.1.18 Patient with a right ulnar club-hand. Note the ulnar deviation of the hand, synostosis of the index and middle fingers and the shortening of the forearm.

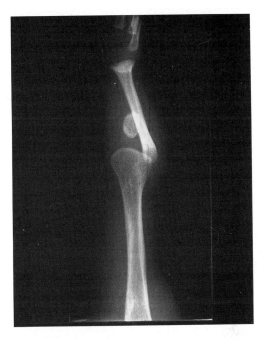

Fig. 8.1.19 Radiograph of an ulnar club-hand. Note the short radius, rudimentary ulna and only three radial digits present.

is some movement present flexion is usually limited to approximately 100°. There is often radiohumeral dislocation. The wrist and hand are usually deviated to the ulnar side, but the carpus is seldom completely dislocated on the distal radius, unlike the situation in radial clubhand. The little, ring and sometimes middle fingers may be absent or hypoplastic. Syndactyly is also common. In a significant number of cases there is some structural abnormality present in the opposite limb, but bilateral ulnar deficiency is uncommon. The condition is not thought to be familial.

The following radiographic appearances may be seen on the earliest films:

1 Hypoplasia: the ulna is complete but short; the distal ulnar epiphysis is present.
2 Partial aplasia: the distal ulna and its epiphysis are missing.
3 Complete aplasia: the whole ulna is missing.

In partial and complete aplasia a fibrocartilaginous anlage may be found at the site of the 'missing' bone and may eventually ossify. Ogden *et al.* (1976) suggest that a significant fibrocartilaginous band exists in many but not all cases. This band inserts into the distal radial epiphysis or the carpus.

Treatment

Despite the ugly appearance, many children have very good functional hands. Ogden *et al.* (1976) advise exploration and excision of the cartilaginous band in the first year of life to prevent progressive deformity. In the author's personal experience, this is by no means always necessary. If the forearm is weak and unstable, fusion of the ulnar remnant to the radius to create a 'one bone' forearm can improve function and is worthwhile. If the forearm is reasonably stable with some pronation and supination, this operation is not indicated as it may reduce function.

AMPUTATION THROUGH THE FOREARM (see also p. 252)

This condition occurs sporadically. It is almost always unilateral and the patient is not severely incapacitated. Elbow flexion is usually powerful and so a below-elbow prosthesis may be fitted. The most useful prosthesis is the sprung split hook. Elbow movement can be arranged to activate the hook. It should be remembered that the prosthesis will only be used to help the normal hand,

and that sophisticated dexterity is not needed. The surgeon may well alienate the patient by insisting on inappropriate skill.

A patient with a long mobile stump may be a candidate for Krukenberg's operation. The original operation required an abdominal skin flap, but recent modifications allow local skin to be used together with a small amount of split skin. The forearm bones are parted and the wrist and finger flexors and extensors are sewn to the ends. Swanson (1974) has advocated the use of Krukenberg's operation in one of the arms of the rare bilateral congenital amputee. The other arm is fitted with a prosthesis and the Krukenberg's arm becomes the dominant one. In children the inevitable ugliness of a Krukenberg's arm is not a problem, appearance being of much less importance than function.

The most useful pincers are about 12.5 cm long. The skin flaps are cut so that normally innervated skin may line the opposing surfaces of the pincers. The biceps and triceps open the radial and ulnar limbs of the pincers respectively. The pronator teres muscle, combined with the wrist flexors, closes the radial limb. The brachialis muscle closes the ulnar limb. If the limbs are left well covered with muscle it is feasible to cover the gaps in the skin with split skin. The pincer grip may be made more precise by angling the limbs with osteotomies. It is wise to do this as a secondary procedure after useful function has been established.

It is quite feasible to fit a dress hand to a Krukenberg's stump. The patient may wear this on social occasions and may remove it for work and recreation.

DUPLICATION OF THE THUMB

Digital duplication may be seen in several forms. It is particularly common in the thumb when the radial member is usually the abnormal one. It is always unilateral, and is not part of any recognized syndrome. The abnormal digit should be excised. If the duplication affects only the terminal phalanx, the result of excising the soft tissue between the double phalanges is better than that seen following excision of one or other phalanx, as the remaining phalanx continues to grow askew, and an ugly deformity ensues.

DUPLICATION OF THE LITTLE FINGER

In contrast, duplication of the little finger is a well recognized feature of several syndromes. It is seen in Laurence−Moon−Biedl syndrome, in trisomy 13 and trisomy 18, and in Ellis−van Creveld syndrome. The abnormal finger should be removed. There is seldom

any doubt about the identity of the digit to be removed: it is usually functionless.

TRIGGER THUMB

This is one of the most common congenital hand deformities. There is no true triggering phenomenon, for the child cannot extend the interphalangeal joint. The majority of cases resolve spontaneously, but a few need to be dealt with at the age of 18 months or as soon after as possible, when the chances of spontaneous resolution are small. Division of the mouth of the flexor sheath allows the tendon to move normally. Residual flexion deformity does not occur (Dinham and Meggitt, 1974).

LOBSTER CLAW HAND

This deformity is commonly familial. Function is almost always surprisingly good. The deformity exists in two forms. In the first form the index, middle and ring rays are deficient. The thumb and little finger rays are short and stiff. It is possible to improve function by deepening the web between the digits using a double Z-plasty. Any carpal or metacarpal elements are removed at the same time. Later one or other of the digits may be rotated at an osteotomy to improve prehension.

In the second type the hand is split down to the carpus between two of the central rays. The other rays are usually abnormal. Function may be improved by operation only if the fingers and thumb are reasonably mobile and strong. The cleft is closed by excising the skin from its border. A tented rectangular flap, base distal, is fashioned from the mesial surface of the larger finger and used to form the web (Barsky, 1951) (Fig. 8.1.20).

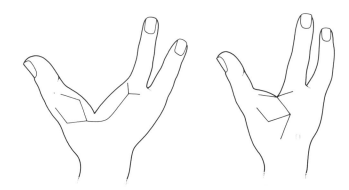

Fig. 8.1.20 Reduction of the gap in lobster claw hand by the Barsky technique (1951).

ABNORMAL MUSCLES

Although seldom described, abnormal muscles in the hand are not uncommon. Extensor digitorum manus brevis causes a swelling on the dorsum of the carpus which resembles a ganglion. It becomes trapped under the distal edge of the extensor retinaculum and becomes painful. In these circumstances it should be removed (Smith and Browne, 1979). A swelling in the palm may be an extension of the palmaris longus muscle. It should be removed if it causes either interference with gripping or pain.

ARTHROGRYPOSIS MULTIPLEX CONGENITA (see also pp. 22 and 62)

This distressing disorder occurs sporadically. There is no evidence of a genetic cause. Affection is variable: some or all of the joints have fixed deformity of varying degree. It is present at birth and does not progress. There is no evidence of sensory or central neurological disorder, but muscle weakness and wasting are severe. The degree of affection is usually symmetrical. It has been shown that the obstruction to movement is usually extra-articular: the capsule is non-elastic and adheres firmly to the neighbouring periosteum (Williams, 1973).

The elbow may have a flexion deformity. In these cases the triceps is almost non-existent, but the biceps is powerful and residual movement is useful and strong. Attempts to improve elbow function fail inevitably, for extension can only be achieved by sacrificing biceps. More commonly the elbow is stiff in extension. The triceps is powerful and the biceps is absent in these cases. Function is poor and surgical reconstruction can be very rewarding. However, before starting a course of operations the surgeon must satisfy himself that he is not going to make the patient worse. The child may walk with crutches, and loss of elbow stiffness in extension may affect his mobility seriously. An experienced physiotherapist should be involved in pre-operative planning and in post-operative rehabilitation.

The most useful procedure for a stiff straight elbow is a posterior capsulotomy and a triceps-to-biceps tendon transfer. A long curved incision is made over the triceps tendon, which is taken across the medial side of the elbow, and then over the biceps tendon. The triceps tendon is divided off the olecranon and the muscle mobilized belly up to the spiral groove. A generous window is made in the medial intermuscular septum beneath the ulnar nerve. The posterior capsule of the elbow is divided from epicondyle to epicondyle to allow the elbow to flex fully. The forearm flexors and extensors are divided in the distal part of the cubital fossa and the biceps tuberosity on the radius is identified. The biceps tendon is inserted into this, and the triceps tendon is passed through the window in the septum and sewn to the biceps tendon in as much tension as possible with multiple mattress sutures. The buttonhole technique is the most secure for this, but there may not be enough length in the triceps tendon to allow this luxury. The elbow is maintained fully flexed during the suturing, and the elbow is splinted in about 100° of flexion for 3 weeks before beginning rehabilitation.

Very occasionally the elbow is stiff in extension in the absence of a triceps. Simple posterior capsulotomy of the elbow gives the child useful passive mobility. Furthermore, in the presence of active forearm flexors, it may be possible to restore some active elbow flexion to these children by means of a combined posterior capsulotomy and a Steindler flexoroplasty. Through a longitudinal medial incision centred over the medial epicondyle, the posterior capsule is first divided to achieve full flexion. The whole flexor origin is then detached from the medial epicondyle: the median nerve marks the lateral boundary of the flexor muscles. The combined belly is mobilized as far as the deep head of the pronator teres. The elbow is fully flexed and the combined flexor origin is sewn as high up the medial intermuscular septum as possible. Care must be taken not to kink the combined belly too sharply, for this will stop any voluntary activity.

The wrist in arthrogryposis multiplex congenita is often stiff in full flexion. It is sometimes possible to improve the wrist by means of a Scaglietti muscle slide, but the operation weakens elbow flexion and the results are disappointing. Much more reliable is proximal row carpectomy. Through a dorsal longitudinal incision the scaphoid, lunate and triquetral (cuneiform) bones are excised. This usually allows the wrist to extend to the neutral position. In exceptional cases it may also be necessary to excise some or all of the distal row. The corrected position is held with crossed Kirschner wires for about 6 weeks.

Flexion deformities of the metacarpophalangeal joints and stiffness of the interphalangeal joints are seldom remediable. Operations simply replace one deformity with another and do not improve function.

CONSTRICTION RINGS

The aetiology of these rings is poorly understood. They occur sporadically and vary from barely perceptible transverse marks to deep annular grooves. In the severe forms the dermis in the depths of the grooves adheres to the periosteum of the underlying bone. Naturally, the neurovascular trunks deep to these severe bands are compromised and distal dystrophy is commonly seen. It is not unusual to see a deep groove around the arm and fixed deformity of the wrist and fingers. This deformity resembles arthrogryposis multiplex congenita and should be treated along the same lines. Complete absence of both sensation and active movement distal to a constriction ring is an indication for amputation. In less severe cases the appearance of the grooves may be improved by multiple Z-plasties. Should the constriction encircle the limb it is wise to do the operation in at least two stages in order to prevent distal oedema.

SYNDACTYLY

This is seen most often between the ring and middle fingers. It is more common in boys. The junction may be skin only or it may involve some or all of the other structures of the fingers. The mild forms are sporadic, but severe forms are seen in several rare inherited syndromes, e.g. orofaciodigital syndrome (girls only), de Lange's syndrome, Goltz's syndrone, Apert's syndrome and Carpenter's syndrome.

In the severe forms hand function is impeded by the syndactyly, and some separation of the fingers must be attempted by the age of 18 months. The results of separation are better if the operation is done at the age of about 5 years, and it is wise to postpone the operation to that age in the mildly affected. It should be remembered that there is not enough skin to cover both separated digits. It is best to arrange the incision so that the more important finger is covered with native skin only. It will grow better and sensation will be better if this can be achieved. The deficiencies of a less important finger may be covered with full thickness skin graft. The web should be constructed with a transverse distal border so as to avoid asymmetric deformation of the fingers with growth.

A square-ended dorsally based flap is made for the web. A curved incision from the corner of the web flap on the less important finger is extended along the dorsum of the syndactyly distal to the apex, making sure that the longitudinal elements of the curved incision do not cross the dorsal skin joints over the interphalangeal joints. The skin flaps thus outlined are raised and a reciprocal incision is made on the palmar aspect of the syndactyly so that the flap can be used to close the defect in the more important finger (Fig. 8.1.21). The gap in the less important finger is filled with a skin graft.

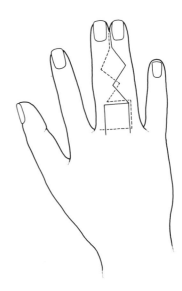

Fig. 8.1.21 Principles of flap construction for syndactyly operation.

MACRODACTYLY

In this rare abnormality one or more digit is enlarged in all dimensions. The digits usually grow faster than the rest of the hand and the disparity gets worse. Each case should be treated on its merits. It is possible to shorten the finger by excising some of the middle phalanx. Its girth may be decreased by removing some part of the digital nerves (which are usually disproportionally enlarged). In children the growth may be slowed by epiphysiodesis. This is not very reliable, however. As a last resort the ugly gigantic digit may be amputated (Tusage, 1967).

CAMPTODACTYLY

This common disorder is congenital and usually familial. There is gradually progressive flexion deformity of the proximal interphalangeal joint. It is usually confined to the little finger, but it sometimes affects several fingers. Severe forms of the condition are seen in many of the skeletal dysplasias and in the inherited collagen disorders, e.g. Marfan's syndrome. In childhood the deformity is correctable if tension in the superficialis tendon is reduced by flexing the wrist. Severe progressive forms may be ameliorated in childhood by lengthening the rogue tendon at its musculotendinous junction. In adults the contracture becomes fixed and a normal digit cannot be restored. If necessary the deformity may be corrected by arthrodesis.

FLEXION CONTRACTURE OF THE THUMB

This deformity usually occurs sporadically, but sex-linked recessive inheritance has also been recorded. The thumb is fully flexed at the metacarpophalangeal joint. The condition is due to hypoplasia of the extensors of the thumb. In the newborn the aim of treatment is the prevention of fixation of the deformity. The thumb should be splinted in extension from birth. Sometimes the power of the extensors gradually improves and splinting may be abandoned at the age of about 6 months. When this does not occur the thumb should be kept extended in a cast until a tendon transfer can be done. The most useful transfer is that of extensor indicis proprius to the dorsum of the thumb.

Should the diagnosis be made later, then fixed contracture will have developed. It should be corrected completely and as expeditiously as possible for function will be extremely poor otherwise. The web is lengthened by a Z-plasty. The adductor muscle must be divided near its origin from the third metacarpal to allow abduction. The deformed metacarpophalangeal joint is corrected by division of the capsule anteriorly. If the extensor tendons are absent, metacarpophalangeal arthrodesis may be necessary to keep the thumb out of the palm, but an extensor indicis proprius tendon transfer may suffice.

FLEXION CONTRACTURE OF THE FINGERS

A similar contracture of the fingers is sometimes seen. The long extensors are deficient and the fingers are fixed at the metacarpophalangeal joints. Treatment is along similar lines to the thumb contracture. No spare extensor tendons, however, may be available for transfer. In such circumstances Littler's technique (1959) is useful. The sublimis tendon from the ring finger is re-routed around the ulnar side of the wrist, across the dorsum of the hand, split into four components and sewn into the extensor hoods of the fingers.

CLINODACTYLY

Radial deviation of a finger, most commonly the little finger, may occur as a solitary familial disorder, or it may be part of a generalized congenital disorder, e.g. Down's syndrome. The deviation is in the middle phalanx where an epiphyseal abnormality, delta phalanx, may be seen. Disability is usually slight and treatment is not required. On occasion, however, the deviation may impede function of other fingers and a corrective osteotomy may be done. The operation should be delayed until near the time of skeletal maturity, for asymmetric growth may otherwise frustrate the intention of the operation. A wedge of bone is excised from the convex side of the deformed phalanx and the position held with crossed Kirschner wires until the osteotomy has united (Burke and Flatt, 1979).

REFERENCES

Alldred A.J. (1963) Congenital pseudarthrosis of the clavicle. *J. Bone Joint Surg.* **45B**, 312–319.

Almquist E.E., Gordon L.H. and Blue A.I. (1969) Congenital dislocation of the head of the radius. *J. Bone Joint Surg. [Am.]* **51A**, 1118–1127.

Barsky A.J. (1951) Congenital anomalies of the hand. *J. Bone Joint Surg.* **33A**, 35.

Bauman G.I. (1932) Absence of the cervical spine. Klippel–Feil syndrome. *JAMA* **98**, 129–132.

Birch-Jensen A. (1949) *Congenital Deformities of the Upper Extremities.* Copenhagen Thesis. Odense. Andelsbogtrykkeriet.

Bonola A. (1956) The surgical treatment of Klippel–Feil syndrome. *J. Bone Joint Surg.* **38B**, 440–449.

Brooks B. (1922) Pathologic changes in muscle as a result of disturbances of circulation. *Arch. Surg.* **5**, 188.

Burke F. and Flatt A. (1979) Clinodactyly; a review of a series of cases. *Hand* **11**, 269–280.

Campbell D. and Wilkinson J.A. (1979) Scapular osteotomy for the treatment of Sprengel's shoulder. *J. Bone Joint Surg.* **61B**, 514.

Cattell H.S. and Filtzer D.L. (1965) Pseudo-subluxation and other normal variations in the cervical spine in children. *J. Bone Joint Surg.* **47A**, 1195–1399.

Dinham J.M. and Meggitt B.F. (1974) Trigger thumbs in children. *J. Bone Joint Surg.* **56B**, 153–155.

Dunn P.M. (1973) Congenital sternomastoid torticollis: an intra-uterine postural deformity. *J. Bone Joint Surg.* **55B**, 877.

Fawcett J. (1913) The development and ossification of the human clavicle. *J. Anat. Physiol.* **47**, 225.

Flatt A.E. (1977) *The Care of Congenital Hand Anomalies.* St Louis, C.V. Mosby.

Gibson D.A. and Carroll N. (1970) Congenital pseudarthrosis of the clavicle. *J. Bone Joint Surg.* **52B**, 629–643.

Gray S.W., Romaine C.B. and Skandalakis J.E. (1964) Congenital fusion of the cervical vertebrae. *Surg. Gynecol. Obstet.* **118**, 373–385.

Green W.T. (1957) The surgical correction of congenital elevation of the scapula (Sprengel's deformity). *J. Bone Joint Surg.* **39A**, 1439.

Grove J. and Goldner J.L. (1974) Contracture of the deltoid muscle in the adult after intramuscular injections. *J. Bone Joint Surg.* **56A**, 817–820.

Henry A. and Thorburn M.J. (1967) Madelung's deformity. *J. Bone Joint Surg.* **49B**, 66–73.

Hensinger R.N., Lang J.E. and MacEwen G.D. (1974) Klippel–Feil syndrome. *J. Bone Joint Surg.* **56A**, 1246–1253.

Hulbert K.F. (1950) Congenital torticollis. *J. Bone Joint Surg.* **32B**, 50–59.

Kelikian H. and Doumanian A. (1957) Swivel for proximal radio ulnar synostosis. *J. Bone Joint Surg.* **39A**, 945–952.

Klippel M. and Feil A. (1912) Anomalie de la colonne vertebrale par absence des vertèbres cervicales: cage thoracique remontant jusqu'à la base du crâne. *Bull. Soc. Anat. (Paris)* **87**, 185.

Lamb D.W. (1977) Radial club hand. *J. Bone Joint Surg.* **59A**, 1–13.

Littler J.W. (1959) The prevention and correction of adduction contracture of the thumb. In De Palma A.F. (ed) *Clinical Orthopaedics.* Philadelphia, J.B. Lippincott, vol. 13.

Lloyd-Roberts G.C. (1971) *Orthopaedics in Infancy and Childhood.* London, Butterworths.

Lloyd-Roberts G.C., Apley A.G. and Owen R. (1975) Reflections upon the aetiology of congenital pseudarthrosis of the clavicle. *J. Bone Joint Surg.* **57B**, 24–29.

Lloyd-Roberts G.C. and Bucknill T.M. (1977) Anterior dislocation of the radial head in children. *J. Bone Joint Surg.* **59B**, 402–407.

Lucas L.S. and Gill J.H. (1947) Birth injury. *J. Bone Joint Surg.* **29**, 367.

MacCon M.B. (1974) *Radial Club Hand. A Review of 106 Cases.* ChM (Orth.) Thesis, University of Liverpool, UK.

MacDonald D. (1969) Sternomastoid tumour and muscular torticollis. *J. Bone Joint Surg.* **51B**, 432–443.

McFarland B. (1936) Congenital dislocation of the head of the radius. *Br. J. Surg.* **24**, 41–49.

Madelung O.W. (1879) Die spontane Subluxation der Hand nach Vorne. *Arch. Klin. Chir.* **23**, 395.

Middleton D.S. (1930) The pathology of congenital torticollis. *Br. J. Surg.* **18**, 188.

Ogden J.A., Kirk Watson H. and Bohne W. (1976) Ulnar dysmelia. *J. Bone Joint Surg.* **58A**, 467–475.

Smith J.S. and Browne P.A. (1979) Extensor digitorum brevis manus. *Hand* **2**, 217–223.

Sprengel O. (1891) Die angeborene Verschiebung des Schulterblattes nach Oben. *Arch. Klin. Chir.* **42**, 545.

Stark E.W. and Borton T.E. (1973) Klippel–Feil syndrome and associated hearing loss. *Arch. Otolaryngol.* **97**, 415–419.

Swanson A.B. (1974) Krukenberg amputation. *J. Bone Joint Surg.* **56B**, 153–155.

Tachdjian M.O. (1972) *Pediatric Orthopedics.* Philadelphia, W.B. Saunders.

Tusage K. (1967) Treatment of macrodactyly. *Plast. Reconstr. Surg.* **39**, 590.

Williams P.F. (1973) The elbow in arthrogryphosis. *J. Bone Joint Surg.* **55B**, 834–840.

Woodward J.W. (1961) Congenital elevation of the scapula. Correction by release and transplantation of muscle origins. *J. Bone Joint Surg.* **43A**, 219–228.

Wynne-Davies R. (1973) *Heritable Disorders in Orthopaedic Practice.* Oxford, Blackwell Scientific Publications.

The Lower Limb

Congenital Shortening and Absence of the Femur

R. King & D.F. Powell

INTRODUCTION

Proximal femoral focal deficiency (PFFD) implies that the proximal femur is lacking in completeness and results in varying degrees of shortness of the extremity. Associated with this are a bulbous thigh (ship ventilatory shape) and flexion, abduction and external

rotation contractures of the hip (Fig. 8.2.1). Historically, cases of congenital short femur, developmental coxa vara and phocomelia have been included with PFFD (Reiner, 1901; Nilsonne, 1928; Freund, 1936; Golding, 1948; Amstutz and Wilson, 1962; Scheer, 1972; Teal, personal communication). Langston (1939) was the first to recognize PFFD as a separate clinical entity. It was essential that a classification be developed that would correlate with the known natural history of PFFD and allow separation into groups for which specific operative recommendations could be made.

CLASSIFICATION

The classification of Aitken *et al.* (1969) satisfied the above criteria but did not include the milder forms of PFFD (Hamanishi, 1980) (Figs 8.2.2 and 8.2.3). The

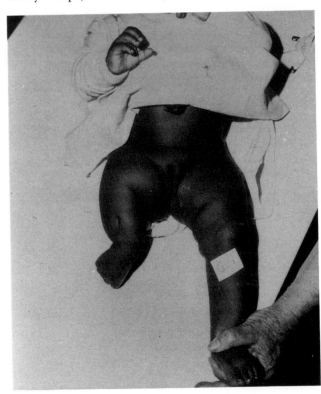

Fig. 8.2.1 Characteristic abduction, flexion and external rotation of the thigh.

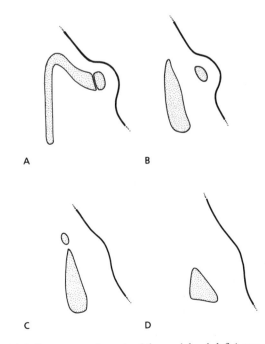

Fig. 8.2.2 Four types of proximal femoral focal deficiency.

223

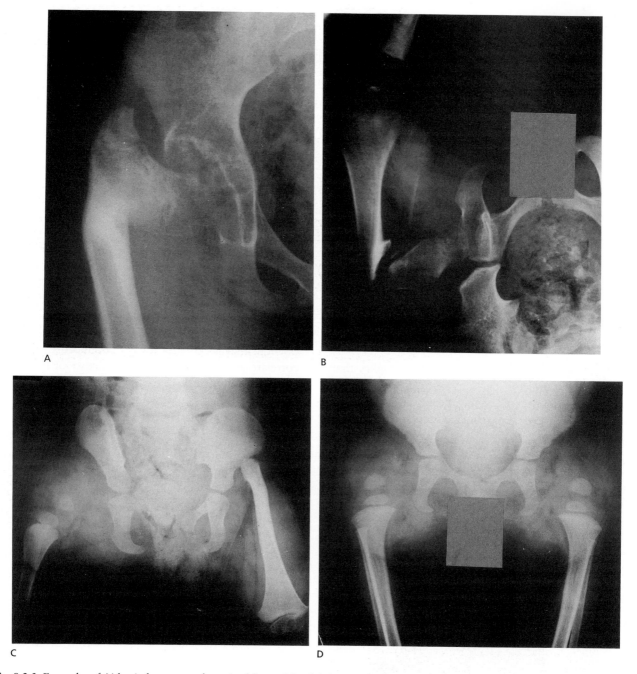

A

B

C

D

Fig. 8.2.3 Examples of Aitken's four types of proximal femoral focal deficiency. Type A has elements of acetabulum and femoral head, as does type B. Types C and D exhibit lack of acetabulum and head of femur.

classification used by these authors divided PFFD into four types, A–D.

1 Type A includes congenital short femur with coxa vara, congenital short femur with bowing and miniaturization of the femur (Figs 8.2.4, 8.2.5 and 8.2.6). An acetabulum is always present, within which is a femoral head. True miniaturization of the femur (less than 40% growth inhibition) and intact knee and hip should be classified other than as true PFFD.

2 Type B presents with an acetabulum and a femoral head, the ossification of which is usually delayed. The proximal shaft of the femur is displaced laterally, but eventually is joined to the head of the femur by a cartilaginous anlage.

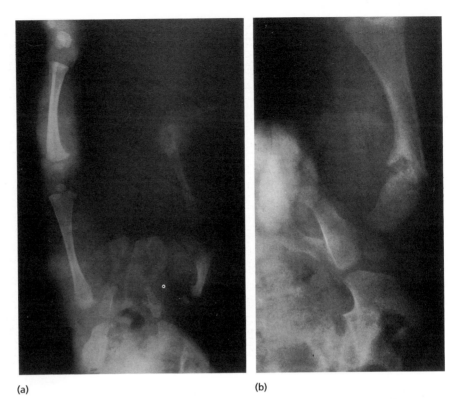

(a)

(b)

Fig. 8.2.4 Type A proximal femoral focal deficiency, representing miniaturization of the femur.

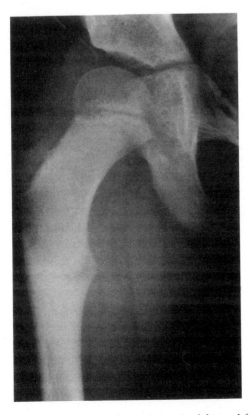

Fig. 8.2.5 Final appearance of type A proximal femoral focal deficiency.

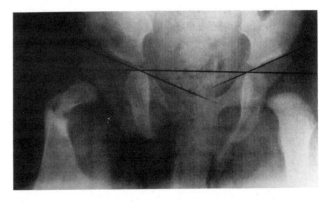

Fig. 8.2.6 Type A proximal femoral focal deficiency showing congenital short femur with bowing.

3 Type C has no acetabulum and hence no femoral head. The shaft of the femur is shortened and usually tends to articulate with the ilium.

4 Type D has neither acetabulum nor a femoral head. The femoral shaft is presented by the condyles of the femur only and represents the most severe deficiency.

The distinction between Types A and B often cannot be made until ossification of the neck and head of the femur occurs (Fixsen and Lloyd-Roberts, 1974; Lange *et al.*, 1978). Magnetic resonance imaging may prove useful in distinguishing these two types (Hillman *et al.*, 1987). It is not uncommon for the ankle on the affected side to lie at the level of the knee joint of the normal side. The fibula is commonly completely absent on the affected side; Nilsonne (1928) reported an incidence of 50%, Aitken *et al.* (1969) 70% and Amstutz and Wilson (1962) 80%.

EMBRYOLOGY

Ossification is commonly delayed in congenital deformities, and this is seen in PFFD. Figure 8.2.7 shows the pelvis at birth, and Fig. 8.2.8 shows the hip 18 months later with the appearance of the ossification centre for the femoral head. Because of this delayed ossification, attempts to obtain pelvifemoral stability by bone grafting from the shaft of the femur to the acetabulum have been described (Langston, 1939; Ring, 1959; Sideman, 1963). Arthrography of the hip has been used to outline the delayed ossification of the femoral head (Lloyd-Roberts and Stone, 1963). This confusion can be resolved when it is realized that the ilium, ischium and pubic symphysis develop from a common cartilaginous anlage. The elements of the head and neck of the femur are actually hewn from this common block of cartilage, and the hip joint appears as a cleft between the head of the femur and what is later to become the acetabulum (Strayer, 1943; Gardner and Gray, 1950; Strayer, 1950; O'Rahilly, 1951; Harrison, 1961; King, 1964; Laurenson, 1964).

Figure 8.2.9 represents a 17 mm embryo (4 weeks) and shows the approximate size of the limb bud and the development of the hip joint at this stage. The ilium, ischium and pubic symphysis still consist of pre-cartilage, and the acetabulum shows little increase in depth. At 22 mm (Fig. 8.2.10) the acetabulum deepens medially

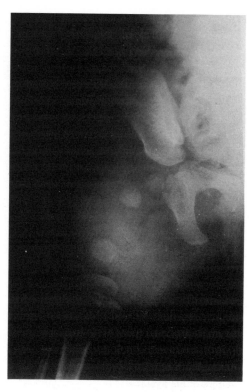

Fig. 8.2.8 Radiograph of the hip 18 months later now shows the appearance of an ossification centre for the femoral head.

and the acetabular cleft is forming. As the lower limb develops in a proximal distal direction, and in view of the embryological development of the acetabulum described, it could possibly be inferred that if an acetabulum is present at birth a femoral head might appear. Conversely, it might be assumed that if no acetabulum is present at birth, no femoral head will appear. These conclusions have been corroborated by a review of personal cases, consultations, and radiographs of over 200 cases of PFFD. When it is established that a femoral head is present, though ossification is delayed, a treatment programme based on the classification previously described can be initiated with confidence, achieving predictable results at an earlier time.

TREATMENT

Lack of pelvifemoral stability, malrotation and leg length inequality present as problem areas in treating PFFD (Bevan-Thomas and Millar, 1967; Aitken *et al.*, 1969; King, 1969; Scheer, 1972; King, 1973; Fixsen and Lloyd-Roberts, 1974; Lange *et al.*, 1978; Panting and Williams, 1978; Koman and Meyer, 1979; Kruger, 1980). These problems can be readily solved by the use of a non-standard prosthesis that includes a wide-

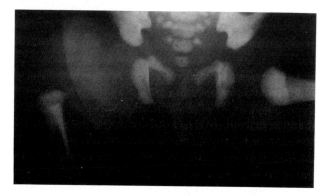

Fig. 8.2.7 Radiograph of a pelvis at birth, showing delay of ossification.

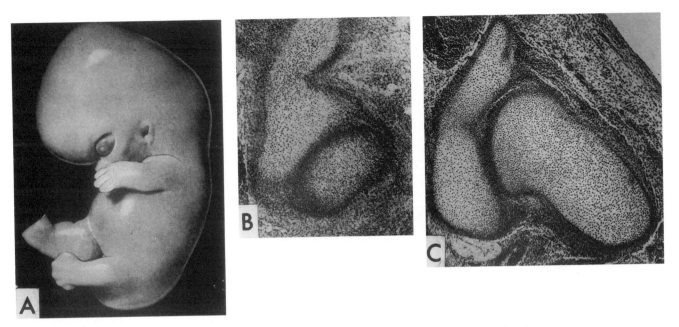

Fig. 8.2.9 A 17 mm embryo and development of the hip joint at this stage. (By kind permission of Luther Strayer.)

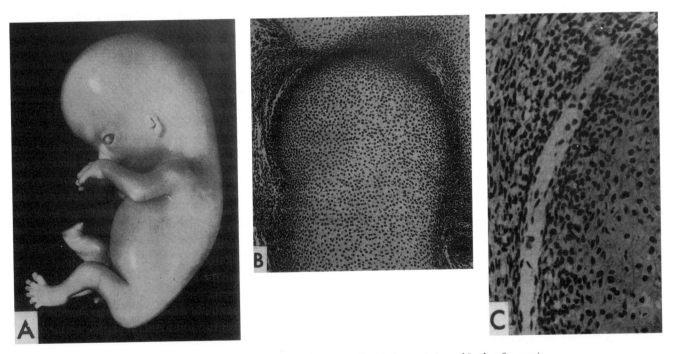

Fig. 8.2.10 A 22 mm embryo and development of the hip at this stage. (By kind permission of Luther Strayer.)

mouthed socket, a platform for support of the foot and outside knee joints (Fig. 8.2.11). Functionally and cosmetically, this prosthesis leaves much to be desired. Panting and Williams (1978) have described non-conventional orthotic and prosthetic devices which are currently being used to correct leg length inequality. Dissatisfaction with the functional and cosmetic aspects of these devices has led to an effort to develop and categorize operative means for each type of deformity.

The contractures of flexion, abduction and external rotation do not need preliminary stretching by traction or surgery. Correcting the elements of the femur to a single skeletal lever seems to relieve these contractures by the resultant shortening from the knee

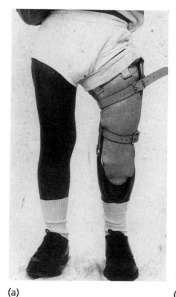

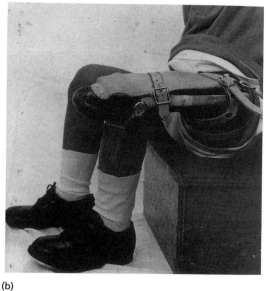

(a)   (b)

Fig. 8.2.11 (a) Standing and (b) sitting views of a patient with a pre-operative non-standard prosthesis.

arthrodesis and soft tissue stripping, particularly for type A (Gillespie and Torode, 1990). There appear to be four basic surgical problems: (i) the need for pelvifemoral stability; (ii) stabilization of the knee joint; (iii) presence of foot; and (iv) leg length inequality. In addition, the proximal musculature may be inadequate (Steel *et al.*, 1987). Usually some degree of resolution of these problems can be made by creation of a skeletal lever.

Generally, the surgical procedures outlined below are recommended.

Hip joint

There are four main procedures used on the hip joint in the operative correction of PFFD: (i) valgus subtrochanteric femoral osteotomy (type A); (ii) single skeletal lever (Fig. 8.2.12); (iii) metaphyseal–epiphyseal synostosis (type B) (Fig. 8.2.13); and (iv) Chiari osteotomy with fusion of the femoral segment to the pelvis (type D) (Fig. 8.2.14).

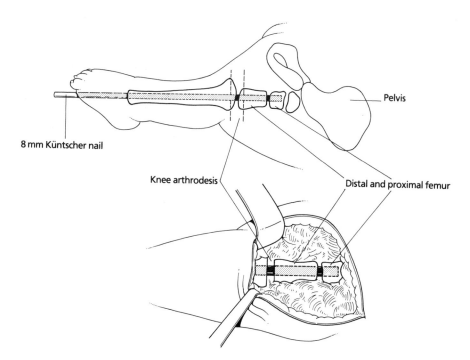

8 mm Küntscher nail

Pelvis

Knee arthrodesis

Distal and proximal femur

Fig. 8.2.12 Creation of a single skeletal lever and performance of knee arthrodesis.

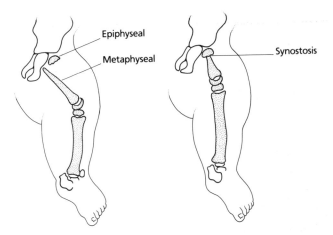

Fig. 8.2.13 Metaphyseal–epiphyseal synostosis.

Knee joint (Figs 8.2.15, 8.2.16, 8.2.17, 8.2.18 and 8.2.19)

Knee arthrodesis in extension is performed at the time of hip surgery and involves two principal procedures. First, articular cartilage is removed from both sides of the knee joint until the bony epiphysis is seen. This does not injure the physis. Secondly, central penetration of the physis of the proximal tibia and distal tibia and femur is performed by an 8 mm Kuntscher nail. The nail is passed retrogradely from the knee fusion site distally, to emerge out of the sole of the foot. The nail is then pushed across the area of knee fusion into the femoral segment.

Ankle and foot

Disarticulation at the ankle joint using the heel pad for end-bearing is done at the time of nail removal. This nail is removed when the knee arthrodesis is solid, usually at 4–6 weeks. Failure of fusion has not been seen using

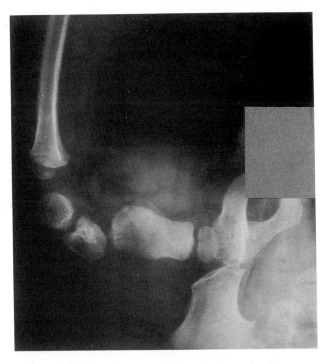

Fig. 8.2.15 Patient P.M. — pre-operative radiograph of type B PFFD.

this technique. Syme's amputation is essentially that described by Wood *et al.* (1965). Careful subperiosteal dissection of the calcaneum is essential to prevent breakdown of the septa of fibroelastic adipose tissue of the heel pad, which are essential for a good weight-bearing stump. The calcaneal apophysis must be removed separately with complete freeing of the Achilles tendon to prevent proximal and posterior migration of the heel pad. Suturing the anterior tibial and extensor tendons into the heel pad can prevent migration and obviate Kirschner wire fixation.

Alternatively, rotation plasty (Van Ness, 1950) can be performed in selected cases instead of Syme's

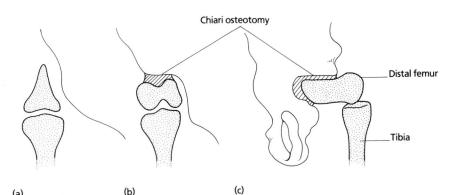

Fig. 8.2.14 Operation in some cases of type D PFFD to use knee as hip joint.

(a)　　　(b)　　　(c)

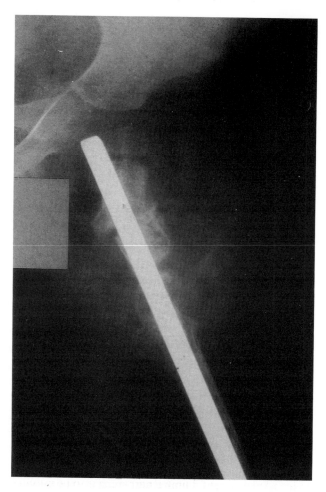

Fig. 8.2.16 Patient P.M. — final realignment of knee fusion and pseudarthrosis to make a single skeletal lever.

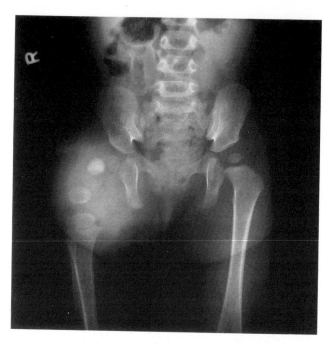

Fig. 8.2.17 Patient H.G. — type B PFFD, pre-operative.

amputation. This involves rotation of the foot 180° so that the toes point posteriorly; rotation is achieved at the distal one-third of the tibia (Fig. 8.2.20). This operation has two main advantages; it allows the foot in plantar flexion to extend the knee and in dorsiflexion to flex the knee, and there is added sensory feedback in the below-knee stump as opposed to the above-knee stump.

Rotation plasty however, has a number of disadvan-

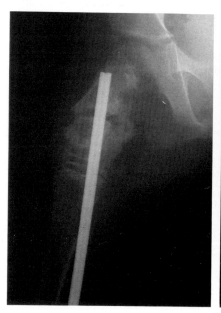
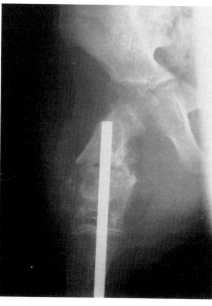

Fig. 8.2.18 Patient H.G. — post-operative, with intramedullary rod in place.

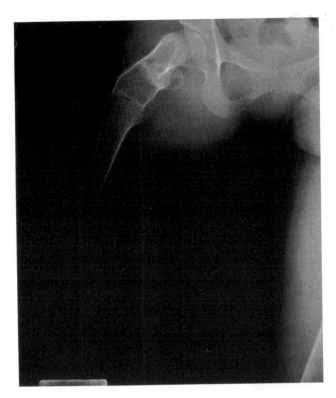

Fig. 8.2.19 Patient H.G. — at skeletal maturity following creation of a single skeletal lever.

tages. It is cosmetically ugly. Kostuik *et al.* (1975) removed toes from the rotated foot to make it more cosmetically acceptable, but this reduces the strength of the foot to move the prosthesis. A maximum of only 90° of flexion of the knee can be obtained, and kneeling is impossible. In addition, there is a tendency to derotate to the original position. This occurs every 3–5 years and requires re-rotation. Kostuik *et al.* (1975) advised doing rotation plasty after the age of 12 years because of re-rotation. The technique of Kritter (1977) tends to eliminate this and probably can be done in pre-school years. Finally, for the operation to be successful, the patient must have a fibula, normal foot and ankle, and preferably a stable hip (Kritter, 1977). (The fibula is absent in approximately 70% of cases of types B, C and D PFFD.) The Van Ness rotation plasty can be used only in unilateral PFFD.

Inequality of leg lengths

Leg length equality can be immediately achieved by application of a non-standard prosthesis. The constant rate of growth inhibition can be reasonably assessed by obtaining sequential scanograms and using Green–Anderson growth charts (Anderson *et al.*, 1963) or the Moseley straight-line graph. Thus, a reasonably accurate determination of the final leg length discrepancy can be made (Amstutz, 1969; Lange *et al.*, 1978; Koman and Meyer, 1979; Pappas and Arthur, 1985). This allows planning of leg length equalization procedures, including femoral lengthening (only if the patient has a stable hip and knee joint), concomitant femoral lengthening and shortening of the opposite femur and epiphyseal arrest of the opposite femur at a propitious time. These procedures apply mainly to type A PFFD, where the majority of patients will maintain a relatively constant 60–80% growth inhibition of the affected limb (Koman and Meyer, 1979). If the average skeletally mature femur measures 44 cm and the shortened femur has a 60% growth inhibition, the length at maturity will be 27 cm. This leaves a shortening of 17 cm, which is a safe maximum that can be accomplished by a series of lengthenings using the Wagner (1978) apparatus and beginning at the age of 8 years.

An alternative is femoral diaphyseal lengthening with the Ilizarov device; more than one lengthening may be required. Subluxation of the knee can be prevented by extending the frame across the knee joint (Figs 8.2.21 and 8.2.22). It is mandatory to have a stable hip and knee joint or disastrous consequences can follow. The parents of the child should be aware of the multiple operations required and the possibility that amputation might still be necessary. It is also essential that a plantigrade foot is present if limb lengthening is to be initiated. Indications for lengthening remain the same despite new diaphyseal lengthening techniques.

If there is more than 60% growth inhibition a knee fusion and Syme's amputation should be done early as previously described (p. 229). A subtrochanteric valgus osteotomy should be performed to correct any varus deformity of less than 100° present before leg lengthening. A 3 cm gain in length may occur with valgization osteotomy. Although the ultimate goal is equalization of leg lengths and adequate pelvifemoral stability, the placing of abnormal pressure on an already smaller femoral head must be avoided. Injudicious efforts to attain leg length equality at all costs can result in chondrolysis or subluxation of the femoral head.

The initial post-operative prosthesis is a non-standard ship ventilator-shaped socket, single-axis knee and solid-ankle cushion-heel foot. A pelvic band with hip control is used to control rotation. With time the ship ventilator shape of the thigh tends to disappear, so that a quadrilateral socket with a silesian bandage and without suction can be prescribed. With time a suction socket can be utilized.

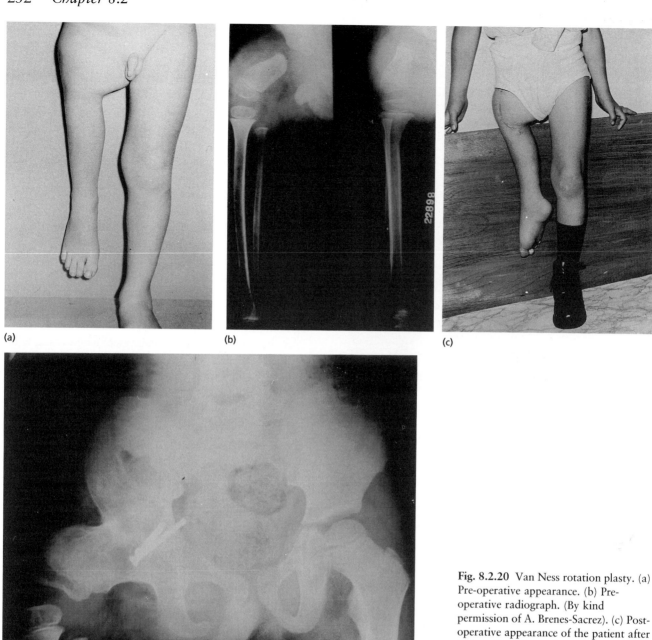

(a)

(b)

(c)

(d)

Fig. 8.2.20 Van Ness rotation plasty. (a) Pre-operative appearance. (b) Pre-operative radiograph. (By kind permission of A. Brenes-Sacrez). (c) Post-operative appearance of the patient after fusion of the femoral segment to the pelvis and Van Ness rotation plasty. (d) Radiograph showing fusion of the femoral segment to the pelvis. (By kind permission of A. Brenes-Sacrez).

Operations for PFFD

TYPE A

The indications for equalizing leg lengths have been described above. Realignment of the coxa vara by osteotomy may be needed for better mechanical leverage.

This should be done at the subtrochanteric level and the osteotomy site held by pins or internal fixation.

TYPE B

Knee fusion and realignment of the fragments to create a single skeletal lever are necessary. The author has not

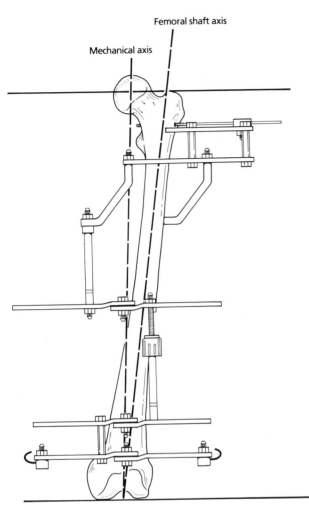

Fig. 8.2.21 Anteroposterior view of the femur with an Ilizarov frame applied.

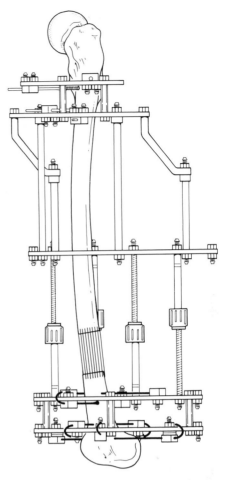

Fig. 8.2.22 Lateral view of the femur after diaphyseal lengthening.

felt that excision of the cartilaginous fragment to achieve bone-to-bone contact is needed. Bone formation occurs at the site of pseudarthrosis when converted to a single lever by arthrodesis of the knee, and bone grafting has not been necessary.

With maturity of the knee fusion (4–6 weeks), the Kuntscher nail is removed from the sole of the foot and a Syme's amputation is performed. The skeletal lever now becomes complete. Epiphysiodesis of the distal femoral epiphysis may be indicated if the projected end of the lever lies below the opposite knee joint.

Much has been said regarding the difficulty of early differentiation of types A and B PFFD (Fixsen and Lloyd-Roberts, 1974; Lange *et al.*, 1978). Push–pull radiographs and cineradiography have been advocated to determine the stability between the shaft of the femur and the hand and neck. Fixsen and Lloyd-Roberts (1974) have shown that the initial plain radiographic appear-

ance of the proximal femoral shaft is valuable in assessing future stability. Thus, three reliable indicators were described: (i) shaft length greater than half the normal side; (ii) presence of a bulbous proximal end; and (iii) absence of proximal femoral sclerosis. As the object is to create pelvifemoral stability, the author has not utilized these for prognostic purposes. As stated previously, magnetic resonance imaging is very useful in differentiating type A from type B PFFD.

If there is no continuity between shaft and head, metaphyseal–epiphyseal synostosis should be undertaken (King, 1973).

TYPE C

As no acetabulum and hence no femoral head are present, fusion of the knee can be used to create a skeletal lever. No attempt is made to create pelvifemoral stability. The femur usually presents as a long segment, and so the ankle joint lies at a level below the opposite knee joint. This will necessitate a below-knee amputation to bring the prosthetic knee joint to the same level. Epiphysiodesis may be needed to produce a stump 5–7.5 cm above the normal knee at maturity. Because the distal tibial epiphysis is sacrificed, this amputation should be done as near growth completion as possible to decrease the chance of overgrowth of the tibia and/or fibula. A non-conventional prosthesis incorporating the foot is used until the decision to amputate is considered, and the patient participates in this decision. These operations result in an above-knee amputation with improved cosmesis, though the patient loses some ability to run, which would be retained in a non-conventional prosthesis.

TYPE D

Limited success can be achieved in obtaining pelvi-femoral stability through a Chiari osteotomy and fusion with the femoral segment in 90° of flexion. This uses the knee joint as a functional hip joint and, coupled with a Van Ness rotation plasty, has offered improved ambulation and stability over using a non-conventional prosthesis. This operation should only be considered in a unilateral case, and it should be remembered that stability may be absent. The iliofemoral fusion may lead to fitting problems secondary to anterior prominence after iliofemoral fusion. Syme's amputation may be preferable to rotation plasty (Steel *et al.*, 1987).

Operation is contraindicated in bilateral cases (Aitken *et al.*, 1969; King, 1973; Aitken, 1975; Panting and Williams, 1978), particularly in the presence of any degree of absence of the upper extremities. Although ambulation is difficult and cumbersome, fitting these patients in non-conventional prostheses that retain the feet does correct the gross short stature. At home, these patients can walk without their prostheses.

Removal of the femoral segment has been advocated to place the tibia in closer relationship to the pelvis to achieve stability, to remove bulk for better prosthetic fitting, and through shortening to equalize prosthetic and normal knee centres (Bevan-Thomas and Millar, 1967). Wentzlaff (1969) in three cases felt that none of these were achieved.

Complications

BENDING OF THE STUMP IN THE PROSTHESIS
(Fig. 8.2.23)

This occurs when the patient has outgrown the prosthesis. The bending may occur as a result of excessive

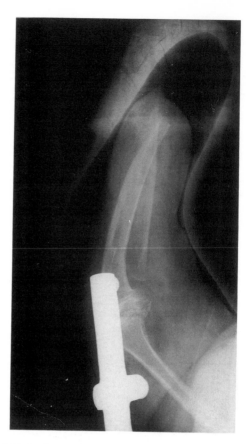

Fig. 8.2.23 Radiograph of a stump in a prosthesis to show bending.

pressure on the posterior aspect of the physis at the knee. This excessive pressure may occur posteriorly as a result of outgrowing the prosthesis and/or of constant pressure on this area of the epiphysis as the skeletal lever motivates the prosthesis. This results in compression and slowing of growth of the posterior aspect of the epiphysis at the knee, with resultant angulation (Heuter–Volkmann principle).

This condition can be corrected by a high osteotomy of the tibia and/or femur and reinsertion of a Kuntscher nail retrogradely down the tibia and out of the heel pad (Fig. 8.2.24). The osteotomy is held by a Kuntscher nail driven proximally across the tibial epiphysis, knee arthrodesis, femoral epiphysis and into the femur. Once the osteotomy is solid, the nail can be withdrawn under local analgesia.

PREMATURE CLOSURE OF THE PROXIMAL AND DISTAL TIBIAL OR DISTAL FEMORAL EPIPHYSIS BY CENTRAL PENETRATION OF THE INTRAMEDULLARY NAIL

No cases have been seen using an 8 mm Kuntscher rod with central penetration of the epiphyses.

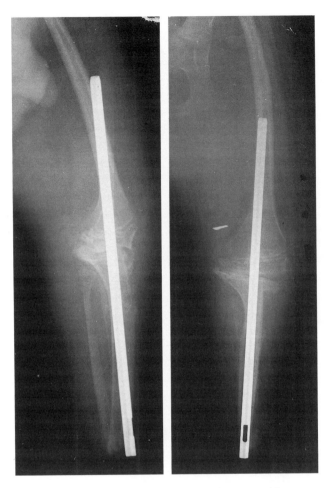

Fig. 8.2.24 Osteotomy of the tibia with realignment of fragments over an 8 mm intramedullary nail.

RE-ROTATION OF THE VAN NESS ROTATION PLASTY

The feet seem to turn back gradually to the original position in about 5 years (Kostuik *et al.*, 1975). This can be corrected by another osteotomy so that the foot points posteriorly. The technique of Kritter (1977) seems to have eliminated this.

POSTERIOR MIGRATION OF THE HEEL PAD IN SYME'S AMPUTATION

This tendency can be lessened by complete removal of the calcaneal apophysis and complete transection of the Achilles tendon attachment. The circulation to the heel flap should not be jeopardized, however, to excise an apophysis that is already displaced high into the posterior and distal one-third of the leg. In these instances the apophysis and Achilles tendon should be left to

migrate; migration in such cases has not been excessive. Suture of the anterior tibial and extensor tendons into the heel pad decreases the tendency to posterior migration.

Unexpected benefits

Trochanteric apophyses have appeared in response to the function of skeletal levers. With maturity and function of the stump the ship ventilator-shaped prosthesis has gradually given way to a quadrilateral socket without suction, and silesian bandage for suspension to a quadrilateral closed end-socket with suction for suspension. Growth of the femoral head and increased circumferential growth of the skeletal lever has had positive benefits. Liposuction may prove useful in decreasing the circumference of the proximal thigh in adolescents or older patients (Kruger, 1990) (Fig. 8.2.25).

CONCLUSIONS

An attempt has been made to use a classification system for PFFD, developed by Aitken *et al.* (1969), that allows for a planned operative approach for each of the four types identified. If an acetabulum is present a femoral head can be expected to develop. Histologically, the material between the proximal and distal femoral elements represents dormant cartilage awaiting mechanical realignment to complete its transformation to bone.

Each case should be evaluated separately, and the type of operative conversion best suited to the elements of the proximal femur present should be performed. It has not been found necessary to correct the contractures by a separate procedure. In the conversions described the contractures of flexion, abduction and external rotation are probably released through the soft tissue dissection and femoral shortening associated with the knee fusion performed at the same time. These conversions should be done as early as possible, preferably between 2 and 3 years of age, to allow maximum remodelling of the proximal femur to occur. The principle of establishing a single skeletal lever by alignment of fragments over an intramedullary rod has thus far proved sound. It has provided pelvifemoral and skeletal stability of the femoral segment, on which existing musculature can act to operate a prosthesis. No closure of physeal lines has been noticed due to the central penetration for epiphyseal plates by an intramedullary rod.

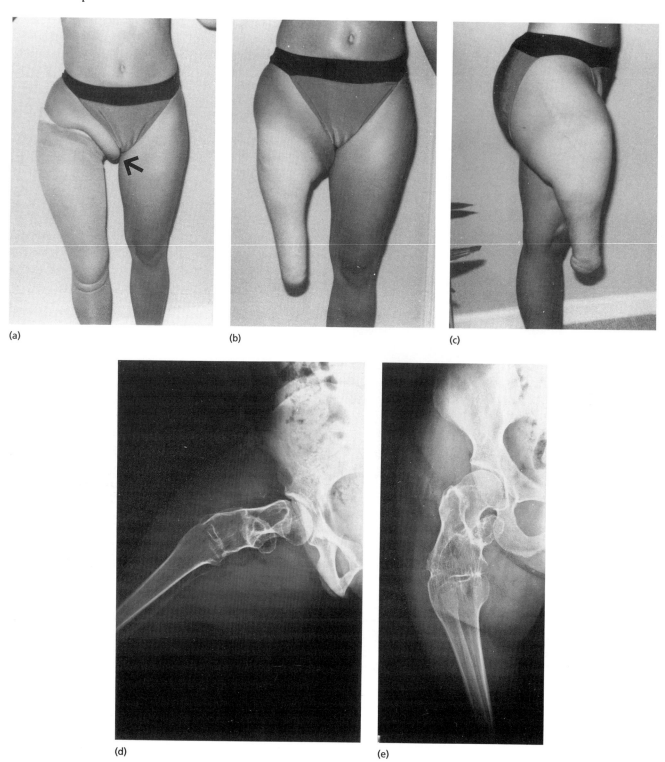

(a)

(b)

(c)

(d)

(e)

Fig. 8.2.25 A 23-year-old woman following knee arthrodesis and Syme's amputation for PFFD. (a–c) Pre-operative appearance with prominent adductor roll. (d, e) Mature arthrodesis with congruous hip and excellent hip function.

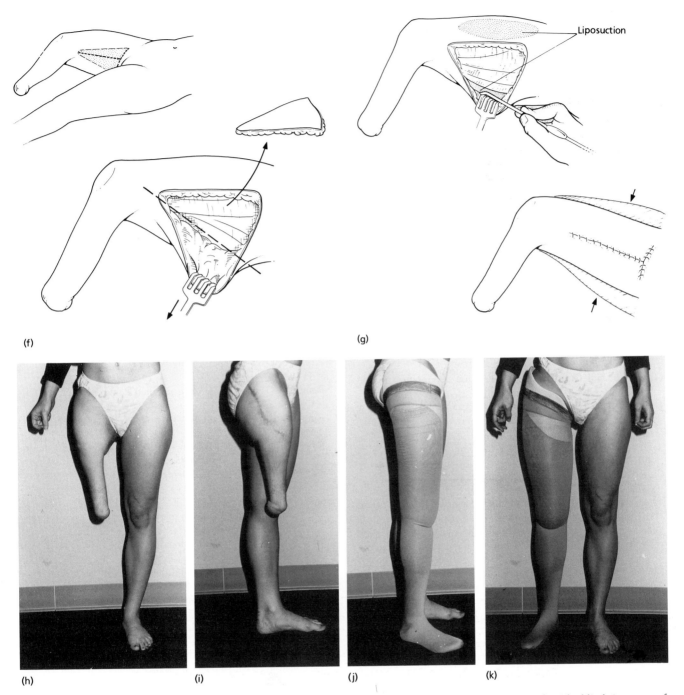

(f)

(g)

(h)

(i)

(j)

(k)

Fig. 8.2.25 (*continued*) (f, g) Operative procedure — medial thigh reduction, lateral scar revision, liposuction of residual limb (courtesy of F.D. Burstein). (h–k) Post-operative appearance and prosthesis fit after removal of 400 ml of fat through liposuction and excision of 40 cm^2 of redundant medial thigh skin.

REFERENCES

Aitken G.T. (1975) Congenital lower limb deficiencies. In American Academy of Orthopedic Surgeons. *Instruction Course Lectures.* St. Louis, C.V. Mosby, vol. 24.

Aitken G.T. (1969) Proximal femoral focal deficiency — definition, classification and management. Symposium, Washington, D.C., National Academy of Sciences.

Amstutz H.C. (1969) The morphology, natural history and treatment of proximal femoral focal deficiency. Symposium, Washington, D.C., National Academy of Sciences.

Amstutz H.C. and Wilson P.D. Jr. (1962) Dysgenesis of the proximal femur (coxa vara) and its surgical management. *J. Bone Joint Surg.* **44A**, 1.

Anderson M., Green W.T. and Messner M.B. (1963) Growth and predictions of the lower extremities. *J. Bone Joint Surg.* **45A**, 1–14.

Bevan-Thomas W.H. and Millar E. (1967) A review of proximal femoral focal deficiencies. *J. Bone Joint Surg.* **49A**, 1376.

Epps C.H. Jr. (1983) Proximal femoral focal deficiency — current concepts. *J. Bone Joint Surg.* **65A**, 768–870.

Fixsen J.A. and Lloyd-Roberts G.D. (1974) The natural history and early treatment of proximal femoral dysplasia. *J. Bone Joint Surg.* **56B**, 86.

Freund E. (1936) Congenital defects of femur, fibula and tibia. *Arch. Surg.* **33**, 349.

Gardner E. and Gray D.J. (1950) Prenatal development of the human hip joint. *Am. J. Anat.* **87**, 163.

Gillespie R. and Torode I.P. (1983) Classification and management of congenital abnormalities of the femur. *J. Bone Joint Surg.* **65B**, 557–568.

Golding R.C. (1948) Congenital coxa vara. *J. Bone Joint Surg.* **30B**, 161.

Hamanishi C. (1980) Congenital short femur. *J. Bone Joint Surg.* **62B**, 307.

Harrison T.J. (1961) The influence of the femoral head on pelvic growth and acetabular form in the rat. *J. Anat.* **95**, 12.

Hillman J.S., Mesgarzadeh M., Revesz G., Bonakdarpour A., Clancy M. and Betz R.R. (1987) Proximal femoral focal deficiency — radiologic analysis of 49 cases. *Radiology* **165**, 769–773.

King R.E. (1964) Proximal femoral focal deficiencies. *Int. Clin. Inform. Bull.* **3**, 1.

King R.E. (1969) Some concepts of proximal femoral focal deficiency. Symposium, Washington, D.C., National Academy of Sciences.

King R.E. (1973) Proximal femoral focal deficiencies. In Tronzo R. (ed) *Surgery of the Hip Joint*, 1st edn. Philadelphia, Lea and Febiger, Ch. 6.

Koman A. and Meyer L. (1979) Current management of proximal femoral focal deficiency. Paper presented to the American Academy of Orthopedic Surgeons, San Francisco, 1979.

Kostuik J.P., Gillespie R. and Hall J.E. (1975) Van Ness rotational osteotomy for treatment of proximal femoral deficiency and congenital short femur. *J. Bone Joint Surg.* **57A**, 1039.

Kritter A.E. (1977) Tibial rotation-plasty for proximal femoral focal deficiency. *J. Bone Joint Surg.* **59A**, 927.

Kruger L. (1980) Lower limb deficiencies. *Clin. Orthop.* **148**, 97.

Kruger L.M. and Stone P.A. (1990) Suction assisted lipectomy — an adjunct to orthopaedic treatment. *J. Pediatr. Orthop.* **10**, 53–57.

Lange D.R., Schoenecker P.L. and Baker C. (1978) Proximal femoral focal deficiency. *Clin. Orthop.* **135**, 15.

Langston H.H. (1939) Congenital defect of the shaft of the femur. *Br. J. Surg.* **27**, 162.

Laurenson R.D. (1964) Bilateral anomalous development of the hip joint. Post mortem study of a human fetus twenty-six weeks old. *J. Bone Joint Surg.* **46A**, 283.

Lloyd-Roberts G.C. and Stone K.H. (1963) Congenital hypoplasia of the upper femur. *J. Bone Joint Surg.* **45B**, 557.

Nilsonne H. (1928) Uber den kongenitalen Femur Defekt. *Arch. Orthop. Unfallchir.* **26**, 138.

O'Rahilly R. (1951) Morphological patterns in limb deficiencies and duplications. *Am. J. Anat.* **89**, 135.

Panting A.L. and Williams P.F. (1978) Proximal femoral focal deficiency. *J. Bone Joint Surg.* **60B**, 46.

Pappas A.M. (1983) Congenital abnormalities of the femur and related lower extremity, malformations. *J. Pediatr. Orthop.* **3**, 45–60.

Reiner M. (1901) Uber den kongenitalen Femurdefekt. *Z. Orthop. Chir.* **9**, 544.

Ring P.A. (1959) Congenital short femur. *J. Bone Joint Surg.* **41B**, 73.

Scheer G.B. (1972) Treatment of proximal focal femoral deficiencies. *Clin. Orthop.* **85**, 292.

Sideman S. (1963) Agenesis femur: report of case. *J. Int. Coll. Surg.* **40**, 152.

Steel H.H., Lin P.S., Betz R.R., Kalamchi A. and Clancy M. (1987) Iliofemoral fusion for proximal femoral focal deficiency. *J. Bone Joint Surg.* **69A**, 837–843.

Strayer L. Jr. (1943) Embryology of the hip joint. *Yale J. Biol. Med.* **16**, 13.

Strayer L. Jr. (1950) Congenital deformities of lower extremity. *Proc. Am. Acad. Orthop. Surg.* **7**, 100.

Van Ness C.P. (1950) Rotation-plasty for congenital defects of femur. *J. Bone Joint Surg.* **32B**, 12.

Wagner H. (1978) Operative lengthening of the femur. *Clin. Orthop.* **136**, 125.

Wentzlaff E.F. (1969) Surgical ablation of the remaining femoral segment in proximal femoral focal deficiency. *Int. Clin. Inform. Bull.* **9**, 1.

Wood W.C., Zlotsky N. and Westin G.W. (1965) Congenital absence of the fibula. *J. Bone Joint Surg.* **47A**, 1159–1169.

Congenital Pseudarthrosis of the Tibia

S.S. Coleman

INTRODUCTION

Congenital pseudarthrosis of the tibia is one of the most enigmatic conditions that faces the paediatric orthopaedic surgeon. Hatzoecher is given credit by Henderson and Clegg (1941) as being the first to describe this unusual problem, and the difficulties in treating it have persisted and remained a major challenge ever since. It exhibits capricious behaviour, its true aetiology is unknown, it manifests itself in many different ways, and it is unpredictable in response to conventional treatment of almost any sort. These frustrations in the past led to amputation of the foot in many patients. For example, Murray and Lovell (1982) published a report on 26 patients followed to near skeletal maturity, and 12 underwent amputation. Recent advances, however, have provided more promising results, though by no means has the therapeutic challenge become simplified. It is the purpose of this chapter to review some of the theories of aetiology, past programmes of treatment, current advances in treatment and future therapeutic considerations.

AETIOLOGY

Theories of the aetiology are numerous, but the exact cause is unknown. Such suggestions as intrauterine trauma, localized vascular abnormalities of the tibia, and constriction due to proliferating fibrous tissue have never been proved. Although associated with neurofibromatosis, a cause and effect relationship has not been established. Causal relationships to localized lesions, e.g. fibrous dysplasia and other benign intraosseous lesions, have been too inconsistent to have any validity. Studies of the removed tissue at the ultrastructural and electron microscopic level have been inconclusive.

CLASSIFICATION

There is no widely agreed, clear-cut classification. The reasons are related to the multiplicity of factors that have some bearing on the cause of this disorder. Most of the classifications are descriptive in character, and except for the following three issues they have no appreciable bearing on either the method of treatment or its outcome. These three substantial factors are: (i) the location of the pseudarthrosis (mid-shaft or lower third); (ii) presence or absence of neurofibromatosis; and (iii) whether the tibia and fibula are both involved in the process.

One important feature of the lesion is whether the abnormality represents pre-pseudarthrosis (anterolateral bow without fracture) or whether a true fracture exists with failure of union and pathological evidence of pseudarthrosis. Clearly, the presence of a deformed but intact tibia and fibula requires different treatment from that for established pseudarthrosis. These different manifestations will be discussed in greater detail with regard to treatment. From a practical standpoint, the above description and classification of the abnormalities in this condition, at least for treatment and prognosis, is as good as any yet promulgated.

TREATMENT

Past therapeutic programmes have almost exhausted all possible methods of achieving osteosynthesis. These have included dual onlay grafts held with screw fixation, (Boyd, 1941) osteotomy and reversal of the entire tibial shaft (Safield and Millar, 1959), 'bypass' grafts taken from the opposite tibia (Mcfarland, 1959), allograft bone, homograft bone, intramedullary rodding (Charnley, 1956), pedicled cross-legged bone graft from the normal tibia to the pseudarthrosis (Farmer, 1952), iliac isograft with intramedullary rodding (Umber *et al.*, 1982), contralateral fibular graft by microvascular technique, ipsilateral fibular pedicled graft (Coleman and Coleman, 1991; Coleman, unpublished data), 'bone transport' techniques (Paley *et al.*, 1990), and various forms of electrical stimulation (Brighton *et al.*, 1975; Bassett *et al.*, 1981; Paterson and Simonis, 1985). At the present time there is simply no procedure that has proved over time to have a clear advantage over any other. As with all complex and difficult problems searching for a solution, however, it is helpful to outline the current most attractive treatment programmes and to attempt to put them into perspective.

Treatment of pre-pseudarthrosis

Pre-pseudarthrosis, which most commonly manifests as a congenital anterolateral bow of the tibia, is the precursor of congenital pseudarthrosis (Fig. 8.2.26). Two features determine treatment: (i) whether the tibia is intact and can be effectively braced for a substantial period of time; and (ii) osteotomy should be avoided if possible; there is a real risk or non-union. A well-fitting,

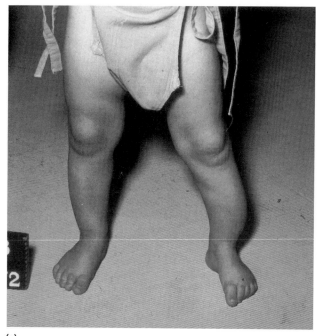

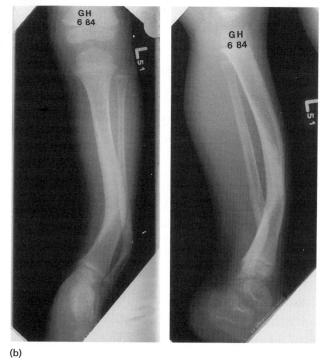

(a)

(b)

Fig. 8.2.26 (a) Typical clinical appearance of pre-pseudarthrosis or congenital anterolateral tibial bow in a 2-year-old boy. (b) Radiographs in another 4-year-old boy.

is essential after osteotomy of the tibia (see p. 245).

Pseudarthrosis follows spontaneous fracture of the deformed tibia, or it may complicate osteotomy (Fig. 8.2.27).

Earlier treatment procedures

Several methods of treatment utilized in the past have been discarded because of conceptual or technical shortcomings. It is important that these be properly relegated to history. The 'reversal' of the tibial shaft (Sofield *et al.*, 1959) was based upon the concept that by reversing the diaphysis of the tibia, good healthy proximal metaphyseal bone would replace the less osteogenic bone at the level of the more distal pseudarthrosis. Failure was common, and this operation is discredited. Dual onlay grafts held by transfixion screws, particularly when allografts were employed, experienced a similar high

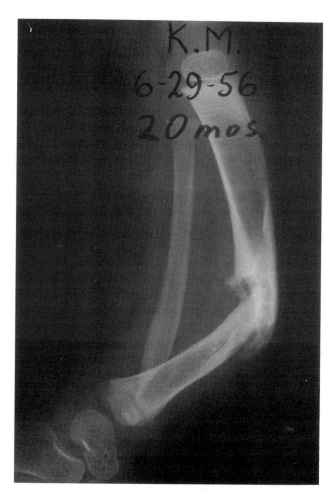

Fig. 8.2.27 Lateral radiograph showing the typical anterolateral bow, wherein a recent fracture at the apex of the bow has occurred. This particular patient had neurofibromatosis.

properly fabricated polypropylene splint is the most acceptable form of treatment for a deformed tibia that is still intact. The child wears the splint whenever up and about, and it must be adjusted with growth. This splint rate of failure of union or re-fracture through screw holes, even if union was achieved. Cross-legged full thickness vascularized skin and bone grafts (Farmer, 1952) never gained popularity because of the complex nature of the procedure and the unpredictable results obtained. The 'bypass' graft described by McFarland (1959) has had a chequered history. It does not directly correct the deformity, and few satisfactory long-term results have been reported. Furthermore, it appears most appropriate for congenital anterolateral bow before the development of true pseudarthrosis.

Current treatment procedures

Because of these dismal results, requiring repeated procedures and often leading to amputation, other operations have gained popularity. Unfortunately, there is still confusion about the best form of treatment, and long-term proven results are lacking. These other forms of treatment are now discussed.

INTRAMEDULLARY PROCEDURES

Intramedullary tibial rodding, utilizing autogenous iliac bone grafting as described by Charnley (1956) was one of the major advances in the currently accepted programmes of operative treatment. Charnley showed that intramedullary fixation eliminated stress-risers, permitted impaction of the fragments, and stabilized short distal fragments by placing the rod across the ankle and subtalar joints. Several recent successful series have been based on these biomechanical and biological concepts.

Intramedullary fixation and autogenous bone grafting, currently popular in the USA, was introduced by Williams (1965), who used the rodding technique for correction of the deformities in osteogenesis imperfecta. The technique was easily adapted to congenital pseudarthrosis (Fig. 8.2.28). By placing the rod through the distal fragment of the tibia, across the ankle through the talus and calcaneum, and then out through the heel, it is possible to pass the rod proximally (retrogradely) into the proximal tibial fragment under careful radiographic control. The proximal portion of the rod crosses the central portion of the proximal tibial physis and is firmly embedded into the proximal epiphysis. A smooth rod reduces the risk of injury to the physis. The rod can be left in the distal tibial epiphysis, or in the case of a short distal tibial fragment, it can lie within the calcaneum, crossing both ankle and subtalar joints. As noted earlier, the rod inevitably migrates proximally out of the tarsal bones and into the tibia (Fig. 8.2.29).

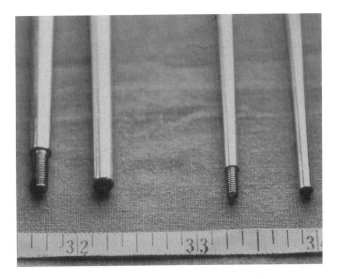

Fig. 8.2.28 Male and female ends of the rods developed by Williams of Australia. Three different sizes and lengths are available (special order).

Recently, Anderson *et al.* (1990) have added a variation wherein a small portion of methylmethacrylate is placed about the proximal (metaphyseal) portion of the rod in order to give greater assurance that the rod will advance proximally (with growth). Long-term follow-up of this modification is not yet available.

RESECTION

Resection of the pseudarthrosis, together with a generous segment of the tibia on either side of the lesion, is based on the concept that the bone and its vasculature are both defective. The resected segment is replaced by an appropriate length of the contralateral fibula, along with its nutrient artery, utilizing a microvascular technique, i.e. the nutrient artery and vein of the donor fibula are anastomosed to available vessels of the abnormal leg. This technique was originally developed in Shanghai, and has been utilized by several groups in the USA, notably that of Weiland (Weiland, 1980; Weiland *et al.*, 1990). Although there have been noteworthy successes with this procedure, there are several negative conceptual features. First, the contralateral normal limb is rendered a 'one-bone' leg. Secondly, the long-term effects on the otherwise normal ankle joint have not been described. These concerns relate principally to the development of ankle valgus due to altered growth of the remnant of distal fibula. As a result of the lack of bony continuity of the fibula, normal stress patterns are not exerted across the ankle mortice (Fig. 8.2.30).

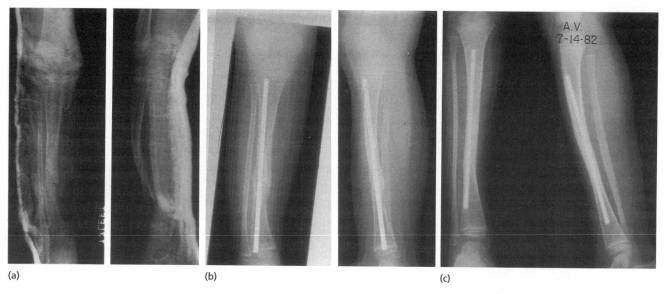

(a)   (b)   (c)

Fig. 8.2.29 Radiographs showing a satisfactory result following treatment by a Williams intramedullary rod and iliac bone grafting. (a) Mid-shaft tibial fracture through pre-existing anterior bow in a 20-month-old boy. (b) Solid union 3 months later. (c) Eighteen months later, at age 3.5 years, persistence of union is evident. Note the growth of the limb as evidenced by the migration of the rod away from the physis.

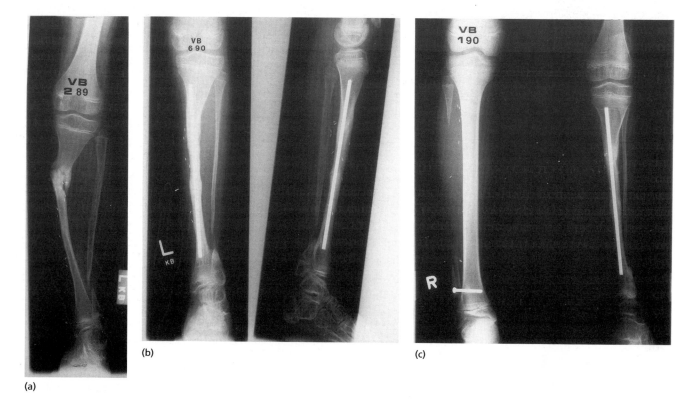

(a)   (b)   (c)

Fig. 8.2.30 Microvascular contralateral fibular graft to replace tibial pseudarthrosis. (a) Failure of the union of proximal anastomosis. (b) This was treated with a Williams intramedullary rod, which produced solid union. (c) Note absence of diaphysis of the opposite fibula and early valgus configuration of the ankle joint.

FIBULAR TRANSPOSITION

Recently, it has been proposed that the ipsilateral fibula be transposed to the adjacent tibia, preserving the vasculature of the fibula by means of a pedicle (Coleman and Coleman, 1991; Coleman, personal communication). The fibula is mobilized at the level of the pseudarthrosis and is transferred and applied to the denuded lateral aspect of the tibia above and below the pseudarthrosis.

It is fixed to the tibia by cerclage wires. A small series of patients shows promising results (Fig. 8.2.31). The major advantage of this technique over that previously described is that the normal contralateral leg is not violated, and a well-vascularized ipsilateral fibula is put to good use. In all cases, synostosis of the distal tibia and fibula is performed in order to prevent the development of ankle valgus and to maintain a horizontal ankle mortice.

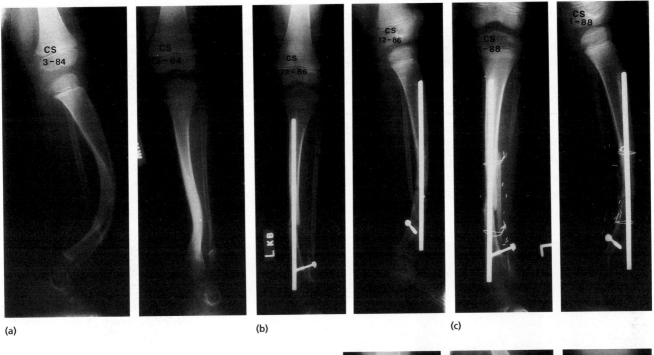

(a)　　　　　　　　　　(b)　　　　　　　　　(c)

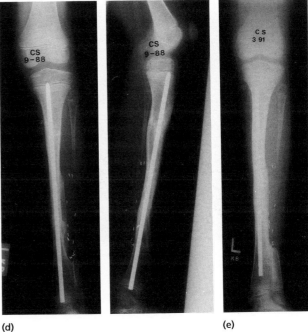

(d)　　　　　　　　　(e)

Fig. 8.2.31 Ipsilateral pedicled fibular graft. (a) Radiograph of the tibia of 4-year-old boy showing the anterolateral (pre-pseudarthrosis) deformity of the tibia with associated pseudarthrosis of the fibula. (b) The patient had neurofibromatosis and the small fibular fragments did not lend themselves well to intramedullary rodding, and therefore synostosis of the distal tibia and fibula was accomplished, in addition to intramedullary rodding and iliac bone grafting of the tibia. (c) Because of failure of tibial union, the ipsilateral fibula was transferred to the tibia, leaving the vascular pedicle intact. (d) The tibial rod was changed, which necessitated proximal tibial osteotomy, but 9 months after the fibular transfer, solid union was evident. (e) Progressive strengthening of the tibial union and acceptable ankle configuration was evident 2.5 years later.

BONE TRANSPORT

There have been several recent reports wherein the Ilizarov principle of 'bone transport' has been employed. In these cases, no substantial invasive procedure is utilized. An osteotomy employing the corticotomy principle is done in the proximal portion of the involved tibia. The Ilizarov technique is used to compress the proximal and distal fragments of the pseudarthrosis (Paley *et al.*, 1990). This compressive effect appears to provide a stimulus to union of the pseudarthrosis, and as the proximal fragment is displaced distally during compression, the proximal corticotomy distraction site is replaced by 'regenerate' bone (Fig. 8.2.32). Correction of any angular deformity can be accomplished at the same time. This is a very attractive approach to a complex problem, but there are several major concerns that must be addressed. These include the lack of long-term evaluation of union of the pseudarthrosis and attention to any fibular abnormality; the technological aspects require substantial sophistication. Furthermore, there is no internal splinting such as that provided by an intramedullary rod to prevent or discourage re-fracture.

This bone transport and compression programme must await longer follow-up before it can be accepted as the most appropriate long-term solution of the treatment of congenital tibial pseudarthrosis.

ELECTRICAL STIMULATION

Several investigators have reported superior results with the addition of one or more methods of electrical stimulation (Brighton *et al.*, 1975; Bassett *et al.*, 1981; Paterson and Simonis, 1985). It has produced rather disappointing results unless correction of deformity by intramedullary rodding and bone grafting has been accomplished either before or in conjunction with the electrical stimulation. As the rate of success is high even without electrical stimulation, it is difficult to assess its true value in treatment of congenital pseudarthrosis.

Coexisting fibular pseudarthrosis

Fibular pseudarthrosis has not been given sufficient attention in the description of most treatment regimens. Fibular pseudarthrosis with an intact tibia leads to pro-

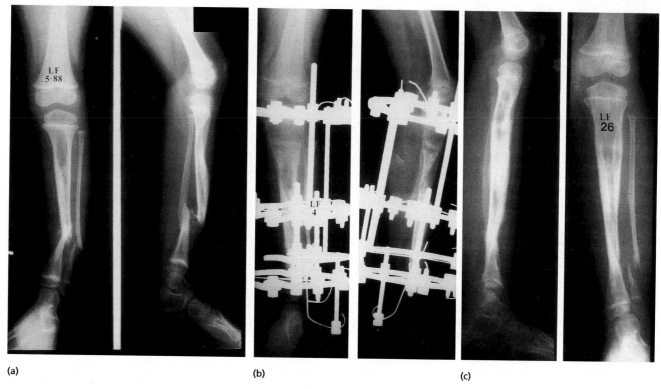

(a)   (b)   (c)

Fig. 8.2.32 Congenital tibial pseudarthrosis treated by the Ilizarov technique. (a) Pseudarthrosis of both tibia and fibula. (b) The large number of circular devices used, with the transfixion wires. (c) Final result (to date) shows solid union of the tibial pseudarthrosis, the persistent presence of the fibular pseudarthrosis and ankle valgus. (Case example and radiographs courtesy of Dr Dror Paley, Baltimore, Maryland, USA.)

gressive ankle valgus, with tilt of the tibial plafond and hypoplasia of the lateral aspect of the distal tibial epiphysis. The methods of managing this problem include: (i) intramedullary rod with bone grafting of the fibula at the same time as the tibia is treated; (ii) securing synostosis of the distal tibia and fibula if the fibula does not lend itself to intramedullary rodding (e.g. medullary cavity too small, as is often seen in neurofibromatosis); (iii) stapling of the medial distal tibial physis, an unproven and unpredictable practice; and, (iv) corrective osteotomy of the distal tibia. The author's preference is to perform synostosis if union of the fibula cannot be accomplished (Fig. 8.2.33). The aim is a stable ankle mortice, with a horizontal tibial plafond.

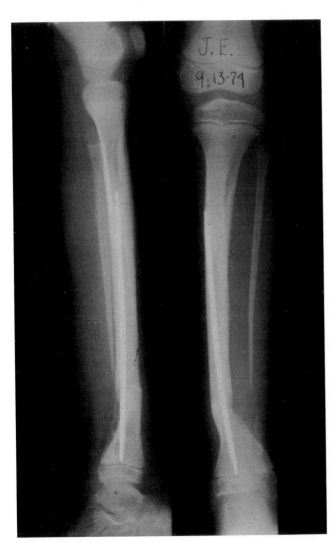

Fig. 8.2.33 The need for distal tibiofibular synostosis is well illustrated in this 10-year-old girl whose fibula is clearly atrophic. Although solid tibial union is the primary goal, preservation of the ankle mortice is also very important.

Post-operative care

The author's post-operative care following conventional intramedullary rodding and autogenous iliac bone grafting consists of applying a 1½ hip spica cast for 3 months. The patient is not allowed to weight-bear and is kept recumbent. The cast is removed and as long as the rod is in its proper position and alignment of the tibia has been maintained, a well-moulded above-knee polypropylene brace is applied and ambulation is permitted, even if clear-cut union has not occurred (Fig. 8.2.34). If the rod has been placed across the ankle and subtalar joint (short distal tibial segment), a solid ankle in the brace is also prescribed. If the rod can be contained in the tibia, then a free ankle and free knee is fabricated into the brace. This brace must be worn for the full growing period of the child. Modifications in length and fit of the brace must be made as needed.

Depending on the age at which union is achieved, the child may outgrow the rod, and periodically it must be replaced. It is essential that it is not removed without being replaced. In the author's experience the internal splint provided by the rod plays an essential role

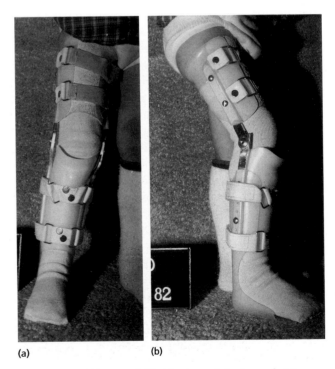

(a)   (b)

Fig. 8.3.34 (a) Front and (b) side views of the brace that is preferred for protection of the tibia before fracture or operation, or for use after the operative procedure and the removal of the cast. The basic orthotic principle is that the very snug fitting pretibial polypropylene shell can be firmly compressed against the anterior aspect of the tibia by Velcro starps.

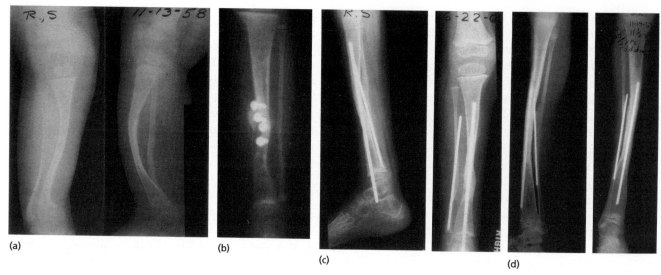

(a)   (b)   (c)   (d)

Fig. 8.2.35 (a) Initial radiograph in a 1-year-old boy with anterolateral bow. (b) A dual onlay graft (maternal bone donor) was a failure. (c) Radiographs of the results of intramedullary rodding and iliac bone grafting 18 months later. Note that the rod is across the ankle and subtalar joints. (d) Nearly 9 years later the tibia and fibula remain united, and the original rods placed several years earlier are now completely contained within the medullary cavities.

in maintenance of correction and guarding against refracture. Usually the rod slowly migrates proximally with growth and ascends from the calcaneum and talus across the ankle joint (Fig. 8.2.35).

If the tibial pseudarthrosis does not unite after rodding and bone grafting, the vascularized ipsilateral fibula can be transferred to the tibia, to bridge the pseudarthrosis. By mobilizing the central three-fifths of the fibula on its vascular pedicle, the fibula can easily be transferred to the tibia and displaced distally so that it bridges the pseudarthrosis and is held there by cerclage wires. The opposing surfaces of the tibia and fibula are sub-periosteally exposed and 'fish scaled'. Autogenous iliac bone is used to reinforce the osteogenic capacity, and tibiofibular synostosis is necessary (Fig. 8.2.33). The intramedullary rod is replaced if appropriate. The cast and brace programme is followed as described above. This programme should be employed before utilization of the contralateral fibula as a microvascular transfer, for the reasons mentioned earlier. The procedure of using the contralateral fibula should be used only when the final option is amputation of the foot after failure of the pedicled ipsilateral fibula transfer.

AMPUTATION

Fortunately, amputation is not often indicated, though there will be an occasional instance when successful preservation of an acceptable and serviceable limb will be best served by removal of the foot at the ankle. The major reasons that lead to this unattractive conclusion are: (i) excessive shortening of the limb due to multiple failed attempts at union; (ii) unacceptable shortening and poor configuration of the foot and poor function of the ankle; and (iii) the request of the parents and child due to 'therapeutic fatigue' (Fig. 8.2.36).

If the foot is removed it should be done by means of disarticulation through the ankle utilizing Syme's principle. An end-bearing stump is created. The pseudarthrosis (properly treated as described before) eventually unites (Fig. 8.2.36). Transmedullary amputation inevitably leads to the need for periodic revisions due to 'overgrowth' of the amputated ends of the transected bone. It should, therefore, be avoided (Fig. 8.2.37).

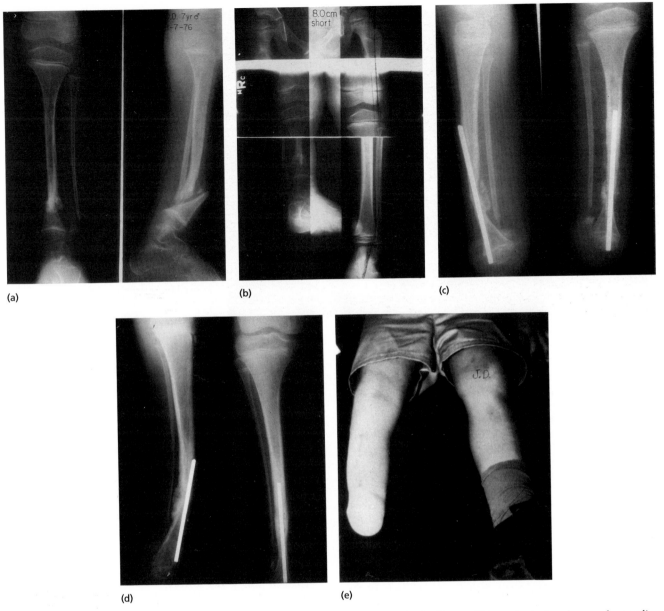

(a)

(b)

(c)

(d)

(e)

Fig. 8.2.36 The rare need for amputation of the foot is illustrated in this radiograph of a 7-year-old boy who had undergone four earlier procedures designed to gain union of the tibia. (a) Atrophy, overriding and obvious pseudarthrosis. (b) Orthoradiograph shows over 7.5 cm of shortening, and the foot was exceedingly small and atrophic. Amputations of the foot was requested by the parents because of excessive shortening, atrophy, small size of foot, and 'therapeutic fatigue'. (c) Eighteen months later the amputation can be seen together with early union of the tibia. (d) Six years later the tibia was solidly united. (e) The end-bearing disarticulation stump (Syme's principle).

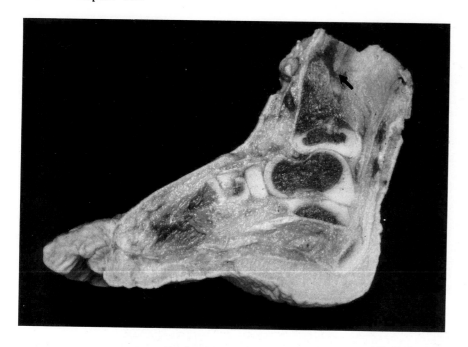

Fig. 8.2.37 Gross specimen of a transmedullary amputation for congenital pseudarthrosis of the tibia. The area of pseudarthrosis is shown by the arrow. This is a much less desirable method of amputation than ankle disarticulation, because of the common need for revisions and the inferior type of prosthesis (non-end-bearing) compared with Syme's principle.

REFERENCES

Anderson D.J., Schoenecker P.L., Rich M.M. *et al.* (1990) The use of the Peter Williams intramedullary rod in treatment of congenital pseudarthrosis of the tibia. *Orthop. Trans.* **14**, 638.

Boyd H.B. (1941) Congenital pseudarthrosis. Treatment by dual bone grafts. *J. Bone Joint Surg.* **23**, 497–510.

Bassett C.A., Caulo N. and Kort J. (1981) Congenital pseudarthrosis of the tibia: treatment with pulsed magnetic fields. *Clin. Orthop. Rel. Res.* **154**, 136–149.

Brighton C.T., Friedenberg Z.B. *et al.* (1975) Direct current stimulation of non-union and congenital pseudarthrosis. *J. Bone Joint Surg.* **57A**, 368–377.

Charnley J. (1956) Congenital pseudarthrosis of the tibia treated by intramedullary nail. *J. Bone Joint Surg.* **38A**, 283–290.

Coleman D.A. and Coleman S.S. (1991) Congenital pseudarthrosis of the tibia with ipsilateral fibular graft. *Orthop. Consult.* **12**, 5.

Farmer A.W. (1952) The use of a composite pedicle graft for pseudarthrosis of the tibia. *J. Bone Joint Surg.* **34A**, 591.

Henderson M.S. and Clegg R.S. (1941) *Proc. Mayo Clin.* **16**, 769.

McFarland B. (1959) Pseudarthrosis of the tibia in childhood. *J. Bone Joint Surg.* **41A**, 1371–1391.

Murray H.H. and Lovell W.W. (1982) Congenital pseudarthrosis of the tibia: a long term follow-up study. *Clin. Orthop. Rel. Res.* **166**, 14–20.

Paley D., Green S., Catagni M. *et al.* (1990) Treatment of congenital pseudarthrosis by the Ilizarov technique. *Orthop. Trans.* **14**, 287.

Paterson D.C. and Simonis R.C. (1985) Electrical stimulation in the treatment of congenital pseudarthrosis of the tibia. *J. Bone Joint Surg.* **67B**, 454–462.

Sofield H.A. and Millar E.A. (1959) Fragmentation, realignment and intramedullary rod fixation of deformities of the long bones in children. *J. Bone Joint Surg.* **41A**, 1371–1391.

Umber J.S., Moss S. and Coleman S.S. (1982) Surgical treatment of congenital pseudarthrosis of the tibia. *Clin. Orthop. Rel. Res.* **166**, 28–33.

Weiland A.J. (1980) Congenital pseudarthrosis of the tibia: treatment with vascularized autogenous fibular grafts. *Johns Hopkins Med. J.* **147**, 89–95.

Weiland A.J., Weiss A.P.C., Moore J.R. and Tolo V.T. (1990) Vascularized fibular grafts in the treatment of congenital pseudarthrosis of the tibia. *J. Bone Joint Surg.* **72A**, 654.

Williams P.F. (1965) Fragmentation and rodding in osteogenesis imperfecta. *J. Bone Joint Surg.* **47B**, 23.

Chapter 9

The Integrated Care of the Limb-Deficient Child

R.H. Luff & S. Sooriakumaran

INTRODUCTION

Limb deficiency is rare in children; it varies in extent from almost undetectable to complete absence and gives rise to handicaps varying from minimal to extremely severe. This chapter deals with the multidisciplinary management of limb deficiency from diagnosis to the 16th birthday; care is directed not only at the patient but also towards parents and siblings, grandparents, carers and school staff. It is thus essential that any service taking on the care of such children has open access to all the professional skills needed — clinical and technical — and is prepared to deal with the wider aspects of counselling and guidance.

PREVALENCE

Partial or complete absence of one or more limbs may occur in isolation or as part of a recognizable syndrome. The respective importance of the various aetiologies depends on the population studied and its social condition. In England for the year 1988, limb deficiency of sufficient severity to warrant referral for prosthetic assessment occurred most commonly from congenital causes in the group aged 0–9 years (13 of 24), but from trauma (48 of 77) in the group aged 10–19 years (Department of Health, 1988).

Congenital

It is difficult to provide a single figure for prevalence as this varies throughout the world and according to the agency collecting information and the criteria used. Most studies on a national basis suggest an incidence of 50 in 100 000 (Evans *et al.*, 1991). In the UK, the incidence of significant limb deficiency, i.e. that requiring assessment for prosthetic or other treatment, is approximately 1 in 4000 live births.

The upper limb is more commonly affected than the lower and the left more commonly than the right. Single deficiencies are most common, but deficiencies affecting two, three or four limbs occur, the rarity increasing with the number of affected limbs. Abnormalities of other systems can occur, and limb deficiency can present as a component of a number of rare syndromes.

Trauma

This is a rare cause of a rare condition. The authors' experience includes loss from road traffic accidents, injury from commercial food processing equipment and bite injury by a gorilla. The presentation and subsequent management is further complicated by substantial burdens of guilt experienced by carers.

Tumour

Limb ablation for neoplasia, usually malignant, is a rare cause and in children is becoming rarer with the appreciation of the need for early diagnosis, the increased efficiency of limb conserving surgery and the improved survival after chemotherapy. When ablation occurs in childhood, it often is at a proximal level. Treatment of these children after limb ablation is often complicated by the effects of chemotherapy and radiotherapy.

Vascular

Massive haemangiomas and lymphatic abnormalities occasionally cause such distress from gigantism of the limb and recurrent ulceration that ablation is unavoidable. Amputation is often performed in a stepwise fashion, ascending the limb. This is seen for instance in Klippel–Trenauney–Weber syndrome (Klippel and Trenauney, 1900; Sooriakumaran and Lal Landham, 1991) in which the massive haemangioma in the leg

249

eventually leads to hip disarticulation. Occasionally, limb loss occurs after essential vascular access in extremely small children; management is often complicated by the intercurrent disease processes.

Drugs

A small number of drugs is implicated in producing limb deformity and deficiency in man: thalidomide, aminopterin, methotrexate and alcohol. Probably the most notorious of these is thalidomide, which produced widespread abnormalities of the limbs, facial skeleton and dentition, giving rise to the characteristic facies of the condition (Millen, 1962) and a wide variety of usually symmetrical deficiencies in the arms and/or legs. The causative mechanisms are unknown. Alcohol when taken in sufficient quantities in early pregnancy produces a characteristic syndrome which occasionally includes major limb reduction deformity (Pauli and Feldman, 1986).

Infections

The only infection believed to be implicated is intra-uterine infection with varicella Zoster virus. A rare complication of this is congenital limb deformity; limb hypoplasia may be marked, together with the formation of only rudimentary digits.

Intrauterine trauma

The relevance of external trauma to the developing fetus is unclear. Abnormalities of the uterine cavity can give rise to limb deficiency, as in so-called amniotic constriction band syndrome (Streeter, 1930).

High-energy irradiation

Ionizing radiation is known to be a cause of limb abnormality and deficiency, as for example after the use of nuclear weapons in Japan. There is no evidence that diagnostic ultrasonography has any such effect.

Nutritional factors

The Bristol University Project into the Causes of Congenital Arm Loss investigated dietary habits in pregnancy and failed to find any conclusive evidence of a nutritional link with arm deficiency. This contrasts with, for example, the evidence relating to neural tube defects. A rare consequence of maternal diabetes mellitus is variable hypoplasia of the lower limb.

CLASSIFICATION OF LIMB DEFICIENCIES

The varied nature of limb deficiencies has led to several attempts at classification, each of which had merits and failings (Frantz and O'Rahilly, 1961; Swanson, 1976). In recent years the International Standards Organization, together with the International Society for Prosthetics and Orthotics, has developed a new and comprehensive classification for congenital limb deficiency and a standardized means of recording clinical and radiological findings (International Standards Organization, 1989).

In essence, the classification records deficiencies as longitudinal or transverse, and then records the actual anatomical structures affected. This classification is strongly recommended to all those dealing with congenital limb deficiency. (Although it may be applied to limb loss from other causes, the standard descriptors for amputation levels, e.g. transtibial, transhumeral, should be applied to limb loss arising from amputation.)

INITIAL MANAGEMENT

Parents and carers

Whatever the cause of limb loss, the parents are invariably and understandably anxious and concerned. As mentioned above, there may be a burden of perceived guilt and there will be concern for the future of the affected child, the risk for further children and the effect of the abnormality on the rest of the family. It is essential that the parents and any siblings are part of the multidisciplinary structure that plans the management and care of the child.

Sympathetic, appropriate and accurate counselling is required. Family perceptions of limb deficiency, in terms of both cause and effect, may be bizarre, but every such view should be expressed so that relevant advice and reassurance may be given. This will entail medical, prosthetic, occupational, therapeutic and social skills and may take up a considerable part of one clinic. Enough time should be allowed for any such consultation. One clinician with an international reputation in the care of such cases makes a practice of providing parents with a tape recording of the first consultation (Day H., personal communication).

Care of the limb-deficient child is often shared between several centres—paediatric, orthopaedic, plastic surgical, rehabilitation—and between several specialist staff. One child known to the authors sees three orthopaedic surgeons concurrently. It is thus vital that all those simultaneously concerned with management of a child are in frequent communication so that conflict of advice and inappropriate timing of treatment is avoided.

In the case of congenital limb deficiency, counselling should start at the moment of diagnosis. Modern diagnostic ultrasonography is of such a high standard in the UK that routine scans are now demonstrating limb deficiency *in utero*. Counselling of the expectant mother is practised by one of the authors and is expected to be become a routine procedure. The authors' experience is that pre-natal diagnosis combined with effective counselling considerably eases the subsequent course of family management and rehabilitation of the child.

Genetic counselling

The possibility of subsequent children being similarly affected is a matter of great and understandable concern to the parents, and often to other members of the family. In only a small minority of cases, however, is there any identifiable genetic component. It is important that any affected family should be offered access to a clinical geneticist to obtain information and advice regarding risk to future siblings and to offspring of the affected child, as it is estimated that 12% of new presentations of congenital limb deficiency correspond to known syndromes (Calzorali *et al.*, 1990) and thus permit accurate risk assessment for siblings and subsequent generations. The syndromes associated with major limb deficiencies are shown in Table 9.1 (Kingston, 1989; Evans *et al.*, 1991).

Chromosomal abnormalities account for another small group, and there is a further heterogenous group, including Poland's, femur/fibula/ulna (FFU) and de Lange's syndromes, which are sporadic and of unknown aetiology.

REHABILITATION

Operative treatment

It must be emphasized that any operative intervention is an integral part of the overall rehabilitation of the child. The indications for operation are:

1 Removal of non-viable tissue.
2 Preservation of tissue at risk.
3 Improvement of function.
4 Improvement of appearance.

In most cases, cosmetic considerations are secondary to those of function; an operation for cosmetic reasons alone is best delayed until the affected child can be fully involved in consent.

Decisions on the timing of an elective operation should

Table 9.1 Syndromes associated with major limb deficiencies

Syndrome	Mode of inheritance
Adams−Oliver Syndrome	Autosomal dominant
Cleft hand and foot syndrome	Autosomal dominant
Holt−Oram syndrome	Autosomal dominant
Roberts' syndrome	Autosomal recessive
Grebe syndrome	Autosomal recessive
Thrombocytopenia and absent radius (TAR syndrome)	Autosomal recessive
Split hand and foot syndrome (inbred)	X-linked recessive

be made on a multidisciplinary basis to take into account the condition itself and the physical, cognitive and emotional development of the child. Life events and crises within the family must also be considered. In general terms, interventions should facilitate bimanual activity (3−6 months) or standing (10−12 months). An operation should be considered in terms of elongation, rotation, transplantation and ablation.

ELONGATION

This is a complex technique, not without complications (Maffuli *et al.*, 1993). As much as 8 cm of lengthening can be achieved in the lower limb; treatment should be undertaken at about 10 years of age and may last for 18 months. It has been applied to congenital tibial dysplasia, proximal femoral focal deficiency (see Chapters 8.1 and 11) and in some upper limb deficiencies.

ROTATION

This is employed to realign limb segments in the complete limb to improve function, e.g. in radial club hand or pollicization, and to realign the remaining limb segments to improve function, e.g. in rotationplasty (Van Nes, 1950) after radical local excision. Derotation is a common complication, and particularly in the lower limb the individual, often adolescent, has severe psychological disturbance. Careful counselling is needed together with long-term support of both the child and the involved family.

TRANSPLANTATION

This is applicable to transverse hand deficiencies in which opposition, and therefore pincer grip, cannot be achieved. Toe-to-hand digital transfer (O'Brien *et al.*, 1978) is clearly applicable to the (rare) isolated traumatic loss of the thumb in childhood. The more common situation of congenital deficiency of the distal hand, however, is complicated by the abnormal anatomy present, and there may be major bone, nerve and circulatory defects. In such cases, digital transfer may be technically impossible. In any case, the function of the whole hand must be considered, as transplantation to produce an isolated digit will result in little improvement in function.

ABLATION

The indications for limb ablation in childhood are: (i) congenital deformity; (ii) trauma; (iii) malignancy; and (iv) vascular insufficiency. This disabling and deforming intervention carries additional problems in childhood over and above those experienced by the adult amputee, because the child undergoes continued skeletal and soft tissue growth. Transdiaphyseal amputation, particularly at the transtibial and transhumeral levels, results in longitudinal bone overgrowth, leading to the need for multiple revisions of the residual limb up to the time of skeletal maturity.

In amputation surgery in children, these levels should be avoided if possible in favour of disarticulation, thus avoiding the inevitable repeated operations and consequent shortening of the residual limb. Thus, in longitudinal fibular deficiency, which often leads to Syme's disarticulation at the ankle, the adult outcome similar to that for an excellent transtibial (below-knee) amputee. It is important to bear in mind that the residual limb will in any case become relatively shorter because of differential growth on the amputated side. There are well-established techniques (Marquardt, 1976) to minimize bone overgrowth if transtibial or transhumeral amputation is unavoidable.

It is essential that good operative practice is followed in amputation in childhood, and this should be a pain-free experience. Proper attention should be paid to the handling of soft tissues, particularly divided nerves and muscle. A well-fashioned myoplasty (Burgess *et al.*, 1971; Neff, 1988) when appropriate will accelerate healing and improve function of the residual limb. Division of visible nerves under tension to allow the cut ends to retract into soft tissue will reduce the incidence of painful neuroma formation and thereby facilitate rehabilitation. Transdiaphyseal bone section can lead to areas of excessive pressure in subsequent rehabilitation, but this can be avoided by careful sculpting of the cut end to produce the largest possible radius of curvature. The skin closure technique does not appear to affect outcome, but the positioning of scars over myoplastic

tissue will improve comfort and avoid adherence to underlying rigid structures.

Prosthetic management

PRINCIPLES

The prosthetic component of rehabilitation in limb-deficient children must be viewed as part of a multidisciplinary exercise in which many skills and experiences are brought to bear on one, often tiny, patient. It should not intimidate the child nor its carers, and decisions must be shared between all those concerned, not least the limb-deficient child and the carers. It is important to establish from the outset that some conditions of limb deficiency are treated best without prosthetic involvement, e.g. cleft hand or radial club hand. These cases need full functional support from professionals experienced in dealing with the issues that arise from time to time and should remain under the care of the nearest appropriate clinic for regular review.

All children with limb deficiency should, as mentioned above, be seen by the relevant specialist service — plastic and reconstructive, orthopaedic, paediatric and neurological, rehabilitation — at the earliest possible time. Each of these will be able to make the necessary therapy assessments and share information, so that the child's management is a collaborative procedure and is as effective and efficient as possible. Unfortunately, it is rare in the UK for these services to be sited close together. Effective communication between the family and all the teams involved is thus essential.

Rehabilitation consists of the dynamic processes provided to an individual who has one or more disabilities, to facilitate the achievement of all goals in physical, mental and social well-being appropriate to that individual. In congenital limb deficiency, this process is often one of habilitation, developing skills not previously present. Every stage in this process must thus take account of the growth and development of the child and its needs, which may be in part determined by peer group pressures and family wishes. The structure of best practice in the UK is described in a recent publication by the Amputee Medical Rehabilitation Society (1992).

UPPER LIMB DEFICIENCY

Upper limb deficiency inevitably results in arm length discrepancy and inability to grasp and manipulate in the midline and in the centre of the visual field. There is also always a cosmetic deficit of varying degree. A well-established limb-using habit may lead to extension of the perceived body image into the prosthesis with concurrent improvement in function. There is much interest in the correct design of prostheses to encourage this interaction between perception and device.

Treatment is planned to achieve: (i) limb-wearing habit; (ii) restoration of limb length and appearance; (iii) grasp in the midline; (iv) concept of terminal function; and (v) manipulative skills.

Diagnosis to 3 months

This period is spent in counselling the parents and in allowing them to become accustomed to the concept of regular clinic attendance. Their questions are answered and the importance of the parental role emphasized. During this period all necessary referrals are made and communication links established. The parents should be fully informed of their options, including contact with special interest and support groups, e.g. Reach.

3–6 months

Growth to this stage usually allows restoration of length and appearance, so that with the maturation of motor skills the child is able to oppose both hands in space in the midline. There is evidence that the necessary motor adjustments to allow purposeful movement develop early in life; it is thus important that limb length is normal to permit this to occur. Such prostheses are usually described as cosmetic or one-piece devices. The smallest will have a mitten hand which is changed to a cosmetic hand as growth continues. The prescription may need adjustment to allow crawling to occur, as the hand position for crawling is different from that used for opposition.

6–12 months

Limb-wearing habit is established and the family are supported in this by contact with a specially trained occupational therapist who is normally based in a prosthetic rehabilitation centre. Regular review is necessary to ensure that correct fitting is maintained, as an ill-fitting limb will be rejected. It is equally important for the parents' self esteem that the cosmetic results of early treatment are as good as possible.

15 months to 3 years

At the beginning of this stage, body-powered terminal function should be introduced so that more sophisticated play function is achieved. The small muscular effort possible at this age requires that terminal devices have low intrinsic friction and very light opening resistance. This imposes design constraints, and parents should be fully informed about these. There is much interest at present in the provision of electrically powered prostheses to very small children (Scott, 1988) which may provide function with much better cosmetic results.

3–5 years

Manipulative skills increase and with increasing growth, greater weight tolerance and longer concentration span most children will use some form of externally (electrically) powered arm. Not all will accept of the benefit of such treatment, and careful assessment, not just of the child but also of the family and its circumstances, and follow-up are needed. Liaison is needed with staff of nurseries and playschools in this period to involve them actively in the child's rehabilitation and to eliminate any concerns about the prosthesis.

5 years onwards

The rehabilitation programme follows the child's development, special needs and abilities and interests. Peer group pressures sometimes result in a change in compliance, change in limb type, or rejection of limb-wearing altogether. This is a changing situation and the family should remain under review in order to respond to the child's wishes as they arise. Increasing growth and strength widen the prosthetic options; complex electronic control is possible ('bionic arms') and a wide range of externally powered and body-powered terminal devices are available. The cosmetic results improve with increasing size, particularly for partial hand deficiency for which very pleasing silicone replacements are now possible.

Wheeled mobility now presents very little challenge to individuals with upper limb deficiency. Bicycles, motorcycles and cars can all be legally adapted to cope with most deficiencies. Liaison between the rehabilitation clinic, licensing and insuring concerns and appropriate companies specializing in adaptations are necessary.

Transverse partial hand deficiencies present particular difficulties for establishing power grip without producing very poor cosmetic results. As the length discrepancy is often minimal and the function of the residual limb is usually very good, no prosthetic treatment other than an opposition plate may be required. There are great problems for deficiencies at the level of the carpus, however, for which there is no good solution at present.

LOWER LIMB DEFICIENCY

Deficiency in the lower limb, irrespective of cause, results in some degree of length discrepancy together with loss of joint motion and muscle power. Just as in the hand, minor degrees of foot abnormality or limb shortening require either no prosthetic treatment or specialized footwear only. When prosthetic treatment is appropriate, the aims of such treatment are to: (i) enable bipedal gait; (ii) correct length discrepancy; (iii) restore joint motion; (iv) normalize gait; and (v) facilitate individual goals. Current prostheses have good cosmetic outcomes together with sophisticated replacement of joint motion and stability. It is not yet possible to replace muscle power in the same way as for the upper limb; there are, however, energy-storing components that benefit some users considerably.

Diagnosis to 9 months

As for upper limb deficiency, this period is usefully spent in counselling, obtaining genetic advice when appropriate and preparing the family for the long-term commitment to prosthetic treatment of the affected child. Questions and uncertainties should be dealt with, particularly in relation to timing, types of prostheses and likely outcomes. It must be kept clearly in mind that affected children should lead an essentially normal life; unless there are intercurrent conditions, life expectancy is not reduced. The family should be closely involved in discussions and decisions and be fully informed of their options, including contact with special interest and support groups, e.g. Steps. This phase leads up to the stage when the child is able to stand with support; the exact timing will thus vary between individuals.

9 months to 3 years

Standing and walking skills are developing so the requirements of prostheses are for light weight, length correction and stability. The fundamental components of any lower limb prosthesis remain unchanged throughout treatment and consist of:

1 Socket—this forms the interface between child and prosthesis and is designed to transmit the forces of standing and walking. In congenital deficiency, it may enclose and stabilize otherwise inadequate joints.

2 Suspension—both gravity and centrifugal forces in gait work to separate the prosthesis from the wearer and need to be resisted. Continuous growth makes suction fitting impossible, so that additional external suspension, as simple and unobtrusive as possible, is needed.

3 Articulations—ideally, every absent joint motion is replaced, but this is often neither technically nor biomechanically feasible. In very small children, length constrains prescription and a minimal 'joint', e.g. the solid ankle-cushion heel, may be necessary to provide movement to permit roll-over in mid-stance. Stability can be provided by joint elimination, alignment, stabilizers, or locking devices.

4 Cosmesis—traditional ('conventional') prostheses have both load-bearing structure and cosmesis provided by their exoskeletal nature. In contrast, the more modern endoskeletal or modular prostheses require external cladding to provide cosmetic finish. This results in a soft feel to the limb; the final external finish may be coloured and textured using stockings, plastic skins, or spray finishes.

3–10 years

With increasing growth and development of motor skills, most children will transfer to the use of modular limb systems. A much wider range of components is available for these in contrast to conventional limb types, though the range of modular systems for the smaller child is still somewhat limited. Frequent review—the authors recommend a maximum interval of 3 months—is necessary to allow for growth, which is by no means constant or predictable, to deal with the repair work inevitable in these heavily used prostheses and to meet changes in need.

10 years onwards

This period is concerned with keeping the prescription in line with rapidly expanding activities. Many children acquire interests in sports whose skills may entail careful re-evaluation of prosthetic needs. When discussing these issues, it is important to realize that there are very few sporting activities closed to the lower limb amputee. Contact with the British Amputee Sports Association may be helpful. It is also important to note that adolescents may be able to drive at the age of 16 years if they are in receipt of certain benefits in the UK; proximal lower limb prostheses may need redesigning to allow for driving.

As mentioned above, operative revision may be necessary from time to time and provides an important opportunity for collaboration between specialist teams. Major revision of the residual limb will certainly necessitate socket revision and may completely change the nature of the prescription. It is axiomatic that this is best achieved by consultation between surgical and rehabilitation teams, so that the child receives optimum care throughout.

COEXISTING UPPER AND LOWER LIMB DEFICIENCY

Very occasionally, and almost always as a result of septicaemia or congenital deficiency, children present with multiple limb involvement. (The thalidomide disaster in 1960 was a clear and fortunately isolated example of drug-induced, complex, multiple limb deficiency.) Such children require highly specialized treatment and not uncommonly need admission to specialist paediatric units to deal with the complexities of their physical, psychological and social needs. This must occur in close proximity to a rehabilitation unit capable of providing the specialized upper and lower limb prostheses that are often necessary.

An important element of the care of such children is the appreciation that their walking ability may be severely restricted as a result of the fatigue associated with prosthetic gait. Early referral for wheelchair and sometimes seating assessment should be made; wheelchair needs should be reviewed as frequently as prosthetic ones, as the same issues of growth, repairs and changing need apply. The thalidomide cases referred to above clearly show that even in the presence of profound multiple limb deficiency, completely independent living is possible in an appropriately adapted environment.

OUTCOME

As described above, the outcome of health care for children with limb deficiency can and should be extraordinarily good, and any deviation from this represents some degree of failure of the caring services. It is essential that all concerned clearly understand that the outcome is not merely dependent on the extent of physical loss, but also on the psychological profile of the child, on the involvement and support by the family and on the cooperation and collaboration of the specialist teams within the caring services.

Although in the lower limb prosthetic restoration of function is needed to stand and walk and most children have excellent outcomes, this is by no means as certain in upper limb loss. Outcomes for such cases demonstrate the difficulties in replacing the sophisticated functions of the hand; assessment, training and support all play a part in assisting these children to benefit from the extra abilities that a prosthesis may provide.

SUMMARY

Major limb loss is fortunately rare in childhood, and orthopaedic surgeons will see few cases in a working lifetime. The results of carefully planned and implemented surgery can be of great benefit to the child, and the outcome of habilitation and rehabilitation should be excellent. This chapter has attempted to show the great importance of communication, cooperation and collaboration between the specialist teams involved in producing the best of outcomes for affected children.

Useful addresses

Reach
The General Secretary
13 Park Terrace
Crimchard
Chard
Somerset TA20 1LA

STEPS
15 Statham Close
Lymm
Cheshire WA13 9NN

British Amputee Sports Association (BASA)
Harvey Road
Aylesbury
Bucks HP21 9PP

REFERENCES

Amputee Rehabilitation, Recommended Standards and Guidelines: A Report by the Working Party of the Amputee Medical Rehabilitation Society (1992). London, Royal College of Physicians.

Bristol University Project into the Causes of Congenital Arm Loss. Joint Publication between University of Bristol and Reach. Available from the General Secretary of Reach.

Burgess E.M., Romano R.L., Zettl J.H. and Schrock R.D. (1971) Amputations of the leg for peripheral vascular insufficiency. *J. Bone Joint Surg.* **53A**, 874–889.

Calzorali E., Manservigi D., Garani G.P., Cocchi G., Magagni C. and Milan M. (1990) Limb reduction defects in Emilia Romagna, Italy: epidemiological and genetic study in 173,109 consecutive births. *J. Med. Genet.* **27**, 353–357.

Department of Health. *Amputation Statistics for England, Wales and Northern Ireland 1988.* Blackpool, Department of Health Statistics and Management Information Division, 1988.

Evans D.R.G., Thakker Y. and Donnai D. (1991) Hereditary and dysmorphic syndromes in congenital limb deficiency: *Prosthet. Orthot. Int.* **15**, 70–77.

Frantz C.H. and O'Rahilly R. (1961) Congenital skeletal limb deficiencies. *J. Bone Joint Surg.* **43A**, 1202–1204.

International Standards Organization. (1989) *ISO 8548−1 1989: Prosthetics and Orthotics − Limb Deficiencies − Part 1: Method of Describing Limb Deficiencies Present at Birth*. Geneva, ISO Central Secretariat.

Kingston H.M. (1989) Dysmorphology and teratogenesis. *BMJ* **298**, 1235−1239.

Klippel M. and Trenauney P. (1900) Du naevus varique osteo-hypertrophique. *Arch. Gen. Med.* **185**, 641−672.

Marquardt E. (1976) Plastiche Operationen bei drohender konchendurchspiessung am kindlichen Oberarmstumpf. Eine Vorlanfige Mittleung. *Z. Orthop.* **114**, 711−714.

Millen J.W. (1962) Thalidomide and limb deformities. *Lancet* **ii**, 599−600.

Neff G. (1988) Above Knee Amputation Surgery. In Murdoch G. (ed.) *Amputation Surgery and Lower Limb Prosthetics*. Oxford, Blackwell Scientific Publications, pp. 117−129.

Maffuli N., Pattinson R.C. and Fixsen J. (1993) Lengthening of congenital limb length discrepancies using callotasis − early experience of the Hospital for Sick Children. *Ann. R. Coll. Surg.* **75**, 105−110.

O'Brien B.M., MacLeod A.M., Sykes P.J., Browning F.S.C. and Threlfall G.N. (1978) Microvascular second toe transfer for digital reconstruction. *J. Hand Surg.* **3**, 123−133.

Pauli R.M. and Feldman P.F. (1986) Major limb malformations following intrauterine exposure to ethanol: two additional cases and literature review. *Teratology* **33**, 273−280.

Scott R.N. (1988) Myoelectric prostheses: state of the art. *J. Med. Eng. Technol.* **12**, 143.

Sooriakumaran S. and Lal Landham T. (1991) The Klippel−Trenauney syndrome. *J. Bone Joint Surg.* **73B**, 178−179.

Streeter G.L. (1930) Focal deficiencies in foetal tissue and their relation to intrauterine amputation. *Contra. Embryol. Carnegie Inst.* **22**, 1−44.

Swanson A.B. (1976) A classification for congenital limb malformations. *J. Hand Surg.* **1**, 8−22.

Van Nes C.P. (1950) Rotationplasty for congenital defects of the femur: making use of the ankle for the shortened limb to control the knee joint of the prosthesis. *J. Bone Joint Surg.* **32B**, 12−16.

Chapter 10

Torsional Deformities of the Lower Extremities

N.H. Harris

INTRODUCTION

Femoral and tibial torsional deformities are a common cause of symptoms for which anxious parents seek medical advice. The children are referred to orthopaedic clinics with a variety of diagnoses, among which are foot deformities, knock knees, bow legs and dislocated hips.

Angular deformities, which may in fact coexist with the torsional deformities, will not be discussed except in so far as they have a bearing on diagnosis. Also excluded are children who have associated abnormalities, e.g. congenital dislocation of the hip, poliomyelitis, cerebral palsy, or spina bifida, all of which may be the cause of, or influence, a torsional deformity.

DEFINITIONS

There arises from a bad and unapt formation of words a wonderful obstruction of the mind.
(*Francis Bacon*, 1561–1626.)

In order to avoid confusion, some of the terms used in this chapter will be defined here.

Transcondylar axis of the femur

This is a horizontal line through the femoral condyles (Fig. 10.1). This axis, together with the shaft axis, constitutes the transcondylar plane (frontal or coronal plane) of the femur.

Angle of femoral anteversion

The angle is formed by the intersection of the transcondylar plane and the plane of the femoral neck (Fig. 10.1). It is a measure of the torsion in the femoral shaft, which normally directs the head and neck anteriorly in relation to the femoral condyles. It is clearly possible for the angle of anteversion to represent torsion in the femoral shaft, neck, or both. The angle is commonly understood to refer to torsion in the femoral neck, however, and the distinction is of no practical importance.

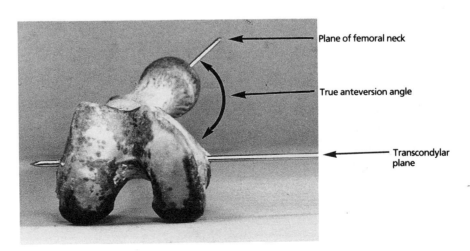

Fig. 10.1 Transcondylar axis of the femur and the angle of anteversion.

Plane of femoral neck

True anteversion angle

Transcondylar plane

Angle of femoral retroversion

The femoral neck is retroverted when it is directed posteriorly to the transcondylar plane. If the angle of anteversion is less than normal for the age, the term 'relative retroversion' is used.

Angle of inclination of the femoral neck

This angle (the neck–shaft angle) is formed by the intersection of the femoral shaft axis with the neck axis.

Angle of acetabular anteversion

The angle is formed by the intersection of the obliquely placed acetabulum and the sagittal plane (Fig. 10.2). When the acetabulum is directed forwards more than normal (and therefore its anterior obliquity is increased), the anteversion angle is increased.

Angle of tibial torsion

The angle is formed by the intersection of the median sagittal plane of the tibia and the coronal plane. The angle is zero when the sagittal plane is directly antero-posteriorly, and both malleoli will then be in the coronal plane with the foot pointing forwards.

PATTERNS OF DEFORMITY

The deformity is referred to as 'simple' when several segments of the limb are rotated in the same direction and 'mixed' when an abnormal primary rotation in one segment is associated with the opposite compensatory deformity in another segment of the same limb. From a practical point of view it is useful to consider two patterns of primary deformity: medial torsion of the limb (femur and tibia), associated with genu varum and an in-toeing gait; and lateral torsion, usually associated with genu valgum, pronated feet and an out-toeing gait. These deformities are usually bilateral, but occasionally unilateral, and may be located in one segment only.

NORMAL DEVELOPMENT OF THE LOWER EXTREMITIES

Intrauterine period

The knees and hips become flexed and the plantar surfaces of the feet face the trunk. In the later months of pregnancy the fetus adopts a knee–chest position; gradually the legs descend on the trunk and rotate 90° internally so that the knees face anteriorly. These changes are associated with increasing anterior inclination of the acetabulum, which continues after birth. During the later months of pregnancy the tibia is rotated medially. Anteversion of the femoral neck is about 5° in the third month, and it increases to about 15° in the fourth months, reaching about 40° at birth.

Newborn infants

The intrauterine position in the later months of pregnancy determines the position of the legs and feet at

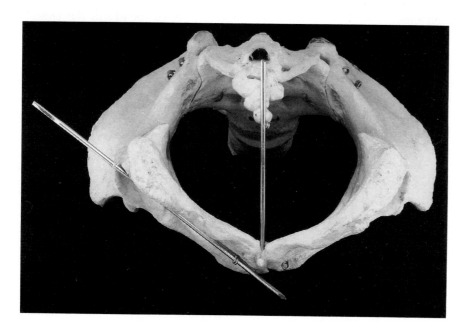

Fig. 10.2 The acetabular anteversion angle. The pelvis is viewed from below and is in the equivalent of the prone position.

birth. The legs usually lie in external rotation with the hip and knee flexed. With the hip extended, external rotation is about 30° more than internal rotation and is associated with about 40° of femoral anteversion. The relatively laterally rotated position of the legs is explained by the fact that forward and medial rotation of the acetabulum is incomplete. The tibia is rotated medially between 5° and 30° and is often associated with mild lateral bowing. The feet are turned inwards but correction beyond neutral is easily obtained.

It is important to appreciate that the posture described is a physiological one and not a true deformity; it will change spontaneously as the infant develops provided that extrinsic factors, e.g. certain sleeping and sitting postures, do not exert their influence. The hips and knees extend gradually and the acetabulum and femur rotate medially. The average acetabular anteversion is 7° compared with 17° in adults, and this correlates with the gradual medial rotation of the lower extremity (McKibbin, 1970). Until recently, when considering the stability of an infant's hip, particular attention has been paid to the degree of femoral anteversion; as pointed out by McKibbin it is clearly important to consider the relationship to the sagittal plane of both the femoral neck and the acetabulum. Now that a technique is available for measuring acetabular anteversion, it may be important to assess its significance with regard to abnormalities of femoral rotation in the presence of a stable hip.

Children

At about 7 years of age passive hip rotation in full extension is about 45° each of internal and external rotation, which is the normal adult range. At the same time as these rotational changes are taking place there is a gradual reduction in the angle of femoral anteversion, the greatest fall occurring during the first 4 years, reaching 12–15° at skeletal maturity (Fig. 10.3). Sommerville (1957) referred to persistent fetal alignment or anteversion of the femoral neck; he pointed out that the normally taut capsule of the extended hip usually moulds away the anteversion present at birth during the early years of life. If the capsule stretches anterior subluxation of the hip may occur and the anteversion may persist. In some instances the capsule remains taut but the anteversion is incompletely moulded away. Tibial torsion also changes, so that there is about 20° of external torsion at the end of the growth period; however, a range of 0–40° is considered to be consistent with normal appearance and function (Hutter and Scott, 1949). Lateral bowing of the tibia corrects at the same time and often passes through a stage of physiological genu valgum (Bohm, 1933).

SOME RELEVANT MECHANICAL FACTORS

Epiphyseal growth may be modified by such factors as heredity, blood supply, infection, trauma, muscle imbalance and joint posture. According to Heuter-Volkmann's law there is an inverse relationship between the pressure across an epiphysis and its rate of growth; increased pressure across the plate will decrease the rate of growth, and conversely a decrease in pressure will increase the rate. Angular and torsional deformities originate in the region of epiphysis. Asymmetrical pressure applied perpendicular to the plate produces an angular deformity, and torque forces applied parallel to the plate result in a torsional deformity. According to

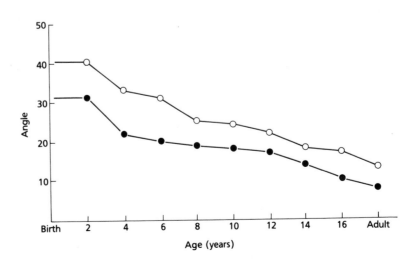

Fig. 10.3 The average normal range of femoral anteversion.

Wolff's law, the femur and tibia will rotate or deviate according to the stresses to which they are habitually subjected. It would seem reasonable to postulate that stresses produced by certain sleeping and sitting postures might be capable of producing torsional deformities of the femur, tibia and foot.

The common coexistence of angulation and torsion in a single bone may be explained by the fact that combined perpendicular and torque forces are applied to the growth plate. Examples of this phenomenon are a common occurrence in clinical practice; thus, physiological lateral bowing of the tibia is generally associated with medial tibial torsion, and conversely genu valgum is usually associated with an increase in lateral tibial torsion. It is generally accepted that isolated angular deformities, e.g. genu valgum, correct spontaneously and seldom produce a therapeutic problem (Farrier and Lloyd-Roberts, 1969). Physiological angular deformities, however, may become unphysiological in the presence of a torsional deformity, because the latter produces abnormal stress on the epiphysis.

AETIOLOGY

It is likely that certain congenital factors play a part in the development of the primary torsional deformity. Thus, abnormal or asymmetrical intrauterine pressure may increase or decrease the normal physiological rotation of the limb that is present at birth, namely external rotation of the hips, medial tibial torsion and lateral convexity (the result of angulation of the distal tibial epiphyseal plate which is oblique and faces medially). Medial tibial torsion, which is a feature of the gorilla and orang-utan, may represent an atavistic reversion or developmental arrest. Lateral torsion of the hip is extremely common in West Indians and racial factors may thus be significant. Hereditary factors may play a part in internal rotation deformities of the hip, for it is not uncommon for several children and one of the parents to have the same deformity; Crane (1959) noted a familial relationship in 21 of 72 patients. Joint laxity, which may be familial, is almost always present in internal rotation deformities of the hip associated with increased anteversion.

It seems reasonable to assume that if a primary aetiological factor in producing a rotational deformity in a newborn is the result of abnormal or asymmetrical pressure, which modifies the normal intrauterine posture, that child may subsequently adopt certain sleeping and sitting postures because it is easier to do so. These are referred to as post-natal malpositions, and if allowed to persist may perpetuate or increase the primary deformity. Fitzhugh (1941) was one of the first to describe the relationship of lower limb deformities with sleeping, sitting and play postures. Clearly, it is possible that children may acquire a rotational deformity, sometimes with an associated angular deformity, as a result of post-natal malposition. Questioning of the parents reveals that most such children were nursed from birth in the prone position because of the policy of the obstetric unit. As indicated earlier, some children will acquire a secondary or compensatory rotational deformity, and perhaps the best example is the lateral rotation of the tibia which compensates for primary medial rotation at the hip. An angular deformity, e.g. genu valgum, may also be acquired because the primary deformity causes an abnormal foot strike, and this in turn results in asymmetrical pressure on the epiphyseal plate.

CLINICAL ASPECTS

From 1962 the author made a study of children with torsional deformities of the lower extremity (Harris, 1972). Serial clinical and radiological examinations were carried out on several hundred children; follow-up continued to the age of 10 years or more, though in some instances the deformity had corrected earlier. The study forms the basis for what follows in the remainder of this chapter.

Post-natal malpositions

The two main groups are prone sleeping and sitting positions. It should be appreciated that there is often a close relationship between sleeping and sitting postures; persistence of certain sleeping postures will undoubtedly result in the child adopting a characteristic posture later on.

PRONE SLEEPING (Table 10.1)

There are a number of variations, each of which produces a characteristic deformity that may affect any segment of the lower extremity, either individually or in combination.

Knee–chest posture (Fig. 10.4)

This is the fetal posture in the later months of pregnancy and is responsible for the physiological position at birth: external rotation of the hip (associated with femoral neck anteversion of 30–40°), medial torsion of the tibia, genu varum, adduction and varus of the forefoot. Persistence of the posture may exaggerate the physiological

Table 10.1 Limb deformities caused by various prone sleeping positions

Posture	Hip	Tibia	Ankle	Foot	
Prone, knee–chest (fetal position)	External rotation	Medial torsion	Equinus	Adduction, varus	Bow legs
Prone, hips extended					
Feet internally rotated	Internal rotation	Medial torsion	Equinus	Adduction, varus	
Feet externally rotated	External rotation	Lateral torsion	Equinus	Valgus	
Frog position					
Prone	External rotation	Lateral torsion	—	Abduction	Knock knees
Supine	External rotation	Lateral torsion	—	Valgus	Knock knees

rotation and produce a deformity (Fig. 10.5). These children subsequently sit in the reverse tailor position (see Fig. 10.12).

Prone with extended hips

The deformities that result will depend on the position of the feet. If they are laterally rotated the hips and tibias develop a similar deformity (Fig. 10.6), and this is associated with relative retroversion of the femoral necks (Fig. 10.7). Angular deformity does not occur. Sometimes the forefoot is abducted and the hindfoot forced into such a degree of valgus that all the features of a calcaneovalgus deformity are demonstrated (Fig. 10.8). If the forefoot is held in the neutral position, equinus at the ankle results and is one of the causes of walking on tiptoe in children (Fig. 10.9). Later on, these children sit in the tailor or cross-leg position. If the feet are medially rotated, the opposite deformity occurs (Fig. 10.10).

Prone frog-leg posture (Fig. 10.11)

The deformities are similar to those resulting from the prone position with extended hips, but in addition genu valgum develops due to shortening of the iliotibial tract and biceps femoris (Fig. 10.11).

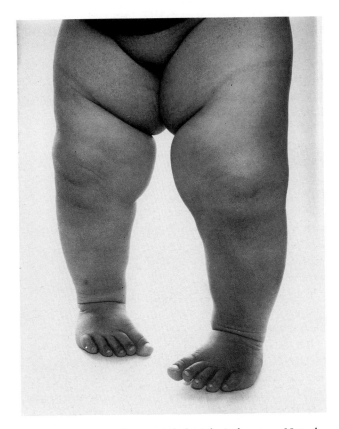

Fig. 10.5 Exaggerated post-natal physiological posture. Note the externally rotated hips, medial tibial torsion, adduction and varus of the forefoot.

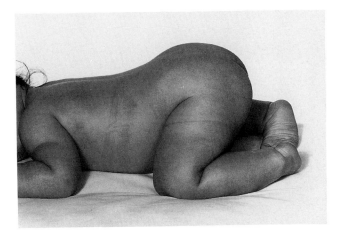

Fig. 10.4 The knee–chest posture.

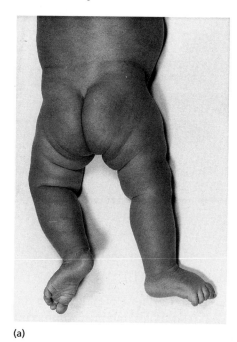
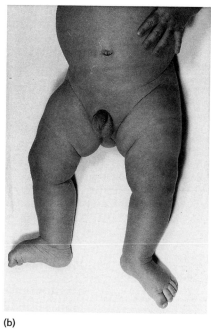

(a)   (b)

Fig. 10.6 Post-natal malposition. (a) Prone with extended hips. (b) Note that the hip, tibia and foot are laterally rotated.

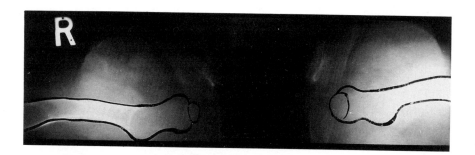

Fig. 10.7 Radiograph showing less than normal anteversion in a 1-year-old child. The angle is 15° (normal, 30–40°).

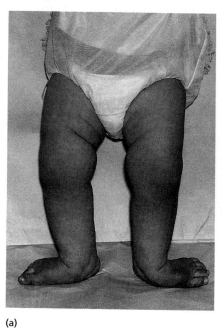
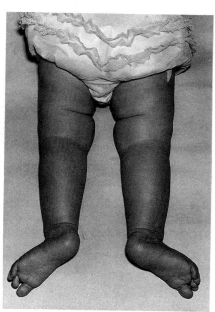

(a)   (b)

Fig. 10.8 Severe deformity resulting from prone lying. (a) Weight-bearing: severe calcaneovalgus deformity. (b) Prone: legs and feet are externally rotated.

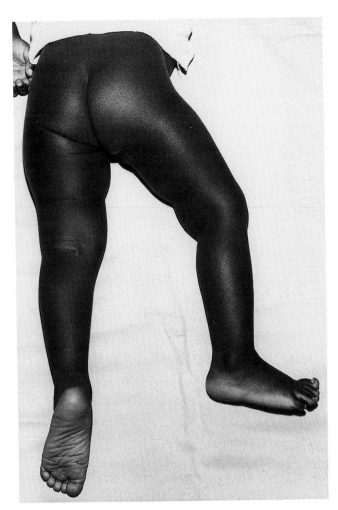

Fig. 10.9 Sleeping posture producing equinus — one of the causes of children walking on tiptoe.

SITTING (Table 10.2)

The posture most commonly associated with deformities is the reverse tailor position. Usually the feet are laterally rotated (Fig. 10.12). The hips in full extension rotate medially to 90° and external rotation is markedly restricted (Fig. 10.13); there is an associated increase in femoral neck anteversion (Fig. 10.14). The children often stand and walk with the patellas squinting inwards because it is easier for them to do so (Fig. 10.15). The tibia may be externally rotated more than normal, usually to compensate for the hip deformity. Bow leg is apparent rather than real, because the tibia is viewed obliquely; if the legs are laterally rotated until the patellas face anteriorly, the bow leg disappears and the pronated feet become more obvious (Fig. 10.16). Occasionally, the feet are medially rotated (Fig. 10.17a); hip deformity is the same but the tibia is medially rotated with an associated forefoot varus (Fig. 10.17b). According to Hutter and Scott (1949) this particular sitting posture is very common in Japan, and the adult population there is known to have an increased incidence of medial tibial torsion. Usually the children have slept prone in the knee−chest position.

ISOLATED PRIMARY EXTERNAL TIBIAL TORSION

A few children have been seen, usually presenting between 6 and 8 years of age, who have a bilateral increased external tibial torsion with an associated and probably secondary postural valgus deformity of the feet (Fig. 10.18). The hips are normal, and close questioning of the parents indicates that these children have not had an abnormal sleeping or sitting posture, and the aetiology is therefore unknown.

Symptoms

Infants may be referred because the mother has noticed that the feet are turned outwards, and sometimes it is noticed that the lower extremity is externally rotated; later these children walk with the legs and feet turned out but at this stage the complaint is usually that the child has flat feet.

In the presence of the internal rotation deformities, one or more of the following symptoms is mentioned by the parent; turns the feet in; falls excessively; clumsy gait; runs awkwardly; aching legs; tires easily; and abnormal shoe wear. In some instances, particularly

Table 10.2 Limb deformities caused by various sitting positions

Posture	Hip	Tibia	Foot
Reverse tailor			
Feet internally rotated (sitting on feet)	Internal rotation	Medial torsion	Adduction, varus
Feet externally rotated	Internal rotation	Lateral torsion	Valgus
Tailor (cross-leg)	External rotation	Medial torsion	Varus

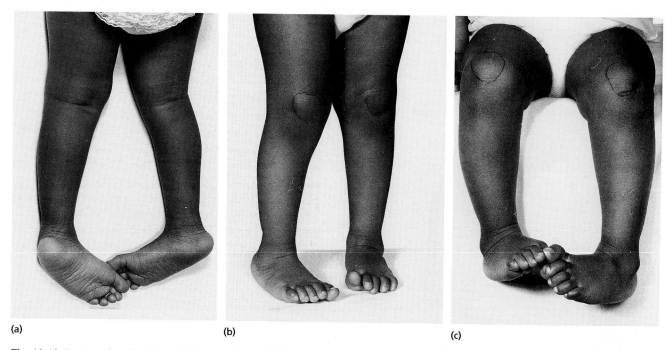

(a)   (b)   (c)

Fig. 10.10 Post-natal malposition. (a) Prone with medially rotated feet. (b) Child stands and walks with in-toeing gait. (c) Sitting with knees 90° flexed to show medial tibial torsion.

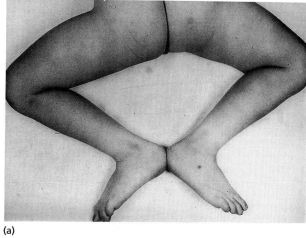

(a)

Fig. 10.11 (a) Prone frog-leg posture. (b) Note valgus deformity of knees and feet.

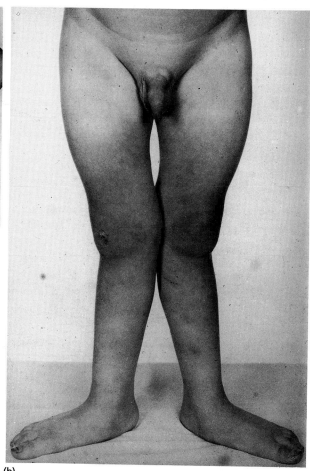

(b)

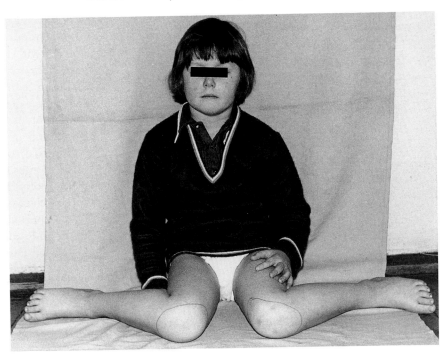

Fig. 10.12 The reverse tailor posture. The feet are laterally rotated.

with girls, the complaint by the parent is principally a cosmetic one. McSweeny (1971) has reported that 13% of all children have an in-toeing gait due to increased anteversion.

Clinical signs

It is important to examine all segments of the lower extremity, including the hips, regardless of the presenting

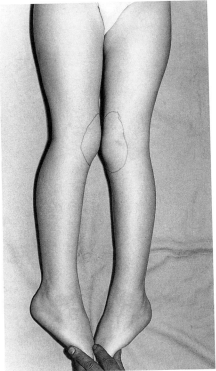
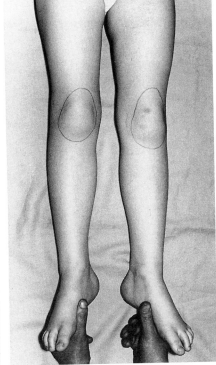

Fig. 10.13 Altered hip rotation.
(a) Exaggerated medial rotation.
(b) Corresponding reduced external rotation.

(a)

(b)

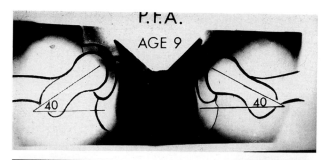

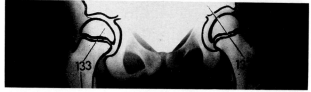

Fig. 10.14 Radiograph showing increased femoral neck anteversion.

symptoms which may, for example, refer to the feet only. First, the child's gait should be observed with the legs and feet fully exposed. The child should then be examined standing, supine and prone, noting the sitting posture normally adopted. Joint laxity can be estimated by examination of the elbows, wrists, fingers and knees. Significant generalized increase in joint laxity has been noted in children with abnormal anteversion. The feet

are observed while the child is standing, looking for the presence of pes planovalgus; if internal rotation is more than 70° with much reduced external rotation, medial femoral torsion is present. The reverse is also true, so that more than 70° of external rotation may indicate some degree of external torsion (retroversion). A rough estimate of the amount of torsional deformity in the femur can be made by measuring the degree of internal and external rotation at the hip in full extension (Fig. 10.19). If internal rotation exceeds external rotation by 30° or more, anteversion is increased; if the reverse applies relative retroversion is present. The estimate is only approximate because the correlation between clinical and radiological measurements is not accurate. Medial and lateral rotation together are usually about 100°; if, for example, internal rotation is 90° and external rotation is 0° or 10°, a significant amount of anteversion is present. It is important to note that not all children with an in-toeing gait and increased internal rotation of the hip in extension have increased anteversion. McSweeny (1971) reported that one-third of such children had normal anteversion and the in-toeing in these children was probably due to abnormal acetabular rotation. Gelberman *et al.* (1987) confirmed McSweeny's findings. It is suggested that soft tissue contracture anterior to the hip joint or shortening of the medial rotators might be the cause.

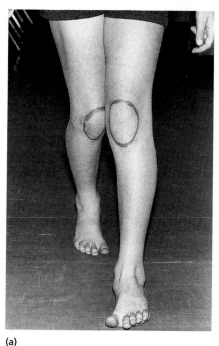

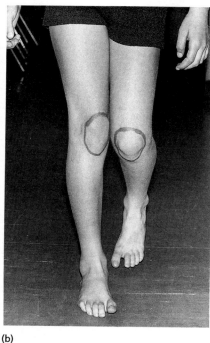

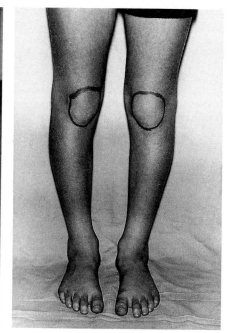

(a)   (b)   (c)

Fig. 10.15 (a) Squinting patella. (b,c) Gait showing medial rotation of knee and foot.

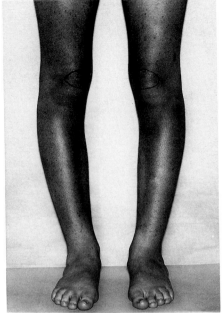
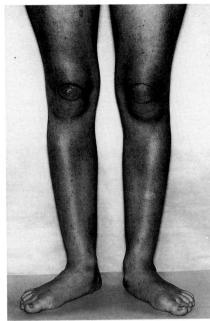

Fig. 10.16 (a) Apparent bow leg when feet pointing directly forwards. (b) Bow leg disappears when knees face anteriorly and pronated feet are now seen.

(a)

(b)

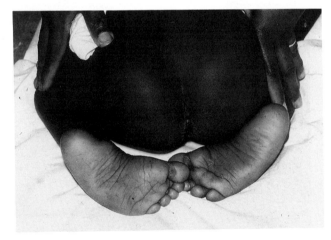

(a)

Fig. 10.17 (a) Sitting on medially rotated feet. (b) Note medial tibial torsion and varus forefoot.

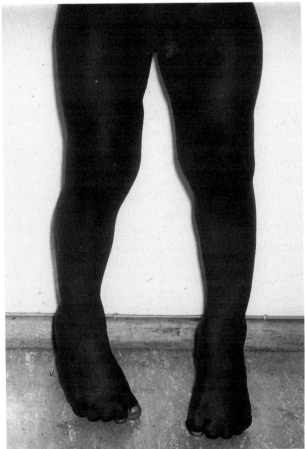

(b)

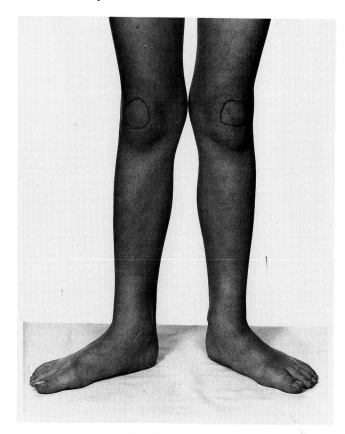

Fig. 10.18 Child showing primary increased external tibial torsion and secondary pronation of feet.

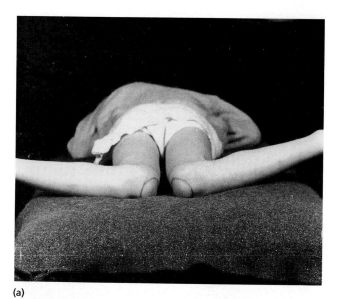

(a)

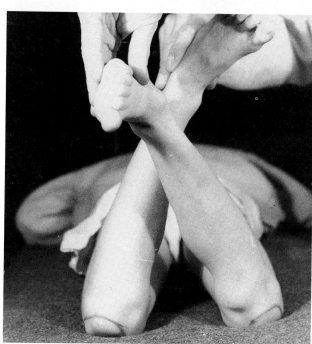

(b)

Fig. 10.19 Method of clinical assessment of anteversion from amount of hip rotation in extension. Patient prone. (a) 90° internal rotation. (b) Approx. 20° external rotation.

A reasonably accurate clinical estimate of tibial torsion is obtained as follows. The child sits on the edge of a table with the knees flexed to 90°; the relationship between the plane of the tibial tubercle and the malleoli is determined and this will indicate the degree of torsion (Fig. 10.20). Alternatively, it may be determined by measuring the angle between the second metatarsal and the tibial tuberosity. As indicated earlier, in some children with medial femoral torsion (increased anteversion) a compensatory increase in external tibial torsion occurs.

Angular deformity, e.g. genu valgum or varum, is looked for while the child is standing. The deformity is often more apparent than real, because the torsional abnormality only permits an oblique view of the tibia. A simple test will indicate whether the deformity is true or apparent: the legs are examined with the feet pointing directly forwards, noting whether the patellas are turned in or out; the feet are then rotated in or out until the knees are directly forwards (Fig. 10.16); if the deformity is not real it will then disappear.

Natural history

It has already been noted that physiological angular deformities, e.g. genu valgum and varum, which always correct spontaneously, may fail to do so if associated with a rotational deformity. In general, there is a tendency towards spontaneous improvement of most rotational deformities provided that extraneous factors,

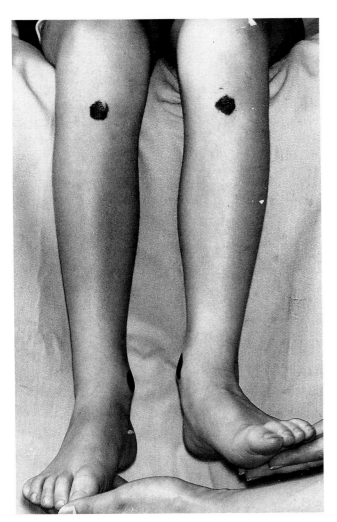

Fig. 10.20 Method for clinical estimation of tibial torsion.

e.g. abnormal sleeping and sitting postures, do not intervene. Deformities that are secondary or compensatory (most often seen in the tibia) seldom if ever correct spontaneously; furthermore, their presence serves as a useful prognostic guide for the primary deformity (usually the hip), indicating that improvement is unlikely to occur.

The author's studies (Harris, 1972) indicate that no more than 5% of medial rotation deformities of the hip will correct to normal; of those that do not correct, 60% will be left with a significantly increased angle of anteversion (over 40°). Fabry *et al.* (1973) confirmed these findings. It is of practical significance to appreciate that after the age of 8 years very little if any change takes place in the angle of anteversion (McSweeny, 1971; Fabry *et al.*, 1973), and it is particularly so if the angle is 50° or more.

Between 90%–95% of lateral rotation deformities of the hip will correct spontaneously to normal by about 3 years of age. Failure to correct results from an abnormal sleeping or sitting posture.

It may be stated with confidence that any deformity will not correct spontaneously after the age of 7 years. If an unselected group of adults is examined, it will be found that about 2% have significant medial tibial torsion severe enough to cause symptoms.

If lateral tibial torsion is primary, usually in association with an abnormal sleeping posture, spontaneous correction occurs provided that the posture changes during the first few years of life. If it is secondary, e.g. compensatory to a medial rotation deformity of the hip, it will not correct.

It is predictable that foot deformities will not correct spontaneously unless improvement occurs first in the associated deformities of the leg.

CLINICAL SIGNIFICANCE OF ROTATION DEFORMITIES

There is considerable speculation, but no hard evidence to support or refute the opinion, that a severe degree of rotational deformity of the adult lower extremity may predispose the hip and knee to the later development of osteoarthritis. In addition, it is said that the foot is likely to develop painful deformities.

The principal functional disturbance in children with internal rotation deformity of the hip, associated with compensatory external rotation of the tibia, is clumsiness when walking and running; the children are likely to complain of aching legs, which is the result of abnormal stress from attempts to correct an abnormal gait. Valgus of the hindfoot combined with forefoot varus and supination are often present and may result in aching feet and a complaint that shoes are rapidly deformed. There appears to be a high incidence of internal rotational deformity of the hip in adolescence with recurrent subluxation of the patella, but whether this is cause or effect is impossible to say. In the author's experience it is the cosmetic disability after skeletal maturity, particularly in girls, that is a major concern for parents. There is no doubt that the appearance can be extremely ugly (Fig. 10.21), and presents the clinician with a dilemma when he has to decide if surgical correction should be undertaken for purely cosmetic reasons.

It is not unreasonable to speculate that abnormal gait patterns that start in childhood and persist into adult life will eventually lead to osteoarthritis of the hip or knee as a result of abnormal stresses on them. Shands (1961) stated that the basic factor is joint incongruity, and that

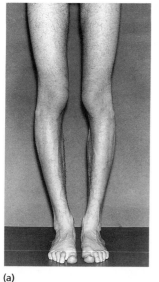
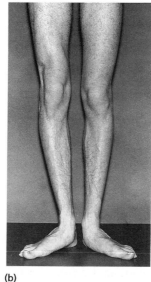

(a)　　　　　　　　(b)

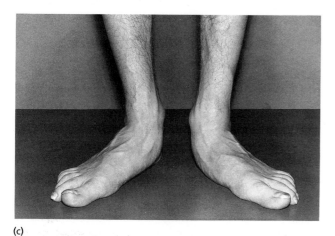

(c)

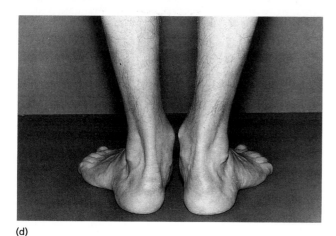

(d)

Fig. 10.21 (a−d) Young adult with residual rotation deformity of the legs and pronated feet.

a major cause of this is increased anteversion of the hip; he is supported in this view by others (Guran *et al.*, 1963; Morscher, 1967; Fabry *et al.*, 1973). Experience of total hip replacement for osteoarthritis has not convinced the author that increased anteversion is a major aetiological factor, though it is an element in hip dysplasia, which is a common cause of osteoarthritis. This opinion is supported by a study of normal and osteoarthritic adult hips in which there was no significant difference between the angle of anteversion in the two groups (Wedge *et al.*, 1989).

Pain in the knee, generally attributed to chondromalacia patellae, is a common symptom in young adults, particularly women; the diagnosis is made on relatively flimsy evidence and treatment is on the whole unrewarding. Clinical studies suggest that one possible cause of the pain is an abnormal gait pattern associated with a supinated forefoot and compensatory valgus hindfoot; not uncommonly the foot deformity is secondary to a torsional abnormality in the femur or tibia, and the result may be a torsional malalignment of the patellofemoral joint (Insall *et al.*, 1976). Further work including anteversion measurements needs to be done, and if the association is subsequently proved the clinical significance of torsional deformity will assume additional practical importance.

RADIOLOGICAL INVESTIGATION

Measurement of femoral torsion

It is not necessary to measure the degree of anteversion unless operative correction is contemplated following clinical assessment; other indications are certain patients with congenital dislocation of the hip and cerebral palsy. Any technique should be accurate and reproducible, and the radiation dose must be low. It is perhaps also important to consider whether or not complex equipment is required and its cost. The available techniques are described below.

FLUOROSCOPIC METHOD (Rogers, 1931)

The patient lies prone, the knee flexed to 90°, and the hip rotated until the femoral neck seen on the image intensifier lies directly in line with the femoral shaft. At this point the angle formed between the tibia and the plane of the table is a measure of the anteversion or retroversion. It is accurate but not as reproducible as other methods, the dose of X-rays is high, and expensive equipment is needed.

AXIAL METHOD (Dunn, 1952)

The technique is based on the theory that if the X-ray beam is directed along the axis of the femoral shaft so that the femoral condyles and neck are superimposed, the angle between the plane of the femoral neck and the transcondylar plane can be measured directly (Fig. 10.22). The patient lies supine, the hip and knee flexed to 90° and held in a special support; the X-ray beam can then be directed longitudinally along the femoral shaft. While it is reasonably accurate and reproducible, a prohibited dose of X-rays is necessary to produce films on which measurements can be made. The high dose of X-rays is avoided if the technique is modified by using axial tomography (Hubbard and Staheli, 1972), but this is more complex and expensive specialized equipment is required.

BIPLANE TECHNIQUE

Numerous workers have described the technique based on the same principle, namely obtaining two projections of the femoral neck from which the apparent anteversion and neck shaft angles may be measured; the two angles are determined from a standard table based on trigonometric considerations (Dunlap *et al.*, 1953; Ryder and Crane, 1953; Magilligan, 1956; Muller, 1956; Budin and Chandler, 1957; Shands and Steele, 1958; Harris, 1965). The technique is accurate, reproducible, does not require a high dose of X-rays, produces good quality films and requires only simple, relatively inexpensive equipment.

The patient lies supine, and for the anteroposterior

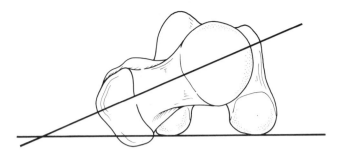

Fig. 10.22 View of the proximal end of the femur to determine the angle of anteversion.

projection the hip must be in neutral position; this is best achieved if the knees are flexed at 90° over the end of the table. From this projection the apparent neck−shaft angle is measured (Fig. 10.23). For the lateral projection, the hips are flexed 90° and abducted to an optimum of 20°, the knees are flexed 90°, the tibias parallel and the hip in neutral rotation. The legs are held in the correct position by a simple apparatus which can be clamped to the table. The horizontal bar is clamped at right angles to the side of the table; it represents the transcondylar plane of the femur and appears as a reference line on the bottom of the radiograph (Fig. 10.24).

The tube is centered 90 cm above the pubic symphysis. Correct positioning will be confirmed if the proximal half of the femoral shaft is parallel to the reference bar. The apparent angle of anteversion can now be measured (Fig. 10.25). The true angle is found by reference to the standard correction table (Fig. 10.26).

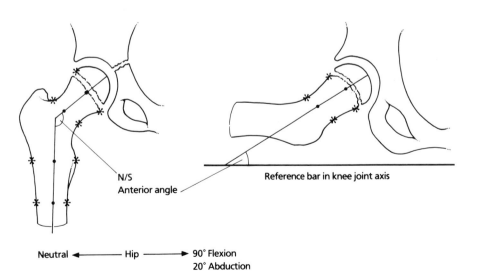

Fig. 10.23 The two radiographic projections for measuring apparent angles of inclination and anteversion.

N/S
Anterior angle

Reference bar in knee joint axis

Neutral ◄——— Hip ———► 90° Flexion
20° Abduction

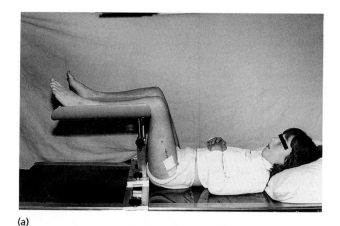

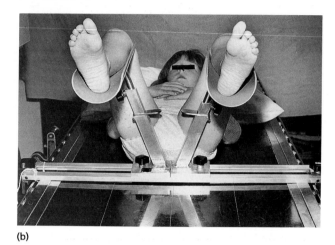

Fig. 10.24 Positioning the apparatus for lateral projection. (a) Hips and knees at 90°. (b) Hips abducted 20°, tibias parallel.

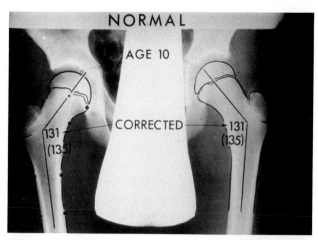

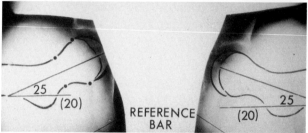

Fig. 10.25 Radiograph showing the two projections.

ULTRASONOGRAPHY

The technique was described by Moulton and Upadlyay (1982). The method has been compared with computed tomographic (CT) measurements in patients and found to be unreliable (Berman *et al.*, 1987). These results appear to have been confirmed by dry measurements (Lausten *et al.*, 1989). Terjesen and Anda (1990), however, reported that the technique is accurate; they pointed out that 10° has to be subtracted from the ultrasonographic value to give comparably accurate measurements by CT scan. Clearly, further studies are required, and if it could be shown to be reproducible and accurate, ultrasonography should be the method of choice for measuring femoral rotation because no radiation is involved.

COMPUTED TOMOGRAPHY

This was described by Hernandes *et al.* (1981). The measurement is simple, very accurate and reproducible, but it is expensive and radiation exposure is higher than with the biplane technique.

The legs and feet have to be immobilized so that no rotation or hip flexion movements occur during the procedure. One slice will depict the femoral neck with the upper border of the greater trochanter. The distal section is taken just below the upper pole of the patella. It is usual to obtain both sides on a single slice. The axis of the femoral neck and transcondylar neck can now be determined without difficulty and the angle of anteversion measured.

Measurement of acetabular anteversion

A relatively simple radiological technique has been described (Crispin *et al.*, 1978). Special apparatus is not required, and the technique is accurate if used for children between the ages of 1 and 14 years. A simpler technique is to use CT (Visser *et al.*, 1982). Acetabular anteversion is determined by measuring the angle formed by a tangent to the anterior and posterior lips of the acetabulum in relation to a perpendicular line through the triradiate cartilage. The measurement is possibly of value in the management of children with congenital dislocation of the hip over 1 year of age (Lloyd-Roberts

Anteversion

	5	10	15	20	25	30	35	40	45	50	55	60	65	70	75	80
100	4/101	9/100	15/100	20/100	25/100	30/98	35/99	40/98	45/97	50/96	55/96	60/94	65/94	70/93	75/92	80/91
105	4/105	10/105	15/104	20/104	25/103	30/103	36/102	41/101	46/100	51/99	56/99	60/97	65/96	70/95	75/94	80/92
110	5/110	10/110	16/109	21/108	26/108	31/107	37/106	42/105	47/104	52/103	57/101	61/100	66/98	71/97	76/95	80/93
115	5/115	11/115	16/114	21/112	27/112	32/111	37/110	43/109	48/107	52/105	57/104	62/102	67/101	71/99	76/96	81/94
120	6/120	11/119	17/118	22/117	28/116	33/115	38/114	44/112	49/110	53/108	58/106	62/104	68/103	72/101	77/98	81/95
125	6/125	12/124	17/123	23/121	28/120	34/119	39/118	44/116	50/114	54/112	59/109	63/106	68/105	73/103	77/100	82/96
130	6/130	12/129	18/127	24/126	29/125	35/124	40/122	46/120	51/117	55/115	60/112	64/109	69/107	73/104	78/101	82/97
135	6/134	13/133	19/132	25/131	31/130	37/129	42/126	47/123	52/120	57/118	61/114	66/112	70/109	74/105	78/102	83/98
140	7/139	13/138	20/137	26/135	32/134	38/132	44/130	49/127	53/124	58/120	62/116	67/115	71/111	75/107	79/103	83/100
145	7/144	14/143	21/142	27/139	33/138	40/136	45/134	51/131	55/128	59/124	63/119	68/117	72/114	76/110	79/104	83/101
150	8/149	15/147	22/146	29/144	35/143	41/141	47/138	52/135	57/133	61/129	65/124	69/120	73/116	77/112	80/106	84/102
155	9/154	17/153	25/151	31/149	38/148	44/146	50/142	55/139	59/136	63/132	67/128	71/124	75/119	78/115	81/108	85/103
160	10/159	19/158	28/157	34/154	41/153	47/151	52/147	57/144	62/140	66/136	69/132	73/128	76/122	79/117	82/111	85/105
165	12/164	23/164	32/161	40/159	47/158	53/156	58/153	63/149	65/144	69/140	72/135	75/130	78/126	81/119	83/113	86/106
170	15/169	27/168	37/166	46/164	53/162	58/159	63/157	67/154	71/150	73/145	76/141	78/134	81/129	83/122	85/116	87/109

(Left axis label: Valgus)

Fig. 10.26 Correction table for determining the angle of femoral anteversion.

et al., 1978). Further studies are necessary, but measurement of acetabular anteversion may be useful for obtaining a more accurate and stable hip following osteotomy for increased anteversion. Equally, it may be important to measure acetabular anteversion before undertaking a femoral rotation osteotomy in the management of congenital dislocation of the hip (Harris, 1976).

Measurement of tibial torsion

It is the author's opinion that for all practical purposes, a sufficiently accurate estimate of tibial torsion can be made by clinical examination, and this method has been used successfully for obtaining good correction by tibial osteotomy. Radiologically, a qualitative assessment may be make by taking a standard lateral projection of the ankle joint and comparing it with a lateral view taken with the malleoli in the same coronal plane — a position obtained by rotating the leg medially. An accurate radiological technique has been described using CT (Jacob *et al.*, 1980); the mean value in a normal cadaveric tibia was found to be 30°.

TREATMENT

The need for treatment, the measures to be adopted and their timing depend on two factors: the natural history and the short-term and long-term effects, both functional and cosmetic. Knowledge of the former is such that the method of treatment and its timing, particularly with regard to operative correction, is reasonably straightforward; thus, by way of example, it may be stated with confidence that it is seldom necessary to offer treatment for external rotation deformities of the hip, almost all of which correct spontaneously by 2−3 years of age. As a general rule, the younger the child the more likely it is that simple measures will produce at least a partial correction; an older child is more likely to have developed compensatory (secondary) deformities, and in such instances treatment becomes complex and an operation is more likely to be necessary.

The short-term effects of treatment are mainly functional and cosmetic, occurring for the most part during the growth period, and are well understood. With regard to the long-term effects, the lack of strong evidence in support of their clinical significance makes it unwise to use such criteria alone for deciding the need for operative correction.

Conservative measures

The following measures are generally applicable, with a few exceptions, to all varieties of rotational deformities.

STRETCHING EXERCISES

Torsional stretching in the opposite direction to the deformity should be taught to the parents. It may help in simple mild deformities in young children, particularly in the hip joint. Furthermore, there is no doubt that anxious parents also benefit, because they like to take an active part in the management of their child's problems.

CORRECTION OF POSTURAL HABITS

The correct sleeping posture should be initiated during the first few months of life, after which it is unlikely that this can be changed. It is the practice in some obstetric units to nurse babies prone; from the point of view of external rotational deformities of the hip and associated foot deformities, this position should be discouraged; side lying offers the same advantages. Tight bedclothes will prevent the infant spontaneously altering sleeping posture, which starts between 4 and 6 months. Bulky nappies are best avoided as they encourage the prone frog-leg position. It is useful to encourage a sitting posture that is the reverse of the deformity; the lower extremities should be maintained in a neutral position by sitting on a small chair or stool.

DENIS BROWNE BOOTEES AND BAR

The splint is useful and is best reserved for severe tibial torsion; if it is used to correct hip deformities there is a danger of stretching the knee ligaments, which may result in an angular deformity, e.g. knock knee. It is a valuable night splint and may help to change or neutralize the effects of the sleeping posture.

SHOES AND INSOLES

Good supporting shoes are clearly important for all children, but they are particularly valuable if the feet are pronated, as they often are in the presence of an internal rotational deformity at the hip and increased external tibial torsion. Extra valgus stiffening is a help, and for the severely pronated foot Helfet's heel seats or cups made from a cast are recommended; alternatively, a Plexidure orthosis made from a cast is popular with chiropodists, and the author's experience with them is favourable. Whichever appliance is used, regular supervision is essential, and generally they should be used at least until skeletal maturity is reached.

Surgical measures

The most valuable procedures are high femoral and tibial osteotomy. The former is used to correct internal rotation deformity (increased anteversion) of the hip, and the latter to correct either internal or external rotation deformity of the tibia. It must be emphasized that the decision to advise an operation is made only after full, careful and repeated examination of the lower extremities—if necessary extending over a 2—3 year period. It is equally important to have full and frank discussions with the parents and the child about the nature of the condition and details about possible surgery. It is the parents who will provide most of the information on which a decision to advise surgery is based.

INDICATIONS

Operation in general should be considered for children with severe deformity that has not significantly improved or corrected spontaneously following the application of simple conservative measures. In order to allow time for improvement to occur, it is advisable to defer operation until about 7—8 years of age; significant functional improvement sometimes takes place, though the structional deformity remains. The important factors, which must be considered together and not in isolation, are as follows.

Functional disability

Information on this aspect will usually be provided by the parents and the school. If there is any doubt a functional assessment should be obtained from the physiotherapy department.

Cosmetic factor

This is largely a question of the abnormal gait pattern. Generally, parents raise this question only with regard to girls. Although it is a highly subjective matter, it is nevertheless an important consideration and should not be ignored.

Excessive shoe wear

The deformation of shoe uppers and wear necessitating repair or new shoes every few weeks is a common presenting symptom. Experience has convinced the author that operative correction of the rotation deformity produces a significant improvement in the gait and degree of shoe wear.

Compensatory deformity

These complex deformities are generally associated with a severe cosmetic and functional disability, and as pointed out earlier, they do not correct spontaneously. Operation should be considered for the primary deformity before the secondary one is too advanced; in this way, operative correction of the latter may be avoided.

Internal rotation deformity of the hip

A useful guide is to consider surgery if the angle of anteversion is 40° or more and if, as usually found, it is associated with 90° of internal rotation and not more that 10° of external rotation of the hip.

External rotation deformity of the hip

It is very rare for operation to be required, because almost all cases will correct spontaneously in the first few years of life. For the few exceptions, it is advisable to wait until the child is a least 7 years of age. Anteversion of 10° or less associated with about 90° of external rotation at the hip would be the criteria for considering operation.

OPERATIVE TECHNIQUE

Several points are worthy of comment in order to reduce errors, minimize the time spent in hospital and assist rapid return of function. With regard to femoral osteotomy, preoperative measurement of the anteversion angle enables the surgeon to achieve an accurate correction; internal fixation of the osteotomy with a Coventry screw and plate avoids the need for immobilization in a plaster spica (Fig. 10.27). Simple skin traction for 2 weeks followed by weight-bearing in the third week is quite safe.

Although both hips can be corrected at the same time, it is preferable to operate on the second one 1−2 weeks later.

The technique recommended for tibial osteotomy is that described by O'Donoghue (1940); it is safe, simple and accurate. The principle of the technique is illustrated in Figs 10.28 and 10.29. Following operation, a long leg cast is required for 6−8 weeks and weight-bearing is safe after 2 weeks. If both femurs and tibias require correction, the author prefers to do the former during

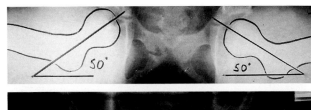
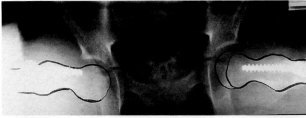
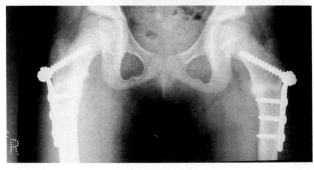

Fig. 10.27 Radiograph showing operative correction of increased anteversion.

one admission and then wait until rehabilitation has been achieved before embarking on the tibias. If two surgeons are available, an alternative is to undertake simultaneous correction of one femur and the opposite tibia and the others 2 weeks later.

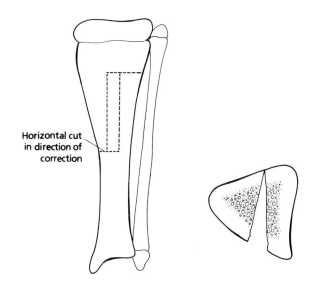

Horizontal cut in direction of correction

Fig. 10.28 Technique for correcting tibial torsion.

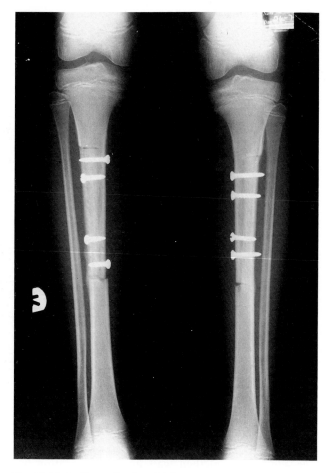

Fig. 10.29 Radiograph after tibial osteotomy.

COMPLICATIONS

In the case of femoral osteotomy the author has not encountered any instances of non-union or failure of the fixation in 110 operations. Inadequate correction has occurred in a few instances; it is purely a technical problem and should be preventable if an accurate estimate of the preoperative anteversion is obtained. In a few patients, reduction of the neck—shaft angle (varus deformity) has occurred, and the result is some degree of temporary shortening; the angle returns to normal in due course.

With regard to tibial osteotomy, a failure to obtain full correction resulted on a few occasions. Delayed union has occurred four times in 37 osteotomies; it is much more likely to occur if the operation is undertaken in children over 10 years of age. Deep infection resulting in bone involvement has occured twice, leading to morbidity of several months, but eventual healing without permanent disability.

RESULTS OF OPERATION

The criteria for judging the success of the operation are functional and cosmetic. The former is difficult to assess, but if there was a significant defect preoperatively then provided full correction is obtained there is always an improvement. Cosmetic improvement is most striking, for which parents invariably express their gratitude. Until the late clinical effects of persistent deformity are more clearly understood, it cannot be said that the operation prevents disabilities in later adult life, though it is the author's opinion that this will indeed prove to be the case.

REFERENCES

Berman L., Mitchell R., and Catz D. (1987) Ultrasound assessment of femoral anteversion. *J. Bone Joint Surg.* **69B**, 268−270.

Bohm M. (1933) Infantile deformities of the knee and hip. *J. Bone Joint Surg.* **15**, 574.

Budin E. and Chandler E. (1957) Measurement of femoral neck anteversion by a direct method. *Radiology* **69**, 209.

Crispin A.R., Harris N.H. and Lloyd-Roberts G.C. (1978) A method for calculating acetabular anteversion in children. *Paediatr. Radiol.* **7**, 155.

Crane L. (1959) Femoral torsion and its relation to toeing-in and toeing-out. *J. Bone Joint Surg.* **41A**, 421.

Dunlap K., Shands A.R. Jr, Hollister L.C. Jr *et al.* (1953) A new method for determination of torsion of the femur. *J. Bone Joint Surg.* **35A**, 289.

Dunn D.M. (1952) Anteversion of the neck of the femur. A method of measurement. *J. Bone Joint Surg.* **34B**, 181.

Fabry F., MaCewan G.D. and Shands A.R. Jr (1973) Torsion of the femur. *J. Bone Joint Surg.* **55A**, 1726.

Farrier C.D. and Lloyd-Roberts G.C. (1969) The natural history of knock-knee in children. *Practitioner* **203**, 789.

Fitzhugh M.L. (1941) Faulty alignment of the feet and legs in infancy and childhood. *Physiother. Rev.* **21**, 239.

Gelberman R.H., Cohen M.S., Desai S.S., Griffin P.P., Salamon P.B. and O'Brien T.M. (1987) Femoral anteversion: a clinical assessment of in-toeing gait in children. *J. Bone Joint Surg.* **69B**, 75−78.

Guran P., Masse P., Bruchon D. *et al.* (1963) Conséquences cliniques de l'antéversion exagérée du cor femoral. *Arch. Fr. Pediatr.* **20**, 856.

Harris N.H. (1965) A method of measurement of femoral neck anteversion and a preliminary report on its practical application. *J. Bone Joint Surg.* **47B**, 188.

Harris N.H. (1972) Rotation deformities and their secondary effects in the lower extremities in children. *J. Bone Joint Surg.* **54B**, 172.

Harris N.H. (1976) Acetabular growth potential in congenital dislocation of the hip and some factors upon which it may depend. *Clin. Orthop.* **119**, 99.

Hernandes R.J., Tachdjian M.O., Poznanski A.K. and Dias L.S. (1981) CT determination of femoral torsion. *Am. J. Radiol.* **137**, 97−101.

Hubbard D.D. and Staheli L.T. (1972) The direct radiographic method of measurement of femoral torsion using axial tomography. *Clin. Orthop.* **86**, 16–20.

Hutter C.G., Jr and Scott W. (1949) Tibial torsion. *J. Bone Joint Surg.* **31A**, 511.

Insall J., Falvo K.A. and Wise D.W. (1976) Chondromalacia patellae. A prospective study. *J. Bone Joint Surg.* **58A**, 1–8.

Jacob R.P., Haertel M. and Stussi E. (1980) Tibial torsion calculated by computerised tomography and compared to other methods of measurement. *J. Bone Joint Surg.* **62B**, 238–242.

Lausten G.S., Jorgesnsen F. and Boesen J. (1989) Measurement of anteversion of the femoral neck: ultrasound and computerised tomography compared. *J. Bone Joint Surg.* **71B**, 237–239.

Lloyd-Roberts G.C., Harris N.H. and Crispin A.R. (1978) Anteversion of the acetabulum in congenital dislocation of the hip: a preliminary report. *Orthop. Clin. North Am.* **9**, 89.

McKibbin B. (1970) Anatomical factors in the stability of the hip joint in the new born. *J. Bone Joint Surg.* **52B**, 148.

McSweeny A. (1971) A study of femoral torsion in children. *J. Bone Joint Surg.* **53B**, 90.

Magilligan D.J. (1956) Calculation of the angle of anteversion by means of horizontal roentgenography. *J. Bone Joint Surg.* **38A**, 1231.

Morscher E. (1967) Development and clinical significance of the anteversion of the femoral neck. *Wiederherstellungschir. Traumatol.* **9**, 107.

Moulton A. and Upadhyay S.S. (1982) A direct method of measuring femoral anteversion using ultrasound. *J. Bone Joint Surg.* **64B**, 469–472.

Muller M.F. (1956) Ischiometrie radiologique. *Rev. Chir. Orthop.* **42**, 124.

O'Donoghue D.H. (1940) Controlled rotation osteotomy of the tibia with special reference to deformities resulting from club foot and poliomyelitis. *South Med. J.* **33**, 1145.

Rogers S.B. (1931) A method for determining the angle of torsion of the neck of the femur. *J. Bone Joint Surg.* **13**, 821.

Ryder C.T. and Crane L. (1953) Measuring femoral anteversion. The problem and the method. *J. Bone Joint Surg.* **35A**, 321.

Shands A.R. Jr (1961) The treatment of osteoarthritis of the hip by conservative measures. *Acad. Med. NJ Bull.* **7**, 312.

Shands A.R. Jr and Steele M.K. (1958) Torsion of the femur: follow-up report of the Dunlap method for its determination. *J. Bone Joint Surg.* **40A**, 803.

Sommerville E.W. (1957) Persistent fetal alignment of the hip. *J. Bone Joint Surg.* **39B**, 100.

Terjesen T. and Anda S. (1990) Ultrasound measurements of femoral anteversion. *J. Bone Joint Surg.* **72B**, 726–727.

Visser J.D., Jonkers A. and Hillen B. (1982) Hip joint measurements with computerised tomography. *J. Paediatr. Orthop.* **2**, 143–146.

Wedge J.H., Munkacsi I. and Loback D. (1989) Anteversion of the femur and idiopathic osteoarthrosis of the hip. *J. Bone Joint Surg.* **71A**, 1040–1043.

Chapter 11
Leg Length Inequality

M. Saleh & M. Bell

INTRODUCTION

Limb length discrepancy may be a result of congenital deformity, acquired disease, or trauma. The consequences of such deformities may be controlled by orthosis or surgery. Until the 1970s operative techniques of limb lengthening were generally unreliable, and small discrepancies (<3 cm) were managed with shoe raises and other orthoses. Large and progressive discrepancies (10 cm or more at maturity), e.g. congenital reduction deformities with or without foot involvement, were managed by amputation. Discrepancies of intermediate size were considered appropriate for operation either lengthening or more commonly contralateral growth arrest or shortening, with up to 6 cm of correction obtainable.

Non-mechanical attempts at lengthening, e.g. growth acceleration by influencing local metabolic changes using chemical, hormonal, vascular, electrical and surgical stimuli, were generally unsuccessful. Some success however, has been attributed to periosteal stripping (Wilde and Baker, 1987). Surgical lengthening, because of the expertise required and the high complication rate, remained the province of a few specialist centres. Newer techniques have become safer and encouraged its more widespread use. For this reason and because of its capacity to correct associated deformity, there has been a reversal in the trend for shortening. The technique involves dividing the bone and gradually distracting it until the desired length is achieved (callus distraction) (De Bastiani *et al.*, 1987; Ilizarov, 1990). Lengthening may also be achieved by distraction of the growth plate, either rapidly by a technique known as distractional epiphysiolysis (Monticelli and Spinelli, 1981) or at a slower rate by a process termed chondrodiatasis (De Bastiani *et al.*, 1986a, b).

INDICATIONS AND TIMING OF SURGERY

Lengthening is mainly performed in the lower limb to provide symmetrical stance. Asymmetrical stance produces symptoms secondary to postural adaptation, e.g. scoliosis, hip adduction and knee flexion or recurvatum deformities on the long side, and equinus deformity on the short side (Fig. 11.1). If the shortening is present from an early age, fixed deformities will prevent normal skeletal and joint development. When the gait is observed a limp and vaulting are apparent with increased energy expenditure. In an adult of average height, a shortening of 3 cm or more that is left uncompensated will lead to fixed deformity in the spine, back pain and an unacceptable limp (Friberg, 1983). In contrast, upper limb lengthening is seldom indicated as it is mainly of cosmetic benefit, though occasionally it is necessary to obtain increased reach for personal hygiene. It is mainly confined to the humerus, as lengthening of both forearm bones is associated with unacceptable levels of functional impairment. When one forearm bone is short, lengthening may be justified to realign the wrist, increase function and improve cosmesis.

The aetiology of conditions leading to shortening that is amenable to operative correction includes a number of congenital and acquired conditions, e.g. hip dysplasia secondary to congenital dislocation of the hip, congenital pseudarthrosis of the tibia, congenital shortening of the femur or hypoplasia of the fibula, poliomyelitis, spina bifida, Ollier's disease, post-irradiation shortening, and trauma or infection producing growth plate disturbance and fracture or malunion. Most procedures are carried out in children (ratio of children : adults 4 : 1), though an increasing number of adults are presenting with fracture-related shortening (Saleh, 1992a). A more recent indication for lengthening has been in children with disproportionate short stature, e.g. achondroplasia, in

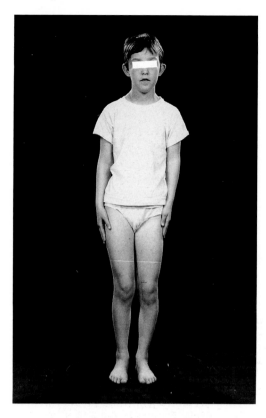

Fig. 11.1 Asymmetrical stance produces symptoms secondary to postural adaptation, e.g. scoliosis, hip adduction and knee flexion or recurvatum deformities on the long side and equinus deformity on the short side.

which the limbs are short in relation to the trunk (Saleh and Burton, 1991).

Lengthening may be carried out at any age, but for practical and biological reasons it is more appropriate in younger patients and before the development of fixed compensatory deformities. Lack of cooperation and small bone size make lengthening difficult before the age of 5 years. Small discrepancies may be most appropriately treated at skeletal maturity to avoid underestimation or overestimation. Staged short lengthenings throughout childhood may be indicated in some conditions, e.g. congenital shortening, to avoid longer lengthenings which carry a higher risk. Woven bone forms after callus distraction but remodels with time, taking on a normal haversian architecture enabling repeat lengthenings to be performed at the same site and reducing the risk of refracture (Saleh *et al.*, 1993).

ASSESSMENT

History

The onset and rate of shortening or deformity and the

availability of previous anthropometric, photographic, or radiographic information should be established. If the discrepancy is long-standing, compliance in the use of orthoses and any previous attempts at operative correction will provide useful information on the likelihood of secondary fixed deformities. Direct questioning should establish whether back, hip and other lower limb symptoms are present, as well as any evidence of neurological compromise. A history of osteomyelitis or radiotherapy may indicate contralateral limb shortening.

A full medical history should be taken to establish anaesthetic and operative risk factors, e.g. cardiopulmonary compromise, blood dyscrasias (as pin sites may be the source of a persistent diathesis), congenital cardiac anomalies (as bacteraemia may develop secondary to a pin site infection) and the presence of antibiotic allergies. Psychosocial factors are important, because treatment may extend over many months or in some cases years. Assessment of the ability of the patient and the family to cope with the stress of lengthening, as well as of schooling, housing and financial needs, must be undertaken as these are valid reasons for considering simpler options than lengthening.

Examination

The lower limbs should initially be examined with the patient standing to assess spinal posture and limb alignment. With corrective blocks placed under the foot leg length may be assessed as well as fixed spinal deformity. Lateral bending is particularly useful. Scoliosis, genu valgus or varus, a valgus heel or equinus foot should be noted. The range of movements and power should be recorded in the hip, knee, ankle and foot. Any joint instability should be noted. The soft tissues are examined for scarring, sinuses and other deformities. Shoe wear should be assessed and a full neurovascular assessment made. Aligning the iliac crests with the patient standing on corrective blocks is the most reliable, simple, clinical test for discrepancy if there is no pelvic hypoplasia (Eichler, 1972) (Fig. 11.2). Tape measurements should also be made from the anterior superior iliac spine to the medial malleolus; however, if the latter is ill-defined or the heel is small the measurement should be taken to the heel. The site of discrepancy may be readily appreciated by flexing both hips and knees to between 70° and 90° and lining up the heels. The discrepancy may be in the heel, tibia, femur, or pelvis. Laboratory-based anthropometric measurements using specifically designed benches, rulers and calipers are also of value.

Upper limb examination follows similar principles and will not be described further.

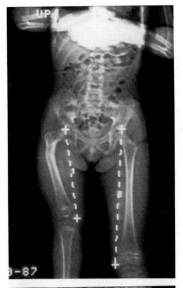

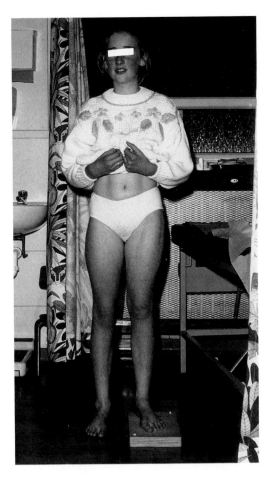

Fig. 11.2 Aligning the iliac crest with the patient standing on corrective blocks is the most reliable simple clinical test for discrepancy if there is no pelvic hypoplasia (Eichler, 1972).

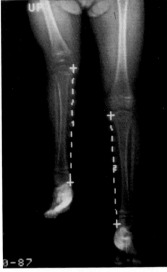

Fig. 11.3 CT scan for measuring limb length. Note the measurement is critically dependent on accurate cursor placement.

Investigations

Limb length may be measured with a variety of radiological techniques, including conventional views that take spot pictures of the hip, knee and ankle, parallel beam views and computed tomography (CT) (Fig. 11.3). Lateral bending radiographs of the thoracolumbar spine are useful to exclude fixed spinal deformity. Anteroposterior and lateral radiographs of the affected segment and standing anteroposterior mechanical axis films of the lower limbs are also useful (Fig. 11.4). In congenital cases or those with joint abnormalities, special views may be required. For hip dysplasia, in addition to anteroposterior and lateral radiographs an anteroposterior view in 20° of abduction and full internal rotation may be useful. For the knee, lateral radiographs in full extension are useful, as are weight-bearing lateral radiographs from mid-tibia to the toes for ankle and foot deformities.

Growth prediction and final discrepancy estimates may be made with anteroposterior wrist radiographs for carpal bone age and anthropometric measurements (Anderson *et al.*, 1963; Moseley, 1977) and from a chart of anthropometric values (Aldegheri and Agostini, 1993). Composite photographs may be used to assess the effects of lengthening and shortening procedures on body proportions (Nicolls and Saleh, 1988; Nicolls, 1988) (Fig. 11.5). Using a built up shoe for a period and monitoring back pain may help to assess the degree of spinal involvement.

TO LENGTHEN OR TO SHORTEN?

It is possible to produce a 2.5–5 cm gain in leg length

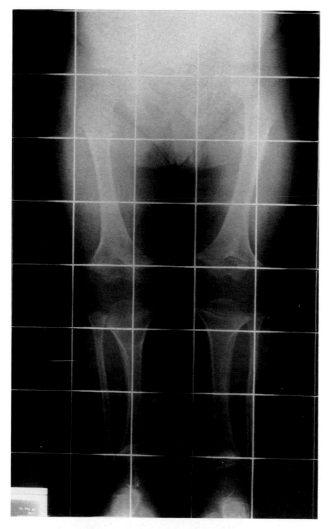

Fig. 11.4 Standing anteroposterior mechanical axis films of the lower limbs against a 5 cm grid.

with very few complications. Therefore, in most cases leg lengthening should be the treatment of choice as opposed to limb shortening. It must be remembered that limb shortening will take place on the so-called 'normal' limb. The development of complications or problems in this limb should be avoided at all costs.

LIMB SHORTENING

Indications

The indications for limb shortening fall into two major categories:

1 The correction of a limb that is too long: this includes groups of conditions that are called local giantism.
  (a) Neurofibromatosis.
  (b) Arteriovenous malformations.
  (c) Hemihypertropies.
  (d) Post-traumatic overgrowth.
2 A short limb in which it is considered unsafe to lengthen.
  (a) A bone that has become short due to exposure to radiation.
  (b) Patients with problems with joints above and below the segment to be lengthened.
  (c) Any limb with significant soft tissue damage with scarring.
  (d) Any limb with vascular compromise.
  (e) The presence of any infection in the bone segment to be lengthened.

GROUP 1

In limbs that are too long, the decision to shorten is the obvious one and the indication to shorten is the same as for lengthening, in that the discrepancy is such that limb equalization should be carried out. If the discrepancy is small, i.e. less than 2 cm, this should be accommodated by a small shoe raise in the first instance. In discrepancies over 2 cm, equalization should be considered and shortening performed if indicated.

GROUP 2

Post-radiotherapy shortening

In the authors' experience of lengthening, people who have had the bone irradiated encounter considerable problems in creating satisfactory regeneration. This leads to poor-quality bone formation, which is brittle and often repeatedly fractures. Under these circumstances limb shortening is a more appropriate procedure to correct limb length.

Leg lengthening in patients with unstable joints

This is likely to end with serious complications. Lengthening the femur in the presence of an unstable hip can lead to hip dislocation. The dislocation compounds the problems of the short limb and so must be avoided at all costs. Once the hip has dislocated it is difficult to recover from this situation, despite the reversal of the lengthening process.

If lengthening is to be considered in an unstable hip, a procedure to stabilize the hip must be carried out before lengthening. The procedure used depends on the underlying hip pathology.

The same considerations apply to instability around the knee. Lengthening of the tibia or the femur can

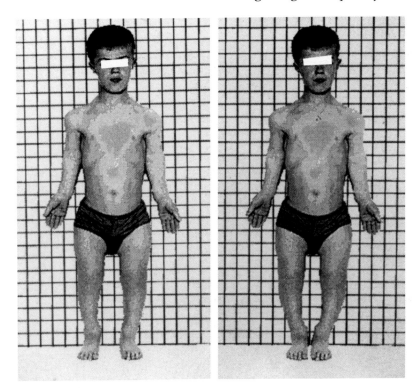

Fig. 11.5 Composite photographs may be used to assess the effects of lengthening and shortening procedures on body proportions (Nicolls and Saleh, 1988; Nicolls, 1990).

result in dislocation of the knee, which must be avoided as relocation of the knee once it has dislocated can be a difficult problem.

Soft tissue damage

At the present time bone regeneration in the technique of callus distraction is very reliable. The major problems that occur are due to soft tissue tension and subsequent soft tissue contractures. If there is any limitation in joint range before lengthening, it will undoubtedly become worse as a result of lengthening. If there has been significant muscle damage, i.e. following trauma, which has resulted in a limitation of joint range, this limitation will increase as a result of lengthening. If the range of knee flexion is 0–90° then leg lengthening is contra-indicated, as the range of knee flexion will certainly be less than 90° at the end of the procedure. Serious consideration to limb shortening should be given under these circumstances.

The same provisos are applicable to the tibia. If there is significant reduction in dorsiflexion of the foot before lengthening, it is inevitable that an equinus deformity of the ankle will develop. Leg lengthening can be carried out under these circumstances with the use of additional frames to stabilize the foot and prevent the deformity occurring.

Vascular compromise

If the limb has impaired circulation of any form, limb lengthening may produce an ischaemic foot. This is not a justifiable risk in the majority of cases, and therefore other methods of limb equalization should be considered for these patients. The same consideration applies to people with neurological impairment in the limb.

Infection

Leg lengthening in a segment that has previously been infected carries the risk that the infection may recur. If it does recur, there is a possibility of an infected non-union at the lengthening site. Consideration must be given to other methods of equalization in these circumstances.

Techniques of limb shortening

Four basic techniques are available for limb shortening:
1 Staples.
2 Epiphysiodesis.
3 Open excision of bone segments.
4 Closed shortening techniques.

CHOICE OF TECHNIQUE

The timing of limb shortening procedures depends on the time at which the discrepancy becomes apparent and when it becomes a functional problem. This is related to the cause of the discrepancy. It is obvious that use of staples and epiphysiodesis is only of value when the epiphyses are still open. The other two techniques can be used when the epiphyses are closed. Care must be taken not to damage the adjacent epiphysis.

To use staples and epiphysiodesis requires regular, careful charting of the patient before operation. Monitoring of the patient's chronological age, bone age and the amount of discrepancy must be carried out. This information should then be plotted on a chart (Moseley, 1977) to enable the surgeon to predict the discrepancy of the limb at skeletal maturity. Other charts have been produced by Aldegheri and Agostini (1993) and Demeglio (personal communication, 1990) in Montpelier.

As a rough guide, a discrepancy that is present at the age of 4 years will double by skeletal maturity. A discrepancy present at 9 years of age will be 20% more at the end of growth.

Most growth in the lower limb takes place around the knee, with the femoral epiphysis contributing approximately 56% to that growth. At puberty the knee contributes approximately 5 cm to overall height. Therefore, in patients who have had their discrepancy carefully monitored it is possible to achieve 5 cm of shortening by epiphysiodesis carried out just before puberty. Epiphysiodesis carried out at an earlier age is unreliable, and staples can be used to slow down growth before carrying out a femoral epiphysiodesis just before puberty.

If the epiphyses are closed then the only techniques available are either to excise a fragment of the bone by an open technique or to use the closed shortening technique described by Winquist and Hansen (1978).

STAPLING (Blount and Clark, 1949)

The main indication for staples is local giantism due to arteriovenous malformations or neurofibromatosis. Both medial and lateral approaches should be used to expose the femoral and tibial epiphyses. The head of the fibula should also be stapled in these cases.

Technique

A longitudinal incision is made over the lateral and medial sides of both the lower femur and upper tibia. The bone on the medial side is exposed by reflecting anteriorly the belly of the vastus medialis muscle. The site of the epiphysis is determined by placing a small pin into the epiphysis and confirming its position by radiography. On the lateral side, the tensor fascia latae is split and the muscle reflected to expose the lateral femoral condyle. A pin is used to identify the epiphysis: it will not go into bone but sinks into the softened cartilage of the epiphysis.

Separate incisions should be made over the upper tibia, both on the medial and lateral side. Care must be taken on the lateral side to identify the common peroneal nerve and protect it.

Once the radiograph has confirmed that the pins are within the epiphysis, staples are then used to straddle the epiphysis. These are distributed evenly across the epiphysis to produce an even growth arrest (Fig. 11.6). A single staple can be used across the head of the fibular epiphysis.

Following stapling a Robert Jones bandage is worn

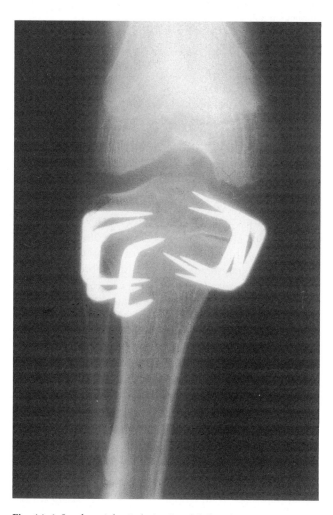

Fig. 11.6 Staple epiphysiodesis. Careful distribution is necessary to produce even growth arrest.

for a period of 2–3 days until the pain subsides, and weight-bearing is then commenced. Partial weight-bearing with crutches is recommended for the first 1–2 weeks. After that the patient should be fully mobile. No restriction should be placed on activities.

Careful out-patient review is essential with regular radiographic follow-up. Review is required to determine: (i) that the stapling is slowing down growth; (ii) there is no migration of the staples from the site; and (iii) no varus/valgus, antecurvatum or recurvatum deformities are appearing, and no bony bridges are forming across the epiphysis to form a permanent epiphysiodesis

Complications

Deformities can occur if the staples are not spread evenly around the epiphysis or if they migrate from the site. The main complication of stapling is the unsightly scars. The staples should be left in until it is demonstrated by the use of straight-line graphs that the perfect time has arrived to carry out a formal epiphysiodesis. The use of staples is recommended in the early stages as the staples can be removed to allow the epiphysis to recover. It may be possible at an early stage to correct leg length discrepancy and then allow normal growth to take place.

EPIPHYSIODESIS

This has been the mainstay of limb equalization in children for many years. It is a reliable method of producing limb shortening, but it is not without its complications. Phemister (1933) first described the technique of taking out a ring of the periosteum from around the epiphysis and using a bone block across the epiphysis. More recently, percutaneous epiphysiodesis has been described (Bowen and Johnson, 1984). An image intensifier is used to identify the epiphysis, which is then marked with a Kirschner wire or a small Steinmann pin. Having identified the epiphysis a small hole is made through the skin and down to bone. The epiphysis is drilled and a burr or curette is inserted into the epiphysis, which is removed piecemeal (Fig. 11.7). Small incisions are made both on the medial and lateral sides. Care must be taken over the fibular epiphysis, and probably an open technique is to be recommended to ensure that no damage occurs to the common peroneal nerve.

Published results suggest this is a very reliable method that produces less deformity and a more complete fusion of the epiphysis than previously described open techniques (Canale and Christian, 1990).

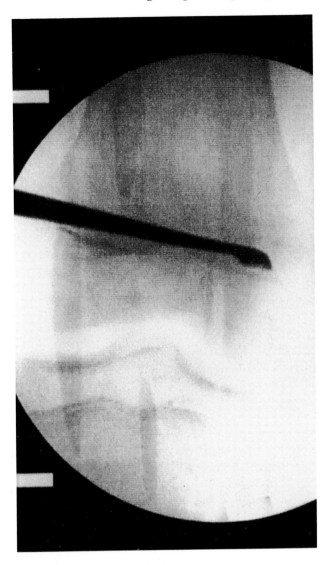

Fig. 11.7 Percutaneous epiphysiodesis.

Epiphysiodesis is a demanding technique. The timing at which epiphysiodesis is carried out is crucial: if carried out too late the discrepancy is not corrected, and if carried out too early a normal limb then becomes the shorter limb. Moseley (1977) described straight line graphs and Demeglio (1990) a set of tables to help surgeons predict the limb length discrepancy and the length of the normal limb at the end of growth. Working backward on the charts, it is possible to determine exactly when to carry out epiphysiodesis to ensure that the discrepancy is corrected.

It must be remembered that epiphysiodesis is carried out at a time determined by bone age rather than chronological age. A number of patients with leg length discrepancies have a bone age that lags behind their chronological age. For this reason, regular radiography of the left hand should be undertaken to evaluate the bone age. It should be stressed, however, that the estimation of bone age is not without a significant degree of error, despite using the tables of Greulich and Pyle (1959). At around the age of puberty the bone age may change rapidly and catch up with the chronological age, therefore greater vigilance is needed at this time to ensure that the window for epiphysiodesis is not missed. Indeed, Demeglio (1990) has stated that epiphysiodesis is usually carried out too late.

During puberty 5 cm of growth occurs around the knee, therefore epiphysiodesis at this time will result in a 5 cm correction of length discrepancy. In girls puberty starts at about 11 years of bone age and in boys at the bone age of 13 years and lasts approximately 2 years. To try to achieve correction of greater than 5 cm by epiphysiodesis carries a greater risk as the timing is more difficult to determine.

To correct a leg length discrepancy of over 5 cm it is best to consider two alternative techniques: first, epiphysiodesis and secondly, limb shortening by open excision of a bone segment.

Complications

The complications of epiphysiodesis are: (i) incomplete correction; (ii) overcorrection; and (iii) production of deformity. Menelaus (1966) reported a 10% overcorrection in his series.

There is a risk that epiphysiodesis may damage the tibial apophysis, which may produce a recurvatum deformity. Care must be taken that an epiphysiodesis is complete, as varus and valgus deformities may otherwise occur.

SHORTENING BY OPEN EXCISION OF BONE SEGMENT

This procedure has been standard treatment in adults for correcting limb length discrepancy for many years. It was considered to be a safe and reliable method compared with lengthening in the early years. It is not without complications, however and those that have been reported include non-union, delayed union, angular deformities of the shortening site and infection, plus all the complications of an open operation. The methods used have varied from 'Z' cut osteotomies in the femur to supracondylar and subtrochanteric osteotomies. The osteotomies have been stabilized with intramedullary nails, condylar blade plates or simple bone plating. Shortening by bony resection may also be performed in the tibia (Broughton *et al.*, 1989).

Wagner (1977) described the technique for the femur

of using an angled blade plate and a metaphyseal excision of bone. He was able to obtain 7–10 cm of shortening. Removing segments greater than 7 cm, however, can produce significant difficulties in getting the two bone ends together. This is because the excess of muscle after removal of bone cannot fit into its skin envelope, producing a hydrostatic effect of preventing the two bones coming into continuity. The use of the AO equipment and compression device enables some of these extensive osteotomies to be dragged together and compressed to form a stable osteosynthesis. This technique has produced a more reliable rate of union. The patient has to endure restricted weight-bearing for many months, however, and a significant quadriceps lag develops as a result of this type of surgery. The quadriceps lag improves after a period of 3 months, however, and all knee motion is regained. A second operation is required to remove the plate before activities can be resumed.

CLOSED SHORTENING

Kuntschner (1958) first introduced intramedullary nails to stabilize femoral fractures. He expanded the techniques for stabilization of the femur following open excision of a segment of bone for femoral shortening. In the 1950s he developed an intramedullary saw to carry out closed shortening of the femur. This advance was taken a stage further by Winquist and Hansen (1978) who, with the help of the Boeing Company in Seattle, developed their own intramedullary saw. They reported their results using the intramedullary saw followed by stabilization of the fracture with closed femoral nailing. The early patients, however, developed rotary malalignment because of the inability to gain total control over the proximal and distal fragments with the early AO nails, but with the development of locking nails this complication is avoidable.

Technique of closed femoral shortening

The first important step is to determine how much shortening is to be achieved. Using this technique it is difficult to achieve much more than 7 cm of shortening. If more than this is attempted, an open technique should be used. Up-to-date radiographs of the femur are required in the anteroposterior and lateral planes. The width of the intramedullary cavity at various levels and the width of the cortex are determined. These are essential measurements. With these measurements the site of the osteotomies can be planned pre-operatively.

Intramedullary saws (Fig. 11.8) are of different sizes ranging from 13 mm to 17 mm (Fig. 11.9). Each saw

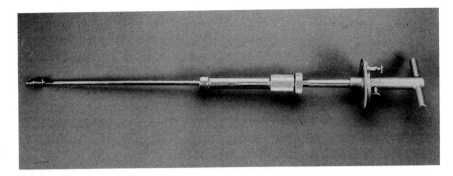

Fig. 11.8 Intramedullary saw.

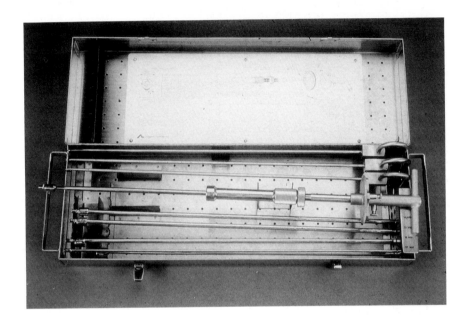

Fig. 11.9 13–17 mm intramedullary saws.

will divide a different thickness of cortex (Fig. 11.10). With knowledge of the width of the cortex and width of the femur, and knowing which saw cuts which diameter and cortical thickness, it is possible to decide the site of the osteotomy and therefore plan to what size the femur has to be reamed. The proximal osteotomy site has to be reamed to a greater extent to accept the larger saw than does the distal osteotomy site.

Standard techniques of closed femoral nailing are used. The femur is broached through a small incision in the buttock, and guide-wires are passed down the femur. A vent is inserted into the distal femoral canal. The femur is reamed to accept the appropriate distal intramedullary saw (Fig. 11.11) and the osteotomy is completed. The site of this division is usually on the junction of the middle and upper thirds of the femur. The site of the proximal osteotomy is then determined and the femur reamed to accept the appropriate size of saw at this level; the osteotomy is completed.

The unscrubbed surgeon manipulates the limbs to displace the femur at the distal osteotomy site. Once this has been achieved, reverse cutting chisels are inserted down the shaft of the femur and hooked onto the free segment of bone. With the use of a slotted hammer and a sharp blow on the intramedullary chisel, it is possible to split the napkin-ring type segment of bone. This is much easier with smaller segments. With larger segments it may be beneficial to use the expanders of Winquist and Hansen (1978). In some cases it is necessary to use a small lateral incision to complete the osteotomy and/or split the segment.

After the segment has been divided and split into two or three fragments, the unscrubbed surgeon manipulates the femur and moves the fragments out of the way so that the two bone ends can be approximated. When the two bone ends are approximated a guide-wire is inserted into the distal segment. Once the guide-wire is in position measurements can be taken to determine the appropriately sized nail, which is then inserted over the guide-wire. While hammering the nail into place, care should

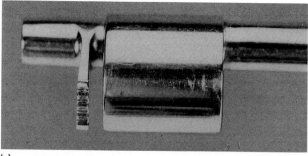

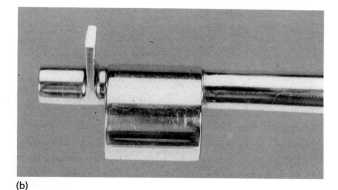

(a)

(b)

Fig. 11.10 The saw blade (a) closed and (b) open.

be taken not to distract at the osteotomy site, and a counter-force must be applied to the knee by the unscrubbed surgeon.

It is also necessary to lock the proximal fragment. If the bone has not been divided below the isthmus of the femur, it may not be necessary to carry out a distal interlock, but if there is any doubt about the rotary stability, distal interlocking should be carried out. The best nail to use at the present time is the AO nail which

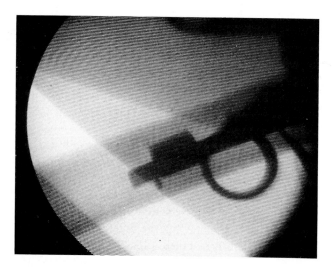

Fig. 11.11 Checking the saw position with the image intensifier.

has a slot in the proximal part of the nail (Fig. 11.12). This allows the nail to be locked proximally, but as weight-bearing takes place further compression at the osteotomy site will be achieved.

Some quadriceps lag results from this procedure but it improves over 2–3 months. The patient can be mobilized quickly, however, and partial weight-bearing is commenced in the first week. Hospitalization is short, approximately 7–8 days. Full weight-bearing is allowed after 1 month if pain allows. Union takes approximately 3 months (Fig. 11.13). In the cases reported so far there have been no instances of non-union using this technique. Rotary malalignment can be avoided by the use of locking intramedullary nails.

Closed tibial shortening

Most shortening should take place in the femur. Shortening of the tibia is much more hazardous. There is a risk of compartment syndrome, and the methods of fixation are less reliable. With the advent of locking tibial nails, however, this technique has become safer. It is possible to achieve approximately 3 cm of shortening in the tibia. The technique used is open excision of the bone segment

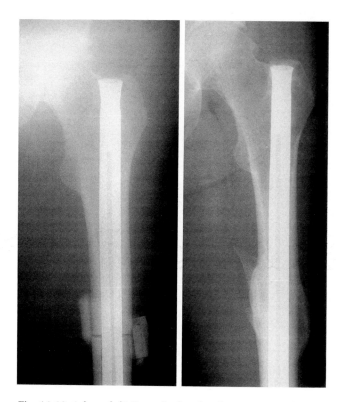

Fig. 11.12 (*above left*) Bone displaced and osteotomy stabilized with a nail.

Fig. 11.13 (*above right*) Healed osteotomy.

as intramedullary saws are not designed for use with the tibia. It is important to be very careful with dissection to preserve the periosteum and muscle attachments to the tibia. The shortening should be carried out as high as possible on the bone at the junction of the upper and middle thirds. Shortening of the mid-shaft and lower third are fraught with danger of non-union. With shortening of the tibia there is a significant risk of muscle lag, which may take some time to recover. There is an indication for splinting the foot in the correct position when first weight-bearing, and early physiotherapy is essential.

Femoral shortening should be carried out if at all possible, despite the problems that may result in slightly uneven knee heights. This is by far the safer and more reliable technique. Reaming the intact femora can result in fat embolism, however (Dahl, personal communication), and therefore careful monitoring is essential in these patients. Pennig (personal communication) has suggested that before reaming an intact femur a small hole should be drilled into the lateral femoral condyle to decompress the femur. He believes this may reduce the incidence of fat embolism.

LIMB LENGTHENING

Historical perspective

Codivilla (1905) published the first account of operative lengthening. The method involved a sudden and strong pull on an os calcis pin after performing an oblique femoral osteotomy. The limb was then held in its corrected position by a plaster cast which included steel bars. Codivilla's technique was refined by Putti (1921), who presented a method of continuous distraction using pins above and below an osteotomy. The pins were connected to a telescopic tube containing a powerful spring and screw. His technique was probably the first using slow distraction between pins that stabilize the bone.

Abbott (1927) popularized tibial elongation and used transfixation with Steinman pins and a device for slow distraction. His apparatus was further modified by several workers. Anderson (1972) described a very large series using a modification of the Abbott device performed from 1933 to 1970 in Edinburgh. These devices were bulky and necessitated prolonged bed-rest for the duration of lengthening and subsequent bony consolidation.

The use of an external fixation frame with a built-in distraction capability by Wagner in 1963 (Wagner, 1971) provided the basis of a much more reliable tech-

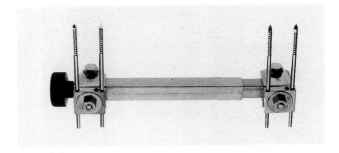

Fig. 11.14 Wagner apparatus for lengthening.

nique (Fig. 11.14). The frame was placed on the side of the leg and connected to the bone by screws which pierce the skin. A screw mechanism was used to provide gradual distraction. A minimum of three operations was required: initial osteotomy and external fixation, plating and grafting of the distraction gap and plate removal (Fig. 11.15). Extensive skin incisions were necessary to insert and remove the plate, and the complication rate was 40% (Wagner, 1971).

Ilizarov, developed a circular frame for fracture stabilization and perfected a technique of distraction lengthening with spontaneous callus formation by the mid-1960s (Ilizarov and Deviatov, 1971; Ilizarov and Trokhova, 1973). His approach was based on a general biological principle that governs the stimulation of tissue growth and regeneration during distraction. He noted that gradual distraction of living tissues created stresses that stimulated and maintained active regeneration on certain tissue structures. This concept is perhaps a more specialized statement of Wolff's law (Wolff, 1892) and has been termed the tension–stress effect (Ilizarov, 1989a, b). Ilizarov coupled these biological principles with the use of a circular frame that allowed correction of deformity in all planes in conjunction with lengthening.

Advances continued to be made, particularly by DeBastiani, who developed two techniques for lengthening using a unilateral external fixation system (Orthofix). *Chondrodiatasis* involves slow stretching of the growth plate with new bone said to be formed by stimulation of its metabolic rate (DeBastiani *et al.*, 1986a, b). The other technique has been named *callotasis* (DeBastiani *et al.*, 1987) and involves division of the cortex of the bone in the metaphyseal region (corticotomy) with preservation of the periosteal envelope. Slow distraction at 1 mm/day is commenced after a delay to allow recovery of the medullary blood supply. This produces an environment conducive to early and spontaneous callus formation without the need for grafting. After remodelling, the structural characteristics of the new bone

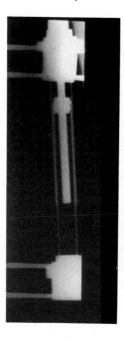 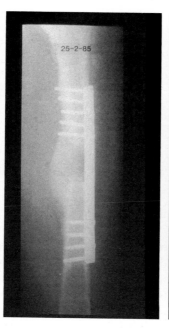 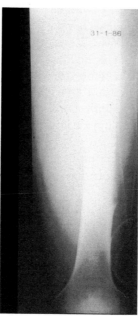

Fig. 11.15 Three main stages of the Wagner technique: distraction, plating and bone grafting and plate removal.

approaches normal (Saleh *et al.*, 1993), compared with the disorganized structure of bone lengthened by the Wagner method (Pesch and Wagner, 1974).

In 1975 Vilarrubias *et al.* recognized not only the need for spontaneous callus formation, but also the importance of soft tissue tension as a rate-limiting step in lengthening as well as a potent cause of joint subluxation. By appropriate percutaneous tendon releases and by holding joints in their most stable configurations, longer lengthenings were achieved (Vilarrubias *et al.*, 1990).

Leg lengthening is still the treatment of choice for the vast majority of cases of leg length inequality. Most leg length discrepancies are due to congenital abnormalities, which can be corrected safely with the present leg lengthening techniques. In a number of situations, however, limb shortening is indicated as described above. Any surgeon who undertakes limb lengthening must be an expert in the relevant techniques and be cognisant with the methods of equalizing leg length; techniques of leg shortening must also be part of the surgeon's armamentarium.

Leg lengthening by callus distraction

Lengthening by callus distraction (callotasis) was a term introduced by DeBastiani *et al.* (1987). An important difference between this technique and that described by Wagner (1971) was a period of waiting after bone division. By waiting until bone healing took place, distraction took place through the area of fracture repair.

The technique has proved to be the most reliable method of achieving an increase in limb length with many fewer complications than with other methods. It is possible to carry out a 10–15% segment lengthening with few major complications. The complications are related more to soft tissue tension and other soft tissue problems rather than to the formation of bone. Bone formation is not a major problem and only very seldom is an additional bone graft required.

If an attempt is made to increase the limb length by more than 15% significant problems can occur due to soft tissue tension. This can lead to deformity, joint contractures and some delay in the formation of a satisfactory regenerate. To overcome the problems of soft tissue tension in extensive limb lengthening, several authors have suggested the use of prophylactic releases. The aim of the releases is to weaken the muscles, which tend to become tight during the lengthening phase. In addition to the releases, splints are used to hold the knee and ankle in the correct alignment in the lengthening phase, to prevent contractures that may result from the increasing soft tissue tension.

TECHNIQUE

Callus distraction is divided into four stages:
1 Application of external fixator and corticotomy: this is followed by a period of between 5 and 10 days of waiting time.
2 Distraction or lengthening phase: here the bone is lengthened at 1 mm/day.
3 Neutralization phase: this is the time when the length-

ening device is locked. It is at this time that there is increasing calcification of the regenerate.

4 Dynamization phase: at this time the lengthening device is unlocked to allow axial compressive forces to be applied through the regenerate. The fixator prevents rotation or varus or valgus stresses being applied to the regenerate. The aim of this phase is to increase the speed at which corticalization of the regenerate takes place.

The type of device used to carry out leg lengthening by callus distraction is not important, provided the device has sufficient strength to prevent deformities occurring and sufficient flexibility to allow bone to regenerate. It is possible to use the Orthofix and Wagner external fixators as well as circular frames like the Ilizarov device. Several important factors are common to all techniques of callus distraction, however, whichever device is used.

If at all possible, the division of bone should be in the metaphysis. In using the Orthofix device on the femur, the pins should be placed in the 1 and 3 or 4 or 1, 2 and 4 positions and the upper pin just above the level of the lesser trochanter. Corticotomy then takes place 1 cm below the distal of the two screws. This forms a most stable situation for support of the corticotomy site. If the 1 and 5 positions are used the corticotomy then takes place lower down the femoral shaft towards the diaphysis, which is not to be recommended. The pins should be inserted almost perpendicular to the shaft, and the fixator body lies parallel to the mechanical axis of the leg to ensure that as the lengthening takes place, deformity does not occur (Figs 11.16 and 11.17).

In the tibia the upper pin should be placed parallel to the tibial plateau. This ensures that when lengthening takes place no deformity occurs. The fibula must be divided and a segment removed. It is preferable to remove the periosteum in addition to a 1 cm segment of bone. If extensive limb lengthening is to be carried out, the fibula should be fixed at the tibia. This can be done by the use of a single Kirschner wire, and there is no need to use a screw. In short lengthenings, fixation of the fibula to the tibia is not essential. If there is any doubt about the integrity of the ankle joint, however, the fibula should be anchored to the tibia (Fig. 11.24).

Corticotomy

The bone should be divided with preservation of the periosteum, which recent work has suggested is the most important structure in the formation of new bone. Damage to the periosteum certainly results in poorer callus formation. Other workers have suggested that preservation of the intramedullary vessels is also important (Paley, 1986).

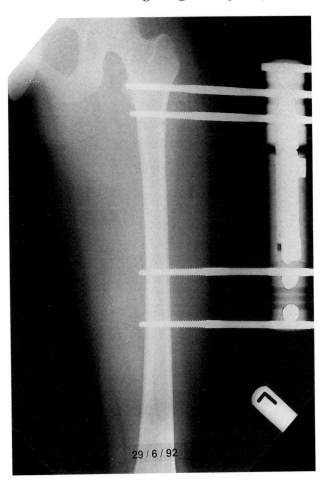

Fig. 11.16 Femoral lengthening. Pins are placed perpendicular to the mechanical axis of the femur. The upper pin is just above the lesser trochanter in the 1 and 3 positions. Corticotomy is approximately 1 cm distal to the second proximal pin.

The authors carry out corticotomy by a small open technique. Once down to the bone, the periosteum is incised and reflected, and using a 3.5 mm drill multiple holes are made in the bone at the site of the corticotomy. Using an osteotome, the drill holes are then connected. If the lengthening device is under tension at this phase, the bone ends will suddenly separate once the corticotomy is complete. By using this technique it is possible to preserve some of the intramedullary vessels and the periosteum. It must be confirmed that the corticotomy is complete, as if it is not distraction will not take place (Fig. 11.17).

After the application of the lengthening device, the range of knee flexion is assessed because as the knee flexes the iliotibial band moves posteriorly. This motion is stopped by the pins. It is often necessary to release the iliotibial band around the distal pins to obtain a full range of knee motion.

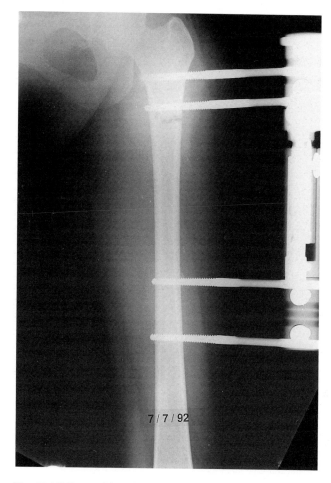

7 / 7 / 92

Fig. 11.17 Femoral lengthening. The upper pin is at the level of the lesser trochanter. The pins are in the 1 and 3 positions. Corticotomy is just distal to the second proximal pin. The drill holes just visible. The fixator body is parallel to the mechanical axis.

Post-operative care.   Post-operative analgesia is essential. Patient-controlled analgesia systems have been shown to be very valuable. The authors place all their patients on CPM machines to obtain as much knee flexion as possible in the post-operative phase. The dressings are left undisturbed for 2 days when they are removed, as are the drains from the corticotomy site. Aggressive physiotherapy is instituted at an early stage to maintain ranges of joint motion. Strict instructions regarding pin sites are given, and cleaning of pin sites is demonstrated.

Distraction phase

The period of waiting after the corticotomy has been carried out appears to be important. A period of 1 week

should elapse before lengthening is commenced in infants and adolescents. In the older patient this should be extended to 10 days. In the very young and those with Ollier's disease, lengthening should be commenced at approximately 5 days. Failure to start lengthening early results in premature consolidation of the corticotomy site. If this occurs, osteoclasis or a further corticotomy has to be performed.

After the period of delay distraction is started at the rate of 1 mm/day. This should be achieved in four segments of 0.25 mm each. There is evidence to suggest that better bone is formed if distraction is continuous throughout the day, but contrary to this, the soft tissues need a period of time to recover following distraction. Taking these two factors into consideration, it appears that the rate of 1 mm in four equal segments of 0.25 mm throughout the day appears to be the optimum rate of distraction.

Work by Matsushita (personal communication) has suggested that lengthening in the evening may be more beneficial to the soft tissues. It has been demonstrated that most growth takes place at night, and this might be related to the surge of growth hormone that occurs in the evening. As a consequence of this, lengthening may be best achieved by continuous lengthening throughout the evening, both for the soft tissues and the production of a good bone regenerate.

After the operation intensive physiotherapy is instituted to maintain joint motion. The decision to use prophylactic splints to prevent contracture depends on personal preference. Radiographs should be obtained 4 days after lengthening has commenced to confirm that the corticotomy site is distracting satisfactorily (Fig. 11.18). If this is so, then the patient can be discharged home. Follow-up is then on an out-patient basis.

The patient should be reviewed every 2 weeks, but if any problems arise between reviews free access to a clinic should be available. Follow-up should include examination by the physiotherapist to ensure that a satisfactory range of joint motion is being maintained. If significant reduction in joint range has occurred, lengthening can either be slowed down, intensive physiotherapy commenced, or dynamic splints applied.

Pin sites should be checked to ensure that they are clean. If not, further nursing input is required to ensure that the patient is cleaning the pin sites satisfactorily. Antibiotics may be required to prevent or to treat overt infection. It may be necessary to carry out a surgical release around the site if the skin becomes tight. If a significant infection of the underlying bone occurs, the

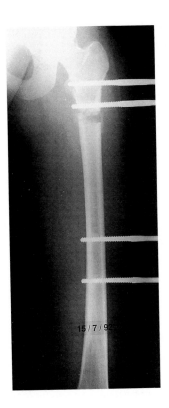

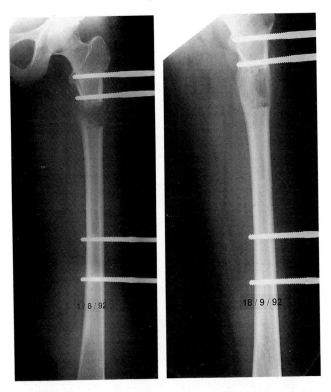

Fig. 11.18 Radiograph 4 days after commencing distraction. The corticotomy site is opening satisfactorily.

Fig. 11.19 (*above left*) Further radiograph 8 days later confirming that distraction is taking place at the corticotomy site and early callus is forming.

Fig. 11.20 (*above right*) Lengthening is completed satisfactorily with development of calcification within the regenerate.

pin may have to be removed and replaced. If pin problems do develop, lengthening may have to be abandoned or the method or type of device changed.

Determination of whether distraction is progressing satisfactorily is made by both clinical and radiological parameters. Clinically, measurements made on the fixator confirm that the gap is increasing between the pins. Further confirmation can be obtained from the measuring device on the fixator. If the pins start to bend this is an indication that a deformity is developing at the lengthening site or that premature consolidation has taken place.

Ultrasonography has been used to monitor the development of new bone formation in the regenerate (Eyres *et al.*, 1993). It can identify the interval between the bone ends and determine the rate at which new bone is filling the gap. It can also be used to determine when the formation of bony regenerate is complete as the indentifiable gap disappears. It has yet to be proved as a useful tool to determine when the bone is sufficiently strong for the fixator to be removed.

Plain radiographs are taken in the anteroposterior plane to confirm that distraction is proceeding satisfactorily (Fig. 11.19), that no deformity is occurring at the

lengthening site, and that the pins have not loosened as a result of infection. Radiographs should be taken every 2 weeks during the lengthening phase, and on a monthly basis after lengthening has been completed and the neutralization and dynamization phase are in progress (Fig. 11.20).

Dual-energy X-ray absorptiometry is also being developed to measure bone mineralization. The early experience with this technique suggests that it will be useful in determining the timing for proceeding to the next phase of lengthening. It provides an index of the bone mineralization of the regenerate, and it is hoped that it will give an accurate indication of the time at which it is safe to remove the fixator, rather than relying on clinical interpretation of a plain radiograph.

Weekly use of dual-energy X-ray absorptiometry can give a measurement of the speed of bone mineralization. If bone mineralization is proceeding too slowly, this suggest's that distraction is being carried out at too fast a rate. Therefore the technique appears to be a useful tool for monitoring the speed at which distraction takes place and allowing adjustments to be carried out.

It is recommended that an overcorrection of 5 mm should be achieved, as slight loss of length can take place during the dynamization phase. CT gives an accurate assessment of limb length (Fig. 11.21).

Neutralization phase

After lengthening has been completed the patient proceeds to the neutralization phase. It is at this time that the regenerate becomes further mineralized. The patient must continue with pin site care and work hard with physiotherapy to maintain joint range. It is recommended that full weight-bearing should be under-taken as far as possible to try to stimulate further mineralization.

The neutralization phase is achieved by locking the Orthofix fixator.

Radiographs are taken at monthly intervals to assess bone mineralization (Fig. 11.22) to determine when it will be safe to allow dynamization to take place. Complete mineralization of the regenerate must have occurred before it is advisable to allow axial load through the regenerate. It is difficult to determine the exact time of allowing axial load through the regenerate, which must be strong enough to take the load without com-pression (which leads to loss of leg length), but the delay should be minimized as this increases the time the fixator will have to remain *in situ*.

The neutralization phase takes approximately the same time as that required to distract the limb.

Dynamization phase

Dynamization is the period when axial load is allowed to pass through the regenerate by unlocking the Orthofix fixator. The fixator prevents varus/valgus and rotational forces from being applied to the regenerate, but axial

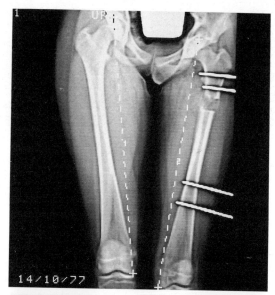

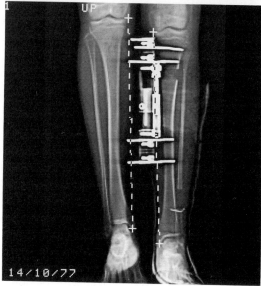

Fig. 11.21 CT scan. This is for determination of the length gained and to accurately identify the time at which to stop lengthening.

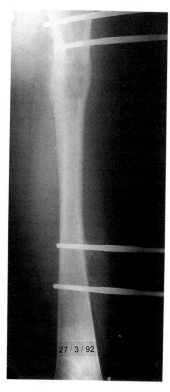

Fig. 11.22 Calcification within the regenerate of sufficient quality to allow dynamization.

load is permitted. It is believed that the axial loading increases the mineralization of the bone and the cortication of the regenerate segment. The time to proceed from neutralization to dynamization phase is sometimes difficult to determine (Fig. 11.23). Before the fixator is dynamized it is important to note the distance between the two inner pins and a reading must be taken from the scale on the lengthening device. After the fixator has been unlocked and axial compression allowed, some 2–3 mm of limb length may be lost. If further length is lost, however, the bone is of insufficient strength to take axial compression. It is suggested that the distraction device is reapplied and a further period of distraction is carried out to achieve the desired length gain. A further period of neutralization is then required before proceeding further to dynamization.

Orthofix have now produced a compression ring that allows dynamization to take place at an earlier stage. This allows only 2 mm of axial movement (Figs 11.24 and 11.25), which prevents excessive loss of length at dynamization but allows earlier passing of axial load through the regenerate.

Further mineralization of the regenerate will take place and it will slowly begin to differentiate into

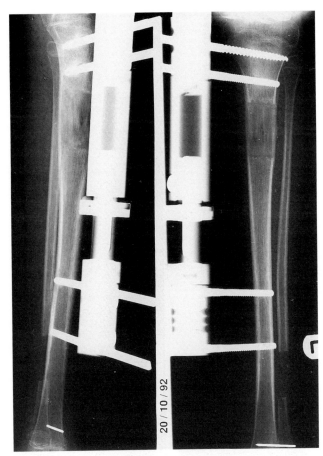

Fig. 11.24 After 1 month of dynamization using the Dynoring, showing increased corticalization of the lateral section of the regenerate.

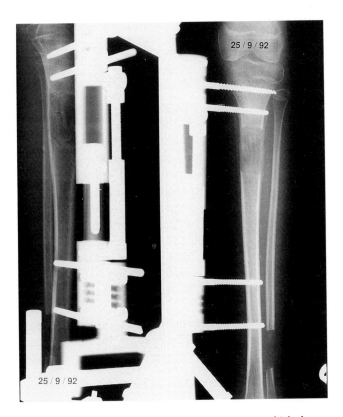

Fig. 11.23 Tibial lengthening, showing the time at which the decision was made to dynamize using the Dynoring.

cortical-type bone. The fixator can be removed when there is evidence of cortication appearing in the regenerate in at least two planes on radiographs taken at 90° to each other. It is at this stage that dual-energy X-ray absorptiometry may help to determine whether bone mineralization is sufficient to allow unprotected weight-bearing on the limb after removal of the fixator. The time from the commencement of the dynamization phase to fixator removal is approximately the same as the neutralization phase.

The timing of fixator removal can be a most difficult decision for the clinician. If there is any doubt as to whether the new bone is sufficiently strong to allow the patient unhindered weight-bearing, it is best to admit the patient to hospital to remove the fixator but leave the pins *in situ*. The patient is then mobilized in the hospital for 24 h. If no change in the position of the pins and no pain or deformity occur, the pins are then removed. If there is any doubt about the strength of the bone within the tibia, a tibial gaiter can be applied to

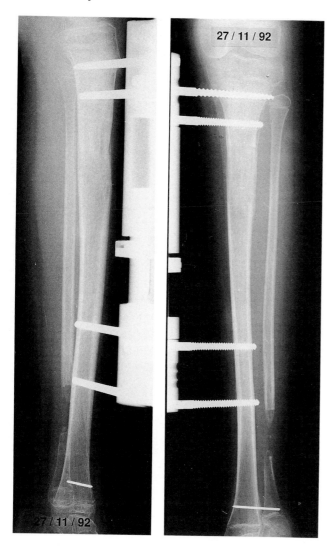

27 / 11 / 92

27 / 11 / 92

Fig. 11.25 Five weeks later showing excellent bone formation. Corticalization is taking place in both planes. The fixator was removed at this stage.

prevent varus and valgus stresses being applied through the newly formed bone.

If, after a sufficiently long period of dynamization, there is no improvement in the quality of bone being formed, this suggests that the regenerate is being protected from stress. Under these circumstances it should be ensured that the fixator is freely mobile and that dynamization is actually occurring. If dynamization is occurring and there is still stress protection, the fixator is too stiff. It is then best to remove the fixator and apply a cast. In some cases where three screws have been used in each clamp, removal of one of the screws will increase the flexibility of the system.

If a cast is used, weight-bearing should be encouraged to promote mineralization and the cast should be removed at an appropriate time. When a cast has to be used with the femur, a hip spica or cast brace with a pelvic band is indicated. Before the fixator is removed, the authors now carry out a dual-energy X-ray absorptiometric scan to assess bone mineralization and ultrasonography to assess the newly formed bone. In a number of instances small holes in the cortex of the regenerate have been found on ultrasonography. These techniques give some indication of whether any additional protection is required after the fixator has been removed.

Fixator removal

Fixator removal can be carried out in the out-patient department for older children, but some younger children benefit from a short general anaesthetic. It is important to clean the wounds around the pins to prevent infection. The pin holes close within 48 h. After the fixator is removed the child should be partially weight-bearing with crutches. This helps to develop confidence and slowly improves the bone quality. The children themselves determine the period of time for which they will use crutches, but a period of 6 weeks is recommended. The bone will continue to remodel, and over a period of 1 year its strength will continue to increase. After 18 months it is difficult to identify the site of bone lengthening (Fig. 11.26).

COMPLICATIONS

Lengthening seldom permanently reduces the joint range. It is important that the range of motion of the knee should always be from 0° to 40°. After removal of the femoral fixator, this range of motion is improved dramatically, and over a period of 1 year almost a full range of joint motion will be regained. It is important to identify any problems occurring at a joint throughout the lengthening phase, and the surgeon must be prepared to slow down lengthening to increase the range of joint motion. Complications that must be avoided are joint subluxation and dislocation. Posterior subluxation of the knee can occur due to tightening of the hamstrings with lengthening.

The classification of complications and their management have been discussed by Paley (1990) and Saleh and Scott (1992). The major complications are discussed below.

Deformity

If deformity occurs during lengthening, this should be

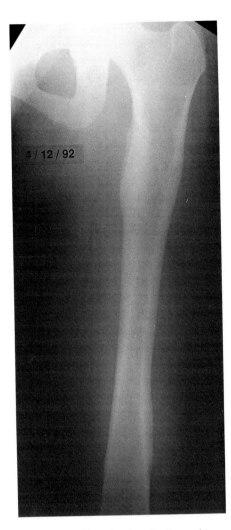

4/12/92

Fig. 11.26 Short femoral lengthening. Radiographic appearance 18 months later. Identification of the site of lengthening is difficult. Recanalization of the regenerate is complete.

corrected as soon as possible. It may be possible to change the external fixation device and at the same time correct the deformity. In other cases it is necessary to change the pins or increase the number of pins to prevent the deformity from recurring. Deformity must be corrected before full consolidation of bone has occurred, otherwise a femoral osteotomy will have to be carried out with a further period of time with a fixator at a later date, to correct the deformity. Up to 10° of varus in the femur is acceptable, but anything more than 5° of valgus in the tibia is unacceptable and must be corrected.

Premature consolidation of corticotomy

This is an early complication that presents with increased difficulty in distracting the lengthening device, associated with bending of the pins. Radiographs will confirm premature consolidation. The patient should be advised to stop attempting lengthening, should be admitted to hospital, and under a general anaesthetic the fixator should be removed and a closed osteoclasis carried out. If this is impossible, the regenerate needs to be divided using a small osteotome, which can be used percutaneously under image intensification control. Lengthening is then commenced immediately in the post-operative phase.

Fusion of fibular osteotomy

Despite removing 1 cm of bone and the periosteum, occasionally the fibular osteotomy will join. If the fibula has been fixed to the tibia this may prevent problems. If the fibula has not been fixed to the tibia, however, the fibula will migrate proximally, which leads to an unstable ankle. Care must be taken to look for and exclude this complication. If identified, excision of a further segment of fibula is indicated.

Pin site sepsis

Throughout all stages of lengthening, pin site sepsis is a problem and most cases do have one or two episodes. Clear and firm instructions should be given regarding cleaning of pin sites, and most cases of sepsis respond to increased cleaning. On a few occasions it may be necessary to use antibiotics to treat sepsis and prevent further sepsis developing.

Soft tissue contractures

These can occur, but if joint ranges are maintained they should be prevented. It may be necessary to carry out an Achilles tendon lengthening if, despite physiotherapy and splinting, an equinus deformity develops. This can be carried out using the Hoke method.

If hamstring tightness occurs it is best to slow down lengthening and institute aggressive physiotherapy, with which measures it is possible to overcome the tightness. If hamstrings do become tight, care must be taken in evaluating the radiographs to ensure that subluxation of the knee does not occur. This is a considerable problem in patients with congenitally short femora.

Neurological sequelae

If lengthening takes place too quickly, there is a possibility of neurological or neurovascular complications. If any tingling or paraesthesia in the foot is identified, the distraction should be reversed. This should release the tension on the nerve and the problem should resolve. Further lengthening should not be continued until complete resolution of symptoms.

Stress fractures

These can occur after the fixator has been removed. This usually indicates that the fixator has been removed too early. The treatment is a period of time in plaster, or if deformity is starting to appear, reapplication of a fixator, allowing dynamization.

Fracture

Fracture does occur after limb lengthening. The use of callus distraction appears to reduce this complication. For this reason, however, protected weight-bearing is indicated immediately after the fixator is removed, for a period of 6 weeks. A return to full sporting activity is not recommended until radiographs show complete recanalization of the regenerated segment.

CASES AT RISK

The patient should lengthen with the knees in full extension. If subluxation of the knee does occur, reversal of the lengthening process is indicated to allow soft tissue tension in the hamstrings to reduce and the knee to relocate.

Dislocation of the hip is a problem that should never occur in lengthening. If the hip is unstable, this should be identified before undertaking the lengthening procedure. If lengthening is still indicated, hip stabilization procedures must be carried out before lengthening. If, after hip stabilization procedures, there is some doubt as to the stability of the hip, then distal lengthening should be performed with a distal corticotomy. Prophylactic releases of the adductors and hip flexors are also indicated. Careful monitoring of the hip throughout the lengthening phase is essential. If serious problems of hip instability are apparent, consideration must be given to limb shortening rather than lengthening.

Procedures that can be used to stabilize the hip are:
1 Placing the fixator across the hip with a hip hinge: this carries considerable risk of damage to the abductor muscles, and stiffness around the hip joint can occur because of lack of mobility at the hip throughout the lengthening phase. It may also compromise the possibility of carrying out hip replacements in the future if any infection of the pins in the pelvis occurs. The pins across the hip should be removed as soon as the length-

ening has been completed to allow hip mobilization to take place as soon as possible. Removal of the pins also reduces the incidence of infection.
2 The other possibilities are specific procedures to the hip itself before lengthening. These include shelf procedures and pelvic osteotomies. The types of osteotomy that should be considered are Chiari's osteotomy and/or triple osteotomies with realignment of the acetabulum.

BONE HEALING INDEX

The time taken from the first application of the fixator and the corticotomy to the removal of the fixator in relation to the length gained is known as the bone healing index, which is expressed as the number of days per centimetre length gained. As a working rule, the figure of 40 days/cm can be quoted. In some conditions, however, this index is longer than 40 days, though in young children and people with Ollier's disease the bone healing index is much shorter. It is also different between the femur and the tibia. In patients with achondroplasia the bone healing index appears to be about 35 days/cm.

Leg lengthening by chondrodiatasis

Many authors in the past have reported attempts to carry out limb lengthening by stretching the physis. It was always felt, however, that the length achieved by distracting the physis was a result of a fracture of the physeal plate. Length was achieved, but as a consequence the physis fused.

DeBastiani *et al.* (1986a; 1986b) developed the technique of chondrodiatasis from experimental work in rabbits, which showed that gentle tension across the physis increased the number of cells in the proliferative phase in the physis. This was the cause of the increased length achieved. It was concluded that the most important factor was the speed of distraction, which was 0.5 mm/day.

Clinically, it has been proved that lengthening can take place at the physis, but after lengthening the physeal plate closes. It is believed that in clinical situations lengthening continues to take place as a result of a fracture rather than increasing cell division in the physis. It is therefore recommended that chondrodiatasis is not attempted until physeal plate closure is imminent.

TECHNIQUE

It is possible to carry out chondrodiatasis on the lower femoral, upper and lower tibial physes. Chondrodiatasis of the distal tibial physis is technically very difficult to achieve, and therefore it is not recommended other than in skilled hands.

Two pins are placed into the epiphysis of the distal femur parallel to the physeal line. Further pins are then inserted into the proximal femur. In the tibia the pins are placed in the epiphysis parallel to the tibial plateau. Two further pins are then inserted into the tibia. The position and the placement of the pins must be monitored with an image intensifier.

Following insertion of the pins distraction is commenced at 0.5 mm/day, usually in two stages, one in the morning and one in the evening. After approximately 5 days it becomes more and more difficult to distract the fixator. There is a sudden episode of pain related to the physis, after which it is easy to distract the lengthening device. It is at this time that the physis fractures. Lengthening is then carried out as for callus distraction, but continuing at 0.5 mm/day (Fig. 11.27). The same attention to detail regarding knee and ankle motion is essential. Pin site care is even more important as the pins in the lower femur often transfix the knee joint. Care is essential to prevent the development of septic arthritis.

Following the distraction phase a period of neutral-

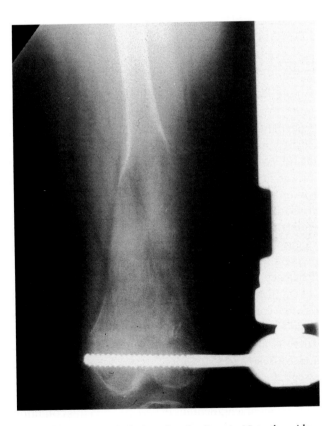

Fig. 11.27 Radiograph during chondrodiatasis. Note the wide callus zone.

ization is needed to allow mineralization of the regenerate. Dynamization follows, as in callotasis. Fixator removal and the indication for fixator removal are as for callotasis.

Limb lengthening with circular frames — Ilizarov technique

Instead of using screws and a single-sided fixator, tensioned Kirschner wires and a circular frame may be used. The principles of the operation are similar to those described for callotasis. The advantage lies in the fact that pre-existing deformity and axial deviation during lengthening may be corrected progressively by appropriate hinge and threaded rod placement (Fig. 11.28). The fine wires provide better purchase in soft and cancellous bone, and the technique may be used to correct concurrent soft tissue deformities, e.g. equinus of the foot (Fig. 11.29) (Hardy *et al.*, 1991; Saleh, 1992b). They are also indicated for unstable joints, as the fixation may be extended across a joint to prevent subluxation.

Circular frames with transfixation wires are less well tolerated and carry an increased risk of nerve or vessel injury; it is more appropriate, therefore, to reserve their use for complicated lengthenings. It is an unnecessary burden for both patient and surgeon in simpler cases in which a predictable result can be achieved with a unilateral frame (Saleh, 1992b; Saleh and Scott, 1992).

Leg lengthening using bifocal techniques

Three bifocal techniques have been described by Ilizarov to correct shortening with deformity or bone loss. Bifocal techniques may be performed using circular frames or specially adapted unilateral frames. Extreme shortening or shortening with metaphyseal deformity may be corrected by bifocal lengthening. Both metaphyses within the segment may be lengthened simultaneously. This technique has certain theoretical advantages, e.g. shorter lengthened segments and better frame stability, leading to more rapid consolidation with fewer soft tissue problems and bony deformity (Saleh and Hamer, 1993).

Diaphyseal osteotomies may also be used to correct deformity. Complicated multilevel, multiplanar corrections with lengthening may only be performed satisfactorily with a circular frame (Fig. 11.30). If the deformity is diaphyseal — unless it is a hypertrophic non-union — the potential for lengthening is poor, and a correction of the angulation is performed immediately with or without bone resection, and lengthening is performed at a healthy metaphyseal site. This technique,

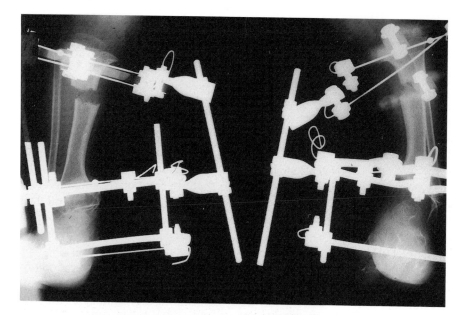

Fig. 11.28 Deformity correction using a circular frame.

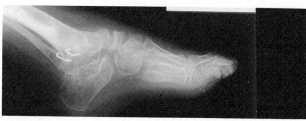

(a)

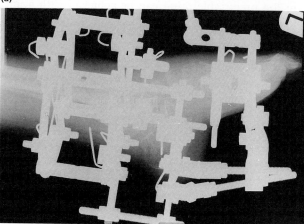

(b)

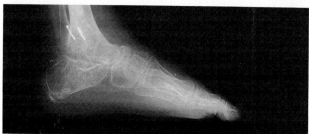

(c)

Fig. 11.29 Correction of concomitant equinus deformity. (a) Before; (b) during; (c) after.

known as compression–distraction, may also be used to close short segments of bone loss acutely. Longer segments are closed by bone transport (Fig. 11.31), in which the middle segment is transported down within the soft tissue envelope (Fig. 11.32) (Saleh, 1992a).

LENGTHENING IN SPECIFIC CONDITIONS

Congenital deficiency

Among the most common cases for lengthening in the authors' practice are patients with congenital length discrepancy. A large variety of uncommon anomalies exists, but perhaps the situation seen most commonly is the following. The femur is short with a normal hip; the knee is in slight valgus caused by a hypoplastic lateral femoral condyle. The tibial spine is flattened as the cruciates are deficient. The tibia is often slightly short with a variable fibula deficiency. The ankle may be in valgus and often is of the ball and socket configuration owing to tarsal coalition. There may be a lateral ray deficiency in the foot.

Lengthening in these patients involves an increased risk of complications. Length gain is limited and is usually stated to be up to 10% of the segment length. There is an increased risk of joint subluxation (Jones and Moseley, 1985), and strategies for prevention are essential. The Vilarrubias technique addresses this high-risk situation, enabling the authors to perform up to 32% segment lengthenings in patients with this condition (Saleh, 1992b). Renzi-Brivio *et al.* (1990) report lengthenings using chondrodiatasis and callotasis of between

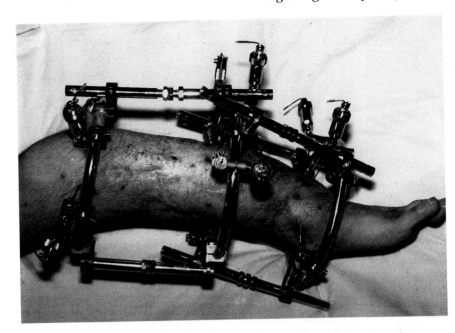

Fig. 11.30 Complex multilevel multiplanar correction with a circular frame.

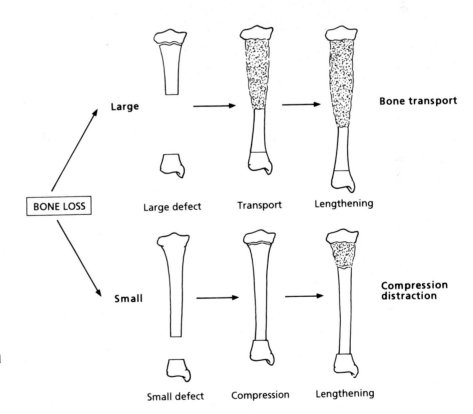

Fig. 11.31 Bone defects may be treated by acute closure and lengthening at an adjacent metaphysis or by bone transport.

4% and 28%. They did not report problems with knee subluxation, but commented that soft tissue surgery may be necessary.

Vascularity of the limb may also be congenitally deficient (Hootnick *et al.*, 1980). This may produce post-lengthening problems of long-term trophic changes, mild exercise intolerance and temperature intolerance (Dutroit *et al.*, 1990). These findings in cases of severe discrepancy need to be balanced with amputation and use of a prosthetic limb (Ferguson *et al.*, 1987).

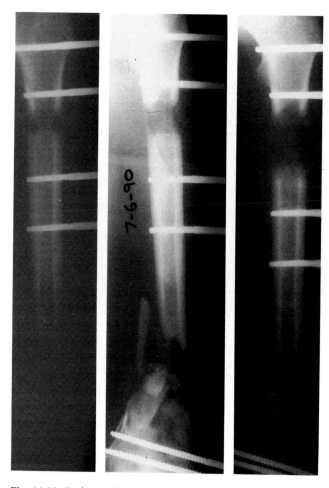

Fig. 11.32 Radiographic series demonstrating bone transport.

Poliomyelitis

Leg length discrepancy is usual in childhood polio-myelitis that has affected only one lower limb (Ratliff, 1959). The amount of discrepancy is related to the pattern of paralysis. When paralysis is confined below the knee, shortening seldom exceeds 4 cm. When all of the limb is paralysed, however, the discrepancy is greater but still seldom exceeds 8.5 cm (Ratliff, 1959). Age at onset has little effect on discrepancy (Stinchfield *et al.*, 1949). The pattern of growth retardation is variable and has been described in detail by Shapiro (1982), who found that growth disturbance was usually maximal for the first 4–5 years after infection, with the rate of discrepancy diminishing after that. Some children, how-ever, continue until cessation of growth with the same degree of annual discrepancy.

Very little has been written in the recent literature about lengthening in poliomyelitis. A significant pro-portion of patients reported in earlier series, however, underwent lengthening for this reason. Macnicol and Catto (1982) reviewed 24 patients 20 years after Anderson technique lengthening for discrepancy in poliomyelitis. All of these patients were active and had a mean of 5.5 cm of lengthening in the tibia. All but one considered the procedure worthwhile, despite the long duration of in-patient treatment. Macnicol and Catto noted that muscle power was maintained in all cases, but that walking speed was markedly reduced compared with a normal population. Walking speed of the length-ened group was not compared with a matched con-trol group of non-lengthened poliomyelitis patients, however, though there is probably no reason why they should differ. It was also noted that 25% of patients had more than 10° of genu valgum and 59% had cold intolerance, the latter finding not unusual in poliomyelitis.

Sofield *et al.* (1958) reviewed 26 patients with polio-myelitis a mean of 22 years after Abbott lengthenings. Most of the patients were satisfied with the operation, but the technique was considered unsatisfactory. Foot problems were exacerbated or even initiated, and unlike the Macnicol and Catto series, they noted that many patients lost a grade of muscle power.

It is reasonable to assume that with modern techniques lengthening will produce good results in patients with poliomyelitis. Those with experience in lengthening note that the tissues are reasonably extensible, and it is likely with modern ambulant techniques that muscle power would be retained. Particular caution, however, should be exercised in two groups of patients. Patients with fixed flexion contractures of the knee, particularly if the quadriceps is weak, are very susceptible to knee sub-luxation. The flexion contracture should be treated first in this group (Leong *et al.*, 1982) followed by lengthening with splinting in extension. The other at-risk group is those patients with weakness around the hip and hip dysplasia. The situation is worsened if the adductors are strong with weak abductors. The hip must be stabilized if lengthening is contemplated, perhaps by techniques described by Lau *et al.* (1986) and Eberle (1982).

Achondroplasia and other restricted growth conditions

Lengthening in short stature is an ethical issue that will not be discussed further here. Patients with restricted growth may have many difficulties with function as well as psychosocial problems (Saleh and Burton, 1991). The magnitude of these problems varies with the society to which the patient belongs. In many countries no pro-visions are made for short-statured people, preventing them from gaining a suitable education, making social-ization very difficult and precluding employment.

Patients with disproportionate short stature, e.g. those with achondroplasia, are most suitable for lengthening procedures. Stature may be increased by up to 30 cm over a period of 2.5 years. More modest gains can be achieved more quickly. Differing strategies may be used for lengthening (Saleh and Sharrard, 1989; Saleh, 1989). Aldegheri *et al.* (1988) initially favoured lengthening of one limb at a time, applying devices to femur and tibia. This has the advantage of keeping the patient on his or her feet but towards the end of a long lengthening the raise on the unlengthened leg may become unmanageable. Aldegheri *et al.* now favour crossed lengthening, i.e. one femur and the contralateral tibia. Vilarrubias *et al.* (1990) apply devices to both tibia's, initially keeping patients in wheelchairs for the lengthening period. It is possible for the patient to withdraw from the programme with this technique without having a major leg length discrepancy. Femoral lengthening is combined with extension osteotomies to correct hyperlordosis.

One group of patients with achondroplasia and pseudoachondroplasia have marked angular deformity and ligamentous laxity. Lengthening in these patients, who may be having difficulty standing and walking, offers hope of considerable improvement in function. Arm lengthening may also be indicated for improved reach as well as cosmesis. While lengthening in the forearm is fraught with risk, humeral lengthening provides very satisfying results.

Trauma and tumour

Segmental loss of bone arising from severe trauma or limb-sparing operations for musculoskeletal tumours has been treated by a variety of techniques including prostheses, vascularized bone grafts and large free grafts. In young patients, complications including prosthetic loosening, donor site morbidity, graft failure and massive graft infection may all occur. Lengthening techniques offer the advantage of transport of a bony segment to fill the defect with the patient's own bone of normal character, thus producing new bone from an osteotomy at a distant site. The procedure requires either the use of an Ilizarov frame or a unilateral device, such as the Orthofix Limb Reconstruction System which has three pin clamps. Bone formation is similar to that achieved in lengthening, and muscle relationships appear undisturbed. The effects of chemotherapy and radiotherapy on callus formation are as yet unknown, but successful reconstructions have been carried out. This technique is also of value in congenital pseudarthrosis of the tibia, where the pseudarthrotic segment can be excised.

CONCLUSIONS

Operative treatment of limb inequality involves making the choice between procedures that lengthen one leg, slow the growth of the contralateral leg, or shorten that leg. Techniques are improving for correction using all of these approaches, and the method must be chosen that suits both the skills and the materials available to the surgeon. The ability of the patient and family to cope with various forms of treatment must also be considered.

If lengthening is performed, improved results are now attainable. An understanding of the biological response of bone and soft tissues to distraction allows the surgeon to anticipate complications before they develop. Similarly, the equipment can be more appropriately selected, e.g. using supplementary fixation to prevent subluxation of abnormal joints. Lengthening is a demanding technique, but with care provides a high level of satisfaction for the patient as well as for the surgeon.

REFERENCES

Abbott L.C. (1927) The operative lengthening of the tibia and fibula. *J. Bone Joint Surg.* 9, 128.

Aldegheri R., Trivella G., Renzi-Brivio L., *et al.* (1988) Lengthening of the lower limbs in achondroplastic patients. *J. Bone Joint Surg.* 70B, 69−73.

Aldegheri R., Agostini S. (1983) A chart of anthropometric values. *J. Bone Joint Surg.* 75B, 86−88.

Anderson M., Green W.T. and Messner M.B. (1963) Growth and predictions of growth in the lower extremities. *J. Bone Joint Surg.* 45A, 1−14.

Anderson W.V. (1972) Lengthening of the lower limb: its place in the problem of limb length discrepancy. *Mod. Trends. Orthop.* 5, 1.

Blount W.P. and Clark G.R. (1949) Control of bone growth by epiphyseal stapling. Preliminary report. *J. Bone Joint Surg.* 31A, 464−478.

Bowen J.R. and Johnson W.J. (1984) Percutaneous epiphysiodesis. *Clin. Orthop. Rel. Res.* 190, 170−173.

Broughton N.S., Olney B. and Menelaus M.B. (1989) Tibial shortening for leg length discrepancy. *J. Bone Joint Surg.* 71B, 242−245.

Canale T.S. and Christian C.A. (1990) Techniques of epiphysiodesis around the knee. *Clin. Orthop. Rel. Res.* 225, 81.

Codivilla A. (1905) On the means of lengthening in the lower limbs, the muscles and tissues which are shortened through deformity. *Am. J. Orthop. Surg.* 2, 353.

DeBastiani G., Aldegheri R., Renzi-Brivio L. and Trivella G. (1986a) Limb lengthening by distraction of the epiphyseal plate: a comparison of two techniques in the rabbit. *J. Bone Joint Surg.* 68B, 545−549.

DeBastiani G., Aldegheri R., Renzi-Brivio L. and Trivella G. (1986b) Chondrodiatasis—controlled symmetrical distraction of the epiphyseal plate: limb lengthening in children. *J. Bone Joint Surg.* 68B, 550−556.

DeBastiani G., Aldegheri R., Renzi-Brivio L. and Trivella G. (1987) Limb lengthening by callus distraction (callotasis). *J. Paediatr. Orthop.* 7, 129–134.

Dutroit M., Rigault P., Padovani J.P., Finidon G., Touzet P. and Durand Y. (1990) The outcome for children treated by limb lengthening for congenital hypoplasia of the lower limbs. *Fr. J. Orthop. Surg.* 4, 14.

Eberle E.F. (1982) Pelvic obliquity and the unstable hip after poliomyelitis. *J. Bone Joint Surg.* 64B, 300–304.

Eichler J. (1972) Methodological errors in documenting leg length and leg length discrepancies. *Der Orthopadie* 1, 14–20.

Eyres K.S., Bell M.J. and Kanis J.A. (1993) New bone formation during leg lengthening. *J. Bone Joint Surg.* 75B, 96–106.

Ferguson C.M., Morrison J.D. and Kenwright J. (1987) Leg-length inequality in children treated by Symes amputation. *J. Bone Joint Surg.* 69B, 433–436.

Friberg O. (1983) Clinical symptoms and biomechanics of lumbar spine and hip joint in leg length inequality. *Spine* 8, 643–651.

Greulich W.W. and Pyle S.I. (1959) *Radiographic Atlas of Skeletal Development of the Hand and Wrist*, 2nd edn. Stanford, California, Stanford University Press.

Hardy J.M. Tadlaoui A., Wirotius J.M. and Saleh M. (1991) The Sequoia circular fixator for limb lengthening. *Orthop. Clin. North Am.* 22, 663–675.

Hootnick D.R., Levinsohn E.M., Randall P.A. and Packard D.S. (1980) Vascular dysgenesis associated with skeletal dysplasia of the lower limb. *J. Bone Joint Surg.* 62A, 1123–1129.

Ilizarov G.A. and Deviatov A.A. (1971) Operative elongation of the leg. *Ortop. Travmatol. Protez.* 32, 20–25.

Ilizarov G.A. and Trokhova V.G. (1973) Operative elongation of the femur. *Ortop. Travmatol. Protez.* 34, 51–55.

Ilizarov G.A. (1989a) The tension–stress effect on the genesis and growth of tissues. Part I: The influence of stability of fixation and soft-tissue preservation. *Clin. Orthop.* 238, 249.

Ilizarov G.A. (1989b) The tension–stress effect on the genesis and growth of tissues. Part II: The influence of the rate and frequency of distraction. *Clin. Orthop.* 239, 263.

Ilizarov G.A. (1990) Clinical application of the tension-stress effect for limb lengthening. *Clin. Orthop.* 250, 8–25.

Jones D.C. and Moseley C.F. (1985) Subluxation of the knee as a complication of femoral lengthening by the Wagner technique. *J. Bone Joint Surg.* 67B, 33–35.

Kuntschner G. (1958) The Kuntschner method of intramedullary fixation. *J. Bone Joint Surg.* 40A, 17–26.

Lau J.H.K., Parker J.L., Hsu L.C.S. and Leong J.C.Y. (1986) Paralytic hip instability in poliomyelitis. *J. Bone Joint Surg.* 68B, 528–533.

Leong J.C.Y., Alade C.O. and Fang D. (1982) Supracondylar femoral osteotomy for knee flexion contracture resulting from poliomyelitis. *J. Bone Joint Surg.* 64B, 198–201.

Macnicol M.F. and Catto A.M. Twenty year review of tibial lengthening for poliomyelitis. *J. Bone Joint Surg.* 64B, 607–611.

Menelaus M.B. (1966) Correction of leg length discrepancy by epiphyseal arrest. *J. Bone Joint Surg.* 48B, 336–339.

Monticelli G. and Spinelli R. (1981) Distractional epiphysiolysis as a method of limb lengthening. III. Clinical applications. *Clin. Orthop.* 154, 274–285.

Moseley C.F. (1977) A straight line graph for leg length discrepancies. *J. Bone Joint Surg.* 59A, 174–179.

Nicolls M.J. (1988) Computer aided manipulation of photographs in leg lengthening. *Audiovis. Media Med.* 13, 13–16.

Nicolls M.J. and Saleh M. (1988) Composite photographs in leg lengthening. *Audiovis. Media Med.* 11, 96–99.

Paley D. (1988) Current techniques of limb lengthening. *J. Paediatr. Orthop.* 8, 73–92.

Paley D. (1990) Problems, obstacles and complications of limb lengthening by Ilizarov technique. *Clin. Orthop.* 250, 81.

Pesch H.J. and Wagner H. (1974) Histomorphologische Betrude de knochen reneration unter distraktion bei der diaphysaren verlangerungs osteotomie *Verh. Dtsch. Ges. Pathol.* 58, 305.

Phemister D.B. (1933) Operative arrest of longitudinal growth in the treatment of deformities. *J. Bone Joint Surg.* 15, 1–15.

Putti V. (1921) The operative lengthening of the femur. *JAMA* 77, 934.

Ratliff A.H.C. (1959) The short leg in poliomyelitis. *J. Bone Joint Surg.* 41B, 56–69.

Renzi-Brivio L., Lavini F. and DeBastiani G. (1990) Lengthening in the congenital short femur. *Clin. Orthop.* 250, 112.

Saleh M. and Sharrard W.J.W. (1989) Leg lengthening in achondroplasia. In Coombs R., Green S. and Sarmiento A. (eds) *External Fixation and Functional Bracing*. London, Orthotext, pp. 329–334.

Saleh M. (1989) Limb lengthening for short stature. *Growth Matters* 1, 2–5.

Saleh M. and Burton M. (1991) Leg lengthening: patient selection and management in achondroplasia. *Orthop. Clin. North Am.* 22, 589–599.

Saleh M. (1992a) Non-union surgery. Part I. Basic principles of management. *Int. J. Orthop. Trauma* 2, 4–18.

Saleh M. (1992b) Technique selection in leg lengthening: the Sheffield practice. *Semin. Orthop.* 7, 137–151.

Saleh M. and Scott B.W. (1992) Pitfalls and complications of leg lengthening: the Sheffield experience. *Semin. Orthop.* 7, 207–222.

Saleh M., Stubbs D., Street R., Lang D. and Harris S. (1993) Histology of human lengthened bone. *J. Paediatr. Orthop.* 2, 16–21.

Saleh M. and Hamer A. (1993) Bifocal lengthening—preliminary results. *J. Paediatr. Orthop.* 2, 42–48.

Shapiro F. (1982) Developmental patterns in lower extremity length discrepancies. *J. Bone Joint Surg.* 64A, 639–651.

Sofield H.A., Blair S.J. and Millar E.A. (1958) Leg lengthening: a personal follow up of forty patients some twenty years after the operation. *J. Bone Joint Surg.* 40A, 311–322.

Stinchfield A.J., Reidy J.A. and Barr J.S. (1949) Prediction of unequal growth of the lower extremities in anterior poliomyelitis. *J. Bone Joint Surg.* 31A, 478–486.

Vilarrubias J.M., Ginebreda I. and Jimeno E. (1990) Lengthening of the lower limbs and correction of lumbar hyperlordosis in achondroplasia. *Clin. Orthop.* 250, 143.

Wagner H. (1971) Operative Beinverlangerung. *Chirurgie* 42, 260.

Wagner H. (1977) Surgical lengthening or shortening of the femur. In Gschwend N. (ed) *Progress in Orthopaedic Surgery*. New York, Springer Verlag.

Wilde G.P. and Baker G.C.W. (1987) Circumferential periosteal release in the treatment of children with leg-length inequality. *J. Bone Joint Surg.* 69B, 817–821.

Winquist R. and Hansen S. (1978) Closed intramedullary shortening of the femur. *Clin. Orthop. Rel. Res.* 136, 54–61.

Wolff J. (1892) Das gesetz der transformation der knochen. Berlin, Verlag von August Hirschwald.

Chapter 12
Juvenile Chronic Arthritis

Chapter 12.1
Medical Aspects

B.M. Ansell

INTRODUCTION

Chronic arthritis in childhood is uncommon. In the UK various epidemiological studies have suggested that 1 in 1000 of the childhood population has an episode of swelling of one or more joints persisting for more than 3 months and for which no specific cause can be found. Only about half of these, however, will progress to chronic arthritis. Similar figures have come from elsewhere in the world, particularly Scandinavia (Kunnamo *et al.*, 1986).

Nomenclature and classification is still unsatisfactory, though there is general agreement that chronic arthritis of childhood comprises a heterogeneous group of conditions, most of which are different from adult sero-positive rheumatoid arthritis (Ansell, 1990a). From the European League against Rheumatism (EULAR) Workshop of 1977, the umbrella term of 'juvenile chronic arthritis' arose, while in the USA the term 'juvenile arthritis' has been used to cover all rheumatic diseases in childhood that have a peripheral or axial arthritis, with the term 'juvenile rheumatoid arthritis' reserved for a group of closely related rheumatic diseases characterized by idiopathic peripheral arthritis (Cassidy *et al.*, 1989). All present classifications use 16 years as the upper age limit for onset, and that there must be persistent arthritis in one or more joints for a minimum of 6 weeks to 3 months. In view of the lack of any diagnostic test, the active exclusion of other defined disorders is essential. These include infections, blood dyscrasias, hypogamma-globulinaemia, the more uncommon connective tissue disorders, Lyme's disease, Reiter's syndrome and many orthopaedic conditions. Classification by mode of onset is probably better at 6 months than at 3 months (Table 12.1.1), while presently disease course classification is being assessed, as this may ultimately prove the best for indicating prognosis.

Table 12.1 Diagnosis of juvenile chronic arthritis

Onset
    Under 16 years
Duration of arthritis
    Minimum of 3 months
Classification by onset
    3−6 months
Systemic   →   Polyarthritis
Polyarticular (five or more joints in first 3 months)
    IgM rheumatoid factor negative
    IgM rheumatoid factor positive
Pauciarticular (less than five joints in first 3−6 months)
    Under 6 years ± antinuclear antibodies; usually girls ± chronic iridocyclitis
    9 years or over, HLA B27 positive; usually boys
    Others

Active exclusion of other well-defined entities, e.g. more uncommon connective tissue disease, infections, malignancy, orthopaedic problems

AETIOLOGY

This is unknown, and pathogenetic mechanisms remain unclear (Lang and Shore, 1990). Numerous immuno-logical abnormalities have been described in these patients, and these would appear to be particularly pronounced during active disease; certain medications, particularly corticosteroids, may have a marked effect on the immune system, complicating interpretation of observed immune aberrations.

Genetic aspects are equally difficult to unravel, but family predisposition has been suggested (Rosenberg and Petty, 1980), while a study of 12 affected sibling pairs showed a significant difference between the observed and expected ratio of siblings sharing two haplotypes (Clemens *et al.*, 1985). In young-onset pauciarticular disease, a strong association between HLA

A2, HLA DR5 and HLA DRw8 has been reported (Albert and Ansell, 1984; Hall *et al.*, 1986). Associations have also been reported with HLA DRw4 and HLA DRw52, with negative associations with HLA DR1 and DR4. Recently, it has been suggested that epitopes sharing between HLA DR5, DRw6, DRw8 and DRw52 may be important in predisposing to disease. That more than one chromosome may be involved is suggested by the antigen increase in HLA DPw2 in pauciarticular disease (Odum *et al.*, 1986; Fernandez-Vina *et al.*, 1994).

The next subgroup that shows strong HLA association is those children who carry IgM rheumatoid factor in their serum; they are clinically and immunogenetically indistinguishable from patients with adult-onset rheumatoid arthritis, and they carry HLA DR4 (Clemens *et al.*, 1983). In seronegative polyarticular onset disease, a strong association was demonstrated with HLA DRw8 in children whose age of disease onset was less than 5 years (Hall *et al.*, 1988). In older onset pauciarticular disease, boys aged 9 years and upwards often carry HLA B27. Some of these will undoubtedly develop classic ankylosing spondylitis. An increased incidence of HLA B27 is also found in both boys and girls in post-dysenteric arthritis. Except for this form of arthritis, including those patients who progress to typical Reiter's syndrome, the initial triggering mechanism is unknown.

Despite a history of sore throats in many children with systemic illness and the occasional finding of rises in AS0 titres and also viral titres, no specific infection has been identified (Tyndall *et al.*, 1984). Although conclusive evidence for a viral aetiology is lacking, the fact that some viruses, e.g. parvovirus or rubella, are capable of initiating an arthropathy suggests there is a need for further consideration with newer technology.

PATTERNS OF DISEASE ACCORDING TO ONSET

Systemic onset

For the diagnosis of systemic juvenile chronic arthritis, persistent intermittent fever associated with at least one other feature, preferably the typical rash, is required, and the later development of arthritis. It accounts for approximately one-fifth of children referred with juvenile chronic arthritis.

The fever is high with one or two daily temperature spikes, often up to 40°C. The other features include the characteristic maculopapular rash, generalized lymphadenopathy, splenomegaly, hepatomegaly (Fig. 12.1.1) or pericarditis. The most common age of onset for this pattern is under 5 years, when boys are affected as

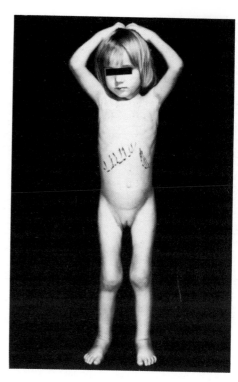

Fig. 12.1.1 Lymphadenopathy and hepatosplenomegaly in a 3-year-old girl who had presented with fever, rash and malaise 10 months previously. Arthritis of the wrists, knees and ankles is already evident.

frequently as girls, but the disease can be seen throughout childhood and, indeed, into adult life; after 5 years of age girls are more commonly affected than boys. Generalized lymphadenopathy, particularly of epitrochlear and axillary nodes, may be so prominent as to suspect lymphoma. Abdominal pain or distension due either to enlarged mesenteric nodes or to serositis can suggest an acute abdominal disorder.

Initially there may be no joint symptoms. The disease may present with minor arthralgia, intermittent bouts of joint swelling or severe polyarthritis; very occasionally, acute neck pain may suggest meningitis. Ultimately, most of these children develop arthritis, the most usual sites being the knees and wrists, followed by the ankles and tarsi (Figs 12.1.1 and 12.1.2). Flexor tendon involvement in the hand, which causes splinting of the metacarpophalangeal joints and loss of movement at proximal interphalangeal joints, is common after a few weeks; at times there is associated swelling of the proximal interphalangeal joints (Fig. 12.1.2). In the first few months of the disease it is rare for other joints to be affected, though if the disease persists actively for more than 1 year extension tends to occur, and by 5 years from onset hip involvement is seen in 40% of patients.

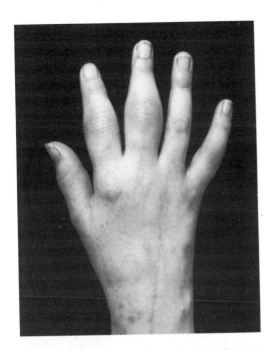

Fig. 12.1.2 Severe swelling of the second and third proximal interphalangeal joints with flexor tenosynovitis in these fingers and also the fifth finger in an 8-year-old girl who had developed systemic juvenile arthritis 3 years previously. Note the typical maculopapular rash extending over the forearm, as well as involvement of the wrist and carpus.

Polyarthritic onset

A polyarthritic onset of juvenile chronic arthritis is defined as the involvement of five or more joints throughout the first 3 months; it can develop at any time in childhood and is seen even before the first birthday. It is more common in girls than boys. A very small proportion of patients, 6% or less, have persistent IgM rheumatoid factor; they tend to be older, aged 10 years and over, and predominantly female. Subgrouping by the presence or absence of IgM rheumatoid factor is usual, as the joint distribution as well as the prognosis appear to be different (Clemens *et al.*, 1983).

Seronegative onset

The distribution of joint involvement is similar irrespective of whether there has been a polyarthritic onset or the polyarthritis has followed a systemic onset. The most commonly involved joints are the knees (60%) followed by the carpi and the wrists, so that there is swelling over the back of the hands extending up to the base of the metacarpals, then the ankles and tarsi (Fig. 12.1.3). Neck involvement is seen in approximately one-third of cases, causing pain and loss of extension, though at times there can be severe torticollis. Torticollis may be a presenting feature; it is occasionally due to atlanto-axial subluxation, but more commonly results from spasm due to unilateral involvement of apophyseal joints or subluxation of C2 on C3. Typical hand involvement consists of arthritis of the proximal and distal interphalangeal joints together with flexor tenosynovitis, the metacarpophalangeal joints usually being splinted by the severity of the flexor tendon swelling. Involvement of the interphalangeal joints of the toes is not uncommon, while early in the course the first metatarsophalangeal joint is involved. This usually occurs in association with hindfoot involvement. Tenosynovitis in the foot is not uncommon (Fig. 12.1.3).

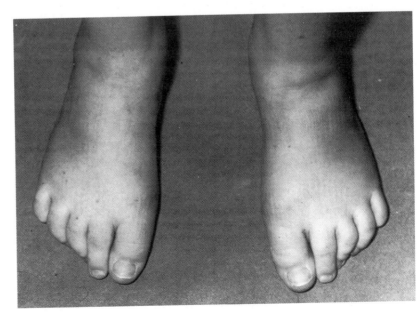

Fig. 12.1.3 Polyarthritic onset of juvenile chronic arthritis at the age of 18 months. Now, 9 months later, there is soft tissue swelling around the ankles and over the tarsi and mid-tarsal joints. Note clawing of the toes and general swelling of great toes, particularly the terminal interphalangeal joints.

When the arthritis persists actively for 1 year or more other joints, notably the elbows, hips, shoulders, metatarsophalangeal and temporomandibular joints, become affected.

IgM rheumatoid factor-positive onset

This tends to affect older children aged 9–10 years and upwards and is more common in girls. The arthritis usually affects the small joints of the hands and feet initially, with soft tissue swelling of the metacarpophalangeal, proximal interphalangeal and metatarsophalangeal joints as well as the wrists and carpi in the first few weeks. Large joints can be involved early, particularly the knees and ankles, but characteristically only in association with the small joints. Elbow nodules, with the same site and histological characteristics as seropositive adult rheumatoid arthritis, are not uncommon.

The importance of the age of onset was suggested by a prospective study (Hanson *et al.*, 1969), in which it was shown that 80% of patients with positive rheumatoid factor tests had an onset between 12 and 16 years. The rheumatoid factor tests can be positive within 6 weeks of the first symptom and in the vast majority by 3 months. Indeed, it is exceptional for the rheumatoid factor tests to become positive after more than 1 year of illness; they remain positive unless slow-acting drugs, e.g. gold, are given for prolonged periods.

In contrast to seronegative arthritis, periostitis along the shafts of the metacarpals, metatarsals and bases of proximal phalanges can occur within a few weeks, and erosions can occur within months of onset, particularly in the hands and feet (Ansell and Kent, 1977). The main reason for separating this subgroup is the persistence of activity, rapid joint destruction and complications. HLA typing has confirmed that these patients carry HLA DR4 in excess and in the same amount as in adult seropositive rheumatoid arthritis (Clemens *et al.*, 1983).

Pauciarticular onset

Pauciarticular arthritis is defined as arthritis of four or fewer joints in the first 3 months and is by far the most common type of presentation. It is further subdivided by age of onset.

YOUNG ONSET (UNDER 6 YEARS)

Such children are usually aged between 1 and 5 years when they first present with arthritis, with girls predominating (Fig. 12.1.4).

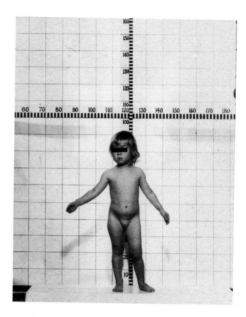

Fig. 12.1.4 Monarticular onset at age 2 years with involvement of the left knee only. Note the position of the leg with slight overgrowth of the affected side, flexion and valgus deformity.

The most commonly involved joints are the knee, ankle and/or elbows, while a single finger with proximal interphalangeal joint swelling and flexor tenosynovitis can occur alone or accompany another joint. Less commonly, the neck or wrist and carpus may be the presenting site. These children often carry antinuclear antibodies; indeed, the presence of antinuclear antibody in the serum is closely associated with the presence or future development of chronic iridocyclitis. Thus, it is essential that they are screened by an ophthalmologist (Kanski, 1989). As previously noted this subgroup, which is unique to childhood, carries HLA A2, DR5 and DRw8. Some will go on to a quiet insidious polyarthritis with the slow addition of one joint after another; as yet there is no specific marker for such patients.

OLDER ONSET (9 YEARS AND OVER)

This affects particularly boys and is characterized by a lower limb arthropathy affecting knees, ankles and hips; this last site is more common in teenagers than in the 9–10-year-olds (Ansell, 1980).

There is often enthesitis which can affect the heel either at the insertion of the plantar fascia or Achilles tendon, or both, as well as the tibial tubercle, patella and greater trochanter. This is sometimes referred to as 'SEA' syndrome (Rosenberg and Petty, 1982).

The frequency with which sacroiliitis develops later is not known, but in one of the author's studies more than

50% had developed it by the 5-year follow-up. A family history of ankylosing spondylitis or arthropathy with sacroiliitis is common; there may be an association with ulcerative colitis or regional enteritis. These patients carry HLA B27 and are usually referred to a spondyloarthropathy.

A previous history of an episode of diarrhoea raises the suspicion of post-dysenteric arthritis or, if there are features such as conjunctivitis and urethritis, of Reiter's syndrome.

It is important to recognize this subgroup because of the varying manifestations and course of the disease (Jacobs *et al.*, 1982).

OTHER ONSET

A small group of girls aged 7–11 years presents with the disease restricted to one or both knees. These girls usually have a normal erythrocyte sedimentation rate and are negative for all autoantibodies; they have a good prognosis.

JUVENILE PSORIATIC ARTHRITIS

These patients also not uncommonly present with pauciarticular arthritis, which tends to spread to an asymmetric polyarthritis that can be locally destructive (Shore and Ansell, 1982). A sausage digit, either finger or toe, with swelling of both interphalangeal joints and flexor tenosynovitis is a common mode of presentation. At this time the child may have no skin lesions, but nail pits are not uncommon. A family history of psoriasis is obtained in 40%. Criteria for juvenile psoriatic arthritis are not yet established (Southwood *et al.*, 1989).

LABORATORY ASPECTS

In systemic disease the Westergren erythrocyte sedimentation rate is usually high, up to 100 mm/h or more. There is polymorphonuclear leucocytosis, often as high as 95% in a 20 000–30 000 white cell count, while platelets may also be considerably raised. The haemoglobin concentration tends to fall to about 10 g/dl; it seldom goes lower than this in the early diagnostic stage, but with persistence of the systemic state for 1–2 years it may fall to 6–7 g/dl. Immunoglobulins, particularly IgG, tend to rise and immune complexes can be detected relatively early by a number of techniques (Moran *et al.*, 1979). IgM rheumatoid factor is absent from the serum, though very occasionally antinuclear antibodies can be detected.

A polyarthritic onset is associated with a moderately raised erythrocyte sedimentation rate, 60–70 mm/h, a slight rise in the total white cell count with polymorphonuclear leucocytosis and a moderate rise in platelet count. Modest rises in all immunoglobulins are not uncommon. IgM rheumatoid factor, as shown by the latex test, sheep cell agglutination test, rheumatoid arthritis haemagglutinin test or other commercial tests, is persistently positive in about 6%. Antinuclear antibodies are occasionally detected, often in those patients with a positive rheumatoid factor test. Other tests, e.g. those for extractable nuclear antigen and antibodies to DNA, are negative and complement levels are normal.

With a pauciarticular onset, the erythrocyte sedimentation rate may be normal or moderately raised, haemoglobin is usually normal—indeed a low value calls for investigation into bleeding from the gastrointestinal tract, e.g. regional enteritis—and white blood cell count and platelet count are normal. Antinuclear antibodies are often present, particularly in girls with an onset below 6 years of age. Rheumatoid factor is negative. There is occasionally IgA deficiency.

RADIOLOGICAL CHANGES

With the exception of osteoporosis, radiological changes tend to be late (Ansell and Kent, 1977). Indeed, in the first few months of illness the main reason for radiological assessment is to exclude other disorders, e.g. leukaemia or epiphyseal anomalies.

In pauciarticular arthritis, growth anomalies start to become obvious after about 6 months, with the epiphyses of the affected joint increasing in size compared with the unaffected opposite joint. Early erosions, that is within 1 year, are seen predominantly in cases with IgM rheumatoid factor. Later radiological change depends on the age of onset and joint involvement and is described under Prognosis (see below).

Magnetic resonance imaging will allow very effective assessment of the soft tissue swelling (Stannard and Fink, 1989).

PROGNOSIS

The overall prognosis in terms of mortality is good. There are two main causes of death: infection early and usually in association with systemic illness, and amyloidosis later. The last condition is also more common in those who have had a systemic onset of disease. The course tends to be unpredictable, and relapses can occur after long periods of remission. The majority of children ultimately go into remission, however, but with varying degrees of residual deformity (Calabro *et al.*, 1976).

No population studies have been undertaken. Outcome in practice is influenced by a number of factors, including the duration of the disease at the time of referral. Thus, in the initial review of patients at the Juvenile Rheumatism Unit at Taplow, UK, 60% of those children seen within 1 year of onset had normal function at the 5-year follow-up, compared with only 25% of those seen later in the course of the disease (Ansell and Wood, 1976). There are, however, certain points common to both groups: those children who had an onset before the first birthday, and to a lesser extent those with an onset between the first and second birthday, had a very much poorer functional outcome, because the younger the child the more difficult it is to prevent the development of contractures and deformities. Approximately half of the patients seen early in the course of systemic disease are improving by the 1-year follow-up, and these tend to do well. The remainder may have persistent systemic illness often exacerbated by intercurrent infection, up to 4–5 years from onset; and in these there is usually associated severe, generalized polyarthritis (Svantesson *et al.*, 1983). Most children with polyarthritis, irrespective of whether it was of systemic or polyarthritic onset, show prolific synovitis.

The most serious joint involvement associated with a poor functional outcome is the hip. This is particularly likely in children who have an onset under the age of 5 years and whose disease persists actively for more than 5 years. Radiologically, these children show alterations in the development of the hip joints (Fig. 12.1.5) (Gallino *et al.*, 1984), and although some restoration of hip joint function is possible (Bernstein *et al.*, 1977), it is still not certain how long such joints will function adequately (Fig. 12.1.6).

A polyarthritic onset can be associated with prolonged activity of the arthritis, and although some cases have a monocyclic course, this tends to be prolonged over several years. Many will recover, however, with few residual effects (Fig. 12.1.7) (Ansell, 1987). About 10% of polyarthritic patients show little palpable synovial

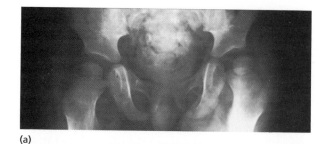

(a)

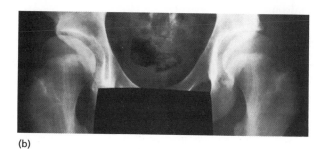

(b)

Fig. 12.1.6 (a) This 2-year-old boy had had an acute onset of systemic Still's disease 8 months previously. At the time of the first radiological examination there was severe spasm in the left hip, so that the apparent increase in size of the epiphysis on that side may be partly positional. The right hip showed loss of movement with discomfort but no spasm. (b) Same boy's hips, now aged 15 years. His disease has been inactive for 8 years and he regards himself as normal. Note, however, the unusual shape of the femoral heads, the straight femoral necks and the narrowing of the joint space on the left side.

thickening, but gradually contract in a manner that leads to a slow but steady loss of function. Involvement of the cervical spine, particularly in the absence of adequate measures to maintain mobility, is associated with failure of development of vertebrae and widespread apophyseal joint fusion. It is not uncommonly associated with failure of development of the lower jaw, irrespective of whether there has been temporomandibular involvement.

Persistent joint involvement is associated radiologi-

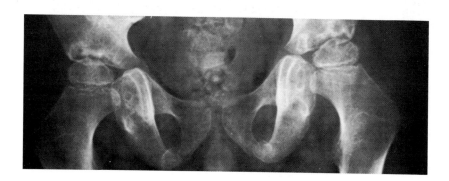

Fig. 12.1.5 A 5-year-old boy who had had a systemic onset of severe juvenile chronic arthritis requiring corticosteroid therapy 3 years previously. Note the shape of the acetabulae together with the cystic changes taking place associated with erosions, narrowing of joint space and overdevelopment of the femoral heads, which have a tendency to upward migration.

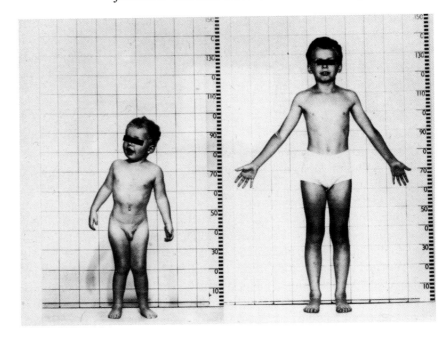

Fig. 12.1.7 This boy presented with polyarthritis at the age of $3\frac{1}{2}$ years. Note the marked torticollis and the tendency to flexion contractures at the knees. After appropriate treatment with splinting, physiotherapy and non-steroidal anti-inflammatory drugs, he improved and the disease became inactive after 3 years. Six years after onset he is straight and leading a completely normal life, without any therapy.

cally with periosteal new bone formation adjacent to involved joints, particularly in the phalanges, as a result of flexor tenosynovitis (Fig. 12.1.8). Overall failure of development of joints is not uncommon in protracted disease. Persistent disease activity is associated with progressive bony change, seen most commonly in the hands, knees, tarsus and cervical spine (Fig. 12.1.9) and later the hips. Asymmetrical growth anomalies are rare unless the onset of the disease is pauciarticular.

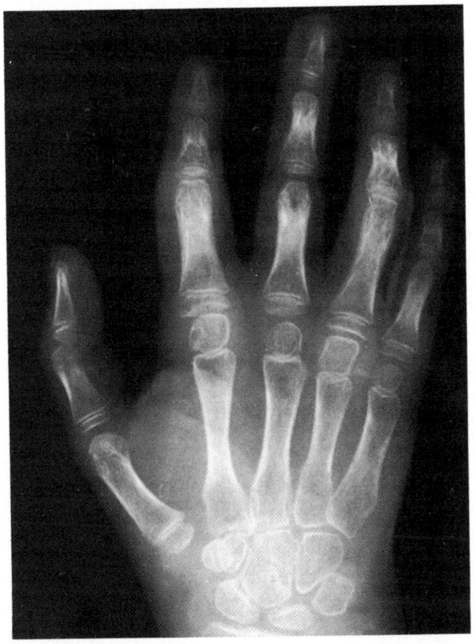

Fig. 12.1.8 Radiograph of the hand of a 10-year-old boy, 8 years after the onset of juvenile chronic arthritis. Note that although there is osteoporosis and angulation of carpal bones and metacarpal heads, there is no gross destruction. There has been periosteal reaction along the second and third proximal phalanges in association with flexor tenosynovitis, which is causing contracture of these fingers. This is in sharp contrast to the radiological change in seropositive disease (see Fig. 12.1.9).

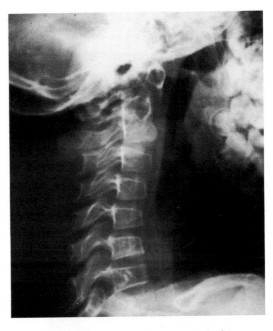

Fig. 12.1.9 Cervical spine involvement in a girl of 11 years of age with juvenile chronic arthritis of 10 years' duration. Note the curious alignment with step-like pattern of vertebrae, the poor development of the vertebrae and the tendency to subluxation of C2 on C3. Early apophyseal joint involvement is obvious at C2/C3 and C3/C4.

Those children with widespread polyarthritis following systemic disease, whose onset of their illness was under the age of 5 years, commonly show overall retardation of growth; this is often exaggerated by the administration of corticosteroid therapy. Those children with a polyarticular onset have less overall retardation (Bernstein *et al.*, 1977). Growth rate improves as the disease goes into remission.

The presence of IgM rheumatoid factor is associated with the early development of erosions and persistent disease activity, so that it is not uncommon to see gross widespread destructive changes within a few years of the onset of seropositive disease (Fig. 12.1.10). Hip involvement is common and causes severe protrusion, Atlantoaxial subluxation is not uncommon, while other joint problems include subluxation at the metacarpophalangeal and metatarsophalangeal joints, destruction of knee epiphyses and the complications of carpal tunnel syndrome, ruptured tendons, etc. Vasculitis is uncommon, as are aortic incompetence (Leak *et al.*, 1981), and lung fibrosis.

Function is usually well maintained in pauciarticular disease, though local deformity of affected joints tends to occur; in this group eye involvement can be more sinister than joint involvement, as if it is unheeded or poorly treated it can lead to blindness. Those 15% of children who develop polyarthritis tend to do particularly badly, not only because of the persistence of activity,

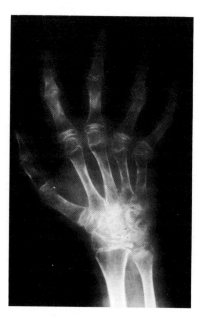

Fig. 12.1.10 Gross erosive changes at the wrist, metacarpi and proximal and distal interphalangeal joints in a 13-year-old girl, $2\frac{1}{2}$ years after the onset of seropositive juvenile rheumatoid arthritis.

but also in the gradual way in which they accumulate more affected joints, so that measures to maintain joint position and control disease activity are instituted late; many of these children also have iridocyclitis.

MANAGEMENT

In all forms of juvenile chronic arthritis, the aim of treatment is to suppress activity and prevent joint deformities. Therapy may need to be continued for many years, but most children can live at home and attend a normal school despite continuing disease activity; only a very small proportion will need to go to special schools. Parents should be encouraged to play a major role in supervising therapy. As juvenile chronic arthritis is relatively rare, it is desirable for the paediatrician and rheumatologist to work with each other and to associate with an ophthalmologist and an orthopaedic surgeon and possibly also an orthodontist. It is also important that the team that looks after such children includes a physiotherapist, occupational therapist and a social worker, all of whom will need to develop special expertise, while access to an orthotist for special needs and a child psychiatrist and an educational psychologist are desirable.

Prolonged bed-rest is to be discouraged, though a sick child with systemic illness will need to spend a considerable time in bed, with due attention being paid to joint position, splinting and physiotherapy. In all children, adequate rest is important, so either a short rest period at midday when at school or on return home is desirable. If the hips and knees are involved, resting is best carried out in a prone position and indeed, with such involvement, a period of prone lying is desirable every day to try and prevent or overcome flexion deformities of the hips and knees. Specially designed prone-lying beds can be used, but this can also be achieved by lying on the floor in front of the television. Rest splints for the wrists, knees and ankles worn at night will also prevent deformities, while work splints can protect joints when in use. Those joints that are particularly worth splinting are the wrist when writing, the neck while doing schoolwork and, if the quadriceps are weak, the knees when walking (Lawton, 1990). Heel cup insoles also maintain a neutral position of the foot. When there is acute spasm or contractures of the hips and knees, skin traction either for prolonged periods throughout the 24-h period or just at night may be desirable. Once deformities are overcome, night skin traction may be a valuable way of preventing recurrence. At times it will be necessary to spare the lower limb joints, in which case gutter crutches or special walking aids may be desirable. Mobility can often be maintained by a bicycle, tricycle, pedal car, or tractor. Remarkable improvement can be achieved in this way in association with appropriate physiotherapy (Fig. 12.1.11) (Ansell, 1981).

Physiotherapy is aimed at preventing muscle wasting, improving muscle and joint function and thereby helping with contractures. It takes the form of a daily exercise programme tailored to individual needs and preferably supervised by the parents with regular advice from the physiotherapist (Jarvis, 1990). Hydrotherapy is beneficial when the hips and knees are involved, and children prefer their exercise programme in water rather than on dry land. In general, with active joint disease competitive sport is discouraged, but the child can join in exercise to music, and cycling and swimming are excellent sports.

Drug treatment

Aspirin is no longer the drug of first choice because of the worry about Reye's syndrome (Hall, 1986). For children under 5 years, ibuprofen is available in suspen-sion. The dose should be 30–40 mg/kg/day given in three or four divided doses. Diclofenac sodium, 3 mg/kg/day, is also available for those under 5 years old, and there is a paediatric suppository containing 12.5 mg. For older children naproxen sodium and piroxicam have the advantage that they can be given twice-daily or once-daily, respectively, which is particularly helpful when children are attending normal school. Should intolerance develop to sodium, tolmetin up to 30 mg/kg/day, may be a suitable alternative. Aspirin is reserved for those children who do not improve on any of the non-steroidal anti-inflammatory drugs available for children and is particularly valuable when there is fever. It should be given at 80 mg/kg/day in divided doses. Side-effects are less common in children than in adults, but there must be appropriate choice of preparation to allow all round control. Children do not usually complain of tinnitus, so overdose has to be suspected if there is nausea, vomiting, hyperpnoea, and this requires estimation of blood salicylate levels; the aim is a blood level of about 2 mmol/l. Parents must

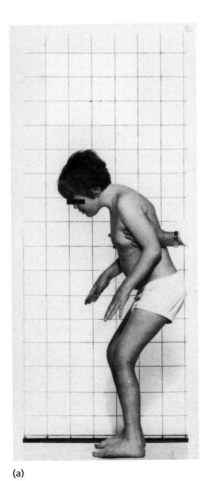

Fig. 12.1.11 (a) A 13-year-old boy, 2 years after a systemic onset of juvenile chronic arthritis. Note the active arthritis with severe deformity. A full conservative regimen with splinting for the wrists, traction for most of the 24-h period for knees and hips and intensive physiotherapy was instituted, together with appropriate drugs to reduce inflammation. (b) Same boy, 3½ years later, off all drugs and able to lead a normal life, but with quite severe residual changes.

(a) (b)

be warned to watch for side-effects and intercurrent infections. In systemic disease, it is wise to check liver function regularly.

Current therapies include the use of intravenous immunoglobulin to control the systemic features (Silverman *et al.*, 1989) and methotrexate (Truckenbrodt and Hafner, 1986). Slow-acting drugs, e.g. antimalarials, gold, or penicillamine, appear to have little role in seronegative polyarthritis (Brewer *et al.*, 1986), except for methotrexate. The multicentre trial in polyarthritis showed that methotrexate, 10 mg/m^2, was the first drug effective in reducing the activity of arthritis over a 6-month period. It should be noted, however, that low doses were no better than placebo (Giannini *et al.*, 1992). Gold, penicillamine, or methotrexate should be added in IgM rheumatoid factor-positive disease as soon as erosions have developed. Gold and penicillamine are equally effective, and both have side-effects that include rashes, proteinuria and bone marrow depression; in addition, penicillamine can cause nausea, anorexia, a lupus-like syndrome and myasthenia gravis. Regular supervision of therapy with blood counts and urine checks are essential throughout therapy, which may last for years. Methotrexate behaves as in adult seropositive disease. Sulphasalazine may also be useful in such cases.

For the spondyloarthropathy group, who are usually older, flurbiprofen and indomethacin may also be considered. Sulphasalazine appears to be useful in some older patients with spondyloarthropathy (Ansell *et al.*, 1991), but not in any other subgroups. Both azathioprine and methotrexate may be helpful in a refractory peripheral arthritis in this subgroup.

Corticosteroids do not affect the ultimate prognosis nor the occurrence of complications, and their use is limited by side-effects. When given on a daily regimen, particularly in divided doses, failure of growth is usual, as is suppression of the hypothalamic—pituitary—adrenal axis and osteoporosis. It is necessary to use them in children with systemica illness who are unresponsive to other therapy and very occasionally in children with polyarthritis who continue to worsen despite a full regimen as previously described. In such cases it is wise to use a single daily dose given in the morning, with a very marked difference in the size of the dose on the following days, e.g. prednisolone, 20 mg alternating with 2 mg; this dose regimen will mean that it takes longer for the disease to come under control, but it does prevent suppression of the hypothalamic—pituitary—adrenal axis. Corticotrophin gel is sometimes preferred, particularly for the management of systemic illness, as it is often easier to withdraw. It should also be given on an alternate-day regimen, however, if cushingoid features and suppression of the hypothalamic—pituitary—adrenal axis are to be avoided. The possibility of reducing spinal osteoporosis by the use of deflazacort when it becomes available will need consideration (Ansell, 1990b).

Local corticosteroids have been increasingly used. The injection of triamcinolone cetonide, 20—40 mg, into the knee in young-onset pauciarticular arthritis has proved invaluable in maintaining position and function (Earley *et al.*, 1988). Hydrocortisone injections into flexor tendon sheath inflammation is also valuable. Other sites, e.g. the wrists, are currently under study.

In general there is little place for the use of cytotoxic drugs, e.g. cyclophosphamide or chlorambucil, as the long-term prognosis with respect to mortality is good, while the potential of this kind of therapy for mutagenesis and oncogenesis is not known. In children who have experienced serious side-effects with other drugs, however, or who have the one potentially fatal complication—amyloidosis—these drugs may need to be considered (Schnitzer and Ansell, 1977).

CONCLUSIONS

Throughout what will be a long and difficult course in many children, it is important that joints are maintained in a functional position, that muscles are allowed to develop and that growth of mind and body is interfered with as little as possible. The tenacity of the parents to keep up a regimen over many years is one of the main aids to success in the long-term care of these children. There will be ups and downs, successes and disappointments, and it is essential that the group of people treating the child speaks with one voice and that each individual member should be approachable as required by the needs of the child at any one time. Given good care, more than 80% of children with this serious illness will be able to take their place in society and lead normal lives.

REFERENCES

Ansell B.M. and Albert E.D. (1985) Joint report: Juvenile chronic arthritis pauciarticular type. In Albert E.D., Baul M.P. and Mayr W.R. (eds) *Histocompatibility Testing 1984*. Berlin, Springer, pp. 368—374.

Ansell B.M. (1980) Juvenile spondylitis and related disorders. In Moll J.M.H. (ed) *Ankylosing Spondylitis*. Edinburgh, Churchill Livingstone, pp. 120—136.

Ansell B.M. (1981) Rehabilitation in juvenile chronic arthritis. *Clin. Rheum. Dis.* 7, 469—484.

Ansell B.M. Juvenile chronic arthritis. *Scand. J. Rheumatol. Suppl.* 66, 47—50.

Ansell B.M. (1990a) Classification and nomenclature. In Woo P., White P. and Ansell B.M. (eds) *Paediatric Rheumatology Update*. Oxford, Oxford University Press, pp. 3–5.

Ansell B.M. (1990b) Corticosteroid therapy. In Woo P., White P.H. and Ansell B.M. (eds) *Paediatric Rheumatology Update*. Oxford, Oxford University Press, pp. 81–84.

Ansell B.M. and Kent P.A. (1977) Radiological changes in juvenile chronic polyarthritis. *Skeletal Radiol.* 1, 129–144.

Ansell B.M. and Wood P.H.N. (1976) Prognosis in juvenile chronic polyarthritis. *Clin. Rheum. Dis.* 2, 397–412.

Ansell B.M., Hall M.A., Loftus J.K. *et al.* (1991) A multicentre pilot study of sulphasalazine in juvenile chronic arthritis. *Clin. Exp. Rheumatol.* 9, 201–203.

Bernstein B.H., Forrester D., Singsen B. *et al.* (1977) Hip joint restoration in juvenile rheumatoid arthritis. *Arthritis Rheum.* 20, 1099–1104.

Brewer E.J., Giannini E.H., Kuzmina N. *et al.* (1986) D-penicillamine and hydroxychloroquine in the treatment of severe juvenile rheumatoid arthritis: results of a USA/USSR double blind placebo controlled trial. *N. Engl. J. Med.* 314, 1269–1276.

Calabro J.J., Holgerson W.G., Sonpal G.M. *et al.* (1976) Juvenile rheumatoid arthritis: a general review and report on 100 patients observed for 15 years. *Semin. Arthritis Rheum.* 5, 257–298.

Cassidy J.T., Levinson J.E. and Brewer E.J. (1989) The development of classification criteria for children with juvenile rheumatoid arthritis. *Bull. Rheum. Dis.* 38, 1–7.

Clemens L.E., Albert E. and Ansell B.M. (1983) HLA studies in IgM rheumatoid factor positive childhood arthritis. *Ann. Rheum. Dis.* 42, 431–434.

Clemens L.E., Albert E. and Ansell B.M. (1985) Sibling pair affected by chronic arthritis: evidence for a genetic predisposition. *J. Rheumatol.* 12, 108–113.

Earley A., Cuttica R., McCullough C. *et al.* (1988) Triamcinolone into the knee joint in juvenile chronic arthritis. *Clin. Exp. Rheumatol.* 6, 153–155.

Fernandez-Vina M., Fink C.W. and Stastny P. (1994) HLA associations in juvenile arthritis. *Clin. Exp. Rheumatol.* 12, 205–214.

Giannini E.H., Brewer E.J., Kuzmina N. *et al.* (1992) Methotrexate in resistant juvenile rheumatoid arthritis: results of a USA/USSR double blind placebo controlled trial. *N. Engl. J. Med.* 326, 1043–1049.

Gallino L., Pountain G., Mitchell N. *et al.* (1984) Development of the hip in juvenile chronic arthritis: a radiological assessment. *Scand. J. Rheumatol.* 13, 310–318.

Hall S.M. (1986) Reye's syndrome and aspirin—a review. *J. Royal Soc. Med.* 79, 596–598.

Hall P.J., Burman S.J. and Laurent M. (1986) Genetic susceptibility to early onset pauci-articular juvenile chronic arthritis: a study of HLA and complement markers in 158 British patients. *Ann. Rheum. Dis.* 45, 464–474.

Hall P.J., Burman S.J., Barash J. *et al.* (1988) HLA and C4 antigens in polyarticular onset sero-negative disease: association of early onset with HLA Drw8. *J. Rheumatol.* 16, 55–59.

Hanson V., Drexler E. and Kornreich H. (1969) The relationship of rheumatoid factor to age of onset in juvenile rheumatoid arthritis. *Arthritis Rheum.* 12, 82–86.

Jacobs J.C., Berdon W.E. and Johnston A.D. (1982) HLA B27 associated spondylo arthropathy in childhood: clinical, pathological and radiological observation in 58 patients. *J. Pediatr.* 100, 521–528.

Jarvis R. (1990) Physiotherapy for juvenile arthritis. In Woo P., White P.H. and Ansell B.M. (eds) *Paediatric Rheumatology Update*. Oxford, Oxford University Press, pp. 90–98.

Kanski J.J. (1989) Screening for uveitis in juvenile chronic arthritis. *Br. J. Ophthalmol.* 73, 225–228.

Kunnamo I., Kallio P. and Pelkonen P. (1986) Incidence of arthritis in urban Finnish children. *Arthritis Rheum.* 29, 1232–1238.

Lang B.A. and Shore A. (1990) A review of current concepts on the pathogenesis of juvenile rheumatoid arthritis. *J. Rheumatol.* 17 (Suppl. 1), 1–15.

Lawton S. (1990) Occupational therapy. In Woo P., White P.H. and Ansell B.M. (eds) *Paediatric Rheumatology Update*. Oxford, Oxford University Press, pp. 99–105.

Leak A.M., Miller-Craig M.W. and Ansell B.M. (1981) Aortic regurgitation in sero-positive juvenile arthritis. *Ann. Rheum. Dis.* 40, 229–234.

Moran H., Ansell B.M., Mowbray J.F. *et al.* (1979) Antigen—antibody complexes in the serum of patients with juvenile chronic arthritis. *Arch. Dis. Child.* 54, 120–122.

Odum N., Morling N., Friis J. *et al.* (1986) Increased frequency of HLA-DPw2 in pauci-articular onset juvenile chronic arthritis. *Tissue Antigens* 28, 245–250.

Rosenberg A.M. and Petty R.E. (1980) Similar patterns of juvenile rheumatoid arthritis within families. *Arthritis Rheum.* 23, 951–953.

Rosenberg A.M. and Petty R.E. (1982) A syndrome of sero-negative enthesopathy and arthropathy in children. *Arthritis Rheum.* 25, 1041–1047.

Schnitzer T.J. and Ansell B.M. (1977) Amyloidosis in juvenile chronic arthritis. *Arthritis Rheum.* 20, 245–252.

Shore A. and Ansell B.M. (1982) Juvenile psoriatic arthritis: an analysis of 60 cases. *J. Pediatr.* 100, 529–535.

Silverman E., Roifman C., Greenwald M. *et al.* (1989) Treatment of severe systemic juvenile rheumatoid arthritis with IV gamma globulin. *Clin. Exp. Rheumatol.* 7, Abstract 41.

Southwood T.R., Petty R.E., Malleson P.N. *et al.* (1989) Psoriatic arthritis in children. *Arthritis Rheum.* 32, 1014–1021.

Stannard M.W. and Fink C.W. (1989) Diagnosis of synovial cyst in children by magnetic resonance imaging. *J. Rheumatol.* 16, 540–541.

Svantesson H., Akesson A., Eberhardt K. *et al.* (1983) Prognosis in juvenile rheumatoid arthritis with systemic onset—a follow up study. *Scand. J. Rheumatol.* 12, 139–144.

Truckenbrodt H. and Hafner R. (1986) Methotrexate in juvenile rheumatoid arthritis. A retrospective study. *Arthritis Rheum.* 29, 801–807.

Tyndall D.A., Bacon T., Parry R. *et al.* (1984) Infection and interferon production in systemic juvenile chronic arthritis. *Ann. Rheum. Dis.* 43, 1–7.

Chapter 12.2
Surgical Aspects

M. Swann

INTRODUCTION

The contents of this chapter are based on the surgical experience gained from treating patients at the Medical Research Council Unit for Juvenile Rheumatism at the Canadian Red Cross Unit, Taplow, UK, which closed in 1987 and subsequently at Wexham Park Hospital, Slough, UK. This work began in 1946 and has steadily gained momentum since then, both in the quality and scope of surgical management.

The advances in available surgical techniques have benefitted at large number of patients with juvenile chronic arthritis. Not least among them is the advent of hip arthroplasty, which has transformed the lives of many of these victims so that they have found themselves as housewives, parents and useful working citizens. This section is concerned with the selection of patients who would benefit from various surgical procedures, but with an awareness that the very nature of the condition makes the selection and procedure more critical than in similar problems created by other diseases. Of all the patients referred to the Juvenile Rheumatism Unit, 10% have subsequently had some surgical procedure, and of these more than half have had multiple procedures. If those patients who have a general anaesthetic for the purpose of examination or intra-articular steroid administration are also included, this amounts to about 25% of all the cases, which number approximately 5000 patients (Fig. 12.2.1).

At the outset it should be stated that much really worthwhile surgery can be undertaken in this field, but only in association with a team masterminding the overall care of the patient. This team should include a paediatric rheumatologist, surgeon, anaesthetist and physiotherapist, while back-up should be provided in many other spheres, including education for the young and rehabilitation and training for older patients. Indeed,

it is totally unwise to embark on any surgical procedure without the appropriate staff and facilities, for without these the patient's life may be at stake. This is not to overdramatize the problems, for even the induction of an anaesthetic can present serious problems.

The work that forms the substance of this chapter has related to the surgical aspects of juvenile chronic arthritis in patients who are 16 years old or less at the time of operation. A close liaison with the rheumatologist in combined clinics has provided the opportunity for selection of patients who will benefit from early surgical intervention, e.g. simple soft tissue procedures. Patients have been selected at an active phase of their disease in a growing skeleton. At the same time this matches the age that defines this particular heterogenous group of diseases, i.e. 16 years or younger at onset. This point is important to appreciate, as it forms the fundamental basis of this practice and it is not, therefore, comparable to other authors' accounts, where this upper age limit is not used. Such reports may often include patients whose disease is inactive and who are well beyond skeletal maturity.

Surgery is an adjunct to the overall medical management of the patient. It may be used early to help to prevent a problem developing, or later when conservative methods are failing. In some patients it will be at the forefront of treatment, particularly in cases referred with an already established deformity.

The diseases of this group produce their effects on the musculoskeletal system in many adverse ways, some of which are primary and a direct result of the disease, and some secondary. Thus, disease in a hip produces a flexion contracture at that joint, while the knee below may develop a flexion contracture that is entirely compensatory. It is clearly ideal to prevent both of these events occurring, but should they do so it is important to identify where the primary fault lies. A timely correction

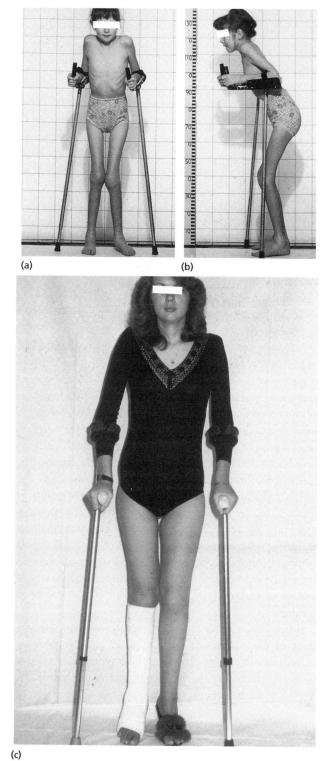

(a)   (b)

(c)

Fig. 12.2.1 (a, b) Patient with polyarthritis shortly after onset, aged 9 years. (c) Same patient, aged 18 years, following bilateral hip replacements when she was 11 years old and subsequent supracondylar osteotomies. Her right foot is in plaster following a triple arthrodesis (see also Fig. 12.2.20) and hence the need for crutches. The patient is now 25 years old and has just had a revision arthroplasty of the left hip.

of the flexion contracture at the hip may result in the double benefit of seeing the knee straighten at the same time.

The impact of juvenile chronic arthritis, as far as the surgeon is concerned, is felt in soft tissue, bones and joints, but whether it is synovitis, a modification of normal epiphyseal growth, or pannus destruction, the end result and the problem that require treatment are compounded by many factors. These must be identified in order to recruit the best procedure available. Thus, as destruction occurs in hip disease, the joint remains stable in as much as the remnants of the femoral head usually remain within the acetabulum. In the knee, however, a considerable degree of subluxation may occur in addition to articular damage, so that anatomical realignment must be attained in addition to the other measures necessary.

SPECIAL PROBLEMS

Age

The common factor among these patients is that they are all young and suffering from polyarthritis. The age span is considerable, however, and in part related to the variant of the disease as described in the previous chapter on the medical aspects of this disease. The surgeon will therefore be asked to deal with children little more than babies at one end of the scale and with the mini-adults who are teenagers with rheumatoid factor-positive disease at the other. In addition, there will be patients who have traversed the stormy years of an active disease process and who are left with residual damage; in some of these, surgical procedures may be applied to alleviate the problems. Patients in this last group are often in their 20s or early 30s and usually require joint reconstruction.

Size

These patients tend to be small in stature, but maintain proportional growth of their trunk and limbs, except where localized disease activity has produced epiphyseal stimulation and overgrowth or conversely premature arrest and thus shortening. Loss of stature may also occur when osteoporosis has led to vertebral collapse. Some patients will have received steroids, with their effect of skeletal shortening, though an awareness of this problem has led to better control of the timing and dose regimen of these drugs when prescribed. Nevertheless, from the surgeon's point of view, the skeletons are small and this problem will be alluded to later when dealing with joint arthroplasties. The bones tend to be porotic and much additional care is required, particularly in anaesthetized patients, to avoid fractures.

Activity of disease

At one end of the scale patients with previous but now inactive disease will be referred for surgery. These are patients whose joint destruction in earlier years has led to increasing problems of superadded degenerative change and deformity. This group presents less of a problem; a large number will be seeking joint replacement, particularly of the hips. In contrast, surgery and its results are masterminded by the disease activity in a particular case, not only at the time of operation but in subsequent follow-up. Much is as anticipated: thus, synovectomy of the knee must be timed during chronic low-grade synovitis before destruction of the articular surface will make the result less than good. While results of soft tissue release of the hips have on the whole been good, some cases have not responded well, and an analysis of the cause reveals that these are patients with continuing high disease activity, a resurgence of activity after remission, or presenting with the dry type of synovitis.

Ideally, perhaps, all patients should be treated in remission, but it appears that this is neither practical nor necessary and the longer term result is not so much affected by disease activity at the time of surgery, but rather by activity at the time of follow-up assessment. The pain or activity in other non-operated joints may make assessment of an operated joint difficult. Nevertheless, the absence of pain, which can be very considerable, must be achieved, and mobility and other parameters are a bonus. Forward planning will take into account that other joints, which are as yet unaffected, may yet become so. Thus, for the most part arthrodesis is seldom performed, even if at a time of assessment for surgery all seems well or relatively well in the other joints.

Anaesthesia

It is of paramount importance that the anaesthetist is aware of the difficulty of intubation and maintaining an airway in these children. The facet joints of the cervical spine are destroyed, and spontaneous bone fusion renders part or all of the cervical spine rigid (Fig. 12.2.2). Exceptionally, subluxation of the atlantoaxial joint tends to occur (Fig. 12.2.3) in seropositive cases, and very occasionally this may also occur at other levels. The problem is compounded by failure of jaw development and stiffness of the temporomandibular joints, so

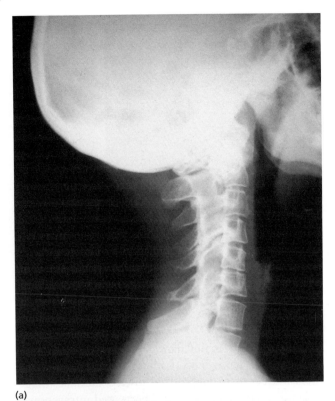

(a)

(b)

Fig. 12.2.2 Patient, aged 18 years, who developed polyarthritis at the age of 9 years. Radiographs show posterior fusion between C2, C3 and C4 and between C5 and C6 (a) in extension (b) in flexion. (The anaesthetist must have recent radiographs of the cervical spine available.)

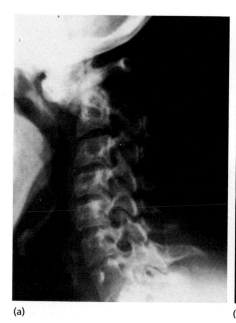

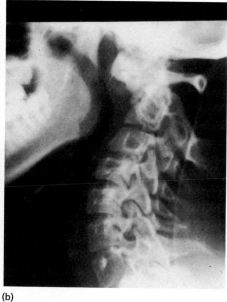

(a)   (b)

Fig. 12.2.3 Patient with seropositive disease, aged 8 years at onset. Admitted as an emergency, aged 16 years, with quadriplegia. Radiographs in (a) flexion and (b) extension reveal irreducible atlantoaxial subluxation and a rigid cervical spine. She was treated conservatively by skull traction and stabilization occurred *in situ*, but without reduction. Nevertheless, she made a full neurological recovery and has since had both hips and both knees replaced, wearing a collar for stressful occasions and receiving ketamine anaesthesia.

that access and maintenance of the airway is most difficult and hazardous. Radiographs of the cervical spine must be up to date and be shown to the anaesthetist.

Until recently, ketamine has been used intravenously as an analgesic and anaesthetic agent to overcome this problem. This had some undesirable side-effects, however, including an increase in intraoperative bleeding as a result of a rise in blood pressure and post-operative hallucinations. The use of this drug has been superseded, except in some cases at the induction of anaesthesia to permit the introduction of an endotracheal tube under fibre-optic guidance. As an alternative the use of a laryngeal mask, as described by Brain (1983), has proved satisfactory. It is the author's present practice to use epidural or spinal anaesthesia for lower limb surgery, and this has been found to be very satisfactory. Fortunately, the lumbar spine is seldom affected in the rheumatic complaints, and access through this route is not difficult. The added advantage of post-operative pain relief can be continued with the use of an epidural catheter.

The use of local anaesthetic alone has not proved satisfactory and can be a frightening experience for a child who may be faced with a number of operations in the future.

From the anaesthetist's point of view, venous access may be difficult because of limb deformity and a paucity of veins. Nevertheless, patients undergoing major surgery will require blood transfusion, so that venepuncture has to be performed. From the surgeon's point of view, adequate time must be allowed for these often prolonged pre-operative preparations in the anaesthetic room.

Bone quality and bone stock

A word of warning to the surgeon is timely at this point. Apart from subarticular bone destruction, which is part of the disease process, the associated hyperaemia causes peri-articular osteoporosis. This in turn may be compounded by disuse atrophy and in some cases steroids have been given. The total effect is not only a small skeletal system, which has already been mentioned, but also a very friable one, demanding great care particularly in the anaesthetized patient. On occasions, the eggshell-thin cortical bone can be cut with a knife. It is recommended that the surgeon himself or a qualified member of staff applies the tourniquet if one is indicated, that extra padding is placed beneath the cuff and that a very careful control is kept of the tourniquet pressure. When a tourniquet is not applied heavy bleeding is sometimes encountered, particularly in hip surgery, and suitable provision must be made for this event. In preparing operating lists extra time must be allowed for these cases.

Prosthetic size

The surgeon must ensure that he has a prosthesis of suitable size before embarking on replacement surgery. Some manufacturers now make a wide range, including mini-prostheses, which is essential for some of the smaller patients. If any doubt exists it is recommended that a radiograph is obtained, with the relevant joint and the prosthesis at the same magnification, so that measurements can be made pre-operatively and a suitable size confirmed (Fig. 12.2.4). Occasionally, it is necessary to have a custom-built prosthesis for a particular case, and this is outlined in more detail later (see p. 327). More sophisticated methods of measurement, e.g. computed tomography, should be employed where relevant and individual cases discussed with the manufacturer.

Motivation and rehabilitation

Motivation is the foundation of success and a prime factor in many facets of orthopaedic surgery, but in none more so than in operations on children crippled by arthritis. Cooperation must first be established; younger children under about 5 years of age lack comprehension of the aims of the operation, and for this reason this age group is unsuitable for procedures such as synovectomy. Rehabilitation following operation must be in a setting where the personnel and facilities are suitable to the patient's needs, preferably in the environment of primary medical care and not isolated in a surgical ward.

UPPER LIMB

Shoulder

Although shoulder involvement is not uncommon, disabling symptoms are rare. As with the elbow, however, pain and limitation of movement may influence the ability of the patient to use crutches. The early onset of shoulder disease in the absence of pain is often masked by compensatory scapular movement, and it is the limitation of movement of other upper limb joints that highlights the shoulder problem. The disease here is curiously bilateral and symmetrical on radiographs. As destruction of the joint surfaces progresses, so by capsular contraction and spasm the humeral head rides up and impinges on the acromion. Sometimes in the more proliferative type of disease the subacromial bursa becomes distended.

The only indication for operative interference is pain. Limitation of movement must be accepted, because there is no operative method of improving this problem.

TREATMENT

The methods available are similar to those employed in other major joints. Aspiration and local injection of steroids into the subacromial bursa, particularly if enlarged, will relieve symptoms in many patients. Manipulation and cast fixation for 8 weeks in a position of function has proved an acceptable method, firm fibrous ankylosis ridding the patient of pain. Alternatively, the joint may be formally fused by operative means (Fig. 12.2.5). There is a danger that the ipsilateral elbow will become stiff while enclosed within the spica intended for the shoulder, and a method must be employed that will allow free elbow movement to continue. The double osteotomy of Benjamin (1969) has been used in several patients who have enjoyed an immediate and sustained relief of pain. Arthroplasty is only appropriate after skeletal maturity, so it is

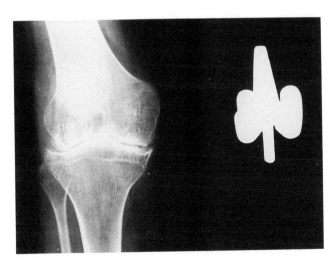

Fig. 12.2.4 Patient, aged 23 years, with seropositive disease with onset at the age of 10 years. A small Attenborough prosthesis is seen alongside the proposed joint. This particular prosthesis has now been superseded.

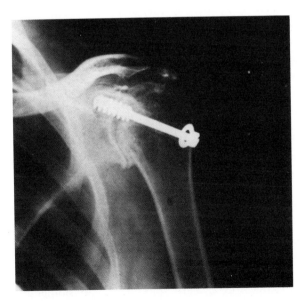

Fig. 12.2.5 Arthrodesis of the left shoulder is readily obtained in a joint with a natural tendency to stiffen.

inapplicable in the age group under consideration. It has been used in a number of cases over the age of 16 years, however, but special precautions need to be taken because of the poor quality and porosity of the bone.

Elbow

The elbow is not only commonly involved in juvenile chronic arthritis, but it often gives rise to troublesome symptoms. The synovitis causes joint destruction, swelling instability and overgrowth of the radial head. The patient complains of severe pain at times, weakness, stiffness, swelling and locking.

Intra-articular corticosteroid, which can be repeated on one or two occasions, may tide the patient over for some time before an operation becomes necessary. Synovectomy should be offered not only where there is persistent thickening and effusion, but unlike in the knee, it can also be used in late cases where there is considerable radiological evidence of damage and significant pain. The operation is performed through medial and lateral incisions, the radial head is removed if it is thought to be contributing to the problem, and the ulnar nerve is transposed, if indicated. Results are rewarding in terms of pain relief in 95% of cases, and some increase in movement has been gained by some patients.

Arthrodesis of the elbow has not been attempted, and where it has occurred spontaneously as part of the disease it has proved very disabling. Arthroplasty in a mature skeleton may be considered if synovectomy has failed and sufficient peri-articular bone remains for firm fixation of the prosthesis. In younger patients and in those lacking bone stock, an interposition arthroplasty using fascia lata or other appropriate material has given a number of worthwhile results. External splinting and supports have so far been the mainstay of treatment in the more disabled cases.

Hand and wrist

The hand and wrist, including the carpus, share a multitude of synovial joints, so it is to be expected that most patients suffering from juvenile chronic arthritis in one of its forms will at some time have at least one of these joints involved. If the synovial sheaths of the flexor and extensor tendons are also included, few patients will escape some manifestation, and if the many growth plates and epiphyseal centres are involved, then the stage is set for severe disability. Probably nowhere else is better rewarded by early splinting and physiotherapy to prevent deformity and stiffness.

TENDON SHEATHS

The synovial sheaths invest both flexor and extensor tendons. Swelling may arise from proliferative synovitis, synovial oedema, or effusion within the sheaths. The bulk produced by the swelling will inhibit movement, while later during resolution adhesions may form. Fortunately, unlike in adult rheumatoid disease, tendon rupture is rare, but occasionally it does occur; the most common tendon to suffer this damage is the extensor pollicis longus, while boutonnière deformity and swan-neck deformity are also seen. In seronegative disease, the start of tendon sheath involvement is often associated with patients who are affected by systemic manifestations of their disease. In seropositive cases, bulky proliferative synovitis occurs, which may lead to carpal tunnel syndrome if it extends above the wrist or to triggering of a finger if it extends more distally.

The treatment of these problems is dictated by their virulence and effect. For example, synovectomy for acute synovitis with a largely oedematous element will give poor rewards and will often lead to recurrence and post-operative adhesions and stiffness. Indeed, the systemic illness of the child will mitigate against operative intervention. These cases will be in hospital and as the disease regresses or can be brought under control, so the tendon sheath involvement will also regress. It is important to maintain gentle active and passive exercises to prevent adhesions as well as functional splinting during this time. When flexor synovial sheath disease activity continues the local use of corticosteroid is beneficial. This is administered as an intrathecal injection of hydrocortisone under anaesthetic as the injections are painful. Occasionally, patients with a persistent thickening from proliferative synovitis in a limited field affecting one or perhaps two fingers will benefit from a simple synovectomy, followed by rapid mobilization. The problems presented by a trigger finger or carpal tunnel compression are dealt with in conventional fashion, with the use of local corticosteroid, or failing a response, operative decompression.

WRIST AND CARPAL JOINTS

These joints are grouped together, as synovitis can lead to joint destruction and deformity at all these sites. The specific effect of synovitis is dictated by the degree, age at onset and the particular extraneous forces about the joint.

The wrist and carpus are very commonly involved, and a flexion deformity begins to develop early. This must be spotted and treated by splinting before contracture and inevitable deformity occur. If remission is early good movement can be anticipated, but at worst (if the carpus fuses) a good functional position will minimize the disability. Cases will be seen where the distal radial and ulnar epiphysis are affected, leading to a change of anatomical relationships at this site. In some patients growth arrest of the ulnar leads to ulnar translocation of the carpus with eventual subluxation. Attempts at correction by splinting alone may generate destructive compression forces between the lunate bone and the radius, in which event ulnar distraction lengthening and bone grafting may be of value. Subluxation of the distal ulna often causes a painful swelling, with some risk of tendon rupture occasioned by pronation and supination. Provided that the distal growth plates are closed, ulnar styloidectomy may be indicated.

In a severely damaged wrist and carpus, pain and deformity will dictate the need for operative intervention. The choice lies between arthrodesis and arthroplasty. The former is well tried and, if the indications are correct, it can be a most successful procedure mimicking that which nature often attempts. Careful appraisal of the whole upper limb position must be made, however, as in some patients who already have stiff shoulders and elbows the retention of a small amount of movement, particularly in radial deviation, may make a disproportionate difference in their quest for independence. Arthroplasty of the wrist is still being developed and the outcome is awaited. Swanson's arthroplasty (see Chapter 18.1) has a place in the treatment of these patients, and the current concern about implant failure and silicone synovitis is less relevant here because large forces across the wrist are not transmitted in this group of patients.

FINGER JOINTS

Involvement of these joints is indicated by spindle-shaped swellings rather than the diffuse swelling of swollen flexor sheaths, though both may occur concurrently (Fig. 12.2.6). Later changes, e.g. stiffening or deformity, will confirm the location of the problem. A variety of derangements may be seen in different patients. The metacarpophalangeal joints may benefit from synovectomy, particularly if one of these joints is predominantly affected. Later, as the joint shows ulnar drift, a realignment procedure is worth undertaking. Silicone arthroplasty of the metacarpophalangeal joints has a place in advanced cases after the completion of growth. The interphalangeal joints are eroded, leading in some cases to ultimate fusion. Erosion of the volar plate may lead to a swan-neck deformity (Fig. 12.2.7). Synovec-

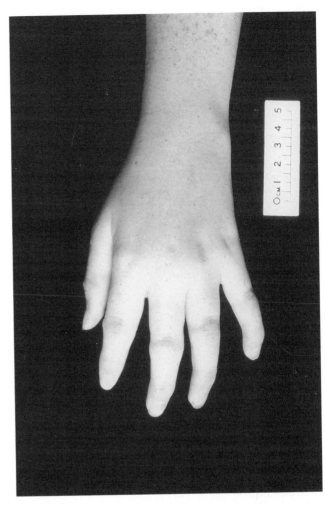

Fig. 12.2.6 Polyarthritis with onset at the age of 6 years. The patient, now aged 13 years, exhibits tendon sheath and joint involvement. Note the ulnar drift of the little finger.

tomy is seldom worth the attempt; the author advocates the use of Silastic implants to stabilize the joints when the problem is severe enough.

LOWER LIMB

Hip

This is the most common joint to attract surgical attention. The hip is often involved early in the natural history of juvenile arthritis, and severe destructive changes occur long before growth has ceased. To the physical inability to get about are added the psychological problems of the sheltered life of a cripple. Early and energetic attempts must be made to prevent the establishment of deformity, particularly while it still remains controllable by conservative means.

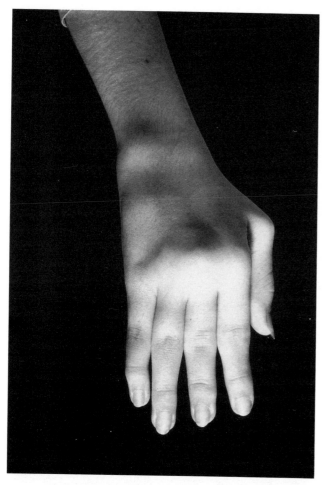

Fig. 12.2.7 Patient, now aged 15 years, with onset of disease at 4 years of age. Note involvement of the joints, swan-neck deformities and subluxation of the ulnar styloid.

With few exceptions, some basic patterns of deformity emerge. The femur becomes flexed, internally rotated and adducted. This attitude is produced progressively by muscle spasm, muscle contracture, joint destruction, capsular contracture and finally fibrous ankylosis. At the same time anteversion and valgus of the neck of the femur may develop and contribute to the problem. Thus, not only may internal rotation be increased but subluxation of the hip joint encouraged (Fig. 12.2.8).

ASSESSMENT

It may be necessary to examine the hip under anaesthetic in order to establish how much apparent contracture is produced by pain and muscle spasm. At the same time, the opportunity can be taken to perform arthrography of the joint, as this may define the presence of a joint space even where one is not apparent on the plain radiograph (Fig. 12.2.9). It is difficult to obtain clear anteroposterior radiographs of the hip when fixed flexion is present, as the anterior lip of the acetabulum is flexed over the femoral head, apparently reducing the joint space. Computed tomography will give additional information, which must be sought if necessary.

TREATMENT

Assuming that some mobility remains, a concentrated programme is started to increase the range of movement and eliminate any contractures. Success in this venture is usually rewarded by an improvement or loss of pain in

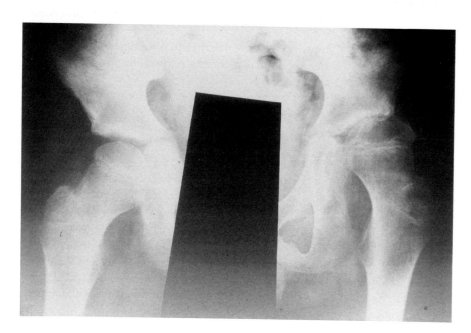

Fig. 12.2.8 Polyarthritis with onset at age 7 years in a patient now aged 12 years. The radiograph shows anteversion and subluxation of the left hip. The patient's bones were suitable for metallic fixation and so corrective varus rotation osteotomy was performed.

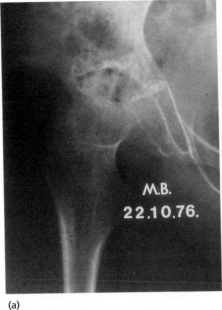
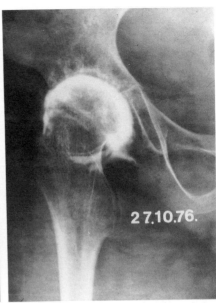

Fig. 12.2.9 Patient with onset of polyarthritis when she was aged 18 months. Bilateral hip disease at the age of 12 years. The left hip required arthroplasty. (a) The right hip has not yet lost shape but the joint space might be obliterated. (b) Arthrogram of the same right hip showing a clear joint space so that a soft tissue release was performed. Reproduced from Arden G.P. and Ansell B.M. (1978) with permission.

(a)   (b)

the affected joint, which can be so severe that it simulates septic arthritis. Lesser degrees are treated by in-patient traction, prone lying and hydrotherapy, while suitable medication controls the pain so that treatment continues in comfort.

Patients with a fixed contracture that is not relieved or improved by conservative means, or in whom the contracture exceeds 20° at the outset, are treated by a soft tissue release. This involves a limited adductor tenotomy through an open groin incision with a tenotomy of the psoas tendon through the same incision. The wound heals without delaying the continuation of traction and physiotherapy, though hydrotherapy is precluded in the immediate post-operative regimen. This procedure has produced some good results without jeopardizing in any way subsequent procedures (Fig. 12.2.10 and Table 12.2.1). More radical procedures have not been found to be any more effective, as it is the psoas muscle that

holds most of an otherwise correctable flexion contracture. The limited soft tissue release usually not only reduces the flexion contracture but also increases the range of motion, pain abates; a number of joints have shown radiological signs of improvement from possible repair by fibrocartilage (Fig. 12.2.11). In some cases it has undoubtedly helped to reduce pressure on the hip during an active phase of the disease, allowing medication and natural resolution to overcome the problem. In a few cases results have been disappointing, but no harm has been done and it has helped the patients temporarily, so that it can be looked on as a holding operation until arthroplasty might be considered. Soft tissue release has been performed as a primary procedure before arthroplasty in patients with marked flexion contracture.

In a number of patients the only solution to their problem unfortunately lies in arthroplasty of the hip. This group includes those with severe joint destruction when the capital epiphysis has closed. Limb growth may still continue from the epiphyses around the knee. More than half of the author's patients continued to grow after this operation and no special problems were encountered from pelvic growth around the acetabular component. Joint replacements in these hips must be total, and because of the porotic bone stock it has been universal practice to use cement. Several prostheses are made for the smaller patients in most manufacturers' ranges. Nevertheless, it is important to be aware of the very small size necessary in patients whose hips have failed to develop because of early-onset disease. These will need to be made by special order in advance. It is

Table 12.2.1 Results of surgery for soft tissue release of hips

Number of patients	52 (33 female, 19 male)
Number of hips	89
Mean age	
Onset of disease	4.1 years
Operation	11.3 years
Mean range of motion	
Pre-operatively	25–74°
Post-operatively	
6 months	8–72°
12 months (89 hips)	5–75°
24 months (46 hips)	2–72°

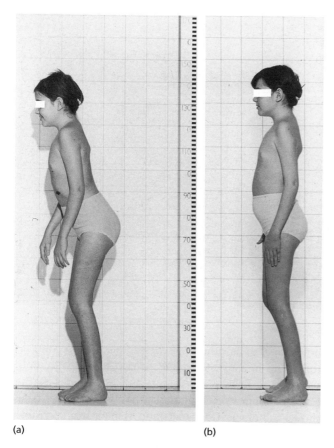

Fig. 12.2.10 A 10-year-old patient with polyarthritis who underwent soft tissue release of the hips. (a) Before operation. (b) After operation, 1 year later.

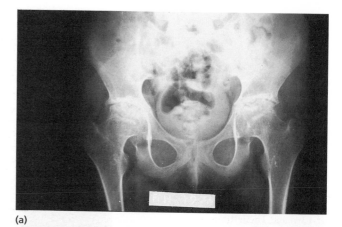

(a)

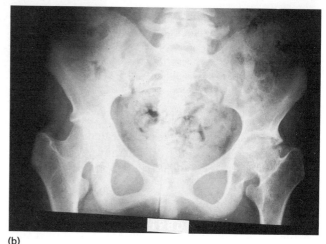

(b)

Fig. 12.2.11 (a) Pre-operative radiograph of the same patient as in Fig. 12.2.10. (b) Post-operative radiograph 1 year later. Note the increased joint space, improved joint surface and general loss of moth-eaten appearance.

best to discuss the methods of measurement with the manufacturers. It is useful to take both anteroposterior and lateral radiographs with a prosthetic model or a radio-opaque ruler at the same magnification.

In many patients growth disturbance with anteversion of the neck is also associated with a deformity of the upper femoral shaft. In plan, it is more elliptical than round with a greater diameter in the sagittal plane. It may be quite impossible to alter this by reaming in order to make a bed for the prosthetic stem, and this fact must be allowed for and accepted (Fig. 12.2.12). The operative approach and method employed will depend on the experience and practice of the individual surgeon.

A review in 1986 of 42 children and 75 hips operated on under 17 years of age showed one loose cup and no infection. A re-review of these cases now in hand, however, reveals that four of these children have since died of amyloid disease and late infection has occurred in four cases. The overall failure rate at 10 years is approaching 30%. Nevertheless, this high-risk group has been relieved of severe pain and a wheelchair existence,

and the majority has enjoyed the opportunity of a good education and many have gained useful employment. In the absence of alternative therapy and with the universal agreement of even those patients whose hips have failed, it would appear worthwhile to continue this practice.

It must be emphasized that in patients with fibrous ankylosis any attempt to dislocate the hip will inevitably be attended by fracture of the porotic femoral shaft. Sometimes the head has to be removed piecemeal with bone nibblers, and copious bleeding is often encountered. Trochanteric osteotomy is not recommended as a means of approach, as the wires applied on closure will cut out the porotic bone. Intertrochanteric osteotomy has no place in the treatment of these patients if internal fixation is not secure enough to obviate the need for protection. An earlier experience resulted in permanently stiff hips post-operatively. It is also unlikely that resurfacing

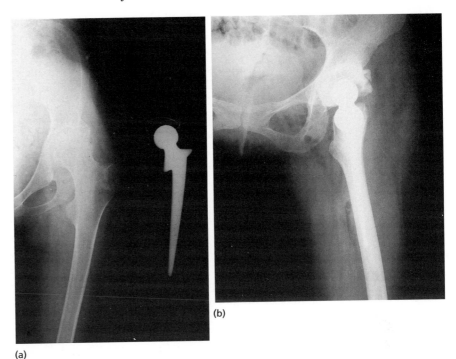

Fig. 12.2.12 Patient with systemic disease with onset at 18 months, now aged 17 years. (a) Hip prosthesis alongside the proposed site of insertion. The dimensions seemed satisfactory but closer appraisal reveals a very narrow medullary cavity and considerable anteversion as well as external rotation. (b) At operation the prosthesis could only be located within the shaft with considerable anteversion.

operations of the hip will be of any value as the femoral head is porotic, destroyed to a considerable depth and often exhibiting avascular necrosis.

Post-operative care of these patients follows that normally practised for such a procedure, and walking with aids is encouraged after 48 h. If both hips are affected benefit will not accrue until both are replaced, and it is the author's practice to do this with a 3-week interval between the operations.

Knee

ASSESSMENT

The knee calls for particularly careful examination to identify the cause of the deformity that demands correction. At best a flexion contracture may be secondary to a similar contracture of the ipsilateral hip, or compensatory to limb length inequality. In these events restoration of normality can be expected, provided that correction of the primary cause is timely. Lateral or rotary deviation is never as benign, however, and even if it is secondary to some other factor, local changes within and around the knee are rapidly induced, precluding quick and simple remedy. This may be illustrated by valgus at the knee secondary to varus at the foot or at the hip. The unequal pressure exerted on the knee epiphyses, combined with the other factors, may produce change that cannot be corrected by simple conservative means.

It is customary to assess the degree of fixed contractures, deformity, stability, swelling from thickened synovium, fluid and range of movement. All these factors are crucial to a decision, but equally so is an evaluation of the adjacent joints and the joints of the contralateral limb. Where flexion contracture is corrected by a soft tissue release, the resulting increase in leg length is greater than when a supracondylar osteotomy is performed. Correction of a fixed valgus at the knee will unbalance a foot that is in fixed varus, and the latter will need correction before the patient walks.

The inflammatory disease produces a sequence of changes within a knee. Pain and swelling, either from synovial oedema and hypertrophy or from an effusion, induce flexion. This is the position of comfort for the knee, but later muscle spasm of the hamstrings maintains the position while the quadriceps muscle wastes and is progressively unable to overcome the problem and actively extend the joint. The surrounding tissues, which include the capsular structures and therefore part of the extensor retinaculum and the all-important posterior capsule, undergo fibrosis and contracture, at first maintaining and later increasing the deformity. There is thus both a flexion and an extension contracture to be overcome.

A fixed flexion contracture will result in abnormal loading contact between the femoral condyle and tibial plateau on weight-bearing. The non-contact surface, apart from its vulnerability to the disease, will also undergo a secondary degenerative change and will be in a poor state to receive weight if correction of the flexion contracture is delayed.

It also appears that the anterior parts of the tibia and femoral growth plates, being relieved of pressure, increase their rate of growth, and will increase the flexion deformity. As this inflammatory process continues, destruction of the cartilaginous articular surfaces occurs, leading to irregularity and often collapse. The intra-articular cruciate ligaments suffer destruction in more virulent disease, but often in less active cases undergo fibrosis and thus may anchor the joint in flexion. Intra-articular adhesions may finally form, binding the two joint surfaces together, notably between an overgrown and deformed patella and the femoral condyle.

It is important to note that many affected knees exhibit posterior subluxation of the tibia. This is produced initially by the pull of the hamstrings when the joint is initially swollen and the capsule distended (Fig. 12.2.13). The popliteus muscle covering the back of the joint would to some extent serve to prevent this subluxation, except for the fact that the muscle is intra-articular and its tendon is invested with synovium. It would therefore be vulnerable to destruction and thus also lose its action of being a medial rotator of the tibia. Later fibrosis maintains the subluxation, particularly if the posterior cruciate ligament is shortened.

In evolving a scheme of treatment for the knee it is essential to evaluate the factors contributing to a given deformity and loss of movement. Thus, a soft tissue release of the posterior structures to correct a flexion contracture is only appropriate if serviceable joint surfaces are thus brought into contact; if not, then supracondylar osteotomy is a better procedure (Fig. 12.2.14).

With the knee at the centre of the limb it is appropriate to consider the general alignment. Although a straight line between the centre of the hip and the ankle should go through the middle of the knee, less attention is usually directed to rotational deformity. Nevertheless, this is important. In juvenile chronic arthritis there is often some internal rotation of the hip, exhibited by the patellae facing inwards towards each other. The psoas muscle, apart from being a powerful flexor of the hip, is also an internal rotator and possibly produces this turn on the femur. The knee and tibia turn into external rotation, so that the ankle is often twisted outwards. Various explanations can be postulated for this. It is compensatory in part for the internal torsion of the femur, the loss of action of the popliteus muscle and tightness of the iliotibial band. When the tarsal joints are stiff, pain relief is experienced by walking with the foot turned out, thus protecting the painful articulations. Persistence of this habit will throw an additional external rotation force on the tibia. Nevertheless, this rotational deformity must be taken into account when corrective

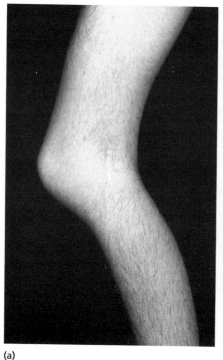

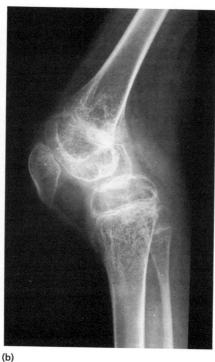

(a)   (b)

Fig. 12.2.13 (a) The knee in a 16-year-old boy with onset of polyarthritis at age 8 years. Note the backward subluxation of the tibia. (b) Radiograph showing the backward subluxation and overgrowth of the patella and osteoporosis.

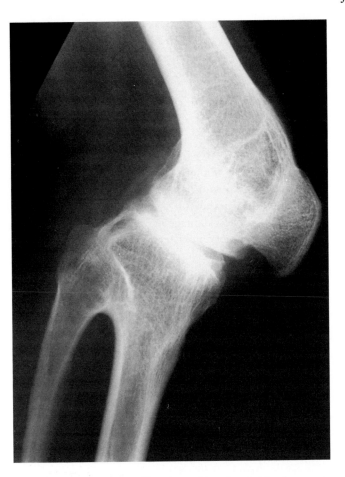

Fig. 12.2.14 An 18-year-old patient with polyarthritis of onset at the age of 3 years; lateral radiographs in the maximum extension obtainable. Correction of the 30° flexion contracture by soft tissue release would be inappropriate, as the worn femoral surface would then take load on weight-bearing. A supracondylar osteotomy was therefore performed in this case. Note the abnormal growth of the patella and its fusion to the femur.

procedures for the knee are planned. As in arthroplasty for rheumatoid arthritis, realignment of the tibia is important in order to maintain the correct line of quadriceps action.

Radiological examination must be considered in the light of some of its limitations. In the young knee it will show nothing of the joint surface, so that the degree of articular destruction cannot be directly appraised. Anteroposterior radiographs must be viewed with the knowledge that with a joint in fixed flexion the joint space appears relatively narrower than in reality, and indeed superimposition of the femoral condyle and tibial plateau may occur in certain planes. Lateral films should be taken in the maximum extremes of flexion and extension; possibly the motion should be viewed on an image intensifier so that the axis of movement can be

evaluated and procedures subsequently avoided which might bring damaged joint surfaces into contact (Fig. 12.2.14). Arthrography will help in defining a joint space where doubt arises; in addition it will outline the suprapatellar pouch indicating its patency. A popliteal cyst may also be displayed. The use of computed tomography or magnetic resonance imaging will give considerable additional information.

Arthroscopy may occasionally be employed, but in many cases the contracture surrounding the knee is such that sufficient distension is not possible to get an adequate view. Nevertheless, in laxer joints arthroscopy may be employed to help evaluate a possible internal derangement, e.g. loose bodies, which are super-added to the inflammatory process and may be paramount in producing symptoms. A synovial biopsy can be obtained at the same time.

In summary, the expectations are that the surgeon will be asked to advise on a knee joint that is painful, swollen and unstable, has a flexion contracture, sometimes a valgus deformity and often with posterior subluxation of the tibia and variable destructive changes within. The demand will be to regain extension, correct the deformity and increase movement and stability. Sometimes emphasis will be placed on reducing the swelling or the effect of hypervascularity on the epiphysis. This opportunity is not lost in reminding surgeons that the prevention of deformity by suitable splinting and physiotherapy in the early stage of joint disease would save considerable time and suffering. No joint is easier to splint than the knee.

OPERATIVE AIMS AND PRINCIPLES

The indications for synovectomy are clearly defined and are dealt with separately (see p. 334). The method chosen to correct a flexion contracture will depend on several factors, among which the extent of the contracture and the state of the joint are the most important considerations. Knee joints may be stiff, held by periarticular capsular contracture, in subluxation and in various stages of destruction. The full spectrum is presented to the surgeon who will advise traction, physiotherapy and splinting for the least involved, and arthroplasty in the more severe cases. It should be reiterated that a flexion contracture should be anticipated and prevented and should therefore be a rare rather than a common problem in these children. Provided that some range of motion is maintained, knees must be able to straighten. The patient can then walk upright without strain and quadriceps fatigue, spare the hips if not already involved, take more weight on the legs and spare the arm joints from weight-relieving on crutches. Allowing full extension at the knee should permit the fitting of a caliper, if indicated.

Whichever method is employed to overcome a flexion deformity at the knee, it must be carried out with care in order to prevent undue traction on the popliteal artery and associated nerves. It should also be recalled that in the presence of a fixed, unyielding posterior hinge that is the joint capsule, outside forces designed to straighten the joint will equally cause compression anteriorly between the tibial plateau and femoral condyle, or posterior subluxation of the tibia on the femur. Serial plasters must be changed frequently and applied without undue force; the wedging technique should never be used. Traction must be applied with the direction of pull in line with the tibia and not with the femur.

TREATMENT

It is convenient to consider the knee to be affected in three progressive stages:
1 Stage 1: knee in which there is a full range of movement and minimal radiological changes.
2 Stage 2: knees with some restriction of movement, even under anaesthesia, and demonstrable radiological changes, but in which a definite joint space remains.
3 Stage 3: gross loss of movement, fixed deformity and marked radiological changes.

Stage 1

Physiotherapy and splinting are indicated to overcome this early stage of disease. An examination under anaesthesia is helpful in confirming the potential for improvement. The limit of fixed flexion that can be safely overcome by serial casts is 25°. It is important that attempts are made not only to eliminate the contracture but also to increase the actual range of motion, for an extension contracture is also present. Although conservative, this treatment can really only be effective if the patient can be supervised in hospital and have daily, prolonged treatment. The presently available methods of traction are best applied under supervision in hospital, though attempts are in hand to design a suitable apparatus to allow traction on an out-patient basis.

Stage 2

If a joint space remains and there is good congruity between the articular surfaces, a soft tissue release of the posterior structures should be considered. This may be used as a primary procedure if, as a result, full correction can be gained or alternatively as a preliminary procedure to remove the tight posterior hinge before serial casts or traction. The operation is best performed via two separate incisions, posteromedial and posterolateral in location. The hamstring muscles are lengthened or divided and a passage made across the back of the posterior capsule so that the neurovascular bundle can be retracted out of the way. The capsule can then be divided under direct vision together with the posterior cruciate ligament if there is backward subluxation of the tibia. If the flexion contracture is considerable, no immediate attempts at full correction of the deformity should be made lest damage occur to the neurovascular bundle. After surgery a plaster cylinder is applied, which is bivalved after 3 days to allow early movement to prevent post-operative stiffness. The cast can be changed in a serial fashion to become progressively straighter and the back shells used during rest and early attempts at walking. The results have been rewarding, for not only has the flexion contracture been reduced but the total range of motion in the joint has also increased (Table 12.2.2).

If a fixed flexion deformity is associated with incongruity of the joint or posterior subluxation, then osteotomy may be deemed more appropriate. The double osteotomy of Benjamin (1969), which is so appropriate for certain cases of adult rheumatoid arthritis, is less so in juvenile chronic arthritis and should therefore only be used on a few occasions. The intra-articular nature of the operation produces adhesions, which in the young tend to bind the joint; subsequent manipulation after bone union may produce a marked inflammatory reaction, haemarthrosis, or bone trauma. The author prefers supracondylar osteotomy with the added advantage that valgus deformity, and to some extent rotation, can be corrected at the same time. This operation is

Table 12.2.2 Results of operations for soft tissue release of the knee

Number of patients	15 (10 male, 5 female)
Number of knees	23
Mean age	
Onset of disease	4.2 years
Operation	12.8 years
Mean range of motion	
Pre-operatively	35−140° (53°)
Post-operatively (mean, 5.2 years)	15−145° (60°)
Flexion contracture	
Pre-operatively	15−80° (34°)
Post-operatively	0−20° (11°)

performed through a small medial incision, leaving a periosteal hinge to prevent displacement. A plaster cylinder is applied with the knee straight, and the patient is encouraged to walk within a few days. This early weight-bearing serves to impact the fragments and to reduce osteoporosis and joint stiffness. The osteotomy has usually united sufficiently to remove the cast after about 5 weeks. The cast can be bivalved and the back half used to preserve the position during rest and early walking. In some cases it has been thought prudent to maintain the correction with a caliper using a cuffed top and double iron with knee hinges.

It should be recognized that an osteotomy entails the production of one deformity to mask another. The femoral division should therefore be made as near the knee as possible, or an ugly 'S' appearance will be produced; at the same time care must be exercised not to damage the lower femoral epiphysis if it is still open. Remodelling at the osteotomy site is efficient, but sometimes the operation may have to be repeated after a growth spurt. If manipulation is thought necessary to hasten knee movement, great care must be exercised lest a supracondylar fracture is produced (Fig. 12.2.15).

Stage 3

If the joint is very badly affected, arthroplasty may be indicated after skeletal maturity (Fig. 12.2.16). The Attenborough and Deane prostheses (Fig. 12.2.4) were the only ones available in a small enough size for some of the author's patients. The longer term results of these, however, as in adult surgery, have been disappointing. Several manufacturers now have small-sized joints available, but unfortunately custom-made knees are prohibitively expensive. So far, the results using the total condylar-type prosthesis appear promising, but the overall experience is limited.

VALGUS DEFORMITY

Several factors contribute to this deformity, and it is important to identify it correctly, because a flexion deformity with some internal rotation of the femur may mimic it. True valgus will occur under a number of circumstances including collapse of the lateral tibial plateau and overgrowth of the lower femoral epiphysis on the medial side. Once initiated the mechanical stress on weight-bearing not only perpetuates but also increases the problem. Radiographs with the patient standing are important and will indicate the line of weight-bearing and degree of instability.

Passive correction of this deformity by conservative

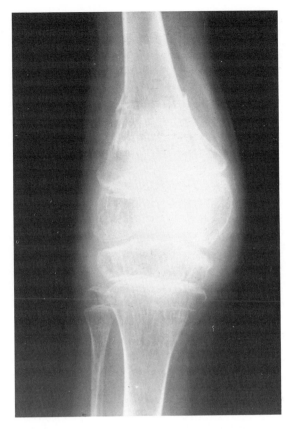

Fig. 12.2.15 Patient aged 12 years with pauciarticular disease which started when he was 4 years old. The radiograph demonstrates a supracondylar fracture produced by gentle manipulation of a porotic knee.

means has little part to play. Forceful attempts to correct the deformity in unyielding structures are not only stressful but also damaging, and division of the lateral joint structure is impractical. Supracondylar osteotomy, which has already been outlined in the treatment of a flexion contracture (see above), is a simple and expedient method of dealing with valgus and is particularly suitable when flexion and valgus are combined. When the cast is applied the leg should be slightly overcorrected, and management subsequently follows that already outlined (see above).

In the growing knee stapling has proved a relatively simple and effective method of correcting both valgus and varus deformities. It does have some disadvantages, however, e.g. ugly scars, and it often proves to be a painful operation with difficulty in regaining movement. Sometimes the bone is too porotic for the staples to take a good hold. It is particularly important to confirm the remaining growth potential in the epiphysis. It is an operation requiring great expertise in the placement of the staples. The rate of correction depends on the speed

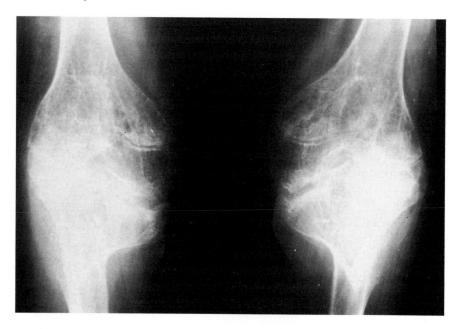

Fig. 12.2.16 Radiograph to show the effect of fulminating disease in a child with polyarthritis persisting for 5 years after the onset of the disease at age 2 years.

of growth, but clinical assessment will confirm the results and timing of the removal of the staples. The indication for the method has been when the intermalleolar distance has exceeded 7 cm. In a few children with growth retardation due to corticosteroids, withdrawal of the drug has led to a late growth spurt and stapling has been successful as late as 13 years of age. Stapling is not recommended to correct leg length inequality when overgrowth is produced by unilateral disease of the knee, as the discrepancy diminishes after synovectomy, when the arthritis heals or becomes bilateral.

SYNOVECTOMY

The knee is a tempting target for synovectomy with its layers of synovial lining commonly affected by the disease and readily accessible to the surgeon. It is the persistence of a synovial swelling from thickening of the membrane or a persistent effusion that attracts attention. This synovial activity seldom produces much pain but does limit movement and leads to flexion contracture, often valgus instability from ligament distension and sometimes epiphyseal overgrowth, particularly of the medial side of the lower femur. The persistence of this activity, despite remission or control of the disease, for at least 6 months is an indication for synovectomy. Radiological assessment of such a joint, unlike in an adult knee, is unhelpful in showing joint destruction; however, it may reveal epiphyseal overgrowth (Fig. 12.2.17). Children with pauciarticular disease do best and those with the adult type with positive rheumatoid factor benefit the least. The very young are unsuitable as

they lack the cooperation and capacity for hard work required to prevent post-operative stiffness, and for this reason an arbitrary lower limit of 5 years of age at the time of operation is made. In summary, the author has found a limited application for synovectomy, as in other joints. A patient with multiple joint involvement who might benefit best demands too many operations at too many sites to consider this method. At the same time, many of these patients are too ill to consider surgery. The natural history of the disease in a particular patient is unpredictable as is the natural progress in any particular joint. Many patients undergo remission with time and medication, so that the author's practice is to offer synovectomy in a therapeutic rather than a prophylactic role. Use of intra-articular corticosteroid is now producing such promising results that the indications for synovectomy are diminishing even more.

The technique of operation uses the preferred approach of the surgeon to remove as much of the synovial lining as possible. If valgus of 20° or more is present, the opportunity to staple an epiphysis should be taken. Early mobilization is essential, but as much emphasis is placed on being able to straighten fully as on bending the knee. A posterior splint, e.g. a plaster slab, should be used at night and during rest periods. If 90° of flexion has not been attained at 2 weeks, formal manipulation under anaesthesia is undertaken; in practice this amounts to nearly half the cases. Manipulation should not on any account be forceful lest supracondylar fractures, haemarthrosis, or an extension lag be produced. Using the simple parameters of degree of pain and range of movement, a satisfactory result can be

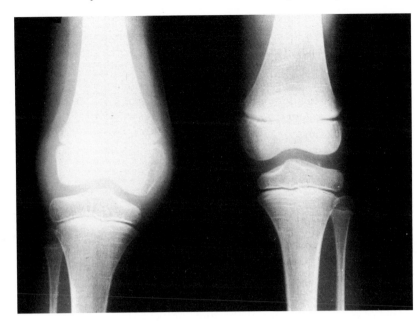

Fig. 12.2.17 An 8-year-old patient with pauciarticular disease. The radiograph shows the effect of unilateral synovitis of the right knee. Soft tissue swelling is noted together with overgrowth of the lower femoral epiphysis.

expected in 90% of knees. Like the experience in adult rheumatoid arthritis, this percentage decreases with time.

ROTATIONAL DEFORMITY OF THE LEG

Reference has been made to internal rotation of the thigh, due to anteversion and psoas action, which leaves the patellas squinting. External rotation is commonly observed at and below the knee, and there are a number of reasons for this. In part it may be compensatory to the position of the thigh, and in some patients it is clearly produced by consistently turning the feet outwards in walking in order to reduce the movement of painful articulation. It is possible that external rotation of the tibia can be produced by contracture of the iliotibial band. Whatever the cause of the torsion or rotation, the line of pull of the quadriceps will be translated laterally, inhibiting the function of this muscle and thus its control of the knee.

In assessing a remedy it is imperative to view the limb as a whole, both in appearance and function. If knee surgery is to be undertaken, correction of any rotary element may be possible at the same time. If not it may be necessary to consider a formal rotation osteotomy or a realignment of the distal quadriceps mechanism.

Foot

The ankle and tarsus are very commonly involved in juvenile chronic arthritis, but fortunately the remedy for many of the problems is by surgical appliances, e.g.

special footwear insoles or calipers, rather than by open operation. All the joints in this region are liable to be affected, though here in particular certain patterns of disease effect specific joints predominantly. Thus, sero-negative arthritis has a predilection for the tarsus, while seropositive disease more commonly affects the forefoot. Those with pauciarticular disease and young male patients, who are in the early stages of ankylosing spondylitis, often suffer from ankle involvement. The synovial sheaths surrounding tendons and the plantar fascia itself may become inflamed, causing tenderness, pain and swelling.

Foot problems arise due to direct involvement of the joints of the foot, or as a result of fixed deformity of the knee, rotation of the leg, or within the foot itself, where failure of function in one element may stress another. For example, stiffness or fusion in the subtalar and mid-tarsal complex may stress and produce pain in the ankle. While identification of the site of joint disease within the foot may be made clear from clinical or radiological assessment, the source of any pain must be clearly identified as it does not necessarily arise from the more obviously radiologically affected joints.

In common with non-rheumatic disorders of the foot, deformity *per se* does not necessarily present a problem if mobility is retained. Fixed deformity, however, is constant in producing symptoms at the points of pressure and at other sites within the foot that become stressed. The clinician should be vigorous in the anticipation and prevention of the onset of deformity and make every effort to keep the foot plantigrade and mobile.

From a practical point of view the main problems experienced in the management of the foot in juvenile chronic arthritis are toe deformities of various sorts, including clawing and hallux valgus, metatarsalgia with painful plantar callosities, mid-tarsal pain and pain and deformity in the hindfoot. This last may be due to either ankle or subtalar joint involvement, or both. There may be differential rates of growth because of epiphyseal involvement, and not uncommonly the feet may differ in size.

EXAMINATION

An obvious problem may immediately present itself, e.g. hallux valgus with an overlying bunion. Often, however, this is not the case, and it is essential for examination to have the patient standing and the whole leg in view. Deformity, pressure points and callosities are noted, together with the posture of the foot, particularly in relation to the limb as a whole. Radiographs should be obtained with the patient standing whenever possible, while various special views can be helpful, e.g. a lateral view of the ankle in both plantar flexion and dorsiflexion to show the possible range of motion. Pedobarographic tracings are helpful in indicating pressure distribution on the foot and serve as a useful record for comparison before and after treatment.

TREATMENT

From the point of view of explanation and management, it is convenient to consider the foot in three parts.

Forefoot and toes

In seronegative disease the interphalangeal joints have taken the brunt of the problem and have responded by inequalities of growth, dislocation and occasionally fusion. It is difficult to prevent these deformities occurring, as splinting the toes is not a practical solution. It is therefore easier to deal with these problems when they arise, and a simple trimming of bone irregularity or excision arthroplasty can afford rapid relief of any problems.

In seropositive disease, the familiar pattern witnessed in adult rheumatic patients is seen. Involvement of the metatarsophalangeal joints leads to their destruction and dorsal dislocation of the base of the proximal phalanx (Fig. 12.2.18). At the same time the toes tend to claw at the interphalangeal joints, while the metatarsal heads are driven plantarwards and painful callosities appear on the sole of the foot. The normal transverse forefoot arch is lost, the foot widens and the gait loses its normal spring, so that the patient tends to plod with the feet turned out. The big toe does not claw like the others, but rather responds by developing a hallux valgus deformity.

The problems range from early, passively correctable clawing of the toes to total destruction of the metatarsophalangeal joint with dislocation and fixed clawing. Patients with early clawing and only minimal radiological changes can be treated conservatively by physiotherapy, metatarsal insoles and occasionally simply tenotomy of the extensor tendons. Single or multiple oblique osteotomies of the metatarsal necks have afforded relief in patients in whom the simpler methods have failed and joint destruction is not marked. These osteotomies unite with angulation, allowing the metatarsal head to rise away from the sole and at the same time relax the pull of the extensor tendons, permitting

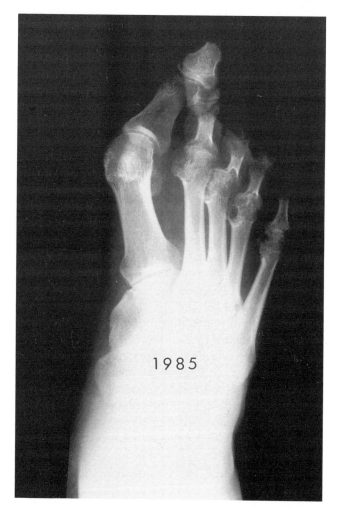

Fig. 12.2.18 Radiograph of a foot in an 18-year-old patient who developed seropositive disease aged 9 years.

the toes to straighten. Early weight-bearing on a shoe is encouraged to minimize post-operative stiffness and to allow weight-bearing to position the divided metatarsal heads.

When dislocation of the metatarsophalangeal joints is complete and articular destruction advanced, forefoot excision arthroplasty is indicated. The method of choice is left to the individual surgeon, but to achieve success it is necessary to excise the joints symmetrically and sufficiently. The end-result should have a fan-like appearance on the radiograph with a marked gap between the divided metatarsal necks and proximal phalanges. Examination after healing should reveal no isolated bone prominence on the sole, while the toes should appear floppy; indeed gait analysis should reveal them to be functionless, their retention being entirely cosmetic.

The great toe requires special attention because of its tendency to develop a hallux valgus deformity. Examination and radiographs will determine the degree of displacement of the first metatarsal and the degree of disease of the metatarsophalangeal joint. The decision can then be made between osteotomy and excision arthroplasty. Several methods of osteotomy have been described, but that of Wilson (1963) commends itself for its simplicity and constant results (Fig. 12.2.19). Keller's arthroplasty (1912) has stood the test of time, but if the other metatarsal heads have been excised then Mayo's operation (Rix, 1968) will produce a more even distribution of weight on the forefoot.

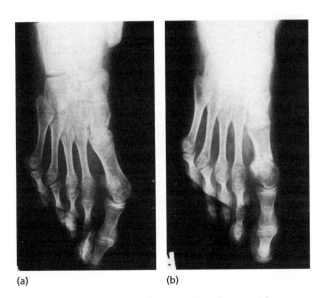

(a)   (b)

Fig. 12.2.19 This patient had seropositive disease with onset at the age of 8 years. (a) Among the toe deformities, the hallus valgus has required treatment. (b) Following a metatarsal osteotomy.

Hindfoot

This excludes the ankle, but otherwise includes all the joints of the tarsus and in particular the triple complex of subtalar, talonavicular and calcaneocuboid joints. These joints are commonly affected by other influences or by primary disease within themselves. No set pattern of deformity occurs, but varus, valgus, pronation, or supination can all occur, depending on a particular stress. Painful collapse of the foot into valgus is most commonly seen, but spasm of the peroneal muscles may equally produce this deformity. A corticosteroid injection can be put into the sinus tarsi. The hindfoot and forefoot usually diverge in the same direction and a careful assessment of any supination or pronation element must be made, as these elements of deformity imply that the patient is walking on the outer or inner side of the foot. This is more important to deal with than pure valgus, which is still compatible with a plantigrade and symptomless foot.

If passive correction is obtainable in the early stages the patient should be given an anaesthetic, and then a plantigrade position obtained and held by a below-knee plaster cast. Four weeks is often sufficient for the retention of the cast, but any sign of relapse can be controlled by a below-knee iron and T-strap. Surgical procedures have not often been required, but occasionally selective mid-tarsal arthrodesis may be indicated, particularly if the talonavicular joint is affected (Fig. 12.2.20) Several patients in the Taplow group have undergone a full triple arthrodesis, and in some patients Dwyer's os calcis osteotomy was helpful.

Ankle

If the ankle and hindfoot joints are included together, 40% of patients with juvenile chronic polyarthritis will develop disease in this area. Fortunately, although pain may be a troublesome feature of ankle joint disease, stability is less of a problem. Disease may directly affect the joint, and occasionally the talus may undergo avascular necrosis secondary to disease in the sinus tarsi, The ankle is often stressed when the other joints of the tarsus have lost mobility. The ankle can be treated like the tarsal joint by a period of immobilization in a below-knee walking cast. Indeed, this is a prudent move as it is sometimes impossible to tell whether it is the ankle or subtalar joint that is producing the symptoms. The choice of operation lies between arthrodesis and some form of arthroplasty. Two of the Taplow patients have had a successful arthrodesis, but arthroplasty has not been performed to date.

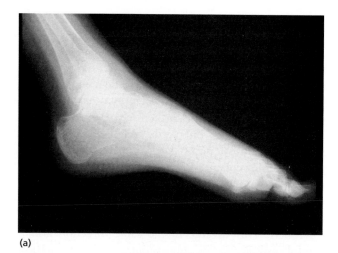

(a)

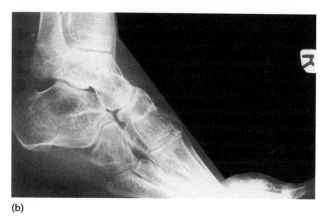

(b)

Fig. 12.2.20 Patient with polyarthritis with onset at age 9 years. (a) Spontaneous triple arthrodesis of the left foot. (b) The right foot was painful and deformed with marked varus, and a surgical triple arthrodesis was later performed on this side.

SOFT TISSUE LESIONS OF THE FOOT

The synovial sheaths of the tendons in the foot and toes are commonly affected by juvenile chronic arthritis, in particular the flexor sheath of the toes and that of the tibialis posterior as it courses around the inner side of the ankle. The Achilles tendon and the plantar fascia are also occasional sites where pain and swelling demand treatment. In all these sites a local injection of corticosteroids under anaesthesia has often been successful in controlling symptoms. Only very occasionally is operative decompression or synovectomy indicated, except in uncontrolled cases.

FRACTURES

Patients with juvenile chronic arthritis are protected from sport-induced trauma because of their inability to participate. Nevertheless, they are more vulnerable to pathological fractures because of the stiffness of their joints and porosis of their bones. This is particularly so in relation to supracondylar fractures of the knee, which is the most common site encountered. The author knows of three occasions when fractures have been produced by manipulation. Immobility rapidly leads to joint stiffness, so that it is important to limit fixation to the minimum necessary and for the least possible time. Ideally, internal fixation might suggest itself, but the porotic nature of the bone makes metallic fixation impractical in most cases.

Several patients have suffered crush fractures of the spine, particularly if they were receiving corticosteroids. No special treatment is indicated, and recovery with remarkable reformation of the vertebrae can be expected.

SPINE

Although spinal problems are common in these patients, there are few conditions amenable to an open operative approach.

The cervical spine has been mentioned in relation to the hazards of general anaesthetics. Atlantoaxial subluxation in seropositive patients may require the support of a collar in its early stages, but greater degrees may require stabilization as is practised in surgery in adults with rheumatoid disease. No known method will prevent fusion of part or all of the cervical posterior facet joints in seronegative disease. The surgeon has a duty to see that this happens in the best possible position, as there is often a tendency to torticollis which if unattended will allow a permanent deformity to be established. These patients should have their necks straightened gently under anaesthesia and be fitted with a firm collar. This is removed for regular physiotherapy followed immediately by reapplication of the collar.

There are no special problems encountered in the dorsal spine, except for vertebral collapse from osteoporosis, which is not amenable to surgical treatment. Ankylosing spondylitis seldom affects the lumbar region before the late teens, and apart from this condition there is an inexplicable sparing of the lumbar region in patients with juvenile chronic arthritis.

Structural scoliosis occurs more commonly in patients with juvenile chronic arthritis than in the normal population. This may arise from postural curves associated with asymmetrical involvement of the lower limb joints causing pelvic tilting. Timely operative relief of the primary cause in the lower limbs has led to a lessening of the spinal curve. Asymmetrical apophyseal joint involvement may also contribute to this problem. In patients with scoliosis, careful appraisal of the underlying pathology should be made, but if the need exists conventional methods of correction and stabilization can be employed.

REFERENCES

Arden G.P. and Ansell B.M. (1978) *Surgical Management of Juvenile Chronic Arthritis*. London, Academic Press.

Benjamin A. (1969) Double osteotomy for the painful knee in rheumatoid arthritis and osteoarthritis. *J. Bone Joint Surg.* **51B**, 694.

Brain A.I.J. (1983) The laryngeal mask — a new concept in airway management. *Br. J. Anaes.* **55**, 801–805.

Keller W.L. (1912) Further observations on the surgical treatment of hallux valgus and bunions. *N Y Med. J.* **95**, 696.

Rix R.R. (1968) Modified Mayo operation for hallux valgus and bunion — a comparison with the Keller procedure. *J. Bone Joint Surg.* **50A**, 1368.

Wilson J.N. (1963) Oblique osteotomy displacement for hallux valgus. *J. Bone Joint Surg.* **45B**, 552.

FURTHER READING

Ansell B.M. and Swann M. (1983) The management of chronic arthritis of children. *J. Bone Joint Surg.* **65B**, 536.

Ansell B.M. and Swann M. (1988) Juvenile arthritis. In Helal B. and Wilson D. (eds) *The Foot*. Edinburgh, Churchill Livingstone, pp. 511–523.

Clarke D.W., Ansell B.M. and Swann M. (1988) Soft tissue release of the knee in children with juvenile chronic arthritis. *J. Bone Joint Surg.* **70B**, 224–227.

Granberry W.M. and Brewer E.J. (1978) The combined pediatric–orthopedic approach to the management of juvenile rheumatoid arthritis. *Orthop. Clin. North Am.* **9**, 481–507.

Mogensen B. (1982) *Hip Surgery in Juvenile Chronic Arthritis*. Thesis, University of Lund.

Pahle J.A., Kass E. and Munthe E. (1978) Orthopaedic surgery for childhood arthritis. *Clin. Rheumatol. Dis.* **4**, 425–442.

Ross A.C., Edgar M.A., Swann M. and Ansell B.M. (1987) Scoliosis in juvenile chronic arthritis. *J. Bone Joint Surg.* **69B**, 175–178.

Ruddlesdin C., Swann M., Ansell B.M. and Arden G.P. (1986) Total hip replacement in children with juvenile chronic arthritis. *J. Bone Joint Surg.* **68B**, 218–222.

Rydholm U. (1986) *Knee Surgery in Juvenile Chronic Arthritis*. Thesis, University of Lund.

Rydholm U. (1990) *Surgery for Juvenile Chronic Arthritis*. Lund, Ortolani.

Soto-Hall R., Johnsson L.H. and Johnsson R.A. (1964) Variations in the intra-articular pressure of the hip joint in injury and disease: a probable factor in avascular necrosis. *J. Bone Joint Surg.* **46A**, 509–516.

Swann M. and Ansell B.M. (1986) Soft tissue release of the hips in children with juvenile chronic arthritis. *J. Bone Joint Surg.* **68B**, 404–408.

Chapter 13
Bleeding Disorders

C. Bulstrode & R.A. Dickson

INTRODUCTION

This chapter is about a group of disorders in which blood clotting fails. There are various mechanisms by which this can occur, and the severity of each particular condition can also alter. Some are inherited, others are acquired.

Patients with bleeding disorders are important to orthopaedic surgeons for two main reasons. First, because their management after acute trauma and elective surgery is complicated by their tendency to bleed. Secondly, because repeated bleeds can result in long-term complications, e.g. bone cysts, muscle fibrosis, nerve palsy and early aggressive arthritis of the affected joints.

In this chapter the genetic basis of inherited bleeding disorders is described, with what is known of the underlying physiology. The common forms of presentation and methods used for diagnosis are then related to the pathological process. Finally, the conservative and operative management of the longer term problem is reviewed in the light of the current high incidence of hepatitis and human immunodeficiency virus (HIV) in those patients with severe haemophilia.

The genetic basis of the disease and the dangers of surgery in haemophiliacs were recognized as early as the second century A.D. It is recorded that the Rabbi Judah, a patriarch, exempted a woman's third son from being circumcised if her two elder sons had previously bled to death after circumcision (Katzemelson, 1958). This observation was either ignored or forgotten in the Western world, however, until the disease was rediscovered and cases described at the end of the 18th century (McKusick and Rapaport, 1958). It is probable that a single mutation in the spermatogenesis of Edward, Duke of Kent (the father of Queen Victoria), resulted in haemophilia affecting a significant number of the male members of the royal families of Europe. The most famous of these, Tsarevitch Alexis, son of Tsar Nicholas II of Russia, was severely affected. His chronic ill health and the justifiable anxiety of his parents over his repeated bleeds may have been the key to the control that Rasputin came to have over the Russian royal family. One of the reasons given for the general dissatisfaction that led up to the Russian Revolution was the influence that the 'mad monk' Rasputin had on the running of the country. It could be said that haemophilia and 20th century political history are inextricably linked.

PHYSIOLOGY AND BIOCHEMISTRY OF CLOTTING

The natural mechanisms concerned with the control of bleeding can be divided into three parts (Fig. 13.1). First, there is a system aimed at physically blocking the escape of blood, immediately after the trauma. Secondly, a system that leads to clot formation, separate from the first, prevents blood loss while repair is going on. Finally, there are mechanisms concerned with the removal of clots once healing is complete and with preventing their inappropriate formation.

Immediate control of blood loss

This mechanism consists of a vascular phase and a platelet phase. The vascular phase is stimulated by physical damage to blood vessel walls and results in reflex vasoconstriction of the free ends of cut blood vessels. Collagen is exposed in the damaged vessel walls and appears to be a powerful stimulus to the accretion of platelets. The constriction of the cut ends of the vessels and the collection of platelets, which stick to each other, stops the initial haemorrhage. Pressure helps this process by reducing the blood pressure locally and by squeezing the vessel walls together, narrowing the gap that needs to be blocked by platelets.

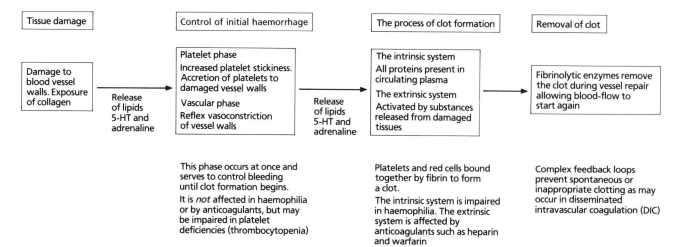

Fig. 13.1 The control of bleeding.

The area of damaged vessel walls and the platelets that have stuck to each other release a whole range of vasoactive amines, e.g. serotonin (5-HT) and adrenaline, which stimulate further vasoconstriction of vessel walls and increase platelet stickiness. They also release lipids which activate enzymes concerned with the formation of the clot. This first mechanism is not affected in haemophilia, but is affected in any disorder where the number or function of platelets is reduced.

Clot formation

The formation of the clot, the second phase in the control of bleeding, is brought about by the transformation of fibrinogen into fibrin. Red cells and platelets are then bound together by long strands of fibrin, creating a temporary but durable structure which prevents further haemorrhage while the tissues are being repaired. The final common pathway for the formation of fibrin is the conversion of prothrombin to thrombin, which in turn brings about the conversion of fibrinogen to fibrin.

Two separate pathways have been identified for the conversion of prothrombin to thrombin, one of which is a cascade of enzymes, all of which are present in plasma, the so-called intrinsic system; the second is a path initiated by substances present in the tissues but not in the plasma. This is the extrinsic system (Fig. 13.2).

INTRINSIC SYSTEM

This consists of a number of precursor proteins present in circulating plasma. Once the first (usually factor XII) has been activated, a cascade begins of one enzyme

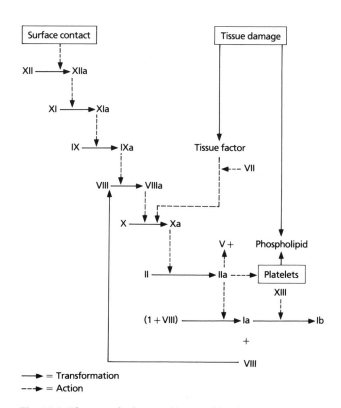

Fig. 13.2 The cascade theory of human blood coagulation.

activating the next (Fig. 13.2), until activated factor X brings about the conversion of prothrombin to thrombin. Factor XII can be activated by contact with a foreign substance, e.g. glass, so this system can be studied and tested in the laboratory. It is the absence or reduction of some of the enzymes involved in this pathway that leads to the various forms of haemophilia. The intrinsic system was originally described as a cascade of factors. Starting with factor XII, it was suggested that the mechanism served to provide a rapid and massive clotting response in the face of injury (Macfarlane, 1964). Subsequent research has shown that there are many more factors than originally thought and that their interaction is a complex web of both positive and negative feedback.

EXTRINSIC SYSTEM

Substances released by damaged tissues activate the extrinsic system, which also results in the activation of thrombin. This system cannot easily be studied in the laboratory, but is the pathway affected by the anti-coagulant drugs, e.g. heparin and warfarin.

Problems in either the extrinsic or intrinsic system can lead to a failure of clotting. In these patients, bleeding after trauma may stop initially (as blood vessels contract and platelets aggregate) but then restarts when a stable clot fails to form.

Removal of clots

Fibrinolytic enzymes start to remove the clot as repair of the blood vessel wall takes place. When the repair is complete, blood starts to flow down the vessel again. The same enzymes are present to ensure that spontaneous and inappropriate clotting does not occur. If these enzymes are deficient or absent, then disseminated intravascular coagulation may occur.

INHERITED DISORDERS OF CLOTTING (HAEMOPHILIA)

Haemophilia A (classic haemophilia) is probably the most common of the severe bleeding disorders. Christmas disease (factor IX deficiency) is much less common. Von Willebrand's disease (a deficiency of factor VIII-type complexes) is probably as common as classic haemophilia, but only a small proportion of cases are severe. Calcium is required for most of the reactions in clotting, so calcium-chelating agents, e.g. ethylene-diaminetetra-acetete (EDTA), are used to prevent blood from clotting in laboratory specimens needed for haemoglobin estimation, but obviously must not be used if clotting studies are to be performed.

Genetics

Both haemophilia A and Christmas disease are sex-linked recessive conditions. This means that genes for both factor VIII and IX are carried on the X chromosome. As they are both recessives they are normally only clinically apparent in the male (XY) where the X chromosome is affected. In females (XX) it is very rare indeed for both chromosomes to be affected, so they may be carriers but seldom manifest the disease. Men with either condition cannot pass it on to their sons (who inherit only a Y chromosome from them), but all their daughters are carriers. There is a 50% chance that the daughters of women carriers will themselves be carriers, and similarly a 50% chance that sons of women carriers will be affected by the disease.

Prevalence

About 5000 patients have been diagnosed with haemophilia in the UK, of whom 2500 are severely affected (with factor VIII levels of less than 2%) (Rizza and Spooner, 1983). The great majority of the severe cases have haemophilia A (factor VIII deficiency). The prevalence of the condition is therefore 16 in 100 000 of the male population; 1 in 7000 liveborn male children in Sweden is a severely affected haemophiliac (Ramgren, 1962a; 1962b). About 30% of cases have no family history, and therefore appear to be new mutations that could not have been prevented by genetic counselling.

Severity

Haemophilia may vary in severity from cases that are only discovered by chance through to cases where severe spontaneous bleeds occur with monotonous regularity. The severity depends on the level of circulating factor, which is normally recorded as a percentage of normal (100%). Patients with over 50% of normal factor levels are regarded as not having haemophilia, as they do not have a significantly increased incidence of bleeding. Between 25% and 35% of normal factor levels patients may not always be diagnosed, as they so seldom have problems. Only patients with factor levels below 25% present problems with surgery. Patients with less than 1% of normal factor tend to bleed spontaneously (Table 13.1). Haemophiliacs who have developed antibodies to factors pose a very serious problem indeed, and surgery should be avoided wherever possible.

ACQUIRED BLEEDING DISORDERS

These should be suspected in patients who have no history (family or individual) of bleeding problems and in whom bleeding is unexpectedly heavy or prolonged. Once it has been decided that the trauma or surgery is not enough in itself to explain the bleeding, then medical causes must be sought. The presence of petechial

Table 13.1 Levels of circulating factor and clinical severity of bleeding

Level of factor (% of normal)	Bleeding pattern
50–100	None
25–50	Bleeding tendency after major injury
5–25	Severe bleeding with operations or minor injury
1–5	Severe bleeding after minor injury, occasionally spontaneous
0	Severe spontaneous bleeds

haemorrhages suggest a platelet/capillary problem, while oozing at drip or injection sites is a clear indication of a clotting problem. Some patients may develop antibodies to factor VIII, often in association with other diseases with an autoimmune basis, e.g. lupus and diabetes. These patients can prove exceptionally difficult to treat.

DIAGNOSIS

Patients with problems in the primary haemostasis system (platelet/capillary defects) commonly present with bleeding immediately from the time of injury. They tend to bleed from minor skin lacerations, mucous membranes and particularly the gastrointestinal tract. Spontaneous bleeds and haemarthroses (bleeding into joints) are rare. Local pressure serves to stop the bleeding. On haematological testing the bleeding time is prolonged and the tourniquet test is positive.

In patients with defects in the secondary phase (coagulation defects) bleeding may restart some considerable time after the injury or continue for an excessive length of time after minor trauma. There may be a clear family history, and in severe cases spontaneous bleeds are characteristic. In contrast to platelet/capillary defects, local pressure may not control the bleeding. The clotting time is generally prolonged and one-stage prothrombin time is normal. Factor defects are diagnosed and their severity measured by specific assay.

Severe haemophiliacs (less than 2% factor) may present as babies or young children with multiple bruises out of proportion to any trauma sustained. The differential diagnosis is bruising secondary to non-accidental injury. Chorionic villous biopsy now allows the diagnosis of haemophilia within the first trimester of pregnancy when termination could be considered. This may reduce the number of severely affected boys born to carrier mothers, but will not affect the 30% whose cases appear to arise from a new mutation.

For a surgeon faced with a patient in whom there is persistent bleeding, local surgical causes must first be excluded, including inadequate attention to haemostasis and infection. A check should then be made for a generalized bleeding problem by taking a full history including family and medication. Examination must include checking for old bruising and for oozing at injection or drip sites. If any of these are present then a haematological opinion should be sought.

CLINICAL PRESENTATION OF HAEMOPHILIA

The age of presentation and type of bleeding depends on the severity of the factor deficiency. Haemophilia seldom presents in the newborn, and cephalhaematomas with bruising from birth trauma are rare. Provided that circumcision is not undertaken, the first bruising appears at 3–4 months when the baby becomes active. As soon as the baby walks at around 1 year, falls will lead to bruising of lips, head and buttocks. There may also be spontaneous bleeds into ankles, knees and even elbows (Rizza and Matthews, 1984). If there are bruises of different ages, then non-accidental injury may be suspected as an alternative diagnosis. Repeated bleeds into joints are both excruciatingly painful and damage the joint itself. The joint may swell and stiffen. The muscles around the joints may waste and the bones become porotic and atrophic. Haemorrhage into muscle is also very painful and may cause such severe swelling that compartment syndromes and nerve palsies result. There may also be spontaneous bleeds from erupting teeth, the gums, the kidneys (leading to haematuria) and the alimentary tract, particularly if gastric irritants are taken. The incidence of bleeds in different parts of the musculoskeletal system is shown in Table 13.2.

Special features of haemophiliac bruising

Haemophiliac bruising may occur after some definite injury, but often there is no known injury. The bruises are lumpy and tend to spread. The skin over the centre of the lump is blanched and free from discoloration. If the bruise is immediately subcutaneous, it is surprisingly mobile. Tension within a haematoma may be severe in places where the skin is tethered, e.g. the scalp, where pressure necrosis of the skin has been described.

Venepuncture and wounds

Surprisingly, venepuncture in severe haemophilia causes little problem. If the antecubital vein is used, pressure

Table 13.2 Relative incidence of acute haemorrhages affecting the musculoskeletal system

	Number of cases	Incidence (%)
Joints		
Knee	318	38.7
Elbow	187	22.7
Ankle	106	13
Shoulder	24	2.9
Wrist	20	2.4
Miscellaneous	14	1.7
Soft tissues		
Iliopsoas	48	5.8
Forearm	31	3.8
Calf	31	3.8
Thigh	30	3.6
Miscellaneous	13	1.6
Total	822	100

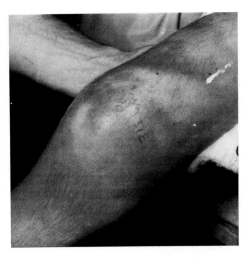

Fig. 13.3 An acute knee haemarthrosis in a haemophiliac patient. The joint is tense and the skin smooth and shiny. The joint is held flexed.

should be applied to the puncture site for several minutes after the removal of the needle with the elbow fully extended to allow firm pressure to be applied.

Bleeds into joints

Bleeds are thought to occur in joints when vessels in the synovial membrane are trapped in the joint. The inflammation and oedema following this trauma then makes the synovium susceptible to further 'nipping' and bleeds. The situation can become self-perpetuating, leading to an acute-on-chronic haemarthrosis/synovitis. The situation can be further complicated by the formation of adhesions across the joint, which tear when the joint is mobilized and lead to further bleeds.

In acute haemarthrosis in a haemophiliac patient the joint is red, hot, swollen and acutely painful (Fig. 13.3). All movement is resisted. If haemophilia has not already been diagnosed or the patient fails to volunteer that he is haemophiliac, the clinical presentation is very similar to that of acute septic arthritis. In a joint where there have been many previous bleeds scarring reduces the amount of swelling and the knee may appear surprisingly normal despite the severe pain felt by the patient.

Bleeding into muscles

In mild haemophilia bleeds into muscles may occur secondary to trauma. In severe cases spontaneous bleeds may also occur. The muscles most commonly affected are the muscles of the calf, thigh, buttock and forearm, as well as the psoas. Repeated bleeds into the calf may

lead to fibrosis, contracture and an equinus deformity. Bleeds into the psoas muscle may track down under the inguinal ligament to the lesser trochanter. Pressure on the femoral nerve in the femoral canal may lead to a transient or even permanent nerve palsy with weakness of the knee extensors. In an acute psoas bleed the abdomen is tender while the hip is held flexed and internally rotated (Fig. 13.4). Any attempt to extend or externally rotate the hip is strongly resisted because of pain. The condition can be confused with acute appendicitis or septic arthritis of the hip if it is not known that the patient is a severe haemophiliac. Bleeding into the forearm flexor compartment may lead to Volkmann's ischaemic contracture (Fig. 13.5). Ultrasonography can be very useful in the diagnosis of a haemophilic bleed. Serial ultrasonographic examinations can be used to monitor the resolution of a bleed (Wilson *et al.*, 1987).

Chronic bleeds

JOINTS

Repeated bleeds into a joint lead to fibrosis of the soft tissues around the joint with the synovial cavity divided into small loculated spaces. Articular cartilage is lost. Without treatment gradual spontaneous arthrodesis occurs, often with considerable pain. Bleeds may then become less frequent but also become difficult to diagnose, as swelling is no longer a marked feature because there is no single synovial cavity to distend. The joint is destroyed by aggressive arthritis. The possible pathways

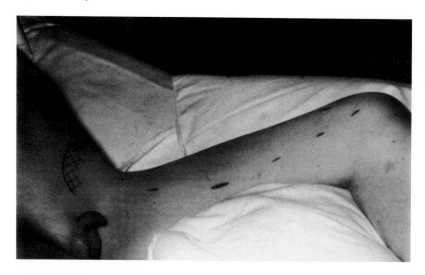

Fig. 13.4 Characteristic clinical picture of an iliopsoas bleed with a femoral nerve lesion. The hip is flexed to relieve discomfort. There is an area of diminished sensation on the thigh and the knee jerk is absent.

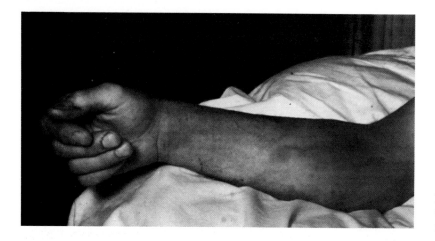

Fig. 13.5 Volkmann's ischaemic contracture of the forearm following a soft tissue bleed into the flexor forearm musculature.

for this are shown in Fig. 13.6. Chronic arthropathy commonly affects the knee joint, and the typical radiographic changes may be noted (Fig. 13.7). It is a cause of avascular necrosis in the hip (Fig. 13.8).

PSEUDOCYSTS

Bleeds into the tendinous attachment of muscles may progress to a pseudocyst. These are said to be present in up to 4.5% of severe haemophiliacs (Ahlberg, 1975). The haematoma may go on to form a multiloculated cyst filled with the tarry degradation products of blood. Instead of resolving, the cyst may grow in size, eroding any bone nearby over a period of years. Further acute bleeds may occur into the cyst and cause rapid enlargement with pain. Eventually, they may erode through skin or viscus, when uncontrolled bleeding or sepsis may cause the death of the patient. The most common site for the cysts is around the femur and ilium.

TREATMENT

Blood and blood products

The failure of clotting may result in considerable blood loss, which may need to be replaced by blood or plasma. Fresh blood and fresh frozen plasma both contain clotting factors. Adequate amounts of factor must be given for a stable clot to be formed, however, so it is usually necessary to give concentrated factor as well.

PREPARATION OF FACTOR VIII AND IX

Human clotting factors are prepared by pooling plasma from many blood donors. Factor VIII can also be obtained from the blood of pigs. In both cases the blood clotting factors are present in very small quantities compared with the other plasma proteins, and a variety of biochemical techniques is used to concentrate the

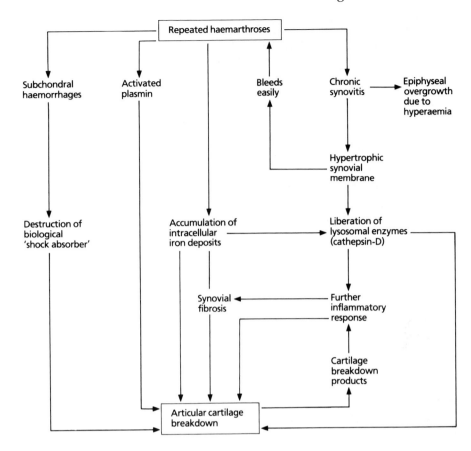

Fig. 13.6 How bleeds lead to arthritis.

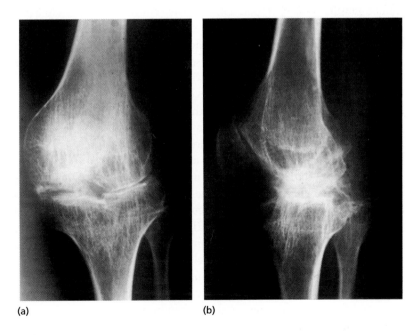

(a)   (b)

Fig. 13.7 (a) Anteroposterior and (b) lateral radiographs of the knee showing chronic haemophiliac arthropathy. There is metaphyseal widening, squaring of the intercondylar notch, flattening of the lower pole of the patella and degenerative changes.

factor at the expense of the other proteins. Nevertheless, factor concentrate contains many other proteins apart from those required for coagulation. Some of the newer products are now relatively pure, but then require the addition of proteins such as albumin to stabilize the factor proteins during preparation and storage. These proteins are potentially antigenic. Once prepared clotting factor concentrate can be dried and stored in a powder

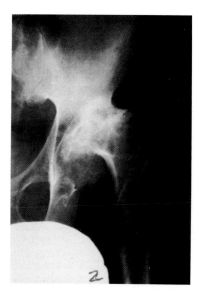

Fig. 13.8 Anteroposterior radiograph of the hip of a haemophiliac patient showing chronic haemophiliac arthropathy with avascular necrosis of the femoral head.

form without losing a significant amount of activity.

It is now known that hepatitis viruses and HIV can be transmitted in blood products. They are particularly likely to be present in anything prepared from pooled human plasma. Factor prepared in this way is now heat-treated and/or detergent-treated to destroy any viral contamination. This process reduces the activity of factor products slightly and increases its cost. Recently, it has been possible to synthesize factor VIII using transgenic techniques in cultured hamster cells containing human DNA. Although factor prepared in this way would be free of any infection, it still contains many antigenic proteins and is currently much more expensive than highly purified factor prepared in the conventional way.

The total amount of factor that needs to be given depends on the body weight of the patient and the amount by which the patients factor levels are to be raised. The half-life of factor VIII is 12 h and of factor IX is 18 h. For small spontaneous bleeds it is normal to try to bring the factor level up to 15% each day. For severe bleeds 30% is more appropriate. Haemophiliac patients normally know how much factor they need in the first instance, and it is then best to take advice from a haematologist.

Patients with antibodies

In patients with antibodies to factor VIII, bleeding cannot easily be controlled because all factor given is destroyed immediately by antibodies. An alternative approach is to use products that bypass the site of action of this antibody, which acts on the blood coagulation cascade. Such products are mainly prothrombin complex concentrates, but the active agents are not exactly known. The substance is not always of value and is both very expensive and potentially hazardous to use. The only other alternatives are to try to swamp the antibodies with very large amounts of factor or to perform plasmaphoresis on the patient to remove the antibodies. This too only provides a very temporary solution to the problem, so surgical, dental and physiotherapy treatments that require factor cover should be avoided whenever possible in these patients.

Acute bleeds

Home treatment has revolutionized the management of acute bleeds in haemophilia. As soon as they are old enough, young people with haemophilia are taught to recognize the first signs of the onset of a bleed, so that their parents and later they themselves can inject factor and abort the bleed as early as possible. This reduces the need for analgesia, as factor replacement appears to have a dramatic effect on the pain produced by a bleed. It also reduces the emergency trips to haemophilia centres to obtain factor and lengthy hospital admissions while the bleed settles down. Unfortunately, there is no clear evidence so far that this enormous, expensive and complex home care programme for haemophilia has reduced the long-term incidence of haemophiliac arthritis, but nevertheless it is the impression of many workers in the field that this condition is both less common and less severe than previously.

Wounds that require suture

It is tempting to apply standard surgical principles to simple wounds, ensuring that they are clean and then closing them. It might be expected that the pressure applied by the sutures might stop the bleeding. Factor cover must still be given, however, otherwise bleeding may continue deep to the suture line, tracking into surrounding tissues and eventually bursting open the wound.

Severe acute bleeds and those bleeds that fail to respond immediately to home factor treatment

These patients need admission to hospital and adequate factor to bring their levels up to at least 30%. The affected limb needs to be immobilized in a position of comfort with, if possible, some compression to the site of the bleed. Strong analgesia may be required to relieve the severe pain. In the early acute phase, immobilization is probably best provided by a Robert Jones bandage rather than a cast, as there is little room for expansion of a cast if swelling continues. There is no evidence that aspiration of the blood from a joint either by arthroscopy or by needle in any way hastens recovery from the bleed. It may even increase the morbidity because of the need for extra factor to cover the period of aspiration or surgery. Although it is very difficult to maintain constant pressure within a bandage for any period of time, the application of a firm bandage does seem to reduce the severity of the bleed and the size of the swelling. This conservative regimen for the management of haemarthrosis results in blood and its degradation products being left in contact with articular cartilage for considerable periods of time, a situation that is known to be damaging. Immobilization is also known to be damaging to articular cartilage, as is excessive pressure within a joint. Nevertheless, any attempt at immediate aspiration and early mobilization can lead to a serious recurrence of bleeding.

The progression of the bleed can be monitored both by measuring the girth of the limb and by ultrasonography. Once the bleeding has stopped the joint immediately becomes less painful and the girth stops increasing. At this point it may be appropriate to reduce the amount of factor being given and to change the Robert Jones bandage to a plaster back-slab. Over the next few days as the swelling starts to decrease, static muscle exercises can be started to rebuild the tone of the muscles around the affected joint. Treatment with ice packs at this stage seems to help resolution of the bleed. Once the limb has returned to its normal girth and is no longer red or hot, gradual mobilization can be started. This phase may be several weeks after the original bleed. The strength and range of movement of the joint is very slowly increased until they reach the same values as before the bleed.

Patients with haemarthrosis of the knee may be left with very weak quadriceps muscles after such prolonged immobilization and can be helped with quadriceps-enhancing splinting when they first start walking again. This splint allows the knee to operate normally, while guarding against a sudden collapse into flexion. Rehabilitation after a bleed in a haemophiliac is a slow and prolonged (Fig. 13.9) process, involving a great deal of in-patient and out-patient time and careful supervision by a skilled physiotherapist. Failure to undertake this rehabilitation programme will result in a stiff, deformed limb. Any attempt to hasten the rehabilitation will be punished by a further bleed.

Chronic bleeds

If conservative treatment fails to prevent repeated bleeding into a joint, operative treatment may need to be undertaken. This should only be considered in a unit with the haematological and surgical experience of dealing with haemophiliac patients. The complications can be severe and the amount of factor required may be very large indeed. It is not normal to offer surgery in patients in whom there is evidence of antibodies to factor VIII. Even using tranexamic acid it may not be possible to control bleeding, however much factor is given. There are isolated reports of a successful outcome of surgery in patients with anti-factor VIII antibodies. Nevertheless, it is normal to avoid operation in patients with antibodies whenever possible.

Synovectomy, either through the arthroscope or open, has proved very useful in reducing the number of bleeds, particularly in the elbow and the knee (Fig. 13.10). There is no evidence, however, that it arrests or even delays the deterioration in the articular cartilage. Operation should only be undertaken using full protection against potential hepatitis or HIV infection. Goggles should be worn and full precautions taken in disposal of all contaminated surgical refuse. Where possible arthroscopy should only be performed using a television camera rather than direct vision to reduce the chance of eye splash.

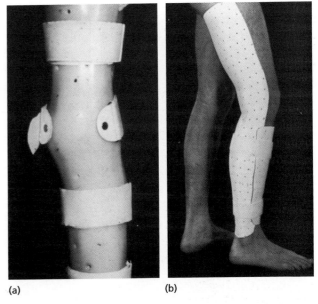

(a)   (b)

Fig. 13.9 (a) Bivalved plastic splint. (b) Quadriceps-enhancing splint. These are used as temporary supports for the knee after immobilization and compression.

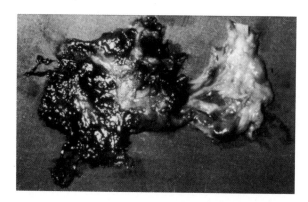

Fig. 13.10 Darkly pigmented, haemosiderin-stained synovium removed from the knee of a haemophiliac patient.

End-stage haemophiliac arthritis

The final stage of haemophiliac arthritis is a destroyed joint. There is considerable bone destruction with an immobile and deformed joint, which is commonly painful. The conservative management of these joints consists of trying to maintain as much movement as possible, particularly in a functional range, while building up muscle power around the joint. Splints can also be used to try to reduce pain. Flexion contractures of the knee can be managed by intensive physiotherapy, reverse dynamic splinting (Fig. 13.11), and a Flow-tron boot (an intermittently inflating pneumatic splint that pro-gressively applies load to straighten the knee. The Flow-tron boot offers the advantage that treatment can be continued at home over a long period of time. Any of these conservative forms of treatment should be supplemented with extra factor cover.

Manipulation under anaesthesia can be useful in the knee when conservative treatment fails to make any further progress. This process needs to be covered with 100% factor during the operation. Every effort should be made to obtain as much extension as possible to allow for locking-out of the knee when walking. A knee splint may then provide considerable support to the patient and enable him to walk with considerably less pain and more confidence. The usual splints used in the author's unit vary from a simple elasticated support bandage, to canvas and leather splints with hinged steel struts, to polypropylene made-to-measure knee splints with locking knee hinges. At the ankle, an ankle/foot orthosis (AFO) polypropylene splint normally used for a foot drop can provide considerable support to a painful, unstable ankle. If this is not adequate, a full caliper may be required.

SURGERY

Major surgery in haemophiliac patients requires careful planning and close liaison between haematologist and surgeon. The patient should be aware of the increased risks of an operation in terms of the increased chance of

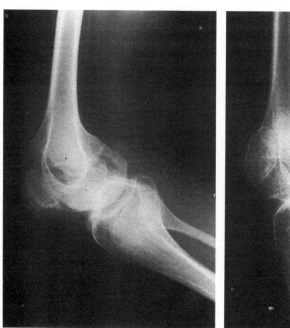

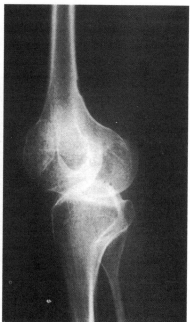

(a)   (b)

Fig. 13.11 (a) A 70° knee flexion contracture in a haemophiliac patient present for 10 years. (b) After 10 days of reversed dynamic slings the knee is straight.

infection, significant bleeding problems, and the reduced chance of a successful outcome compared with similar surgery performed on non-haemophiliac patients. A careful check must be made to ensure that the patient has no antibodies (inhibitors) to factor VIII and the hepatitis and HIV antibody status should be known. It is probably not wise to undertake an operation in the later stages of full-blown acquired immune deficiency syndrome, as there is some evidence to suggest that it may accelerate the course of the disease by reducing the patient's resistance to infection (Green *et al.*, 1990).

Ankle

In the ankle, arthrodesis is the operation of choice. In the author's unit this operation is now performed through a small lateral incision by driving a 2 cm diameter woodworker's brace and bit through the fibula at the level of the ankle joint across to the medial malleolus. Drilling is repeated, tilting the drill bit slightly posteriorly and superiorly to ensure complete obliteration of the tibiotalar joint. The fragments of bone collected from the drill bit are then packed back into the cavity created with extra bone graft from a bone bank if necessary. This procedure minimizes trauma to the ankle and leaves the anterior and posterior margins of the ankle joint intact. This provides considerable stability to the arthrodesis while it is consolidating.

Knee

Various operations have been described in the knee. Patellectomy can provide some relief of pain in patients in whom patellofemoral arthritis is the predominant feature. Arthrodesis of the knee is not often used, as other major joints in the lower limb are commonly involved with arthritis (Fig. 13.12). Successful knee replacements have been described from several units, but the complication rate is high and the lack of long-term results in haemophiliac patients poses a considerable problem for decisions about the management of younger patients.

Hip

In the hip, total replacement of the joint offers the only viable solution as arthrodesis is seldom indicated, given the involvement of other joints. The results of total hip replacement are not as good even as those recorded for hip replacement in young patients who do not have haemophilia, and in the author's unit where 39 total hip replacements have been performed with a median follow-up of just under 8 years, five of the 22 surviving hips have already been revised and three more are likely to require revision in the near future. The 50% survival of hips in this series is therefore unlikely to prove to be more than 10 years. Nevertheless, the very severe pain and disability from which these patients suffer means that the option of a total joint replacement must always be considered.

Pseudocysts

A pseudocyst may need operative removal if it is increasing inexorably in size or if it is eroding bone to such an extent that a pathological fracture has occurred (Fig. 13.13). Neither aspiration, drainage, nor enucleation of pseudocysts is successful. The pseudocyst tends to recur

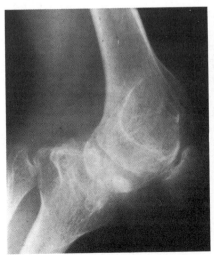
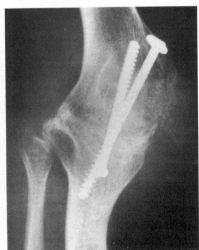

Fig. **13.12** (a) Lateral radiograph of the knee of a haemophiliac patient with severe knee arthropathy. (b) Following arthrodesis in a functional position using internal fixation.

(a)   (b)

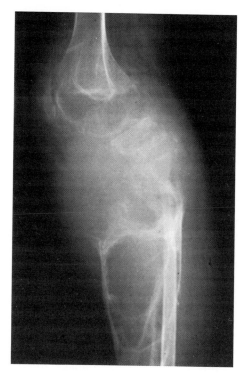

Fig. 13.13 Lateral radiograph of the upper tibia showing a large, expanding haemophiliac cyst.

and may become infected with disastrous consequences. The only surgical option is complete excision of the pseudocyst with its fibrous wall. The operation and post-operative period require 100% factor cover. No drains are used and bandaging with pressure pads is used to obliterate the space while healing occurs.

CONCLUSIONS

Haemophilia poses significant problems for orthopaedic surgeons and in the management of severe arthritis. The management of these cases is expensive, time consuming and fraught with problems. It is probably best left to units specializing in this type of work, where the haematologist and surgeon can work closely together on the problems encountered. The key to management is slow but sure rehabilitation under good factor cover. Undue surgical zeal or hasty rehabilitation is rewarded with a deterioration in the patient's condition, which may cost him his life.

Acknowledgements

The author's thanks are due to Dr Rizza, Director of the Oxford Regional Haemophilia Centre, who devoted so much time to trying to make this text interesting, comprehensible and factually correct.

REFERENCES

Ahlberg A.K.M. (1975) On the natural history of haemophilia pseudo-tumour. *J. Bone Joint Surg.* **57A**, 1133.

Green W.B., DeGriore L.T. and White G.C. (1990) Orthopaedic surgery in HIV positive haemophiliacs. *J. Bone Joint Surg.* **72A**, 2–6.

Katzemelson J.L. (1958) Haemophilia with special reference to the Talmud. *Hebrew Med. J.* **1**, 165.

Macfarlane R.G. (1964) An enzyme cascade in the blood clotting mechanism and its function as a biochemical amplifier. *Nature* **202**, 498–499.

McKusick B.A. and Rapaport S.I. (1962) History of classical haemophilia in a New England family. *Arch Intern Med* **110**, 144.

Ramgren O. (1962a) Haemophilia in Sweden. *Acta Med. Scand. Suppl.* **379**, 37–60.

Ramgren O. (1962b) A clinico- and medico-social study of haemophilia in Sweden. *Acta Med. Scand. Suppl.* **379**, 111–190.

Rizza C.R. and Matthews J.M. (1984) Clinical features of clotting factor deficiencies. In Biggs R. and Rizza C.R. (eds) *Human Blood Coagulation, Haemostasis and Thrombosis.* 3rd edn. Oxford, Blackwell Scientific Publications, pp. 121–169.

Rizza C.R. and Spooner R.J.D. (1983) Treatment of haemophilia and related disorders in Britain and Northern Ireland during 1976–80: report on behalf of the directors of haemophilia centres in the United Kingdom. *BMJ* **286**, 929–933.

Wilson D.J., McLardy-Smith P.D., Woodham C.H. and MacLaron J.C. (1987) Diagnostic ultrasound in haemophilia. *J. Bone Joint Surg.* **69B**, 103–107.

FURTHER READING

Biggs R. and Rizza C.R. (1984) *Human Blood Coagulation, Haemostasis and Thrombosis.* 3rd edn. Oxford, Blackwell Scientific Publications.

Bloom A. and Thomas D.P. (1987) *Haemostasis and Thrombosis.* 2nd edn. Edinburgh, Churchill Livingstone.

Biggs R. (1977) Haemophilia treatment in the United Kingdom from 1969–1974. *Br. J. Haemotol.* **35**, 481–504.

Darby S.C., Rizza C.R., Doll R., Spooner R.J.D., Stratton I.M. and Thakrar B. (1989) Incidence of AIDS and excess of mortality associated with HIV in haemophilia centres in the United Kingdom. *Br. Med. J.* **298**, 1064–1068.

Graham J.B. (1980) Genetic control of factor 8. *Lancet* i, 340–342.

Ingram G.I.C. (1976) Variations in the reaction between thrombin and fibrinogen and their effects on the prothrombin time. *J. Clin. Pathol.* **8**, 318–323.

Kerr C.B. (1965) Genetics of human blood coagulation. *J. Med. Genet.* **2**, 254–303.

World Health Organization. (1972) *Inherited Blood Clotting Disorders.* World Health Organization Technical Report no. 504, p. 14.

Section 2
General Orthopaedics

Chapter 14
Metabolic Bone Disease

A. Fairney

INTRODUCTION

Metabolic bone disease is a term used to embrace a group of generalized bone disorders associated with abnormalities of the formation and metabolism of bone. In this chapter an outline of the cell biology and function of bone is given, followed by the clinical description of different types of metabolic bone disease, linked to this background where possible. A section related to the biochemical investigation of metabolic bone disease is also included.

CELL BIOLOGY OF BONE

Bone is an active tissue that is continually undergoing structural and metabolic changes. Its surface is bathed in bone fluid which is different from the whole body extracellular fluid. Morphologically, bone consists of an organic matrix, which contains bone cells, nerves, blood vessels and marrow, and within which bone mineral is deposited. It has two main functions: the mechanical support and protection of the body, and the maintenance of normal mineral metabolism.

About 99% of the body calcium is present in the skeleton and 1% is present in the blood, extracellular fluid and tissues. In addition, bone is present in two different forms, namely compact or cortical bone, and trabecular bone. Cortical bone, which is particularly found in long bones, is 80–90% calcified and has mainly a mechanical and protective function. Trabecular bone, which is particularly found in the vertebrae, is 15–25% calcified and has mainly a metabolic function.

Bone cells

The different types of cells found in bone control its formation, composition and resorption. There are three main types, namely osteoblasts, osteoclasts and osteo-cytes (Fig. 14.1). In addition, fibroblasts are found in the periosteum, marrow and around blood vessels, and myeloproliferative cells in the bone marrow.

OSTEOBLASTS

These are the bone-forming cells. They are uniform in size, mononuclear and have basophilic cytoplasm. These cells lie in single layers close to the osteoid of newly formed bone and have a high content of alkaline phosphatase. Osteoblasts may be resting, when they appear spindle-shaped and flattened, or active, when they appear larger and plump. They have many functions, which include the synthesis of collagen and of some of the non-collagenous constituents of the bone matrix, in addition to contributing to the mineralization of bone.

The plasma membrane of the osteoblast has receptors for parathyroid hormone and the nucleus of the osteoblast has receptors for oestrogen. These cells originate from a bone marrow stromal cell or connective tissue mesenchymal cell.

OSTEOCLASTS

These are large, multinucleated cells which are found on bone-resorbing surfaces. They lie in small depressions called Howship's lacunae and have ruffled borders that are applied to the bone surface. The cytoplasm is vacuolated and the osteoclasts contain enzymes responsible for the resorption of bone. These enzymes are secreted into the extracellular bone-resorbing compartment which they acidify. As a result, the low pH dissolves the bone crystals and the enzymes degrade the exposed matrix, providing calcium and phosphate in the plasma and hydroxyproline from collagen in the urine (Chambers, 1985).

The osteoclast membrane contains calcitonin receptors but not parathyroid hormone receptors. The

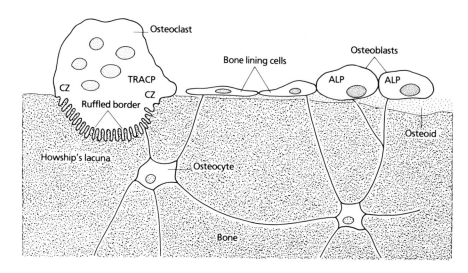

Fig. 14.1 Bone cell types. TRACP, tartrate-resistant acid phosphatase; CZ, clear zone; ALP, alkaline phosphatase. Reproduced from Martin *et al.* (1988) with permission.

osteoclast precursor is a cell of the mononuclear phagocyte system and is a bone marrow-derived cell. There is an interesting relationship between osteoblasts and osteoclasts, and it is thought that osteoblasts initiate osteoclastic bone resorption.

OSTEOCYTES

These are the most common type of cell found in bone and are of variable appearance. They are osteoblasts that become totally entrapped in the matrix being synthesized. The newly formed matrix becomes mineralized so that the osteocyte is surrounded by a mineralized wall. A characteristic of osteocytes is the presence of several long, tapering cell processes. The extension and fusion of these processes governs the formation of a canalicular network. There is disagreement about the function of this type of cell; however, they may be concerned with the passage of bone fluid through a canalicular system to allow mineral exchange, and to allow passage of substances that are concerned with regulation of osteoblast and osteoclast function.

BONE REMODELLING

This is a lifelong event. It is the skeletal process intimately related to mineral homoeostasis and probably serves to remove and replace effete bone. The remodelling sequence of bone (Fig. 14.2) is initiated by osteoclastic resorption (resorptive phase) followed by the absence of osteoclasts or osteoblasts (reversal phase). Subsequently, osteoblasts appear within the resorption bay (Howship's lacuna) and synthesize matrix (formative phase) until a new packet of bone called the osteon is produced.

In non-growing young adults the amounts of matrix resorbed and synthesized are in equilibrium. In older individuals, the amount of new bone is less than the amount removed, resulting in a net decrease in skeletal mass.

Matrix

The framework of the bone is known as the matrix, and it has both collagenous and non-collagenous constituents. Approximately 90% of the organic matrix of an adult bone is collagen and 10% is non-collagenous.

The collagen of the matrix has a complex chemical structure consisting of three polypeptide chains wound into a triple helix. Each chain contains approximately 1000 amino acids, and there are many genetically different collagens. Type I, which is low in carbohydrate, has fewer than ten hydroxylysine residues per chain and occurs only in bone. Each polypeptide chain is synthesized from the procollagen molecule within the fibroblasts or osteoblasts of bone. Collagen is broken down by collagenases to hydroxyproline and hydroxylysine, which are excreted in the urine. The stability of collagen decreases with age. The procollagen extension peptides may be measured in serum as a marker of bone formation.

The non-collagenous part of the matrix is mainly protein containing a number of different constituents. These substances are physiologically important. In immature bone the matrix is woven in arrangement, but as the bone matures it becomes lamellar in form. When unmineralized, the matrix is usually referred to as osteoid.

Table 14.1 shows the amounts of non-collagenous

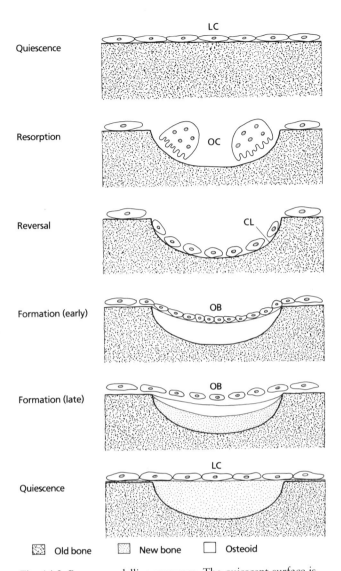

	LC
Quiescence	
Resorption	OC
Reversal	CL
Formation (early)	OB
Formation (late)	OB
Quiescence	LC

Old bone   New bone   Osteoid

Fig. 14.2 Bone remodelling sequence. The quiescent surface is covered by flat bone lining cells (LC). The resorption surface has osteoclasts (OC) lying in Howship's lacuna. In the reversal phase, uncharacterized mononuclear cells smooth the surface and deposit the cement line (CL). In early formation, osteoblasts (OB) deposit osteoid on the cement line. In late formation, mineralization has occurred between the cement line and the osteoid seam. Quiescence is restored at completion of the cycle, with bone lining cells (LC) on the surface. Reproduced from Martin *et al.* (1988) with permission.

Table 14.1 Representative values for the amount of non-collagenous proteins present in compact bone. The amounts given are composite representative values as a percentage of total non-collagenous protein and are based on amounts found in the compact bone of a number of species, including human, bovine and rabbit bone. Reproduced from Triffitt (1987) with permission

	Content (% w/w)
Sialoprotein	9
Bone Gla protein (osteocalcin)	15
Matrix Gla protein	2
Phosphoproteins	9
Osteonectin	23
Proteoglycans	4
Albumin	3
a_2HS-glycoprotein	5
Others	30

apatite surfaces, and the possibility of a role in mineralization has therefore been postulated. Serum levels of osteocalcin are elevated in some bone disease states, particularly those concerned with increased bone turnover and increased osteoblast function. This protein is related to other vitamin K-dependent proteins that are concerned with blood coagulation. More recently, a similar Gla protein has been identified, known as matrix Gla protein. Bone Gla protein and matrix Gla protein share some sequence homology but differ both in size and tissue distribution (Hauschka *et al.*, 1989).

Another bone protein, called osteonectin, is the most abundant non-collagenous bone protein. Osteonectin has a molecular weight of 32 000 Da and is found in developing bone and as a secretory product of cultured osteoblasts. It binds to calcium, mineral hydroxyapatite and collagen and is therefore also thought to be concerned with mineralization. The possible use of osteonectin in the assessment of patients with metabolic bone disease is unknown. Osteonectin is not bone specific and has been identified in platelets. Therefore, plasma for measurement of osteonectin has to be carefully prepared without platelet activation.

Bone mineral

Bone mineral may be amorphous or crystalline in form. Calcium and phosphate are initially deposited as calcium phosphate salts, which are subsequently transformed to hydroxyapatite crystals. These crystals are small and impure and are initially laid down between the collagen fibres of the bone matrix. The crystalline surface for exchange of other bone-seeking elements, e.g. strontium and lead, is very large. The area of the surface and the

proteins in compact bone. Two of the most important ones are bone Gla protein, also known as osteocalcin, and osteonectin (Triffitt, 1987).

Osteocalcin is a bone protein of molecular weight 6800 Da, containing three γ-carboxyglutamic acid (Gla) residues. This protein is synthesized by the osteoblasts, its synthesis being vitamin K-dependent. The function of osteocalcin is unclear, but the Gla residues bind to bone process of crystalline mineral exchange decrease with age. The exact mechanism of mineralization is still not fully understood but probably takes place in membrane bound vesicles (Russell *et al.*, 1986).

The interface between the pre-existing mineralized bone and the uncalcified osteoid is known as the calcification front. This is the site of active mineralization and intense phosphatase activity (Fig. 14.3). Tetracycline given to a patient before bone biopsy labels the site of active mineralization when bone is examined histologically. The osteoid begins to calcify about 10 days after deposition of mineral at the calcification front. Fast calcification of 50−70% of the osteoid takes place in the first few hours after deposition and slower calcification of 30−50% of the osteoid takes place over the next few months. Mineral is known to replace water in the bone matrix, but the mineralization of the osteoid is never fully complete. The rate of mineralization declines with age.

FUNCTION OF BONE

Bone has two main functions, which are biochemically and endocrinologically related. These are skeletal homoeostasis, involving the mechanical support and protection of the body, and mineral homoeostasis, which involves the maintenance of normal mineral metabolism.

Skeletal homoeostasis

This includes the control of bone growth, its maintenance by mechanical stress and remodelling of bone, in addition to the support and protection of the body. Bone develops in embryo in two environments: within membranes, such as the flat bones of the skull, and in the cartilage.

The majority of bones are formed in cartilage and are termed endochondral bones. This type of bone formation begins in a centre of ossification. The primary centre appears in the shaft of the bone and there are secondary centres in the epiphyses. The process of ossification involves vessels penetrating the cartilage followed by osteoblasts forming osteoid, which subsequently becomes mineralized. To allow for articulation and longitudinal growth, a small zone of cartilage is retained at the end of each bone between the epiphysis and metaphysis. At skeletal maturity this epiphyseal plate ossifies, the epiphyses close and growth in length ceases.

Skeletal growth and development differ widely in women compared with men, resulting in a variation in height, weight and frame size, which bears a relationship to the risk of osteoporotic fractures in women in later life. An appreciation of the concept of the development of peak bone mass, defined as the highest value of bone mass that an individual attains during a lifetime, is important. This is because of the loss of bone that accompanies ageing in women. The peak bone mass, as assessed by bone density measurements, is reached about 10 years after maximum height of the skeleton has been attained. Its value is influenced by genetic, environmental and mechanical factors (Fig. 14.4).

Black women have a higher bone density than white women, and there is a correlation between the bone density of mothers and that of their daughters. Genetic influences make a major contribution to variations in adult bone density. Environmental factors, e.g. dietary calcium intake, hormonal status, physical activity and body weight, interact to allow or prevent expression of the bone density genotype. Analysis of twin data suggests that a single gene or set of genes is responsible for this genetic effect.

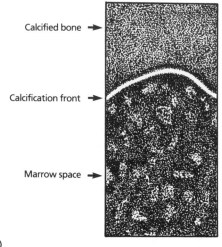

Calcified bone →

Calcification front →

Marrow space →

(a)

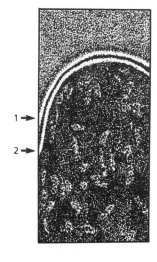

1 →

2 →

(b)

Fig. 14.3 Diagrams of two pieces of undecalcified iliac crest (magnification ×100). (a) A tetracycline fluorescent line labels active mineralization at the calcification front. (b) An additional effect of tetracycline given approximately 10 days later. Two lines (1) and (2) of mineralization are seen in (b).

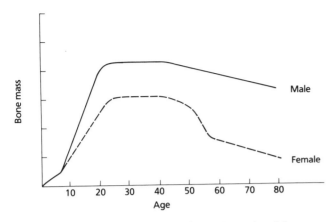

Fig. 14.4 Changes in bone mass with age. Reproduced from Cooper (1989) with permission.

Physical activity influences the growth and density of the skeleton. Animal studies have shown that bone responds to compression by increasing bone mass, and inactivity is associated with bone loss, as after bed-rest and space travel. The mechanism by which physical stimuli are transduced into a series of biological signals leading to bone remodelling is at yet undetermined.

After growth has stopped, internal remodelling of the bone continues by osteoclastic bone resorption followed by osteoblastic bone formation in a cyclical manner. Remodelling occurs at three distinct sites: the endosteal surfaces, causing changes in size of the marrow cavity, the Haversian systems and the periosteal surface of bone to increase the external diameter. Young healthy adults remodel 10% of their skeleton annually, and histologically the extent of active remodelling can be assessed by the number of osteoid borders and resorption cavities seen in the bone.

Bone remodelling is controlled by osteotropic growth regulatory factors such as transforming growth factor and insulin-like growth factors I and II generated locally in bone. These factors, which are important for the coupling of bone formation to bone resorption, promote chemotaxis of osteoblast precursors and enhance the formation of mineralized bone by the osteoblasts. Subsequently, secondary soluble signals are produced by the osteoblasts in response to mediators, e.g. interleukin 1, parathyroid hormone, tumour necrosis factor and 1,25-dihydroxycholecalciferol (1,25(OH)$_2$D$_3$). The identity of these signals is unknown, but they subsequently provoke the osteoclasts to resorb bone (Centralla and Canalis, 1985; Canalis *et al.*, 1988; Mohan and Baylink, 1991).

Mineral homoeostasis

The composition of bone is maintained by bone cells, which act under hormonal control. Because of the predominantly mineral composition of bone, this process is often referred to as mineral homoeostasis.

There is an important exchange of calcium between the bone tissue fluid and extracellular fluid. In an average adult, approximately 25 mmol (1 mmol = 40 mg) of calcium are taken in food each day, of which 5 mmol are absorbed and 20 mmol lost in the faeces. This absorbed calcium contributes towards the plasma calcium concentration, the normal value being 2.15−2.55 mmol/l, varying slightly for different methods and different laboratories. Calcium is present in the plasma as an ionized form (47%) and a protein-bound form (46%). In addition, a small amount is complexed to other substances. The total calcium value is therefore easily affected by changes in plasma proteins, particularly albumin, but it is the ionized calcium fraction that is important for stimulating changes in secretion of calcium-regulating hormones.

The circulating calcium in the plasma equilibrates with the calcium in the skeleton, which totals about 25 000 mmol. The exchange of calcium between bone fluid and extracellular fluid may be as great as 300 mmol/day, and each day approximately 250 mmol of calcium are filtered through the kidney. Reabsorption of 245 mmol takes place in the renal tubule, so that the urinary loss of 5 mmol/day of calcium equals the amount absorbed in the intestine. In a growing subject, however, more calcium is absorbed from the intestine than is excreted in the urine.

The metabolism of phosphate in the body is less well defined than that of calcium. It is absorbed in the upper part of the small intestine and excreted via the kidney. Certain forms of rickets and renal failure are associated with excess urinary loss of phosphate.

Three main hormones affect mineral metabolism: parathyroid hormone, vitamin D (cholecalciferol) and calcitonin. Other hormones that are known to affect bone, such as growth hormone, thyroxine, the sex hormones and adrenocortical hormones, act on skeletal rather than mineral homoeostasis. In addition, humoral substances, e.g. prostaglandins and osteoclast-activating factor, affect the composition of bone by a local action.

PARATHYROID HORMONE

This is a polypeptide hormone containing 84 amino acid residues and is secreted by the parathyroid gland. It has two precursor forms, namely a pre-prohormone and a prohormone whose functions are as yet unknown. The crucial part of the molecule for biological and hormone receptor activity is the 1–34 amino acid sequence. Parathyroid hormone is secreted in response to changes in ionized calcium concentrations in the blood and circulates in heterogeneous forms. These circulating forms are mainly *N*-terminal or *C*-terminal fragments of the hormone. The *N*-terminal fragments are the most active biologically and disappear from the circulation quickly, whereas the *C*-terminal fragments are biologically inactive and disappear from the circulation much more slowly (Fig. 14.5).

The hormone has three main actions:

1 It acts on bone to increase bone resorption, and therefore calcium is mobilized from bone to support the calcium concentration in the serum as necessary.

2 Parathyroid hormone acts on the kidney to increase phosphate clearance and decrease calcium clearance.

3 It acts as a trophic hormone for 1-hydroxylation in the kidney to produce 1,25 dihydroxycholecalciferol (Habener *et al.*, 1984).

At the cellular level parathyroid hormone activates the adenylate cyclase–cyclic AMP-protein kinase A cascade in the bone and kidney target cells. The parathyroid hormone receptor is a glycoprotein that trans-

duces extracellular signals by interacting with a specific GTP binding protein (termed G_s) which activates adenylate cyclase. Each G protein is composed of one distinct α-unit and a β-unit that is common to other G proteins. Patients with pseudohypoparathyroidism type 1a have reduced biological activity of the α-unit and the G_s protein (Fig. 14.6).

In 1989 parathyroid hormone-related protein (PTHrP) was isolated and cloned. This previously unrecognized hormone can reproduce all the essential features of the syndrome of humoral hypercalcaemia of malignancy. Eight of the first 13 amino acid residues of the molecule are homologous with those of parathyroid hormone, allowing it to act via the parathyroid hormone receptor. It therefore may produce hypercalcaemia, hypophosphataemia and an increased urinary cyclic AMP concentration. This peptide has been identified both in malignant and normal tissues, and it seems likely that it has a physiological role in fetal calcium metabolism (Orloff *et al.*, 1989; Fraser, 1989).

VITAMIN D

This refers to a group of fat-soluble sterols which are found in humans in two main forms: vitamin D_2, or ergocalciferol, which is made synthetically by irradiation of ergosterol from plants and vitamin D_3, or cholecalciferol, which occurs naturally. Vitamin D_2 is used to fortify foods, and vitamin D_3 occurs in foods such as fish and is synthesized in the skin by the action of ultraviolet light on 7-dehydrocholesterol via a thermolabile precursor.

The basic vitamin D molecule is a steroid with the B ring opened out. To attain physiological activity, the molecule is hydroxylated in the 25 position in the liver and in the 1 position in the kidney. The renal metabolite formed, $1,25(OH)_2D_3$ (Fig. 14.7) is the major active metabolite. It facilitates the absorption of calcium from the intestine and acts on bone to permit normal mineralization. This metabolite also has actions on the renal tubule and muscle. Both vitamins D_2 and D_3 are hydroxylated before action, but the D_3 metabolites are more active than those of D_2. Additional hydroxylated metabolites of vitamin D are well documented. They include 24,25-dihydroxycholecalciferol, the exact role of which is unclear. The formation of $1,25(OH)_2D_3$ occurs in response to changes primarily in serum phosphate and serum calcium concentration. For example, a low serum calcium value probably acts via parathyroid hormone to stimulate increased formation of $1,25(OH)_2D_3$, which increases intestinal calcium absorption (Reichel *et al.*, 1989).

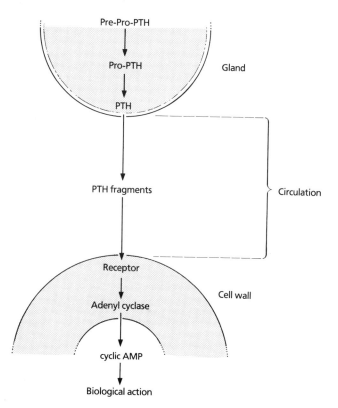

Fig. 14.5 The different forms of parathyroid hormone.

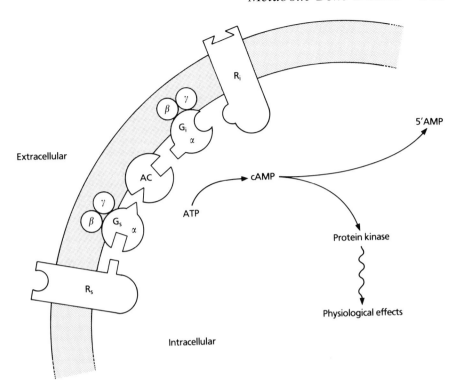

Fig. 14.6 Outline of the adenylate cylase system. R_s and R_i, stimulatory and inhibitory receptors; G_s and G_i, the stimulatory and inhibitory guanine nucleotide-binding regulatory proteins. AC denotes the catalytic unit adenylate cyclase. Reproduced from Levine (1993) with permission.

It is now known that the synthesis of $1,25(OH)_2D_3$ does not occur exclusively in the kidney. Ectopic $1,25(OH)_2D_3$ is produced in sarcoidosis and tuberculosis and during pregnancy when the placental and decidual cells synthesize this hormone. The mechanism of action of $1,25(OH)_2D_3$ is similar to that of other steroid hormones, and the steroid receptor complex either initiates the synthesis of specific RNA encoding proteins or mediates a selective repression of gene expression. The structure of the receptor shows homology with the DNA binding domain of the other steroid hormone receptors and the *V-erb A* oncogene.

The $1,25(OH)_2D_3$ receptor is expressed in many tissues not primarily related to mineral homoeostasis. Furthermore, $1,25(OH)_2D_3$ has an effect on the differentiation and proliferation of haematopoietic cells, and this function extends to an effect on the growth of certain cancer cells.

CALCITONIN

This is a polypeptide hormone containing 32 amino acid residues and which chemically contains an *N*-terminal disulphide bridge. It is secreted by the C cells of the thyroid gland which are derived from the neutral crest. Pharmacologically, it has a potent hypocalcaemic action due to inhibition of bone resorption. It also has an action on the renal tubule so that it produces hypo-

phosphataemia. In combination with other factors it exerts a regulatory effect on calcium balance and skeletal mass. It controls bone remodelling and the uptake, storage and excretion of calcium, particularly in situations involving high calcium demand, e.g. bone growth, pregnancy and lactation.

Calcitonin has been identified in several species and in these different forms has been used therapeutically. These drugs have a low level of toxicity and have been widely used in disorders of bone remodelling and bone loss (Azria, 1989).

METABOLIC BONE DISEASES

Classification

Metabolic bone diseases can be classified according to their basic abnormality of bone structure and function. Because the morphology and function of bone are so interrelated, however, a distinct classification is impossible. The main diseases may be grouped as follows:

1 Disorders of the matrix.
  (a) Congenital, e.g. osteogenesis imperfecta; Marfan's syndrome.
2 Disorders of the cells.
  (a) Imbalance between osteoblasts and osteoclasts, i.e. osteoporosis.
  (b) Overactivity of both cells, i.e. Paget's disease.

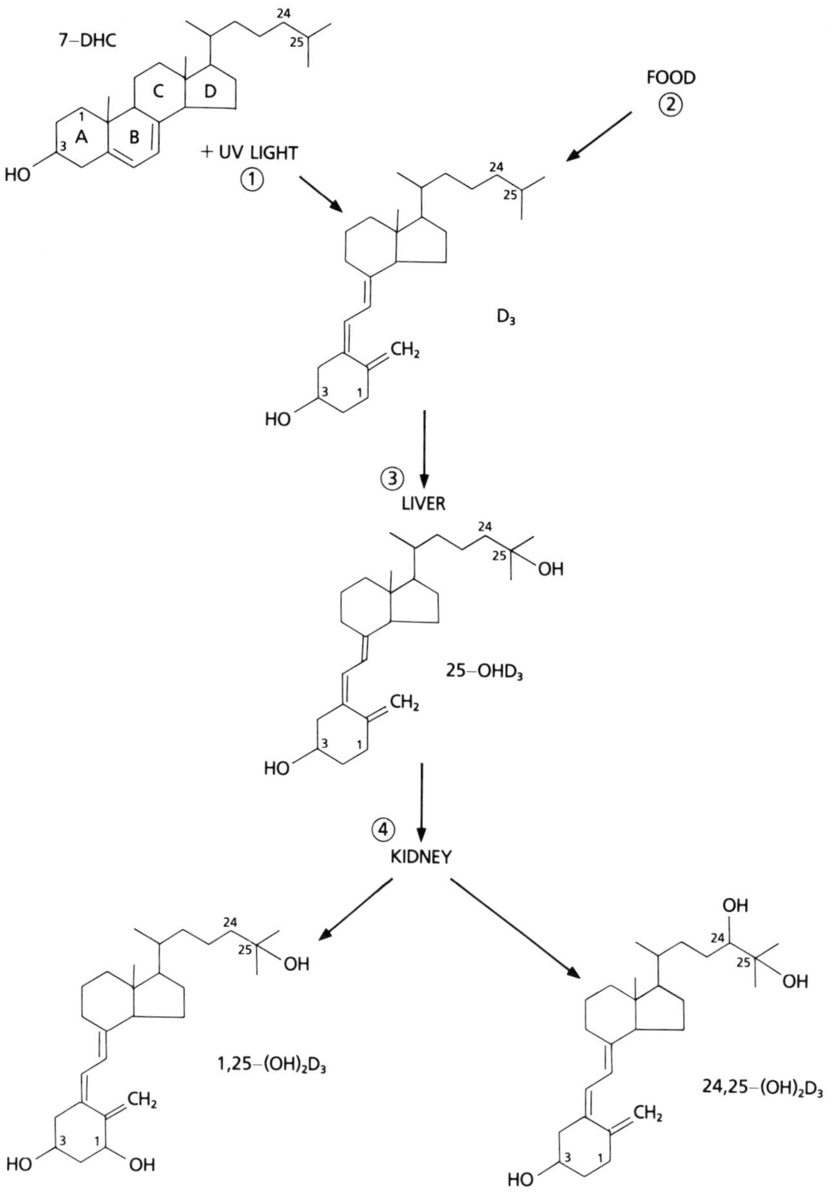

Fig. 14.7 Metabolic pathway of vitamin D. 7-DHC, 7-dehydrocholesterol; D_3, cholecalciferol; $25(OH)D_3$, 25-hydroxycholecalciferol; $1,25(OH)_2D_3$, 1,25-dihydroxycholecalciferol; $24,25(OH)_2D_3$, 24,25-dihydroxycholecalciferol. Numbers 1–4 indicate the sites at which clinical abnormalities may occur.

(c) Increased osteoclastic bone resorption, i.e. malignant hypercalcaemia.

(d) Decreased osteoclast activity, i.e. osteopetrosis.

3 Disorders affecting mineral metabolism.

(a) Abnormalities of vitamin D metabolism.

(b) Disorders of the parathyroid glands.

Congenital disorders of the bone matrix

These are inborn errors of metabolism affecting either the collagenous or the non-collagenous part of the matrix. These disorders may predominantly give skeletal manifestations, as in osteoporosis imperfecta, or present with skeletal manifestations which are a comparatively small part of a generalized clinical disorder, as in Marfan's syndrome, Ehlers–Danlos syndrome and the more uncommon disorders homocystinuria, alkaptonuria and Menkes' syndrome. The disorders affecting the non-collagenous part of the matrix are mainly confined to the mucopolysaccharidoses. With recent biochemical advances, the biochemical understanding and subsequent subtyping of all these disorders has become very complex. A detailed account of these syndromes is therefore beyond the scope of this chapter, but interested readers are referred to the textbooks in the list of further reading, as well as the following specific references: Prockop *et al.*, 1979; Pyeritz and McKusick, 1981; Prockop and Kivirikko, 1984; Sykes and Smith, 1985; Kreig *et al.*, 1988.

OSTEOGENESIS IMPERFECTA

This is a rare inherited disorder, also known as brittle bone disease, in which there is an abnormality in the synthesis or structure of type I collagen. The disorder is characterized by osteopenia, recurrent fracture, deformity and often abnormal teeth. Following recent biochemical and molecular studies, the disease may be classified into four main types. The essential features of each type are shown in Table 14.2. Children with osteogenesis imperfecta are of normal intelligence; the radiological findings are often very bizarre with gross bony deformities and thin bones, so that the whole shaft may appear cystic. Laboratory biochemical tests are usually normal, and there is no established medical therapy.

MARFAN'S SYNDROME

This is a dominantly inherited disorder now known to be caused by mutations in a single fibrillin gene on chromosome 15. It is characterized by skeletal deformity, arachnodactyly, dislocated lenses and aortic dilatation (Tsipouras *et al.*, 1992).

The skeletal abnormalities manifest as a very tall thin patient. This type of abnormality is particularly seen in the fingers, termed arachnodactyly. The chest may be deformed, the limbs long compared to the trunk and the palate high arched. In addition, the patients are loose jointed and have excessively long big toes. The main cause of death is aortic valve disease. There is very little that can be offered to improve the skeletal abnormalities.

HOMOCYSTINURIA

This is a rare, recessively inherited disorder resulting in deficiency of the enzyme cystathionine synthetase so that homocysteine accumulates, which seems to produce skeletal abnormalities. Patients with this disorder exhibit widespread vascular lesions, dislocation of the lenses, skeletal abnormalities and some degree of mental abnormality. The skeletal abnormalities resemble those of Marfan's syndrome, though the increased joint mobility is absent. The patients may have large hands and bones, fair hair and a malar flush. Diagnosis is confirmed by increased amounts of homocystine in the urine. Some patients respond to treatment with pyridoxine.

EHLERS–DANLOS SYNDROME

This is a rare disorder characterized by stretchy skin, fragility of the skin and joint laxity. It may give rise to dislocations and spinal malalignment. There are different subtypes according to the clinical features and biochemical aetiology.

MUCOPOLYSACCHARIDOSES

This term encompasses a group of disorders affecting the skeleton which are due to accumulation of mucopolysaccharides in the lysosomes. They are disorders of metabolic breakdown rather than of synthesis. The different syndromes have been classified according to the biochemical defect, but the best known are those

Table 14.2 Classification of osteogenesis imperfecta. Adapted from Scriver *et al.*, 1989

Type	Clinical features	Inheritance	Biochemical defects
I	Normal stature Blue seleras Hearing loss in 50%	Autosomal dominant	Decreased production of type I procollagen
II	Lethal in perinatal period with gross deformities	Autosomal dominant	Rearrangements in the the fibrillar collagen genes for procollagen I
III	Progressively deforming bones with moderate deformity at birth Very short stature	Autosomal recessive	Mutation preventing incorporation of α_2 chain into procollagen
IV	Normal scleras Mild-to-moderate bone deformity	Autosomal dominant	Point mutations in the α_2 chains

previously referred to by the names of Hurler, Hunter and Morquio. Hurler's syndrome is the most severe with dwarfism, a typical facies, snuffling, chest deformity and enlarged abdomen with hepatosplenomegaly. Radiology shows an abnormally shaped skull, enlarged flattened sella turcica, beaking of the vertebrae, kyphosis and abnormally shaped long bones. The radiological appearance of the phalanges is bullet shaped. Hunter's syndrome is a milder form of this disorder. Morquio's syndrome is particularly known for its orthopaedic features. The children are of normal intelligence, but become deformed and dwarfed. They have short necks, barrel chests, a flexed stance and knock knees.

Some of these patients excrete excess amounts of mucopolysaccharides in the urine. Therapy is being directed towards antenatal diagnosis or replacement of the appropriate enzymes concerned with mucopolysaccharide metabolism.

FIBROUS DYSPLASIA

This is a sporadic condition characterized by expanding fibrous lesions of bone forming mesenchyme. The lesions may be monostotic, when they develop in the second or third decade of life or polyostotic, when they occur before 10 years of age. The lesions cause fracture or deformity, and the skull and long bones are most often affected. The polyostotic form may be associated with café-au-lait spots and hyperfunction of one or more endocrine glands, when it is refered to as McCune–Albright syndrome. The bone lesions have a ground glass appearance on radiographs.

Osteoporosis

Osteoporosis is a common disorder of bone, particularly occurring in elderly patients. It was first documented in 3000 BC, but it was not until comparatively recently that the extent of the abnormality in older women has been fully appreciated (Cummings *et al.*, 1985).

The term osteoporosis has in the past been loosely used to include all states in which there is a reduction in the amount of calcified bone, regardless of whether or not it is associated with fractures. In addition, some clinicians incorrectly use the term osteoporosis synonymously with post-menopausal reduction in bone mass. It is therefore important to carefully define what is meant by osteoporosis. It should also be clearly differentiated from osteomalacia, in which there is a reduction in mineralization of the bone. Osteoporosis and osteomalacia may occur together in the elderly population of the UK.

DEFINITION

Osteoporosis is a term used to describe a state in which there is reduced bone mass for the appropriate age, sex and rate of an individual, and which is associated with a risk of fracture. Osteopenia is a term used to describe increased radiolucency seen on radiographs and which may occur in osteoporosis or osteomalacia. Some clinicians use the term osteopenia however, to describe the reduced bone mass that occurs as a prerequisite to osteoporosis. Osteoporosis may occur as an extension of the physiological reduction of bone mass that arises after the menopause, or less commonly may occur secondary to other disorders, e.g. Cushing's syndrome or corticosteroid therapy.

Histologically, osteoporotic bone is classically described as having a reduction in trabecular bone mass in relation to the total area of the histological section, with a normal ratio of mineral to organic bone matrix. Radiologically, osteoporotic reduction in bone mass is seen as increased radiolucency of the bones, particularly the vertebrae. Apart from the identification of fractures, however, the radiological definition of osteoporosis is relatively inaccurate as a loss of greater than 30% of bone mineral is apparently necessary before the trained radiologist can detect osteopenia. Reduction of bone mass is now more accurately detected by bone densitometry. At the Consensus Development Conference on the prophylaxis and treatment of osteoporosis in 1990, osteoporosis was defined as a disease characterized by low bone mass, microarchitectural deterioration of bone tissue leading to enhanced bone fragility, and a consequent increase in fracture risk (Consensus Development Conference, 1991).

BONE MASS AND OSTEOPOROSIS

The turnover of skeletal calcium varies with age, the gain in bone mineral content being most rapid during infancy and adolescence. Despite rapid bone formation at an earlier age in adolescent girls than in boys, there is a lower bone mass per kg body weight in young women than in young men. This may be a contributing factor to the higher incidence of osteoporosis in elderly women. Apart from the sex of the patient, other factors contributing to the degree of bone loss occurring in later life include diet, ethnic origin, socioeconomic status, physical activity and geographical environment. Bone loss is also age related. It is known that the bone of vertebral bodies begins to decrease at 25–30 years of age. The bone loss eventually affects most of the skeleton in all subjects, though the bone loss occurs earlier in women than in men. In women, bone loss is accelerated by the menopause. Tall subjects are also known to lose bone less rapidly than short subjects. Black people have more bone and a heavier skeleton at all ages than white people. There is decreased new bone formation in children and young adults from an impoverished environment compared with those from a better nourished environment.

Genetic factors may also be involved in the tendency to bone loss, as comparatively low levels of vertebral density have been observed in pre-pubertal children with XO gonadal dysgenesis, certain Chinese and Japanese children, Anglo-Saxon women and American Inuit. Childhood osteopenia is also associated with abnormal haemoglobinopathies and pseudo-pseudohypoparathyroidism. Polymorphism in the vitamin D receptor gene is responsible for up to 75% of the total genetic effect on bone density in healthy individuals (Morrison *et al.*, 1994).

The structural integrity of bone is influenced by external mechanical forces and skeletal muscle mass. Therefore, a relatively sedentary lifestyle probably contributes to the aging process of bone loss. In addition, age-related changes in the intestinal absorption of calcium and parathyroid hormone secretion may perpetuate the accelerated progressive decrease in osteoblast activity. This decrease in quantity of bone matrix with age correlates well with other clinical evidence of ageing in the connective tissues, e.g. the skin.

From the above information, the conclusion reached is that white, post-menopausal women are most at risk of developing osteoporosis. The risk is often enhanced by certain life styles, e.g. cigarette smoking and alcohol abuse. The last factors may act by affecting oestrogen metabolism or by directly suppressing osteoblast function.

AETIOLOGY

The most common type of osteoporosis is that found in post-menopausal women. Numerous other conditions, however, have been documented as being associated with osteoporosis. Clinically, osteoporosis may therefore be divided into primary and secondary types (Table 14.3). Although primary osteoporosis is particularly associated with the accelerated bone loss that occurs after the menopause, it is a multifactorial disorder. Thus, all women become menopausal, but not all women develop osteoporosis. The major risk factors for osteoporosis have now been identified (Table 14.4).

Involutional osteoporosis begins in middle age and may also be subdivided into two types (Table 14.5). The essential features of this subdivision suggest that the two types may have a different aetiology. Type I, or post-

Table 14.3 Classifications of causes of osteoporosis. Reproduced from Peck *et al.* (1987) with permission

Primary osteoporosis
Juvenile
Idiopathic (pre-menopausal women; middle-aged or young men)
Involutional osteoporosis

Secondary osteoporosis (partial list)
Endocrine diseases
  Hypogonadism
  Ovarian agenesis
  Hyperadrenocorticism
  Hyperthyroidism
  Hyperparathyroidism
  Diabetes mellitus
  Acromegaly

Gastrointestinal diseases
  Subtotal gastrectomy
  Malabsorption syndromes
  Chronic obstructive jaundice
  Primary biliary cirrhosis
  Severe malnutrition
  Anorexia nervosa
  Alactasia

Bone marrow disorders
  Multiple myeloma and related disorders
  Systemic mastocytosis
  Disseminated carcinoma

Connective tissue diseases
  Osteogenesis imperfecta
  Homocystinuria
  Ehlers–Danlos syndrome
  Marfan's syndrome

Miscellaneous causes
  Immobilization
  Chronic obstructive pulmonary disease
  Chronic alcoholism
  Chronic heparin administration
  Rheumatoid arthritis

Table 14.4 Major risk factors for primary osteoporosis. Reproduced from Peck *et al.* (1987) with permission

Age (advanced)
Sex (female)
Race (Caucasian and Asian)
Habitus (petite or thin)
Menopause (premature, surgically induced)
Family history (positive)
Lifestyle
  Cigarette smoking
  Alcohol abuse
  Physical exercise limited
  Calcium intake inadequate

Table 14.5 Types of involutional osteoporosis. Reproduced from Riggs and Melton (1983) with permission

	Type I	Type II
Age (years)	51–70	>70
Sex ratio (F/M)	6:2	2:1
Type of bone loss	Mainly trabecular	Trabecular and cortical
Rate of bone loss	Accelerated	Not accelerated
Fracture sites	Vertebrae (crush), distal radius	Vertebrae (multiple wedge), hip
Parathyroid function	Decreased	Increased
Calcium absorption	Decreased	Decreased
Metabolism of 25-hydroxy vitamin D to 1,25 dihydroxy vitamin D	Secondary decrease	Primary decrease
Main causes	Factors related to menopause	Factors related to ageing

menopausal osteoporosis, affects women soon after the menopause and often results in vertebral and Colles' fractures. This type is associated with microscopic changes of the trabecular plates and accelerated bone loss (Fig. 14.8) Type II, or ageing-associated, osteoporosis occurs in men and women aged 70 years or older and is associated with the slow phase of bone loss and hip fractures.

DIAGNOSIS

History

Patients with osteoporosis are often completely asymptomatic and give little evidence of widespread bone disease. Alternatively, a history of pain and/or loss of height may be elicited. The pain may be of two types. There may be localized pain associated with a vertebral fracture. This pain characteristically radiates anteriorly around the flank into the abdomen, legs, or pelvis. Alternatively, patients may complain of dull aching in the back, which is localized to a site slightly lateral of the vertebral column with no radiation. This pain is aggravated by sudden movements, e.g. sneezing, and is relieved by rest. Generalized skeletal pain and root pain are very uncommon in osteoporosis, and often the patient is completely asymptomatic despite a vertebral compression fracture. In addition, patients may complain of loss of height over the years, which is related to the vertebral compression as wedging of the vertebral bodies takes place.

Clinical features (Woolf and Dixon, 1988)

On examination, there may be tenderness localized to the area of deformed vertebrae. The main clinical findings, however, relate to the loss of stature due to vertebral compression and fracture. The patient's height is less than that found some years previously, if that is known. Accurate measurements of height are therefore an important guide to the progression of the osteoporosis. The diminished stature is accompanied by shortening of the trunk, so that the arms and legs appear disproportionately long. The reduction in suprapubic length means that the pubis to heel distance, minus crown to pubis distance, is greater than 5 cm. Also the pubis to heel distance remains 50% of the finger-tip span. Due to loss of height there is a lower dorsal kyphosis which is often termed the dowager's or widow's hump. Subsequently, as the spine compresses, there is a downward angulation of the ribs and significant narrowing of the normal gap between the lower ribs and iliac crest. This produces abdominal distension and prominent horizontal skin creases in an 'accordion'-like manner. There is a loss of the anterior lumbar curve producing a forward pelvic tilt associated with a shuffling unsteady gait. There is an increased incidence of fractures in patients with osteoporosis, particularly sited at the distal end of the radius and the femoral neck (Royal College of Physicians, 1989).

Some types of secondary osteoporosis deserve further comment.

Juvenile osteoporosis. Osteoporosis also occurs uncommonly in children and adolescents. It has certain unusual features that help to make the diagnosis. Patients

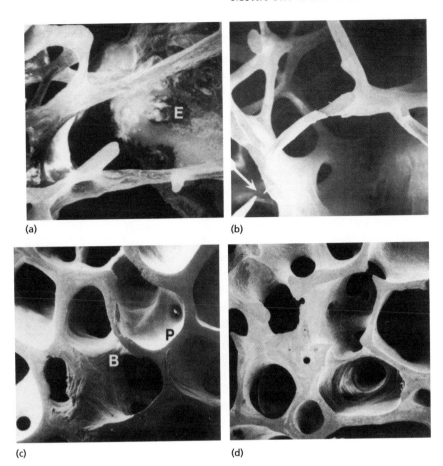

Fig. 14.8 (a, b) Low-power scanning electron micrographs of iliac crest biopsies from two women with osteoporosis, aged 61 and 47 years, respectively, with multiple vertebral compression fractures. Autopsy samples from (c) a 44-year-old normal man and (d) a 75-year-old normal woman who had suffered sudden death. Note that the lack of trabecular bone in the biopsy shown in (a) allows a clear view of the endosteal surface (E) of one of the cortices P, trabecular plate; B, trabecular bar. Field width, 2.6 mm in each case. Reproduced from Dempster *et al.* (1986) with permission.

commonly complain of pain at the ends of long bones, e.g. the ankle. There is reduced growth rate and later the typical spinal deformities of adult osteoporosis occur. Radiologically, the cortices of the bones are thin, and there may be partial fractures of the metaphyses. The vertebral changes may be difficult to differentiate radiologically from osteomalacia, and true fractures of the long bones are common. The disorder seems to be self-limiting. Some authors consider that juvenile osteoporosis is identical to juvenile epiphysitis, or Scheuermann's kyphosis, as these patients also present with wedge-shaped vertebrae and kyphosis.

Immobilization osteoporosis. This is a common form of osteoporosis which often goes unnoticed because it is asymptomatic and localized. It may occur in a generalized form following prolonged immobilization due to paralysis and has received more attention following the observation that astronauts produce changes in calcium balance after periods of weightlessness. There is controversy about the exact way in which bone tissue is lost in immobilization. It is known, however, that exercise stimulates bone formation, so with immobilization some essential stimulus to the osteoblast may be removed.

Corticosteroid-induced osteoporosis. Cushing's syndrome or long-term treatment with corticosteroids, as in asthma and connective tissue disorders, may produce osteoporosis. The corticosteroids suppress osteoblast function, block intestinal calcium absorption and increase urinary calcium excretion. This disorder particularly affects the axial skeleton. The relationship between dose and duration of therapy and clinical osteoporosis in patients on steroid therapy is unclear. There may also be osteoporosis of the skull, which is unusual in other forms of osteoporosis. Also, when fractures occur they heal with abundant callus formation giving a particular 'cotton-wool' appearance on radiographs. Prevention of this type of osteoporosis is obviously by reduction in the dose of corticosteroids, but this is not always possible (Smith, 1990).

SPECIAL INVESTIGATIONS

Pathology

The predominant feature of osteoporosis is the lack of abnormal haematological and biochemical findings. Classically, the serum calcium, phosphate and alkaline phosphatase, and urinary hydroxyproline values are normal. Elevation of serum alkaline phosphatase values only occur following fractures or when there is associated osteomalacia in the same patient. More recently, research into the aetiology of osteoporosis has shown that there may be abnormally low values of serum 1,25(OH)$_2$D$_3$ in patients with osteoporosis (Riggs and Melton, 1983).

Radiology

It is often difficult for even a very experienced radiologist to differentiate osteoporosis from normal, age-related bone loss and from other disorders, e.g. osteomalacia. Apart from the assessment of spinal deformities and detection of fractures and vertebral wedging, radiology as a diagnostic tool in osteoporosis has largely been superseded by measurement of bone mineral density. Some specific radiological findings, however, are landmarks of osteoporosis. In the vertebrae there is accentuation of end-plate shadows (Fig. 14.9), with preservation of the vertebral trabeculae of the bone and with biconcave compression of one or more vertebrae (Fig. 14.10) with expansion of the intervertebral discs. Erosion of the cortex of the bone is rare. As the disease process

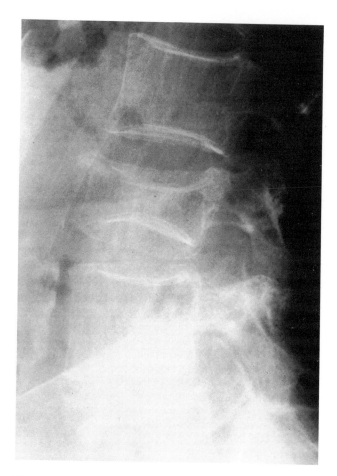

Fig. 14.10 Concave osteoporotic lumbar vertebrae.

progresses, pressure of the intervertebral discs may produce localized herniations into the vertebral body, giving rise to Schmorl's nodes. Progression of the osteopenia leads to wedging or compression fracture of a vertebral body. This is particularly seen on radiographs of the thoracic spine. It is important to note that in the radiological vertebral wedging seen in osteoporosis, the apex of the wedge is usually anterior.

Radiological examination of peripheral bones may show cortical thinning with the appearances of diffuse demineralization. In the pelvis and femora, however, there is usually a thin rim of well-mineralized cortex and decreased trabecular bone. There may be less osteophytosis than usual for the age of the patient and a relative increase in calcification of the aorta compared with the radiolucency of the bones.

An index of the severity of the osteoporotic process may be obtained by measuring the cortical thickness of the femur, metatarsal, metacarpal or phalangeal bones and comparing the thickness of both cortices. If it is less than 45% of the width of the shaft of the bone, this is evidence of significant osteopenia.

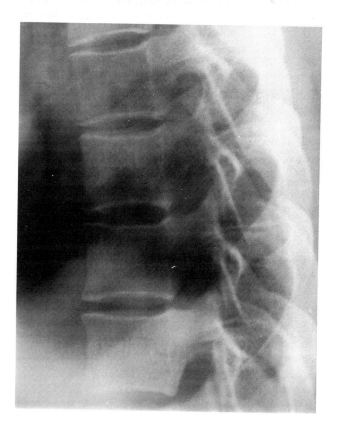

Fig. 14.9 Accentuation of the end-plate shadows of vertebral bodies in osteoporosis.

Bone densitometry

Measurement of bone density is becoming an essential procedure in the diagnosis and treatment of osteoporosis. At specialized centres or in health screening clinics, bone density measurements can determine whether the bone density is below that expected for a patient with respect to age, sex, race and weight of the subject. Patients with below-normal bone density may therefore be at risk of developing osteoporosis, or if fractures are already present have the diagnosis confirmed (Fig. 14.11). In addition, serial measurements are useful to assess the response to treatment (Johnston *et al.*, 1989).

TREATMENT

Significant advances in the management of patients with osteoporosis have been made over recent years. This aspect of osteoporosis may be considered under three categories: prevention, treatment of those at risk and those with overt osteoporosis.

The prevention of osteoporosis is largely achieved by ensuring that women, particularly when young, develop a high peak bone mass by means of a diet adequate in calcium coupled with exercise and avoidance of risk factors, e.g. smoking and an excess alcohol intake. There is some evidence that oestrogen in the oral contraceptive pill may provide some protection against osteoporosis. Subsequently, peri-menopausal women or those with positive risk factors, e.g. a family history or corticosteroid therapy, should be offered a bone mineral density measurement. If the value is greater than 1 SD below normal, they should be offered hormone replacement therapy at the menopause. If the result is within 1 SD of normal the measurement should be repeated in 3 years' time. Women receiving hormone replacement therapy should have annual mammography and thorough investigation of any abnormal vaginal bleeding. Patients usually begin on low-dose oestrogen preparations (conjugated oestrogen, 0.625 mg/day for 26 days) with a progestagen on days 15−26 of the month, and continue for at least 5 years. Trials of a combined oestrogen−progesterone preparation are in progress to avoid menstrual bleeding. Hormone replacement therapy is contraindicated in women who have had carcinoma of the breast.

Some patients with overt osteoporosis with fractures are suitable for hormone replacement therapy if they are within 10 years of the menopause. If not, and if there is pain associated with the fractures, treatment with other antiresorptive drugs is now very promising. Calcitonin has been widely used by injection, and trials of intranasal preparations are now in progress. The drug has the added advantage of producing a central pain-relieving effect as well as preventing further bone loss. In addition, 3-monthly cyclical regimens of oral bisphosphonates (disodium etidronate) and calcium are also being investigated. Although fluoride stimulates bone formation, its place in the treatment of osteoporosis remains controversial because of the incidence of side-effects when used at a high dose. A minimum intake of calcium, 800 mg/day, is recommended for all adult women, increasing to 1500 mg/day after the menopause if possible (Avioli and Heaney, 1991).

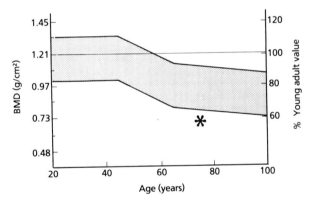

Fig. 14.11 Bone density result (using LUNAR dual energy X-ray absorptiometry) on a 76-year-old woman with vertebral osteoporosis. Diagram shows mean bone mineral density (BMD) (g/cm²) for L2−L4 compared to % of young adult reference range which is the expected peak bone mass for a subject 20−40-years-old, of the same sex and nationality. The patient value shown (*) is 0.667 g/cm² which is less than 60% of 4 SD below the young adult peak value. The fracture risk doubles with each decrease of 1 SD. Therefore this patient has a risk of fracture 16 times greater than that of a young adult female. The tinted area on the diagram shows the change in BMD with age (mean ± 1 SD). The patient value is 71% of that expected of her age. (Reproduced by courtesy of Mrs E. Thomas, St. Mary's Hospital, Bone Densitometry Unit, London.)

Paget's disease

Paget's disease was first described by Sir James Paget in 1877. It is a disorder that produces focal enlargement and deformity of the skeleton and was originally thought to be an inflammatory disorder, being termed osteitis deformans. It is characterized by excessive bone resorption and subsequent excessive bone formation due to overactivity of bone osteoclasts and osteoblasts. The disorder may be monostotic or polyostotic.

INCIDENCE

Many patients are asymptomatic, so that accurate studies

of the incidence of the disorder are difficult to find. Autopsy studies, however, reveal an incidence of approximately 3.5% in England, though a great variation in the incidence has been reported throughout the world. Paget's disease occurs most commonly in Great Britain, Australia, New Zealand and Germany, and is rare in India, China, Japan, the Middle East, Africa and Scandinavia. It occurs particularly in middle-aged and elderly subjects, men being affected more than women. The incidence of the disorder increases with age, so that by 80 years of age the incidence may reach approximately 10%. The disorder sometimes occurs in more than one member of a family.

AETIOLOGY

Although the disease was originally thought to be inflammatory in origin, for many years the aetiology of the gross bone resorption and new bone formation has been ill-understood. At least 20% of patients have positive family histories, and genetic analysis suggests an autosomal dominant pattern of inheritance. There is ethnic and geographic clustering, so that for example in Lancashire, UK, 6.3–8.3% of subjects over 55 years of age in several towns have signs of Paget's disease on radiographs. It is also possible that Paget's disease has a viral aetiology. Inclusions that resemble viral nucleocapsids have been described in the nuclei and cytoplasm of osteoclasts of pagetic sites. The virus particles resemble members of the paramyxovirus family, e.g. respiratory syncytial virus or measles virus.

DIAGNOSIS

History

Patients with Paget's disease may be completely asymptomatic, particularly if only a monostotic form of the disease is present. In more extensive forms of the disorder, however, the patient may complain of crippling deformities, pain, exhaustion due to secondary effects on the vascular system, and symptoms related to nerve compression, e.g. deafness. The pain is usually dull and boring in nature. It is related to the site of the disease. If present in the pelvis and vertebrae, the pain is exacerbated by weight-bearing and is worse at night. Very occasionally it is sharp and radiating. The pain may be related to stretching of the nerve endings in the periosteum of the enlarging bone or to stimulation of nerve endings in the hyperaemic marrow. Pain may also be related to microfractures in the pagetic bone, or to other disorders of joints, e.g. osteoarthritis, that occur simultaneously in the same patient.

Clinical features

On examination there may be severe deformities of the skeleton, particularly affecting the skull, pelvis and legs. The skull may be enlarged, particularly in the occipital and frontal regions, as noted by measuring the circumference. This is due to increased thickness of the bony cortex of the skull. The enlarged bones often give obvious facial deformities and sometimes the increased weight of the head makes it difficult for the patient to hold the head erect. In addition, the pagetic bony remodelling weakens the base of the skull so that there may be collapse onto the cervical spine. There may be deafness and abnormalities of balance when the temporal bone is involved, by direct involvement of the inner ear or compression of the eighth nerve. Visual abnormalities due to optic nerve compression are rare. Enlargement or deformity of the jaw may cause severe displacement of the teeth and other dental problems. Involvement of the vertebrae can produce neurological signs from neural compression, and also difficulty in walking and paraparesis. The tibia and fibula are commonly involved in Paget's disease, the tibia being anteriorly and laterally bowed. Signs of Paget's disease in the upper extremities are comparatively rare.

Two main complications may occur in this disorder: fractures and malignancy. Fractures are characteristically transverse and may not be necessarily complete. An incomplete fissure fracture need not result from trauma and often is a precursor of a complete fracture, e.g. in the tibia or femur. The femoral fractures are often subtrochanteric, in contrast to those of the femoral neck seen in older subjects without Paget's disease.

A malignant change in pagetic bone may occur in as many as 10% of patients with polyostotic disease. Of patients over 40 years of age found to have bone sarcoma, 20% have Paget's disease. The sarcoma usually presents with pain and swelling in bone that is already pagetic. In contradistinction to the distribution of the basic disease, sarcomas are not uncommonly found in the humerus. The tumours are of varying histological type and herald a very poor prognosis for the patient. One unusual type of sarcoma, giant cell tumour, usually involves the calvarium or facial bones and carries a much better survival rate than other histological types of sarcoma.

Some other complications of Paget's disease are worthy of mention. Extramedullary haemopoiesis may occur either in the reticuloendothelial system, e.g. the spleen, or in other sites, e.g. the thymus and kidneys. Some patients may have hypercalciuria and are therefore likely to form renal calculi. In the osteolytic and mixed phases of the disorder there is a marked increase in blood flow through involved extremities. This is due to increased perfusion of pagetic bone, and as a result there is an elevated skin temperature over the affected areas. In elderly patients with generalized disease, cardiac output is also increased to such an extent that congestive cardiac failure may occur. Arterial calcification is commonly found in patients with Paget's disease, and intracardiac calcification is more common than normal. There is an association between pseudoxanthoma elasticum and Paget's disease, supporting the view that there might be a widespread disorder of connective tissue.

INVESTIGATIONS

Pathology

Biochemical investigations of patients with even generalized Paget's disease show normal concentrations of serum calcium, phosphorus and parathyroid hormone. Urinary calcium excretion is only increased if there are fractures or immobilization of the patient. The values obtained for both serum and urinary hydroxyproline are increased, and the amount of urinary hydroxyproline excreted correlates with the extent of the Paget's disease. In addition, elevation of serum alkaline phosphatase activity is characteristically seen in this disease. The values obtained may be astronomically high, are of bony origin and correlate well with the urinary hydroxyproline concentration. The patients with the highest levels of the serum alkaline phosphatase activity, e.g. greater than ten times the upper limit of normal, typically have involvement of the skull.

Histological examination of pagetic bone shows three different pictures according to the progression and phase of the disease. In the first, or 'hot', phase there is osteolysis and intense resorption of the existing bone. Multinucleated osteoclasts are found in large numbers at the bones surfaces. The bone resorbed is replaced by fibrous tissue. In the second, or mixed, phase spicules of bone are deposited in a disorganized fashion. The osteoclasts become less numerous, and more osteoblasts are seen associated with the newly formed bone in a mosaic pattern. In the third, or 'cold', phase bone formation is dominant with the presence of numerous osteoblasts. The new bone that is formed is disorganized and weak.

Radiology

Radiological evidence of Paget's disease is typically seen in the skull, vertebrae, pelvis and lower limbs. In the skull the disorder produces two major patterns. The earliest of these, which may often be asymptomatic, has been called osteoporosis circumscripta. The absorption of the inner and outer tables of the skull gives rise to circumscribed radiolucent areas. The second pattern occurring later shows deposition of new bone in a patchy fashion among the radiolucent areas. In addition, particularly the frontal and occipital bones show a dense and enlarged radiological appearance. Gradually, the whole of the calvarium becomes thickened and the classic 'cotton-wool' appearance on the skull radiograph is seen (Fig. 14.12).

As mentioned above, the enlarged skull may affect the cervical spine; a radiograph of the base of the skull may therefore show platybasia. In the lumbosacral spine, the vertebral bodies may be enlarged with thick margins and central, coarse, vertical striations. The height of a vertebral body may be significantly decreased and the spine is not uniformly affected. The radiological changes seen in the extremities show deformity with increased bone density (Fig. 14.13).

When complications occur, the fractures are characteristically transverse. Incomplete microfissures are often seen before a complete fracture. Bone scans are the most sensitive means of identifying pagetic sites; however, the scan is non-specific and may be positive in degenerative disease or with metastatic lesions.

TREATMENT

Most patients with Paget's disease do not require treatment because they are asymptomatic; however, there

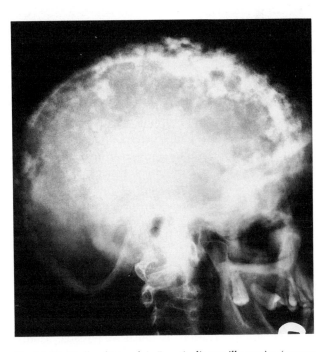

Fig. 14.12 Skull radiograph in Paget's disease illustrating 'cotton-wool' appearance.

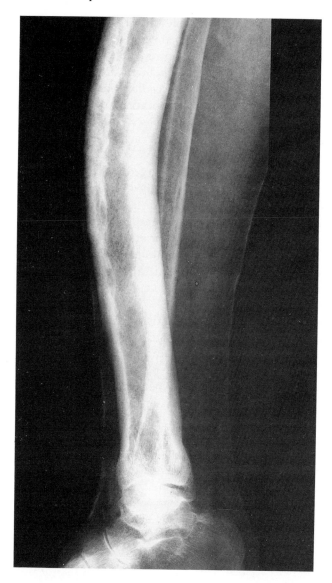

Fig. 14.13 Extensively deformed tibia in Paget's disease.

are certain definite indications for treatment. These include severe bone pain corresponding to areas of pagetic bone, cardiac failure, hypercalcaemia and recurrent renal calculi as a result of Paget's disease. It is debatable whether features such as multiple fractures, skeletal compression of nerve tissue, extensive disability due to the disease and the prevention of malignant change definitely warrant treatment.

Various types of treatment have been tried, some with a considerable measure of success. The pain may be initially controlled by simple analgesics, and orthopaedic surgery may be required when gross distortion of the bone gives rise to compression symptoms. It is essential to avoid immobilization as much as possible as this predisposes to hypercalcaemia and hypercalciuria.

Two major types of agent are available to suppress disease activity. These are calcitonin and bisphosphonates. Calcitonin acts directly on osteoclasts to reduce bone resorption and may be given as porcine, salmon, or human calcitonin by intramuscular or subcutaneous injection. It also has a pain-relieving effect. Trials using an intranasal preparation are in progress. The bisphosphonates are analogues of pyrophosphate and inhibit bone resorption by binding to hydroxyapatite crystals and inhibiting their growth and dissolution. Five different types of bisphosphonates have been tested clinically, e.g. disodium etidronate which is given orally. The newer compounds, which do not impair calcification of newly formed bone, are more potent and can be given intravenously.

Disorders associated with abnormalities of vitamin D

It has been known since the early part of this century that rickets is a disease due to a dietary deficiency, and Chick *et al.* (1922) showed the curative effect of sunlight, artificial ultraviolet light and cod-liver oil in children with rickets after the First World War. For many years it was thought that the antirachitic substance was vitamin D itself, and it was not until comparatively recently that the beautiful metabolic pathway for vitamin D was discovered. This has clarified the cause of many of the different types of bone disease associated with lack or resistance to vitamin D.

Clinical abnormalities associated with disorders of the supply or metabolism of vitamin D are predominantly deficiency states. Hypervitaminosis D is a rare condition and presents with clinical signs and symptoms of hypercalcaemia long before any evidence of bone disease is observed. Hypovitaminosis D is due to many causes (Fig. 14.7, p. 362), and deficiency may arise at several sites in the vitamin D metabolic pathway. Initially, the clinical features of vitamin D-deficient bone disease will be described, together with information on the investigations and diagnosis. Later in the chapter details pertinent to different aetiological types of vitamin D deficiency are given (p. 375).

The clinical manifestations of hypovitaminosis D fall into two distinct types depending on whether the patient is still growing or not. These are rickets in children and osteomalacia in adults, though they are essentially the same disorder.

RICKETS

In rickets the failure of calcification due to vitamin D deficiency is most severe in the parts of the skeleton where bone growth is most rapid, e.g. the metaphyses of the long bones. The growth rates of particular bones vary with age; at birth the skull grows fast, during the first year of life growth is most rapid in the upper limbs and ribs, and after 2 years of age growth in the legs is fast. These anatomical variations in bone growth velocity determine the sites of the clinical deformities produced in rickets. In order to compensate for the vitamin D deficiency secondary hyperparathyroidism occurs. Deformities arising before the age of 4 years largely correct themselves if the rickets heal, but deformities occurring after the age of 4 years usually remain permanent, e.g. short stature or bow legs (Fig. 14.14). Sometimes rickets is only manifest at puberty in conjunction with the growth spurt. The adult manifestations of vitamin D deficiency, such as Looser's zones, are very rarely seen in children.

Clinical features

The clinical findings depend on whether the child is examined early in the development of the disease or seen later, when the clinical features are much more severe and deformities marked.

Early rickets presents with overproduction of cartilage at the metaphysis, so that there are hard fusiform swellings at the bone ends, e.g. the wrists. Pain is uncommon at this stage except in the knees on weight-bearing.

More severe rickets shows bony deformities and a myopathy affecting muscle function. In the early months of life the skull is deformed with frontal bossing and posterior flattening where the child's head has been resting on the pillow. Later, at about 1 year of age, there is bilateral collapse of the chest wall giving Harrison's sulcus and also swelling of the ends of the ribs causing a 'rickety rosary'. After attempting to walk the rachitic child develops bow legs and knock knees.

The myopathy of severe rickets is seen in infants who on examination are weak and floppy. In older children a proximal myopathy is observed involving the hips and shoulders, so that there is a waddling gait, difficulty in walking upstairs and in raising the arms above the head. It quickly responds to treatment in 2−3 weeks.

Investigations

The serum calcium and phosphate concentrations are reduced quite early in the disorder, the phosphate reduction being partly due to the secondary hyperparathyroidism. In addition, there is elevation of serum alkaline phosphatase activity from osteoblast hyperactivity. In children, care must be taken to interpret alkaline phosphatase values in comparison with an age-matched normal range. Vitamin D deficiency, regardless of its aetiology, produces a generalized aminoaciduria in children and the serum 25-hydroxy vitamin D value is often low.

The radiological findings in rickets are characterized by a widening of the growth plate and an irregular appearance at the end of the metaphysis. These are manifest by a cupping concavity at the ends of long bones, e.g. the ulnar (Fig. 14.15). The radiological changes may fluctuate, so that the lesions may heal and recur successively giving Harris lines of arrested growth and transverse regions of irregular bone structure. If the rachitic changes are very severe, undercalcified subperiosteal bone tissue gives the shafts of the long bones a fuzzy outside margin surrounded by a fine line of periosteum. In children the signs of secondary hyperparathyroidism are irregular erosions of subperiosteal bone around certain metaphyses, particularly the femoral neck, medial side of the proximal humeral ends and other regions of maximal bone remodelling. The bone cysts and subperiosteal erosions in the phalanges seen in

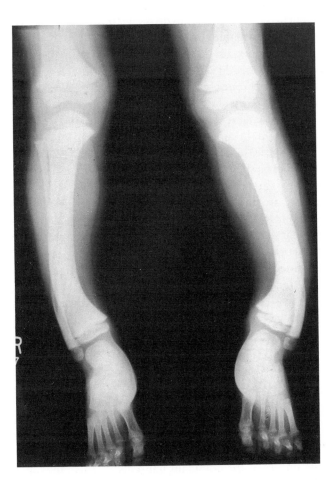

Fig. 14.14 Permanent deformity in healed rickets.

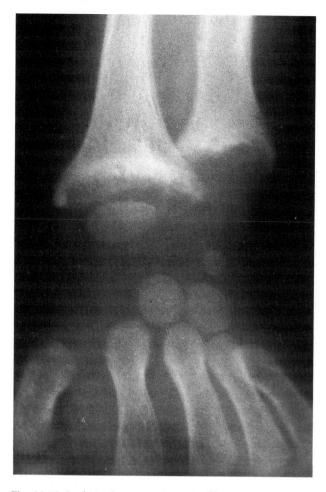

Fig. 14.15 Rachitic changes at the ends of the radius and ulnar.

adults due to hypersecretion of parathyroid hormone are not usually seen in children.

OSTEOMALACIA

This is often difficult to diagnose clinically, because the slow turnover of bone in adults compared with the growing bone of children gives rise to less definite signs. Clinical signs of disorders known to be associated with osteomalacia, however, may give a clue, indicating the need for a careful search for osteomalacia.

Clinical features

Patients may complain of generalized pain that disappears on lying still and can be elicited by pressure, coughing, or turning. Pain occurs particularly in the lumbar vertebrae, causing low back pain which may extend to the ribs and lower limbs. Involvement of the spine may cause kyphosis. The proximal myopathy seen in adult osteomalacia may produce muscle weakness, stiffness and difficulty in walking that is so severe that the patient is thought to have a neurological disorder. Osteomalacia may occur as a sequel to childhood rickets, in which case the patient will be short. Very occasionally the associated hypocalcaemia may be so severe as to cause symptoms of tetany. Clinical features of a disorder accompanying osteomalacia, e.g. malabsorption and renal failure, should not be forgotten.

Investigations

The biochemical changes in adult osteomalacia are often less clear than those in patients with rickets. The serum calcium level may be normal or low, the phosphate level normal or low and the alkaline phosphatase activity raised. Elevated alkaline phosphatase values of non-bony origin, particularly in the elderly, should be excluded by isoenzyme estimations or other biochemical measurements. In addition, values for serum 25-hydroxy vitamin D may be low, depending on the site of abnormality producing vitamin D deficiency. Measurements of serum 1,25-dihydroxy vitamin D are not yet generally available for clinical practice.

The radiological findings are characterized by Looser's zones, or pseudo- or Milkman's fractures. These are ribbon-like zones of rarefaction or demineralization occurring particularly in the shafts of long bones, pubic rami and lateral edge of the scapula (Figs 14.16, 14.17 and 14.18). In contrast to the multiple microfractures of Paget's disease, Looser's zones occur on the concavity of long bones such as the femur and are wider and usually single. The bones otherwise appear normal, and these zones are thought to be traumatic in origin. If the osteomalacia is of long standing and severe, other radiological signs may be apparent. These are an alteration of vertebral shape so that the bodies are uniformly and symmetrically squashed into a biconcave contour, often referred to as codfish vertebrae. There may be bending of the shafts of the long bones and in extreme cases the pelvis may be pushed in at the sacrum and both acetabular causing a triangular 'trefoil' shape.

In contrast to rickets, secondary hyperparathyroidism is often seen in severe osteomalacia. Subperiosteal erosions, particularly on the radial side of the middle phalanges of all the fingers, are commonly observed. At a later stage, if the erosions affect the terminal phalangeal shaft, collapse of the bone occurs causing pseudo-clubbing. The changes in the phalanges affect the working fingers of the dominant hand most. There may also be cysts in the long bones, erosion of the vault of the

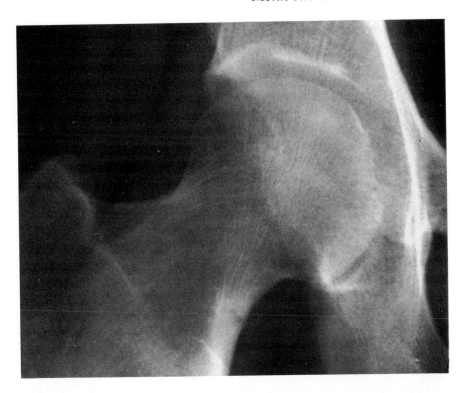

Fig. 14.16 Looser's zone on the femoral neck in osteomalacia.

skull and a widening of the spaces at the pubic and sacroiliac joints.

Bone biopsy and histological examination of bone are not necessary for the routine diagnosis of rickets and osteomalacia. In elderly subjects, in whom it may be difficult to diagnose osteomalacia without direct examination of the bone, there is a place for bone biopsy to differentiate between osteomalacia and osteoporosis. In osteomalacia there is excess osteoid due to defective mineralization of the matrix (Fig. 14.19).

SPECIAL TYPES OF RICKETS AND OSTEOMALACIA

Additional information is useful when trying to determine the aetiology of this type of bone disease.

Nutritional rickets and osteomalacia

This type of bone disease occurs in the UK, particularly in the elderly and in the Asian immigrant population. Although usually referred to as nutritional, the disorder is probably multifactorial in origin.

The elderly are often housebound or frail, so that they are unable to go out in the sunshine on their own, and in addition often take a diet with a low vitamin D content. Up to 30% of elderly patients with fractures of the neck of the femur have osteomalacia. Often elderly patients have a mixed picture of osteomalacia and osteoporosis.

It is important to diagnose the osteomalacia component of this bone disease, because at the present time osteomalacia is more easily treated than osteoporosis.

Immigrant patients also show a combination of poor dietary vitamin D intake and defective cutaneous synthesis of cholecalciferol. Asian women often stay at home indoors more than native British women of a comparable age, and in addition many Asian immigrants eat their native diet which includes chapattis. Chapatti flour has a high phytate content which decreases calcium absorption from the intestine. The exact efficiency of skin synthesis of vitamin D in coloured races is unclear, and it is interesting to note that it is the Asian, not the West Indian, immigrants who usually present with osteomalacia or rickets. The major risk factor for the migrant population is the drastic reduction in solar exposure coupled with the persistence of a very low vitamin D intake.

Gastrointestinal and biliary disorders

Gastrointestinal disorders may be associated with impaired absorption of calcium and also of vitamin D and its metabolites. Symptoms related to the underlying malabsorption syndrome may not always be obvious, and the bone disease may be the only presenting manifestation of an occult malabsorption syndrome.

Rickets and osteomalacia may occur with any of the

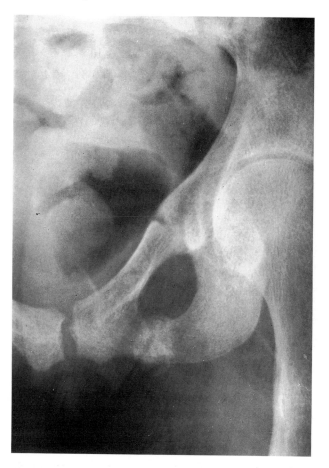

Fig. 14.17 Looser's zones in the pubic rami of a patient with post-gastrectomy osteomalacia.

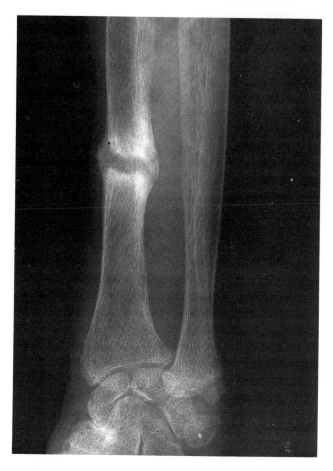

Fig. 14.18 Fracture in the radius of an elderly woman with osteomalacia.

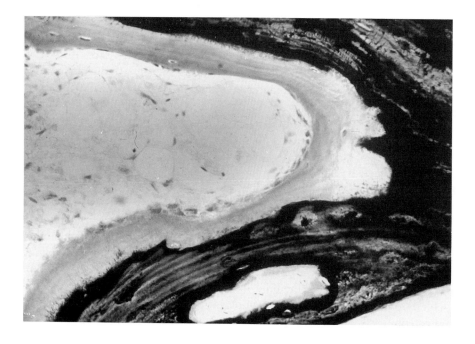

Fig. 14.19 Histological section of bone biopsy in osteomalacia. Dark mineralized trabecular bone and a wide area of uncalcified osteoid are shown.

recognized forms of malabsorption syndrome. Bone disease is uncommon in pancreatic disease, however, but is found in up to 50% of patients with gluten-sensitive enteropathy. Children with this disorder also have delayed puberty, a hypochromic microcytic anaemia that is unresponsive to iron, and show an atrophic mucosa on a small intestinal biopsy. Osteomalacia following gastrectomy is much more common than is generally appreciated. This may be due to poor dietary intake or self-imposed restrictions of dairy products to avoid diarrhoea and dumping syndrome, rapid transit of food, impaired absorption of vitamin D and calcium, and phosphate depletion due to excessive use of phosphate-binding antacids.

In biliary cirrhosis in adults and biliary atresia in children, bone disease is common and low serum 25-hydroxy vitamin D values are often found. In chronic alcoholism the bone disease observed is usually due to a direct effect of alcohol on bone rather than to the liver disease *per se*. Also in liver disease in general, the bone disorder is more likely to be osteoporotic in type rather than osteomalacia (Compston, 1986).

Renal bone disease

For many years the term 'renal rickets' has been used to describe the association of rickets with renal disease of some kind. As knowledge of renal and bone disease has advanced, the use of the term 'renal rickets' has led to considerable aetiological confusion. The use of this term should now be abolished.

Renal bone disease is of two broad types depending on whether the aetiology involves primarily the renal tubule or the renal glomerulus, designated as renal tubular osteodystrophy and renal glomerular osteodystrophy, respectively. Renal tubular osteodystrophy is not necessarily associated with abnormalities of vitamin D metabolism, but because of its close clinical association with rickets and osteomalacia, it will be described after renal glomerular osteodystrophy.

Renal glomerular osteodystrophy. This is often simply referred to as renal osteodystrophy and may be associated with all forms of pathology causing chronic renal failure. In this disorder there is a failure of production of $1,25(OH)_2D_3$ and phosphate retention. The basic abnormalities in chronic renal failure that affect the bones are an acquired impairment of intestinal calcium absorption, secondary hyperparathyroidism and defective maturation of osteoid and mineral parts of the skeleton. These abnormalities are occasionally reversed by chronic haemodialysis, but are usually refractory to dialysis and may actually progress in an accelerated way during treatment. The renal glomerular bone disorders cover a wide spectrum of abnormalities including osteomalacia, osteitis fibrosa, osteopenia, osteosclerosis, subperiosteal new bone formation and ectopic calcification.

The alterations in vitamin D metabolism and associated malabsorption of calcium stimulate parathyroid hyperplasia. This produces elevated circulating values of parathyroid hormone in order to correct the hypocalcaemia, and is termed 'secondary hyperparathyroidism'. The parathyroid response eventually may assume such large proportions that despite acquired or induced hypercalcaemia, parathyroid hormone secretion continues at an excessive rate. This autonomous secretory state has been termed 'tertiary hyperparathyroidism'.

Patients with chronic pyelonephritis, polycystic kidneys and obstructive uropathy are more predisposed to renal bone disease than patients with chronic glomerulonephritis or renal disease. Osteomalacia associated with renal disease is also more common in Europe than in the USA and Australia. There are very wide variations in the incidence of symptomatic bone disease in patients with end-stage renal disease, and patients who live longer with renal failure are more likely to develop renal osteodystrophy. The patients with most symptoms are those whose bone lesion is predominantly osteomalacia rather than osteitis fibrosa.

The signs of renal osteodystrophy are particularly well seen on radiological examination. Secondary hyperparathyroidism is confirmed by subperiosteal bone resorption in the phalanges, medial margin of the proximal tibia and distal ends of the clavicles. A skull radiograph often demonstrates a mottled ground-glass appearance with a mixed picture of osteosclerotic and osteolytic lesions. Large cystic 'brown tumours' may be present in the long bones, phalanges, metacarpals, ribs and skull. Histologically, these are solid giant cell tumours that are brown due to deposition of haemosiderin. In long-standing renal disease, particularly in younger patients, osteosclerosis is seen. This abnormality has an axial distribution and characteristically gives rise to the 'rugger jersey' spine, in which there are alternating bands of increased bone density and relatively lower density (Fig. 14.20). It progresses to give totally sclerotic vertebral bodies. Patients with radiological evidence of osteitis fibrosa are known to have very high serum parathyroid hormone levels.

Children with renal failure are particularly prone to developing renal osteodystrophy and show qualitative and quantitative differences from the osteodystrophy seen in adults with renal failure. The striking abnormalities are in the growth plates of the long bones, and the

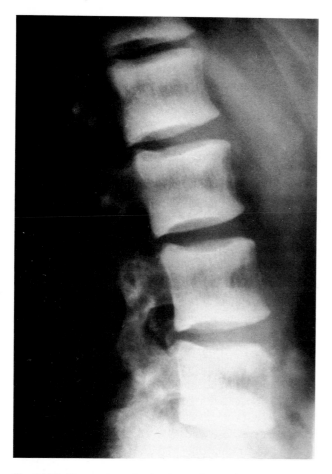

Fig. 14.20 'Rugger jersey' spine in renal osteodystrophy.

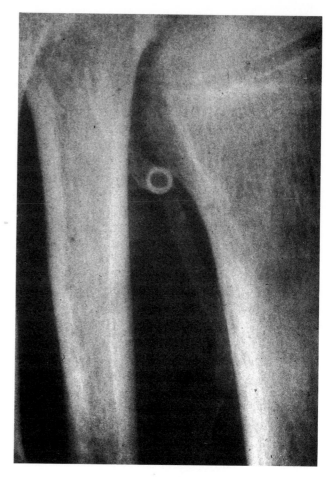

Fig. 14.21 Arterial calcification associated with renal osteodystrophy.

radiological signs are similar to those described generally for rickets. The lesions may progress to cause epiphyseal slipping and severe skeletal deformities.

Soft tissue calcification is becoming a more common complication of chronic renal failure. It may be metastatic or dystrophic, correlates with hyperphosphataemia and usually accompanies severe osteitis fibrosa. Sometimes it is associated with vitamin D and calcium treatment or the correction of uraemic acidosis. The calcification causes severe symptoms and particularly occurs in arteries (Fig. 14.21), eyes, periarticular tissue, skin, subcutaneous tissue and viscera. The so-called 'red-eye' syndrome of renal failure is due to acute infection and inflammation associated with conjunctival calcification.

Osteomalacia may occur particularly in patients with end-stage renal disease who are being treated by dialysis. This has been termed dialysis osteomalacia and is related to the presence of excess aluminium in the water used to prepare the dialysate and to aluminium in the phosphate binders. Aluminium is known to interfere with the mineralization of bone and possibly to have direct effects on osteoblast function. Patients with this type of osteomalacia may be treated with the chelating agent desferrioxamine mesylate.

Renal tubular osteodystrophy. This has many different aetiologies. All aetiological types are uncommon, but three of the more common ones are described below.

Pseudo-vitamin D deficiency or *vitamin D-dependent rickets* type I and II are rare inborn errors of vitamin D metabolism. Despite an adequate vitamin D intake, these patients have the clinical, radiological and biochemical features of classic vitamin D deficiency. In type I the presumed defect is of the renal 25-hydroxy vitamin D 1-hydroxylase enzyme, and the patients have low circulating 1,25-dihydroxy vitamin D values. The disorder manifests itself before the age of 2 years and is probably inherited as an autosomal recessive disease. Type II disease may be clinically associated with alopecia, epidermal cysts and oligodontia. In this type of rickets, the patients have very high levels of serum $1,25(OH)_2D_3$ and intracellular defects involving the interaction of vitamin D with its receptor (Marx and Barsony, 1988).

The clinical syndromes in which there is *hypophosphataemia* and *rickets* may be acquired or congenital in aetiology. The acquired forms include altered renal tubular function as in renal Fanconi's syndrome, which is characterized by defects in proximal tubule transport leading to impaired reabsorption of glucose, phosphate, amino acids and bicarbonate. Inherited hypophosphataemic vitamin D-resistant rickets was first described by Albright and is inherited as an X-linked dominant trait. The patients are short, but careful treatment with large amounts of phosphate and high doses of $1,25(OH)_2D_3$ may produce normal growth. The basic defect is an inherited abnormality of phosphate transport by the renal tubule and other transport tissues, e.g. the gut. There is an increased urinary phosphate clearance, and the maximum tubular reabsorptive capacity for phosphate is reduced. The disorder begins in infancy with predominant bony deformities but no muscle weakness. The children are dwarfed with short legs and have typical abnormalities of the face and skull. The facies shows a prominent forehead, and the anterior–posterior measurement of the skull is long. Biochemical investigations show normocalcaemia, hypophosphataemia and no amino aciduria. Radiologically, the characteristic changes of rickets are seen. The vaues for serum $1,25(OH)_2D_3$ are normal.

Adult-onset hypophosphataemic osteomalacia is a rare disorder in which there is no family history of rickets or osteomalacia and which occurs in a previously healthy young adult. The aetiology is unknown, but this type of osteomalacia can be associated with non-endocrine tumours of soft tissues, e.g. neurofibromatosis, or fibrous dysplasia. Patients present with a rapid onset of bone pain and proximal muscle weakness and are found to have hypophosphataemia. Radiological and histological examination confirms the presence of osteomalacia.

Hypophosphatasia is a rare disorder that gives rise to rickets or osteomalacia. It is characterized by a reduction of activity in the tissue-non-specific (liver/bone/kidney) isoenzymes of alkaline phosphatase, but normal activity of the intestinal and placental isoenzymes. The disease may present in childhood or adult life, and the diagnosis is made on the radiological and biochemical findings.

Tumour osteomalacia

There has been recent interest in the rare occurrence of tumour-associated rickets and osteomalacia. The syndrome is characterized by remission of the bone disease after resection of the coexisting tumour. Patients usually present with bone and muscle pain, muscle weakness and occasionally recurrent fractures of long bones. There is hypophosphataemia and low circulating $1,25(OH)_2D_3$ values. It is likely that the tumour produces a humoral substance that affects proximal renal tubule function. The tumours involved are often of mesenchymal origin, e.g. sclerosing haemangiomas, non-ossifying fibromas and giant cell tumours.

Anticonvulsant osteomalacia

The hepatic metabolism of cholecalciferol depends on hepatic microsomal mixed function oxidases. These enzymes may be induced by drugs such as barbiturates and phenytoin, and the antituberculous drug rifampicin. Some patients on anticonvulsants develop osteomalacia. The mechanism has not been conclusively related to the abnormal metabolism of vitamin D, however, though these patients respond well to vitamin D treatment.

TREATMENT

The treatment of rickets and osteomalacia depends on the aetiology of the condition. It ranges from improved diet, increased exposure to sunshine and low or high vitamin D supplements, to administration of synthetic analogues of vitamin metabolites, such as $1\alpha(OH)D_3$ and $1,25(OH)_2D_3$.

Patients with nutritional rickets and osteomalacia should be encouraged to go out in the sunshine as much as possible and to eat a vitamin D replete diet (up to 400 IU/day of cholecalciferol). Details of the vitamin D content of foods may be obtained from McCance and Widdowson's The Composition of Foods 1991 (Holland *et al.*, 1991). Vitamin D supplements at a dose of 500–5000 IU may be given. If the patient responds there is an increase in muscle strength in a few days. Initially, bone pain may become worse and there is a temporary increase in serum alkaline phosphatase activity known as the phosphatase flare. The values for plasma calcium and phosphate increase, the parathyroid hormone values fall and estimations of 25-hydroxy vitamin D rise (Fig. 14.22). Radiological improvement does not start to become apparent for 1 month and histological improvement may take many months.

For patients with other types of vitamin D deficiency, e.g. malabsorption, the primary cause should be corrected; alternatively high doses of vitamin D–greater than 40 000 IU/day–or synthetic analogues may be given in microgram quantities as recommended in the

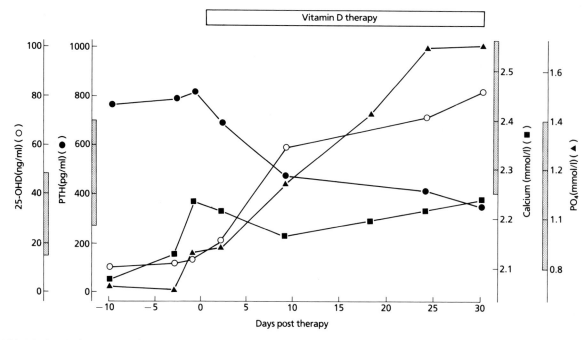

Fig. 14.22 Biochemical response of a patient with osteomalacia to vitamin D therapy.

British National Formulary (1994). For patients with renal glomerular osteodystrophy treatment consists of haemodialysis or transplantation for the renal failure itself and also the prevention or reduction of hyper-phosphataemia with phosphate-binding agents and administration of the 1-hydroxylated derivatives of vitamin D to counteract the effects of renal failure. Unfortunately, aseptic necrosis of bone, particularly of the femoral head, may occur after transplantation in patients on corticosteroids. For patients with metastatic calcification or tertiary hyperparathyroidism, para-thyroidectomy may be appropriate.

Patients with hypophosphataemic rickets do not respond to phosphate supplements alone and usually require large doses of vitamin D or treatment with $1,25(OH)_2D_3$. Patients with adult-onset hypophospha-taemic osteomalacia, however, do often respond to phosphate supplements alone. Anticonvulsant osteo-malacia responds to microgram quantities of $25(OH)D_3$ or the dihydroxy analogues. Tumour osteomalacia is usually cured by removal of the tumour.

Disorders of the parathyroid glands

Parathyroid disease is relatively common among endo-crine disorders and is now more widely recognized than before. This is due to the growing awareness of the physiology of parathyroid hormone and because of the more frequent estimations of serum calcium since the advent of multichannel biochemical analysers.

Disorders of the parathyroid glands may be due to overactivity or underactivity. Hyperparathyroidism may be primary or secondary, when there is hyperplasia of the glands to compensate for some forms of prolonged hypocalcaemia (see p. 377). In addition, secondary hyperparathyroidism may progress to an autonomous state with hypercalcaemia. This is termed tertiary hyper-parathyroidism. Underactivity of the parathyroid glands may be due to deficient secretion of parathyroid hormone itself, referred to as hypoparathyroidism, or an abnor-mality in the metabolism or function of the hormone, which is termed pseudohypoparathyroidism.

PRIMARY HYPERPARATHYROIDISM

This most commonly occurs between the third and fifth decades of life and is two to three times more common in women than in men. Patients may continue for many years with minimal symptoms and undetected disease, or alternatively the clinical manifestations may occur very suddenly. Very occasionally patients may present with hypercalcaemic dehydration and coma in para-thyroid crisis. Asymptomatic hyperparathyroidism is now recognized more widely, and consequently the inci-dence of primary hyperparathyroidism may approach 1 in 1000 persons.

The most common aetiology is a benign adenoma of one gland which is predominantly composed of chief cells. It is usually of monoclonal origin. In 10–15% of cases, there is hyperplasia of all four glands, but carcinoma of the parathyroid glands is rare (3% of patients with primary hyperparathyroidism). Adenomas may also occur in ectopic sites, e.g. the thymus, thyroid gland, pericardium and retro-oesophageal areas.

Primary hyperparathyroidism may be familial and associated with other well-defined endocrinopathies. These hereditary disorders may be divided into two genetically distinct syndromes. The first syndrome, referred to as multiple endocrine neoplasia type I, consists primarily of tumours of the parathyroid glands, pituitary gland and pancreas, and may be associated with Zollinger–Ellison syndrome. The second syndrome, referred to as multiple endocrine neoplasia type II, consists of medullary carcinoma of the thyroid gland, phaeochromocytoma and parathyroid adenomas. These syndromes may be associated with a primary dysplasia of neuroectoderm.

Clinical features

The clinical manifestations of the disorder reflect the sequelae of hypercalcaemia, e.g. malaise, lethargy and nausea, or are manifestations of the hyperparathyroidism itself. Classically, they have been described as 'stones, bones, abdominal groans and psychic moans'. The most common features are either renal or skeletal, though the skeletal changes, e.g. osteitis fibrosa cystica, are now less common than 20 years ago. This probably reflects earlier detection of the disorder.

The renal effects of primary hyperparathyroidism can be divided into two types: anatomical and functional. The anatomical effects include nephrolithiasis or nephrocalcinosis, together with their sequelae, e.g. urinary tract infections. The functional manifestations are the tubular and glomerular disorders resulting from the deleterious effects of sustained hypercalcaemia. The prolonged hypercalcaemia is particularly associated with abnormalities of proximal tubular function, e.g. amino aciduria and glycosuria. Patients with severe bone disease do not usually develop renal stones and vice versa.

The classic bone changes in primary hyperparathyroidism are known as osteitis fibrosa cystica. When these changes are present pain is often severe and localized to the site of the lesion. The most important changes are found in the hands where subperiosteal bone resorption may be so severe in the terminal phalanges as to cause pseudo-clubbing.

There are often well-recognized clinical features associated with primary hyperparathyroidism. Neuromuscular symptoms may affect the legs so that patients may complain of difficulty in climbing stairs and rising from a chair. There may be symptoms of depression, personality changes, loss of memory and even sometimes progression to psychosis. Often patients are unaware of depression until after treatment, when the improvement becomes obvious. Gastrointestinal symptoms of peptic ulcer are often associated with primary hyperparathyroidism. A few of these patients later turn out to have Zollinger–Ellison syndrome, and the peptic ulcer symptoms improve after treatment of the hyperparathyroidism. Pancreatitis has a well-documented association with primary hyperparathyroidism; it may be acute or chronic, when it is usually accompanied by pain. Several types of joint disorder may occur. These include chondrocalcinosis with or without attacks of pseudo-gout. Patients are more prone to develop hypertension.

Patients with asymptomatic hyperparathyroidism must be distinguished from those with familial hypocalciuric hypercalcaemia. The latter patients have other affected members in their families and hypercalcaemia may be detected in siblings in the first decade of life.

Investigations

Measurement of the serum calcium level in a sample of blood taken from a fasting patient with minimal stasis shows persistent hypercalcaemia. It is doubtful whether normocalcaemic hyperparathyroidism is a true entity. The serum inorganic phosphate level is usually low unless the glomerular filtration rate is lowered, when the serum inorganic phosphate level rises to become normal or even high. There is often hypercalciuria, and blood alkaline phosphatase and hydroxyproline values are only elevated when there is definite bone involvement.

It is often difficult to determine whether the cause of asymptomatic hypercalcaemia is hyperparathyroidism, particularly when there are no skeletal or renal signs. If persistent hypercalcaemia is present, the lack of response of the serum calcium to the cortisone suppression test (Fig. 14.23) may be helpful in sorting out hyperparathyroidism from other causes of hypercalcaemia.

Measurements of parathyroid hormone (using an intact molecule assay) are helpful in the differential diagnosis of hypercalcaemia and in confirming a clinically suspected case of hyperparathyroidism. Care should be taken when interpreting the values obtained, as although in the presence of an adenoma the value may be within the normal range, it may be inappropriately high in the presence of hypercalcaemia. It should

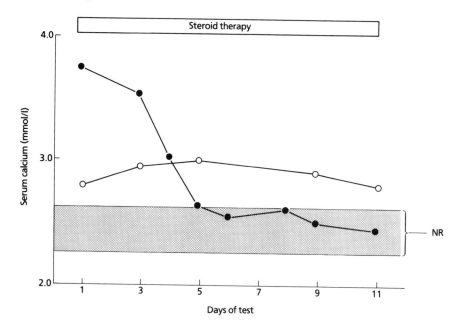

Fig. 14.23 Responses of patients with myeloma (solid circles) and primary hyperparathyroidism (open circles) to the cortisone suppression test.

be noted that if the serum calcium value is high, the secretion of parathyroid hormone should be suppressed. Serum calcium concentration should always be measured at the same time as a parathyroid hormone estimation. Measurements of the hormone can also be of use in localizing a tumour, as they can be performed on samples obtained from selective venous catheterization of the neck. The highest value is obtained from the site anatomically nearest to the site of the tumour.

The classic radiological changes of osteitis fibrosa cystica in the hands show subperiosteal erosions of the radial aspect of the middle phalanges (Fig. 14.24). The erosions may also involve the terminal phalanges and can be detected at the end of the clavicle at the acromio-

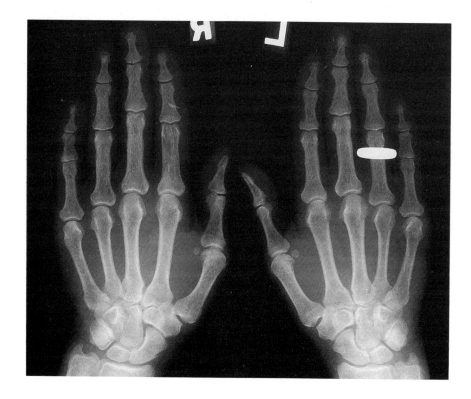

Fig. 14.24 Subperiosteal bone resorption, particularly in the middle phalanx of the index finger of the left hand in primary hypoparathyroidism.

clavicular joint, pubic symphysis and sacroiliac joints. These findings are pathognomonic of increased secretion of parathyroid hormone and are also found in secondary hyperparathyroidism. Two types of cysts may be seen in the bones on radiology. These are true bone cysts, in which there is a fluid-filled cavity lined with fibrous tissue, often occurring under the periosteum (Fig. 14.25). The other cysts are brown tumours consisting of poorly mineralized woven bone containing bone cells and haemosiderin, which makes them brown. Another classic sign is loss of the lamina dura around the teeth, which is seen in about 80% of patients with primary hyperparathyroidism.

During the past 50 years, the pattern of bone disease in primary hyperparathyroidism has changed, so that osteitis fibrosa cystica is less common and a more subtle bone change is now often seen on radiographs. This is a diffuse form of osteopenia, which resembles osteoporosis and may be severe enough to give rise to vertebral crush fractures. It differs from the osteopenia of elderly women as it is not homogeneous, so there is reduced bone density alternating with bone of normal intensity, producing a mottled appearance in bones such as the skull. Osteosclerosis seldom occurs in primary hyperparathyroidism.

Treatment

Primary hyperparathyroidism is treated by exploration of the neck and removal of the adenoma or hyperplastic glands. Careful post-operative management is required to cope with the common transient hypocalcaemia or post-surgical hypoparathyroidism. After correction of the hyperparathyroidism the brown tumours heal, but the true bone cysts do not. It is unclear whether surgery is needed for patients with asymptomatic hyperparathyroidism as opinions among surgeons differ. In these patients, however, it is wise to assess renal function and eliminate the presence of renal calculi and urinary tract infection. If renal function is significantly impaired or renal calculi are present, surgical treatment should be undertaken. If the patient is managed conservatively, renal function tests should be performed and bone density monitored. The treatment of secondary and tertiary hyperparathyroidism is referred to in the section on vitamin D disorders (see p. 377).

HYPOPARATHYROIDISM

This is a rare disorder that is most commonly due to damage to parathyroid tissue following thyroid surgery. The bone changes are comparatively small, but this disorder is interesting as in the very rare pseudo-forms the aetiology can be partly explained by abnormalities of the metabolic pathway of parathyroid hormone.

The clinical features of hypoparathyroidism may be grouped into those due to the severe hypocalcaemia and those associated with the underlying cause. Hypocalcaemia of the degree found in hypoparathyroidism causes marked neurological, ectodermal and dental signs and symptoms. There may be tetany often preceded by paraesthesiae in the hands, feets and around the mouth. The muscular spasms occurring may not only be carpopedal in type but affect other sites, e.g. the larynx, causing stridor. Patients often complain of cramp and muscle stiffness, and they can exhibit psychotic behaviour and other psychiatric symptoms. There is often a history of long-standing fits and on examination there may be papilloedema and choreiform muscle movements.

Examination of the skin shows a dry, scaly condition. The nails are brittle, the hair coarse and the eyebrows

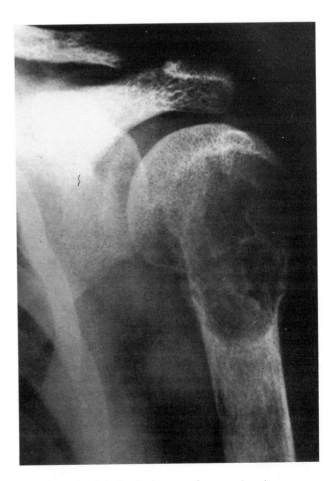

Fig. 14.25 Cystic lesion in the upper humerus in primary hyperparathyroidism.

may be sparse. Subcapsular cataracts may be observed, and there is enamel hypoplasia of the teeth. The teeth often erupt late, and the jaws are typically short and wide. Electrocardiography shows a prolonged QT interval, which is sometimes associated with cardiomegaly and congestive cardiac failure. The specific clinical features of the individual types of hypoparathyroidism are described below. They include, for example, candidiasis as seen in idiopathic hypoparathyroidism.

The diagnosis of hypoparathyroidism is confirmed by low serum calcium, high serum phosphate and normal plasma protein concentrations. In hypoparathyroidism the serum parathyroid hormone value is low, and the urinary cyclic AMP response to parathyroid hormone may be used to differentiate between true and pseudohypoparathyroidism.

The types of hypoparathyroidism may be classified according to their aetiology:

1 True hypoparathyroidism.
  (a) Surgical.
  (b) Idiopathic.
  (c) Neonatal.
  (d) Miscellaneous.
2 Pseudohypoparathyroidism.
  (a) Type I.
  (b) Type II.
3 Pseudopseudohypoparathyroidism.

True hypoparathyroidism

Surgical. This may be transient or permanent and also of varying degrees, e.g. complete, partial, or latent. It occurs most commonly after surgery involving the thyroid gland, and many years ago was usually due to accidental removal of the parathyroid glands along with thyroid tissue. This is very seldom the case now, and post-operative hypoparathyroidism is usually due to interference with the parathyroid blood supply when mobilizing the thyroid gland or underlying parathyroid tissue *in situ*. Transient hypocalcaemia following thyroid surgery is more common than is fully appreciated.

In some series it has been reported that post-operative tetany may occur in as many as 60% of patients, the aetiology being a sudden post-operative fall in serum calcium level rather than a particularly low serum calcium value *per se*. This particularly occurs after surgery for thyrotoxicosis, where the serum calcium may have been elevated pre-operatively and when handling of the thyroid gland at operation may have produced secretion of calcitonin.

Parathyroid surgery is also often followed by transient or permanent hypoparathyroidism. This may occur after removal of a large primary adenoma that is associated with three remaining atrophied glands. Alternatively, it is the practice for some surgeons to perform a total parathyroidectomy for parathyroid hyperplasia, causing tertiary hyperparathyroidism. The resulting hypoparathyroidism is then corrected with calcium and vitamin D supplements. Surgical hypoparathyroidism may also arise after total laryngectomy for carcinoma of the larynx.

Idiopathic. This type of hypoparathyroidism is rare and may present early in life, either during childhood or adolescence. Both presentations may be associated with a family history. Some cases of idiopathic hypoparathyroidism are associated with candidiasis, pernicious anaemia and endocrinopathies, e.g. Addison's disease. This suggests an autoimmune aetiology, and this concept is supported by reports of detection of antibodies to parathyroid tissue in some cases of idiopathic hypoparathyroidism.

Neonatal. Physiological hypoparathyroidism occurs in newborn infants, but in some babies this may be so severe as to cause dangerous hypocalcaemia; it may also extend into the early infant years. The condition may be transient or permanent and is seen more commonly in babies that are premature or have mothers with diabetes or hyperparathyroidism. In addition, neonatal hypoparathyroidism may be associated with developmental abnormalities of related anatomical structures, e.g. the third and fourth pharyngeal pouch syndrome (DiGeorge's syndrome). The babies may present with neonatal convulsions.

Miscellaneous. There are other, miscellaneous, causes of hypoparathyroidism, e.g. massive doses of external radiation to the neck and deposition of iron in the parathyroid tissue. The latter occurs in haemochromatosis and in patients with iron overload syndromes following multiple blood transfusions for disorders such as thalassaemia.

Pseudohypoparathyroidism

This term describes a heterogeneous syndrome characterized by biochemical hypoparathyroidism, increased plasma levels of parathyroid hormone and peripheral unresponsiveness to parathyroid hormone. It is a rare hereditary disorder which was first described by Albright *et al.* in 1942. The clinical features are similar to those found in hypoparathyroidism, but in addition there is a family history of the disorder. The mode of inheritance has been suggested as an X-linked dominant trait.

Patients with this disorder have an abnormal appearance with a short neck and a round face. In addition they are short in height, often intellectually retarded, and classically have short fourth or fifth metacarpals or metatarsals. The bones may be more dense than normal on radiographs, and have exostoses or adjacent subcutaneous calcification. Associated hypothyroidism and defects in taste and smell have been described as part of the syndrome.

Despite hypocalcaemia and hyperphosphataemia, circulating parathyroid hormone levels are high. The pathological defect seems to be in the metabolic pathway between the formation of the hormone and its action at the cellular level in the renal tubule and bone (see Fig. 14.6, p. 361). Parathyroid hormone (or extract) produces large increases in urinary cyclic AMP excretion in normal or hypoparathyroid subjects and a minimal response in patients with pseudohypoparathyroidism (Fig. 14.26). It was originally assumed that the defect was in the parathyroid hormone-sensitive adenylate cyclase in the bone and kidney. Further studies, however, have shown that some patients with clinical features of pseudohypoparathyroidism produce a normal cyclic AMP response to parathyroid hormone, but not an increase in urinary phosphate as might be expected. An attempt has therefore been made to divide this syndrome into two types: pseudohypoparathyroidism type I, characterized by a decreased cyclic AMP and urinary phosphate response to parathyroid hormone, and pseudohypoparathyroidism type II, characterized by a normal cyclic AMP but decreased urinary phosphate response to parathyroid hormone.

These types may be further subdivided according to the function of their stimulatory and inhibitory receptors (Rs and Ri) and the stimulatory and inhibitory guanine nucleotide-binding regulatory proteins (Gs and Gi) of the adenylate cyclase system. The clinician is often confused by the existence of another related syndrome, termed pseudopseudohypoparathyroidism. This disorder shows the skeletal abnormalities of pseudohypoparathyroidism but is not accompanied by any biochemical changes. It is now thought to be due to deficient Gs activity.

Treatment

Although the sequence of parathyroid hormone is known and the hormone has been synthesized, there is no preparation available for therapeutic purposes. The treatment of the hypoparathyroid syndromes therefore consists of correcting the hypocalcaemia by means of calcium supplements, together with vitamin D.

Thyroid disease affecting bone

The thyroid gland has an important effect on bone by means of its hormones thyroxine (T4), tri-iodothyronine (T3) and calcitonin. These hormones predominantly affect skeletal homoeostasis, but they have some effects on mineral homoeostasis as well.

THYROID HORMONE DEFICIENCY

Deficiency of T4 and T3 in children causes retardation of growth and maturity of the skeleton. In congenital thyroid deficiency, causing the clinical syndrome of cretinism, there is a severe delay in the appearance of ossification in the epiphyses, particularly in the femurs. When ossification eventually occurs, there is an irregular pattern of multiple foci which later coalesce giving a stippled appearance called epiphyseal dysgenesis. The occurrence of dysgenesis in a particular centre of ossification can be used to date the onset of the hypothyroidism. The hypothyroid dwarf retains infantile skeletal proportions, and children with thyroid hormone deficiency have delayed dentition and loss of deciduous teeth. Because of the delayed ossification the bone has a porous appearance, and the decreased bone density is reflected by low activity of serum alkaline phosphatase. The excretion of calcium, phosphate and hydroxyproline in the urine is low. The serum calcium level is usually normal or only slightly decreased.

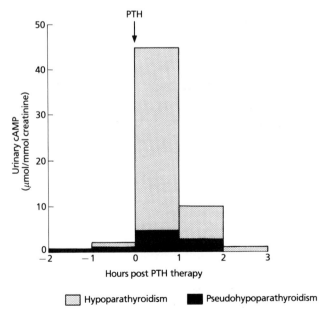

Fig. 14.26 Urinary cyclic AMP changes in pseudohypoparathyroidism.

THYROID HORMONE EXCESS

Increased secretion of thyroid hormones in children produces an acceleration of growth and accelerated maturation of the bone. In some children there may be early eruption of the teeth and because of the increased growth they are often tall. In adults there is increased activity of osteoblast and osteoclast function. The serum alkaline phosphatase value may be increased. Very occasionally thyroid acropachy is observed; this is a form of hypertrophic osteoarthropathy. There is subperiosteal swelling, but no new bone formation as in hypertrophic pulmonary osteoarthropathy. The changes are usually seen in the metacarpals and phalanges. The bony changes, accompanied by soft, diffuse swelling of adjacent tissues, are often associated with pretibial myxoedema and exophthalmos. This usually occurs after the hyperthyroidism has been treated.

In hyperthyroid states there is an increased excretion of calcium and phosphate in the urine, but urolithiasis is surprisingly uncommon. In approximately 20% of cases the serum calcium level is raised, probably due to increased bone resorption. This mild hypercalcaemia is not usually clinically important and corrects itself with treatment of the hyperthyroidism. Other than the changes described above significant skeletal changes are seldom seen in hyperthyroidism. Women with hyperthyroidism and thyroxine-treated women with low serum thyrotrophin-releasing hormone values are at risk of developing osteoporosis.

CALCITONIN EXCESS

Large amounts of calcitonin are secreted in association with medullary carcinoma of the thyroid. This is a tumour of the thyroid that may have a familial incidence and be associated with phaeochromocytoma, hyperparathyroidism and certain neuroectodermal clinical features, e.g. polypoid neuromas of the lips and tongue. Despite secreting large amounts of calcitonin, patients with this tumour have no readily recognizable abnormality of skeletal and mineral metabolism. Most of the patients are normocalcaemic.

Hypercalcaemia of malignancy

Hypercalcaemia is a common complication of malignancy. It may occur in approximately 30% of patients with advanced breast cancer and in 20% of patients with lung cancer. Calcium is released from the bone into the extracellular fluid by increased bone resorption due to factors from the malignant cells that stimulate the osteoclasts. In addition, there is increased calcium reabsorption in the proximal renal tubules, possibly as a result of renotrophic factors produced by the malignant tumour. The tumours that produce hypercalcaemia may be divided into three clinical groups. These are haematological malignancies, e.g. myeloma and lymphomas which produce lymphokines, and solid tumours with metastases that may directly erode bone themselves or produce osteoclast stimulatory factors, e.g. prostaglandins and interleukin 1. In addition, solid tumours may be associated with bone resorption and hypercalcaemia because of the production of transforming growth factors and parathyroid hormone-related peptide. This peptide is derived from a gene on chromosome 12 that is distinct from the gene for parathyroid hormone on chromosome 11.

CLINICAL FEATURES

The clinical features of hypercalcaemia are diverse and vary according to the duration of the raised serum calcium level and the rapidity of its change. Patients with hypercalcaemia may become drowsy and lethargic and may complain of hallucinations and headaches. Alternatively, when the hypercalcaemia is mild and of long standing, relatives of the patient may notice aggressive behaviour with some paranoid features. The patients are often anorexic and constipated. They have polyuria, and with severe hypercalcaemia there is vomiting which is often difficult to control.

Examination shows a hypotonic muscle weakness and depressed tendon reflexes. Localizing neurological signs are rare unless related to the underlying malignant disease, but in severe hypercalcaemia (serum calcium concentration >4 mmol/l) the patient becomes confused, disoriented and later comatose. There is often tachycardia and sometimes hypertension.

Biochemical investigations show a raised serum calcium level which at times may be alarmingly high. The serum phosphate value may be low and the alkaline phosphatase activity raised, depending on the presence or absence of osseous metastases. There may be an inability to concentrate the urine and in patients with hypercalcaemia not related to increased parathyroid hormone secretion, metabolic alkalosis has commonly been observed. Haematological investigations may show evidence of widely spread malignant disease and after long-standing hypercalcaemia, nephrocalcinosis may be seen on radiographs. Because of the accompanying malignant disease, however, the clinical signs related to the malignancy usually become manifest before the long-term effects of hypercalcaemia are observed. The

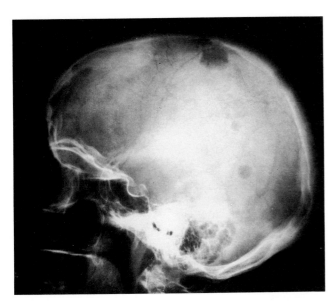

Fig. 14.27 Osteolytic metastatic deposits in the skull.

main radiological findings, therefore, usually show evidence of widespread osteolytic bone metastases (Fig. 14.27) or signs of a primary tumour, e.g. a carcinoma of the bronchus on chest radiography. An electrocardiograph may show shortening of the QT interval, and in severe hypercalcaemia cardiac arrest may occur. There is a progressive slowing of the electroencephalographic recording as the serum calcium values rise; however, the findings can sometimes mimic those due to cerebral metastases.

TREATMENT

Hypercalcaemia may be so severe (serum calcium >4.0 mmol/l) as to be life-threatening or less severe, when treatment is directed at the alleviation of symptoms.

In severe hypercalcaemia, the basis of emergency treatment is rigorous correction of dehydration by means of normal saline infusions to increase calcium excretion. These should be coupled with careful attention to electrolyte imbalance as potassium depletion may occur. If there is evidence of fluid overload, furosemide may be necessary. Most cases of severe hypercalcaemia respond promptly to enthusiastic rehydration. If severe hypercalcaemia continues, however, the bisphosphonate drugs are now considered to be the most effective agents to supplement fluid replacement. Three intravenous preparations are available, and a single infusion of pamidronate disodium, 30 mg over 2 h, has produced good results (Heath, 1991). Intravenous phosphate has been used in the past, but it is dangerous and carries a long-term risk of extraskeletal calcification. Corticosteroids are particularly useful in patients with myeloma and leukaemia (see Fig. 14.23, p. 382) but in other forms of malignancy, the response to steroids is unpredictable. Calcitonin produces only a relatively modest reduction in serum calcium concentration, though this treatment is comparatively free from side-effects.

Treatment of less severe hypercalcaemia is primarily by correction of dehydration, together with some other appropriate agent for treatment of the underlying malignancy. The bisphosphonates, and possibly cytotoxic drugs such as gallium nitrate and cisplatin which are cytotoxic to osteoclasts, may be used.

Osteopetrosis

This is the best known of a group of disorders now referred to as sclerosing bone dysplasias. It is also known as marble bone disease and was first described in 1904 by Albers-Schonberg. There are two distinct clinical forms of the disease: the autosomal dominant or benign type, and the autosomal recessive or malignant form, which if untreated is fatal in infancy or early childhood. Generalized osteosclerosis may initially present with nasal symptoms and cranial nerve palsies due to involvement of the skull. The skeleton is uniformly dense and the ends of the long bones are widened to produce an 'Erlenmeyer flask' deformity. In this disorder there is defective osteoclast function, so that skeletal reabsorption is impaired. Treatment of the severe forms involves marrow transplantation or possibly use of $1,25(OH)_2D_3$ and calcium. Recently, an autosomal recessive syndrome of osteoporosis with renal tubular acidosis and cerebral calcification associated with a deficiency of carbonic anhydrase II has been described.

Metabolic bone disease in the elderly

Metabolic bone disease commonly occurs in elderly patients. It can be difficult to differentiate between the different types, particularly osteomalacia and osteoporosis. Table 14.6 is provided to compare the features of the four most common forms of bone disease found in elderly patients.

BIOCHEMICAL INVESTIGATIONS

This section is intended as a short guide for the investigation of patients with metabolic bone disease. It contains advice on the practicality and role of the various tests available.

Table 14.6 Bone disease in the elderly

Diagnosis	Pathology	History	Important clinical features	Radiographic appearance	Biochemistry (serum)		Bone biopsy
Osteomalacia	Reduced mineral content	Generalized pain Difficulty in walking	Kyphosis Muscular weakness	Looser zones Codfish vertebrae Subperiosteal erosions	Ca P ALP* D†	N or ↓ N or ↓ ↑ ↓	Excess unmineralized osteoid
Osteoporosis	Reduced bone mass	Loss of height Little or localized pain Liability to fracture	Kyphosis Loss of height	Accentuation of vertebral end-plate shadows Codfish vertebrae Anterior vertebral wedging Schmorl's nodes	Ca P ALP D	N N N N	Reduced amount trabecular bone
Paget's disease	Disorganized overactivity	Asymptomatic or intense dull pain Deformity Deafness	Severe deformity of skull, pelvis and legs Deafness	Transverse fissure fractures 'Cotton-wool' skull Increased density and deformed long bones	Ca P ALP D	N N ↑ ↑ N	Overactive disorganized bone
Malignant disease	Malignant deposits	Localized pain Hypercalcaemic symptoms Pathological fracture	Localized tenderness General signs of malignant disease	Localized osteolytic lesions Vertebral deposits with posterior wedging	Ca P ALP D	N or ↑ N or ↑ ↑ N	Malignant cells in normal bone

* ALP = Serum alkaline phosphatase value.
† D = Serum 25-hydroxy vitamin D value.

Measurement and interpretation of serum calcium concentration

In the laboratory, clinical problems may be classified according to the result of an initial serum calcium estimation. Patients suspected on clinical evidence of having metabolic bone disease may be divided into three groups: those who are hypercalcaemic, those who are hypocalcaemic and those who are normocalcaemic. It is not always easy to define either hypercalcaemia or hypocalcaemia precisely, because reference ranges differ according to methodology and there may be changes in *in vivo* calcium partition.

There are three separate fractions of calcium in plasma. They are distributed so that approximately 50% of the plasma calcium is ionized, 40% is protein bound in the form of calcium albuminate, and up to 10% is complexed mainly to citrate, phosphate and bicarbonate. No physiological significance has been ascribed to the complexed and protein-bound fractions, and it is generally assumed that only the ionized fraction is physiologically active and under hormonal control.

TOTAL CALCIUM

A wide variety of techniques is available for measuring

total serum calcium levels. It is important that samples for serum calcium estimation should be taken under standard conditions and that simultaneous serum protein concentrations should be taken into account when interpreting results. Blood should be taken without venous stasis and when the patient is fasting. The tourniquet, if used, should be released when the needle is in the vein, and a pause of 10 sec should be allowed before blood is withdrawn because venous occlusion increases the serum protein concentration. The effect of serum protein concentration, particularly albumin, on total serum calcium levels is very significant, but reservations have been expressed about the validity of correcting serum calcium for protein concentration because of the implicit assumption that protein binding of calcium is uniform. Many of the studies describing plasma calcium corrections make no comparison with ionized calcium levels. Nevertheless, when gross changes in plasma protein concentrations are observed, as in nephrotic syndrome and liver disease, correction of the measured serum calcium level or knowledge of the degree of hypoalbuminaemia is essential.

Serum calcium results may be corrected for variations in albumin concentration in the following way. For each 1 g/l that a patient's plasma albumin level is below 40 g/l, a correction factor of 0.02 mmol/l is added to the total calcium concentration. Alternatively, for each 1 g/l that the albumin level is above 40 g/l, the correction factor is subtracted (Editorial, *BMJ*, 1977).

IONIZED CALCIUM

The ideal calcium fraction to be measured for the clinical assessment of patients is the ionized portion. Unfortunately, this estimation is beyond the scope of most routine laboratories at present. Until a robust method is available, this deficiency cannot be rectified. Even then meticulous attention to detail in the collection and handling of samples will be required. The main problem encountered is the influence of pH on the protein binding and the consequent change in the ionized calcium fraction with altered pH of the sample.

SCHEMES FOR INVESTIGATING PATIENTS

Despite the problems in ascertaining if a patient is truly hypercalcaemic or hypocalcaemic, patients with abnormalities in serum calcium levels and those apparently normocalcaemic patients suspected on clinical grounds of having metabolic bone disease must be investigated further. For this purpose, three schemes of investigation are presented (Figs 14.28, 14.29 and 14.30). These are simplified schemes, but should enable the majority of clinical problems involving metabolic bone disease to be resolved. The starting point for the schemes is the total serum calcium concentration, though as a first step before extensive investigation is attempted, allowance should be made for abnormal serum albumin concentration. It is also wise to confirm the abnormality in serum calcium with a second specimen, ensuring that this is taken under ideal conditions with minimal venous stasis after an overnight fast.

Biochemical tests of calcium metabolism

PHOSPHATE

The measurement of serum phosphate essentially means determination of inorganic phosphate. As large amounts of organic phosphates are present in erythrocytes it is important to separate the serum from the red blood cells as soon as possible to obtain accurate results. Certain substances, e.g. heparin, methicillin, powdered pituitary and tetracyclines, have been reported to increase serum phosphate concentration, and aluminium hydroxide, adrenaline, ether anaesthesia and insulin to decrease it. Provided that there is no impairment of distal renal tubular function and the patient has been on a normal diet, serum phosphate values are a helpful indicator of increased or decreased parathyroid function. These changes reflect the effect of parathyroid hormone on urinary phosphate excretion. Physiological factors also affect phosphate excretion. The normal range for children is higher than for adults, this being an important consideration when investigating possible paediatric hypophosphataemic bone disease. In addition, adult values are lower than normal during the menstrual period, after meals and in elderly men. Blood samples for phosphate estimation, and also for calcium and albumin measurement, should be collected when the patient is fasting.

PHOSPHATE TOLERANCE TEST

In the diagnosis of hypophosphataemia associated with rickets and osteomalacia, an oral phosphate tolerance test may be a more sensitive diagnostic index than a low plasma phosphate level. This is a simple test to perform; in normal subjects, following a load of sodium phosphate powder, 6.9 g in 200 ml of water, the maximum rise in patients with familial hypophosphataemia not receiving vitamin D is 0.25 ± 0.04 mmol/l.

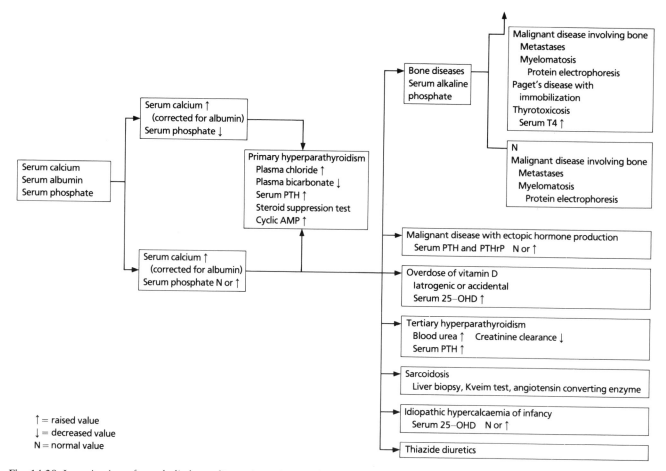

Fig. 14.28 Investigation of metabolic bone disease in patients with hypercalcaemia.

ALKALINE PHOSPHATASE

Alkaline phosphatase is secreted by osteoblasts and the serum concentration rises when osteoblasts are activated. This enzyme is also synthesized by liver and secreted into the bile.

Serum alkaline phosphatase values are elevated in childhood, the highest concentrations occurring during the first year of life and at puberty. At puberty, girls have significantly lower values than boys; a peak of activity at about 13 years of age has been observed in boys. Another age-dependent change is the increase in serum alkaline phosphatase activity in women during the fifth and sixth decades of life, and increased concentrations are found during the healing of fractures, particularly in the elderly.

In pathological conditions, the highest serum alkaline phosphatase values are usually associated with Paget's disease. The increased osteoblastic activity found in rickets and osteomalacia of any aetiology also causes increased serum alkaline phosphatase activity. Serum alkaline phosphatase activity is normal in the majority of patients with primary hyperparathyroidism, but is usually raised when there is radiological evidence of subperiosteal bone resorption.

Surgical treatment of primary hyperparathyroidism is often followed by an initial rise in alkaline phosphatase activity in healing of the bony lesions. Other conditions that may increase serum alkaline phosphatase activity include infiltration of bone by malignant disease and osteosarcoma. The difficulty in deciding whether raised alkaline phosphatase activity indicates bone or liver disease, particularly in malignant conditions, may be solved by the use of serum 5'-nucleotidase and γ-glutamyltransferase as indices of liver dysfunction or by differential measurement of bone and liver alkaline phosphatase isoenzymes. Serum alkaline phosphatase activity is normal in osteoporosis, osteogenesis imperfecta and osteopetrosis. Low serum alkaline phosphatase activity may be found in the inherited condition of hypophosphatasia, which may simulate rickets radiologically. Increased urinary excretion of phosphoethanolamine is also usually found in this disorder.

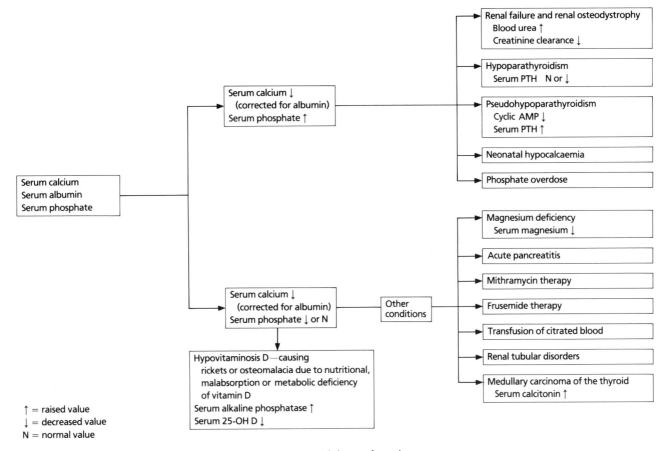

Fig. 14.29 Investigation of metabolic bone disease in patients with hypocalcaemia.

ACID PHOSPHATASE

Bone, or tartrate-resistant, acid phosphatase is abundant in osteoclasts and increased activity in the serum may be detected in a wide variety of conditions. These include metastatic malignant disease, Paget's disease and hyperparathyroid bone disease. Measurement of this enzyme is not used on a routine clinical basis, but the recent development of radioimmunoassays that are specific for this isoenzyme should provide a better method for assessing osteoclastic bone resorption in the future.

VITAMIN D AND ITS METABOLITES

Assays for two metabolites are available as follows.

25-Hydroxy vitamin D

Estimations show a marked seasonal variation which affects the interpretation of clinical results. This assay is useful in confirming rickets and osteomalacia due to vitamin D deficiency (except when of renal origin) and in diagnosing hypervitaminosis D.

For the oral 25-hydroxycholecalciferol absorption test, $25(OH)D_3$ may be administered orally and the serum concentration measured during the following 24 h. This test is valuable in establishing the cause of rickets and osteomalacia in gastrointestinal disease.

1,25-Dihydroxy vitamin D

Methods to measure 1,25-dihydroxy vitamin D in serum are now available in specialist centres. They are labour intensive and difficult, however, as they require extraction, chromatography and detection of this vitamin D metabolite by radioimmunoassay or radioreceptor assay. These assays are only required to diagnose renal osteodystrophy, for therapeutic monitoring of 1,25-dihydroxy vitamin D levels and in the investigation of hypercalcaemia possibly due to extrarenal synthesis of 1,25-dihydroxy vitamin D.

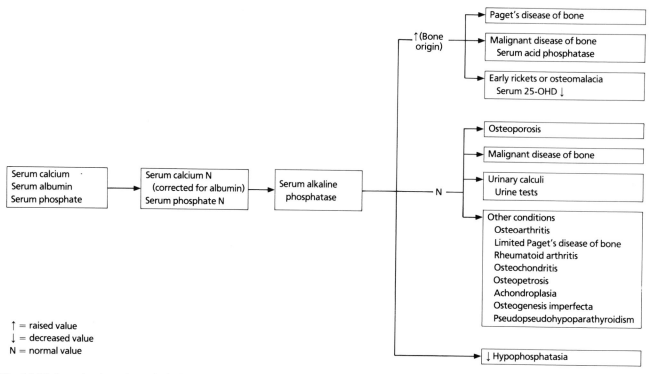

Fig. 14.30 Investigation of metabolic bone disease in patients with normocalcaemia.

PARATHYROID HORMONE

Assays of parathyroid hormone are now more readily available, but there is still lack of uniformity of results between different laboratories. Until recently, assays for parathyroid hormone lacked sensitivity, and the C-terminal assays gave misleading results in patients with renal insufficiency. The two-site immunoradiometric assays, which measure intact 1–84 parathyroid hormone, now provide differentiation between normal, depressed and elevated values of parathyroid hormone and are not subject to interference from C-terminal fragments.

Parathyroid hormone results are of value only if considered in conjunction with serum calcium and phosphate values. Inappropriately high values of serum parathyroid hormone for a particular serum calcium result are found in primary and tertiary hyperparathyroidism, though some patients with hypercalcaemia due to primary hyperparathyroidism have normal serum parathyroid hormone levels. In such cases the estimation of parathyroid hormone in samples obtained by neck vein catheterization may aid the detection and localization of a parathyroid tumour. Elevated serum parathyroid hormone values are also found in secondary hyperparathyroidism, as in chronic renal failure and nutritional rickets. The importance of parathyroid hormone-related protein as a humoral factor in hypercalcaemia associated with malignancy is now well recognized. Although the development of assays for parathyroid hormone-related protein in specialized centres is well advanced, however, these measurements are not yet available for routine diagnostic use.

CALCITONIN

Although calcitonin values may be high in umbilical cord and maternal sera or after parturition and in chronic renal failure, the use of calcitonin assays for routine clinical purposes is limited. Their importance is confined to the diagnosis and management of the rare medullary carcinoma of the thyroid and detection of relatives of patients at risk of developing familial medullary carcinoma of the thyroid and phaeochromocytoma. Despite a high serum calcitonin concentration, patients with medullary carcinoma of thyroid are often normocalcaemic. In addition, calcitonin may prove to be useful as a tumour marker in a variety of non-thyroid tumours, and the assay can be used in conjunction with secretagogues, e.g. pentagastrin or a calcium infusion, to detect latent hypercalcitoninaemia. Unfortunately at present, calcitonin assays suffer the same drawback as parathyroid hormone assays; these include the heterogeneity of reagents and lack of uniformity of results between different laboratories.

MAGNESIUM

Seventy percent of magnesium in normal human serum is unbound, but knowledge about the control of magnesium metabolism, particularly by the calcium-regulating hormones, is very confused. The clinical need for magnesium estimations usually arises in patients with tetany who do not respond to parenteral calcium therapy. In such patients, particularly newborn infants, hypomagnesaemia may be the cause of the symptoms. In adults, the most common causes of hypomagnesaemia are massive intestinal resection and prolonged diarrhoea (Brautbar and Gruber, 1986).

STEROID SUPPRESSION TEST

This test may be useful in the differential diagnosis of hypercalcaemia of obscure origin. It necessitates administration of hydrocortisone, 150 mg/day orally (or equivalent dose of prednisolone) for 10 days, after which the dose is gradually reduced. Serum calcium, total protein and albumin are measured before the test and on days 5, 7, 8, 9 and 10. In virtually all patients with primary hyperparathyroidism, the serum calcium level remains elevated, and suppression of serum calcium to the normal range makes a diagnosis of hyperparathyroidism very unlikely. Exceptions do occasionally occur; for example, some suppression may be seen in patients with hyperparathyroidism and concomitant radiologically evident bone disease, and failure of suppression may be seen in malignant disease with ectopic parathyroid hormone production. Now that assays for intact parathyroid hormone are available, the need for this test is much less.

CYCLIC AMP

Parathyroid hormone causes an increase in the rate of excretion of cyclic AMP in the urine, and in primary hyperparathyroidism the urinary excretion of cyclic AMP may be increased.

In pseudohypoparathyroidism, the urinary cyclic AMP response to exogenous parathyroid hormone is markedly diminished, consistent with renal unresponsiveness to parathyroid hormone. The diagnosis of pseudohypoparathyroidism is therefore made by the infusion of 200 USP units of parathyroid hormone and measurement of the changes in urinary or plasma cyclic AMP. In addition, the serum parathyroid hormone concentration is increased in pseudohypoparathyroidism.

URINARY HYDROXYPROLINE

The 24-h urinary excretion of total hydroxyproline may be used as an index of bone resorption in adults. Urine samples must be collected when the patient is on a low-gelatine diet, and as a result this test has not been extensively used. Raised values may occur in Paget's disease, osteomalacia, malignant disease involving bone, hyperthyroidism and fibrous dysplasia. The excretion of hydroxyproline after a 12-h fast is not influenced by the previous day's diet. Therefore, the ratio of hydroxyproline:creatinine in fasting urine may also be used as an index of bone resorption.

Recently, measurement of the urinary excretion of the collagen pyridinium cross-links (hydroxylysylpyridinoline and lysylpyridinoline) has been shown to be a more sensitive marker of bone resorption than hydroxyproline. Further method development is required, however, before this test is suitable for routine use.

OTHER URINE TESTS

Examination of the urine offers little diagnostic assistance in disorders of calcium metabolism other than for renal stones, where it is essential to diagnose cystinuria and hyperoxaluria, and for measurement of calcium excretion in familial hypocalciuric hypercalcaemia.

MISCELLANEOUS SUPPORTIVE TESTS

Certain other standard biochemical tests are very often required to support the use of chemical tests of calcium metabolism, e.g. measurements of serum urea, electrolytes, chloride and creatinine. There are also certain tests concerned with calcium metabolism, e.g. calcium balance studies and tubular reabsorption of calcium and phosphate, which although they often yield interesting results, provide little additional diagnostic information when trying to solve routine calcium problems.

Development of specific bone cell biochemical markers is a very active current field of research. It is likely that osteoblast markers, e.g. osteocalcin, bone alkaline phosphatase and procollagen I extension peptide, and osteoclast markers, e.g. tartrate-resistant acid phosphatase and pyridinoline cross-links, will soon be in routine use (Deftos, 1991).

BONE BIOPSY

Bone may be examined histologically by means of a bone biopsy. This is usually taken from the iliac crest by percutaneous trephine. An adequate specimen for histological purposes is 1–2 cm long and 5–10 mm thick. Bone is technically difficult tissue to deal with, and examination by biopsy assumes a high degree of uniformity throughout the body. The tissue is examined qualititatively and quantitatively. Undecalcified tissue gives most information and a variety of stains, such as silver, may be used to show up different types of tissue. Tetracycline is deposited in the bone at the site where mineralization is taking place when this compound is in the blood. The tetracycline shows up as a fluorescent line and remains as a permanent feature in the bone until the bone is resorbed (Malluche and Faugère, 1986).

Quantitative examination is particularly laborious as the histologist usually has to use manual methods with his own eye as the sensing device. An eyepiece graticule is used to quantitate different sample fields for, for example, area of osteoid, periosteal perimeter and area of resorption spaces. The computerized quantitation of bone, histomorphometry, is now available. Bone histology is a highly specialized branch of histopathology and is only available in certain centres.

REFERENCES

Albright F., Burnett C.H., Smith P.N. *et al.* (1942) Pseudohypoparathyroidism—an example of the 'Seabright–Bantam syndrome' *Endocrinology* **30**, 922–932.

Avioli L.V. and Heaney R.P. (1991) Calcium intake and bone health. *Calcif. Tissue Int.* **48**, 221–223.

Azria M. (1989) *The Calcitonins — Physiology and Pharmacology.* Basel, Karger.

Brautbar N. and Gruber H.E. (1986) Magnesium and bone disease. *Nephron* **44**, 1–7.

British Medical Association and Royal Pharmaceutical Society of Great Britain. (1994) *British National Formulary Number 27.* London, Pharmaceutical Press.

Canalis E., McCarthy T. and Centralla M. (1988) Growth factors and the regulation of bone remodeling. *J. Clin. Invest.* **81**, 277–281.

Centralla M. and Canalis E. (1985) Local regulators of skeletal growth: a perspective. *Endocr. Rev.* **6**, 544–551.

Chambers T.J. (1985) The pathobiology of the osteoclast. *J. Clin. Pathol.* **38**, 241–252.

Chick H., Dalyell E.J., Hume M. *et al.* (1922) The aetiology of rickets in infants. *Lancet* **ii**, 7–11.

Compston J.E. (1986) Hepatic osteodystrophy: vitamin D metabolism in patients with liver disease. *Gut* **27**, 1073–1090.

Consensus Development Conference. (1991) Conference Report: prophylaxis and treatment of osteoporosis. *Osteoporosis Int.* **1**, 114–117.

Cooper C. (1989) Epidemiological aspects of osteoporosis and age

related fractures. In Ring E.F.J., Evans W.D. and Dixon A.S. (eds) *Osteoporosis and Bone Mineral Measurement.* York, Institute of Physical Sciences in Medicine, pp. 7–16.

Cummings S.R., Kelsey J.L., Nevitt M.C. and O'Dowd K.J. (1985) Epidemiology of osteoporosis and osteoporotic fractures. *Epidemiol. Rev.* **7**, 178–208.

Deftos L.J. (1991) Bone protein and peptide assays in the diagnosis and management of skeletal disease. *Clin. Chem.* **37**, 1143–1148.

Dempster D.W., Shane E., Horbert W. and Lindsay R. (1986) A simple method for correlative light and scanning electron microscopy of human iliac crest bone biopsies: qualitative observations in normal and osteoporotic subjects. *J. Bone Miner. Res.* **1**, 15–21.

Editorial. (1977) Correcting the calcium. *BMJ* **1**, 598.

Fraser W.D. (1989) The structural and functional relationships between parathyroid hormone-related protein and parathyroid hormone. *J. Endocrinol.* **122**, 607–609.

Habener J.F., Rosenblatt M. and Potts J.T. Jr. (1984) Parathyroid hormone, biochemical aspects of biosynthesis, secretion, action and metabolism. *Physiol. Rev.* **64**, 985–1053.

Hauschka P.V., Lian J.B., Cole D.E.C. and Gundberg C.M. (1989) Osteocalcin and matrix Gla protein: vitamin K dependent proteins in bone. *Physiol. Rev.* **69**, 990–1047.

Heath D. (1991) The treatment of hypercalcaemia of malignancy. *Clin. Endocrin.* **34**, 155–157.

Holland B., Welch A., Unwin I., Buss D., Paul A. and Southgate D.A.T. (1991) McCance and Widdowson's The Composition of Foods, 5th edn. London and Cambridge, The Royal Society of Chemistry and MAFF.

Johnston C.C., Melton L.J., Lindsay R. and Eddy D.M. (1989) Clinical indications for bone mass measurements. *J. Bone Miner. Res.* **4** (Suppl. 2), 1–28.

Krieg T., Hein R., Hatamochi A. and Aumailley M. (1988) Molecular and clinical aspects of connective tissue. *Eur. J. Clin. Invest.* **18**, 105–123.

Levine M.A. (1993) Parathyroid hormone resistance syndromes. In *Primer on the Metabolic Bone Diseases and Disorders of Mineral Metabolism*, 2nd edn. American Society for Bone and Mineral Research. New York, Raven Press, pp. 194–200.

Malluche H.H. and Faugère M.C. (1986) *Atlas of Mineralized Bone Histology.* Basel, Karger.

Martin T.J., Ng. K.W. and Nicholson G.C. (1988) Cell biology of bone. *Baillieres Clin. Endocrinol. Metab.* **2**, 1–30.

Marx S.J. and Barsony J. (1988). Tissue-selective 1,25-dihydroxyvitamin D_3 resistance: novel applications of calciferols. *J. Bone Miner. Res.* **3**, 481–487.

Mohan S. and Baylink D.H. (1991) Bone growth factors. *Clin. Orthop. Rel. Res.* **263**, 30–48.

Morrison N.A., Qi J.C., Tokita A. *et al.* (1994) Prediction of bone density from vitamin D receptor alleles. *Nature* **367**, 284–287.

Orloff J.J., Wu T.L. and Stewart A.F. (1989) Parathyroid hormone-like proteins: biochemical responses and receptor interactions. *Endocr. Rev.* **10**, 476–495.

Peck W.A., Riggs B.L. and Bell N.H. (1987) *Physicians Resource Manual on Osteoporosis—a Decision Making Guide.* Washington D.C., National Osteoporosis Foundation.

Prockop D.J. and Kivirikko K.I. (1984) Heritable diseases of collagen. *N. Engl. J. Med.* **311**, 376–386.

Prockop D.J., Kivirikko K.I., Tuderman L. and Guzman N.A. (1979) Biosynthesis of collagen and its disorders. *N. Engl. J. Med.* **301**, 13–23.

Pyeritz R.E. and McKusick V.A. (1981) Basic defects in Marfan syndrome. *N. Engl. J. Med.* **305**, 1011–1012.

Reichel H., Koeffler P. and Norman A.W. (1989) The role of the vitamin D endocrine system in health and disease. *N. Engl. J. Med.* **320**, 980–991.

Riggs B.L. and Melton J. (1983) Evidence for two distinct syndromes of involutional osteoporosis. *Am. J. Med.* **75**, 899–901.

Royal College of Physicians. (1989) *Fractured Neck of Femur — Prevention and Management*. London, Royal College of Physicians of London.

Russell R.G.G., Caswell A.M., Hearn P.R. and Sharrard R.M. (1986) Calcium in mineralised tissues and pathological calcification. *Br. Med. Bull.* **42**, 435–446.

Scriver C.R., Beaudet A.L., Sly W.S. and Valle D. (1989) *The Metabolic Basis of Inherited Disease*, 6th edn. New York, McGraw-Hill.

Smith R. (1990) Corticosteroids and osteoporosis. *Thorax* **45**, 573–578.

Sykes B. and Smith R. (1985) Collagen and collagen gene disorders. *Q. J. Med.* **56**, 533–547.

Triffitt J.T. (1987) The special proteins of bone tissue. *Clin. Science* **72**, 399–408.

Tsipouras P., Del Mastro R., Sarfarazi M. *et al.* (1992) Genetic linkage of the Marfan syndrome, ectopia lentis, and congenital contractural arachnodactyly to the fibrillin genes on chromosomes 15 and 5. *N. Engl. J. Med.* **326**, 905–909.

Woolf A.D. and Dixon A.S.J. (1988) *Practical Problems in Medicine*: *Osteoporosis: a Clinical Guide*. London, Dunitz.

FURTHER READING

Albright F. and Reifenstein E.C. (1948) *The Parathyroid Glands and Metabolic Bone Disease*. Baltimore, Williams and Wilkins.

American Society for Bone and Mineral Research (1990) *Primer on the Metabolic Bone Diseases and Disorders of Mineral Metabolism*, 1st edn.

Avioli L.V. and Krane S.M. (1990) *Metabolic Bone Disease*, 2nd edn. Philadelphia, W.B. Saunders.

Besser G.M. and Cudworth A.G. (1987) *Clinical Endocrinology — an Illustrated Text*. London, Gower Medical Publishing.

Doherty M., Deighton C. and Compston J.E. (eds) (1994) Rheumatology, part 3. Metabolic bone disease. *Med. Int.* **22** (suppl.).

Kanis J.A. (1991) *Pathophysiology and Treatments of Paget's Disease of Bone*. London, Dunitz.

Riggs B.L. and Melton L.J. (1992) The prevention and treatment of osteoporosis. *N. Engl. J. Med.* **327**, 620–627.

Scriver C.R., Beaudet A.L., Sly W.S. and Valle D. (1989) *The Metabolic Basis of Inherited Disease*, 6th edn. New York, McGraw-Hill.

Wilson J.D. and Foster D.W. (1985) *Williams Textbook of Endocrinology*, 7th edn. Philadelphia, W.B. Saunders.

Chapter 15
Bone and Joint Infections

N.H. Harris

INTRODUCTION

Knowledge of the pathological changes and the natural history is the basis of treatment for most disease processes, and this applies particularly to bone and joint infections. Certain anatomical factors, however, help our understanding of the later pathological changes. It is thus appropriate to discuss first certain of these relevant anatomical features.

Long bones

Figure 15.1 represents the end of a child's long bone. The vascular pattern during growth and the blood flow in the region have been described in detail by Trueta and Harrison (1953) and Trueta (1957). Epiphyseal arteries anastomose with each other and are directed into the epiphysis and towards the joint surface in the form of a series of arcades. The metaphyseal arteries form inter-connecting anastomoses in the subsynovial tissues before they enter the bone (circus articuli vasculosi of Hunter). After entering the bone they turn towards the epiphyseal plate. There is no arching system of anastomoses as in the epiphysis, but one of branching vessels. Before the establishment of the growth plate at about 1 year of age, the metaphyseal vessels perforate the plate and form a free anastomosis with the epiphyseal vessels. This is sometimes referred to as the fetal pattern. After about 1 year of age the fully developed growth plate acts as a barrier, preventing significant communication between the two sets of vessels. The metaphyseal vessels, however, do anastomose freely with those in the diaphysis, which in turn arise from the nutrient arteries.

During growth haemopoietic red marrow is present in the epiphysis and metaphysis. In adults it is restricted to a zone of the epiphysis under the articular cartilage and the metaphysis. From the point of view of localization of infection, a fundamental fact is that only the red marrow

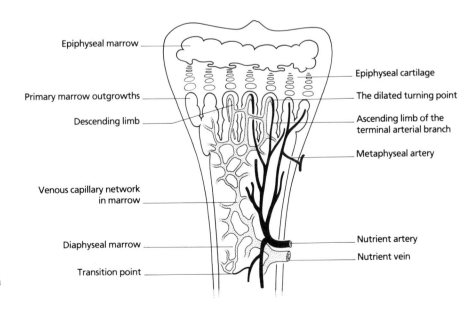

Fig. 15.1 End of a child's long bone. Note the vascular pattern in the metaphysis and adjacent diaphysis of an immature bone.

Labels in figure: Epiphyseal marrow; Primary marrow outgrowths; Descending limb; Venous capillary network in marrow; Diaphyseal marrow; Transition point; Epiphyseal cartilage; The dilated turning point; Ascending limb of the terminal arterial branch; Metaphyseal artery; Nutrient artery; Nutrient vein.

397

contains large, thin-walled venous sinusoids, or venous lakes as they are sometimes called. They form an anasto-mosing meshwork of intensely vascular channels. These vascular spaces are fed by comparatively small afferent vessels. It follows that the blood flow will slow down when it reaches the venous sinusoids and thus form an ideal site for the multiplication of pathological bacteria. It is significant that the area incorporating this vascular pattern in the metaphysis corresponds with the distribution of bone sepsis in the early stages of acute osteomyelitis. The yellow fatty marrow normally only contains capillaries of normal size.

The articular cartilage comes into contact with the capillary vessels at its periphery and with vessels from the epiphyseal circulation on the deep surface. Vessels pass through the subchondral bone and give rise to capillary loops at the deep surface in the calcified basal layers of the cartilage. Other relevant anatomical considerations may be listed as follows:

1 In certain sites the metaphyseal region is intracapsular, thus facilitating the direct spread of infection from the bone through the very thin metaphyseal cortex into the joint. Examples of such sites are hip, knee, distal femoral epiphysis and elbow.

2 During growth the metaphysis, because of its vascular pattern, is the part of the bone that is most vulnerable to minor trauma.

3 The diaphysis receives its blood supply through one or more nutrient arteries, which subdivide after entering the bone. The inner cortex is mainly supplied from this source.

4 The outer cortex is supplied from the periosteal circulation; if any source of blood supply to cortical bone is jeopardized a collateral supply is available. The cortical capillary lattice communicates with the radially arranged vessels from the medulla and with the periosteal vessels. Under these circumstances the cortical capillary system could receive blood from either source should the need arise.

5 In children the deeper layer of the periosteum is highly vascular and is only loosely attached to the bone. In adults the periosteum becomes progressively more adherent to the bone with age.

Vertebral column

Pathological and clinical features of infections involving the vertebral bodies and disc spaces are conditioned by certain anatomical features, principally due to the vascular supply (Wiley and Trueta, 1959). The arterial supply follows the embryological pattern; thus, for example, one intercostal artery supplies two vertebrae

(the lower half of one and the upper half of the vertebra below). Infections will therefore involve the adjacent parts of two vertebrae and the intervening cartilaginous disc. Vessels from the vertebral, intercostal and lumbar arteries penetrate the numerous foramina in the cortex of the bodies and ramify in the marrow. There is a rich anastomosis of the vessels on the posterior aspect of the bodies, and the vessels also penetrate the cortex and anastomose with the segmental vessels. Specialized vascular tufts have been demonstrated in the cartilaginous end-plates, and it is thought that this is where the infection is first localized. The nucleus pulposus and the annulus fibrosus (except at its periphery) are vascular at all edges.

In the majority of patients infection reaches the vertebra through one of the many arteries that enter the body, but it is theoretically possible that the venous system is the route involved. The venous drainage of the vertebral column has been well described by Henriques (1947), who described the internal venous plexus of Batson (1940) and its communication with the venous system of the vertebral systemic veins. Henriques pointed out that if tumour cells can pass through the chest wall and pelvic veins to the vertebral venous plexus, then it is not unreasonable to assume that infection can pass by the same route.

Early narrowing of the disc space, which is such a characteristic radiological feature of vertebral body infection, is probably the result of damage to the cartilaginous end-plate following impairment of the blood supply from the metaphysis. The damage will allow herniation of the disc material through it.

ACUTE PYOGENIC INFECTION OF LONG BONES

Pathogenesis

AETIOLOGY AND BACTERIOLOGY

The term osteomyelitis was first coined by Nelaton (1844). Haematogenous osteomyelitis is a more accurate description, because it describes the fact that there is accompanying bacteraemia or septicaemia. A primary focus of infection is not often found, but the usual sites are nasopharyngeal, a tooth socket, or skin, and the focus will predispose to bacteraemia. In infants, infection may reach the blood through the umbilical cord.

Infection of bones may also occur as a direct result of inoculation from a penetrating wound in a compound fracture, after surgery using implants, and directly from an adjacent infected ulcer as with a varicose ulcer overlying the tibia.

Infants and children are very much more commonly affected than adults, confirming that haematogenous osteomyelitis usually involves rapidly growing bones where there is a rich blood supply; it is for this reason that localization occurs in the metaphysis of long bones. Very occasionally the infection starts in the diaphysis.

Butler (1940) pointed out the high incidence before 1930, and in his review of 500 patients between 1919 and 1937 the mortality was 25%. After 1930 the incidence declined and this was attributed to improved nutrition and housing. The mortality did not alter, because there was no available method of treating septicaemia. In 1944 penicillin was effectively used for the first time (Trueta and Morgan, 1954), and in this report of 100 patients the mortality was zero. It was assumed that the disease would disappear or that if it did occur, curing it would not be a problem. Both these assumptions have proved to be wrong (Winters and Cahen, 1960; Gilmour, 1962). The morbidity remains relatively high, and this may be related to late diagnosis.

There are a number of predisposing factors, the most common of which is trauma, with common occurrence in the lower limbs of children. The fragile metaphyseal vessels are damaged resulting in thrombosis and stasis which establishes an ideal culture medium. The predisposing factors in infants are predominantly umbilical sepsis, delivery by caesarian section and jaundice. Premature infants are more prone to septicaemia. Immunodeficiency from whatever cause is most commonly seen in children, but also in adults who have had dialysis or renal transplantation (Spencer, 1986). In adults there is usually a predisposing cause, e.g. diabetes, chemotherapy for malignant disease, or failure of the neutrophil response in aplastic anaemia and leukaemia, and more recently acquired immune deficiency syndrome (Roca and Yoshikawa, 1979). Murray (1960) reported the rapid silent progression of infection and extensive bone destruction in patients on systemic steroid therapy. Sickle-cell anaemia is a known predisposing cause of osteomyelitis, particularly due to *Salmonella* infection (Golding *et al.*, 1959); the disease is often multifocal, and it is the blocking of the marrow blood vessels by degraded sickle cells that presents bacteria with an ideal site for multiplication. *Salmonella* food poisoning outbreaks are much more common than hitherto, and it is as well, therefore, to bear in mind the possibility of osteomyelitis arising in these patients.

The most common infecting organism is coagulase-positive *Staphylococcus aureus*; coagulase-negative *Staphylococcus* is occasionally responsible but generally in the less acute infections. *Haemophilus influenzae* is responsible in about 20% of cases, and other Gram-negative organisms occur perhaps more often than is supposed—namely *Escherichia coli*, *Proteus* sp., *Pseudomonas* sp., *Salmonella* sp. and *Brucella* sp. The possibility of an unusual organism should always be considered, particularly in adults, when there is an associated illness such as diarrhoea and urinary infection, and in compound fractures and after implant surgery. β-haemolytic streptococci are commonly isolated pathogens in neonates.

PATHOLOGICAL CHANGES

The sequence of events following establishment of infection in the metaphysis can be closely correlated with the anatomical considerations discussed earlier.

Inflammatory exudates rapidly accumulate, raising the intraosseus pressure; venous return is obstructed leading to stasis and thrombosis of vessels. Death of bone results from the direct effect of bacterial toxins and vascular impairment in the cortex and periosteum; it is likely that these changes will have occurred by about the third day of the illness. The peripheral branches of the nutrient artery are secondarily thrombosed by spread of infection from the venous side of the vascular loops (Fig. 15.1), and if the infection is not controlled the nutrient artery itself may thrombose. Suppuration and bone absorption follow rapidly, producing a further rise in pressure. Pus soon breaks through the thin metaphyseal cortex to form a subperiosteal abscess; if the metaphysis is intracapsular as in the hip joint, pyoarthrosis results. In infants, infection can spread to involve the epiphysis and also the joint; the hip is the most common site and it has commonly undergone subluxation or dislocation when the infection is diagnosed. Thrombosis of vessels may cause an aseptic necrosis of the epiphysis. Whatever the mechanism the epiphysis may be partially or completely destroyed (these joint changes will be further discussed in the section on septic arthritis on p. 411).

In children the growth plate acts as a barrier to the spread of infection. Primary epiphyseal osteomyelitis does very occasionally occur in children over 18 months of age, however, as reported by Rosenbaum and Blumhagen (1985) and Srensen *et al.* (1988).

In adults there is no barrier to the spread of infection to the subarticular bone and the joint; spread to form a subperiosteal abscess is rare because of the more fibrous nature of the periosteum and its firm adherence to the cortex. In fact, intramedullary spread may occur quite rapidly throughout the length of the diaphysis.

After the third or fourth day the vascular layer of the

periosteum is stripped from the cortex, thus denuding the outer layer of its blood supply which, combined with the impairment of blood flow to the inner cortex, is likely to result in sequestrum formation. This becomes isolated from living tissue by pus and impairs the effectiveness of antibiotics.

Stripping of the periosteum is soon followed by the development of new bone which forms the involucrum. Rapid and early development of massive periosteal new bone is characteristically seen in infants because of the highly vascular nature of the periosteum. Once sequestra and an involucrum have been allowed to form, chronic disease has developed, and this will be discussed later (see p. 407).

It must be stressed that effective treatment, whether it is with antibiotics alone or combined with surgical drainage, depends on a proper understanding of the pathological changes that have been described. The fundamental change that occurs during the first 2−3 days of the illness, and which is common to all age groups, is vascular impairment, which leads to a varying degree of bone necrosis and sequestrum formation. Chronic disease will follow unless effective treatment is given in the early stages.

Clinical features

Effective treatment depends on early diagnosis, which in turn depends on careful history-taking and examination. Although a family doctor is likely to see only a few such patients in a lifetime of practice, the possibility of such a diagnosis must always be borne in mind in acutely ill infants and children with limb pain.

Typically, in the more acute form of the disease, a child will present with a sudden onset of severe pain at the site of the lesion associated with systemic manifestations and fever. The examining doctor should be alert to the fact that previously administered antibiotics may mask the signs and symptoms; furthermore, the presentation in infants is quite different, in that there is often no systemic illness, and this may also be the case in the elderly. A few infants will present with acute septicaemic illness.

The most important localizing sign is acute local tenderness and some swelling, and this will be more easily found where the bone is relatively superficial. The child will resent interference, and if there is doubt the examination should be repeated about 1 h later.

The affected limb will be immobile, presenting as pseudoparalysis, and this is a particularly important sign in infants when associated with swelling and pain on passive movement. The adjacent joint may be swollen, and it will often be impossible to decide if it is primarily or secondarily infected. An infant's joint can be moved passively, unlike in older children where the infected joint is quite rigid.

If a fluctuant abscess is clinically detectable, generally this indicates that the infection has existed for several days.

It is as well to remember that in adults, the usually associated illnesses, e.g. rheumatoid arthritis, may confuse the picture, and so it is sensible to constantly think of the possibility of a bone infection when considering the differential diagnosis.

Investigations

The erythrocyte sedimentation rate is usually but not invariably raised in the early stages, and it is often as high as 100 mm in the first hour. The higher it is above 40 mm the more likely the infection is to be pyogenic rather than tuberculosis. The total and differential white blood counts are often normal in the first 24 hours (Harris, 1960); sometimes the total blood count may be normal but the differential count reveals polymorphonuclear leucocytosis. A variable degree of anaemia occurs, due to the septicaemia.

Blood cultures are positive in about 50% of cases (Harris, 1960); blood samples should be taken as soon as possible after suspecting the diagnosis and three samples should be used after suitable intervals. Antibiotics that have been given before taking blood samples are likely to reduce the chances of obtaining a positive culture. Most laboratories will provide a verbal report after 24 h. The technique and diagnostic value of determining anti-staphylococcal antibody titres have been reported (Lack and Towers, 1962). Anti-α-haemolysin (normal range up to 4 units/ml) and anti-Panton−Valentine leucondin (normal range up to 8 units/ml) are the most useful and both should be determined, but they are probably of little diagnostic value during the first 2−3 weeks of the illness. It is useful, however, to differentiate staphylococcal from tuberculous infections, particularly in deeply placed lesions, e.g. in the spinal column.

Radiographs are generally negative in the first 7−10 days, except that non-specific swelling of the soft tissues may be visible. In infants, however, a periosteal reaction may be seen after a few days (Fig. 15.2). The early recognizable changes in the bone are patchy osteolytic areas in the metaphysis and associated periosteal new bone formation extending over a variable length of the diaphysis (Fig. 15.3). In neonates, the hip joint is the most common site of infection, and early signs are

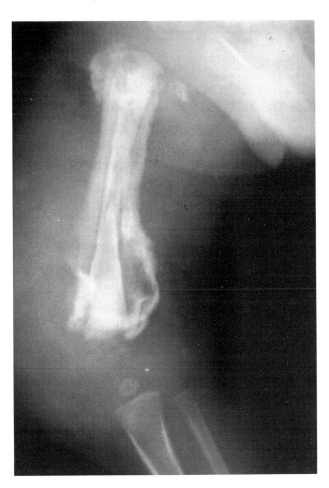

Fig. 15.2 Acute osteomyelitis in the femur of an infant. Note the typically extensive periosteal new bone.

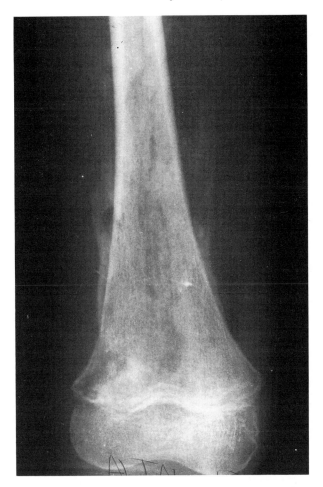

Fig. 15.3 Typical radiographic appearance of acute osteomyelitis. Note the periosteal new bone and bone erosions in the metaphysis.

patchy metaphyseal osteolysis with or without lateral subluxation. The diagnosis in these infants is often late, and to avoid mistakes a routine hip radiograph should be taken in all infants suspected of having osteomyelitis, whatever the site.

A bone scan may be helpful in the first 48 h. It is important to request a blood pool or vascular phase and a delayed skeletal image. In the presence of osteomyelitis both are positive, but in a soft tissue infection, e.g. cellulitis, only the vascular phase is positive.

The only reliable diagnostic investigation is aspiration or exploration for pus, which has the additional merit of providing material for culture and sensitivity testing, and from which a result can be obtained in 24 h. Aspiration is useful in deeply placed infections, e.g. in the spine. Exploration, however, is more reliable and if the diagnosis remains in doubt no harm will result. On occasions a surgeon may regret not operating and adopting a 'wait and see policy'.

Differential diagnosis

The only conditions likely to present difficulties are minor trauma and cellulitis. In the past, acute poliomyelitis and acute rheumatism were often the first diagnoses, but these conditions are now very seldom seen in clinical practice.

It is worth noting, in view of the relatively high incidence, that non-accidental injury in infants commonly affects the metaphyseal region of long bones and in the early stages may be indistinguishable from an infected lesion.

Treatment

There is general agreement that if complications such as early recurrence of infection and chronic disease are to be avoided, effective treatment must start within a few days of the illness. Trueta and Morgan (1954) were the first to point out that effective treatment should start within 3 days of illness. It follows that successful treatment depends on early diagnosis; if this can be achieved, then treatment will start before ischaemic changes have occurred.

GENERAL MEASURES

These are self-evident and include complete bed-rest with adequate splinting of the affected parts, and analgesics and intravenous fluids in acutely ill patients.

ANTIBIOTICS

The subject has been reviewed by Blockey and McAllister (1972), Gillespie (1981) and Scales and Arnoff (1984). Since Trueta and Morgan (1954) reported the effectiveness of penicillin and early operative drainage, it has become clear that antibiotics control the septicaemia and reduce the mortality from a pre-antibiotic rate of 25% to zero.

A further significant change has taken place since about 1950, namely that there has been a steady rise in the incidence of penicillin-resistant staphylococci isolated from patients with osteomyelitis. In the author's series of 84 patients, the organism was cultured in 64 patients, and 35% of the isolates were resistant (Harris, 1962). During the same period the number of complications, e.g. sequestra and chronic disease, rose considerably, and most of the reported series indicate an

incidence of about 30% (Fig. 15.4). It was also noteworthy that in 11 of the 27 complications there was a delay in starting effective antibiotic therapy due to the presence of penicillin-resistant *Staphylococcus* sp. In Mann's (1963) series of 100 patients, 55% of the staphylococci were resistant to penicillin, and in seven of the 13 complications the initial antibiotic was ineffective for the same reason.

The results of these and other studies make it clear that a major cause of complications is ineffectiveness of the initial antibiotic due to resistant organisms. In order to reduce morbidity, the antibiotic must act against penicillin-resistant staphylococci and be administered at the earliest possible moment after the start of the illness in adequate doses and for a sufficient length of time. It should ideally have the following properties:

1 Effective against the most likely pathogen—coagulase-positive *Staphylococcus* sp. and *Streptococcus* sp. in infants.
2 Bactericidal properties to reduce the possibility of recurrence.
3 Low toxicity, permitting prolonged therapy if necessary.
4 Capable of administration by oral and parenteral routes.
5 Formation of resistant strains must be rare.
6 Production of effective blood and tissue concentrations.

Initial therapy (before the sensitivity of the organism is known) in infants consists of flucloxacillin sodium, 200 mg/kg/day, and benzylpenicillin (penicillin G),

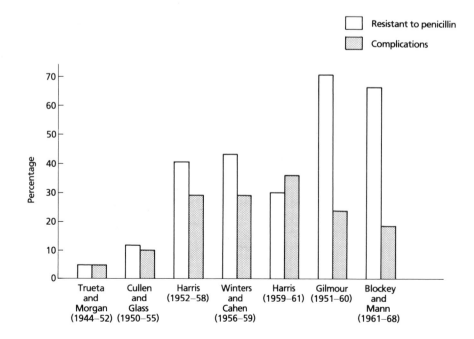

Fig. 15.4 Correlation between the incidence of penicillin-resistant staphylococci and complications.

250 000 units/kg/day; the first few doses should be parenteral. The oral dose can be adjusted to flucloxacillin, 100 mg/kg/day, and if the organism is resistant, fusidic acid is recommended. For children flucloxacillin, 250 mg/6 h, alone is sufficient. If *E. coli, Pseudomonas* sp., *Proteus* sp., or *Haemophilus* sp. is suspected, carbenicillin sodium (which also acts against Gram-positive staphylococci) is the most appropriate drug and is given in doses of 200–400 mg/kg/day combined with gentamicin sulphate. If a *Salmonella* infection is suspected, amoxycillin combined with gentamicin, 7.5 mg/kg/day, are the best drugs to use. Once the organism has been isolated and its sensitivity determined, the appropriate antibiotics are continued orally for 6 weeks. Undoubtedly, if treatment starts very early before bone changes have occurred, 3 weeks of antibiotics will be sufficient. The best guide is the clinical state of the patient—pyrexia and local signs, e.g. tenderness and swelling. The erythrocyte sedimentation rate is a reliable guide and if regular readings show it is falling, this is probably an indication that infection has been eliminated.

Difficulty arises in patients who are allergic to penicillin, for they are also usually allergic to the cephalosporins, which under normal circumstances are a good alternative to penicillin. The available alternatives are fusidic acid, lincomycin hydrochloride and erythromycin.

OPERATIVE TREATMENT

An operation in acute osteomyelitis is an adjunct to antibiotic therapy. Operative drainage of a bone and the subperiosteal abscess effectively decompresses the medulla and reduces the risk of vascular impairment and its consequences, e.g. bone necrosis and sequestrum formation. It has the added advantages of providing material for culture and sensitivity testing, rapid relief of pain, and assisting the access of antibiotics to the focus of infection.

Sir Harry Platt provided a good working principle that remains valid today: 'A small incision down to the metaphysis at the point of tenderness and puncture of the bone by a series of small drill holes will save many limbs and lives. If the diagnosis is not confirmed the patient will suffer no harm.'

It was said in the previous section that most acute infections will be cured by antibiotics alone, provided that certain conditions are met. Operation, however, must not be reserved for complications, e.g. chronic disease, and it has an important part to play in the early stages of the condition in selected patients, namely those whose infections are not controlled by antibiotic therapy after 36–48 h (Harris, 1962; Mollan and Piggot, 1977; Arnoff and Scales, 1983; Galasko, 1989). Contrary views have been expressed, notably by Mann (1963) and Gillespie (1981).

The following guidelines are proposed. After admission of the patient, a decision must be made as to whether to perform immediate drainage (usually for therapeutic but occasionally also for diagnostic reasons) or to wait to observe the response to antibiotic therapy. The decision should be based on the length of history before admission, previously administered antibiotics by the general practitioner, the general condition of the patient and the severity of the local signs. In a few patients the illness may have started a few days earlier, and antibiotics may have been given which mask the true severity of the condition. The constitutional reaction may be severe, accompanied by severe local pain and tenderness, and a palpable, fluctuant, abscess may exist. In such circumstances, after a large initial dose of antibiotics and intravenous fluids if appropriate, it is not unreasonable (some would say obligatory) to perform immediate drainage.

Technique of drainage

Aspiration of an abscess is unreliable and may be difficult in very deep infections, and furthermore it may have to be repeated. Open drainage is the ideal technique and should be performed under general anaesthesia, preferably with a tourniquet.

An incision is made over the metaphysis, and wide stripping of the soft tissues is unnecessary. After removal of the subperiosteal pus, several drill holes are made into the metaphysis; guttering of the bone is not necessary. It is safe to close the wound without drainage.

Infantile long-bone infections are an exception, and an operation is seldom necessary in this age group, despite the gross radiological changes that are often seen; however, if there is a large local abscess it should be drained.

The principle of early operation is based on the pathological changes during the first few days of the illness. Anatomical and pathological factors are fundamental to a proper understanding of the natural history of the disease, and unless it is appropriate all treatment becomes empirical.

PRIMARY SUBACUTE PYOGENIC OSTEOMYELITIS

This type of infection is insidious in onset, without a

systemic reaction, and there is no history of previous acute attacks or recently administered antibiotics. It is now the most common form of presentation and was first described by Harris and Kirkaldy-Willis in 1965. The subject has also been reviewed by King and Mayo (1969), Green *et al.* (1981) and Roberts *et al.* (1982).

Pathogenesis

This type of infection is probably the result of the interaction of a low-virulence organism and the host's resistance. The organism is usually a coagulase-positive *Staphylococcus* sp., but occasionally a coagulase-negative *Staphylococcus* sp. has been isolated. Although the organism reaches the bone via the blood stream, there is no septicaemia. The infection is localized to the metaphysis in some cases as in the acute form of the disease, but the diaphysis is not uncommonly primarily involved and may give rise to difficulties in diagnosis.

Primary subacute pyogenic osteomyelitis principally affects children and young adults. The typical lesions are not seen in infants, though as described earlier, the infantile form of osteomyelitis usually presents as a subacute illness, as indeed do vertebral infections in adults.

The lesions can be conveniently divided into those with and those without abscess formation. When an abscess occurs there may be minimal reaction in the surrounding bone (an osteolytic lesion), and it usually occurs in the metaphyseal region; sometimes the growth plate is breached and the epiphysis will then become involved. In other instances there is considerable surrounding sclerosis and periosteal reaction; this type usually occurs in the diaphysis and is often referred to as a Brodie's abscess (Brodie, 1836). The term 'Brodie's abscess' is used rather loosely to describe a form of chronic osteomyelitis secondary to a previous acute attack. Sir Benjamin Brodie, however, described a classic, primary, low-grade bone abscess.

In lesions without pus formation, patchy necrosis occurs in the diaphysis with or without metaphyseal involvement and cortical sequestration. In other instances, a sclerosing non-suppurative lesion occurs in the diaphysis without sequestration or abscess formation, and is sometimes referred to as Garré's osteomyelitis. The cortical cancellous bone is thickened and the medullary cavity is partly obliterated by new bone; it is rare to obtain a positive culture from this lesion. It has been referred to more recently as chronic sclerosing osteomyelitis (Kopits and Debuskey, 1977; Collert and Isacson, 1982; Mollan *et al.*, 1984).

Clinical features

The onset is insidious and the principal complaint is intermittent attacks of pain over several days or weeks. Spontaneous remission, often of long duration, is not unknown. The diagnosis is usually delayed for some weeks after the onset of symptoms. A constitutional reaction is very rare, as is a pyrexia. In most instances, local swelling and tenderness are evident.

Investigations

The erythrocyte sedimentation rate, total and differential white blood count are usually normal and are therefore unreliable guides to the nature of the lesion. Blood culture is invariably sterile. The anti-staphylococcal antibody titres are of value provided that it is remembered that false-negatives occur in 8% of all grades of infection.

RADIOLOGY

Several radiologically distinct types may be recognized, and the appearance can be reasonably well correlated with the distinctive pathological lesions described above; more than one type may occur in a single bone.

A Brodie's abscess (Fig. 15.5) is most commonly seen in the tibial diaphysis. The lesion is surrounded by a zone of dense sclerosis and a variable periosteal reaction. A larger osteolytic lesion with minimal sclerotic and periosteal reaction, but no sequestra and a round or irregular outline, occurs in metaphyseal lesions and most often in the distal tibia (Fig. 15.6). Other locations are the os calcis (Fig. 15.7), the proximal humerus (Fig. 15.8) and distal radius (Fig. 15.9); multiple lesions sometimes occur (Fig. 15.10). In other instances multiple osteolytic lesions occur as part of a diffuse reaction in the diaphysis (Fig. 15.11). A more localized diaphyseal lesion also occurs (Fig. 15.12). Patchy diaphyseal necrosis accompanied by a periosteal reaction and cortical sequestration will sometimes resemble Ewing's sarcoma when it involves only the diaphysis (Fig. 15.13). The other lesion without abscess formation is primary sclerosing Garré's osteomyelitis, which characteristically shows much thickening of cortical cancellous bone and partial obliteration of the medullary cavity (Fig. 15.14).

Radioactive isotope scanning is a helpful procedure, though in isolation it must not be relied on for making a definitive diagnosis.

EXPLORATION

Diagnostic exploration, which is the only certain method

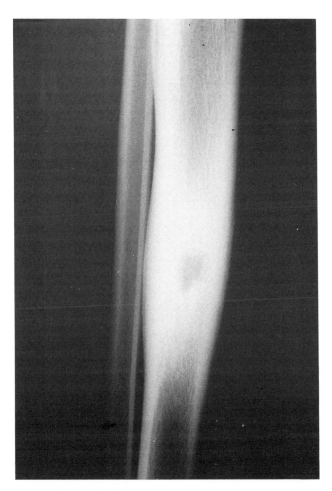

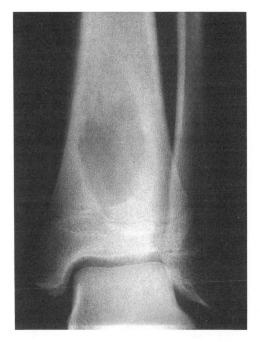

Fig. 15.6 Brodie's abscess. Note the large osteolytic staphylococcal lesion with minimal sclerotic and periosteal reactions.

Fig. 15.5 Brodie's abscess. 2-year history of pain in the tibia diagnosed as an osteoid osteoma. Note the osteolytic lesion surrounded by a zone of sclerosis and periosteal new bone.

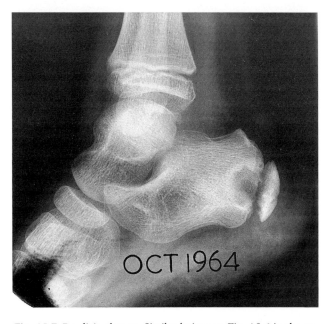

Fig. 15.7 Brodie's abscess. Similar lesions to Fig. 15.6 in the os calcis.

of confirming the diagnosis of the lesion (which may not resemble a characteristic inflammatory condition on the plain radiograph), is to remove material for culture and histology if appropriate. It is particularly advisable to proceed in this way if a tumour is suspected, and it is also of critical importance to try to culture an organism. Where a bone abscess is present, exploration will form part of the normal therapeutic measures.

Differential diagnosis

The varied radiological appearance of these lesions often leads to difficulty in diagnosis, and in particular the following lesions should be considered.

TUBERCULOSIS

In both diseases infection may spread across the growth plate to involve the epiphysis, but it much more commonly does so in tuberculosis. Decalcification and minimal or no periosteal reaction are typical features of the latter.

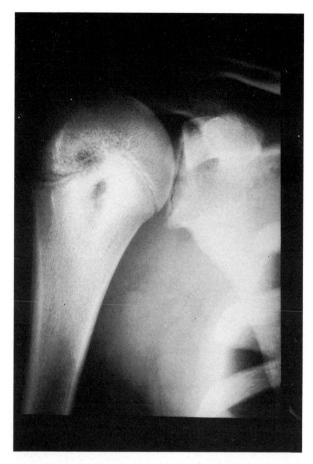

Fig. 15.8 Brodie's abscess. Similar lesions to Fig. 15.6 in the proximal humerus.

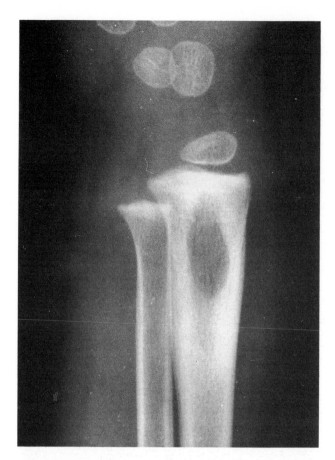

Fig. 15.9 Brodie's abscess. Similar lesions to Fig. 15.6 in the distal radius.

OSTEOID OSTEOMA

It may be impossible to confidently distinguish this lesion from a small subacute bone abscess. The history of night pain, usually relieved by aspirin, and a normal erythrocyte sedimentation rate would be more in favour of an osteoid osteoma.

PRIMARY MALIGNANT BONE TUMOUR (E.G. EWING'S SARCOMA)

Clinical and radiological features are indistinguishable, and biopsy is obligatory.

OSTEOCLASTOMA

This occurs at the end of a long bone after fusion of the epiphysis. The radiological appearance of expansion and thinning of the cortex are typical features; however, a biopsy is essential if there is the slightest doubt about the diagnosis.

MISCELLANEOUS

Other conditions that may present difficulties are simple bone cysts, non-osteogenic fibroma and fibrous dysplasia. Biopsy is the only way to resolve the problem.

Treatment

This aspect has been reviewed by Ross and Cole (1985). Patients seldom show a constitutional reaction, and a period of strict bed-rest is generally not necessary. Relief of pain is more easily achieved, however, if the involved part can be immobilized by appropriate splinting.

ANTIBIOTICS

These are given in accordance with the principles described earlier for acute osteomyelitis. Antibiotics alone are indicated in those patients in whom there is no obvious bone cavity or an abscess. For diffuse diaphyseal lesions a course of 4–6 months of treatment is advised, but generally 6 weeks is sufficient.

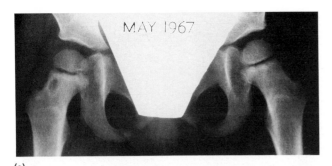

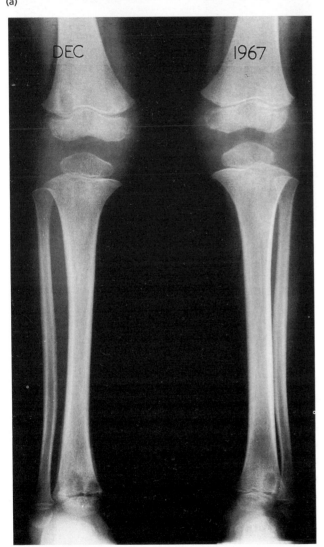

Fig. 15.10 (a, b) Multiple infected (coagulase-negative) staphylococcal lesions in the right proximal and distal femoral metaphysis, and the proximal and distal metaphysis of both tibias.

OPERATIVE DRAINAGE

This is indicated in patients in whom an abscess is present, and in such cases a bone cavity can usually be

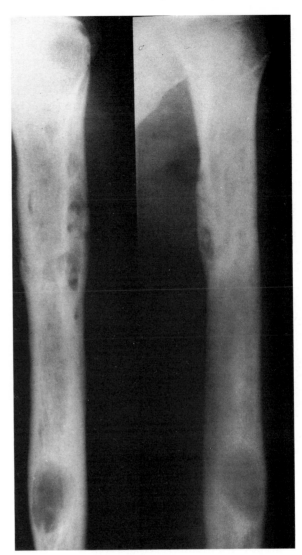

Fig. 15.11 A diffuse diaphyseal subacute staphylococcal infection. Note that the periosteal reaction is minimal. At operation granulation tissue but no pus was found. No antibiotics had been given when this radiograph was taken 26 days after the onset.

seen on the radiograph. Operative drainage is also advisable if a joint is involved and in those patients who fail to improve with conservative treatment. As indicated earlier, operation must be undertaken if there is doubt about the diagnosis, in which case material is taken for biopsy; at the same time if there is a cavity in the bone, this should be thoroughly curretted.

CHRONIC OSTEOMYELITIS

Pathogenesis

Chronic infection of bone is usually a sequel to acute

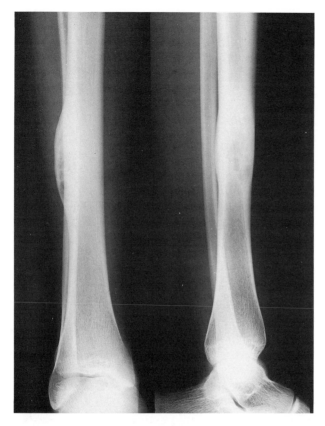

Fig. 15.12 Primary subacute diaphyseal lesion. Note the multiple abscess cavities.

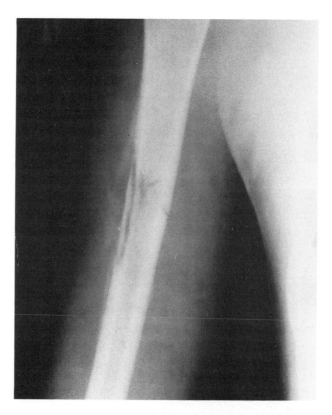

Fig. 15.13 This 12-year-old child complained of pain for 1 month. Note that the patchy osteolytic areas and periostitis are confined to the diaphysis.

osteomyelitis that has been imperfectly treated or treated late after diagnosis of an acute infection. It is much less common in the UK than 20 years ago, but it remains a familiar problem in developing countries.

Chronic osteomyelitis is perhaps seen with increasing frequency following a compound fracture, particularly when the tibia is involved; not uncommonly it occurs if some form of internal fixation has been used, and less commonly it may occur after internal fixation for a closed fracture. In the latter case, chronic infection becomes established because the initial infection is diagnosed late and/or effective treatment is not given once the diagnosis has been made. Deep infection after joint replacement (discussed in detail on p. 421) occurs in a similar way, that is, the initial acute infection is either diagnosed days or weeks after it has become established or alternatively, the treatment prescribed is inappropriate.

Isolation of the causative organism is less predictable than in acute infections. A wide range of organisms may be responsible, but the most common is coagulase-positive *Staphylococcus* sp. More than one organism may be present, however, and *E. coli* and *Pseudomonas* sp. may coexist with the *Staphylococcus* sp.

PATHOLOGICAL CHANGES

The changes described here are those seen following previous infection; they are to some extent modified in post-traumatic and joint replacement patients.

Essentially, there is a combination of bone erosion, cortical and subperiosteal new bone formation, and sequestrum and abscess formation. The relative amount of each will vary from one patient to another. One of the striking features of chronic disease is the irregularly thickened cortex due to the periosteal new bone formation — the involucrum. If the periosteal reaction fails or is impaired due to loss of blood supply, then in the acute stage an osseous defect and pseudarthrosis may occur. The involucrum is perforated by cloacae, through which pus discharges into one or more sinuses.

The osteoblastic activity associated with osteoclastic resorption produces dense, relatively avascular bone. There is also a variable amount of dense avascular scar tissue surrounding the abscess cavities, which may contain sequestra. The skin over the involved bone, particularly over the tibia, is often of poor quality and adherent, and where a sinus exists it is excoriated. The dense

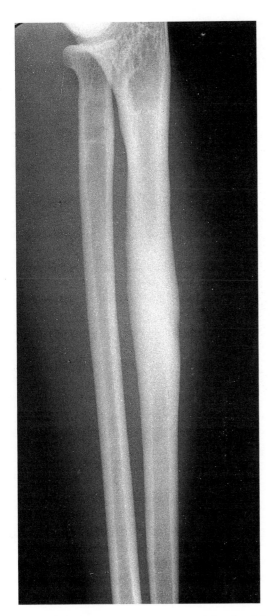

Fig. 15.14 Sclerosing Garré's osteomyelitis of the ulna. Note the typical localized cortical thickening with smooth margins.

avascular bone and scar tissue act as a barrier to the effective diffusion of antibiotics.

COMPLICATIONS

A pathological fracture may occur if involucrum formation is defective for some reason. The bone is vulnerable to such an occurrence after radical surgery, and this must be recognized when considering the post-operative care.

Amyloid disease was at one time the most common sequel to long-standing chronic sepsis, but it is seldom if ever seen now in the UK.

Two forms of malignant change occur very occasionally: either an epidermoid carcinoma or a sarcoma that is endosteal in origin.

Clinical features

SECONDARY TO ACUTE OSTEOMYELITIS

The patient presents with a history of a previous acute attack of osteomyelitis months or years previously, and there may have been several attacks of pain, local abscess formation and a discharging sinus; between attacks the infection is quiescent. In some instances the discharging sinus has persisted from the first onset.

The patient is generally not ill, and pyrexia seldom occurs. One or more discharging sinuses are present, and the poor-quality skin is often adherent to the underlying bone. There may be an obvious abscess and the bone is greatly thickened. In developing countries, extensive involvement of the diaphysis may occur and will sometimes be associated with either pseudarthrosis or a large bone defect.

Radiographs are useful not only for diagnosis but also for demonstrating sequestra, abscess cavities and whether or not active infection is present. The involved bone is greatly thickened and sclerotic, with irregular translucent areas representing bone erosion (Fig. 15.15). Sequestra may be obvious and appear as fragments of dense bone, either on the surface or within an abscess cavity, which appears as a lytic area surrounded by dense sclerotic bone (Fig. 15.16). A cloaca is indicated by a focal cortical defect. Tomography may be necessary to demonstrate sequestra and an abscess cavity. Acute infection is suggested by the presence of fresh periosteal new bone formation. An isotope scan is helpful for demonstrating an acute recurrence, as may be an iridium-labelled white cell scan.

FOLLOWING A FRACTURE

Osteomyelitis may follow infection of the wound in a compound fracture, and it is usually the result of inadequate treatment of the infection. The original wound may fail to heal or if it has healed it breaks down days, weeks or months later.

The development of osteomyelitis is one of the recognized hazards of internal fixation of a closed fracture. It is perhaps more common, and certainly more extensive, after intramedullary fixation than following insertion of a plate and screws. The patient presents with features that are similar to those described earlier, but with the added complication that a fracture is present and often

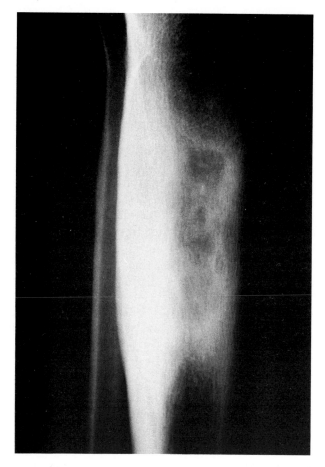

Fig. 15.15 Chronic osteomyelitis. Note sclerotic bone and translucent areas.

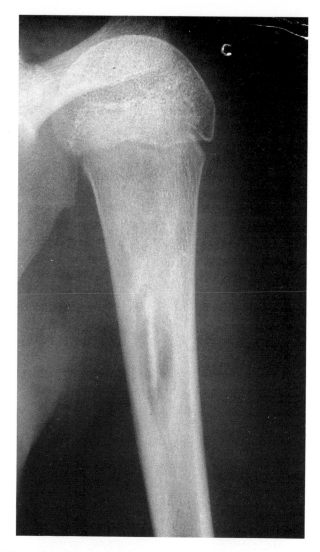

Fig. 15.16 Chronic osteomyelitis secondary to acute osteomyelitis. Note the sequestrum contained within an abscess cavity.

un-united; usually there is a variable degree of skin loss, and an implant may be present.

Although the presence of infection may be obvious, it is sometimes difficult to be certain that the bone is involved; thus, it may not be easy to distinguish fracture callus from new bone formation due to infection. If periostitis is extensive and a sequestrum is present, infection is the most likely cause. An isotope scan is a useful investigation when the diagnosis is in doubt. Locally increased uptake at the fracture site does not necessarily indicate infection, but if it extends some distance along the diaphysis then infection is probable.

Treatment

PREVENTION

Chronic disease should be a rarity if the principles of treatment enunciated for acute osteomyelitis are followed. The problem in compound fractures is somewhat different. Prevention depends largely on well-established principles, namely avoidance of internal fixation in a contaminated wound, thorough debridement of non-viable tissue, gentle handling of tissues, elimination of haematomas, careful skin closure without tension, and if necessary skin grafting to cover defects; if appropriate an external fixator should be used to control the fracture. Antibiotics should be given, but it must be stressed that their availability does not mean that these principles can be ignored. It not uncommonly happens that despite the use of these measures a deep wound infection occurs. If spread to the bone and fracture site is to be prevented, it is essential to drain the wound on the slightest suspicion that pus may be present. It is clearly essential to remove the dressing and inspect the wound at regular intervals.

ESTABLISHED INFECTION

The object of treatment is to remove all necrotic bone and soft tissue, restore bone continuity and correct skin defects where appropriate. Chronic infection following previous acute osteomyelitis is now rare; more often it is a post-traumatic problem involving the tibia. In either event, operative treatment will be necessary and a number of pre-operative measures should be adopted. They are: correction of anaemia; determination of the nature of the organism and its antibiotic sensitivity; and starting the administration of the antibiotic before operation and continuing for about 6 months afterwards.

Operative treatment has been discussed in some detail by Rowling (1970), Yoshimura *et al.* (1989), Fitzgerald *et al.* (1985), and Daoud and Saighi-Bouaouina (1989); only general principles will be discussed here.

Sinuses and surrounding unhealthy skin must be excised. Excision of necrotic bone including sequestra needs to be as complete as possible, and this is best judged by the appearance of bleeding bone; all scar and any other tissue of doubtful viability must be excised. Wide saucerization of the bone, provided that a strong involucrum has formed, enables the dead space to be reduced to a minimum. Any residual dead space or cavity should be packed with gentamicin beads; experience has shown that this is the most effective method of sterilizing infected bone and significantly increases the incidence of primary healing. The beads may be left *in situ* for several weeks.

Once infection has been eliminated, attention can be directed to treating the skin and bone defects, usually at a second stage. The skin problem and dead space may be dealt with by local muscle flaps, e.g. gastrocnemius and soleus in the tibia, or microvascular free tissue transfer. Bone defects are dealt with by a variety of techniques including cancellous grafts (Papineau *et al.*, 1976) when safe closure of the wound is unlikely, corticocancellous grafts and vascularized bone grafts. In patients with non-union of fractures and bone defects, an external fixator should be used to maintain stability during healing. These often complex procedures need careful planning and discussion with patients, who should be made aware that in some instances the only alternative may be amputation.

ACUTE PYOGENIC JOINT INFECTION

Pyogenic arthritis may be primary when the organism reaches the joint via the bloodstream. As with osteomyelitis, there is initial septicaemia from a focus of infection elsewhere. There are a number of predisposing factors: premature infants are much more prone to septicaemia, and umbilical sepsis is probably another source of some neonatal joint infections. Immunodeficiency, either innate or as may be seen in renal transplant units, is a factor that may be easily missed unless it is routinely considered. Joints affected by rheumatoid arthritis, particularly in patients receiving steroids, are probably more vulnerable to infection, but the diagnosis is often made late because the possibility of infection as a cause of rapid joint deterioration is not considered.

The causative organisms are similar to those found in acute osteomyelitis.

In neonates, joints (most commonly the hip) are usually infected secondarily by direct spread of infection from a bone focus. This is possible because of the free communication of metaphyseal and epiphyseal vessels before the growth plate is fully established. In children, where the metaphysis is intracapsular, direct spread to the joint will usually occur. In adults, infection may occasionally spread to a joint from the end of a long bone. The adult hip joint, however, may be involved by spread of infection from pelvic organs, e.g. the bladder; the route of infection is through the pelvic venous plexus into which venous drainage from the hip occurs (Henriques, 1958).

Pathological changes

The changes were described by William Hunter in 1743, and they are the same whether the joint is involved primarily or secondarily. In the former, however, it is rare to find organisms in the synovial fluid because they are rapidly taken up by the synovium; in the latter, when a bone focus ruptures into the joint, it is more usual to find the causative organism.

The synovial membrane becomes acutely inflamed, and periarticular structures are similarly involved. A purulent effusion accumulates rapidly; it is rich in leucocytes and fibrin. The early stages are followed later by organization of the exudates; adhesions are produced in the synovial recesses and periarticular structures, and they are responsible for the loss of joint motion that often follows.

A far more serious effect is the variable degree of articular cartilage destruction. The process is a rapid one, and the full thickness may be lost in a matter of a few days, at first in areas subject to maximum pressure. Lack (1959; 1961) showed that rapid chondrolysis is due principally to activation of the blood proenzyme plasminogen, converting it to plasmin.

Plasminogen activators are released by pathogenic cocci and leucocytes into the inflammatory exudates.

The fibrin in joints that have been subjected to trauma or infection absorbs plasmin, and any excess is removed by the plasmin inhibitor that is normally present in joint tissues. This normal physiological defence mechanism breaks down when excess plasmin is released.

Bacterial toxins have a direct action on the chondrocytes. The normal lubricating effect of synovial fluid is lost because the infection interferes with the production of hyaluronic acid.

The final outcome will, of course, depend on prompt diagnosis and effective treatment. In a child's joint a variable degree of articular cartilage destruction and some loss of motion or fibrous ankylosis with fixed deformity may occur. The last event is much less common in the adult. Spontaneous fusion is by no means invariable, as indicated by Bulmer (1966), who reported 11 instances out of 47 hips.

Additional structures are at risk in infants, namely the epiphysis, growth plate and metaphysis; this is particularly so with regard to the hip joint. The cartilaginous epiphysis may be completely or partially destroyed by the infection or by vascular necrosis from thrombosis of its nutrient vessels, and indeed may sequestrate; it is on the extent of this damage that the final shape of the articular surface depends. The growth plate may be damaged, but in fact it is more resistant to infection than the epiphysis. Premature fusion of the epiphysis may follow, with interference to longitudinal growth, but it does not prevent regeneration of the epiphysis (Banks and Compere, 1941).

It is important to note that in the early stages of the infection, a radiograph may suggest that these structures have been destroyed; in fact, the appearance may well be due to reversible decalcification.

The effect on the infants' hip requires special mention. Dislocation or subluxation is a known sequel during the first few days of the illness; the accumulation of inflammatory exudate raises the intracapsular pressure, the capsule and ligaments are softened, and muscle spasm causes the joint to adopt a flexed and adducted position which contributes to the dislocation. A further consequence is that the ectopic femoral head fails to develop. Necrosis of the capital epiphysis and femoral neck may result from ischaemia and/or infection. Damage to the growth plate may occur with survival of the epiphysis, and the result is pseudarthrosis with coxa vara and shortening of the limb by up to 10 cm. It is noteworthy that the epiphyseal plate of the greater trochanter makes a significant contribution to longitudinal growth; in certain circumstances, therefore, the amount of shortening may be less than expected.

Other sequelae are premature or asymmetrical closure of the proximal femoral epiphysis, complete destruction of the epiphysis and femoral neck (usually associated with dislocation) and epiphysitis producing a variable degree of destruction and leading to deformity — usually coxa magna.

The sequelae in the knee joint are loss of half of the femoral or tibial epiphysis and the metaphysis, causing a varus or valgus deformity and some impairment of longitudinal growth. Damage to articular cartilage will lead to secondary osteoarthritis, but spontaneous fusion is rare.

Infants

CLINICAL FEATURES

The first classic description was given by Smith (1874). The subject has been reviewed by Obletz (1960), Lloyd-Roberts (1960), Paterson (1970) and Wilson and Di Paola (1986).

The patient is often ill, with septicaemia, and a reliable history is usually not available. Diagnosis is never easy and will largely depend on awareness that the condition may exist. The importance of early diagnosis is evident from the pathological changes, for delay leads to irreversible joint destruction.

Septicaemia is suggested by failure to thrive, irritability, cyanosis during feeding, failure to maintain weight, the presence of umbilical sepsis, a fall in the haemoglobin concentration and pyrexia. It is important to recognize that a constitutional reaction and pyrexia are quite often absent.

The joint becomes swollen, red and tender and any attempted passive movement causes extreme pain. A sudden loss of movement of a limb (pseudoparalysis) may be the presenting feature. Muscle spasm produces joint deformity, which in the hip is usually flexion, adduction and external rotation, and in the knee fixed flexion. With regard to the hip, it is wise to assume that dislocation has occurred or is imminent, because it is impossible to elicit the usual physical signs due to pain and muscle spasm. It is always a sensible precaution to routinely examine the hips each day in infants with septicaemia. It is also important to bear in mind that antibiotics may have been given previously for treatment of a septic focus, and before the diagnosis is suspected, and therefore the expected signs may be masked.

INVESTIGATIONS

These are the same as for acute osteomyelitis; the white blood count is normal and the erythrocyte sedimentation rate is usually raised. Useful radiological features in the early stages are widening of the joint spaces and soft tissue swelling. The hip joint may show lateral displacement or dislocation, and this is not necessarily a late feature. The proximal end of the femur or iliac portion of the acetabulum may show evidence of a focus of osteomyelitis, but if present it is likely that the joint infection is many days old (Fig. 15.17). Reversible decalcification of the ossific nucleus and metaphysis may give a false impression that the epiphysis has been destroyed (Fig. 15.18).

Reduced density of the epiphysis usually indicates hyperaemia. If normal density persists in the presence of surrounding osteoporosis, however, this may be the earliest sign of avascular necrosis. Such changes are unlikely to occur in the first 10–14 days. Some of the earlier sequelae are illustrated in Figs 15.19, 15.20 and 15.21.

Joint aspiration is the usual investigation and must be done as a matter of urgency when the diagnosis is suspected, and the pus sent for culture and sensitivity testing.

Children

The presentation is usually an acute illness with pyrexia and all the symptoms and signs seen in infants. Similar investigations do not present any special features.

Adults

The subject has been reviewed by Bulmer (1966), who reported a series of 50 patients with infection of the hip joint, and Kelley *et al.* (1970). The special features are that many patients, particularly older ones, have a reduced constitutional reaction similar to that seen in infants, and the onset may be insidious. The signs are loss of joint motion due to pain and muscle spasm. The diagnosis is unlikely if some passive joint movement can be obtained; swelling and tenderness are invariably present.

Another presentation is migrating polyarthralgia followed later by a septic arthritis of one or more joints.

The erythrocyte sedimentation rate is usually raised, but the white blood count is not helpful. Radiology is of little value in the early stages, though soft tissue swelling may be noted. The earliest significant change is loss of articular cartilage as shown by narrowing of the joint space (Fig. 15.22a), and this may be seen as early as the seventh day. Later, a variable degree of bone destruction may be seen (Fig. 15.22b).

Reference was made earlier to the fact that a joint

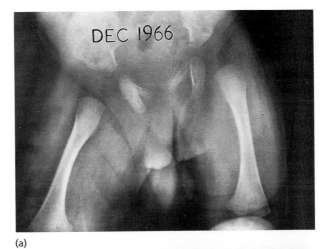

(a)

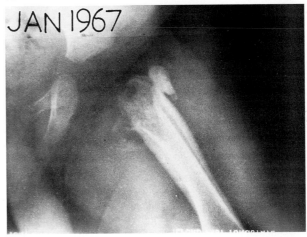

(b)

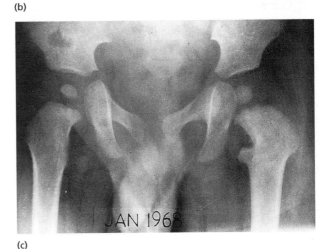

(c)

Fig. 15.17 (a) Infantile septic arthritis of the left hip. Note the swelling of the thigh and widened joint space. The cartilaginous capital epiphysis is probably displaced laterally. (b) 2 weeks later; note the focus of infection in the proximal femoral metaphysis accompanied by extensive periosteal new bone. (c) 6 months later a normally placed epiphysis has appeared.

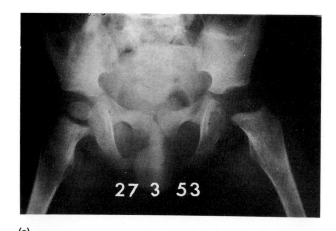

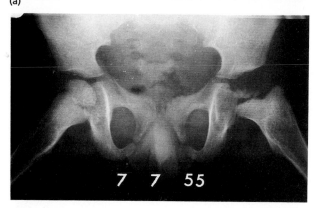

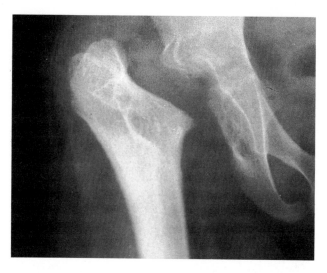

Fig. 15.20 Old septic arthritis in infancy. Note the destroyed head and neck.

Fig. 15.18 (a) Septic arthritis in the left hip. Note the apparent destruction of the capital epiphysis. (b) 2 years later, the epiphysis is visible.

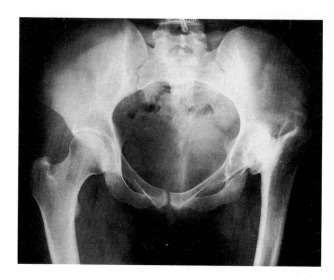

Fig. 15.21 Septic arthritis with destruction of the left femoral neck.

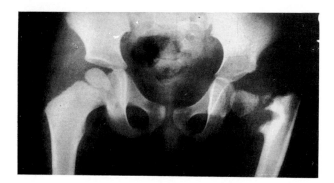

Fig. 15.19 Severe coxa vara following septic arthritis.

rheumatoid disease; such joints are rapidly destroyed (Fig. 15.23).

Differential diagnosis

TRAUMA

In infants and young children metaphyseal fracture and epiphyseal injuries, single or multiple, are commonly seen in non-accidental injury. The condition closely mimics acute septic arthritis; however, there are no signs of septicaemia and radiographs help to make the diagnosis.

affected by rheumatoid arthritis is more susceptible to septic arthritis, which may follow an intra-articular steroid injection. The diagnosis is often missed (Russell and Ansell, 1972), because it is thought that the sudden increase in pain and swelling is an exacerbation of the

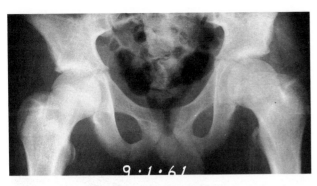

(a)

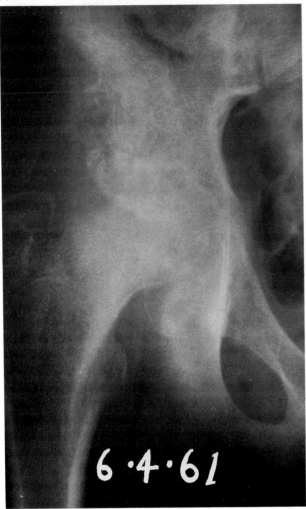

(b)

Fig. 15.22 (a) Primary acute septic arthritis of the right hip in a boy of 13 years. Note the narrowed cartilage space. (b) 3 months later the joint has been destroyed.

ACUTE OSTEOMYELITIS

The two conditions may co-exist, particularly in the infants' hip. On other occasions it may not be easy to differentiate a non-inflammatory effusion in a joint adjacent to a septic bone focus. Septic arthritis will be excluded by the presence of a reasonable range of joint motion.

TRAUMATIC SYNOVITIS

This is a particularly common condition affecting children's hips. Limitation of passive joint motion is minimal except for internal rotation, which always produces considerable pain and spasm. There is no local tenderness or swelling, and the erythrocyte sedimentation rate is normal.

GOUT

This is very common in adults and may affect the joint. The periarticular tissues are swollen and tender, and the overlying skin is often warm and red. There is a joint effusion, and motion is restricted by pain. Tophi may be present, and uric acid levels are usually but not invariably raised. A radiograph may show a punched-out, subarticular osteolytic area (Fig. 15.24).

CHONDROCALCINOSIS

This gives rise to difficulty, but a radiograph is helpful; Hamblen *et al.* (1966) have reviewed the subject.

SUBACUTE PYOGENIC JOINT INFECTION

It is important to note that as with osteomyelitis, a joint infection may have a subacute presentation. This is usually seen in adults, but may occur in children and has been reported in infants.

Clinically, there is no systemic reaction; the joint will be swollen, tender and painful to move, but total loss of motion is unusual. The erythrocyte sedimentation rate is raised. The organism in these cases is of low virulence, and it is rare to obtain a positive culture.

In patients in whom there is a history of a trauma or a recent operation has been performed, e.g. a meniscectomy, the diagnosis may be missed unless subacute infection is considered as a possibility; reflex sympathetic dystrophy is often the first diagnosis. Joint aspiration and examination of the pus will help to avoid mistakes.

Treatment

In general, if effective treatment starts within the first 4 days of the illness, structural damage will be avoided.

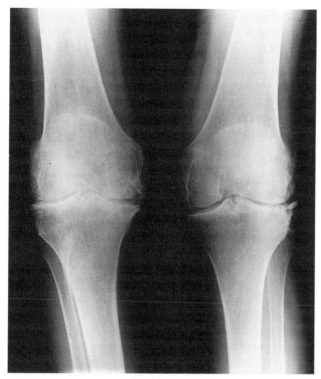

(a)

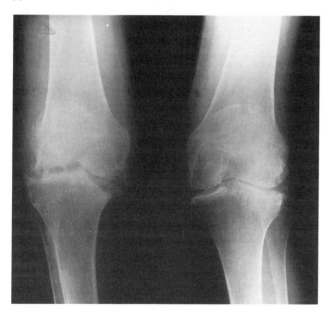

(b)

Fig. 15.23 (a) Rheumatoid knee joints in which septic arthritis developed spontaneously in the right and was diagnosed as an exacerbation of the rheumatoid disease. (b) Some months later showing the gross destructive changes of the articular surface and subchondral bone.

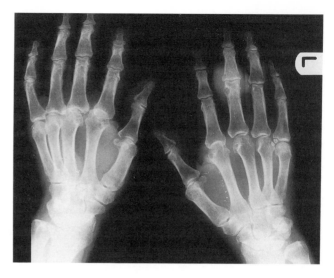

Fig. 15.24 Gout. Note the typical subarticular cystic areas.

INFANTS

The administration and choice of antibiotic are governed by the same principles as for acute osteomyelitis, and the dose is based on the weight of the infant. Parenteral therapy is most appropriate in the early stages.

Aspiration is both diagnostic and therapeutic and must be used as soon as the diagnosis is suspected; a suitable antibiotic is sometimes inserted into the joint. Aspiration is not the method of choice for the hip joint; early, thorough, decompression of the hip is of critical importance if complications are to be avoided. Dislocation is more common in those hips treated by aspiration than after operative drainage (Samilson *et al.*, 1958). Open drainage has the added advantage that the capital epiphysis can be inspected.

Preventing a dislocation can be achieved by immobilizing the hip in abduction (the Lorenz position) using one of the many types of splint designed for this purpose (Lloyd-Roberts, 1960). If the hip is dislocated when the diagnosis is first made, reduction is a matter of great urgency if permanent damage of the epiphysis is to be avoided. Gentle positioning of the leg into abduction is all that may be required. Force must not be used, and if necessary reduction can be achieved by gradual abduction with traction over a period of days. Immobilization must continue until there is good evidence that healing has occurred.

If there is any doubt about the state of the capital epiphysis because it is not visible on a radiograph, arthrography should be performed when the infection has been eliminated.

LATE SURGERY

Hip

This subject has been discussed in detail by Choi *et al.* (1990). A wide variety of changes may occur and these were discussed earlier. The object of treatment is to salvage a stable, preferably mobile, joint and reduce the shortening. For a late-diagnosed dislocation, an attempt at closed manipulation should first be made; it is surprising how well the hip develops even in late cases. If closed manipulation fails, open reduction is undertaken provided that all danger of recrudescence of the infection has passed, usually 18 months to 2 years after the onset.

In patients with resolving ischaemic changes or delay in the appearance of the ossific nucleus, immobilization in abduction should continue until re-ossification has occurred.

For subluxation either acetabuloplasty or proximal femoral osteotomy will be necessary to restore stability.

For progressive valgus deformity (because of asymmetrical premature closure of the lateral part of the growth plate) the treatment is epiphysiodesis of the medial part of the plate. A leg length discrepancy may be corrected by lengthening of the tibia or epiphysiodesis of the contralateral distal femoral growth plate.

Coxa vara is treated by an appropriate osteotomy. If the deformity is associated with pseudarthrosis, an intertrochanteric abduction osteotomy (perhaps with bone grafting) will stimulate union and correct the deformity. A similar operation may stabilize the joint when a capital epiphysis has been destroyed and the femoral neck remains in the acetabulum.

For hips with destruction of the femoral head and neck, the most suitable palliative procedure is trochanteric arthroplasty (Hunka *et al.*, 1982); a leg equalization procedure may also be required.

Knee

A supracondylar osteotomy may be required to correct an angular deformity; it is best done at least 2 years after elimination of the infection and when it is certain that partial epiphyseal loss is real and not merely apparent. If there is significant shortening, i.e. 5 cm or more, an appropriate leg equalization procedure should be performed.

ADULTS

It is particularly important to make certain that the joint is immobilized in the correct functional position because of the increased risk of fibrous or bony ankylosis. Aspiration and installation of antibiotics are the accepted methods of treatment, but for the hip joint arthrotomy is more appropriate. It is wise to continue antibiotics and protect the weight-bearing joint until a stable, pain-free state has been achieved.

In the event of permanent damage to the articular surface, the salvage operations available are arthrodesis, excision arthroplasty and joint replacement. The last option may be justifiable in the hip, for example, if at least 1 year has passed since the primary infection.

SPINAL INFECTIONS

The subject has been reviewed by Griffiths and Jones (1971) and Digby and Kersley (1979). Infection may occur at any age, but is somewhat more common in the adult and is very rare in infants. The vertebral body is much more commonly affected than the posterior neural arch, and about two-thirds of the infections involve the lumbar spine.

The most common organism is coagulase-positive *Staphylococcus* sp.; others that have been isolated include *Pseudomonas pyocyanea*, *E. coli*, *Salmonella* sp. and *S. typhi*. Spinal brucellosis has been reviewed by Lifeso *et al.* (1985). The organisms reach the spine by haematogenous spread from a septic focus elsewhere. There is in addition a communication between the pelvic veins and the vertebral venous plexus (Batson, 1940); undoubtedly pelvic sepsis and operations on the bladder, for example, in the presence of urinary infection may occasionally spread to the spine.

Pathological changes

The initial focus is in the vertebral body close to the end-plate whence spread occurs to adjacent bone and the disc. Necrosis of the latter usually results from impairment of the blood supply and possibly also from the direct action of bacterial toxins. Sequestration may occur. Cancellous bone of the vertebral body seldom sequestrates. Collapse of bone occurs and this appears as progressive anterior wedging. Simultaneously, the disc space becomes progressively narrowed. Abscess formation is common and at first is paravertebral. It will track to the renal angle from the thoraco lumbar level and also to the psoas sheath.

Although compression of the spinal cord by pus and necrotic disc material can occur and lead to paraplegia, it is much less common than with tuberculosis. A characteristic feature not seen in tuberculous infection is relatively early new bone formation on the lateral and anterior aspects of the vertebral body. There is a natural tendency for the adjacent vertebral bodies to undergo spontaneous fusion.

Symptoms and signs

In a high proportion of patients, particularly in the elderly, the infection runs a relatively mild course. The onset is insidious with intermittent attacks of back pain and minimal or no constitutional reaction. The history is often of several weeks duration; muscle spasm and limitation of movement are often absent. The picture resembles that seen in a tuberculous infection, even to the extent of presenting with angular kyphosis. Less commonly, the onset is acute with pyrexia and a constitutional reaction. Severe localized pain and muscle spasm cause loss of movement, and perhaps nerve root pain may develop. Pain referred to the chest, abdomen and leg may lead to misdiagnosis. Paraplegia is rare, and careful neurological examination should always be undertaken in suspected cases.

Investigations

These are the same as described for acute osteomyelitis of long bones. Anti-staphylococcal antibody titres are useful in patients with an insidious onset because they are positive in over 90% of proven staphylococcal investigations and therefore are of assistance in distinguishing it from tuberculosis. Titres for *S. paratyphi* and *Brucella*

sp. antibodies should also be measured in suspected spinal infections.

With regard to radiology, the earliest signs 3–4 weeks after onset are disc space narrowing with poor definition of the vertebral end-plate or erosions (Fig. 15.25). Lateral tomography may show minimal lesions more clearly (Fig. 15.25). A certain amount of vertebral body collapse occurs later and causes anterior wedging (Fig. 15.26), and a paravertebral abscess may be noted (Fig. 15.27). New bone formation is a characteristic feature (Fig. 15.28) and helps to distinguish it from tuberculosis. The healing phase is indicated by anterior buttress formation and sclerosis of the vertebral body, which may progress to spontaneous fusion (Fig. 15.29). An isotope bone scan is positive but non-specific.

Needle biopsy controlled by image intensifier is a very useful diagnostic test, and in the hands of the expert is a safe and straightforward procedure. If it fails or for some reason is impractical, or if urgent decompression is required, then open biopsy should be performed.

Differential diagnosis

A staphylococcal infection of the low-grade type is often indistinguishable from tuberculosis, and no one single feature differentiates them. Other conditions are lesions affecting the vertebral body that produce a variable degree of collapse and wedging. They include trauma, compression, Scheuermann's kyphosis, collapse due to osteoporosis from whatever cause, Paget's

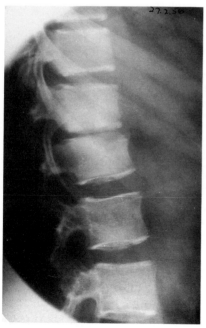

(a)

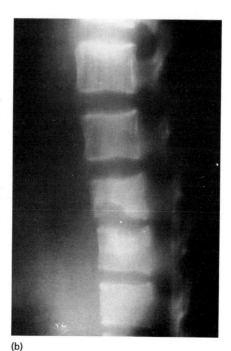

(b)

Fig. 15.25 (a) Acute osteomyelitis in D10–D11. Note the narrow disc space and erosion of the vertebral body. (b) Tomogram to show the extent of the lesion.

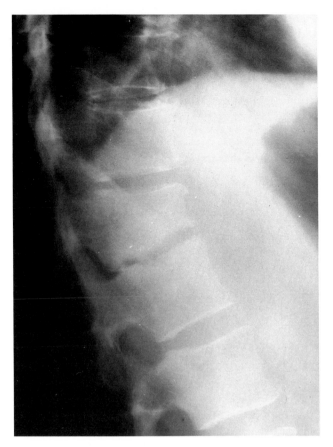

Fig. 15.26 Acute osteomyelitis. Note the anterior wedging due to partial collapse of the vertebral body and the destroyed disc.

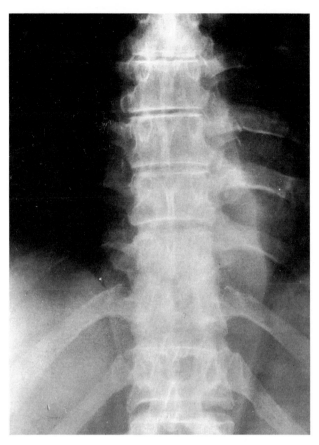

Fig. 15.27 Acute osteomyelitis. Note the paravertebral abscess from a D10–D11 staphylococcal lesion 6 months from onset and treated at first as tuberculous.

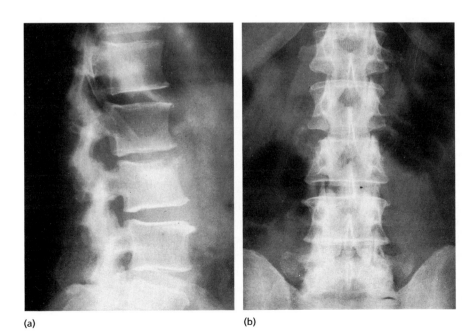

(a)

(b)

Fig. 15.28 (a, b) Acute osteomyelitis. Note the characteristic new bone formation and narrow disc space, which together suggest a pyogenic rather than a tuberculous infection.

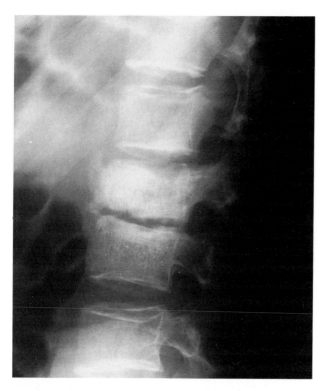

Fig. 15.29 Acute osteomyelitis. The healing stage. Note the sclerosis of the vertebral body and anterior buttress formation.

disease, secondary neoplasm, myeloma, haemangioma, Hodgkin's disease and eosinophilic granuloma. In all these conditions the disc space is preserved, in contrast to inflammatory disease in which it is always narrowed.

Treatment

It must be stressed that isolation of the causative organism is an essential prerequisite for successful treatment. This is particularly so with patients with an insidious onset when tuberculosis cannot easily be excluded.

The affected part should be immobilized and simple bed-rest is usually sufficient, though for the cervical spine a supporting collar would be appropriate.

The principles of antibiotic therapy are the same as those already discussed, but a longer course of treatment is usually prescribed, namely for about 3 months.

Aspiration of an abscess is recommended both for diagnostic and therapeutic purposes. Surgical drainage should seldom be necessary and is best reserved for patients with a large abscess not adequately controlled by aspiration and antibiotics, and particularly if there are signs of paraplegia. There is no place for wide surgical excision and fusion to restore stability, which usually occurs spontaneously.

In the course of the infection, certain criteria are used to determine the need for continued treatment; they are serial determinations of erythrocyte sedimentation rate and good quality radiographs to show such favourable signs as absence of erosions and new bone formation producing a buttress between adjacent vertebral bodies (Fig. 15.29).

Intervertebral disc infections

Primary infection of a disc in adults has been described (Kemp *et al.*, 1973). The presentation is back pain and nerve root irritation without much constitutional reaction. The thoracic spine is the most common site. Abscess formation is unusual, but inflammatory granulation tissue may extend into the subarachnoid space to cause paraplegia.

The earliest radiological sign is narrowing of the disc space with later subchondral sclerosis of the adjacent vertebral bodies; bony bridging between adjacent vertebral bodies represents the healing phase. Isotope scanning is a useful diagnostic aid (Kemp *et al.*, 1973).

Antibiotic therapy cures the condition if given in the early stages, but later operative clearance of the disc space may be necessary and this is certainly so if paraplegia exists.

Spinal infection secondary to a diagnostic or operative procedure

Garcia and Grantham (1960) reported 26 cases in a series of a 100 patients with a diagnosis of vertebral osteomyelitis. Lumbar puncture and discography are two procedures that may be followed by infection unless strict aseptic precautions are taken. Laminectomy and spinal fusion are very seldom complicated by osteomyelitis.

Benign lesion of an intervertebral disc space in children (discitis: see also Chapter 4, p. 118)

PATHOLOGY AND NATURAL HISTORY

The condition has been discussed by Smith and Taylor (1967). The usual age of presentation is 2–6 years, and it is essentially benign in nature. It usually involves the lumbar spine. The aetiology is uncertain, but it is thought to be either a viral or staphylococcal infection. The causative agent reaches the disc by a haematogenous route, and the pathological process starts in the cartilaginous end-plate and readily gains access to the nucleus pulposus and spreads to involve the vertebral body. The disc is reduced in height by loss of water-binding capacity and breakdown of intercellular matrix. Suppuration does not occur, nor does extravertebral extension.

Erosion of end-plates and ballooning of the disc into the vertebral body may be followed by some bone destruction, but anterior wedging does not occur. Reactive new bone formation develops. About 2 months after onset the healing phase starts with restoration, partial or complete, of the disc, and the bone will become sclerotic. Residual anterior beaking of the vertebral body is sometimes seen, but fusion is extremely rare. Recovery is invariable in the course of a few months.

SYMPTOMS AND SIGNS

The child presents with vague back pain, a reluctance to walk, anorexia, vomiting, and a normal or slightly raised temperature. Examination reveals muscle spasm, limitation of movement and local tenderness. Hamstring spasm may restrict hip motion in some patients. The erythrocyte sedimentation rate is only slightly raised and the white cell count is normal; blood culture is invariably negative.

The earliest radiological sign is narrowing of the disc space, erosion and cavitation of the end-plate and some bone destruction in the vertebral body (Fig. 15.30). Evidence of healing after about the sixth week of the illness is manifested by reconstruction of the end-plate, sclerosis and increased height of the disc space (Fig. 15.30).

TREATMENT

During the acute phase bed-rest is all that is required to relieve pain; the length of time depends only on the presence of pain and general condition of the child. There is no evidence that antibiotics influence the course of the infection, though it is nevertheless common practice to give a 3–4 week course of an anti-staphylococcal agent.

The natural healing process described above will take place whether or not bed-rest is prescribed.

JOINT IMPLANT INFECTIONS

For the purpose of this section, only infections after a total hip replacement will be considered, but the principles apply also to the knee and, in fact, any major joint replacement.

Over the last 20 years an enormous literature has built up on this subject, which is not surprising considering the potentially catastrophic and disabling effect of the complication after what has become a very common standard procedure. General aspects have been reviewed by a number of authors, namely Hunter and Dandy (1977), Fitzgerald *et al.* (1977), Gristina and Kolkin (1983), Surin *et al.* (1983) and Klenerman (1984).

Incidence

In the early years of joint replacement the deep infection

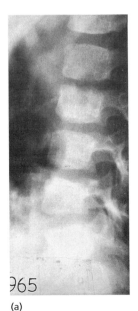

Fig. 15.30 (a) A benign disc space infection in L1–L2. Note the disc space narrowing and the end-plate erosion. (b) The later films show sclerosis of the body, restoration of the end-plate and a gradual increase in the height of the disc.

965

(a)

DEC 1965   OCT 1966

(b)

rate was as high as 12–15%. Since the advent of prophylactic measures and a better understanding of the risk factors, the rate has fallen to less than 2% in most centres. If surgery is performed in an ultra-clean operating environment and if prophylactic antibiotics are used, a deep sepsis rate of less than 1% can be achieved (Lidwell, 1986).

Definitions

Deep infection is one in which purulent material exists beneath the deep fascia, involves the joint and surrounds the prosthesis. An early infection is one that occurs within 3 months of the operation and is usually acute. A later infection is one that occurs 1 year or more after the operation and is usually subacute.

Aetiology

The most likely cause of an acute infection is from an airborne source. The largest proportion of pathogenic bacteria enter the wound from unscrubbed personnel moving about the operating theatre (Burke, 1963). A non-sterile surgical technique will be responsible in a few cases.

It has been suggested that wound contamination may also be responsible for late infections; it is postulated that the organism involved is of low-grade virulence (L forms) and may lie dormant for long periods.

Haematogenous spread is responsible for some late infections; in these cases there has been no previous wound problem, the hip has remained asymptomatic, and the infection is acute in onset. There may or may not be an obvious source of infection. Some early deep infections may also be haematogenous in origin, and the primary source of infection is either the respiratory tract, skin, teeth, or urinary tract.

There is no doubt that patients who have had a prosthesis inserted are more susceptible to deep infection following transient and systemic bacteraemia that may follow such procedures as removal of teeth and instrumentation of the urinary tract.

The organisms involved are varied; in addition to the commonly found Gram-positive *Staphylococcus* spp. and *Streptococcus* spp., Gram-negative organisms such as *E. coli*, *S. albus* and coagulase-negative streptococci are sometimes isolated. Infection caused by coagulase-negative staphylocci, e.g. the normal skin commensal *S. epidermidis*, is more common than previously supposed.

Other factors that increase the risk of deep infection are as follows. There is no doubt that biomaterials alter the host defence mechanisms (Gristina *et al.*, 1980), the tissue response is greater with metal-on-metal articulations, and the macrophage response is inhibited by methylmethacrylate. It is likely that the implant increases the host susceptibility to infection for an indefinite period after the operation. Haematoma and debris, e.g. bone and cement fragments, increase the risk of infection. There appears to be an increased risk of late deep sepsis in those patients who have a superficial wound discharge with a positive bacteriological culture following the operation, and in whom the wound heals before the patient leaves hospital (Surin *et al.*, 1983).

If complications occur, e.g. a dislocation, and surgical intervention is required, there is an increased risk of deep infection. Previous operation on the hip, particularly if it was followed by wound infection, significantly increases the deep infection rate. Patients with rheumatoid arthritis are more susceptible to infection, but steroids are probably not a risk factor, nor is diabetes. The longer the operation lasts (in excess of 2.5 h), the greater the risk of infection.

Diagnosis

The major difficulty is distinguishing between superficial and deep infection, and it should be remembered that if the patient has been receiving prophylactic antibiotics it is likely that the normal signs of infection will be masked. Infection localized to the suture line is probably superficial. Persistent erythema with oedema and induration is likely to result from a deep infection, and this will be confirmed if significant discharge occurs. It is easy to be misled by the fact that a deep infection is not necessarily accompanied by discharge, and indeed superficial manifestations are sometimes absent.

Pain may result from either mechanical loosening or infection, and of course these two may coexist. If due to infection, the pain is generally of gradual onset in late infections and aggravated by weight-bearing and to some extent temporarily relieved by antibiotics.

In early acute infections, pyrexia is usual but is often absent in late infections. The erythrocyte sedimentation rate is a reliable indicator, but if normal it does not exclude infection, particularly if antibiotics have been given. A persistently raised erythrocyte sedimentation rate in late deep infections is an important diagnostic sign and helps to distinguish the pain due to mechanical loosening. The total and differential white cell counts are an unreliable indicator of infection, particularly the late subacute type.

Plain radiographs are of no diagnostic value in the early acute stages; an isotope scan will be positive in the early post-operative months (usually to about 1 year) in the absence of infection. In late infections plain radiographs may show signs of mechanical loosening, e.g. radiolucencies wider than 2 mm at the cement–bone or cement–prosthesis interface, endosteal resorption of bone, fracture of the cement, or migration of the components. Infection may be the cause of loosening but the changes are not specific. A strongly positive isotope scan is indicative of infection, particularly in the early blood pool or vascular phase. A positive gallium scan is obtained in infection but not loosening.

Aspiration of the joint will give a positive result in most patients, particularly if antibiotics have not been recently administered. Any material sent for examination should also be cultured anaerobically.

Prophylactic measures

Active foci of infection should be looked for and eliminated before total hip replacement; a good example is an infected varicose ulcer or foot infection. Poor nutrition and anaemia must be corrected before operation, and this is particularly important in the elderly.

Prophylactic antibiotics are a powerful weapon for preventing infection (Hill *et al.*, 1981) and should be given routinely. They will not be effective, however, unless started a few hours before the operation. It is wise to give them for a minimum of 36 h and some would say 7 days. Flucloxacillin is recommended, or one of the cephalosporins if a broad-spectrum drug that acts against some Gram-negative organisms is required. Patients should be warned and general practitioners must be aware that it is a sensible precaution to administer prophylactic antibiotics for dental extractions and certain urinary tract operations.

Antibiotic-impregnated cement allows elution of the drug into the tissues surrounding the implant (where its presence is of critical importance) and also into the bloodstream. The technique was first reported by Buchholz and Engelbrecht in 1970. In recent years it has been standard practice to use cement containing gentamicin, 0.5–1 g to 40 g of powdered cement. Extensive studies have revealed considerable variation (3 weeks to 5 years) in the period during which a bactericidal concentration persist in the tissues. It is most unlikely that haematogenous infection that occurs 1 year or more after operation will be prevented by use of this cement. The subject has been reviewed by Trippel (1986). It seems to be generally agreed now that gentamicin does not have a mechanical effect on cement. There is some evidence to suggest that use of this material is more effective than systemic antibiotics in the

prevention of deep infection (Josefsson *et al.*, 1981). In view of the conflicting reports, the conclusion must be that it is obligatory to use either systemic antibiotics or the impregnated cement for prophylaxis; undoubtedly some surgeons will continue to use both methods. Lynch *et al.* (1987) have shown that impregnated cement significantly lowers the incidence of deep infection following revision operations (which have a higher rate of infection than primary procedures).

A detailed study for the Medical Research Council by Lidwell *et al.* (1982; 1983; 1986) produced strong evidence that operating in a theatre with an ultra-clean area and wearing conventional clothing reduced the incidence of deep infection to half that in a standard environment, and where body-exhaust suits were worn the incidence was reduced to less than one-quarter.

Most surgeons now accept that operating in an ultra-clean area is desirable but not essential because the same low sepsis rate (less than 1%) can be achieved by use of prophylactic antibiotics (and or impregnated cement) and the newer type of impervious operating gowns.

At operation a meticulous aseptic technique, gentle handling of the tissues, thorough removal of debris before closing of the wound and prevention of haematoma formation are standard prophylactic measures, whatever additional techniques are used.

Treatment

Acute infection during the early weeks after an operation is best treated by drainage of the wound (from which culture of the organisms may be obtained) combined with systemic antibiotics. Problems arise in making a prompt diagnosis because prophylactic antibiotics mask the usual signs; it is important in such cases to start the treatment as soon as deep infection is suspected and even if the signs are minimal. Antibiotics are unlikely to control the infection. Prompt surgical drainage may prevent the deep infection from becoming established in some cases.

An acute haematogenous infection occurring late is usually associated with a severe systemic reaction. In addition to the usual general measures, intensive intravenous antibiotic therapy is required. When the acute illness has resolved, consideration must be given to removal of the prosthesis and all the cement, if the deep infection is to be eliminated and significant loss of bone stock prevented.

Exchange arthroplasty is now an established procedure for any patient requiring removal of a prosthesis. A one-stage procedure (including reinsertion of a prosthesis) was advocated by Buchholz *et al.* (1981).

It consisted of meticulous attention to removal of all cement and involved debris, use of antibiotic-impregnated cement and systemic antibiotics. In the first series the success rate was 77% and later 90% success was reported. In general it is probably safer to use a two-stage procedure (Salvati *et al.*, 1982). The first stage is thorough debridement and gentamicin-impregnated beads are inserted; large doses of antibiotics are given between the two stages. The timing of the second stage will depend on numerous factors including the virulence of the organism and the degree of bone destruction; it will vary from a few weeks to 1 year in some cases.

Revision operation for an infected prosthesis (and indeed also for non-infected cases) should only be performed by a surgeon experienced in implant work, and it is not appropriate for the occasional operator.

The only salvage procedure available is excision arthroplasty (Girdlestone pseudarthrosis). It is used when exchange arthroplasty fails and in those patients in whom infection is combined with severe loss of bone stock. The operation will generally relieve pain, but function is often worse than before the initial joint replacement (Petty and Goldsmith, 1980; McElwaine and Colville, 1984). In most instances the infection is eliminated, but in a few sinus formation recurs, and this is particularly so if all the cement is not removed.

BONE AND JOINT TUBERCULOSIS

The incidence of this condition has fallen steadily in the developed world; in 1978−1979 it was 0.34 in 100 000 of the indigenous population of England and Wales, compared with 29 in 100 000 of ethnic groups from the Indian Subcontinent. Tuberculosis remains a serious problem in developing countries. The infection is a classic manifestation of an interaction between the host and the tubercle bacillus, *Mycobacterium tuberculosis*. Anything that lowers natural resistance, e.g. malnutrition, will act as a predisposing factor. If affects mostly children and young adults.

The most susceptible parts of the skeleton are regions of growth, e.g. epiphyseal and metaphyseal zones in children, and bones containing haemopoietic marrow, e.g. the vertebral bodies in adults.

For descriptive and therapeutic purposes the various regions may be classified as follows:
1 Extra-articular disease: this is a focal bone lesion which does not encroach on a joint surface. Examples are metaphyseal lesions of long bones, a lesion in the femoral neck, greater trochanter, rib and sternum, and dactylitis (spina ventosa).
2 Intra-articular disease: essentially this is primarily a lesion of the synovium with or without marginal erosions involving the articular cartilage. An intracapsular bone focus may spread to involve the joint.
3 Vertebral infections.

Pathological changes

No bone or joint is immune, but the most common sites involved are the spine followed by the hip and knee. Skeletal foci occur as a result of haematogenous spread to reticuloendothelial tissue from a lesion in the lungs or lymphatic nodes. Not uncommonly there are associated foci in other organs, e.g. the kidney.

The pathological process is essentially a destructive one; in joints the manifestation is exudative and in bone it is proliferative. Initially, there is a vascular stage followed by a chronic avascular one. The inflammatory process involves bone, cartilage, synovium and fascia; it has the ability to pass across a cartilaginous growth plate from a metaphyseal focus into the epiphysis, a process that is very rare in pyogenic infections.

Obliterative endarteritis results in sequestration. The lowered oxygen tension in the lesion may be responsible for the organisms passing into a resting phase and becoming relatively resistant to antibiotics, remaining dormant for years. Bone trabeculae are destroyed and necrotic tissue and exudate form an abscess. Fibrous tissue replaces the destroyed bone. At the periphery is a highly vascular zone that causes relative decalcification of the bone; it is this process that gives the radiological appearance of increased density some distance from the focus of infection.

In a joint, the synovium and subchondral bone are mainly affected at first. A metaphyseal lesion is usually associated with joint involvement. Pus and necrotic tissue collect in the joint cavity. Unlike in pyogenic infection the normal protective mechanism is inhibited, and fibrin accumulates and adheres to the joint surface. The articular cartilage remains intact for a relatively long period because again unlike in pyogenic infections, there is very little accumulation of plasmin due to the presence of a high concentration of plasmin inhibitor and an absence of plasminogen activator (Lack, 1959). Eventually, the articular cartilage becomes softened and ulcerated from the spread of tuberculous granulations over the surface and from subchondral involvement.

Course and natural history

Without antituberculous drugs the infection runs a characteristically slow course with extensive destruction of bone and cartilage. An abscess enlarges and may track a considerable distance from the primary site; if it extends to the skin the sinus may become secondarily infected with pyogenic bacteria. The abscess wall gradually becomes thickened with mature fibrous tissue, and the caseous central zone may become calcified. The natural healing process, which begins before the destructive phase is finished, may be hindered by the presence of an abscess and dense scar tissue.

In the later stages of joint infection, fibrous ankylosis occus; bone fusion is unusual provided that some articular cartilage is preserved. Fibrotic infiltration of the capsule and synovium will produce a contracture.

Therapy is to a large extent based on knowledge of the local impediments to healing. They may be summarized as follows:

1 The lesion at the time of presentation is relatively avascular, so that the passage of antibiotics is impaired. Caseous material inhibits antibiotic activity.
2 Healing is prevented by tuberculous debris, sequestra and abscess formation.
3 Fibrous ankylosis of a joint is relatively insecure, and recurrence of infection is possible.
4 Necrotic tissue, e.g. sequestra, may contain macrophages with ingested live tubercle bacilli, which can remain quiescent for years.
5 A rigid cavity containing tuberculous granulation tissue is a cause of delayed healing.

Complications

Early diagnosis and effective treatment should prevent the following complications, which were common in the pre-antibiotic era: total or partial joint destruction followed by fibrous ankylosis, often in a poor functional position; joint contracture with a variable degree of bone and cartilage destruction; joint subluxation or dislocation; and paralysis in spinal disease.

Prognosis

In general the natural response of the individual, which in turn depends on the effectiveness of the reticuloendothelial system, will determine the outcome. The prognosis is worse in the presence of malnutrition and an associated lesion in other systems.

Antituberculous drugs, combined if necessary with operation to remove the impaired healing factors, has enormously improved the prognosis by significantly reducing mortality and morbidity.

Clinical features

The onset is insidious, and there is often very little in the way of a constitutional reaction. Pain is the presenting symptom, increasing in severity as time passes and not generally relieved by rest. The affected part swells and is tender. A history of previous pulmonary infection or a positive family history may be obtained.

Examination reveals low-grade pyrexia, significant muscle atrophy and impaired joint motion associated with muscle spasm causing deformity, which later leads to a contracture. An abscess may be palpable and is often at some distance from the focus of infection. An associated lesion in other systems must be excluded. Neurological signs in the limbs may be found in spinal infections, which are discussed later.

Investigations

The erythrocyte sedimentation rate is markedly raised and serial readings are a useful indication of the effect of therapy. A negative tuberculin skin test probably excludes a tuberculous infection. The sputum and urine must be routinely examined and cultured. A joint effusion or abscess should be aspirated for culture and sensitivity testing. Resort to biopsy including a lymph node is occasionally necessary in some joint infections when rheumatoid arthritis and pyogenic infection are difficult to exclude.

Good-quality plain radiographs are not only helpful for diagnostic purposes but they influence the choice of treatment, particularly operative treatment. Tomography and isotope scanning are useful adjuncts to plain radiographs.

An important early radiological sign in a joint infection is a widespread rarefaction of the juxta-articular bone, associated with increased density of soft tissues, indicating the presence of an abscess, which sometimes contains calcified material. The cartilage space is relatively well preserved in the early stage because the articular cartilage is intact, and this distinguishes it from pyogenic infection and rheumatoid arthritis (Fig. 15.31). Later, marginal bone erosions are seen at the site of the capsular reflection, and this is followed by a variable degree of articular cartilage and subchondral bone destruction producing joint narrowing (Fig. 15.32).

The bone lesion is typically a well-defined area of bone destruction indicated by irregular cavitation with minimal surrounding reaction, e.g. a zone of sclerosis and periosteal reaction, as is usually seen in pyogenic infections. The process may extend across the growth plate into the epiphysis (Fig. 15.33). A square-shaped

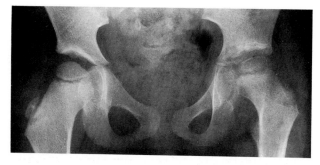

Fig. 15.31 Early stages of a tuberculous left hip. Note decalcification of the bone and increased density of the adjacent soft tissues, suggesting an abscess which was confirmed.

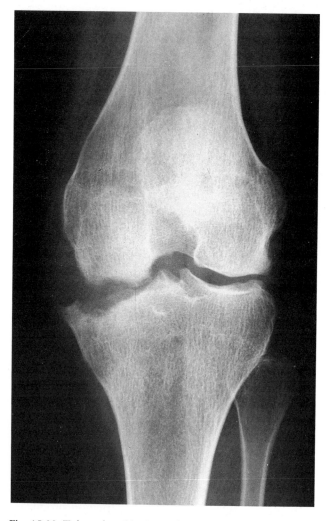

Fig. 15.32 Tuberculous hip. Note the marginal erosions and destruction of articular cartilage on the medial side.

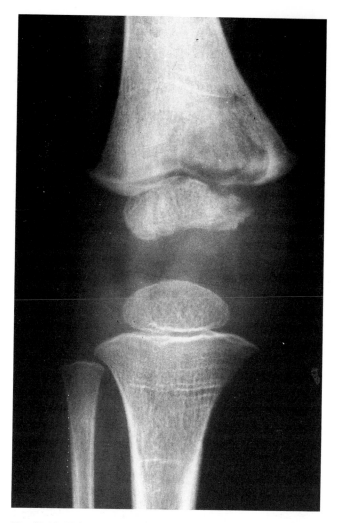

Fig. 15.33 Tuberculous hip. Note the erosion of bone, which involves the epiphysis, and the absence of sclerosis, which differentiates it from a pyogenic infection.

epiphysis and coarse intramedullary trabeculation is typical of synovial involvement of the knee joint (Fig. 15.34).

In the later stages inactivity will be suggested by the absence of rarefaction, increasing sclerosis which sometimes may indicate secondary pyogenic infection, calcification in an abscess and bony ankylosis (Fig. 15.35). Tuberculous dactylitis has a typical appearance (Fig. 15.36), as does the rare cystic type (Fig. 15.37).

Treatment

The aim is to eradicate the disease and preserve function, and as far as joints are concerned this means a useful range of painless motion and stability. If there is a choice between a mobile and an ankylosed joint, the decision must to some extent depend on the country of origin and social customs. In less well-developed countries where medical services are poor, an ankylosis is probably best. If, for religious or other reasons, squatting and kneeling are important, then a mobile joint is preferable.

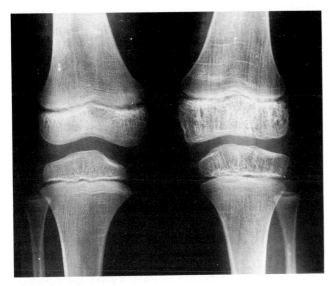

Fig. 15.34 Tuberculous synovitis of the left knee. Note the coarse trabeculation and square shape of the femoral epiphysis.

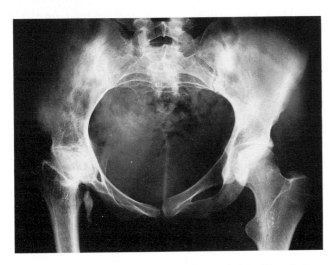

Fig. 15.35 The late stage of a tuberculous right hip. Note the loss of articular cartilage, sclerosis and calcification. Calcification in an abscess and ankylosis of the joint suggest a healed lesion.

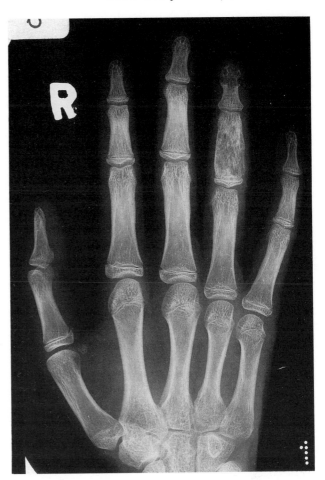

Fig. 15.36 Tuberculous dactylitis affecting the middle phalanx of the ring finger. Note that typically the joints are spared, the medulla is expanded and the cortex thinned.

In general, however, eradication of disease and a return to normal function will largely depend on the stage at which definitive treatment is provided. The course of the disease and its response to treatment is most accurately assessed by careful clinical examination, serial determinations of erythrocyte sedimentation rate and radiography.

GENERAL MEASURES

Local rest of a joint is by simple splinting in a position of function or traction, as appropriate, and early controlled mobilizing exercises are advised. Joint lubrication and the nutrition of articular cartilage are maintained by movement and weight-bearing. The latter should begin as soon as there is evidence of healing.

CHEMOTHERAPY

At least 85% of patients will be cured by effective antituberculous drugs (Medical Research Council 1973a, b; 1974a, b). This only holds true, however, if the drugs are started during the early vascular stage of the disease. There is no doubt that combined drug therapy prevents the emergence of resistant strains. Short courses of 6–9 months are recommended and it is usual to start the following first line drugs:
1 Rifampicin, 10–20 mg/kg/day up to a maximum of 600 mg.
2 Isoniazid, 5–10 mg/kg/day up to a maximum of 300 mg.

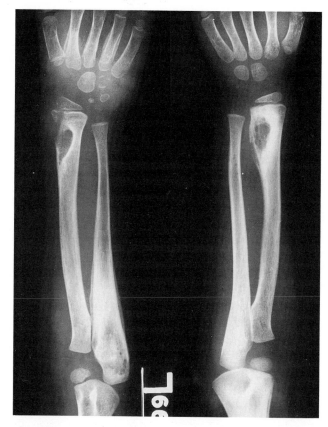

Fig. 15.37 Cystic tuberculosis of the distal radius. Note the typical oval shape with a sharply defined margin. The bone is expanded with a periosteal reaction, and the cortex is eroded at one point.

3 Ethambutol, 15 mg/kg/day up to a maximum of 1200 mg.

These drugs are best given in one daily dose together with vitamin B6, 25 mg/day. Ethambutol is discontinued after 3 months. A small percentage of patients (10−15%) will not respond adequately, due either to drug resistance or to the lesion being relatively avascular and containing caseous material and sequestra. A number of patients will therefore require operative treatment.

OPERATION

There are two principal operative procedures. The first is eradication of the disease, which means removal of all diseased and necrotic tissue, with the objective of restoring normal function, that is, a mobile, painless and stable joint. This approach is appropriate for localized extra-articular and some intra-articular lesions, but only if the articular cartilage is reasonably well preserved. The same applies to partial synovectomy, which is particularly useful for the knee joint.

The other operative procedure is resection, which involves removal of all involved structures until healthy tissue is reached. This method of treatment is usually reserved for more advanced cases. In the knee joint, for example, fusion of the joint is to be expected and in the hip either pseudarthrosis, fusion, or total replacement.

Indications

In an extra-articular lesion, operation is usually necessary in order to obtain material for culture and to confirm the diagnosis. As a general rule for joint lesions, operation is best reserved for those patients who have failed to respond favourably a short time after starting chemotherapy. It should also be undertaken for drainage of a large abscess, when the diagnosis is uncertain, and in the later stages of the disease when it is most unlikely that chemotherapy can be totally effective.

Clearly, operation will be necessary after elimination of the infection if there is residual pain, stiffness and instability. In such instances several procedures are available, e.g. joint replacement, arthrodesis, excision arthroplasty and osteotomy.

Technique

Details vary according to the joint involved, but the general principles are as follows:
1 Wide exposure and excision of all sinuses.
2 Thorough evacuation of the abscess.
3 Total excision of all necrotic tissue and sequestra, converting the avascular lesion into a vascular area.
4 Residual bone defects can be packed with autogenous bone graft.
5 Involved synovium or tendon sheath should be excised.
6 As far as possible, elimination of any dead space and use of suction drainage.
7 Early mobilization of joints after initial rest in a position of function.

In the early stages of hip disease, treatment should result in a mobile, pain-free joint. In those cases where there is serious damage to the articular cartilage, a firm fibrous union may be the best end result. In other patients, excision arthroplasty (Tuli and Mukherjee, 1981) or the relatively new procedure of interpositional arthroplasty using multilayered amnion (Vishwakarma and Khare, 1986) are appropriate. Total hip replacement is a reasonable procedure in carefully selected cases in which infection is quiescent and when the patient is particularly concerned to preserve mobility, as is the case in some developing countries where social custom often dictates the treatment; encouraging results have been reported by Kim *et al.* (1986).

The most reliable treatment for a destroyed joint if relief from pain and stability are all-important is undoubtedly arthrodesis, usually by an extra-articular technique.

In the early stages of knee joint disease, chemotherapy followed by early controlled mobilization using a continuous passive motion machine is probably the treatment of choice. Synovectomy is a useful procedure in selected patients, but generally it is followed by a variable degree of stiffness. Arthrodesis is a reliable procedure for destroyed painful and unstable joints. A supracondylar osteotomy is used to correct a flexion contracture.

Tuberculosis of the spine (see also Chapter 21)

This was reviewed recently by Griffiths (1987). Although spinal infections are much less common in the UK than hitherto, nevertheless 150 new cases occur each year — 40% of which are Europeans and the remainder are patients from the Indian subcontinent. The spine is involved in more than half of all patients with skeletal tuberculosis. The effect of the declining incidence in North America and Western Europe is a lack of awareness of the condition, which often results in late diagnosis. In all patients with a spinal lesion in whom infection is a possibility, it is important to have a high index of suspicion that tuberculosis could be the cause.

PATHOLOGY

A classic description of the pre-antibiotic morbid anatomy was given by Seddon (1935). Any part of the spine may be affected, but tuberculosis is most common in the dorsal region.

Multiple level involvement occurs, and some lesions are much more obvious than others. The vertebral body is the usual site of involvement, but very occasionally the posterior elements are involved, either simultaneously with the body (Travlo and Toit, 1990) or in isolation (Babhulkar *et al.*, 1984). The arrangement of the blood vessels determines the pattern of the vertebral body involvement. The initial focus is usually paradiscal, affecting adjacent end-plates of one segment and leading to impaired nutrition of the disc, which is eventually destroyed.

Another type is diffuse central osteitis leading to collapse and late disc involvement. Sometimes it starts as an anterior or lateral quadrant focus with collapse. Two very rare types are neural arch disease and a tuberculous epidural granuloma without bone involvement.

The pathological changes do not differ from the description given in an earlier section (see p. 424). Typically, abscess formation occurs early. Bone is eroded, fragmented and softened leading to collapse and deformity abscess soon extrudes in various directions. Spread to the side of the vertebral body produces a paravertebral abscess; in the upper cervical spine it will form a retropharangeal abscess, and at the mid or lower cervical level it presents in the posterior triangle. In the dorsal spine it may either pass extrapleurally to simulate an empyema or along the intercostal space to form a chest wall abscess. From the lower dorsal spine it will pass to the loin and simulate a perinephric abscess. From the lumbar spine it enters the psoas sheath and may present either in the groin or the pelvis. If the pus extends anteriorly beneath the common ligament, erosion of the anterior aspect of several bodies may occur. Posterior extrusion will compress the spinal theca and cause paraplegia.

Deformity has two principal effects, namely damage to the spinal cord and reduction in chest capacity. Vertebral body collapse leads to ankylosis, which may be anterior (kyphos) or lateral. Telescoping of the facets will prevent significant subluxation when angulation occurs. If the facets permit forward and downwards subluxation, acute paraplegia may result. The greater the number of vertebral bodies involved, the greater the deformity. Deformity will increase the stress on the area of infection and delay healing. A relatively small amount of destruction in the dorsal region produces significant angulation, while the opposite is the case in the lumbar region.

In childhood disease, destruction of the metaphyseal region and vertebral body results in cessation of growth in length; the posterior elements continue to grow normally, resulting in anterior angulation. Even if the infection is quiescent the deformity will increase due to the differential growth factor (Figs 15.38 and 15.39).

PARAPLEGIA

Early diagnosis, chemotherapy and radical surgery have combined to reduce the incidence of paraplegia. There are parts of the world, however, where late diagnosis and infection are common and indeed many patients first present with paraplegia. The overall incidence is 20–30% of cases.

It is now usual to distinguish two types, namely paraplegia with active disease (early or late onset) and after the disease has healed (Hodgson and Yau, 1967).

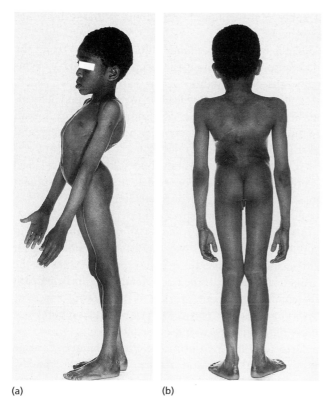

(a)   (b)

Fig. 15.38 (a, b) Tuberculosis of the dorsal spine in a child with severe deformity.

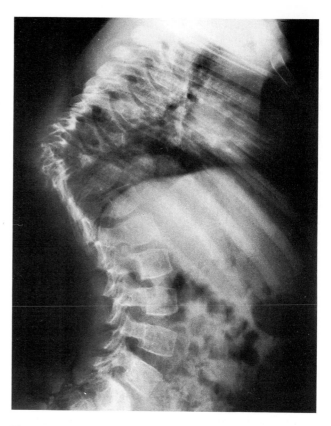

Fig. 15.39 Radiograph to show the effect of differential growth.

Active disease

In any individual patient there is often more than one cause of paraplegia. In most it is due to anterior extradural compression by an abscess or sequestrated disc material and bone. Extrinsic pressure may be from oedema or granulation tissue that extends around the dura and simulates a spinal tumour; an epidural granuloma occurs occasionally in the absence of a bone lesion. Inflammatory tissue occasionally involves and penetrates the dura, and an intradural extramedullary abscess will then compress the cord (Hodgson *et al.*, 1967). It has been postulated but not proved that thrombosis of spinal arteries is a cause of paraplegia.

Recrudescence of active disease after years of quiescence causes paraplegia as a result of compression of a susceptible spinal cord that is much reduced in thickness. In a small number of patients paraplegia may be of sudden onset due to an angulation deformity associated with subluxation. Paraplegia is particularly common in disease of the lower cervical spine in older children and adults, and also in disease affecting the posterior elements; almost all of these patients will present with paraplegia.

Inactive disease

In these cases the paraplegia is always associated with acute angulation and the spinal cord is kinked and tightly stretched over a bony ridge in the floor of the spinal canal; the cord has usually undergone a variable degree of atrophy and degeneration from chronic ischaemia. A further causative factor could be constructive compression from fibrosis of the dura.

PROGNOSIS

With regard to prognosis of the paraplegia, the longer the duration the worse the outlook. Recovery does sometimes occur, however, after 1−2 years. Paraplegia in extension, and particularly if partial with some voluntary control, has a more favourable prognosis. Severe sensory loss and sphincter paralysis indicate a poor prognosis.

CLINICAL FEATURES

Children present with general malaise, backache and stiffness, adults with backache and no root symptoms. Local tenderness, muscle spasm, loss of movement and a

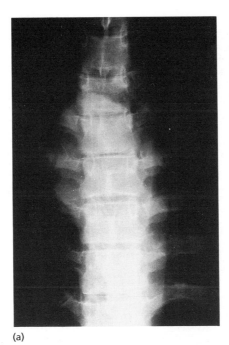
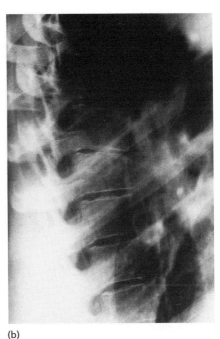

Fig. 15.40 (a, b) Early tuberculous infection of the dorsal spine. Note the narrow D5−D6 disc space and a small paravertebral abscess.

(a)

(b)

palpable abscess at a distance from the focus of infection are the relatively non-specific physical signs. All patients with suspected spinal infection, and indeed any spinal pathology, must have a careful neurological examination.

INVESTIGATIONS

These are similar to other tuberculous lesions, but needle biopsy is a valuable diagnostic aid. The earliest radiological sign is narrowing of the disc space without a bone lesion (Fig. 15.40); vertebral body involvement is indicated by a variable degree of collapse and angulation (Fig. 15.41). A paravertebral abscess is commonly present (Fig. 15.42). Multiple lesions are best visualized by routine use of isotope scanning.

TREATMENT

As a result of a number of controlled trials set up by the UK Medical Research Council to determine the most reliable method of treatment, numerous reports were published (Medical Research Council, 1973a, b, 1974a, b, 1976). All patients received 18 months of chemotherapy. Patients were either ambulant with no restraints or had a plaster jacket. Other patients had bed-rest for 6 months, limited focal surgery to evacuate pus and sequestra, radical excision by wide exposure

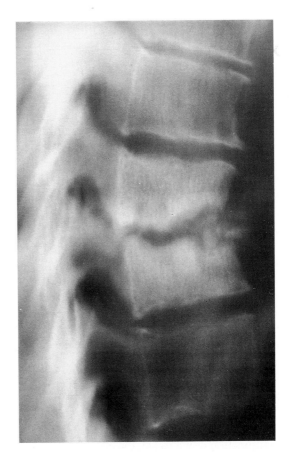

Fig. 15.41 Tuberculous infection of the spine. Note the vertebral body erosion and partial collapse.

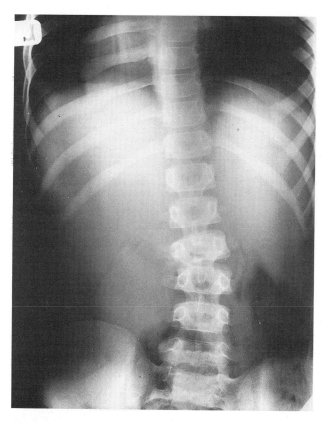

Fig. 15.42 Tuberculous infection of the spine. Note the large right psoas abscess.

and direct anterior approach, and bridging of the gap with an autogenous bone graft as pioneered by Hodgson and Stock (1960) and others (Kirkaldy-Willis and Thomas, 1965; Jackson, 1971).

The regimen that included radical operation gave 89% successful results; 93% healed by bone fusion and with minimal deformity. The other regimens all gave 82% to 85% satisfactory results.

It is accepted that in countries with limited medical facilities the ambulatory routine with chemotherapy is the method of choice. In other countries patients should have radical operation if there is severe destruction and abscess formation, if the disease progresses despite chemotherapy, and if there is any doubt about stability. Radical operation eradicates the focus of infection, avascular tissue and the abscess, leaving a vascular bed into which an autogenous strut graft (from rib or iliac crest) is placed to maintain stability.

The approach to C1 and C2 is transoral; for C3 to C7 the standard anterior approach is used. For the cervicothoracic junction down to D4, the approach is along the anterior border of the right sternocleidomastoid muscle, extending to include a midline sternal splitting incision.

D4 to L2 are approached through a left thorocotomy incision; the thoracolumbar level is approached through the bed of the tenth rib and the lumbar spine is best exposed through a left oblique retroperitoneal approach.

Paraplegia was at one time almost always treated by either anterolateral decompression or the more direct anterior approach with radical excision; some surgeons continue to advocate these techniques. Since Pattinson (1986) reported an 84% success rate with chemotherapy alone, however, this is probably the method of choice in most patients. It should be emphasized that laminectomy has no place in the treatment of paraplegia, except possibly in those rare instances when it is due to neural arch disease. Laminectomy should then be followed by a posterior fusion.

SOME UNCOMMON BONE AND JOINT INFECTIONS

Some of these conditions do not occur in the UK, and those that do are very rare. Mandel *et al.* (1979) gave a detailed account of these conditions.

Syphilis

In infants and young children the infection is congenital and characteristically presents as metaphysitis and osteoperiostitis that is bilateral and symmetrical, or as symmetrical hydrarthrosis of the knee, sometimes referred to as Clutton's joint (Rasool and Govender, 1989). In adults the principal lesion is osteoperiostitis and gumma formation; the lesions are a tertiary manifestation of acquired disease.

METAPHYSITIS

Several metaphyses are involved, the most common site being the distal radius and the proximal medial aspect of the tibia (Winberger's sign). A zone of bone destruction with a loss of trabeculae occurs in the juxtaepiphyseal part of the metaphysis (Fig. 15.43) and is associated with diffuse periostitis. A pathological fracture through the metaphysis sometimes occurs.

Severe local pain is the presenting symptom, and the affected part is enlarged and tender. Positive serological tests help to distinguish the condition from acute osteomyelitis. Some of the skeletal changes may mimic nonaccidental injury. The possibility of congenital syphilis should be considered if destructive bone lesions are present.

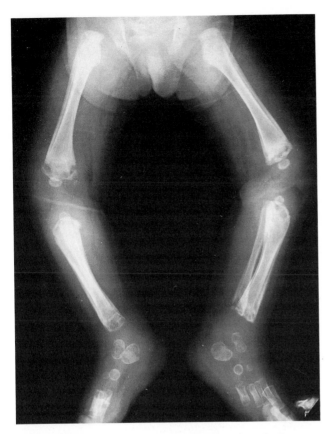

Fig. 15.43 Congenital syphilitic metaphysitis. Note the bone destruction in the juxtaepiphyseal part of the metaphysis and the periostitis.

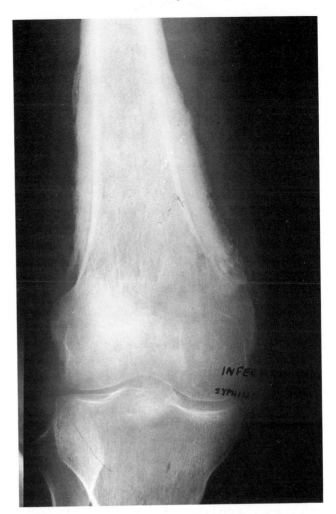

Fig. 15.44 Osteoperiostitis. Note the diffuse periostitis.

OSTEOPERIOSTITIS

Usually there are multiple lesions and the tibia is most often affected. There is either diffuse infiltration with inflammatory granulation tissue or a more localized lesion; a variable amount of bone destruction and new bone formation occurs, but sequestration does not occur.

The presenting symptom is a deep boring type of pain, waking the patient at night. Examination reveals a diffuse or localized tender swelling.

The radiological appearance shows a number of different features, namely a diffuse periostitis with an 'onion-peel' appearance, dense new bone formation producing cortical thickening, and areas of decreased density representing bone destruction (Fig. 15.44). Pyogenic osteomyelitis or a primary metaphyseal bone tumour have to be differentiated, and positive serology is a help in this regard.

CLUTTON'S JOINT

This condition presents as a symmetrical non-painful hydrarthrosis of the knee in children. The effusion is clear, serology is positive, and the child will show other stigmata of syphilis.

GUMMA

This is seen in adults and appears on a radiograph as a well-defined, 'punched out' area in the cortex or medulla. It is associated with subperiosteal new bone (Fig. 15.45).

TREATMENT

All lesions, particularly congenital types, respond well to standard antibiotic therapy.

Yaws

This treponemal infection closely resembles syphilis and is seldom seen in the UK. It is principally found in Africa

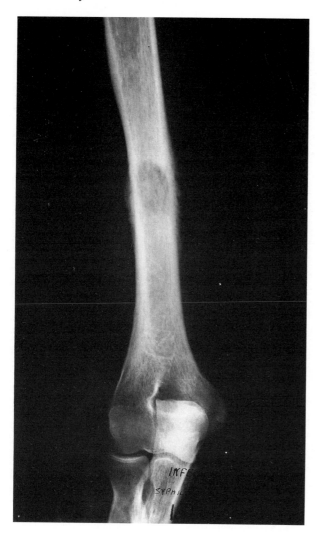

Fig. 15.45 A gumma. Note the 'punched-out' medullary lesion and periosteal new bone.

and the Far East. The pathological and skeletal manifestations are indistinguishable from those of adult syphilis; congenital infection does not occur.

Salmonella osteomyelitis

Osteomyelitis develops in less than 1% of patients with typhoid fever and usually occurs many months or even years after apparent recovery. The organism enters the bloodstream after multiplying in the intestinal wall. It occurs sometimes without a previous history of typhoid fever. Sickle-cell disease is a very common predisposing factor (Engh *et al.*, 1971; Adeyokunnu and Hendrickst, 1980); 70% of osteomyelitis in patients with sickle-cell disease is due to *Salmonella* infection.

The infection develops at the site of microvascular bone infarcts following bacteraemia. The bones most

affected are the vertebrae, ribs, sternum and tibia. Septic arthritis is rare. The lesions are similar to those seen in pyogenic osteomyelitis. In children it is usually the metaphysis of a long bone that is affected, and the infection may cross the epiphyseal plate to involve the epiphysis and spread to involve the diaphysis where a periosteal reaction occurs. In adults multiple lesions occur in the diaphysis with minimal periosteal reaction, and sequestration is unusual, as is an involucrum (Fig. 15.46). In the spine there is either a destructive lesion of the body and disc with a paravertebral abscess or increased density and a normal disc (Fig. 15.47). Eventually, ankylosis of the involved vertebra occurs.

In sickle-cell disease infected lesions are often multiple and symmetrical, the involucrum is prominent, and osteonecrosis is seen in the metaphyses around the knee joint and the diaphyseal cortex. A typical appearance is seen in the hand (Fig. 15.48).

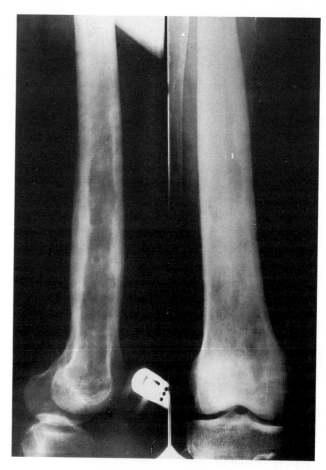

Fig. 15.46 *Salmonella* infection involving the lower femoral diaphysis. Note the minimal periosteal reaction and erosion of the inner cortex.

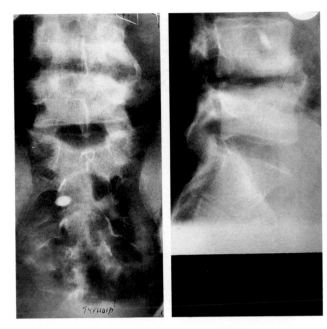

Fig. 15.47 *Salmonella* infection. Note the partial loss of disc space and extensive new bone formation.

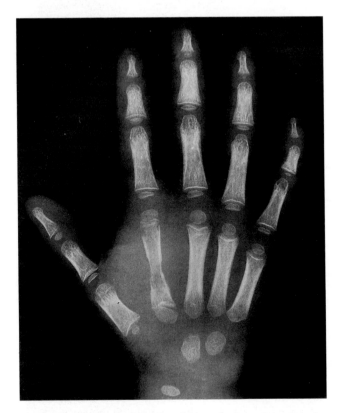

Fig. 15.48 *Salmonella* infection of the second metacarpal shaft. The child also has sickle-cell anaemia. Note the features of a hyperplastic marrow — coarse trabecular pattern, medullary expansion and cortical thinning.

CLINICAL PICTURE

This resembles that seen in pyogenic osteomyelitis, the condition is usually subacute. The organism can be recovered from the lesion and/or the bloodstream in most patients, and the agglutination test will also establish the diagnosis. A blood count with a specific request to look for sickle cells should be requested in appropriate patients, and it is also necessary to request a skeletal survey.

TREATMENT

This does not differ significantly from pyogenic osteomyelitis; antibiotics such as ampicillin are given after sensitivity tests have been done.

Brucellosis

Three species of *Brucella* infect humans — *B. melitensis*, *B. abortus* and *B. suis*. The organism enters the body through the lymphatic system and then passes into the bloodstream and localizes in those organs that contain an abundance of reticuloendothelial tissue. Granulomatous nodules, an abscess and caseation occur.

The onset is either acute or insidious. The presenting features are aching pain, headaches, general weakness, sweating and an irregular fever, all of which may last for weeks or months. Any bone or joint may be involved, but most commonly the spine in adults and a joint, particularly the hip, in children. A spine infection usually occurs in the 40–60-year age group and principally affects the lumbar region; about 12% of patients have cord compression.

An agglutination reaction of 1/80 is diagnostic. Blood, pus and joint fluid will provide a positive culture in the acute stage.

The radiographic findings are as follows. Joint changes are non-specific and are indistinguishable from those seen in tuberculosis. The long bone changes resemble those of subacute pyogenic osteomyelitis, including irregular osteolytic lesions with minimal periosteal reaction. The vertebral changes resemble those seen in tuberculosis, but bone and disc destruction is not so extensive. Early bone reaction, e.g. osteophytic outgrowths, may in due course produce intervertebral bridging, and any paravertebral abscess is minimal (Fig. 15.49). The condition responds to a course of tetracycline.

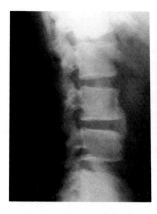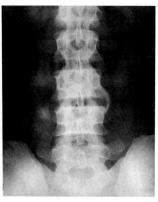

Fig. 15.49 Brucellosis of L4–L5. Note the minimal bone destruction, well-preserved disc space and intervertebral bridging.

Hydatid disease

The disease has been reviewed by Lewis *et al.* (1975). Bone infestation by the organism *Echinococcus granulosus* constitutes about 2% of the organs that may be affected. The life cycle will not be discussed here.

The essential lesion is a cyst with a lining membrane that is capable of producing daughter cysts. The sites commonly involved are the spine, sacrum and pelvis. Growth of the lesion is very slow, and it spreads along the medulla and gradually erodes the trabeculae but does not expand the cortex. If the cortex is breached the lesion then expands in the soft tissues. A pathological fracture may occur.

CLINICAL PICTURE

The lesion remains silent for many years. The presenting symptoms are pain from pressure of the enlarging cyst, swelling and a pathological fracture. Vertebral infection is often accompanied by neurological signs.

RADIOLOGICAL FEATURES

The appearance is that of an irregular multilocular cyst without cortical expansion, periosteal reaction, or sclerosis. The cortex is later thinned and breached (Fig. 15.50). In the spine the vertebral body and disc will show evidence of destruction, and typical paraspinal extension and involvement of ribs occurs. Computed tomography and magnetic resonance imaging are helpful in indicating the extent of the disease.

Such conditions as aneurysmal bone cyst, solitary cyst, giant cell tumour and chondrosarcoma have to be differentiated. Several laboratory diagnostic tests are available, namely Casoni's test, a complement fixation test and a precipitation test.

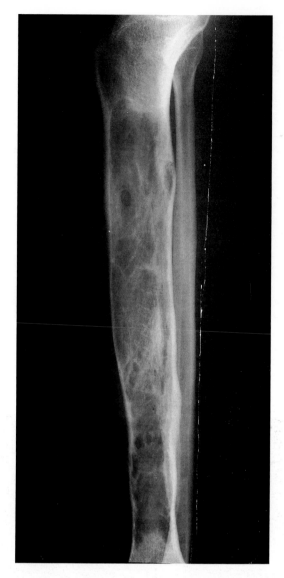

Fig. 15.50 Hydatid disease. Note that the tibia is expanded by multilocular cysts; the cortex is thinned and a periosteal reaction is absent.

TREATMENT

The best chance of obtaining a cure is by a combination of radical operation, irrigation with scolecidal agents such as 0.5% silver nitrate, and chemotherapy with albendazole, 10 mg/kg/day (Szypryt *et al.*, 1987).

Leprosy (Hansen's disease)

This is a systemic condition due to *Mycobacterium leprae*, which involves skin, peripheral nerves and bone. Two types of lesion involve bone.

Specific destructive osteitis occurs from either a tuberculoid response with the formation of a granuloma or a lepromatous reaction. Typically, the lesions are large, usually involving the fingers. There may be trabecular destruction with no periosteal reaction in the subarticular region and some cortical erosion. A granuloma produces the pseudo-osteitic change without reactive sclerosis.

The other type of lesion is a non-specific neuropathic bone condition secondary to loss of sensation following nerve involvement. It is most often seen in the feet. Atrophic ulcer develops followed by secondary infection with bone and joint destruction typical of Charcot's disease (Fig. 15.51).

Peripheral nerves, e.g. the common peroneal and ulnar nerves, are commonly affected, producing varying degrees of paralysis.

TREATMENT

Initial treatment is always medical, using appropriate bactericidal drugs. Operation is helpful in some of the trophic foot lesions. Excision of dead and infected tissue will allow healing of trophic ulcers. Decompression of involved nerves (Chaise and Roger, 1985) will aid

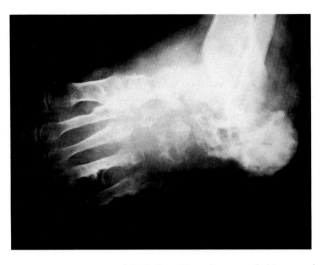

Fig. 15.52 Mycetoma of the hallux. Note the expanded bone and cystic defects.

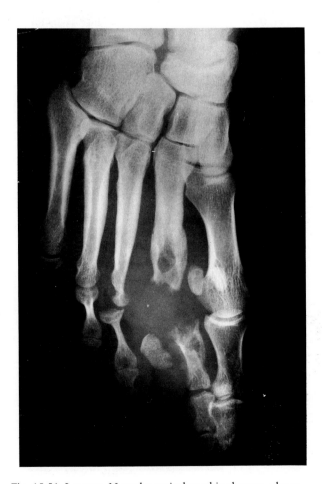

Fig. 15.51 Leprosy. Note the typical trophic changes—bone destruction associated with an osteitis.

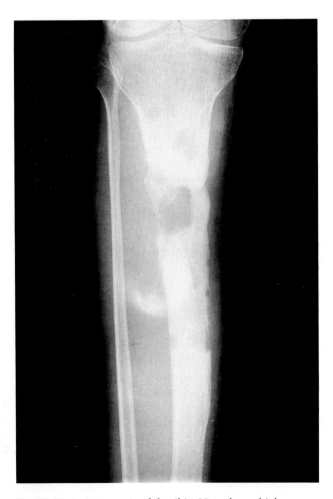

Fig. 15.53 Actinomycosis of the tibia. Note the multiple translucent areas giving a honeycomb appearance; some reactive sclerosis is present.

recovery of paralysis and may prevent neuropathic foot problems.

Mycetoma

This is an infection that is prevalent in the Tropics. It is due to two groups of organisms, namely maduromycetes and actinomycetes. It is referred to by some as madura foot because of its anatomical and geographical location. The organisms live in the soil and enter the body through a skin abrasion. When the foot is involved the infection may be superficial with nodules and discharging sinuses; if the plantar fascia is penetrated the bone becomes secondarily involved with much resultant swelling and discharging sinuses. The infection may spread within the muscle sheaths. Secondary pyogenic infection is common. The bone lesion is either localized as large cystic cavities or as a diffuse condition with abscesses and bone destruction.

The patient presents with a grossly swollen extremity, multiple sinuses, foul smelling discharge and ulcerated skin. In a typical foot infection the radiograph will show blurred and distorted soft tissue margins, with cortical defects in the bones and marginal sclerosis. The bone expands producing numerous cystic defects, and there is

a periosteal reaction (Fig. 15.52). Sequestra do not occur.

TREATMENT

Essentially, chemotherapy is used to combat the fungal and secondary pyogenic infection. Operation in the localized form of the disease may be necessary later (Maghoub, 1976).

Actinomycosis

The infection is caused by the anaerobic *Actinomyces* spp. The bones most commonly affected are the mandible due to extension from the oropharynx, the rib and vertebra from a pulmonary lesion, and the pelvis from a caecal lesion. Very occasionally, a primary bone focus occurs.

The lesion is essentially a granuloma with abscess formation that presents as a hard mass with a discharging sinus. Material for examination must be cultured anaerobically. The radiograph will show that the bone has a 'honeycomb' appearance due to bone destruction and reactive sclerosis (Fig. 15.53). There is usually a periosteal reaction.

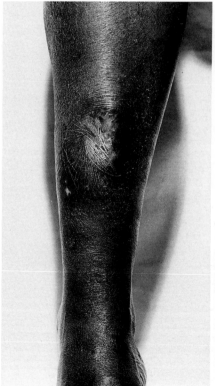 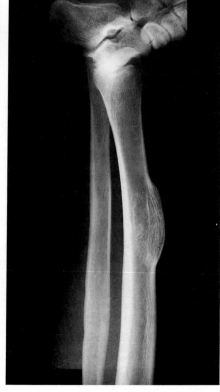

Fig. 15.54 (a) Tropical ulcer—chronic scar tissue overlying thickened bone. (b) Note the localized thickened cortex on the anterior surface of the tibia.

(a)   (b)

The usual treatment is a prolonged course of penicillin, and operation is seldom necessary.

Tropical ulcer

This is a chronic infection involving the tibia. It occurs only in developing countries. The aetiology is uncertain, but trauma and poor nutrition are predisposing factors. *Borrelia vincenti* and *Fusiformis fusiformis* (Vincent's organisms) are often isolated, though a mixed flora is common. The organism enters the tissues through a minor skin abrasion, often overlying the tibia. A painful superficial ulcer develops which gradually involves deep structures down to and including the bone, leading to profuse discharge and granulation. Malignant change can occur. Spontaneous healing of the ulcer is followed by recurrent skin breakdown (Fig. 15.54). The underlying bone is affected by periosteal new bone and cortical sequestration may occur.

Treatment is usually a combination of operative excision, skin grafting and antibiotics.

REFERENCES

Adeyokunnu A.A. and Hendrickst R.G. (1980) *Salmonella* osteomyelitis in childhood. *Arch. Dis. Child.* **55**, 175–184.

Arnoff S.C. and Scales P.V. (1983) Treatment of childhood skeletal infections. *Pediatr. Clin. North Am.* **30**, 271–280.

Babhulkar S.S., Tayade W.B. and Babhulkar S.K. (1984) Atypical spinal tuberculosis. *J. Bone Joint Surg.* **66B**, 239–242.

Banks S.W. and Compere E.L. (1941) Regeneration of epiphyseal cartilage. *Ann. Surg.* **114**, 1076–1084.

Batson O.V. (1940) The function of the vertebral veins in the spread of metastases. *Ann. Surg.* **112**, 138–149.

Blockey N.J. and McAllister T.A. (1972) Antibiotics in acute osteomyelitis in children. *J. Bone Joint Surg.* **54B**, 299–309.

Brodie S.W.B. (1836) *Pathological and Surgical Observations on the Diseases of the Joints.* London, Longman, p. 354.

Buchholz H.N. and Engelbrecht H. (1970) *Uber Die Antibiotica Bei Veomischurg Mit Dem Kunsthauz.* Palacos Chirurg.

Buchholz H.N., Elson R.A., Engelbrecht H. *et al.* (1981) Management of deep infection of total hip replacement. *J. Bone Joint Surg.* **63B**, 342–353.

Bulmer J.H. (1966) Septic arthritis of the hip in adults. *J. Bone Joint Surg.* **48B**, 289–298.

Burke J.F. (1963) The identification of the sources of staphylococci contaminating the surgical wound during operation. *Ann. Surg.* **158**, 898–904.

Butler E.C.B. (1940) Complications and late results of acute haematogenous osteomyelitis. *Br. J. Surg.* **110**, 261.

Chaise F. and Roger B. (1985) Neurolysis of the common peroneal nerve in leprosy. *J Bone Joint Surg.* **67B**, 426–429.

Choi I.H., Pizzutillo P.D., Bowen J.R. *et al.* (1990) Sequelae and reconstruction after septic arthritis of the hip in infants. *J Bone Joint Surg.* **72A**, 1150–1165.

Collert S. and Isacson J. (1982) Chronic sclerosing osteomyelitis (Garré). *Clin. Orthop.* **164**, 136–140.

Daoud A. and Saighi-Bovaovina A. (1989) Treatment of sequestra. Pseudarthrosis in defects of long bones of children who have chronic haematogenous osteomyelitis. *J. Bone Joint Surg.* **71A**, 1448–1468.

Digby J.M. and Kersley J.B. (1979) Pyogenic non-tuberculosis spinal infection. *J. Bone Joint Surg.* **61B**, 47–55.

Engh C.A., Hughes J.L., Abrams R.C. *et al.* (1971) Osteomyelitis in the patient with sickle cell disease. *J. Bone Joint Surg.* **53A**, 1–15.

Fitzgerald R.H. Jr., Nolan D.R., Ilstrup D.M., Scoy R.E. Van, Washington J.A. and Coventry M.B. (1977) Deep wound sepsis following total hip replacement. *J. Bone Joint Surg.* **59A**, 847–855.

Fitzgerald R.H. Jr., Ruttle P.E., Arnold P.G. *et al.* (1985) Local muscle flaps in treatment of chronic osteomyelitis. *J. Bone Joint Surg.* **67A**, 175–185.

Galasko C.S.B. (1989) The management of bone and joint infection. *Br. J. Hosp. Med.* **42**, 32–44.

Garcia A.J.R. and Grantham S.A. (1960) Haematogenous vertebral osteomyelitis. *J. Bone Joint Surg.* **42A**, 429–436.

Gillespie W.J. and Mayo K.M. (1981) The management of acute haematogenous osteomyelitis in the antibiotic era. *J. Bone Joint Surg.* **63B**, 126–131.

Gilmour W.N. (1962) Acute haematogenous osteomyelitis. *J. Bone Joint Surg.* **44B**, 841–853.

Gledhill R.B. (1973) Subacute osteomyelitis in children. *Clin. Orthop.* **96**, 57–69.

Golding J.S.R., MacIver J.E. and Wint L.N. (1959) The bone changes in sickle cell anaemia and its genetic variants. *J. Bone Joint Surg.* **41B**, 711–718.

Green N.E., Beauchamp R.D. and Griffin P.P. (1981) Primary subacute epiphyseal osteomyelitis. *J. Bone Joint Surg.* **63A**, 107–14.

Griffiths D.L.L. (1987) Tuberculosis of the spine. *Curr. Orthop.* **1**, 179–184.

Griffiths M.E.D. and Jones D.M. (1971) Pyogenic infection of the spine. *J. Bone Joint Surg.* **53B**, 383–391.

Gristina A.G. and Kolkin J. (1983) Total joint replacement and sepsis. *J. Bone Joint Surg.* **65A**, 128–134.

Gristina A.G., Costerton J.W., Leake E. *et al.* (1980) Bacterial colonization of biomaterials. *Orthop. Trans.* **4**, 355.

Hamblen D.L., Currey H.L. and Key J.J. (1966) Pseudogout simulating acute suppurative arthritis. *J. Bone Joint Surg.* **48B**, 51–55.

Harris N.H. (1960) Some problems in the diagnosis and treatment of acute osteomyelitis. *J. Bone Joint Surg.* **42B**, 535–541.

Harris N.H. (1962) The place of surgery in the early stages of acute osteomyelitis. *BMJ* **1**, 1440.

Harris N.H. and Kirkaldy-Willis W.H. (1965) Primary subacute pyogenic osteomyelitis. *J. Bone Joint Surg.* **47B**, 526–532.

Henriques C.Q. (1947) The veins of the vertebral column and their role in the spread of cancer. *Ann. R. Coll. Surg. Engl.* **1**, 51.

Henriques C.Q. (1958) Osteomyelitis as a complication of urology. *J. Bone Joint Surg.* **46B**, 19.

Hill C., Flanant R., *et al.* (1981) Prophylactic cefazolin versus placebo in total hip replacement. *Lancet* **i**, 795.

Hodgson A.R. and Stock F.E. (1960) Anterior spinal fusion for tuberculosis of the spine. *J. Bone Joint Surg.* **42A**, 295–310.

Hodgson A.R. and Yau A. (1967) A clinical study of 100 consecutive cases of Pott's paraplegia. *Paraplegia* **5**, 1–16.

Hodgson A.R., Skinsnes O.K. and Leong C.V. (1967) The

pathogenesis of Pott's paraplegia. *J. Bone Joint Surg.* **49A**, 1147–1156.

Hunka L., Said S.E., MacKenzie D.A. *et al.* (1982) Classification and surgical management of severe sequelae of septic hips in children. *Clin. Orthop.* **171**, 30–36.

Hunter G. and Dandy D. (1977) The natural history of the patient with an infected total hip replacement. *J. Bone Joint Surg.* **59B**, 293–297.

Jackson J.W. (1971) Surgical approaches to the anterior aspect of the spinal column. *Ann. R. Coll. Surg. Engl.* **48**, 83.

Josefsson G., Lindberg L. and Wicklander B. (1981) Systemic antibiotics and gentamicin-containing bone cement in the prophylaxis of postoperative infections in total hip arthroplasty. *Clin. Orthop.* **159**, 194.

Kelly P.J., Martin W.J. and Coventry M.B. (1970) Bacterial (suppurative) arthritis in the adult. *J. Bone Joint Surg.* **52A**, 1595–1602.

Kemp M.B.S., Jackson J.W., Jerimiah J.D. *et al.* (1973) Pyogenic infections occurring primarily in intervertebral discs. *J. Bone Joint Surg.* **66B**, 645–650.

Kim Y.Y., Ahn B.H., Bae D.K. *et al.* (1986) Arthroplasty using the Charnley prosthesis in old tuberculosis of the hip. *Clin. Orthop.* **211**, 116–121.

King D.M. and Mayo K.M. (1969) Subacute haematogenous osteomyelitis. *J. Bone Joint Surg.* **51B**, 458–463.

Kirkaldy-Willis E.H. and Thomas T.G. (1965) Anterior approaches in the diagnosis and treatment of infections in the vertebral bodies. *J. Bone Joint Surg.* **47A**, 87–110.

Klenerman L. (1984) The management of the infected endoprosthesis. *J. Bone Joint Surg.* **66B**, 645–651.

Kopits S.E. and Debussey H. (1977) Primary chronic sclerosing osteomyelitis. *Johns Hopkins Med. J.* **140**, 241.

Lack C.H. (1959) Chondrolysis in arthritis. *J. Bone Joint Surg.* **41B**, 384–387.

Lack C.H. (1961) Chondrolysis. *Ann. Phys. Med.* **6**, 93.

Lack C.H. and Towers A.G. (1962) Serological tests for staphylococcal infection. *BMJ* **2**, 1227.

Lewis J.W. Jr., Koss W. and Kerstein M.D. (1975) A review of echinococcal disease. *Ann. Surg.* **181**, 390–396.

Lidwell O.M. (1986) Clean air at operation and subsequent sepsis in the joint. *Clin. Orthop.* **211**, 91–102.

Lidwell O.M., Lowbury E.J.L., Whyte W. *et al.* (1982) Effect of ultraclean air in operating rooms on deep sepsis in the joint after total hip or knee replacement. *BMJ* **285**, 10–14.

Lidwell O.M., Lowbury E.J.L., Whyte W. *et al.* (1983) Ventilation in operating rooms. *BMJ* **286**, 1214.

Lifeso R.M., Harder E. and McCorkell S.S. (1985) Spinal brucellosis. *J. Bone Joint Surg.* **67B**, 345–351.

Lloyd-Roberts G.C. (1960) Suppurative arthritis in infancy. *J. Bone Joint Surg.* **42B**, 706–720.

Lynch M., Esser M.P., Shelley P. *et al.* (1987) Deep infection in Charnley friction arthroplasty. *J. Bone Joint Surg.* **69B**, 355–360.

McElwaine J.P. and Colville J. (1984) Excision arthroplasty for infected total hip replacement. *J. Bone Joint Surg.* **66B**, 168–171.

Maghoub E.L.S. (1976) Medical management of mycetoma. *Bull. World Health Organ.* **54**, 303.

Mandel D.B. (1979) *Principles and Practise of Infectious Diseases*, New York, Wiley.

Mann T.S. (1963) Some aspects of acute haematogenous osteitis in children. *BMJ* **11**, 1561.

Medical Research Council Working Party on Tuberculosis of the Spine. (1973a) A controlled trial of ambulant out-patient treatment and in-patient rest in bed in the management of tuberculosis of the spine in young Korean patients on standard chemotherapy. *J. Bone Joint Surg.* **55B**, 678–697.

Medical Research Council Working Party Report on Tuberculosis of the Spine. (1973b) A controlled trial of plaster-of-Paris jackets in the management of ambulant out-patient treatment of tuberculosis of the spine in children on standard chemotherapy. *Tubercle* **54**, 261.

Medical Research Council Working Party on Tuberculosis of the Spine. (1974a) A controlled trial of debridement and ambulatory treatment in the management of tuberculosis of the spine in patients on standard chemotherapy. *J. Trop. Med. Hyg.* **77**, 72.

Medical Research Council Working Party on Tuberculosis of the Spine. (1974b) A controlled trial of anterior spinal fusion and debridement in the surgical management of tuberculosis of the spine in patients on standard chemotherapy. *Br. J. Surg.* **61**, 853.

Medical Research Council Working Party on Tuberculosis of the Spine. (1976) A five year assessment of controlled trials of in-patient and out-patient treatment and of plaster-of-Paris jackets for tuberculosis of the spine in children on standard chemotherapy. *J. Bone Joint Surg.* **58B**, 399–411.

Mollan R.A.B. and Piggot J. (1972) Acute osteomyelitis in children. *J. Bone Joint Surg.* **59B**, 2–7.

Mollan R.A.B., Craig B.F. and Biggart J.E. (1984) Chronic sclerosing osteomyelitis. *J. Bone Joint Surg.* **66B**, 583–585.

Murray R.O. (1960) Radiological bone changes in Cushing's syndrome and steroid therapy. *Br. J. Radiol.* **33**, 1.

Nelaton A. (1844) Eléments de Pathologie Chirurgicale. Paris.

Obletz B.F. (1960) Acute suppurative arthritis of the hip in the neonatal period. *J. Bone Joint Surg.* **42A**, 23–30.

Papineau L., Pilon L., Alfageme A. *et al.* (1976) Chronic osteomyelitis of long bones. *J. Bone Joint Surg.* **58B**, 138.

Paterson D.C. (1970) Acute suppurative arthritis in infancy and children. *J. Bone Joint Surg.* **52B**, 474–482.

Pattinson P.R.M. (1986) Pott's paraplegia. *Paraplegia* **24**, 77.

Petty W., Goldsmith S. (1980) Resection arthroplasty following total hip arthroplasty. *J. Bone Joint Surg.* **62A**, 889–896.

Rasool M.N., Govender S. (1989) The skeletal manifestations of congenital syphilis. *J. Bone Joint Surg.* **71B**, 752–755.

Roberts J.M., Drummond D.S., Breed A.L. *et al.* (1982) Subacute haematogenous osteomyelitis in children. *J. Pediatr. Orthop.* **2**, 249.

Roca R.P. and Yoshikawa T.T. (1979) Primary skeletal infections in heroin users. *Clin. Orthop.* **644**, 238.

Rosenbaum D.M. and Blumhagen J.D. (1985) Acute epiphyseal osteomyelitis in children. *Radiology* **156**, 89.

Ross E.R.S. and Cole W.L. (1985) Treatment of subacute osteomyelitis in childhood. *J. Bone Joint Surg.* **67B**, 443–448.

Rowling D.E. (1970) Further experience in the management of chronic osteomyelitis. *J. Bone Joint Surg.* **52B**, 302–307.

Russell A.S. and Ansell B.H. (1972) Septic arthritis. *Ann. Rheum. Dis.* **31**, 40.

Salvati E.A., Chefofsky K.M., Brause B.D. *et al.* (1982) Reimplantation in infection. A 12 year experience. *Clin. Orthop.* **170**, 62.

Samilson R.L., Bersani F.A. and Watkins M.B. (1958) Acute suppurative arthritis in infants and children. *Pediatrics* **21**, 798.

Scales P.V. and Arnoff S.C. (1984) Antimicrobial therapy of childhood skeletal infections. *J. Bone Joint Surg.* **66A**,

1487–1492.

Seddon M.J. (1935) The morbid anatomy of caries of the thoracic spine in relation to treatment. *Lancet* **ii**, 355.

Smith T. (1874) On the acute arthritis of infants. *St Bart's Hosp. Rep.* **10**, 189.

Smith R.F. and Taylor T.K.F. (1967) Inflammatory lesions of intervertebral discs in children. *J. Bone Joint Surg.* **49A**, 1508–1520.

Spencer J.D. (1986) Bone and joint infections in a renal unit. *J. Bone Joint Surg.* **68B**, 489–493.

Srenson T.S., Hedeboe E.R. and Christensen E.A. (1988) Primary epiphyseal osteomyelitis in children. *J. Bone Joint Surg.* **70B**, 818–820.

Surin V.V., Sundholm K. and Backman L. (1983) Infection after total hip replacement. *J. Bone Joint Surg.* **65B**, 412–418.

Szypryt E.P., Morris D.L. and Mulholland R.C. (1987) Combined chemotherapy and surgery for hydatid bone disease. *J. Bone Joint Surg.* **69B**, 141–144.

Travlo J. and Toit G. (1990) Spinal tuberculosis: beware the posterior elements. *J. Bone Joint Surg.* **72B**, 722–723.

Trippel S.B. (1986) Antibiotic-impregnated cement in total hip arthroplasty. *J. Bone Joint Surg.* **68A**, 1297–1302.

Trueta J. (1957) Normal vascular anatomy of the human femoral head during growth. *J. Bone Joint Surg.* **39B**, 358–394.

Trueta J. and Harrison M.H.M. (1953) Normal vascular anatomy of the femoral head in adult man. *J. Bone Joint Surg.* **64B**, 446.

Trueta J. and Morgan J.D. (1954) Late results in the treatment of one hundred cases of acute haematogenous osteomyelitis. *Br. J. Surg.* **169**, 29.

Tili S.M. and Mukherjee S.K. (1981) Excision arthroplasty for tuberculosis and pyogenic arthritis of the hip. *J. Bone Joint Surg.* **638**, 29–32.

Vishwakarma G.K. and Khare A.K. (1986) Amniotic arthroplasty for treatment of the hip. *J. Bone Joint Surg.* **68B**, 68–74.

Wiley A.M. and Trueta J. (1959) Vascular anatomy of the spine and relationship to pyogenic vertebral osteomyelitis. *J. Bone Joint Surg.* **41B**, 796–809.

Wilson N.I.L. and Di Paola M. (1986) Acute septic arthritis in infancy and childhood. *J. Bone Joint Surg.* **68B**, 584–587.

Winters J.L. and Caren I. (1960) Acute haematogenous osteomyelitis. *J. Bone Joint Surg.* **42A**, 691–704.

Yoshimura M., Shimada T., Matsuda M. *et al.* (1989) Treatment of chronic osteomyelitis of the leg by peroneal myocutaneous island flap and transfer. *J. Bone Joint Surg.* **71B**, 593–596.

Chapter 16
Pathology of Aseptic Bone Necrosis

M. Catto

INTRODUCTION

Aseptic bone necrosis is becoming an increasingly common cause of disability. It is a common complication of intracapsular fracture of the neck of the femur, which is a special hazard in the enlarging elderly population (Silman, 1992; Anderson *et al.*, 1993). It is a risk not only to tunnellers working in compressed air but also to divers employed in the exploitation of offshore oil. It gives rise to articular symptoms in some patients receiving therapeutic steroids and particularly in those on immunosuppressive therapy following organ and bone marrow transplantation. Some long-term survivors of malignant lymphoma and leukaemia also develop iatrogenic bone necrosis. In addition to necrosis associated with these and other well-accepted causes, e.g. sickle cell disease and Gaucher's disease, so-called idiopathic necrosis, chiefly of the femoral head, has been reported since 1960 in ever-increasing numbers in North America and Europe. Work is being carried out in many centres to identify the predisposing factors in this puzzling group.

The widespread use of prosthetic replacement of joints and the investigation in some centres of the early stages of necrosis by core biopsy (Ficat and Arlet, 1968; Ficat, 1985) have allowed pathologists to establish a generally accepted pattern of morphological changes, which has led to more accurate interpretation of radiographs. The sequence of events that gives rise to these morphological changes is more speculative and controversial.

In order to avoid repetition, this section begins with a general account of the recognition and patterns of bone necrosis. Any differences in pattern are touched on subsequently when the individual associations with aseptic necrosis are described. The more controversial aspects are discussed at the end of the chapter. The pathology of Perthes' disease is included in Chapter 5, and that of osteochondritis dissecans in Chapter 6.

RECOGNITION OF BONE NECROSIS

The death of bone does not alter its radiological density, so plain radiographs are not helpful in diagnosis. The only exception is if the affected part is efficiently immobilized for at least 4–6 weeks, e.g. in treatment of a fracture of the talus or scaphoid bone. Living bone then becomes porotic due to osteoclastic bone resorption. Since there are no living cells in the necrotic tissue, the dead bone cannot undergo resorption and so appears relatively denser (Santos, 1930; Phemister, 1934) (Fig. 16.1).

The term bone necrosis implies not only death of a focus of bone trabeculae but also of the intertrabecular marrow. Necrosis occurs most commonly at sites of predominantly fatty marrow, probably due to its poorer blood supply compared with that of haemopoietic marrow. Experimental evidence suggests that cells of haemopoietic marrow die within 6–12 h and osteocytes within 12–48 h of removal of their blood supply, while fatty marrow survives for perhaps as long as 5 days. Histological changes of necrosis first develop from about 48 h in cells of the haemopoietic marrow; the loss of osteocytes from the lacunae, which indicates death of the bone itself, tends to be slower and may not be complete for 2–4 weeks (Catto, 1965a). This means that histological examination of a core biopsy of, for example, the femoral head after intracapsular fracture may be unhelpful, not only because of sampling problems but if it is taken soon after injury, the presence of osteocytes does not necessarily indicate that the bone is living.

REVASCULARIZATION AND REPAIR

Repair processes may be regarded as occurring in two phases. First, when the dead bone abuts on live marrow, capillaries and undifferentiated mesenchymal cells grow

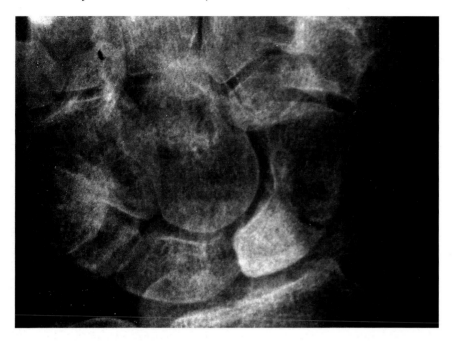

Fig. 16.1 Fractured scaphoid bone treated for 4 weeks in a plaster cast. The bone proximal to the fracture line appears dense in comparison with the carpal bones, which are porotic as a result of immobilization.

into the dead marrow spaces while accompanying macrophages mop up dead fat and cellular debris. Secondly, the mesenchymal cells may then differentiate into osteoblasts or fibroblasts. Under favourable circumstances marrow revascularization is followed by laying down of new bone, chiefly on the surface of dead spongy trabeculae (Fig. 16.2). These sandwich-like trabeculae may persist for a long time, acting as histological markers for the extent of previous bone death, and if sufficiently thickened they may produce increased radiological density. Thus, the first radiographic evidence of previous necrosis may be patchy sclerosis due to repair (Bobechko

and Harris, 1960). The osteoclastic resorption of dead bone in an active patient is often long delayed, except in the dense bone of the subchondral plate. At any time during the repair process when conditions are less favourable, although revascularization of the marrow may continue, osteoblasts do not differentiate and the dead bone tends to become surrounded by dense fibrous tissue.

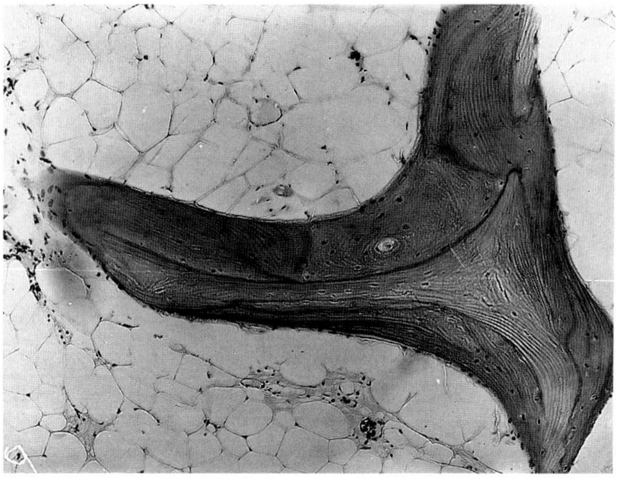

The lesions of bone necrosis are conveniently divided into two groups depending on the part of the bone involved. The medullary lesions are symptomless, while the juxta-articular lesions are potentially disabling; the joint surface may collapse and secondary degenerative changes in the joint follow.

MEDULLARY NECROSIS

This occurs particularly in association with dysbarism and the haemoglobinopathies, occasionally in Gaucher's disease, and in patients treated with steroids or without any known predisposing cause. The lower femoral shaft and the upper shaft of the tibia and humerus are most commonly affected, often bilaterally.

The extent of the necrosis varies from small foci to large areas involving most of the width of the medullary cavity and sometimes also the endosteal cortex. Medullary necrosis itself produces no radiological change and sometimes, in steroid-treated patients, there is little formation of bone in the repair process so that radiologically unsuspected areas of bone necrosis may be discovered at necropsy (Fig. 16.3a). In lesions that have

Fig. 16.2 Dead trabecula with empty bone lacunae surrounded by new living bone, forming a 'sandwich' trabecula. (H&E, ×95.)

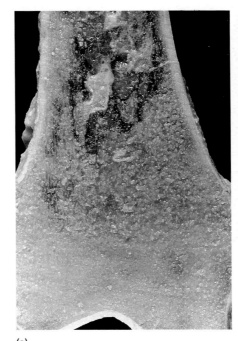
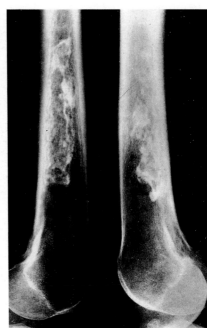

Fig. 16.3 (a) Irregular area of medullary bone necrosis surrounded by haemorrhagic marrow and fibrous tissue. This was an unexpected finding at necropsy in a renal transplant patient with a negative skeletal survey. (b) Extensive old medullary necrosis in the lower end of both femora in a man who had stopped working in compressed air 30 years previously. Reproduced from Davidson (1976) by permission of Dr J.K. Davidson and Elsevier, Amsterdam.

(a)　　　　　　　　　　(b)

been present for a long time, any remaining dead marrow appears yellowish, opaque and sometimes flecked with calcium. It tends to be surrounded by a serpiginous capsule of dense greyish, glistening collagen which may be patchily calcified. Bone trabeculae at the margin of the collagen are often broadened by the previous apposition of living bone on the dead trabeculae. Thickening of trabeculae by new bone may be sufficient to be identified in clinical radiographs and, when the endosteal part of the cortex is involved, new bone contributes to the increased cortical width that has sometimes been described. The generally accepted interpretation of these morphological findings is that there has been partial revascularization of the dead marrow with incomplete, arrested repair. The dominant radiological change is calcification, and when this occurs in the serpiginous collagen bordering dead tissue the wavy line of increased density has been likened to a coil of smoke (Fig. 16.3b).

Calcified enchondromas may be difficult to distinguish radiologically, though they tend to show a less well-defined margin, the calcification appearing as rounded compact masses rather than the linear strands characteristic of partially revascularized medullary bone necrosis. Bone islands consist of ovoid or oblong areas of cortical bone with sharply defined margins, which usually remain unchanged for years but due to remodelling may show increased uptake on radionuclide bone scans. They are found most often in the medullary part of the end of the humerus and femur, and occasionally give rise to difficulty in differential diagnosis from the early,

more irregular patches of sclerosis caused by trabecular thickening.

Reports of a number of cases of sarcoma arising in association with medullary bone necrosis have been published. Most tumours occurred in middle-aged or elderly men with multiple areas of medullary bone necrosis. About two-thirds of the patients lack any predisposing cause for the bone necrosis (Frierson *et al.*, 1987) (Fig. 16.4). The most common association is with dysbarism, and of four patients reviewed by Galli (Galli *et al.*, 1978) the most recent exposure to compressed air was 17 years before the tumour presented, indicating the long induction period. Most of the reported tumours were fibrosarcomas or malignant fibrous histiocytomas, and almost all of the patients died with pulmonary metastases a mean of 18 months after diagnosis. It has been postulated that histiocytic proliferation, which is part of the chronic reparative process, undergoes malignant transformation (Michael and Dorfman, 1976).

The incidence of malignant change in bone necrosis is not known, but it is presumably small. While repeated radiographs or bone scans are not justified, patients with known medullary necrosis should be warned to report if they develop pain at the site of the lesion.

JUXTA-ARTICULAR NECROSIS

While there are some minor differences in the patterns of response to juxta-articular bone necrosis depending

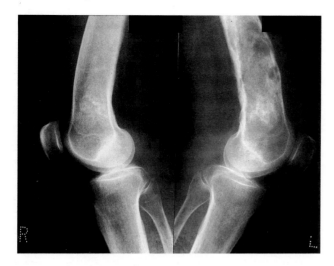

Fig. 16.4 Bilateral old calcified medullary infarcts in the distal femora of a woman aged 57 years. No predisposing cause was known. A malignant fibrous histiocytoma is associated with the infarct on the left side.

on its cause, the general picture and the sequence of events are similar. Attention is drawn to any variation in pattern or reaction in the appropriate section.

The anterosuperolateral part of the femoral head and the central dome of the humeral head are most often affected, and following structural failure, symptoms in the weight-bearing hip joint are most prominent. The femoral condyles, the talus, scaphoid bone, capitate bone and capitulum of the humerus are less often involved. In some conditions, e.g. dysbaric or post-transplant necrosis, several bones may be affected, often symmetrically. It is convenient to divide the natural history of juxta-articular necrosis into three stages.

Stage 1: before the onset of structural failure and collapse

At this stage the patient is usually symptom-free and the joint contour is completely normal. Magnetic resonance imaging or scintigraphy (see p. 451) may reveal the presence of necrosis before any radiological change is observed. Except in immobilized patients, irregular mottled areas of increased density may be the first radiological evidence of abnormality, and these later tend to coalesce to form a more compact sclerotic line across the bone end marking the junction between living and dead bone. Serial radiographs have shown that the dense line, once formed, seldom alters its position (Fig. 16.5). On examination by the naked eye, the joint contour is normal and the articular cartilage bluish, smooth, glistening and of normal thickness. As in adults the synovial fluid nourishes the articular cartilage except for the small amount deep to the calcified tidemark, this is usually the only site from which chondrocytes are lost.

Beneath the articular cartilage is a variable depth of opaque, yellow, necrotic marrow and bone trabeculae devoid of osteocytes. Sometimes calcification occurs within the dead marrow. Vascular granulation tissue or

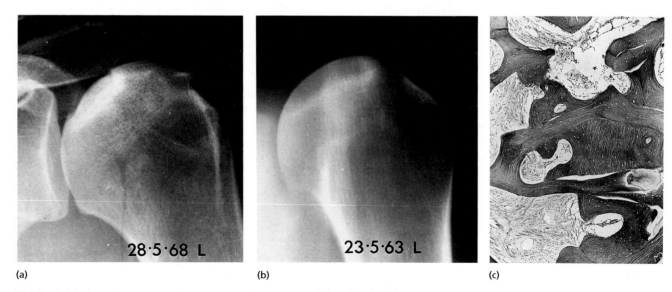

(a) (b) (c)

Fig. 16.5 (a) Dense line demarcating the extent of remaining subchondral dead bone in the humeral head of a tunnel worker. (b) Radiographs were taken yearly and the patient was symptomless until structural failure with collapse of the joint surface occurred 5 years after his initial radiograph. Reproduced by permission of Dr J.K. Davidson. (c) Dense line resulting from the laying down of massive amounts of new bone on the surface of dead trabeculae. The joint surface and remaining subchondral dead bone is to the left. (H&E, ×55.)

greyish, glistening, dense collagen separates this dead tissue from the underlying living bone. Within this border zone of fibrovascular tissue and for some distance deep to it, the dead bone trabeculae may be broadened by the formation of new living bone on their surfaces (Fig. 16.5c). The quantity of new bone varies in both the amount formed on individual trabeculae and the depth to which it extends. Mottled areas of increased density and the sclerotic line are both due to a true increase in radiological density resulting from the apposition of living bone on the surface of dead trabeculae. The trabeculae tend to be thickest where they abut on dense collagen (Fig. 16.5c), and as they extend from this zone they gradually regain their normal thickness and a full complement of osteocytes.

The broadening and strengthening of the trabeculae of cancellous bone may be regarded as a reactive remodelling response to compressive stresses (Sevitt, 1981). It is interesting to note that when femoral neck fractures were treated by prolonged immobilization and the head thus protected from these stresses, revascularization was accompanied by resorption of dead bone and porosis and the articular cartilage degenerated (Santos, 1930; Sherman and Phemister, 1947). While in active patients, the repair process in spongy bone is thus characterized by the formation of new bone, the slower revascularization of the more compact bone of the subchondral plate is accompanied by osteoclasis, which is only later followed by new bone formation (Glimcher and Kenzora, 1979a; Sevitt, 1981).

In most conditions the commonly accepted interpretation of these morphological changes is that bone necrosis has been followed by some revascularization and incomplete repair. When the junction between dead and living tissue is formed by a band of dense, poorly vascularized collagen, it seems reasonable to suggest that the advancing revascularization front has halted (Catto, 1976; Springfield and Enneking, 1976), though osteoblasts may still be forming bone on the deep surface and osteoclasts resorbing dead bone within the collagen.

Stage 2: structural failure followed by collapse

The most reliable indication of structural failure is the sudden onset of pain, and this may occur before any evidence of trabecular fracture is identifiable radiologically.

The trabecular fracture always occurs in dead bone and is often immediately beneath the subchondral plate, partially separating a shallow articular sequestrum which has been likened to an eggshell. This subchondral fracture gives rise to a crescent line of increased radiolucency running parallel to the joint surface (Norman and Bullough, 1963). Demonstration of structural failure may be particularly difficult in the hip joint. At first an anteroposterior view may show a normal contour, but lateral views, particularly those taken in the frog-leg position, more readily demonstrate the trabecular fracture, which often occurs in the anterior quadrant of the femoral head and is seen in profile in this view (Fig. 16.6). Traction to the limb often accentuates the crescent line.

Initially the contour of the joint surface appears smooth and unchanged; it is easily indented by pressure, and springs back to its original shape when the pressure is removed. A wrinkle later appears in the articular cartilage at the margin of the dead zone, and this is followed by cracks and fissures (Fig. 16.7a) and sometimes by tearing at the edge of the sequestrum, so that a hinged flap of articular surface forms (Fig. 16.7b). Once cracks or fissures allow communication between the dead bone and the joint space, creamy yellowish bony detritus, resulting from grinding of the dead bone and marrow, may escape into the synovial fluid and stimulate reactive synovitis. Fibrocartilage sometimes forms on the undersurface of the sequestrum.

Trabecular fractures sometimes occur deeper in the necrotic bone than immediately below the subchondral plate. The crescent line is not seen radiologically, and the first evidence of structural failure is alteration in the contour of the bone end, as is seen also when collapse follows subchondral fracture. In the femoral head a step appears beneath the acetabular lip and often also at the

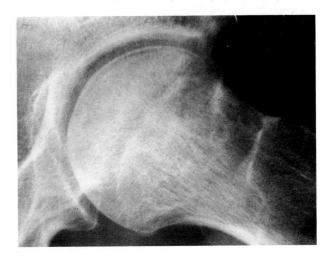

Fig. 16.6 'Radiolucent crescent sign' indicating subarticular fracture through dead bone in a compressed air worker. Reproduced from Davidson (1976) by permission of Dr J.K. Davidson and Elsevier, Amsterdam.

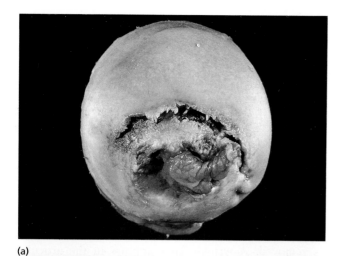

(a)

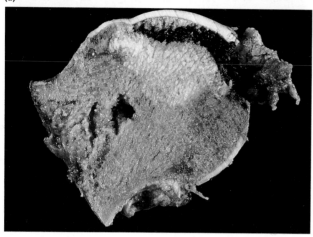

(b)

Fig. 16.7 (a) Although there is a subarticular fracture through dead bone, the contour of the femoral head appears normal. The well-preserved articular cartilage has cracked above the fovea. (b) There is a step near the lateral margin of the joint surface and a hinged flap, consisting of normal-looking articular cartilage with a fringe of subchondral dead bone, has separated. There is a wedge of bone necrosis deep to the subchondral fracture. The patient had received a renal transplant 1 year previously.

margin of the fovea (Fig. 16.8). The uncollapsed margin of the bone end may produce a ring-like ridge around the sunken dome (Fig. 16.9). These changes are often followed by osteophyte formation at the living margin of the joint (see below).

At this stage the area of dead bone may appear dense due to calcification of dead marrow (Sissons *et al.*, 1992) (Fig. 16.10) or of debris within the marrow spaces (Springfield and Enneking, 1976) as well as to compaction and fragmentation of trabeculae (Sevitt, 1981). A radiolucent line sometimes develops at the junction between dead and living bone, immediately adjacent to the dense line. This results from osteoclastic

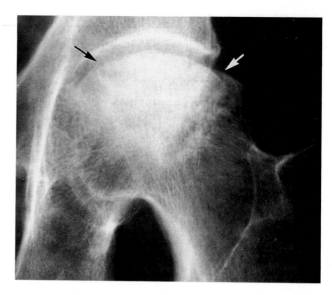

Fig. 16.8 Idiopathic necrosis of the femoral head. There is one step in the contour of the femoral head beneath the acetabular margin (white arrow) and another more medially (black arrow). The sequestrum has sunk into the femoral head. The joint space is well preserved. Reproduced from Davidson (1976) by permission of Elsevier, Amsterdam.

resorption of dead bone as it passes through the collagenous front. The replacing collagen is poorly vascular and may become fibrocartilaginous. Endochondral ossification of the fibrocartilage may occur on the revascularized deep surface. If the overlying dead bone is ground away the fibrocartilage may be exposed and form a new, though functionally inferior, joint surface (Milgram, 1984). Occasionally the original hinged

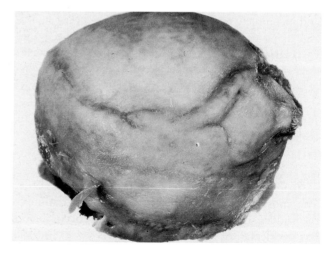

Fig. 16.9 Fracture of dead trabeculae has occurred deeper in the femoral head of a compressed air worker. The separated sequestrum has sunk down into the surrounding head, which forms a ridge around it. Reproduced from Davidson (1976) by permission of Elsevier, Amsterdam.

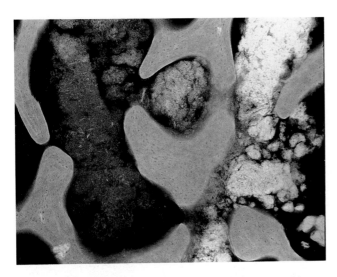

Fig. 16.10 Microradiograph of an undecalcified section of juxta-articular osteonecrosis including the margin of the infarct where revascularization is occurring on the right. Here rounded aggregates of increased density represent calcification which is less marked to the left, nearer the centre of the dead zone. Reproduced from Sissons *et al.* (1992) by permission of Professor H.A. Sissons and Springer-Verlag.

articular sequestrum becomes tenuously reattached by the in-growth of fibrocartilage among the stumps of its dead trabeculae (Fig. 16.11).

Stage 3: development of secondary osteoarthritis

Following collapse of the joint surface osteophytes form; the viable margin of the bone end remodels as a result of

capillary invasion of the deep surface of the articular cartilage and subsequent endochondral ossification. Whether capillary invasion is stimulated by alteration in the shape of the joint surface or by revascularization of any underlying dead bone is debatable. Osteophytic lipping may also occur at the opposing joint face. Even when these changes have developed, the joint space may remain well preserved due to the relatively unchanged cartilage covering the dead bone. This implies that these degenerative changes are secondary to bone necrosis. Later, however, the radiological appearances may be more difficult to distinguish from primary osteoarthritis (Fig. 16.12).

BONE NECROSIS WITH SECONDARY OSTEOARTHRITIS COMPARED WITH PRIMARY OSTEOARTHRITIS WITH SECONDARY BONE NECROSIS

In one hospital practice, bone necrosis is reported to underlie about 20% of total hip replacements undertaken for arthritis; both hips are affected in about 75% of these patients (Bullough and Di Carlo, 1990). When serial radiographs showing the initial necrosis and subsequent progression are unavailable, suspicion of preceding necrosis is aroused by a history of a sudden onset of pain during physical activity and by unexpected and rapid collapse and disintegration of the femoral head. The gross appearance, which tends to confirm the presence of previous necrosis, is the loss of the convex profile of the femoral head. This may be replaced by a

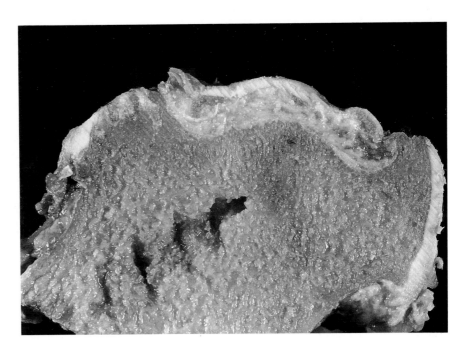

Fig. 16.11 This 25-year-old girl developed pain in both hips 1 year after a renal transplant. A sequestrum separated and this was followed by progressive collapse of the femoral head. At operation the articular cartilage had reattached by fibrocartilage to the remaining living bone. Only a few small pockets of dead bone remained.

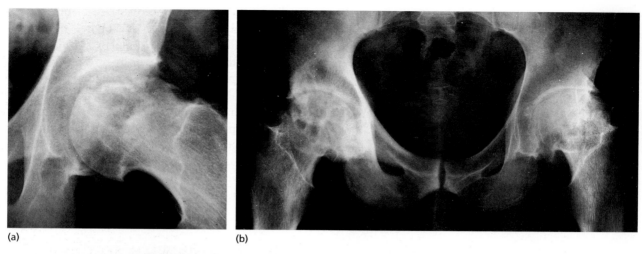

(a)   (b)

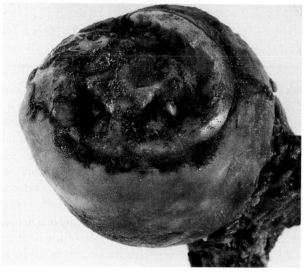

(c)

Fig. 16.12 This labourer developed hip pain while working in compressed air. (a) He was later found to have a shallow fragmented articular sequestrum in each femoral head (b) Eight years after the onset of pain the sequestrum had disappeared and severe bilateral osteoarthritis with loss of joint space had developed. (c) The articular sequestrum disintegrated leaving a shallow crater surrounded by a rim of densely sclerotic, eburnated live bone. On section of the head several degenerative 'cysts' were present. Reproduced from Davidson (1976) by permission of Dr J.K. Davidson and Elsevier, Amsterdam.

flat crater surrounded by a rim of densely sclerotic eburnated bone (Fig. 16.12), or when necrosis has been extensive, by a deep saddle-shaped deformity of the remaining stump of bone (Bullough and Di Carlo, 1990) (Fig. 16.13). Residual fragments of dead bone or cartilage on or within a collagenous bed may line the crater or saddle, marking the junction of remaining living bone with unrevascularized and now disintegrated dead tissue.

In contrast, bone necrosis that follows rather than precedes osteoarthritis is reported in about 6% of femoral heads removed at arthroplasty (Ilardi and Sokoloff, 1984). It is seen in primary osteoarthritis and also accompanying the later stages of rheumatoid disease, but is seldom recognizable radiologically (Sissons *et al.*, 1992). One or more sharply defined yellow areas may be seen on the exposed eburnated bone of the convex surface of the femoral head (Fig.

16.14). On section these well-demarcated small necrotic wedges, which are usually less than 1 cm in depth, may be bordered by a reddish rim of granulation tissue and often abut on a subarticular pseudocyst (Ilardi and Sokoloff, 1984). The necrotic bone trabeculae, like the adjacent living ones, are greatly thickened by appositional bone, confirming that necrosis has followed the sclerosis and eburnation of the joint surface probably as a result of a locally diminished vascular supply in areas subjected to high compressive stress.

INVESTIGATION OF BONE NECROSIS

Interpretation of the radiographic appearances following bone necrosis is based on a well-established sequence of pathological changes as described above. The first evidence of necrosis, however, is not recognizable in

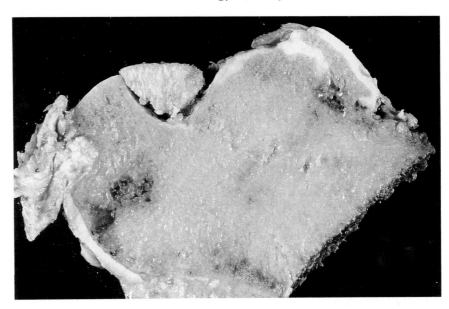

Fig. 16.13 All the dead subchondral bone, except for a small loose wedge, has been ground away leaving a deep depression. Medially the exposed bone surface is sclerotic. Elsewhere fibrocartilage has formed a new surface covering the remaining living bone.

plain films in mobile patients until 6 months or more after the onset of ischaemia (Bayliss and Davidson, 1977). More prompt diagnosis might help the clinician to decide on the most appropriate treatment for an intra-articular fracture of the femoral neck. Furthermore, the results of treatment in patients with non-traumatic bone necrosis are enhanced if surgery is carried out before structural failure and collapse of the joint surface develop. This opportunity arises, for example, in the clinically silent hip of a patient with known idiopathic or steroid-associated necrosis in the contralateral

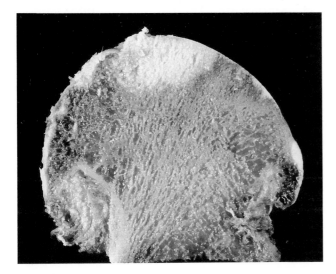

Fig. 16.14 The articular surface consists of exposed sclerotic bone with a series of small pale wedges of dead bone. Marginal osteophytes are prominent. Reproduced from Sissons *et al.* (1992) by permission of Professor H.A. Sissons MD and Springer-Verlag.

hip. These clinical considerations have led to a search for diagnostic methods that give an early indication of bone necrosis.

Bone and marrow scintigraphy

Scintigraphy has been used for about 40 years in the attempted pre-radiographic diagnosis of bone necrosis, particularly as it affects the femoral head (Arden and Veal, 1953). Radionuclides of phosphorus (^{32}P) and strontium (^{85}Sr, ^{87}Sr) were first employed, but ^{99m}technetium-labelled diphosphonates give better resolution and a very low radiation dose to the skeleton and are now the most popular radionuclides for bone scanning (Bonnarens *et al.*, 1985). Uptake immediately after injection of the radionuclide reflects blood flow; at the time of imaging 3 h later, it is thought to relate to bone formation. The radionuclide localizes along mineralized surfaces, probably due to adsorption onto the calcium of newly-formed hydroxyapatite crystals (Jones *et al.*, 1976; Lausten and Christensen, 1989). At first bone or marrow scans should show absent or decreased uptake, but once repair is underway uptake increases above the normal level. Bone marrow scans depend on phagocytosis of the radionuclide-labelled particles by marrow macrophages. Scans with ^{99m}technetium sulphur colloid are seldom used, however, as uptake was found in less than half the femoral heads of a control series of elderly patients without fracture. Better uptake has been reported using antimony colloid (Turner, 1983) or smaller particles (Tawn and Watt, 1989).

Evaluation of a suspected abnormal bone or marrow scintiscan is based on comparison with a normal contralateral hip. The method is thus more reliable in the assessment of femoral head vascularity following fracture or dislocation than when an asymptomatic hip is compared with one already affected by idiopathic or steroid-associated necrosis. In general, a post-traumatic decrease in uptake indicates an increased risk of bone necrosis and late segmental collapse, but in some cases an avascular area later revascularizes (D'Ambrosia *et al.*, 1978; Tawn and Watt, 1989). Indeed, the finding of a zone of reduced uptake may not of itself be a firm indication for primary prosthetic replacement (Drane and Rudd, 1985). Conversely, although the scintiscan may detect blood flow to an area, it does not predict either the adequacy or the permanence of the vascular supply (D'Ambrosia *et al.*, 1978).

Scintigraphy is a sensitive but non-specific investigation, and the results must be assessed in the light of the clinical and radiological findings. 'Cold' areas of decreased radionuclide uptake may be caused, for example by deposits of metastatic cancer or myeloma or follow infection or radiation, while 'hot' areas are associated with any cause of increased vascularity or bone formation.

Single photon emission computed tomography (SPECT)

The use of SPECT assists the identification of photon-deficient defects by separating underlying and overlying scintigraphic activity into sequential tomographic images. In this way the site of interest is well seen and the sensitivity of planar scintigraphy is increased from 55% to 85%. In the hip SPECT eliminates activity from the acetabulum and from the reparative front which grows in a cup-like fashion from adjacent live tissue. The photopenic and presumably dead area may be recognizable for as long as 18 months (Collier *et al.*, 1985). The method is also of use in identifying necrosis at the knee (Gupta *et al.*, 1987).

Computed tomography

The early stage of bone necrosis of the femoral head is not readily recognized on computed tomography (CT). Assessment requires appreciation of rather subtle changes in the range of normal trabecular patterns in axial slices. The normal typically thick, weight-bearing trabeculae as they arch towards the subchondral plate are seen on cross-section as a star or asterisk, and clumping and fusion of the peripheral part of the rays is associated with repair following revascularization

(Dihlmann, 1982). CT is helpful, however, in the later stage in revealing more clearly than magnetic resonance imaging (see below) the extent of the subchondral trabecular fracture and slight flattening and collapse, particularly of the anterior part of the articular surface.

Conventional tomography is now seldom used in the investigation of bone necrosis.

Magnetic resonance imaging

Magnetic resonance images are derived from radio frequency signals produced by hydrogen nuclei in the tissue when the patient is placed in a strong magnetic field and subjected to radio frequency pulses. The investigation has many advantages. It is not invasive, does not entail the use of ionizing radiation and so far appears to be free of any biological hazard. Furthermore, it produces high soft tissue contrast resolution, and, as distinct from CT, images of equal resolution are obtainable in all planes (Jergesen *et al.*, 1985). The changes in the femoral head have been most extensively investigated, and it is generally agreed (Jergesen *et al.*, 1990a; Markisz *et al.*, 1987; Beltran *et al.*, 1988; Mitchell *et al.*, 1987a; Hauzeur *et al.*, 1989; Lee *et al.*, 1990) that magnetic resonance imaging is the most sensitive and specific method, other than biopsy, of recognizing non-traumatic bone necrosis at the stage when radiographs are still negative. In published series the diagnosis of necrosis by magnetic resonance imaging has been confirmed by core biopsies and by the development of typical radiological changes. Not all the morphological changes that underlie the signal variations (Bassett *et al.*, 1987; Mitchell *et al.*, 1987b; Lang *et al.*, 1988; Jergesen *et al.*, 1990b) are yet fully elucidated, because core biopsy affords little material and whole femoral heads are removed at a late stage.

The normal medullary cavity of the upper femur emits a strong (white) magnetic resonance signal where it contains abundant hydrogen-rich fatty marrow, whereas the cortical bone, subchondral bone plate and the epiphyseal scar, with fewer and less mobile hydrogen ions, give a weaker signal (black). In the early stage of necrosis the signal intensity of the marrow may appear to decrease in a zonal or focal pattern. Sometimes more diffuse abnormalities are also attributed to bone marrow oedema. Indeed, it has been suggested that the diffuse oedema pattern even in the absence of focal changes may predict necrosis (Turner *et al.*, 1989). Unfortunately, the typical changes on magnetic resonance imaging take time (Speer *et al.*, 1990), sometimes weeks, to develop, and they are thought to depend on the replacement of dead marrow by a reparative process

(Ruland *et al.*, 1992). As a result this investigation is less valuable than scintigraphy in assessing the state of the femoral head following acute femoral neck fracture or dislocation (Speer *et al.*, 1990; Lee *et al.*, 1990).

At the reactive interface between dead and revascularized viable tissue, more than 90% of necrotic femoral heads develop a non-specific, low-signal band the same as that which marks the sclerotic margin of a bone tumour. On T2-weighted (long-sequence) images, however, this is seen to consist of a narrow, low-signal outer component probably related to thickened trabeculae, with an inner high-signal component that may represent granulation, fibrous, or chondroid tissue (Fig. 16.15) (Mitchell *et al.*, 1987b; Lang *et al.*, 1988). This 'double line' is thought to be a specific indicator of bone necrosis (Mitchell *et al.*, 1989). At an early stage the area cupped by the low-signal band is iso-intense with fat, and these patients are said to respond well to treatment by core biopsy (see below) (Mitchell *et al.*, 1989). The size of the area outlined by the band, which presumably represents residual dead tissue, is not surprisingly of prognostic importance. Whether treated by core decompression (Beltran *et al.*, 1990) or untreated (Takatori *et al.*, 1993), femoral heads with only a small dead area in the medial anterosuperior zone are much less likely to develop collapse of the necrotic segment than those where more than half the head is necrotic.

Magnetic resonance imaging is of great value in high-risk patients in the diagnosis of 'idiopathic' necrosis of the femoral head in the pre-radiological stage; also, due to its multiplanar capabilities, it accurately reveals the precise site and extent of bone death, which is often greater than expected from plain films. In the later stages, however, the combination of plain films and computed tomography may be more helpful in picking up subtle flattening of the joint surface, in assessing joint space narrowing (Lee *et al.*, 1990), and in identifying trabecular fractures which on magnetic resonance imaging may be difficult to distinguish from granulation tissue (Mitchell *et al.*, 1987b).

'Functional exploration of bone' (Ficat, 1985)

Serre and Simon (1961) were the first clinicians to use intraosseous venography in the investigation of idiopathic femoral head necrosis in humans. They noted that necrosis was associated with raised bone marrow pressure, and since then a three-phase invasive investigation devised by Arlet and Ficat for the pre-radiological diagnosis of femoral head necrosis has been adopted in several centres (Fig. 16.16). It has been suggested that necrosis is probable if the baseline pressure, the stress test, or the intramedullary venogram is abnormal (Ficat, 1985), but that a firm diagnosis can only be made on the basis of the histology of the bone cores. The more widespread use of magnetic resonance imaging should diminish the need for invasive techniques in the recognition of early bone necrosis.

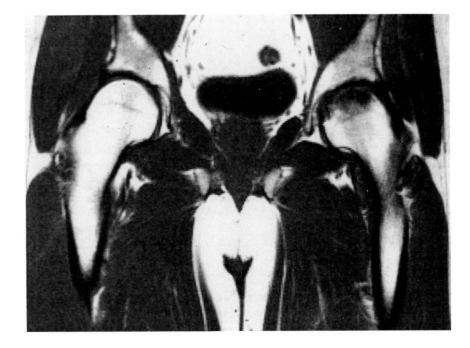

Fig. 16.15 Magnetic resonance imaging shows normal high signal intensity of the fatty marrow of the right femoral head with a faint low intensity band marking the epiphyseal scar. The signal intensity is diminished in a zonal pattern affecting the superolateral part of the left femoral head; this is due to bone necrosis. Reproduced by kind permission of Dr N. Raby.

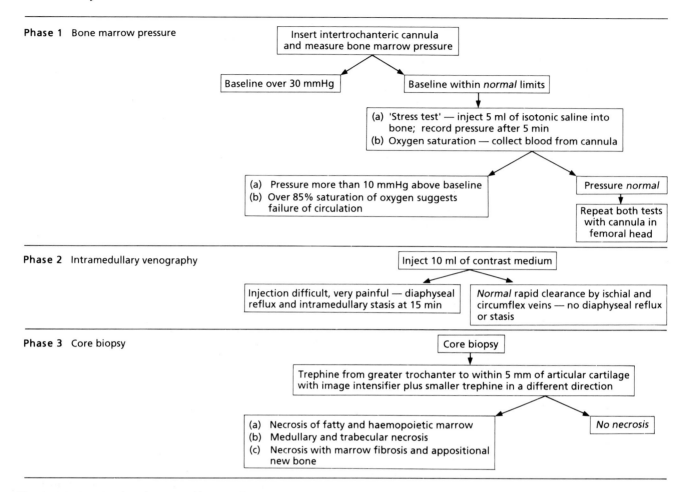

Phase 1 Bone marrow pressure

Insert intertrochanteric cannula
and measure bone marrow pressure

Baseline over 30 mmHg

Baseline within *normal* limits

(a) 'Stress test' — inject 5 ml of isotonic saline into
bone; record pressure after 5 min
(b) Oxygen saturation — collect blood from cannula

(a) Pressure more than 10 mmHg above baseline
(b) Over 85% saturation of oxygen suggests
failure of circulation

Pressure *normal*

Repeat both tests
with cannula in
femoral head

Phase 2 Intramedullary venography

Inject 10 ml of contrast medium

Injection difficult, very painful — diaphyseal
reflux and intramedullary stasis at 15 min

Normal rapid clearance by ischial and
circumflex veins — no diaphyseal reflux
or stasis

Phase 3 Core biopsy

Core biopsy

Trephine from greater trochanter to within 5 mm of articular cartilage
with image intensifier plus smaller trephine in a different direction

(a) Necrosis of fatty and haemopoietic marrow
(b) Medullary and trabecular necrosis
(c) Necrosis with marrow fibrosis and appositional
new bone

No necrosis

Fig. 16.16 'Functional exploration of bone'. After Ficat, 1985.

BONE NECROSIS FOLLOWING TRAUMA

Fracture always results in local damage to blood vessels
of bone and thus to a limited amount of bone death. In
some sites, due to the anatomy of the blood supply,
more extensive bone necrosis occurs. The common sites
of necrosis are the femoral head, the body of the talus
and the scaphoid bone; in each case the dead bone is
intra-articular and has little soft tissue attachment.
Occasionally, the humeral head, the lunate bone, the
capitate bone or the navicular bone is affected. Material
for pathological examination has been obtained chiefly
from the femoral head.

Femoral head necrosis following intracapsular fracture

Most intracapsular femoral neck fractures occur in
elderly patients, particularly in women. In this age
group with a tendency to osteoporosis, the fracture
often follows relatively minor falls contributed to by
medical problems, e.g. poor eyesight, muscle weakness
and dizziness or unsteadiness secondary to medication
(Cooper *et al.*, 1987; Anderson *et al.*, 1993). While
some surgeons continue to rely chiefly on internal fixation (Hunter, 1983), an increasing number of frail
patients over 70 years old with fully displaced fractures
are now treated by primary arthroplasty, partly because
their poor bone stock makes it difficult to retain efficient
internal fixation and second operations significantly
increase the mortality rate (Sikorski and Barrington,
1981).

Children and young adults usually suffer subcapital
femoral neck fractures following major trauma, e.g. a
road traffic or riding accident. Necrosis in children also
sometimes follows slipping of the capital epiphysis or
energetic manipulation and extreme frog-leg immobilization of congenital dislocation of the hip (Buchanan
et al., 1981) (see Chapter 5).

RADIOLOGICAL DIAGNOSIS

Necrosis of the femoral head has long been recognized as a complication, particularly of displaced fractures, but its early diagnosis is difficult. Bone marrow (Tawn and Watt, 1989) or bone scintigraphy (Ruland *et al.*, 1992) give the earliest indication of necrosis, though their prognostic value is limited (see pp. 451 and 452). When patients were treated by lengthy immobilization in traction, necrosis might be recognized on plain films after about 6 weeks by a *relative increase in density* (see Fig. 16.1, p. 444) of the unchanged dead bone of the femoral head in comparison with the disuse porosis of the adjacent living bone of the pelvis and shaft (Phemister, 1934). This sign is still useful in children after the fracture has been treated by immobilization in a hip spica, but with the widespread use of internal fixation of the fracture and early mobilization of adult patients a relative increase in density indicating necrosis is seen only when fixation has failed.

Areas of *true increased density* in high-quality serial radiographs may be sought (Bayliss and Davidson, 1977) as evidence of revascularization and the apposition of new living bone on the scaffold of dead trabeculae, but care is needed in distinguishing these from progressive impaction of trabeculae at the fracture site, from local callus and occasionally from calcification of dead marrow. It may not be possible to diagnose necrosis radiologically until the fracture has united and there is structural failure with collapse of the joint surface. While this has been recognized as early as 6 months, in most patients it does not appear for more than 1 year and sometimes as late as 2.5 years or more after fracture. The classic picture of collapse may be preceded by loss of sphericity of the femoral head and slight flattening of the anterosuperior segment (Frangakis, 1966).

Some authors still misleadingly describe femoral head necrosis as 'developing late'. It must be emphasized that the necrosis occurs at the time of injury and attempted reduction and fixation; it is the clinical and radiological diagnosis that may not be reached until collapse of the weight-bearing joint surface occurs, months or years later.

BLOOD SUPPLY TO THE FEMORAL HEAD

Intracapsular fractures of the neck of the femur have a constant pattern; they extend from the epiphyseal scar at the junction between the superior aspect of the neck and the articular cartilage along the ascending trabeculae to the calcar, a spike of which may be included in the head fragment (Klenerman and Marcuson, 1970). When the fracture is displaced it seems inevitable that the very important superior retinacular vessels (Trueta and Harrison, 1953) will be damaged as they lie on the neck before penetrating the bone at the margin of the articular cartilage (Fig. 16.17). Viability and the potential for revascularization then depend on any remaining blood supply from the inferior group of vessels, which may also be torn, and from those of the ligamentum teres. While the vessels of the ligamentum teres are of no importance for the vascularity of the femoral head under

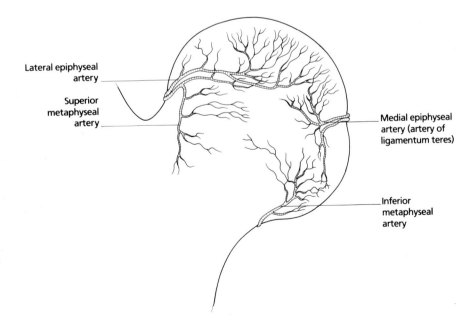

Fig. 16.17 Blood supply to the femoral head (after Trueta and Harrison, 1953). The lateral epiphyseal arteries and superior metaphyseal arteries together form the important superior retinacular arteries.

Lateral epiphyseal artery
Superior metaphyseal artery
Medial epiphyseal artery (artery of ligamentum teres)
Inferior metaphyseal artery

normal circumstances, they may be an important source of revascularization of the partially necrotic femoral head (Sevitt, 1964; Catto, 1965a), and then show enlargement and more frequent filling (Mussbichler, 1970).

Undisplaced fractures are likely to suffer less severe damage to retinacular vessels, but those with intact capsules may be particularly vulnerable to raised intra-articular pressure following traumatic haemarthrosis. Some investigators suggest that the pressure is sufficient to produce tamponade and venous obstruction, thereby reducing the already jeopardized blood flow to the femoral head (Crawfurd *et al.*, 1988; Harper *et al.*, 1991). This may be improved by joint aspiration (Kristensen *et al.*, 1989).

INCIDENCE OF NECROSIS AND PATTERN OF REVASCULARIZATION

Less than one-third of femoral heads removed at arthroplasty or necropsy are completely viable (Sevitt, 1964; Catto, 1965a; Calandruccio and Anderson, 1980). Necrosis of the femoral head is not an 'all or nothing' phenomenon, however, and more than half of the necrotic femoral heads contain some viable bone, almost always as a wedge based on the fovea (Fig. 16.18). This varies from a few millimetres in depth to virtually all the head inferior to the upper margin of the fovea. Necrosis is thus most common in the anterosuperolateral sub-chondral region of the head.

Revascularization may occur relatively rapidly if there is a large remaining wedge of viable marrow in the subfoveal region, but when the femoral head is completely necrotic extension of new vessels from the sub-foveal region is minimal. Revascularization is then almost entirely dependent on in-growth of vessels from across the fracture line, and although there is active proliferation of new vessels on the neck side, this is usually a slow process (Sevitt, 1964). Spread across the fracture line may be interrupted by movement at the fracture site or by continuing impaction of the necrotic head, while good contact between the bone ends may be prevented by the presence of fragmented bone, soft tissue, or blood clot. Organization of this material results in fibrosis, which may unite the bone ends but tends to inhibit in-growth of new vessels into the head (Sevitt, 1964).

Whether revascularization spreads from the subfoveal region, from across the fracture line, or from both directions, the superolateral subchondral region of the femoral head is almost always the last area to regain a blood supply (Fig. 16.19).

NECROSIS AND FRACTURE HEALING

While necrosis of the femoral head used to be blamed for failure of union of the fracture, more emphasis is

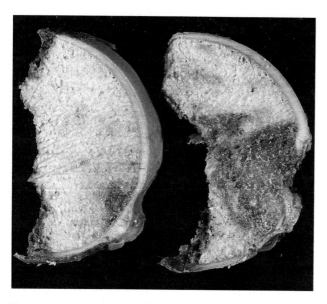

Fig. 16.18 Much of the femoral head is necrotic, opaque and white. A wedge of remaining viable bone is based on the fovea.

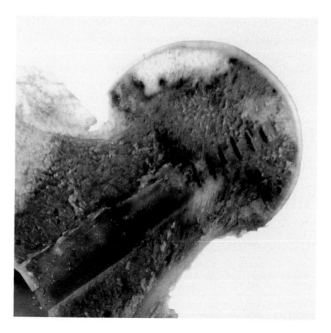

Fig. 16.19 The fully displaced intracapsular fracture has united. At necropsy a small amount of dead bone is still seen in the subchondral region. There was evidence microscopically that a large wedge of subfoveal bone had survived.

now placed on mechanical factors. In the absence of an accurate quantitative method of determining femoral head viability *in vivo*, the mechanical and vascular factors involved seem inseparable. While it is common sense that a fracture is more likely to unite when callus forms on both sides of the fracture line, it is also clear that when callus forms only in the neck good reduction and stable fixation are essential. Given these conditions, about 75% of intracapsular fractures will unite (Barnes *et al.*, 1976).

There is some evidence to suggest that union without subsequent collapse is more likely when the femoral head is only partially necrotic (Catto, 1965a). There may thus be a difference in prognosis between completely and partially necrotic femoral heads. Unfortunately, although many different techniques including arteriography, venography, radionuclide scans and magnetic resonance imaging have been developed to try to assess the state of the femoral head following fracture, none has been wholly successful.

FACTORS INFLUENCING LATE COLLAPSE OF THE FEMORAL HEAD

Late collapse of the femoral head is usually recognized more than 6 months following fracture and mostly before the end of the second year (Barnes *et al.*, 1976; Jacobs, 1978; Calandruccio and Anderson, 1980), though it may appear later. It is not seen in clinically non-united fractures, but occurs in about 25% of united fractures in women and in about 15% in men (Barnes *et al.*, 1976). As might be expected, late collapse occurs less commonly in undisplaced fractures, in both adults and children than in partially or fully displaced fractures (Table 16.1).

While a moderate degree of valgus reduction helps to produce a more stable position and increases the rate of fracture union, a severe degree of valgus displacement has been shown in several surveys to increase greatly the risk of developing femoral head collapse in both displaced and undisplaced fractures (Garden, 1971; Barnes *et al.*, 1976). Smith (1959) noted that extreme valgus positioning of the femoral head during arthroplasty caused the femoral head to stop bleeding, perhaps as a result of increased tension occluding the ligamentum teres vessels; either this mechanism or increased vascular damage (Calandruccio and Anderson, 1980) might explain the association.

It is difficult to assess the influence of different types of fixation device on the development of late collapse, because wide variations of incidence are reported using the same device in different groups of patients. Surveys have found no significant difference in the incidence of late collapse in relation to the method of fixation (Barnes *et al.*, 1976; Calandruccio and Anderson, 1980). Opinion is divided as to whether early reduction reduces the incidence of late collapse (Massie, 1973; Barnes *et al.*, 1976; Calandruccio and Anderson, 1980).

PATTERN OF LATE COLLAPSE OF THE FEMORAL HEAD

In cases of late collapse a major part, if not all, of the femoral head dies at the time of the fracture; often when the femoral head is removed years later a large part remains unrevascularized. In many of these femoral heads revascularization depends almost entirely on in-growth of blood vessels across the fracture line, there being little if any contribution from vessels of the ligamentum teres (Fig. 16.20). When necrosis is incomplete or revascularization is more extensive, it is the antero-superolateral segment of the femoral head that remains dead (Catto, 1965b).

Structural failure may occur in dead bone both at its junction with living bone and sometimes also in the subchondral region. It is clear, however, that in some cases the only site of trabecular fracture is in the subchondral region (Catto, 1965b; Sevitt, 1981) (Fig. 16.20).

Attention has been drawn to the differences between traumatic and non-traumatic necrosis (Springfield and Enneking, 1976; Glimcher and Kenzora, 1979b). Following fracture the amount of bone necrosis is often greater, the line of structural failure is sometimes deeper at the junction of living and necrotic tissue, and calcified marrow debris is scantier. There are many similarities, however, and radiologically the conditions may be indistinguishable (Park, 1976).

Once late collapse occurs, osteophytes develop at the living margin of the femoral head, often with lipping of the acetabular margin. At first the joint space is well preserved, but it diminishes when the articular sequestrum disintegrates.

Table 16.1 Avascular necrosis (late collapse) in united femoral neck fractures

Study	Undisplaced (%)	Displaced (%)
Calandruccio and Anderson (1980)	14	40
Barnes *et al.* (1976)	16	28
Canale and Bourland (1977)*	0	45

* This study involved children under 17 years of age.

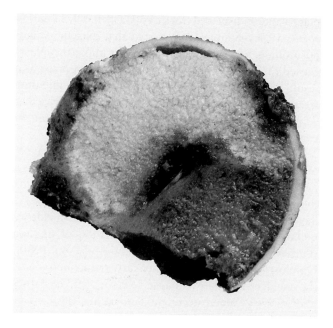

Fig. 16.20 This elderly woman developed pain in the hip 3 years after an intracapsular fracture of the femoral neck which united. A major part of the femoral head removed at arthroplasty a few months later was still necrotic. A subarticular fracture through dead bone had partially separated the articular cartilage, which was of normal thickness. The inferomedial part of the head had revascularized, as had a small island of bone at the fovea. Reproduced from Davidson (1976) by permission of Elsevier, Amsterdam.

In this elderly group of patients the amount of disability varies greatly and bears little relation to the severity of the radiographic changes. Interestingly, of 181 patients with late segmental collapse reported by Barnes *et al.* (1976), almost 25% were symptom-free while 30% were severely disabled, those who were fit enough having undergone prosthetic replacement surgery.

Dislocation of the hip

About 95% of dislocations of the hip are posterior. They usually occur in car accidents when the knee hits the dashboard, and with the hips flexed at 90° the femoral head is driven posteriorly out of the acetabulum. In more severe injuries the posterior lip of the acetabulum may be fractured. The incidence of femoral head necrosis has been reported as 10% (Nicoll, 1952) and 26% (Brav, 1962). It is more common when the acetabulum is fractured (probably in association with greater soft tissue damage), following open reduction, and when reduction is delayed for more than 24 h (Donaldson *et al.*, 1968; Barquet, 1982).

The inevitable rupture of the ligamentum teres is unlikely to produce necrosis of any part of the head, because the subfoveal bone is supplied by anastomoses from the superior retinacular arteries (Sevitt and Thompson, 1965). The important retinacular vessels may be damaged, however, by avulsion of the capsule at the base of the neck or by constriction by the capsule if the femoral head buttonholes through it. Post-mortem arteriographic injection of the vessels from a dislocated, totally necrotic femoral head showed that the superior retinacular vessels were not filled (Sevitt and Thompson, 1965).

Fracture of the talus

Diagnosis of necrosis of the talus following injury depends on the recognition of a relative increase in density 6–8 weeks after non-weight-bearing immobilization of the injury. To assess this it is important to have an anteroposterior view of the talus that is not overlapped by the posterior tibial malleolus (Graham and Wood, 1976). The presence of a blood supply may be indicated by the development of immobilization porosis of the bone or of a subchondral zone of radiolucency in the proximal talus. This is also an indicator of revascularization of dead bone once fracture union has occurred (Hawkins, 1970). Aseptic necrosis is relatively uncommon following undisplaced fractures of the neck or body of the talus. As the severity of the injury to soft tissue increases, so does the incidence of necrosis; it is seen in about 36% of patients with fracture of the neck and subtalar dislocation (Graham and Wood, 1976).

Following reduction, union of the fracture usually occurs and revascularization may follow, though it sometimes takes several years to complete and still leaves the patient with stiffness and discomfort in the subtalar joint. Collapse has been reported more than 2 years after injury (Graham and Wood, 1976).

Fracture of the scaphoid bone

Bone necrosis following fracture through the waist of the scaphoid bone probably occurs in about 10–15% of patients (Graham and Wood, 1976). It is rare following hair-line fractures and common following more severe injuries with displacement and mid-carpal dislocation. Almost all the vessels that supply the scaphoid bone enter in the ligamentous area and in the region of the tubercle; very occasionally a small vessel may enter the proximal pole. Necrosis usually affects the proximal fragment and may be recognized as a 'cold' area on scintigraphy soon after fracture or by the development of a relative increase of radiographic density after 4–8 weeks in a plaster cast (Fig. 16.1, p. 444). The fragment becomes more porotic as revascularization spreads, and if the process is incomplete collapse of the necrotic pole and degenerative joint disease may follow.

Fracture of the capitate bone

The capitate bone has a vulnerable blood supply (Vander Grend *et al.*, 1984), and necrosis of its proximal pole may follow a fracture with or without accompanying carpal dislocation, may develop in association with chronic occupational or athletic stress (Bolton-Maggs *et al.*, 1984), or may occur spontaneously. Delay in diagnosis and reduction of the fracture increases the risk of necrosis, but immobilization usually leads to fracture healing and subsequent revascularization (Rand *et al.*, 1982).

BONE NECROSIS ASSOCIATED WITH WORK IN COMPRESSED AIR (DYSBARIC OSTEONECROSIS)

In recent years, partly due to the offshore oil industry and the increase in underground tunnelling associated with new transport systems, there has been a sharp rise in the number of people exposed to hyperbaric conditions. This has been paralleled by increasing concern about the prevalence of potentially disabling and often late-presenting bone necrosis in otherwise healthy young men, despite adherence to accepted decompression schedules (Kindwall *et al.*, 1982). Bone necrosis occurs most often in tunnellers or caisson workers and less commonly in divers. It has not been reported in staff working in medical hyperbaric chambers (Ledingham and Davidson, 1969). Only a few cases of disabling osteonecrosis have been reported in aviators exposed to a low-pressure environment at high altitudes in unpressurized aircraft (Markham, 1967), and bone necrosis is very rare in low-pressure chamber operators (Allen *et al.*, 1974).

Medullary lesions are found in the lower end of the femur (see Fig. 16.3b, p. 445), the upper end of the tibia, the neck of the humerus and the neck of the femur in that order of frequency, while juxta-articular lesions are more common in the shoulder than in the hip. The knee and ankle are hardly ever affected, and lesions are chiefly confined to the long bones. Only occasionally are sites such as the lunate bone (Kawashima *et al.*, 1978), the talus (O'Doherty *et al.*, 1989) and the spine involved. Screening radiographs should include views of the shoulder in internal and external rotation, antero-posterior views of the hip joints, and anteroposterior and lateral views of the knee to include not only the upper third of the tibia but as much of the lower end of the femur as possible. An additional lateral view of the hip joint is useful in demonstrating the early radiolucent crescent line (Davidson, 1976) (see Fig. 16.6, p. 447).

Compressed air workers

WORKING METHODS

Compressed air is used in the construction of tunnels under rivers or across harbours to prevent water seeping through the ground and flooding the workings. The pressure required to prevent this depends partly on the height of the water above the tunnel and partly on the porosity of the ground. Pressures are usually less than about 400 kPa (4 atmospheres) absolute. Men working on a tunnel enter a manlock, which is rapidly raised to the pressure of the working chamber. When the shift is completed, usually after 8 h, the men re-enter the manlock and are slowly decompressed to atmospheric pressure. The time taken on this decompression lengthens with both an increase in working pressure and an increased exposure time. The aim of the legally binding tables used to calculate decompression procedures is to minimize the risk of workers developing decompression sickness. This may be in the form of joint pain (type I decompression sickness), often referred to as the bends or if less severe as the niggles, or it may result in more serious constitutional upset (type II) (Melamed *et al.*, 1992) with pallor, sweating, vomiting and symptoms of cardiovascular or respiratory distress, and occasionally paraplegia. If symptoms appear after re-entry into free air, the workman is recompressed in a medical recompression chamber.

FREQUENCY OF BONE NECROSIS

The overall frequency of bone necrosis in 2534 compressed air workers registered with the Medical Research Council decompression sickness panel in Newcastle is 17.6% (444 men) (Davidson, 1989); the distribution of the lesions is shown in Fig. 16.21. While most of the lesions are clinically silent shaft lesions, 36% are juxta-articular and at least one-third of these go on to produce symptoms due to structural failure and collapse of the joint surface. Severe disablement is most likely in those workers with hip joint collapse. About one-third of the lesions are bilateral, and more than half of the affected workers have more than one radiological lesion. The incidence of bone necrosis varies in different work

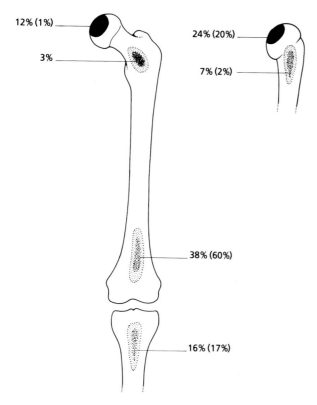

Fig. 16.21 Sites of bone necrosis in tunnellers (data without parentheses) and divers (data within parentheses) (Davidson, 1989).

projects, and many factors, e.g. shift lengths, total number of shifts worked and maximum pressure experienced, are important. Incidence rates based on radiology are underestimates, and scintigrams suggest that lesions may be present though radiographs are normal (Gregg and Walder, 1981).

Divers

WORKING METHODS

Professional divers may work from a diving bell, be connected to the surface by continuous air lines, or remain at pressure for many days during so-called saturation dives. They usually work shorter shifts at greater pressures than compressed air workers, because the pressure increases by approximately 100 kPa (1 atmosphere) for each 10 m of depth. Recreational divers using self-contained underwater breathing apparatus (scuba divers) run less risk of bone necrosis, as exposure time is usually relatively short and they tend not to go beyond depths of about 60 m (about 600 kPa pressure). In contrast, experimental simulated dives have been made as deep as 615 m (about 6000 kPa pressure).

FREQUENCY OF BONE NECROSIS

The reported incidence of bone necrosis varies greatly depending largely on the degree of supervision and the stringency of the decompression process. The overall prevalence in Japanese shellfish divers, who at that time were ignorant of correct decompression procedures, was about 50% (Ohta and Matsunaga, 1974). This is in contrast to the figure of about 4% under the well-supervised conditions of diving in the British Royal Navy (Harrison, 1971) and in commercially employed North Sea divers (Decompression Sickness Central Registry, 1981). The sites of the lesions in 207 North Sea divers are illustrated in Fig. 16.21. Aside from the overall lower incidence, the striking difference in comparing divers with compressed air workers is that only 21% of the former compared with 36% of the latter develop the potentially disabling juxta-articular lesions; of these about 15% progress to structural failure. Involvement of the femoral head is rare. As in the compressed air workers more than one-third of the lesions are bilateral and more than half the divers have multiple lesions.

Factors relating to bone necrosis

PRESSURE

Bone necrosis is unlikely to develop in men working in compressed air at pressures below 117 kPa and in divers confined to depths of 30 m or less (Decompression Sickness Central Registry, 1981). As the pressure increases the risk of developing bone lesions also increases (Ohta and Matsunaga, 1974); in commercial divers in the UK the prevalence of osteonecrosis rose from less than 2% in those who had dived to 100 m or less, to 22% in those who had dived to 300 m (Decompression Sickness Central Registry, 1981).

DECOMPRESSION SICKNESS

The prevalence of osteonecrosis in both compressed air workers (Davidson, 1976; Lam and Yau, 1992) and commercial divers (Decompression Sickness Central Registry, 1981) is higher in those who have suffered one or more attacks of decompression sickness. It must be emphasized, however, that both compressed air workers and divers may develop bone necrosis without ever having required therapeutic recompression. The relationship between bone necrosis and acute decompression sickness remains controversial. The relationship may not be direct, but the two may share a common pathway

(Chryssanthou, 1978). It seems clear that decompression tables that minimize the number of episodes of acute decompression sickness unfortunately do not prevent bone necrosis.

NUMBER OF EXPOSURES

Although bone necrosis has been reported on several occasions after a single exposure to hyperbaric conditions, as in three survivors who escaped from the submarine Poseidon after it sank in 37 m of water (James, 1945), in general increasing numbers of exposures increase the risk. About half of seasoned compressed air workers with some years of experience have radiographic evidence of necrosis (McCallum, 1974), while the prevalence in commercially employed divers rises from less than 1% under 4 years' experience to more than 10% at 12 years (Decompression Sickness Central Registry, 1981). The prevalence in Japanese shellfish divers rose from 15% at 19 years old to 76% in those over 40 years old (Ohta and Matsunaga, 1974). Age itself, as distinct from experience, is probably not important, but obesity may be a predisposing factor (Decompression Sickness Central Registry, 1981; Lam and Yau, 1992). Individual susceptibility must play a large part, but unfortunately there is no means of predicting which individuals will develop bone lesions.

Aetiology and pathogenesis of dysbaric osteonecrosis

Investigation of the aetiology and pathogenesis of dysbaric osteonecrosis has been hampered by the delay in the clinical and radiological diagnosis and by the lack of a satisfactory animal model (Gregg and Walder, 1986). The dramatic fall of incidence of bone necrosis in compressed air workers in the USA following the introduction in 1963 of tables using extended decompression times, and in the lower incidence of necrosis in well-supervised British naval and commercial divers compared with the unprotected Japanese shellfish divers, provides good circumstantial evidence that imperfectly controlled decompression is important in the pathogenesis. During decompression, nitrogen dissolved in the tissues is cleared by the bloodstream, and as a result of the pressure gradient across the alveoli is removed in the expired air. Ultrasonic monitors have shown, however, that showers of 'silent' bubbles may form during decompression without producing any of the manifestations of decompression sickness (Evans et al., 1972). While these decompressions may be 'safe' in relation to decompression sickness, they may not be safe in relation to the development of bone necrosis.

Bone may be more prone to necrosis than other tissues because of the relatively slow rate of gas exchange in the fatty marrow, which remains supersaturated for a long time following decompression and thus allows persistent and profuse intravascular and extravascular gas bubbles to produce ischaemia, particularly if there are repeated insults. The compressive effect of bubbles on blood vessels is probably enhanced by the rigidity of the surrounding bony structures, while the poor collateral circulation in some sites in bone renders them particularly susceptible to ischaemia. It has been suggested that bone necrosis may also be caused by fat emboli, produced either by disruption of adipose tissue and fatty marrow by gas bubbles or by breaking of lipoprotein linkages at the blood–bubble interface. A number of other complex mechanisms, e.g. red blood cell sludging, platelet aggregation and haemoconcentration, perhaps play a part. Swelling of marrow fat cells during decompression has been shown in rabbits (Thomas and Walder, 1984) and may be a contributory factor either directly by increasing pressure on blood vessels within the bony framework or indirectly by slowing blood flow and so promoting an increase in bubble size (Gregg and Walder, 1986). Most of the postulated mechanisms are directly or indirectly related to bubble formation.

Morbid anatomical studies of fatalities in compressed air workers and divers have not greatly helped in elucidating the pathogenesis of bone necrosis, though they have sometimes revealed radiologically unsuspected necrosis. Histological features suggestive of intravascular bubbles have been seen in animals (Colonna and Jones, 1948) and in man some weeks or months after the last exposure to compressed air; they are sometimes (Kawashima et al., 1978) but not always associated with bone necrosis. There seems little doubt that gas bubbles may be present in blood vessels following 'safe' decompressions; however, many factors, including their number, size and duration, the type of tissue affected and its vascular pattern, may determine whether their presence alone or in combination with other mechanisms is sufficient to cause bone necrosis. A more detailed discussion of the pathogenesis is to be found in a number of papers (Chryssanthou, 1978; Hallenbeck and Anderson, 1982; Gregg and Walder, 1986).

Types of bone lesions

A radiological classification of bone lesions was prepared by the UK Medical Research Council Decompression Sickness Panel (Davidson and Griffiths, 1970), and because of repeated examinations it has been possible to watch the development and progress of some lesions.

MEDULLARY LESIONS

The symptomless medullary lesions in the head, neck and shaft of the long bones are seen as dense areas that have an irregular outline and appear to consist of thickened and fused trabeculae. These may progress to the more commonly seen irregular calcified areas, which appear first as linear streaks and are best seen on lateral views; they later often develop to form oblong areas occupying the whole width of the medullary cavity (see Fig. 16.3b). They represent chiefly calcification in the collagenous tissue surrounding dead bone.

JUXTA-ARTICULAR LESIONS

These are potentially disabling and may also appear as small, irregular, dense areas adjacent to the intact joint surface, or as rounded opacities that tend to fuse to give a subchondral segment of increased density or 'snowcap' appearance, particularly in the humeral head. These appearances seem to result from the superimposition, in different cuts of the bone end, of trabeculae thickened by appositional new bone on remaining foci of dead bone (Catto, 1976) (Fig. 16.22). A dense 'linear opacity' may traverse the bone end close to the joint surface (see

Fig. 16.5) or extend in a deep cone into the neck and shaft (Fig. 16.23). It may be difficult to recognize in the hip without tomography or a frog-leg view because of the acetabular shadow. The dense line marks the extent of the remaining subchondral zone of dead bone which sometimes, following extensive revascularization, represents only a small part of the original dead tissue (McCallum *et al.*, 1966).

The general pattern of these juxta-articular lesions is similar to that previously described (p. 445). Although the necrotic zone may form a single compact subarticular mass, however, there is sometimes the impression that it has arisen through the confluence of smaller foci (Welfling, 1971), suggesting that a major vascular supply is not cut off. The dense line may be particularly sharply defined, due not only to arches of appositional new bone on the surface of dead trabeculae at the junction of dead and living tissue (see Fig. 16.5c), but sometimes also to calcification of the intervening collagen, which is a more common feature in dysbaric than in post-traumatic bone necrosis. Radiographs can remain unchanged over many years (see Fig. 16.5), though bone scans using ^{99m}technetium diphosphonate sometimes still show activity, suggesting continuing repair (Gregg and Walder, 1981).

The pain associated with structural failure is often of sudden onset in the shoulder, but is usually insidious in the hip. A radiolucent subchondral crescent sign (see

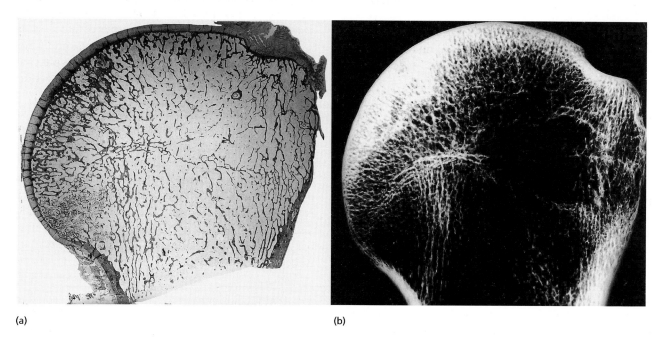

(a)   (b)

Fig. 16.22 Broad 'sandwich' trabeculae (a) surround small pockets of remaining dead subchondral bone and (b) produce localized subchondral sclerosis on the slab radiograph. This type of picture gives rise to the 'snowcap' lesion in clinical radiographs. Reproduced by permission of Elsevier, Amsterdam.

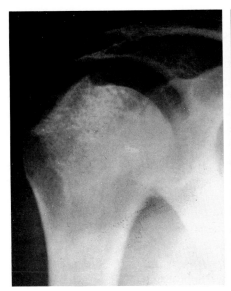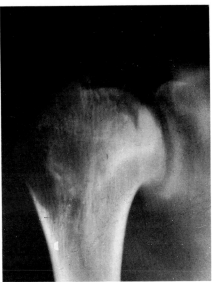

Fig. 16.23 This man was exposed to compressed air only twice on consecutive days and on each occasion suffered type I bends. Two years later he presented with pain in both shoulders. Collapse of the articular surface is seen with step formation. The tomogram shows fragmentation of the articular sequestrum, and the extent of the dead bone is outlined by the dense line extending into the neck. Reproduced from Davidson (1976) by permission of Dr. J.K. Davidson and Elsevier, Amsterdam.

Fig. 16.6) or an extensive, shallow, and sometimes fragmented, articular sequestrum may be evident radiologically (Fig. 16.23; see also Fig. 16.12a). As the joint surface collapses a well-defined step often appears and osteophytes later develop, being particularly prominent at the inferior margin of the humeral head. The joint space usually remains unchanged till late, when degenerative changes also develop in the acetabulum or glenoid fossa; eventually the appearances may be difficult to distinguish from those of primary osteoarthritis (see Fig. 16.12). In general, even when humeral lesions are painful, there is not severe limitation of movement, whereas the more rare femoral lesions may be crippling.

Unfortunately, it is impossible to predict which juxta-articular lesions will progress to structural failure and collapse. Radiologically equivocal and apparently early dense areas may develop structural failure and sequestrum formation within a few months of diagnosis (Walder, 1974), and sometimes pain appears within 18 months of the first exposure to compressed air (Davidson, 1976). In some patients followed up for at least 12 years, however, juxta-articular lesions have remained unchanged (Davidson, 1976), and in others structural failure as well as new subchondral lesions have occurred as late as 10 years after stopping work in compressed air (Gregg and Walder, 1981; Van Blarcom et al., 1990). This long delay in clinical presentation may complicate claims for financial compensation. Collapse is probably not inevitable even when large areas of juxta-articular bone have died (Davidson, 1976).

Management

Bone grafting of juxta-articular lesions that have already collapsed has not proved beneficial (McCallum et al., 1966). While hip joint replacement gives a good result, there is concern as to the functional life of the prosthesis in these relatively young and active men. Workers with symptomless shaft lesions are permitted to continue working in compressed air and to carry out normal diving, though unduly hazardous diving is curtailed. There is no certain evidence that this group is more likely than others to develop juxta-articular lesions (Decompression Sickness Central Registry, 1981). Those with juxta-articular lesions are usually not allowed to work in compressed air over 124 kPa, and divers are advised to stop or are confined to shallow depths using 100% oxygen. In some projects restrictions are also placed on the type of physical labour undertaken in order to try to minimize the risk of structural failure. Scintigraphy using [99m]technetium-labelled methylene diphosphonate has been used experimentally (Gregg and Walder, 1980) and clinically (Pearson et al., 1982) to allow earlier, pre-radiographic diagnosis of dysbaric osteonecrosis. It has been suggested that in the annual surveillance of divers, after an initial radiographic skeletal survey, scintigraphy might be a suitable method of regular follow-up. Only sites with increased uptake would then require radiography or other confirmatory investigations.

IDIOPATHIC NECROSIS OF THE FEMORAL HEAD IN ADULTS

This type of aseptic bone necrosis excludes causes such as trauma, radiation, work in compressed air, the haemoglobinopathies and Gaucher's disease. Several conditions have been reported in association with so-called idiopathic necrosis. These include: alcoholism; gout and hyperuricaemia; disorders of fat metabolism; obesity; systemic lupus erythematosus and other collagen disorders; haemostatic disorders; and minor congenital malformation of the hip.

Although patients on long-term steroid therapy were included in the early published large series of cases (Patterson *et al.*, 1964; Merle d'Aubigné *et al.*, 1965), they are now regarded as a separate group sometimes with rather different presenting radiological appearances and pathology. They are discussed separately on p. 466.

Idiopathic necrosis of the femoral head was seldom described before 1960, but since then reports of several large series of patients have been published in Europe and North America, though there are relatively few reports in the UK where this still seems to be a less common condition. The cause of the apparent increase in cases is uncertain; some authors have attributed it to an increased clinical awareness of the condition, others to the more widespread use of steroid therapy and to increased alcohol abuse.

Clinical features

More than 80% of patients are male, and while there is a wide age range the peak incidence is between 30 and 60 years of age. Aching pain is usually the first symptom, often in the groin but sometimes referred to the thigh and knee. It may be of sudden onset, but often is more gradual and intermittent. At first it is relieved by rest and only in the late stages is there night pain. Internal rotation and abduction are often painful and limited, while flexion is usually little affected. Radiographs may be negative when the patient first presents, but magnetic resonance imaging should reveal the dead marrow. Several authors (Marcus *et al.*, 1973; Springfield and Enneking, 1976; Hungerford and Zizic, 1978; Ficat, 1985) have designated different stages in the evolution of the condition (Table 16.2).

The reported prevalence of bilateral involvement varies, but on average is about 50%; this increases with time. While treating the presenting symptomatic hip, clinicians have looked for and have closely studied the early pre-radiological (stage 0 and I) changes in the second hip (Marcus *et al.*, 1973; Lee *et al.*, 1980) with the aid of the three-phase functional exploration described on p. 453. While non-invasive magnetic resonance imaging should reduce the diagnostic application of the method, its continued use is likely in those centres that find a marked therapeutic advantage from forage in the stage before collapse has occurred (see p. 471). The impression is that, in contrast to post-traumatic necrosis, the natural history of idiopathic necrosis is usually one of relentless progression through the various stages with little successful spontaneous regression (Springfield and Enneking, 1976; Glimcher and Kenzora, 1979b; Lee *et al.*, 1980). The length of time between the recognition of necrosis and the development of the subchondral fracture varies from a few months to several years (Marcus *et al.*, 1973; Lee *et al.*, 1980).

Table 16.2 Staging of idiopathic necrosis of the femoral head

Marcus *et al.* (1973)		Ficat (1985)	
I	Asymptomatic: increased isotope uptake, normal or irregular mottled density, normal joint surface, diagnosis by core biopsy	0	Silent hip, symptomless and no radiographic change—other side affected
II	Asymptomatic: well-defined infarct with thick surrounding rim	I	Sudden pain in groin, some limitation of internal rotation and abduction; radiograph normal or subtle trabecular blurring
III	Mild symptoms and crescent sign	II	Worsening symptoms, patchy or linear sclerosis—intact head
IV	Episodic pain, femoral head flattening	III	Subchondral fracture, crescent line, segmental flattening
V	Disabling pain and osteoarthritis but infarct still recognizable		
VI	Incapacitating restrictions of movement: severe osteoarthritis now radiologically indistinguishable from primary type	IV	Loss of articular cartilage, marginal osteophytes—osteoarthritis superimposed on deformed head

(Stages III and IV in Ficat (1985) grouped as: Irreversible)

Structural changes

The morphological changes follow the general pattern that has already been described, but there are some points of special interest. The amount of necrotic bone is said to be less than that commonly found after trauma (Springfield and Enneking, 1976) and the repair processes slower and with less osteoblastic differentiation (Glimcher and Kenzora, 1979b). Some revascularization occurs before the process ceases and the dense line becomes apparent radiologically, demarcating the remaining necrotic bone which usually occupies about 25% or less of the femoral head. Fracture almost always occurs in the dead subchondral bone, producing the radiological crescent line and separating a shallow articular sequestrum. Once collapse of the femoral head begins, fragmented bone trabeculae may be seen in the marrow spaces.

Calcification of dead marrow also occurs and may increase with time. It is most striking at the junction of the dead tissue with the collagenous revascularization front, where it sometimes forms rounded aggregates and contributes markedly to the increased radiological density (Sissons *et al.*, 1992). Failure of more complete revascularization has been attributed to clogging of the marrow spaces with the calcified material (Springfield and Enneking, 1976). Attempted removal of the calcified material at the margin between dead and living tissue is associated with osteoclastic resorption of dead trabeculae, and as a result a line of decreased radiological density may develop proximal to the dense line.

Contributory factors

So many different conditions have been described in association with 'idiopathic' necrosis of the femoral head that it has been suggested that very few cases can still be considered to be truly idiopathic (Cruess, 1978; Jacobs, 1978). It is, however, difficult to assess whether an occasionally coexisting condition is a predisposing factor or simply coincidental, and even when there appears to be a strong association this has to be considered in relation to the incidence of the condition in the general population. A minor congenital anomaly has been suggested as a predisposing factor in osteonecrosis affecting the femoral head or the knee. About half the patients of Merle d'Aubigné *et al.* (1965) showed some slight radiological anomaly of the hip, most often mild coxa valga, but the incidence in the general population is uncertain.

A history of alcoholism has been reported in 15–74% of patients with idiopathic necrosis of the femoral head (Patterson *et al.*, 1964; Boettcher *et al.*, 1970) and has been reported as the most common association in the idiopathic group. The figure of 17% in one Swiss series, however, was not significantly higher than the incidence of alcoholism in the general population (Zinn, 1971). Looked at in another way, from 29% to 5% (Orlić *et al.*, 1990) of alcoholics from treatment centres develop bone necrosis, and the degree of increased risk may be related to their intake (Matsuo *et al.*, 1988). In the alcoholic group both femoral heads are commonly affected (73% in Hungerford and Zizic's (1978) series) and some patients develop necrosis in other sites, e.g. the humeral head, upper tibia and lower femoral shaft (Jones, 1971; Jacobs, 1978; Orlić *et al.*, 1990).

Several reports have been published of femoral head necrosis related to gout (Boettcher *et al.*, 1970), and McCollum *et al.* (1970) found that about 40% of their patients with femoral head necrosis had clinical gout or symptomless hyperuricaemia. None showed gross deposits of urates, but in some scattered urate crystals were identifiable in alcohol-fixed synovium. The mechanism by which bone necrosis might be brought about by gout or hyperuricaemia remains obscure.

There has been much interest in alterations in lipid metabolism in patients with osteonecrosis. The abnormalities are varied and include hypercholesterolaemia and raised serum levels of triglycerides and β-lipoproteins. In one family, hyperlipoproteinaemia has been associated with radiological evidence of necrosis of the femoral head over four generations (Palmer *et al.*, 1981). Obesity and clinical or latent diabetes have also been associated. While hyperlipidaemia has been found in as many as 80% of patients with idiopathic femoral head necrosis (Jacobs, 1978), in other series the incidence was no greater than in a control group (Hartmann, 1971).

It is intriguing that relatively few instances of femoral head necrosis have been linked with known vascular disease. It is suggested that vasculitis accounts for the few patients with femoral head necrosis in lupus erythematosus untreated with steroids (Siemsen *et al.*, 1962). Femoral head necrosis has been reported occasionally following both polycythaemia and slow thrombosis of the lower aorta (Leriche's syndrome) (Hughes *et al.*, 1971), while emboli have been held responsible for bone necrosis at different sites in two patients with infective endocarditis. Investigation of blood coagulation by a battery of tests in patients with idiopathic necrosis of the femoral head has shown abnormal but inconsistent results (Boettcher *et al.*, 1970).

Occasionally, necrosis of the femoral head develops without predisposing factors in the late stage of pregnancy or after delivery (Arlet *et al.*, 1982; Pellici *et al.*, 1984), during maintenance dialysis (Langevitz *et al.*, 1990) or in patients infected with human immuno-deficiency virus (Gerster *et al.*, 1991; Chevalier *et al.*, 1993). Both the pathogenesis of the necrosis and the significance of these observations are unclear.

The cause of idiopathic necrosis remains uncertain and is probably multifactorial, more than one associated disorder, e.g. gout, alcoholism and steroid medication, being found in about one-quarter of patients (Jacobs, 1978). It is striking that almost all patients suffer from some kind of systemic illness (Boettcher *et al.*, 1970; Zinn, 1971; Kenzora and Glimcher, 1985).

BONE NECROSIS ASSOCIATED WITH STEROID THERAPY

The term 'steroid arthropathy' (Sweetnam *et al.*, 1960) probably includes two different conditions. The first is bone necrosis, which may occur in previously normal joints following systemic steroid therapy. The second occurs in joints already damaged by rheumatoid arthritis or osteoarthritis and most commonly follows repeated intra-articular injections of steroids. A similar picture is often attributed to the excessive use of analgesics (Murray and Jacobson, 1971; Solomon, 1973; Newman and Ling, 1985), e.g. indomethacin, phenylbutazone and salicylates, this so-called analgesic arthropathy is less widely accepted. Whichever drugs are involved, the usual slowly progressive joint destruction of the primary condition may be unexpectedly accelerated with a rapidly progressive but relatively painless collapse and disorganization of the joint similar to a neuropathic arthritis. It is thought to result from unappreciated osteochondral fractures (Murray and Jacobson, 1971) or fractures of porotic trabeculae (Solomon, 1973) in association with a diminution of the normal protective pain responses.

Pathological examination of end-stage femoral heads from patients with analgesic arthropathy has not been helpful in establishing the primary event. The absence of bone necrosis at this late stage does not necessarily exclude preceding primary bone necrosis, for the dead bone may have crumbled away, while the presence of necrotic bone may be secondary to joint fracture rather than the primary event. It seems unwise to assume that rapid deterioration in a damaged joint during treatment with steroids or other analgesics is necessarily the result of bone necrosis.

Pietrograde and Mastromarino (1957) first described the association of systemic steroid therapy with bone necrosis in a patient with pemphigus. Although the pathogenesis remains controversial (see p. 469) over the years the circumstantial evidence for the link has become overwhelming; steroid treatment is now recognized as a common precursor of bone necrosis, particularly in young patients. The condition is characterized by the common involvement of several bones with joint collapse. Sometimes there is relatively little reparative bone formation, which leads to late diagnosis.

While necrosis is occasionally reported in Cushing's syndrome (Fisher and Bickel, 1971), most cases are iatrogenic. They occur in many different conditions and follow a variety of treatment schedules. These include the long-term regimen of immunosuppressive therapy after organ transplant (see below) or high-dose, short courses (O'Brien and Mack, 1992) used most often to reduce post-surgical cerebral oedema (Taylor, 1984; Sambrook *et al.*, 1984). Very occasionally a patient receiving soft tissue (Roseff and Canoso, 1984) or intra-articular steroid injections develops necrosis in distant joints (Laroche *et al.*, 1990). Prolonged systemic treatment and high doses (Felson and Anderson, 1987) each increase the risk of osteonecrosis, but there is disagreement as to whether total dose or fluctuation in tissue levels is more important. Individual susceptibility is undoubtedly a major but unpredictable factor.

Post-transplantation bone necrosis

Bone necrosis was first recognized as a complication of the immunosuppressive regimen in renal transplant patients by Starzl *et al.* (1964). A few cases have also been described following heart transplantation (Burton *et al.*, 1978; Isono *et al.*, 1987) and in allogeneic bone marrow recipients, particularly those with severe graft-*versus*-host disease (Enright *et al.*, 1990; Mascarin *et al.*, 1991).

The incidence of radiologically recognized necrosis following renal transplantation has been reported to vary between 3% and 41%. In most series, as in cardiac transplantation, it has been about 20%. A decrease in steroid dose may be associated with a fall in the incidence of bone necrosis (Harrington *et al.*, 1971; Davidson *et al.*, 1985). The introduction of cyclosporin A to the immunosuppressive regimen in the early 1980s permitted a reduction in the maintenance dose of steroids and in parallel with the fewer episodes of rejection also decreased the number of high-dose steroid boluses. The prevalence of symptomatic bone necrosis has dropped to about 1–3% (Landmann *et al.*, 1987; Lausten *et al.*, 1988) in patients followed for a minimum of 2 years. The condition is likely to be underestimated, however, in any series where investigation is confined to symptomatic patients. Unsuspected lesions may be found at operation or necropsy (Pierides *et al.*, 1975; Catto, 1976) (Figs 16.24 and 16.25; see also Fig. 16.3a). While renal bone disease was found in many of the early patients with renal transplants (Ibels *et al.*, 1978), its severity is reported to have diminished with improved medical management of pre-transplant patients, on dialysis (Kenzora and Glimcher, 1985).

In some patients the first evidence of necrosis is the onset of joint pain, which much be distinguished clinically from pyrophosphate arthropathy and the rather ill-defined musculoskeletal pain from which these patients may suffer. About half the patients with bone necrosis develop pain within 1 year and three-quarters or more within 2 years of transplantation, though occasionally necrosis may appear after 6 years or more (Davidson *et al.*, 1985).

The femoral head is most often affected, and in about 75% of these patients both sides are involved (Fig. 16.24). The next most common lesions are in the

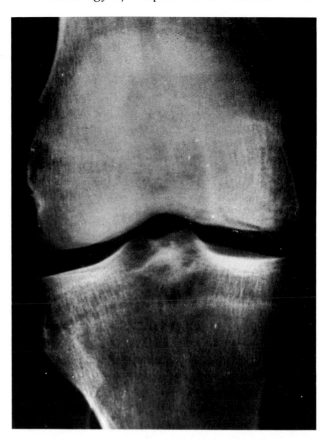

Fig. 16.25 This 23-year-old girl developed pain in her right knee about a year after a renal transplant. The radiograph showed flattening of the medial condyle and a subarticular fracture. At operation subchondral bone necrosis without structural failure was also found in the lateral condyle. Necrosis of both femoral heads was also present. Reproduced by permission of Dr J.K. Davidson.

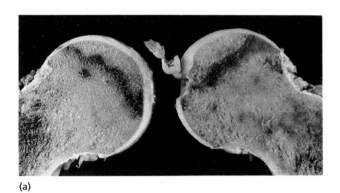

(a)

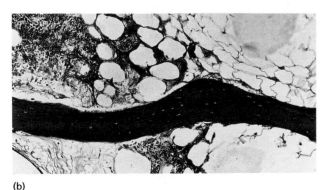

(b)

Fig. 16.24 (a) Necropsy of this patient who died 18 months after renal transplantation showed subchondral necrosis of the femoral heads outlined by haemorrhagic marrow. There was no structural failure. No abnormality was recognized on clinical or slab radiographs because there was almost no reactive proliferation of bone on the surface of the dead trabeculae. (b) Necrotic fatty marrow is seen on the right and fibrin-soaked haemopoietic marrow and fibrous tissue on the left.

humeral head (Cruess, 1985) and in the femoral condyles, giving rise to knee joint effusion (Fig. 16.26). The tibial plateaux, the talus, the capitulum of the humerus, the proximal radius and ulna, the distal tibia, the scaphoid, lunate and navicular bones or the metatarsal head and patella may be involved (Milgram and Riley, 1976). Most patients have more than one joint affected, and about half have more than one site involved. In general, lesions are most common in the weight-bearing joints, and necrosis of the femoral head causes the most disabling and persistent symptoms. Medullary lesions are seldom reported in radiological surveys, but may be found at necropsy (Catto, 1976).

Bone necrosis in malignant lymphoma and childhood leukaemia

Bone necrosis is reported in survivors of malignant lymphoma treated with steroids combined with multi-

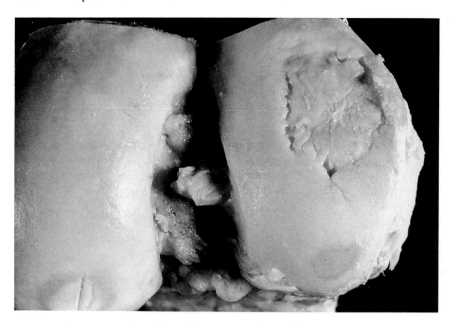

Fig. 16.26 This renal transplant patient was found at necropsy to have osteonecrosis of his lateral femoral condyle with formation of an articular sequestrum which was slightly depressed and showed early tearing of the covering articular cartilage.

agent chemotherapy and/or radiotherapy for advanced disease or recurrence (Ihde and DeVita, 1975; Thorne *et al.*, 1981; Prosnitz *et al.*, 1981; Rossleigh *et al.*, 1986). This is perhaps surprising in view of the intermittent nature of the treatment and in many cases the small total dose of steroid. Osteonecrosis is about half as common in non-Hodgkin's lymphoma as in Hodgkin's disease (Rossleigh *et al.*, 1986) when it usually affects about 1–4% (Thorne *et al.*, 1981; Engel *et al.*, 1981), though occasionally as many as 10% (Prosnitz *et al.*, 1981) of treated survivors. The femoral head is the most common site and both sides are involved in more than half the cases causing considerable disability in a young, active group of patients. About 20% of osteonecrotic lesions occur in the humeral head.

Bone necrosis may be recognized in children with acute lymphocytic leukaemia at the time of diagnosis, during relapse, or at autopsy and is then attributed to packing of the marrow spaces with tumour. Some reports, however, link bone necrosis with the therapy of acute lymphocytic leukaemia (Felix *et al.*, 1985). In one series a few patients, under 5%, on maintenance therapy during the first remission developed symptomatic necrosis, and no doubt the figure would rise if asymptomatic patients were screened (Murphy and Greenberg, 1990). All the patients with necrosis were in a high-risk group treated for 1 month with intensive dexamethasone therapy; those on standard protocols without dexamethasone did not develop bone necrosis. Unfortunately, these young patients may become severely disabled and wheelchair-bound due to involvement and subsequent collapse at multiple sites. As it is estimated that up to

70% of patients with acute lymphocytic leukaemia will be cured of their disease (Murphy and Greenberg, 1990), there must be concern that the number of cases will increase.

It seems likely that steroids are implicated in the development of bone necrosis in both malignant lymphoma and acute lymphocytic leukaemia, but radiotherapy and multi-agent chemotherapy (Harper *et al.*, 1984; Marymont and Kaufman, 1986) may have a synergistic effect, as very occasionally each alone has been associated with bone necrosis.

Bone necrosis in systemic lupus erythematosus

Bone necrosis occurring in the course of systemic lupus erythematosus was described by Dubois and Cozen in 1960. In about 90% of affected patients multiple joints are involved (Darlington, 1985; Fishel *et al.*, 1987), often symmetrically; the femoral head is the most common site. The reported prevalence of bone necrosis has ranged from 3% to as high as 52% (Zizic *et al.*, 1985); about a quarter of cases are symptomless and only picked up on radiological screening (Klippel *et al.*, 1979; Zizic *et al.*, 1985). The great majority of patients have been treated with steroids as is true also of the more uncommon patients (Klippel *et al.*, 1979) with bone necrosis associated with rheumatoid arthritis (Watanabe *et al.*, 1989). It is tempting to implicate vasculitis and an increased tendency to thrombosis, well-accepted features of systemic lupus erythematosus, as contributory factors in steroid-treated patients and as the cause of necrosis in the remainder (Dubois and

Cozen, 1960). Although vasculitis has occasionally been described in synovium (Siemsen *et al.*, 1962; Labowitz and Schumacher, 1971), it has not been demonstrated (Leventhal and Dorfman, 1974) convincingly in bone. Treatment with steroids is now generally regarded as a more important factor in the production of bone necrosis than the disease process itself.

Structural changes

The involvement of several joints and the coexistence of juxta-articular and separate irregular metaphyseal areas of dead bone are reported to be characteristic of steroid-associated necrosis (Milgram, 1990). In some patients, as is common in other conditions, the first evidence of necrosis on plain films may be early patchy bone sclerosis, or later a well-defined dense line separating dead from living bone. In others, however, and particularly in about 75% of renal transplant patients, the first radiological sign in the femoral or humeral head is structural failure as recognized by the crescent line (p. 447) of subchondral trabecular fracture or by flattening of the joint surface. Collapse and rapid destruction of weight-bearing areas promoted by metabolic bone disease may follow, while the dead area may appear more dense due to mechanical impaction of dead trabeculae or calcification of dead tissue.

The sequence of morbid anatomical changes is similar to that already described. Particularly following renal transplantation, however, it is less common to see dense collagen and thick 'sandwich' trabeculae at the junction of dead and living tissue. Instead the junction (even in necrosis of some years' duration) may be haemorrhagic and outlined by congested haemopoietic marrow, sometimes suggesting that necrosis is extending (Catto, 1976) (see Fig. 16.24). While mesenchymal cells may proliferate at the margins of the necrotic zone with production of a little loose fibrous tissue, usually few osteoblasts are seen and and the amount of new bone formed is scanty, thus explaining the lack of radiologically recognizable repair sclerosis in some cases (Glimcher and Kenzora, 1979b) (see Figs 16.24 and 16.25). Medullary necrosis and juxta-articular lesions without structural failure may be found unexpectedly at necropsy or occasionally at operation (see Figs 16.3a and 16.24a). The features of steroid-associated necrosis at the knee are described on p. 475.

PATHOGENESIS OF IDIOPATHIC OR STEROID-ASSOCIATED NECROSIS

The causes of non-traumatic bone necrosis are contentious, probably multifactorial and often operate against a background of systemic disease (Jacobs, 1978; Hungerford and Zizic, 1983; Jones, 1985; Cruess, 1986; Mankin, 1992; Solomon, 1985). The postulated mechanisms and possible sequence of events are discussed briefly below, and Table 16.3 relates these to some of the varied diseases and conditions associated with bone necrosis.

Microfracture of subchondral bone

As an early radiological feature of bone necrosis in many steroid-treated patients is collapse of the joint surface, and osteoporosis is a known complication of hypercortisonism, it was suggested that the subarticular, radiologically lucent line might represent localized bone resorption and subchondral porosis (Solomon, 1973), aggravated in some of renal transplant patients by hyperparathyroidism (Ibels *et al.*, 1978). Necrosis might then be secondary to fracture of weakened but viable trabeculae, which fail to unite due to a decrease in

Table 16.3 Some postulated mechanisms in the production of bone necrosis

Interruption of arterial supply
Fracture, dislocation, slipped capital femoral epiphysis, congenital dislocation of the hip post-treatment

Capillary occlusion by embolism or thrombosis
Dysbarism (nitrogen bubbles, fat emboli?)
Corticosteroids (fat emboli?)
Alcohol (fat emboli?)
Sickle cell disease (abnormal red blood cells)
Polycythaemia vera (red blood cells)
Gaucher's disease?

Injury to vessel wall
Radiation injury
Vasculitis, e.g. in systemic lupus erythematosus
Gaucher's disease (angiospasm?)

Intraosseous capillary tamponade
Gaucher's disease (bloated macrophages)
Corticosteroids (enlarged marrow fat cells)
Alcohol (enlarged marrow fat cells)
Dysbarism (enlarged marrow fat cells and gas bubbles)

Direct damage to osteocytes
Radiation injury
Corticosteroids?

osteoblastic activity. The presence of subarticular necrosis without fracture is evidence against this hypothesis (see Fig. 16.24), and it is now more generally accepted that fracture usually follows necrosis rather than the reverse.

Direct cell toxicity

Kenzora and Glimcher (1985) theorize that the concomitant systemic illness found in many patients has a direct deleterious effect on bone cells which, on the addition of corticosteroid therapy in susceptible patients, becomes irreversible, leading to cell death in anatomically vulnerable sites. Osteocyte death following massive intracellular accumulation of lipids has followed very high doses of corticosteroids in rabbits (Kawai *et al.*, 1985). This finding, however, cannot be uncritically accepted as an explanation for the significantly increased diffuse osteocyte loss without marrow necrosis that has been reported in the subchondral bone of renal transplant patients compared with age-matched controls (Humphreys *et al.*, 1989), nor can it be assumed that diffuse osteocyte loss, which is also a common finding in the femoral head of elderly patients, is necessarily a preliminary to frank infarction of bone and marrow.

Fat embolism

Repeated showers of fat emboli are regarded by several authors as a likely cause of bone necrosis (Jones, 1971; Cruess, 1978; Fisher, 1978) and over many years Jones (1985) has collected a range of supportive circumstantial evidence for this pathogenesis. Clinical signs of fat embolism have been reported in many of the conditions associated with osteonecrosis, and three mechanisms have been suggested (Jones, 1985). The emboli may be disseminated from a fatty liver as in alcoholism and hypercortisonism, from disruption of marrow fat in sickle-cell disease and pancreatitis, or result from destabilization and coalescence of plasma lipoproteins as postulated in dysbarism. Fat emboli within bone may perhaps initiate focal intravascular coagulation and so produce bone necrosis (Jones, 1992).

In rabbits, corticosteroid-induced fat emboli and injected iodized oil fluid injection (Lipiodol) have all been shown to localize in the subchondral blood vessels of the femoral and humeral head but are not always associated with bone necrosis (Jones and Sakovich, 1966; Fisher, 1978). Repeated lymphangiography with Lipiodol has not been associated with human osteonecrosis (Hartmann, 1971). Subchondral arteriolar fat emboli have also been demonstrated by some authors in the bones of patients with aseptic necrosis, while others have either failed to demonstrate them, have been unconvinced of their significance, or have found them in apparently normal femoral heads (Solomon, 1985). Furthermore, there is technical difficulty in distinguishing intravascular fatty globules from normal or artefactual marrow fat.

Vascular occlusion or narrowing

Although idiopathic necrosis of the femoral head is thought by many to result from a direct disturbance of the blood supply, the site of this in the vascular tree and the mechanism by which it is brought about are not clear. Vascular thrombosis is seldom found histologically. Occasionally, changes similar to giant cell arteritis have been described in the soft tissue attachments of the femoral head (Merle d'Aubigné *et al.*, 1965). Vasculitis is a known complication of steroid therapy, but it was not recognized clinically in a large series of patients (Fisher and Bickel, 1971) nor in rabbits given high doses of corticosteroids.

Superselective angiography of the medial circumflex artery, however, in steroid-treated patients with normal hips and in those with pre-radiological necrosis showed impairment of extra-osseous blood-flow with apparent limited penetration of the artery into the femoral head in some patients in both groups (Atsumi and Kuroki, 1992). Sometimes small branching vessels were seen, presumably related to revascularization. Post-mortem perfusion of the femoral head in a similar group of patients also revealed abnormalities of the vascular pattern; in some cases microscopy showed obliterative changes in intra-osseous and capsular vessels (Spencer and Brookes, 1988). The significance of these findings remains unclear. It has been noted that impairment of arterial blood flow may be secondary to raised bone marrow pressure (Hungerford and Lennox, 1985) rather than a primary event.

Intra-osseous small vessel tamponade

It has been suggested (Johnson, 1964) that as the fatty marrow is held within the rigid bony framework an increase in its volume, whether from oedema, enlarged lipocytes, tumour or Gaucher's cell infiltration, may raise the intra-osseous pressure sufficiently to compress capillaries and sinusoids and bring about ischaemia with bone and marrow necrosis. The situation in bone has been likened to the 'compartment syndrome' in soft tissue which, if it is not decompressed, results in muscle necrosis (Hungerford and Lennox, 1985). While marrow fat cells in experimental animals given high doses of corticosteroids (Wang *et al.*, 1977) or of alcohol (Solomon, 1985) increase significantly in size and intra-osseous pressure may rise, bone necrosis has not resulted and it remains uncertain whether the pressure generated in man is sufficient to initiate the postulated sequence of events.

TREATMENT

There is general agreement that treatment of juxta-articular necrosis is more likely to be successful if it is undertaken before structural failure occurs. There is controversy, however, as to the most effective treatment (Colwell, 1989; Hungerford, 1989). Several centres use Arlet and Ficat's three-stage functional investigation of the hip (p. 453). The core biopsy is regarded not simply as a diagnostic measure but as an important therapeutic step, 'decompressing' the bone and so lowering bone marrow pressure. Patients treated by forage (core decompression) at stage I or II and then followed for a minimum of 5 years showed overall a clinical success rate of 90% and only 21% developed progressive radio-logical changes (Ficat, 1983). The results are rather better in patients treated during stage I than stage II (Stulberg, 1990; Ficat, 1983). In other hands results, though better than following conservative management (Stulberg *et al.*, 1991), were less good and 50–60% of patients later developed joint collapse and needed further surgery (Kenzora, 1985; Hopson and Siverhus, 1988; Lausten and Mathieson, 1990). Patients con-tinuing steroid treatment after forage are particularly likely to develop progressive changes (Tooke *et al.*, 1988). Bone grafting by inserting a strut of tibial or fibular cortex along the track of the core biopsy has been advocated (Marcus *et al.*, 1973), and it has been suggested that a vascularized pedicle graft of cancellous bone may be more advantageous biologically, if not mechanically. Electrical stimulation has also been tried.

Once collapse of the femoral head has occurred, two main lines of treatment have been undertaken. Osteo-tomies both varus and valgus have had some success, particularly in patients under 55 years old without metabolic bone disease (Maistrelli *et al.*, 1988). In most centres, however, hemiarthroplasty has been more popular, total hip replacement being reserved for the late stage when both sides of the joint show advanced degenerative disease. In general, results of arthroplasty for osteonecrosis tend to be less satisfactory than those carried out for primary osteoarthritis, perhaps because of poor bone stock.

GAUCHER'S DISEASE

Gaucher's disease most often develops in children, adolescents and young adults and runs a protracted course. The condition is most common in Ashkenazi (European) Jews in whom it is the most usual genetic disorder. It is transmitted as an autosomal recessive trait and is due to deficiency of the lysosomal enzyme gluco-cerebroside hydrolase, which results in the accumulation of its insoluble substrate glucosylceramide in the cells of the macrophage–monocyte system. The most reliable diagnosis is made by finding a markedly depressed level of the enzyme in the patient's peripheral blood leucocytes (Beutler and Saven, 1990).

The gene for the enzyme has been identified on chromosome 1 in the region of q21, and at least three common mutations appear to have some prognostic significance. Patients homozygous for mutation 1226 are reported to have the best prognosis, and indeed may be entirely asymptomatic (Zimran *et al.*, 1989). Of the three clinically distinct phenotypes, type 1 affects about 90% of patients. It lacks the neurological involvement of types 2 and 3, but is associated with orthopaedic complications which cause considerable morbidity.

The clinical manifestations of type 1 Gaucher's disease result from the accumulation of the large polyhedral macrophages rich in glucosylceramide in the liver, spleen and bone marrow. In bone this produces focal radio-lucent areas, or if marrow involvement is more diffuse and extensive, cortical thinning and flask-shaped meta-physes, both carrying a risk of pathological fracture. Not surprisingly, the extent of marrow involvement revealed by magnetic resonance imaging is greater than that recognized on plain films, and the method has the advantage over computed tomography of producing coronal images. It has been suggested that complications of fracture and necrosis are more likely in patients with widespread marrow replacement (Rosenthal *et al.*, 1986). Some patients dramatically develop sudden, exquisitely painful acute 'bone crises' (Bell *et al.*, 1986; Yosipovitch and Katz, 1990) which, like those of sickle cell disease (see p. 473), are difficult to differentiate from acute pyogenic osteomyelitis. The condition may follow a virus infection (Mankin *et al.*, 1990) or perhaps is due to intramedullary haemorrhage (Horev *et al.*, 1991). The episode usually subsides within a few days (Beighton *et al.*, 1982), but is followed by radiological evidence of infarction, most often involving a large segment of the medullary cavity and sometimes also the endosteal cortex of a long bone or the pelvis. Most long bone infarcts, however, are not preceded by a bone crisis but are asymptomatic and recognized radiologically as foci or more extensive areas of sclerosis. These appearances result from calcification of dead marrow rather than from appositional new bone formation, as revascularization is usually slight, though radionuclide scans may show increased uptake.

More important to the patient than medullary necrosis is juxta-articular involvement which, in both adults and children, most commonly affects one or both femoral heads (Amstutz, 1973) or occasionally the humeral head (Rourke and Heslin, 1965), the femoral or tibial condyles, talus, or capitulum. In children necrosis of the femoral head produces a picture similar to Perthes' disease (Todd and Keidan, 1952) (see Chapter 5), but slow reconstitution may be followed by further episodes of necrosis in adult life and subsequent osteoarthritic changes. In adults the pattern of necrosis in the femoral head is similar to that of idiopathic osteonecrosis (p. 465), but there may be little reactive bone sclerosis (Jaffe, 1972). Necrosis of the femoral head has also been described in Fabry's disease (Boettcher *et al.*, 1970), a lipid storage disorder rather similar to Gaucher's disease.

The means by which necrosis is brought about in Gaucher's disease is uncertain, but the most popular suggestion is that the bloated macrophages so pack the marrow spaces that intra-osseous sinusoids are compressed (Jaffe, 1972). Certainly, the marrow pressure is raised (Solomon, 1985). Other possibilities are that the cells block the lumina of vessels in the marrow, as they are known to do in the liver and spleen, and that marrow necrosis is followed by collagenous scarring, which in its turn may promote further ischaemia and bone death.

Orthopaedic treatment has been largely concerned with dealing with pathological fractures, and the sometimes difficult prosthetic replacement of damaged joints, often in unusually young and active patients. An exciting development (Barton *et al.*, 1991; Beutler, 1991; Mankin, 1993) has been enzyme replacement by repeated intravenous infusions of commercially produced, macrophage-targeted, mannose-terminated enzyme, which has improved patients' well-being and after a time has reduced the stores of lipid in liver, spleen and probably also in the bone marrow. Both bone biopsy (Barton *et al.*, 1992) and magnetic resonance imaging (Johnson *et al.*, 1992) suggest a return of the bone marrow towards normal. Investigation of the effect of this expensive and prolonged treatment continues, but it is hoped that soon complete and lasting correction of the underlying abnormality may be brought about by gene transfer (Beutler, 1991; Mankin, 1993).

CHRONIC PANCREATITIS

Subarticular necrosis of the femoral or humeral heads (Gerle *et al.*, 1965) or the talus (Baron *et al.*, 1984) and medullary infarcts have been described in patients with chronic relapsing pancreatitis, but they are rare. It is thought that during an attack of pancreatitis, lipase and other enzymes liberated into the peritoneal fluid are taken up in lymphatics and reach the bloodstream by the thoracic duct. When the enzymes reach adipose tissue, fat cells are broken down into fatty acids, which take up calcium. Only if necrosis of the fatty marrow is widespread does bone necrosis occur.

A proportion of patients with bone necrosis associated with pancreatitis are alcoholics, and it is difficult to be certain of the relative importance of the two factors (Jacobs, 1978).

SICKLE CELL DISEASE

More than 100 abnormal haemoglobins have now been identified, but HbS, found chiefly in patients of Afro-Caribbean ancestry, is the only one to give rise to the sickling phenomenon and so to bone necrosis. The term *'sickle cell disease'* implies the presence of two abnormal allelomorphic genes related to haemoglobin formation, at least one of which is the sickle cell gene. The group includes not only sickle cell anaemia (S/S) but also the combination of HbS with other abnormal haemoglobins such as HbC (S/C), HbD (S/D) or with the thalassaemia gene (S/β Thal) common in the Mediterranean littoral. The term *'sickle cell trait'* refers to the presence of the sickle cell gene in association with normal adult haemoglobin (A/S). These individuals may develop red cell sickling when exposed to conditions of extreme hypoxia; alcohol appears to promote sickling. Bone necrosis has only very occasionally been reported (Nachamie and Dorfman, 1974; Lally *et al.*, 1983; Frierson *et al.*, 1987). The diagnosis of bone necrosis in patients of Afro-Caribbean or Mediterranean origin should lead to screening for sickling.

Pathogenesis of bone lesions

HbS owes its pathogenicity to the fact that when deoxygenated, the substitution of valine for glutamic acid in one of the amino acid sequences results in a ring-like malformation which locks adjacent molecules of haemoglobin together, stacking them in rows. If a sufficient proportion of the haemoglobin in the cell is in the S form the cell assumes the characteristic sickle shape. The more rigid sickled cells that form under hypoxic conditions may pass on into better oxygenated tissues where most 'unsickle' and return to normal. Eventually, with repeated sickling and unsickling, their membrane becomes damaged and sickling becomes permanent. As sickled cells flow less readily and increase blood viscosity, they may become trapped at capillary junctions and in sinusoids; this results in increasing stasis and local hypoxia, further sickling, and finally vascular occlusion. If the condition persists endothelial damage and infarction follow. When thrombosis occurs it is probably a secondary change. The irreversibly sickled red cells are more fragile than normal and have a shorter life, so that haemolytic anaemia develops.

Radiological examination may show the resultant compensatory hyperplasia of the haemopoietic marrow in the flat bones and long bone metaphyses as osteoporosis with cortical thinning and a widening of the medulla and intertrabecular spaces. The marrow hyperplasia is often less marked in the mixed haemoglobinopathies (S/C, S/D and S/β Thal) than in sickle cell anaemia (S/S).

Patterns of bone necrosis

ACUTE INFARCTIONS OR BONE CRISES

These are characterized by acute episodes of pain and tenderness, sometimes with fever and leucocytosis. The ill-effects may be diminished by prompt diagnosis, hydration, oxygen administration and exchange transfusion. The so-called hand–foot syndrome (dactylitis) which occurs in children, usually between 6 and 24 months, is often the first clinical evidence of sickle cell disease (Worrall and Butera, 1976; Theis and Owen, 1988) and tends to appear as fetal haemoglobin decreases and HbS increases. The dorsum of the hands or feet becomes swollen, oedematous and painful, perhaps because the vessels in the haemopoietic marrow of the small tubular bones are particularly susceptible to vasoconstriction due to cold (Stevens et al., 1981). The symptoms subside without treatment in 1–2 weeks.

Several bones are often affected, sometimes symmetrically. In the early stages, while bone marrow aspiration shows marrow necrosis (Charache and Page, 1967), radiological examination is normal, and indeed no evidence of infarction may ever become apparent. In some cases at about 2 weeks, subperiosteal new bone formation appears along with some patchy erosion of the cortex due to the in-growth of granulation tissue from the surviving periosteal circulation (Weinberg and Currarino, 1972). The broadened bone may later remodel and return to normal, but sometimes growth

ceases temporarily with resultant stunting, the central part of the growth plate supplied by diaphyseal vessels being chiefly affected while the periphery survives (Cockshott, 1963). The marrow may re-populate or be replaced by fibrous tissue.

Acute marrow infarcts may affect patients of all ages and involve many sites, e.g. the spine, face, skull, ribs, or sternum as well as the long bones (see below). When marrow infarction involves the bone end, there may be associated joint pain and effusion, while large infarcts sometimes give rise to fat or bone marrow emboli.

The differential diagnosis between acute bone infarcts and the much rarer osteomyelitis (Keeley and Buchanan, 1982; Theis and Owen, 1988) is often difficult particularly as infection of necrotic marrow occasionally complicates both dactylitis in infants and long bone infarcts in older children. Osteomyelitis may involve several bones and be bilateral and symmetrical. The patient appears more ill and toxic, the acute symptoms fail to resolve, and increasing soft tissue swelling may be followed by fluctuation (Epps et al., 1991). Bone and bone marrow scans are seldom helpful apart from drawing attention to the involvement of multiple sites, and diagnosis depends on positive bacteriological cultures from blood or bone. In most reports staphylococci are much less often implicated than *Salmonella* spp. (Adeyokunnu and Hendrickse, 1980; Ebong, 1986; Bennett and Namnyak, 1990), which is thought to enter the bloodstream from large intestine damaged by local ischaemia. There is often no previous history of typhoid infection. In areas where typhoid is endemic, prophylactic chloramphenicol may be given to patients in an acute bone crisis.

NECROSIS OF LONG BONE SHAFTS

The presentation and natural history of long bone necrosis varies markedly with age. More than 90% of diaphyseal infarcts associated with an acute, painful bone crisis occur in children under 9 years old (Bohrer, 1970). While a few patients develop a pathological fracture, the infarct usually resolves and then bone scans and radiographs return to normal. The femur and tibia (Bohrer, 1970) and humerus (Keeley and Buchanan, 1982) are most often affected, and about one-quarter of lesions are bilateral and symmetrical. The shaft close to the metaphysis is particularly vulnerable. This metadiaphyseal site accounts for most localized lesions and is often most severely affected when the whole length of the shaft is infarcted. The same problem of differential diagnosis from osteomyelitis applies to this group as to infants with dactylitis.

Diaphyseal lesions in older children and adults are often silent clinically and are only recognized as incidental, unexpected findings at radiological or, particularly in the case of medullary infarcts, at post-mortem examination (Diggs, 1967). In these older patients, radioisotope scans and radiological changes do not return to normal. Magnetic resonance imaging may be helpful in distinguishing recent medullary infarcts from chronic, old, fibrotic ones (Rao *et al.*, 1986). Some foci of long-standing marrow necrosis appear sclerotic due to calcification of encapsulating fibrous tissue and dead marrow and to the formation of appositional new bone on the surface of dead trabeculae. Sclerotic areas in ribs, vertebrae, or the pelvis may mimic Paget's disease or osteoblastic metastases. Widespread cortical necrosis tends to result in broadening of the shaft by incorporation of subperiosteal new bone and narrowing of the medullary cavity by endosteal new bone (Diggs, 1967). Delicate concentric cylinders of bone may result from a reparative subperiosteal reaction and give the radiological appearance of 'a bone within a bone'. The structural changes may be difficult to interpret, particularly when there has been more than one episode of necrosis with incomplete repair.

JUXTA-ARTICULAR BONE NECROSIS

The femoral head is the most common site of juxta-articular bone necrosis and has the greatest potential for producing pain and disability. Sickle cell disease is the most common cause of femoral head necrosis in children (Milner *et al.*, 1991). The radiologically diagnosed prevalence in symptomatic patients of all ages is between 3% (Iwegbu and Fleming, 1985; Theis and Owen, 1988) and 5% (Lee *et al.*, 1981). When asymptomatic patients are screened, this rises to about 10% (Milner *et al.*, 1991) and in adults may reach 40% (Ware *et al.*, 1991).

Necrosis of the femoral head in children and adolescents produces a radiological picture similar to that of classic Perthes' disease (see Chapter 5). The whole epiphysis or, more commonly, only a segment in the antero-superior region may be affected. Spontaneous healing with restitution of a normal-looking femoral head is most likely to occur in young patients with only segmental involvement. In older children or those with necrosis of the whole epiphysis the femoral head becomes flat, broad and mushroom-like, with a wide femoral neck but a well-preserved joint space. Perhaps partly as a result of further episodes of necrosis, 20% of adults who were known to have suffered capital necrosis in childhood were found to be pain-free on long-term review (Hernigou *et al.*, 1991).

In adults, the pattern of necrosis and subsequent collapse is similar to that seen following intracapsular fracture or idiopathic necrosis (Diggs and Anderson, 1971; Middlemiss, 1976), though the histological appearances may be a complex pattern of haemorrhage and episodes of necrosis with interrupted repair (Sherman, 1959). The amount of disability from degenerative joint disease varies greatly and does not necessarily correspond to the severity of radiological changes. Before surgery the importance of the skeletal symptoms must be assessed in relation to the patient's activity, because this may be seriously curtailed as a result of anaemia and heart failure. Furthermore, joint replacement may be complicated by excessive haemorrhage and subsequent haematological crises, as well as by early mechanical and septic loosening of the prosthesis and infection of the infarct, leading to a failure rate of 50% at 5 years (Hanker and Amstutz, 1988).

Necrosis of the humeral head is rare in children. In adults it may give rise to a radiological picture of patchy sclerosis due to bone repair (Chung *et al.*, 1978) with structural failure of the subchondral bone plate and some collapse of the head. Occasionally, the knee joint or the talus is affected. While sickle cell disease may be cured by bone marrow transplantation (Kodish *et al.*, 1990), this tends to be reserved for severely affected patients because it carries a 5–10% mortality rate and the risk of graft-*versus*-host disease.

RADIATION OSTEODYSPLASIA

Damage to bone may result from the ingestion of radionuclides or from external radiation, though the latter is more uncommon since megavoltage therapy replaced orthovoltage therapy. Only the most severely affected patients develop actual bone necrosis, which probably results from both direct cellular damage and vascular narrowing.

The most usual sites of radiologically recognizable radiation osteodysplasia are in the pelvis and upper femur of women treated for gynaecological malignancy and in the bones around the shoulder following post-mastectomy radiation to the axilla. Bone formation is more inhibited than resorption, and small radiolucencies in the bony cortex result from failure of filling in of resorption areas around the Haversian spaces. In the medulla the marrow spaces may be replaced by fibrous tissue that is patchily calcified. Abnormal woven or lamellar bone may form on the surface of some trabeculae while others are more slender than normal. The chief importance of the resulting irregular patches of increased and decreased radiodensity is that they should not be assumed to represent metastases from the originally treated carcinoma.

Bone included in the radiation field may fracture months or years after treatment and often without radiological evidence of underlying osteodysplasia. The femoral neck is most often affected with a slow slip into varus, and histology shows that this 'stress' fracture is not usually associated with pre-existing necrosis; sometimes osteoporosis appears to be the cause.

Collapse of the superoanterior part of the femoral head is an uncommon sequel to the fracture, but is sometimes seen without any previous injury. It is not necessarily preceded by bone necrosis, but may result from fracture through porotic bone trabeculae with subsequent sinking down of the joint surface (Catto, 1976).

OSTEONECROSIS OF THE KNEE

Secondary osteonecrosis

Secondary osteonecrosis of the knee may be associated with steroid therapy following organ transplantation (Ahuja and Bullough, 1978) (Figs 16.25 and 16.26), rheumatoid arthritis, systemic lupus erythematosus (Aglietti *et al.*, 1983), or sickle cell anaemia. The patient usually complains of the gradual onset of pain in the knee which involves the *lateral* condyle of the femur in about 60% of cases. In about 50% of patients the contralateral knee, which is often pain-free initially, is found to be affected at the same time or later (Pollack *et al.*, 1987). Patchy subchondral lucency may be seen in the femoral condyle with alteration in the joint contour (Fig. 16.25) and shedding of a sequestrum into the joint. While the appearances have some resemblance to osteochondritis dissecans (Chapter 6) the fragment is usually larger, and collapse of the joint surface is progressive (Hall and Hume, 1970; Aichroth *et al.*, 1971). Sometimes the loose body is driven down into the necrotic condyle.

Spontaneous osteonecrosis

The clinical findings of secondary osteonecrosis contrast with the much larger group of patients without a known predisposing cause. In spontaneous osteonecrosis of the knee the patient is normally a healthy woman of 60 years or more who complains of the dramatically sudden onset of severe pain in the knee, almost always over the weight-bearing area of the *medial* femoral condyle. The lateral condyle (Marmor, 1984) or the medial tibial plateau (Houpt *et al.*, 1982) is only

occasionally involved. There is exquisite local tenderness, sometimes with an effusion, and some restriction of flexion and extension.

At the onset of symptoms the radiological appearances are usually normal, but scintigraphy shows a focally intense increased uptake (Bauer, 1978). This localized pattern helps to differentiate the condition from other causes of knee pain, e.g. osteoarthritis with its less marked and more diffuse uptake, and also from meniscal tears (Lotke and Ecker, 1985). Discrete, well-defined low-signal areas in the subchondral region contrast with high signals from the surrounding normal fatty marrow on magnetic resonance imaging. The demonstration of bone marrow changes (Pollack *et al.*, 1987; Bjorkengren *et al.*, 1990) reinforces the scintigraphic findings and helps to make the diagnosis when no abnormality develops subsequently on radiography. Magnetic resonance imaging also gives a clearer picture of the extent of the lesion, which is often larger than plain films later suggest. Scintigraphy and magnetic resonance imaging may draw attention to silent disease in the contralateral knee, though this is uncommon in the spontaneous compared with the secondary cases (Pollack *et al.*, 1987).

The first detectable radiological change is a thin subchondral line of radiolucency on lateral views, with perhaps slight flattening of the normal contour of the condyle on weight-bearing. The subchondral translucency later becomes more apparent, and surrounding sclerosis due to reactive bone formation develops. In a few patients there is rapid collapse of the medial joint space with a marked varus deformity.

STRUCTURAL CHANGES

A spectrum of changes is seen in the knees at arthrotomy. At an early stage there may be only a localized oval depression of the condylar surface with some discoloration of the cartilage. Later the shallow articular sequestrum tends to become partly separated as a hinged flap by the confluence of small peripheral tears. Finally, it may fragment and separate completely from the underlying bone. The depth of dead bone beneath the sequestrum varies, and it seems less likely to be substantial in patients with spontaneous osteonecrosis (Houpt *et al.*, 1982) than in those with steroid-associated disease. Revascularization is associated with the in-growth of granulation and fibrous tissue and with the formation of appositional new bone on the surface of dead trabeculae, which is sometimes sufficient to produce a rim of sclerosis around the remaining dead bone. There is, however, a likelihood that revascularization will be incomplete and dead bone will be ground away leaving a shallow or deep crater with a base of fibrocartilage containing fragments of dead bone (Ahuja and Bullough, 1978). Adjacent articular cartilage is then likely to show degenerative changes.

PROGNOSIS

The initial acute pain tends to subside within 6–15 months, but the clinical course depends chiefly on the size of the lesion (Lotke and Ecker, 1988; Al-Rowaih *et al.*, 1991). Those patients who initially have scintigraphic and magnetic resonance findings of osteonecrosis but do not develop radiological changes and those whose lesions measure less than 3.5 cm^2 or occupy less than half the condylar width tend to have a better prognosis. Some lesions heal spontaneously with restricted weight-bearing; others later develop degenerative changes in the joint, but these are usually relatively mild

in comparison with the more severe and rapidly progressive arthritis associated with larger sequestra. It has been suggested (Rozing *et al.*, 1980) that osteonecrosis may be the underlying cause of more cases of osteoarthritis of the knee than is generally realized.

'OSTEOCHONDROSES' ('OSTEOCHONDRITIS') (Brower, 1983)

The so-called osteochondroses are a heterogeneous collection of eponymous conditions which usually involve an epiphysis or apophysis of the immature skeleton, often at the time of its greatest growth activity. The onset of symptoms tends to be earlier in girls than boys. The lesions have in common radiological changes of sclerosis, fragmentation and decrease in size of the ossification centre. Some conditions progress to osteoarthritis, while others appear to be self-healing with

Table 16.4 Some so-called osteochondroses

Syndrome	Site	Age peak and sex	Comment	Pathogenesis
Sever	Calcaneum	9–11 years old	Radiological fragmentation and sclerosis of secondary ossification centre in calcaneum is normal in weight-bearing child. Painful heel not related to radiological changes	Variant of normal
Köhler	Navicular bone	3–7 years old M:F–5:1	Uncommon, may be bilateral. Sclerotic fragmented, flattened bone—thin wafer but usually reconstitutes without disability. Look for another cause for pain and local swelling	Fragmented ossification centre may be incidental radiographic finding and normal variant. A few may be genuine examples of bone necrosis
Scheuermann	Vertebral epiphysis, commonly lower thoracic sometimes also upper lumbar	13–17 years old No constant sex preference	Several vertebrae affected (3–5), irregular vertebral body borders with wedging, kyphosis and mild scoliosis	Repeated stress during adolescence leading to microfracture of weak vertebral end plate with herniation of disc tissue into vertebral body. No bone necrosis. Wedging due to loss of disc cushion
Blount	Medial/proximal tibia	1–3 years old Occasional in adolescents	Bowing of proximal tibia with sharp angulation and metaphyseal beaking, unilateral or asymmetrical. (c.f. physiological bowing, smooth curve, bilateral and symmetric, resolves.)	Stress and compression → abnormality of endochondral ossification

Table 16.4 *Continued*

Syndrome	Site	Age peak and sex	Comment	Pathogenesis
Osgood–Schlatter	Tibial tubercle	10–15 years old, particularly athletic boys	Bilateral 25% — fragmented tuberosity — soft tissue swelling — thickening of patellar tendon	Avulsion fracture along attachment of patellar tendon to developing tibial tuberosity or chronic tendonitis with heterotopic ossicles
Sinding–Larsen–Johansson	Lower pole patella	10–14 years old	Traction at proximal attachment of patellar tendon. Radiographic bony fragments and soft tissue swelling	Avulsion fracture
Kienböck	Lunate bone	20–40 years old — rare under 15, usually male	Involves dominant hand in manual workers may → osteoarthritis at the radial—lunate interface	?Repeated traumatic compression fracture of bone, may be associated with short ulna with compression against radius only
Freiberg	Metatarsal head especially second	10–15 years old M:F—1:3	Uncommon, bilateral in 10% fracture → deformity, loose bodies → arthritis of MP joint	Repeated stress leading to subchondral fracture. Often associated with hallux valgus or short first metatarsal
Panner	Capitulum humerus	4–16 years old Usually boys	Seldom bilateral may → epiphysis condensed and fragmented but usually reconstitutes without disability — radial head may enlarge due to hyperaemia	Repeated stress Young baseball pitchers — 'little leaguer's elbow'
Calvé	Vertebral body	Young children	Collapse and sclerosis of vertebral body. Vertebra plana — 'coin on edge' vertebra. Some regeneration but reconstitution often incomplete	Eosinophil granuloma — very occasionally due to Hodgkin's disease or other tumours

reconstitution of the bony contour. These lesions were originally thought to result from vascular insufficiency which produced primary bone necrosis, but it is now believed that in many, necrosis is secondary to trauma, which is often mild, repeated stress rather than a single acute episode. In some conditions no necrosis is seen, the radiological changes being due to some other cause, e.g. eosinophil granuloma in Calvé's disease of the vertebra, or to a variant of normal as in Sever's disease of the calcaneum (Table 16.4). In all limb lesions it is important to obtain radiographs of the asymptomatic side for comparison. It would seem appropriate to abandon the eponyms and the term osteochondrosis, and where the cause of necrosis remains uncertain, to refer to idiopathic necrosis of the site. Histological material from most of these conditions is relatively scanty (Jaffe, 1972; Milgram, 1990) and even when available for study may throw little light on the pathogenesis. Perthes' disease is dealt with in Chapter 5.

SOME UNSOLVED PROBLEMS

Why do dead bone trabeculae fracture?

Fracture usually occurs near to or immediately below the subchondral plate or at the junction of dead and living bone. Either or both of these sites may be involved irrespective of the cause of the necrosis.

There is controversy as to whether trabecular fractures are the result of resorption associated with repair or of the failure of trabeculae to withstand mechanical stress. The rational planning of treatment depends on the answer. Attempts have been made to encourage revascularization by limiting weight-bearing or by bone grafting in the hope that this process would be complete before trabecular fracture occurred. It has been suggested, however, that better clinical results might follow the prevention of revascularization (Glimcher and Kenzora, 1979c) as has been reported in experiments in dogs (Johnson and Crothers, 1976).

SUBCHONDRAL FRACTURE

Observations on the repair of experimentally produced femoral head necrosis in rabbits, and examination of core biopsies from patients with uncollapsed idiopathic necrosis of the femoral head (Springfield and Enneking, 1976), have emphasized that revascularization of the subchondral bone plate at the margin of dead bone is accompanied by osteoclastic resorption, dead bone being removed before new living bone is laid down. In rabbits the disproportionate loss of bone at this site persisted for 18 months (Kenzora *et al.*, 1978). It has been suggested that the weakened subchondral plate fractures first, and this is followed by secondary fracture of dead trabeculae. While this could well be the initiating event in examples of collapse in the early years, it is more difficult perhaps to explain long-delayed fractures in dysbaric osteonecrosis (see Fig. 16.5, p. 446).

It is known that trabecular stress fractures occur and repair in living bone (Todd *et al.*, 1972), but when dead bone trabeculae fracture they cannot heal. This mechanism may account for some of the subchondral fractures (Köberle and Constant, 1979) that are sometimes confined to an area remote from the site of revascularization of the subchondral plate (Solomon, 1985).

FRACTURE AT THE JUNCTION OF DEAD AND LIVING BONE

Fracture of dead trabeculae close to their junction with 'sandwich' trabeculae broadened by the apposition of new living bone has been explained as a result of concentration of mechanical stresses with rotary and axial loading forces, producing a shear fracture at the site (Calandruccio and Anderson, 1980). Fibrous tissue usually marks the junction between dead and living tissue, and the dead trabeculae within this may undergo osteoclastic resorption. While this resorption is often regarded as the cause of trabecular fracture, it has also been interpreted as a reaction secondary to motion and deformation of trabecular fractures initiated by disintegration of the subchondral plate (Glimcher and Kenzora, 1979b).

Why is revascularization often incomplete?

While it seems clear that dead bone and marrow can completely revascularize, in many cases the process halts before it is completed. Where trabecular fracture is found at the junction between dead and living bone, for example as is sometimes seen deep in the femoral head following healing of intracapsular fractures of the femoral neck, this secondary fracture may be interpreted either as the result of resorption of dead bone following the halting of revascularization or as the cause of its cessation. Certainly, trabecular discontinuity is associated with collagenization of the revascularization front and sometimes with the development of a fibro-cartilaginous layer which effectively separates dead from living bone and is a barrier to further spread of the repair processes (Calandruccio and Anderson, 1980). It is still uncertain, however, whether trabecular fracture or collagenization is the first event, and in any case trabecular fracture cannot explain the failure of complete revascularization in intact juxta-articular necrosis or in medullary lesions.

In many conditions, and very markedly in dysbaric osteonecrosis, the junction between dead and living bone is marked by a radiologically dense line. This proliferated new bone may form arches joining together the 'sandwich' trabeculae on the revascularized side of the junction (see Fig. 16.5c, p. 446). These arches may provide the most effective mechanical and structural support, but have also been postulated as a causal factor in the arrest of the repair process (Weatherly *et al.*, 1977). The failure of repair in idiopathic necrosis of the femoral head has been attributed to clogging of the marrow by calcified material (Springfield and Enneking, 1976).

Another possible explanation for failure of complete revascularization, for example in the femoral head, is that there is a natural limit to the amount of dead bone that can be revascularized. Although Sevitt (1981) has illustrated two completely revascularized femoral heads removed 10 years after intracapsular fracture, by this time it is difficult to establish whether the whole femoral head or only a part of it was originally dead.

Perhaps the most appealing explanation of failure of complete revascularization is that the process may be interrupted by further episodes of necrosis. Repeated exposure to the hyperbaric environment, repeated episodes of red cell sickling and (accepting that steroids are indeed responsible for bone necrosis) the continuous administration of steroids following transplantation, are among the conditions that might be expected to promote further episodes of necrosis. Morphological evidence of recurrent necrosis has been reported in Perthes' disease (McKibbin and Ralis, 1974) and in idiopathic necrosis of the femoral head (Springfield and Enneking, 1976; Inoue and Ono, 1979). While it may be easy to recognize that two separate areas of bone have become necrotic at different times (McCallum *et al.*, 1966), it is more difficult to be certain that revascularization has been interrupted by another ischaemic episode as joint collapse may disrupt vessels (Catto, 1976).

REFERENCES

Adeyokunnu A.A. and Hendrickse R.G. (1980) *Salmonella* osteomyelitis in childhood. A report of 63 cases seen in Nigerian children of whom 57 had sickle cell anaemia. *Arch. Dis. Child.* **55**, 175–184.

Aglietti P., Insall J.N., Buzzi R. and Deschamps G. (1983) Idiopathic osteonecrosis of the knee: aetiology, prognosis and treatment. *J. Bone Joint Surg.* **65B**, 588–597.

Ahuja S.C. and Bullough P.G. (1978) Osteonecrosis of the knee. A clinicopathological study in twenty eight patients. *J. Bone Joint Surg.* **60A**, 191–197.

Aichroth P., Branfoot A.C., Huskisson E.C. *et al.* (1971) Destructive joint changes following kidney transplantation. *J. Bone Joint Surg.* **53B**, 488–494.

Allen T.H., Davis J.C. and Hodgson C.J. (1974) U.S. Air Force experience in hypobaric osteonecrosis. In Beckman E.L. and Elliott D.H. (eds) *Dysbarism-Related Osteonecrosis*. Symposium, US Department of Health, Education and Welfare, pp. 17–18.

Al-Rowaih A., Lindstrand A., Björkengren A., Wingstrand H. and Thorngren K.-G. (1991) Osteonecrosis of the knee: diagnosis and outcome in 40 patients. *Acta Orthop. Scand.* **62**, 19–23.

Amstutz H.A. (1973) The hip in Gaucher's disease. *Clin. Orthop.* **90**, 83–89.

Anderson G.H., Raymakers R. and Gregg P.J. (1993) The incidence of proximal femoral fractures in an English county. *J. Bone Joint Surg.* **75B**, 441–444.

Arden G.P. and Veall N. (1953) The use of radioactive phosphorus in early detection of avascular necrosis in the femoral head in fractured neck of femur. *Proc. R. Soc. Med.* **46**, 344–346.

Arlet J., Mazières B. and Netry C. (1982) Osteonecrosis of the femoral head and pregnancy. *Clin. Rheumatol.* **1**, 95–103.

Atsumi T. and Kuroki Y. (1992) Role of impairment of blood supply of the femoral head in the pathogenesis of idiopathic osteonecrosis. *Clin. Orthop.* **277**, 22–30.

Barnes R., Brown J.T., Garden R.S. *et al.* (1976) Subcapital fractures of the femur. *J. Bone Joint Surg.* **58B**, 2–24.

Baron M., Paltiel H. and Lander P. (1984) Aseptic necrosis of the talus and calcaneal insufficiency fractures in a patient with pancreatitis, subcutaneous fat necrosis and arthritis. *Arthritis Rheum.* **27**, 1309–1313.

Barquet A. (1982) Avascular necrosis following traumatic hip dislocation in childhood. Factors of influence. *Acta Orthop. Scand.* **53**, 809–813.

Barton N.W., Brady R.O., Dambrosia J.M. *et al.* (1991) Replacement therapy for inherited enzyme deficiency—macrophage-targeted glucocerebrosidase for Gaucher's disease *N. Engl. J. Med.* **324**, 1464–1470.

Barton N.W., Brady R.O., Dambrosia J.M. *et al.* (1992) Dose-dependent responses to macrophage-targeted glucocerebrosidase in a child with Gaucher's disease. *J. Pediatr.* **120**, 277–280.

Bassett L.W., Mirra J.M., Cracchiolo A. III and Gold R.H. (1987) Ischemic necrosis of the femoral head. Correlation of magnetic resonance imaging and histologic sections. *Clin. Orthop.* **233**, 181–187.

Bauer G.C.H. (1978) Osteonecrosis of the knee. *Clin. Orthop.* **130**, 210–217.

Bayliss A.P. and Davidson J.K. (1977) Traumatic osteonecrosis of the femoral head following intracapsular fracture. Incidence and earliest radiological features. *Clin. Radiol.* **28**, 407–414.

Beighton P., Goldblatt J. and Sacks S. (1982) Bone involvement in Gaucher disease. In Desnick R.J., Gatt S. and Grabowski G.A. (eds) *Gaucher Disease. A Century of Delineation and Research.* New York, Alan R Liss, pp. 107–129.

Bell R.S., Mankin H.J. and Doppelt S.H. (1986) Osteomyelitis in Gaucher disease. *J. Bone Joint Surg.* **68A**, 1380–1388.

Beltran J., Herman L.J., Burk J.M. *et al.* (1988) Femoral head avascular necrosis: MR imaging with clinical-pathologic and radio-nuclide correlation. *Radiology* **166**, 215–220.

Beltran J., Knight C.T., Zuelzer W.A. *et al.* (1990) Core decompression for avascular necrosis of the femoral head: correlation between long-term results and pre-operative MR staging. *Radiology* **175**, 533–536.

Bennett O.M. and Namnyak S.S. (1990) Bone and joint manifestations of sickle cell anaemia. *J. Bone Joint Surg.* **72B**, 494–499.

Beutler E. (1991) Gaucher's disease. *N. Engl. J. Med.* **325**, 1354–1360.

Beutler E. and Saven A. (1990) The misuse of marrow examination in the diagnosis of Gaucher disease. *Blood* **76**, 646–648.

Björkengren A.G., Al-Rowaih A., Lindstrand A., Wingstrand H., Thorngren K.G. and Pettersson H. (1990) Spontaneous osteonecrosis of the knee: value of MR imaging in determining prognosis. *AJR Am. J. Roentgenol.* **154**, 331–336.

Bobechko W.P. and Harris W.R. (1960) The radiographic density of avascular bone. *J. Bone Joint Surg.* **42B**, 626–632.

Boettcher W.G., Bonfiglio M., Hamilton H.H. *et al.* (1970) Non-traumatic necrosis of the femoral head; part 1—relation of altered hemostasis to etiology. *J. Bone Joint Surg.* **52A**, 312–329.

Bohrer S.P. (1970) Acute long bone diaphyseal infarcts in sickle cell disease. *Br. J. Radiol.* **43**, 685–697.

Bolton-Maggs B.G., Helal B.H. and Revell P.A. (1984) Bilateral avascular necrosis of the capitate. A case report and review of the literature. *J. Bone Joint Surg.* **66B**, 557–559.

Bonnarens F., Hernandez A. and D'Ambrosia R. (1985) Bone scintigraphic changes in osteonecrosis of the femoral head. *Orthop. Clin. North Am.* **16**, 697–703.

Brav E.A. (1962) Traumatic dislocation of the hip. Army experience and results over a twelve year period. *J. Bone Joint Surg.* **44A**, 1115–1134.

Brower A.C. (1983) The osteochondroses. *Orthop. Clin. North Am.* **14**, 99–117.

Buchanan J.R., Greer R.B., III and Cotler J.M. (1981) Management strategy for prevention of avascular necrosis during treatment of congenital dislocation of the hip. *J. Bone Joint Surg.* **63A**, 140–146.

Bullough P.G. and Di Carlo E.F. (1990) Subchondral avascular necrosis: a common cause of arthritis. *Ann. Rheum. Dis.* **49**, 412–420.

Burton D.S., Mochizuki R.M. and Halpern A.A. (1978) Total hip arthroplasty in the cardiac transplant patient. *Clin. Orthop.* **130**, 186–190.

Calandruccio R.A. and Anderson W.E., III (1980) Post-fracture avascular necrosis of the femoral head. Correlation of experimental and clinical studies. *Clin. Orthop.* **152**, 49–84.

Canale S.T. and Bourland W.L. (1977) Fracture of the neck and intertrochanteric region of the femur in children. *J. Bone Joint Surg.* **59A**, 431–444.

Catto M. (1965a) A histological study of avascular necrosis of the femoral head after transcervical fracture. *J. Bone Joint Surg.* **47B**, 749–776.

Catto M. (1965b) The histological appearances of late segmental collapse of the femoral head after transcervical fracture. *J. Bone Joint Surg.* **47B**, 777–791.

Catto M. (1976) Pathology of aseptic bone necrosis. In Davidson J.K. (ed) *Aseptic Necrosis of Bone.* Amsterdam, Elsevier, pp. 3–100.

Charache S. and Page D.L. (1967) Infarction of bone marrow in the sickle cell disorders. *Ann. Intern. Med.* **67**, 1195–1200.

Chevalier X., Larger-Piet B., Hernigou P. and Gherhardi R. (1993) Avascular necrosis of the femoral head in HIV-infected patients. *J. Bone Joint Surg.* **75B**, 160.

Chryssanthou C.P. (1978) Dysbaric osteonecrosis. Etiological and pathogenetic concepts. *Clin. Orthop.* **130**, 94–106.

Chung S.M.K., Alavi A. and Russell M.O. (1978) Management of osteonecrosis in sickle-cell anemia and its genetic variants. *Clin. Orthop.* **130**, 158–174.

Cockshott W.P. (1963) Dactylitis and growth disorders. *Br. J. Radiol.* **36**, 19–26.

Collier B.D., Carrera G.F., Johnson R.P. *et al.* (1985) Detection of femoral head avascular necrosis in adults by SPECT. *J. Nucl. Med.* **26**, 979–986.

Colonna P.C. and Jones E.D. (1948) Aeroembolism of bone marrow. An experimental study. *Arch. Surg.* **56**, 161–171.

Colwell C.W. (1989) The controversy of core decompression of the femoral head for osteonecrosis. *Arthritis Rheum.* **32**, 797–800.

Cooper C., Barker D.J.P., Morris J. and Briggs R.S.J. (1987) Osteoporosis, falls and age in fracture of the proximal femur. *BMJ* **295**, 13–15.

Crawfurd E.S.P., Emery R.J.H., Hansell D.M., Phelan M. and Andrews B.G. (1988) Capsular distension and intracapsular pressure in subcapital fractures of the femur. *J. Bone Joint Surg.* **70B**, 195–198.

Cruess R.L. (1978) Experience with steroid-induced avascular necrosis of the shoulder and etiologic considerations regarding osteonecrosis of the hip. *Clin. Orthop.* **130**, 86–93.

Cruess R.L. (1985) Corticosteroid-induced osteonecrosis of the humeral head. *Orthop. Clin. North Am.* **16**, 789–796.

Cruess R.L. (1986) Osteonecrosis of bone. Current concepts as to etiology and pathogenesis. *Clin. Orthop.* **208**, 30–39.

D'Ambrosia R.D., Shoji H., Riggins R.S. *et al.* (1978) Scintigraphy in the diagnosis of osteonecrosis. *Clin. Orthop.* **130**, 139–143.

Darlington L.G. (1985) Osteonecrosis at multiple sites in a patient with systemic lupus erythematosus. *Ann. Rheum. Dis.* **44**, 65–66.

Davidson J.K. (1976) Dysbaric osteonecrosis. In: Davidson J.K. (ed.) *Aseptic Necrosis of Bone.* Amsterdam, Elsevier, pp. 147–212.

Davidson J.K. (1989) Dysbaric disorders: aseptic bone necrosis in tunnel workers and divers. *Baillières Clin. Rheumatol.* **3**, 1–23.

Davidson J.K. and Griffiths P.D. (1970) Caisson disease of bone. *X-ray Focus* **10**, 2–11.

Davidson J.K., Tsakiris D., Briggs J.D. and Junor B.J. (1985) Osteonecrosis and fractures following renal transplantation. *Clin. Radiol.* **36**, 27–35.

Decompression Sickness Central Registry (1981) Aseptic bone necrosis in commercial divers. *Lancet* **ii**, 384–388.

Diggs L.W. (1967) Bone and joint lesions in sickle cell anemia. *Clin. Orthop.* **52**, 119–143.

Diggs L.W. and Anderson L.D. (1971) Aseptic necrosis of the head of the femur in sickle cell disease. In Zinn W.M. (ed.) *Idiopathic Ischemic Necrosis of the Femoral Head in Adults.* Stuttgart, Georg Thieme, pp. 107–111.

Dihlmann W. (1982) CT analysis of the upper end of the femur: the asterisk sign and ischemic necrosis of the femoral head. *Skeletal Radiol.* **8**, 251–258.

Donaldson W.F., Rodriguez E.E., Skovran M. *et al.* (1968) Traumatic dislocation of the hip in children. *J. Bone Joint Surg.* **50A**, 79–87.

Drane W.E. and Rudd T.G. (1985) Femoral head viability following hip fracture: prognostic role of radionuclide bone imaging. *Clin. Nucl. Med.* **10**, 141–146.

Dubois E.L. and Cozen L. (1960) Avascular (aseptic) bone necrosis associated with systemic lupus erythematosus. *JAMA* **174**, 966–971.

Ebong W.W. (1986) Acute osteomyelitis in Nigerians with sickle cell disease. *Ann. Rheum. Dis.* **45**, 911–915.

Engel I.A., Straus D.J., Lacher M., Lane J. and Smith J. (1981) Osteonecrosis in patients with malignant lymphoma: a review of twenty-five cases. *Cancer* **48**, 1245–1250.

Enright H., Haake R. and Weisdorf D. (1990) Avascular necrosis of bone: a common serious complication of allogeneic bone marrow transplantation. *Am. J. Med.* **89**, 733–738.

Epps C.H. Jr, Bryant d'O.D. III, Coles M.J.M. and Castro O. (1991) Osteomyelitis in patients who have sickle-cell disease. *J. Bone Joint Surg.* **73A**, 1281–1294.

Evans A., Barnard E.E.P. and Walder D.N. (1972) Detection of gas bubbles in man at decompression. *Aerosp. Med.* **43**, 1095–1096.

Felix C., Blatt J., Goodman M.A. and Medina J. (1985) Avascular necrosis of bone following combination chemotherapy for acute lymphoblastic leukemia. *Med. Pediatr. Oncol.* **13**, 269–272.

Felson D.T. and Anderson J.J. (1987) A cross-study evaluation between steroid dose and bolus steroids and avascular necrosis of bone. *Lancet* **i**, 902–905.

Ficat R.P. and Arlet J. (1968) Diagnostic de l'ostéonécrose femoro-capitale primitive au stade 1 (stade pré-radiologique). *Rev. Chir. Orthop.* **54**, 637–648.

Ficat R.P. (1983) Treatment of avascular necrosis of the femoral head. In Hungerford D.S. (ed.) *The Hip. Proceedings of the Eleventh Open Meeting of the Hip Society.* St Louis, CV Mosby, pp. 296–305.

Ficat R.P. (1985) Idiopathic bone necrosis of the femoral head. Early diagnosis and treatment. *J. Bone Joint Surg.* **67B**, 3–9.

Fishel B., Caspi D., Eventov I., Avrahami E. and Yaron M. (1987)

Multiple osteonecrotic lesions in systemic lupus erythematosus. *J. Rheumatol.* **14**, 601–603.

Fisher D.E. (1978) The role of fat embolism in the etiology of corticosteroid-induced avascular necrosis. *Clin. Orthop.* **130**, 68–80.

Fisher D.E. and Bickel W.H. (1971) Corticosteroid induced avascular necrosis. A clinical study of seventy-seven patients. *J. Bone Joint Surg.* **53A**, 859–873.

Frangakis E.K. (1966) Intracapsular fracture of the neck of the femur. *J. Bone Joint Surg.* **48B**, 17–30.

Frierson H.F., Fechner R.E., Stallings R.G. and Wang G.-J. (1987) Malignant fibrous histiocytoma in bone infarct. Association with sickle cell trait and alcohol abuse. *Cancer* **59**, 496–500.

Galli S.J., Weintraub H.P. and Proppe K.H. (1978) Malignant fibrous histiocytoma and pleomorphic sarcoma in association with medullary bone infarcts. *Cancer* **41**, 607–619.

Garden R.S. (1971) Malreduction and avascular necrosis in subcapital fractures of the femur. *J. Bone Joint Surg.* **53B**, 183–197.

Gerle R.D., Walker L.A., Achord J.L. *et al.* (1965) Osseous changes in chronic pancreatitis. *Radiology* **85**, 330–337.

Gerster J.C., Camus J.P., Chave J.P., Koeger A.C. and Rappoport G. (1991) Multiple site avascular necrosis in HIV infected patients. *J. Rheumatol.* **18**, 300–302.

Glimcher M.J. and Kenzora J.E. (1979a) The biology of osteonecrosis of the human femoral head and its clinical implications. I. Tissue biology. *Clin. Orthop.* **138**, 284–309.

Glimcher M.J. and Kenzora J.E. (1979b) II. The pathological changes in the femoral head as an organ and in the hip joint. *Clin. Orthop.* **139**, 283–312.

Glimcher M.J. and Kenzora J.E. (1979c) III. Discussion of the etiology and genesis of the pathological sequelae; comments on treatment. *Clin. Orthop.* **140**, 273–312.

Graham J. and Wood S.K. (1976) Aseptic necrosis of bone following trauma. In Davidson J.K. (ed) *Aseptic Necrosis of Bone.* Amsterdam, Elsevier, pp. 101–146.

Gregg P.J. and Walder D.N. (1980) Scintigraphy versus radiography in the early diagnosis of experimental bone necrosis with special reference to caisson disease of bone. *J. Bone Joint Surg.* **62B**, 214–221.

Gregg P.J. and Walder D.N. (1981) A study of old lesions of caisson disease of bone by radiography and bone scintigraphy. *J. Bone Joint Surg.* **63B**, 132–137.

Gregg P.J. and Walder D.N. (1986) Caisson disease of bone. *Clin. Orthop.* **210**, 43–54.

Gupta S.M., Foster C.R. and Kayani N. (1987) Usefulness of SPECT in the early detection of avascular necrosis of the knees. *Clin. Nucl. Med.* **12**, 99–102.

Hall M.C. and Hume D.M. (1970) Separation of massive avascular osteocartilaginous fragment of femoral condyle following renal transplantation. *J. Bone Joint Surg.* **52A**, 550–555.

Hallenbeck J.M. and Andersen J.C. (1982) Pathogenesis of the decompression disorders. In Bennett P.B. and Elliott D.H. (eds) *The Physiology and Medicine of Diving*, 3rd edn. London, Baillière Tindall, pp. 435–440.

Hanker G.J. and Amstutz H.C. (1988) Osteonecrosis of the hip in the sickle-cell diseases: treatment and complications. *J. Bone Joint Surg.* **70A**, 499–506.

Harper P.G., Trask C. and Souhami R.L. (1984) Avascular necrosis of bone caused by combination chemotherapy without corticosteroids. *BMJ* **288**, 267–268.

Harper W.M., Barnes M.R. and Gregg P.J. (1991) Femoral head blood flow in femoral neck fractures. An analysis using intraosseous pressure measurement. *J. Bone Joint Surg.* **73B**, 73–75.

Harrington K.D., Murray W.R., Kountz S.L. *et al.* (1971) Avascular necrosis of bone after renal transplantation. *J. Bone Joint Surg.* **53A**, 203–215.

Harrison J.A.B. (1971) Aseptic bone necrosis in naval clearance divers: radiographic findings. *Proc. R. Soc. Med.* **64**, 1276–1278.

Hartmann G. (1971) The possible role of fat metabolism in idiopathic ischemic necrosis of the femoral head. In Zinn M. (ed) *Idiopathic Ischemic Necrosis of the Femoral Head in Adults*. Stuttgart, Georg Thieme, pp. 140–144.

Hauzeur J.P., Pasteels J.L., Schoutens A. *et al.* (1989) The diagnostic value of magnetic resonance imaging in non-traumatic osteonecrosis of the femoral head. *J. Bone Joint Surg.* **71A**, 641–649.

Hawkins L.G. (1970) Fractures of the neck of the talus. *J. Bone Joint Surg.* **52A**, 991–1002.

Hernigou P., Galacteros F., Bachir D. and Goutallier D. (1991) Deformities of the hip in adults who have sickle-cell disease and had avascular necrosis in childhood. A natural history of fifty-two patients. *J. Bone Joint Surg.* **73A**, 81–92.

Hopson C.N. and Siverhus S.W. (1988) Ischemic necrosis of the femoral head: treatment by core decompression. *J. Bone Joint Surg.* **70A**, 1048–1051.

Horev G., Kornreich L., Hadar H. and Katz K. (1991) Hemorrhage associated with 'bone crisis' in Gaucher's disease identified by magnetic resonance imaging. *Skeletal Radiol.* **20**, 479–482.

Houpt J.B., Alpert B., Lotem M. *et al.* (1982) Spontaneous necrosis of the medial tibial plateau. *J. Rheumatol.* **9**, 81–90.

Hughes E.C. Jr, Schumacher H.R. and Sbarbaro J.L. Jr (1971) Bilateral avascular necrosis of the hip following Leriche syndrome. *J. Bone Joint Surg.* **53A**, 380–382.

Humphreys S., Spencer J.D., Tighe J.R. and Cumming R.R. (1989) The femoral head in osteonecrosis. A quantitative study of osteocyte population. *J. Bone Joint Surg.* **71B**, 205–208.

Hungerford D.S. (1989) The role of core decompression in the treatment of ischemic necrosis of the femoral head. *Arthritis Rheum.* **32**, 801–806.

Hungerford D.S. and Lennox D.W. (1985) The importance of increased intraosseous pressure in the development of osteonecrosis of the femoral head: implications for treatment. *Orthop. Clin. North Am.* **16**, 635–654.

Hungerford D.S. and Zizic T.M. (1978) Alcoholism associated ischemic necrosis of the femoral head. Early diagnosis and treatment. *Clin. Orthop.* **130**, 144–153.

Hungerford D.S. and Zizic T.M. (1983) Pathogenesis of ischemic necrosis of the femoral head. In Hungerford D.S. (ed) *The Hip. Proceedings of the Eleventh Open Scientific Meeting of the Hip Society*. St Louis, CV Mosby, pp. 249–262.

Hunter G.A. (1983) The rationale for internal fixation and against hemiarthroplasty. In Hungerford D.S. (ed.) *The Hip. Proceedings of the Eleventh Open Scientific Meeting of the Hip Society*. St Louis, CV Mosby, pp. 34–41.

Ibels L.S., Alfrey A.C., Huffer W.E. *et al.* (1978) Aseptic necrosis of bone following renal transplantation. *Medicine* **57**, 25–45.

Ihde D.C. and DeVita V.T. (1975) Osteonecrosis of the femoral head in patients with lymphoma treated with intermittent combination chemotherapy (including corticosteroids). *Cancer* **36**, 1585–1588.

Ilardi C.F. and Sokoloff L. (1984) Secondary osteonecrosis in osteoarthritis of the femoral head. *Hum. Pathol.* **15**, 79–83.

Inoue A. and Ono K. (1979) A histological study of idiopathic avascular necrosis of the head of the femur. *J. Bone Joint Surg.* **61B**, 138–143.

Isono S.S., Woolson S.T. and Schurman D.J. (1987) Total joint arthroplasty for steroid-induced osteonecrosis in cardiac transplant patients. *Clin. Orthop.* **217**, 201–208.

Iwegbu C.G. and Fleming A.F. (1985) Avascular necrosis of the femoral head in sickle-cell disease. *J. Bone Joint Surg.* **67B**, 29–32.

Jacobs B. (1978) Epidemiology of traumatic and non-traumatic osteonecrosis. *Clin. Orthop.* **130**, 51–67.

Jaffe H.L. (1972) In *Metabolic, Degenerative and Inflammatory Diseases of Bones and Joints.* Philadelphia, Lea & Febiger, pp. 506–522.

James C.C.M. (1945) Late bone lesions in caisson disease: 3 cases in submarine personnel. *Lancet* **ii**, 6–8.

Jergesen H.E., Heller M. and Genant H.K. (1985) Magnetic resonance imaging in osteonecrosis of the femoral head. *Orthop. Clin. North Am.* **16**, 705–716.

Jergesen H., Heller M. and Genant H. (1990a) Signal variability in magnetic resonance imaging of femoral head osteonecrosis. *Clin. Orthop.* **253**, 137–149.

Jergesen H., Lang P., Moseley M. and Genant H. (1990b) Histologic correlation in magnetic resonance imaging of femoral head osteonecrosis. *Clin. Orthop.* **253**, 150–163.

Johnson J.T.H. and Crothers O. (1976) Revascularization of the femoral head. A clinical and experimental study. *Clin. Orthop.* **114**, 364–373.

Johnson L.A., Hoppel B.E., Gerard E.L. *et al.* (1992) Quantitative chemical shift imaging of vertebral bone marrow in patients with Gaucher disease. *Radiology* **182**, 451–455.

Johnson L.C. (1964) Histogenesis of avascular necrosis. In *Proceedings of the Conference on Aseptic Necrosis of the Femoral Head.* St. Louis, National Institutes of Health, pp. 55–77.

Jones A.G., Francis M.D. and Davis M.A. (1976) Bone scanning: radionuclide reaction mechanisms. *Semin. Nucl. Med.* **6**, 3–18.

Jones J.P. Jr (1971) Alcoholism, hypercortisonism, fat embolism and osseous avascular necrosis. In Zinn W.M. (ed) *Idiopathic Ischemic Necrosis of the Femoral Head in Adults.* Stuttgart, Georg Thieme, pp. 112–132.

Jones J.P. Jr (1985) Fat embolism and osteonecrosis. *Orthop. Clin. North Am.* **16**, 595–633.

Jones J.P. Jr (1992) Intravascular coagulation and osteonecrosis. *Clin. Orthop.* **277**, 41–53.

Jones J.P. Jr and Sakovich L. (1966) Fat embolism of bone. A roentgenographic and histological investigation with use of intra-arterial lipiodol in rabbits. *J. Bone Joint Surg.* **48A**, 149–164.

Kawai K., Tamaki A. and Hirohata K. (1985) Steroid-induced accumulation of lipid in the osteocytes of the rabbit femoral head. A histochemical and electron microscopic study. *J. Bone Joint Surg.* **67A**, 755–763.

Kawashima M., Torisu T., Hayashi K. *et al.* (1978) Pathological review of osteonecrosis in divers. *Clin. Orthop.* **130**, 107–117.

Keeley K. and Buchanan G.R. (1982) Acute infarction of long bones in children with sickle-cell anemia. *J. Pediatr.* **101**, 170–175.

Kenzora J.E. (1985) Treatment of idiopathic osteonecrosis: the current philosophy and rationale. *Orthop. Clin. North Am.* **16**, 717–725.

Kenzora J.E. and Glimcher M.J. (1985) Accumulative cell stress: the multifactorial etiology of idiopathic osteonecrosis. *Orthop.*

Clin. North Am. **16**, 669–679.

Kenzora J.E., Steele R.E., Yosipovitch M.D. *et al.* (1978) Experimental osteonecrosis of the femoral head in rabbits. *Clin. Orthop.* **130**, 8–46.

Kindwall E.P., Nellen J.R. and Spiegelhoff D.R. (1982) Aseptic necrosis in compressed air tunnel workers using current OSHA decompression schedules. *J. Occup. Med.* **24**, 741–745.

Klenerman L. and Marcuson R.W. (1970) Intracapsular fractures of the neck of the femur. *J. Bone Joint Surg.* **52B**, 514–517.

Klippel J.H., Gerber L.H., Pollak L. and Decker J.L. (1979) Avascular necrosis in systemic lupus erythematosus – silent symmetric osteonecrosis. *Am. J. Med.* **67**, 83–87.

Köberle G. and Constant R.B. (1979) Avascular necrosis or late segmental collapse? *Clin. Orthop.* **141**, 310–311.

Kodish E., Lantos J., Siegler M., Kohrman A. and Johnson F.L. (1990) Bone marrow transplantation in sickle-cell disease. *Clin. Res.* **38**, 694–700.

Kristensen K.D., Kiaer T. and Pedersen N.W. (1989) Intraosseous PO$_2$ in femoral neck fracture; restoration of bloodflow after aspiration of hemarthrosis in undisplaced fractures. *Acta Orthop. Scand.* **60**, 303–304.

Labowitz R. and Schumacher H.R. Jr (1971) Articular manifestations of systemic lupus erythematosus. *Ann. Intern. Med.* **74**, 911–921.

Lally E.V., Buckley W.M. and Claster S. (1983) Diaphyseal bone infarctions in a patient with sickle cell trait. *J. Rheumatol.* **10**, 813–816.

Lam T.H. and Yau K.P. (1992) Dysbaric osteonecrosis in a compressed air tunnelling project in Hong Kong. *Occup. Med.* **42**, 23–29.

Landmann J., Renner N., Gächter A., Thiel G. and Harder F. (1987) Cyclosporin A and osteonecrosis of the femoral head. *J. Bone Joint Surg.* **69A**, 1226–1228.

Lang P., Jergesen H.E., Moseley M.E., Block J.E., Chafetz N.I. and Genant H.K. (1988) Avascular necrosis of the femoral head: high-field-strength MR imaging with histologic correlation. *Radiology* **169**, 517–524.

Langevitz P., Buskila D., Stewart J., Sherrard D.J. and Hercz G. (1990) Osteonecrosis in patients receiving dialysis: report of two cases and review of the literature. *J. Rheumatol.* **17**, 402–406.

Laroche H., Arlet J. and Mazières B. (1990) Osteonecrosis of the femoral and humeral heads after intra-articular corticosteroid injections. *J. Rheumatol.* **17**, 549–551.

Lausten G.S. and Christensen S.B. (1989) Distribution of ^{99m}Tc-phosphate compounds in osteonecrotic femoral heads. *Acta Orthop. Scand.* **60**, 419–423.

Lausten G.S. and Mathiesen B. (1990) Core decompression for femoral head necrosis: prospective study of 28 patients. *Acta Orthop. Scand.* **61**, 507–511.

Lausten G.S., Jensen J.S. and Olgaard K. (1988) Necrosis of the femoral head after renal transplantation. *Acta Orthop. Scand.* **59**, 650–654.

Ledingham I.A. and Davidson J.K. (1969) Hazards in hyperbaric medicine. *BMJ* **3**, 324–327.

Lee C.K., Hansen H.T. and Weiss A.B. (1980) The 'silent hip' of idiopathic ischemic necrosis of the femoral head in adults. *J. Bone Joint Surg.* **62A**, 795–800.

Lee M.J., Corrigan J., Stack J.P. and Ennis J.T. (1990) A comparison of modern imaging modalities in osteonecrosis of the femoral head. *Clin. Radiol.* **42**, 427–432.

Lee R.E., Golding J.S.R. and Serjeant G.R. (1981) The radiological features of avascular necrosis of the femoral head in homozygous sickle cell disease. *Clin. Radiol.* **32**, 205−214.

Leventhal G.H. and Dorfman H.D. (1974) Aseptic necrosis of bone in systemic lupus erythematosus. *Semin. Arthritis Rheum.* **4**, 73−93.

Lotke P.A. and Ecker M.L. (1985) Osteonecrosis of the knee. *Orthop. Clin. North Am.* **16**, 797−808.

Lotke P.A. and Ecker M.L. (1988) Current concepts review. Osteonecrosis of the knee. *J. Bone Joint Surg.* **70A**, 470−473.

McCallum R.I. (1974) Osteonecrosis in tunnel and caisson workers. In Beckman E.L. and Elliott D.H. (eds) *Dysbarism-Related Osteonecrosis.* Symposium. Washington, US Department of Health, Education and Welfare, pp. 3−6.

McCallum R.I., Walder D.N., Barnes R. *et al.* (1966) Bone lesions in compressed air workers. *J. Bone Joint Surg.* **48B**, 207−235.

McCollum D.E., Mathews R.S. and O'Neil M.T. (1970) Aseptic necrosis of the femoral head. *South. Med. J.* **63**, 241−253.

McKibbin B. and Ralis Z. (1974) Pathological changes in a case of Perthes' disease. *J. Bone Joint Surg.* **56B**, 438−447.

Maistrelli G., Fusco U., Avai A. and Bombelli R. (1988) Osteonecrosis of the hip treated by intertrochanteric osteotomy. *J. Bone Joint Surg.* **70B**, 761−766.

Mankin H.J. (1992) Current concepts. Non-traumatic necrosis of bone (osteonecrosis). *N. Engl. J. Med.* **326**, 1473−1479.

Mankin H.J. (1993) Gaucher's disease: a novel treatment and an important breakthrough. *J. Bone Joint Surg.* **75B**, 2−3.

Mankin H.J., Doppelt S.H., Rosenberg A.E. and Barranger J.A. (1990) Metabolic bone disease in patients with Gaucher's disease. In Avioli L.V., Krane S.M. (eds) *Metabolic Bone Disease,* 2nd edn. Philadelphia, WB Saunders Company, pp. 730−752.

Marcus N.D., Enneking W.F. and Masson R.A. (1973) The silent hip in idiopathic necrosis. *J. Bone Joint Surg.* **55A**, 1351−1366.

Markham T.N. (1967) Aseptic necrosis in a high altitude flier. *J. Occup. Med.* **9**, 123−126.

Markisz J.A., Knowles R.J.R., Altcheck D.W., Schneider R., Whalen J.P. and Cahill P.T. (1987) Segmental patterns of avascular necrosis of the femoral heads: early detection with MR imaging. *Radiology* **162**, 717−720.

Marmor L. (1984) Osteonecrosis of the knee: medial and lateral involvement. *Clin. Orthop.* **185**, 195−196.

Marymont J.V. and Kaufman E.E. (1986) Osteonecrosis of bone associated with combination chemotherapy without corticosteroids. *Clin. Orthop.* **204**, 150−153.

Mascarin M., Giavitto M., Zanazzo G.-A. *et al.* (1991) Avascular necrosis of bone in children undergoing allogeneic bone marrow transplantation. *Cancer* **68**, 655−659.

Massie W.K. (1973) Treatment of femoral neck fractures emphasizing longterm follow up and observations on aseptic necrosis. *Clin. Orthop.* **92**, 16−62.

Matsuo K., Hirohata T., Sugioka Y., Ikeda M. and Fukuda A. (1988) Influence of alcohol intake, cigarette smoking and occupational status on idiopathic osteonecrosis of the femoral head. *Clin. Orthop.* **234**, 115−123.

Melamed Y., Shupak A. and Bitterman H. (1992) Current concepts: medical problems associated with underwater diving. *N. Engl. J. Med.* **326**, 30−35.

Merle d'Aubigné R., Postel M., Mazabraud A. *et al.* (1965) Idiopathic necrosis of the femoral head in adults. *J. Bone Joint Surg.* **47B**, 612−633.

Michael R.H. and Dorfman H.D. (1976) Malignant fibrous histiocytoma associated with bone infarcts. Report of a case. *Clin. Orthop.* **118**, 180−183.

Middlemiss H. (1976) Aseptic necrosis and other changes occurring in bone in the haemoglobinopathies. In Davidson J.K. (ed) *Aseptic Necrosis of Bone.* Amsterdam, Elsevier, pp. 271−300.

Milgram J.W. (1984) Reparative cartilaginous callus in subarticular osteonecrosis of bone. *Clin. Orthop.* **186**, 272−283.

Milgram J.W. (1990) *Radiologic and Histologic Pathology of Nontumorous Diseases of Bones and Joints.* Northbrook, Illinois. Northbrook Publishing Company Inc., pp. 1027−1050.

Milgram J.W. and Riley L.H. Jr (1976) Steroid induced avascular necrosis of bones in eighteen sites. A case report. *Bull. Hosp. Joint Dis.* **37**, 11−23.

Milner P.F., Kraus A.P., Sebes J.I. *et al.* (1991) Sickle cell disease as a cause of osteonecrosis of the femoral head. *N. Engl. J. Med.* **325**, 1476−1481.

Mitchell D.G., Rao V.M., Dalinka M.K. *et al.* (1987a) Femoral head avascular necrosis: correlation of MR imaging, radiographic staging, radionuclide imaging and clinical findings. *Radiology* **162**, 709−715.

Mitchell D.G., Joseph P.M., Fallon M. *et al.* (1987b) Chemical-shift MR imaging of the femoral head: in vitro study of normal hips and hips with avascular necrosis. *AJR Am. J. Roentgenol.* **148**, 1159−1164.

Mitchell D.G., Steinberg M.E., Dalinka M.K., Rao V.M., Fallon M. and Kressel H.Y. (1989) Magnetic resonance imaging of the ischemic hip. Alterations within the osteonecrotic, viable and reactive zones. *Clin. Orthop.* **244**, 60−77.

Murphy R.G. and Greenberg M.L. (1990) Osteonecrosis in pediatric patients with acute lymphoblastic leukaemia. *Cancer* **65**, 1717−1721.

Murray R.O. and Jacobson H.G. (1971) *The Radiology of Skeletal Disorders.* Edinburgh, Churchill Livingstone.

Mussbichler H. (1970) Arteriographic findings in necrosis of the head of the femur after medial neck fracture. *Acta Orthop. Scand.* **41**, 77−90.

Nachamie B.A. and Dorfman H.D. (1974) Ischemic necrosis of bone in sickle cell trait. *J. Mt. Sinai Hosp.* **41**, 527−536.

Newman N.M. and Ling R.S.M. (1985) Acetabular bone destruction related to non-steroidal anti-inflammatory drugs. *Lancet* **ii,** 11−14.

Nicoll E.A. (1952) Traumatic dislocation of the hip joint. *J. Bone Joint Surg.* **34B**, 503.

Norman A. and Bullough P. (1963) The radiolucent crescent line: an early diagnostic sign of avascular necrosis of the femoral head. *Bull. Hosp. Jt. Dis.* **24**, 99−104.

O'Brien T.J. and Mack G.R. (1992) Multifocal osteonecrosis after short term high-dose corticosteroid therapy: a case report. *Clin. Orthop.* **279**, 176−179.

O'Doherty D.P., Lowrie I.G. and Gregg P.J. (1987) Caisson disease of the talus: brief report. *J. Bone Joint Surg.* **69B**, 847−848.

Ohta Y. and Matsunaga H. (1974) Bone lesions in divers. *J. Bone Joint Surg.* **56B**, 3−16.

Orlić D., Jovanovic S., Antičević D. and Zečević J. (1990) Frequency of idiopathic aseptic necrosis in medically treated alcoholics. *Int. Orthop.* **14**, 383−386.

Palmer A.K., Henzinger R.N., Costenbader J.M. and Bassett D.R. (1981) Osteonecrosis of the femoral head in a family with hyperlipoproteinemia. *Clin. Orthop.* **155**, 166−171.

Park W.M. (1976) Spontaneous and drug-induced aseptic necrosis. In Davidson J.K. (ed) *Aseptic Necrosis of Bone.* Amsterdam, Elsevier, pp. 213−269.

Patterson R.J., Bickel W.H. and Dahlin D.C. (1964) Idiopathic avascular necrosis of the head of the femur. A study of fifty two cases. *J. Bone Joint Surg.* **46A**, 267–282.

Pearson R.R., Macleod M.A., McEwan A.J.B. and Houston A.S. (1982) Bone scintigraphy as an investigative aid for dysbaric osteonecrosis in divers. *J. R. Nav. Med. Serv.* **68**, 61–68.

Pellici P.M., Zolla-Pazner S., Rabhan W.N. and Wilson P.D. Jr (1984) Osteonecrosis of the femoral head associated with pregnancy. Report of three cases. *Clin. Orthop.* **185**, 59–63.

Phemister D.B. (1934) Fractures of the neck of the femur, dislocations of hip and obscure vascular disturbances producing aseptic necrosis of head of femur. *Surg. Gynecol. Obstet.* **59**, 415–440.

Pierides A.M., Simpson W., Stainsby D. *et al.* (1975) Avascular necrosis of bone following renal transplantation. *Q. J. Med.* **44**, 459–480.

Pietrogrande V. and Mastromarino R. (1957) Osteopatia da prolungata trattamento cortisonico. *Ortop. Traumatol.* **25**, 791–810.

Pollack M.S., Dalinka M.K., Kressel H.Y., Lotke P.A. and Spritzer C.E. (1987) Magnetic resonance imaging in the evaluation of suspected osteonecrosis of the knee. *Skeletal Radiol.* **16**, 121–127.

Prosnitz L.R., Lawson J.P., Friedlander G.E., Farber L.R. and Pezzimenti J.F. (1981) Avascular necrosis of bone in Hodgkin's disease patients treated with combined modality therapy. *Cancer* **47**, 2793–2797.

Ragnarsson J.I., Ekelund L., Karrholm J. and Hietala S.-O. (1989) Lowfield magnetic resonance imaging of femoral neck fractures. *Acta Radiol.* **30**, 247–252.

Rand J.A., Linscheid R.L. and Dobyns J.H. (1982) Capitate fractures. A longterm follow-up. *Clin. Orthop.* **165**, 209–216.

Rao V.M., Fishman M., Mitchell D.G. *et al.* (1986) Painful sickle cell crisis. Bone marrow patterns observed with MR imaging. *Radiology* **161**, 211–215.

Roseff R. and Canoso J.J. (1984) Femoral osteonecrosis following soft tissue corticosteroid infiltration. *Am. J. Med.* **77**, 1119–1120.

Rosenthal D.I., Scott J.A., Barranger J. *et al.* (1986) Evaluation of Gaucher disease using magnetic resonance imaging. *J. Bone Joint Surg.* **68A**, 802–808.

Rossleigh M.A., Smith J., Straus D.J. and Engel I.A. (1986) Osteonecrosis in patients with malignant lymphoma. A review of 31 cases. *Cancer* **58**, 1112–1116.

Rourke J.A. and Heslin D.J. (1965) Gaucher's disease. Roentgenologic bone changes over 20 years interval. *AJR Am. J. Roentgenol.* **94**, 621–630.

Rozing P.M., Insall J. and Bohne W.H. (1980) Spontaneous osteonecrosis of the knee. *J. Bone Joint Surg.* **62A**, 2–7.

Ruland L.J. III, Wang G.-J., Teates C.D., Gay S. and Rijke A. (1992) A comparison of magnetic resonance imaging to bone scintigraphy in early traumatic ischemia of the femoral head. *Clin. Orthop.* **285**, 30–34.

Sambrook P.N., Hassall J.E. and York J.R. (1984) Osteonecrosis after high dosage: short-term corticosteroid therapy. *J. Rheumatol.* **11**, 514–516.

Santos J.V. (1930) Changes in the head of the femur after complete intracapsular fracture of the neck. *Arch. Surg.* **21**, 484–530.

Serre H. and Simon L. L'ostéonécrose primitive de la tête fémorale chez l'adulte. (1961) *Acta Rheum. Scand.* **7**, 265–286.

Sevitt S. (1964) Avascular necrosis and revascularisation of the femoral head after intracapsular fractures. *J. Bone Joint Surg.* **46B**, 270–296.

Sevitt S. (1981) *Bone Repair and Fracture Healing in Man.* Edinburgh, Churchill Livingstone.

Sevitt S. and Thompson R.G. (1965) The distribution and anastomoses of arteries supplying the head and neck of the femur. *J. Bone Joint Surg.* **47B**, 560–573.

Sherman M. (1959) Pathogenesis of disintegration of the hip in sickle cell anemia. *South. Med. J.* **52**, 632–637.

Sherman M.S. and Phemister D.B. (1947) The pathology of ununited fractures of the neck of the femur. *J. Bone Joint Surg.* **29**, 19–40.

Siemsen J.K., Brook J. and Meister L. (1962) Lupus erythematosus and avascular bone necrosis. *Arthritis Rheum.* **5**, 492–501.

Sikorski J.M. and Barrington R. (1981) Internal fixation versus hemi-arthroplasty for the displaced subcapital fracture of the femur: a prospective study. *J. Bone Joint Surg.* **63B**, 357–361.

Silman A.J. (1992) Epidemiology in orthopaedics in the 1990s. In Catterall A. (ed) *Recent Advances in Orthopaedics.* Edinburgh, Churchill Livingstone, pp. 1–13.

Sissons H.A., Nuovo M.A. and Steiner G.C. (1992) Pathology of osteonecrosis of the femoral head. A review of experience at the Hospital for Joint Diseases, New York. *Skeletal Radiol.* **21**, 229–238.

Smith F.B. (1959) Effects of rotatory and valgus malpositions on blood supply to the femoral head. *J. Bone Joint Surg.* **41A**, 800–815.

Solomon L. (1973) Drug-induced arthropathy and necrosis of the femoral head. *J. Bone Joint Surg.* **55B**, 246–261.

Solomon L. (1985) Mechanisms of idiopathic osteonecrosis. *Orthop. Clin. North Am.* **16**, 655–667.

Speer K.P., Spritzer C.E., Harrelson J.M. and Nunley J.A. (1990) Magnetic resonance imaging of the femoral head after acute intracapsular fracture of the femoral neck. *J. Bone Joint Surg.* **72A**, 98–103.

Spencer J.D. and Brookes M. (1988) Avascular necrosis and the blood supply of the femoral head. *Clin. Orthop.* **235**, 127–140.

Springfield D.S. and Enneking W.F. (1976) Idiopathic aseptic necrosis. In Ackerman L.V., Spjut H.J. and Abel M.R. (eds) *Bones and Joints.* Baltimore, Williams and Wilkins, pp. 61–87.

Starzl T.E., Marchioro T.L., Porter K.A. *et al.* (1964) Renal homotransplantation. Late function and complications. *Ann. Intern. Med.* **61**, 470–497.

Stevens M.C.G., Padwick M. and Serjeant G.R. (1981) Observations on the natural history of dactylitis in homozygous sickle cell disease. *Clin. Pediatr.* **20**, 311–317.

Stulberg B.N., Bauer T.W. and Belhobek G.H. (1990) Making core decompression work. *Clin. Orthop.* **261**, 186–195.

Stulberg B.N., Davis A.W., Bauer T.W., Levine M. and Easley K. (1991) Osteonecrosis of the femoral head: a prospective randomized treatment protocol. *Clin. Orthop.* **268**, 140–151.

Sweetnam D.R., Mason R.M. and Murray R.O. (1960) Steroid arthropathy of the hip. *BMJ* **1**, 1392–1394.

Takatori Y., Kokubo T., Ninomiya S., Nakamura S., Morimoto S. and Kusaba I. (1993) Avascular necrosis of the femoral head. Natural history and magnetic resonance imaging. *J. Bone Joint Surg.* **75B**, 217–221.

Tawn D.I. and Watt I. (1989) Bone marrow scintigraphy in the diagnosis of post traumatic avascular necrosis of bone. *Br. J. Radiol.* **62**, 790–795.

Taylor L.J. (1984) Multifocal avascular necrosis after short-term high-dose steroid therapy. *J. Bone Joint Surg.* **66B**, 431–433.

Theis J.C. and Owen R. (1988) Skeletal complications in sickle cell disease in the UK. *J. R. Coll. Surg. Edinb.* **33**, 306–310.

Thomas I.H. and Walder D.N. (1984) The effect of compressed air on marrow fat cell size in the rabbit femur. *J. Bone Joint Surg.* **66B**, 290.

Thorne J.C., Evans W.K., Alison R.E. and Fornasier V. (1981) Avascular necrosis of bone complicating treatment of malignant lymphoma. *Am. J. Med.* **71**, 751–758.

Todd R.C., Freeman M.A.R. and Pirie C.J. (1972) Isolated trabecular fatigue fractures in the femoral head. *J. Bone Joint Surg.* **54B**, 723–728.

Todd R.M. and Keidan S.E. (1952) Changes in the head of the femur in children suffering from Gaucher's disease. *J. Bone Joint Surg.* **34B**, 447–453.

Tooke S.M.T., Nugent P.J., Bassett L.W. *et al.* (1988) Results of core decompression for femoral head osteonecrosis. *Clin. Orthop.* **228**, 99–104.

Trueta J. and Harrison M.H.M. (1953) The normal vascular anatomy of the femoral head in adult man. *J. Bone Joint Surg.* **35B**, 442–461.

Turner D.A., Templeton A.C., Selzer P.M., Rosenberg A.G. and Petasnick J.P. (1989) Femoral capital osteonecrosis: MR finding of diffuse marrow abnormalities without focal lesions. *Radiology* **171**, 135–140.

Turner J.H. (1983) Post-traumatic avascular necrosis of the femoral head predicted by pre-operative technetium-99 antimony-colloid scan. An experimental and clinical study. *J. Bone Joint Surg.* **65A**, 786–797.

Van Blarcom S.T., Czarnecki D.J., Fueredi G.A. and Wenzel M.S. (1990) Does dysbaric osteonecrosis progress in the absence of further hyperbaric exposure? A ten year radiologic follow-up of 15 patients. *AJR Am. J. Roentgenol.* **155**, 95–97.

Vander Grend R., Dell P.C., Glowczewskie F., Leslie B. and Ruby L.K. (1984) Intraosseous blood supply of the capitate and its correlation with aseptic necrosis. *J. Hand Surg.* **9A**, 677–680.

Walder D.N. (1974) Management and treatment of osteonecrosis in divers and caisson workers. In Beckman E.L. and Elliott D.H. (eds) *Dysbarism-Related Osteonecrosis.* Symposium. Washington, US Department of Health, Education and Welfare, pp. 195–199.

Wang G.-J., Sweet D.E., Reger S.I. and Thompson R.C. (1977) Fat-cell changes as a mechanism of avascular necrosis of the femoral head in cortisone treated rabbits. *J. Bone Joint Surg.* **59A**, 729–735.

Ware H.E., Brooks A.P., Toye R. and Berney S.I. (1991) Sickle cell disease and silent avascular necrosis of the hip. *J. Bone Joint Surg.* **73B**, 947–949.

Watanabe Y., Kawai K. and Hirohata K. (1989) Histopathology of femoral head osteonecrosis in rheumatoid arthritis: the relationship between steroid therapy and lipid degeneration in the osteocyte. *Rheumatol. Int.* **9**, 25–31.

Weatherly C.R., Gregg P.J., Walder D.N. *et al.* (1977) Aseptic necrosis of bone in a compressed air worker. *J. Bone Joint Surg.* **59B**, 80–84.

Weinberg A.G. and Currarino G. (1972) Sickle cell dactylitis: histopathologic observations. *Am. J. Clin. Pathol.* **58**, 518–523.

Welfling J. (1971) Hip lesions in decompression sickness. In Zinn W.M. (ed.) *Idiopathic Ischemic Necrosis of the Femoral Head in Adults.* Stuttgart, Georg Thieme, pp. 103–106.

Worrall V.T. and Butera V. (1976) Sickle cell dactylitis. *J. Bone Joint Surg.* **58A**, 1161–1163.

Yosipovitch Z. and Katz K. (1990) Bone crisis in Gaucher's disease: an update. *Isr. J. Med. Sci.* **26**, 593–595.

Zimran A., Sorge J., Gross E., Kubitz M., West C. and Beutler E. (1989) Prediction of severity of Gaucher's disease by identification of mutations at DNA level. *Lancet* **ii**, 349–352.

Zinn W.M. (1971) Clinical picture and laboratory findings. Results of a Swiss multi-centre study. In Zinn W.M. (ed.) *Idiopathic Ischemic Necrosis of the Femoral Head in Adults.* Stuttgart, Georg Thieme, pp. 9–33.

Zizic T.M., Marcoux C., Hungerford D.S., Dansereau J.V. and Stevens M.B. (1985) Corticosteroid therapy associated with ischemic necrosis of bone in systemic lupus erythematosus. *Am. J. Med.* **79**, 596–604.

Chapter 17
Rheumatoid Arthritis and Related Diseases

Chapter 17.1
Pathology

P.J.L. Holt

INTRODUCTION

The inflammatory chronic polyarthritides are a spectrum of diseases with clinical and pathological similarities, some of which may be highly characteristic allowing classification, in crude terms, by the different proportion of features found in each disease. Such features include the rheumatoid nodule, terminal interphalangeal synovitis in psoriatic arthropathy, raised titres of antibodies to native DNA in systemic lupus erythematosus and, in a negative sense, the relative necessity for the presence of the histocompatibility antigen HLA B27 before making a diagnosis of ankylosing spondylitis. Synovitis, which is the prime pathological change producing arthritis in these conditions, usually does not differ greatly between different diseases and aetiological processes. The damage done by the synovitis may be markedly different, however, cartilage destruction and bone erosion being much more pronounced in rheumatoid factor-positive rheumatoid arthritis. Moreover, these are not static diseases; some features change as the disease fluctuates, e.g. the rheumatoid nodule and level of anti-DNA antibodies, while others are permanent, e.g. the histocompatibility antigen HLA B27. Thus, the initial diagnosis may be only tentative until evolution of the disease features leads to a clearer clinical picture. The clinical investigator sees patients and reviews specimens at various stages of this spectrum and is asked to produce a coherent pathogenic schema from incomplete and varying data. The rather unscientific basis by which these clinical diagnoses are arrived at can be seen from the disparate criteria used for the diagnosis of rheumatoid arthritis (Ropes *et al.*, 1958; revised Arnett *et al.*, 1988) (Table 17.1.1), though in fairness these criteria were originally designed primarily for epidemiological classification.

The use of the term 'rheumatoid arthritis' implies that arthritis is an essential feature, and the above criteria lay great stress on the articular changes. The non-articular systemic aspects, however, are equally likely to influence morbidity, and as long ago as 1949 Ellman introduced the term 'rheumatoid disease' to change the clinical emphasis from the joints to systemic disease. This is not a semantic question, as the concept of rheumatoid disease implies that articular features may be absent or minor while systemic disease may be severe. Furthermore, at the extremes of the rheumatoid spectrum, overlap with other diseases, e.g. systemic lupus erythematosus and polyarteritis nodosa, occurs in both clinical and pathological features (Gardner, 1992).

As these are diverse diseases, it is perhaps more useful to discuss the aetiopathogenesis of the various changes found, which when put together make up a syndrome, rather than to discuss the pathogenesis of a disease syndrome as such.

In considering pathogenesis, some attempt must be made to distinguish between primary and secondary events. Thus, many of the alterations in immunological and biochemical features probably have little pathological significance, certainly as presently understood. They do, however, attract much attention.

In essence, the pathology of rheumatoid disease can be considered in three parts:

1 Synovitis giving rise to cartilage, bone, tendon or ligament destruction.

2 Vasculitis with widespread secondary changes due to ischaemia and resulting fibrosis. The tendency to fibrosis may in fact be enhanced in rheumatoid disease, hence the characteristic tendency to nodule formation. Vasculitic changes underlie many of the systemic features of this disease.

3 Secondary changes, e.g. rises in immunoglobulin and acute phase reactants, whose immediate interest is as markers of disease activity but whose prime importance may be as modulators of inflammation and thus disease activity: anaemia and conditions such as Sjögren's syndrome and chronic uveitis (in children) and acute uveitis

Table 17.1.1 American Rheumatism Association criteria for the diagnosis of rheumatoid arthritis

Ropes *et al.*, 1958	Arnett *et al.*, 1988
1 Morning stiffness	1 Morning stiffness for more than 1 h
2 Pain on motion or tenderness in a joint	2 Arthritis in three or more joint areas
3 Swelling of joint due to fluid or soft tissue	3 Arthritis of hand joints
4 Swelling of second joint	4 Symmetrical arthritis
5 Symmetrical joint swelling, i.e. involving right and left	5 Rheumatoid nodules
6 Typical rheumatoid nodules	6 Typical radiographic changes (hand or wrist)
7 Typical radiographic changes including periarticular osteopenia	7 Serum rheumatoid factor
8 Positive test for serum rheumatoid factor	
9 Synovial fluid forming poor mucin clot with dilute acetic acid	
10 Characteristic synovial histology	
11 Characteristic histology of rheumatoid nodule	
Criteria 1–5 must be present for at least 6 weeks	Criteria 1–4 must be present for at least 6 weeks
If seven of these criteria are present the diagnosis is classic rheumatoid arthritis; if five are present, it is definite rheumatoid arthritis; if three are present, probable rheumatoid arthritis.	No differentiation into type of arthritis
Note: These features have no weighting.	

(in adults), where an association with certain types of inflammatory arthritis is found, though why this happens is unknown. The rheumatoid factors and lymphocyte abnormalities will be treated in this section, as at present there is little evidence that they initiate the diseases.

These features will be studied separately, though they may of course occur concurrently.

SYNOVITIS

Synovial reaction

This is thought to be the earliest event in most cases of rheumatoid disease and in all cases of chronic inflammatory arthritis. For a variety of reasons, however, studies of the early pathological change in humans are few. Where available, these agree with those found in animal models. The early macroscopic changes and subsequent progression have been assessed by arthroscopy of knees at various stages of the disease and compared with the clinical features.

Initial vascularization is followed by hyperplasia and pannus formation, initially of the meniscii and later of the articular cartilage. At all stages the changes in the meniscii are more advanced and severe than those in the cartilage. Radiological changes are relatively late. The use of magnetic resonance imaging may provide earlier and better documentation of the articular changes. Kulka *et al.* (1955) and Schumacher (1975) have described early lesions which appear at the junction of synovial tissue and cartilage. Here dilatation of the capillaries

and venules together with endothelial changes of necrosis and thrombosis occur (Fig. 17.1.1). Thus, vascular events are early and prominent, to be obscured later by the grosser secondary reactions. The evolution of early synovial hyperaemia and hyperplasia may occur either episodically or progressively and is dependent on vascular budding, possibly as a result of the angiogenetic factor found in synovial fluid (Brown *et al.*, 1980). A similar vasoproliferative factor has been found in neoplastic tissue and in macrophages and lymphocytes.

The endothelium of the post-capillary venules develops a high cell type, probably due to cytokines (tumour necrosis factor α and γ interferon). Inflammatory synovial fluid will produce this response. Receptors on the activated endothelial cells provoke leucocyte adhesion and the relevant lymphocytes are targeted to the appropriate organ (in this case the synovium) because of receptors on their surfaces. This is a specific action and not due to random targeting of lymphocytes. Exudation of fluid with tissue oedema and synovial effusion follow, leucocytes marginate in response to slowing of the blood flow and migrate through vessel walls to infiltrate the tissues. It must be emphasized, however, that synovial hypertrophy usually precedes immunocyte infiltration.

The synovial reaction is made up of a heterogeneous collection of cells derived from several sources, particularly the blood and synovial tissues. The major disparity between synovium and synovial fluid is the relative lack of polymorphonuclear cells in the first tissue and their common occurrence in the second tissue. The principal

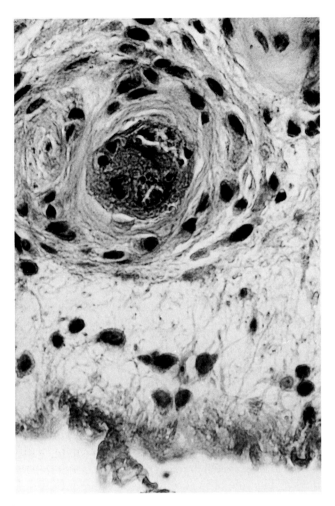

Fig. 17.1.1 Rheumatoid arthritis — synovial perivasculitis. Synovial cells (top) with oedematous subsynovial connective tissue containing arteriole, occupied by recent thrombus and surrounded by macrophages, occasional lymphocytes and excess new collagen. (H&E, ×350.)

infiltrating cells are small lymphocytes, which become arranged in the tissues either diffusely or in nodular patterns around the blood vessels, bearing a superficial resemblance to lymph nodes. In some cases, however, particularly when synovitis is well established, a polymorphonuclear reaction may predominate. Later with established inflammation, proliferation of blood vessels and fibroblasts occurs under the influence of locally produced mediators, e.g. angiogenetic factor and connective tissue-activating peptide, leading to the formation of connective tissue which provides a support for the cellular element. Angiogenesis is a necessary prerequisite for the proliferation of the synovial membrane, for which macrophage cytokines are responsible. The result of the cellular infiltration and tissue hypertrophy is a synovium thickened from the original membrane a

few cells thick to form frond-like villi 1 cm high and up to 2 mm in diameter. Thus, not only does the synovium now contain many inflammatory cells, it also has a markedly increased secretory surface area and the villi are prone to detachment, adding to the joint fluid detritus.

At least two types of synovial cell (synoviocyte) can be identified, mainly by morphology:
1 Type A — about one-third of the total — which appear to correspond to phagocytic cells elsewhere.
2 Type B, which have the structure and function of synthesizing cells and probably produce hyaluronate, collagenase, proteolytic enzymes and proteoglycan proteases, together with inhibitors, e.g. α_2-macroglobulin, and other constituents of tissue and synovial fluid.

Intermediate cell types (type C) have also been described (Barland *et al.*, 1962; Williamson *et al.*, 1966). More recent work has used surface markers to differentiate cell types (Burmeister *et al.*, 1983), though it is recognized that cell function may vary from time to time. In addition lymphokines, prostaglandins and other chemical mediators are produced. The variable, but often intense, infiltration of lymphocytes and plasma cells is capable of producing large quantities of polyclonal immunoglobulin, only a proportion of which is antiglobulin (rheumatoid factor) (Smiley *et al.*, 1968).

Inflamed synovium thus represents a source of many destructive and regulatory agents, most of which eventually pass into the synovial fluid and blood. Normal synovial fluid, which can be regarded as a transudation of serum to which macromolecules, notably hyaluronic acid, have been added by normal synovial cells, becomes increasingly an inflammatory exudate with a wide diversity of added components in increasing quantities. The effects of this can only be judged in a crude manner, because the analysis of individual reaction pathways is at present difficult, particularly when considered in isolation. The synovial cells may respond to a variety of agents, some of which are non-specific and it has been suggested that rheumatoid lymphocytes may escape from the normal suppression exerted by the increasing levels of prostaglandin found in inflammatory tissue, this being one of the factors leading to the development of chronic rheumatoid synovitis (Morley, 1976). Other lymphocyte suppressors, e.g. C-reactive protein, may be less effective.

The work of Karsh *et al.* (1981) seems to have demonstrated that continuing synovitis is dependent on recirculating lymphocytes. Thoracic duct drainage in humans leads to a marked reduction in circulating lymphocytes, synovial lymphocyte infiltration and clinical arthritis. Re-infusion of the separated lymphocytes shows that they tended to be sequestered in the diseased joints and associated with the recrudescence of active arthritis. The type or number of lymphocytes that recirculate through the synovial tissue is unknown, though most studies suggest that about 75% are T cells; the apparent relative lack of B cells may be because these progress to plasma cells. It is of interest, however, that although the proportions of different types of circulating blood lymphocytes appear to be normal, an increased number of activated lymphocytes can be found both in the circulation (where up to 10% may show evidence of activation) and in the synovial fluid (Eghtedari *et al.*, 1980). The significance of these cells is uncertain, but extracts of synovial tissue, synovial cells and synovial fluid have all been shown to cause activation of rheumatoid blood lymphocytes *in vitro* (Bacon *et al.*, 1973; Kinsella, 1973; Crout *et al.*, 1976). This activation may represent a non-specific stimulation (or lack of lymphocyte suppression, i.e. regulation) and is found to correlate with disease activity. It is noteworthy that the circulating blood mononuclear leucocytes in rheumatoid disease tend to spontaneously produce IgM rheumatoid factor and that if these cells are artificially and non-specifically stimulated, they have a much greater tendency to produce IgM rheumatoid factor than normal peripheral blood lymphocytes (Koopman and Schrohenloher, 1980). Otherwise, *in vitro* tests of lymphocyte function in rheumatoid arthritis have revealed little variation from normal.

A special type of synovial reaction may occur at the erosion front where inflamed synovium comes into contact with articular cartilage and a rather characteristic dendritic cell appears. This cell has been found to contain collagenase along its dendritic processes (Woolley *et al.*, 1978). More recently, the same group has emphasized the accumulation of mast cells in this area, which among other things can cause bone resorption.

The changes found in the synovium may be patchy and vary with time; in particular, as healing occurs the cellular infiltrate becomes less pronounced and fibrous tissue predominates.

Synovial fluid

As a result of the cellular proliferation and increased surface area of the synovium, there is exudation of fluid forming a synovial effusion. The fluid is variably inflammatory in nature, dependent on the degree of synovial reaction, and quite distinct from the effusions found in traumatic joints. Thus, the fluid may be turbid, thin with low viscosity, clots may occur and the total white cell count ($20-50 \times 10^9/l$) is raised; most of the cells will be polymorphs, though mononuclear cells and rhagocytes or rheumatoid arthritis (RA) cells also occur (Fig. 17.1.2). This last type are leucocytes found most profusely in rheumatoid synovial fluids, but also in other inflammatory fluids, and they contain cytoplasmic inclusions and can be shown to contain IgM rheumatoid factor (Hollander *et al.*, 1965). The extent to which polymorphs migrate to the inflamed joint has been estimated by Hollingsworth *et al.* (1967) to exceed $10^9/$ day (equivalent to the total blood content) in a joint fluid containing 25 000 granulocytes/ml — an average figure. The characteristics of synovial fluid vary with disease activity and time, thus, in the first 6 weeks of rheumatoid synovitis the fluid may be predominantly lymphocytic, only later becoming polymorphonuclear (Gatter and Richmond, 1975). Immune complexes are often present in the synovial fluid, resulting in complement activation and the release of chemotactic factors (Winchester *et al.*, 1970; Ward, 1975), leading to the further ingress of inflammatory cells.

Further examination of the synovial fluid shows it to be biochemically greatly altered from normal. Thus, the hyaluronic acid that is largely responsible for the normal viscosity of synovial fluid is depolymerized, presumably due to the effect of enzymes released from the synovial A cells and other phagocytic cells. The consequences of this depolymerization are not fully understood, but a 'thin' watery synovial fluid is a good indicator of inflammation. The role of hyaluronic acid in joint lubrication is not clear, but it may be more important for the integrity of the cartilage, in particular the superficial layers. The molecular constituents of inflamed synovial fluid are interesting in that they show a relative increase in higher molecular weight constituents, due partly to increased synovial vessel permeability and partly to the increased local synthesis of immunoglobulins.

The examination of synovial fluid has been well reviewed (Currey and Vernon-Roberts, 1976; Freemont and Denton, 1992). In general it can be said that examination of the fluid helps to divide the arthritides into:

1 Non-inflammatory (including traumatic or bleeding and clotting defects when blood may be present).
2 Microcrystalline (uric acid or calcium pyrophosphate crystals).
3 Inflammatory, e.g. in rheumatoid disease.
4 Infective, where the organism may be seen or cultured. More recently, attempts to define the disease process, the rate of destruction and perhaps the prognosis have been carried out with limited but encouraging results (Freemont *et al.*, 1991).

The early appearance of polymorphs, with their poten-

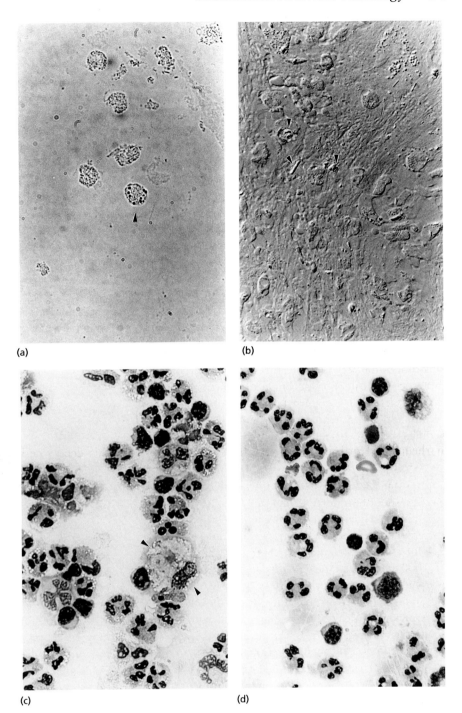

Fig. 17.1.2 Synovial fluid cytology. Wet preparations: (a) rhagocyte unstained; (b) pyrophosphate crystals (Normanski phase). Jenner–Giemsa stains: (c) cytophagocytic polymorphs; (d) classic synovial fluid in rheumatoid arthritis — mainly neutrophils, some small, medium and large lymphocytes, occasional erythrocytes.

tial oxidative and proteolytic enzymes, is found in most forms of acute inflammatory arthritis. These polymorphs have limited ability to recirculate and are thus trapped within the synovial cavity. The potential enzyme activity may be controlled in two ways: either neutralization by inhibitor systems or ingestion of the polymorphs by macrophages. Enzyme inhibitors are present but may be saturated. More recently, it has been recognized that these polymorphs undergo time-dependent programmed senescence and death (apoptosis) and can then be recognized and phagocytosed intact by macrophages, forming cytophagocytic mononuclear cells without the release of the contained enzymes. Thus both mechanisms — enzyme inhibition and inflammatory cell phagocytosis — will reduce and may limit or terminate the inflammatory reaction.

Cytophagocytic mononuclear cells have been most closely associated with seronegative arthritis and are known as Reiter cells. They occur in other fluid spaces, pleura and peritoneum. The factors regulating polymorph apoptosis are largely unknown; however, this process may occur in other cells, e.g. lymphocytes, and plays a part in controlling immune reactions.

Raised intra-articular pressure

The effect of intra-articular pressure on joint function is important. In normal joints the pressure is subatmospheric, but as the fluid volume increases the pressure increases, particularly on exercise. Thus, the normal positive/negative pressure cycle within the joint is lost, and this almost certainly affects cartilage nutrition. There is no evidence that pressure between the layers of normal articular cartilage is ever deleterious, however, in diseased joints with abnormal cartilage and synovial fluid, increasing pressure can produce damage. Although the mechanisms of damage are not clear, abnormal lubrication, the very high pressures that can occur, thin cartilage and osteoporotic bone all contribute. These changes are well recognized in the 'robust' type of rheumatoid patient who continues using inflamed joints, perhaps because of high pain tolerance, resulting in marked periarticular cyst formation (Castillo *et al.*, 1965; De Haas *et al.*, 1974). As synovial fluid volume in normal joints increases, so the intra-articular pressure increases out of proportion, and this pressure increase is even more marked in chronically inflamed joints, probably because of the thickened capsule and consequent lack of elasticity (compliance). Pressures in the range of 1000 mmHg can be recorded. Under pressure the synovial fluid is forced through weak areas of the cartilage, and acting hydrodynamically on the underlying bone produces a cavity that is later filled with fat and fibrous tissue (Fig. 17.1.3). The result is an epiphyseal bone pseudo-cyst or geode (literally a 'cavity within a stone'), which can sometimes be seen on radiographs but sometimes dramatically on computed tomograms or magnetic resonance scans and always implies a defect in the overlying cartilage.

Raised intra-articular pressure, either of acute or chronic nature, may lead to the formation of para-articular fluid collections in the soft tissue, the best known being a popliteal cyst, followed by escape of fluid into the calf to cause pseudo-thrombophlebitis. Encapsulated collections of synovial fluid are also found around other joints, however, particularly those of the fingers, elbows and shoulders. One of the immediate benefits of resting the inflamed joint is to reduce fluid production

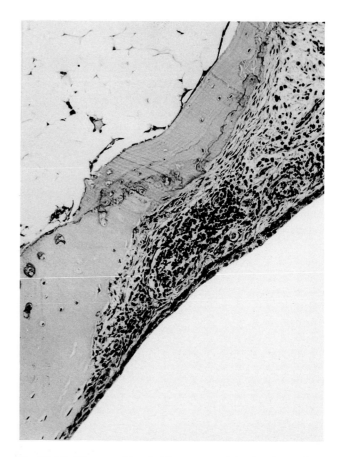

Fig. 17.1.3 Rheumatoid arthritis—pannus. Margin of articular cartilage undergoing degradation and progressive replacement by cellular inflammatory tissue containing many lymphocytes and plasma cells. (H&E, ×70.)

and the hydrodynamic pressure following exercise. The adoption by an inflamed joint of a flexed position is in part an attempt to reduce the intra-articular pressure by maximizing the intra-articular space.

As pointed out, the pressure inside an inflamed joint may reach pressures far higher than those within an inflamed capillary, producing a capillary shut down or ischaemia, which may be of varying duration depending on the cycle of intrasynovial pressure. At a crude level, fluctuation of the oxygen partial pressure in synovial fluid during exercise cycles with recurrent hypoxia has been shown. Relative intra-articular anoxia, despite increased vascularity, represents the high cost of metabolic activity and the impedance to the blood flow of raised intra-articular pressure. Obliteration of the capillary blood flow is easily obtained at the intra-synovial pressures occurring with a quite small effusion.

Oxygen-derived free radicals are toxic and have been shown to damage biomembranes and molecules, a wide variety of cells, erythrocytes, endothelial cells and tissue constituents, e.g. hyaluronic acid and collagen. Inhibition of antiproteinases has been demonstrated, and this removes one of the protective mechanisms of the joint against proteinases, which are thought to be responsible for cartilage destruction.

That free radicals can damage important molecules and indeed make them more immunogenic can be shown for IgG, DNA and possibly collagen. It is possible that production of superoxide anion radicals by neutrophils may be reduced by anti-inflammatory drugs, in particular corticosteroids.

Tenosynovitis

The synovitis of tendon sheath linings is essentially similar to that found within joints. There are, however, a number of variations: it occurs within a closely sealed space and, by mechanical impedance, or following fibrosis and adhesion between parietal and visceral synovial layer or of adjacent tendons, results in impaired movement of the tendons. Infiltration of the tendons varies from a few cells to large areas of fibrinoid necrosis and 'nodule' formation which may result in tendon rupture; however, the mechanisms of tendon rupture are not clear. Destruction of tendon by the surrounding inflammation is probable, but in conditions such as systemic lupus erythematosus rupture can occur with little evidence of inflammation and is usually attributed to local vasculitis. Enlargement of the synovial sheaths, sometimes with rupture, forms the characteristic dorsal sheath effusions of rheumatoid disease. Intra-articular ligaments, e.g. the cruciate and long head of biceps, may be similarly surrounded, invaded and destroyed by synovial tissue. In some situations the inflammatory reaction, by producing periosteal hyperaemia, can lead to periostitis of the underlying bone.

Although chronic synovitis is characteristically found in the inflammatory arthropathies, transient mild synovitis may be found in osteoarthritis and following trauma, such as occurs in hyperextension injuries of the fingers in basketball players and battered children.

Articular cartilage

This consists essentially of a framework of collagen fibres made up of highly cross-linked fibrils, and it is thus relatively insoluble. Within this sponge-like mesh is the ground substance, which is mainly proteoglycan and is highly soluble, and the fluid phase and chondrocytes it contains. The fibre orientation, size and constituent proteoglycans vary throughout articular cartilage, but have an orderly organization. The collagen is responsible for anchoring the proteoglycans on which the turgor, flow and creep of articular cartilage depend. Access of enzymes, principally from the inflamed synovial fluid but probably also from chondrocytes, rapidly results in loss of proteoglycan and the cartilage loses its resilience. Although mature collagen is relatively inert, the proteoglycans have a short half-life; the exact period is uncertain but estimates vary from 8 days in the rabbit (Mankin and Lippiello, 1969) to 250–600 days in humans (Maroudas, 1974). It is probable that the varying estimates reflect the marked heterogeneous distribution of proteoglycans with varying half-life in different regions of cartilage.

Minor changes in the chemistry of collagen occur with ageing. Changes in the chemical composition of the proteoglycan occur throughout life and influence the water content of the cartilage. The cartilage structure is highly organized, and its integrity is highly dependent on the intact surface layer. Once disruption of this layer occurs the underlying cartilage is vulnerable. The extent of adaptation of cartilage between the highly congruous bone ends is limited and the resulting wear causes self-perpetuating destruction. These changes, which are irreversible, occur well before radiological evidence is available (nuclear magnetic resonance imaging may improve this).

Involvement of articular cartilage in rheumatoid disease is always secondary to synovial inflammation produced by different mechanisms at different sites (Dingle, 1979). Some mechanisms depend on direct contact between synovial cells and cartilage, in others there is degradation at a distance by enzymes produced by the synovium or by soluble mediators from the synovium acting on chondrocytes, which then results in cartilage destruction.

Chondrocytes within the cartilage may be responsible for local proteoglycan destruction by the production of proteinases following stimulation by catabolin (probably interleukin-1β) which is produced by synovium. This is particularly marked near the massed cells of the pannus. In recent years the chondrocytes have increasingly become the focus of attention as a cause of cartilage breakdown, either because of excessive synthetic function producing abnormal growth with shear strains in the cartilage, or as a source of destructive enzymes.

Proteoglycan degradation occurs early; the metalloproteases that have been demonstrated in cartilage are one means of initiating proteoglycan degradation (Sapolsky *et al.*, 1975). The source of these enzymes is uncertain and they may, like other enzymes, be always present together with inhibitors *in situ*, but not functional until the inhibitory effect is removed, again by means that are not clear. Plasmin (for which plasminogen activator is present in inflammatory synovial tissue) is one possible way in which enzyme inhibitors could be removed. Conversely, the quantities of protease released following the death of the enormous numbers of polymorphs in synovial fluid may be too much for the available inhibitors to deal with, and the excess enzymes may then remain uninhibited and active. Elastase and cathepsin D released from polymorphs have been shown to bring about proteoglycan breakdown. As degradation of the proteoglycan polymers proceeds, the smaller fragments are further digested by lysosomal enzymes within polymorphs and similar cells.

Simultaneously with the digestion of proteoglycan, collagen degradation occurs. Collagen is a highly cross-linked structure at the intermolecular level and is thus difficult to solubilize. The initial step in digestion is due to proteinases attacking the non-helical region, which contains the intermolecular cross-links. This effectively destroys the cross-linking and leads to solubilization. The denatured collagen is then easily digested by collagenases present in macrophages and synovial cells (Harris and Krane, 1974).

At the synovial−cartilage junction, proliferating synovium penetrates deep to the cartilage and also spreads over the surface of the adjacent cartilage to form a pannus (Figs 17.1.3 and 17.1.4). The first lesion forms the characteristic angular erosion, seen on radiographs, which undermines the cartilage and separates it from the subchondral bone, which is in turn excavated (Figs 17.1.4 and 17.1.5). This hypertrophied synovium can

be shelled out of the cavities produced. The cartilage destruction at the angular erosion front seems to be due to the presence of collagenases secreted locally by the dendritic cells shown in this region by Woolley *et al.* (1978). Immunoreactive collagenase is not found elsewhere in the cartilage or synovium, though synovial tissue cultures will produce collagenase in large quantities (Dayer *et al.*, 1976). Away from the area of the erosion front, immune complexes have been demonstrated in the superficial layers of articular cartilage, though they are imprecisely defined (Cooke *et al.*, 1975; Jasin, 1985). It would be convenient to think that the pannus was due to chemotaxis of synovial cells and immunocytes, as a result of the presence of immune complexes in the cartilage; however, as immune complexes are not found beneath the pannus, this is not proved (Shiozawa *et al.*, 1980). The whole mechanism of formation and localization of the pannus, the angular erosion and probably most of the pathways of articular destruction await further study (Salisbury and Nottage, 1985).

Distant from contact with any synovial tissue, articular cartilage may show changes in its surface, usually consisting of loss of the amorphous surface gel and thinning of the superficial layers of cartilage, with depolymerization of matrix proteoglycans and irregular depressed areas (Holt, 1975). The sequential changes have not, for obvious reasons, been studied in humans. The resilience of the cartilage is lost, its mechanical properties deteriorate, and fragmentation (commencing at the surface) occurs (Fig. 17.1.5). Replacement of cartilage is by

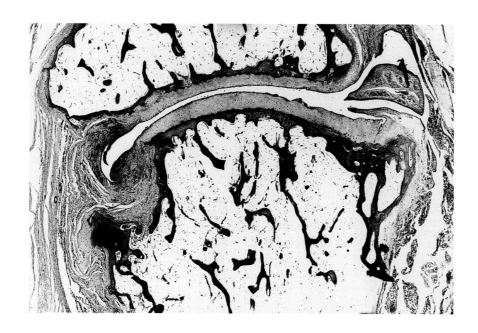

Fig. 17.1.4 Rheumatoid arthritis — synovitis of the proximal interphalangeal joint. Angular erosion (left) undermining cartilage and involving bone; elsewhere the articular cartilage is relatively intact. Periarticular osteopenia. (H&E, ×6.5.)

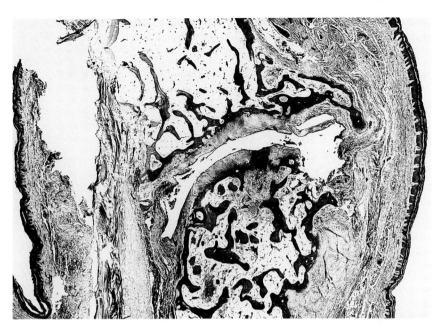

Fig. 17.1.5 Rheumatoid arthritis — synovitis of the terminal interphalangeal joint. More advanced stage with destruction and penetration of articular cartilage to form small subchondral cyst (geode). Secondary osteoarthrosis. (H&E, ×4.5.)

fibrosis, and the new tissue produced obviously has quite different characteristics from the original structures, though the types of cartilage overlap.

Normal articular cartilage consists predominantly of collagen type II, but replacement occurs with both type I and type II collagens. The normal architecture is not reformed. Interpretation of the significance of these changes, however, is subject to the difficulties of the technical methods at present available and outside the scope of the present discussion. These changes, certainly in the early histological stages, are quite different from those found in osteoarthritis, where although there may be a mild intermittent and probably localized inflammation, significant generalized inflammation is not found.

The cartilage, being radiotranslucent, is represented on radiographs by the distance between the bone ends, which diminishes with cartilage loss. The early stages of angular erosion, however, are not seen radiologically, and thus the pathological changes are always much more advanced than the radiological ones. The early destruction of articular cartilage, which is largely irreversible, cannot be over-emphasized and indicates the necessity to determine the aggressiveness of treatment at an early stage.

Subchondral bone

Although not usually apparent clinically and probably of little practical importance, early inflammatory changes can be found in the subchondral bone. Inflammation leads to periarticular osteopenia, hyperaemia of the periosteum and thickening of the bone shafts adjacent to the joint, resulting in the persisting cylindrical phalanges of juvenile arthritis and the asymmetrical periostitis characteristic of psoriasis and Reiter's syndrome. Localized hyperaemia in young joints may lead to precocious epiphyseal development and advanced ossification with subsequent early cessation of bone growth. This picture is more commonly seen with low grade and intermittent inflammation and is characteristic of the recurrent monoarthritis of haemophilia. By adult life the bone growth has usually regained symmetry, though stigmata such as Harris's line and abnormal secondary ossification centres may remain. More generalized osteopenia may result from treatment, particularly with corticosteroids, and relative immobility.

Bone resorption is dependent on osteoclastic activity to first remove calcium before collagenases can degrade the collagen matrix. Both prostaglandins and cytokines released from mononuclear leucocytes and immunocytes are able to stimulate osteoclastic activity. 1,25-dihydroxycholecalciferol (vitamin D) plays a part in increasing bone turnover. This active metabolite of vitamin D is produced by the activated synoviocytes of the inflamed joint. Its local and systemic significance is still to be evaluated; however, 1,25-dihydroxycholecalciferol has direct effects on the cells of the immune system and acts in many ways like a cytokine.

Estimates suggest that 50% of bone mass has to be lost before this loss is radiologically apparent. The most sensitive measure of bone loss is the fall in trabecular bone mass; however, this is a relatively small proportion of the total bone mass and is difficult to measure.

Isotopic methods and computed tomography have been used, but they tend to be difficult to standardize.

VASCULITIS

The prevalence of this feature as a clinical entity is uncertain, but as suggested above, vasculitis is thought to be a prominent and early event in the course of the synovial lesions, and any of several forms may occur simultaneously in a patient. Gardner (1992) has suggested that there are three main forms of vasculitis, depending on whether medium, small, or terminal arteries are involved. The changes are found in many tissues other than the synovium, often without associated clinical features.

Necrotizing arteritis

The pathology is similar to, and may be indistinguishable from, that of polyarteritis nodosa (Fig. 17.1.6). Segmental panarteritis affects medium and small arteries; luminal thrombosis and adventitial cellular infiltrate can affect any tissue producing widespread, varied and often severe syndromes. Neuropathies, typically mononeuritis (foot or wrist drop), mesenteric infarction, or parenchymal lung changes, are problems that may result from this type of arteritis.

Subacute arteritis

In subacute arteritis, the small arteries are surrounded and invaded by lymphocytes and fibrosis, often excessive, occurs. As blood flow is unimpaired, ischaemia is uncommon and little functional change results. This type of arteritis probably underlies nodule formation.

Fibromuscular hyperplasia (obliterative endarteritis)

This takes the form of an acellular fibrosis and proliferation of the intima, the internal elastic lamina remaining intact, leading to gradual occlusion of the lumen. Thrombosis may occur within the lumen, and this picture is very characteristic of digital arteritis.

The above varieties of arteritis often coexist and the resulting clinical features vary from neuropathies, to ulceration of the skin, to parenchymal tissue damage. All are prevalent in patients with rheumatoid disease, particularly those with severe disease and with high titres of antiglobulins (rheumatoid factor). The prognosis is worse in patients with any of the forms of vasculitis (Erhardt *et al.*, 1989). It should be noted that the evidence for systemic vasculitis is much less impressive

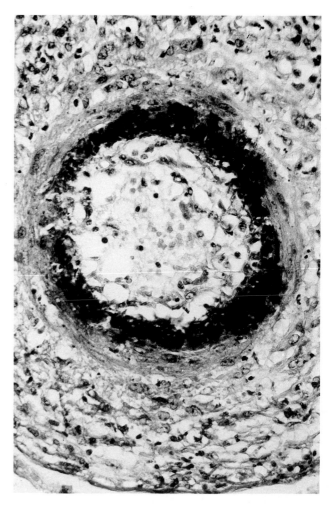

Fig. 17.1.6 Long-standing rheumatoid disease — necrotizing vasculitis. Necrosis of wall of medium-sized visceral muscular artery. Accumulation of plasma protein ('fibrinoid') in intima and necrosis of media. (MSB, ×200.)

in several otherwise identical forms of synovitis, e.g. in psoriasis.

Nodule formation

The most characteristic feature of vasculitis is the rheumatoid nodule, which has long been recognized as the hallmark of rheumatoid disease, though it only occurs in about 15% of cases. Early description of the histology (Collins, 1937) has been amplified by electron microscope studies (Cochrane *et al.*, 1964) and studies of the enzymes produced in nodules (Harris, 1972; Harris *et al.*, 1975).

Although the full pathogenesis is unknown, from the anatomical sites at which nodules are found it can be deduced that pressure or trauma must be an important factor. Similar nodules may be found in heel pads — a site of high trauma — in normal people, however, and particularly in insulin-requiring diabetic patients, where the associations with immunological factors are less clear (author's unpublished data).

Of the four basic types of immune reaction, immune complex-mediated inflammation (Arthus' or type III reaction) is thought to be the one most likely to be the cause of the vasculitis. In this, IgM and IgG rheumatoid factors, which are invariably found in these patients (Theofilopoulos, 1974) form complexes, either by self-aggregation or by fixing IgG, that are capable of being deposited on the wall of blood vessels. This has been supported by the demonstration of IgG, IgM and complement C3 in affected vessels (Conn *et al.*, 1972) and the presence of circulating immune complexes in the serum. The increased incidence of cryoglobulins in patients with vasculitis has been well documented; however, as most of these cryoglobulins have been demonstrated at unphysiological temperatures their *in vivo* significance is uncertain.

The chemotactic effect resulting from complement activation mediators attracts polymorphs and augments the local inflammation in the vessel wall that produces the vasculitis. The factors, other than perhaps trauma and cold, that lead to complex localization in vessels are obscure, though interest has increasingly centred around vasoactive amines, perhaps arising from sensitized basophils and mast cells and causing increased local permeability and 'stickiness' of blood cells to the blood vessels. The prostacyclins, which are normally found in vascular endothelium and some of which inhibit platelet adhesion, may have a similar effect on immune complexes.

The features of rheumatoid nodules represent a vigorous exudation and proliferation of connective tissue around vessels. This intense fibrous reaction is highly characteristic of rheumatoid arthritis and can be seen in a transient form around rheumatoid nail fold infarcts, but not in those occurring in systemic lupus erythematosus or other vasculitic conditions. In the centre of the nodule necrosis occurs with degenerating collagen fibres, cell walls and other debris, which is a highly specific feature. The necrosis probably results from a combination of micro-infarcts and the release of proteinases and collagenases by the ensuing cellular infiltrate (Harris, 1972; Harris *et al.*, 1975). Surrounding this central necrosis is a palisade of histiocytes, radially arranged with multinucleate giant cells. The outer layers are of fibrous tissue attaching the nodules to adjacent tissue.

Although most commonly seen in the skin, similar nodules have been described on the vocal chords, cardiac valves and in the lungs and pleura. Because of the fibrous nature of mature nodules, regression, even with otherwise successful medical treatment, is rare. Surgical removal is often partial with a strong tendency to recurrence. The usual forms of episcleritis, though resembling a nodule, lack the fibrous reaction and are more cellular in nature, usually resolving with treatment and leaving little permanent damage.

Parenchymal tissue changes

The lung lesions are readily detected, but are important because their significance is often not appreciated. Thus, intrapulmonary granulomas either alone or associated with pneumoconiosis (Caplan, 1953) or other irritant dusts may be unassociated with arthritis but are usually associated with rheumatoid factor. The larger, well-demarcated nodules can be sampled by needle biopsy if there is other evidence of rheumatoid disease, otherwise the diagnosis of intrathoracic neoplasm may be made erroneously. The association of interstitial pulmonary fibrosis with rheumatoid factor has led to the concept of 'rheumatoid lung'. This may not be a separate entity and is similar to other types of interstitial pulmonary fibrosis. Clinically, fine dry râles are heard without a cough, unless secondary infection has occurred. Decreased diffusing capacity of carbon monoxide is found. The condition is only slowly and variably progressive, the final outcome ranging from clinically insignificant impairment to intractable pulmonary failure. When associated with arthritis the main limitation is locomotor deficiency. Non-specific infections and a tendency to chronic bronchitis are not uncommon. The part played by recurrent chest infection and smoking in the production of the chronic pulmonary fibrosis is unknown. Distinguishing the pulmonary changes induced by gold, penicillamine and methotrexate, which have a serious prognosis if treatment is continued, is often difficult. More recently an increased incidence of bronchiectasis has been found in rheumatoid arthritis.

Pleural effusions and fibrosis are common but of little significance. Pleural effusions are usually small, but occasionally large effusions occur. Aspiration may show a low glucose content and rheumatoid cells. The main importance of the rheumatoid cells (or lupus cells in systemic lupus erythematosus) is that if their nature is not recognized, when they are found in the pleural aspirate at the outset of rheumatoid disease, the cellular morphology raises the possibility of pulmonary neoplasia. Involvement of the pulmonary arterioles is a rare cause of pulmonary hypertension.

Granulomas within the heart are usually symptomless, though occasionally heart block supervenes. Involvement of the valves seldom leads to haemodynamic problems, though recent echocardiographic investigations have demonstrated not only rather rigid, but also rather floppy valves. Echocardiography may also reveal small pericardial effusions and pericardial thickening, which are common findings at autopsy. Very occasionally pericardial thickening, with or without an effusion, is sufficient to cause tamponade.

Renal changes due to rheumatoid disease are debated, and if they occur are of little significance. The changes are non-specific, though it has been suggested that glomerular filtration rates decline more rapidly than in a normal ageing population. The effect of therapy on the kidney is still not clear; thus, aspirin has been shown to cause increased renal tubular epithelial cell desquamation. Renal papillary necrosis is occasionally found, but to what extent this is due to the disease and to what extent to the analgesics used is unresolved; of the latter, it seems to be largely associated with phenacetin-containing drugs. All the prostaglandin inhibitory drugs may interfere with renal clearance of sodium, even to the extent of precipitating heart failure and hypertension; this is reversible.

Amyloidosis may be found in many organs, but it is only in the kidney that it usually presents a clinically significant problem as nephrosis and/or hypertension, particularly in the childhood forms of inflammatory arthritis. The glomerulus is the main site of involvement, the amyloid being deposited on the basement membrane. Vascular deposits and tubular involvement are also found. The prognosis for this rare form of renal failure is poor, treatment being relatively ineffective. Fortunately, it is uncommon (perhaps increasingly so) in a clinically significant form. Renal vein and inferior vena cava thrombosis are well-recognized complications of renal amyloid deposition. Tubular defects of little significance are found in Sjögren's syndrome.

In the alimentary tract, only Sjögren's syndrome is closely associated with rheumatoid disease. It is usually slowly progressive, acute symptoms being rare. The parotid and submandibular glands are not usually greatly enlarged, except in cases with an acute onset. The mouth, nose, eyes and often ears are dry, resulting in secondary caries, difficulty in chewing and swallowing, anosmia, conjunctivitis and 'glue ear'. The salivary glands are infiltrated with lymphocytes, and similar changes are easily seen in labial mucosal biopsies, which can be used to make a diagnosis. Sjögren's syndrome may affect other secretory surfaces, e.g. the vagina and bronchial tree, in the latter case resulting in a mild bronchitic picture. Involvement of the stomach, pancreas, gall bladder and liver is more controversial and probably of little clinical significance.

SECONDARY CHANGES

Humoral

The combination of a target organ with ready access, i.e. synovium and synovial fluid, have led to interesting studies of the immunopathogenesis of inflammatory joint disease (Panayi, 1993). Rheumatoid factor, or more accurately antiglobulins, exist in several forms. The classic rheumatoid factor is of IgM antibody type and consequently has an excellent capacity to form aggregates and is easily detected by agglutination techniques, e.g. that used in the sheep cell agglutination test (Rose−Waaler test) or latex fixation test. These tests lead to the major division into seronegative and seropositive (rheumatoid factor-positive) inflammatory arthritis. This division has many attractions, influencing diagnostic options, complications, treatment and prognosis. In these tests, the antigen used is IgG and the classic reaction can be represented as IgM rheumatoid factor−IgG. In this reaction IgG can be either free or tissue-associated; in the latter case the associated structure, e.g. a cell, may be involved in the ensuing immunological reaction (Fig. 17.1.7). The reaction of serum IgM rheumatoid factor−IgG is a weak one and needs alteration of the IgG molecule in order to occur. Higher avidity rheumatoid factors, however, can be obtained by culturing the peripheral blood lymphocytes of rheumatology patients (Vaughan *et al.*, 1976). The result of having heterogeneous rheumatoid factor molecules with different binding strengths (avidities) is not known. It is likely that some or all high-avidity rheumatoid factor molecules will be tissue-bound and not detected, and similarly some will be tightly bound in the serum and not measured by the above tests unless the complexes are dissociated before assay in the test system. These latter molecules are one form of 'hidden rheumatoid factor'.

Although the incidence of complications is closely associated with the titre of IgM rheumatoid factor, attention has turned to other types of rheumatoid factor, in particular an IgG type, which is not easily detected by agglutination techniques (and is another form of 'hidden rheumatoid factor'). IgG rheumatoid factor is present in both seropositive and seronegative patients with rheumatoid disease and forms self-association complexes both with other molecules of IgG rheumatoid factor and with IgG. These complexes are small and soluble and

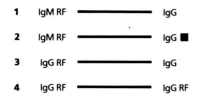

Fig. 17.1.7 Rheumatoid factor (antiglobulin) complexes. IgM rheumatoid factor is the classic rheumatoid factor; IgG rheumatoid factor is the non-haemagglutinating 'hidden' rheumatoid factor. The square denotes a cell or other structure to which immunoglobulin is attached. (1) Classic rheumatoid factor reaction. (2) Cell surface deposition of rheumatoid factor complex. (3) Non-haemagglutinating rheumatoid factor complex. (4) Self-associating small rheumatoid factor complex.

are therefore often associated with complications due to vasculitis. The main types of rheumatoid factor complexes that can be found are illustrated in a simplified schema (Fig. 17.1.7).

Although statistically linked with prognosis and diagnosis in rheumatoid diseases (Cats and Hazeudet, 1970), it must be remembered that in small titres classic IgM and IgG rheumatoid factors are found in a high proportion of the 'normal' population, this proportion increasing with age in both sexes, and transiently after non-specific infections or other antigenic stimulation. Only one-third of IgM rheumatoid factor-positive people have rheumatoid disease (Lawrence, 1977) and the diagnostic significance is thus greater in the young and when the titre is higher.

Although having diagnostic and prognostic significance, the role of rheumatoid factor, which must be regarded as an autoantibody, in pathogenesis has not been fully defined despite considerable effort. The presence of rheumatoid factor in an immune complex situation results in the formation of larger complexes, which are associated with more complement molecules—this can be readily demonstrated *in vitro*. This type of complex is much more readily phagocytosed and removed. Thus, one function of antiglobulins may be in limiting the circulating immune complexes and mopping up the altered IgG produced within the joint, either by phagocytes in synovial fluid and tissue or, if the altered IgG escapes into the circulation, by removal in the reticuloendothelial system, e.g. of liver and spleen. The rheumatoid process is thus limited to being an extravascular immune complex disease, principally of the joint. By comparison, systemic lupus erythematosus is primarily an intravascular immune complex disease.

The inherent tendency of patients with rheumatoid disease to produce IgM-type antibodies to many immunogens, in contradistinction to the IgG antibodies

of systemic lupus erythematosus, has long been known. Recent work has suggested that the function of the reticuloendothelial system is often impaired in rheumatoid disease, and that the extent of this impairment may be important in determining the incidence of complications. Improved function of the reticuloendothelial system following plasmapheresis or treatment has coincided with a fall in the circulating immune complexes (Williams *et al.*, 1979) and temporary clinical improvement.

The evidence of vascular disease is to be found in the early stages of nodule formation, synovitis and the nail-fold lesions already mentioned. The presence of circulating immune complexes has been amply demonstrated by a variety of techniques, but like all such tests they may not demonstrate the important complexes, which would be utilised, and thus removed, at sites of tissue damage, but are more in the nature of epiphenomena or overspill. Raised complement components C3 and C4 are found in the serum. These elevated levels probably reflect an acute phase type of reaction similar to the rise in fibrinogen and C-reactive protein found in inflammation. Evidence of increased breakdown (turnover) of these complement components, however, has been available for a long time (Zvaifler, 1969; Versey *et al.*, 1973). The deposition of immune complexes together with complement in the articular cartilage has already been mentioned. Deposits are also found in the synovial tissue. There is little evidence, however, of specific complement deposition elsewhere, even in the systemic complications such as vasculitis. As a result of complement activation, leucocyte chemotaxis occurs and activation of the lysosomes can then lead to local damage, particularly if this activation and release of lysosomal enzymes occur in a confined space so that the released enzymes cannot escape or be readily inactivated.

Rheumatoid factor is by definition an antibody directed against immunoglobulin. The antigenic sites are on the Fc or tailpiece of the immunoglobulin molecule and are multiple and partly under genetic control. Thus, the reaction between autologous IgG and rheumatoid factor is stronger than in the heterologous situation. To become antigenic the mature IgG molecule has to be slightly altered. How normal IgG molecules are changed is not clear, but Johnson *et al.* (1974) have demonstrated that patients with rheumatoid disease have increased levels of circulating IgG whose spatial configuration is abnormal and which consequently probably become antigenic. The site at which this alteration occurs is unknown but may be within sites of inflammation, e.g. the joint, or follow involvement in an immune reaction and would be one way in which the autoimmune process could be perpetuated. Glycosylation of proteins is reduced in rheumatoid arthritis and some chronic infections, and this includes IgG. This abnormal IgG may represent an immunogen in susceptible patients. Other factors are necessary for the autoimmune process, however, in particular to determine the target selected (Parekh *et al.*, 1985).

Genetic features are obviously important here, and the earlier work on twins and families (Lawrence, 1977) has been given a more fundamental basis by the advent of histocompatibility testing in which the strikingly high incidence of HLA DRW4 in rheumatoid arthritis had been shown (Stastny, 1978). This is in marked contrast to the findings in juvenile chronic arthritis, where the incidence of HLA DRW4 is reduced below normal, and other D locus haplotypes are found to be associated with different clinical patterns of childhood disease (Stastny and Fink, 1979). The continued search for genetic markers has suggested that further associations may arise, for example between HLA DRW3 and severe forms of arthritis and reaction to treatment (Table 17.1.2). That extrapolation from adult rheumatoid diseases to the childhood chronic arthritides may not be appropriate is further illustrated by the significance of antinuclear factors, which in young children strongly suggest that chronic uveitis may be present and not that systemic lupus erythematosus is likely.

Although rheumatoid factor is a characteristic feature

Table 17.1.2 Association of histocompatibility antigens and rheumatic disease. B, D and TM0 histocompatibility haplotypes (measured by various techniques)

Histocompatibility antigen	Type of rheumatic disease
HLA B5	Behçet's syndrome
HLA B8	Strength of immune response
HLA B27	Reactive arthritides, ankylosing spondylitis, acute uveitis
HLA DR2	Sjögren's syndrome
HLA DR3	Systemic lupus erythematosus, severe rheumatoid arthritis, toxic reactions to treatment, Sjögren's syndrome
HLA DR4	Rheumatoid arthritis ↑, juvenile chronic arthritis ↓
HLA DR5	Juvenile chronic arthritis ↑
HLA DR6	Juvenile chronic arthritis ↑
HLA DR8	Juvenile chronic arthritis ↑
HLA TM0	Juvenile chronic arthritis ↑ ++

↑   Increased.
↓   Decreased.
++   Markedly.

of rheumatoid arthritis as pointed out above, it is not diagnostic.

Antibodies directed against collagen or its fragments have been described in rheumatoid arthritis and other diseases; however, the incidence varies widely between different reports and thus the true significance of these antibodies in humans is not clear. Autoimmunity to collagen type II, which is almost exclusively found in articular cartilage, is very characteristic of rheumatoid arthritis, though it is only found in a small percentage (10–15%) of patients where it may occur as a result of the arthritis rather than as a precursor. It seems probable, however, that breakdown of the parent molecules in the inflamed tissue would create antigenic particles. The synthesis of small amino acid chains corresponding to segments of the collagen molecule has demonstrated clear-cut epitopes reacting with patient sera. In animal experiments the ability of immunity to collagen to provoke arthritis seem more clear-cut (Morgan, 1990). A genetic component to the development of auto-immunity to collagen has been demonstrated. Auto-immunity to proteoglycan has been demonstrated, but the results are not clear-cut, these being rather difficult molecules to investigate.

Cellular immunity

The strict division into cellular and humoral immunity is artificial, there being marked interaction between T lymphocytes (cellular immunity) and B lymphocytes (humoral immunity), however, it has practical value as T and B lymphocytes can be separately identified and assayed. Although much work has been undertaken with peripheral blood and synovial T lymphocytes in rheumatoid disease, on the whole little change from normal has been found. Technical difficulties increase the problem of lymphocyte assay and account for much of the variability in the results. The work of Karsh *et al.* (1981) suggests that lymphocytes are necessary for continuation of the rheumatoid process, and the ability to develop rheumatoid disease in agammaglobulinaemia (Good *et al.*, 1957) suggests that T lymphocytes may be the more significant type of lymphocyte. T lymphocytes normally exert a controlling function (helper CD4, suppressor CD8[+]) over the immunoglobulin-producing B cells. In addition, T lymphocytes have the ability to act directly either by producing cytotoxicity of cells, which are usually identified by viral antigens, or by the production of mediators which influence other cells, e.g. macrophages and osteoclasts, or produce the vascular changes of inflammation and osteopenia.

The work of Chattopadhyay *et al.* (1979) indicates

that there is a lack of suppressor T cells in rheumatoid synovial tissue; in contrast, helper cell activity was normal as compared to peripheral blood, thus allowing unfettered immunoglobulin production by the B cells. This has been discussed earlier in relation to the synovial reaction. The difficulty of obtaining good control tissues is well known, and further work in this area is obviously necessary.

Cytokines

These cell regulators are small proteins produced by immunocytes, macrophages and other cells. The synovium and synovial fluid contain considerable quantities of cytokines. They are principally a form of cellular intercommunication between immunocytes, but also influence other cells, usually in proximity. Although increasing numbers of cytokines are being described, they are produced by three main cell types: T lymphocytes; macrophages (including type A synoviocytes); and fibroblastic cells (including type B synoviocytes). Most of the synovial fluid cytokines are produced by the synovial tissue. In rheumatoid arthritis, however, the synovial fluids show a relative deficiency of T cell-derived cytokines, and abnormalities of cytokine production have been shown in both synovial fluid and peripheral blood T cells. Thus, immune dysregulation is widespread and not confined to the joint. Cytokines have activating and inhibiting effects on cells of variable duration and to some extent are interdependent. Although individual functions have been assigned to identified cytokines, the complicated interplay of cytokines and cells *in vivo* is not well understood. Natural inhibitors are found in tissues. In general the inflammatory response is amplified by cellular proliferation and activation.

The number of cytokines is continually being extended. Interleukin 2, interleukin 3, interleukin 4 and interferon γ are produced by T cells, while interleukin 1, interleukin 6 and tumour necrosis factor are produced by macrophages (Krane *et al.*, 1988; Arend and Dayer, 1990; Duff, 1993). At present transforming growth factor β appears to be the most potent down-regulator of T lymphocytes in the synovial fluid. Cytokine expression is particularly marked at the cartilage−pannus junction in patients with rheumatoid arthritis as distinct from the normal cartilage−pannus interface (Chu *et al.*, 1992).

Cytokine research has developed rapidly, but the effects of cytokines are still poorly understood, partly because they have different effects on different cells and indeed the effect in a given cell type may vary at different times. Both synergism and antagonism between these mechanisms is being demonstrated. It has therefore been difficult to understand the *in vivo* significance of changes in individual cytokines. Although thought to act primarily on cells involved in the immune response, e.g. lymphocytes and macrophages, they also act on vascular endothelium, interstitial tissue and bone. More general effects are to promote the acute phase responses, prostaglandin production and fever. The effect on haemopoeisis is not clear.

A recent development in the mediator field has been the demonstration of inflammation following the release of substance P, a neurotransmitter released by afferent nerve terminals. This may explain the symmetry of certain types of arthritis and the lack of inflammatory arthritis in limbs paralysed before the onset of arthritis. Inhibition or potentiation of cytokine action is a potentially useful way of up-grading or down-grading the immune system and treating inflammatory arthritis.

Acute phase proteins

A variety of proteins is found to be elevated, usually reflecting the severity of the inflammation and waxing and waning with it. They are called acute phase proteins (or reactants) because they are found in raised quantities shortly after the onset of inflammation. This appears to be a non-specific reaction and the extent of increase varies between different elements. Fibrinogen and C-reactive protein are well known, but others occur in the α_1-globulin and α_2-globulin region on electrophoresis; haptoglobin, complement components (principally C3 and C4), caeruloplasmin, serum amyloid A (SAA) and antiproteases, e.g. α_1-antitrypsin and α_2-antitrypsin may all be raised. The extent of these increases varies from 50% for caeruloplasmin to a 1000-fold for C-reactive protein. The consequence of this non-specific response is probably to deal more effectively with inflammation. Thus, increased fibrinogen will allow for better clotting, caeruloplasmin rises to provide superoxide dismutase activity, haptoglobin will bind to haemoglobin released from erythrocyte breakdown and the anti-enzymes will reduce the escaping protease activity released by cell death. The acute phase proteins may also regulate the immune response. Some of these functions can be illustrated by C-reactive protein.

C-REACTIVE PROTEIN

This plasma protein was found in 1930 to precipitate polysaccharide extracts of pneumococci. It is practically undetectable in health but rises dramatically in response to any type of inflammation and equally rapidly falls as the inflammation diminishes. Synthesis occurs in the liver, probably stimulated by leucocyte interleukin 1 and 6 products and prostaglandin E_1. C-reactive protein can bind to both soluble and particulate products of dying cells, e.g. those of necrotic tissue, and can then activate the classic complement pathway as actively as IgG antibodies (Kaplan and Volanakis, 1974), resulting in phagocytosis and removal. Thus, one function of C-reactive protein is to act as a scavenger for the breakdown products normally produced in the body but enhanced at times of inflammation. Although inflammatory reactions follow intracutaneous injections of C-reactive protein in certain conditions, it is unlikely that this protein is a prime participant in the inflammatory response. The role of C-reactive protein as a regulator of lymphocyte function has been suggested by the demonstration of its presence on the surface of lymphocytes. Various results have been found, and this question is still unresolved.

PROSTAGLANDINS

These are a heterogeneous group of compounds with a variety of physiological and pharmacological effects. They are found in most cellular tissues, though the types and concentrations vary from tissue to tissue. Thus, vasodilatation, increased vascular permeability, pain (which in some cases is primarily due to an enhancement of the effect of histamine and bradykinin) and osteoclastic bone reabsorption have been demonstrated, and the last may be of importance in formation of bone erosions. Prostaglandins play a part in leucocyte chemotaxis as well as themselves being produced by leucocytes. The presence of prostaglandins in tissue is difficult to determine because of their instability. They have been demonstrated in synovial fluid in proportion to the cellular concentration, however, suggesting but not proving that they arise from invading leucocytes (Higgs *et al.*, 1974). It is probable that prostaglandin precursors are derived from unsaturated fatty acids, e.g. arachidonic acid, which is stored as a phospholipid in the cell membrane of, for example, a macrophage, until released and converted by a series of enzyme steps to prostaglandins, thromboxanes, or prostacyclin (Fig. 17.1.8). All these substances are relatively unsaturated and are presumably primarily active locally rather than systemically. Prostacyclins and thromboxanes seem to be partly antagonistic, prostacylin being enzymically produced in endothelial cells and thromboxanes in platelets; one reduces thrombosis and the other increases it. The effect of prostaglandins on the immune system is

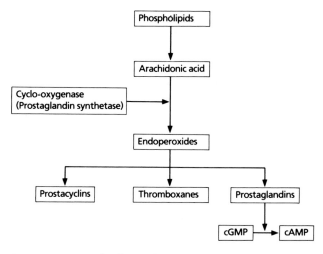

Fig. 17.1.8 Prostaglandin synthesis.

complicated and produced primarily via their effect on cyclic nucleotides. They have either inhibiting or stimulating effects on cellular activity. These effects may be reversed at higher or lower concentration, partly explaining the variation found in *in vitro* results. In certain immune reactions lymphocytes are normally suppressed by prostaglandins, lack of this suppression being one of the postulated mechanisms for the chronicity of the immune disease (Morley, 1976).

The vogue for prostaglandin synthetase inhibitor drugs, e.g. aspirin and propionic acid derivatives, owes much to the prominence of prostaglandins in inflammation and the demonstration by Ferreira (1972) that although prostaglandins themselves are relatively weak pain producers, they markedly increased the pain produced by kinins.

KININS

The kinins are a series of small polypeptides which are present as their precursors, plasma and tissue prekallikrein; on activation these become kallikrein which, in turn, acts on the inactive plasma kininogens (prekinins) to form active kinins. Activation of kininogen conversion is possible by a variety of pathways. Urate crystals will activate Hageman factor, and other intraarticular debris, e.g. collagen from degenerating articular cartilage, may have a similar effect. Proteolytic enzymes, of which there are ample in the inflamed joint, will also activate kallikrein. Immune complexes of rheumatoid factor and IgG have been shown to deplete kininogen (Epstein *et al.*, 1969), also indicating activation of the kinin pathway. The most important of the kinins is bradykinin.

As a group the kinins produce capillary vasodilatation and permeability, and pain (enhanced by prostaglandins) and may be chemotactic for leucocytes. While the precursors are present in large quantities in many tissues, the kinins formed are readily destroyed, so that their activity is localized and measurements difficult. Free kinins have been found in the synovial fluid of inflamed joints.

FIBRIN

Activation of the clotting sequence, as well as initiating kallikrein formation, results in fibrin formation. The fibrin clots formed in active rheumatoid disease are often of poor quality but are easily found throughout the synovial space, and this is largely due to the inefficient fibrinolytic mechanism within the joint. The persistence of fibrin within the synovial cavity may act as an irritant, and although no evidence of an immunological response to blood products has been detected in humans, chronic inflammation has been induced by fibrin in animals (Glynn, 1968). The 'rice bodies' of chronically inflamed joints consist of fibrin and collagen. In addition, bleeding into the joint from the inflamed synovium is probably more common than is usually recognized, particularly with exercise including physiotherapy (Bennett *et al.*, 1972), and this may increase the inflammatory response to an already inflamed joint.

AETIOLOGY OF RHEUMATOID DISEASE

The association of aetiological factors in the rheumatic diseases is a good example of a chicken and egg situation. Should the disease be defined according to its clinical and pathological features or to its initiating factors and inherited susceptibilities?

The infective theories for the aetiology of rheumatic diseases have been briefly reviewed by Bennett (1978). He suggested that four general mechanisms could operate:

1 Multiplication of an agent within the joint space.
2 Infectious agent or its derived antigens localized within the joint space initiates immune response.
3 Infectious agent or its derived antigens are at a distant site but the immune response provoked causes arthritis.
4 Infectious agents produce 'arthritogenic toxins'.

The first group would consist of pyogenic infections and such viruses as smallpox. The second group is typified by rubella and certain of the *Mycoplasma* infections that are found naturally in animals or have been used to initiate experimental models of animal arthritis. In the third group are found the 'reactive' arthritides,

namely those following infection distant to the joint but with cross-immunity with joint and other tissues, resulting in arthritis and other systemic features of disease. Typical examples are Reiter's syndrome following *Shigella* infection or *Salmonella* infections, or non-specific urethritis. Ankylosing spondylitis may fall in this class. Rheumatic fever due to cross-reactivity with streptococcal antigens would be another example. In this group there is evidence of an increased genetic susceptibility. The fourth group has an uncertain place in human pathology.

Arthritis has been well documented in Lyme's disease, where a specific organism has been found. At various times *Mycoplasma*, human T-cell lymphotrophic virus type 1 (HTLI), rubella, parvoviruses, mycobacteria and fungal organisms have been suspected, either because of direct infection or due to altered immune responses of the invaded cell. The concept of superantigens has arisen, i.e. bacteria and viruses that as intact organisms and without prior processing can stimulate a large population of T cells, probably non-specifically.

A new discovery is that of heat shock proteins, which are neoproteins expressed on the surface of cells in response to stress (Winrow *et al.*, 1990). These proteins are highly conserved in nature and present in many animal species. Mycobacteria and fungal organisms are the prime candidates for an external source of these proteins, to which an immune response is raised. This immune response may then react with synovial cells, which express similar heat shock proteins under stress.

Despite circumstantial evidence—largely from epidemiological investigations (Lawrence, 1977)—no definite organism or vector has been found for the most common form of arthritis: rheumatoid arthritis or its childhood equivalents. Perhaps one of the most pertinent observations is that sera from patients with rheumatoid arthritis contain an antibody that reacts with a nuclear antigen extracted from human lymphoblast cell lines infected with Epstein—Barr virus (Alspaugh and Tan, 1976). It appears that the rheumatoid lymphocyte is more readily infected by this virus, which may then prolong the life-span of the infected cell. The function of this 'immortalized' cell is not clear.

Parvoviruses, particularly B19 strain, have been demonstrated in the course of a form of arthritis that is usually of short duration and sometimes associated with the transient appearance of an antiglobulin antibody. Similarities between viral glycoprotein and the B chains of HLA DW4, DW14 (subtypes of DR4) and DR1 MHC molecules have been detected and suggest that molecular mimicry could produce altered responses to the viral infection in genetically susceptible patients. Even when an infective agent has been implicated, however, the relative importance of it in the immune response is usually unclear.

Although the nature of the putative infective agent is unknown, associations with histocompatibility antigens in rheumatoid arthritis have been found (Stastny, 1978; Stastny and Fink, 1979) (see Table 14.1.2). One of the most striking features to arise from this type of work is the close association between the reactive arthritides and possession of HLA B27 antigens. Other associations have been found for Sjögren's syndrome (HLA DW3) and Behçet's syndrome (HLA B5). The background incidence of some histocompatibility antigens varies widely throughout the world. This is well illustrated by HLA B27 which is rare in Japan (less than 1%) compared with an incidence of about 7% in Caucasians and an even higher incidence in certain North American Indians. Thus, the relative risk of developing diseases varies throughout the world; however, as this variation is less marked than the variation in gene markers, it follows that where the incidence of gene markers is low then the relative risk of developing disease in persons possessing these markers is higher.

Histocompatibility antigens may be important in other ways. Thus, the strength of the immune response evoked or the liability to develop autoimmune disease may be linked to regions in chromosome 6, indicating an inherited tendency to develop more severe autoimmune disease. The form this takes is in part determined by other chromosome 6 regions or chance contact with environmental agents, e.g. infection. As most infections are ubiquitous, it is likely that most people contact them and may develop temporary disease, but only those that are susceptible go on to the chronic disease state. This susceptibility varies throughout life, with increasing age, with declining regulation of the immune system and a progressive tendency to autoimmune disease, as marked by the appearance of more autoantibodies. These are a major variable, though peaks in the incidence curves suggest other variables, one of which is the hormonal changes of puberty and the menopause.

At the present time patients with well-defined features of disease are being grouped according to the different genetic markers known, to see if a correlation can be found between different markers, and hence an association between pathogenetic pathways and the resulting clinical course. By this means it may become apparent that clinically similar diseases are in fact dissimilar, require different handling and are susceptible to different complications, in particular with regard to treatment (Panayi *et al.*, 1978).

CONCLUSIONS

Consideration of the wide variety of pathogenetic mechanisms available shows that the diverse pictures found clinically may result from a varying mixture of pathological mechanisms in people genetically susceptible and aided by such factors as occupation, gender and age of onset. Until a clearer understanding of these pathways of tissue destruction and regeneration is available, treatment and prognosis will be based on empirical rather than scientific guidelines.

Acknowledgement

The photomicrographs have been provided by Professor D.L. Gardner, Dr A.J. Freemont and Mr J. Denton.

REFERENCES

Alspaugh M.A. and Tan E.M. (1976) Serum antibody in rheumatoid arthritis reactive with a cell associated antigen. Demonstrated by precipitation and immunofluorescence. *Arthritis Rheum.* 19, 711–719.

Arend W.P. and Dayer J.M. (1990) Cytokines and cytokine inhibitors are antagonists in rheumatoid arthritis. *Arthritis Rheum.* 33, 305–315.

Arnett F.C., Edworthy S.M., Block D.A. *et al.* (1988) The American Rheumatism Association 1987 revised criteria for the classification of rheumatoid arthritis. *Arthritis Rheum.* 31, 315–324.

Bacon P.A., Cracchiolo A. and Bluestone R. (1973) Cell mediated immunity to synovial antigens in rheumatoid arthritis. *Lancet* ii, 699–702.

Barland P., Novikoff A.B. and Hamerman D. (1962) Electron microscopy of the human synovial cell. *J. Cell Biol.* 14, 207–220.

Bennett J.C. (1978) The infectious aetiology of rheumatoid arthritis. *Arthritis Rheum.* 21, 531–538.

Bennett R.M., Hughes G.R.V., Bywaters E.G.L. *et al.* (1972) Studies of a popliteal synovial fistula. *Ann. Rheum. Dis.* 31, 482–486.

Brown A.R., Weiss J.B., Tomlinson I.W. *et al.* (1980) Angiogenetic factor from synovial fluid resembling that from tumours. *Lancet* i, 682–685.

Burmeister G.R., Dimitriu-Bona A., Waters S.J. and Winchester R.J. (1983) Identification of three major synovial lining cell populations by monoclonal antibodies directed to Ia antigens and antigens associated with monocytes, macrophages and fibroblasts. *Scand. J. Immunol.* 17, 69–82.

Caplan A. (1953) Certain unusual radiological changes occurring in the chest of coal miners suffering from rheumatoid arthritis. *Thorax* 8, 29–37.

Castillo B.A., El Sallab R.A. and Scott J.T. (1965) Physical activity, cystic erosions and osteoporosis in rheumatoid arthritis. *Ann. Rheum. Dis.* 24, 522–527.

Cats A. and Hazeudet H. (1970) Significance of positive tests for rheumatoid factor in the prognosis of rheumatoid arthritis. *Ann. Rheum. Dis.* 29, 254–260.

Chattopadhyay C., Chattopadhyay H., Natvig J.B. *et al.* (1979) Rheumatoid synovial lymphocytes lack concanavalin A-activated suppressor cell activity. *Scand. J. Immunol.* **10**, 479–486.

Cochrane W., Davies D.V., Dorling J. *et al.* (1964) Ultramicroscopic structures of the rheumatoid nodule. *Ann. Rheum. Dis.* **23**, 345–363.

Collins D.H. (1937) The subcutaneous nodule of rheumatoid arthritis. *J. Pathol. Bacteriol.* **45**, 97–115.

Conn D.L., McDuffie F.C. and Dyck P.J. (1972) Immuno-pathologic study of sural nerves in rheumatoid arthritis. *Arthritis Rheum.* **15**, 135–143.

Cooke T.D., Hurd E.R., Jasin H.E. *et al.* (1975) Identification of immunoglobins and complement in rheumatoid articular collagenous tissues. *Arthritis Rheum.* **18**, 541–551.

Crout J.E., McDuffie F.C. and Ritts R.E. (1976) Induction of peripheral blood lymphocyte transformation by autologous synovial fluid lymphocyte and synovial fluid. *Arthritis Rheum.* **19**, 523–531.

Currey H.L.F. and Vernon-Roberts B. (1976) Examination of synovial fluid. *Clin. Rheum Dis.* **2**, 149–177.

Dayer J.M., Krane S.M., Russell G.G. *et al.* (1976) Production of collagenase and prostaglandins by isolated adherent rheumatoid synovial cells. *Proc. Natl. Acad. Sci.* **73**, 945–949.

De Haas W.H.D., de Boer W., Griftioen F. *et al.* (1974) Rheumatoid arthritis of the robust reaction type. *Ann. Rheum. Dis.* **31**, 81–85.

Dingle J.T. (1979) Recent studies on the control of joint damage. Heberden Oration 1978. *Ann. Rheum. Dis.* **38**, 201–214.

Duff G.W. (1993) Cytokines and anti-cytokines. *Br J Rheumatol.* **32** (Suppl 1), 15–20.

Eghtedari A.E., Bacon P.A. and Collins A. (1980) Immunoblasts in synovial fluid and blood in the rheumatic diseases. *Ann. Rheum. Dis.* **39**, 318–322.

Epstein W.V., Tan M. and Melmon K.L. (1969) Rheumatoid factor and kinin generation. *Ann. N.Y. Acad. Sci.* **168**, 173–187.

Erhardt C.C., Mumford P.A., Venable P.J. and Maini R.N. (1989) Factors predicting a poor life prognosis in rheumatoid arthritis: an eight year prospective study. *Ann. Rheum. Dis.* **48**, 7–13.

Ferreira S.H. (1972) Prostaglandins, aspirin-like drugs and analgesia. *Nature* (*N. Biol.*) **240**, 200–203.

Freemont A.J. and Denton J. (1992) Juvenile arthritis. In Gresham G.A. (ed) *Atlas of Synovial Fluid Cytopathology.* Dordrecht/Boston/London, Kluwer Academic Publishers 117–119.

Freemont A.J., Denton J., Chuck A., Holt P.J.L. and Davies M. (1991) Diagnostic value of synovial fluid microscopy: a reassessment and rationalisation. *Ann. Rheum. Dis.* **50**, 101–107.

Gardner D.L. (ed) (1992) *The Pathological Basis of the Connective Tissue Diseases.* London, Edward Arnold.

Gatter R.A. and Richmond J.D. (1975) Predominance of synovial fluid lymphocytes in early rheumatoid arthritis. *J Rheum.* **2**, 340–345.

Glynn L.E. (1968) The chronicity of inflammation and its significance in rheumatoid arthritis. *Ann. Rheum. Dis.* **27**, 105–121.

Good R.A., Rotstein J. and Mozyietti W.F. (1957) The simultaneous occurrence of rheumatoid arthritis and agammaglobulinaemia. *J. Lab. Clin. Med.* **49**, 343–350.

Harris E.D. Jr. (1992) A collagenolytic system produced by primary cultures of rheumatoid nodule tissue. *J. Clin Invest.* **51**, 2973–2976.

Harris E.D. Jr. and Krane S.S. (1974) Collagenases. *N. Engl. J. Med.* **291**, 557–560.

Harris E.D. Jr., Faulkner C.S. III and Brown F.E. (1975) Collagenolytic systems in rheumatoid arthritis. *Clin. Orthop.* **110**, 303–316.

Higgs G.A., Vane J.R., Hart F.D. *et al.* (1974) The effects of anti-inflammatory drugs on prostaglandin concentration in synovial fluid from patients with rheumatoid arthritis. In Robinson H.J. and Vane J.R. (eds) *Prostaglandin Synthetase.* London, Raven Press, pp. 165–171.

Hollander J.L., McCarthy D.J. Jr., Astorga G. *et al.* (1965) Studies on the pathogenesis or rheumatoid joint inflammation. *Ann. Intern. Med.* **62**, 271–280.

Hollingsworth J.W., Siegel E.R. and Creasey W.A. (1967) Granulocyte survival in synovial exudate of patients with rheumatoid arthritis and other inflammatory joint diseases. *Yale J. Biol. Med.* **39**, 289–296.

Holt P.J.L. (1975) Joint cartilage: physiology and changes in arthritis. In Holt P.J.L. (ed) *Current Topics in Connective Tissue Diseases.* Edinburgh, Churchill Livingstone, pp. 24–47.

Holt P.J.L. (1990) The classification of juvenile chronic arthritis. *Clin. Exp. Rheumatol.* **8**, 331–334.

Jasin H.E. (1985) Autoantibody specificities of immune complexes sequestered in articular cartilage of patients with rheumatoid arthritis and osteoarthritis. *Arthritis Rheum.* **28**, 241–248.

Johnson P.M., Watkins J., Scopes P.M. *et al.* (1974) Differences in serum IgG structures in health and rheumatoid disease. *Ann. Rheum. Dis.* **33**, 366–370.

Kaplan K.M. and Volanakis J.E. (1974) Interaction of C-reactive protein complexes with the complement system. I. Consumption of human complement associated with the reaction of C-reactive protein and pneumococcal C polysaccharide and with the choline phosphatide, lecithin and sphingomyelin. *J. Immunol.* **112**, 2135–2147.

Karsh J., Klippel J.H., Plotz P.H. *et al.* (1981) Lymphoresis in rheumatoid arthritis: a radiological trial. *Arthritis Rheum.* **24**, 867–893.

Kinsella T.D. (1973) Induction of autologous lymphocyte transformation by synovial fluids from patients with rheumatoid arthritis. *Clin. Exp. Immunol.* **14**, 187–191.

Koopman W.J. and Schrohenloher R.C. (1980) Enhanced *in vitro* synthesis of IgM rheumatoid factor in rheumatoid arthritis. *Arthritis Rheum.* **23**, 985–992.

Krane S.M., Goldring M.B. and Goldring S.R. (1988) Cytokines. In *Cell and Molecular Biology of Vertebrate Hard Tissues.* Ciba Foundation Symposium No. 136. London, Ciba Foundation, 239–256.

Kulka J.P., Bocking D., Ropes M.W. *et al.* (1955) Early joint lesions of rheumatoid arthritis. *Arch. Pathol.* **59**, 129–141.

Lawrence J.S. (1977) *Rheumatism in Populations.* London, Heinemann.

Mankin H.J. and Lippiello L. (1969) The turnover of adult rabbit articular cartilage. *J. Bone Joint Surg.* **51A**, 1591–1600.

Maroudas A. (1974) Transport through articular cartilage and some physiological implications. In Ali S.Y., Elves M.W. and Leaback D.H. (eds) *Normal and Osteoarthritic Cartilage.* London, Institute of Orthopaedics, pp. 33–47.

Morgan K. (1990) What do anti-collagen antibodies mean? *Ann. Rheum. Dis.* **49**, 62–65.

Morley J. (1976) Prostaglandins as regulators of lymphoid cell function in allergic inflammation: a basis for chronicity in rheumatoid arthritis. In Dumonde D.C. (ed) *Infection and Immunology in the Rheumatic Diseases*. Oxford, Blackwell, pp. 511–519.

Panayi G.S. (1993) The immunopathogenesis of rheumatoid arthritis. *Br. J. Rheumatol.* 32 (Suppl. 1), 4–14.

Panayi G.S., Wooley P. and Batchelor J.R. (1978) Genetic basis of rheumatoid disease: HLA antigens, disease manifestations and toxic reaction to drugs. *BMJ* 2, 1326–1328.

Parekh R.B., Dwek R.A., Sutton B.J. *et al.* (1985) Association of rheumatoid arthritis and primary osteoarthritis with changes in the glycosolution pattern of total serum IgG. *Nature* 316, 452–457.

Ropes M.W., Bennett G.A., Cobb S. *et al.* (1958) Revision of diagnostic criteria for rheumatoid arthritis. *Bull. Rheum. Dis.* 9, 175–176.

Salisbury M.D. and Nottage W.M. (1985) A new evaluation of gross pathological changes and concepts of rheumatoid articular cartilage degeneration. *Clin. Orthop. Rel. Res.* 199, 243–247.

Sapolsky A.I., Woessner J.F. Jr and Howell D.S. (1975) A photometric assay for protease digestion of the proteoglycan subunit. *Anal. Biochem.* 67, 649–654.

Schumacher H.R. (1975) Synovial membrane and fluid morphological alterations in early rheumatoid arthritis. Microvascular injury and virus-like particles. *Ann. N.Y. Acad. Sci.* 256, 39–64.

Shiozawa S., Jasin H.E. and Ziff M. (1980) Absence of immunoglobins in rheumatoid cartilage–pannus junctions. *Arthritis Rheum.* 23, 816–821.

Smiley J.D., Sachs C. and Ziff M. (1968) *In vitro* synthesis of immunoglobin by rheumatoid synovial membrane. *J. Clin. Invest.* 47, 624–632.

Stastny P. (1978) HLA-D and Ia antigens in rheumatoid arthritis and systemic lupus erythematosus. *Arthritis Rheum.* 21, S139–S143.

Stastny P. and Fink C.W. (1979) Different HLA-D associations in adult and juvenile rheumatoid arthritis. *J. Clin. Invest.* 63, 124–130.

Theofilopoulos A.N., Burtonboy G., Lospalluto J.J. *et al.* (1974) IgM rheumatoid factor and low molecular weight IgM: an association with vasculitis. *Arthritis Rheum.* 17, 272–284.

Vaughan J.H., Chihara T., Moore T.L. *et al.* (1976) Rheumatoid factor-producing cells detected by direct haemolytic plaque assay. *J. Clin. Invest.* 58, 933–941.

Versey J.M.B., Hobbs J.R. and Holt P.J.L. (1973) Complement metabolism in rheumatoid arthritis. 1. Longitudinal studies. *Ann. Rheum. Dis.* 32, 557–564.

Ward P.A. (1975) Complement dependent phlogistic factors in rheumatoid synovial fluids. *Ann. N.Y. Acad. Sci.* 256, 169–176.

Williams B.D., Pussell B.A., Lockwood C.M. *et al.* (1979) Defective reticuloendothelial system function in rheumatoid arthritis. *Lancet* i, 1311–1314.

Williamson N., James K., Ling N.R. *et al.* (1966) Synovial cells: a study of the morphology and an examination of protein synthesis of synovial cells. *Ann. Rheum. Dis.* 25, 534–546.

Winchester R.J., Agnello V. and Kunkel H.E. (1970) Gammaglobulin complexes in synovial fluids of patients with rheumatoid arthritis. *Clin. Exp. Immunol.* 6, 689–706.

Winrow V.R., McLean L., Morris C.J. and Blake D.R. (1990) The heat shock protein response and its role in inflammatory disease. *Ann. Rheum. Dis.* 49, 128–132.

Woolley D.E., Harris E.D. Jr., Mainardi C.I. *et al.* (1978) Collagenase immunolocalisation in cultures of rheumatoid synovial cells. *Science* 200, 773–775.

Zvaifler N.J. (1969) Breakdown products of C_3 in human synovial fluid. *J. Clin. Invest.* 48, 1532–1542.

Chapter 17.2
Clinical Aspects and Treatment

M.H. Seifert

INTRODUCTION

The rheumatic diseases include a wide variety of disorders, which in terms of patient referrals form one of the largest disease groups encountered in medicine. There is now a much more concise classification of these diseases and many new ones have been recognized. Clinical diagnosis and treatment have become highly sophisticated and research has flourished. Despite the progress in unravelling the rheumatic diseases their aetiology often remains obscure. Only those diseases likely to be encountered by the practising orthopaedic surgeon will be described, and the reader is therefore advised to consult other rheumatology texts for details of less common rheumatic disease and for more detailed description of the diseases found in this chapter (Kelley *et al.*, 1993, McCarty, 1993).

RHEUMATOID ARTHRITIS

This is the pivot of the rheumatic diseases, and it can be said that only when rheumatoid arthritis has been excluded should the diagnosis of any other rheumatic disease be considered. Females are affected more commonly than males, in a ratio of 2.5:1; the reason for this is not known, though it is likely to be hormonally related.

Onset

The disease is systemic and its onset is often heralded by malaise, fever and fatigue. It may begin at any time from the first few weeks of life until the ninth decade, but the peak time of presentation is 35–45 years.

The hormonal aspect of the disease is also illustrated by its presentation around the time of the menopause, the acute exacerbations that follow pregnancy and termination, and the remissions that commonly occur during pregnancy. Classically, the disease presents as symmetrical polyarthritis occurring in the small joints of the hands and feet. Presentation as monarthropathy or in asymmetrical larger joints, however, is well recognized, and therefore it is necessary to keep in mind the possible diagnosis of rheumatoid arthritis when faced with any inflammatory arthropathy.

Presentation

A number of presentations can be expected.
1 *Slowly progressive polyarthritis*: this gradually becomes worse daily over a period of weeks or months with swelling developing in one and then another joint.
2 *Episodic polyarthritis*: acute swelling of one joint spontaneously resolves with an asymptomatic interval between. The intervals gradually become shorter until frank polyarthritis develops. This is the palindromic form of onset (Mattingly *et al.*, 1981).
3 *Monarticular or oligoarticular arthritis*: usually a larger joint is swollen and only later will a polyarthritis develop.
4 *Fulminating polyarthritis*: more commonly found in elderly patients. If the onset of the disease is acute with widespread joint involvement and a marked systemic upset, these patients often have a favourable prognosis. If the disease is insidious in onset with slowly progressive destructive change and initially only a few joints involved, the prognosis is less favourable.

Most patients, however, seem to fit into a third type of onset with the disease running an irregular course with exacerbations and remissions, and the prognosis of this is variable.

From the follow-up of large series of patients over a number of years, the following generalizations can be made of patients with definite rheumatoid arthritis presenting to a hospital clinic.
1 About 25% have a short-lived disease that results in

no persisting arthritis or disability.

2 Twenty-five per cent have a disease that remits with only a mild persisting disability.

3 Forty-five per cent develop persistent arthropathy punctuated by remissions and exacerbations and leading to progressive deformity of a variable degree.

Ten per cent have a severe disability resulting in gross deformities and restriction to bed or chair for the rest of their lives (Duthie *et al.*, 1964).

Symptoms

As in most joint diseases associated with inflammation, periods of inactivity cause the affected joints to become stiff, and this is particularly found in the early morning. In the active disease the length of early morning stiffness may be used as a measure of disease severity. Patients report that they awake in the early morning with their hands flexed and knees stiff. After prolonged inactivity such as sitting they may, because of joint stiffness, have difficulty in rising and later climbing stairs. Table 17.2.1 lists the symptoms of early rheumatoid arthritis.

Signs

Early in the disease there may be little abnormal to find on physical examination apart from tenderness on deep palpation in the affected joints. Later, the signs of inflammation—tenderness, swelling, heat and redness—become more evident. The metacarpophalangeal and proximal phalangeal joints are the most commonly involved followed by the wrists, particularly over the ulnar styloid, and metatarsophalangeal (MTP) joints, then knees, shoulders, elbows, ankles, mid-tarsal joints, cervical spine and the temporomandibular joints. Table 17.2.2 lists the signs of early rheumatoid arthritis.

In early disease, swelling of the proximal phalangeal joints may cause rings to tighten, and it is a common early complaint that these have had to be enlarged or removed. Tenosynovitis is common, affecting both flexor and extensor tendons, and may be a presenting sign. Palmar erythema and increased sweating of the palms and soles (hyperhydrosis) is also a common manifestation

Table 17.2.1 Symptoms of early rheumatoid arthritis

Early morning joint stiffness
Joint swelling
Polyarthralgia
Weight loss
Fever
Malaise and fatigue

Table 17.2.2 Signs of early rheumatoid arthritis

Joint swelling—symmetrical
Joint tenderness on deep palpation
Limited motion
Tenosynovitis
Muscle atrophy
Autonomic dysfunction (hyperhydrosis and palmar erythema)
Carpal tunnel syndrome

of the autonomic dysfunction present. Swelling around the wrist may produce signs of median nerve compression in the carpal tunnel, this having been described as a presentation of the disease (Chamberlain and Corbett, 1970).

Articular involvement

The diathrodal joints are the ones that become inflamed in this disease, and initial swelling due to synovitis is most marked over extensor surfaces where the capsule of the joint is distensible. It is conventional to describe the joints from the head downwards.

TEMPOROMANDIBULAR JOINTS

It has been estimated that 71% of patients with rheumatoid arthritis have involvement of these joints, causing pain and difficulty with chewing. Circular tomography has shown erosive change of the condylar head.

CERVICAL SPINE (see Chapter 21, pp. 740–744)

Involvement of the atlantoaxial joint in rheumatoid arthritis is more common than is generally recognized (Meijers *et al.*, 1984). The transverse ligament of the atlas becomes attenuated, and erosion of the odontoid peg occurs with subsequent instability at this level and pressure on the cervical cord. Patients quite often do not complain of much pain or headache, and the problem is not discovered unless the cervical spine is viewed on a lateral radiograph in full flexion and extension; tomography may also be required. Subluxation occurs at other levels of the cervical spine. If the separation of the anterior surface of the odontoid peg from the posterior surface of the anterior arch of the atlas is more than 2.5 mm in women or 3 mm in men, the condition is pathological. Vertical subluxation may also occur. Magnetic resonance imaging of the cervical spine is very helpful in diagnosing atlantoaxial subluxation and other problems in the cervical spine, and if necessary any images in the coronal, sagittal, or axial plane can be obtained (see Chapter 30.1).

Symptoms when they do occur consist of occipital headaches, neck weakness and long tract signs. When severe, quadriplegia and even death may result. Patients with this degree of cervical spine involvement have severe articular disease and are, therefore, likely to be candidates for surgery. It is, therefore, mandatory to obtain radiographs of the cervical spine in these patients before anaesthesia.

SHOULDER JOINT

This may be involved quite early in the disease, and synovial swelling at the glenohumeral joint is a presenting sign. With advanced disease very marked limitation of movement may occur. Acromioclavicular joint involvement is the major cause of pain in the shoulder region of these patients. Magnetic resonance imaging is the most sensitive investigation of lesions around the shoulder joint and has contributed greatly to the differential diagnosis of disease in this area.

ELBOW

Involvement of this joint causes severe disability, and boggy synovial swelling can be associated with gross restriction of movement and ulnar nerve entrapment.

HAND AND WRIST

These joints show the most characteristic findings in rheumatoid arthritis and are seldom spared.

As previously mentioned, the early rheumatoid hand shows signs of hyperhidrosis and palmar erythema; there is also minimal synovial swelling of the proximal interphalangeal and metacarpophalangeal joints. At the wrist there may be limitation in movement with tenderness and swelling over the ulnar styloid. An early and sometimes presenting sign is swelling along the flexor sheaths resulting in 'trigger finger'. As well as the flexor tendons, extensor tendons may be involved and cause linear swelling on the dorsum of the hand indistinguishable from synovial hypertrophy. With advanced disease and prolonged synovial inflammation, the more classic appearance of rheumatoid deformity develops (Fig. 17.2.1).

Dorsal interossei muscles waste, so that the metacarpophalangeal joints become more pronounced. Wasting of the abductor pollicis brevis muscle occurs due to compression of the median nerve at the wrist (carpal tunnel syndrome). The characteristic ulnar deviation is

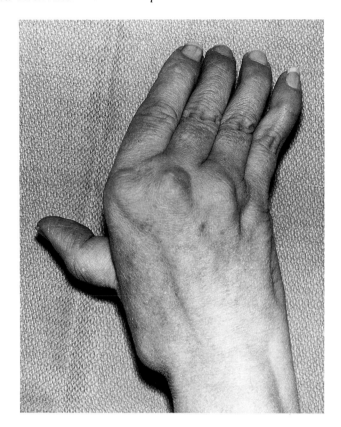

Fig. 17.2.1 Synovial thickening in rheumatoid arthritis.

by no means unique to the diagnosis of rheumatoid arthritis, and other conditions, e.g. reflex sympathetic dystrophy and Parkinson's disease, may produce similar changes. The pathogenesis of the ulnar drift is complex and has been well described (Swezey, 1971/1972). In summary, the collateral ligaments stretch and the ulnar fibrocartilaginous plate slips palmwards. There is then palmward pull of the base of the proximal phalanges by the strong flexor muscles and the characteristic volar subluxation occurs. Extensor tendons stretch and ulnar drift of the fingers occurs as their tendons slide laterally into the groove on the ulnar side of the joint. Further joint deformities result in hyperextension of the proximal interphalangeal joint, flexion of the terminal interphalangeal joint, swan-neck deformity and flexion of the proximal interphalangeal joint with hyperextension of the terminal interphalangeal joint—boutonnière or button-hole deformity. Hyperextension of the distal phalanx of the thumb is another characteristic deformity, the 'Z-shaped' thumb.

Extensor tendon rupture is most common in the region of the ragged ulnar head. The overlying tendons become frayed and the fifth tendon followed by the fourth, third and second then rupture. It may be remembered, however, that these dropped fingers may be caused by weakening and lengthening of the extensor tendons by the dislocation, and occasionally by an entrapment neuropathy of the radial nerve at the elbow. With more advanced disease extensive deformity may occur but only very occasionally is any bony ankylosis produced.

SPINE AND HIPS

There is little clinical evidence of lower spinal involvement in rheumatoid arthritis, and sacroiliitis is not a symptomatic feature. The hips are a source of pain and limited movement, but pronounced involvement is not common. When it does occur it can be very disabling. It has been said that protrusio acetabuli occurs only in rheumatoid arthritis and other inflammatory joint disease; however, it can sometimes be found in patients with osteoarthritis. It should not be forgotten that another cause of hip disease in rheumatoid arthritis is the avascular necrosis that can occur in patients receiving high-dose steroids. Fortunately, the more conventional lower doses of steroids in use today seldom cause this problem.

KNEES

The knee is commonly affected and may be a presenting sign, particularly if bilateral involvement is found. A characteristic flexion contracture develops with a marked valgus deformity, a feature being tricompartment disease. Instability due to involvement of the cruciate and medial collateral ligaments is troublesome. The presence of a popliteal cyst should be carefully sought and is more often detected with the patient lying prone and palpating the popliteal fossa. Rupture of a popliteal cyst into the calf should be suspected in any patient with rheumatoid arthritis presenting with acute calf pain; it can often be mistaken for a deep vein thrombosis. Popliteal cysts may become tender and hard, and descend into the calf, often due to a valve-like mechanism allowing synovial fluid to flow into the cyst from the knee joint, but not to return (Genovese *et al.*, 1972). When the cyst ruptures sudden severe pain develops in the calf, and this is accompanied by swelling and tenderness with ankle oedema and a positive Homans' sign. An arthrogram is necessary to make the diagnosis (Fig. 17.2.2), but when available magnetic resonance imaging is particularly valuable and the diagnostic accuracy is very good.

ANKLES AND FEET

The ankle joint has relatively less synovial tissue than

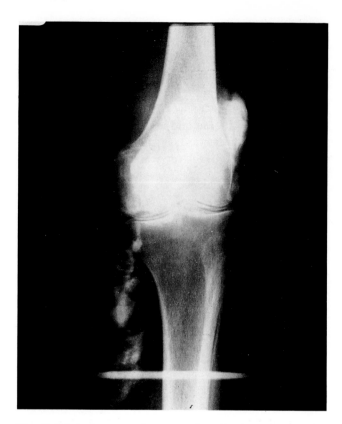

Fig. 17.2.2 Arthrogram of a ruptured popliteal cyst in rheumatoid arthritis.

the knee and is, therefore, much less involved, most problems in this region being due to disease of the subtalar joint (Dixon, 1971). Pain in the ankle joint is usually due to tendinitis of the peroneal and posterior tibial tendons. When synovial hypertrophy occurs, marked bulging appears anteriorly and laterally to the joint margin. A combination of ankle and subtalar joint inflammation is suggestive of rheumatoid arthritis.

Rheumatoid arthritis may present in the feet, and tenderness of the metatarsal heads should be sought if the disease is suspected. The metatarsal arch of the foot typically collapses, resulting in weight-bearing occurring on the second, third and fourth metatarsal head rather than the first and fifth; with tightness of the plantar fascia a pes cavus deformity occurs causing the toes to 'cock up'. Painful callosities develop over metatarsal heads following subluxation and ulcers over the dorsal surfaces of the involved toes. Lateral deviation of the first metatarsal phalangeal joint is common with subsequent bunion formation.

Extra-articular involvement

It should not be forgotten that rheumatoid arthritis also

involves other systems besides joints, and for this reason the term 'rheumatoid disease' is often favoured to describe all the manifestations of this complex collection of symptoms and signs. The extra-articular manifestations are usually of a minor nature as far as the patient's symptoms are concerned, but may develop into major complications leading to death in the severely affected.

RHEUMATOID NODULES

These are always associated with IgM rheumatoid factor, so that in its absence any subcutaneous nodule would be suspect. Only on histology can the nodule be definitely said to be due to rheumatoid arthritis. The most characteristic site is the extensor surface of the forearm, and there the nodules are often multiple (Fig. 17.2.3). When formed along the forearm they are commonly fixed to the periosteum, but they may also be palpated within an olecranon bursa. Nodules may be found around the knee and in other areas of pressure, e.g. the back of the skull, at the bridge of the nose in patients wearing tight glasses and over the sacrum. In the last area breakdown and ulceration is a troublesome complication. In fact, such breakdown may occur in any subcutaneous nodule with obvious ulcer and septic complications. Other sites for nodule formation are over tendons of the hands, causing triggering of the fingers, and in the pleura and lung, mimicking neoplasms. Typical nodule formation is described in the larynx and on the vocal chords. Nodules may be found in the pericardium and myocardium and even in the sclera of the eye.

The size of the nodule may vary with the state of the disease, sometimes disappearing entirely with disease remission.

OCULAR MANIFESTATIONS

The importance of ocular manifestations in rheumatoid arthritis is due to the common lack of clinician awareness of these complications and also because the patient is so preoccupied with the joint disease that serious eye complications can develop before they are noticed. All the eye complications present with a red eye (Hazleman and Watson, 1977).

Episcleritis is quite common and occurs in other connective tissue diseases. It is acute, sometimes painful, but usually self-limiting lasting for about 10 days.

Scleritis (Fig. 17.2.4) is more important, and if neglected can lead to blindness. It is painful and leads to thinning of the sclera so that the blue colour of the choroid shows through. Scleromalacia perforans is an unusual complication of necrotizing scleritis in patients with long-standing rheumatoid disease. A rheumatoid nodule situated in the sclera sloughs, causing eventual loss of the eye.

Keratoconjunctivitis sicca occurs in 10% of patients with rheumatoid disease, but again is only noted when the patient is directly asked whether there is dryness or grittiness in the eyes. When it occurs with dryness of the mouth and peripheral arthropathy it is called Sjögren's syndrome (see below).

PULMONARY MANIFESTATIONS

Pulmonary complications of rheumatoid disease are rare but important (Macfarlane *et al.*, 1978). Rheumatoid nodules may occur in the lung at any stage of the disease and are usually associated with subcutaneous rheumatoid nodules elsewhere, but can obviously cause a diagnostic dilemma when they occur as single lesions. If

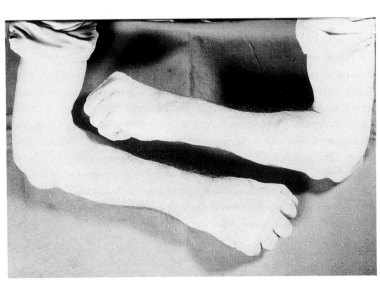

Fig. 17.2.3 Multiple rheumatoid nodules on the extensor aspect of the forearm.

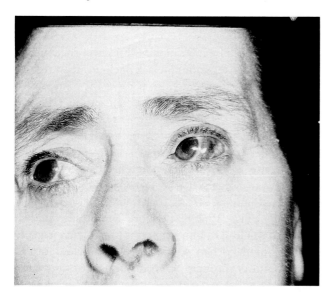

Fig. 17.2.4 Scleritis in rheumatoid arthritis.

associated with pneumoconiosis the condition has been termed Caplan's syndrome. A more common complication is the development of pleurisy with or without a pleural effusion, this being found more commonly in men. Typically, the effusion, which is an exudate, has an elevated protein content and a reduced glucose level. Again, diagnostic problems can arise and it is important to differentiate from tuberculous infection and neoplasm.

Perhaps the most uncommon pulmonary complication of rheumatoid disease is diffuse interstitial fibrosis, this again being more common in men. It is associated with subcutaneous nodules and high titres of rheumatoid factor.

CARDIAC INVOLVEMENT

The most common cardiac manifestation of rheumatoid disease is pericarditis, and as this tends to be asymptomatic diagnosis is usually made at autopsy. With the use of echocardiography, however, the incidence of pericardial effusions has been shown to be 55% in chronic rheumatoid nodular arthritis and 15% in non-nodular cases (Bacon and Gibson, 1974). The only other significant cardiac involvement is when rheumatoid granuloma causes distortion of valve cusps with resulting valvular insufficiency, or conduction defects due to infiltration of the conducting system and myocardium. These last complications are rare.

NEUROMUSCULAR INVOLVEMENT

Neuromuscular involvement in rheumatoid disease is quite common and probably occurs in at least 10% of patients. Muscle weakness is a common but not profound symptom in patients with active polyarthritis. Myositis due to vasculitis may be found on biopsy, and wasting of muscle due to steroid or anti-malarial treatment is also recognized, though in none of these are muscle enzymes elevated. The major nerve deficits are due to the following.

Neuropathy

This may be a pure sensory neuropathy usually affecting the feet in a stocking distribution and occurring more commonly in seropositive men who have had the disease for more than 10 years. They complain of burning pain, electric shock sensations and numbness, and can be shown to have loss of sensation to vibration, light touch and pin prick; position sense is retained. When a motor component is added the distribution is in all four limbs peripherally and the onset is acute. The abrupt onset of wrist or foot drop is indistinguishable from mononeuritis multiplex and an arteritis of the vasa nervosum is found on biopsy. The prognosis is grave.

Cervical myelopathy

Subluxation of the cervical spine has been discussed, and when cord compression develops the result is a neurological emergency. The loss of position sense, increased deep tendon reflexes and the presence of pathological reflexes with flexor muscle spasm suggest that the neurological symptoms are due to cord compression. Bladder and bowel dysfunction is ominous.

Entrapment neuropathies

The compression of the median nerve in the carpal tunnel has been mentioned as a presenting symptom in rheumatoid disease; in more advanced disease this is quite common. The ulnar nerve can be affected at the wrist and elbow and less commonly the posterior interosseous branch of the radial nerve is compressed as it passes over the lateral epicondyle causing wrist drop. The anterior tibial nerve can be entrapped by a popliteal cyst, and posterior tibial nerve compression can cause pain and paraesthesiae in the heel and medial part of the foot, the so-called tarsal tunnel syndrome. The cause of the entrapment neuropathies is inflammation and large effusions occurring in enclosed spaces, thus encroaching on the nerve.

RHEUMATOID VASCULITIS

The vasculitis that develops in rheumatoid disease may be classified under two headings. Inevitably these types of vasculitis may overlap.

Obliterative endarteritis

This is found particularly in digital vessels and is responsible for nail-fold lesions, cutaneous lesions of the finger or toe pulps and Raynaud's phenomenon. These small haemorrhagic lesions may ulcerate, and very occasionally gangrene develops. The histology is non-inflammatory and the lesions are often asymptomatic.

Inflammatory vasculitis

This type of inflammatory vasculitis is associated with polyneuritis, skin infarction and ulceration. A high level of rheumatoid factor and rheumatoid nodules together with pericarditis is a feature. In extreme cases visceral ischaemia leading to infarction has been reported. 'Malignant rheumatoid disease' is more common in men and is usually fatal.

LYMPHADENOPATHY

Localized lymph node enlargement in the region of an inflamed joint is more common than expected and may lead to diagnostic confusion. Biopsy usually shows non-specific lymphoid hyperplasia, though the appearance of giant follicular lymphoma has been reported. Generalized lymphadenopathy is rare and should suggest reticulosis.

ANAEMIA

This is a common feature in patients with rheumatoid disease; it responds poorly to therapy and probably has a number of causes. The administration of anti-rheumatic drugs over many years inevitably causes blood loss, but the aetiology in rheumatoid arthritis is more complicated than this simple explanation. The anaemia is normocytic and normochromic and the serum iron level is low. Unlike iron deficiency anaemia, the total iron binding capacity is also low with, on bone marrow examination, adequate iron, but poor haemoglobinization of red cells. The factors that lead to the failure of iron uptake by the red cells are ill understood (Bennett, 1977).

Felty's syndrome

Felty reported five patients with deforming rheumatoid arthritis, splenomegaly and neutropenia in 1924. Other features include lymphadenopathy, skin pigmentation, chronic leg ulceration, thrombocytopenia and haemolytic anaemia. It is still not clear whether this is a variant of rheumatoid disease or an entity in itself. The neutropenia may lead to recurrent infections. The syndrome occurs in less than 5% of patients with rheumatoid disease, and the splenomegaly may precede or follow neutropenia. Splenectomy is not advised as a treatment except in cases of severe haemolytic anaemia or thrombocytopenia (Spivak, 1977).

SJÖGREN'S SYNDROME

The association of dry eyes (keratoconjunctivitis sicca), dry mouth (xerostomia) and a connective tissue disease (50% being patients with rheumatoid arthritis) is termed Sjögren's syndrome. When this exists without a connective tissue disease it is called sicca syndrome. It is more common in women and may be found in 10–15% of patients with rheumatoid arthritis. As well as dry eyes and mouth the vagina and tracheobronchial tree are also characteristically dry. A Schirmer's test and rose bengal staining of the cornea are positive (Moutsopoulos *et al.*, 1980).

LABORATORY FINDINGS

A number of investigations can be performed on a patient suspected of having rheumatoid arthritis. None is specific and none can replace sound, clinical judgement, accurate history-taking and examination. Too often the patient is subjected to numerous and repeated investigations in the hope that the diagnosis can be made in the presence of a hurried and scanty physical examination. Laboratory investigations are most valuable as a guide to the severity of the disease, management and possibly prognosis.

Haematology

The anaemia of rheumatoid arthritis has been discussed; about 25% of patients have 10 g/dl or less of haemoglobin. As well as the anaemia of chronic disease, blood loss may occur from the use of salicylates and other anti-inflammatory drugs.

The erythrocyte sedimentation rate is conventionally measured by the Westergren method. It is expected to be elevated, and although lagging slightly behind, usually parallels disease activity. Sudden rapid and unexplained elevations of erythrocyte sedimentation rate should alert the clinician to the possibility of joint infection.

Serology

Rheumatoid factor need not be present to make a diagnosis of rheumatoid arthritis; in about 20% of patients it never appears. Conversely, it may be present in a number of other conditions, ranging from 90% in Sjögrens syndrome and 30% in systemic lupus erythematosus to chronic diseases, e.g. pulmonary fibrosis, syphilis and sarcoidosis (Bartfield, 1969). It is also found in about 5% of normal people, particularly the elderly. The significance of rheumatoid factor is that in general, the higher it is the poorer the prognosis and the greater the likelihood of complications, e.g. nodules, vasculitis and severely destructive joint disease. Occasionally, antinuclear factor is present, but usually in a low titre. This has little individual significance in adults with rheumatoid arthritis. Similarly, serum levels of complement are usually normal or very occasionally high; this again is not significant.

In the synovial fluid of patients with rheumatoid arthritis, complement levels are reduced while levels are elevated or normal in seronegative joint disease. Other findings in the synovial fluid, e.g. inclusion bodies or ragocytes and elevated white cell counts, are non-specific.

Histology

The findings on synovial biopsy are non-specific. The diagnosis of the disease cannot be made on synovial histology alone. The usefulness of needle biopsy or open biopsy of inflamed synovium is in non-articular involvement, when other diseases, e.g. tuberculosis or pigmented villonodular synovitis, are to be excluded.

RADIOLOGICAL FEATURES

Most of the findings in specific joints have been discussed with the description of the clinical picture. Certain cardinal radiological features, however, are required to make the diagnosis of rheumatoid arthritis on a radiograph (Table 17.2.3). Again, radiographic findings are only helpful when the clinical findings are suggestive of the disease.

Table 17.2.3 Radiological features of rheumatoid arthritis

Soft tissue swelling
Periarticular osteoporosis
Marginal erosions
Joint space narrowing
Deformity

In general it is important to obtain radiographs of both hands, wrists and feet in all patients with a suspected diagnosis of rheumatoid arthritis. It is sometimes advisable to include radiographs of the pelvis, knees and cervical spine in a routine screen of the disease. Soft tissue swelling around joints, whether due to synovial fluid or inflamed synovium, can usually be seen, and rheumatoid nodules are often identifiable radiographically. Periarticular osteoporosis is an early radiographic sign and can sometimes be detected more easily if the film is viewed from a distance. Generalized osteoporosis develops at more advanced stages of the disease.

Marginal erosions characteristically occur where the synovium reflects on the articular cartilage, and if looked on in different views may appear cystic. Different projections may be necessary to demonstrate erosions. The ulnar styloid is a common area in which early erosive change occurs. Joint space narrowing typically occurs over the whole area of the involved joint, probably due to cartilage 'dehydration' as a result of enzymic degradation. It is important not to interpret joint space narrowing in oblique views. Weight-bearing views are helpful in lower limb joints.

Joint deformity is a late finding in rheumatoid disease and can be gross (Fig. 17.2.5). In a small percentage of patients with advanced disease, bony ankylosis develops in the carpal and tarsal joints.

TREATMENT OF RHEUMATOID ARTHRITIS

Treatment of rheumatoid arthritis is aimed at alleviation of local and general inflammation, prevention of tissue damage, prevention of deformity and preservation of function, and the reversal of phenomena threatening organ function, e.g. mononeuritis, myocarditis and lung disease.

Patient education

It is very important to educate the patient about the disease. Most patients have a vague knowledge of rheumatoid arthritis and do not appreciate that the

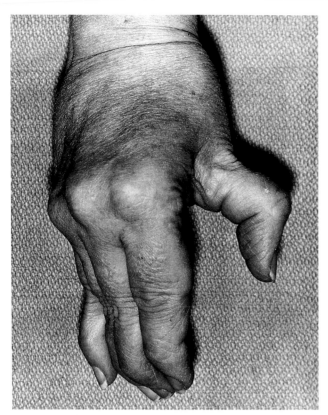

Fig. 17.2.5 Typical joint deformities in rheumatoid arthritis.

disease may partially remit and exacerbate spontaneously. Many believe they will inevitably become disabled, and this causes intense anxiety and depression. The patient should be instructed on realistic goals to control the disease, to relieve symptoms, preserve joint function and enable a realistic lifestyle to be maintained. Patients should be warned that many of the drugs used in the treatment of rheumatoid arthritis take weeks or even months to show any signs that the disease is improving.

Systemic rest

There is a body of evidence to suggest that physical rest can rapidly alleviate an acute flare of rheumatoid disease. The nature of the disease with fever, weight loss, anaemia, lymphadenopathy and visceral involvement dictates that more systemic involvement than inflamed joints is apparent, and periods of rest varying from 2–4 h during the day to admission and bed-rest in hospital are advisable.

Physical therapy

The aims of physical therapy are to maintain a range of motion in the joints, to minimize disuse atrophy of muscle, deformity and excessive articular trauma, and to provide local rest.

Preservation of the range of motion in joints is best obtained by the patient moving all joints gently through a full range of movements once daily. This exercise is best performed after the initial joint stiffness has died down or after a hot bath. Patients should be instructed in how to prevent joint deformity, e.g. sleeping in as near an anatomical position as possible and avoiding the placing of pillows under painful knees. Gentle isotonic or isometric exercises should be performed, and all vigorous exercises avoided.

Joint protection can be encouraged by splinting. Splints are particularly valuable in relieving pain from inflamed joints. Splints should be removed once each day to encourage exercise.

Application of heat or cold to involved areas often relieves pain and muscle spasm, and a home visit should always be encouraged.

Medical treatment

There are two main goals in the medical treatment of patients with rheumatoid arthritis. The first is to alleviate the pain and swelling of involved joints, and this has been greatly improved by the development of an increased number of effective non-steroidal anti-inflammatory drugs. The second aim is to modify the course of the disease. This can be effected by using disease-modifying anti-rheumatoid drugs, e.g. gold, penicillamine, anti-malarial drugs and sulphasalazine. With the increased use and experience of these second-line drugs, the necessity for using steroids has been greatly reduced and their consequent troublesome side-effects should no longer be a threat. A further group of drugs is also recognized as useful in the long-term treatment of rheumatoid arthritis; these are the immuno-regulatory agents, e.g. azathioprine and methotrexate.

NON-STEROIDAL ANTI-INFLAMMATORY DRUGS

There has been a great increase in the number of effective non-steroidal anti-inflammatory drugs (NSAIDs) available over the past 20 years, resulting in fewer patients experiencing difficulty in relief of pain and stiffness, and a reduction in joint swelling with less damage to involved joints and therefore less early orthopaedic intervention.

Although salicylates in the form of soluble asprin can be shown to have a rapid therapeutic effect, and they have long been the mainstay of the early treatment of rheumatoid arthritis, patients rapidly become intolerant of their toxic side-effects, which include tinnitus, deafness and gastric ulceration. The choice of NSAID tends to be empirical, but it is advisable to be familiar with a few preparations and to be aware that patients might respond to one group of NSAIDs, e.g. the propionic acid derivatives (ibuprofen and naproxen), but not to another, e.g. the phenylalkanoic acid derivatives (indomethacin and diclofenac). There is evidence that despite the control of pain and inflammation by NSAIDs, the disease still progresses in the majority of patients.

IDENTIFICATION OF PATIENTS WITH PROGRESSIVE DISEASE

Numerous clinical and laboratory variables have been shown to correlate with aggressive disease activity.
1 Older age at onset of disease.
2 Female sex.
3 Presence of nodules.
4 High titre of rheumatoid factor.
5 Severity of joint erosions when patient is first seen.
  Measurement of acute phase responses, e.g. erythrocyte sedimentation rate and C-reactive protein provide an approximate guide to disease activity.

INDICATIONS FOR DISEASE-MODIFYING THERAPY

The decision to treat patients with disease-modifying agents is based on the presence of persistent synovitis, laboratory criteria and the development of erosive damage on radiographs (Table 17.2.4). After a trial of NSAIDs lasting 4–6 months and using adequate doses of different groups of NSAIDs has failed to bring the disease under control, disease-modifying therapy should be initiated.

CHOICE OF DISEASE-MODIFYING DRUG

Fortunately, NSAIDs can continue to be prescribed while disease modifying drugs have time to work. Their symptomatic effects are greater than and additive to the effects of NSAIDs and analgesics. They are thought to alter the natural history of the condition in the long term.

Table 17.2.4 Indications for disease-modifying therapy

Clinical evidence of synovitis
Morning stiffness for more than 1 h
Inadequate response to NSAIDs
Erosive disease on radiographs
Raised erythrocyte sedimentation rate or C-reactive protein

Gold salts and penicillamine are the most commonly used disease-modifying drugs in the UK. They take up to 3 months before improvement is recognized, and therefore NSAIDs should continue but be slowly withdrawn as the effect of the disease modifier takes hold. Because regular blood tests for marrow suppression and urine tests for proteinuria are required, it is conventional for an experienced clinician to supervise the monitoring of these toxic drugs.

Intramuscular gold in the form of sodium aurothiomalate, 50 mg/week for 10 weeks, then 50 mg/month, and penicillamine, 125 mg/day increasing slowly to 1 g/day have similar profiles of toxicity, which include:
1 skin rash;
2 stomatitis;
3 proteinuria;
4 thrombocytopenia;
5 aplastic anaemia (rare).

Oral gold as auranofin is less effective than intramuscular gold, but has a lower incidence of side-effects, diarrhoea being the most troublesome. Doses are 3 mg twice daily increasing to 9 mg/day if the response is inadequate. If ineffective after 4–6 months the drug should be withdrawn as no benefit is then likely.

Anti-malarials are also used as disease-modifying agents because of their low incidence of side-effects. Rare cases of retinal toxicity have been recorded, however, and can be identified early by ophthalmological screening. The dose of hydroxychloroquine sulphate is 400 mg/day for 6 months, reducing to 200 mg/day for a further 6 months in those patients who respond. Few rheumatologists would continue to use this drug for more than 2 years.

Sulphasalazine is now accepted as a useful-slow-acting anti-rheumatic drug in rheumatoid arthritis. It has many of the characteristics of other disease-modifying anti-rheumatoid drugs, e.g. gold and penicillamine, and because it needs less supervision and monitoring for side-effects after the first 3 months it is becoming the disease-modifying drug of first choice for progressing rheumatoid arthritis. It produces improvement in clinical and laboratory parameters of disease activity and a slow action of 2–3 months before any beneficial effect is noted. Side-effects, though common, are not too troublesome and usually consist of nausea, vomiting and abdominal symptoms, and dizziness and instability; these are reduced if the enteric-coated formulation of the drug is used. Hypersensitivity in the form of skin rashes, hepatic changes and agranulocytosis is also recognized and is likely to occur early in the use of the drug rather than later. A reduction in dose usually limits these side-effects, and serious adverse events requiring cessation of therapy are uncommon. The dose of sulphasalazine is 500 mg/day for 1 week building up each week by 500 mg/day until a total of 2 g/day is reached at 4 weeks; the dose can be increased if necessary.

Immunosuppressant and cytotoxic drugs such as azathioprine, methotrexate, chlorambucil and cyclophosphamide are generally used in patients with progressive rheumatoid arthritis associated with vasculitis who are resistant to other disease-modifying drugs or who experience troublesome side-effects from them. With close monitoring the potentially serious short-term haematological side-effects, which are generally dose-related, predictable and potentially avoidable, can be avoided. Cytotoxic therapy is tailored to the needs of individual patients, and an appropriate dose is adjusted until a satisfactory clinical response is achieved or the patient is moderately immunosuppressed. In clinical practice this is reflected by mild leucopenia and lymphopenia. This suppression of white blood cells may have disavantages for elective orthopaedic procedures, and as a rule patients should stop immunosuppressive drugs 1 week before surgery. Methotrexate is currently proving a worthwhile immunosuppressant for patients with rheumatoid arthritis, and a dose of 7.5–10 mg/week is effective. As well as monitoring immunosuppression in patients on methotrexate, evidence of abnormal liver function and pulmonary fibrosis should also be sought.

The main concern regarding the use of cytotoxic drugs for long-term therapy is the risk of chromosomal damage and an increased long-term risk of malignancy. Cyclophosphamide in particular is associated with a fourfold increase in the risk of late malignancy.

CORTICOSTEROIDS

There is still controversy over the use of corticosteroids in the treatment of rheumatoid arthritis. They are dramatic in their effectiveness in improving the symptoms and signs of synovitis in rheumatoid arthritis, but their use is limited because of long-term side-effects, in particular osteoporosis. There is a difference of opinion as to when to use corticosteroids in the management of rheumatoid arthritis. Some clinicians use a low-dose regimen of less than 7.5 mg/day while awaiting the delayed effects of disease-modifying drugs. Others use much higher doses only as a last resort when all other treatments have failed. Significant adrenal suppression is less likely to occur if the corticosteroids are taken early rather than later in the day, and doses of less than 7.5 mg/day are less likely to produce osteoporosis. Sudden

drops in the dose of corticosteroid can precipitate an acute flare of rheumatoid arthritis, and the patient should be weaned off the drug very gradually at approximately 1 mg/day at monthly intervals.

The operative treatment of corticosteroid-treated patients with rheumatoid arthritis is particularly fraught with problems, e.g. impaired wound healing, increased risk of infection, post-operative hypotension and wound dehiscence. Consultation with a rheumatologist is particularly advisable well before surgery in such patients, as even minor changes in corticosteroid therapy, e.g. conversion to an alternate day regimen or to a daily morning regimen may reduce these risks. Another major area of controversy is 'cover' over periods of illness and operation. In those patient taking over 7.5 mg/day of prednisone/prednisolone in the morning, and in particular in those taking divided daily doses, careful monitoring of blood pressure and renal function is important, and in overwhelming infection, supplementation is vital. Over periods of elective surgery, individual practice is again variable. Increasingly, anaesthetists are finding that with careful post-operative monitoring and recovery rooms, requirements for intravenous corticosteroid are not as great as in previous years.

In patients who are taking 5 mg/day or more of prednisone/prednisolone, it is important that their normal daily prednisone dose is replaced by the equivalent dose of intravenous hydrocortisone hemisuccinate. Much will depend on the time of the operation, i.e. morning or afternoon, and on the scale of surgery. For most patients who have taken their normal steroid or have had the intravenous equivalent, 100 mg intravenously with the premedication will be sufficient, provided that following surgery they receive further 100 mg intravenous supplements twice daily while unable to take their normal oral dose. Where post-operative infection occurs, there may be a need for moderately increased daily corticosteroid therapy, but in cases of hypotension, consideration should always be given to other possible causes rather than the simple attribution to insufficient corticosteroid cover. Of prime importance in patients with rheumatoid arthritis at the time of surgery, and in particular with corticosteroid-treated patients, is the need for adequate fluid intake.

INTRA-ARTICULAR STEROIDS

There is further controversy about the aspiration and injection of corticosteroids into joints. With a non-touch technique and strict aseptic precautions it is very rare to introduce sepsis into a rheumatoid joint. Aspiration and injection certainly relieve pain and reduce synovitis in a troublesome joint, and provided the joint is not treated more often than every three months, no long-term adverse effects should occur. Methyl prednisolone or triamcinolone are generally used because of their low aqueous solubility and tendency to remain within the joint. Suspected septic arthritis and evidence of infection elsewhere, e.g. in the urinary or upper respiratory tracts, are absolute contraindications.

OTHER DISEASES OF CONNECTIVE TISSUE

Systemic lupus erythematosus

The orthopaedic surgeon has to be able to differentiate between this disease and rheumatoid arthritis because arthritis or arthralgia is its most common manifestation. Over the past few years great advances have been made in the serological diagnosis of this multisystem disease and in its treatment. Despite this, its aetiology remains unknown. As in rheumatoid arthritis the disease is more common in women than in men (ratio of 9:1). The peak age of presentation is in the second and third decades, and the disease is more common in blacks. Although rare, there seems to be an increasing incidence of new cases, probably associated with more highly sophisticated diagnostic techniques, more use of drugs causing a lupus-like syndrome and more awareness of the disease in general. The disease is characterized by either acute fulminating crises or slow progression punctuated by periods of exacerbation and remission. These exacerbations are attended by fever, malaise, weight loss and anorexia.

MUSCULOSKELETAL INVOLVEMENT

Arthritis or arthralgia is the usual presenting symptom in 93% of patients. Small joints are more commonly involved and pain in these is usually disproportionately greater than would be expected from the signs. Morning stiffness occurs in about 50% of patients. The arthritis is symmetrical, and in long-standing cases a joint deformity superficially similar to that of rheumatoid arthritis may develop. The deformity should not be confused with that in rheumatoid arthritis because of the obvious absence of contractures and ankylosis. The cause of the deformity is correctable subluxation of the small joints due to a combination of capsular laxity and tendon involvement. Radiology shows no erosive change, and synovial fluid analysis and biopsy are not helpful. Aseptic necrosis, usually in weight-bearing joints, has been reported in 5% of patients with systemic lupus erythematosus and is not always associated with steroid therapy.

SKIN DISEASE

Skin, hair and mucous membranes are involved in 85% of patients with systemic lupus erythematosus. Although the butterfly rash is characteristic of the disease it occurs in only 41% of patients. The rash is light-sensitive and may occur on other exposed areas. Other rashes include the pruritic papular rash of discoid lupus erythematosus occurring in the butterfly area and over the scalp and ears. In 10% of patients vasculitis of the skin occurs. This is distributed over the upper arms, and particularly on the nail-folds and palms of the hands. More troublesome ulcers may develop in the lower limbs and livedo reticularis (a mild vasculitis) is extremely common.

Alopecia can occur with discoid lupus erythematosus and more profusely in systemic disease, particularly along the frontal line of the forehead. Raynaud's phenomenon is present in 20% of patients and may precede the disease for many years.

RENAL DISEASE

This is present in 50−60% of patients and presents early in the disease. Most of these cases are treatable and non-progressive, so that only haematuria and/or proteinuria is present. In 25% of patients with renal disease the picture is more severe, and on histology diffuse proliferative disease is the most aggressive type of nephritis.

CARDIAC DISEASE

In 25% of patients pericarditis occurs and is commonly associated with pulmonary disease. Myocarditis and endocarditis also occur. The characteristic Libman−Sacks endocarditis involves the inferior aspect of the mitral valve.

PULMONARY DISEASE

This occurs in 30% of patients and takes the form of a unilateral pleural effusion. Fibrosis is found in some patients and abnormalities of pulmonary function are expected.

CENTRAL NERVOUS SYSTEM DISEASE

In 60% of patients neuropsychiatric features are found.

Seizures and organic psychoses are the most commonly encountered problems.

OCULAR DISEASE

'Cytoid bodies' or exudates together with retinal haemorrhages are the most troublesome ocular manifestations, though conjunctivitis is the most common.

LABORATORY FINDINGS

Haematology

One or more of the following abnormalities is present at some time in systemic lupus erythematosus.
1 Anaemia: this may be monocytic, normochromic, or less commonly haemolytic.
2 Leucopenia: fewer than 4000 white blood cells/mm^3 are found in two-thirds of patients.
3 Thrombocytopenia: between 100 000 and 150 000 platelets/mm^3 are found in about one-third of patients.
4 Erythrocyte sedimentation rate: this is moderately to markedly raised in most patients.

Immunology

The lupoid cell can be demonstrated in synovial fluid, pleural fluid and blood, but its presence does not necessarily correlate with disease activity. The lupoid cell test has been largely replaced by anti-nuclear antibody screening and DNA antibody binding tests.

When the anti-nuclear antibody is found, serum antibodies are present to a number of nuclear antigens and these can occur in other chronic rheumatic diseases. The test is, therefore, not specific for systemic lupus erythematosus. Antibodies to double-stranded DNA (anti-DNA antibodies) are the most specific marker for systemic lupus erythematosus (Hughes, 1971) DNA binding levels are usually a good indication of disease activity. Serum complement level is perhaps an even better indication of the activity of the disease, the most useful components being C3 and C4. A lowered complement level is indicative of renal disease.

Urine examination

This should be performed on all patients with systemic lupus erythematosus, proteinuria and haematuria being obvious indications of renal disease. Creatinine clearance and blood urea measurement are also helpful.

Synovial fluid examination

Apart from demonstration of low complement levels, synovial fluid analysis is of no value.

Skin biopsy

On directed immunofluorescence of non-exposed skin as well as exposed skin, a 'band' of immunoglobulins and complement components can be demonstrated at the dermal/epidermal junction in 70% of patients.

TREATMENT

The initial treatment will vary depending on the severity of the disease. If there is a rapid onset of symptoms with positive anti-DNA antibody titres and low serum complement levels, more aggressive treatment should be initiated. Generally, the patient should be made aware of the nature of the disease and given reassurance that medical attention will always be available. The patient should be able to recognize signs and symptoms of disease activity, e.g. arthralgia or skin rashes, heralding a flare. Avoidance of the sun with sun screens should be encouraged, and rest should also be included in the treatment. If there are dermatological manifestations anti-malarial therapy with hydroxychloroquine significantly improves the skin. Anti-inflammatory drugs help the arthritis and can also be of value in the pericarditis and pleural effusions that occur.

The use of oral steroids in high doses, however, is necessary in active disease with the gradual lowering of the dose of steroids as the activity subsides—a maintenance dose of prednisolone, 10–20 mg, is often required.

With very severe renal and central nervous system disease, immunosuppression with cyclophosphamide may be necessary.

Scleroderma (progressive systemic sclerosis)

Although an uncommon condition, progressive systemic sclerosis nevertheless usually presents with pain and stiffness in joints and vascular changes, thus directing the patient to the orthopaedic surgeon. The sex incidence is 3:1 in favour of females, and although rare in childhood, it can affect most other ages, the peak being at 30–50 years of age. The aetiology remains obscure.

The onset is insidious, with vascular feature predominating. Raynaud's phenomenon may precede the onset of skin changes by months or years, and this is followed by symmetrical painless oedema and then gradual thickening of the skin over the dorsum of the hands and feet. As the disease progresses all the limbs are involved and finally the trunk. The skin is thickened, leathery in texture and causes restriction to the underlying structure and an expressionless immobile facies. Telangiectasia consisting of dilated capillary loops and venules also occurs over the hands and face, and calcinosis occurs subcutaneously with resulting ulceration over fingertips and bony prominences.

GASTROINTESTINAL DISEASE

Gastrointestinal involvement causes loss of oesophageal motility, and this is often an early feature and quite symptomless. When they do occur, symptoms consist of sticking of dry food and a dull ache in the substernal region. Oesophagitis may develop later. Small intestinal dilatation and hypomotility can also occur · and are associated with malabsorption.

PULMONARY DISEASE

This is second in prevalence to oesophageal involvement and occurs late in the disease. Interstitial pulmonary fibrosis causing a dry cough and dyspnoea is the most prominent feature, and disturbances in pulmonary function are expected.

CARDIAC DISEASE

Cardiac involvement is much less common and usually secondary to pulmonary involvement. Myocardial fibrosis and (uncommonly) pericarditis have been described.

RENAL DISEASE

Disease of the kidney is responsible for the majority of deaths from progressive systemic sclerosis, and the development of hypertension indicates an unfavourable prognosis.

MUSCULOSKELETAL INVOLVEMENT

These symptoms range from arthralgia and morning stiffness in early cases to inflammatory arthritis, which is uncommon. The joint symptoms are associated with the most prominent skin involvement, and later in the disease the joint deformities that occur are due to the involvement of tendon sheaths.

LABORATORY FINDINGS

There is no pathognomonic test for progressive systemic sclerosis. The erythrocyte sedimentation rate is moderately raised and there may be mild anaemia. Antinuclear antibodies of a speckled type are found in about 50% of patients.

RADIOLOGICAL FEATURES

These are very helpful in the diagnosis of progressive systemic sclerosis. Oesophageal hypomotility on barium swallow is a helpful early sign. On radiographs of the hands and feet resorption of the distal tufts and subcutaneous calcification is a very characteristic, though later, feature (Fig. 17.2.6).

TREATMENT

This is a difficult disease to treat, and the effectiveness of treatment is difficult to assess, partly because of the variability of its severity and rate of progression and also because spontaneous improvement may occur after several years. Treatment is generally systemic, e.g. vasodilators for Raynaud's phenomenon and more recent calcium antagonists, e.g. nifedipine, prostaglandin E infusions and prostacyclin. For treating the disease itself no drug or combination of drugs has been proved to be of value in adequately controlled prospective trials. Anti-inflammatory agents and corticosteroids have proved to be disappointing. Immunosuppressive therapy with

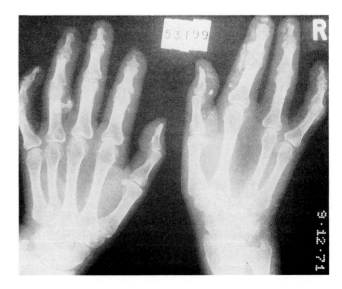

Fig. 17.2.6 Resorption of the distal tufts of index fingers and soft tissue calcification in progressive systemic sclerosis.

azathioprine, cyclophosphamide or chlorambucil has also proved disappointing, and there is no general agreement on the effectiveness of these agents.

Polyarteritis nodosa

This disease of connective tissue is characterized by inflammation and necrotizing arteritis in the walls of small and medium-sized arteries. The aetiology is unknown and the disease occurs three times more commonly in men than in women, with a mean peak age of 40 years. Because of the varied nature of the arteritis, the clinical features depend on the extent and site of involvement. General symptoms, e.g. fever, malaise and weight loss, are usually present and it is these, together with an unexpected multisystem involvement, that should alert the clinician. Thus, hypertension and kidney disease with involvement of the cardiovascular system, e.g. myocardial infarction or pericarditis, symptoms of 'acute abdomen', central nervous system signs, or foot or wrist drop might suggest the disease. Also prominent are bronchial asthma, skin rashes or nodules, orchitis, musculocutaneous symptoms and eye disease. It will be seen that few of these problems will direct the patient to the orthopaedic surgeon, but muscle tenderness and arthralgia are common. The diagnosis is usually confirmed on biopsy of an involved organ, the presence of small or medium-sized vessels being required in the specimen. In the laboratory an elevated erythrocyte sedimentation rate is to be expected, there is usually a polymorphonuclear leucocytosis and sometimes eosinophilia. Renal investigations are also important.

There is a strong association between polyarteritis nodosa and hepatitis B antigen, with 25–40% of patients carrying the antigen. This interesting association is the first of a virus–antibody immune complex in a connective tissue disease. Treatment with corticosteroids is the initial approach, but the addition of a cytotoxic agent, e.g. cyclophosphamide, sometimes results in a striking remission.

Polymyositis and dermatomyositis

These are diffuse inflammatory disorders of striated muscle of unknown cause. Dermatomyositis is an inflammatory muscle disease with a characteristic skin rash, while the rash is absent in polymyositis. There is no fundamental difference between the two diseases except for the skin rash and a greater risk of malignancy in dermatomyositis. Females are more commonly affected, and all age groups are susceptible. The disease is of importance to orthopaedic surgeons because it overlaps other connective tissue diseases and because it presents with muscle weakness, pain and swelling.

MUSCLE DISEASE

Proximal muscle groups of the shoulder and pelvic girdle are characteristically involved, though involvement of the anterior neck muscles causing difficulty in raising the head may be an early symptom. The onset is usually insidious, though rapid onset accompanied by constitutional upset and oedematous, indurated muscles can occur. Contracture and shortening of muscle is a late manifestation of the disease, as is calcinosis of muscles that results from severe bouts of myositis.

SKIN MANIFESTATIONS

In 40% of patients the typical rash of dermatomyositis occurs. This is a dusky purplish eruption in a 'butterfly' distribution over the face and extensor surfaces of joints. Periorbital oedema is a feature, and a lilac-coloured rash over the upper eyelids is diagnostic.

JOINT MANIFESTATIONS

A symmetrical transient synovitis may initially be present and be confused with rheumatoid arthritis.

OTHER FEATURES

Other connective tissue disorders such as rheumatoid arthritis, systemic lupus erythematosus and progressive systemic sclerosis may be associated with polymyositis; Sjögren's syndrome and Raynaud's phenomenon may precede the disease.

Coexisting malignancies occur in about 20% of patients with polymyositis alone, but the incidence is higher if the skin manifestations are present, particularly if florid. Malignancy is less common in younger patients, but nevertheless should be sought, the most common sites being lung, uterus, ovary, breast and prostate.

DIAGNOSIS

Routine laboratory investigations reveal an elevated erythrocyte sedimentation rate in 50% of cases. Leakage of muscle enzymes from diseased muscle is not always evident, but levels of creatinine phosphokinase, serum aspartate aminotransferase and aldolase may be elevated in the acute disease and are useful indicators of disease activity.

Muscle biopsy from clinically involved sites is important, though involvement may be patchy and disappointing false-negatives are reported. Electromyography is also an essential investigation in polymyositis, as differentiation from a non-inflammatory myopathy can be clearly made. Prognosis varies with age and is worse in the older age group, partly but not only due to malignancy. The highest proportion of deaths occurs within the first 2 years of diagnosis. Deaths are usually associated with pneumonitis due to aspiration pneumonia.

TREATMENT

Steroids in varying doses are the drugs of choice, and combination with suppressive agents can be tried.

SERONEGATIVE SPONDARTHRITIDES

The term seronegative spondarthritis describes the following diseases.
1 Ankylosing spondylitis.
2 Reiter's disease.
3 Psoriatic arthritis.
4 Enteropathic arthritis.
5 Ulcerative colitis.
6 Crohn's disease.

The members of this group of diseases have the following characteristics which justify their place as a group separate from the other arthropathies.
1 Absence of rheumatoid factor and therefore rheumatoid nodules.
2 Inflammatory peripheral arthritis.
3 Sacroiliitis, usually associated with ankylosing spondylitis.
4 Clinical overlap between the diseases.
5 A familial aggregation and an association with the histocompatibility antigen HLA B27.

Rheumatoid factor is absent from almost all cases of these diseases, and when present only represents the 5% prevalence in the 'normal' population. The descriptions of the diseases in this group will clearly indicate the close overlap that they exhibit clinically.

As well as the similarity that exists between these diseases, there is a tendency to familial aggregation, i.e. there is a significant increase in the prevalence of the disease among families compared with control populations (Kellgren, 1964). Familial association has also been found in this group of patients, and this means that there is evidence of more than one disease from this group appearing within a single family (Moll *et al.*, 1974). Association of the HLA B27 antigen with ankylosing spondylitis has underlined these previously recognized disease associations.

Ankylosing spondylitis

This is an inflammatory joint disease with a predilection for the cartilaginous joints of the axial skeleton. With the recognition of the presence of HLA B27 in 96% of patients with this disease (Brewerton *et al.*, 1973a), there is evidence that the disease is more common than previously thought, and subclinical or *forme fruste* varieties exist.

The disease usually begins between the ages of 20 and 40 years with the presenting symptom being backache, though in up to 30% of cases the disease presents in peripheral joints. The backache is worse in the early morning and is associated with stiffness, which tends to ease both during the day and with mild physical activity. Towards the end of the day or after excessive physical activity, however, the stiffness may once more increase. This is initially due to muscle spasm and inflammation and can, therefore, respond to treatment with anti-inflammatory agents and localized heat. Sometimes the first manifestation of the disease is a totally stiff lumbar spine.

Physical examination may reveal very few signs in the early stages, though direct palpation or springing of the sacroiliac joints can produce pain.

LUMBAR SPINE

Straightening of the lumbar spine and the loss of normal lumbar lordosis is an early physical sign causing quite marked limitation of movement despite minimal symptoms. Minor limitations of movement can be measured by the Schober test, in which the distance between the fifth lumbar spinous process and a mark 10 cm above this is measured after flexion; the normal increase in linear distance is 4 cm or more, and less than this is significant. The traditional fingertip to floor measurement is unsatisfactory, because with a good range of movement in the hips some patients can touch the floor with a totally ankylosed lumbar spine.

THORACIC SPINE AND CHEST

Chest pain and tenderness of the thoracic spine generally cause symptoms 5–6 years after the onset of the disease. The limited expansion of the chest and chest pain on inspiration are due to involvement of costochondral junctions, and costovertebral and sternoclavicular joints. These joints may be tender on palpation. With more advanced disease a dorsal kyphosis develops and chest expansion is reduced to less than 50% of normal. It should be remembered that chest expansion decreases with age and is less in women (Moll and Wright, 1972).

CERVICAL SPINE

Ankylosing spondylitis is an ascending disease, so that after reaching the thoracic spine the cervical spine may become involved. Although symptoms occasionally occur initially in the cervical spine, it is rare for the disease to be confined to this area.

Cervicodorsal kyphosis develops causing a fixation in anterior flexion with neck pain and restriction in the field of vision, so that the provision of prismatic spectacles to allow for forward vision may be necessary.

PERIPHERAL JOINTS

Although characteristically a disease of the axial skeleton, 30% of patients present with disease of peripheral joints. These joints are usually the hips and shoulders with bilateral involvement. Much less commonly the knees, wrists and ankles and even small joints of the hands become asymmetrically involved. Hip involvement may be far more incapacitating than a rigid spine, and flexion contractures at the hip result in flexion at the knee to maintain an 'erect' posture.

ASSOCIATED CONDITIONS

In addition to the other seronegative spondarthritides that may complicate ankylosing spondylitis, disease may develop in other systems apart from the musculoskeletal one.

Cardiac disease

Aortic incompetence, cardiomegaly and conduction defects are the most common cardiac manifestations and occur in about 4% of patients with advanced disease. A much higher incidence (25%) of disease at the aortic root is found at autopsy, the pathology being similar to that found in syphilitic aortitis.

Iritis

This may be a complication in about 25% of patients. It is not related to severity, but to the length of the disease. It is much more commonly associated with peripheral joint involvement, preceding the joint disease in some cases. Recurrent attacks, which are usually unilateral, may lead to glaucoma or blindness.

Pulmonary disease

Irregular fibrosis of the upper lobes occurs in some patients and this may be associated with cyst formation. Tuberculosis must, therefore, be excluded. Despite the rigidity of the chest wall, however, pulmonary function is not greatly reduced, probably because of the increased diaphragmatic breathing.

Neurological disease

Atlantoaxial subluxation may develop spontaneously, but is usually associated with minor trauma. Fractures may occur at both levels in the cervical spine, particularly at C5/C6. Cauda equina lesions have been described and are suggested if the patient develops urinary incontinence, impotence, absence of ankle jerks and perineal numbness.

RADIOLOGICAL FEATURES

Very early disease may show no evidence of radiological change; soon, however, blurring of the bony margins occurs in the sacroiliac joints and in the majority of cases is bilateral. Later sclerosis occurs on the 'ilium' side of the joint and in advanced disease the sacroiliac joints become obliterated or are represented by a shadow. The presence of sacroiliitis is crucial to the diagnosis of ankylosing spondylitis, as in its absence a definite diagnosis is not possible. For the best radiological results a full posteroanterior view of the pelvis is advised. An early feature may be diffuse osteoporosis of the spine with loss of the normal lordotic curve. Superficial erosive changes occur later in the disease and have been suggested as the cause of the squaring of the vertebrae that occurs in ankylosing spondylitis (Fig. 17.2.7). Romanus and Yden (1955) showed that erosions at the upper and lower ends of the anterior vertebral edge cause a flattening of the vertebral body (Romanus lesions). Parovertebral ossification or bony bridging of syndesmophytes occurs later in the disease and is typically found at the dorsolumbar junction on the lateral aspect of the vertebral body. When widespread, syndesmophytes lead to the characteristic bamboo spine. Much later the vertebral column becomes totally ankylosed, and at this stage damage arises from fracture of the spine and atlantoaxial subluxation.

DIAGNOSIS

Because of the inflammatory nature of the disease the erythrocyte sedimentation rate is elevated in those

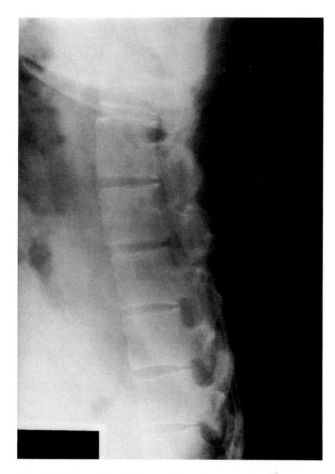

Fig. 17.2.7 Squaring of the vertebrae (Romanus lesion) in ankylosing spondylitis.

patients with active disease, and by definition rheumatoid factor is expected to be negative. When ankylosing spondylitis is suspected it is well to rule out the other seronegative spondarthritides associated with this disease.

The close association of the HLA B27 tissue type and ankylosing spondylitis has previously been mentioned, but its use as an indiscriminate screening test for diagnosis in patients with back pain is inappropriate. About 20–50% of the general population have back pain and as 6% of those will have HLA B27, only 1 in 5 of this HLA B27-positive subgroup will have ankylosing spondylitis. It has been suggested (Editorial, 1977) that tissue typing has a limited role in the diagnosis of ankylosing spondylitis and should be reserved for specific diagnostic problems, e.g. chronic backache in a young adult with inflammatory bowel disease and patients with juvenile ankylosing spondylitis.

As well as radiography as an aid to diagnosis, scintiscanning has a place in identifying sacroiliitis before the development of radiological changes.

DIFFERENTIAL DIAGNOSIS

The majority of cases of low backache occurring in young men will not be due to ankylosing spondylitis, and the differential diagnosis will be that of almost any type of back pain. As has been mentioned, it is worthwhile excluding other causes of seronegative inflammatory back pain.

TREATMENT

Active physiotherapy is important in the treatment of ankylosing spondylitis, and patients should be taught the importance of regular exercises early after diagnosis of their disease. The exercises include breathing exercises and hip extension exercises to promote and maintain mobility. Some physiotherapy departments conduct regular group classes for such patients and hydrotherapy sessions are encouraged. Drug treatment for ankylosing spondylitis is based on the use of non-steroidal anti-inflammatory drugs; steroids have no place. Phenylbutazone, 100 mg three times daily, is still available for use in ankylosing spondylitis if prescribed from hospital, though its use is not permitted for other rheumatic diseases because of its potential side-effects on the bone marrow. Naproxen and indomethacin are also valuable anti-inflammatory agents in the disease, having been shown to be effective and with fewer side-effects than phenylbutazone.

Reiter's disease

This is classically considered to be a syndrome consisting of non-specific urethritis, conjunctivitis and polyarthritis following bacterial dysentery or sexual exposure. Since the original description by Hans Reiter in 1916, mucosal ulceration, circinate balanitis and keratoderma blennorrhagica have been added as features of the syndrome, and in addition reports have been made of cardiac and neurological involvement. Reiter's disease is, therefore, now considered as a symptom complex (Keat and Rowe, 1991).

Reiter's disease is 50 times more common in males than in females, and most cases occur between the ages of 16 and 35 years, the disease has, however, been reported in children. The aetiology remains obscure, but it is still widely regarded as a post-infectious or 'reactive' arthritis that affects those genetically predisposed. *Shigella* sp., *Salmonella* sp. and *Yersinia* sp. have all been identified as possible agents in the dysenteric onset of the disease. *Mycoplasma* sp. and *Chlamydia* sp. have also been isolated from ocular and urethral lesions. As has been mentioned, there is an increased incidence of other seronegative spondarthropathies in relatives with Reiter's disease and a hereditary predisposition, strongly suggested by the presence of HLA B27 in 75% of patients with Reiter's disease (Brewerton *et al.*, 1973b) compared with 4–6% of the general population.

CLINICAL MANIFESTATIONS

These may not necessarily all be present at the same time, and the clinician is advised to question thoroughly the patient who has 'forgotten' previous attacks of urethritis or conjunctivitis. Similarly, other manifestations of the symptom complex may develop at a future date. The clinical manifestations of the disease are listed in Table 17.2.5.

Arthritis and tendinitis

This may be the most prominent symptom, as the first features, urethritis and conjunctivitis, are usually mild enough to be missed by the patient. The arthritis is acute, asymmetrical, polyarticular and mostly confined to the joints of the lower limbs. When present in the knee joints, gross effusions may develop. Any asymmetrical arthritis presenting acutely in a young man requires a diligent search for other manifestations of Reiter's disease. After an initial period of polyarthritis the arthritis settles in a few joints only. Characteristically, inflammation at tendinous insertions and periostitis may cause heel pain, plantar fascitis and Achilles tendinitis. Back pain arising from soft tissues or from sacroiliitis is also a feature, and after 5 years 50% of patients with the disease have established sacroiliitis. The arthritis settles after about 2 weeks and then subsides entirely after 3 months. In chronic severe cases, residual joint deformity in the form of spondylitis, heel pain and forefoot arthritis may develop. Metatarsophalangeal joint subluxation and 'sausage' swelling of the toes are characteristic.

Urethritis

As previously mentioned, this may be asymptomatic and

Table 17.2.5 Clinical features of Reiter's disease

Arthritis and tendinitis
Urethritis
Conjunctivitis and iritis
Mucocutaneous lesions
Other manifestations

require prostatic massage and the examination of early morning urine specimens for shreds of mucoid material. More occasionally, the urethritis is very severe and is associated with haematuria. It should be pointed out that in the dysenteric form of Reiter's disease, urethritis remains a common complication.

Conjunctivitis and iritis

Conjunctivitis may be mild and transient and missed by the patient. It is more usually bilateral and associated with a sterile discharge. Iritis occurs in 5–10% of patients during their first attack and has been found in as many as 20–50% of patients with the disease, sometimes occurring without attacks of arthritis. More unusually keratitis occurs with frequent attacks of iritis.

Mucocutaneous lesions

Painless ulcerated lesions (circinate balinitis) occurring around the external meatus and corona of the penis are quite commonly found. In uncircumcised men it is necessary to retract the foreskin for closer examination. In the buccal and palateal mucosa similar painless superficial ulceration may be apparent. Frequent examination is required, as these lesions are transient in nature.

Much more obvious but less commonly, pustular lesions occur on the soles of the feet and palms of the hands. These are initially brown macules that develop into pustules and then become hyperkeratoid. The last lesions closely resemble psoriasis both macroscopically and microscopically and may progress further to cause subungual hyperkeratosis (Fig. 17.2.8). These skin lesions, called keratoderma blennorrhagica, may also occur less commonly in the dysenteric form of Reiter's disease and are self-limiting, usually clearing within weeks.

Other manifestations

Constitutional upsets, e.g. fever and weight loss, may occur early and can be abrupt in onset. Cardiac abnormalities, e.g. arrhythmias, are well recognized and in chronic disease aortic incompetence has been reported. Very uncommonly pulmonary and neurological involvement have been found.

LABORATORY FEATURES

There is no specific laboratory test for Reiter's disease. In most patients, erythrocyte sedimentation rate is raised and remains so during the active phase. There may be

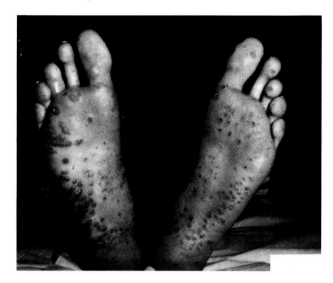

Fig. 17.2.8 Keratoderma blennorrhagia in Reiter's disease.

mild hypochromic anaemia and leucocytosis is expected. In 75% of patients HLA B27 is positive (Brewerton *et al.*, 1973b), and it is these patients who have associated ankylosing spondylitis. In non-specific urethritis the percentage of patients with HLA B27 falls to 9%, in other words close to the level found in the normal population. It would seem, therefore, that the presence of HLA B27 positivity in a patient with non-specific urethritis increases the likelihood of developing full-blown Reiter's disease, and in those patients with Reiter's disease who have HLA B27 there is an increased likelihood of ankylosing spondylitis. The measurement of HLA B27 in these patients would, therefore, have some prognostic significance. The synovial fluid is characteristically turbid with a high leucocyte count and is sterile. Levels of complement in the fluid are found to be normal, in contrast to the low levels found in rheumatoid arthritis.

RADIOLOGICAL FEATURES

Early in the disease no radiological abnormalities except soft tissue swelling can be demonstrated, and in mild cases no radiological abnormalities ever occur. In more severe cases and with repeated attacks the following may appear on radiographs.
1 Osteoporosis around involved joints.
2 Erosive changes.
3 Periostitis along metatarsals, phalanges of the feet, tarsal bones and pubis.
4 Calcaneal spurs.
5 Sacroiliitis, which may be unilateral.

6 Isolated 'spur' formation on single vertebrae in a skip fashion.

DIFFERENTIAL DIAGNOSIS

Because only two of the three primary manifestations of the disease may be present, or a previous history of urethritis or conjunctivitis is not obtained, it may be difficult to make a diagnosis. The acute nature of the arthritis suggests an infectious cause, gout, or pseudo-gout. Infection with *Neisseria gonorrhoeae* has in the past been suggested as a cause of Reiter's disease, and urethral culture may be positive for this organism. The acute arthritis associated with gonorrhoea, however, is very different from that of Reiter's disease. This disease is more common in women, usually settles in one joint and the skin lesions are pustular and haemorrhagic. Furthermore, acute gonococcal arthritis responds rapidly to appropriate antibiotic therapy (Seifert *et al.*, 1974). Ankylosing spondylitis, psoriatic arthritis and the enteropathic arthropathies should also be excluded before a final diagnosis of Reiter's disease is accepted.

PROGNOSIS

Long-term studies have suggested that about 10% of patients have active disease 20 years after their first attack. In a few cases chronic erosive arthritis and recurrent attacks of acute arthritis, uveitis and spondylitis are the outcome. Most acute attacks, however, settle within 2−3 months.

TREATMENT

As in ankylosing spondylitis, Reiter's disease responds to indomethacin, naproxen and phenylbutazone but if systemic features, e.g. weight loss and fever develop, bed-rest and further investigation are required. Soft tissue lesions and tendon involvement are common in Reiter's disease and respond to local corticosteroid injections. Aspiration of involved joints is also beneficial.

Psoriatic arthritis

Controversy has persisted for many years around the association between arthritis and psoriasis, but it is now accepted that about 7% of patients with psoriasis have evidence of an inflammatory arthropathy. Moll and Wright (1973) have classified the disease into five clinical groups.
1 Classic psoriatic arthritis with distal interphalangeal joint involvement.

2 Severely deforming type with ankylosis and in some arthritis mutilans.

3 Clinically similar to rheumatoid arthritis but without rheumatoid factor.

4 Monarthritis or asymmetrical arthritis.

5 An ankylosing spondylitis-type of arthritis representing 5% of all types of psoriatic arthritis.

A combination of the above patterns may also be found. The type or extent of the arthritis itself is not usually related to the severity of the psoriasis, though the mutilans type is associated with long-standing skin disease.

As a rule, the skin lesions precede the arthritis, though in some cases the onset is synchronous and in others the arthritis appears first. In patients who have not yet developed skin lesions the pattern of joint involvement is of great diagnostic help. In most patients persistent skin disease exists with intermittent flare of synovitis. Nail involvement occurs in 80% of patients with psoriatic arthritis compared with 30% in patients with psoriasis alone. The most common changes are pitting, subungual hyperkeratosis, transverse ridging and generalized discoloration of the nail (Fig. 17.2.9). These changes are not characteristic of psoriasis, and fungal infection should always be excluded. Evidence of psoriasis is not always obvious in a patient with undiagnosed inflammatory polyarthropathy, and the clinician is urged to search for psoriasis on the back, in the internal cleft, in the umbilicus and in the scalp. These areas may be associated with patches of psoriasis of which the patient is oblivious.

LABORATORY FEATURES

There are no specific laboratory tests for psoriasis. It is obvious that rheumatoid factors will be absent. Although commonly stated that uric acid is elevated in psoriasis, thus complicating the differential diagnosis, reports from large series suggest that hyperuricaemia is not a common finding in psoriasis and psoriatic arthritis (Lambert and Wright, 1977). Histocompatibility typing is not helpful in the differential diagnosis of psoriatic arthropathy; however, in those patients with sacroiliitis, HLA B27 is considerably increased, though there is a normal prevalence in those patients with peripheral arthritis only.

RADIOLOGICAL FEATURES

The radiological picture in psoriatic arthritis is helpful in confirming the clinical diagnosis. There may be little to see in early mild attacks, but later more specific features develop. Erosions are marginal along the phalangeal shaft and a scalloped appearance develops.

'Whittling' of the phalanges at their distal ends and resorption of the terminal phalangeal tufts are characteristic. Periostosis occurs along the shafts of the metacarpal and metatarsal bones. There is a predilection for terminal interphalangeal joints and calcification of the nails. In more destructive disease ankylosis of interphalangeal joints occurs and complete resorption of the joints results in arthritis mutilans. Sacroiliac and apophyseal joint involvement is indistinguishable from the radiological appearance in ankylosing spondylitis.

DIFFERENTIAL DIAGNOSIS

It is important to search for unrecognized patches of psoriasis in a patient with inflammatory polyarthropathy. Reiter's disease may be extremely difficult to exclude as the skin lesions are identical both macroscopically and histologically. Asymmetrical causes of distal interphalangeal joint disease, e.g. osteoarthritis, particularly when in the early inflammatory phase, are very similar to the distal interphalangeal involvement in psoriatic arthritis. At a later stage the radiological appearance of Heberden's nodes may be very confusing. Gout is yet another inflammatory joint disease that must be excluded.

Psoriasis may develop in a patient with seropositive nodular rheumatoid arthritis, as both are relatively common diseases. Sometimes a seronegative polyarthropathy cannot be fully classified, and it is then that long-term follow-up is required to determine the nature of the disease. Most cases of psoriatic arthritis are mild and do not cause the gross disabilities usually associated with the other inflammatory polyarthropathies.

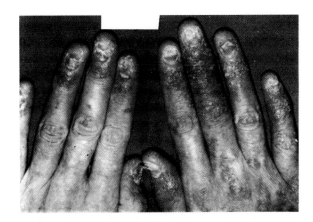

Fig. 17.2.9 Nail changes in psoriatic arthritis.

TREATMENT

A variable relationship seems to occur between the treatment of psoriasis and the treatment of psoriatic arthritis. The introduction of dithranol combined with ultraviolet A light in the treatment of psoriasis has been of considerable benefit to a number of patients. Psoriatic arthritis seems to respond well to local corticosteroids, for isolated joints, and to naproxen or indomethacin for widespread disease. When the disease is destructive, as in rheumatoid arthritis, intramuscular gold can be useful. Methotrexate has also been found to be beneficial in the disease and improves both the arthritis and the skin disease. A more effective but troublesome drug for the treatment of severe disease is cyclosporin, which requires very careful monitoring for side-effects.

Monoarthritis associated with psoriasis tends to respond well to corticosteroid injection and the use of radio-isotopes in people of suitable ages. Operative synovectomy is also a useful procedure and more effective than in rheumatoid arthritis.

REITER'S DISEASE AND PSORIATIC ARTHRITIS ASSOCIATED WITH HIV INFECTION

There has been an increasing incidence of patients infected with HIV presenting with acutely swollen joints. HIV itself has not been implicated as the cause of this acute arthritis, though the virus has been cultured from synovial fluid and therefore presents a potential hazard when aspirating these joints in HIV-infected patients. Patients can present with reactive arthritis, presumably from a reaction to the various organisms proliferating as a result of immunosuppression. The treatment of this reactive arthritis is the same as for Reiter's disease. Psoriasis and psoriatic arthritis can also be present in HIV-infected patients, again requiring caution when aspirating joints and treating the patient. Patients previously only mildly affected with psoriasis may develop extensive skin disease as the symptoms of immunodeficiency develop (Buskila *et al.*, 1990).

Enteropathic arthritis

Certain inflammatory bowel diseases are associated with both peripheral and spondylitic arthropathy. It is also apparent that skin and eye lesions may be associated, consequently allying them even closer to the other sero-negative spondarthritides.

Ulcerative colitis and regional enteritis have long been known to be associated with inflammatory arthropathy, and whether there is some connection with underlying intestinal infection and the development of anticolon antibodies is not clear. The development of sacroiliitis and spondylitis is in keeping with the increased incidence of HLA B27 in some of these patients.

CLINICAL FEATURES

The peripheral arthritis associated with these diseases is of a large joint type, it is transient, asymmetrical and non-deforming. When the spine is involved, however, classic ankylosing spondylitis develops and all the complications of the latter may become apparent.

Between 10% and 20% of patients with ulcerative colitis and regional enteritis may develop peripheral arthropathy (Haslock and Wright, 1973). There are bouts of arthritis with either monarticular involvement or a few joints only involved. Attacks are crescendo in nature and sometimes migratory, usually lasting for a duration of under 1 month. One attack per year is expected and is associated with a flare of the intestinal disease. Attacks of erythema nodosum often accompany these episodes, particularly in ulcerative colitis.

Ankylosing spondylitis occurs in at least 5−7% of these patients, its course being entirely different from the peripheral arthritis, because if present it persists. It does not parallel, and in some cases antedates, the inflammatory bowel disease.

TREATMENT

Treating the intestinal disease affects the peripheral arthritis, which tends to abate as the intestinal inflammation is eased. Non-steroidal anti-inflammatory drugs also help the peripheral joint involvement. The accompanying spondylitic arthropathy is treated in the same way as ankylosing spondylitis. Sulphasalazine, often used for the intestinal disease, also has a beneficial effect on the joint disease and can be used in the absence of obvious intestinal inflammation.

CRYSTAL-INDUCED ARTHROPATHIES

The two diseases that will be described are associated with the deposition of crystals in joints.

Gout

The term gout is derived from the Latin *gutta*—drop—the ancient belief being that 'foul' humours dropped into the weakened joints.

The disease represents about 6% of rheumatic disease seen in a hospital clinic and 90% of sufferers are men.

The first attack is usually in the fifth decade and very uncommonly in a prepubertal boy. When the disease occurs in women it does so in the post-menopausal period. It is a familial disease that is conventionally divided into primary gout and secondary gout.

PRIMARY GOUT

This term is applied to those cases that result in hyperuricaemia due to a heritable error of metabolism causing an over-production or retention of uric acid. Purine biosynthesis and/or renal excretion of uric acid is disturbed, and the resulting hyperuricaemia is associated with acute attacks of arthritis. The origin of hyperuricaemia in these patients is ill-understood, though the genetic aetiology of some rare conditions, e.g. Lesch–Nyhan syndrome and glycogen storage disease, are fully understood.

SECONDARY GOUT

This follows the development of hyperuricaemia due to some other, usually acquired, disorder. The causes of secondary gout include:
1 myeloproliferative disease and reticuloses;
2 chronic haemolytic states;
3 drugs (diuretics, pyrazinamides, salicylates in small doses);
4 starvation, ketoacidosis, acute alcoholism;
5 chronic glomerulonephritis and pyelonephritis;
6 hypothyroidism.

CLINICAL FEATURES

The progressive history of a patient with gout can be divided into four stages. Initially, there is asymptomatic hyperuricaemia, a period when unknown to the subject the serum uric acid level is raised. The presence of hyperuricaemia is only recognized after detection on routine screening for reasons other than gout. Although there is an increased risk of gout in patients with hyperuricaemia, after further investigation it is usual not to treat this asymptomatic finding. In a proportion of patients, however, crystals of sodium urate precipitate into a joint and an attack of acute gouty arthritis ensues. When this has abated a period of freedom from arthritis, intercritical gout, may occur. Throughout this period hyperuricaemia persists. Some sufferers have one or two attacks of gout yearly, while other have attacks in varying joints, these attacks becoming more frequent and troublesome over the years. Eventually chronic gouty arthritis develops, with joints no longer recovering between acute attacks and with the gradual development of deforming arthritis and tophi.

ACUTE GOUTY ARTHRITIS

The picture of a hot, red, exquisitely tender first metatarsophalangeal joint is classic. In more than 70% of cases this is the joint that is initially involved, though other joints in the foot and less commonly the knees and hands may be involved (Grahame and Scott, 1970). The presentation is largely monarticular and if polyarticular is asymmetrical. The patient is characteristically awoken, having previously been in good health, with excruciating pain in the involved joint. This is of increasing intensity and reaches a peak within hours.

The affected joint is reddened, shiny and swollen with associated dilated superficial veins. It is impossible to wear socks or shoes and even the weight of a sheet is unbearable. The great toe is erythematous, but in an involved knee there is less discoloration, effusion being a more prominent sign. Without treatment resolution takes days or even weeks. As the swelling subsides, desquamation of the overlying skin is noted. Attacks of acute gout may be spontaneous but can also be precipitated by local trauma, e.g. a blow to the joint, or after excessive walking, during systemic illness, e.g. myocardial infarction, and also following operations.

Treatment of acute gout

Acute gout is due to the deposition of monosodium urate crystals into involved joints, which results in acute inflammation in those joints. Treatment of the acute attack is to reduce the effects of inflammation. Immobilizing the acutely inflamed joint has an initial effect, and the aspiration of crystals with synovial fluid if possible also helps. Drugs, however, play an important role in easing the inflammation. Traditionally, colchicine was the drug of choice in acute gout, but because of its well-known tendency to produce diarrhoea it is not as popular as before. Doses of 0.5 mg are given at 2-hourly intervals until the attack subsides or side-effects occur. Intravenous colchicine is said to work more effectively without toxicity in doses of 1 mg for acute attacks, but care must be taken to avoid extravasation. More commonly, indomethacin or naproxen are used, indomethacin in an initial daily dose of 200 mg and naproxen most effectively as naproxen sodium, 825–1375 mg. These doses are large ones, and many attacks of gout will resolve with much smaller doses if the medication is taken as soon as the patient is sure of an attack. To ensure early treatment, gouty patients should keep a supply of tablets with them, particularly when travelling away from home. Treatment with reduced doses should be continued for 4–5 days after a major attack has subsided and then discontinued, but minor attacks can often be aborted by just one tablet. Many of the other NSAIDs have been shown to be effective in the treatment of gout.

CHRONIC GOUTY ARTHRITIS

This occurs after repeated attacks of gout in the involved joint, but may be found in joints not previously troubled by arthritis. Deposition of sodium urate in the joint results in a destructive arthropathy which is asymmetrical and often involves the small joints of the hands (Fig. 17.2.10). On close examination the white mass of sodium urate may be seen underlying the thinned skin, and these areas of tophi may discharge. Although recurrent ulceration is common, infection is fortunately rare. Approximately one-fifth of gouty subjects develop tophi. Other areas in which they develop besides periarticular subcutaneous tissue include the helix of the ear, along tendon sheaths and the olecranon and prepatellar bursae. About 15% of patients with gout develop renal stones, which when consisting of pure uric acid are radiolucent. These calculi may lead to renal disease, and renal failure is probably the most common cause of death.

LABORATORY FEATURES

The diagnosis of gout is a classic one, often with a very classic history. Serum uric acid should be raised at some stage in the disease, and the identification of uric acid crystals in synovial fluid is diagnostic. Histological examination of tophi and classic radiological features are also helpful.

Serum uric acid levels

Attacks of gout occur when levels of serum uric acid change. It is still not known why there is this apparent fluctuation in serum uric acid level. It is not mandatory to have an elevated level of serum uric acid during an attack of acute gout. If the serum uric acid is elevated, it is necessary to establish that this is not secondary to drugs, e.g. salicylate in small amounts or diuretics. For this reason it is advisable to establish serum uric acid measurements during the intercritical phase of the disease and preferably when the patient is taking no medication likely to cause hyperuricaemia. It should be stressed that hyperuricaemia found in a patient presenting with a painful joint does not necessarily mean that the patient has gout. Before subjecting the patient to unnecessary treatment, the association between the two must be established.

Identification of crystals of monosodium urate

With an obvious effusion, e.g. in the knee, synovial fluid is available for examination. With effusions in small joints, aspiration in the presence of pain is much more hazardous. The presence of urate crytals in the synovial fluid confirms the diagnosis. The specimen of fluid should not be anticoagulated when collected and on light microscopy characteristic needle shaped monosodium urate crystals may be identified. Under polarized

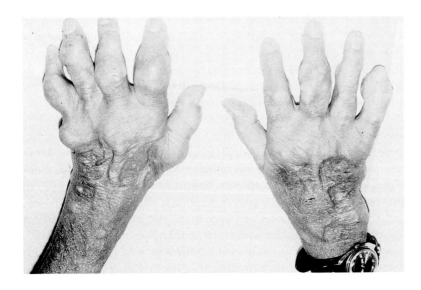

Fig. 17.2.10 Destructive arthropathy and tophi of chronic gout.

light microscopy, however, the crystals can be identified within polymorphs or lying freely in the fluid and showing strongly negative birefringence.

Examination of tophi

It is important to fix in absolute alcohol any surgical specimen that requires examination for urate crystals, otherwise these crystals will disperse. Specimens of tophi and synovial tissue may be examined in this way and monosodium urate crystals identified under polarized light microscopy.

RADIOLOGICAL FEATURES

Apart from the soft tissue swelling during an acute attack, there are no radiological abnormalities in the early stages of the disease. With the development of chronic gouty arthritis, characteristic features appear. The bony defects have a sharply defined, punched-out lytic appearance with sclerotic margins. An 'overhang margin' is highly characteristic of gout (Fig. 17.2.11). Typical areas of asymmetrical involvement occur in the feet, mostly in the heads of the phalanges.

DIFFERENTIAL DIAGNOSIS

Several arthropathies may be confused with gout.
1 Pseudo-gout.
2 Rheumatoid arthritis.
3 Osteoarthritis.
4 Psoriatic arthritis.
5 Infectious arthritis.
6 Acute bursitis (bunion).

As will be discussed below, pseudo-gout characteristically shows deposition of calcium pyrophosphate dihydrate crystals in the involved joints. Men and women are equally affected and the first metatarsophalangeal joint is seldom involved. Chondrocalcinosis is seen on radiographs.

Rheumatoid arthritis should be excluded, particularly when a palindromic onset is present. Osteoarthritis seldom causes confusion, though it may often be found in gouty subjects.

Perhaps the most important differential diagnosis is between a septic joint and an acute gouty joint. Each may be mistaken for the other, and examination of synovial fluid will be the only decisive investigation; however, a careful clinical history of onset and previous attacks is helpful. Acute bursitis of the first metatarsophalangeal joint is commonly mistaken for gout, and if the patient has taken small amounts of aspirin for the

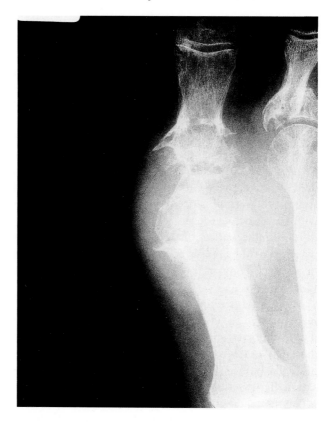

Fig. 17.2.11 Chronic gout showing the characteristic 'overhang margin'.

pain, the resultant hyperuricaemia confuses the issue further.

TREATMENT

Treatment for hyperuricaemia is indicated in several circumstances. One absolute indication is evidence of renal disease caused by uric acid deposition in the kidneys, in which case allopurinol is the drug of choice. Strong indications include attacks occurring more than three times a year, uric acid levels over 500 mmol/l, tophaceous deposits, or polyarticular gout attacks. In these circumstances and in the absence of renal disease, probenecid (a uricosuric drug) may be prescribed in a dose of 0.5 g twice daily to four times daily, but allopurinol, 300 mg/day in the morning, is now the drug most commonly used. Uric acid levels should be checked subsequently to ensure that the dose is correct, and to ensure that the patient is taking the drug. Before commencing treatment for hyperuricaemia, the patient should be started on prophylactic treatment for gout, which should be continued for approximately 1 month. Attacks of gout are more frequent when starting probenecid or allopurinol, and patients are usually ungrateful if not warned to take prophylactic gout medication. Breakthrough attacks are uncommon after the first month, and very rare after 3 months.

As hyperalimentation and obesity are common factors in the production of gout, most gout sufferers should be given the option of reducing weight rather than a lifetime of tablets. A considerable number respond well to weight reduction, which has other beneficial effects, and do not then require treatment for hyperuricaemia. All gouty patients should be advised of the necessity for a high daily fluid intake to reduce the chance of uric acid stones. Allopurinol is occasionally indicated in patients with high uric acid levels without gout, particularly in those with the tendency for stone formation, and for this reason should be prescribed for marked hyperuricaemia in patients living in hot dry climates, e.g. the Middle East.

Allopurinol is known to cause an erythematous skin reaction in 0.5−1% of patients, and probenecid is a useful alternative in this situation. Gout secondary to diuretic therapy is a problem of increasing importance, particularly in patients with severe cardiac decompensation. In this situation, hyperuricaemia of major degree is common, and gout is often seen in the cardiac clinic. As the incidence of allopurinol syndrome with fever, renal and hepatic damage is thought to be greater in patients with cardiac decompensation, allopurinol should not be routinely prescribed to patients with major hyperuricaemia on diuretics until gouty attacks occur. Azapropazone, 600 mg twice daily, is a suitable alternative in this situation, as it is an effective remedy for gout and a potent uricosuric agent.

Pseudo-gout

As implied, this condition is associated with acute or chronic joint disease clinically mimicking the poly-arthropathy produced by the deposition of crystals of monosodium urate in joints. The significant difference is that the crystals deposited in pseudo-gout are calcium pyrophosphate dihydrate. Associated with the presence of calcium pyrophosphate crystals is a characteristic calcification detected in the cartilage of affected joints, the term chondrocalcinosis being used to describe this radiographic appearance. Although almost all patients with calcium pyrophosphate crystal-induced arthritis show calcification of cartilage on radiographs of the involved joint, the converse is not necessarily true.

CLINICAL FEATURES

Pseudo-gout is marginally more common in men than in women (ratio 1.5:1), and most patients are in their sixth decade. Large joints, e.g. the knee (Fig. 17.2.12), shoulder and wrist, are commonly involved and only very occasionally is the first metatarsophalangeal joint affected. Attacks last from a few days to several weeks and are often precipitated by trauma, surgery, or acute illness. Although the joint is hot and inflamed, the severe pain of uric acid gout is absent and desquamation of the skin does not occur. Perhaps a more systemic upset, e.g. malaise and low-grade fever, occurs with pseudo-gout than with gout, and attacks are more prolonged (McCarty, 1977). Osteoarthritic changes are present in the majority of patients with calcium pyrophosphate crystal deposition disease and are probably an important sequel to this.

Several disease associations have been reported and as the limited list in Table 17.2.6 indicates this may be primarily because the patients are from an elderly population.

LABORATORY FEATURES

Synovial fluid

The pathognomonic feature is the demonstration of

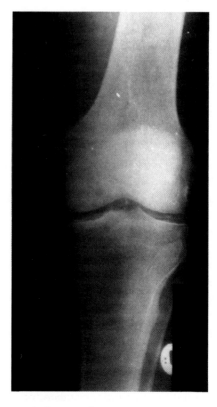

Fig. 17.2.12 Calcification of menisci in pseudo-gout.

Table 17.2.6 Diseases associated with pseudo-gout

Diabetes mellitus
Hyperuricaemia (plus gout)
Hyperparathyroidism
Haemochromatosis

---

calcium pyrophosphate dihydrate crystals in the synovial fluid. These crystals are rhomboidal in shape and often within polymorphs. Under polarized light microscopy they show weakly positive birefringence.

Synovial biopsy

A synovial biopsy specimen preserved in alcohol will show calcium pyrophosphate dihydrate crystals if synovial fluid is not available.

RADIOLOGICAL FEATURES

Punctate and linear radiodensities occur in fibrous or hyaline (articular) cartilage, the most commonly involved site being the fibrocartilaginous menisci of the knee. Other involved fibrocartilaginous structures are in the radioulnar joint, pubic symphysis, the glenoid and acetabular labia and the intervertebral discs. For this reason it is advisable to screen a patient for calcium pyrophosphate deposition with the following four radiological views: (i) anteroposterior view of each knee; (ii) anteroposterior view of the pelvis; (iii) and postero-anterior view of the wrists. A more extensive survey will not help.

DIFFERENTIAL DIAGNOSIS

Those diseases that have to be excluded when making the diagnosis of uric acid gout should also be considered among those to be excluded for the diagnosis of calcium pyrophosphate crystal disease.

TREATMENT

Anti-inflammatory drugs and joint aspiration help, but of course lowering uric acid level has no effect.

MISCELLANEOUS DISEASES

Polymyalgia rheumatica and giant cell arteritis

This disease is likely to present in an orthopaediac clinic because of the development of generalized pain and stiffness in the muscles of the shoulder and pelvic girdle. The upper back and neck are also involved. The syndrome may be an early manifestation of rheumatoid arthritis or latent malignancy, but more often no association is found, the only hazard being the possible development of giant cell arteritis and its associated danger of blindness. Because of their close association these two diseases are considered together.

Polymyalgia rheumatica is not a rare condition, being reported in some series as commonly as gout and half as commonly as rheumatoid arthritis in patients over 70 years of age; it is therefore suprising that it has only recently been widely recognized. It is three times more common in women than in men, and the sufferer is usually over the age of 60 years.

CLINICAL FEATURES

The clinical history is very characteristic. Usually the patient is over 60 years of age. The onset is often acute, and characteristically the patient complains of non-specific muscle pains around the neck and shoulders, lower back, buttocks, or thighs. Early morning stiffness, particularly around the shoulders, is a hallmark of the disease and may be so pronounced that the patient has to roll out of bed. A feeling of general malaise, low-grade fever, weight loss, night sweats and depression are well-recognized features.

Giant cell arteritis is present on biopsy of the temporal artery in approximately 30% of patients with polymyalgia rheumatica who have no temporal artery symptoms, and it is found in 90% of patients with classic symptoms of tenderness over the temporal arteries. When acute temporal artery tenderness is a presenting feature, giant cell arteritis is easily diagnosed. The artery may be thickened, nodular and have overlying erythema; the pulse may be absent. Involvement may be bilateral or unilateral. Although the temporal artery is the most obvious because of its superficiality, causing tenderness on the head and headaches, other cranial arteries present alternative symptoms. Sudden unilateral blindness, diplopia, claudication in the masseter muscle when chewing, tingling in the tongue and even stroke may be present (Healey and Wilke, 1977).

LABORATORY FEATURES

There is no specific diagnostic test for polymyalgia rheumatica, though the erythrocyte sedimentation rate is expected to be raised, often over 100 mm in the first hour. Anaemia is also common and may be related to disease activity. Elevation of liver alkaline phosphatase has been reported (Glick, 1972) but no characteristic abnormal findings are demonstrated on liver biopsy.

DIAGNOSIS

The vexed question as to whether to biopsy the temporal arteries of patients with polymyalgia rheumatica has not been answered. It is important to know whether the patient is in danger of developing giant cell arteritis, and thus potentially endangering sight. The use of temporal arteriography to indicate a suitable biopsy site has proved to have a low sensitivity and give false-positive results (Sewell *et al.*, 1980). At least 2 cm of artery should be studied and multiple sections examined. As indicated earlier, even with classic tender temporal arteries, 10% of biopsies prove negative.

DIFFERENTIAL DIAGNOSIS

Other diseases in which an elevated erythrocyte sedimentation rate and generalized muscle pains are prominent must be excluded. Multiple myelomatosis, rheumatoid arthritis of the elderly, polymyositis and occult carcinoma should all be excluded. In cases of doubt, a trial period of prednisolone, 10 mg, as a therapeutic test may be carried out.

TREATMENT

Patients with definite clinical evidence of giant cell arteritis require urgent treatment with adequate doses of corticosteroid, prednisone/prednisolone, 30 mg/day in the morning, being an adequate starting dose for all but the very severely affected. Response to such a dose should be rapid, both clinically and with reduction of the erythrocyte sedimentation rate, and this dose should be continued for at least 10 days. With complete response, the dose of corticosteroid may then be reduced to 20 mg/day in the morning, which should be maintained for about 4 weeks. Depending on continuing clinical improvement, the dose may be gradually reduced over the next 6 months until a maintenance dose of 10 mg on alternate mornings or 5 mg/day in the morning is achieved, and this should be maintained for a period of 1 year from onset.

In giant cell arteritis without symptoms of polymyalgia, the physician is very dependent on the erythrocyte sedimentation rate for ensuring that clinical remission is maintained on as low a dose of steroid as is reasonable. In patients with polymyalgic symptoms, it is much easier to assess clinical remission and to keep the patient's steroid dose at a level that allows full normal activities with minimal symptoms. Considerable variation in dose requirements are common, and in patients in whom there is felt to be a significant risk of blindness, an immediate dose of prednisolone, 60 mg, is recommended, followed by 30 mg/day in the morning. Regular supervision is required both to monitor clinical remission and erythrocyte sedimentation rate and to assess that an adequate steroid dose is maintained.

In polymyalgia rheumatica uncomplicated by features of giant cell arteritis, therapeutic practice is variable, with daily doses of prednisolone from 7.5 mg to 15 mg being recommended, and with comparable reductions to 5 mg/day in the morning being made. Treatment should not be necessarily withheld until the results are to hand. A mistaken diagnosis can always be corrected later, but visual loss due to giant cell arteritis can seldom be reversed.

Failure of response to minimal doses of corticosteroid is not uncommon, and where the clinical picture is typical of giant cell arteritis or polymyalgia rheumatica and investigations do not support other diseases, the corticosteroid dose should be doubled.

REFERENCES

Bacon P.A. and Gibson D.G. (1974) Cardiac involvement in rheumatoid arthritis: an echocardiographic study. *Ann. Rheum. Dis.* **33**, 20–24.

Bartfield H. (1969) Distribution of rheumatoid factor activity in non-rheumatoid states. *Ann. N.Y. Acad. Sci.* **168**, 30.

Bennett R.M. (1977) Haematological changes in rheumatoid disease. *Clin. Rheum. Dis.* **3**, 433–465.

Brewerton D.A., Caffrey M., Hart F.D. *et al.* (1973a) Ankylosing spondylitis and HLA 27. *Lancet* **i**, 904–907.

Brewerton D.A., Caffrey M., Nicholls A. *et al.* (1973b) Reiter's disease and HLA 27. *Lancet* **ii**, 996.

Buskila D., Gladman D.D., Langevitz P. *et al.* (1990) Rheumatologic manifestations of infection with the human immunodeficiency virus (HIV). *Clin. Exp. Rheumatol.* **8**, 567–573.

Chamberlain M.A. and Corbett M. (1970) Carpal tunnel syndrome in early rheumatoid arthritis. *Ann. Rheum. Dis.* **29**, 149.

Dixon A. St. J. (1971) The rheumatoid foot. In Hill A.G.S. (ed) *Modern Trends in Rheumatology.* London, Butterworth, vol. 2, pp. 158–173.

Duthie J.J., Brown P.E., Truelove L.H. *et al.* (1964) Course and prognosis in rheumatoid arthritis. *Ann. Rheum. Dis.* **23**, 193–204.

Editorial (1977) Ankylosing spondylitis and its early diagnosis. *Lancet* **ii**, 591–592.

Genovese G.R., Jayson M.I.V. and Dixon A. St. J. (1972) Protective value of synovial cysts in rheumatoid knees. *Ann. Rheum. Dis.* **31**, 179.

Glick, E.N. (1972) Raised serum alkaline phosphatage levels in polymyalgia rheumatica. *Lancet* **ii**, 328.

Grahame R. and Scott J.T. (1970) Clinical survey of 354 patients with gout. *Ann. Rheum. Dis.* **29**, 461–468.

Haslock I. and Wright V. (1973) The musculoskeletal complications of Crohn's disease. *Medicine (Baltimore)* **52**, 217–225.

Hazleman B.L. and Watson P.G. (1977) Ocular complications of rheumatoid arthritis. *Clin. Rheum. Dis.* **3**, 501–526.

Healey L.A. and Wilske K.R. (1977) Manifestations of giant cell arteritis. *Med. Clin. North Am.* **61**, 261–270.

Hughes G.R.V. (1971) Significance of anti-DNA antibodies in SLE. *Lancet* **ii**, 861.

Keat A. and Rowe I. (1991) Reiter's syndrome and associated arthritides. *Rheum. Dis. Clin. North Am.* **17**, 25–41.

Kelley W.N., Harris E.D., Ruddy S. and Sledge C.B. (1993) *Textbook of Rheumatology.* Philadelphia, W.B. Saunders Company.

Kellgren J.H. (1964) The epidemiology of rheumatic diseases. *Ann. Rheum. Dis.* **23**, 109–122.

Lambert J.R. and Wright V. (1977) Serum uric acid levels in psoriatic arthritis. *Ann. Rheum. Dis.* **36**, 264–267.

McCarty D.J. (1977) Calcium pyrophosphate dihydrate crystal deposition disease (pseudogout syndrome)—clinical aspects. *Clin. Rheum. Dis.* **3**, 61–89.

McCarty D.J. (1993) *Arthritis and Allied Conditions.* Philadelphia, Lea and Febiger.

MacFarlane J.D., Dieppe P.A., Rigden B.G. *et al.* (1978) Pulmonary and pleural lesions in rheumatoid disease. *Br. J. Dis. Chest* **72**, 288–300.

Mattingly S., Jones D.W., Robinson W.M. *et al.* (1981) Palindromic rheumatism. *J. R. Coll. Physicians Lond.* **15**, 119–123.

Meijers K.S.E. *et al.* (1984) Cervical myelopathy in rheumatoid arthritis. *Clin. Exp. Rheumatol.* **2**, 239–245.

Moll J.M.H. and Wright V. (1972) An objective clinical study of chest expansion. *Ann. Rheum. Dis.* **31**, 1.

Moll J.M.H. and Wright V. (1973) Familial occurrence of psoriatic arthritis. *Ann. Rheum. Dis.* **32**, 181.

Moll J.M.H., Haslock I., MaCrae I.F. *et al.* (1974) Associations between ankylosing spondylitis, psoriatic arthritis, Reiter's disease, the intestinal arthropathies and Behçet's syndrome. *Medicine (Baltimore)* **53**, 343–364.

Moutsopoulos H.M. *et al.* (1980) Sjögrens syndrome (Sicca syndrome) current issues. *Ann. Intern. Med.* **92**, 212–226.

Romanus R. and Yden S. (1955) Pelvo-spondylitis ossificans. In Rheumatoid or Ankylosing Spondylitis: a Roentgenological and Clinical Guide to its Early Diagnosis (especially Anterior Spondylitis). Copenhagen, Munksgaard, p. 22.

Seifert M.H., Warin A.P. and Miller A. (1974) Articular and cutaneous manifestations of gonorrhoea. Review of sixteen cases. *Ann. Rheum. Dis.* **33**, 140–146.

Sewell J.R., Allison D.J., Tarin D. *et al.* (1980) Combined temporal arteriography and selective biopsy in suspected giant cell arteritis. *Ann. Rheum. Dis.* **39**, 124–128.

Spivak J.L. (1977) Felty's syndrome: an analytical review. *Johns Hopkins Med. J.* **141**, 156–162.

Swezey R.L. (1971/1972) Dynamic factors in deformity of the rheumatoid arthritic hand. *Bull. Rheum. Dis.* **22**, 640.

Chapter 18

Surgical Management of Rheumatoid Arthritis

Chapter 18.1
The Upper Limb

A.B. Swanson & G. de Groot Swanson

INTRODUCTION

There is little disagreement on the use of surgery in the later stages of rheumatoid arthritis when deformity and loss of function have occurred. Decisions regarding surgical management of soft tissue involvement, however, are controversial. The surgeon who manages the rheumatoid arthritic patient ımust understand the pathological course of the disease in order to make appropriate decisions. The clinical stages of rheumatoid arthritis are:

1 acute, or inflammatory;
2 subacute, or proliferative;
3 chronic, with deformities resulting from soft tissue destruction; and
4 fixed deformities of the skeletal system.

The course of rheumatoid disease is marked by remissions and recurrences, and its most familiar target is the synovium. Various joints or tendon sheaths may demonstrate the different stages of synovitis at the same time.

The destruction of joints and connective tissue is mainly the result of synovitis. If synovitis persists, it may overgrow the bone and cartilage as a pannus and eventually result in (i) capsular distension, (ii) cartilage destruction, (iii) subcortical erosions, (iv) ligament loosening, and (v) eventual joint disintegration. However, degenerative changes become an important part of the disease process as the joint loses its lubricative efficiency, and loss of normal anatomical alignment and increased articular wear develop.

This section will deal with the surgical management of rheumatoid arthritis in the upper limb as it involves joints and tendons. The surgical techniques for reconstruction of joint lesions requiring implant arthroplasty are discussed separately in Chapter 20.1.

SYNOVECTOMY IN THE HAND AND WRIST

It is difficult to document the results of surgical synovectomy because of the great variations in the natural course of the disease and in the stages of the disease in the same individual, which preclude obtaining proper double-blind studies. The rheumatoid process has usually three possible courses. The first is characterized by initial inflammatory activity followed by spontaneous recovery within the first 2 years. The second course is cyclic in nature, and recurrence of disease causes repeated damage to the joint. The third course is characterized by continuous and unrelenting activity of the disease, with almost certain joint destruction. It is a well-established fact that synovectomy alone, without joint reconstruction, can be of no benefit when it is performed in the late stages of the disease, when disorganization of the joint is associated with erosive lesions and dislocation of joints. In cases in which there is persistent articular swelling without radiographic evidence of joint destruction or erosions, however, and in which the generalized disease process is not unremitting, synovectomy can be beneficial (Fig. 18.1.1). It is also a well-known fact that there may be a recurrent synovitis in 20–50% of the cases following synovectomy. If synovial inflammation persists in the presence of good medical therapy, however, and particularly if it worsens, synovectomy in the hand and wrist should be considered. Synovectomy procedures aim to remove pathological synovium, prevent synovial invasions of tendons and ligaments, preserve the joint cartilage and bone, relieve obstruction to movement and gliding, improve stability and relieve pain.

Despite considerable reservation as to the benefits of synovectomy in the small joints of the hand, the authors are thoroughly convinced that early synovectomy of soft tissue structures in the hand and forearm is an absolute surgical requirement if there is evidence of restricted

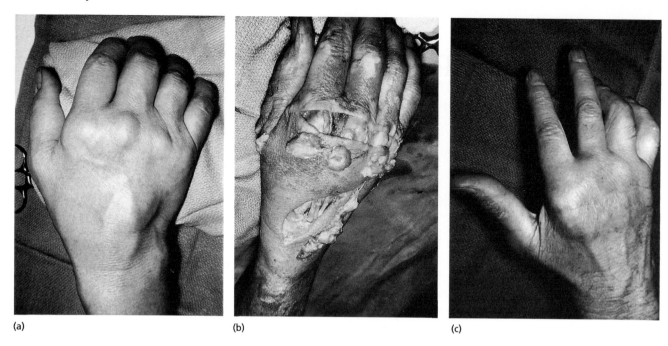

(a)   (b)   (c)

Fig. 18.1.1 (a, b) Hand of a 40-year-old male with rheumatoid arthritis in which there is severe synovitis of the metacarpophalangeal joints and the wrist with minimal deformity. (c) Six years after surgery the patient has had some progression of deformity in the metacarpophalangeal joints but has had a much improved hand. Synovectomy without additional reconstructive procedures is rarely indicated. (Reproduced from Swanson, 1973, by kind permission of C.V. Mosby Co.)

tendon gliding or nerve compression. Acute tenosynovitis may be the first sign of a rheumatoid disturbance and may precede articular symptoms. The histopathology of the synovial reaction of both tendon sheaths and joints is identical. The hypertrophied synovium may completely fill the synovial sheath and accumulate, particularly in the areas adjacent to retinacular ligaments or pulley structures. Tendon dysfunction is caused by the mechanical blockage of the adherent synovia or by involvement of the tendon itself, resulting in tendon nodules or ruptures.

The extensor tendons and wrist

Synovitis of the wrist occurs in about 60% of patients with rheumatoid arthritis. The extensor tendons are significantly involved in 30% of cases, with an incidence of 4% of tendon ruptures in the patients examined.

Synovial covering of the extensor tendons occurs mainly under the dorsal carpal ligaments. When severely hypertrophied, the synovia may extrude both distally and proximally, and the actual synovial involvement is usually greater than is noted clinically (Fig. 18.1.2). Frequently the radio-ulnar, radiocarpal and intercarpal joints are also affected. Synovectomy should be thorough but not radical. Theoretically the entire synovium should be removed, but technically, complete removal is not

possible without causing excessive damage to the tendon surface by stripping of the adherent synovia.

OPERATIVE TECHNIQUE

Incisions over the dorsum of the hand and wrist should avoid including narrow-based flaps that could result in skin necrosis in this area. The preferred incisions are shown in Fig. 18.1.3a. If the distal radio-ulnar joint is to be included in the operative procedure, as is most frequently the case, the incision is then carried proximally along the distal 6 or 7 cm of the ulna. Dissection is carried down to the extensor retinacular ligament, preserving as many dorsal veins as possible; only the transverse communicating venous branches are ligated and the integrity of the longitudinal veins is maintained. The superficial branches of both the ulnar and radial nerves are identified and preserved. The retinacular ligament is incised as shown in Fig. 18.1.3b, and elevated from the underlying extensor compartments as a rectangular flap based radially on the second compartment.

A synovectomy of the extensor indicis, extensor digitorum and extensor digiti minimi is carried out by stripping the synovium from the tendons. Sharp dissection should be avoided to prevent cutting or scarring of the tendons' surfaces. The extensor pollicis longus tendon is elevated from its bed and Lister's tubercle is

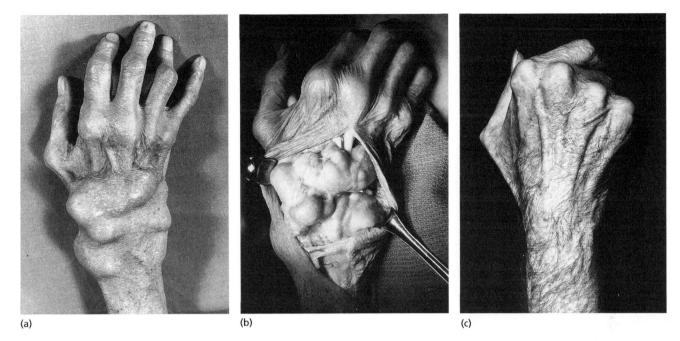

(a)   (b)   (c)

Fig. 18.1.2 (a) Severe dorsal synovitis of the wrist secondary to rheumatoid arthritis in a 60-year-old man. (b) Marked hypertrophy of the synovium surrounding the extensor tendons. These masses are frequently filled with fibrinous rice bodies. (c) Five-year postoperative follow-up, with no recurrence at the wrist. The patient has had progression of the digital deformities. (Reproduced from Swanson, 1973, by kind permission of C.V. Mosby Co.)

smoothed off. The dorsal carpal ligament is incised and sharply elevated as a distally based flap to expose the radiocarpal and intercarpal joints (Fig. 18.1.3c). Traction on the hand will facilitate the exposure and a synovectomy can be done with a small pituitary-type rongeur. Zones of erosion in the exposed bones should be freed of their synovial invasion. It is impossible to do a complete synovectomy in this area, and no radical attempts should be made. On closure, the extensor retinacular ligament is relocated (Fig. 18.1.3d). In advanced cases an implant arthroplasty of the radiocarpal joint may be indicated (see Chapter 20.1).

The transverse retinacular ligament is longitudinally incised over the sixth dorsal compartment to expose the extensor carpi ulnaris and the distal radio-ulnar joint. A synovectomy of this joint is then carried out. If indicated, as is often the case in the ulnar head syndrome, the ulnar head is resected and can be capped with a silicone implant. The physiological advantages of this procedure and the technique are discussed in Chapter 20.1.

When there is evidence of synovial involvement of the first extensor compartment, which contains the extensor pollicis brevis and the abductor pollicis longus, a decompression of this compartment is carried out. The transverse retinacular ligament is incised longitudinally after careful retraction of the veins and of the superficial

radial nerves, and a synovectomy is performed. Decompression of the tendons is probably more important than radical synovectomy.

Usually a solution of hydrocortisone is injected onto the synovectomized areas before closure of the skin. The skin is closed with interrupted sutures, and small silicone rubber drains are inserted into the wound. A bulky conforming dressing is applied and the limb is elevated for 2 or 3 days. Active motion of the fingers is usually started after 1 or 2 days and encouraged to the limits of the patient's pain and fatigue. After 3–5 days the patient is fitted with a dynamic brace that has finger extension loops to assist moving the tendons of muscles which are often weak after longstanding deformity, and to prevent formation of adhesions. The brace is worn continuously until good movement and strength have been obtained. Motion of the wrist can usually be started within 2 weeks after surgery.

Rupture of extensor tendons occurs more frequently in the tendons to the fifth and fourth digits and in the extensor pollicis longus. Repair is usually accomplished by a side-to-side transfer to intact tendons. Occasionally, when all tendons are ruptured, the extensor carpi ulnaris may be transferred to the extensor tendons, or the flexor digitorum sublimis (superficialis) to the middle or ring finger may be used in this repair by transferring it

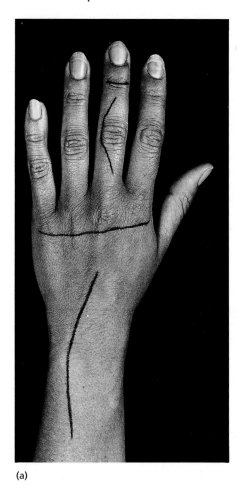

(a)

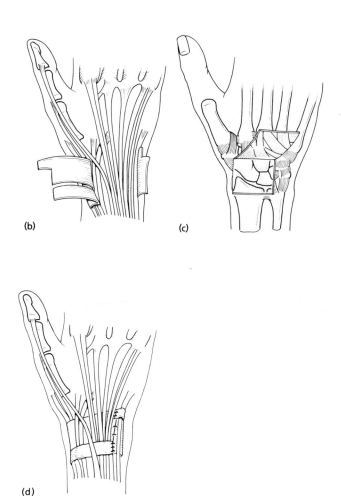

(b)   (c)

(d)

Fig. 18.1.3 (a) The recommended incisions to expose the extensor aspects of the fingers, hand and wrist. (b) Flaps of the extensor retinaculum, used when extensive synovectomy of the dorsal aspect of the wrist is performed. (c) Capsuloligamentous structures are elevated as a distally based flap from underlying radius and carpal bones to expose the joints. (d) The distal flap is placed over the wrist joint under the extensor tendons. The proximal portion is placed over the tendons to check possible bowstringing effect. EPL tendon is left subcutaneous. The extensor carpi ulnaris can be maintained over the ulna by a flap made from the retinaculum. The ulnar portion of the retinaculum can be used to maintain in position a dorsally dislocating distal ulna after reconstruction of the distal radio-ulnar joint. (b.c.d. redrawn with permission from Swanson and de Groot Swanson, 1991).

dorsally through the interosseous membrane into the extensor compartment. This type of procedure is needed very infrequently in the authors' experience. The extensor indicis is a good transfer for the ruptured extensor pollicis longus. The use of the brace is generally started 2 weeks after repair of ruptured tendons and maintained for 4–8 weeks or until good movement and strength have been obtained.

The flexor tendons

Significant synovitis of the flexor tendons is present in 38% of rheumatoid patients and may be present in the carpal tunnel, the palm and the fingers. It occurs at an early stage of the rheumatoid disease, and the only symptoms may be a feeling of morning stiffness and aching pain in the palm, wrist and forearm. Later, swelling and synovial hypertrophy at the wrist cause pain, weakness of grip and limitation of both finger flexion and extension. Commonly there may be involvement of the median nerve, but symptomatic and objective evidence of nerve compression is present in only a small percentage of the hands. There may also be involvement of the ulnar nerve, which is due in part to flexor synovitis within the canal of Guyon and in part to subluxation of carpal bones.

At the wrist level, there may be evidence of swelling proximal to the carpal tunnel. Crepitation, felt over the palmar aspect of the wrist on active finger flexion, is a reliable sign. In the palm, flexor synovitis may present as palpable tender swellings at the level of the metacarpal heads, with palpable crepitation on flexion and extension of the digits. In the fingers, synovial hypertrophy and nodules may be palpated on active flexion and extension of the digit. Entrapment of tendons within the flexor sheath may occur, and a trigger phenomenon or locking of the digit in flexion or in extension may be present. This phenomenon is present when there is a small lesion within the flexor tendon in the digit and also when there is a synovial invasion around the tendon substance. The patient may feel the snapping of the tendon against the sheath. If the synovial hypertrophy is extensive, or if the finger is locked in extension, joint stiffness will occur. In the early stages the joints may still be intact, and the loss of flexion can be localized to the tendon mechanism when the joints can still be passively moved into flexion. Later, associated joint stiffness in extension may develop, especially at the proximal interphalangeal joint. Flexor tendon synovitis, because of the pain resulting from blockage of tendons either through the presence of nodules or hypertrophic synovitis at the pulley systems, is a more common cause of failure of joint flexion than joint involvement itself. In the authors' opinion most cases of interphalangeal joint extension deformity and swan neck deformity originate as a flexor tendon synovitis. Attempts to flex the fingers are painful, and the patient will carry out digital flexion only at the level of the metacarpophalangeal joints through the action of the intrinsic muscles. A type of 'intrinsic habit' is developed. The intrinsics have a greater advantage for function in the intrinsic-plus position of flexion of the metacarpophalangeal joint and extension of the proximal interphalangeal joint, and a vicious circle for the development of the swan neck deformity results (Tubiana, 1969).

These patients frequently have associated metacarpophalangeal and proximal interphalangeal joint deformities that require articular surgery. The flexor tendons should be released in a primary procedure, and the surgery of the joint should be done during a second operation.

OPERATIVE TECHNIQUE

The flexor synovectomy is carried out proximal to distal through staged incisions until all mechanical blockage of the flexor tendons has been identified and relieved. The procedure should begin with an incision in the palm and wrist, similar to the approach used in a carpal tunnel release (Fig. 18.1.4). The incision is designed so that both the carpal tunnel and Guyon's canal can be exposed while the palmar branch of the median nerve is avoided. The transverse carpal ligament is incised longitudinally and the flexor tendons are identified. Traction

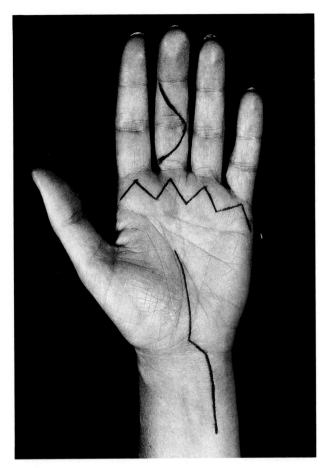

Fig. 18.1.4 Commonly used incisions to expose the flexor aspect of the wrist, hand and digits.

on them will demonstrate the degree of restriction to the flexor tendons. The synovium is carefully removed to avoid injury to the tendon surfaces. A limited synovectomy is done around the median nerve in a longitudinal fashion, including the area of the motor branch to the thenar musculature. The authors occasionally will incise the perineurium, but overzealous circumferential stripping of the nerve is avoided to prevent injury to its vascular supply (Fig. 18.1.5). The synovectomy should be complete on the flexor digitorum superficialis tendons. However, the flexor digitorum profundus tendons are frequently adherent to one another, and no excessive dissection should be done to free them.

The dissection may be carried into the subcutaneous space ulnad to the transverse carpal ligament to expose the ulnar artery and nerve in Guyon's canal. In several cases the authors noted a definite impingement of the ulnar nerve, especially of the descending motor branches. We believe that atrophy of the intrinsic muscles, which is frequently seen in rheumatoid arthritis, may very well

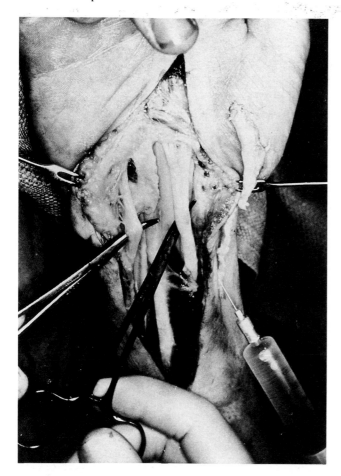

Fig. 18.1.5 Exposure of the median and ulnar nerves after a flexor synovectomy of a rheumatoid wrist. A strip of the transverse carpal ligament that has been resected is shown to the right of the incision. (Reproduced from Swanson, 1973, by kind permission of C.V. Mosby Co.)

be related to an entrapment syndrome involving the motor branches of the ulnar nerve at the wrist.

If the fingers cannot be easily pulled down into the palm and their joints are passively movable, a distal restriction of the flexor tendons must be exposed (Fig. 18.1.6). A 'W' incision is made distal to the distal palmar crease to expose individually, by blunt dissection, the flexor sheaths and tendons of the fingers. Occasionally a localized synovial hypertrophy will be found immediately proximal to, and underneath, the proximal pulley. The proximal pulley is preserved unless it appears to be entrapping the tendons. The flexor sheath is incised along its radial border and the flexor tendons are pulled up into the wound in an attempt to obtain finger flexion. The flexor digitorum superficialis and the flexor digitorum profundus tendons may be adherent to each other in this area. If the tendons are adherent to the flexor sheath, they must be thoroughly mobilized. Fre-

quently, the flexor digitorum superficialis tendon is most severely involved. Severe attrition or, occasionally, rupture of this tendon may be found; in such cases the flexor sublimis tendon is pulled down and resected at the wrist. Nodules within the tendon substance may be present and should be locally removed if they appear to be threatening the continuity of the tendon. They are excised by careful longitudinal dissection, with care being taken to spare all tendon substances. The tendon is then re-approximated with 6/0 silk or Dacron sutures. Traction on the flexor profundus tendon should completely flex the digit unless there is joint stiffness.

If traction of the flexor profundus tendon does not effect interphalangeal flexion of the digit, further distal obstruction is present. The digital flexor mechanism is exposed as shown in Fig. 18.1.4. Lateral incisions on the radial side of the index finger or on the ulnar side of the little finger are not recommended because of the possibility of inadvertent injury to the digital nerve. The tendon sheath is incised longitudinally, and synovectomy is performed in the area opposite the proximal phalanx. Occasionally nodules will be found in the flexor profundus tendon distal to the flexor sublimis tendon bifurcation; they can be removed, as noted above.

If hyperextension deformity of the proximal interphalangeal joint of more than 10° is present, a slip of the flexor sublimis tendon can be used to perform a tenodesis to hold the proximal interphalangeal joint in approximately 20° of flexion as shown in Fig. 18.1.7. This procedure has been used successfully for more than 30 years in the authors' clinic to correct a swan neck deformity when the digit is approached from the palmar aspect.

Synovectomy of the flexor tendons must be comprehensive, and full excursion of the tendon should be obtained before the procedure is completed. A corticosteroid solution is injected around the tendons before closure. The skin is re-approximated with interrupted sutures, and small silicone drains are inserted. A voluminous conforming dressing is applied, including a palmar plaster wrist splint. Elevation of the upper extremity is maintained with a sling for 2–5 days. A dynamic brace is then provided to hold the fingers in corrected position while the patient carries out a prescribed exercise programme; this is especially important if the proximal pulleys have been incised. The brace can help prevent ulnar deflection of the flexor tendons. This splint is worn continuously for 4–6 weeks. Any required additional surgical reconstruction of finger joints is usually done 6–8 weeks after the patient has recovered from tendon surgery.

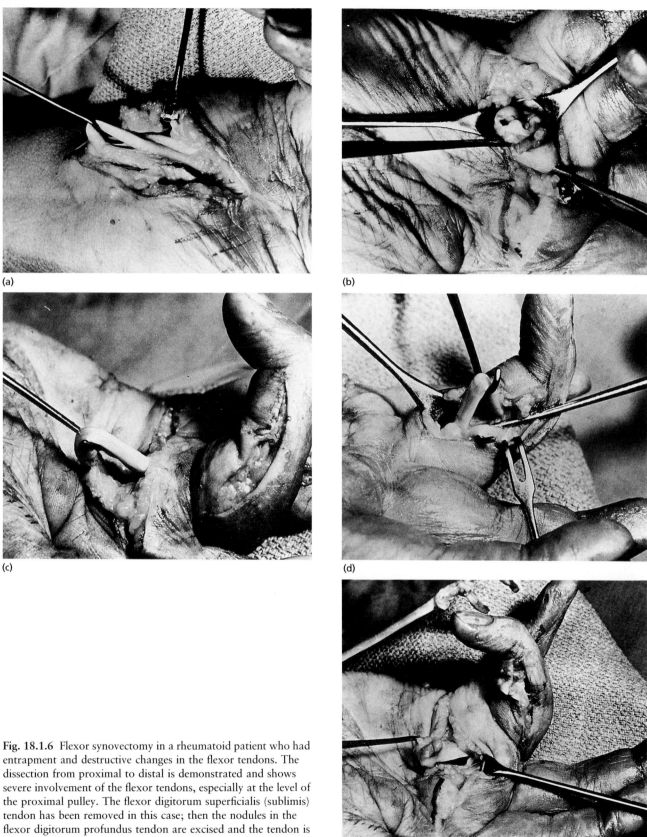

(a)

(b)

(c)

(d)

Fig. 18.1.6 Flexor synovectomy in a rheumatoid patient who had entrapment and destructive changes in the flexor tendons. The dissection from proximal to distal is demonstrated and shows severe involvement of the flexor tendons, especially at the level of the proximal pulley. The flexor digitorum superficialis (sublimis) tendon has been removed in this case; then the nodules in the flexor digitorum profundus tendon are excised and the tendon is repaired. (Reproduced from Swanson, 1973, by kind permission of C.V. Mosby Co.)

(e)

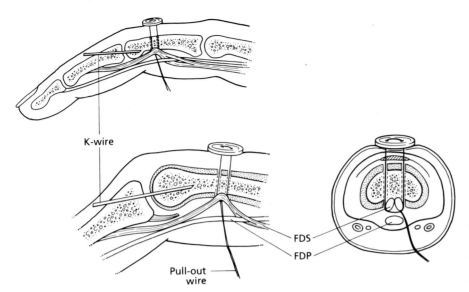

K-wire

FDS
FDP

Pull-out
wire

Fig. 18.1.7 Methods used in tenodesis of
the flexor digitorum sublimis tendon to
the proximal phalanx. In tenodesis
procedures it is best to attach the tendon
directly into bone. A Kirschner wire
should be used to temporarily fix the
proximal interphalangeal joint at the
desired angle of flexion. If the sublimis
tendon must be resected, the stump of the
tendon is used for the tenodesis. If the
sublimis tendon is retained, it can be
tenodesed to the proximal phalanx just
proximal to the bifurcation for the flexor
digitorum profundus tendon. FDS =
flexor digitorum sublimis; FDP = flexor
digitorum profundus. (Reproduced from
Swanson, 1973, by kind permission of
C.V. Mosby Co.)

The finger joints

The reconstructive surgeon who would undertake synovectomy of these small joints must be able to weigh the advantages against the disadvantages. If the patient will eventually require articular reconstruction, it would be preferable to wait and proceed in one operation. If multiple joint involvement is present, or if a late stage of the disease is present with active progression, synovectomy should not be considered. Synovectomy procedures for the digital joints are most frequently done in our clinic in association with reconstructive surgery of other joints. Synovectomy of the proximal interphalangeal joints has frequently been done at the same time as implant resection arthroplasty of the metacarpophalangeal joints.

There are basically two groups of patients in whom synovectomy can be of value. The first group consists of patients who have a small number of joints involved, such as one or two proximal interphalangeal joints without deformity, and evidence of persistent localized dorsal synovitis. A dorsal incision is made over the proximal interphalangeal joint, the hypertrophied synovium is removed from the dorsal pouch and the central tendon is resutured. The second group of patients have some mild or moderate deformity without joint subluxation. Restoration of the anatomy and rebalancing of muscular forces must be done at the same time as the synovectomy in these cases.

METACARPOPHALANGEAL JOINT

Involvement at the level of the metacarpophalangeal

joint will require correction of both ulnar drift and the tendency towards palmar subluxation. In these cases Zancolli's (1968) procedure is preferred, which includes:
1 a capsular reconstruction of the metacarpophalangeal joint with a dorsal capsulodesis;
2 a transverse section of the extensor tendon at the metacarpophalangeal joint, with tenodesis to the base of the proximal phalanx;
3 section of the intertendinous connections between the middle and ring fingers;
4 release of the ulnar intrinsic muscles of the third, fourth and fifth digits; and
5 reinforcement of the radial interosseus muscles of the second and third digits.
Straub (1959) and others have also performed soft tissue reconstructions in similar cases, with transfer of the ulnar interosseous tendons to the distal portion of the collateral ligament on the radial aspect of the adjacent digits.

Longstanding synovitis of the metacarpophalangeal joint may result in deformation of the joint surfaces into what has been described as a cup-and-saucer deformity. The base of the proximal phalanx widens and deepens centrally to receive the head of the metacarpal. The result is a relatively stable and mobile 'natural' arthroplasty, which is most commonly seen in the index and middle fingers. If these joints provide adequate motion and are pain free, no further surgery is indicated. However, occasionally, resection arthroplasty may be worthwhile. Adequate bone stock must be present in the metacarpals to receive the stems of the implants. Occasionally there is inadequate bone stock to receive the finger joint implant, especially in the little and ring fingers, due to severe bone absorption. The Tupper (1989) type of resection arthroplasty is then used for these joints. This procedure consists of detaching the palmar plate at its proximal origin, bringing it as a flap between the bone ends to the dorsal surface of the resected metacarpal shaft, and suturing it through a drill hole in the dorsal bone cortex. The collateral ligaments can also be reattached.

PROXIMAL INTERPHALANGEAL JOINT

Patients with synovial hypertrophy of the proximal interphalangeal joint, associated with mild or moderate boutonnière or swan neck deformity in which there is no radiographic evidence of erosive disease, may be candidates for soft tissue reconstructive procedures providing there is only a minimal degree of associated joint contracture. However, if subluxation, severe contracture or erosive disease of the joint is present, fusion of the joint is preferred. A primary implant resection arthroplasty and reconstruction of the tendon mechanism is usually not indicated in rheumatoid arthritis. Furthermore, flexible implant arthroplasty of both the metacarpophalangeal (MP) and proximal interphalangeal joints of the same digit should not be done.

Because treatment of the proximal interphalangeal and distal interphalangeal joints varies according to their degree of disability and other associated articular disturbances, an attempt has been made to classify their treatment as shown in Table 18.1.1.

The reconstructive procedures for reconstruction of the extensor mechanism in swan neck and boutonnière deformities are similar whether an implant is used as an adjunct to resection arthroplasty or not; the indications, surgical techniques and postoperative care for these various procedures are discussed in detail in Chapter 20.1, along with alternative methods of treatment (e.g. dermadesis, arthrodesis).

DISTAL INTERPHALANGEAL JOINT

Rheumatoid disabilities of the distal interphalangeal joints may be either primary or secondary to a collapse deformity of the digit. Localized synovectomy of the distal interphalangeal joint is seldom necessary; however, in certain cases it can be done. Through a transverse incision, the joint is exposed on each side of the extensor tendon and the synovium is removed with small instruments. The joint should be temporarily fixed with a Kirschner wire for both proximal interphalangeal and distal interphalangeal synovectomy procedures if deformity is present or the tendon repair requires it.

If the distal joint is unstable, subluxated or deviated, or shows evidence of joint destruction, fusion procedures are the treatment of choice. Contractures of the joint may be treated by soft tissue release and temporary Kirschner wire fixation, which may allow some amount of useful residual movement. Slight flexion movements of the distal interphalangeal joints are very important in finely coordinated activity, but in the presence of good movement of the proximal joints, fixation of a distal interphalangeal joint in a functional position may not be a great loss. Arthrodesis procedure of the distal interphalangeal joint is carried out through a transverse skin incision made directly over the joint, incising the extensor mechanism. The base of the distal phalanx is shaped in a concave fashion, with an air drill, to receive the rounded head of the middle phalanx. This ball-and-socket type of relationship positions the joint in the desired angle and provides good bone contact. A Kirschner wire is placed longitudinally in a retrograde fashion across the joint and may be bent *in situ* to approximately 10° of flexion. The joint is then compressed tightly, and small bone chips may be inserted in the fusion area. The Kirschner wire is then cut, leaving approximately 5 mm extruding from the fingertip. The wire is left in place for 6 weeks or more. It is removed when there is radiographic evidence of bone healing.

Reconstructive procedures for distal interphalangeal joint deformities secondary to proximal interphalangeal joint involvement are discussed in Chapter 20.1.

The thumb ray

CLASSIFICATION AND MECHANISM OF DEFORMITIES

A longstanding experience in the evaluation of the rheumatoid thumb has led to an attempt to classify its disabilities as shown in Table 18.1.2.

A sound understanding of the mechanism of deformities is important to select the proper treatment.

Boutonnière deformity

This is the most common collapse deformity of the thumb in rheumatoid arthritis (5% of rheumatoid hands). It is caused primarily by arthritic involvement of the metacarpophalangeal joint. Initially, the joint capsule and extensor apparatus around the metacarpophalangeal joint are stretched out by the synovitis process. The extensor pollicis brevis tendon and adductor expansion are displaced ulnarward. The lateral thenar expansions are displaced radially. The attachment of the extensor pollicis brevis tendon to the base of the proximal phalanx

Table 18.1.1 Treatment of proximal interphalangeal (PIP) and distal interphalangeal (DIP) joints

---

SWAN-NECK DEFORMITY OF PIP JOINT
Without involvement of MP joint
Initial deformity of PIP joint:
    Local injections (corticosteroids or other agents)
    Flexor tendon synovectomy, with or without tenodesis of flexor
        digitorum superficialis tendon (Fig. 18.1.7)
    Intrinsic tendon release, with or without flexor tendon
        synovectomy

Flexible deformity of PIP joint:
    Dermadesis at PIP joint (Fig. 18.1.8)
    Relocation of lateral tendons, with or without elongation of
        central tendon (Fig. 18.1.9)
    Tenodesis of flexor digitorum superficialis tendon, with flexor
        synovectomy

Rigid, subluxated or dislocated PIP joint:
    Resection of joint with relocation of lateral tendons, with
        implant arthroplasty (very rarely)
    Resection of joint and fusion

Treatment of DIP joint when required in any of the above
    conditions:
    Temporary pinning in neutral position if passively corrected
    Fusion if severely damaged or flexed

With involvement of MP joint
Flexible deformity of PIP joint:

Treatment of MP joint	*Treatment of PIP joint*
Synovectomy with proximal release of intrinsic tendons	Manipulation with temporary Kirschner wire fixation in flexion if required
Relocation of subluxated joint, with proximal release of intrinsic tendons	Manipulation with temporary Kirschner wire fixation in flexion if required, *or* dermadesis
Joint resection with proximal release of intrinsic tendons, with implant arthroplasty	Manipulation to 50° flexion with temporary Kirschner wire fixation, *or* relocation of lateral tendons with or without elongation of central tendon

Rigid, subluxated or dislocated PIP joint:

Treatment of MP joint	*Treatment of PIP joint*
Joint resection with implant arthroplasty	Relocation of lateral tendons with elongation of central tendon
	Joint resection with fusion

Treatment of DIP joint if required in any of the above conditions:
    Temporary pinning in neutral position if passively correctable
    Fusion if there is severe flexion deformity or articular change

BOUTONNIÈRE DEFORMITY OF PIP JOINT
Initial deformity of PIP joint:
    Local injections (corticosteroids or other agents), splinting
    Synovectomy
Flexible deformity of PIP joint (Fig. 18.1.10):
    Reconstruction of central tendon ⎤
    Elongation of lateral tendons ⎥ with or without
    Combined above procedures   ⎦ synovectomy
Rigid deformity of PIP joint:
Without bone erosions
    Joint release, with reconstruction of central tendon and
        elongation of lateral tendons
    Joint resection with reconstruction of tendons, with implant
        arthroplasty (very rarely)
    Distal release of lateral tendons
With bone erosions
    Joint resection with reconstruction of central and lateral
        tendons, with implant arthroplasty (very rarely)
    Joint resection and fusion
Subluxated or dislocated PIP joint:
    Joint resection with reconstruction of central and lateral
        tendons, with implant arthroplasty (very rarely)
    Joint resection and fusion
DIP joint treatment if required in any of above conditions:
    Distal release of lateral tendons
    Fusion
MP joint treatment if required is the same as described above
    under swan neck deformity

STIFF OSTEOARTHRITIC PIP JOINT
Non-dislocated PIP joint:
    Joint resection with implant arthroplasty
Subluxated or dislocated PIP joint:
    Joint resection with implant arthroplasty
    Joint resection and fusion
DIP joint treatment if required in either condition:
    Fusion if needed

---

is lengthened and becomes ineffective. The ability to extend the metacarpophalangeal joint is decreased and results in a flexion deformity of the proximal phalanx. The extensor pollicis longus tendon and the extensor insertions of the intrinsic muscles apply all their power to the distal phalanx and secondarily produce hyperextension of the interphalangeal joint. Pinch movements further aggravate the deformity and a vicious circle is established: the more the flexion of the metacarpophalangeal joint, the greater the tendency for the interphalangeal joint to hyperextend and the thumb ray to collapse. In time, as contractures develop, the deformity becomes fixed. Destructive articular changes compound the deformity, and disorganization and subluxation of the joint may occur.

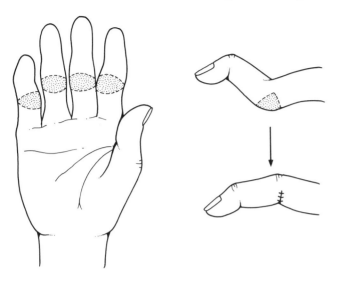

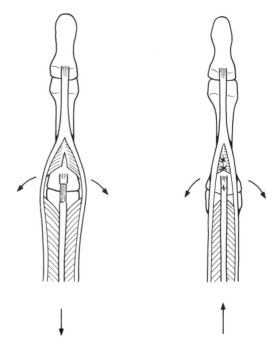

Fig. 18.1.8 The dermadesis procedure for correction of a mild flexible hyperextension deformity in weak hands. An elliptical wedge of skin is excised from the flexor aspect of the proximal interphalangeal joint, taking care to avoid the underlying nerves and vessels. Enough skin should be removed to create a flexion contracture of approximately 20°. (Reproduced from Swanson, 1973, by kind permission of C.V. Mosby Co.)

Fig. 18.1.10 Repair of the extensor mechanism in a boutonnière deformity. The stretched-out central tendon is advanced distally and it is reinserted to the base of the middle phalanx by passing sutures through a small drill hole in the bone.

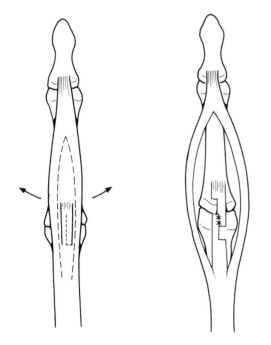

Table 18.1.2 Classification of the disabilities of the rheumatoid thumb

---

Postural deformities
Longitudinal collapse deformities:
    Boutonnière (primary metacarpophalangeal joint disturbance)
    Swan neck (primary carpometacarpal joint disturbance)
    Other
Fixed positional deformities:
    Adducted retropositioned thumb
    Other

Unstable, stiff or painful joints
Interphalangeal joint
Metacarpophalangeal joint
Carpometacarpal joint

Tendon disabilities (contracture, displacement, rupture)
Flexor pollicis longus
Extensor pollicis longus
Extensor pollicis brevis
Abductor pollicis longus
Intrinsics

Fig. 18.1.9 Technique for elongation of the central tendon and relocation of the lateral tendons in a swan neck deformity. The central tendon is separated from the dorsally displaced lateral tendons, which are allowed to relocate palmad. The central tendon is step-cut transversely and dissected proximally, thereby lengthening it. The cut ends of the central tendon are re-approximated in a lengthened position with interrupted sutures, with the knots buried.

Swan-neck deformity

A swan-neck deformity of the thumb is usually initiated by destructive changes at the carpometacarpal joint. It is present in 9% of rheumatoid thumbs, and is far more common in osteoarthritic thumbs. When restriction of motion occurs at the base of the thumb, compensatory movements that occur at the distal joints to provide thumb function result in instability and deformity of the swan neck type. Similarly, when motion of the trapeziometacarpal joint during abduction becomes painful, the patient avoids abduction and an increasing adduction contracture develops. If there is an effusion in the joint, further loosening of the capsule occurs allowing subluxation of the metacarpal. As a result the normal movements required in pinch become increasingly painful and the distal joints are used to compensate for the lack of movement at the base of the thumb. The result is hyperextension of the interphalangeal joint, but more frequently hyperextension of the metacarpophalangeal joint and further adduction of the first metacarpal. A vicious circle of deformity is therefore established. The more the adduction contracture of the metacarpal, the greater the tendency for the metacarpophalangeal joint to hyperextend and the thumb ray to collapse. Occasionally, severe erosive changes in the carpometacarpal joint and absorption of the trapezium occur. This decompresses the joint and the severity of the deformity is decreased.

Adducted retropositioned thumb

This deformity is seen in less than 5% of rheumatoid patients and presents difficult treatment problems. Typically, the thumb metacarpal is retropositioned, adducted and externally rotated. It appears that the deformity is initiated by a synovitis at the carpometacarpal joint. Awkward positioning of the thumb on a flat board during acute illness can result in a permanent deformity. The ability of the extensor pollicis longus muscle to adduct and externally rotate the metacarpal is predominant. Palmar and radial subluxation of the metacarpal off the trapezium occurs. Consequently, the patient has difficulty abducting the metacarpal and may develop an abduction deformity at the metacarpophalangeal joint by stretching the ulnar collateral ligament in grasp activities.

Instability, stiffness or pain

These may occur at the interphalangeal, metacarpophalangeal or carpometacarpal joint as isolated deformities in rheumatoid arthritis. They result from synovial invasion and erosive changes of the bone or may be seen in association with other deformities. These deformities are accentuated with other deformities.

Tendon disabilities

Tendon disabilities in the rheumatoid thumb may be related to muscle contracture, tendon displacement, adhesions or ruptures, similar to those seen in the other digits in the rheumatoid hand.

The extensor pollicis longus tendon is the most commonly ruptured tendon in the rheumatoid thumb; this occurs most often within the third extensor compartment in the area of Lister's tubercle. The rupture of this tendon results in a sudden drop of the thumb metacarpophalangeal joint and some loss of extensor power at the distal phalanx. The deformity may be confused with the boutonnière deformity, which is also an extrinsic minus problem; the hyperextension of the distal joint is, however, not as prominent. The lack of extension of the metacarpophalangeal joint is usually associated with less flexion contracture and, most importantly, the long extensor tendon cannot be prominently palpated on the back of the hand in forced extension and retroposition of the thumb.

Rupture of the flexor pollicis longus is not rare and must be thought of in any hyperextended interphalangeal deformity of the thumb. This often occurs at the entrance of the digital flexor canal. Careful examination of active flexion will differentiate the hyperextended interphalangeal joint of the thumb from that of the ruptured flexor pollicis longus.

Ruptures of the abductor pollicis longus and extensor pollicis brevis are rare. Disability of the intrinsics usually results from their displacement and secondary contracture caused by synovial invasion and stretching of the dorsal hood of the metacarpophalangeal joint of the thumb. The intrinsic attachment to the dorsal hood is consequently displaced palmarly and this results in a distortion of its normal function.

SURGICAL TREATMENT OF DISABILITIES OF THE THUMB

The most frequently used methods in the authors' clinic for surgical treatment of thumb disabilities include implant arthroplasty for the carpometacarpal, metacarpophalangeal and interphalangeal joint; capsulodesis or fusion of the metacarpophalangeal joint; and hemitenodesis or fusion of the interphalangeal joint.

Thumb basal joints

Patients with rheumatoid arthritis may have severe absorptive changes of the trapezium and base of the metacarpal, which produce a result not unlike resection arthroplasty. If the joint is reasonably stable, mobile and pain free, no surgery is indicated. However, some patients have a dislocation of the metacarpal off the trapezium in addition to severe erosive and absorptive bone changes and ligamentous loosening at the base of the thumb. It is important to realign the thumb ray but the destructive changes may be too great to allow implant arthroplasty or other stabilizing procedures. In these cases, the authors have resected the base of the metacarpal and partially resected the carpus so that the base of the metacarpal can be reduced in position. The metacarpal is held in position of function with a temporary Kirschner wire fixation. A pain-free, reasonably stable fibrous ankylosis results. This has allowed us to perform other procedures necessary at the metacarpophalangeal and interphalangeal joints, such as fusion or arthroplasty. The indications, surgical technique and postoperative care for implant reconstruction of the thumb basal joints are discussed in Chapter 20.1.

The metacarpophalangeal joint

Adduction of the first metacarpal. If severe and untreated, this will imbalance the thumb and seriously affect the result of resection arthroplasties of the trapezium. If the angle of abduction between the first and second metacarpals does not reach at least 45° or more, the origin of the adductor pollicis muscle must be released from the third metacarpal through a separate palmar incision.

Hyperextension of the metacarpophalangeal joint. This contributes to the adduction tendency of the metacarpal and prevents proper abduction of the metacarpal and seating of the trapezium or trapeziometacarpal implant. If the metacarpophalangeal joint hyperextends less than 10°, no treatment is necessary except to apply the postoperative cast so that the metacarpal is abducted and not the proximal phalanx. If the metacarpophalangeal joint hyperextends from 10° to 20°, a Kirschner wire is placed obliquely across the joint while it is held in 10° of flexion. The wire is extracted when the cast is removed 4–6 weeks after surgery. This fixation facilitates maintenance of abduction of the metacarpal during the healing phase. If hyperextension of the metacarpophalangeal joint is greater than 20°, stabilization is an absolute necessity either by palmar capsulodesis or fusion. In patients who have a 30–40° flexion of the metacarpophalangeal joint of the thumb, a capsulodesis is the operation of choice to save the available flexion. These procedures should be performed at the same time as the implant is inserted. If the swan neck deformity is severe with no flexion available at the metacarpophalangeal joint, fusion of this joint and temporary fixation of the distal joint in extension are performed.

Capsulodesis for swan neck deformity. If hyperextension of the metacarpophalangeal joint is present to more than 20° and flexion of the joint is possible to only 30–40°, the joint being otherwise stable with good articular surfaces, a palmar capsulodesis procedure is indicated (Fig. 18.1.11). This procedure has worked well in correction of hyperextension deformity if attention is paid to obtaining a firm union between the palmar plate and the bone.

Boutonnière deformity. A boutonnière deformity of the thumb is usually not associated with arthritis of the basal joints of the type that would require implant arthroplasty. However, when this situation does occur, fusion of the metacarpophalangeal joint and release of the extensor pollicis longus at the distal joint may be performed at the same time as the implant procedure for the thumb basal joints.

Synovectomy can also be performed for the metacar-

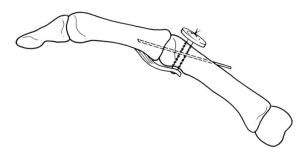

Fig. 18.1.11 Capsulodesis of thumb metacarpophalangeal joint; the palmar aspect of the joint is exposed through a lateral incision. Proximal membranous insertions of the palmar plate are incised. The tendinous attachments on the sesamoid bones are left intact. Periosteum is stripped from the volar aspect of the metacarpal neck. Two small drill holes are made vertical to bone and converted into a cavity with a small curette. The dorsal aspect of the palmar plate is roughened and fixed in the bony depression with a pull-out wire suture exiting dorsally over the button. Tension of the palmar plate flap must allow 10–15° of flexion of the metacarpophalangeal joint. Joint flexion is maintained with a Kirschner wire for 6 weeks. The pull-out wire is removed after 3 weeks. (Reproduced from Swanson, 1973, by kind permission of C.V. Mosby Co.)

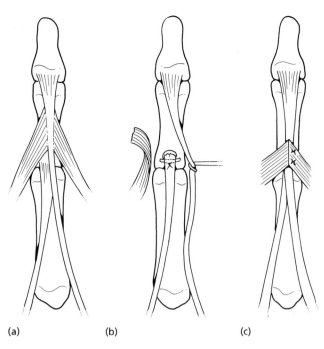

(a)   (b)   (c)

Fig. 18.1.12 Reconstruction of the extensor mechanism of the metacarpophalangeal joint of the thumb. (a) Dorsal expansions of intrinsic muscles are incised along both sides of the extensor pollicis longus tendon. The extensor pollicis brevis tendon is released from the base of the proximal phalanx. (b) Extensor pollicis brevis tendon is reinserted to bony concavity made in the base of the proximal phalanx by passing 3/0 Dacron suture through a small drill hole made in the bone. Knots are inverted and the tension carefully adjusted. (c) The extensor pollicis longus tendon is advanced distally and similarly sutured to the base of the proximal phalanx. Extensor expansions of intrinsic muscles are brought over area and sutured to each other.

pophalangeal joint of the thumb in cases of boutonnière deformity. If the metacarpophalangeal joint is only minimally contracted (less than 10° of fixed flexion contracture) and there is no evidence of erosive joint disease, synovectomy of the metacarpophalangeal joint with preservation of the joint surfaces and careful reconstruction of the extensor mechanism can be a useful procedure. The technique for reconstruction of the tendon mechanism is similar to that described for implant arthroplasty of the metacarpophalangeal joint (see Chapter 20.1) and is illustrated in Fig. 18.1.12. The metacarpophalangeal joint is fixed in 0° of extension with a Kirschner wire for a period of 4 weeks. If the distal joint is destroyed, implant arthroplasty or fusion in the appropriate position is indicated. If the distal joint is adequate but presents a hyperextension deformity with contracture of the extensor pollicis longus tendon, it is lengthened or simply transected distally to decrease the extensor power at the distal joint. The distal joint is

then pinned in 10° of flexion with a small Kirschner wire for a period of 4–6 weeks until the tendons have healed.

Implant resection arthroplasty. Implant resection arthroplasty of the metacarpophalangeal joint of the thumb is indicated for severely destroyed joints with associated stiffness of the distal or basal joints and in boutonnière deformities in which the metacarpophalangeal joint is destroyed and the distal joint requires fusion. This procedure has provided adequate stability and the increased movement of flexion has been important especially for fine coordinated movements. The indication, operative technique and postoperative care for this procedure are described in Chapter 20.1.

Arthrodesis. Arthrodesis of the metacarpophalangeal joint of the thumb is indicated in cases of severe joint destruction by rheumatoid arthritis, provided there is adequate mobility at the distal and basal joints. Fusion of the metacarpophalangeal joint to simplify the articular chain system of the thumb ray by subtracting a joint can also be of great importance in balancing a severe collapse deformity of either the boutonnière or the swan neck type, when the distal and basal joints are adequate. The joint is exposed through a longitudinal dorsal incision and the extensor hood is longitudinally incised through the middle. The head of the metacarpal is shaped convexly to fit the concavity formed at the base of the proximal phalanx. A longitudinal wire is placed in a retrograde fashion through the entire thumb ray and is bent in place by flexing the joint to the desired position (Fig. 18.1.13). The fusion must be performed with the

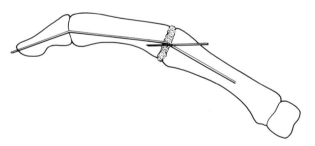

Fig. 18.1.13 Fusion of the metacarpophalangeal thumb joint. The metacarpal head is shaped convexly to fit concavity made at the base of the proximal phalanx. Longitudinal wire is placed retrogradely through the interphalangeal and metacarpophalangeal joints and bent in place to the desired position. Cancellous bone fragments are used as graft. Small wire is placed obliquely across the metacarpophalangeal joint and sectioned subcutaneously. This is removed after 6–8 weeks or left in place indefinitely. Longitudinal wire is removed after 6 weeks. (Reproduced from Swanson, 1973, by kind permission of C.V. Mosby Co.)

thumb in a functional position of 10° of flexion, 5° of abduction and slight pronation as required. A few fragments of cancellous bone can be inserted as a graft between the bone ends. A small Kirschner wire is introduced obliquely across the joint to further stabilize it and the bone ends are firmly compressed together. The wire is sectioned subcutaneously and removed after 6–8 weeks or left in place indefinitely. The longitudinal wire is removed without difficulties after 6 weeks. This procedure is usually successful because good bone contact and fixation are easily obtained in this joint.

The interphalangeal joint

In rheumatoid arthritis, severe erosive changes of the interphalangeal joint result in angulation deformity and subluxation, as seen in 35% of the cases. Arthrodesis of this joint is indicated and, occasionally, bone grafting will be necessary when severe bone absorption is present. A single relatively large (1.57 mm) intramedullary wire and a 0.89-mm cross-pin to further assure the fixation are used. It is important to obtain good bone-to-bone contact and to maintain the fixation until firm healing can be demonstrated radiologically, usually 6–10 weeks after surgery.

Occasionally, a flexible hyperextension deformity of the interphalangeal joint occurs that seems to be related to a palmar plate and collateral ligament relaxation. The patient may be able to actively flex the joint, but on strong pinch, severe hyperextension occurs that results in considerable disability. A flexor tenodesis procedure (Fig. 18.1.14) can prevent hyperextension and still

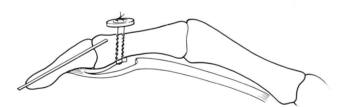

Fig. 18.1.14 Flexor tendon hemitenodesis of the thumb interphalangeal joint. Slip of flexor pollicis longus is prepared, leaving its distal attachment intact. Periosteum is stripped from the volar aspect of the neck of the proximal phalanx; two small drill holes are made through bone in a vertical direction and converted with a curette to form a small cavity to receive the tendon slip. Flexor slip is secured in position, using a pull-out suture exiting dorsally over a button to obtain 10–15° of flexion of the interphalangeal joint. A small Kirschner wire is placed across the joint to maintain desired flexion. The pull-out wire is removed after 3 weeks and the Kirschner wire after 6 weeks. (Reproduced from Swanson and Swanson, 1975, by kind permission of C.V. Mosby Co.)

allow flexion; this procedure may be used instead of arthrodesis of the distal joint, especially if lateral stability is present and the joint surfaces are intact.

In a small number of cases presenting moderate erosive changes with secondary ligamentous instability and pain, implant arthroplasty of the interphalangeal joint of the thumb has been performed (see Chapter 20.1).

THE ELBOW

Classification of the arthritic elbow

Based on his experience and that gathered from the literature, one of the authors (ABS) has attempted to classify the treatment of the rheumatoid elbow according to the severity of the clinical and radiological findings, and to correlate the treatment method for each group as follows:

TYPE I

The elbow presents pain, weakness, flexion contracture of less than 15° and persistent synovitis; there are minimal palpable crepitations at the elbow with very little or no loss of function. Radiographs may reveal subchondral porosis, minimal joint narrowing or are negative. Treatment should be medical; occasionally an intra-articular injection of steroids is indicated. These elbows may recover spontaneously.

TYPE II

The elbow presents pain on all motions, weakness, flexion contracture of 15–30°, persistent synovitis and chronic painful synovial involvement with crepitation at the radiohumeral joint. Radiographs show minimal narrowing of the joint with subchondral porosis and joint erosion. The suggested treatment is synovectomy through a lateral approach facilitated by radial head resection and implant replacement.

TYPE III

The elbow presents pain on all motions, crepitation, weakness, persistent synovitis and flexion contracture greater than 30°, with or without ulnar nerve symptoms. Radiographs show osteoporosis, joint narrowing and irregularity, with multiple erosions. The recommended treatment is synovectomy and débridement of the joint through a lateral approach facilitated by radial head resection and implant replacement. If there is evidence of ulnar nerve involvement, as seen in less than 10% of cases, an additional medial incision taking care to preserve the ulnar collateral ligament is indicated to complete the medial synovectomy. The ulnar nerve may be released or translocated. These cases could require an interposition arthroplasty.

TYPE IV

The elbow presents pain on all motions, weakness, severe crepitation, instability and flexion contracture or lateral deviation deformities, with or without ulnar nerve symptoms. Radiographs show osteoporosis, moderate-to-severe joint irregularities, multiple erosions and cystic changes. The suggested treatment is arthroplasty (interposition or resection type) with ligamentous reconstruction as needed.

TYPE V

The elbow presents pain on all motions, crepitation, flexion contracture, severe instabiliy and subluxation. Radiographs show severe bone absorption, cystic erosions, cystic changes and a 'knife and fork' deformity. The recommended treatment is resection arthroplasty or implant replacement.

Elbow synovectomy

Some form of involvement of the elbow joint is present in two-thirds of the rheumatoid arthritic patients presenting for hand surgery. These elbow lesions often have an insidious onset, and the patient remains unaware of their development until crepitation and limitation of motion of the radiohumeral joint are noted clinically. Crepitation at the proximal radio-ulnar and radiohumeral joints may be palpated with the elbow relaxed and flexed to about 90°. The examiner places one hand at the distal end of the forearm of the patient to give firm support and control, while the thumb of the other hand is placed at the radiohumeral joint and the fingers are placed at the medial side of the elbow joint. With the hand holding the forearm, the full range of passive pronation and supination movement is performed, and the presence of crepitation can easily be felt by the thumb as it is applied over the radiohumeral joint. The same method is used to palpate synovial thickening or effusion around the elbow joint.

The radiohumeral joint almost always shows destructive changes at surgery if there is significant synovitis, even though radiographs may appear normal. Several authors have noted that severe degenerative changes may be present in the radiohumeral joint while the articulation of the humerus on the olecranon is relatively

well preserved. When painful crepitation is first felt at the radial head, early synovectomy of the elbow joint is indicated to relieve pain and retard or prevent further cartilaginous and joint destruction. In an elbow synovectomy the radial head should be removed to obtain a wider exposure of the joint, allowing a thorough resection of synovial tissue and thus an increased range of motion and relief of pain. A second medial incision is used if there is evidence of synovial thickening medially. Other authors prefer both a medial and lateral incision on a posterior transolecranon approach to perform a complete synovectomy. An uncommon but important complication from proliferative synovitis at the elbow is entrapment of the posterior interosseous nerve. It is essential to recognize this lesion and decompress the nerve, often with a synovectomy. The improved motion after elbow synovectomy is due primarily to the excision of the radial head and secondarily to the removal of the synovial tissue. Although resection of the radial head appears to be a simple answer to the disturbance at the radiohumeral joint, it can result in definite problems.

When the radial head is resected, muscle pull and extrinsic forces stretch the interosseous membrane, the annular and quadrate ligaments producing proximal displacement of the radial shaft. This also happens in external rotation torque of the forearm on the humerus. Re-establishment of contact between the capitellum and the remainder of the radius generally occurs due to the proximal displacement of the radius, and in some cases to new bone formation. This proximal displacement of the radial shaft frequently results in stretching and widening of the distal radio-ulnar joint, followed by limitation of wrist motion, radial deviation of the hand and prominence of the distal end of the ulna. These derangements result in pain, instability, weakness and tenderness at the distal radio-ulnar joint. Stretching of the interosseous membrane also limits the range of motion, especially supination. When only the radial head is resected, the structures that could prevent development of the above deformity are the interosseous membrane, the annular and quadrate ligaments and the scar tissue formed at the site of the bone resection. However, following simple resection arthroplasty, the extremity must be immobilized with the wrist in ulnar deviation until the scar tissue is mature enough to maintain the radial shaft in its correct position; the prolonged immobilization and the resultant scar tissue contracture ultimately decrease the expected range of motion. In rheumatoid arthritis, postoperative complications at the wrist joint after radial head resection may be overlooked because frequently the distal radio-ulnar joint is also affected, and any further pathology is imputed to the generalized disease.

The normal valgus angle of the elbow is due to the shape of the humeral trochlea and further angulation is limited by the radial head, which plays an important role in the stability of the elbow in the face of lateral stress. When it is resected, the valgus deviation is increased by the loss of bone support at the lateral side of the elbow and also because the lateral muscles of the forearm are stronger flexors of the elbow than those of the medial side. One reason for this is that the more proximal origin of the brachioradialis muscle is on the humerus. If the annular and quadrate ligaments are partially destroyed, as in some cases of rheumatoid arthritis, or when an excessively large segment of the proximal end of the radius is removed, the tendency towards deformity is increased. These complications can be prevented by leaving the annular and quadrate ligaments intact when the radial head is resected. The space left by the resection should be filled with a space-occupying implant as described in Chapter 20.1.

THE SHOULDER

The painful shoulder presented as an isolated symptom in an otherwise normal patient receives a great deal of attention because of the patient's complaints and the severe loss of function that frequently accompanies bursitis in the area. However, in the arthritic patient whose sphere of functional activity has been largely restricted by involvement of multiple joints, disabilities of the shoulder joint are often ignored by both the patient and the physician. Severe disability of this joint is accompanied by marked destructive changes, but the patient will usually not complain unless he experiences severe crepitation or instability. Therefore, the evaluation of the upper extremity should start first with the elbow, then the shoulder, and the hand last, to bring into light problems about the shoulder that the patient might ignore because he has placed so much emphasis on his hand deficiencies. An armamentarium of surgical procedures has been developed to correct more obvious problems in the joints of the hand and lower extremity, but the surgical treatment of the arthritic shoulder has not received much attention.

Loss of shoulder movement may result secondarily in severe limitation of normal functional activity of the hand and elbow and in the shoulder–hand syndrome, which can destroy the function of the entire extremity if it is severe. Evaluation and treatment of shoulder disabilities must be included in the definition of an integral rehabilitation and reconstructive surgery programme for the arthritic upper extremity.

Dynamic physiology of shoulder joint

The shoulder is the proximal joint of the upper extremity and is the most mobile of all joints in the human body. Its joints allow movement in three planes in space and also motion in a combination of these planes:
1 flexion and extension in the sagittal plane;
2 abduction and adduction in the frontal plane;
3 flexion and extension in the horizontal plane while the arm is abducted to 90°;
4 axial rotation, which is the result of movements performed relative to any two of the three axes;
5 circumduction, which combines the movements of all three axes, its amplitude being defined as the cone of circumduction. The shape of this cone will vary according to the amplitude of movement of each of the three components.

RANGE OF MOTION

Movements of flexion and extension, performed in the sagittal plane, normally range from 180° of flexion to 50° of extension. Movements in the frontal plane usually range from 50° of adduction to 180° of abduction. Motions of the upper limb in the horizontal plane take place about a vertical axis and range from an angle of 30° posterior to the vertical plane of the body to an angle of 140° anterior to this plane. Axial rotation of the arm normally measures from 90° of external rotation to 90° of internal rotation.

Movements that may be required of the shoulder in activities of daily living are complex. Bringing the hand to the face or placing the hand behind the head may require abduction and lateral rotation of more than 90°. When a person puts on a coat unassisted, the first sleeve is usually placed with the arm in flexion and abduction and the second with the arm in extension and internal rotation. Movement of the hand to the front of the body usually requires rotation and extension of the arm, and placing it behind the body usually requires rotation and abduction. The position of function of the shoulder varies according to its purpose and is suggested to be from 40° to 20° of flexion, 50° to 20° abduction, and 30° to 50° internal rotation.

ANATOMICAL CONSIDERATIONS

It seems appropriate that the physiology and anatomy of the shoulder joint be discussed, at least in part, because of the tremendous importance they play for anyone attempting to devise reconstructive and rehabilitation programmes.

The shoulder girdle could be described as comprising five joints:

1 the glenohumeral joint, which is between the humerus and the glenoid surface of the scapula;
2 the subdeltoid joint, which is not an anatomical joint but consists of two musculotendinous surfaces moving on each other (it is mechanically linked to the gleno-humeral joint because it is moved by any movement in that area);
3 the scapulothoracic joint, which is not a true anatomical joint but has great physiological importance in allowing the arm to achieve a full range of motion;
4 the sternoclavicular joint; and
5 the acromioclavicular joint.

The glenohumeral joint is a true ball-and-socket articulation. The head of the humerus is shaped like a third of a sphere and faces superiorly, medially and posteriorly in the glenoid cavity. The glenoid cavity of the scapula is less deep than the convexity of the humeral head; however, it is deepened by the glenoid labrum, which is a surrounding ring of fibrocartilage. The upper humerus has two tuberosities (greater and lesser) for muscular attachments that are separated by the bicipital groove. The humeral head is surrounded by a capsule reinforced by ligamentous bands arising from the glenoid labrum (glenohumeral ligaments) and the coracoid process (coracohumeral ligament). This capsule is loose enough to allow the remarkable range of motion present in the normal shoulder. However, it is tightened up on movement of the joint to provide stability and maintain the relative position of the articular surfaces. Synovial tissue completely lines the inner surface of the capsule, invests the bicipital tendon and lines the bursae around the joint, the most notable being the subdeltoid bursa.

The peri-articular muscles, which cross the joint transversely, act as active ligaments and are important in securing the coaptation of the articular surfaces. These muscles are the supraspinatus, the subscapularis, the infraspinatus, the teres minor and the tendon of the long head of the biceps. Coaptation of the glenohumeral joint is also accomplished by the long muscles as they cross the joint. Dislocation of the humeral head in the infra-glenoid direction is prevented in part by the action of the short head of the biceps, the coracobrachialis, the long head of the triceps, the deltoid muscle and the clavicular head of the pectoralis major muscle.

Superior dislocation of the humeral head, which may be caused by excessively strong contraction of the long muscles across a disorganized joint, is prevented by the presence of the coraco-acromial arch and contraction of the supraspinatus muscle. The subdeltoid bursa forms a cleavage between the deltoid muscle and the underlying peri-articular short cuff muscles. Adhesions in this area will prevent the important gliding required to achieve abduction and will consequently restrict motion. During abduction, the greater tuberosity is pulled superiorly and medially by the action of the supraspinatus muscles, allowing the head of the humerus to slip under the coraco-acromial arch. This point is extremely important in the pathomechanics of the arthritic shoulder.

Fortunately, the scapulothoracic joint is not often involved in the arthritic process. Its function becomes increasingly important as movement of the glenohumeral joint is decreased, since it will provide a compensatory movement of the arm when the glenohumeral joint is stiffened. However, it adds very little motion to the total movement of the joint when the glenohumeral joint is loose and unstable. Adequate function of the scapulothoracic joint is dependent on the condition of its surrounding muscles: the serratus anterior, trapezius, rhomboid and underlying subscapularis, teres minor and major and supraspinatus and infraspinatus muscles.

The sternoclavicular joint may be involved in the arthritic process and may limit movement of the shoulder girdle through pain and/or incongruity and instability. Proper mobility of this joint is important because it allows movement of the clavicle in all three planes. Its dysfunction will usually secondarily affect the shoulder girdle, but only in its extremes of movement.

The acromioclavicular joint is frequently involved in the arthritic processes, and its dysfunction may also limit potential shoulder motion through pain, incongruity and instability. Stiffness of this joint will prevent movement of the shoulder girdle in its extremes of range of motion. The stability of the acromioclavicular joint depends mainly on the coracoclavicular ligaments. The coraco-acromial ligament, which passes horizontally between the coracoid process and the acromion, participates in the formation of the superior coraco-acromial arch, which checks the position of the humeral head in the vertical and superior direction.

Motor muscles affecting the scapular movement are the trapezius, rhomboid, levator scapulae, serratus anterior and pectoralis minor muscles. The serratus anterior and the trapezius muscles form a coupling to initiate abduction at the scapulothoracic joint. The abduction at the glenohumeral joint is initiated by the important coupling formed by the deltoid and the supraspinatus muscles. The supraspinatus muscle forces the humeral head against the glenoid cavity and compensates for the tendency towards the superior dislocation produced by the deltoid muscle. The supraspinatus keeps the articular surfaces in apposition and is therefore the starting muscle for abduction. The abducting efficiency of the deltoid increases as the angle of abduction increases, and it takes over once abduction has been initiated by the supraspinatus muscle. The movement of the early stage of abduction from between 0° and 90° is concentrated at the glenohumeral joint. The second phase of abduction involves the other joints of the shoulder girdle. However, there can be no artificial division of these movements because all the joints of the shoulder girdle and their controlling muscles are active to some degree during all phases of abduction. The movements of flexion are also divided between the glenohumeral and scapulothoracic joints and are controlled by movements of the deltoid, coracobrachialis, pectoralis major, trapezius and the serratus anterior muscles.

Rotation movements of the shoulder are important to move the hand in front of the trunk anteriorly and laterally; these mediolateral movements are necessary to move the hand across the table, as in eating and writing. The medial rotators at the shoulder are the latissimus dorsi, teres major, subscapularis and pectoralis major muscles. The lateral rotators are the infraspinatus and teres minor muscles. The scapula is also involved in rotation; lateral rotation is accomplished by the rhomboids and trapezius, and medial rotation by the serratus anterior and pectoralis minor muscles.

Adduction is produced by the two muscular couplings: the rhomboids and teres major, and the long head of the triceps and the latissimus dorsi. Extension movements at the glenohumeral joint are accomplished by the teres major and teres minor muscles, the posterior fibres of the deltoid and the latissimus dorsi. Extension at the scapulothoracic joint is accomplished by the rhomboids, trapezius and latissimus dorsi muscles.

Treatment of disease processes about joints of the shoulder girdle

BURSITIS AND TENDINITIS

Inflammatory changes involving the subdeltoid bursa and the bicipital tendon are frequently found in the general population as separate entities without necessary development of arthritis of the shoulder. However, the arthritic processes that occur in the glenohumeral joint are almost always associated with involvement of these structures. Synovitis occurring within the shoulder joint cannot be controlled by treatment of the peri-articular structures alone. Physical therapy programmes are extremely important to maintain the gliding mechanisms necessary for shoulder movement and to prevent capsular and muscular contractures. Hence a comprehensive exercise programme for maintenance of shoulder movement should be prescribed early for every arthritic patient. Local injections of corticosteroids into the shoulder joint, bicipital tendon and subdeltoid bursa can provide some temporary relief and can be particu-

larly important in facilitating the physical therapy programme.

Surgical excision of soft tissue structures of the shoulder joint is probably of little benefit in the total picture of this arthritic disability. Synovectomy of the shoulder joint is usually not done because so many other joints of seemingly greater priority demand surgical attention and because it is almost impossible to perform a complete synovectomy and restore the joint. Rarely, severe synovial involvement of the subdeltoid bursa may require local resection.

Acromioclavicular joint

The acromioclavicular joint is commonly involved in the shoulder joint problem but also may show evidence of involvement secondarily in traumatic arthritis or osteoarthritis. Local tenderness and pain on movement, especially adduction of the arm, and radiographic evidence of destructive changes mark the diagnosis. Conservative measures such as the injection of anti-inflammatory drugs, medical treatment and physical therapy are frequently of benefit. Excision of the clavicle distal to the coracoclavicular ligaments may be indicated if the disabling symptoms are localized to this area.

Sternoclavicular joint

Arthritic destruction of the sternoclavicular joint is rare; however, this joint may show evidence of primary involvement in both rheumatoid and osteoarthritic patients. If this lesion cannot be treated by conservative measures, resection of the inner end of the clavicle proximal to the costoclavicular ligaments and a synovectomy can be done. This procedure can be very hazardous because of the underlying vascular structures.

Glenohumeral joint

Soft tissue surgery for arthritic changes in the glenohumeral joint is rarely indicated. As previously noted the subacromial bursa is rarely involved as an isolated problem. Associated attrition and disruption of the supraspinatus tendon, as well as the biceps tendon, are common. Fixed contractures in adduction and internal rotation, especially in the patient confined to a wheelchair, make it difficult to re-establish a useful range of motion. Superior subluxation of the head of the humerus against the coraco-acromial arch is common and it can only be treated by joint surgery, including arthroplasty. Occasionally a very severe synovitis process may be present and synovectomy of the joint is useful mainly to relieve pain. In patients who have multiple joint involve-

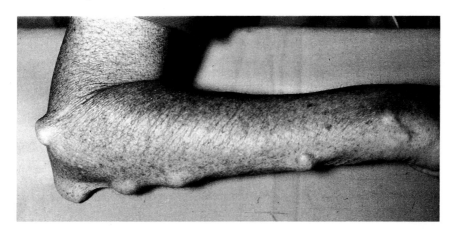

Fig. 18.1.15 Severe rheumatoid nodules in a seropositive 70-year-old rheumatoid patient. These lesions are of both functional and cosmetic concern for the patient. (Reproduced from Swanson, 1973, by kind permission of C.V. Mosby Co.)

ment and in whom shoulder joint pain is not a prominent problem, the authors would give first priority to the reconstruction of the other joints; the hand and elbow are usually operated on before the shoulder in these cases. Successful surgery of the shoulder requires an experienced surgeon, who also understands the need for an organized and prolonged rehabilitation programme, and a cooperative patient. Implant replacement procedures are discussed in Chapter 20.1.

RHEUMATOID NODULES

The rheumatoid nodule is a characteristic lesion of rheumatoid arthritis and occurs in approximately 20% of patients. The nodules are usually developed in areas of chronic external irritation, such as over the knees and elbows (Fig. 18.1.15). They may become large and cystic, may destroy the overlying skin, or may become infected and drain. The nodule consists of a fibrovascular granulation tissue with large concentrations of chronic inflammatory cells. As the nodule matures, fibrinoid degeneration occurs, and its necrotic centre is surrounded by a fibroblastic tissue. The distinctive microscopic feature of the nodule is palisading of fibroblasts around the central area of necrosis. These nodules are an example of the arthritis that occurs secondarily to the auto-immune response of the disease. Patients often request the removal of these bothersome lesions both because of cosmetic concern and because of the pain on pressure that occurs and occasional breakdown and drainage. The lesions may be adherent to the overlying skin and occasionally may be in the area of underlying nerves. They should be dissected out bluntly. When they occur in the finger, they may involve the digital nerves,

and careful dissection is required. When they occur at the fingertip, they may displace and destroy the pulp fat. The wounds should be drained, since the dead space created may be an area for haematoma development. These nodules recur frequently, and the patient should be informed of this potentiality.

Soft tissue procedures, including synovectomy for the upper extremity, can be useful in properly selected patients. The operative techniques necessary for a good result require the careful attention of the surgeon who would care for the arthritic patient.

REFERENCES

Straub L.R. (1959) The rheumatoid hand. *Clin. Orthop.* **15**, 127–139.

Swanson A.B. (1973) *Flexible Implant Resection Arthroplasty in the Hand and Extremities.* St Louis, C.V. Mosby.

Swanson A.B. and de Groot Swanson G. (1975) Thumb disabilities in rheumatoid arthritis: Classification and treatment. In: *American Academy of Orthopaedic Surgeons Symposium on Tendon Surgery in the Hand.* St. Louis, C.V. Mosby, pp. 233–254.

Swanson A.B. and de Groot Swanson G. (1991) Flexible implant arthroplasty of the radiocarpal joint. *Ser. Anthrop.* **2**, 78–84.

Swanson A.B. and de Groot Swanson G. (1994) Complications of arthroplasty and joint replacement at the wrist. In: Epps Jr. C.H. (ed.) *Complications in Orthopaedic Surgery.* Philadelphia, J.B. Lippincott Co., pp. 957–995.

Tupper, J.W. (1989) The metacarpophalangeal volar plate arthroplasty. *J. Hand Surg.* **14A** (Part 2), pp. 371–375.

Tubiana R. (1969) The mechanisms of deformities of the fingers due to musculotendinous imbalance. In Tubiana R. (ed.) *The Rheumatoid Hand.* Groupe d'Étude de la Main, Monograph no. 3. Paris, L'Expansion Scientifique Française, pp. 133–141.

Zancolli E. (1968) *Structural and Dynamic Bases of Hand Surgery.* Philadelphia, J.B. Lippincott Co.

Chapter 18.2

The Lower Limb

P.J. Abernethy & W.A. Souter

INTRODUCTION

In the early 1960s, when interest was first aroused in the surgery of rheumatoid arthritis, the surgical armamentarium for dealing with lower limb problems was extremely limited. Thirty years later with the advent of joint replacement the surgical approach has changed out of all recognition. Reconstruction of the lower limb in rheumatoid patients is now one of the most exciting challenges facing the orthopaedic surgeon and moreover one which, given adequate patient selection and meticulous attention to the details of operative technique and post-operative management, should yield dramatically successful and worthwhile results.

Although the patient may suffer from extensive upper and lower limb joint pathology, most patients wish their lower limbs to be treated first in order to establish a degree of walking independence. On rare occasions this approach may have to be modified in order to allow the patient to use walking aids which may be necessary following surgery to the lower limb joints.

The surgical armamentarium and the general principles of management of rheumatoid disease are nowhere better illustrated than in relation to the knee joint. It would therefore seem appropriate that our review of lower limb surgery should commence with this joint.

THE KNEE

The knee is the most commonly affected major joint in rheumatoid arthritis. Fleming *et al.* (1976) showed that one or both knees eventually become affected in 90% of patients with bilateral involvement in 30−35% of patients.

The early phases of involvement are characterized by thick boggy swelling of the synovium including the suprapatellar pouch whilst the development of a flexion deformity usually signifies some degree of cartilage damage. Initially such a knee will have a springy feel on passive extension but later the deformity becomes rigid and at this stage can be corrected only by surgical intervention. Once bone erosion is established the knee will usually exhibit a degree of axial malalignment. Valgus deformity is most common, varus deformities do occur and often both are combined with some element of posterior subluxation. The stages of progressive radiological deterioration are illustrated in Fig. 18.2.1. In stages 1 and 2 of the disease surgery may be resorted to in an attempt to abort the inflammation and hopefully prolong the life of the joint. In the later stages of the disease when irrevocable destruction has already occurred, reconstructive surgery may yield very worthwhile results. The surgical armamentarium includes synovectomy, osteotomy, hemi-arthroplasty, total joint replacement and arthrodesis.

Synovectomy

Synovectomy was first introduced by Volkman at the end of the nineteenth century and later established in clinical practice by Swett (1923). Total synovectomy of the knee joint cannot be done without an extensive anterior and posterior approach which is better avoided. The accepted practice is for an approximate 85% clearance to be carried out through a more limited anterior incision. Not only is synovium incompletely removed at the time of surgery but there is good-evidence to show that the synovium which is excised regenerates rapidly. Goldie (1971) was able to carry out 14 elective arthrotomies between 1 and 3 years after synovectomy. Although some of the features compatible with rheumatoid pathology were present, e.g. multiple layers of synovial cells with excess vascularity and lymphocytic infiltration, encouragement could be taken from the relative absence of villi and the normal pH of the synovial fluid. Mitchell and Shepard (1971) studied

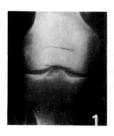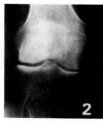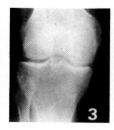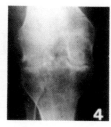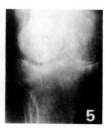

Fig. 18.2.1 Staging of joint erosion in rheumatoid arthritis. (1) Soft tissue swelling and osteoporosis. (2) Marginal erosions and/or minimal joint space narrowing. (3) Definite narrowing of joint space. (4) Joint space reduced to a mere line and erosions penetrating subchondral plate. (5) Total disorganization of joint and loss of normal condylar contours.

elective biopsies of synovium and cartilage taken at intervals from 2 months to 5–6 years post-synovectomy and they demonstrated that the configuration of the regenerated synovium was remarkably normal at 2 months. Moreover, the appearance of chondrocytes under electron microscopy steadily returned to normal within 7 months. The serosal layers, however, were highly collagenized with very little cellular infiltration.

The results of synovectomy must be related to the natural history of rheumatoid disease but in a condition that is punctuated by good and bad spells over variable periods of time it is difficult to assess the precise value of this operation. Because of this, uncontrolled trials tend to be viewed somewhat sceptically yet the results obtained in a number of these demonstrate certain points so consistently that their findings can probably be regarded as reasonably valid. Vainio (1966) reviewed 201 cases of knee synovectomy and found satisfactory relief of pain and swelling in 68% of these patients. He noted that results of surgery were very much related to the state of the articular surfaces at the time of the operation. This, however, is what might also be expected even if synovectomy was valueless, i.e. that the best preserved joints would last longest. These findings have been substantiated over the years by many other authors including Gariepy *et al.* (1966), Geens *et al.* (1969), Laurin *et al.* (1974), Gschwend *et al.* (1977) and Taylor and Hill (1978). The preservation of the articular cartilage, however, is no absolute guarantee of a good long-lasting result and in long-term review 18% of well-preserved knees went on to deteriorate (Laurin *et al.*, 1974). Geens in 1969 looked at several reviews dating from 1923–1967. These included the work of Vainio, London, Stevens, Whitfield, Jakubowski and Conaty. Of all 500 cases considered, 80% had improvement after synovectomy and 20% did not.

In an attempt to match the results of synovectomy with the natural history of the condition, controlled trials were undertaken in the UK in 1976 and in the USA in 1977. Both trials studied the effect of synovectomy

of the metacarpophalangeal joints and the knee joint. Neither showed that any benefit could be demonstrated in metacarpophalangeal joints. In the case of the UK trial in relation to the knee, joint pain, soft tissue swelling and tenderness were significantly less at 3 years post-synovectomy. The results in the USA knee group were less conclusive with only soft tissue swelling being significantly less in the synovectomized group.

The commonest indication in current operative practice for synovectomy would be in a patient with a well-preserved knee joint with hypertrophic synovitis and persistent pain and swelling which had proved resistant to medical treatment over a period of at least 6 months. It is also of value in juvenile chronic arthritis of the mono- or pauci-articular varieties rather than in the poly-articular form of the disease (Jacobson *et al.*, 1985; Rydholm *et al.*, 1986).

The open operation is best performed through a longitudinal anterior incision. There is no need to divide the vastus medialis insertion. Using the Erkes technique (Abbot and Carpenter, 1945) the vastus medialis is elevated from the medial intermuscular septum and then retracted laterally with the whole of the quadriceps mechanism and the patella. The suprapatellar pouch is then enucleated and the synovium stripped from the anteromedial and anterolateral aspects of the joint. Meticulous clearing of synovium is required from the margin of the articular cartilage and in and around the collateral and cruciate ligaments. It is preferable to preserve the menisci because of their load-attenuating properties. Post-operative mobilization using a knee mobilizing machine is instituted and if the patient's knee flexion is not steadily approaching 90° within 2 weeks a gentle manipulation under general anaesthetic should be considered.

With its easier rehabilitation the less invasive procedure of arthroscopic synovectomy carried out through multiple portals is now established as the operation of choice.

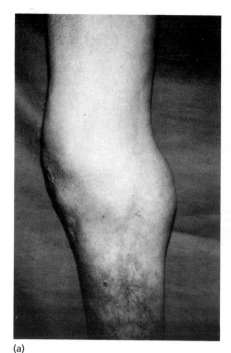 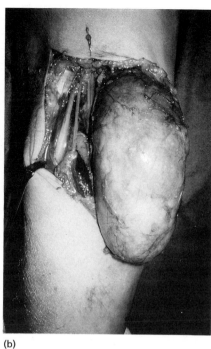

(a)   (b)

Fig. 18.2.2 (a) Large popliteal cyst; (b) findings at surgery. (Reproduced with permission from Abernethy P.J., 1989.)

POPLITEAL CYSTS

In rheumatoid disease these are usually semimembranosus bursae. Jason and St Dixon (1970) and Pinder (1973) have suggested that anterior synovectomy is an appropriate way of dealing with these cysts. Occasionally it may be necessary to consider local excision of the cyst if it becomes very large (Fig. 18.2.2). On these occasions it can be filled with hundreds of fibrin bodies. However in order to prevent recurrence this should be combined with an anterior synovectomy or a joint replacement, otherwise one is simply removing the 'egg' and leaving the 'chicken'.

These cysts can rupture giving rise to acute pain in the calf and are frequently misdiagnosed as deep venous thrombosis. An arthrogram of the knee under these circumstances will show leakage of the dye into the calf which is pathognomonic of cyst rupture.

SURGERY IN THE LATER STAGES OF RHEUMATOID ARTHRITIS

Posterior release

Flexion contractures are common in this group of patients. Although patients are partly dependent on the function in the upper limbs when bilateral flexion deformities of 40° or more develop, they are very likely to become confined to a wheelchair. Flexion deformities that are unaccompanied by posterior subluxation of the

tibia on the femur may be corrected by serial plaster casts. If the joint itself is significantly eroded then correction is usually achieved at the time of total joint replacement when a posterior capsular release can contribute significantly to the correction of the deformity.

In cases where patients have been bedridden or chairbound and have flexion contractures of 90° or more, posterior release may have to be carried out prior to joint replacement surgery. This can be done through a lazy S incision in the popliteal fossa followed by posterior capsular release combined with hamstring lengthening if necessary. Following release it is important that the skin flaps should not be under undue tension. If this is a concern then the knee can be left slightly flexed and subsequently straightened by physiotherapy or serial casting.

Osteotomy

It is doubtful if osteotomy has any place in the management of an inflammatory pan arthritis. Correction is only logical where a load can be transferred to a normal joint compartment. Results of osteotomy are disappointing and unpredictable but Benjamin (1969) reported on double osteotomy of the distal femur and proximal tibia. The femoral division is carried out intra-articularly through the upper border of the articular cartilage and the tibia is divided not more than 2.5 cm distal to the joint. Plaster immobilization is maintained for 5 weeks and the knee is then gently manipulated under general anaesthesia. Pain relief apparently can be obtained in approximately 75% of patients. The operation does not appear to have achieved wide acceptance due mainly to a fear of significant loss of movement or non-union at the osteotomy sites.

MacIntosh double hemi-arthroplasty

This is mentioned largely for historical interest as it formed an important milestone in the development of knee surgery in rheumatoid arthritis. The insertion of metal discs of variable thickness on to carefully resected tibial plateaus were used for knees which had reached severe grade 3 or grade 4 levels of radiological deterioration (see Fig. 18.2.1). Despite early enthusiastic and extensive reviews by MacIntosh and Hunter in 1972 and by Hastings and Hewitson in 1973, where good to excellent results were found in 75% and 87% of cases respectively, the operation was complicated by a tendency for the discs to migrate and also with an unacceptable recurrence of pain due to bone erosion in one or other femoral condyle. There is no doubt that total knee replacement can achieve a more complete and long-lasting degree of pain relief and for these reasons the use of the MacIntosh hemi-arthroplasty has now largely been abandoned.

Total knee arthroplasty (see Chapter 20.4)

There is no indication for uni-compartmental replacement in rheumatoid disease because of the widespread pathology throughout the joint. Total knee arthroplasty has become the most commonly required operation for the rheumatoid knee joint. Because of the frequency of knee involvement (Fleming *et al.*, 1976) it has also become the most commonly replaced joint on the rheumatoid service at the Princess Margaret Rose Orthopaedic Hospital in Edinburgh. (Abernethy, 1990).

THE DESIGN OF PROSTHESES

Routine use of rigid hinge prostheses has now largely been abandoned because it has been realized that these fully constrained joints fall very short of the sophisticated biomechanics of the normal knee. In the event of loosening or infection the pathology may be so extensive that further reconstruction may not be possible. The potential disaster of an infected cemented hinge has become only too well known with several mid-thigh amputations being recorded in the literature. There may be rare occasions when they can be used in revisional surgery where adequate stability cannot be achieved using unlinked components. In this respect the alternative use of a partially constrained linked prosthesis such as the Kinematic rotating hinge may be considered by some. In the event of failure further reconstruction or fusion may be extremely difficult to achieve. The advantages of rotating hinged devices over rigid hinges remains theoretical rather than practical.

The current practice now relates to the use of unlinked condylar prostheses. One-piece tibial components are generally favoured and the high-density polyethylene tibial component is now incorporated into a metal tray to reduce the tendency to plastic deformation. The use of a central tibial stem is most widely favoured to minimize varus valgus and rotational stresses. Recent developments allow the use of modular stems of varying lengths and thicknesses to give operative flexibility when dealing with bone deficiencies so common in the rheumatoid group.

The question of whether the posterior cruciate ligament should be retained is still widely debated. There are some who would doubt its significant functional role in the absence of the anterior cruciate ligament (Goodfellow and O'Connor, 1977). Others feel that it can play a significant contribution to the absorption of shearing stresses within the joint (Walker, 1989). In some rheumatoid knees the degree of deformity is such that soft tissue balancing cannot be achieved without sacrificing the posterior cruciate ligament.

If the tibial component is dished there is constraint between the femoral and tibial components. As a result more stresses will be transferred to the bone cement interface with the possibility of increased loosening (Walker, 1989). Making the tibial surface flatter, however, to reduce the contact area between the two components leads to an increase in the sliding contact which in turn increases the chance of polyethylene wear (Bartel *et al.*, 1968). Utilizing a slightly dished semi-constrained tibial component enables a compromise to be reached between these two problems. Newer implants are now available which allow the surgeon to switch from a posterior cruciate preserving to a posterior cruciate substituting design of modular plastic insert which fit into standard metal tibial trays.

INDICATIONS FOR SURGERY

Knee replacement arthroplasty is indicated essentially for the treatment of severe pain that usually interferes with patients' everyday activities and disturbs their sleep. More relative indications include instability, stiffness and deformity particularly in those younger patients with juvenile chronic arthritis. The patient's age is important in relation to the longevity of the implant but in rheumatoid arthritis operation is often offered at a younger age despite the poor quality of the patient's bone. It is felt that the reduced activity of these patients can afford a significant degree of joint protection and overall the function and durability of the operation outweighs the grim alternative of a wheelchair existence.

AIMS OF SURGERY

The condylar prosthesis should be used as a spacer as illustrated in Fig. 18.2.3. The femoral component should be implanted at 7° of valgus with reference to the anatomical axis of the femur and the tibial component implanted at 90° to the longitudinal axis of the tibia in both the anteroposterior and lateral planes. The artificial joint line should be parallel to the floor and it is also important to restore the normal mechanical axis of the limb which aligns the centre of the hip, the knee and the ankle (Fig. 18.2.4).

OPERATIVE TECHNIQUES

The incidence of wound necrosis can be reduced by the use of a midline incision. In the event of previous surgery then the previous incision should be utilized. If there was more than one incision then as a general rule the most lateral incision should be utilized. The capsule is incised through a medial parapatellar incision. The patella is everted and the lateral half of the fat pad excised to give access to the lateral tibial plateau. An appropriate jigging system is then utilized to cut an equal extension and flexion gap to allow the introduction of variable thickness tibial components to provide stability throughout the whole range of available movements.

There is much argument about the role of patellar replacement in total knee arthroplasty. Ranawat (1986) has considered the advantages and disadvantages of patella replacement, generally supporting the concept of patellar re-surfacing. Abraham *et al.* (1988), however, found there was no advantage in patellar re-surfacing. It is the authors' view that the patella should be replaced in the rheumatoid population. In one series from the Edinburgh arthritis surgical service, 275 total condylar knee replacements were carried out in an essentially rheumatoid population of whom approximately half had had their patella re-surfaced. This group had less anterior knee pain and better stability with less reduction of bone stock in the longer term compared to those whose patella was not re-surfaced (Wheelwright *et al.*, 1990). Whether re-surfaced or not the patella must track easily and lie within the femoral groove during passive flexion and extension of the knee. No support should be applied by the surgeon's thumb during the testing of these movements and if the patella does not track easily in this manner it is necessary first to resect any fibrous synovial folds lying within the lateral recess of the knee. If this fails to improve the tracking then an extended lateral release from within the knee should be carried out under direct vision. If possible the superior lateral geniculate vessels should be preserved to help maintain patellar vascularity.

If both knees need to be replaced, due consideration can be given to synchronous replacements of the knees in those patients who are deemed fit enough to withstand two major procedures. It has been reported that there are no increased complications when this is carried out and the period of hospitalization can be significantly reduced (Morrey *et al.*, 1987).

SPECIAL TECHNICAL PROBLEMS

Severe malalignment

Axial realignment can usually be achieved by adequate soft tissue release on the contracted side of the joint.

To correct a fixed valgus deformity it is necessary to

Fig. 18.2.3 Use of condylar prosthesis as a spacer. (a) Normal joint with tight ligaments. (b) Eroded joint with slack ligaments. (c) Replaced joint, prosthesis acting as a spacer to restore ligament length.

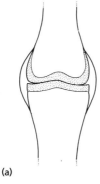
(a)

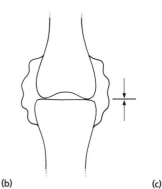
(b)

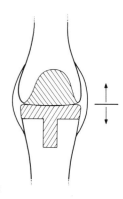
(c)

the medial ligament has not been achieved by radical excision of the osteophytes on the medial femoral and tibial margins (Fig. 18.2.5). The most difficult form of malalignment in the rheumatoid knee is the flexed knee associated with a valgus and external rotation deformity of the tibia. This deformity may also require resection of the posterior cruciate ligament.

Stiff knee

The problem in these cases is how to manage the extensor apparatus. This must be released in order to gain access to the joint in a flexed position and can often be achieved by freeing all the scar tissue from the suprapatellar pouch and the medial and lateral gutters. The capsule should be stripped carefully from the medial aspect of the tibia combining this with external rotation of the tibia to allow the extensor mechanism to dislocate laterally. Failure to achieve this may require the use of a VY release of the quadriceps tendon where an oblique limb can be added to the proximal end of the medial parapatellar incision. This is then advanced at the end of the procedure to allow more knee flexion. Rehabilitation of these knees is extremely difficult and prolonged owing to a significant extensor lag.

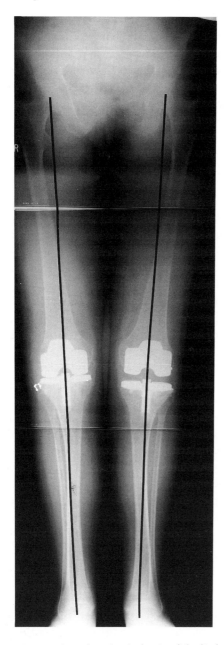

Fig. 18.2.4 Restoration of mechanical axis of the limb following the insertion of bilateral condylar replacements of the Kinematic variety. Thicker spacer used in the left knee to restore normal ligament length. (Reproduced with permission from Abernethy P.J. 1989.)

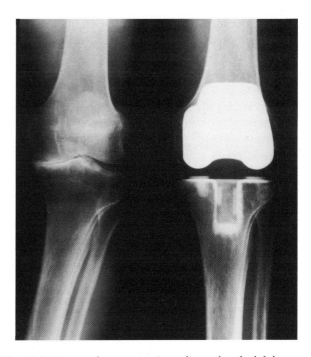

Fig. 18.2.5 Pre- and post-operative radiographs of a left knee demonstrating the correction of severe varus deformity which can be achieved using a condylar prosthesis provided adequate medial release is undertaken at the time of surgery.

release the posterolateral capsule from the tibia, divide the iliotibial band and the popliteus tendon and if this is insufficient the lateral collateral ligament can be released from its femoral attachment.

Release of the medial capsular structures and the pes anserinus from the tibial metaphysis may be necessary to correct a fixed varus deformity if sufficient slack in

Bone deficiency

The tibial component should be implanted on to a flat tibial bone surface. With bony deficiencies caution is required in the amount of tibial plateau which should be resected in order to achieve this. The compressive strength diminishes rapidly with resections of more than 1 cm of bone. The alternative is to remove less bone and to fill the defects with polymethyl methacrylate. This is best reserved for small defects as it is not an ideal substance for this purpose (Brooks *et al.*, 1984). Local bone harvested from the chamfer cut or the resected posterior femoral condyles is readily available to fill focal deficiencies in primary total knee arthroplasty.

With larger central defects consideration may be given to the use of morselized femoral head allograft and this should be combined with the use of a longer stem to allow the stress to bypass the area of deficient bone. If there is no intact peripheral rim of bone present the resulting deficiency can be dealt with by the use of a modular wedge fitted to a standard baseplate. Alternatively, if the defect is too large to be dealt with in this way a custom-built tibial component incorporating the appropriate wedge could be used. These, however, are expensive and often do not fit the defect accurately at the time of operation. Most workers now prefer to use femoral head allograft under these circumstances. The peripheral defect is trimmed with a saw to produce a flat surface onto which the femoral head is temporarily fixed using Kirschner wires. The head is then cut with a saw to produce a flat surface onto which the tibial component can be fixed (Fig. 18.2.6). The long-term fate of these segmental allografts is as yet uncertain. Altchek *et al.* (1989) reported on 14 patients with an average follow-up of more than 4 years. They claimed that all the bone grafts appeared to have been consolidated in this group. Dorr *et al.* (1986) reported that out of 24 knees observed for 6 years after treatment with bone grafting two had failed.

POST-OPERATIVE MANAGEMENT

If there is any doubt about wound healing the authors feel it is preferable to immobilize the knee in an extension splint for a few days before starting active movement. In most cases, however, the authors favour the use of a knee mobilizing machine which greatly facilitates the early recovery of knee motion. Most studies suggest, however, that in the longer term the final range of movement is unchanged (Romness and Rand, 1988).

RESULTS

There are relatively few long-term reports on the results of knee arthroplasty in patients with rheumatoid arthritis. In a series of 29 total knee replacements in 17 patients with rheumatoid arthritis all under the age of 40, Sarokanan *et al.* (1983) reported that 90% were completely relieved of their discomfort at 5 years average follow-up. Twenty-one per cent required re-operation for patellar re-surfacing. There was one case of deep infection. They concluded that the relief of pain and quality of functional improvement which could be achieved outweigh the risks of total joint replacement

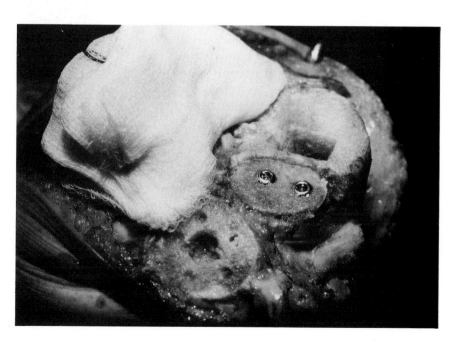

Fig. 18.2.6 Femoral head bulk allograft used to augment peripheral deficiency of the lateral tibial plateau. (Reproduced with permission from Abernethy P.J., 1990.)

in this young population. Ewald and Christie (1987) reported on 72 total knee replacements in 50 patients between the ages of 20 and 45. Again 90% of patients were pain-free at 3.8 years follow-up and of these two had had re-operation for patellar loosening and there was one case of deep infection. Stuart and Rand (1988) reported on 44 total knee replacements in 26 rheumatoid arthritic patients all under the age of 40. Excellent or good results were found in 86%.

275 total condylar knee arthroplasties carried out in a group of Edinburgh patients predominantly with rheumatoid disease and followed up for a mean duration of 6.4 years were assessed using the Hospital for Special Surgery scoring system. Dramatic pain relief was obtained in over 90% of these cases although this score does deteriorate slightly with time. The mean pre-operative total flexion range of 75° increased to 90° after surgery. Only two cases of tibial loosening occurred during this period (Wheelwright *et al.*, 1989).

COMPLICATIONS

Infection (see also Chapter 15)

The reported rate of post-operative infection ranges between 0 and 4%. In those cases without draining sinuses or Gram negative infections the possibility of re-implantation can be entertained. The consensus of opinion is that this should be done as a staged procedure. The arthroplasty is removed and the joint carefully debrided. A block of antibiotic cement is implanted to maintain the distraction between the ends of the bones and maintain the length of the collateral ligaments (Fig. 18.2.7).

High rates of prosthetic salvage are reported for periods of up to 5 years following this technique (Rand and Bryan 1983; Insall, 1986). This has been one of the authors' (PJA) experience using this technique and there have been no failures to date in 15 re-implantations of whom 10 have been followed for over 5 years. The average range of flexion, however, is reduced in these cases.

Where re-implantation is felt to be unwise, arthrodesis can be considered. Under these circumstances compression arthrodesis using multiple-pin fixation in a bi-planar fashion is the preferred method. The pins should be retained for a minimum of 8–10 weeks if possible. Using this technique some authors report an 80% fusion rate following removal of infected condylar type prostheses (Rand and Bryan, 1986; Rand *et al.*, 1987). In the event of difficulty in achieving arthrodesis a long intramedullary nail rod extending from hip to

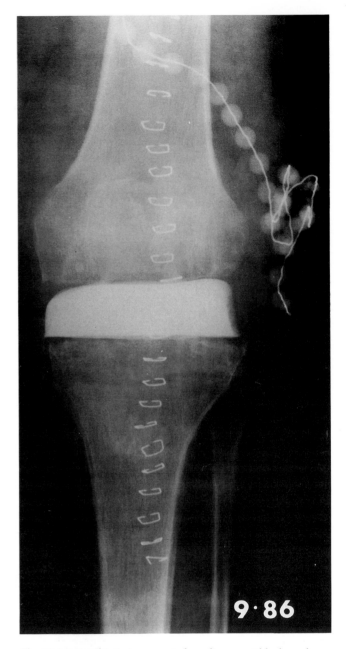

Fig. 18.2.7 Antibiotic impregnated acrylic cement block used as a spacer between the bone ends following removal of infected knee prosthesis. Garamycin beads also utilized.

ankle may be considered provided that the infection has been controlled.

Patellar complications

Patellar instability after operation can be due to tight lateral structures and adequate attention must be given to lateral release under these circumstances. If the limb is aligned in valgus mal-tracking can also occur. Internal rotation of either the tibial or the femoral components will also lead to an increase in the Q angle and again pre-dispose to subluxation. These malalignments require correction in order to resolve the instability.

Patellar fracture has been widely reported with a greater incidence in the re-surfaced than un-resurfaced patellae. Non-operative treatment can be used successfully to deal with those fractures associated with an intact extensor mechanism. In those cases associated with disruption of the extensor mechanism or prosthetic loosening operation is required, but the results of procedures such as reconstructing the patella or carrying out partial or complete patellectomy may give satisfactory results in under 50% of cases (Grace and Rand, 1991).

Peroneal nerve palsy

This occurs in 3% of patients and it is the authors' experience that all eventually recover but can take up to 6 months to do so. Because of the particular risk of this complication in patients with a major valgus deformity the authors recommend performing a lateral popliteal nerve release through a separate incision in all such cases.

UNCEMENTED PROSTHESIS

Although there is considerable interest in the application of uncemented knee prostheses, Ryd (1986) has shown a significant incidence of subsidence in all types of uncemented tibial components on long-term evaluation. This problem is more significant in those with rheumatoid arthritis and for this reason the authors feel that cemented components are preferable in this group of patients.

THE HIP

Although the hips are affected in some 10% of rheumatoid patients (Vainio and Pulkki, 1961), Bryan and Bickel (1971) emphasized that no other joint when affected has so often changed an ambulant rheumatoid patient into a bed-ridden cripple. Consequently the importance of total hip replacement in completely transforming the prognosis for such patients can hardly be overstated. Although total joint arthroplasty is the most commonly performed and effective operation available for rheumatoid hip pathology, it would seem appropriate to look briefly at some of the other surgical procedures that have been utilized in the management of rheumatoid disease.

Synovectomy of the hip has had its advocates but because of its rather variable results and the ever-persistent fear that it might precipitate avascular necrosis of the head of the femur it plays an insignificant role in the modern management of the rheumatoid hip joint.

Upper femoral osteotomy has no significant part to play in the management of an inflammatory arthritis.

Hemi-arthroplasty is also inapplicable since it only addresses one side of the diseased joint and the metallic head of this type of implant cannot be contained by the soft exposed bone in the acetabular floor and a painful migrating femoral head is almost inevitable. For similar reasons cup arthroplasty has no part to play in the modern management of the rheumatoid hip.

Arthrodesis is certainly not a suitable solution in view of the restriction of movement that may already exist or may develop in other lower limb joints. Moreover, it would throw intolerable stresses on the ipsilateral knee leading to its eventual destruction.

Excision arthroplasty is virtually obsolete as regards the primary treatment of the rheumatoid hip except perhaps where surgery has been undertaken merely to relieve pain in a wheelchair-bound patient. It does retain an important place as a relatively safe line of retreat in the infected total hip replacement where revision to another total hip is deemed unwise or where this procedure has itself failed. Under such circumstances excision arthroplasty can provide a remarkably pain-free functional hip but if it is to do so the line of resection should be done as smoothly as possible along the inter-trochanteric line and any projecting acetabular margins should be removed. Post-operative skin or skeletal traction should be maintained for 6 weeks after which the patient can be mobilized fully weight-bearing. In many cases a weight-relieving caliper will be found helpful particularly where multiple hip surgery has resulted in loss of bone stock. Full compensation for the telescoping of the pseudarthrosis through the use of a heel and sole raise (usually about 3−4 cm) is required. Permanent use of a walking aid to control the Trendelenburg gait is the usual sequel to this operation.

Total hip replacement

With the development of total hip replacement by McKee and Charnley in the early 1960s the surgical armamentarium for the arthritic hip was suddenly transformed. Surgery could now be recommended in appropriate cases in the firm knowledge that a first-class functional result could be achieved in the vast majority of cases (Charnley and Cupic, 1973).

INDICATIONS

The most common indication for operative treatment of the rheumatoid hip is severe pain that has not been adequately controlled by medical treatment. Aggressive deformity and loss of movement may also be less common indications for joint replacement. Any evidence that such deformities are exacerbating ipsilateral or contralateral knee involvement, with the so-called long-leg arthropathy of Dixon and Campbell-Smith (1969) enhances the urgency for operation lest what has initially been a single joint problem becomes compounded into a need for multi-joint replacement.

Severe bilateral adduction deformities may be a mandatory indication for operation especially in female patients where such deformities may constitute a major marital problem, giving rise to very distressing pain during sexual intercourse. This in itself may constitute a very valid indication for undertaking hip replacements in a female patient at an age when one would not normally wish to embark on such an irrevocable step.

OPERATIVE TECHNIQUE

In general the operative procedure in the rheumatoid patient is very similar to that employed in the osteoarthritic patient (see Chapter 20.2).

However, we should concentrate on some of the problems that are particularly associated with the rheumatoid patient. Many of the patients may be extremely osteoporotic and great care must be exercised in handling the limb particularly during dislocation of the hip to prevent a fracture of the shaft of the femur or damage to the ipsilateral knee joint.

In order to guard against femoral shaft fractures the neck can be divided *in situ* and the head removed by inserting a corkscrew extractor.

The operation can usually be done without trochanteric osteotomy and this approach is to be preferred since during the re-wiring of an osteoporotic trochanter there is a real danger that the bone may become completely fragmented. In most standard operations either the Hardinge or posterior approaches are commonly employed. Nevertheless, where the exposure proves difficult and access is confined it is still preferable to remove the trochanter and safeguard the shaft of the femur from the danger of fracture or from perforation due to malposition of the femoral reamers. Particular difficulties with the exposure can be encountered in severe cases of protrusio acetabuli, in those with an extreme flexion deformity or in revisional arthroplasty.

When the acetabular floor is extremely thin removal of fibrous tissue with a curette is all that is required. Perforation of the floor should be avoided under these circumstances. Anchoring holes for the cement should be made into the ischium, ilium and the superior ramus of the pubis. The most important aspect of the operative technique is to achieve lateralization of the femoral head to restore the anatomical centre of rotation. In turn this moves the weight-bearing vector laterally until it is again directed into the body of the ilium where the load is partly attenuated. Failure to achieve adequate lateralization will result in protrusion of the prosthesis. Lateralization may be achieved in several ways, namely by the use of a double cement mix (Eftekhar, 1978), the strength of which may be enhanced by the use of gauze mesh incorporated into the cement (Harris and Jones, 1975; Hastings and Parker, 1975). Although these techniques can provide a satisfactory short-term result, the emphasis is now on using techniques that will build up the deficient acetabular floor using bone grafts. These bone grafts may be used as multiple morselized segments cut from the excised femoral head or from the iliac crest and placed over the thin acetabular floor (McCollum *et al.*, 1980) in conjunction with a cemented or uncemented acetabular component (Fig. 18.2.8). If there is a large medial wall deficiency a single solid bone graft fashioned from the femoral head may be used to reconstruct the medial wall (Heywood, 1980). If the roof of the acetabulum is deficient then it can be reconstructed by screwing on segments of the patient's femoral head or similar allograft bone to reconstruct the roof. Some reports suggest that there is significant graft resorption in longer follow-up in these cases (Mulroy and Harris, 1990).

Where the acetabular floor has become completely fragmented or destroyed but the rim of the acetabulum remains intact the use of a reconstruction plate or an acetabular ring of the Eichler or Harris-Oh type may prove useful (Eichler, 1973). These rings abut against the intact periphery of the acetabulum while their convergent teeth suspend the acetabular cup in the desired position (Fig. 18.2.9).

In the presence of severe osteoporosis with a very capacious femoral medullary canal, larger femoral components can be utilized and great care should be exercised in positioning the femoral component in the correct angle of anteversion and in centralizing the tip of the stem within the femoral canal to achieve a circumferential cement mantle.

Uncemented hip arthroplasty (Chapter 20.3)

In recent years there has been much interest in the role

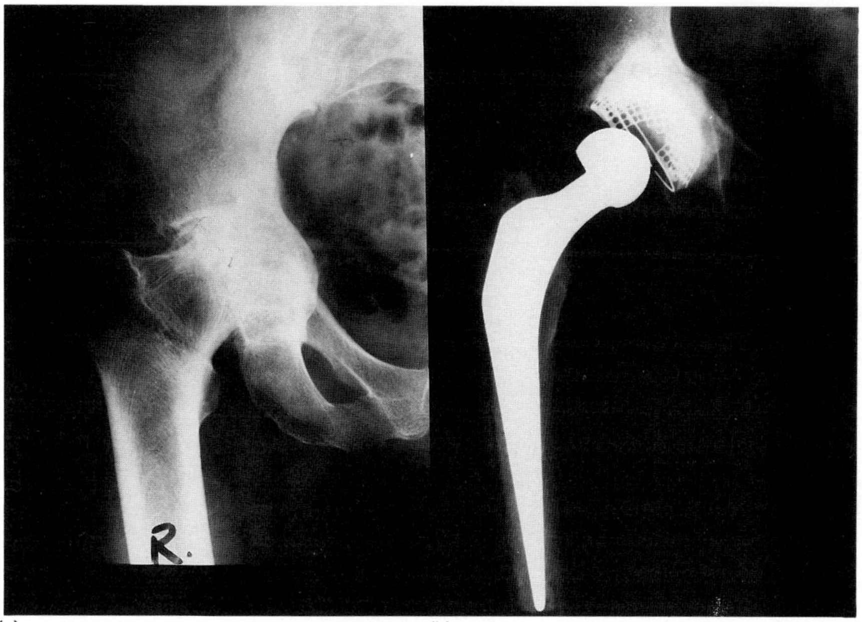

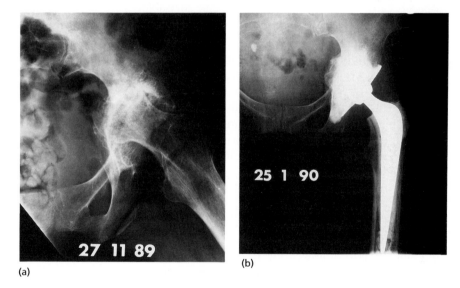

Fig. 18.2.8 (a) Protrusio acetabuli. (b) Total hip replacement with lateralization of the acetabular component achieved by the use of morselized segments of the patient's femoral head. Further augmentation by acetabular mesh is no longer considered necessary.

(a)   (b)

Fig. 18.2.9 (a) Marked protrusio acetabuli. (b) Lateralization of the prosthetic cup achieved by the use of an acetabular ring. The deficient floor has been grafted with morselized bone from the patient's femoral head.

(a)

(b)

of uncemented arthroplasty. This is theoretically particularly attractive when implantation is considered in the younger patient with rheumatoid arthritis (Fig. 18.2.10). The relatively poor fixation afforded by osteoporotic bone combined with the post-operative difficulties in weight protection of the replaced joint in those patients with severe involvement of the upper limbs suggests that rheumatoid arthritis remains a relative indication for their present use. To date no long-term advantage for their use has been clearly demonstrated and at the present time the authors believe that the cemented hip arthroplasty remains the operation of choice for the majority of rheumatoid patients.

POST-OPERATIVE CARE

No special measures need to be taken with the rheumatoid patient except those that may be dictated by arthritic involvement of other joints. When there is significant ipsilateral knee flexion deformity it may be necessary to ensure that for periods throughout the day the hip is maintained in the maximum correction achieved at surgery. This may be done either through periods of prone lying or by the use of a special bed, the foot of which can be lowered at knee level so that the thigh and trunk remains horizontal. In a few cases where trochanteric re-attachment must be regarded as

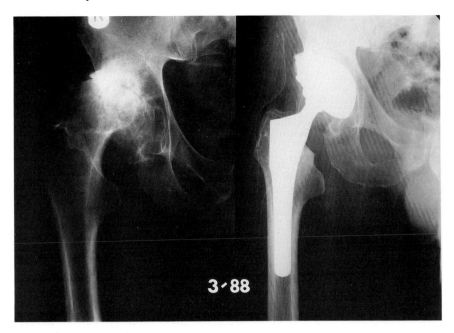

Fig. 18.2.10 Uncemented porous coated anatomic hip replacement in a 30-year-old patient with rheumatoid arthritis.

suspect because of poor bone quality it may be advisable to delay mobilization for 3 weeks. Normally a rheumatoid patient may be allowed out of bed as usual on the second to fifth post-operative day depending on the surgeon's personal preference or the individual patient's pain threshold. Where there is severe rheumatoid involvement of the upper limb a high walking frame or platform crutches may have to be provided to give additional support. In 1970 Welch and Charnley reported 95% complete pain relief in 307 hips with an average follow-up of 32.3 months.

Poss *et al.* (1984) reported on the 6–11-year results of total hip arthroplasty in rheumatoid arthritis where they found a 96% satisfactory clinical result with a mean follow-up of 7 years. Unger *et al.* in 1987 reported on a similar series followed for 10–17 years with an average follow-up period of 12 years. These patients had 80% satisfactory results. The revision rate for mechanical loosening was 13% and for sepsis was 4%. In spite of the prevalence of osteoporosis in rheumatoid patients the incidence of loosening is probably considerably less than in osteoarthritic patients because of the greatly reduced stresses to which the replacements are likely to be subjected in patients disabled with polyarthritis (Gschwend, 1980).

COMPLICATIONS

Dislocation

The overall incidence of dislocation of the hip is between 2 and 3%. According to Poss *et al.* (1984) the risk of a single episode of dislocation is no higher in rheumatoid arthritis than in other arthropathies. Kahan *et al.* (1981) reveal that the greatest risk of dislocation is within the first 5 weeks after surgery. However, late dislocations do occur especially in the rheumatoid group and Kahan observed recurrences in over 60% of those with late dislocations and only 40% of those dislocating within the first 5 weeks.

Non-operative treatment in a spica cast can stabilize two out of three patients. Thus only one out of every 100 patients undergoing total hip arthroplasty will require revision directly due to instability (Morrey, 1991). Where impingement has been excluded and the instability found to be minimal the simplest solution may be the use of a polyethylene wedge screwed onto the rim of the original cup (Olerud, 1985). Where there is severe instability or where there is significant malpositioning of the cup or stem then due consideration should be given to revision of the offending component. In those rheumatoid patients who dislocate after a number of years there is often a wide range of rotation and hip flexion with the formation of a large pseudocapsule which may be important in the aetiology of the dislocation (Kaplin *et al.*, 1987). They have recommended trochanteric advancement in these difficult circumstances. Seventeen of 21 of these hips had no further dislocations following this procedure.

Deep venous thrombosis

Patients with rheumatoid arthritis are thought to have a lower risk of thrombo-embolic disease after hip replacement (Sikorski *et al.*, 1981). The incidence is said to be reduced by the use of the posterior approach, the avoidance of a trochanteric osteotomy and the use of spinal anaesthesia. The routine use of prophylactic anticoagulation drugs in the rheumatoid patient has still not been clarified mainly because of the low incidence of fatal pulmonary embolis (Thorburn *et al.*, 1980).

Infection (see also Chapter 15)

Although the immediate post-operative deep infection rate is not significantly increased in this condition there is much evidence to support the fact that late infection is 2−4 times more common in rheumatoid arthritis (Fitzgerald *et al.*, 1977; Poss *et al.*, 1984). In the authors' opinion this late infection frequently results from haematogenous spread from distant septic foci. Nixon (1983) has shown that systemic steroids also contribute to the increased risk of infection. Antibiotic prophylaxis should be used at the time of surgery. Because of the risk of haematogenous spread it is probably advisable to protect the hip with antibiotics for the rest of the patient's life should any infective problem arise. For similar reasons any urological instrumentation or dental filling or extraction should also be covered. Infection may be difficult to diagnose. Radiographic changes may be suggestive but are rarely diagnostic and a raised erythrocyte sedimentation rate and C-reactive protein may reflect the rheumatoid disease rather than an infection within the hip. A C-reactive protein level of more than 20, however, is unlikely to be due to rheumatoid disease *per se*. Gallium-67 citrate scans can be used and often show an increased uptake under these circumstances. The most important assessment is aspiration of the hip to establish a definite bacteriological diagnosis. If the culture is negative but there are still strong grounds for suspecting infection then the aspiration should be repeated in consultation with a bacteriologist regarding further investigation and management. It is fundamentally important to define the infecting organism so that the appropriate antibiotic treatment can be prescribed in combination with operation.

The prosthesis, cement and granulation tissue should all be removed, at which time tissue specimens should be sent to the bacteriology laboratory if the pre-operative aspirations have remained sterile. If the infection proves to be of the Gram-negative type, particularly that due to *Pseudomonas*, or if any associated sinuses subsequently fail to heal, then the patient may be better left with a Girdlestone. Otherwise due consideration should be given to re-implantation. If the decision is taken to re-implant this may be carried out immediately or delayed for weeks or even months. Salvati *et al.* (1982) have compared the published results of a variety of techniques that use one- or two-stage re-implantations and concluded that a good result was more likely after two-stage re-implantation. Re-implantation is carried out by using antibiotic impregnated cement and systemic antibiotics are continued for 6 weeks after surgery.

Fitzgerald and Jones (1985) have shown that a short time interval between the resection arthroplasty and the re-implantation was identified as a factor adversely influencing the results. They recommended a delay of 12 months between the two procedures. In rheumatoid disease where the patients autoimmune system is compromised the authors feel it is preferable to carry out a two-stage re-implantation. A long delay of several months may be considered a particular hardship in a rheumatoid patient with multiple joint involvement and a compromise may have to be reached on timing of the second operation.

Between the excision and the re-implantation antibiotic impregnated beads were usually left between the bone ends and post-operative traction was applied for a period of 6 weeks. In our practice this technique is now being superseded by the use of a moulded antibiotic impregnated acrylic hemi-arthroplasty which, after hardening, can be inserted into the upper femur and acetabulum (Duncan and Beauchamp, 1991). This acts as a spacer holding the bone ends apart prior to re-implantation. It allows traction to be abandoned and also allows the patient to gently mobilise and to sit out of bed in a chair during this period.

THE ANKLE AND HINDFOOT

Vidigal *et al.* (1975), in a survey of 204 feet of patients with definite rheumatoid arthritis, noted radiological changes in 176 forefeet and 133 hindfeet, involving 124 midtarsal, 64 subtalar and 52 ankle joints.

Rheumatoid pathology may manifest itself in the ankle and hindfoot in a number of ways. This may include tenosynovitis, nodule formation in the Achilles tendon, acute synovitis of the ankle joint itself or late destruction of the ankle. The subtalar and midtarsal joints are also subject to synovitis and as a result a slowly progressive and fixed valgus deformity of the hindfoot commonly occurs. Less frequently a very mobile unstable valgus deformity develops as a result of local erosion within the subtalar joint. A further important cause of this deformity may be rupture of the tibialis posterior tendon occurring as a result of synovial infiltration.

The subtalar and midtarsal joints tend to be involved fairly early in rheumatoid disease and although synovitis of these joints may be acutely painful, more commonly their destruction to the point of virtual ankylosis may occur relatively silently and the patient may not be seen in the surgical clinic until a fully established valgus deformity is present. In some instances severe valgus deformities at the subtalar joint can be combined with tilting of the talus within the ankle mortice producing an erosion at the point of contact between the supralateral aspect of the talus and the tibial surface. The talus can sometimes abut against the tip of the lateral malleolus and induce a stress fracture of the lower fibula. Furthermore, the severe valgus deformity can result in the patient walking on the navicular. When the navicular subluxes off the head of the talus the patient can even walk on the head of the talus, creating problems with local skin ulceration.

Where the deformity remains correctable the pain may be controlled by the use of an orthosis such as a German leather anklet worn inside the patient's shoe. Attention may have to be given to the use of velcro straps to obviate the difficulty of fastening a lacing orthosis by patients whose fingers are affected. An alternative device may be the use of a double below-knee iron with square heel sockets incorporating an elastic wedge into the heel of the shoe and a rocker bottom sole to aid forward propulsion. Cosmetic moulded polyethylene ankle foot orthoses may also be used in these circumstances provided that they are well fitted.

Operative management

TENDON INVOLVEMENT AROUND THE ANKLE

Synovial infiltration resulting from rheumatoid involvement of the small bursa at the insertion of the Achilles tendon may weaken the attachment of the tendon and precipitate rupture. Bursectomy should obviate this danger. More troublesome is the phenomenon of nodule formation within the substance of the tendon often occurring about 2.5–5 cm above its insertion. These nodules are often palpable and may be quite sizeable and may result in rupture of the tendon. Ultrasound may allow visualization and localization of smaller nodules. Excision of these nodules is advisable to prevent tendon rupture and if the resulting defect in the tendon appears ominous it may be advisable to re-enforce the tendon with distally based reflected strips

from its proximal segment as described by Bosworth (1956) and Lindholm (1959).

Acute rheumatoid inflammation of the synovial sheaths around the ankle may also occur. The sheaths of the tibialis posterior and the peronei seem particularly liable to be involved. Synovial hypertrophy may be very obvious as a fusiform swelling anteriorly or behind one or both malleoli. In the presence of significant disease passive stretching of the involved tendons may invoke acute pain. Tenosynovectomy carried out through a straight anterior or a curved incision behind one or both malleoli should be effective in relieving pain and preventing subsequent tendon rupture (Fig. 18.2.11). This is particularly important in relation to the tibialis posterior where its rupture produces a rapid and severe valgus deformity of the foot.

If rupture has recently occurred then reconstruction of the tibialis posterior should be considered using the technique described by Jahs (1982), who recommended suture of the flexor digitorum longus to the distal stump of the ruptured tibialis posterior tendon.

SYNOVITIS OF THE ANKLE JOINT

Epidemiological studies show that the ankle joint tends to be involved much less commonly and much later in the course of the disease than the subtalar and midtarsal joints. Nevertheless acute synovitis of the ankle when it does occur can be extremely disabling and if conservative measures fail operative synovectomy may be considered. Very little has been written about the efficacy of ankle synovectomy but Jakubowski (1973) reviewed a series of 34 cases in which he claimed good results in 24, satisfactory results in eight and poor results in two Gschwend (1980b) reported on 20 patients who had synovectomy of the ankle joint with a mean follow-

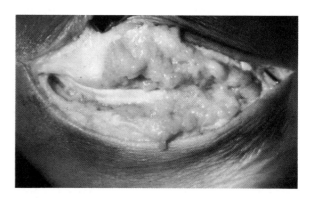

Fig. 18.2.11 Marked proliferative synovitis of peroneal tendons in rheumatoid arthritis.

up of 4.4 years. It should be noted that associated tenosynovectomy was performed in 16 of these patients. Of these patients 15 were free from pain at follow-up but in these cases it is difficult to attribute the success of the procedure to the synovectomy of the joint as opposed to the tenosynovectomy.

Mohing *et al.* (1983) reported on 81 ankle synovectomies in 62 patients using multiple incisions to gain access to the joint. Only 16% were carried out for stage I changes (see Fig. 18.2.1). The results in these patients were good. In the group as a whole however, only 64% of the patients had no pain on activity and 65% had reduction in swelling.

OPERATIVE MANAGEMENT OF THE DESTROYED ANKLE

When this does occur it can be associated with very severe pain and restriction of movement. Sometimes this can be combined with an equinus deformity which tends to throw the knee into hyperextension. On some occasions the foot assumes a valgus attitude in combination with dorsiflexion in which case a flexion deformity is induced at the knee. It is relatively rare for the ankle to be affected in isolation and often there are significant changes at the subtalar and midtarsal joint levels. Under those circumstances it is attractive to consider the possibility of relieving pain and restoring motion to the ankle by ankle arthroplasty. Movement of the ankle joint would allow attenuation of some of the impact forces during the push-off phase of gait or when rising from a chair. This would reduce the loading across the ipsilateral knee and hip and this may be of particular importance in the presence of arthroplasties of these joints.

TOTAL ANKLE REPLACEMENT

During the 1970s there was considerable enthusiasm for ankle arthroplasty. Many prostheses were described; most were constrained and reproduced uni-axial movement only. Examples of these were the ICLH (Imperial College London Hospital) design, the TPR (Thompson–Parkridge–Richards) prosthesis (Fig. 18.2.12) and the Mayo type. In 1985 Bolton-Maggs *et al.* reported on 41 of the ICLH ankle prostheses with a mean follow-up of 5.5 years. Of 34 arthroplasties carried out for rheumatoid disease only six were considered to be satisfactory. Five had already undergone arthrodesis for loosening and eight ankles showed moderate to severe pain. Lachiewicz *et al.* (1984), reporting on 15 uni-axial arthroplasties mainly of the Mayo type in rheumatoid patients, found that 11 ankles had developed radiolucent lines and six components showed evidence of subsidence within a mean follow-up of 39 months.

It was felt that poly-axial prostheses would permit more unconstrained motion and allow some supination and pronation. Kirkup (1985) described the results of 20 poly-axial Smith prostheses of which 15 were reviewed at a mean of 7 years. At that stage six were painfully loose and two had been revised. Nine ankles had little or no pain although two of those had ankylosed. Kirkup has subsequently reported on his experience with the Bath poly-axial prosthesis and of 57 of these devices 86% were *in situ* at an average follow-up of 4.2 years but only 63% were free of pain or only experienced discomfort after activity. Most joints showed radiolucent lines on radiography (Kirkup, 1990).

Despite the need for ankle replacement in the rheumatoid patient the long-term results of the various de-

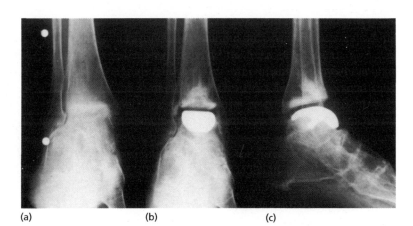

Fig. 18.2.12 (a) Severe rheumatoid destruction of a right ankle. (b) Anteroposterior and (c) lateral projections of the same ankle following replacement with a TPR prosthesis.

(a)   (b)   (c)

vices have demonstrated frequent complications such as loosening (Fig. 18.2.13), instability, prosthetic migration, impaired wound healing and infection. Hamblen (1985), in an editorial review for the *British Journal of Bone & Joint Surgery*, concluded that the ankle could not reliably be replaced by the available prostheses. It should be pointed out that in the event of failure there is considerable loss of bone stock making arthrodesis extremely difficult. In the authors' view total ankle replacement is only indicated as a possible treatment in the elderly and rather inactive rheumatoid patient, particularly in the presence of significant subtalar and midtarsal disease provided that there is still a symmetrical ankle mortice and no significant valgus of the hindfoot. This remains the consensus view of most surgeons working in the field.

ANKLE ARTHRODESIS

For most surgeons ankle arthrodesis is now the procedure of choice to deal with a significantly eroded ankle joint. This is certainly true of the younger and more active patients. Over 20 different methods of ankle arthrodesis have been described, the most common of which employ the use of compression, strut or sliding tibial grafts and dowel or auger techniques (Fig. 18.2.14). Each of these techniques has its devotees. Although Mazur *et al.* (1979) have shown a better gait pattern after fusion of the osteoarthritic ankle than with replacement it is doubtful whether this is true in rheumatoid patients who inevitably have multi-joint involvement of the foot. Because of the problems arising from

arthroplasty, however, ankle arthrodesis remains the procedure of choice for the great majority of rheumatoid patients with significantly destroyed ankle joints. It is not always easy to be certain that the pain is arising from the ankle rather than the subtalar joint. Under these circumstances it is helpful to assess the patient's pain and function before and after an injection of local anaesthetic into the ankle joint. Whichever operative technique is selected it is important that the ankle is ankylosed in neutral or slight dorsiflexion as the midtarsal joint is capable of more plantar flexion than dorsiflexion.

Vahvanen (1969) had no infections in his series of ankle fusions but commented that pseudo-arthrosis was more common after using cancellous bone grafting techniques. Rackman *et al.* (1990), however, found that bone grafting techniques of this type were successful in all of their group of 11 ankles in whom arthrodesis had been achieved in this way in association with the use of an anterior staple. Moran *et al.* (1991) reviewed a series of 30 ankle arthrodeses mainly carried out using a variety of compression techniques. Twelve ankles had skin breakdown and subsequent infection. Of these ankles 18 united after a primary attempt at fusion, six had pain-free fibrous unions and six required further operations for pseudarthroses. They used a modified Mazur scoring system and commented that they achieved good or excellent results in 14 and only four patients had residual pain in the ankle. All these authors regarded the procedure as an effective mode of treatment for the rheumatoid ankle.

Stauffer (1983) summarized the disadvantages of

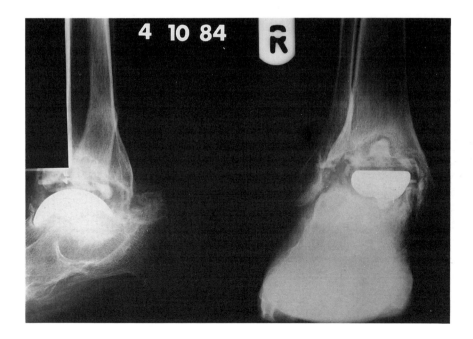

Fig. 18.2.13 Loose TPR ankle arthroplasty showing marked lucencies around the tibial component. Marked collapse of the talus is observed in the lateral view. A stress fracture of the fibula has occurred.

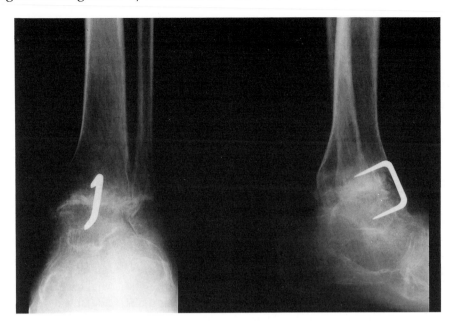

Fig. 18.2.14 Ankle arthrodesis achieved by the use of cancellous bone grafting and fixation by an anterior staple.

ankle arthrodesis. There was an overall non-union rate of 10–20% and on average the ankle took 5.5 months to ankylose. The prolonged immobilization presents difficulties for the average rheumatoid patient. He further commented on the excess stress thrown onto the adjacent joints. Despite this the authors feel that ankle arthrodesis is a more appropriate form of treatment than ankle arthroplasty in the majority of cases.

OPERATIVE MANAGEMENT OF THE TARSAL JOINTS

Talonavicular arthrodesis

This is a useful procedure when the patient presents with pain over the talonavicular joint and radiographs confirm that there is erosion confined to this joint. On other occasions this pathology may be associated with a passively correctable valgus deformity. Under either circumstance a localized talonavicular fusion may be effective (Fig. 18.2.15). The operation is done through a localized medial longitudinal incision centred over the joint and following clearance of the joint cavity the tubercle of the navicular can be excised and used as a bone graft. The alternative is to use iliac crest bone and in both instances the joint is held with staples most easily inserted with a powered device. The patient is mobilized in plaster for approximately 3 months.

Elbaor *et al.* (1976) reviewed 35 cases carried out in Boston and over 90% had marked reduction in symptoms. This operation is felt to prevent subsequent valgus malalignment of the foot.

Subtalar fusions

Rather uncommonly one may be faced with an unstable hindfoot which collapses into gross valgus on weight-bearing but which remains passively fully correctable. At surgical exploration such patients may be found to have a very large, laterally based wedge erosion of the subtalar joint. These cases can be treated very effectively

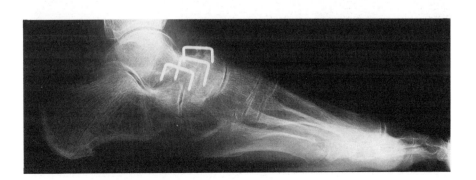

Fig. 18.2.15 Localized talonavicular fusion with staple fixation.

by maintaining full correction with a cortico-cancellous bone graft after the manner of Grice (1955). The fixation may be improved further by the insertion of a cancellous screw through the neck of the talus deep into the body of the calcaneum (Fig. 18.2.16). Weight-bearing in plaster may be allowed as soon as the wound has healed and the cast retained for 12 weeks from the date of operation.

Triple fusion

With a painful fixed plano-valgus deformity of the foot associated with significant erosion of the subtalar and midtarsal joints a triple arthrodesis would be the procedure of choice. Here the deformity is corrected by removal of a medially based wedge of bone between the talus and the calcaneum and between the talus and the navicular. This procedure can be difficult in a very valgus rheumatoid foot and rather than carrying out the operation through a single oblique lateral incision it may be of assistance to expose the talonavicular joint through a separate medial incision. It is of great importance to achieve a plantigrade foot and the use of staples is helpful in maintaining the fixation. In this respect the powered Shapiro stapler can be an extremely useful instrument. A period of 12 weeks of plaster immobilization is usually necessary following the procedure.

THE FOREFOOT

The forefoot is the region of the foot most commonly affected by rheumatoid disease and is also the area for which operative management is most frequently employed. Early phases of involvement of the metatarsophalangeal joints is characterized by inflammatory changes with synovial hypertrophy. This in turn leads to severe clawing of the toes due to dorsal subluxation of the metatarsophalangeal joints and subsequent flexion at the proximal interphalangeal joint level (Fig. 18.2.17). The plantar fat pad is displaced distally to expose the metatarsal heads to the plantar skin. Furthermore the pressure of the shoe on the dorsally displaced toes forces the metatarsal heads down into the sole so that marked callosities are formed over the overlying skin and render walking extremely painful. Similarly, corns form over the prominence of the flexed proximal interphalangeal joints and these lesions are particularly liable to ulcerate. The big toe frequently develops a severe valgus deformity with bunion formation at the metatarsophalangeal joint. This is particularly likely to occur in association with a valgus deformity of the hindfoot. In a much smaller number of patients the interphalangeal joint of the hallux may be involved and becomes characteristically dorsiflexed so that the weight is no longer borne on the terminal pulp of the toe but on the exposed condyles of the distal end of the proximal phalanx with the formation of painful calluses. This in combination with the deformity in the toe makes it impossible for the patient to wear ordinary shoes.

In the early phase of involvement symptoms can largely be alleviated by the use of an insole to relieve the pressure on the plantar prominences. Use of the insole can cause increase in pressure on the dorsum of the toes, however, and under these circumstances specially designed shoes with increased depth are required to accommodate the toe deformities.

With a fit patient and the presence of an established deformity there should be no hesitation in recommending operative treatment as excellent results can be anticipated.

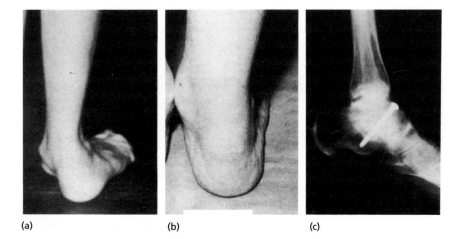

(a)   (b)   (c)

Fig. 18.2.16 (a) Pre-operative appearance of an unstable but correctable valgus hindfoot in a patient with rheumatoid arthritis. (b) Clinical correction following modified Grice procedure. (c) Post-operative radiograph.

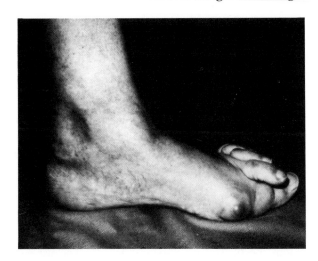

Fig. 18.2.17 Severe rheumatoid involvement of left forefoot. Note dorsal dislocation of the lesser toes, and the hallux valgus deformity with large bunion.

Operations on the rheumatoid forefoot

In most cases the authors feel that it is better not to recommend operation unless it is felt a forefoot resection arthroplasty is required. Operation on isolated toes can be disappointing because of the progressive nature of the disease. However, there are occasions when the disease seems to be inactive or very slowly progressive and a problem may exist in relation to a prominent metatarsal head, a single claw toe deformity or to a hallux valgus deformity. Under these circumstances it is acceptable to deal with these problems in isolation but it is important to point out to the patient that this should be regarded as a holding procedure and that further operations may well be required later.

METATARSAL OSTEOTOMY

When a painful callosity develops over a single metatarsal head and there is no fixed deformity at the metatarsophalangeal joint then a simple oblique osteotomy through the neck of the metatarsal may be appropriate. This was first described by Meisenbach (1916) but more recently popularized by Helal (1975). Although this can lead to non-union it does not seem to create a problem for the patient in most instances. The dorsal displacement of the metatarsal head can however, result in overloading of the adjacent metatarsal heads with the development of similar symptoms at these sites.

PROXIMAL PHALANGECTOMY

A cock-up deformity of the toe in rheumatoid disease is often best dealt with by excision of the proximal third of the proximal phalanx with a dorsal capsular release of the metatarsophalangeal joint. Alternatively a fusion of the proximal interphalangeal joint could be considered.

ISOLATED HALLUX VALGUS DEFORMITY

At an early stage where there is an isolated hallux valgus deformity perhaps associated with a pronated foot, but where the remaining toes are normal, arthrodesis of the metatarsophalangeal joint has been considered by some (Newman and Fitton, 1983). The authors feel this has the disadvantage of transferring stress onto the distal interphalangeal joint which can result in a hyperextension deformity at this level. The alternative of a Keller procedure has the disadvantage of transferring the load to the remaining rays which could be troublesome particularly if they subsequently become affected by rheumatoid disease. In this situation an intramedullary silicone hinge prosthesis may provide the best solution to the problem (Swanson *et al.*, 1979).

FOREFOOT RESECTION ARTHROPLASTY

Where general forefoot involvement has become established the treatment of choice under these circumstances is one of the variants of metatarsal head resection (Hoffman, 1912; Fowler, 1959; Clayton, 1963). The authors still prefer the technique that was learnt many years ago from the late Douglas Savill and which has been described in the literature by Kates *et al.* (1967). The heads of the 1st–5th metatarsals are excised through a plantar approach to give a smooth curve in a slightly oblique line across the stumps of the metatarsal necks. The sesamoid bones are removed from the volar surface of the hallux and the corrected position of the latter is secured by retrograde insertion of a Kirschner wire which remains *in situ* for 3 weeks (Fig. 18.2.18). The redundant skin is excised from the distal skin flap and subsequent wound closure produces a dermodesis effect on the lesser toes and it also re-positions the fat pad beneath the metatarsal necks. Bed-rest is maintained for 3 weeks at which time the Kirschner wires are removed and, if the condition of the wound permits, mobilization in rigid wooden soled sandals is commenced. The patient will usually be able to graduate to the use of ordinary shoes within 6–10 weeks of operation. After a metatarsal head resection it should be remembered that the foot sizes will have probably been reduced by 1–1½ sizes.

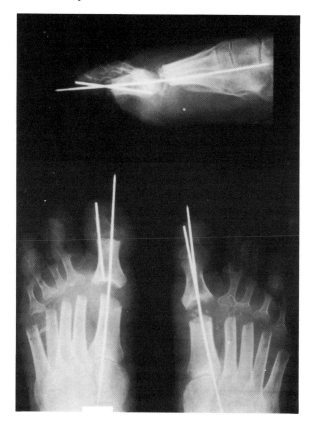

Fig. 18.2.18 Post-operative radiographs of rheumatoid feet following bilateral metatarsal head resection and fusion of the interphalangeal joints in both big toes. Note the long Kirschner wires routinely used after metatarsal head resection to maintain corrected position of the big toes and the short accessory Kirschner wires which are used to stabilize the fusion at the interphalangeal joints.

As the breadth of the foot is often large in relation to its length it may be necessary to find extremely broad fittings in the new size. If this is not possible then surgical shoes can be provided.

Faithful and Savill (1971) reviewed the results of metatarsal head resection in 77 patients (147 feet). 118 feet were regarded as having achieved a Grade I rating defined by the authors as unlimited pain-free walking in normal shoes, 14 were regarded as Grade II results where they had some residual pain requiring the continued use of insoles, while 15 were relegated to Grade III rating on the basis of persistent pain not relieved by conservative measures so that further surgery was probably indicated. Of the patients 80% had had their symptoms satisfactorily abolished and were wearing normal shoes. Using a variety of techniques for forefoot resection, moderate to good results were recorded in 88% of cases by Amuso *et al.* (1971), 83% by Barton (1973) and 84% by Watson (1974).

Barton (1973) highlighted the all-too-frequent problem of delayed wound healing of the plantar wound, this being observed in 23 out of 65 cases—an incidence of 35%. Because of this, and in order to facilitate earlier weight-bearing, some surgeons prefer to perform the operation through three longitudinal dorsal incisions, sited over the first metatarsal and over the second and fourth web spaces (Larmon, 1951). Such an approach, however, lacks the potential dermodesis of the plantar incision while longitudinal contracture on the dorsal scar may act as a deforming force tending to produce a recurrence of the original pathology. However, at 6 months after operation there seems to be little difference between the results of surgery whether carried out through the plantar or dorsal approach. The use of a single transverse dorsal incision has fallen into some disfavour due to the tendency for the wound to dehisce during the recovery period.

Although metatarsal head resection provides very satisfactory symptomatic relief, it must be regarded as equivalent to a physiological amputation because very few patients exhibit any active toe function during walking (Fowler, 1959; Clayton, 1963; Kates *et al.*, 1967). In recent years there has been a tendency to look for a more functional solution to the problem of the rheumatoid forefoot. One such solution has been the attempt to maintain the function of the big toe by carrying out an arthrodesis of the first metatarsophalangeal joint (Watson, 1974). For the reason described above we are not advocates of this procedure. A more rewarding approach would seem to be the use of a stemmed Swanson silastic spacer in the first metatarsophalangeal joint (Swanson *et al.*, 1979; Thomas 1979, 1989). The single-stemmed hemi-arthroplasty should not be used as there have been several reports of breakage and of severe abrasion with silicone-induced synovitis occurring as a result. The double-stemmed devices appear to be more hardy but should be used with caution until the result of long-term follow-ups become more readily available. One particularly useful application, however, would be in the case where there is a stiff first metatarsophalangeal joint and a hyper-extension deformity at the interphalangeal joint of the great toe. In this situation the interphalangeal joint can be fused, fixed with staples or an oblique pin to leave free the medullary canal for the insertion of the stem of the silastic prosthesis.

From time to time the surgeon may be faced with a rheumatoid foot in which toe deformities are so extreme and the clawing of the interphalangeal joints so rigid that a reasonable result from metatarsal head resection is unlikely to be obtained. In these circumstances the surgeon should have no hesitation in resorting to ablation of the toes as recommended by Flint and Sweetnam (1960). The authors, however, feel that it is preferable to amputate the toes through the metatarsal necks and not through the metatarsophalangeal joints themselves otherwise recurrence of callus formation under the remaining metatarsal heads is very likely to occur. This procedure can be virtually guaranteed to produce a very comfortable and functional foot. Moreover it is a very much safer operation than metatarsal head resection which should never be attempted if there is a hint of vasculitis in the toes lest gangrene of the digits may be precipitated (Kates *et al.*, 1967).

MULTIPLE JOINT SURGERY

In view of the success of operative treatment in individual joint problems it was inevitable that multi-joint surgery would be attempted in the management of widespread deformities in the lower limbs (Johnson, 1975; Jergensen *et al.*, 1978; Espley and Herbert, 1981). This type of surgery has now become established in the operative repertoire of those concerned with the treatment of the rheumatoid patient.

Many different patterns of joint involvement may be encountered. The patient usually develops a characteristic posture with flexion deformities of the hips and knees and a marked compensatory lumbar lordosis. This posture is a very exhausting one to maintain and inevitably the deformities tend to be of increasing severity. Superimposed upon the hip and knee problems there may be severe disease of the forefoot or hindfoot which necessitate additional surgery at these sites. Moreover, the lower limbs cannot be thought of in isolation since arthritic involvement of the upper limbs may greatly reduce a patient's ability to use walking aids during the convalescent period following lower limb reconstruction.

Multi-joint surgery may have to be undertaken as a straight sequence of operations in patients presenting with severe erosive disease and deformity in several joints simultaneously. A staggered programme of surgery is carried out in those patients whose disease gradually destroys an increasing number of joints. In this latter type of case, the patient's functional performance may run an undulating course, surgery being required at intervals to maintain it at acceptable or optimal levels. The patient, however, does have the benefit of rehabilitating only one or two joints at a time rather than being subjected to multiple joint surgery during the same period of hospitalization (Souter, 1978).

The aim of multi-joint surgery is principally to relieve pain. For many of these patients any movement, even in a wheelchair or especially any attempt at weight-bearing, may be agonizing. It is also important to restore stability and correct deformities so that the patient can regain an erect posture and begin to mobilize again without expenditure of vast amounts of energy.

The functional level achieved will vary according to the pre-operative severity of the disability.

Patient selection is of fundamental importance in this type of surgery. Those patients undergoing multi-joint surgery during one period of hospitalization must be made aware that they may be in hospital for several months. It is also important that the surgeon should discuss with the patient the results that may be expected from the surgery. In this respect, precise studies are not available and there is considerable difficulty in standardizing assessment techniques to demonstrate exactly what is achieved by these multiple procedures. Jergensen *et al.* (1978) reported that none of 16 patients undergoing bilateral hip and knee replacement returned to work. Souter (1978), reviewing 38 patients with a follow-up from 18 months to 9 years, found those who had undergone reconstructive surgery in three or more lower limb joints had encouraging results with regard to pain status, walking ability and social independence as illustrated in Table 18.2.1. Clearly the results with regard to pain relief are excellent and although the gains in walking ability and social independence are less dramatic, the authors would submit that they are still sufficient to warrant the immense time and effort involved in the rehabilitation of these patients.

In designing the operative programme it is the authors'

Table 18.2.1 Results of multiple joint surgery in lower limbs

Symptoms	No. of patients	
	Pre-operatively	Post-operatively
Pain status		
Pain-free	—	23
Severe pain	38	3
Walking ability		
1 km or more	1	11
Unable, or indoors only	30	10
Social independence		
Light or part-time work or full range of housework	1	8
Unemployable but fairly mobile	6	17
Largely confined to the house	33	15

practice to start where appropriate with surgery to the forefoot as this gives great symptomatic relief while taxing the patient only very minimally. Furthermore, it is important to eradicate any skin ulcers or infected lesions that may be present as a result of foot deformity. Finally the incidence of skin breakdown is probably greater in the foot than in the remainder of the lower limb and it is therefore prudent to carry out this operation prior to the implantation of proximal joint prostheses. Hip reconstruction should follow next in sequence because it is felt that it is easier for the patient to rehabilitate two hip replacements in the presence of painful deformed knees than vice versa. Hip replacement will allow the correction of the proximal limb contractures, the spinal lordosis and to a great extent will equalize the limb lengths. The surgeons and the patients should have now established a mutual rapport which will allow the much greater hurdles of knee surgery to be faced with more confidence (Fig. 18.2.19). Finally, surgery at the hindfoot level may be necessary to render the foot plantar grade.

THE IMPORTANCE OF TEAM MANAGEMENT IN RHEUMATOID SURGERY

With all the programmes of operative treatment outlined above, the actual operations constitute only one facet of the therapy. Patients often have severe systemic disease and careful supervision of their medical management by a skilled rheumatologist is fundamental to the overall success of the venture. Following some of these procedures and especially after multiple operations to the lower limbs, there is often a long road ahead of the patient before adequate walking ability is regained. Thus the services of physiotherapists experienced in this field are essential. Later in the course of the rehabilitation, the occupational therapist has a vital role with regard to functional assessment and the supply of gadgets that can help with such daily tasks as dressing, eating, bathing and toilet. Throughout the period of hospitalization, the social worker may do much to alleviate the personal family and financial worries of the patient. Finally, at the stage of discharge from hospital the general practitioner, the patient's relatives and the domiciliary paramedial services all have an essential role to play.

Through the exhibition of the various surgical weapons described in the foregoing pages and by bringing the many and varied skills of the multidisciplinary professional team to bear on the problems of the severely crippled rheumatoid patient, the prospects for rehabilitating many such cases to a remarkable degree of inde-

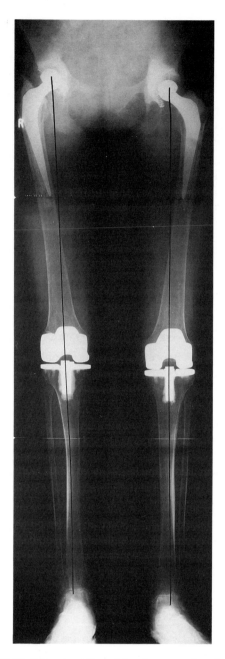

Fig. 18.2.19 Following bilateral forefoot resection, four joint replacement of the lower limbs has been carried out. Note that the mechanical axes of the limbs has been restored. The symptomatic erosion of the left ankle subsequently required ankle arthrodesis.

pendence or even in some cases to gainful employment have been transformed out of recognition from what they were prior to the introduction of joint replacement surgery.

REFERENCES

Abbott L.C. and Carpenter W.F. (1945) Surgical approaches to the knee joint. *J. Bone Joint Surg.* **27**, 277.

Abernethy P.J. (1989) Surgery for rheumatoid arthritis: 2. Lower limb. ii Surgery of the knee. *Curr. Orthop.* **3**, 150−156.

Abernethy P.J. (1990) Surgery of the rheumatoid knee. *Ann. Rheum. Dis.* **49**, Suppl 2, 830−836.

Abraham W., Buchanan J.R., Dawbert H., Grier B., Keefer J. and Wilton S. (1988). Should the patella be re-surfaced in total knee arthroplasty? Efficacy of patellar re-surfacing. *Clin. Orthop.* **236**, 128−134.

Altchek D., Sculco P. and Rawlings B. (1989) Autogenous bone grafting for severe angular deformity in total knee arthroplasty. *J. Arthro.* **4**, 151.

Amuso S.J., Wissinger H.A., Margolis H.M. *et al.* (1971) Metatarsal head resection in the treatment of rheumatoid arthritis. *Clin. Orthop.* **74**, 94.

Bartel D.L., Bicknel V.L. and Wright T.M. (1986) The effect of conformity thickness and material on stresses in ultra high molecular components for total joint replacement. *J. Bone Joint Surg.* **68A**, 1041.

Barton N.J. (1973) Arthroplasty of the forefoot in rheumatoid arthritis. *J. Bone Joint Surg.* **55B**, 126.

Benjamin A. (1969) Double osteotomy for the painful knee in rheumatoid arthritis and osteoarthritis. *J. Bone Joint Surg.* **51B**, 694.

Bolton-Maggs B.G., Sudlow R.A. and Freeman, M.A.R. (1985) Total ankle arthroplasty — a long term review of the London Hospital Experience. *J. Bone Joint Surg.* **67B**, 785−790.

Bosworth D.M. (1956) Repair of defects in the tendo-Achillis. *J. Bone Joint Surg.* **38A**, 111.

Brooks P.J., Walker P.S. and Scott R.D. (1984) Tibial component fixation in deficiencies of tibial bone stock. *Clin. Orthop.* **184**, 302.

Bryan R.S. and Bickel W.A. (1971) Vitallium mould arthroplasty and femoral prosthetic replacement in the surgical management of rheumatoid arthritis in the hip. *Orthop. Clin. North Am.* **2**, 687.

Charnley J. and Cupic Z. (1973) The nine and ten year results of the low friction arthroplasty of the hip. *Clin. Orthop.* **95**, 9.

Clayton M.L. (1963) Surgery of the lower extremity in rheumatoid arthritis. *J. Bone Joint Surg.* **45A**, 1517.

Dixon A. St J. and Campbell-Smith S. (1969) Long leg arthroplasty. *Ann. Rheum. Dis.* **28**, 359.

Dorr L.D., Ranawat C.S. and Sculco P. (1986) Bone grafts for tibial defects in total knee arthroplasty. *Clin. Orthop.* **205**, 153.

Duncan C.P. and Beauchamp C.P. (1991) Total joint replacement for the management of chronic hip infection. *J. Bone Joint Surg.* **73B** (Suppl. 1), 48.

Eftekhar N.S. (1978). *Principles of Total Hip Arthroplasty.* St Louis, C.V. Mosby Co., p. 463.

Eichler J. (1973) Ein Vorschlag zur operativen Behandlung der Protrusio Acetabuli. *Arch. Orthop. Unfallchir.* **75**, 76−80.

Elbaor J.E., Thomas W.H., Weinfeld M.S. and Potter T.A. (1976) Talonavicular arthrodesis for rheumatoid arthritis of the hindfoot. *Orthop. Clin. North Am.* **7**(4), 821.

Espley A.J. and Herbert M. (1981) The replacement of both hip and knee joints in rheumatoid arthritis. *J. R. Coll. Surg. Edin.* **26**, 214.

Ewald F.C. and Christie M.J. (1987) The results of cemented total knee replacement in young patients. *Orthop. Trans.* **11**, 442.

Faithful D.K. and Savill D.L. (1971) Review of the results of excision of the metatarsal heads in patients with rheumatoid arthritis. *Ann. Rheum. Dis.* **30**, 201.

Fitzgerald R.H. and Jones D.R. (1985) Hip implant infection, treatment with resection arthroplasty in late total hip arthroplasty. *Am. J. Med.* **78**, Suppl 6(B), 225.

Fitzgerald R.H., Nolan D.R., Ilstrup D.M. *et al.* (1977) Deep wound sepsis following total hip arthroplasty. *J. Bone Joint Surg.* **9A**, 847−855.

Fleming A., Benn R.T. and Corbett M. (1976) Early rheumatoid disease II. Patterns of joint involvement. *Ann. Rheum. Dis.* **35**, 361.

Flint M. and Sweetnam R. (1960) Amputation of all toes. A review of forty-seven amputations. *J. Bone Joint Surg.* **42B**, 90.

Fowler A.W. (1959) A method of forefoot reconstruction. *J. Bone Joint Surg.* **41B**, 507.

Gariepy R., Demers R. and Laurin C.A. (1966) The prophylactic effect of synovectomy of the knee in rheumatoid arthritis. *Can. Med. Assoc. J.* **94**, 1349.

Geens S. (1969) Synovectomy and debridement of the knee in rheumatoid arthritis. Part I. Historical review. *J. Bone Joint Surg.* **51A**, 617.

Geens S., Clayton M.L., Leidholt J.D. *et al.* (1969) Synovectomy and debridement of the knee in rheumatoid arthritis. Part II. Clinical and roentgenographic study of thirty one cases. *J. Bone Joint Surg.* **51A**, 626.

Goldie I.F. (1971) Pathomorphologic features in original and renegerated synovial tissues after synovectomy in rheumatoid arthritis. *Clin. Orthop.* **77**, 295.

Goldie I.F. (1974) Synovectomy in rheumatoid arthritis. A general review and an eight year follow up of synovectomy in 50 rheumatoid knee joints. *Semin. Arthritis Rheum.* **3**, 219.

Goodfellow J. and O'Connor J. (1977) Kinematics of the knee and prosthetic design. *J. Bone Joint Surg.* **59B**, 119.

Grace J.N. and Rand J.A. (1991) In Morrey B.F. (ed) *Joint Replacement Arthroplasty.* Edinburgh, Churchill Livingstone.

Grice D.S. (1955) Further experience with extra-articular subtalar arthrodesis. *J. Bone Joint Surg.* **36A**, 246.

Gschwend N. (1980a) *Surgical Treatment of Rheumatoid Arthritis.* Philadelphia, W.B. Saunders.

Gschwend N. (1980b) The surgical treatment of rheumatoid arthritis. Springer-Verlag, Stuttgart.

Gschwend N., Winer J. and Boni A. (1977) *Clinical Results of Synovectomy in Rheumatoid Arthritis.* Darmstadt, Steinkopff.

Hamblen D. (1985) Can the ankle be replaced? *J. Bone Joint Surg.* **67**, 689−690.

Harris W.H. and Jones W.N. (1975) The use of wire mesh in total hip replacement surgery. *Clin. Orthop.* **109**, 117.

Hastings D.E. and Hewitson W.A. (1973) Double hemiarthroplasty of the knee in rheumatoid arthritis. A surgery of fifty consecutive cases. *J. Bone Joint Surg.* **55B**, 112.

Hastings D.E. and Parker S.M. (1975) Protrusio acetabuli in rheumatoid arthritis. *Clin. Orthop.* **108**, 76.

Helel B. (1975) Metatarsal osteotomy for metatarsalgia. *J. Bone Joint Surg.* **57B**, 187.

Heywood A.W.B. (1980) Arthroplasty with a solid bone graft for protrusio acetabuli. *J. Bone Joint Surg.* **62B**, 332.

Hoffman P. (1912) An operation for severe grades of contracted or clawed toes. *Am. J. Orthop. Surg.* **9**, 441.

Insall J.N. (1986) Infection of total knee arthroplasty. In *American Academy of Orthopaedic Surgeons Institute Course Lectures.* St Louis, C.V. Mosby, vol. 25, pp. 319−324.

Jacobson S., Levinson J. and Crawford A. (1985) Late results of synovectomy in juvenile rheumatoid arthritis. *J. Bone Joint Surg.* **67A**, 1−8.

Jahs M.H. (1982) Spontaneous rupture of the tibialis posterior tendon. Clinical findings, tenographic studies and new technique of repair. *Foot and Ankle* **3**, 158–166.

Jakubowski S. (1973) Synovektomie des oberen Sprunggelenks. *Orthopäde*, **2**, 79.

Jason M.I.V. St and Dixon A. (1970) Valvular mechanics in juxta articular cysts. (1070). *Ann. Rheum. Dis.* **29**, 415–420.

Jergensen H.E., Poss R. and Sledge C.B. (1978) Bilateral total hip and knee replacement in adults with rheumatoid arthritis. An evaluation of function. *Clin. Orthop.* **137**, 120.

Johnson K.A. (1975) Arthroplasty of both hips and knees in rheumatoid arthritis. *J. Bone Joint Surg.* **57A**, 901.

Kahan M.A., Bakenberry R.H. and Reynolds I.S.R. (1981) Dislocation following total hip replacement. *J. Bone Joint Surg.* **63B**, 7.

Kaplin S.J., Thomas W.H. and Poss R. (1987) Trochanteric advancement for recurrent dislocation after total hip arthroplasty. *J. Arthroplasty* **2**, 119–124.

Kates A., Kessel L. and Kay A. (1967) Arthroplasty of the forefoot. *J. Bone Joint Surg.* **49B**, 552.

Kirkup J. (1985) Richard Smith arthroplasty. *J. Soc. Med.* **78**, 301.

Kirkup J. (1990) Rheumatoid arthritis and ankle surgery. *Ann. Rheum. Dis.* **49**, 837–844.

Lachiewicz R.F., Inglis A.E. and Ranawat C.S. (1984) Total ankle replacement in rheumatoid arthritis. *J. Bone Joint Surg.* **66A**, 340–343.

Larmon W. (1951) Surgical treatment of deformities of rheumatoid arthritis of the forefoot and toes. *Q. Bull. Northwest. Univ. Med. School* **25**, 37.

Laurin C.A., Desmarchais J., Daziano L. *et al.* (1974) Long term results of synovectomy of the knee in rheumatoid arthritis. *J. Bone Joint Surg.* **56A**, 521.

Lindholm A. (1959) A new method of operation in subcutaneous rupture of the Achilles tendon. *Acta Chir. Scand.* **117**, 261.

MacIntosh D.L. and Hunter G. (1972) The use of the hemiarthroplasty prosthesis for advanced osteoarthritis and rheumatoid arthritis of the knee. *J. Bone Joint Surg.* **54B**, 244.

McCollum D.E., Nunley J.A. and Harrelson J.M. (1980) Bone grafting in total hip replacement for acetabular protrusio. *J. Bone Joint Surg.* **62A**, 1065.

Mazur J.M., Schwartz E. and Simons S.R. (1979) Ankle arthrodesis: long term follow up with gait analysis. *J. Bone Joint Surg.* **61A**, 964.

Meisenbach R.O. (1916) Metatarsal osteotomy. *Am. J. Orthop. Surg.* **14**, 206.

Mitchell N.S. and Shepard N. (1971) The effects of synovectomy on synovium and cartilage in rheumatoid arthritis. In Cruess R.L. and Mitchell N.S. (eds) *Surgery of Rheumatoid Arthritis*. Philadelphia, J.B. Lippincott, p. 5.

Mohing W., Kohler G. and Coldewey J. (1982) Synovectomy of the ankle joint. *Int. Orthop.* **6**, 117.

Moran G.C., Pinder I.M. and Smith R.S. (1991) Ankle arthrodesis in rheumatoid arthritis. *Acta Orthop. Scan.* **62**(6), 538–543.

Morrey B.F., Adams R.A., Illstrup D.M. and Bryan R.S. (1987) Complications and mortality associated with bilateral and uni-lateral total knee arthroplasty. *J. Bone Joint Surg.* **69A**, 484–488.

Morrey B.F. (1991) (ed.) *Joint Replacement Arthroplasty*. Edinburgh, Churchill Livingstone, p. 861.

Mulroy R.D. and Harris W.H. (1990) Prohibitive failure rate of femoral head autograft in total hip replacement for acetabular deficiency by 12 years. *Transaction of 57th Annual Meeting of American Academy of Orthopaedic Surgeons*. New Orleans.

Newman R.J. and Fitton J.N. (1983) Conservation of metatarsal heads in the surgery of rheumatoid arthritis. *Acta Orthop. Scand.* **54**, 417–422.

Nixon J.E. (1983) Failure patterns after total hip replacement. *Br. Med. J.* **286**, 166–170.

Olerud, K. (1985) Recurrent dislocation status post total hip replacement. *J. Bone Joint Surg.* **67B**, 402.

Pinder I.M. (1973) The treatment of popliteal cysts in the rheumatoid knee. *J. Bone Joint Surg.* **55B**, 119–125.

Poss R., Malloney J.P., Ewald F.C., Thomas W.H., Batte M.J., Hartness C. and Sledge C.B. (1984) 6–11 year results of total hip arthroplasty in rheumatoid arthritis. *Clin. Orthop.* **182**, 109.

Ranawat C.S. (1986) Patello-femoral joint in total condylar arthroplasty the pros and cons based on a 5–10 year follow up. *Clin. Orthop.* **236**, 128–134.

Rand J.A. and Bryan R.S. (1983) Re-implantation for the salvage of infected total knee arthroplasty. *J. Bone Joint Surg.* **65A**, 1081–1086.

Rand J.A. and Bryan R.S. (1986) The outcome of failed knee arthrodesis following total knee arthroplasties. *Clin. Orthop.* **205**, 82.

Rand J.A., Bryan R.S. and Chao E.Y.S. (1987) Failed total knee arthroplasty treated by arthrodesis of the knee using the Ace–Fisher apparatus. *J. Bone Joint Surg.* **69A**, 39.

Romnes D.W. and Rand J.A. (1988) The role of continuous passive motion following total knee arthroplasty. *Clin. Orthop.* **226**, 34–37.

Ryd L. (1986) Micromotion in knee arthroplasty. Roentgenstereophotogammetric analysis of tibial component fixation. *Acta Orthop. Scand.* **57**, Suppl 220.

Rydholm U., Elbargh R., Ramstam J., Schroeder A., Svantesson H. and Lidgren L. (1986) Synovectomy of the knee in juvenile chronic arthritis, **686**, 2, 223.

Salvati E.A., Chekofsky K.M., Brause B.D. and Wilson P.D. Jr. (1982) Re-implantation in infection—a 12 year experience. *Clin. Orthop.* **170**, 62.

Sarokhan A.G., Scott R.D., Thomas W.T., Sledge C.B., Ewald F.C. and Cloos D.W. (1983) Total knee arthroplasty in juvenile rheumatoid arthritis. *J. Bone Joint Surg.* **65A**, 1071–1081.

Sikorski J.M., Hampson W.G. and Staddon G.E. (1981) The natural history and etiology of deep vein thrombosis after total hip replacement. *J Bone Joint Surg.* **63B**, 171–177.

Souter W.A. (1978) Multijoint surgery in the lower limbs in rheumatoid arthritis. Paper presented at 14th Congress, Societe International de Chirurgie Orthopaedique et de Traumatologie, Kyoto.

Stauffer R.N. (1983) In Evarts (ed.) *Surgery of the Musculo-Skeletal System*. Edinburgh, Churchill Livingstone, vol. 3, pp. 115–142.

Stuart M.J. and Rand J.A. (1988) Total knee arthroplasty in young adults who have rheumatoid arthritis. *J. Bone Joint Surg.* **70A**, 84.

Swanson A.B., Lumsden R.M. and Swanson G. de G. (1979) Silicone implant arthroplasty of the great toe. *Clin. Orthop.* **142**, 30.

Swett P. (1923) Synovectomy and chronic infectious arthritis. *J. Bone Joint Surg.* **5**, 110.

Taylor A.R. and Hill A.G.S. (1978) Synovectomy and surgical management of rheumatoid arthritis. *Clin. Rheum. Dis.* **4**, 287.

Thomas W.H. (1979) Rheumatoid arthritis of the ankle and foot. In: *The American Academy of Orthopaedic Surgeons, Instructional Course Lectures, Vol XXVIII*. St Louis, C.V. Mosby, p. 325.

Thomas W.H. (1989) Reconstructive surgery and rehabilitation of the ankle and foot. In Kelly W.N., Harris E.D., Ruddy S. *et al.* (eds) *Textbook of Rheumatology*. Philadelphia, W.B. Saunders.

Thorburn J., Louden J.R. and Valance R. (1980) Spinal and general anaesthesia and total hip replacements: the frequency of deep venous thrombosis. *Br. J. Anaesth.* **52**, 11−17.

Unger A.S., Inglis P.E., Ranawat C.S. and Johanson N.A. (1987) Total hip arthroplasty in rheumatoid arthritis. *J. Arthroplasty* **II**, 191−197.

Vahvanen V. (1969) Arthrodesis of the T.C. or pantal joints in R.A. *Acta Orthop. Scand.* **40**, 642−652.

Vainio K. (1966) Synovectomie du genou dans les arthrites rhumatismales. *Med. Hyg.* **738**, 616.

Vidigal E., Jacoby R.K., Dixon A. St. J., Radcliffe A.H. and Kirkup J. (1975) The foot in chronic rheumatoid arthritis. *Ann. Rheum. Dis.* **34**, 292−297.

Walker P.S. (1989) Requirements for successful total knee replacement — design considerations. *Orthop. Clin. North Am.* **20**, 15.

Watson M.S. (1974) A long term follow up of forefoot arthroplasty. *J Bone Joint Surg.* **56B**, 527.

Welch R.B. and Charnley J. (1970) Low friction arthroplasty of the hip in rheumatoid arthritis and ankylosing spondylitis. *Clin. Orthop.* **72**, 22.

Wheelwright E.W., Strachan R.K. and Abernethy P.J. (1989) Paper presented to British Orthopaedic Association, Oxford.

Wheelwright E.W., Strachan R.K. and Abernethy P.J. (1990) Paper presented to the British Orthopaedic Association, Glasgow.

Chapter 19
Femoral and Tibial Osteotomy for Osteoarthritis

P. Maquet

INTRODUCTION

Osteoarthritis occurs as the consequence of a disturbance of the balance that normally exists between the resistance of the articular cartilage and bone, and their mechanical stressing: articular pressure has become too high to be withstood by the tissues. Either the compressive stresses in the joint are actually increased or the resistance of the tissues is lowered by biological factors which we do not yet understand.

In many instances of hip and knee osteoarthritis, reducing the articular pressure significantly results in clinical and radiological improvement. This was demonstrated by Pauwels for the hip (Pauwels, 1959, 1973) with long-term follow-up results and by the author for the knee (Maquet, 1984) and the hip (Maquet, 1985). This approach to the problem, however, is more demanding but it is also more stimulating intellectually than a total replacement. To succeed it requires understanding of the mechanics of the joint, clear indications and precise operative technique.

THE HIP

During walking the force R transmitted across the hip joint is the resultant or vectorial sum of the force K exerted on the articulation eccentrically by the mass of the body minus the supporting leg, and the muscular force M necessary to balance K (Fig. 19.1). Force K acts on the hip through a lever arm h', force M through a longer lever arm h. The contribution of the abductor muscles to the force transmitted across the joint, therefore, is more than body weight. The resultant R evokes compressive stresses in the joint. As shown by Pauwels (1973), the outline of the subchondral sclerosis in the roof of the acetabulum indicates the magnitude and distribution of the articular compressive stresses. In a normal hip, a subchondral sclerosis of even width

throughout suggests articular pressure evenly distributed over the weight-bearing surface of the joint (Fig. 19.2a). A dome-shaped subchondral sclerosis constitutes the very first sign of primary osteoarthritis resulting from biological failure: the pressure is increased in the centre

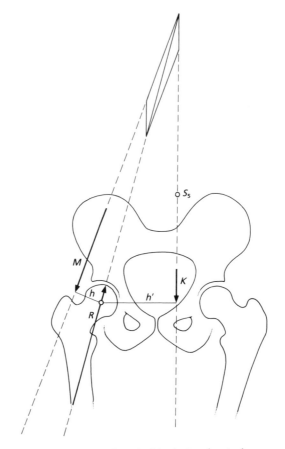

Fig. 19.1 Forces exerted on the hip during the single support period of gait. S_5, centre of gravity of the body minus the supporting leg; K, force exerted by this mass; h', lever arm of force K; M, force exerted by the abductor muscles counterbalancing K; h, lever arm of M; R, force transmitted across the hip joint (= counterforce to the resultant of K and M).

587

of the weight-bearing surface and decreases towards the periphery. The articular tissues are no longer able to distribute pressure evenly (Fig. 19.2b). In osteoarthritis developing with subluxation of the hip, a dense triangle at the edge of the acetabulum corresponds to the outline of the stress diagram. The pressure is maximum at the edge of the acetabulum; medially part of the surface contact of the joint may transmit no weight (Fig. 19.2c). In osteoarthritis with protrusio acetabuli the triangle is medial, in the depths of the socket (Fig. 19.2d).

The goal of surgery consists of decreasing the articular pressure sufficiently to make it tolerable to the tissues. In principle, the articular pressure can be decreased by diminishing the force transmitted across the joint or by enlarging the force-transmitting surface of the joint or,

even more efficiently, by combining both possibilities (Pauwels, 1959).

Decreasing force *R*

THE HANGING-HIP PROCEDURE (VOSS–PAUWELS)

Tenotomy of the abductor, adductor and ilio-psoas muscles decreases the force *R* transmitted across the joint without modifying the articular weight-bearing surface (Fig. 19.3). The hanging-hip procedure is indicated whenever there is no concentration of pressure either at the edge or in the depths of the acetabulum, in other words when the weight-bearing surface of the joint is not decreased. The prerequisites for this pro-

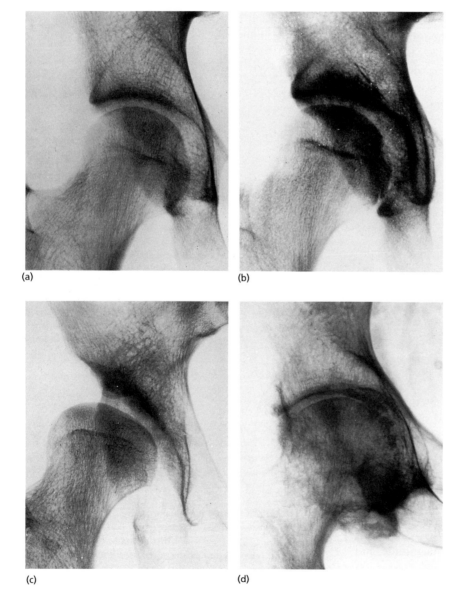

(a)

(b)

(c)

(d)

Fig. 19.2 Distribution of the articular compressive stresses. (a) Normal joint; (b) primary osteoarthritis; (c) osteoarthritis in subluxated joint; (d) protrusio acetabuli.

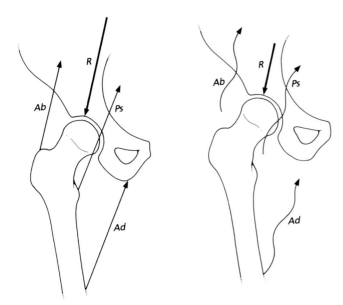

Fig. 19.3 Decreasing force *R* transmitted across the joint by dividing tendons. *Ab* = abductor muscles; *Ad* = adductor muscles; *Ps* = ilio-psoas muscle. (Redrawn after Pauwels, 1959.)

cedure to have a good chance of success are that:
1 the articular surfaces are congruent in any position of the hip;
2 there is no dense triangle at the edge or in the depths of the acetabulum.

When these prerequisites are met, the results of this very simple procedure are often spectacular.

Case example (Fig. 19.4). A 78-year-old female patient

Table 19.1 Range of hip movement in a 78-year-old female patient before and 9 years after a hanging-hip procedure

	Before	After 9 years	Gain
Flexion	75°	100°	35°
Extension	0°	10°	
Adduction	5°	35°	30°
Abduction	5°	5°	
Int. rotation	−5°	45°	95°
Ext. rotation	10°	55°	

complained of a painful hip with considerable limitation of its range of movement (Table 19.1) and a severe limp. The radiograph showed the absence of a joint space (Fig. 19.4a), and a dome-shaped subchondral sclerosis was visible. Cysts were present in the roof of the socket. A hanging-hip procedure was carried out and the patient was relieved of pain immediately. At the 9-year follow-up, the hip remained pain-free. The range of movement had improved considerably (Table 19.1) and the patient walked without a limp. The radiograph showed the reappearance of a joint space (Fig. 19.4b). The subchondral sclerosis was thinned, and extended over a wide area, indicating an enlarged weight-bearing surface. The cysts had disappeared.

However, carrying out a hanging-hip procedure when a dense triangle is present in the roof of the socket, i.e. when the weight-bearing surface of the joint is decreased, regularly results in failure. In such circumstances the weight-bearing surface of the joint has to be enlarged.

Fig. 19.4 (a) Before and (b) 9 years after a hanging-hip procedure carried out in a 78-year-old female patient. (After Maquet, 1985.)

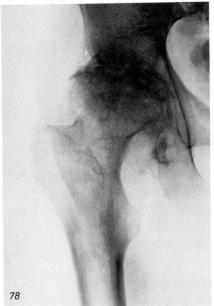

(a)

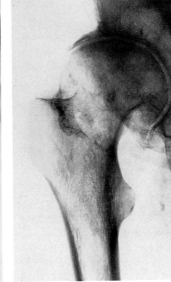

(b)

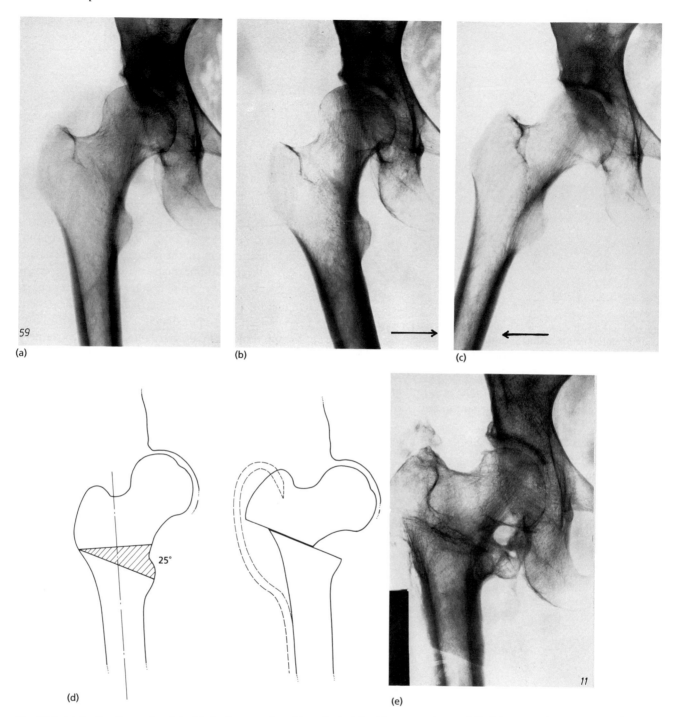

Fig. 19.5 (a) A−P radiographs of the hip in the neutral position, (b) in full adduction and (c) in full abduction, (d) preoperative diagram, (e) eleven-year-follow-up. (After Maquet, 1985.)

Enlarging the weight-bearing surface of the joint and decreasing force *R*

Pre-operatively, to assess the possibility of enlarging the articular weight-bearing surface, three A−P radiographs of the joint are required: one in the neutral position (Fig. 19.5a), one in full adduction (Fig. 19.5b) and one in full abduction (Fig. 19.5c) of the leg. In all three the beam must be centred on the femoral head with the leg internally rotated. Moreover, an overall view of the pelvis enables one to assess the opposite hip and to determine the degree of an adduction contracture. Lateral views complete the radiographic examination.

In the case of the 59-year-old patient illustrated in Fig.

19.5 the articular surfaces of the hip are congruent in full abduction. This suggests that a varus intertrochanteric osteotomy can be considered. This must be confirmed by a diagram (Fig. 19.5e) and, if some doubt remains, by additional radiographs under anaesthesia. In the present instance a varus osteotomy was actually carried out with an excellent result (Fig. 19.5d).

VARUS INTERTROCHANTERIC OSTEOTOMY (PAUWELS I)

Varus intertrochanteric osteotomy generally lengthens the lever arm *h* of the abductor muscles *M* by displacing the greater trochanter laterally (Fig. 19.6). This is particularly significant when dealing with a coxa valga. Varus intertrochanteric osteotomy also changes the direction of the abductor muscles *M* by increasing their inclination to the vertical, thus opening the angle formed by the lines of action of the forces *K* and *M*. Both opening this angle and lengthening the lever arm *h* of force *M* decrease the resultant force *R*. Moreover, the line of action of *R* is displaced medially into the socket. The medial displacement of *R* enlarges the weight-bearing part of the contact surfaces of the joint. Increasing the weight-bearing surface and decreasing the force transmitted across the joint result in considerable diminution of the articular compressive stresses and in their more even distribution.

The prerequisites for a varus intertrochanteric osteotomy for an osteoarthritic hip with a dense triangle at the edge of the acetabulum are:

1 congruence of the articular surfaces in abduction;
2 a coxa valga.

The operation must be planned on a tracing of the hip from the A−P radiograph in the neutral position. The wedge to be resected in order to achieve congruence is measured and the medial displacement necessary to keep the femoral shaft in its previous position in relation to the pelvis is determined (Pauwels, 1959; Maquet, 1985). The procedure is carried out exactly as planned. The patient moves and puts partial weight on the operated leg immediately after surgery. In severe cases, when no joint space remains, walking with two crutches is recommended for 6 months, and with one crutch for six additional months. This partial unloading is aimed at sparing the tissues during their remodelling.

Case example (Fig. 19.7). A 51-year-old female patient presented with a painful hip, limitation of its range of movement (Table 19.2) and limp. The radiograph showed the joint space was narrowed and there was a dense triangle at the edge of the acetabulum (Fig. 19.7a). A 17° varus intertrochanteric osteotomy was planned (Fig. 19.7c) and carried out. At the 14-year follow-up the clinical result remained excellent (Table 19.2) and the radiographic picture was improved: a wide joint

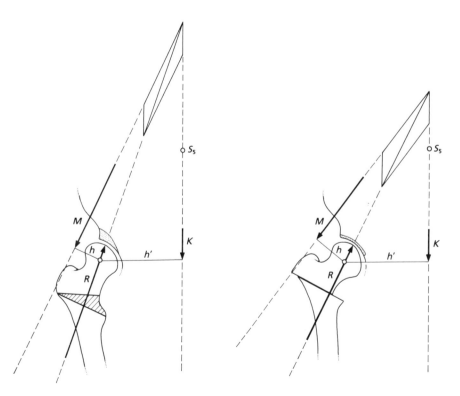

Fig. 19.6 Varus intertrochanteric osteotomy. Abbreviations as in Fig. 19.1.

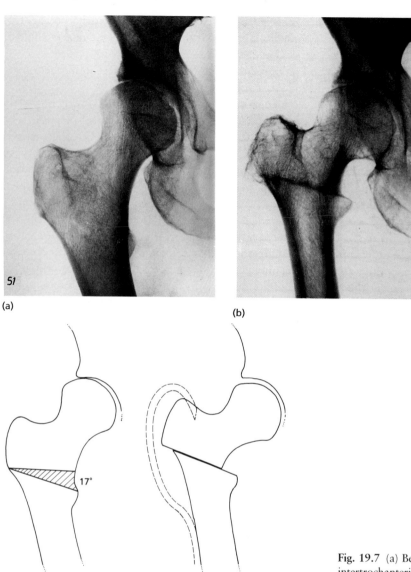

(a)

(b)

(c)

17°

Fig. 19.7 (a) Before and (b) 14 years after a varus intertrochanteric osteotomy carried out in a 51-year-old female patient. (c) Planning. (After Maquet, 1985.)

Table 19.2 Range of hip movement in a 51-year-old female patient before and 14 years after varus intertrochanteric osteotomy

	Before	After 14 years	Gain
Flexion	90°	140°	55°
Extension	−5°	0	
Adduction	5°	40°	70°
Abduction	15°	50°	
Int. rotation	5°	45°	85°
Ext. rotation	5°	50°	

space and a subchondral sclerosis of even width throughout suggested an even distribution of the articular compressive stresses (Fig. 19.7b).

However, in the absence of a coxa valga, a varus intertrochanteric osteotomy may not change the lever arm *h* of the abductor muscles much (Maquet, 1990). In such instances, displacing the greater trochanter laterally is more efficient.

LATERAL DISPLACEMENT OF THE GREATER TROCHANTER (MAQUET)

Lateral displacement of the greater trochanter lengthens the lever arm *h* of the abductor muscles *M* and changes the direction of their line of action as well (Fig. 19.8). This results in opening the angle formed by the lines of action of the forces *K* and *M*. Consequently, the resultant force *R* is decreased and its line of action is displaced medially into the acetabulum, thus enlarging the weight-bearing surface of the joint. For a hip with a normal neck-shaft angle, lateral displacement of the greater trochanter exerts the same mechanical effect as does a varus intertrochanteric osteotomy for a coxa valga: decrease of the force transmitted across the joint and increase of the force-transmitting surface.

Case example (Fig. 19.9). The procedure was carried out on a 33-year-old female patient with osteoarthritis of a hip secondary to avascular necrosis of the femoral head (Fig. 19.9a). Eleven years after the 2 cm lateral displacement of the greater trochanter the clinical result remained excellent: no pain, full range of movement (Table 19.3), normal gait and unrestricted walking capacity. The radiograph showed the dense triangle in the roof of the acetabulum (Fig. 19.9a) had been replaced by a thin ribbon of dense bone of even width throughout, delineating a wide joint space (Fig. 19.9b).

VALGUS INTERTROCHANTERIC OSTEOTOMY (PAUWELS II)

In advanced cases of osteoarthritis both the acetabulum and the femoral head are markedly deformed. A medial

Table 19.3 Range of hip movement in a 33-year-old female patient before and 11 years after lateral displacement of the greater trochanter

	Before	11 years after	Gain
Flexion	90°	115°	30°
Extension	5°	10°	
Adduction	5°	30°	60°
Abduction	25°	60°	
Int. rotation	5°	50°	75°
Ext. rotation	0°	30°	

osteophyte develops over the medial aspect of the femoral head, pushing the head laterally (Pauwels, 1973). The articular surfaces are no longer congruent and the joint space disappears. Adduction of the leg may show better congruence of the articular surfaces (Fig. 19.10). A valgus intertrochanteric osteotomy can then be considered. The possibility of achieving congruence of the joint surfaces is determined by drawing from a tracing of the A–P radiograph in the neutral position. The wedge to be resected to ensure congruence may be larger than the possible pre-operative amplitude of adduction. At the end of surgery the articular surfaces should gape somewhat laterally.

Valgus intertrochanteric osteotomy (Fig. 19.11) consists of removing an intertrochanteric wedge with a

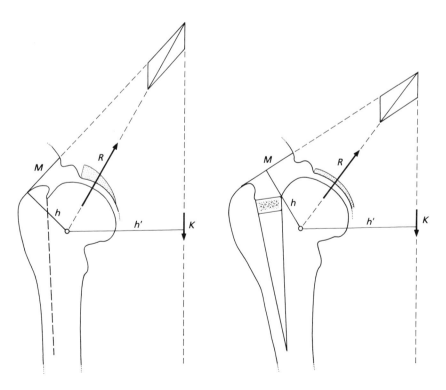

Fig. 19.8 Lateral displacement of the greater trochanter. Abbreviations as in Fig. 19.1.

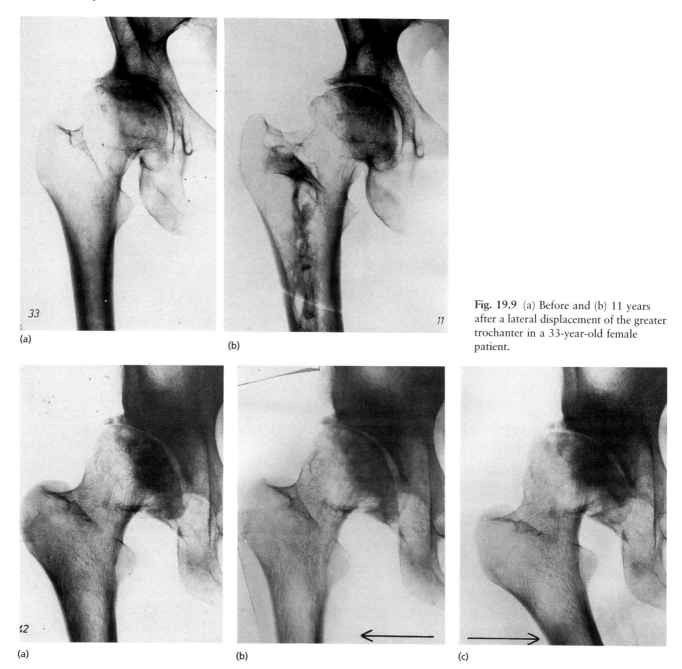

Fig. 19.9 (a) Before and (b) 11 years after a lateral displacement of the greater trochanter in a 33-year-old female patient.

Fig. 19.10 (a) A−P radiographs in the neutral position, (b) in full abduction and (c) in full adduction. (After Maquet, 1985.)

lateral base. The procedure decreases articular pressure by involving the medial osteophyte developed over the femoral head in the weight-bearing surface of the joint, thus significantly increasing the weight-bearing surface. Decrease of the force transmitted across the joint is achieved additionally by dividing the tendons of the adductor, abductor and ilio-psoas muscles. Displacement of the abductor muscles pushed laterally by the femoral head bulging out of the socket may contribute

to the decrease of the force R by lengthening the lever arm h of force M, and to the medial displacement of the line of action of R by changing the direction of force M.

The prerequisites for deciding to carry out a valgus intertrochanteric osteotomy are:

1 a dense triangle at the edge of the acetabulum;
2 improved congruence of the articular surfaces in full adduction whereas the incongruence becomes worse in abduction.

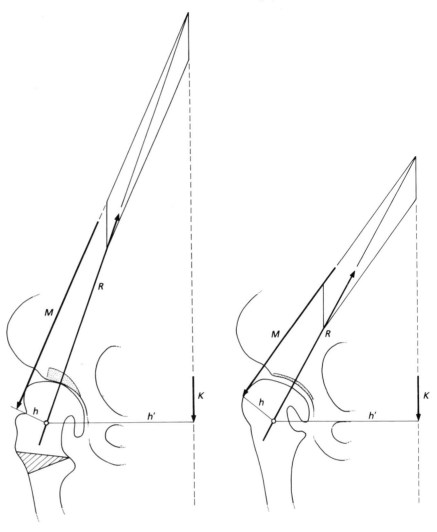

Fig. 19.11 Valgus intertrochanteric osteotomy. Abbreviations as in Fig. 19.1.

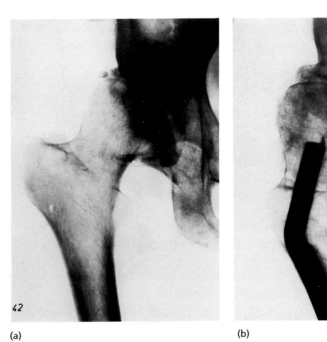

Fig. 19.12 (a) Before and (b) 24 years after a valgus intertrochanteric osteotomy combined with a tenotomy carried out in a 42-year-old female patient.

(a)

(b)

Case example (Fig. 19.12). A 42-year-old female patient complained of hip pain day and night with a limited range of movement (Table 19.4) and a limp. Very marked subchondral sclerosis at the edge of the socket suggested increased and concentrated articular pressure (Fig. 19.12a). After careful planning a 30° intertrochanteric wedge was resected. A good result was obtained. At the 24-year follow-up the hip remained pain-free. The range of movement had improved (Table 19.4). Limping was hardly noticeable. The radiograph showed the subchondral sclerosis was even throughout and extended over a wide area suggesting a considerable diminution and an even distribution of the articular compressive stresses over a large weight-bearing surface (Fig. 19.12b).

Protrusio acetabuli

Osteoarthritis with protrusio acetabuli is an indication for a hanging-hip procedure as long as there is no dense triangle in the depths of the acetabulum. If such a medial triangle is present a valgus osteotomy is recommended. Force R and its counterforce R' can be resolved into a longitudinal component L or L' and a transverse com-

Table 19.4 Range of hip movement in a 42-year-old female patient before and 24 years after valgus intertrochanteric osteotomy

	Before	24 years after	Gain
Flexion	60°	85°	20°
Extension	5°	0°	
Adduction	10°	45°	25°
Abduction	30°	20°	
Int. rotation	0°	0°	0°
Ext. rotation	45°	45°	

ponent Q or Q' as long as both R and R' are resolved along the same directions (Fig. 19.13). In protrusio acetabuli the transverse component Q', which pushes the femoral head inwards, seems to overcome the resistance of the articular tissues. The magnitude of component Q' can be reduced by decreasing the force R' as a whole. This is achieved by a tenotomy of the abductor, adductor and ilio-psoas muscles. The magnitude of component Q' is further diminished by decreasing the inclination of the line of action of force R' to the vertical. This is achieved by a valgus osteotomy.

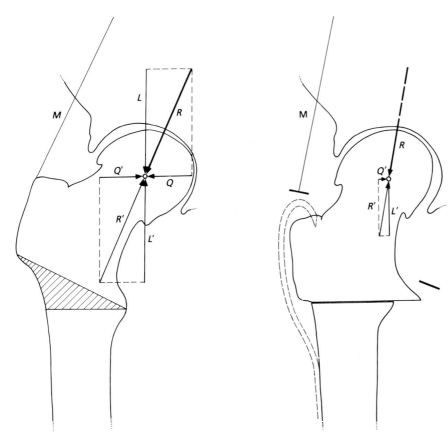

(a)　　　(b)

Fig. 19.13 Resolution of force R into a longitudinal L and a transverse component Q. The same for the counterforce R'. (a) Protrusio acetabuli; (b) after a valgus osteotomy and tenotomy. (Redrawn after Pauwels, 1973.)

Case example (Fig. 19.14). A 58-year-old female patient complained of severe pain in a hip with considerable limitation of its range of movement. The initial radiograph showed the femoral head to be bulging into the pelvis (Fig. 19.14a). A valgus osteotomy was combined with a hanging-hip procedure. Ten years later the clinical and radiological result remained good (Fig. 19.14b).

Contraindication to femoral osteotomy

When the joint surfaces cannot be made congruent in either position (Fig. 19.15), none of the surgical procedures thus described should be considered. They would be doomed to failure because, in such instances, there is no possibility of enlarging the weight-bearing surface of the joint.

The importance of the mechanical effect

The results of the procedures described above are consistently good as long as the indications are correct. They are consistently poor when the procedures have not achieved congruence of the joint surfaces and thus have not decreased the joint pressure significantly (Watillon *et al.*, 1978). Dividing the bone is not enough. It is imperative to decrease joint pressure.

Cases have been described in which a spectacular result was obtained on one side by shortening the opposite leg, thus rotating the acetabulum about the femoral head of the former side with the same effect as a valgus osteotomy (Maquet, 1985). In such instances, almost experimental, the good result can be attributed only to an increase of the articular weight-bearing surface and certainly not to a division of the bone as such.

THE KNEE

Femoro-tibial joints

The force transmitted across the femoro-tibial joint during walking is the resultant force R or vectorial sum of the force P exerted on the joint eccentrically by the mass of the body minus the supporting lower leg and foot, and the muscular force M necessary to balance P (Fig. 19.16). During the single support period of gait force M is at first anterolateral, then lateral and finally posterolateral, always opposite to the line of action of P in relation to the knee. Force R normally acts at the centre of the knee (Maquet *et al.*, 1967) and evokes compressive stresses in the joint. These compressive stresses are fairly evenly distributed over both tibial plateaus in a normal knee, as shown by the subchondral scleroses underlining the plateaus (Fig. 19.17). In osteoarthritis developing on or into a varus deformity, force R is displaced medially with increase and concentration of the stresses in the medial aspect of the knee (Fig. 19.18). This results in a dense triangle underlining the medial plateau in the A–P radiograph (Fig. 19.19). In osteoarthritis with a valgus deformity force R is displaced laterally with increase of joint pressure in the lateral

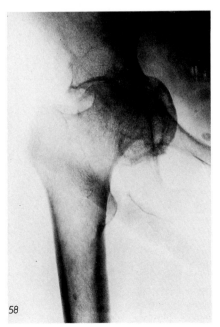
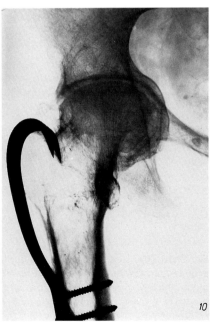

Fig. 19.14 (a) Before and (b) 10 years after a valgus intertrochanteric osteotomy plus tenotomy carried out in a 58-year-old female patient.

(a)   (b)

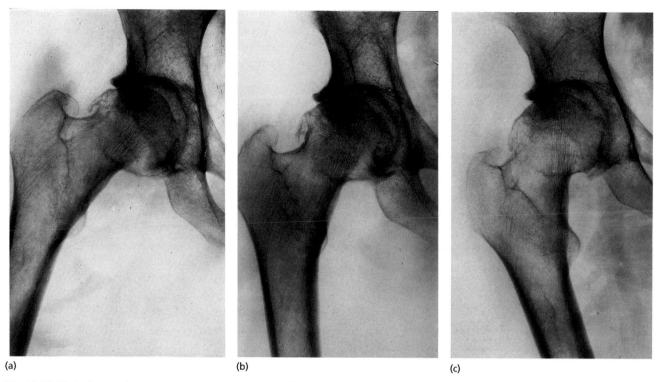

Fig. 19.15 No indication for an osteotomy or a tenotomy. (After Maquet, 1985.) Full abduction (a), neutral position (b), full adduction (c).

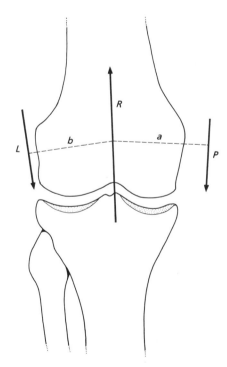

Fig. 19.16 Forces exerted on the knee during the single support period of gait. *P* = force exerted by the mass of the body minus the supporting lower leg and foot; *a* = lever arm of force *P*; *L* = force exerted by the muscles to counterbalance *P*; *b* = lever arm of force *L*; *R* = force transmitted across the joint (= counterforce to the resultant of *P* and *L*).

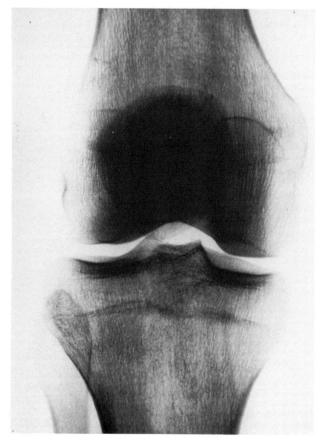

Fig. 19.17 The symmetrical subchondral scleroses underlining the tibial plateaux suggest an even distribution of the articular compressive stresses over large weight-bearing surfaces. (After Maquet, 1985.)

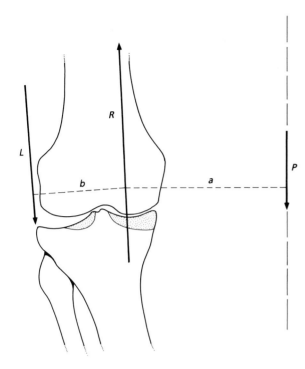

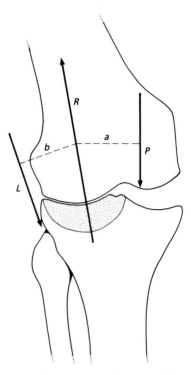

Fig. 19.18 Medial displacement of force *R*. Abbreviations as in Fig. 19.16.

Fig. 19.20 Lateral displacement of force *R*. Abbreviations as in Fig. 19.16.

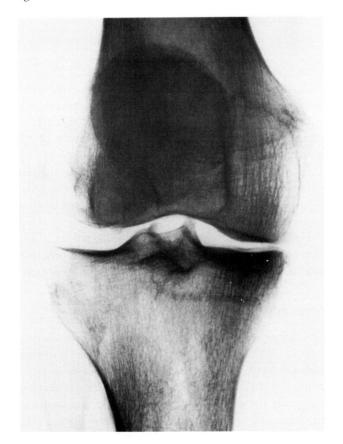

Fig. 19.19 Dense triangle beneath the medial plateau in osteoarthritis with a varus deformity.

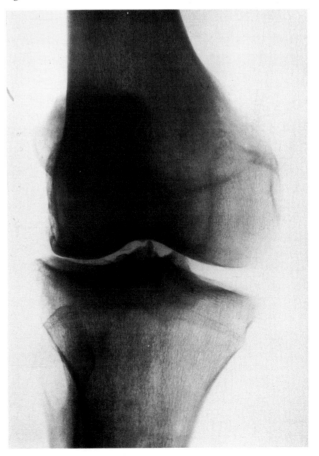

Fig. 19.21 Dome-shaped sclerosis beneath the lateral plateau in osteoarthritis with a valgus deformity.

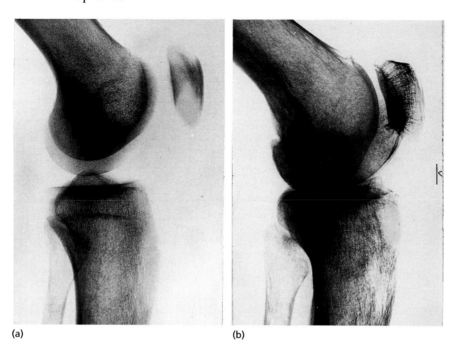

(a)   (b)

Fig. 19.22 Lateral view of (a) a normal knee and of (b) a knee with a flexion contracture (from Maquet, 1984).

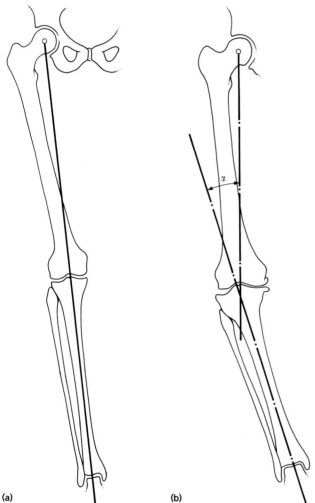

(a)   (b)

Fig. 19.23 Measuring a varus deformity. (a) Normal knee; (b) varus knee.

aspect of the joint (Fig. 19.20). An upside-down sclerotic dome underlines the medial aspect of the lateral plateau (Fig. 19.21). The fundamental difference between the distribution of the stresses in the varus and in the valgus deformity has been explained based on the geometrical features of the deformed knees (Maquet, 1984). In a lateral view the tibial plateaus of a normal knee are underlined by a subchondral sclerosis of even width throughout (Fig. 19.22a). In a flexion contracture the compressive stresses are concentrated posteriorly. A dense triangle underlines the posterior aspect of the plateaus (Fig. 19.22b).

A procedure aimed at reducing the articular pressure should replace force *R* to the centre of the knee in order to distribute *R* evenly over weight-bearing surfaces as large as possible.

Flexion contracture is generally corrected as a first step of the surgical procedure by dividing the posterior capsule through both a medial and a lateral approach.

OSTEOARTHRITIS WITH A VARUS DEFORMITY

The deformity is measured as accurately as possible on a long A−P radiograph showing the whole leg from the femoral head to the ankle. This radiograph is taken while the patient is putting full weight on the leg. Normally the centre of the femoral head, the centre of the knee and the centre of the ankle are aligned (Fig. 19.23a). A line thus is drawn from the centre of the femoral head to the middle of the transverse diameter of the bone at the level of the considered osteotomy (the

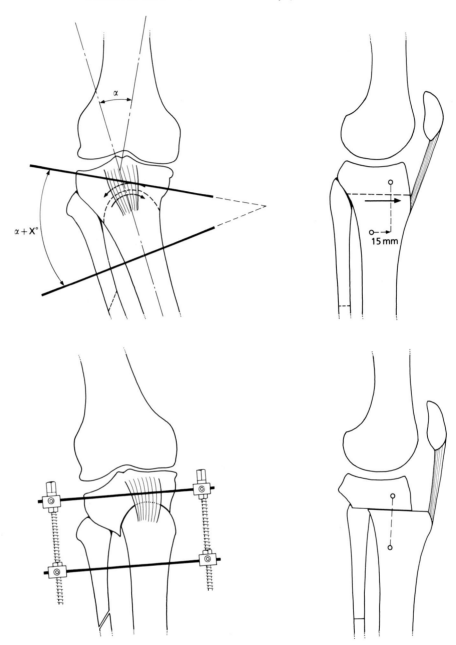

Fig. 19.24 Overcorrection of a varus knee.

upper tibia for a varus knee, the supracondylar aspect of the femur for a valgus knee generally). Another line is drawn from this point to the centre of the ankle. The angle formed by the two lines measures the deformity (Fig. 19.23b). The surgical procedure is planned graphically on a tracing from the A−P radiograph in standing.

To recentre force *R* a varus deformity should be overcorrected to compensate for the weakness of the muscles which seems to be the most frequent cause of osteoarthritis with a varus deformity. It appears that an overcorrection of between 3° and 6° gives the best results at 10 years or more follow-up (Maquet *et al.*,

1982; Goutalier *et al.*, 1987). For a varus knee an osteotomy of the upper end of the tibia is generally the best choice, as demonstrated geometrically (Maquet, 1984).

Steinmann pins are inserted proximally and distally to the osteotomy site. They form the angle corresponding to the planned correction (Fig. 19.24). A barrel-vault osteotomy with the anterior tuberosity in the concavity of the cylindrical cut is then carried out. The fragments are displaced until the Steinmann pins are parallel and the distal fragment of the tibia is shifted forwards to achieve an anterior displacement of the tibial tuberosity.

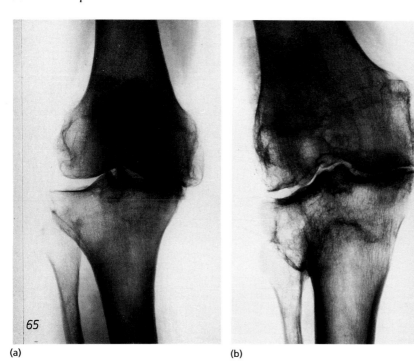

(a)   (b)

65   11

Fig. 19.25 Osteoarthritis of a knee with a varus deformity in a 65-year-old patient, (a) before and (b) 11 years after an overcorrecting tibial osteotomy.

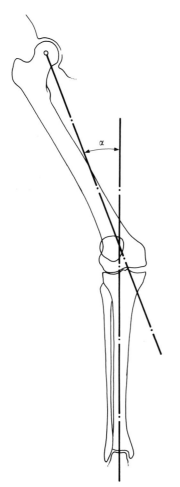

α

Fig. 19.26 Measuring a valgus deformity. (After Maquet, 1984.)

No tourniquet, or immobilization is required. The patient is advised to put weight on the operated leg from the second day. The Steinmann pins are removed after 2 months and bony union is evident.

Case example (Fig. 19.25). A 65-year-old female patient presented with severe osteoarthritis in the medial compartment of both knees: narrowing of the joint space, and increase of the sclerosis beneath the medial tibial plateau (Fig. 19.25a). The varus deformity of the right knee was 20°. A valgus barrel-vault osteotomy of the tibia was carried out. At the 11-year follow-up the knee remained pain-free with a full range of movement. In the radiograph taken in the standing position a wide joint space had reappeared, the two tibial plateaus were underlined by a sclerosis of even width throughout (Fig. 19.25b). This means an even distribution of joint pressure over large weight-bearing surfaces. The left knee was operated on similarly with an equally good result.

OSTEOARTHRITIS WITH A VALGUS DEFORMITY

The valgus deformity is measured in the same manner as the varus deformity (Fig. 19.26). The valgus deformity should be slightly overcorrected (by 1° to 2°) by means of a supracondylar osteotomy of the femur. The reason for choosing a femoral osteotomy in a valgus deformity is geometrical and has been demonstrated elsewhere (Maquet, 1984).

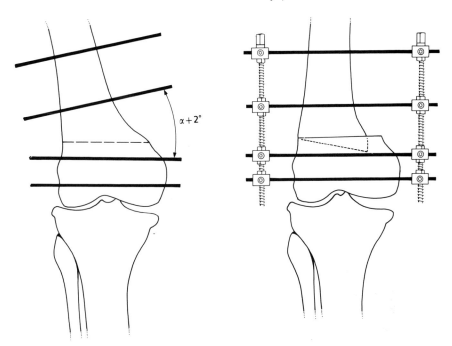

Fig. 19.27 Distal femoral osteotomy in osteoarthritis predominant in the lateral compartment with valgus deformity.

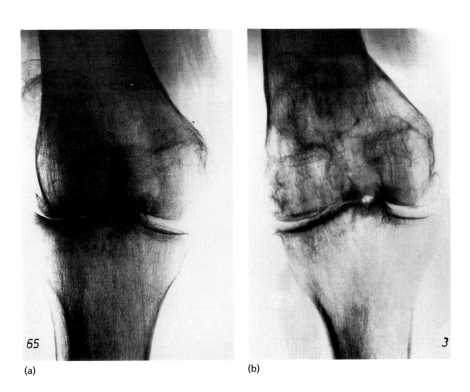

Fig. 19.28 Osteoarthritis with a valgus deformity in a 65-year-old patient (a) before and (b) 3 years after a supracondylar osteotomy of the femur.

(a)   (b)

Surgery is also planned graphically here (Fig. 19.27). The fragments are fixed under compression by four Steinmann pins, two in the diaphysis and two in the condyles, and two compression devices each equipped with four mobile units. The patient starts walking with weight-bearing from the second day. The pins are removed after 2 months.

Case example (Fig. 19.28). A 65-year-old obese female patient presented with severe osteoarthritis of the lateral aspect of the knee and a 16° valgus deformity. The lateral joint space was narrowed and underlined by a dome-shaped sclerosis (Fig. 19.28a). A supracondylar osteotomy of the femur was carried out slightly over-correcting the deformity. At the 3-year follow-up the

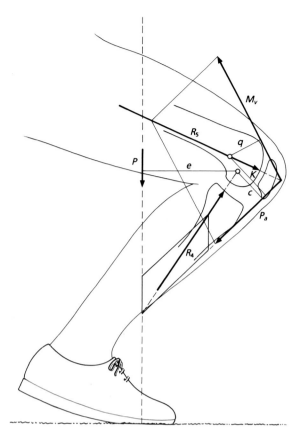

Fig. 19.29 Forces exerted on the knee joint as projected on a sagittal plane. P = force exerted by the mass of the body minus the lower leg and foot; e = lever arm of force P; P_a = force exerted by the patellar tendon; c = lever arm of force P_a acting on the femoro-tibial joint; R_4 = force transmitted across the femoro-tibial joint (= counterforce to the resultant of P and P_a); k = lever arm of force P_a acting on the patello-femoral joint; M_v = pull of the quadriceps tendon; q = lever arm of force M_v; R_5 = force transmitted across the patello-femoral joint (= counterforce to the resultant of M_v and P_a).

knee was pain-free with a full range of movement. The radiograph taken in the standing position showed a lateral joint space had developed and the subchondral scleroses beneath the plateaux were of even width throughout (Fig. 19.28b).

The clinical results and the radiological changes suggest a redistribution of the compressive stresses over the largest possible surfaces as long as the overcorrection is sufficient to replace the resultant force R to the centre of the knee. The subchondral scleroses tend to become symmetrical and the structure of the cancellous bone beneath both tibial plateaux becomes normal again. These changes for the best do not occur when the overcorrection is insufficient (Maquet *et al.*, 1982).

Arthroscopy shows the reappearance of cartilage in the areas where previously the bone was eburnated as a

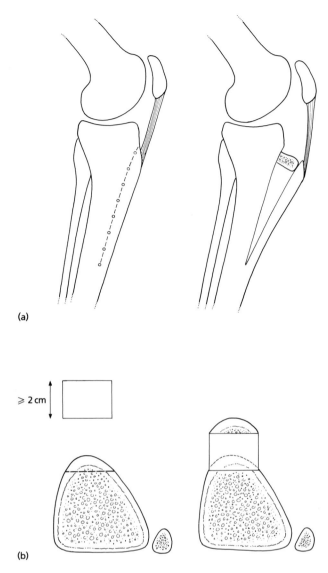

Fig. 19.30 Anterior displacement of the tibial tuberosity. (After Maquet, 1984.)

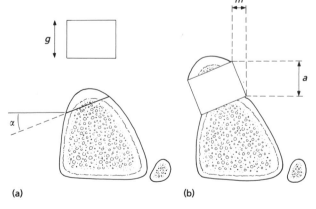

Fig. 19.31 (a) Anterior versus (b) anterior and medial displacement of the tibial tuberosity (cross-section). (After Maquet, 1984.)

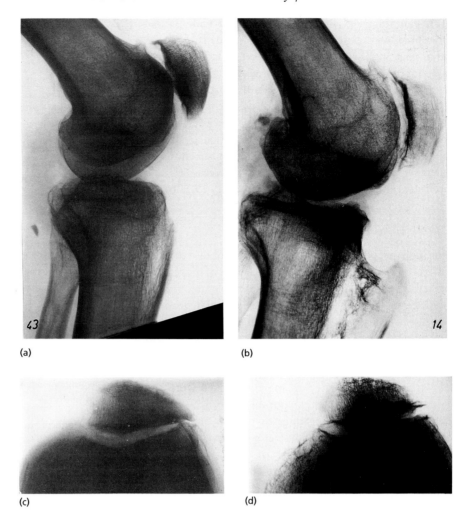

(a)

(b)

(c)

(d)

Fig. 19.32 Patello-femoral osteoarthritis in a 47-year-old male patient (a) before and (b) 14 years after an anterior and medial displacement of the tibial tuberosity. Skyline view (c) before and (d) 14 years after surgery.

result of overpressure. This is fibro-cartilage as demonstrated histologically (Fujisawa *et al.*, 1976). Such a regeneration is not observed when overcorrection has not been achieved.

Patello-femoral joint

The force R_5 pushing the patella against the femur results from the upwards and backwards pull of the quadriceps tendon M_v and the downwards and backwards pull of the patella tendon P_a (Fig. 19.29). The patella tendon P_a acts on the femoro-tibial joint with the lever arm c and on the patello-femoral joint with the lever arm k. Force R_5 normally is distributed over the medial and lateral facets of the patella proportionally to the articular surfaces of these facets so that the compressive stresses are evenly distributed throughout.

Displacing the tibial tuberosity forwards significantly (by at least 2 cm) at the top of a long shingle (so as not to lower the patella) decreases the resultant force R_5 by lengthening the lever arm c of the patella tendon and, above all, by opening the angle formed by the pull of the quadriceps tendon M_v and that of the patella tendon P_a.

The surgical procedure consists of separating the crest of the tibia with the tuberosity from the remainder of the bone. The tuberosity is maintained displaced forwards by inserting a bone graft behind the attachment of the patella tendon (Fig. 19.30). Again no tourniquet or immobilization is required. The patient walks with weight-bearing from the second day.

If the patella is subluxated laterally the bone is divided obliquely so as to displace the tuberosity medially as well as forwards (Fig. 19.31). Recentring the patella in the intercondylar groove enlarges the weight-bearing surface of the joint by involving again the medial facet in the transmission of the patello-femoral compressive force.

Case example (Fig. 19.32). A 43-year-old male patient presented with patello-femoral osteoarthritis. The patella was high riding and subluxated laterally. The subchondral sclerosis was increased considerably (Fig. 19.32a). The tibial tuberosity was displaced anteriorly and medially. At the 14-year follow-up the knee remained pain-free with a full range of movement and no limp. The radiograph showed the articular surface of the patella was underlined by a thin subchondral sclerosis demonstrating a significant decrease and an even distribution of the joint pressure (Fig. 19.32b).

CONCLUSION

Through properly planned osteotomies about the hip and the knee, there often exists a possibility of decreasing articular pressure sufficiently to make it tolerable for the tissues. This possibility of decreasing articular pressure depends on the geometry of the affected joint. Therefore, no standard method can be recommended. The surgical procedure must be customized for each individual instance, planned on paper pre-operatively, and carried out accurately. Subjected to manageable pressure the bone and cartilage react favourably: the exaggerated subchondral sclerosis regresses to normal and a joint space reappears which demonstrates the development of cartilage. These objective signs of decreased articular pressure appear after spectacular clinical improvement of the condition which is equivalent to healing. However, these clinical and radiological changes fail to materialize if articular pressure was not sufficiently decreased as a result of a wrong indication or poorly planned surgery.

REFERENCES

Fujisawa Y., Masuhara K., Matsumoto N., Mii N., Fujihara H., Yamaguchi T. and Shiomi N. (1976) The effect of high tibial osteotomy. An arthroscopic study of 26 knee joints. *Clin. Orthop. Surg.* (Jpn) 11, 576–590.

Goutalier D., Hernigou Ph., Medevielle D. and Debeyre J. (1987) Devenir à plus de dix ans de 93 ostéotomies tibiales effectuées pour gonarthrose interne sur genu-varum (ou l'influence prédominante de la correction angulaire frontale). *Rev. Chir. Orthop.* 72, 101–113.

Maquet P., Simonet J. and de Marchin P. (1967) Biomécanique du genou et gonarthrose. *Rev. Chir. Orthop.* 53, 11–138.

Maquet P., Watillon M., Burny F., Andrianne Y., Rasquin C. and Donkerwolcke M. (1982) Traitement conservateur de l'arthrose du genou. *Acta Orthop. Belg.* 48, 204–261.

Maquet P. (1984) *Biomechanics of the Knee with Application to the Pathogenesis and the Surgical Treatment of Osteoarthritis.* Berlin, Springer-Verlag.

Maquet P. (1985) *Biomechanics of the Hip as Applied to Osteo-Arthritis and Related Conditions.* Berlin, Springer-Verlag.

Maquet P. (1990) Importance de la position du grand trochanter. *Acta Orthop. Belg.* 56, 307–322.

Pauwels F. (1959) Directives nouvelles pour le traitement chirurgical de la coxarthrose. *Rev. Chir. Orthop.* 45, 681–702.

Pauwels F. (1973) *Atlas zur Biomechanik der gesunden und kranken Hüfte.* Berlin, Springer-Verlag.

Watillon M., Hoet F. and Maquet P. (1978) Les ostéotomies de Pauwels. Analyse de 804 cas d'ostéotomie. *Acta Orthop. Belg.* 44, 248–279.

FURTHER READING

Maquet P. (1963) Considérations biomécaniques sur l'arthrose du genou. Un traitement biomécanique de l'arthrose fémoro-patellaire. L'avancement du tendon rotulien. *Rev. Rhum. Mal. Osteo-artic.* 30, 779–783.

Maquet P. (1969) Biomechanics and osteoarthritis of the knee. SICOT 11e Congrèss Mexico. (1970) Conférences, symposiums et communications particulières publiés par. *J. Del chet.* Bruxelles, Imprimerie des sciences, 1970, pp. 317–357.

Maquet P. (1974a) Le sourcil cotyloïdien matérialisation du diagramme des contraintes dans l'articulation de la hanche. *Acta Orthop. Belg.* 40, 150–165.

Maquet P. (1974b) Coxarthrose protrusive. Etude biomécanique et traitement. *Acta Orthop. Belg.* 40, 166–171.

Maquet P. (1976a) Advancement of the tibial tuberosity. *Clin. Orthop.* 115, 225–230.

Maquet P. (1976b) Réduction de la pression articulaire de la hanche par latéralisation chirurgicale du grand trochanter. *Acta Orthop. Belg.* 42, 266–271.

Maquet P. (1978) La latéralisation chirurgicale du grand trochanter. *Acta Orthop. Belg.* 44, 192–196.

Marchin P. de, Maquet P. and Simonet J. (1963) Considérations biomécaniques sur l'arthrose du genou. Quelques remarques sur les radiographies. *Rev. Rhum. Mal. Osteo-artic.* 30, 775–776.

Merle d'Aubigné R. (1970) Cotation chiffrée de la fonction de la hanche. *Rev. Chir. Orthop.* 56, 481–486.

Müller W. (1929) *Biologie der Gelenke.* Leipzig, Barth, p. 113.

Pauwels F. (1935) Der Schenkelhalsbruch ein mechanisches Problem. *Z. Orthop. Chir.* 63 (Suppl).

Pauwels F. (1963) Importance of biomechanics in orthopedics. SICOT 9th Congress Vienna. Postgraduate course. Verlag der Medizinische Akademie. E 1–30.

Pauwels F. (1973) Kurzer Überblick über die mechanische Beanspruchung des Knochens und ihre Bedeutung für die funktionelle Anpassung. *Z. Orthop.* 111, 681–705.

Radin E., Maquet P. and Parker H. (1975) Rationale and indications of the 'hanging hip' procedure. *Clin. Orthop.* 112, 221–230.

Radin E. (1986) The Maquet procedure. Anterior displacement of the tibial tubercle. *Clin. Orthop.* 213, 241–248.

Voss C. (1956) Die temporäre Hangenhüfte. *Münch. Med. Wschr.* 98, 1.

Chapter 20
Joint Replacement

Chapter 20.1

Joint Reconstruction in the Hand and Wrist

A.B. Swanson & G. de Groot Swanson

INTRODUCTION

Restoration of pain-free function to unstable, stiff or dislocated joints continues to present a challenge to the reconstructive surgeon. The development of joint implants for the hand and wrist has furthered the possibilities for joint reconstruction and is one of the important breakthroughs in this field. When indicated, however, soft tissue reconstruction, simple resection arthroplasty and joint arthrodesis remain useful procedures in the vast armamentarium of surgical options.

IMPLANT RESECTION ARTHROPLASTY

Basic concepts

In 1962, an Orthopaedic Research Department was instituted at Blodgett Memorial Medical Center (Grand Rapids, Michigan) to develop implants for arthroplasty of the small joints of the extremities. The basic concept of implant resection arthroplasty was developed on the premises that a non-fixed, flexible, low-modulus implant could adapt to the biomechanical variances of loading forces to help distribute and decelerate the loads to the contiguous bone and therefore could be useful as an adjunct to resection arthroplasty procedures. The ideal design was developed after years of flex and load testing, and was named the 'distributing-load flexible hinge'.

The flexible hinge implant acts as a dynamic spacer to maintain internal alignment and spacing of the reconstructed joint and as an internal mold that supports the healing capsuloligamentous system around the implant while early motion is started. Joint stability is achieved through reconstruction of the ligamentous and musculotendinous systems. The implant becomes stabilized by the 'encapsulation process', and no permanent fixation is required. Controlled post-operative motion in a dynamic brace is important to guide the orientation of the healing capsular structures to obtain a functional balance of mobility and stability in the desired arc and alignment. The basic concept can be summarized as: 'bone resection + implant + encapsulation = functional joint'. The useful adaptability of the capsuloligamentous stabilization should further be emphasized. When increased mobility is desired, such as in the finger joint arthroplasty, early motion is started. When greater stability than mobility is desired, such as in the carpal bones, radiocarpal joint or first metacarpophalangeal joint reconstructions, the post-operative immobilization is carried out for longer.

Stability of a reconstructed joint cannot be dependent on any implant if it is to be tolerated on a long-term basis and must be achieved through reconstruction of the extrinsic capsular ligamentous and musculotendinous systems. The smooth flexible implant is completely included in the encapsulation process. Contrary to rigid implants, the flexible hinge and unfixed stems allow proper distribution of forces over a broader area and allow adjustments to the required axis of rotation with little resistance. The implant life is therefore increased and the bone is less likely to react at the implant interface when the forces are within its strain tolerance. Favourable bone remodelling around silicone flexible hinged implants has been noted as evidenced by maintenance of the shape of the cut end of the bone with metaphyseal cortical thickening and production of new bone around the intramedullary stems. Excessive bone resorption and 'pencilling' of the cut bone end as often seen after simple resection arthroplasty does not occur (Fig. 20.1.1).

GROMMET BONE LINERS

Flexible hinge silicone implant arthroplasty has received wide acceptance as the preferred method for reconstructive surgery of the finger joints. However, fracture

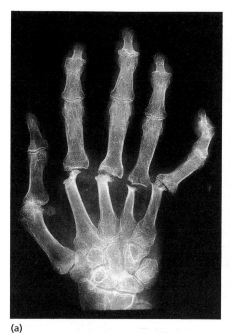

(a)

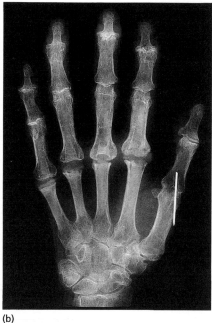

(b)

Fig. 20.1.1 Comparative radiographs of right and left hand of the same patient with rheumatoid arthritis 5 years after surgery. (a) Simple resection arthroplasty of metacarpophalangeal joints of index, middle, ring and little fingers was carried out on the right hand. Note marked remodelling of amputated metacarpal ends. (b) Flexible implant arthroplasty of four metacarpophalangeal joints and fusion of thumb metacarpophalangeal joint was carried out on the left hand. Note maintenance of squared-off appearance of bone ends and controlled bone remodelling around implant stems. Note fracture of implant on long finger; the patient presented no clinical changes. The contour of the bone ends has been maintained, as compared to progressive pencilling seen in the opposite hand, because the implant continues to maintain joint space and integrity of capsular structure and bone. (Reproduced with permission from Swanson and de Groot Swanson, 1982a.)

or cutting of the implant by sharp bone edges and implant abrasion can occur, particularly in patients with severe rheumatoid disease, recurrent synovitis, incomplete correction of deformities or abusive patterns of daily activity. A high performance (HP) silicone elastomer with improved resistance to tear propagation was developed in 1974. The fracture rate of HP silicone hinged implants was approximately 5% at the level of the fingers and wrist, and was reported to be as high as 25% by other clinics. To correct this problem, a research project was initiated in 1976 to develop bone liners (grommets) to shield the implant midsection. A laboratory study, *in vivo* animal trials and human clinical studies were carried out to evaluate ingrowth and press-fit fixation, semicircular and circumferential designs, and nine different materials (porous polyethylene, proplast, pyrolytic carbon, stainless steel, stainless steel mesh, ion-bombarded cobalt-chromium, smooth cobalt-chromium, titanium and glutaraldehyde-prepared bovine pericardium). The titanium press-fit circumferential design provided the best implant protection and bone response. Approximately 2000 circumferential titanium grommets have been used in the authors' clinic for the first metatarsophalangeal joint, since 1985, and the metacarpophalangeal joints since 1987; excellent implant protection and good bone tolerance have been obtained to date (Fig. 20.1.2).

PARTICULATE SYNOVITIS

In 1985, the authors reported that particulate synovitis and cystic bone changes can occur around abraded silicone implants due to the so-called 'frustrated macrophage', which, after ingesting particles, releases a variety of osteolytic enzymes. This phenomenon was seen particularly with carpal bone implants overloaded with excessive compressive and shear stresses, implant oversize or subluxation, carpal instability and excessive activity. These problems occurred more often with HP silicone elastomer implants (25%) than with the original silicone elastomer (3%). Particle related synovitis occurs less frequently with flexible hinged implants such as the finger, wrist and double-stemmed toe. The use of titanium grommets has decreased implant wear and further improved the durability of the latter procedures.

The synovitis and non-septic osteolysis associated with hip and knee total joint procedures are recognized as a particle problem and can occur around a number of implant materials including teflon, cobalt chrome, titanium (metal-to-metal), methylmethacrylate, carbon, and particularly polyethylene. It is felt that while HP silicone is more tear resistant, it is also more likely to generate wear particles from abrasion when used for spacer implants (carpal bones and single-stem toe), and that the reactions could be related to the physical size of particles, and not their chemical composition. In 1985, the authors resumed the use of carpal bone implants made of conventional silicone elastomer (CSE). In 1986,

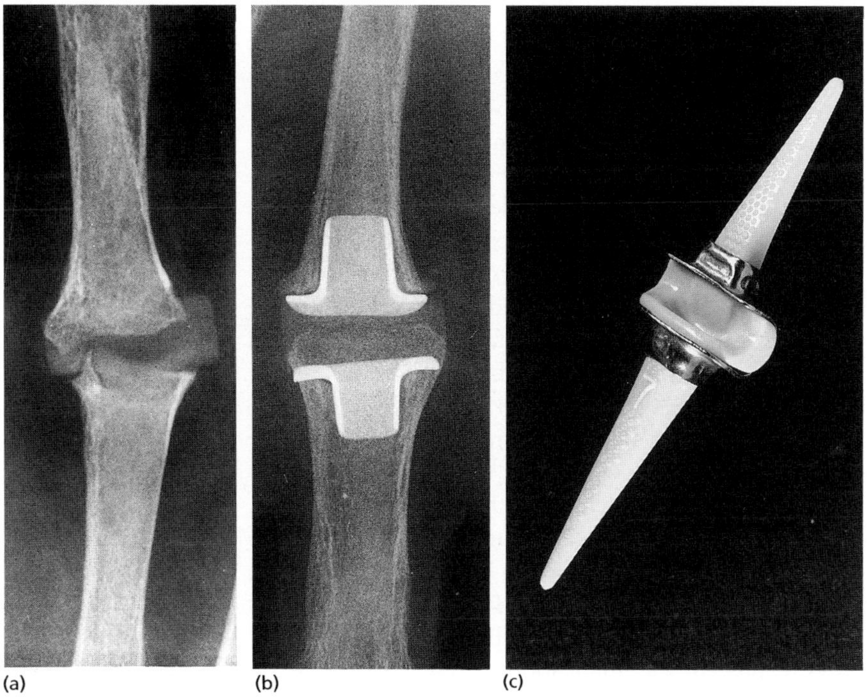

Fig. 20.1.2 (a) Radiograph of metacarpophalangeal joint arthroplasty showing cutting effect of sharp bone edge into the silicone implant. (b) Radiograph 24 months after metacarpophalangeal joint revision arthroplasty with proximal and distal half grommets (initial design). (Reproduced with permission from Swanson and de Groot Swanson, 1987a). (c) Titanium circumferential grommets (final design) protect bone/implant interface.

(a)　　　(b)　　　(c)

the authors also developed titanium spacer implants which have been used since that time with very promising results.

Although there have been a few reports in the literature suggesting a relationship between silicone implants and a broad spectrum of connective tissue diseases, systemic illness and autoimmune phenomena, the causal relationship has not been proven. It is known that patients with rheumatoid arthritis are at increased risk of developing lymphomas, leukaemia and myelomas possibly due to the immunological abnormality of rheumatoid arthritis. The participation of antigen-specific lymphocytes or antibodies in silicone particle-induced macrophage reactions has not been demonstrated in ongoing studies. Animal and human autopsy studies have shown that if migration of silicone particles occurs, it is limited to regional lymph nodes with no evidence of systemic dissemination.

The authors have undertaken an in-depth research study on the particle problem with the engineering and biology departments of a local university. They are using an *in vitro* model to try to duplicate the macrophage reaction in an effort to further understand and find solutions to the particle-induced reactions which can occur from metals, plastics or elastomers.

SALVAGEABILITY

Salvageability of an arthroplasty procedure implies preservation of bone and soft tissues so that a secondary procedure can be performed. The capsuloligamentous structures around any flexible implant can be reconstructed to improve the stability, alignment and durability of the arthroplasty, and revision procedures to further reinforce, release or realign the capsule and ligaments when necessary are easily performed. Because the implants are not firmly attached to bone, replacement is a relatively simple procedure. Furthermore, if a fracture of an implant develops or removal becomes necessary, a functioning resection arthroplasty remains. The bone stock removal is minimal, and bone absorption is rare so that an arthrodesis procedure with a bone graft can easily be accomplished. If synovitis is present, synovectomy and implant removal or replacement should be considered.

Surgical considerations and staging

If arthroplasty is to be considered, the patient must be cooperative and in good general condition. The skin and neurovascular status must be adequate, and the elements necessary to produce a functional musculotendinous system must be available, along with adequate bone stock to receive and support the implant. Adequate facilities must also be available for the operative and post-operative therapy.

Long-standing synovitis of the metacarpophalangeal joint may result in a 'cup-and-saucer' deformity. The base of the proximal phalanx widens and deepens centrally to receive the head of the metacarpal. If the joints have adequate motion and are pain-free, no further surgery is indicated. In patients with severe progressive rheumatoid arthritis (arthritis mutilans) who have inadequate bone stock to support the implant, a simple resection arthroplasty or arthrodesis with a bone graft is indicated. In the Tupper resection arthroplasty, the palmar plate is detached at its proximal origin, brought as a flap between the bone ends and sutured to the dorsal cortex of the resected metacarpal. The collateral ligaments can also be reattached.

Patients who are candidates for associated reconstructive procedures of weight-bearing joints of the lower extremity and who will require walking with crutches should have reconstruction of their upper extremities delayed. Excessive manual labour and awkward hand weight-bearing, such as seen in some crutch walkers, should be avoided after surgery. If crutch walking cannot be avoided, special platform-type crutches should be used to prevent the application of damaging forces to the newly reconstructed finger joints. Reconstruction of a foot and hand can be carried out at the same stage by two surgical teams.

In the presence of multiple joint involvement in the hand, knowledge of the pathogenesis of deformities is essential to recognize the cause of deformity and select the appropriate treatment method and staging. The metacarpophalangeal joint is the key joint for finger function. However, because of their interdependence, deformities of the proximal interphalangeal joints may compromise the results of metacarpophalangeal joint reconstruction. Collapse deformities of the wrist can affect the distal balance of the hand by interfering with the function of the extrinsic muscles of the fingers. In metacarpophalangeal joint disabilities associated with severe wrist involvement, the wrist should be treated first. In the rheumatoid hand, tendon repair and synovectomy of tendon sheaths must be done 6–8 weeks before arthroplasty of the metacarpophalangeal joints. However, if the extensor tendons are ruptured and the metacarpophalangeal joints are dislocated, arthroplasty of these joints is carried out before wrist and tendon reconstruction. If both the metacarpophalangeal and proximal interphalangeal joints are involved, the former joint is usually treated first. In swan-neck deformity, surgery of the metacarpophalangeal and proximal interphalangeal joints is performed at the same stage. In boutonnière deformity, the proximal interphalangeal joint is reconstructed first. Implant arthroplasty of both the metacarpophalangeal and proximal interphalangeal joints is not recommended.

Several different procedures are often performed on the same extremity during one surgical stage, depending on the tourniquet time available. An operation of an extremity should not exceed 2 hours of tourniquet time; a stellate ganglion block is recommended if the time should exceed 1–1½ hours. Pre-cooling of the arm with ice packs, as recommended by Tajima and our clinic, can safely prolong the tourniquet time to as long as 3 hours.

LOCAL HYPOTHERMIA BLANKET TECHNIQUE

The ice blanket is constructed of flannel cloth, adhesive straps, and reusable cold gel packs. The gel packs are inserted into separate pockets along the length of the blanket to provide limb cooling while avoiding direct

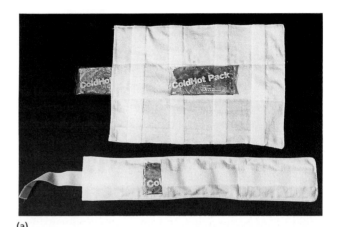

(a)

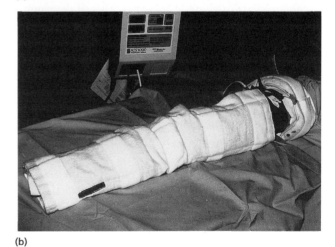

(b)

Fig. 20.1.3 Hypothermia blanket technique. (a) Long (six pockets) and short (three pockets) ice blankets are fitted with cold gel packs and frozen at −12°C. (b) Application of the short blanket above the tourniquet and of the long blanket proximally while anaesthesia is administered. (Reproduced with permission from Swanson *et al.*, 1991).

skin contact of the cold packs. The long blanket is fitted with six cold packs, and the short blanket with three packs (Fig. 20.1.3a). The blankets are cooled in the freezer section of a standard refrigerator at −12°C.

The long ice blanket is wrapped circumferentially around the upper extremity from the shoulder to the fingers to cool the arm for approximately 45 min before tourniquet inflation. When the patient is brought to the operating theatre, the ice blanket is briefly removed to apply the pneumatic tourniquet. The short ice blanket is then applied above the tourniquet and the long blanket is reapplied below while anaesthesia is being administered (Fig. 20.1.3b). The short blanket is left in place throughout surgery and the long blanket is removed to proceed with skin preparation and application of drapes. Following exsanguination with an Esmarch's bandage, the tourniquet is inflated to 70−100 mmHg above the patient's systolic blood pressure.

MEASURES TO PREVENT INFECTION

Implant arthroplasty procedures may be destroyed by infection. Prevention of contamination of an open wound by virulent organisms and the degree of tolerance of the host and tissues to their presence are important factors. The tissues must be handled with an atraumatic technique and kept moist with saline irrigations throughout the procedure to maintain their viability. Postoperative haematomas and dead spaces must be avoided.

The procedures are carried out under strict sterile conditions in an operating room equipped with a laminar air-flow. The patient is given 1 g of Ancef (cefazolin sodium) intravenously pre-operatively and then 1 g intravenously every 8 hours for 24 hours. If the patient is allergic to penicillin, the above is substituted with 600 mg of Cleocin (clindamycin phosphate).

THE HAND

Finger joint distributing-load flexible hinge

This is a one-piece intramedullary stemmed implant made of high-performance silicone elastomer (Wright Medical Technology Inc., Arlington, Tennessee). This material has a 400% greater tear propagation resistance than any previous material. The finger joint flexible hinge has been mechanically tested to up to 600 million flexion repetitions to 90° without showing evidence of material failure. It is available in 11 anatomical sizes (00−9) and can be used as an adjunct to resection arthroplasty of the metacarpophalangeal, proximal and distal interphalangeal joints.

Metacarpophalangeal joint of the fingers

IMPLANT ARTHROPLASTY

Indications

The indications for implant arthroplasty of this joint are painful rheumatoid or post-traumatic disabilities:
1 fixed or stiff metacarpophalangeal joints;
2 radiographic evidence of joint destruction or subluxation;
3 ulnar drift, not correctable by surgery of soft tissues alone;
4 contracted intrinsic and extrinsic musculature and ligament system; and
5 associated stiff interphalangeal joints.

Operative technique (Fig. 20.1.4)

A dorsal transverse skin incision is made over the necks of the metacarpals. The dissection is carried down to expose the extensor tendons. The dorsal veins that lie between the metacarpal heads are carefully released by blunt longitudinal dissection and are retracted laterally. The extensor hood is exposed to the base of the proximal phalanx. Its radial portion is usually stretched out and the extensor tendon dislocated ulnarward. A longitudinal incision is made in the extensor hood fibres parallel to the extensor tendon on its ulnar aspect. In the index and little fingers, the approach is made between the extensor communis and proprius tendons. The hood fibres and capsule are dissected from the underlying synovium and retracted to the radial side to expose the joint. A comprehensive soft tissue release is performed to allow the base of the proximal phalanx to be displaced above the metacarpal. The ulnar collateral ligament is released from its phalangeal insertion in all fingers. In the index finger the latter structure is included in the capsuloligamentous reconstruction. The radial collateral ligament insertions are preserved whenever possible; in the index finger and occasionally in the middle finger this ligament is reattached to the base of the proximal phalanx and/or the metacarpal as described later. The soft tissue release around the head of the metacarpal and base of the proximal phalanx allows exposure of the bone ends.

The neck of the metacarpal is exposed and transected with an air drill or motor saw leaving part of the metaphyseal flare. Care should be taken to avoid splintering the bone. The head of the metacarpal is removed with the hypertrophied synovium. A rongeur is useful to complete the synovectomy. If the joint is severely

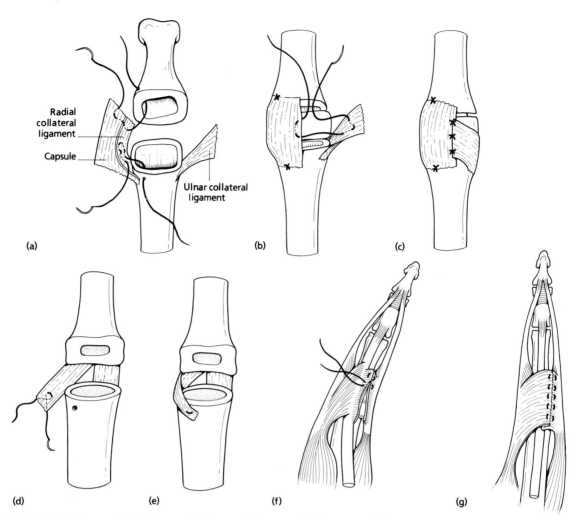

Radial
collateral
ligament

Capsule

Ulnar collateral
ligament

(a)   (b)   (c)

(d)   (e)   (f)   (g)

Fig. 20.1.4 (a) In index and middle fingers, the intramedullary canal of the proximal phalanx is reamed in a rectangular shape placed high on the dorsal ulnar side and low on the palmar radial side. Radial collateral ligament and related structures are sutured through the drill hole made in the dorsoradial aspect of the metacarpal. Distal reattachment to the proximal phalanx may also be needed. Sutures are placed before grommets and implant insertion. (b, c) Ulnar collateral ligament sutured to ulnar edge of capsule (a, b, c redrawn with permission from Swanson and de Groot Swanson, 1989). (d, e) Reconstruction of inadequate radial collateral ligament with a distally based flap made of the radial half of the palmar plate. Remaining radial collateral ligament and capsule are incorporated in the repair. The flap is sutured to the dorsoradial aspect of the cut end of the metacarpal (d, e redrawn with permission from Swanson, 1973a). (f) Closure of extensor hood with inverted knots. (g) Reefing of extensor hood to centralize extensor tendon.

subluxed, the metacarpal head is removed before soft tissue release.

The cartilage at the base of the proximal phalanx of the digits is resected, including marginal osteophytes or severe deformities. More bone may be removed to increase the joint space. All cartilage is removed because progressive cartilage degeneration could result in recurrent synovitis.

After the bone ends are resected, the palmar plate is released off the base of the phalanx and often completely resected in all but the index finger where it can be incorporated in the radial collateral ligament repair as described later.

The ulnar intrinsic tendon is pulled up into the wound with a blunt hook and sectioned at the myotendinous junction if contracted. However, in the index finger, this tendon normally applies a supinatory force and must always be preserved to avoid a pronation tendency.

Rheumatoid patients often have an inadequate first dorsal interosseous muscle or have a tendency for pronation deformity of the index finger and occasionally the middle finger. Reconstruction of the radial collateral ligament is important to correct the lateral and rotatory alignment, and to improve lateral stability for pinch. At this stage, the distally divided ulnar collateral ligament of the index finger is dissected proximally, taking care to maintain its attachment on the metacarpal.

This proximally based ulnar collateral ligament flap will be used for the capsuloligamentous reconstruction (Fig. 20.1.4a, b, c). The radial collateral ligament is sectioned off the base of the proximal phalanx and dissected *en bloc* with the overlaying capsule to prepare a proximally attached flap. At closure, these structures are sutured to the radio-dorsal aspect of the proximal phalanx. A similar procedure is occasionally performed for the middle finger. If the radial collateral ligament is inadequate, the proximally divided radial half of the palmar plate is dissected to its attachment on the phalanx to prepare a distally based flap that will be incorporated in the radial collateral ligament repair (Fig. 20.1.4d, e).

In all fingers, the flexor sheath is incised longitudinally in its dorsal aspect and the flexor tendons are pulled up with a blunt hook; a partial synovectomy and tendon sheath release are performed as needed. After skin closure, the joints and tendon sheaths are injected with Thiotepa and Decadron.

The abductor digit minimi musculotendinous unit is exposed on the ulnar aspect of the fifth metacarpophalangeal joint, pulled up with a blunt hook, and sectioned, avoiding the ulnar digital nerve. Preferably, the cut end of the abductor digiti minimi is attached to the flexor digiti minimi tendon immediately underneath it. This provides important flexor power to the fifth metacarpophalangeal joint.

The metacarpal intramedullary canal is prepared in a rectangular fashion with a broach-and-air drill with a leader point bur to prevent perforation through the cortex. Too much reaming of the canals should be avoided. The medullary canal of the fourth metacarpal is often narrow and must be carefully reamed.

Test implants are used to select the correct size implant. The stem should fit well into the canal and the mid-section should abut against the bone end. The ends of the stems should not abut the end of the reamed medullary canals and are shortened as needed. On rare occasions, if the cut of the stem is too wide to glide into the distal end of the reamed canal, the canal may be further reamed distally or a smaller implant used. The largest implant possible should be used (usually sizes 4−8). When using grommets, the implant size is usually smaller than the size used without grommets.

The medullary canal of the proximal phalanx is similarly reamed. The bone must not be splintered, and sharp points or rough surfaces should be smoothed. Proper fit of the implant is verified; with the joint in extension, there should be no impingement of its mid-section. If there is, soft tissue release or bone resection has not been adequate. In the index finger, the intra-

medullary canal of the proximal phalanx is reamed in a proper rectangular and axial configuration to stabilize the grommet and implant stems and help maintain slight supination (Fig. 20.1.4a). The rectangular shape is oriented high on the ulnodorsal side and low on the radiopalmar side. In contrast, in the little finger, a position of slight pronation is desired, and the medullary rectangle is positioned high on the radiodorsal side and low on the ulnopalmar side.

The circumferential grommet is a press-fit bone liner contoured to fit the shape of the implant mid-section and stems (Fig. 20.1.2). No special bone preparation is required. The grommets are centred in the intramedullary canals and the shoulders should fit the bone ends without protruding laterally. The grommets are pushed in place with a flat instrument without distorting them. If the grommet does not fit easily, further reaming is required. The grommet sizes correspond to the implant sizes. A grommet size smaller than the implant is never used. With the sizer implant and grommets in place, the mobility of the joint is tested. Grommets or bone ends should not impinge on the implant mid-section. Sufficient bone stock must be present to support the grommet which must be fitted into metaphyseal bone. In certain cases of severe metacarpophalangeal joint dislocation, when more bone must be removed to bring the finger into extension, the implant should be used without grommets. Often grommets are not used in the fifth metacarpophalangeal joint because of poor bone stock and soft tissue coverage. Grommets should not be used in arthritis mutilans. When grommets are not used, the cut-end of the bones are carefully smoothed with a diamond bur.

Sutures for reattachment of the ligaments and capsule are placed before insertion of grommets and implant. The radial collateral ligament of the index finger (occasionally the middle finger) is advanced dorsally and sutured to the base of the proximal phalanx with a 2−0 Dacron suture passed through a 1 mm drill hole made on the radiodorsal aspect of the cut end of the phalanx (Figs 20.1.4a, b, c). The overlaying radial capsule is included in this repair. Proximal reattachment to the metacarpal may also be needed; a 3−0 Dacron suture is used at this level. If the radial collateral ligament is inadequate, a distally based flap made of the radial half of the palmar plate is incorporated in the repair and similarly sutured to the radiodorsal aspect of the cut end of the metacarpal along with the residual collateral ligament and capsule (Fig. 20.1.4d, e). The first dorsal interosseous muscle fibres become dorsally advanced with this repair. Although the procedure seems to slightly limit flexion of the metacarpophalangeal joint, it is important to correct pronation deformities and to increase lateral and vertical stability for pinch.

The wound is thoroughly irrigated with a triple antibiotic solution containing neomycin, polymyxin and bacitracin. The implant is first inserted in the medullary canal of the metacarpal and then into the proximal phalanx using blunt instruments and a 'no-touch' technique. With the implant and grommets in place, the sutures for the radial collateral reconstruction are securely tied with inverted knots as the finger is held in slight supination and abduction; proper tension of the radial collateral ligament and capsule is obtained. The distally released ulnar collateral ligament and capsule are sutured to the ulnar edge of the radial collateral ligament and capsule with the same sutures (Fig. 20.1.4b, c).

The extensor hood is closed with 3 to 5 4−0 Dexon sutures inverting the knots (Fig. 20.1.4f, g). The stretched out radial portion of the extensor hood is reefed in overlapping fashion to centralize the extensor tendon over the joint, using one or two 3−0 Dacron sutures, and 4−0 Dexon sutures inverting the knots. In the index and middle fingers it is important not to overcorrect the extensor tendon radially to avoid a pronation tendency. In cases of severe or long-standing flexion deformity, the extensor tendon should also be reefed longitudinally to correct any residual extensor tendon lag. Exceptionally, an extensor tendon tenodesis to the base of the proximal phalanx is indicated; the suture is passed through a small-drill hole made in the bone. The juncturae tendinae which have been divided during extensor tendon release are reapproximated with 4−0 Dexon sutures. Perfect balance of the extensor mechanism is essential.

The skin incision is closed with interrupted 5−0 nylon sutures; four small drains made from strips of silicone elastomer sheeting are inserted into the wound under the skin. Betadine gauze or non-adherent dressing such as rayon is applied over the wound. A voluminous hand-conforming dressing is applied, avoiding pressure on the radial side of the index. A narrow plaster splint is included on the palmar aspect. Dacron batting is placed transversely across the palm and longitudinally over the dorsal and palmar aspects of the forearm, wrist, hand and fingers. Sheet wadding or Webril is then applied circumferentially. A narrow plaster or wooden splint is applied to the palmar aspect. Sheet wadding is passed longitudinally between the fingers to maintain their radial position. The entire dressing is finally wrapped with a conforming non-constrictive bandage, such as Kling.

Post-operative care and bracing

Immediate and continuous elevation of the hand and the forearm during the post-operative course is very important. On the first post-operative day the drains are usually removed and a high profile dynamic brace (Cygnus Systems, Grand Rapids, Michigan) is applied unless there is unusual swelling. The rubber band slings are placed on the proximal phalanges to guide the alignment of the digits into a slight radial direction to prevent recurrent ulnar drift (Fig. 20.1.5). The tension of the rubber bands should be tight enough to support the digits and yet loose enough to allow 70° of active flexion: this is particularly true of the little finger, which may have weak flexion power. The authors prefer to limit flexion of the index and middle fingers to 45−60° because less motion enhances the stability. The thumb outrigger is usually applied because of the tendency for the patient to bring the thumb over the fingers on flexion and thus aggravate the tendency towards ulnar drift. If there is a tendency towards pronation of the metacarpophalangeal joint of the index finger, additional outrigger bars are applied to provide a supinatory force to the joint. The extension portion of the brace is worn day and night for the first 3 weeks, alternating with specific flexion exercises started the day after surgery. Starting on the second week, if there is flexor weakness

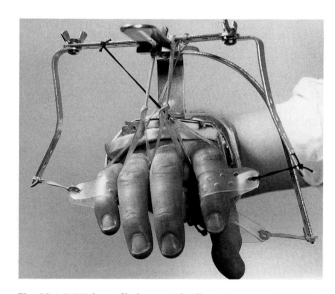

Fig. 20.1.5 High profile brace with all outriggers attached. The finger slings maintain radial correction of the fingers. A string is used for the index finger for 2−3 weeks to favour joint stability over mobility. An additional sling is placed on the middle phalanx of the index and little fingers to create a rotatory torque in favour of supination for the index and pronation for the little finger. (Reproduced with permission from Swanson *et al.*, 1990.)

and good extension, the extensor sling can be removed for 1–2 hours a day to achieve greater active flexion of the metacarpophalangeal joints. In patients who have normal proximal interphalangeal joints, small padded aluminium splints are taped on the dorsum of these joints to help localize all flexion force at the metacarpophalangeal joint. At 3 weeks, a flexion outrigger may be worn for 30 min three times a day to flex the metacarpophalangeal joints passively. Other traction devices designed to improve flexion in the presence of adequate extension include flexor slings applied to the proximal phalanges, or rubber bands attached from glued-on nail hooks, pulling to a special wrist strap. The extension portion of the brace is usually worn at night only, starting on the fourth post-operative week for another 3 weeks or longer if needed.

It is advisable for the patient to use the hand protectively during the early post-operative phase. The post-operative rehabilitation programme must be continued for at least 3 months after surgery because of the tendency of these joints to tighten up. It is best to gradually, rather than abruptly, discontinue the exercises and wise to follow a weekly self-evaluation of the range of motion. Following this, the patient can safely use his or her hand for activities of daily living and vocational skills. However, the patient should continue to exercise and splint as necessary for up to 1 year after surgery. Further reading on this important rehabilitation programme is strongly suggested.

A very cooperative patient following a good rehabilitation programme can obtain an excellent range of motion following the implant resection arthroplasty method (Fig. 20.1.6).

Metacarpophalangeal joint of the thumb

IMPLANT ARTHROPLASTY

Indications

The indications for implant arthroplasty of the metacarpophalangeal joint of the thumb are painful rheumatoid, degenerative and post-traumatic disabilities with severe destruction of the joint and: (i) associated stiffness of distal joint or basal joints, and (ii) boutonnière deformity when the metacarpophalangeal joint is destroyed and the distal joint needs fusion. This procedure has provided adequate stability and the increased flexion has been important, particularly for fine coordinated movements.

Operative technique

The metacarpophalangeal joint is exposed through a dorsal, gently curved skin incision. The extensor hood is incised parallel to the extensor pollicis longus on the radial side. Dissection is carried between the extensor pollicis longus and brevis tendons preserving the attachment of the extensor pollicis brevis to the proximal phalanx. The joint capsule is incised transversely. Prep-

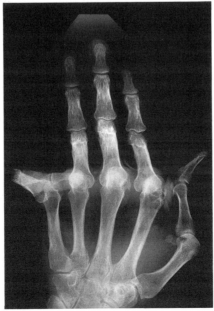 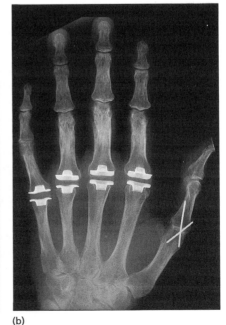

Fig. 20.1.6 (a) Pre- and (b) post-operative radiograms showing circular grommets as an adjunct to flexible implant resection arthroplasty of metacarpophalangeal joints with severe rheumatoid involvement. The thumb metacarpophalangeal joint was fused. (a)　　　　(b)

aration of the bone to receive the implants and grommets is similar to that described for the metacarpophalangeal joints of the fingers (p. 613). The collateral ligaments are left intact whenever possible; if released, they are reattached to bone as described for the proximal interphalangeal joint (Fig. 20.1.9d, e). Implant size 3–6 are usually used. The palmar plate is seldom released. Before insertion of grommets and implant, a 3–0 Dacron suture is passed through a small drill hole made in the base of the proximal phalanx to centralize the extensor pollicis brevis over the joint (Fig. 18.1.11, p. 553). The extensor pollicis longus is advanced distally and tenodesed to the base of the proximal phalanx with the same suture. The extensor hood is sutured, and imbricated over both tendons using inverted knots. If the extensor pollicis brevis tendon is released, it is later reinserted to a bony concavity made in the base of the proximal phalanx by passing 3–0 Dacron sutures through small drill holes made in the bone.

Post-operative care

A conforming dressing is applied for 3–5 days. The thumb metacarpophalangeal joint is maintained in 0° of extension for 3–4 weeks with a taped-on padded aluminium splint. No special exercises are prescribed after splint removal except for normal functional adaptations. Forceful activities should be avoided for 6–8 weeks.

ALTERNATIVE PROCEDURES FOR THE
METACARPOPHALANGEAL JOINT OF THE THUMB

Mild-to-moderate boutonnière deformity of less than 10° of fixed flexion contracture of the metacarpophalangeal joint can be treated by preserving the joint surfaces and using the same tendon reconstruction technique as for the implant arthroplasty. The joint is fixed in 0° of extension with a Kirschner wire for a period of 4 weeks. If the distal joint is destroyed implant arthroplasty or fusion is indicated. If the distal joint is adequate but presents a hyperextension deformity the extensor pollicis longus tendon is lengthened or simply transected distally to decrease the extensor power at the distal joint. The distal joint is then pinned in 10° of flexion with a small Kirschner wire for 4–6 weeks.

Treatments for hyperextension deformities of the metacarpophalangeal joint of the thumb are described on p. 000.

A fusion of the metacarpophalangeal joint of the thumb is indicated in cases of severe joint destruction by rheumatoid arthritis and to simplify the articular chain

in severe collapse deformities provided there is adequate mobility at the distal and basal joints.

Interphalangeal joint of the thumb

Arthrodesis is usually the preferred treatment for instability of the interphalangeal joint of the thumb; bone grafting is necessary if bone resorption is severe.

In a small number of cases presenting adequate bone stock and ligamentous stability, implant resection arthroplasty of the interphalangeal joint has been performed using a single-stemmed or a small flexible hinge silicone implant as an articular spacer to preserve some pain-free motion; this can be important in certain prehensile activities, particularly when other joints are disabled.

A flexible hyperextension deformity of the distal interphalangeal joint with good lateral stability and intact articular surfaces can be corrected with a flexor tendon hemitenodesis to prevent hyperextension while allowing some flexion (Fig. 20.1.7).

Proximal interphalangeal joint

Treatment of the proximal interphalangeal joint varies with the type and severity of deformity presented and associated deformities of contiguous joints as listed in Table 20.1.1. The joint can be stiff with or without lateral deviation, or there can be either a swan-neck or a boutonnière deformity.

Patients with a mild or moderate boutonnière or swan-neck deformity and no radiographic evidence of joint destruction may be candidates for soft tissue reconstructive procedures providing there is only a

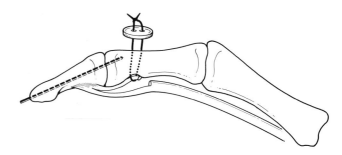

Fig. 20.1.7 Flexor hemitenodesis of the thumb interphalangeal joint. The distally based flexor pollicis longus slip is drawn into the concavity made on the palmar aspect of the neck of the proximal phalanx with wire to obtain 10–15° flexion of the interphalangeal joint. The wire was removed at 3 weeks. Kirschner wire fixation of the distal joint was maintained for 6 weeks. (Redrawn with permission from Swanson and de Groot Swanson, 1975.)

Table 20.1.1 Treatment of interphalangeal joint disabilities with or without involvement of the metacarpophalangeal joints

SWAN-NECK DEFORMITY OF PIP JOINT

Without involvement of MP joint

Initial deformity of PIP joint
  Local injections (corticosteroids or other agents)
  Flexor tendon synovectomy with or without tenodesis of flexor
    digitorum superficialis tendon
  Intrinsic tendon release with or without flexor tendon
    synovectomy

Flexible deformity of PIP joint
  Dermadesis at PIP joint
  Relocation of lateral tendons with or without elongation of
    central tendon
  Tenodesis of flexor digitorum superficialis tendon with flexor
    synovectomy

Rigid, subluxated or dislocated PIP joint
  Resection of joint with relocation of lateral tendons and
    implant arthroplasty (rarely)
  Resection of joint and fusion

Treatment for DIP joint when required in any of these conditions
  Temporary pinning in neutral position if passively correctable
  Fusion if severely damaged or flexed

With involvement of MP joint

Flexible deformity of PIP joint

Treatment of MP joint	*Treatment of PIP joint*
Synovectomy with proximal release of intrinsic tendons	Manipulation with temporary Kirschner wire fixation in flexion if required
Relocation of subluxated joint, with proximal release of intrinsic tendons	Manipulation with temporary Kirschner wire fixation in flexion if required, *or* dermadesis
Joint resection with proximal release of intrinsic tendons, and implant arthroplasty	Manipulation to 50° flexion with temporary Kirschner wire fixation, *or* relocation of lateral with or without elongation of the central tendon

Rigid, subluxated or dislocated PIP joint:

Treatment of MP joint	*Treatment of PIP joint*
Joint resection with implant arthroplasty	Relocation of lateral tendons with elongation of central tendon
	Joint resection with fusion

Treatment of DIP joint if required in any of the above conditions:
  Temporary pinning in neutral position if passively
    correctable
  Fusion if flexion deformity is severe or articular damage
    exists

BOUTONNIÈRE DEFORMITY OF PIP JOINT

Initial deformity of PIP joint
  Local injections (corticosteroids or other agents) or splinting
  Synovectomy

Flexible deformity of PIP joint
  With or without synovectomy
  Reconstruction of central tendon
  Elongation of lateral tendons
  Combination of above two procedures

Rigid deformity of PIP joint
  Without bone erosion
  Joint release with reconstruction of central tendon and
    elongation of lateral tendons
  Joint resection with reconstruction of tendons with implant
    arthroplasty (rarely)
  Distal release of lateral tendons
  With bone erosions
  Joint resection with reconstruction of central tendon and lateral
    tendons, with implant arthroplasty (rarely)
  Joint resection and fusion

Subluxated or dislocated PIP joint
  Joint resection with reconstruction of central tendon and lateral
    tendons, with implant arthroplasty (rarely)
  Joint resection and fusion

Treatment of DIP joint if required in any of these conditions
  Distal release of lateral tendons
  Fusion

STIFF OSTEOARTHRITIC PIP JOINT

Non-dislocated PIP Joint
  Joint resection with implant arthroplasty

Subluxated or dislocated PIP joint
  Joint resection with implant arthroplasty
  Joint resection with fusion

Treatment for DIP joint if required in either of these conditions
  Fusion if needed

Source: Swanson, 1973.
MP, metacarpophalangeal; PIP, proximal interphalangeal; DIP, distal interphalangeal.

minimal joint contracture. Adjustment of the tension of the central and lateral tendons is essential to correct deformities. Joint fusion is indicated in the presence of subluxation, severe contracture or erosive disease, and inadequate radial collateral ligament. Implant arthroplasty of the proximal interphalangeal joint is

rarely done in swan-neck deformity and only occasionally used for isolated boutonnière deformity.

SWAN-NECK DEFORMITY

In swan-neck deformity, flexor synovitis is treated first.

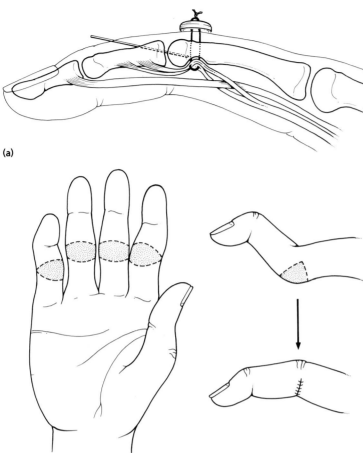

(a)

(b)

Fig. 20.1.8 (a) Tenodesis of flexor digitorum sublimis (FDS). The FDS tendon is drawn into the concavity made on the palmar aspect of the neck of the proximal-phalanx just distal to the bifurcation of the FDS tendon with the wire suture exiting over a button. The tension has been adjusted to allow 20–30° extension lag of the proximal interphalangeal joint. Kirschner wire fixation for 6–8 weeks. Wire suture removed in 4–5 weeks. (b) Dermadesis: elliptical wedge of skin sufficient to create 20° flexion contracture is excised from the flexor aspect of the proximal interphalangeal joint preserving underlying vessels and nerves. Kirschner wire fixation for 3 weeks. Splinting in flexion for 6 weeks. (Redrawn with permission from Swanson, 1973a.)

If the joint surfaces are preserved, adequate release of the dorsal capsule, collateral ligaments and palmar plate, relocation of the lateral bands palmarly, and procedures to check the hyperextension deformity are indicated. In moderate swan-neck deformity, Zancolli's and Littler's checkrein procedures are useful. In flexible hyperextension deformity of the proximal interphalangeal joint without involvement of the metacarpophalangeal joint, tenodesis of the flexor digitorum sublimis can be performed at the same time as a flexor synovectomy (Fig. 20.1.8a). In mild flexible deformity in weak hands, dermadesis is indicated (Fig. 20.1.8b). The joint is immobilized in 20° of flexion with a taped-on aluminium splint for 10 days, followed by active flexion exercises. Hyperextension of the joint must be avoided in the first 3–6 weeks to favour a flexion contracture. In combined involvement of the metacarpophalangeal and proximal interphalangeal joints, both joints are repaired at the same surgical stage. In severe swan-neck deformity the joint is fused. Flexion deformities of the distal interphalangeal must be corrected at the same time to obtain proper balance of the digit (Table 20.1.1).

BOUTONNIÈRE DEFORMITY

In combined involvement of the metacarpophalageal and proximal interphalangeal joints, the boutonnière deformity is repaired first. If the joint surfaces are preserved and contracture is minimal, joint release, synovectomy, reconstruction of the central tendon and dorsal relocation of the lateral bands are indicated. Repair of the extensor mechanism and collateral ligament system is similar to that described for implant arthroplasty of the proximal interphalangeal joint. The proximal interphalangeal joint is splinted in extension for 3–6 weeks. The distal joint should be allowed to flex freely. Active flexion–extension exercises are started 10–14 days after surgery, alternating with an extension splint worn at night for about 10 weeks, or until the joint is stable. If the distal joint cannot be flexed passively, the lateral tendons are released proximal to the insertion of Landsmeer's ligament. Joint fusion is preferred in rheumatoid arthritis.

IMPLANT ARTHROPLASTY

Indications

This procedure is indicated for painful, degenerative, or post-traumatic deformities with destruction or sub-luxation of the proximal interphalangeal joint and stiffness that cannot be corrected with soft tissue reconstruction alone. The presence of adequate bone, soft tissue and muscle/tendon balance are essential pre-requisites. An intact flexor tendon mechanism is essential for active flexion of the joint. Because these patients often present adhesions between the flexor digitorum superficialis and profundus tendons, the flexor mechanism should be inspected and released as needed through a separate transverse palmar incision.

An implant arthroplasty of the proximal inter-phalangeal joint is preferred for an isolated disability. For disabilities of both the index and middle fingers in a working man, fusion of the proximal interphalangeal joint of the index finger in 20–40° of flexion and implant arthroplasty of the proximal interphalangeal joint of the middle finger is preferred. Flexion of the proximal interphalangeal joints of the ring and little fingers is very important for grasping small objects and function should be restored if possible. Implant arthro-plasty of contiguous joints (e.g. MP and PIP) is not recommended and implant arthroplasty of the proximal interphalangeal joint is very rarely indicated in rheuma-toid deformities.

Operative technique (Fig. 20.1.9): *Stiff PIP joint without collapse deformity*

A gentle 'C'-shaped incision is made over the dorsum of the joint so that the skin suture line does not lie directly over the tendon repair (Fig. 20.1.9a). In the little and index fingers, the incision is placed away from the presenting surface. The dorsal veins are respected. If associated flexor tendon surgery is also indicated, a midlateral incision or palmar incision is used. A 'central tendon sparing' technique is used. The exposure is made between the lateral band and central tendon on both sides of the joint (Fig. 20.1.9b). The collateral ligaments and palmar plate are released only proximally to dis-locate the joint laterally for exposure (Fig. 20.1.9c). In severe involvement of both sides of the joint, which would interfere with reconstruction of the radial col-lateral ligament, arthrodesis should be considered because stability of the radial collateral ligament is essential to resist the ulnar deviating forces applied during prehension.

The head of the proximal phalanx is resected at the metaphyseal flare and the intramedullary canal is pre-pared as described for the metacarpophalangeal joint. Using the sizing set, the largest acceptable implant is selected (sizes 0–3, and most often size 1). The mid-section of the implant should seat well against the smoothed bone ends, and with the joint in extension there must be no impingement. Additional bone resection and/or soft tissue release are performed as needed. Grommets are not used at the level of the proximal interphalangeal joint.

Sutures (4–0 Dacron) are placed in 0.5 mm drill holes made in the proximal phalanx for reconstruction of the collateral ligament system (Fig. 20.1.9c). If the distal attachment of the radial collateral ligament appears weakened, it can be reinforced with a suture passed through a drill hole made in the base of the middle phalanx. The implant is then inserted in a similar fashion to that described for the metacarpophalangeal joint. The ligaments are firmly reattached to the proximal phalanx with proper tension to obtain good lateral stability and alignment and to allow passive motion from full extension to 70° of flexion. The lateral bands are then sutured back to the central band with inverted knots (Fig. 20.1.9e).

The skin incision is sutured and drained. The operative dressing must protect the integrity of the radial collateral ligament and prevent ulnar deviation. Following recon-struction of the index proximal interphalangeal joint, a small splint is placed on the radial side of the finger.

Post-operative care

Guarded active flexion/extension exercises are started the day after surgery because the central tendon attach-ment has not been disturbed. It is important to protect the repaired collateral ligaments from lateral deviating forces for 6 weeks. In the index finger, this is achieved with a small dynamic splint placed on the radial side of the finger (Fig. 20.1.10a). Buddy splinting to an intact radial digit (e.g. ring to middle finger) is useful for the lateral digits (Fig. 20.1.10b). During the flexion exer-cises, the movement must be localized at the proximal interphalangeal joint with a number of devices (e.g. Finger Crutch: AliMed, Dedham, Mass.) that support the metacarpophalangeal joint in extension (Fig. 20.1.10c). Grasping devices (e.g. Grip-X: AliMed) are used for isometric exercises to increase flexor muscle strength while maintaining finger alignment. Following this procedure, the expected motion ranges from −10° to 0° and 30° to 70° flexion (Fig. 20.1.11). Extension lag can be treated with night-time extension splinting. If

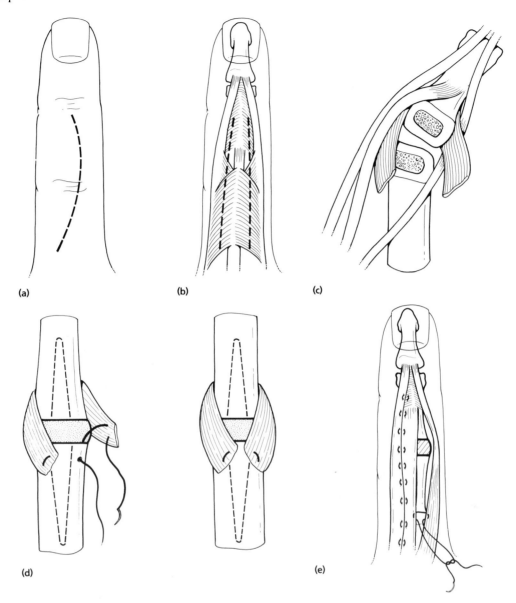

(a)   (b)   (c)

(d)   (e)

Fig. 20.1.9 Proximal interphalangeal joint implant arthroplasty. (a) Skin incision. (b) Exposure made between lateral band and central tendon on both sides of joint. (c) Collateral ligaments and palmar plate released proximally to dislocate joint laterally for exposure. (d) Sutures passed through drill holes in proximal phalanx for reattachment of collateral ligaments. (e) Lateral bands sutured to central tendon.

necessary, after 3 weeks, passive motion may be indicated and is achieved with manual passive exercises or flexion devices that are applied as the palmar surface of the proximal phalanx is supported to prevent meta-carpophalangeal joint flexion. Rubber-band traction can be attached from a sling placed on the middle phalanx or from finger nail hooks to the palmar attachment of the brace or a Velcro wrist strap. It may be indicated to splint the distal interphalangeal joint in extension during the flexion exercises to further concentrate the motion at the proximal interphalangeal joint.

Undue pressure on the dorsal skin flap must obviously be avoided during the post-operative course. In some cases, swelling can persist for several months and can be decreased with finger wrapping techniques.

If the distal interphalangeal joint is fused, the skin around the fixation pin must be kept clean and protected with Betadine ointment and an elastoplast, and bumping or motion of the pin must be avoided to prevent loosening or pin-tract infection. Fixation pins are usually removed after 6–8 weeks.

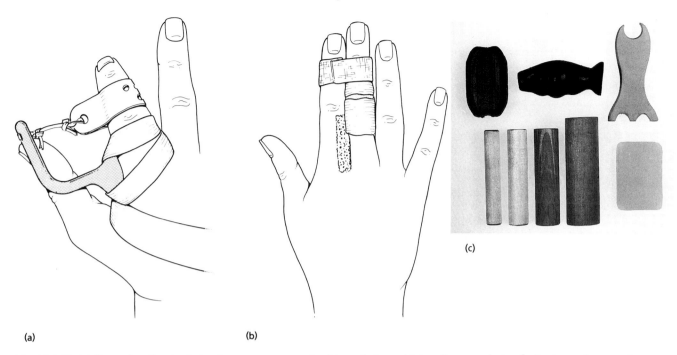

Fig. 20.1.10 (a) Dynamic splint for index finger protects proximal interphalangeal joint alignment during flexion/extension exercises. (b) Buddy splinting to intact digit. (c) Variety of exercise devices, including the finger crutch (top right) and a Grip-X (top centre). (Redrawn with permission from Swanson and de Groot Swanson, 1991a.)

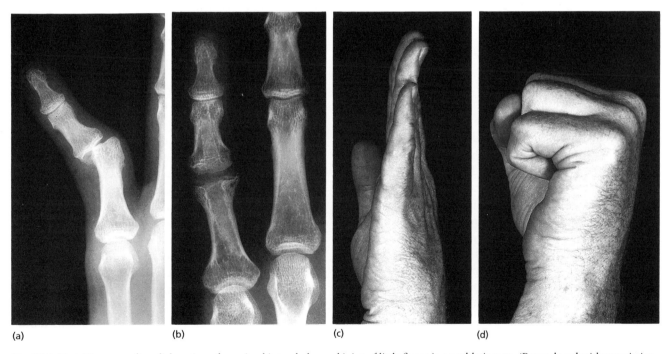

Fig. 20.1.11 (a) Longstanding dislocation of proximal interphalangeal joint of little finger in an athletic man. (Reproduced with permission from Swanson and de Groot Swanson, 1991a.) (b) Radiograph showing excellent position and tolerance of implant. (c, d) Twenty years post-operatively the patient maintains excellent pain-free flexion and extension.

THE CARPUS

The carpal bone implants were designed to act as articulating spacers to maintain the relationship of the adjacent carpal bones following resection of the scaphoid, lunate, or trapezium and have been used in the author's clinic since 1965. Bone remodelling around these implants has been excellent in the majority of cases. Silicone particle-induced cystic changes can occur, however. These reactive problems occurred more often around scaphoid and lunate implants than around thumb basilar implants.

The authors now use spacer implants made of conventional silicone elastomer (trapezium, condylar, scaphoid and lunate) and of titanium (convex condylar, scaphoid, lunate and single-stem toe).

Revision procedures may be indicated for symptomatic progression of disease to other carpal articulations, implant subluxation or fracture, or bone cyst formation. These procedures can include synovectomy, removal or replacement of the implant, curettage of cysts with cancellous bone grafting, selective intercarpal bone fusions, implant arthroplasty or arthrodesis of the radiocarpal joint. Good results have usually followed revision surgery.

The thumb basal joints

Any reconstructive surgery of the thumb must consider the entire ray, its balanced musculotendinous system and the position, mobility and stability of all three articulations. Each joint may be affected primarily, or secondarily, by imbalances of the other joints as seen in the boutonnière and swan-neck deformities.

The problems presented at the basal joints of the thumb differ in osteoarthritis and rheumatoid arthritis. Accurate evaluation of the location of the arthritic involvement and alignment of adjacent bones are essential in selecting the appropriate treatment. The disease can involve the trapeziometacarpal joint alone or can also affect the peritrapezial or other carpal bone articulations, with or without absorption or displacement of adjacent carpal bones. Treatment methods can be selected from the following: resection arthroplasty of the trapeziometacarpal joint, with or without a convex or concave condylar implant, and resection of the entire trapezium with or without a trapezium implant.

Implant resection arthroplasty of the basal joints of the thumb helps maintain a smooth articulating joint space with improved joint stability, mobility, pain relief and strength. Selection of the appropriate treatment, meticulous operative technique including capsuloligamentous stabilization, medialization of the implant and correction of associated deformities of the thumb ray, are essential for a good result. Trapezium implants made of conventional silicone elastomer (CSE) are preferred in cases of pantrapezial involvement in patients with osteoarthritis. In isolated trapeziometacarpal involvement in patients with osteoarthritis, titanium convex condylar implants are recommended. In patients with rheumatoid arthritis, or cases of severe erosive osteoarthritis, convex or concave condylar CSE implants or simple resection arthroplasty are preferred (Fig. 20.1.12).

TRAPEZIUM IMPLANT RESECTION ARTHROPLASTY

Indications

Trapezium implant (CSE) resection arthroplasty is indicated in cases of degenerative or post-traumatic arthritis presenting localized pain and palpable crepitation at the base of the thumb on the 'grind test' (circumduction with axial compression of the thumb) and radiographic evidence of pantrapezial arthritic changes. Associated thumb ray deformities must also be corrected. This procedure is contraindicated when there is severe displacement, absorption, or involvement of contiguous carpal bones.

Operative technique (Fig. 20.1.13)

The approach is made through a dorsoradial skin incision (Fig. 20.1.13a). Branches of the superficial radial nerve are carefully preserved and longitudinal veins are spared. The distal portion of the first dorsal compartment retinaculum is incised longitudinally. The dissection is carried between the abductor pollicis longus and extensor pollicis brevis tendons. The radial artery branch is exposed, mobilized and protected by proximal retraction with a small rubber tubing (Fig. 20.1.13b). The joint capsule is incised in a 'T' fashion and the capsular flaps are elevated off the underlying bone. The trapezioscaphoid and trapeziometacarpal joints are identified. Traction on the thumb allows further freeing of the dorsal capsular attachments around the trapezium. It is important to stay close to the bone during the dissection to avoid injury to the artery, underlying tendons, or capsule.

The trapezium is sectioned into pieces and removed piecemeal including its ulnar distal projection between the first and second metacarpals. Small flecks of bone are left with the underlying capsule to preserve the palmar capsuloligamentous support. Traction on the thumb or distal retraction with a two-prong rake on the

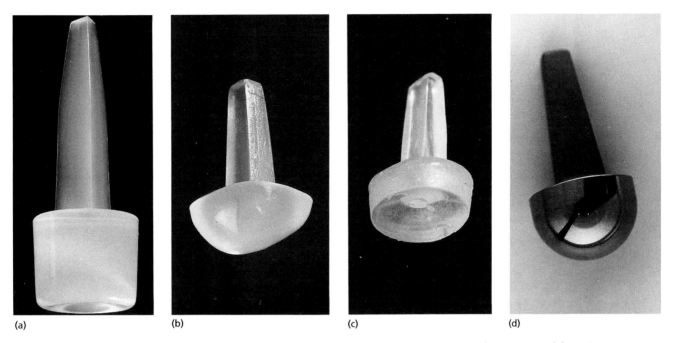

(a) (b) (c) (d)

Fig. 20.1.12 Silicone (CSE) implants for reconstruction of the thumb basal joints: (a) trapezium; (b) convex condylar; (c) concave condylar; (d) and titanium convex condylar. (Reproduced with permission from Swanson and de Groot Swanson, 1991c.)

base of the metacarpal facilitates the exposure. Osteophytes or irregularities on the distal end of the scaphoid, trapezoid or bases of the first and second metacarpals are trimmed. The trapezium must be positively identified to prevent removing portions of adjacent bones. If the trapezoid is shifted radially, a portion of its radial aspect is removed to allow good seating of the implant over the scaphoid facet. The base of the first metacarpal is squared off, leaving most of its cortical and subchondral bone intact. To prevent perforation through its sidewall, the intramedullary canal is probed first with a thin broach and then prepared in a triangular shape using burs with a small leader point to fit the implant stem. If the canal is enlarged, bone chips are inserted to provide intramedullary stability of the stem. The proper size implant should fit the trapeziectomy space and allow stable circumduction of the thumb; the collar should sit squarely on the metacarpal base and the implant should be well medialized over the distal scaphoid. Implant sizes 2 and 3 are most commonly used. Before implant insertion, the wound is thoroughly irrigated to remove all debris.

A secure capsuloligamentous reconstruction around the implant is essential to stabilize it over the scaphoid. The flexor carpi radialis tendon is exposed in the forearm, and a 7–8 cm tendon slip is developed from its radial third. The slip is dissected distally to the fibro-osseous canal, pulled into the trapeziectomy site, and freed to its insertion on the second metacarpal which is carefully preserved. The radial artery must be carefully protected throughout the procedure. Transverse lacerations of the tendon slip must be avoided. The techniques for capsuloligamentous reinforcement using the flexor carpi radialis tendon slip and capsular closure are shown in Fig. 20.1.13c, d and e. In some cases, additional sutures are placed through the proximal end of the first metacarpal to securely close the distal capsule.

After suturing of the capsular flaps, the abductor pollicis longus is advanced distally on the metacarpal and the extensor pollicis brevis is tenodesed to the abductor tendon insertion over the metacarpal to help abduction and restrict its hyperextension action on the first metacarpophalangeal joint. The first dorsal compartment is loosely closed over the abductor pollicis longus and extensor pollicis brevis tendons. The extensor pollicis longus tendon is left subcutaneous.

The incision is closed and drained with care to protect the branches of superficial radial nerve. A conforming dressing, including an anterior and posterior plaster splint, is applied. The arm is kept elevated and the drains are removed in 48 h. After 3–4 days, a short-arm thumb-spica cast is applied and worn for 6 weeks; sutures are removed through a window in the cast at 3 weeks. Guarded motion, including pinch and grasp

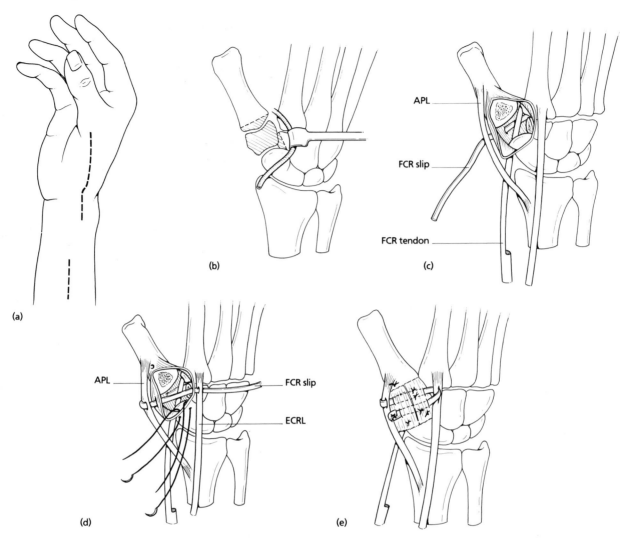

Fig. 20.1.13 (a) Incision centred over trapezium, parallel to extensor pollicis brevis tendon, has short transverse arm over distal wrist crease to continue proximally. The flexor carpi radialis tendon is exposed through a separate incision. (b) Radial artery branch is identified and protected. The trapezium is removed, the base of the first metacarpal resected, and partial trapezoidectomy is performed. (c) A slip is made of flexor carpi radialis (FCR) tendon (preserving metacarpal insertion), and passed under FCR tendon, and laterally through radial capsule and abductor pollicis brevis muscle. (d) Flexor carpi radialis (FCR) tendon slip is passed medially through abductor pollicis longus tendon (APL), lateral capsule across trapezoidectomy site, through medial capsule, under radial artery branch and through distal portion of extensor carpi radialis (ECRL). 3–0 Dacron sutures are passed through capsular reflections off scaphoid for capsular closure. (e) Implant is inserted and slip folded under dorsal capsule, looped through APL and sutured. Capsular reflections sutured proximally and distally. APL is advanced distally on metacarpal. (Redrawn with permission from Swanson and de Groot Swanson, 1991c.)

activities using various exercise devices, are then started (Fig. 20.1.14).

TRAPEZIOMETACARPAL IMPLANT ARTHROPLASTY

Indications

Implant arthroplasty of the trapeziometacarpal joint with a convex condylar CSE silicone implant is indicated in rheumatoid arthritis and severe erosive osteoarthritis with basilar joint involvement associated with severe displacement, resorption or fusion of the contiguous carpal bones. A concave condylar implant is used when there is inadequate bone stock to allow shaping of the trapezium to receive a convex implant. A titanium convex condylar implant is preferred for isolated involvement of the trapeziometacarpal joint in patients with osteoarthritis. The technique is similar for the various implants.

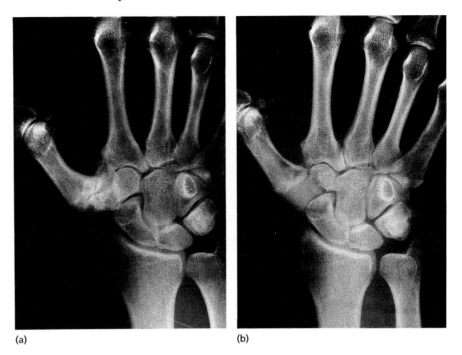

Fig. 20.1.14 (a) Pantrapezial degenerative arthritis with subluxation of the carpometacarpal joint. (b) Result 13 years after trapezium implant arthroplasty with the original silicone elastomer. Note trapezoidectomy, excellent host tolerance and implant position. The patient is pain-free and has an excellent clinical result. (Reproduced with permission from Swanson and de Groot Swanson, 1991a.)

(a)　　　　(b)

Operative technique (Fig. 20.1.15)

The surgical approach and preparation of the first metacarpal are similar to those described for the trapezium implant (p. 624). The capsule is incised longitudinally over the radial side of the trapeziometacarpal joint. Approximately 2–4 mm of the base of the metacarpal and the articulating projection of the trapezium to the

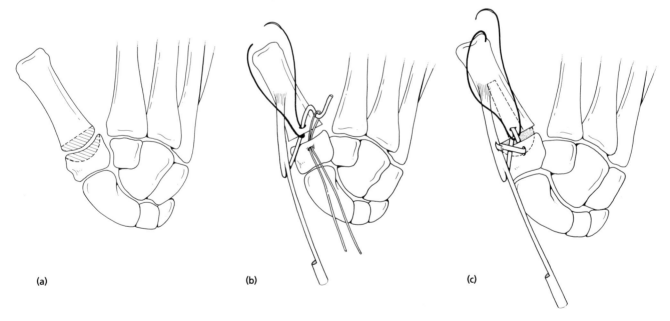

(a)　　　　(b)　　　　(c)

Fig. 20.1.15 (a) Base of metacarpal excised, concavity shaped in distal facet of trapezium and medullary canal prepared in triangular shape. (b) An 8 cm slip made of lateral third of abductor pollicis longus (APL) tendon is passed under the APL tendon and looped through the 2–3 mm drill hole in the radiodorsal aspect of the metacarpal from the inside out with a wire loop. The slip is then passed through the hole in the medial aspect of the trapezium from the inside out ('in-and-out' technique). Two drill holes are made in the base of the metacarpal to pass 3–0 Dacron sutures for capsular closure. (c) The remaining tendon slip is securely interwoven and sutured to reinforce capsular closure. The distal end of the slip is passed through the abductor pollicis longus and sutured to the radial capsule advancing APL distally. (Redrawn with permission from Swanson and de Groot Swanson, 1991c.)

second metacarpal are resected. The distal facet of the trapezium is shaped in a concavity slightly larger than the head of the convex condylar implant (Fig. 20.1.15a). Enough bone should be removed to create a joint space of approximately 4 mm and to allow 45° radial abduction of the first metacarpal. The implant stem is inserted in the medullary canal of the first metacarpal. A distally based slip of abductor pollicis longus tendon is interwoven through the metacarpal, trapezium, capsule, and abductor pollicis longus tendon insertion to provide an excellent checkrein to radial subluxation of the base of the metacarpal (Fig. 20.1.15b, c). The abductor pollicis longus insertion is advanced distally and any associated deformities of the thumb ray must be corrected. Because of the narrow joint space, the usual range of motion obtained with the trapezium implant cannot be expected. However, this technique can provide a stable, pain-free, functional thumb joint (Fig. 20.1.16).

Special considerations

Adduction of the first metacarpal and hyperextension of the metacarpophalangeal joint promote lateral subluxation of the carpometacarpal joint and contracture of the adductor pollicis muscle resulting in a swan-neck collapse deformity. Correction of hyperextension at the metacarpophalangeal joint is essential to prevent implant subluxation.

Adduction contracture of the first metacarpal. If the angle of abduction between the first and second metacarpals does not reach at least 45°, the origin of the adductor pollicis muscle should be released from the third metacarpal through a separate palmar incision.

Hyperextension deformity of the metacarpophalangeal joint. If the metacarpophalangeal joint hyperextends less than 10°, no treatment is necessary except to apply the post-operative cast so that the metacarpal is abducted and not the proximal phalanx. If the metacarpophalangeal joint hyperextends from 10° to 20°, it is pinned in 10° of flexion for 4–6 weeks. If hyperextension is greater than 20° with near normal flexion and good lateral stability of the joint, a palmar capsulodesis of the metacarpophalangeal joint may be indicated to preserve available flexion and restrict the hyperextension (Fig. 20.1.17). Fusion of the joint should be done for hyperextension deformities with no available flexion, lateral instability due to collateral ligament disruption or articular destruction. Implant arthroplasty of the metacarpophalangeal joint is not indicated in this situation.

Operative recommendations

Important considerations in reconstruction of the thumb basal joints include:
1 Separate indications for the use of trapezium, convex (silicone or titanium) and concave condylar implants.
2 Proper medialization of the trapezium implant on the

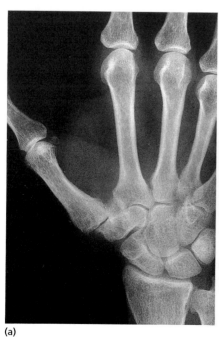

(a)

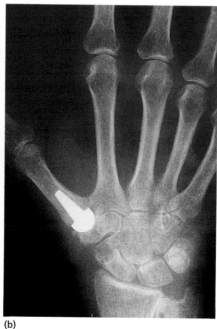

(b)

Fig. 20.1.16 (a) Degenerative arthritis and subluxation of the trapeziometacarpal joint. (b) Four years after trapeziometacarpal joint arthroplasty with a titanium convex condylar implant, the patient has good pain relief and functional result. (Reproduced with permission from Swanson and de Groot Swanson, 1991c.)

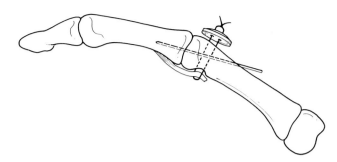

Fig. 20.1.17 Palmar capsulodesis: palmar aspect of joint exposed through lateral incision. Proximal membranous insertion of palmar plate incised preserving tendinous attachment to sesamoid bone. The periosteum is stripped from the palmar aspect of the metacarpal neck; two drill holes are made and converted into a small concavity with the curette. The detached proximal end of the palmar plate is drawn into the concavity with the pullout wire and the tension adjusted to obtain 10–15° metacarpophalangeal joint flexion. Pullout wire was removed at 3 weeks. Kirschner wire fixation for 6 weeks. (Redrawn with permission from Swanson, 1973a.)

scaphoid facet and of the condylar implant on the trapezium surface. Partial trapezoidectomy and resection of exostoses at the base of the first metacarpal assure stable implant seating.

3 Firm capsuloligamentous reconstruction with a slip of flexor carpi radialis tendon for trapezium implants, and a slip of abductor pollicis longus tendon for condylar implants.

4 Precise preparation of the intramedullary canal and insertion of additional bone chips around the implant stem, should the canal be enlarged, are essential for stability and bone remodelling.

5 Simultaneous correction of associated imbalances of the thumb ray.

Carpal scaphoid and lunate

Treatment of necrosis, fracture or fracture dislocation and subluxation of the scaphoid or lunate includes a wide variety of procedures, e.g. conservative methods, localized bone grafting, excision or implant replacement, intercarpal fusions, or wrist implant arthroplasty or fusion. Proper evaluation of the specific problems presented, including severity of disease (Tables 20.1.2 and 20.1.3), patient's age and functional requirements is essential in selecting the best treatment.

The carpal bone implants act as articulating spacers to maintain the relationship of the adjacent carpal bones following local resection procedures while preserving wrist mobility. Their use allows stabilization of associated intercarpal instability to prevent collapse and settling of the carpus. These implants have essentially the same shape as their anatomical counterpart, the concavities being more pronounced to provide greater stability. The scaphoid implants are available in five sizes, and because of mirror-image differences, models for the left and right wrist are available; lunate implants are available in five sizes. Implants made of titanium are preferred to the conventional silicone elastomer implants. High-performance silicone elastomer implants are not recommended for carpal bone replacements (p. 610). Fixation of silicone implants with sutures or Kirschner wires is no longer used.

Ligamentous instability and carpal collapse are frequently associated with pathology of the scaphoid or lunate and may be a contraindication to the implant procedure unless a stable relationship of the carpal bones can be re-established with appropriate intercarpal fusions. Cancellous bone, preferably obtained from the ilium, is used; resected bone, if healthy, can also be used. Firm internal fixation is obtained with staples, Kirschner or threaded wires, or preferably a Herbert bone screw. Cysts in contiguous bones should be curretted and bone grafted at the time of the procedure. The palmar ligaments should be preserved during carpal bone excision by leaving a small wafer of the palmar part of the bone, or they should be repaired if weakened. The implant must not be oversized and should not be used if space is inadequate. Carpal bone implant replacement is not indicated in cases of advanced pathology. In these cases wrist implant arthroplasty or fusion is preferred.

SCAPHOID

Indications

Use of a scaphoid implant may be considered upon diagnosis of the following clinical conditions:
1 acute fractures (comminuted or grossly displaced);
2 pseudarthrosis, especially with small proximal fragment;
3 Preiser's disease;
4 avascular necrosis of a fragment;
5 failures due to previous surgery.
This procedure is contraindicated when there is:
1 the possibility of conservative treatment;
2 generalized arthritis of the wrist;
3 severe carpal instability with inadequate or irretrievable ligament or bone support to stabilize the implant;
4 long-standing disease with inadequate space to receive the implant.

Table 20.1.2 Classification for scaphoid pathology and treatments

Stage	Pathology	Treatment options
I	Acute scaphoid fractures Acute scaphoid fracture/dislocation	Immobilization Open or closed reduction
II	Non-union of scaphoid	Bone graft Bone stimulator
III	Avascular necrosis of a fragment with Carpal height collapse 0–5% Lunate dorsiflexion minimal (R–L angle, 0–10°)	Partial scaphoid implant replacement Scaphoid implant replacement
IV	Comminuted or grossly displaced fracture Avascular necrosis with scaphoid degenerative arthritic changes Subluxation of scaphoid with degenerative arthritic changes Non-union of scaphoid with cystic changes with Carpal height collapse 5–10% Lunate dorsiflexion minimal to moderate (R–L angle, 10–30°) Mild degenerative arthritic changes of contiguous bones (particularly between lunate and capitate)	Scaphoid implant replacement with/without intercarpal fusions
V	Stage IV pathology of scaphoid with Carpal height collapse >10% Lunate dorsiflexion moderate to severe (R–L angle >30°) Mild to moderate degenerative arthritic changes of contiguous bones	Scaphoid implant replacement with intercarpal fusions Proximal row carpectomy Fusion proximal carpus to radius Hemi-arthroplasty
VI	Stage IV pathology of scaphoid or previous surgery with Carpal height collapse >15% Lunate dorsiflexion severe (R–L angle >30°) Severe intercarpal and radiocarpal degenerative arthritic changes	Total wrist implant arthroplasty Wrist arthrodesis Ulna impingement treatment as required

Source: Swanson A.B. *et al.*, 1986. (R–L angle: radio-lunate angle).

Surgical technique (Fig. 20.1.18)

An 8–10 cm dorsoradial longitudinal incision is made across the radiocarpal joint midway between the tip of the radial styloid and Lister's tubercle. Dissection is carried to the retinaculum, taking care to preserve the longitudinal veins and branches of the superficial radial nerve. The extensor retinaculum is incised over the extensor pollicis longus tendon, and elevated from the third compartment radially to expose the second compartment (Fig. 20.1.18b). The extensor carpi radialis longus and brevis tendons are mobilized to their insertion for retraction. The extrinsic extensors of the fingers are mobilized ulnarward. The dorsocarpal wrist ligament and capsule are incised in a T-shape and, with the wrist flexed, elevated from the radius by sharp dissection

staying close to bone to preserve adequate tissues for reattachment (Fig. 20.1.18c). The wrist extensor tendons are retracted radially to identify the scapholunate junction and the capitate, and then ulnarward to visualize the distal portion of the scaphoid and its articulations with the trapezoid, trapezium and radius. If necessary, intraoperative radiograms can help identify the carpal bones. The scaphoid is removed piecemeal avoiding injury to the underlying palmar ligaments. A thin bony wafer is left in the palmar ligaments to assure their important continuity (Fig. 20.1.18d). If the scaphoid distal pole is completely removed, there will be a hole left in the palmar ligaments through which the implant could protrude. Before implant insertion, the integrity of the palmar ligaments is assessed; these are reefed or repaired as necessary.

Table 20.1.3 Classification for avascular necrosis of lunate and treatments

Stage	Pathology	Treatment options
I	Sclerosis of lunate with 　Minimal symptoms 　Normal carpal bone relationships	Splinting and rest Revascularization Ulna and radius lengthening/shortening
II	Sclerosis of lunate with cystic changes with 　Clinical symptoms 　Normal carpal bone relationships	Lunate implant replacement Ulna and radius lengthening/shortening
III	Sclerosis, cysts, and fragmentation of lunate with 　Scaphoid-radius angle 40−60° 　Carpal height collapse 0−5% 　Carpal translation minimal	Lunate implant replacement with/without 　intercarpal fusions
IV	Sclerosis, cysts, fragmentation of lunate with 　Scaphoid-radius angle <70° 　Carpal height collapse 5−10% 　Carpal translation moderate	Lunate implant replacement with intercarpal 　fusions
V	Sclerosis, cysts, fragmentation of lunate with 　Scaphoid-radius angle >70° 　Carpal height collapse >10% 　Carpal translation severe 　Cystic changes in contiguous bones	Lunate implant replacement and intercarpal 　fusions Wrist arthrodesis Ulna impingement treatment as required
VI	Sclerosis, cysts, fragmentation of lunate with 　Scaphoid-radius angle >70° 　Carpal height collapse >15% 　Carpal translation severe 　Cystic changes in contiguous bones 　Significant intercarpal and radiocarpal 　　degenerative arthritic changes	Total wrist implant arthroplasty Wrist arthrodesis Ulna impingement treatment as required

Source: Swanson A.B., Maupin B.K., de Groot Swanson G. *et al.*, 1985.

The adjacent carpal bones are evaluated for presence of arthritic and cystic changes, cartilage loss, surface irregularities, and instability patterns. In the presence of collapse deformities or instability, associated intercarpal bone fusions are important to improve the distribution of forces across the wrist joint. Rotation of the lunate must be corrected and the carpus stabilized with fusion of the lunate to the capitate and/or triquetrum and hamate.

Approximately 1 cm of the posterior sensory branch of the posterior interosseous nerve is resected to provide some sensory denervation of part of the carpal area. Care is taken to avoid injury to the small arteries and veins in the area.

Implant sizing is started with the smallest trial size implant. It is important to avoid using an oversized implant as this could result in excessive implant force-loading and displacement. The titanium implant is stabilized as shown in Fig. 20.1.18e, f. The stability of the silicone implant, if used, is maintained by the integrity of the capsuloligamentous structures. The implant position and stability are verified on passive wrist motion. Before inserting the implant, the wound is thoroughly irrigated with saline solution to remove all debris. The implant should be handled with blunt instruments.

The dorsocarpal ligament is sutured with 2−0 Dacron sutures passed through two small drill holes made in the dorsal distal radius before implant insertion (Fig. 20.1.18d). The repair is firmly secured with additional Dacron and Dexon sutures inverting the knots. A strip of extensor retinaculum can be used to reinforce the dorsal carpal ligaments if necessary. The retinaculum is sutured over the extensor tendons except for the extensor pollicis longus, which is left free in the subcutaneous tissues (Fig. 20.1.18g). The incision is closed in layers and drained. A secure conforming dressing including a palmar splint is applied.

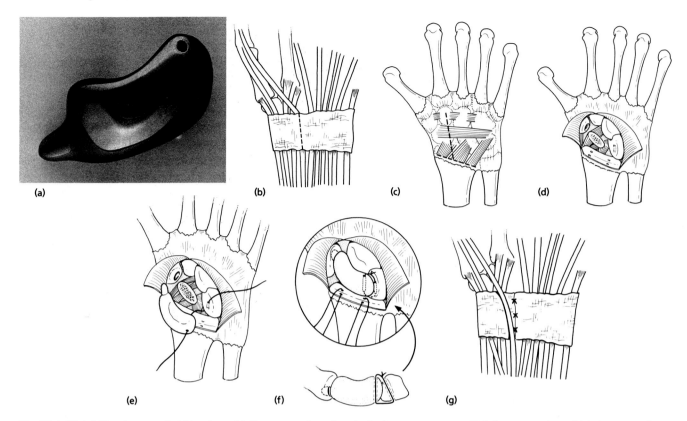

Fig. 20.1.18 (a) Titanium scaphoid implant. (b) Extensor retinaculum incised over extensor pollicis longus tendon which is retracted radially. Extensor carpi radialis brevis and longus tendons can be retracted ulnarly, radially or from each other as needed. (c) Dorsocarpal ligament incised in a T-shape with vertical extension over scaphoid in direction of trapezoid and horizontal extension over distal radius at insertion of dorsal capsule. (d) Scaphoid resected leaving small bony wafer to preserve continuity of radiocarpal ligaments. A bony shelf is made on the under-surface of the trapezium for stabilization of the implant distal pole. A suture hole is made through the lunate for passage of the fixation suture. Two drill holes are made in the distal radius to pass sutures for closure of dorsocarpal ligament. (e) Implant distal pole stabilized in the bony shelf made in the trapezium undersurface. Proximal pole stabilized with 2−0 Dacron suture passed through the lunate with a wire loop, and implant suture hole. (f) As the 2−0 Dacron suture is securely tightened, the implant becomes firmly reduced in position. (g) Extensor retinaculum is closed over extensor tendons, except for extensor pollicis longus which is left in the subcutaneous tissues. (Redrawn with permission from Swanson *et al.*, 1994.)

Post-operative care

The extremity is kept elevated for 1 or 2 days, and shoulder and finger movements are encouraged. A long-arm thumb spica cast is applied for 4 weeks and a short-arm spica cast is used for an additional 4 weeks. After intercarpal fusions the cast is used for 8−12 weeks. Skin sutures are removed at 3 weeks through a cast window. At 8 weeks, isometric gripping exercises are started to strengthen the extrinsic and intrinsic muscles. Use of the wrist is usually resumed at 12 weeks. Excessive or abusive motion must be avoided after carpal bone replacement (Fig. 20.1.19).

LUNATE

Indications

Use of a lunate implant may be considered upon diagnosis of the following clinical conditions:
1 avascular necrosis — Kienböck's disease;
2 longstanding dislocations;
3 localized osteoarthritic changes; and
4 resistance to conservative treatment.

The contraindications to this procedure are similar to those described for the scaphoid implant arthroplasty (p. 629).

Surgical technique (Fig. 20.1.20)

A dorsal longitudinal incision across the radiocarpal

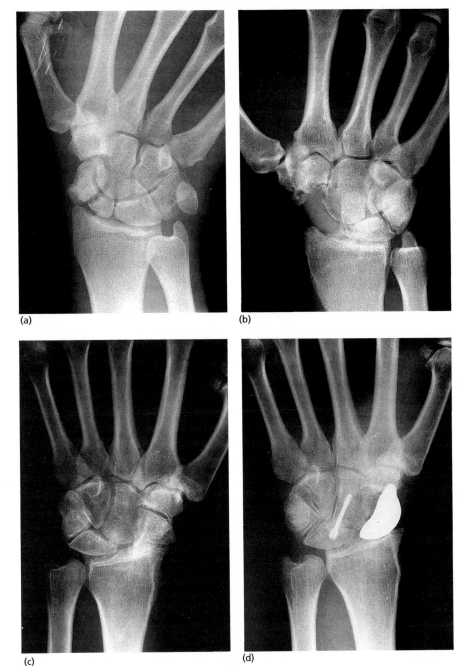

Fig. 20.1.19 (a) Pre-operative radiograph showing non-union of scaphoid bone of 3 years' duration in a 21-year-old athletic male (reproduced with permission from Swanson, 1973). (b) Radiograph 20 years after scaphoid implant arthroplasty with original silicone elastomer. Note excellent bone tolerance. The patient has a pain-free wrist, 120 pounds grip strength and excellent functional result. (c) Pre-operative radiograph showing SLAC wrist with severe osteoarthritic changes at the scaphoradial articulation, and between the lunate/capitate and triquetrum/hamate. There is a good joint space between the lunate and radius. (d) Post-operative radiograph showing a titanium scaphoid implant replacement with arthrodesis between the lunate, capitate and hamate. A Herbert screw was used to secure the lunate to capitate fusion. The patient has an excellent functional result. (b, c, d from Swanson *et al.*, 1994.)

area and centered at Lister's tubercle is used to expose the lunate bone. A transverse skin incision may be used in some of the uncomplicated cases, particularly in the female. A volar approach is recommended when the lunate bone is dislocated volarly. The superficial sensory branches of the radial and ulnar nerves are carefully preserved. The extensor retinaculum is incised over the extensor pollicis longus tendon which is mobilized for radial retraction. The extensor carpi radialis longus and brevis are retracted radially. The extensor digitorum communis tendons are retracted ulnarward. With the wrist flexed, the dorsocarpal ligament is incised in a 'T' shape and elevated close to bone (Fig. 20.1.20b). Adequate dissection is necessary to identify properly the capitate, triquetrum, scaphoid, radius and lunate. Roentgenograms are taken, if necessary, for anatomical orientation.

The lunate is removed piecemeal, avoiding injury to the dorsal and palmar carpal ligaments. A thin bony wafer is left in the palmar ligaments to preserve their

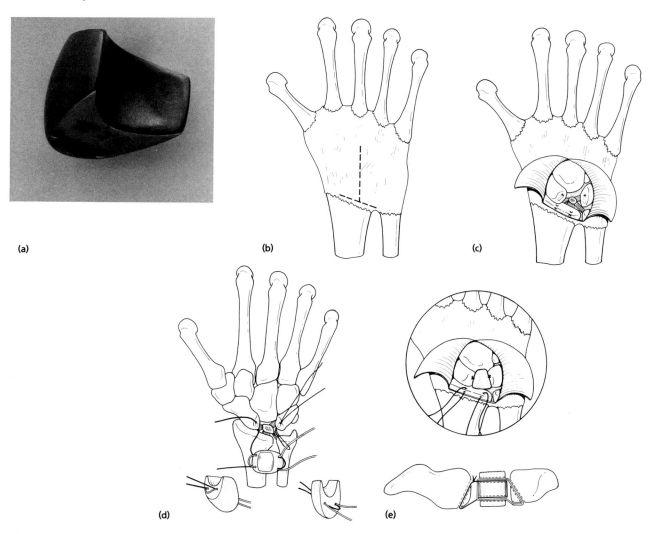

(a)

(b)

(c)

(d)

(e)

Fig. 20.1.20 (a) Titanium lunate implant has two transverse holes for suture fixation (redrawn with permission from Swanson A.B. and de Groot Swanson G., 1985). (b) The dorsocarpal ligament is incised in a 'T' shape with the vertical extension placed over the lunate in the direction of the capitate, the horizontal extension is placed at the insertion of the dorsal capsule on the distal radius. (c) Lunate resected leaving small bony wafer to preserve integrity of radiocarpal ligaments. Small holes are made through the articular surface of the proximal pole of scaphoid and triquetrum in a palmar direction to pass 2−0 Dacron sutures for implant fixation. Two drill holes are made in the distal radius to pass sutures for closure of dorsocarpal ligament. (d) A 2−0 Dacron suture is passed through scaphoid and looped through the implant starting with the palmar suture hole and exiting through the dorsal hole. Another 2−0 Dacron suture is similarly passed through triquetrum and looped through the implant. Sutures are pulled through the holes in the bones with a wire loop. The short flat implant surface articulates with the scaphoid and the long flat surface articulates with the triquetrum. (e) As the 2−0 Dacron suture is tightened, the implant becomes firmly reduced in position. Two 2−0 Dacron sutures are placed through the small drill holes in the distal dorsal radius for closure of the dorsocarpal ligament. (c, d, e redrawn with permission from Swanson and de Groot Swanson, 1993.)

important continuity; their integrity must be verified and obtained to prevent palmar subluxation of the implant. If the lunate bone is totally removed, there will be a defect between the two strong bands of the palmar ulnocarpal and radiocarpal ligaments, which are attached on each side of the lunate. A tendon graft or a slip of the flexor carpi radialis tendon can be used if direct reapproximation of these structures is impossible.

The associated bones are evaluated for presence of arthritic changes, loss of cartilage, surface irregularities, cystic changes, and collapse patterns. Traction and compression of the hand across the wrist joint can help appreciate instability patterns, particularly vertical rotation of the scaphoid. In the presence of collapse patterns or instability of the carpus, associated limited carpal bone fusions are very important to improve the distribution of forces across the wrist joint. Rotary subluxation of the scaphoid must be corrected and the carpus stabilized either by triscaphe or scaphocapitate fusion using an iliac bone graft. The scaphocapitate fusion is preferred when there are cystic changes in the capitate. Because of the great tendency for rotation of the scaphoid, intercarpal bone fusions are carried out in the majority of cases.

Approximately 1 cm of the posterior sensory branch of the posterior interosseous nerve is resected to provide some sensory denervation of part of the carpal area.

Implant sizing is started with the smallest trial size implant. It is important to avoid using an oversized implant as this could result in excessive implant force-loading and displacement. Small drill holes are made in the triquetrum and scaphoid to suture the implant as shown in Fig. 20.1.20c, d, e. The implant position and stability are verified on passive wrist motion. No sutures are used through silicone implants and their stability is maintained through the integrity of the capsuloligamentous system.

The dorsocarpal ligament is sutured with 2−0 Dacron sutures passed through two small drill holes made in the dorsal distal radius before implant insertion (Fig. 20.1.20c). The repair is firmly secured with additional Dacron and Dexon sutures with inverted knots. A strip of extensor retinaculum can be used to reinforce the dorsal carpal ligaments if necessary. The retinaculum is sutured over the extensor tendons except for the extensor pollicis longus, which is left free in the subcutaneous tissues. The wound is closed in layers and drained. A conforming dressing, including anterior and posterior plaster splints, is applied.

Post-operative care

The extremity is elevated for 1−2 days, and the patient is instructed to move the shoulder and fingers. Plaster immobilization is worn for a total of 8 weeks. A long-arm thumb spica cast is applied 1−2 days after surgery depending on the amount of swelling present. If a cast has been applied at surgery, it should be bivalved. Skin sutures are removed after 2−3 weeks through a window in the cast. At 4 weeks, a short-arm cast is applied and worn for another 4 weeks. The cast may be tightened or changed, as needed. The rehabilitation programme includes isometric gripping exercises to strengthen the extrinsic and intrinsic muscles of the hand and forearm and shoulder movements. Use of the wrist is usually resumed at 8 weeks, unless an intercarpal fusion was performed, which may require a longer recovery time. Post-operative roentgenograms are taken at intervals to evaluate the position of the implant and the bone status (Fig. 20.1.21).

SURGICAL RECOMMENDATIONS

The following considerations are essential to obtain long-term good results in carpal bone implant arthroplasty.

1 Patient selection — in the young, active or hard-labouring patient, associated procedures including limited intercarpal fusions, motion restriction by soft tissue capsular reconstruction, and strictly supervised post-operative care and instructions are important. Alternative non-implant procedures such as soft tissue reconstruction or arthrodesis may be considered.

2 Identification of pre-operative collapse or instability patterns, bone cysts and arthritis of other intercarpal joints.

3 Meticulous surgical technique.

4 Stabilization of collapse deformities. A scapho-trapezio-trapezoid or a scaphocapitate fusion is recommended in lunate implant arthroplasty. If there is lunate instability in a wrist requiring scaphoid implant arthroplasty, a lunocapitate or lunotriquetrum fusion is indicated. Intercarpal fusions are carried out with a cancellous bone graft (preferably iliac bone) and internal fixation.

5 Subchondral bone cysts must be treated at the same time by curretage and cancellous bone grafting.

6 The implant must not be oversized and if the space is inadequate it should not be used.

7 The titanium implants have suture holes for stabilization to adjacent bones. Stability of silicone implants is maintained by the capsuloligamentous structures; wires or sutures are not used.

8 Plaster cast immobilization for a minimum of 8 weeks and avoidance of excessive or abusive motion post-operatively.

The authors believe that lunate and scaphoid implant arthroplasties are useful procedures. Long-term good results can be achieved if the pathologic condition is well identified, the severity of disease is not too advanced, and the proper surgical indications and techniques are followed.

THE WRIST

Disabilities of the wrist are common and severe in rheumatoid arthritis, and also occur in osteoarthritis and following fractures and dislocations. The radiocarpal, distal radio-ulnar and intercarpal joints can be affected individually or in combination. Selection of the appropriate treatment depends on the site and extent of involvement, instability, deformity, arthritic destruction and the patient's requirements (Table 20.1.4). The wrist

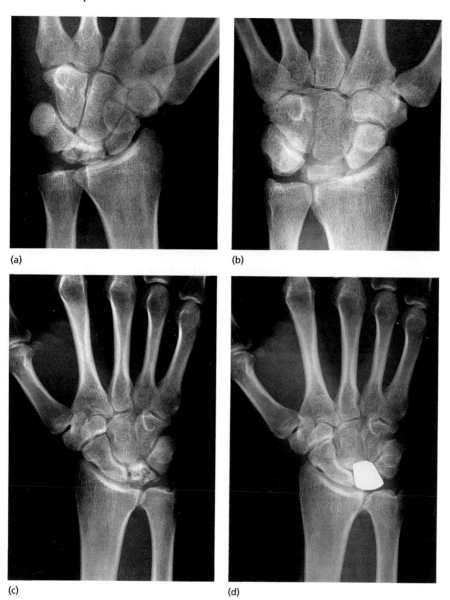

(a)

(b)

(c)

(d)

Fig. 20.1.21 (a) Pre-operative radiograph showing Kienböck's disease in a 21-year-old man (reproduced with permission from Swanson and de Groot Swanson, 1985). (b) Twenty years after lunate implant arthroplasty with the original silicone elastomer there is excellent maintenance of carpal bone structure and stability. This very active man is symptom-free (reproduced with permission from Swanson *et al.*, 1994). (c) Pre-operative radiograph showing grade II lunate pathology. (d) Radiograph 5 years after lunate titanium implant arthroplasty. (c and d reproduced with permission from Swanson and de Groot Swanson, 1991a.)

is the key joint for hand function. Proper transmission of muscle forces from the forearm to the digits requires a stable wrist. However, a mobile wrist is important to position the hand in functional adaptations and to move objects toward the body in activities of daily living. Wrist flexion is particularly important if the fingers or proximal joints are disabled. Reconstructive procedures of the wrist must provide reasonable stability, strength and mobility to assist in hand adaptations.

RADIOCARPAL JOINT

A double-stemmed, flexible-hinge implant for the radiocarpal joint was first developed in 1967. The barrel-shaped midsection is slightly flattened on its dorsal and volar surfaces and the core of the implant has a Dacron reinforcement for axial stability and resistance to rotatory torque. Since 1974, the implant has been made in five sizes of high performance silicone elastomer. Implant design modifications have included a wider midsection and a shorter distal stem (Fig. 20.1.22). Titanium bone liners (grommets) have been developed and used since 1982 to protect the implant's midsection from shearing forces and improve the durability.

Indications

Wrist implant arthroplasty is indicated in cases of arthritic or traumatic disability resulting in:

Table 20.1.4 Classification for wrist arthritis and treatments. (Courtesy of A.B. Swanson, 1985)

Age	Pathology	Treatment options
I	Transient synovitis, pain and weakness without instability or deformity in radiocarpal, intercarpal and distal radio-ulnar joints and tendons	Physical treatment: protection, splinting, therapy Medical treatment: injection steroids and/or alkylating agents
II	Persistent synovitis, pain and weakness without instability or deformity in radiocarpal, intercarpal and distal radio-ulnar joints; tendon involvement present	Synovectomy of tendons, joints; capsular stabilization of wrist joint and tendon rebalancing
III	Distal radio-ulnar deformity and destruction with stable radiocarpal joint	Partial or total resection of distal ulna with ligament and tendon reconstruction with/without ulnar head implant Shortening of ulna and reconstruction of stability with capsuloligamentous and tendon repair
IV	Arthritis limited to stable radiocarpal joint	Fusion of proximal row carpus to radius Hemi-arthroplasty of radiocarpal joint Total joint arthroplasty Treat distal radio-ulnar joints as needed
V	Arthritis limited to radiocarpal joint with ulnar translation instability	Fusion of proximal row to radius Fusion of segment distal ulna to radius with osteotomy of proximal ulnar diaphysis with/without ulnar head implant Hemi-arthroplasty — semiconstrained Total joint arthroplasty Treat distal radio-ulnar joint as needed
VI	Subluxation of radiocarpal joint Severe intercarpal and radiocarpal arthritis Destruction of proximal carpal row Stiffness of wrist Tendon balance achievable	Total joint arthroplasty Total joint arthrodesis Treat distal radio-ulnar joint as needed
VII	Severely unstable wrist Loss of bone in carpus and distal radius Progressive bone destruction (Mutilans type) High physical activity requirements of patient Tendon balance not achievable	Total joint arthrodesis Treat distal radio-ulnar joint as needed

1 instability of the wrist due to subluxation or dislocation of the radiocarpal joint;
2 severe deviation of the wrist causing musculotendinous imbalance of the digits;
3 stiffness or fusion of the wrist in a non-functional position; and
4 stiffness of a wrist when movement is a requirement for hand function.

The procedure is contraindicated in the presence of opened epiphyses, inadequate skin, bone, or neurovascular systems, irreparable tendon damage, and in uncooperative individuals. The authors do not recommend this method for patients who are excessively active.

Surgical technique (Fig. 20.1.23)

A straight longitudinal incision is made over the dorsal wrist, taking care to preserve the superficial sensory nerves. The extensor retinaculum is incised as shown in Fig. 20.1.23a and synovectomy of the extensor compartments is performed. The dorsal capsuloligamentous structures are carefully reflected from the radius and the carpal bones preserving a distally based flap (Fig. 20.1.23b). A part of the proximal carpal row is usually absorbed and the remnants are displaced palmarward on the radius. A proximal row carpectomy is performed and the proximal edge of the capitate is squared off. In certain cases, part of the scaphoid capitate and triquetrum bones can be left. Injury to the underlying tendons and neurovascular structures should be avoided.

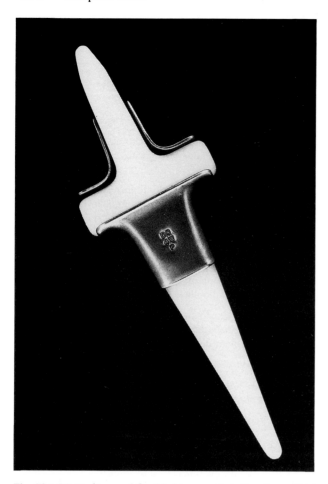

Fig. 20.1.22 Radiocarpal flexible hinge made in five sizes of high performance silicone elastomer. Titanium grommets are available in corresponding sizes. Distal stem shown at top. (Reproduced with permission from Swanson and de Groot Swanson, 1991b.)

The end of the radius is squared off to fit against the distal carpal row. The distal row of carpal bones should be left intact because of their importance in maintaining the stability of the metacarpal bases (Fig. 20.1.23c). The radiocarpal subluxation should be completely reduced.

The intramedullary canal of the radius is prepared to receive the proximal implant stem. If there has been a marked radiocarpal dislocation with soft tissue contracture, it is preferable to shorten the distal radius rather than remove more of the carpal bones. The distal stem of the implant fits through the capitate bone into the intramedullary canal of the third metacarpal. The intramedullary canal of the third metacarpal is prepared by carefully passing a wire or thin broach through the capitate bone and the base of the metacarpal and into its canal. A Kirschner wire can be passed into the metacarpal and out through its head to verify the intramedullary orientation. The final reaming is carried out with an air drill with a smooth point bur to prevent

perforation through the lateral cortex. The distal implant stem, which should not extend beyond the proximal metaphysis of the third metacarpal, is shortened as needed.

The proper-sized implant is determined with trial implants. Adequate bone preparation and soft tissue release allows passive motion without buckling or impingement of the implant. The bone ends should be smooth and abut the implant's midsection. A 1–1.5 cm joint space is usually required. The distal radius and base of the capitate are further shaped to allow a precise press-fit of the grommets. The distal radius and base of the capitate are further shaped to allow a precise press-fit of the grommets. The distal grommet is placed dorsally and the proximal grommet palmarly. The grommet sizes correspond to the implant sizes. A grommet size smaller than the implant is never used. With the grommets in place, the implant sizer is inserted, and joint flexion/extension and proper axial alignment are assessed.

The distal ulna is usually resected and may be capped with a silicone ulnar head implant. Stabilization of the distal radio-ulnar joint is essential to provide wrist stability and is obtained by attaching the sixth compartment retinaculum to the interosseous membrane or radius (see Fig. 20.1.25b).

Repair of both the palmar and dorsal capsuloligamentous structures around the implant is critical. The palmar ligaments are reefed proximally and/or distally, according to where they are loose. The proximal palmar reefing is performed by passing 2–0 Dacron sutures through two small drill holes made in the palmar distal edge of the cut end of the radius. The distal palmar reefing is performed by passing a 2–0 Dacron suture through a small drill hole made in the cut end of the capitate bone (Fig. 20.1.23d, e). Sutures for reattachment of the dorsal capsuloligamentous flap are passed through small drill holes in the dorsal cortex of the distal radius. All sutures are passed before grommets and implant insertion. The wound is thoroughly irrigated and the grommets are press-fitted. The proximal stem of the wrist implant is first inserted into the intramedullary canal of the radius. The distal stem is then introduced through the capitate into the intramedullary canal of the third metacarpal (Fig. 20.1.23f). The dorsal carpal ligament is firmly sutured over the implant (Fig. 20.1.23g). The mobility of the wrist is tested. No more than 20° of extension and flexion and 10° of ulnar and radial deviation should be possible on passive manipulation. An excessive range of motion, which may increase the potential for implant failure, does not significantly improve wrist function. If necessary, the capsule is tightened laterally with sutures passed through the radial

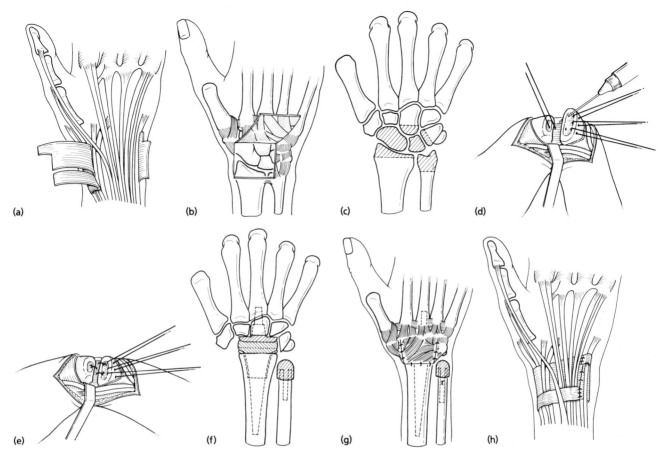

Fig. 20.1.23 (a) Extensor retinaculum incised to form radial-based flap between first and second compartments. Narrow distal flap used for relocation of extensor carpi ulnaris tendon in reconstruction of ulnar head. (b) Capsuloligamentous structures are elevated as a distally based flap from underlying radius and carpal bones. (c) Usual areas of bone resection. (d, e) Palmar capsuloligamentous structures are reefed proximally and/or distally as required with 2−0 Dacron sutures passed through the drill holes made in the palmar cortex of the distal radius and/or capitate. Sutures for reattachment of dorsal capsuloligamentous flap are passed through the drill holes in the dorsal distal radius. (f) Proximal stem of the implant fits into the intramedullary canal of radius and distal stem inserted through capitate into the intramedullary canal of the third metacarpal, not to extend beyond the proximal metaphysis. The distal grommet is placed dorsally, and the proximal grommet palmarly. The ulnar head implant is in place. (g) Capsuloligamentous flap sutured over the implant. (h) Retinacular flap positioned under extensor tendons. Proximal retinacular flap sutured over extensor tendons to prevent bow-stringing. EPL tendon is left subcutaneous. Narrow distal flap used as a pulley to relocate extensor carpi ulnaris tendon over the distal ulna. (a, b, c, f, g, h redrawn with permission from Swanson and de Groot Swanson, 1991b; d redrawn with permission from Swanson *et al.*, 1984; e redrawn with permission from Swanson and de Groot Swanson, 1991a.)

and ulnar cortex of the radius. Adequate capsuloligamentous repair is essential for proper function and durability of the implant.

The distal extensor retinaculum flap is brought over the wrist joint under the extensor tendons and sutured in place as shown in Fig. 20.1.23h. The proximal retinacular flap is sutured over the extensor tendons except the extensor pollicis longus which is left subcutaneous. If necessary, the wrist extensor tendons are shortened or transferred to obtain wrist extension without deviation. The extensor tendons of the digits are repaired as necessary. Reconstruction of the distal radio-ulnar joint is completed with a retinacular flap from the sixth dorsal compartment to relocate dorsally the extensor carpi ulnaris tendon.

Closure and post-operative care

The wound is closed in layers and drained. A voluminous conforming hand dressing is applied, including a palmar splint, with the wrist in neutral position. The extremity is elevated for 1−2 days. A dorsally well-padded short arm cast, with the wrist in neutral position, is then applied and fitted with outriggers to hold rubber-band slings to support finger extension if digital tendons have been repaired. This is worn for 4–6 weeks to assure stability of the wrist. A dorsal window is made in the cast for wound inspection and suture removal.

Following cast removal, an exercise programme is begun to achieve 20° flexion and extension and 10° radial and ulnar deviation. The patient should be restricted from excessive or abusive activity. Passive stretching exercises are not recommended.

Because this method requires no cement fixation nor significant bone resection, the implant can be removed or replaced as necessary, or the procedure can be converted to an arthrodesis by bone grafting. The authors believe that the wrist flexible implant resection arthroplasty method has a useful place in the reconstruction and rehabilitation programme of the upper extremity (Fig. 20.1.24).

DISTAL RADIO-ULNAR JOINT

In 1966, one of the authors (ABS) developed a silicone intramedullary stemmed, cuffed ulnar head implant to cap the end of the resected ulna in an effort to preserve the anatomical relationships and physiology of the distal radio-ulnar joint following ulnar head resection. The goal of this procedure is to preserve ulnar length to help prevent ulnar carpal shift and provide greater wrist stability. The ulnar head implant provides a smooth articular surface for the radio-ulnar and carpo-ulnar joints, and for the overlying extensor tendons. It decreases the incidence of bone overgrowth of the resected bone end and allows reconstruction of the distal radio-ulnar joint, stabilization of the distal ulna and dorsal rerouting of the extensor carpi ulnaris tendon.

The implant is fabricated in eight sizes from high performance 100 silicone elastomer. The stem of the implant has an attached, non-absorbable, polyester retention cord to secure the implant in position at the time of surgery. The last one-third of the stem is covered with polyester velour to provide fixation of the stem in the intramedullary canal by ingrowth.

Indications

The ulnar head implant replacement arthroplasty may be considered for disabilities of the distal radio-ulnar joint in rheumatoid, degenerative and post-traumatic dysfunctions of this joint. Specific indications include presence of pain and weakness of the wrist joint not improved by conservative treatment and instability of the ulnar head with radiographic evidence of dorsal subluxation and erosive changes. The procedure can also be used to correct sequelae of a failed simple ulnar head resection.

Surgical technique (Fig. 20.1.25)

A 6–8 cm longitudinal incision centred over the ulnar head is made, taking care to preserve the dorsal cutaneous branch of the ulnar nerve. The extensor retinaculum of the sixth dorsal compartment is incised

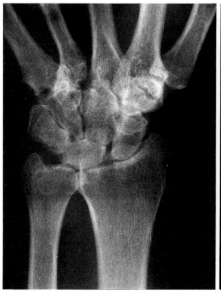
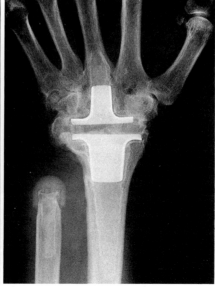

(a)   (b)

Fig. 20.1.24 (a) Pre-operative radiograph showing rheumatoid involvement of the wrist. (b) Radiograph 7 years after surgery shows proximal and distal titanium grommet around stems of flexible hinge wrist implant. Note good bone production around grommets and implant stems. Distal radio-ulnar joint reconstructed with silicone cap. The patient maintains an excellent pain-free functional result. (Reproduced with permission from Swanson and de Groot Swanson, 1991b.)

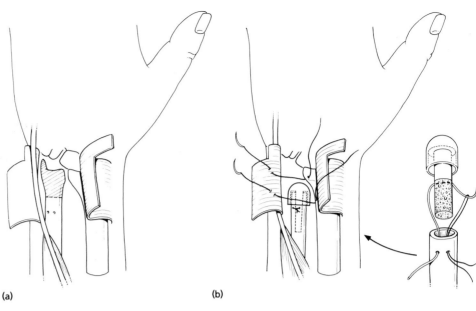

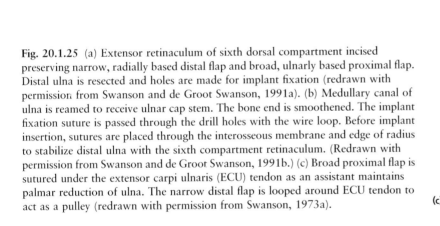

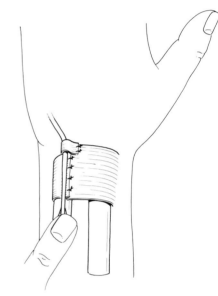

Fig. 20.1.25 (a) Extensor retinaculum of sixth dorsal compartment incised preserving narrow, radially based distal flap and broad, ulnarly based proximal flap. Distal ulna is resected and holes are made for implant fixation (redrawn with permission from Swanson and de Groot Swanson, 1991a). (b) Medullary canal of ulna is reamed to receive ulnar cap stem. The bone end is smoothened. The implant fixation suture is passed through the drill holes with the wire loop. Before implant insertion, sutures are placed through the interosseous membrane and edge of radius to stabilize distal ulna with the sixth compartment retinaculum. (Redrawn with permission from Swanson and de Groot Swanson, 1991b.) (c) Broad proximal flap is sutured under the extensor carpi ulnaris (ECU) tendon as an assistant maintains palmar reduction of ulna. The narrow distal flap is looped around ECU tendon to act as a pulley (redrawn with permission from Swanson, 1973a).

as shown in Fig. 20.1.25a. Synovectomy of the dorsal compartments, if indicated, may be carried out at the same time. The extensor carpi ulnaris, which is usually subluxated palmarward off the ulnar head, is retracted. Retractors are placed under the ulnar neck to protect the underlying structures and the bone is sectioned at the neck with an air drill or motor saw. The periosteum is not stripped off the distal ulna but muscular attachments on the anterior surface of the ulna are released over the distal 2 cm. The ulnar head and attached synovial sac are removed *en bloc* and synovectomy of the joint is completed. The cut edge of the distal ulna and bony

irregularities that may be present, especially at the undersurface of the ulna, are smoothed. The intramedullary canal of the ulna is prepared.

An appropriate implant is selected so that the stem will fit snugly into the intamedullary canal and the cuff, loosely over the bone. Occasionally digital extensor tendons are ruptured as a result of the ulnar head irregularities and must be repaired. The implant is inserted and secured to the end of the ulna with the pre-tied polyester suture to prevent the slight tendency for the implant to extrude from the intramedullary canal in the early post-operative course (Fig. 20.1.25b).

The retinaculum of the sixth dorsal compartment is used as a check ligament to hold the dorsally subluxated ulna in a reduced position. Before implant insertion, the broad proximal ulnarly based retinacular flap is placed under the extensor carpi ulnaris tendon and 2−0 Dacron sutures are placed through the base of the retinacular flap and through the interosseus ligament, close to the radius ulnar border, or through small drill holes in the radius if the local tissues are inadequate (Fig. 20.1.25b). After the implant is tied in position, the retinacular closure is completed as an assistant maintains the palmarward reduction of the ulna (Fig. 20.1.25c). It is important to release the extensor carpi ulnaris tendon proximally and distally to allow free excursion. The narrow distal retinacular flap is used to form a pulley around the extensor carpi ulnaris tendon to maintain it over the dorsum of the ulnar head. The wound is closed and drained in the usual manner. A voluminous conforming hand dressing including a plaster palmar splint is applied with the hand in slight dorsiflexion.

Post-operative care

On the third post-operative day the drain is removed and, if there is no swelling, a short-arm cast or splint is applied in the same position to protect the wrist from excessive activity for 3−6 weeks. The best immobilization is obtained by using a long-arm cast with the forearm in supination. However, most rheumatoid patients are quite inactive so that lesser immobilization is adequate.

REFERENCES

Swanson A.B. (1973a) *Flexible Implant Resection Arthroplasty in the Hand and Extremities.* St Louis, C.V. Mosby Co.

Swanson A.B. and de Groot Swanson G. (1975) Thumb disabilities in rheumatoid arthritis: classification and treatment. In: American Academy of Orthopaedic Surgeons, *Symposium on Tendon Surgery of the Hand.* St Louis, C.V. Mosby, pp. 233−254.

Swanson A.B. and de Groot Swanson G. (1982a) Flexible implant resection arthroplasty in the upper extremity. In: Flynn J.E. (ed.) *Hand Surgery,* 3rd edn. Baltimore, Williams and Wilkins, pp. 382−409.

Swanson A.B. and de Groot Swanson G. (1987a) The complex hand—treatment considerations and priorities of finger deformities. *Rheumatology* 11, 6−27.

Swanson A.B. and de Groot Swanson G. (1989) Arthroplasty in the Rheumatoid Hand. In: D.W. Lamb, G. Hooper and K. Kuczynski (eds). *The Practice of Hand Surgery,* 2nd edn. Oxford, Blackwell Scientific Publications, pp. 565−590.

Swanson A.B. and de Groot Swanson G. (1991a) Flexible implant resection arthroplasty in the upper extremity. In Jupiter J.B. (ed.) *Flynn's Hand Surgery,* 4th edn. Baltimore, Williams and Wilkins, pp. 342−386.

Swanson A.B. and de Groot Swanson G. (1991b) Flexible implant arthroplasty of the radiocarpal joint. *Sem. Arthrop.* 2, 78−84.

Swanson A.B. and de Groot Swanson G. (1991c) Implant arthroplasty for the thumb basal joints. *Sem. Arthrop.* 2, 91−98.

Swanson A.B. and de Groot Swanson G. (1993) Implant resection arthroplasty in the treatment of Kienböck's disease. *Hand Clinics* 9, 483−491.

Swanson A.B., de Groot Swanson G. and Maupin B.K. (1984) Flexible implant arthroplasty of the radiocarpal joint—surgical technique and long-term study. *Clin. Orthop.* 187, 94−106.

Swanson A.B., Maupin B.K., de Groot Swanson G., Ganzhorn R.W. and Moss S.H. (1985) Lunate implant resection arthroplasty—long term results. *J. Hand Surg.* 10A, 1013−1024.

Swanson A.B., de Groot Swanson G., Maupin B.K. *et al.* (1986) Scaphoid implant resection arthroplasty—long term results. *J. Arthrop.* 1, 47−62.

Swanson A.B., de Groot Swanson G. and Leonard J. (1990) Postoperative rehabilitation programs in flexible implant arthroplasty of the digits. In Hunter J., Schneider L., Mackin E. and Callahan A. (eds) *Rehabilitation in the Hand,* 2nd edn. St Louis, C.V. Mosby, pp. 885−890.

Swanson A.B., Livengood L.C. and Sattel A.B. (1991) Local hypothermia to prolong safe tourniquet time. *Clin. Orthop.* 264, 200−208.

Swanson A.B., de Groot Swanson G. and Hendron J.H. (1994) Complications of arthroplasty and joint replacement at the wrist. In: Epps Jr C.H. (ed.) *Complications in Orthopaedic Surgery,* 3rd edn. Philadelphia, J.B. Lippincott Co., pp. 957−995.

FURTHER READING

Isomäki, H.A., Hakulinen P., Joutsenlahti V. (1978) Excess risk of lymphomas, leukemia and myeloma in patients with rheumatoid arthritis. *J. Chronic Dis.* 31, 691.

Madden J.W. and Peacock E.E., Jr (1971) Studies on the biology of collagen during wound healing: dynamic metabolism of scar collagen and remodeling of dermal wounds. *Ann. Surg.* 174, 511−520.

Nalbandian R.M., Swanson A.B. and Maupin B.K. (1983) Long-term silicone implant arthroplasty—implications of animal and human autopsy findings. *JAMA* 250, 1195−1198.

Nalebuff E.A. (1983) Rheumatoid hand surgery—update. *J. Hand Surg.* 8(2), 678−682.

Swanson A.B. (1965) Pathomechanics of the swan-neck deformity. *J. Bone Joint Surg.* 47A, 636.

Swanson A.B. (1966) A flexible implant for replacement of arthritic or destroyed joints in the hand. *NY Univ. Inter-Clin. Inform. Bull.* 6, 16−19.

Swanson A.B. (1968) Silicone rubber implants for replacement of arthritic or destroyed joints in the hand. *Surg. Clin. North Am.* 48, 1113−1127.

Swanson A.B. (1969) Finger joint replacement by silicone rubber implants and the concept of implant fixation by encapsulation. *Ann. Rheum. Dis.* (suppl.) 28, 47−55.

Swanson A.B. (1970a) Arthroplasty in traumatic arthritic joints in the hand. *Orthop. Clin. North Am.* 1, 285−298.

Swanson A.B. (1970b) Silicone rubber implants for the replacement of the carpal scaphoid and lunate bones. *Orthop. Clin. North Am.* 1, 299−309.

Swanson A.B. (1972a) Disabling arthritis at the base of the thumb: treatment by resection of the trapezium and flexible silicone implant arthroplasty. *J. Bone Joint Surg.* **54A**, 456–471.

Swanson A.B. (1972b) Flexible implant arthroplasty for arthritic finger joints: rationale, technique and results of treatment. *J. Bone Joint Surg.* **54A**, 435–455.

Swanson A.B. (1973b) Flexible implant arthroplasty for arthritic disabilities of the radiocarpal joint. *Orthop. Clin. North Am.* **4**, 383–394.

Swanson A.B. (1973c) Implant arthroplasty for disabilities of the distal radioulnar joint. *Orthop. Clin. North Am.* **4**, 373–382.

Swanson A.B. (1973d) Implant resection arthroplasty of the proximal interphalangeal joint. *Orthop. Clin. North Am.* **4**, 1007–1029.

Swanson A.B. (1976) Flexible implant arthroplasty in the hand. *Clin. Plast. Surg.* **3**, 141–157.

Swanson A.B. (1981) A grommet bone liner for flexible implant arthroplasty. *Bull. Prosth. Res., Rehab. Engin. Res. Devel.,* *BPR10–35*, **1**, 108–114.

Swanson A.B. (1982) Bone remodeling phenomena in flexible (silicone) implant arthroplasty in the metacarpophalangeal joints—long-term study. Kappa Delta Award Presentation, 49th Annual Meeting of the American Academy of Orthopaedic Surgeons, January 21, 1982, New Orleans, Louisiana. *Orthop. Rev.* **11**, 129–131.

Swanson A.B. and de Groot Swanson G. (1976) Disabling osteoarthritis in the hand and its treatment. In *Symposium on Osteoarthritis.* St Louis, C.V. Mosby, pp. 196–232.

Swanson A.B. and de Groot Swanson G. (1982b) Flexible implant arthroplasty of the radiocarpal joint: surgical technique and long-term results. In Inglis A. (ed.) *The American Academy of Orthopaedic Surgeons Symposium on Total Joint Replacement of the Upper Extremity.* St. Louis, C.V. Mosby, pp. 301–316.

Swanson A.B. and de Groot Swanson G. (1982c) Arthroplasty of the thumb basal joints. In Leach R.E., Hoaglund F.T. and Riseborough E.J. (eds) *Controversies in Orthopaedic Surgery.* Philadelphia, W.B. Saunders, pp. 36–57.

Swanson A.B. and de Groot Swanson G. (1983) Osteoarthritis in the hand. *J. Hand Surg.* **8**(2), 669–675.

Swanson A.B. and de Groot Swanson G. (1984a) Flexible implant arthroplasty in the rheumatoid metacarpophalangeal joint. *Clin. Rheum. Dis.* **10**, 609–629.

Swanson A.B. and de Groot Swanson G. (1984b) Flexible implant resection arthroplasty in the upper extremity. In Tubiana R. (ed.) *Traité de Chirurgie de la Main,* vol. 11. Paris, Masson, pp. 446–481.

Swanson A.B. and de Groot Swanson G. (1985a) Flexible implant arthroplasty of the digits—long-term results. *Acta Orthop. Bel.* **41**, 679–698.

Swanson A.B. and de Groot Swanson G. (1985b) Arthroplasty of the thumb basal joints. *Clin. Orthop.* **195**, 151–160.

Swanson A.B., de Groot Swanson G. (1987b) Reconstruction of thumb basal joints—development and current status of implant techniques. *Clin. Orthop.* **220**, 68–85.

Swanson A.B. and de Groot Swanson G. (1988) Implant arthroplasty in the carpal and radiocarpal joints. In Lichtman D.M.

(ed) *The Wrist and it's Disorders.* Philadelphia, W.B. Saunders, pp. 404–438.

Swanson A.B., de Groot Swanson G., Maupin B.K., Hynes D.E. and Jindal P. (1989) Failed carpal bone implant arthroplasty: causes and treatment. *J. Hand Surg.* **14A** (2), 417–424.

Swanson A.B. and de Groot Swanson G. (1990) Reconstructive surgery for the rheumatoid hand. In *The CIBA Collection of Medical Illustrations,* Vol. 8 (Part II) *Musculoskeletal System* (Netter F.H., illustrator) Summit N.J., Ciba-Geigy Corp., pp. 219–232.

Swanson A.B. and Herndon J.H. (1977) Flexible (silicone) implant arthroplasty of the metacarpophalangeal joint of the thumb. *J. Bone Joint Surg.* **59A**, 362–368.

Swanson A.B. and Matev I.B. (1970) The proximal interphalangeal joint in arthritic disabilities and experiences in the use of silicone rubber implant arthroplasty in the upper extremity. *J. Bone Joint Surg.* **52A**, 1265.

Swanson A.B., de Groot Swanson G., Hehl R.W., Waller T.J. and Boeve N.R. (1971) Pathogenesis of rheumatoid deformities in the hand. In Cruess R.L. and Mitchell N. (eds) *Surgery of Rheumatoid Arthritis.* Philadelphia, J.B. Lippincott, pp. 143–158.

Swanson A.B., Meester W.D., de Groot Swanson G. *et al.* (1973) Durability of silicone implants—an in vivo study. *Orthop. Clin. North Am.* **4**, 1097–1112.

Swanson A.B., Herndon J.H. and de Groot Swanson G. (1978) Complications of arthroplasty and joint replacement of the wrist. In Epps C.H. (ed.) *Complications in Orthopaedic Surgery.* Philadelphia, J.B. Lippincott, pp. 873–904.

Swanson A.B., de Groot Swanson G. and Watermeier J.J. (1981) Trapezium implant arthroplasty—long term evaluation of 150 cases. *J. Hand Surg.* **6**, 125.

Swanson A.B., de Groot Swanson G. and Frisch E. (1983) Flexible (silicone) implant arthroplasty in the small joints of the extremities: concepts, physical and biological considerations, experimental and clinical results. In Rubin L. (ed.) *Biomaterials in Reconstructive Surgery.* St. Louis, C.V. Mosby, pp. 595–623.

Swanson A.B., de Groot Swanson G. and Winfield D.L. (1984a) The pronated index finger deformity in the rheumatoid hand. *Bull. Hosp. Joint Dis.* **44**, 498–510.

Swanson A.B., Nalbandian R.M., Zmugg T.J., Williams D., Jaeger S., Maupin B.K. and Swanson G. de G. (1984b) Silicone implants in dogs—a ten-year histopathologic study. *Clin. Orthop.* **184**, 293–301.

Swanson A.B., Maupin B.K., Gajjar N.V. and de Groot Swanson G. (1985) Long-term review of flexible implant arthroplasty in the proximal interphalangeal joint of the hand. *J. Hand Surg.* **10A**, 796–805.

Swanson A.B., Poitevin L.A., de Groot Swanson G. and Kearney J. (1986) Bone remodeling phenomena in flexible implant arthroplasty in the metacarpophalangeal joints (Kappa Delta Award Presentation). *Clin. Orthop.* **205**, 254–267.

Tajima T. (1983) Considerations on the use of the tourniquet in surgery of the hand. *J. Hand Surg.* **8** (Part 2), 799–802.

Tupper J.W. (1989) Arthroplasty of the metacarpophalangeal volar plate arthroplasty. *J. Hand Surg.* **14A** (2), 371–375.

Chapter 20.2
Cemented Total Hip Replacement

R.S.M. Ling & A.J. Timperley

INTRODUCTION

In the history of surgery, no operative procedure has had such an immediate and widespread impact as that of cemented total hip arthroplasty. The reasons for this are many. Before its introduction, the unpredictability of the results of osteotomy, the morbidity of arthrodesis, particularly in the elderly, and the prolonged convalescence from both were all problems that confronted the practising surgeon involved in managing osteoarthritis of the hip. These were followed by an operation that apparently could regularly achieve the pain relief of arthrodesis with the movement of the best of osteotomies, and, moreover, with a convalescence appreciably shorter and less demanding than either. For both patient and surgeon, the early results of the new operation were a revelation, the extent of which can be appreciated only by those increasingly few surgeons who can recall the practice of the 1950s and early 1960s.

It was hardly surprising that, once introduced, its use spread rapidly and widely. This is not to suggest that there is no longer a place for proximal femoral osteotomy or arthrodesis in the treatment of the arthritic hip, for, assuredly, there is. However, for the majority of patients requiring operative treatment for arthritic hips, total replacement is now the procedure of choice. The prevalence of arthritis of the hip, and thus the numbers of patients presenting for the operation, the latter's capacity to produce spectacular results, the gulf, in clinical terms, between success and failure, its cost, and the morbidity and cost of its complications ensure a high profile for the operation now and in the foreseeable future.

The significance of the procedure, however, does not depend purely on the transformation that it wrought for patients. Surgeons soon realized that the technology involved in cemented total hip arthroplasty could be applied successfully to other joints, with the result that, today, there is hardly a joint in the appendicular skeleton for which a cemented replacement has not been implanted. This fact, together with the early success and later problems of cemented hip arthroplasty, were largely responsible for the rapid emergence of the multidisciplinary approach to joint replacement that characterized the 1970s and 1980s. This involved, and continues to involve, not only surgeons, but also engineers, tribologists, materials scientists, metallurgists, polymer chemists and pathologists, and spawned an industry with an annual turnover of millions of pounds. Moreover, cemented hip arthroplasty became perhaps the first operation to have political significance, its spectacular and obvious results leading to demands for this type of surgery that became, in some countries, an embarrassment to health-care providers and thus to politicians.

HISTORY

Philip Wiles (Wiles, 1958) of the Middlesex Hospital in London must be credited with the introduction of the first *total* hip replacement. He devised a stainless steel femoral head attached to what was, in effect, the upper end of a modified nail-plate of the type used for the fixation of trochanteric fractures. The head was mated with a stainless steel acetabulum secured by screws. A small number of these implants was used in the 1930s for patients suffering from Still's disease. Follow-up was prevented by the war, but this implant was really the forerunner of total hip replacement as we know it today.

Wiles' implant was fixed without cement. Cement was used by Wiltse and his colleagues (1957) experimentally in the 1950s, and Haboush of New York reported in 1953 (Haboush, 1953) on its use for the fixation of a form of replacement for the femoral head and neck. It was, however, Charnley of Wrightington (1961) and McKee and Watson-Farrar (1966) of Norwich (Fig. 20.2.1) who made the operation into the practical proposition for orthopaedic surgeons that it

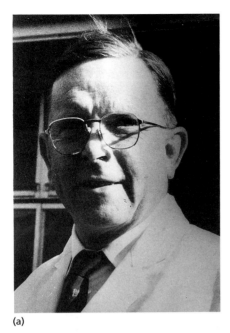
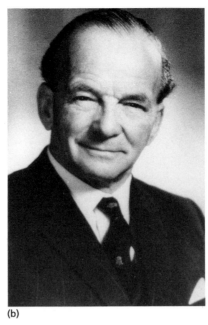
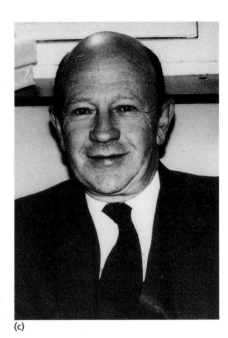

(a)   (b)   (c)

Fig. 20.2.1 (a) The late Sir John Charnley, (b) the late G.K. McKee and (c) J. Watson Farrar.

subsequently became. Charnley was the first to use acrylic cement to anchor the stem of an intramedullary femoral prosthesis (Charnley, 1960), and Mckee and Watson-Farrar the first to use cement for the fixation of the acetabular cup.

LOGISTICS

In 1989, in the UK under the National Health Service, approximately 40 000 total hip arthroplasties were performed as well as between 6000 and 7000 revisions (British Orthopaedic Association Survey, 1990). A significant number were, in addition, carried out privately. In the USA, approximately 120 000 primary total hip arthroplasties and 24 000 revisions are at present being performed annually. These figures give some idea of the enormous surgical workload worldwide that replacement of the hip represents. As Coventry (1991) has said 'Total hip arthroplasty, indeed, might be the operation of the century'.

FORCES TO BE SUSTAINED BY THE ARTHROPLASTY

It is important for the surgeon to have some idea of the forces to which the components of an artificial hip joint are exposed during the activities of daily living. Paul (1976) and Crowninshield *et al.* (1978) were among the first to calculate the magnitudes and directions of the

resultant forces at the normal hip during gait, and with activities such as rising from a sitting position, ascending and descending stairs (Table 20.2.1). Compared with the forces experienced by the hip in two-legged stance, those developed during single-leg stance activities are extremely high, primarily because many of the muscles involved in maintaining the equilibrium of the hip during single-leg stance (e.g. the abductors) act through very short lever arms (Fig. 20.2.2). Direct measurement of these forces in the normal hip is not possible, for obvious reasons, at least with current technology. Once an implant has been used to replace either the femoral head or both components of the hip, however, appropriate instrumentation of the femoral component can allow the direct measurement of the strain developed in the

Table 20.2.1 Magnitude of hip joint resultant force (in multiples of body weight; after Paul, 1976)

Activity	Max. resultant force
Level walking	
slow	4.9
normal	4.9
fast	7.6
Up stair	7.2
Down stair	7.1
Up ramp	5.9
Down ramp	5.1

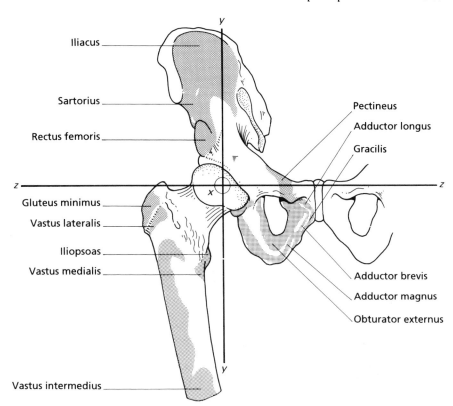

Fig. 20.2.2 Diagram to show the short lever arm of the abductors and the *x*, *y* and *z* components of hip joint force.

Labels on figure: Iliacus, Sartorius, Rectus femoris, Gluteus minimus, Vastus lateralis, Iliopsoas, Vastus medialis, Vastus intermedius, Pectineus, Adductor longus, Gracilis, Adductor brevis, Adductor magnus, Obturator externus

neck of the component during gait, from which the forces applied to the femoral head can be calculated. Rydell (1966) was the first to use such techniques when the femoral head alone had been replaced, while English and Kilvington (1979), utilizing a telemeterized system, were the first to provide such data from a total hip arthroplasty.

Paul (1976), Berme and Paul (1979) and Crowninshield *et al.* (1978) all emphasized the fact that, throughout the gait cycle, not only were there forces acting vertically downwards on the femoral head (the *y* component; see Fig. 20.2.2), but also forces tending to twist the femoral head on the femoral neck (the *x* component; see Fig. 20.2.2). Such forces act backwards during the initial stage of the gait cycle, immediately after heel strike, and forwards during the latter part of the gait cycle, immediately before toe-off. The posteriorly directed component of joint force becomes greatly increased with activities such as getting up from a chair or stair climbing, when the flexed hip is being extended and at the same time the body weight is being lifted (i.e. the body is being 'pushed up') against gravity by the hip. Calculations have suggested that this component of joint force may then reach from three times (Berme and Paul, 1979) to between five and six times (Crowninshield *et al.*, 1978) body weight. Berme and Paul depicted the effect such torsional forces might have on the femoral com-

ponent of a total hip arthroplasty (Fig. 20.2.3), and the '*in vivo*' torsional moments on the femoral head were directly measured in the more recent and very sophisticated *in vivo* strain gauge investigations of Davey *et al.* (1988) and Bergmann (1992) and their colleagues. These workers concluded that the 'out of plane' (i.e. torsional) moment on the femoral head during stair climbing might reach between 22 and 30 Nm. Even more recently, Brand *et al.* (1993) have both calculated and measured the hip joint forces in the same individual. The calculated forces were generally higher than those derived from the *in vivo* strain measurements, though the discrepancy was small. Their conclusions were that the peak resultant forces were in the range of 2.5–3.5 times body weight when walking at a freely selected speed, and the out of plane (i.e. twisting) forces 0.6–0.9 times body weight. These should probably be taken as the most accurate representation of the forces that have to be sustained by a total hip arthroplasty during level walking. They produce not only bending and twisting of the femoral component under cyclical load, but also complex loading of the acetabulum with very high loads on the posterior acetabular wall with activities such as stair-climbing or getting up from a chair.

Practical clinical observations that confirm the importance of torsional forces include the direction of plastic deformation (Fig. 20.2.4; Wroblewski, 1979)

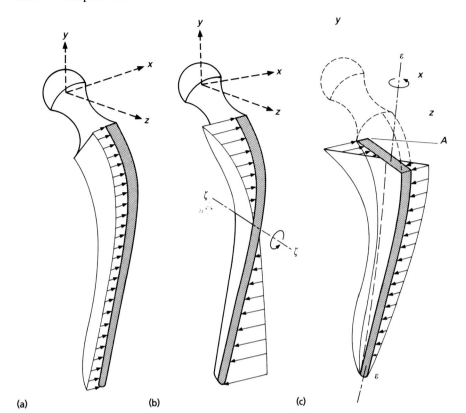

Fig. 20.2.3 The effect of the posteriorly directed component of hip joint force on the femoral component. (Redrawn from Berme and Paul, 1979.)

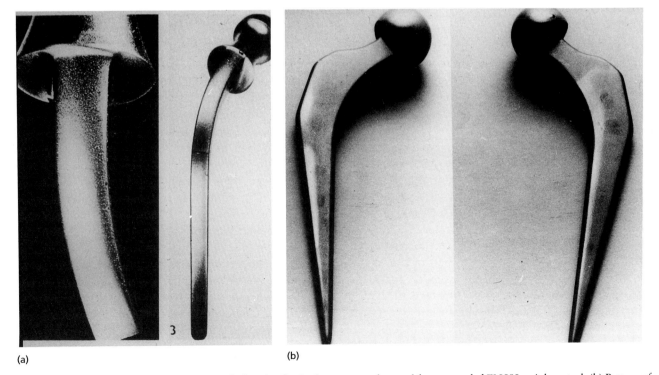

Fig. 20.2.4 (a) Plastic deformation of an original Charnley flat-back stem manufactured from annealed EN58J stainless steel. (b) Pattern of burnishing on a matt-surfaced Exeter stem indicating the action of torsional forces.

sometimes seen in femoral components manufactured from EN58J stainless steel (a ductile alloy) — always backwards; and the patterns of burnishing seen on matt-surfaced femoral components in association with localized endosteal bone lysis. Such patterns (Anthony *et al.*, 1990), produced by fretting of the stem surface against cement, always involve the medial half of the posterior surface of the stem, and lateral half of the anterior surface, and almost exactly reproduce Berme and Paul's diagram (Fig. 20.2.3).

As far as running and jumping are concerned, it is absolutely clear that such activities must be associated with marked increases in the forces applied to the femoral head. In this context, it is as well for the surgeon to be aware of the major deficiencies of the best artificial hip joint by comparison with the normal hip, the destruction of which has in the first place led the patient to seek surgery. The fact that in the normal hip there is no interface between living and inanimate structures is so obvious as hardly to require emphasis. Conventional total hip arthoplasty involves the sacrifice of the femoral head, a structure of great mechanical sophistication, and its replacement with a solid ball of alloy or ceramic of great structural stiffness. The trabecular systems of the femoral head constitute one of the main shock absorbers of the hip (Radin *et al.*, 1970), so that their sacrifice in this way adversely affects peak-load attenuation. Furthermore, the frictional properties of the bearing of the normal hip are about 70 times better than those of the best of current artificial joints. Moreover, there is, in the normal hip, no mechanism akin to impingement of the neck of the femoral component of an artificial joint against the margin of the cup. Such impingement is a further source of shock loading to the interface between implant and bone. Finally, the artificial hip does not have the benefits of the same levels of protective and proprioceptive sensation that grace the normal hip. Taking all these matters together, it is clear that excessive levels of physical activity on the part of patients who have received total hip arthroplasties are risky, to say the least. The point has never been made better than by Charnley, who, in his very first paper on total hip arthroplasty (1961), wrote: 'Objectives must be reasonable. Neither surgeons nor engineers will ever make an artificial hip joint which will last 30 years and at some time during this period enable the patient to play football'.

IMPLANT FIXATION AND TOTAL HIP REPLACEMENT

All orthopaedic surgeons know that satisfactory function following total hip replacement is dependent upon adequate fixation of the components of the arthroplasty to the femur and pelvis. There are certain fundamental facts concerning implant fixation to the human skeleton that are relevant whether cement is being used or not (Ling, 1986), and it is important that these are understood before considering implant fixation specifically related to cemented total hip arthroplasty. They can briefly be summarized as follows:

1 In engineering terms, there is no such thing as absolute fixation of an implant to bone (Swanson, 1977). There will always be *some* movement between them under load, even though its amplitude is miniscule and its precise site uncertain. That this theoretical assertion is true has been confirmed by two types of investigation. First, the sophisticated radiological technique of roentgen stereophotogrammetric analysis (RSA), originally described by Selvik (1974), and second, the direct measurement, in autopsy specimens, of micro-movement between implant and bone in hips known to have functioned asymptomatically *in vivo* (Maloney *et al.*, 1989; Engh *et al.*, 1992). The lower limit of resolution of RSA is of the order of 200 μm, whereas that of the direct measurement techniques is as little as 1.0 μm (Engh *et al.*, 1992).

RSA has shown that there are two types of movement between implant and bone: reversible or inducible displacement, and migration (Baldursson *et al.*, 1980; Green *et al.*, 1983; Mjoberg *et al.*, 1984). Reversible displacement is the recoverable movement that takes place between the weight-bearing and non-weight-bearing phases of each gait cycle (i.e. the loaded and unloaded states of the implant). Migration is the relative movement, over time, between the non-weight-bearing phases of successive gait cycles, and is not recoverable. Since migration is a phenomenon occurring over time, it cannot be measured in autopsy laboratory studies, whereas the reversible displacement in response to cyclical loading can. The amplitude of such reversible axial displacements, occurring between the femoral component and the proximal femoral cortex in autopsy retrievals and under loads comparable to those experienced '*in vivo*' in implants confirmed by subsequent histological examination to be well fixed, may reach 40 μm (Maloney *et al.*, 1989; Engh *et al.*, 1992) whether the femoral component is fixed with cement or by ingrowth of bone into porous surfaces. 40 μm is approximately four times the diameter of a human red blood cell, and a little less than the diameter of the narrowest human hair. Such figures have to be interpreted in the knowledge that the autopsy situation differs mechanically from that existing *in vivo*, primarily in that the action of muscles attached to the femur has not been realistically modelled *in vitro*. The magnitudes of cyclical displacements under load *in vitro* may therefore be somewhat lower than those actually occurring *in vivo*.

Exactly where this reversible axial displacement is occurring is uncertain. With a cemented femoral component, it might be distributed between movement occurring at the stem–cement interface, movement occurring within the cement, movement occurring at the cement–bone interface, and movement occurring within the cancellous bone, if any, separating the cement from the endosteal surface of the cortex. Charnley (1970) developed the thesis of the elasticity of the cement–bone bond in a chapter entitled 'The theory of mechanical fastenings in bone surgery' in his book *Acrylic Cement in Orthopaedic Surgery*. All trainees in orthopaedics should read this chapter, in which there is, incidentally, the first description of what subsequently has become known as 'osseointegration'.

Reversible displacement and migration are not necessarily related. All implants exhibit reversible displacement with the cyclical loading of everyday activities, but not all exhibit migration, though many may do so at various stages of their in-service life (Karrholm, 1989; Ryd, 1992). Neither of these types of movement are necessarily associated with symptoms (see later) on the part of the patient.

2 The initial fixation of *all* skeletal implants, from a single screw to the most complex of joint replacement components, depends upon the establishment of an initial mechanical interlock between the implant (including cement, if cement is being used) and the host bone.

3 The operating surgeon is wholly responsible for the establishment of that interlock, the strength of which depends on the tools and techniques that are employed during the course of the operation and on the strength of the bone that is involved in the interlock.

4 The strength of that interlock, created by the surgeon, in relation to the loads applied through the activities of the patient, determines the scale of movement between the implant and bone with each application of load during the first few post-operative months. This scale of movement is crucial for the nature of the junctional tissues that will subsequently develop between the implant and the bone.

5 Through the mechanical and vascular assault on the bone during the preparation of the implant site, the surgeon inevitably produces a peri-implant zone of bone necrosis. Even with the exceedingly delicate techniques used by the Branemark school (Albrektsson *et al.*, 1981) in the preparation of implant sites in the mandible and maxilla for the subsequent reception of endosteal dental implants, this zone of bone necrosis is never less than 100 µm in width. The techniques used by orthopaedic surgeons in the preparation of the femur and acetabulum during hip arthroplasty are, to say the least, grossly traumatic in comparison. As a consequence, the peri-implant site bone necrosis is more extensive. It must not be forgotten that many authors have shown that reaming the femoral canal effectively devascularizes the inner two-thirds of the femoral cortex (Sevitt, 1981). Thus, at the conclusion of the operation, the implant (including cement, if cement has been used) is 'fixed' to dead bone.

6 The mechanical and vascular assault at the implant site associated with the installation of the implant provokes an inflammatory response on the part of the patient as the first stage in the removal of the dead bone and the healing of the implant bed. The outcome of this process is the establishment of what may reasonably be termed the junctional tissues that will come to separate the implant from living bone during the in-service life of the implant. The nature of the junctional tissues that have been described in relation to both cemented and uncemented implants varies from direct contact between implant and living bone with no intervening cellular layer (osseointegration) (Albrektsson *et al.*, 1981; Linder and Hansson, 1983; Malcolm, 1990; Jasty *et al.*, 1990) to the presence of layers of fibrous tissue, sometimes up to 2 mm thick, separating the implant from living bone (Willert *et al.*, 1974; Freeman *et al.*, 1982; Cook *et al.*, 1991). Osseointegrated and fibrous interfaces may coexist in the same implant. This is probably the rule with uncemented ingrowth systems (Engh *et al.*, 1992), and may be with cemented ingrowth systems. The implant is stabilized in the bone by the junctional tissues, and therefore the mechanical behaviour of the latter is important. In the long term, implant fixation by osseointegration with direct bone-implant contact is regarded by Branemark *et al.* (1977) as superior both mechanically and biologically to fixation in fibrous tissue. Hori and Lewis (1982) pointed out the low elastic modulus of the latter. Thus, fibrous layers that intervene between implant and bone will inevitably increase the amplitude of cyclical movement between the two during the activities of daily living. This may have undesirable consequences (see below).

7 The control of the healing of the initial peri-implant necrosis is evidently of fundamental importance. There is now overwhelming evidence that the response of the skeleton to the insertion of an artificial joint component (given that the latter is manufactured from a non-reactive material) and the repair of the implant site necrosis depend, in practice, primarily on mechanical rather than material factors (Linder and Lundskog,

1974; Uhthoff, 1973; Uhthoff and Germain, 1977; Albrektsson *et al.*, 1981; Pilliar *et al.*, 1981, 1988; O'Carroll *et al.*, 1985; Linder *et al.*, 1988; Ling, 1986, 1989; Spector *et al.*, 1990). These mechanical factors are those that control movement between implant and bone during the early post-operative period, in other words, the balance between the strength of the initial mechanical interlock, created solely by the operating surgeon, and the loads applied by the activities of the patient. Only when the amplitudes of such movements under cyclical loads are below some as yet undetermined minimum, of the order of 50–100 µm, is the environment created that will allow bony healing of the implant bed (Albrektsson *et al.*, 1981; Pilliar *et al.*, 1988). The prime importance of operative technique in creating such an environment is obvious. Bioactive coatings, such as hydroxylapatite, make the mechanical factors less critical (Soballe *et al.*, 1992), but do not allow them to be ignored. As Linder has pointed out (1989), osseo-integration 'should be regarded not as an exclusive reaction to a specific implant material, but as the expression of a non-specific and basic healing potential in bone'. It is *entirely the surgeon's responsibility* to create the mechanical environment in which this healing potential can be fully expressed.

8 Bone turnover and bone remodelling do not cease simply because of the insertion of the components of an artificial joint. Adequate mechanical stress is the major stimulus for the maintenance of skeletal mass. Major changes in the mechanical environment to which the pelvis and femur are exposed inevitably follow the insertion of an artificial hip joint. These are reflected in the response made by living bone in the implant bed, through which load is transferred respectively to the endosteal surfaces of the femur and the acetabulum, that, in turn, respond to the new mechanical environment. The steady turnover of bone means that the bone in contact with the implant 1 year after the operation is not the same bone that is in contact with the implant 10 years after the operation. The inference is that all the factors that control bone turnover may influence continuing implant fixation.

This brief recapitulation of some of the basic facts of implant fixation should make it clear to the reader that the common tendency to place the subject, in its application to the hip, in an almost adversarial context— 'cement vs. cementless'—may, as Linder has said (1989) '. . . well miss the essence of the problem, because both cemented and uncemented implants have been shown to be anchored in bone, provided proper healing conditions prevail'.

CEMENT AND TOTAL HIP REPLACEMENT

Acrylic bone cement is probably the most abused bio-material, literally and figuratively, in use in the field of joint replacement. Ever since it was first used systematically at the hip by Charnley (1960) and by McKee and Watson-Farrar (1966), it has generated controversy, and still does. A striking finding on looking through the literature of cemented hip arthroplasty is the fact that, at 10 years of follow-up, there is no less than a ten-fold difference between the best and worst published figures for aseptic femoral component loosening (Sutherland *et al.*, 1982; Older, 1984; Hamilton and Joyce, 1986; Pavlov, 1987; Fowler *et al.*, 1988). Such findings suggest that the way cement is used may be of great importance, but nevertheless, many surgeons blamed the failures of cemented hip arthoplasty on fundamental failings of cement as a biomaterial. The concept of 'cement disease' emerged (Jones and Hungerford, 1987) with a catalogue of supposedly adverse properties of the material such that the unthinking surgeon might be forgiven for feeling that cement had no further place in hip arthroplasty. Among the failings of the material were the suggestions that it killed bone chemically and thermally, that it inevitably produced fibrous tissue, was not strong enough, was too brittle, caused cardiovascular collapse, attracted macrophages, interfered with leucocyte function, etc.

Cement became regarded as the 'weak link' in total hip arthroplasty. This concept was reinforced in 1979 with the revelation by Charnley (1979) that there was a five-fold increase in the rate of migration of cemented acetabular cups when the results in the same series of patients at 5 years of follow-up were compared with those at 10 years. These findings, coupled with the poor results of cemented arthroplasty in younger patients (Chandler *et al.*, 1981; Dorr *et al.*, 1983), were responsible for the swing away from cemented arthroplasty that took place during the early 1980s in some parts of the world.

More recently, however, it has been realized that uncemented arthroplasties are far from trouble free, being associated with a tiresome incidence of thigh pain (Campbell *et al.*, 1992; Barrack *et al.*, 1992) and an increasing incidence of endosteal bone lysis (Schmalzried *et al.*, 1992) formerly thought to be primarily a complication of cemented arthroplasties. It has also become clear that bone ingrowth into porous surfaced cementless femoral components is not as common as had been anticipated (Cook *et al.*, 1991), primarily because of the difficulty of obtaining a primary mechanical interlock that is strong enough to control interface movement during the early post-operative period. Moreover, the achievement of bone ingrowth is no guarantee against thigh pain (Barrack *et al.*, 1992) or loosening (Jasty *et al.*, 1991).

The recognition of these problems with some cement-free devices emerged at the same as it was becoming increasingly clear that refinements in the techniques of using cement were capable of greatly improving the results of cemented arthroplasties (Wroblewski and van der Rijt, 1984; Roberts *et al.*, 1986; Timperley *et al.*, 1992), even in younger patients (Barrack *et al.*, 1992; Wroblewski and Siney, 1992) and in revisions (Rubash and Harris, 1988; Gie *et al.*, 1993). The improvement has been seen primarily with regard to the performance of the cemented femoral component. Although improvements in the techniques of cement fixation of the acetabular component have certainly occurred, these have not had such evidently satisfactory outcomes as they have in the femur. This has led to the concept of the 'hybrid hip' (Harris and Maloney, 1989), in which a cemented femoral component has been combined with an uncemented socket. The experience of Charnley, however, referred to above, and of Morscher and his colleagues (1984, 1988), has made it clear that no conclusions should be drawn with regard to the outcome of acetabular cup fixation without a follow-up of at least a decade. There is, moreover, some evidence beginning to emerge that wear of the polyethylene socket may be increased in cementless hips associated with metal-backing of the cup (Ritter, 1992, personal communication).

IMPLANT FIXATION USING CEMENT IN TOTAL HIP ARTHROPLASTY

Traditionally, cement in its relationship to total hip arthroplasty has been spoken of as functioning as a 'grout'. The definition of a grout given in the *Shorter Oxford Dictionary* is 'a thin fluid mortar for filling interstices'. Such a definition does not adequately describe acrylic cement as it should be used today in total hip arthroplasty, where it subserves two functions. First, it is the means whereby the implant is 'fixed' to the bone, and second, it is part of the fundamental mechanism of load transmission into the femur and pelvis. Unless the surgeon views it in this way, he may tend to treat the material without the care that is necessary for the consistent achievement of satisfactory results in cemented hip arthroplasty.

As with any other implant, the initial fixation of acrylic cement to bone depends upon the establishment

of a mechanical interlock between the bone and the cement. The unique feature of acrylic cement that allows it to obtain such mechanical interlock with bone is its ability, in the dough state, to take an incredibly detailed cast of any surface with which it comes into contact. Polymerization then locks that cast into the bone and into the cement. Figure 20.2.5 shows the surface of the acrylic cement surrounding a femoral component of a total hip arthroplasty from a patient who died of a ruptured aortic aneurysm 10 days after operation. The bone has been dissolved away from the cement surface, revealing the astonishingly detailed 'mirror image' of the internal surface of the femur that the cement has taken in achieving mechanical interlock. Not even a custom-made implant could ever achieve such an intimate reflection of the internal structure of the femur.

Cement as a material

Bone cement as it is used most commonly at present is self-curing poly methyl methacrylate. It is generally supplied to the operating theatre in 40 g sterile packs of powdered polymer granules and separate glass phials of 20 g of the monomeric methyl ester of methacrylic acid. The polymer may or may not contain a co-polymer, depending upon the brand of cement. In addition, the pack contains, as a rule, a radio-opacifier that is usually zirconium oxide or barium sulphate, together with small amounts (2–3%) of benzoyl peroxide that acts as the activator to the free-radical-assisted polymerization reaction. The fluid component contains, as well as the monomer, small amounts (approximately 2%) of an initiator, a tertiary amine, usually dimethyl para-

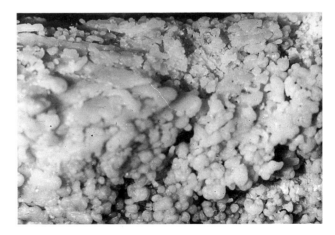

Fig. 20.2.5 Surface of acrylic cement from which the femur has been dissolved away to show the astonishingly accurate cast of the endosteal surface of the femur that has been taken by the cement in the dough stage.

toluidune, and a few parts per million of an inhibitor (usually ascorbic acid or hydroquinone) to prevent spontaneous polymerization of the monomer.

The powder and fluid components are mixed to form a dough. The monomer dissolves the exterior of the co-polymer beads with the release of residual benzoyl peroxide and also takes the polymer into solution. The benzoyl peroxide causes polymerization of the monomer to start, and there is an increase in the viscosity of the dough. The time course of the viscosity changes varies according to the brand of cement. Polymerization of the monomer is an exothermic reaction, the amount of heat being generated depending on the amount of monomer polymerizing (Jefferiss *et al.*, 1975). As polymerization proceeds, the dough is gradually changed with rising viscosity from a fluid to a solid, the whole process, which is very temperature sensitive, taking from 8 to 13 minutes in an ambient temperature of 20°C.

MECHANICAL PROPERTIES

An enormous amount of laboratory work has been done in many centres throughout the world in connection with the mechanical properties of acrylic cement. The interested reader is referred to the review of Saha and Pal (1984) for an excellent summary of this work in connection with the static and fatigue properties of the material.

In essence, acrylic cement is an amorphous polymer that is fundamentally weak in tension (approximately 25 MPa), relatively strong in compression (75 MPa) with an elastic modulus between those of cancellous and cortical bone (Lee *et al.*, 1973). Even heat-cured acrylic (perspex), which is stronger than self-cured acrylic cement, is fundamentally weak in tension. The mechanical properties of cement may be significantly affected by a number of variables, some of which are under the control of the operating surgeon (Halawa *et al.*, 1978). For example, laminations and blood entrapment may seriously weaken cement. In practical use, however, the most important factors leading to the reliable function of cement are, first, to provide it with adequate physical constraint by bone, and second, to endeavour to maintain compression as the dominant mode of loading.

As with all polymers, temperature changes have a major effect on the mechanical behaviour of cement, affecting its viscoelastic properties to a greater extent than its elastic properties (Lee *et al.*, 1990). The change from room to body temperature, for example, produces approximately a 15% reduction in elastic modulus and a three-fold increase in the rate of tensile creep. The viscoelastic behaviour of cement confers upon it load-

spreading, shock-absorbing and decoupling properties that might be thought advantageous in joint replacement surgery.

Anxieties over the relatively low-tensile fatigue strength of cement have led to attempts to improve its fatigue behaviour by eliminating porosities through vacuum mixing or centrifugation (Wixson, 1992). There is no doubt whatsoever that these procedures do increase significantly the fatigue life of cement in the laboratory. Whether they prolong the life of cemented hip arthroplasties in practice is as yet unknown. Furthermore, the excellent long-term results obtained by some surgeons without vacuum mixing or centrifugation will make a relevant controlled trial a statistical nightmare.

VOLUMETRIC CHANGES AT POLYMERIZATION

This is a complex matter. The liquid monomer contracts by just over 20% by volume when it polymerizes. Since monomer makes up one-third of the volume of the cement dough, polymerization changes alone might be expected to result in contraction of approximately 6–7% by volume. However, polymerization is also accompanied by the production of heat, and a variable rise in temperature. The latter will cause thermal expansion. There are thus two processes occurring simultaneously, one of which causes expansion and the other contraction. Furthermore, the increase in temperature may be responsible for the expansion of any voids in the dough containing air or monomer vapour, with further changes in the overall volume. There must be marked differences in heat production and dissipation at different sites in relation to the implant, depending on the local amounts of cement and conducting abilities of the surrounds. The alloy femoral component, of course, constitutes a major 'heat sink'.

The final volume of cement, after cooling, probably represents a small overall shrinkage by comparison with the volume of dough. Such shrinkage may be mechanically significant where 'microinterlock' (see below) has not been achieved by the operating surgeon.

BIOCOMPATIBILITY

The biocompatibility of acrylic cement has been heavily criticized on a number of grounds, of which the most common are the following:

Local and systemic toxicity

Hullinger (1962) demonstrated years ago in tissue culture that pure methyl methacrylate monomer was cytotoxic. The direct exposure of cells in culture to continuing high concentrations of pure monomer, however, is very different from the exposure of the host bone to monomer during the performance of total hip arthroplasty. Linder (1977) has shown that the acute chemical trauma produced by acrylic cement dough adds nothing to the mechanical and vascular trauma already produced by the preparation of the implant site.

From the systemic standpoint, absorbed monomer has been blamed for the adverse cardiovascular effects sometimes reported using acrylic cement. There is no doubt whatsoever that monomer is absorbed into the central circulation during total hip arthroplasty. It is, however, then rapidly metabolized to methacrylic acid (Crout *et al.*, 1979) and this subsequently enters the tricarboxylic acid cycle via methacrylyl co-enzyme A, then following the same pathway as valine (Crout *et al.*, 1979, 1982). There is no relationship between the time course of the changing concentrations of monomer or methacrylic acid in the central venous circulation and cardiovascular changes that may be seen following the insertion of cement, and no evidence to implicate monomer as their cause.

The exotherm of polymerization

The effects of the exothermic reaction of the polymerization of acrylic cement dough are controversial, to say the least, but have been another fruitful field for the criticism of the material. Some (Huiskes, 1979; Mjoberg *et al.*, 1984; Mjoberg, 1986) have taken the view that thermal necrosis of bone secondary to the exotherm of polymerization is a major problem with the use of acrylic cement, and is a contributor to loosening. Others (Jefferiss *et al.*, 1975; Reckling and Dillon, 1977) have concluded that it is of less significance, pointing out that any thermal effect exerted by polymerizing cement follows not only the mechanical and vascular assault of implant site preparation, but also such chemical trauma that the monomer may exert. They also emphasized the point that the amount of heat generated by the polymerization of acrylic cement depends on the amount of monomer polymerizing, the polymerization of 1 gram-molecular weight of monomer (that happens to be 100 g) having a heat output of 13 000 cals. The temperature developed at the interface between bone and cement depends not only on the amount of heat produced, but also on the rate at which it can be dissipated. The latter, in turn, depends upon the thermal properties of the tissues in contact with the cement. Cement polymerizing in air (an insulator) can lose heat only slowly, and therefore the cement surface may become hot. The

asperities of cement shown in Fig. 20.2.6 are no more than 2−3 mm in diameter, with a maximal volume of less than 15 mm^3. This volume of cement dough produces at polymerization no more than 0.65 calorie (Jefferiss *et al.*, 1975) and is therefore incapable of producing a significant rise in temperature locally at the interface.

The significance of the exotherm of polymerization as far as the production of loosening is concerned will remain a matter for controversy until a randomized controlled trial of the use of conventional and low temperature curing cement has been performed.

The tissue reaction to cement

It has been asserted on more than one occasion in the past that the histological reaction to acrylic cement is always that of fibrous tissue formation (Willert *et al.*, 1974; Vernon-Roberts and Freeman, 1976; Freeman *et al.*, 1982). Charnley (1970) was the first to deny this years ago and now direct contact between cement and living bone without the intervention of fibrous layers has been described by a number of authors, including Linder and Hansson (1983), Malcolm (1990) and Jasty *et al.* (1990). This is the consequence of the creation at the time of the operation of a mechanical environment between cement and bone that allows the expression of the basic healing potential of bone. The fact that such direct contact can persist over many years, allowing bone turnover without interface breakdown, does suggest that, whatever experimental evidence there is to the contrary, the biocompatibility of acrylic cement in bulk form in this situation cannot be in real doubt. In particulate form, of course, the situation is different, but this applies no less to all the other biomaterials used in hip arthroplasty (see below).

A most important observation (Maloney *et al.*, 1989) in relation to bone repair adjacent to cement has been the observation that, in well-fixed specimens, the scale of micromovement between the cemented femoral component and the femoral cortex in autopsy retrievals has been of the same order as that in freshly cemented autopsy specimens, utilizing contemporary cementing techniques. This means that the repair response to the implanted cement has not weakened the initial mechanical interlock.

Pre-operative planning and surgical exposure in cemented total hip arthroplasty

PRE-OPERATIVE PLANNING

Pre-operative planning with the use of templates appropriate for the prosthesis that is to be employed is a useful exercise in assessing the size of the implants that are likely to be needed, and their probable positioning as necessary for restoration of leg length. It helps the surgeon to plan for any necessary augmentation of bone deficiencies and may draw attention to other potential difficulties to be encountered during the course of the operation.

SURGICAL EXPOSURE FOR CEMENTED TOTAL HIP ARTHROPLASTY

The precise surgical exposure to be used is very much a matter for the surgeon's choice. The surgeon should be familiar with the main anterior, anterolateral, lateral and posterior exposures. What matters is that the exposure employed should give a full and free view of the acetabulum and proximal femur, since it is not possible to utilize contemporary cementing techniques properly through limited access. Over vigorous retraction should be avoided. Pre-operative planning should lead to anticipation of situations in which both the anterior and posterior aspects of the acetabulum or proximal femur need to be exposed. Such cases are generally revisions with loss of bone stock that requires augmentation by grafting.

If the patient is to be operated upon when lying on his or her side, the pelvis must be properly stabilized on the operating table, and the lumbar lordosis should not be obliterated by overflexing the contralateral hip. If this mistake is made, the cup is likely to be retroverted when the lordosis reappears after the operation, and dislocation may ensue.

Cementing technique in primary interventions

Cementing technique is concerned with the way in which the initial mechanical interlock between cement and bone is established. The importance of the initial mechanical interlock in controlling implant micromovement, and therefore the structure of the junctional tissues, has already been emphasized. Charnley himself clearly recognized this. He realized that his own findings in respect of the histology of the cement–bone interface were at variance with what was then current thinking, i.e. that cement was always associated with a fibrous layer. He explained the difference thus (Charnley, 1979): 'It is postulated that sound mechanical fixation (resulting from good cement technique) is responsible for the absence of thick layers of collagenised fibrous tissue intervening between cement and bone'. The importance of cementing technique is obvious.

Interlock may be achieved with the trabeculae of cancellous bone, described by Miller *et al.* (1978b) as 'microinterlock', or with the gross features of the bony cavity—'macrointerlock'—or with both, the latter being desirable where possible.

Much experimental work has been performed in many laboratories throughout the world in an effort to develop methods of improving the strength of the initial interlock that can be achieved between cement and bone. In general, these investigations have shown that the maximal shear strength of the interface is achieved when cement of reduced viscosity is forced under pressure into the trabecular spaces of strong cancellous bone that have been thoroughly cleaned of all clots and tissue debris (Halawa *et al.*, 1978; Krause *et al.*, 1980, 1982). Such methods have regularly achieved, in the laboratory setting, fourfold increases in the shear strength of the interface by comparison with the use of standard techniques.

Most of this experimental work was carried out in cadaver models, where there is no bleeding. During an actual hip arthroplasty, however, bleeding from the bone surface may be tiresome. Bleeding pressures in the medullary canal of up to 36 cm of water have been recorded (Heyse-Moore and Ling, 1982) during hip arthroplasty. Benjamin *et al.* (1987) have shown, in a laboratory study, that bleeding pressures of levels regularly found in the femur during hip arthroplasty are capable of displacing Simplex cement dough away from bone at any time up to 6 min after the beginning of mixing. These findings are important. They cast doubt on the conclusions from laboratory studies of cementing techniques in cadavers or laboratory models that do not include bleeding. Furthermore, they have implications for the practical use of cement. Unless the cement dough is held against the bone surface under pressures that exceed the bleeding pressure within the bone until the viscosity of the cement is high enough, on its own, to resist the bleeding, the latter may compromise the interface (Benjamin *et al.*, 1987; Bannister and Miles, 1988). This is a particularly important matter in revision surgery, where the opportunities for the achievement of microinterlock may be limited because of compromise of bone stock.

CEMENTING TECHNIQUE IN THE FEMUR

Cementing techniques in the femur can be divided into two broad groups (Ling, 1991). What might be termed traditional techniques are those in which the penetration of the bone by the cement is achieved primarily by the interface pressure that is generated by the femoral component as it is driven into the femur. Contemporary techniques are those in which pressurization of the cement into the endosteal bone of the femur is achieved by the use of suitable instrumentation before the insertion of the femoral component. Any extra penetration generated by the latter is a bonus.

It is absolutely essential for the operating surgeon to understand two basic points, whether opting for traditional or contemporary techniques:
1 During the insertion of the femoral component, the cement−bone interface pressure is directly related to the viscosity of the cement (Fagan, 1984) (Fig. 20.2.6). The

important corollary is that the insertion of the femoral component into cement of reduced viscosity cannot generate any significant bone−cement interface pressure, leaving the interface potentially open to disruption from bleeding at the bone surface. Failure to recognize this point is a real cause of premature failure from loosening.
2 If an intramedullary plug is being used, the cement−bone interface pressures during stem insertion are maximal distally (Markolf and Amstutz, 1976; Oh *et al.*, 1978; Fagan, 1984). Modifications of technique are necessary to obtain satisfactory interface pressures in the proximal third of the femur (see below).

Femoral canal preparation

The most serious error during the preparation of the femoral canal is the removal of too much cancellous bone. While loose and weak cancellous bone should be removed with a brush, the canal must not be entirely stripped of cancellous bone, since this then creates what is, in effect, a revision situation in a primary intervention, with no chance of achieving microinterlock. The danger is most obvious when the surgeon is preparing to insert a stem that is too large for the canal in question.

Femoral pressurization

Satisfactory pressurization of the femoral canal can only be achieved by first converting it into a 'closed space'. This requires the obliteration of the canal distally, about 2 cm beyond the point at which the tip of the prosthesis will eventually reside, and some method of occluding the proximal opening of the canal while still allowing access to the canal for the injection of cement.

An intramedullary plug is the easiest way to occlude the canal distally. The fit must be very tight. Once the plug has been inserted, the canal should be cleaned, using a pressurized lavage system, and then dried. The latter is best achieved by packing the canal with 5 cm ribbon gauze soaked in ten volumes % hydrogen peroxide, or by using iced saline. The canal is then ready for cement insertion, which may be carried out in one of three ways:
1 Digitally and orthograde, using the 'two thumb' method and relatively viscous cement. An exhaust vent is necessary. The technique is most appropriate following trochanteric osteotomy, when the shape of the upper femur lends itself well to pressurization in this way.
2 Orthograde insertion of the cement by the 'suck-down' technique, in which suction is applied to the exhaust vent as digital cement insertion proceeds. This

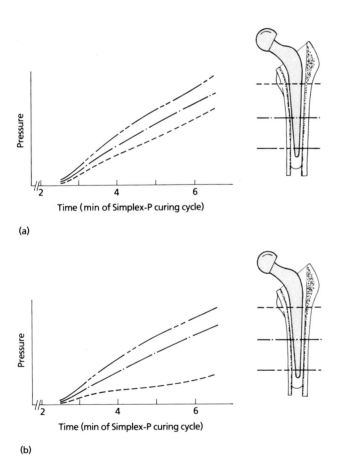

Fig. 20.2.6 The relative pressures produced at sample positions (a) medial and (b) lateral on the cement−bone interface during the insertion of an Exeter stem in to a plugged cavity at different times of the cement during the curing cycle and therefore different viscosities.

technique has two drawbacks. It may lead to more effective filling of the distal canal than the proximal, and sizeable air bubbles may be carried down with the cement unless great care is taken with the digital packing while the suction is active.

3 Retrograde filling of the canal using a cement gun with a spout long enough to reach the plug. This technique requires considerable attention to detail, and filling should be done under direct vision. The latter requires a full exposure of the proximal femur. A suitable proximal cement seal should be available that will fit over the spout. Once the canal has been filled, the gun spout is amputated immediately distal to the seal, and the latter is impacted into the proximal opening of the femur, occluding it and then allowing pressurization of the femur by the continued injection of cement into the closed cavity (Fig. 20.2.7). During this process, if done properly, there should be a steady extrusion of medullary fat through the cortical wall of the proximal femur. Unless the distal plug and the proximal seal are tight, i.e. the canal really has been made into a closed space, the method is best avoided. Satisfactory pressurization of the proximal canal cannot be achieved without a properly fitting seal. Without the latter, the risk of filling the distal canal more effectively than the proximal is very real.

Once the surgeon has mastered this technique, it has much to offer. It does need attention to detail, and unless the surgeon understands the method and is prepared to practice it correctly, he will do better by using method 1 above.

Femoral component insertion

The femoral component should not be inserted until the viscosity of the cement dough has risen sufficiently to prevent any contamination of the interface by bleeding. The later stem insertion is left, the better, provided of

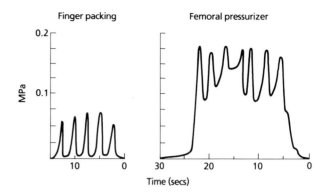

Fig. 20.2.7 Pressure recordings from within the medullary canal proximally and medially during finger packing of cement compared with the use of the proximal femoral seal pressurizer.

course that it is not left too late. Accurate insertion of an appropriately sized stem is necessary for the creation of a complete cement mantle around the stem, a matter of importance for the long-term function of the arthroplasty (see below). As the stem is being inserted, the surgeon should occlude the exit from the canal around the advancing stem. During stem insertion, proximal cement–bone interface pressures are low unless this manoeuvre is carried out (Fig. 20.2.8). Distal cement–bone interface pressures are high during stem insertion (Markolf and Amstutz, 1976; Oh *et al.*, 1978; Fagan, 1984).

Once the stem has reached its final position, the proximal canal should be sealed round the proximal stem, using an appropriate seal, and pressure maintained on the seal until the cement has polymerized (Fowler *et al.*, 1988). Polymerization can be accelerated at this stage by using a pre-warmed stem (Dall *et al.*, 1986b). The stem must not be moved while polymerization is awaited.

If the surgeon leaves stem insertion too late, and is unable to insert it completely, he should take a high-

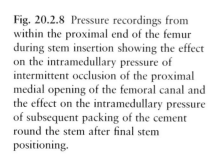

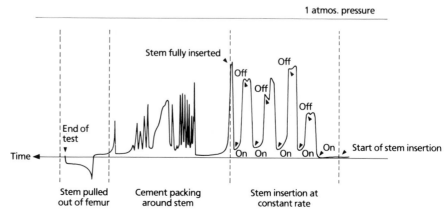

Fig. 20.2.8 Pressure recordings from within the proximal end of the femur during stem insertion showing the effect on the intramedullary pressure of intermittent occlusion of the proximal medial opening of the femoral canal and the effect on the intramedullary pressure of subsequent packing of the cement round the stem after final stem positioning.

speed burr and enlarge and extend the internal dimensions of the cement mantle until there is sufficient room for the stem. The cavity should then be dried, a small further mix of cement inserted, and the stem driven in. The new cement bonds to the old in this situation, providing the cavity is dry. This is quicker, easier and safer than attempting to remove all the cement before starting again, and does not compromise the bone stock in the femoral canal.

CEMENTING TECHNIQUE IN THE ACETABULUM

There is considerable controversy over the best method of preparing and cementing the acetabulum. Nevertheless, the principle of obtaining both microinterlock and macrointerlock applies to the acetabulum just as much as it does to the femur. Microinterlock throughout the whole acetabulum is virtually impossible to achieve without removing the subchondral cortical plate, and the superficial cortex of the floor just above the tear drop. Many surgeons prefer to leave the cortical bone, and rely on obtaining microinterlock in the walls and roof of drill holes or fixation pits made through the cortical subchondral plate. There is however a school of thought (to which the authors belong, as well as Amstutz *et al.*, 1991, and Kerboul, 1985) that believes decortication is appropriate where possible, as long as the subchondral cancellous bone is not severely osteopenic, with preservation of the cortical layer immediately above the tear drop. The unsolved technical problem is to obtain microinterlock near the margins of the cavity, since if the ingress of particulate debris is to be resisted, it is here that direct contact between cement and living bone is required.

There is no concensus over the best combination of fixation pits and drill holes. Curettes and Capener-type long-handled gouges are useful for creating fixation pits, especially in the ischium.

There is no doubt that full bony cover for the acetabular component is necessary (Sarmiento *et al.*, 1990). Augmentation of the acetabulum by grafting may be required to achieve this. Autogenous grafts from the femoral head or the iliac crest are appropriate, using the techniques described by Marti and Besselaar (1981). Deficiencies of the medial wall are best dealt with using the grafting technique of Slooff *et al.* (1984).

Once the surgeon has prepared the acetabular cavity and created full bony cover for the acetabular cup, with cancellous allografting on the socket floor as necessary, the cavity must be cleaned and dried. Pressure lavage followed by packing with gauze soaked in 10 vols % hydrogen peroxide is the authors' preference. The gauze is held under pressure in the socket until the cement dough is ready for insertion and then removed to allow the dough to be packed manually into the drill holes and fixation pits. Some form of pressurization for the whole acetabular cavity is then appropriate. The acetabular pressurizer described by Lee and Ling (Lee and Ling, 1974) is effective when correctly used, and can be combined with the subsequent insertion of a flanged cup (Oh *et al.*, 1985; Shelley and Wroblewski, 1988) in an effort to maintain pressure up until polymerization. As in the femur, the cup should not be introduced until the viscosity of the cement is high enough to resist, on its own, bleeding from the bone surface.

Eccentric cups and thin walled polythene cups should not be used and metal backing, of possible though not certain advantage in theory, has given no advantage in practice and may well be deleterious from the standpoints of socket wear and loosening.

THE JUSTIFICATION FOR THE USE OF CONTEMPORARY CEMENTING TECHNIQUES

In the femur

In vitro experimental studies comparing the stability of cemented and uncemented components have shown that, whereas comparable axial stability can be achieved with or without cement, contemporary cementing offers a significant advantage as far as torsional stability is concerned (Burke *et al.*, 1991; Callaghan *et al.*, 1992). Similar conclusions were reached from *in vivo* animal experiments by Vanderby *et al.* (1989). RSA studies have shown that properly cemented femoral components exhibit less early migration than cementless components (Karrholm *et al.*, 1992), even when the latter were coated with hydroxyl apatite. There are a number of clinical series that have now been reported showing how contemporary cementing improves the outcome for cemented femoral components (Wroblewski and van der Rijt, 1984; Roberts *et al.*, 1986; Timperley *et al.*, 1992; Barrack *et al.*, 1992; Wroblewski, 1993). The study of Timperley *et al.* is of particular significance, since in the series that they reported only one surgeon and one type of prosthesis were involved.

In the acetabulum

The improvements in results in the socket from the use of contemporary cementing has not been as marked as in the femur. Nevertheless, for those surgeons who do use cement in the socket, these techniques have shown themselves to be useful.

Cementing technique in revision surgery

The major problem with the use of cement in revision surgery lies in the loss of bone stock that is so frequently associated with loosening. There may be little or no residual cancellous bone in the femoral canal, the walls of which may be extremely thin or non-existent in places. The surface of the wall of the canal is usually smooth and shiny, presenting little chance of achieving microinterlock through conventional cementing techniques. These bone stock problems frequently make it impossible to obtain the level of implant stability that is necessary for the subsequent development of direct contact between cement and living bone.

In 1984, Slooff *et al.* (1984) reported on the use of a technique in which bone stock deficiencies in the acetabulum were made up with impacted allograft chips, onto which cement was then pressurized. This produced 'microinterlock' between the cement and allograft chips. The results with this method have proved satisfactory to date. A similar technique has now been reported in the femur (Gie *et al.*, 1993), with extremely rewarding reconstitution of bone stock in association with clinical outcomes that approach those for primary interventions, even where the bone stock is heavily compromised. The longest follow-up of the method in the femur does not at present exceed 7 years, but nevertheless it shows promise. The impaction of the allograft chips with this technique is crucial in achieving adequate stability, and experimentally, the proper use of cement improves stability further (Schreurs *et al.*, 1991). The major technical point with these techniques, however, aside from the ability to achieve stability, is that the graft is fixed to the implant, cement being regarded as part of the latter. In effect, therefore, the cement is being coated with graft, so that movement between graft and implant is minimized. This distinguishes the technique from those in which similar grafts are used with uncemented components, where there is inevitably movement between the implant and the graft.

IMPLANT DESIGN IN CEMENTED HIP ARTHROPLASTY

The design criteria for the components of a cemented hip arthroplasty are superficially straightforward. First and most obviously, the device must provide for a suitable range of movement at the articulation. Second, it must transmit the loads generated at the articulation into the femur and pelvis in a reliable manner without causing pain, bone destruction or adverse bone remodelling. Third, it must subserve these functions over years, and preferably for the lifetime of the patient. Finally, if circumstances arise that dictate that the device should be removed, this should be achievable without major damage to the host such that the subsequent replacement of the device becomes a surgical 'Waterloo'.

These apparently simple criteria have spawned a staggering number of different designs that increases year by year. For each, the designers will claim advantages based usually on theoretical, cadaveric and computer simulation studies. For a few, such claims are backed up by long-term clinical performance reports. What the tiro should appreciate, however, is that even the most reliable implant is discredited by incompetent surgery, and that surgery of a high level of expertise can mask unfavourable implant design features, at least up to the medium term. Moreover, all implants, good or bad, are eventually destroyed by persistently unrealistic levels of physical activity on the part of the patient.

The femoral component

LOAD TRANSMISSION

Since the function of the femoral component in hip arthroplasty is to transmit the loads generated at the articular surface into the femur, it is useful, as a preliminary to a consideration of femoral component design, to examine the structure of the normal femoral head and the way in which the trabecular systems of the latter transmit loads into the femoral diaphysis. The subchondral cortical bone of the femoral head is extremely thin (Fig. 20.2.9), and this thin cortical layer continues down into the femoral neck, only becoming thicker in this region as it receives *from within and from above down* the insertions of the medial weight-bearing trabecular system. The superior trabecular arch, often spoken of as the tensile trabeculae of the femoral head, insert in a similar way into the thin cortical bone immediately below the greater trochanter. This bone similarly becomes gradually thicker as successive trabeculae run into it. Although the superior trabecular arch is often regarded as being in tension, Fig. 20.2.10, taken from St. Clair Strange's classic book *The Hip*, makes it quite clear that this trabecular system must normally be loaded in compression.

Thus, both medially and laterally, the proximal diaphyseal cortex is loaded from within through the trabecular systems of the femoral head. It naturally follows that, after total hip arthroplasty, the most nearly physiological way of loading the proximal femur would be by utilizing these same trabecular systems. This can be achieved by the surface replacement or so-called 'double

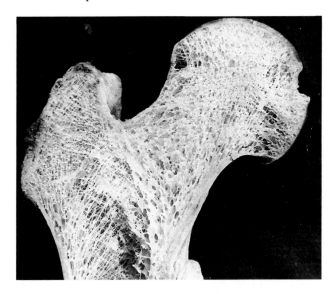

Fig. 20.2.9 Coronal section of the upper femur to demonstrate thin subchondral cortical bone and emphasize the trabecular arrangements.

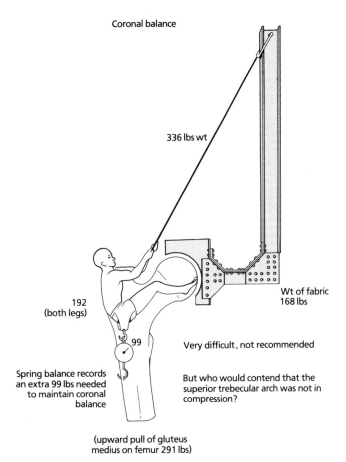

Fig. 20.2.10 Diagram to illustrate compressive loading of the superior trabecular arch — (after St Clair Strange).

cup' type of arthroplasty reported by Freeman (1978) and by Amstutz *et al.* (1977). Unfortunately, this procedure was associated with a number of complications (Freeman, 1984) that led to it being abandoned by many surgeons. There can be no doubt, however, that if the technical and materials problems associated with the technique could be solved, it would reappear as the most physiological form of total hip replacement, and the only one in which the peak-load attenuating function of the femoral head could be retained. At the same time, it would entirely overcome the actual and perceived problems relating to stress shielding of the proximal femur with conventional stemmed arthroplasties.

Load transmitted from the hip joint to the head of a stemmed type of femoral component passes down the stem, across the stem–cement interface, through the cement, across the cement–bone interface and then into any trabecular bone layer that may persist between the cement and the cortex, finally passing, thereby into the endosteal surface of the cortex itself. Such loads are not only axial, but also torsional. The precise sites at which load is actually shed from the stem to the femur depend upon a number of factors that include the technique of the operation to install the stem, the geometry of the stem itself, and the nature of the interfaces between stem and bone. In particular, soft tissue at the interfaces interferes with the direct transmission of load into bone.

The maintenance of cortical mass and integrity depends upon adequate mechanical stimulation through load transmission. If the component geometry and interface structure in any given case are such that a substantial part of the load entering the proximal end of the stem by-passes the proximal femur, then stress shielding of the proximal femur in some degree is the outcome (Fig. 20.2.11). The latter is seen at its most marked where a very stiff, porous coated, uncemented stem becomes osseointegrated in the mid-diaphysis (Engh *et al.*, 1992). Such profound levels of stress shielding are not seen with cemented stems because of the presence of the relatively low modulus layer of cement between the stem and the bone that also acts, in virtue of its viscoelastic properties, as a load-spreader and a decoupler. Nevertheless, both proximal diaphyseal bone loss (McCarthy *et al.*, 1991) and distal diaphyseal hypertrophy may be seen with cemented stems, particularly where proximal cementing is defective (Fig. 20.2.12), and indicates an increase in distal transmission of load, simply because the cement has never properly engaged the proximal endosteal trabeculae. Timperley *et al.* (1992) showed that one of the effects of contemporary as opposed to traditional cementing techniques was the complete abolition of subsequent diaphyseal hyper-

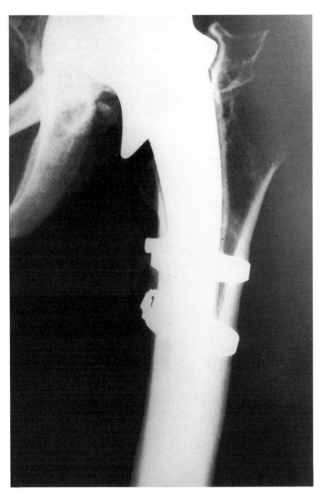

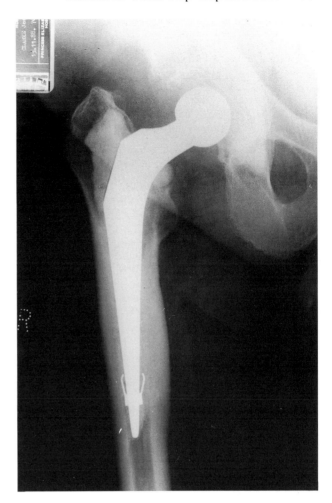

Fig. 20.2.11 Uncemented Thompson stem with proximal stress shielding in association with distal fixation in a small medullary canal.

Fig. 20.2.12 Diaphyseal hypertrophy with cement.

trophy, even when the same stem geometries were being used by the same operator. This can only be because of the greatly improved cement injection into the trabeculae of the proximal femur with contemporary techniques, and a consequent improvement in proximal load transmission to the endosteal cortex.

While the loads generated at the articular surface contribute substantially to the overall loads to be sustained by the femur, it is important to realize that substantial loading comes also through the activity and attachment of muscles. Munih *et al.* (1992) have recently developed Pauwels' thesis that one of the main functions of muscle is to minimize the effects of bending moments on long bones. At the hip, the most important muscle group from this standpoint is the so-called 'pelvic deltoid' (Fig. 20.2.13) described by Henry (1973). This muscle is made up of three-quarters of gluteus maximus together with tensor fascia lata, and acts, through its insertion

into the ilio-tibial tract, as a major lateral tension band for the femur. It is one among a number of muscles that influence the deformation of the femur *in vivo* (Rybicki *et al.*, 1972; Rohlmann *et al.*, 1982). Such deformation thus does not depend purely on the structural stiffness of the femur alone, a fact that raises serious questions over the concept of 'isoelasticity' in femoral component design. It means, moreover, that an attitude of healthy scepticism is appropriate when considering any work dealing with femoral stresses in which muscular activity has not been realistically modelled, either in the laboratory or by the computer.

FEMORAL COMPONENT GEOMETRY

This has always been a very controversial subject. Fashions have changed with time, and new designs have not always represented progress. Until the mid-1970s,

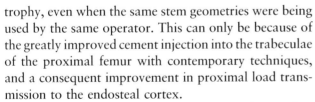

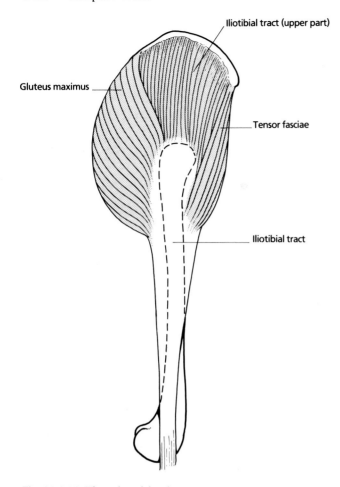

Fig. 20.2.13 The pelvic deltoid.

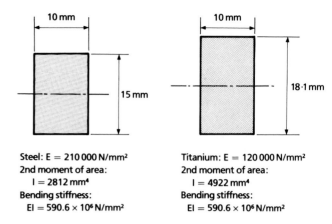

Steel: E = 210 000 N/mm²
2nd moment of area:
 I = 2812 mm⁴
Bending stiffness:
 EI = 590.6 × 10⁶ N/mm²

Titanium: E = 120 000 N/mm²
2nd moment of area:
 I = 4922 mm⁴
Bending stiffness:
 EI = 590.6 × 10⁶ N/mm²

Fig. 20.2.14 Diagrams to show the second moment of area of two femoral components made respectively of stainless steel and titanium with their respective bending stiffness.

femoral components were generally relatively small and manufactured from stainless steel or cast chrome cobalt molybdenum alloy, having a fatigue strength of the order of 220–330 MPa. Many were derived from the Austin-Moore and Thomson type stems that had originally been introduced for replacement of the femoral head without the use of cement. Reports of stem fractures did not start to appear in the literature until the early and mid-1970s (Patterson and Brown, 1972; Charnley, 1975; Collis, 1977). These led to the introduction of high-fatigue-strength alloys (fatigue strength 550–700 MPa) for stem manufacture and to design changes that resulted in substantial increases in stem section. The most extreme example was the CAD, a stem of such section that breakage was eliminated—a relief to the manufacturers. To the chagrin of surgeons, however, loosening increased (Thomas *et al.*, 1986), for reasons that are discussed below.

The main variables in femoral component geometry are as follows:

General configuration

Femoral components can broadly be divided into those in which the stem is curved throughout, exemplified by the McKee-Arden, Muller, Weber and Howse designs, and those in which the stem is straight, exemplified by the Charnley, Muller 'Dual lock' and Exeter designs. A further subdivision is formed by those in which the curve is in two planes, such as the Link SP or APR stems.

In general, cemented stems are intended to be totally surrounded by a sheath of cement. The exception to this is the Muller straight 'Dual lock' type of stem, in which direct contact between the stem and the endosteal cortex of the femur is envisaged medially and laterally, with cement intervening between the two anteriorly and posteriorly. The cement sheath is, in fact, divided into two when this type of stem is used as recommended.

Flexural rigidity

The flexural rigidity or structural stiffness of the stem depends upon the elasticity of the alloy from which stem is manufactured, and the disposition of that alloy throughout the length of the stem. It is obtained by multiplying the elastic modulus of the alloy (E) by the second moment of area (I) of the cross-sectional shape of the stem section. The latter (Fig. 20.2.14) is given by the formula I = base × height cubed divided by 12. In this instance, height is the mediolateral dimension of the stem, and base its anteroposterior dimension. It is important to appreciate the influence of the *cube* of the height in this formula. This means that variations in the height (i.e. width) of the stem have a disproportionately great effect on its structural stiffness by comparison with the elastic modulus of the alloy.

Since the cross-sectional area of the stem generally changes throughout its length, so does its structural stiffness.

Length

There is an almost infinite variation between approximately 120 mm and 300 mm. The tendency to use very long stems with cement was originally recommended in the 1970s (Tonnis and Asai, 1976) and later popularized particularly in revision surgery by Scheller and D'Errico (1982) in the early 1980s. It is now passing, largely because of the difficulties such devices may cause when they fail. There is no known optimum length of stem. As Stuhmer (G. Stuhmer, personal communication, 1983) has said, a stem should be 'as long as necessary and as short as possible'.

Surface finish

Surface finish is relevant in two respects: load transmission and debris production.

A mechanical bond between stem and cement is only possible by mechanical interlock between the asperities on a matt stem surface and cement. Pre-coating the stem with cement enhances the strength of the interlock, but the pre-coating process used in current manufacturing does so only to a limited degree (D. Anuta, personal communication, 1992) by comparison with laboratory techniques (Barb et al., 1982; Ahmed et al., 1984). The surface roughness of currently used matt-surfaced stems varies from 0.3 to more than 5 µm, whereas the surface roughness of a polished stem is approximately 0.01 µm, a difference of one to two orders of magnitude by contrast with the matt-surfaced stems (Fig. 20.2.15). The smoothest of the matt-surfaced stems feels very smooth to the touch, but is actually very rough in surface finish terms.

There is a major difference of opinion with regard to whether or not the stem should be bonded to the cement (Harris, 1992; Ling, 1992). Theoretical analyses using the finite element method provide conflicting opinions (Harrigan and Harris, 1991; Lu et al., 1992) and the matter will only be solved by long-term follow-up studies. In this context, it is interesting that a number of stems in use in the early 1970s had highly polished surfaces, especially the Charnley 'flatback' and the Exeter. Fashion and manufacturing costs subsequently led to a change to matt-surfaced stems of varying roughness and these became almost universal. Some

authors (Fowler et al., 1988; R.C. Johnston, personal communication, 1992; Dall et al., 1993; Timperley et al., 1993; Neumann et al., 1994) have found this change to have been a retrograde step as far as the long-term performance of the stem is concerned. Polishing the stem surface ensures that there will be no bond between the stem and the cement, and it is possible that this may be favourable (Bannister and Miles, 1988; Fowler et al., 1988) as far as the long-term integrity of the cement–bone interface is concerned.

It is certain that, once the stem–cement bond fails, and there is evidence that it regularly does so (see later), fretting between the matt-surfaced stem and cement is a potent source of particulate debris (Lee et al., 1990).

The presence of a collar or flange

Large proximal collars are intended to transmit load directly to the cut surface of the femoral neck and can be shown, with difficulty (Markolf et al., 1980), to do so in the laboratory. Once a computer has been suitably instructed that the collar *does* transmit load to the cut surface of the femoral neck, then appropriate finite element studies (Crowninshield et al., 1980, 1981; Lewis et al., 1984) not surprisingly indicate that such loading increases the strain under load in the proximal and medial femoral cortex. The evidence that with cemented stems, the collar loads the proximal femur effectively in clinical practice, however, does not at present exist. Moreover, it is certain that the proximal and medial femoral cortex *can* be effectively loaded (Ling, 1992) utilizing femoral components that are devoid of a collar of any sort.

Micromotion between the undersurface of the collar and the underlying bone and cement is inevitable in clinical practice, and therefore debris production by fretting of the undersurface of the collar against the adjacent materials is likely (Ling, 1992; Lee et al., 1993). This is probably the main cause of the loss of calcar height often reported with cemented femoral components.

Smaller collars or flanges are intended to transmit load to the proximal end of the cement sheath. Again, however, the undersurfaces of such structures may be a source of fretting and debris production.

Even the smallest of collars does fundamentally alter the way the stem responds to loads applied to the head, and imposes the 'calcar pivot' (Gruen et al., 1979) phenomenon on the stem.

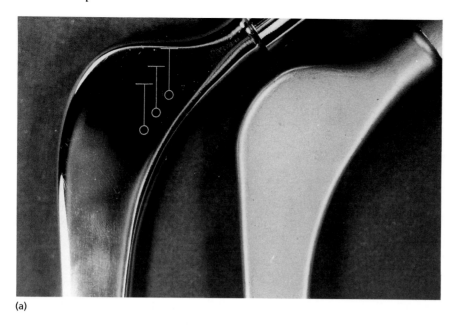

(a)

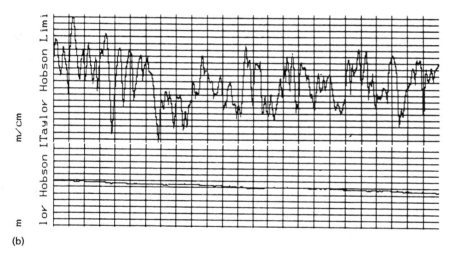

(b)

Fig. 20.2.15 (a) Matt and polished stems. (b) Talysurf traces to show relative roughness of matt and polished surfaces. The vertical scale is 2 μm/cm and the horizontal scale is 100 μm/cm.

Stem taper

The anatomical constraints of the inside of the proximal femur dictate that all femoral components will be to some extent tapered in shape. The taper obviously influences the second moment of area of successive segments of the stem, and therefore their structural stiffness. Although all stems exhibit some taper, very few utilize the inherent properties of the taper as part of their mechanisms of fixation and load transmission. In engineering practice, the taper is one of the most reliable methods of transmitting both axial and torsional forces between one member and another. The taper can only function to transmit load if it can engage, i.e. the male component of the taper must move into the female. Archibald (1991) has examined the characteristics of the

taper in its application to femoral component function. An essential is that the tip of the stem must not be end-bearing, and there must be no structural feature on the stem surface that interferes with the capacity of the taper to engage. There may be practical advantages to the utilization of the principle of the taper in femoral component design (Fowler *et al.*, 1988; Miles *et al.*, 1990; Gie *et al.*, 1993).

Head size

Since the introduction of cemented total hip arthroplasty, there has been much debate concerning the most appropriate size for the femoral head. For metal on plastic bearings, the most common diameter in use worldwide has been 32 mm. Charnley (1979) was the first to suggest that a substantially smaller head diameter (22 mm) would be an advantage from the standpoints of frictional torque and volume of wear debris. Latterly, evidence has begun to accumulate that an intermediate size (26 or 28 mm) may be the optimal (Morrey and Ilstrup, 1989; Hoeltzel *et al.*, 1989; Amstutz *et al.*, 1991), and an increasing number of implants now utilize these diameters. An intermediate size may also be appropriate for metal on metal bearings (Muller, 1992).

Offset, neck length and neck angle

These variables are all related, as shown in Fig. 20.2.16. Offset is defined as the horizontal distance between the midline axis of the stem and the centre of the femoral head. Misorientation of the stem within the femoral canal means that the functional offset (the horizontal distance between the midline axis of the femoral canal and the centre of the femoral head) and the offset of the stem will not be the same.

Modularity

This attractive concept in its application to cemented stems involves fashioning the neck of the implant proximally into the male component of a Morse taper. The female component is contained within the femoral head. The advantages are twofold. The surgeon can select the head size that he feels is appropriate for a particular patient. In revision procedures for loose cups where the femoral component remains soundly fixed, a new femoral head can be fitted to the taper of the neck

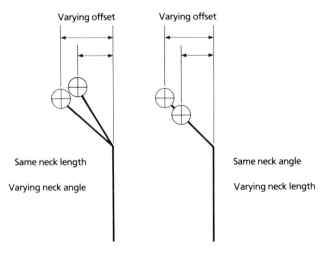

Fig. 20.2.16 The difference between neck length, offset and neck angle.

without changing the soundly fixed stem. The drawbacks mainly relate to the use of the method with dissimilar alloys. It is now common to find titanium alloy stems mated with cobalt-chrome heads. Collier *et al.* (1992a,b) have shown that this may be dangerous because of the effects of corrosion between dissimilar alloys.

The acetabular component

ACETABULAR COMPONENT GEOMETRY

By comparison with the femoral component, the number of variations in high-density polyethylene socket design has been relatively few, and the major controversies that persist relate primarily to the presence or absence of metal backing and of extended lips.

Experience has shown that two features of socket geometry are definitely undesirable: thin walls and eccentricity of the inside diameter with respect to the outside.

Thin-walled sockets can no longer justifiably be used because they are associated with increased loosening rates. This is in part due to the fact that the thin polythene cannot carry the loads safely (Bartel *et al.*, 1986; Hoeltzel *et al.*, 1989) and in part because thin-walled sockets lead to higher stresses in the surrounding cement and acetabular bone (Pedersen *et al.*, 1982). The capacity to utilize a thick socket wall without greatly increasing the outside diameter of the socket is one of the major advantages of smaller heads for the femoral component.

Eccentric sockets guarantee that a turning moment over and above that generated by frictional torque will always be acting at the interface between the socket and the cement (Mittelmeier *et al.*, 1986). Furthermore, any misorientation of the socket may lead to marked variability in the thickness of the high-density polyethylene in the weight-bearing areas, with unfavourable stress distributions that can contribute to loosening.

Metal-backing

Metal backing of the polythene acetabular cup was first introduced by Harris (Harris, 1971) with the idea of making it possible to exchange a worn polythene liner without removing a still soundly fixed metal-back. Later, theoretical studies utilizing the finite element method (Carter *et al.*, 1982; Pedersen *et al.*, 1982; Bartel *et al.*, 1983) provided evidence that metal-backing might favourably influence the absolute stress level and the distribution of stress in both the cement and the bone. Harris and White subsequently (1982) produced clinical evidence that was held to support the use of metal-backing. More recently, however, Ritter *et al.* (1990), in a careful follow-up study, have shown that metal-backing is associated with an increased incidence of loosening. Moreover, Dalstra and Huiskes (1991), in a recent three-dimensional finite-element study, were unable to confirm the theoretical benefits of metal-backing demonstrated in the previous two-dimensional and axi-symmetric studies mentioned above.

The interface between the polythene liner and the metal-back represents a potential source of fretting and debris formation (Collier *et al.*, 1992a, b), and overall, metal-backed sockets can no longer be recommended for cemented total hip arthroplasties.

Extended lips

Extended lips or skirts on the lateral and posterolateral aspects of the socket in an effort to improve stability of the head within the socket were first seen on the Exeter design in the early 1970s. The same feature subsequently appeared on the Osteonics cup. Later, Charnley (1979) introduced the long posterior wall (LPW) socket with the same idea in view, and now such flanges or lips are commonly seen in a number of designs.

Subsequent experience with the Exeter **cup** made it clear that, with the skirt in the lateral position, impingement of the neck of the femoral component against the skirt was common in full flexion and abduction, and the momentary increases in torque generated at the cement—bone interface in association with impingement might contribute to loosening. Murray (1992) came to the same view with respect to the LPW cup, and found, moreover, that the latter conferred no real benefit with respect to stability. The real value of these features is thus in doubt unless the surgeon has the ability to position them exactly where they are needed to improve stability without causing impingement.

Pressurization flanges

An extended polythene flange right round the margin of the cup was introduced by Charnley in the late 1970s (Shelley and Wroblewski, 1988) with the twin aims of improving cement pressurization, particularly near the margins of the acetabulum, and improving the accuracy of placement of the cup within the acetabulum. A later development of the same theme was the 'Ogee' cup. There is now good evidence that this type of technology is of real value clinically, and further developments on the same theme are likely in the future.

THE RESULTS OF CEMENTED HIP ARTHROPLASTY

The literature on this subject is now vast and cannot be covered in detail here. For a comprehensive coverage of the subject, the reader is referred to Amstutz *et al.* (1991), and to Timperley and O'Dwyer (1993). Some aspects of the matter do require comment, however.

Timperley and O'Dwyer (1993) have pointed out the difficulties of comparing the different published series as far as the clinical and radiological outcomes of the operation are concerned. Often the absence of a definition of 'success' or 'failure' of one or both components means that quoted figures are frequently not comparable. Some authors quote re-operation rates as a percentage of the whole series, including those dead and lost to follow-up (Hamilton and Joyce, 1986; Fowler *et al.*, 1988), while others express the rate as a proportion of the number of patients traced for review (Brady and McCutchen, 1986; Dall *et al.*, 1986a). Some papers report on a group of patients selected from the original series by various arbitrary criteria (Eftekhar and Tzitzikalakis, 1986; Wroblewski, 1986; Wejkner *et al.*, 1988; Mulroy and Harris 1990a), and others include in the failure rate cases thought to be loose on radiological grounds (Stauffer, 1982; Pavlov, 1987).

Survivorship analysis was introduced into orthopaedics by Dobbs (1980) in an effort to analyse data when the time of failure is not known for all patients. The outcome of survivorship studies depends upon the definition of 'failure', and assumes that patients who died or were lost to follow-up had the same probability of failure as those that were not withdrawn from the series. Such studies also assume that the survival probabilities for each time interval remain constant throughout the series. Misleading conclusions may be drawn from survivorship studies if confidence intervals are not quoted for survival rates (Lettin *et al.*, 1991).

Tables 20.2.2—20.2.9 are drawn from the work of Timperley and O'Dwyer (1993) and represent the data from 31 sets of published results, presented in a way that attempts to standardize the methods of calculation of failure rates for the separate components and overall, both clinically and radiologically. The tables separate those series in which results can reasonably be compared with results from other series from those that cannot. The number of removed components (Tables 20.2.2, 20.2.3 and 20.2.8) is given as a percentage of the sum of the number of implants removed plus the number known to have been *in situ* at the time of death. Those lost to follow-up are excluded from the calculation on the assumption that the probability of failure in this group

Table 20.2.2 Overall revision rates (from Timperley and O'Dwyer, 1993)

Author	Year	Average follow-up	Mechanical failure (%)	Infection (%)	Total failure (%)	Hip type
Comparable series						
Wejkner	1988	5.2	4.5	7.7	14.1	Charnley
Beckenbaugh and Ilstrup	1978	5.8	2.4	1.5	7.0	Charnley
Hozack *et al.*	1990	6.8		0.6	4.5	Charnley
Johnstone and Crowninshield	1983	10.0	1.0	3.1	4.1	Charnley
Salvati *et al.*	1981	10.0	3.2	2.2	5.4	Charnley
Sutherland *et al.*	1982	10.0	22.0	3.0	25.0	Muller
McCoy *et al.*	1988	10.2	4.0	2.0	6.0	Charnley
Reikeras	1982	10.2	18.1	1.4	19.6	Muller
Stauffer	1982	10.3	8.8	1.4	12.2	Charnley
Jacobsson *et al.*	1990	11.0	5.9	2.9	8.8	Charnley
Older	1986	11.0	3.7	0.5	4.1	Charnley
Cupic	1979	11.5	3.9	4.8	8.2	Charnley
Lachiewicz *et al.*	1986	11.5	2.2	0.0	2.2	Harris
Wejkner	1988	11.6	8.4	8.8	17.2	Charnley
Jacobsson *et al.*	1990	11.9	12.4	2.9	15.2	McKee−Farrar
Fowler *et al.*	1988	13.4	14.3	3.3	17.6	Exeter
August *et al.*	1986	13.9			12.6	McKee−Farrar
Kavanagh *et al.*	1989	15.0	9.3	1.2	11.1	Charnley
Pavlov	1987	15.0		1.9	14.5	Charnley−Muller
Welch *et al.*	1988	16.0	15.5	1.0	16.5	Charnley
Gie *et al.*	1993	16.4	14.9	2.4	17.3	Exeter
Ling	1992	16.5	13.8	2.0	15.8	Exeter
Wroblewski	1986	16.6				Charnley
Non-comparable series						
Hamilton and Joyce	1986	5.4	2.7	0.9	3.5	Charnley
Dall *et al.*	1993	7.5	12.4	1.2	13.7	Charnley 2nd Gen.
Eftekhar and Tzitzikalakis	1986	8.0	2.4	0.9	3.3	Charnley
Dall *et al.*	1993	8.8	7.6	1.9	9.5	Charnley 1st Gen.
Brady and McCutchen	1986	10.0	5.9	2.9	8.8	Charnley
Mulroy and Harris	1990	11.2	6.7		7.0	CAD/HD-2
Dall *et al.*	1986	12.0	14.2		14.2	Charnley
McCoy *et al.*	1988	15.3	5.0		5.0	Charnley

Spaces have been left where it is not possible or inappropriate to calculate a figure.

is the same as in those who were reviewed. The mechanical failure rate relates to components removed as a result of component failure rather than incidental pathology such as ectopic bone formation. The total failure rate is therefore not always the sum of the mechanical failure and failure from infection rates.

As far as radiological results are concerned, the authors' definition of a radiological term is given wherever this was expressed in the original paper. The figure given is usually a percentage of the radiographs available at the final review, excluding those cases that had been revised. Spaces in the tables indicate that insufficient radiological data was given in the original papers for inclusion in the tables.

What is clear is that the best results of cemented total hip arthroplasty are remarkably satisfactory, even with basic cementing techniques, and moreover, hold up well with time.

COMPLICATIONS OF CEMENTED HIP ARTHROPLASTY

Cardiovascular complications of using acrylic cement

In the early days of the use of acrylic cement, cardiovascular collapse was sometimes seen shortly after the femoral component was driven into the cement in the femur. The phenomenon occurred more commonly in femoral head replacement for subcapital fracture than in elective total hip arthroplasty. The matter has been fully

Table 20.2.3 Stem revisions (from Timperley and O'Dwyer, 1993)

Author	Year	Average follow-up	Fractured prosthesis (%)	Aseptic loosening	Total revised (%)	Stem type
Comparable series						
Wejkner	1988	5.2	1.6	3.2	12.5	Charnley
Beckenbaugh and Ilstrup	1978	5.8	0.3	1.5	3.9	Charnley
Hozack *et al.*	1990	6.8		3.8	4.4	Charnley
Johnstone and Crowninshield	1983	10.0	0.7	0.7	4.1	Charnley
Salvati *et al.*	1981	10.0	1.1	1.1	5.4	Charnley
Sutherland *et al.*	1982	10.0	4.3	13.0	19.0	Muller
McCoy *et al.*	1988	10.2	1.0	3.0	6.0	Charnley
Reikeras	1982	10.2		16.7	18.1	Muller
Stauffer	1982	10.3	1.7	4.7	7.4	Charnley
Jacobsson *et al.*	1990	11.0		2.9	5.9	Charnley
Older	1986	11.0	2.3	1.4	4.1	Charnley
Cupic	1979	11.5	0.3	1.4	6.4	Charnley
Lachiewicz *et al.*	1986	11.5	0.0	2.2	2.2	Harris
Wejkner	1988	11.6	3.0	4.4	13.8	Charnley
Jacobsson *et al.*	1990	11.9	0.0	8.6	11.4	McKee–Farrar
Fowler *et al.*	1988	13.4	7.0	2.1	12.5	Exeter
August *et al.*	1986	13.9				McKee–Farrar
Kavanagh *et al.*	1989	15.0	2.4	5.1	9.9	Charnley
Pavlov	1987	15.0				Charnley–Muller
Welch *et al.*	1988	16.0	6.2	3.1	11.3	Charnley
Gie *et al.*	1993	16.4	7.5	3.5	13.4	Exeter
Ling	1992	16.5	4.5	2.6	8.9	Exeter
Wroblewski	1985	16.6				Charnley
Non-comparable series						
Hamilton and Joyce	1986	5.4	0.0	0.0	2.5	Charnley
Dall *et al.*	1993	7.5	0.5	8.7	10.9	Charnley 2nd Gen.
Eftekhar and Tzitzikalakis	1986	8.0	0.7	0.7	2.3	Charnley
Dall *et al.*	1988	8.8	4.2	2.3	8.3	Charnley 1st Gen.
Brady and McCutchen	1984	10.0	1.8	2.4	7.6	Charnley
Mulroy and Harris	1990	11.2		1.9	4.8	CAD/HD-2
Dall *et al.*	1986	12.0	7.1	4.1	12.2	Charnley
McCoy *et al.*	1988	15.3		5.0	5.0	Charnley

Spaces have been left where it is not possible or inappropriate to calculate a figure.

reviewed by James (1984), to whose work the interested reader is referred.

James has pointed out that blood pressure changes after cement insertion are, as a rule, no greater than those occurring after other noxious surgical stimuli, that patients with mild uraemia and hypertension are particularly susceptible to hypotension after the insertion of cement, and that the latter may cause more marked hypotension in a patient who is hypovolaemic.

Avoiding serious blood pressure changes requires careful and continuous monitoring of the blood pressure, preferably using an intra-arterial cannula, adequate analgesia, the correct use of vasoactive drugs, and the avoidance of hypovolaemia at the time of cement insertion.

The evidence as it stands now implicates the embolization of thromboplastins in femoral medullary fat and the products of femoral reaming into the pulmonary vascular bed, with the subsequent aggregation of platelets and the liberation therein of vasoactive amines, as the most likely cause of minor blood pressure changes associated with femoral cementing. Reducing the risks from this phenomenon involves, as well as the measures mentioned above, thorough lavage of the femoral canal and retrograde filling of the canal with cement from a cement gun (Sherman *et al.*, 1983; Byrick *et al.*, 1989).

Table 20.2.4 Stem radiology (from Timperley and O'Dwyer, 1993)

Author	Year	Average follow-up	Subsidence (%)	Definition	Calcar loss (%)	Definition
Hamilton and Joyce	1986	5.4	10.0	>2 mm		
Beckenbaugh and Ilstrup	1978	5.8			16.1	>2 mm
Brady and McCutchen	1986	10.0	3.8	>1 mm	22.3	>1 mm
Johnstone and Crowninshield	1983	10.0			19.4	Discernible
Salvati *et al.*	1981	10.0			11.1	>2 mm
Sutherland *et al.*	1982	10.0	23.0	>5 mm	16.0	Prox. loss
Reikeras	1982	10.2			7.5	
Stauffer	1982	10.3			14.0	Any
Older	1986	11.0			21.0	Discernible
Cupic	1979	11.5			78.0	Any
Lachiewicz *et al.*	1986	11.5	13.2		21.0	>3 mm
Dall *et al.*	1986	12.0	35.7	Any	46.0	Any
Fowler *et al.*	1988	13.4	26.1	>2 mm within mantle	8.5	>2 mm
Kavanagh *et al.*	1989	15.0	12.4	>2 mm		
Gie *et al.*	1993	16.4	32.0	>2 mm within mantle	16.0	>2 mm
Ling	1992	16.5	25.0	>2 mm within mantle	7.5	>2 mm
Wroblewski	1986	16.6	29.0		44.0	Any

A blank has been left where information is not supplied.

Table 20.2.5 Stem radiology (from Timperley and O'Dwyer, 1993)

Author	Year	Average follow-up	Endosteal lysis (%)	Cortical hypertrophy (%)	Cement fracture (%)
Hamilton and Joyce	1986	5.4	3.5		4.8
Beckenbaugh and Ilstrup	1978	5.8		1.2	8.8
Salvati *et al.*	1981	10.0			9.3
Stauffer	1982	10.3			7.8
Older	1986	11.0		18.0	21.0
Mulroy and Harris	1990	11.2	6.8		
Dall *et al.*	1986	12.0	2.4	27.3	14.3
Fowler *et al.*	1988	13.4	8.1		8.5
August *et al.*	1986	13.9	50.0		
Kavanagh *et al.*	1989	15.0			12.4
McCoy *et al.*	1988	15.3			22.9
Gie *et al.*	1993	16.4	13.0	48.0	25.0
Ling	1992	16.5	15.0	45.0	17.5

A blank has been left where information is not supplied.

Table 20.2.6 Stem radiology (from Timperley and O'Dwyer, 1993)

Author	Year	Average follow-up	Lucency (0%)	Lucency 0–50%	Lucency 50–100%	Lucency >100%
Salvati *et al.*	1981	10.0	50.0			
Mulroy and Harris	1990	11.2		23.3%	0.0%	1.0%
Dall *et al.*	1986	12.0	85.0	12.0%	3.6%	
Kavanagh *et al.*	1989	15.0	32.8			8.8%
McCoy *et al.*	1988	15.3	43.0			
Gie *et al.*	1993	16.4	62.0	36.0%	2.0%	0.0%
Ling	1992	16.5	67.5	32.5%	0.0%	0.0%

A blank has been left where information is not supplied.

Table 20.2.7 Socket revisions (from Timperley and O'Dwyer, 1993)

Author	Year	Average follow-up	Revised loose (%)	Revised total (%)
Comparable series				
Wejkner	1988	5.2	1.0	8.6
Beckenbaugh and Ilstrup	1978	5.8	0.9	3.3
Hozack *et al.*	1990	6.8	2.2	2.8
Brady and McCutchen	1986	10.0	2.4	5.9
Johnstone and Crowninshield	1983	10.0	0.3	3.4
Salvati *et al.*	1981	10.0	1.1	3.2
Sutherland *et al.*	1982	10.0	8.0	11.0
McCoy *et al.*	1988	10.2	0.0	3.0
Reikeras	1982	10.2	8.0	9.4
Stauffer	1982	10.3	2.4	5.1
Jacobsson *et al.*	1990	11.0	5.9	8.8
Older	1986	11.0	1.4	1.8
Cupic	1979	11.5	2.2	7.0
Lachiewicz *et al.*	1986	11.5	2.2	2.2
Wejkner	1988	11.6	2.4	10.4
Jacobsson *et al.*	1990	11.9	8.6	14.3
Fowler *et al.*	1988	13.4	5.2	8.5
August *et al.*	1986	13.9		
Kavanagh *et al.*	1989	15.0	3.6	5.4
Pavlov	1987	15.0		
Welch *et al.*	1988	16.0	6.2	7.2
Gie *et al.*	1993	16.4	6.7	9.3
Ling	1992	16.5	6.3	8.5
Wroblewski	1986	16.6		
Non-comparable series				
Hamilton and Joyce	1986	5.4	0.7	1.3
Dall *et al.*	1993	7.5	4.7	6.5
Eftekhar and Tzitzikalakis	1986	8.0	1.0	1.9
Dall *et al.*	1993	8.8	1.9	3.8
Mulroy and Harris	1990	11.2	3.8	4.8
Dall *et al.*	1986	12.0	4.1	6.1
McCoy *et al.*	1988	15.3		5.0

A blank has been left where it is not possible or inappropriate to calculate a figure.

Intra-operative vascular and nerve injury

VASCULAR INJURIES

Ratliff (1984) summarized the features of 32 patients who sustained vascular injuries during the course of total hip arthroplasty. The injuries were classified into five main groups:

1 Laceration of a main vessel outside the pelvis. These injuries were confined to cases in which the anterolateral approach had been used.

2 Laceration of a main vessel inside the pelvis. Cases with very thin or defective medial acetabular walls are at particular risk.

3 Thrombosis of a major vessel ascribed either to trauma from the heat of polymerizing bone cement, or to the assumption of extreme positions of the leg during dislocation or femoral reaming.

4 False aneurysm, generally caused by spicules of acrylic cement attached to the acetabular component eroding through the external iliac, femoral or medial circumflex femoral arteries. The same mechanism, i.e. erosion of an arterial wall by a spicule of cement, can also produce thrombus formation from intimal damage, and later arterial embolism.

5 Arteriovenous fistula between the medial circumflex femoral artery and the posterior aspect of the femoral vein.

Table 20.2.8 Socket radiology (from Timperley and O'Dwyer, 1993)

Author	Year	Average follow-up	Line-free socket (%)	Demarcated socket (%)
Beckenbaugh and Ilstrup	1978	5.8	1.2	12.5
Hozack *et al.*	1990	6.8	37.0	16.0
Brady and McCutchen	1986	10.0		6.1
Johnstone and Crowninshield	1983	10.0		35.0
Salvati *et al.*	1981	10.0	20.4	11.1
Stauffer	1982	10.3	27.7	41.1
Older	1986	11.0	63.0	17.0
Lachiewicz *et al.*	1986	11.5		7.9
Dall *et al.*	1986	12.0	57.0	8.3
Fowler *et al.*	1988	13.4	2.5	
Kavanagh *et al.*	1989	15.0	8.8	27.7
McCoy *et al.*	1988	15.3	29.0	
Gie *et al.*	1993	16.4	17.0	34.1
Ling	1992	16.5	18.2	39.4
Wroblewski	1986	16.6		31.0

A blank has been left where information is not supplied.

Table 20.2.9 Socket radiology (from Timperley and O'Dwyer, 1993)

Author	Year	Average follow-up	Migration (%)	Definition of migration
Hamilton and Joyce	1986	5.4	2.6	Any
Beckenbaugh and Ilstrup	1978	5.8	6.5	Complete lucencies >1 mm
Hozack *et al.*	1990	6.8	13.7	Complete lucencies >1 mm or migration >5 mm
Dall *et al.*	1993	7.5	3.0	Severe changes indicative of loosening
Eftekhar and Tzitzikalakis	1986	8.0	0.7	Any migration + complete lucency >2 mm
Dall *et al.*	1993	8.8	1.9	Severe changes indicative of loosening
Johnstone and Crowninshield	1983	10.0	3.6	Discernible
Salvati *et al.*	1981	10.0	3.7	Progressive
Sutherland *et al.*	1982	10.0	23.0	>5 mm
Stauffer	1982	10.3	11.3	Complete line >1 mm or any migration
Jacobsson *et al.*	1990	11.0	14.6	Complete lucency >2 mm or migration >2 mm
Older	1986	11.0	8.0	>2 mm in Zone 3
Mulroy and Harris	1990	11.2	39.8	Continuous lucency or migration
Lachiewicz *et al.*	1986	11.5	21.1	Any
Wejkner	1988	11.6	10.7	Complete demarcation >1 mm
Jacobsson *et al.*	1990	11.9	10.9	Complete lucency >2 mm, migration >2 mm
Dall *et al.*	1986	12.0	14.3	Any
Fowler *et al.*	1988	13.4	23.0	Lucency >2 mm in Zone 3
August *et al.*	1986	13.9	40.0	>5 mm
Kavanagh *et al.*	1989	15.0	8.8	Movement or cement fracture
Pavlov	1987	15.0	22.0	
McCoy *et al.*	1988	15.3	5.7	Any change in position
Welch *et al.*	1988	16.0	10.5	Moved or complete demarcation >2 mm
Gie *et al.*	1993	16.4	37.5	Lucency >2 mm in Zone 3
Ling	1992	16.5	39.4	Inferior gap or tilting
Wroblewski	1986	16.6	22.1	Any movement

NEUROLOGICAL INJURIES

Prospective EMG studies (Weber *et al.*, 1976) and intra-operative somatosensory evoked potential monitoring (Stone *et al.*, 1985; Black *et al.*, 1991) reveal that neurological injury in association with total hip arthroplasty is common, but generally subclinical. The reported incidence of clinically detectable nerve injury varies between 0.7% (Weber *et al.*, 1976) and 3.7% (Wilson and Scales, 1973), generally being higher in revision surgery and in primary procedures performed for CDH (Schmalzried *et al.*, 1991).

The sciatic nerve is most commonly affected, though injuries to the femoral, lateral popliteal and obturator nerves have also been reported (Ratliff, 1984). In Ratliff's series, the main causes of complete sciatic paralysis were division of the nerve, excessive traction on the nerve (due to levers behind the acetabulum in two cases), penetration of the femoral shaft by prosthesis and cement and a wire surrounding the nerve. Some cases cannot be satisfactorily explained.

Careful post-operative neurological examination is necessary to identify lesser degrees of nerve injury, supplemented, where necessary, by electrical investigation.

PREVENTION

The prevention of neurological and vascular injuries in association with hip arthroplasty requires an appreciation of the type of case in which they are likely to occur, a sound grasp of the anatomy surrounding the hip, a free exposure with the avoidance of excessive retraction, and care.

MANAGEMENT

Vascular injuries

Torrential haemorrhage during hip arthroplasty should be dealt with by immediate firm packing of the wound. Expert vascular assistance should be obtained without delay. Subacute vascular injuries presenting post-operatively require the opinion and help of a vascular surgeon.

Nerve injuries

Intra-operative realization that a peripheral nerve injury has occurred is unusual unless a nerve has been directly divided and the fact is recognized by the surgeon. Under these circumstances, immediate repair should be undertaken.

If a peripheral nerve lesion is recognized post-operatively, it is essential to clarify its cause without delay. This is in the patient's interests, but is also becoming important medico-legally. A neurological opinion is necessary, with appropriate investigations to follow. Re-exploration of the wound may be needed to clarify matters, and to undertake repair if this is feasible. Expertise in peripheral nerve surgery should be available for such procedures.

Intra-operative femoral fracture

INCIDENCE

The incidence of intra-operative femoral fracture in cemented total hip arthroplasty is 1% or less in primary interventions, rising to 3.2% in revisions (Barrington *et al.*, 1984).

PROPHYLAXIS

Prevention of these accidents should be the first aim of the surgeon. Pre-operative planning should alert the surgeon to possible difficulties, and identify any sources of structural weakness in the femur that may predispose to femoral fracture.

Great care in dislocating the hip when the femur is weakened is essential. Full soft tissue releases must be performed *before* attempts are made to dislocate the hip. The head should always be lifted out of the socket by means of a hook around the neck, and not forced out by torsional forces applied to the distal part of the leg. It is wise not to remove any pre-existing plates and screws from the upper femur until the head has been dislocated. If such hardware is removed prior to dislocation, the added weakness and stress concentrating effect of the empty screw holes may precipitate a fracture.

MANAGEMENT

In the opinion of the authors, the management of this difficult problem has been greatly simplified by the technique of impaction cancellous grafting combined with cement, described for use in femoral revision surgery by Gie *et al.* (1993). Stabilization of the fracture externally by plates with unicortical screws, or the Mennem plate (Mennem, 1989), combined if necessary with circlage, allows the impaction grafting to be carried out. This greatly increases the stability, and the grafts prevent cement from getting into the fracture line. Rapid union can be anticipated, together with a stable implant.

Dislocation

Early dislocation following total hip arthroplasty is not only a major setback to the confidence of the patient, but a potentially disastrous complication. Fortunately, with proper care before, during and after the operation, it can be rendered extremely rare.

INCIDENCE

The reported incidence varies from 0.5 to 8% (Hamblen, 1984a; Amstutz and Kody, 1991), being highest in revision surgery.

PREDISPOSING FACTORS

Factors relating to the implant itself include head size, neck–shaft angle, head–neck diameter ratio, socket depth and geometry, and 'captivity'. These all influence the stage at which the neck impinges against the rim of the socket and starts to lever the head out.

For any given implant, the orientation of the components is of major importance. Misorientation of either component may predispose to dislocation and recurrent dislocation, and is the most common factor associated with recurrent dislocation. Misorientation of the cup may be due to malalignment of the patient on the operating table, particularly if the lateral decubitus position is being used. The lumbar lordosis must not then be obliterated by flexing the contralateral hip. This may lead to retroversion of the cup when the lordosis is re-established.

Tissue laxity and poor musculature, including trochanteric migration, may contribute to instability.

Ectopic cement and osteophytes may provide a fulcrum for impingement and consequent dislocation if they are not removed at the time of surgery.

Stupidity, confusion, failure on the part of the patient to perceive pre-operative instructions for the management of the hip in the post-operative period, and careless handling of the patient may all predispose to dislocation.

PROPHYLAXIS

Adequate pre-operative instruction concerning the way in which the patient should treat the hip in the post-operative period and ensuing 3 months is vital. The instructions should bear in mind the approach to be used. High-risk patients (the very old, the confused, the frail and the stupid) are best not operated upon by the posterior approach, through which the risks of dislocation are somewhat increased.

Pre-operatively, accurate component positioning is the single most important factor in the prevention of dislocation.

Post-operatively, there must be proper care in relation to the type of implant employed and to the approach used. Dislocation following the posterior approach is usually posterior, and occurs following impingement in flexion and internal rotation. Conversely, dislocation following the anterior or anterolateral approach tends to occur anteriorly after impingement in external rotation and extension. Patients must be made to realize these facts and learn to avoid impingement in the way they handle their limb for the first 3 months.

MANAGEMENT

Early post-operative dislocation should be treated by reduction and then mobilization in a protective brace that will limit the movement responsible for the dislocation. Six weeks in a single short hip spica with knee hinges and below-knee steels is appropriate for irresponsible patients, or where there is any question of component malalignment. Traction following reduction of a dislocation is to be avoided. It may actually distract the hip, and prevents the redevelopment of muscle that is necessary for proper control of the limb. Ectopic bone prophylaxis should be given after an early post-operative dislocation has been reduced (see below).

If the dislocation recurs, its cause must be very carefully analysed. With significant component malposition, re-operation will become necessary, and the surgeon may also consider using components with a larger head size if the patient is old. The Olerud technique (Olerud and Karlstrom, 1985) of socket augmentation should only be used in low-demand patients. In these, it works well.

Chronic re-dislocators present an extremely difficult problem that should not be tackled without very careful analysis of all the predisposing factors.

Infection

This matter is dealt with in Chapter 15 and will not be mentioned further here.

Thromboembolism

Thromboembolic complications of hip arthroplasty are common, in the absence of adequate prophylaxis (the incidence of deep vein thrombosis is 60–80%), and potentially life threatening (Fordyce and Ling, 1992) — the risk of fatal pulmonary embolism is 1–10%. No surgeon can now realistically involve himself in hip replacement surgery without instituting an effective regime of prophylaxis. The matter will soon become of medico-legal significance (Parker-Williams *et al.*, 1991).

Although low-molecular-weight heparin is popular in some quarters (Routledge and West, 1992) and reduces the risk by 60–70% the authors have seen serious bleeding complications with its use. They prefer to rely on the A–V impulse system (Novamedix, Andover) that has been shown in a randomized controlled trial (Fordyce and Ling, 1992) to be extremely effective in preventing clinically significant venous thrombosis following hip arthroplasty. Its use, moreover, carries no morbidity. Combining this device with elevation of the foot of the bed, the use of graduated compression stockings, and anti-platelet stickiness drugs by mouth is the regimen now in use at the Princess Elizabeth Orthopaedic Hospital, Exeter.

Once deep venous thrombosis or pulmonary embolism has been diagnosed, there is little doubt that the patient should be anticoagulated, and the regimen continued for 3 months.

Ectopic bone

The major importance of ectopic bone formation lies in the restriction of movement that may occur as a consequence. This can spoil an otherwise very satisfactory outcome from the arthroplasty.

INCIDENCE

The reported incidence varies widely from 5% to 30%. Without prophylaxis, approximately 4–5% of patients will develop sufficient ectopic bone to limit movement (Hamblen, 1984b) and another 10–15% will show some ossification without symptoms.

CAUSE

Although there are many theories, its real cause is unknown. There are, however, a number of predisposing factors, some of which suggest an individual susceptibility. For example, patients who develop ectopic bone following hip arthroplasty have over a 90% chance of developing an identical degree of ectopic bone on the opposite side following arthroplasty (DeLee and Charnley, 1976).

PREDISPOSING FACTORS

These include hypertrophic osteoarthritis in males,

ankylosing spondylitis, medial osteoarthritis in either sex, ectopic bone following previous hip surgery (Ritter and Sieber, 1985), and extensive spinal osteophytosis (Blasingame *et al.*, 1981).

DIAGNOSIS

The diagnosis cannot be made on plain radiographs until the ossification is visible. These patients, however, sometimes run a slightly uncomfortable post-operative course, with a little swelling and sometimes reddening of the wound together with a low-grade pyrexia but no concrete evidence of infection. A technetium scan at this stage will show increased uptake before there are any signs of ectopic bone on plain films. Unexplained pain is a common symptom.

PROPHYLAXIS

There are only two effective ways of preventing ectopic ossification after hip arthroplasty: irradiation (Coventry and Scanlon, 1981) or the use of indomethacin. The latter is much more simple to give, and there are now a number of papers that attest to its efficacy (Ritter and Sieber, 1985; Cella *et al.*, 1988; Schmidt *et al.*, 1988). The authors' practice is to start indomethacin 25 mg b.d. the night before operation and to give it in this dosage for 5 days altogether, combined with cimetidine or a similar drug.

TREATMENT

If mature ectopic bone is causing sufficient trouble, surgical excision covered by indomethacin prophylaxis is the most appropriate treatment. The indomethacin should be given in a higher dosage than for routine prophylaxis, and should be continued for at least 2 weeks.

The excision of large masses of ectopic bone can be a formidable procedure, and the surgeon should be prepared to expose both the back and the front of the hip if necessary.

Loosening

The statistics in this section on results of cemented hip arthroplasty make it clear that aseptic loosening remains the most important complication of cemented total hip arthroplasty. The literature on the subject is now vast, and the matter is complex, so that a full discussion is beyond the scope of this chapter. The interested reader is referred to Lee and Ling (1984), Ling (1986), Black

(1988a) and Campbell *et al.* (1991) for further consideration of the subject. Figure 20.2.17 summarizes in diagrammatic form much of what follows.

DEFINITION

The *Concise Oxford Dictionary* describes the meaning of the word 'loose' as 'not rigidly fixed'. The use of the word 'loose' thus implies that the implant is not 'fixed'. On the other hand, it is known now (see above) that soundly fixed implants do actually move cyclically and reversibly in relation to the bone with each application of load, and are not therefore 'rigidly fixed'. Yet they are known not to be 'loose'. Though it would be convenient to be able to define some arbitrary limit of movement between implant and bone above which the implant could be regarded as being 'loose', in the present state of knowledge, this is impossible.

The matter is a semantic minefield, so that there is a need for a pragmatic rather than an absolute definition for what is acceptable movement between implant and bone. In the authors' opinion, the best definition to date is still the one given years ago by Swanson (1977) '. . . a cyclic displacement of the prosthetic component relative to the bone is acceptable if its magnitude does not progressively increase with repeated applications of load and if it does not give rise to pain or the presence of unacceptable quantities of debris'. To this should be added the rider that it should not destroy bone. If the cyclical movement is acceptable, fixation must be regarded as adequate. Loosening can then be defined as 'failure of adequate fixation'.

With regard to the absolute levels of movement that may be involved, Green *et al.* (1983) showed that reversible displacement of 500 μm or less in the femur was always asymptomatic, and 1000 μm might be. If it was not, however, it always increased with time. Lucent lines were associated with increased reversible displacement. Reversible displacement could sometimes disappear with time, i.e. be reduced to below the lower limit of detection by the methods that were used (200 μm), suggesting that implant stability may increase with time, presumably as the junctional tissues mature and bony remodelling takes place. All that can be said at present is that the limiting axial movement in the femur that distinguishes 'loose' from 'not loose' is somewhere between 40 and 500 μm.

Migration occurring early and rapidly carries a poor outlook, and must indicate bone resorption. Progressive migration therefore means progressive bone resorption, and may indicate future loosening (Ryd, 1992). On the other hand, the absence of early migration does not necessarily mean that satisfactory long-term function is certain, primarily because the damaging effects of wear usually take some years to make themselves felt.

Radiological loosening is defined on the basis of

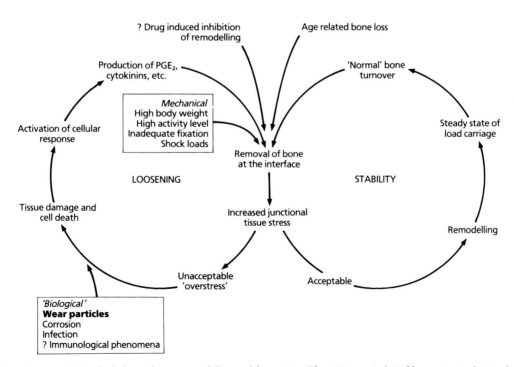

Fig. 20.2.17 Flow chart to show the balance between stability and loosening. The 'vicious circle' of loosening is depicted on the left.

progression of radiolucent lines at the cement—bone interface combined with progressive migration of the implant.

THE CAUSE

In basic terms, loosening will take place when the stresses applied to the junctional tissues and bone supporting the device persistently exceed their strength. Fixation strength depends not only on the nature of the junctional tissues, but on their extent, and on the strength of the bone that supports them. The strongest possible junctional tissue structure (osseointegration) is of no avail if the bone supporting it fails or is removed, for any reason. The stresses applied to the fixation are a reflection of the activity levels of the patient, together with the effects of shock interface loading that may be produced by impingement of the prosthetic components occurring at the extremes of movement. The latter becomes more important as wear of the socket takes place, since this reduces the permitted range of movement before impingement.

The dependence of junctional tissue structure on surgical technique at the primary operation has already been emphasized. Fibrous interfaces are in part a sequel to defective primary surgery, and the excessive micromotion that follows. An essential condition for the effective long-term control of micromotion between implant and bone is the establishment, as a consequence of the methods used at the primary operation, of direct contact between implant (i.e. cement with a cemented device) and bone over an area that is sufficient to carry the anticipated loads, without the creation of dangerously high levels of stress in the junctional tissues or bone.

Once this has been achieved, failure becomes a consequence of the actual or relative removal of bone that is supporting the junctional tissues. The consequence of such a process, if loads remain unchanged, is an increase in the stresses in the junctional tissues and bone that remain to support the device. With further removal of bone, the increase in stress in the residual supporting structures may come to exceed their fatigue strength, and there is then a mechanical failure, the consequence of which is generally a further increase in reversible micromovement, fibrous replacement and migration, culminating in loosening.

These considerations suggest that early failure (within the first 10 years) is most likely to be due to defective primary surgery, gross overload, or destruction of bone from infection. Late failure is connected with the factors that result in the removal of bone from the support of the implant.

REMOVAL OF BONE THAT SUPPORTS THE IMPLANT

Understress secondary to changes in stress distribution consequent upon the presence of the implant

As yet, bony remodelling from such understress (Engh et al., 1992) has not been shown to produce loosening. Its presence, however, may greatly complicate a revision operation when loosening does occur, and it is possible that in the very long term, it may prove to be important.

Reduction or failure of bone turnover

Bone turnover affects the bone that supports the implant just as any other bone in the skeleton. Any factor that interferes with bone formation while leaving bone resorption unchanged will lead to a net removal of bone. Age-related bone loss falls into this category, but as yet, has not been definitely shown to be responsible for loosening, though does increase the internal diameter of the medullary canal with time (Smith and Walker, 1964; Ruff and Hayes, 1982), particularly in women. Particulate debris has been shown to inhibit osteoblast function *in vitro* (Lanza et al., 1991) and drugs that inhibit bone formation, e.g. steroids or certain non-steroidal anti-inflammatory agents, may also be of importance.

Cellular activity at the implant—bone interface

Many authors have now shown that the activity of mononuclear cells at the implant—bone interface can greatly be increased by a number of factors and lead to bone destruction. Willert and his colleagues were the first to draw attention to this phenomenon (Willert and Semlitsch, 1976, 1977). Tissue damage and cell death (from overstress), infection, the products of corrosion and possibly immunological factors may all contribute. Far and away the most important, however, is the influence of particulate debris at the implant—bone interface. The size of the particles is probably more important than their chemical nature, the crucial matter being the ability of the particle to be phagocytosed by macrophages. This leads to activation of the macrophage (Murray and Rushton, 1992) with the elaboration of bone resorbing factors (including proteinases, collagenase, prostaglandins, interleukin-1, tumour necrosis factor, osteoclast activating factor and transforming growth factor; Apple et al., 1990) that act either directly or by stimulating osteoclasts to resorb bone. There is evidence that macrophages and foreign body giant cells on their own can also resorb bone (Athanasou et al., 1992), though probably only slowly. Large particles, too big to be phagocytosed, may become engulfed by foreign body giant cells, and granulomata may form.

The influence of particulate debris is probably the most important factor, in practical terms, in the bone destruction that underlies the genesis of late loosening (Campbell *et al.*, 1991).

THE SOURCE OF PARTICULATE DEBRIS

The articulation itself is an obvious source of wear debris, primarily of high-density polythene where the socket is manufactured from this material. Recently, however, it has become recognized that fretting is a major source of particulate debris. Fretting is defined (Black, 1988b) as 'wear produced by small interpart motions'. Large amounts of debris can be produced in this way, and the particle size may be very small. This means that the particles so produced are easily phagocytosed and transported, and their surface area is high in relation to their mass, increasing their potential biological activity. The amount of movement needed to produce debris in this way is exceedingly small, and is probably reached by the normal interpart motions occurring during normal use of a soundly fixed implant. Recently, the stem–cement interface (Anthony *et al.*, 1990; Lee *et al.*, 1993) has been recognized as a source of metal and acrylic cement debris from fretting, but the fact is that every interface and every coating (Campbell *et al.*, 1991; Collier *et al.*, 1992a, b) is a potential source of debris from this mechanism. Furthermore, fine metal debris so produced may find its way into the articulation, scratch the surface of the head of the femoral component, and thereby be responsible for increased wear of polythene at the articulation. Widespread distribution of such metallic debris has recently been reported by Langkamer *et al.* (1992), and the potential biological consequences are worrying.

THE ACCESS OF PARTICULATE DEBRIS TO THE JUNCTIONAL TISSUE

It is not difficult to see how debris can gain access to the junctional tissues at the latter's margins in the joint cavity. Polythene debris may dissect its way round the periphery of the interface on the acetabular side (Schmalzried *et al.*, 1992a), starting at the margins of the cup, where osseointegration is very hard to achieve using cement, and produce destruction of bone as it goes. In the femur, Malcolm (1990) found evidence of the presence of polythene debris at all areas of the bone–cement interface where this was fibrous, but not where there was direct contact between cement and bone. Such direct contact in the femur may therefore provide a barrier to the direct entry of debris.

What has been more difficult to understand is the appearance of localized lysis in relation to the more distal portions of the femoral component, with apparently intact interfaces elsewhere and proximally (Anthony *et al.*, 1990; Maloney *et al.*, 1990). Anthony *et al.* found fine acrylic and metal debris in the lytic lesions, as well as polythene. Maloney *et al.* originally described only acrylic debris, and this was ascribed to acrylic cement fracture, but a later re-examination of the specimens subsequently revealed polythene in addition (Schmalzried *et al.*, 1992b). A difficulty in interpreting reports on the types of debris present in lytic lesions is the fact that acrylic debris is dissolved out in the preparation of paraffin sections (Anthony *et al.*, 1990). Large fragments of acrylic then appear as voids in conventional H&E stained sections, but very fine debris may be missed unless fresh-frozen sections have been stained with a fat stain that is taken up by acrylic, or particles of barium or zirconium radio-opacifier can be identified.

Anthony *et al.* (1990) provided strong evidence that the acrylic and metal debris had been produced locally by fretting between the stem and cement, and that the polythene had gained access to the endosteal surface of the femur by travelling distally in the thin fibrous layer that frequently separates stem from cement (Fornasier and Cameron, 1976). Any cement mantle defect would then provide a route to the endosteal surface of the femur from this interface, through which the polythene and locally produced acrylic and metal debris might pass. Every case of localized lysis that they reported was proven at surgery to be associated with a cement mantle defect. Such a phenomenon provides a ready and credible explanation for the often observed fact that lytic lesions tend to occur where the metal of the stem is very close to the endosteal surface of the femur—just such sites at which mantle defects might be expected (Fig. 20.2.18). This explains also why very large stems may become associated with lysis.

The hydrostatic and mechanical properties of fibrous layers (Hori and Lewis, 1982) are such that repeated compressive loading exerts a pump-like action that could drive particulate debris slowly along the fibrous layer or its boundaries. Fretting at the stem–cement interface gradually increases the internal dimension of the cement mantle as the cement is sacrificed. This leads to a steady increase in the amplitude of movement of the stem within the cement, particularly in torsion. Eventually, substantial pressure effects are produced that serve to increase the pumping of fluid and debris, together with any bone resorbing factors that may be present, throughout the spaces that communicate with the joint. Anthony *et al.* recorded pressure changes amounting to almost

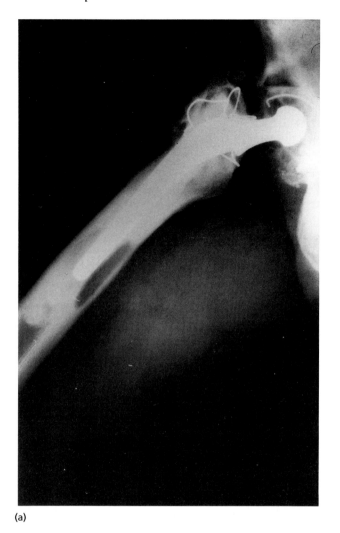

(a)

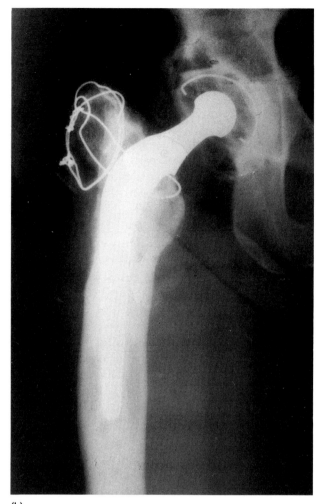

(b)

Fig. 20.2.18 Localized lytic lesion with cement mantle defect.

200 mmHg occurring in a lytic lesion in response to minimal passive movement of the hip. Very much higher pressures would be produced by active use of the hip. It takes little imagination to visualize the catastrophic effects that this may have on the bony supports for the implant. Such mechanisms probably underlie the phenomenon of aggressive granulomata after hip arthroplasty (Tallroth *et al.*, 1989).

The importance of a complete cement mantle in preventing the access of debris to the endosteal surface of the femur by this route is obvious. The reduction of debris production by fretting between stem and cement is best achieved, in the current state of knowledge, by using stems that have polished surfaces. Pre-coating is not regularly effective.

DIAGNOSIS

Persistent pain following hip arthroplasty suggests either that the pre-operative pain was not actually arising in the hip, or the presence of infection. Recurrence of pain after a pain-free period following arthroplasty suggests the possible onset of loosening. Establishing the cause of pain felt at the root of the thigh or in the buttock is not always straightforward, particularly in patients who also suffer from low back disorders. In such cases, a therapeutic trial of an injection of 0.25% marcaine into the hip joint space, under image intensifier control, is often extremely helpful.

Although early loosening may be devoid of abnormal physical signs, particularly if only the socket is involved, a suggestive finding is thigh or groin pain on forced internal rotation of the hip.

Scintigraphy and arthrography have often been used in an attempt to diagnose loosening (Van Rens and Slooff, 1984) but the single most valuable investigation is careful scrutiny of good quality sequential radiographs displayed simultaneously on a wide screen viewing box. Progressive radiolucent lines or lysis, or a progressive change in the position of the implant, make the diagnosis likely. A normal sedimentation rate and C-reactive protein help to exclude infection, but the latter can rarely be totally excluded until the results of operative cultures are available.

MANAGEMENT

This complex matter is beyond the scope of this chapter. The golden rule is, however, to revise before bone stock loss becomes serious. This implies regular radiographic follow-up, that should be regarded as an essential routine for all units involved in hip arthroplasty.

Femoral component fracture

Fracture of the femoral component was an important and distressing complication of total hip arthroplasty in the 1970s and the early 1980s and attracted a considerable literature (Lee and Ling, 1984). Its incidence has been reduced dramatically by modern stem design coupled with the introduction of high fatigue strength alloys and contemporary cementing techniques. Its only practical importance now lies in the fact that arthroplasties from the era of the 1970s and early 1980s will still continue to present from time to time with stem fractures.

CONCLUSIONS

The crucial factors for satisfactory long-term function of a hip arthroplasty, whether cemented or cementless, are the control of the structure and maintenance of the junctional tissues with their bony supports, the production and effects of particulate debris, and the avoidance of gross overload. Sound primary surgery utilizing modern cementing techniques and an implant of proven performance ensure satisfactory junctional tissue structure and acceptable loading. The major tasks for the future lie in developing methods of reducing the production of particulate debris and controlling its effects, and in educating patients to treat their implants with respect.

REFERENCES

Ahmed A.M., Raab S. and Miller J.E. (1984) Metal/cement interface strength in cemented stem fixation. *J. Orthop. Res.* **2**, 105–118.

Albrektsson T., Branemark P.-I., Hansson H.-A. and Lindstrom J. (1981) Osseointegrated titanium implants. Requirements for ensuring a long-lasting, direct bone-to-implant anchorage in man. *Acta Orthop. Scand.* **52**, 155–170.

Amstutz H.C. and Kody M.C. (1991) Dislocation and subluxation. In Amstutz H.C. (ed.) *Hip Arthroplasty.* New York, Churchill Livingstone, pp. 429–447.

Amstutz H.C., Clarke I.C., Christie J. and Graff-Radford A. (1977) Total hip articular replacement by internal eccentric shells. *Clin. Orthop.* **128**, 261.

Amstutz H.C., Yao J., Dorey F.J. and Gruen T.A. (1991) Acrylic fixation-stem and socket replacement: results, principles and technique. In Amstutz H.C. (ed.) *Hip Arthroplasty.* New York, Churchill Livingstone, pp. 239–270.

Anthony P.P., Gie G.A., Howie C.R. and Ling R.S.M. (1990) Localised endosteal bone lysis in relation to the femoral components of cemented hip arthroplasty. *J. Bone Joint Surg.* **72B**, 971–979.

Apple A.M., Sauder W.G., Siverhuss W., Hopson C.N. and Herman J.H. (1990) Prosthesis associated pseudomembrane-induced bone resorption. *Br. J. Rheum.* **29**, 32–36.

Archibald D.A.A. (1991) The role of self-locking tapers in stem fixation. M. Phil. Thesis, University of Strathclyde.

Athanasou N.A., Quinn J. and Bulstrode C.J.K. (1992) Resorption of bone by inflammatory cells derived from the joint capsule of hip arthroplasties. *J. Bone Joint Surg.* **74B**, 57–62.

August A.C., Aldam C.H. and Pynsent P.B. (1986) The McKee–Farrar hip arthroplasty—a long-term study. *J. Bone Joint Surg.* **68B**, 520–527.

Baldursson H., Hansson L.I., Olsson T.H. and Selvik G. (1980) Migration of the acetabular socket after total hip replacement determined by roentgen stereophotogrammetry. *Acta Orthop. Scand.* **51**, 535.

Bannister G.C. and Miles A.W. (1988) The influence of cementing technique and blood on the strength of the bone-cement interface. *Eng. Med.* **17**, 131–134.

Barb W., Park J.B., Kenner G.H. and von Recum A.F. (1982) Intramedullary fixation of artificial hip joints with bone cement precoated implants. I. Interfacial strengths. *J. Biomed. Mater. Res.* **16**, 447–458.

Barrack R.L., Jasty M., Bragden C., Haire T. and Harris W.H. (1992) Thigh pain despite bony ingrowth into uncemented femoral stems. *J. Bone Joint Surg.* **74A**, 507–510.

Barrington T.W., Johansen J.E. and McBroom R. (1984) Fractures of the femur complicating total hip replacement. In Ling R.S.M. (ed.) *Complications of Total Hip Replacement.* Edinburgh, Churchill Livingstone, pp. 30–40.

Bartel D.L., Wright T.M. and Edwards D. (1983) The effect of metal-backing on the stresses in polyethylene acetabular components. In *The Proceedings of the Eleventh Open Scientific Meeting of the Hip Society.* St Louis, C.V. Mosby, pp. 216–228.

Bartel D.L., Bicknell V.L. and Wright T.M. (1986) The effect of conformity, thickness and material on stresses in ultra-high molecular weight components for total joint replacement. *J. Bone Joint Surg.* **68A**, 1041–1051.

Beckenbaugh R.D. and Ilstrup D.M. (1978) Total hip arthroplasty.

A review of three hundred and thirty-two cases with long follow-up. *J. Bone Joint Surg.* **60A**, 306.

Benjamin J.B., Volz R.G., Gie G.A., Ling R.S.M. and Lee A.J.C. (1987) Cementing technique and the effects of bleeding. *J. Bone Joint Surg.* **69B**, 620–624.

Bergmann G., Graichen F. and Rohlmann A. (1992) Loading of hip implants by torsional moments. *Trans. Orthop. Res. Soc.* **17**, 19.

Berme N. and Paul J.P. (1979) Load actions transmitted by implants. *J. Biomed. Eng.* **1**, 268–272.

Black D.L., Reckling F.W. and Porter S. (1991) Somatosensory-evoked potential monitored during total hip arthroplasty. *Clin. Orthop.* **262**, 170–177.

Black J. (1988a) Fixation. In *Orthop Biomat Res Prac*. New York, Churchill Livingstone, pp. 267–283.

Black J. (1988b) Friction and wear. In *Orthop Biomat Res Prac*. New York, Churchill Livingstone, pp. 213–233.

Blasingame J.P., Resnick D., Coutts R.D. and Danzig L.A. (1981) Extensive spinal osteophytosis as a risk factor for heterotopical formation after total hip arthroplasty. *Clin. Orthop.* **161**, 197.

Brady L.P. and McCutchen J.W. (1986) A ten-year follow-up study of 170 Charnley total hip arthroplasties. *Clin. Orthop.* **211**, 51–54.

Brand R.A., Pedersen D.R., Davy D.T., Kotzar G.M., Heiple K.G. and Goldberg V.M. (1993) Comparison of hip joint force calculations and measurements in the same patient. *J. Arthrop.* In press.

Branemark P.-I., Hansson B.O., Adell R., Breine U., Lindstrom J. and Hallen O. (1977) Osseointegrated implants in the treatment of the odentulous jaw: experience from a ten year period. *Scand. J. Plast. Reconstr. Surg.* **11** (Suppl. 16).

British Orthopaedic Association Survey (1990) British Orthopaedic Association, Royal College of Surgeons, London.

Burke D.W., O'Connor D., Zalenski E.B., Jasty M. and Harris W.H. (1991) Micromotion of cemented and uncemented femoral components. *J. Bone Joint Surg.* **73B**, 33–37.

Byrick R.J., Bell R.S., Kay J.C., Waddell J.P. and Mullen J.B. (1989) High volume, high pressure pulsatile lavage during cemented hip arthroplasty. *J. Bone Joint Surg.* **71A**, 1331–1336.

Callaghan J.J., Fulghum C.S., Glisson R.R. and Stranne S.K. (1992) The effect of femoral stem geometry on interface motion in uncemented porous-coated total hip prostheses. *J. Bone Joint Surg.* **74A**, 839–848.

Campbell A.C.L., Rorabeck C.H., Bourne R.B., Chess D. and Nott L. (1992) Thigh pain after cementless hip arthroplasty. Annoyance or ill omen? *J. Bone Joint Surg.* **74B**, 63–66.

Campbell P., Clarke I.C. and Kossovsky N. (1991) Clinical significance of wear debris. In Amstutz H.C. (ed.) *Hip Arthroplasty*. New York, Churchill Livingstone, pp. 550–570.

Carter D.R., Vasu R. and Harris W.H. (1982) Stress distributions in the acetabular region. II. Effects of cup thickness and metal backing of the total hip acetabular component. *J. Biomech.* **15**, 165.

Cella J.P., Salvata E.A. and Sculco T.P. (1988) Indomethacin for the prevention of heterotopic ossification following total hip arthroplasty: effectiveness, contra-indications and adverse effects. *J. Arthrop.* **3**, 229–234.

Chandler H.P., Reineck F.T., Wixson R.L. and Mcarthy J.C. (1981) Total hip replacements in patients younger than thirty years old. *J. Bone Joint Surg.* **63A**, 1426–1434.

Charnley J. (1960) Anchorage of the femoral head prosthesis to the shaft of the femur. *J. Bone Joint Surg.* **42B**, 28–30.

Charnley J. (1961) Arthroplasty of the hip—a new operation. *Lancet* **i**, 1129.

Charnley J. (1970) The theory of mechanical fastenings in bone surgery. In *Acrylic Cement in Orthopaedic Surgery*. Edinburgh, Churchill Livingstone.

Charnley J. (1975) Fracture of femoral prostheses in total hip replacement. *Clin. Orthop.* **111**, 105.

Charnley J. (1979a) *Low Friction Arthroplasty of the Hip. Theory and Practice*. Berlin, Springer-Verlag.

Charnley J. (1979b) Long term radiological results. In *Low Friction Arthroplasty of the Hip*. Berlin, Springer Verlag, p. 84.

Charnley J. (1979c) Cement-bone interface. In *Low Friction Arthroplasty of the Hip. Theory and Practice*. Berlin, Springer-Verlag, p. 36.

Collier J.P., Mayor M.B., Jensen R.E., Surprenant V.A., Surprenant H.P., McNamara J.L. and Belec L. (1992a) Mechanisms of failure of modular prostheses. *Clin. Orthop.* **285**, 129–139.

Collier J.P., Surprenant V.A., Jensen R.E., Mayor M.B. and Surprenant H.P. (1992b) Corrosion between the components of modular femoral hip prostheses. *J. Bone Joint Surg.* **74B**, 511–517.

Collis D.K. (1977) Femoral stem failure in total hip replacement. *J. Bone Joint Surg.* **59A**, 1033–1041.

Cook S.D., Barrack R.L., Thomas K.A. and Hadad R.J. (1991) Tissue growth into porous primary and revision femoral stems. *J. Arthroplasty* Suppl. 6, S37–47.

Corkill J.A., Lloyd E.J., Hoyle P., Crout D.H.G., Ling R.S.M., James M.L. and Piper R. (1976) Toxicology of methylmethacrylate. The rate of disappearance of methylmethacrylate in human blood 'in vitro'. *Clin. Chim. Acta* **68**, 141.

Coventry M. (1991) Foreword. In Amstutz H.C. (ed.) *Total Hip Arthroplasty*. New York, Churchill Livingstone, p. xi.

Coventry M.B. and Scanlon P.W. (1981) The use of radiation to discourage ectopic bone. *J. Bone Joint Surg.* **63A**, 201.

Crout D.H.G., Corkill J.A., James M.L. and Ling R.S.M. (1979) Methylmethacrylate metabolism in man. The hydrolysis of methylmethacrylate to methacrylate acid during total hip replacement. *Clin. Orthop.* **141**, 90.

Crout D.H.G., Lloyd E.J. and Singh J. (1982) Metabolism of methylmethacrylate: evidence for metabolism by the valine pathway of catabolism in rat and in man. *Xenobiotica* **12**, 821–829.

Crowninshield R.D., Johnstone R.C., Andrews J.G. and Brand R.A. (1978) A biomechanical investigation of the human hip. *J. Biomech.* **11**, 75.

Crowninshield R.D., Brand R.A., Johnstone R.C. and Milroy J.C. (1980) The effect of femoral stem cross-sectional geometry on cement stresses in total hip reconstruction. *Clin. Orthop.* **146**, 71–77.

Crowninshield R.D., Brand R.A., Johnstone R.C. and Pedersen D.R. (1981) An analysis of collar function and the use of titanium in femoral prostheses. *Clin. Orthop.* **158**, 270–277.

Cupic Z. (1979) Long-term follow-up of Charnley arthroplasty of the hip. *Clin. Orthop.* **141**, 28–43.

Dall D., Learmonth I., Solomon M., Miles A. and Davenport M. (1993) Mechanical loosening of Charnley femoral stems—a comparison between the long-term results of first generation and subsequent generations stems. *J. Bone Joint Surg.* **75B**, In press.

Dall D.M., Grobbelaar C.J., Learmonth I.D. and Dall G. (1986a) Charnley low-friction arthroplasty in South Africa. *Clin. Orthop.* **211**, 85–90.

Dall D.M., Miles A.W. and Juby G. (1986b) Accelerated polymerisation of bone cement using pre-heated implants. *Clin. Orthop.* **211**, 148–150.

Dalstra M. and Huiskes R. (1991) The influence of metal-backing in cemented cups. *Orthop. Trans.* **15**, 459.

Davey D.T., Kotzar G.M., Brown R.H. *et al.* (1988) Telemetric force measurements across the hip joint after total arthroplasty. *J. Bone Joint Surg.* **70A**, 45–50.

DeLee J.G. and Charnley J. (1976) Radiological demarcation of cemented sockets in total hip replacement. *Clin. Orthop. Rel. Res.* **121**, 20–32.

Dobbs H.S. (1980) Survivorship of total hip replacements. *J. Bone Joint Surg.* **62B**, 168–173.

Dorr L.D., Takei G.K. and Conaty J.P. (1983) Total hip arthroplasties in patients less than forty-five years old. *J. Bone Joint Surg.* **65A**, 474–479.

Eftekhar N.S. and Tzitzikalakis G.I. (1986) Failures and re-operations following low-friction arthroplasty of the hip. *Clin. Orthop.* **211**, 65–78.

Engh C.A., O'Connor D., Jasty M., McGovern T.F., Bobyn J.D. and Harris W.H. (1992) Quantification of implant micromotion, strain shielding and bone resorption with porous-coated anatomical medullary locking femoral prostheses. *Clin. Orthop.* **285**, 13–29.

English T.A. and Kilvington M. (1979) 'In vivo' records of hip loads using a femoral implant with a telemetric output (a preliminary report). *J. Biomed. Eng.* **1**, 111.

Fagan M.J. (1984) A finite element analysis of femoral stem design in cemented total hip replacement. PhD Thesis, University of Exeter.

Fordyce M.J.F. and Ling R.S.M. (1992) A venous foot pump reduces thrombosis after hip replacement. *J. Bone Joint Surg.* **74B**, 45–49.

Fornasier V.L. and Cameron H.U. (1976) The femoral stem–cement interface in total hip replacement. *Clin. Orthop.* **116**, 248–252.

Fowler J., Gie G.A., Lee A.J.C. and Ling R.S.M. (1988) Experience with the Exeter hip since 1970. *Orthop. Clin. North Am.* **19**, 477–489.

Freeman M.A.R. (1978) Some anatomical and mechanical considerations relevant to the surface replacement of the femoral head. *Clin. Orthop.* **134**, 19.

Freeman M.A.R. (1984) The complications of double cup replacement of the hip. In Ling R.S.M. (ed.) *Complications of Total Hip Replacement*. Edinburgh, Churchill Livingstone, pp. 172–200.

Freeman M.A.R., Cameron H.U. and Brown G.C. (1978) Cemented double-cup arthroplasty of the hip: a five year experience with the ICLH prosthesis. *Clin. Orthop.* **134**, 45.

Freeman M.A.R., Bradley G.W. and Revell P.A. (1982) Observations upon the interface between bone and polymethylmethacrylate cement. *J. Bone Joint Surg.* **64B**, 489–493.

Gardiner R.C. and Hozack W.J. (1994) Failure of the cement–bone interface. *J. Bone Joint Surg.* **76B**, 49–52.

Gie G.A., Linder L., Ling R.S.M., Simon J.-P., Slooff T.J.J.H. and Timperley A.J. (1993) Impacted cancellous allografts and cement for revision total hip arthroplasty. *J. Bone Joint Surg.* **75B**, 14–21.

Green D.L., Bahniuk E., Liebelt R.A., Fender E., and Mirkov P. (1983) Biplane radiographic measurements of reversible displacements (including clinical loosening) and migration of total joint replacements. *J. Bone Joint Surg.* **65A**, 1134–1143.

Gruen T.A., McNeice G. and Amstutz H.C. (1979) 'Modes of Failure' of cemented stem-type femoral component. *Clin. Orthop. Rel. Res.* **141**, 17–27.

Haboush E.J. (1953) A new operation for arthroplasty of the hip. *Bull. Hosp. J. Dis.* **13**, 242.

Halawa M., Lee A.J.C., Ling R.S.M. and Vangala S.S. (1978) The shear strength of trabecular bone from the femur and some factors affecting the shear strength of the cement-bone interface. *Arch. Orthop. Trauma Surg.* **92**, 19.

Hale D., Lee A.J.C., Ling R.S.M. and Hooper R.M. (1990) The production of acrylic cement and metal debris by the femoral component in cemented total hip replacement. *J. Bone Joint Surg.* **72B**, 1090.

Hamblen D.L. (1984a) Dislocation. In Ling R.S.M. (ed.) *Complications of Total Hip Replacement*. Edinburgh, Churchill Livingstone, pp. 82–99.

Hamblen D.L. (1984b) Ectopic ossification. In Ling R.S.M. (ed.) *Complications of Total Hip Replacement*. Edinburgh, Churchill Livingstone, pp. 100–109.

Hamilton H.W. and Joyce M. (1986) Long-term results of low-friction arthroplasty performed in a Community Hospital, including a radiologic review. *Clin. Orthop. Rel. Res.* **211**, 55–64.

Harrigan T.P. and Harris W.H. (1991) A three-dimensional non-linear finite element study of the effects of cement-prosthesis debonding in cemented femoral total hip. *J. Biomech.* **23**, 1047.

Harris W.H. (1971) A new total hip implant. *Clin. Orthop. Rel. Res.* **81**, 105–113.

Harris W.H. (1992) Is it advantageous to strengthen the cement–metal interface and use a collar for cemented femoral components of total hip replacements? *Clin. Orthop.* **285**, 67–72.

Harris W.H. and White R.E. (1982) Socket fixation using a metal-backed acetabular component for total hip replacement. *J. Bone Joint Surg.* **64A**, 745–754.

Harris W.H. and Maloney W.J. (1989) Hybrid total hip arthroplasty. *Clin. Orthop.* **249**, 21–29.

Henry A.K. (1973) Extensile exposure. *Extensile Exposure* **182**.

Heyse-Moore G.H. and Ling R.S.M. (1982) Current cement techniques. In Marti R.K. (ed.) *Progress in Cemented Hip Surgery and Revision*. Amsterdam, Excerpta Medica, 71–86.

Hoeltzel D.A., Walt M.J., Kyle R.F. and Simon F.D. (1989) The effects of femoral head size on the deformation of ultrahigh molecular weight polyethylene acetabular cups. *J. Biomech.* **22**, 1163–1173.

Hori R.Y. and Lewis J.L. (1982) Mechanical properties of the fibrous tissue found at the bone–cement interface following total joint replacement. *J. Biomed. Mat. Res.* **16**, 911–927.

Hozack W.J., Rothman R.H., Booth R.E., Balderston R.A., Cohn J.C. and Pickens G.T. (1990) Survivorship analysis of 1041 Charnley total hip arthroplasties. *J. Arthrop.* **5**, 41–47.

Huiskes R. (1979) Some fundamental aspects of human joint replacement. Analyses of stresses and heat conduction in bone-prosthesis structures. *Acta Orthop. Scand. Suppl.* 185.

Hullinger L. (1962) Untersuchungen uber die Wirkung von Kunstharzen (Palacos und Ostamer) in Gewebkulturen. *Arch. Orthop. Unfallchir.* **54**, 54.

Jacobsson S.A., Djerf K. and Wahlstrom O. (1990) A comparative study between McKee–Farrar and Charnley arthroplasty. *J. Arthrop.* **5**, 9–14.

James M.L. (1984) Anaesthetic and metabolic complications. In Ling R.S.M. (ed.) *Complications of Total Hip Replacement*. Edinburgh, Churchill Livingstone, pp. 1–17.

Jasty M., Bragden C.R., Maloney W.J., Haire T. and Harris W.H. (1991) Ingrowth of bone in failed fixation of porous-coated femoral components. *J. Bone Joint Surg.* **73A**, 1331–1337.

Jasty M., Maloney W.J., Bragden C.R., Haire T. and Harris W.H. (1990) Histomorphological studies of the long-term skeletal responses to well-fixed cemented femoral components. *J. Bone Joint Surg.* **72A**, 1220–1229.

Jefferiss C.D., Lee A.J.C. and Ling R.S.M. (1975) Thermal aspects of self-curing polymethylmethacrylate. *J. Bone Joint Surg.* **57B**, 511.

Johnstone R.C. and Crowninshield R.D. (1983) Roentgenolic results of total hip arthroplasty. *Clin. Orthop.* **181**, 92.

Jones L.C. and Hungerford D.S. (1987) Cement disease. *Clin. Orthop. Rel. Res.* **181**, 92–98.

Karrholm J. (1989) Roentgen stereophotogrammetry. A review of orthopaedic application. *Acta Orthop. Scand.* **60**, 491–503.

Karrholm J., Malchau H., Snorrason F. and Herberts P. (1992) Femoral component fixation in total hip arthroplasty. *Trans. Orthop. Res. Soc.* **17**, 291.

Kavanagh B.F., Dewitz M.A., Ilstrup D.M., Stauffer R.N. and Coventry M.B. (1989) Charnley total hip arthroplasty with cement. Fifteen year results. *J. Bone Joint Surg.* **71A**, 1496–1503.

Kerboul M. (1985) The routine operation. In Postel M., Kerboul M., Evrard J and Courpied J.P. (eds) *Total Hip Replacement*. Berlin, Springer-Verlag, pp. 18–35.

Krause W., Krug W. and Miller J. (1980) Cement–bone interface—effect of cement technique and surface preparation. *Orthop. Trans.* **4**, 204.

Krause W.R., Krug W. and Miller J. (1982) Strength of the cement–bone interface. *Clin. Orthop. Rel. Res.* **163**, 290–299.

Lachiewicz P.F., McCaskill B., Inglis A., Ranawat C.S. and Rosenstein B.D. (1986) Total hip arthroplasty in juvenile rheumatoid arthritis. *J. Bone Joint Surg.* **68A**, 502–508.

Langkamer V.G., Case C.P., Heap P., Taylor A., Collins C., Pearse M. and Solomon L. (1992) Systemic distribution of wear debris after hip replacement. A cause for concern? *J. Bone Joint Surg.* **74B**, 831–839.

Lanzer W.L., Crane G.K., Davidson J.A. and Howard G.A. (1991) In vitro human bone cell proliferation: the effects of implant particulates and elevated temperature. Paper read at the 37th Annual Meeting of the Orthopaedic Research Society.

Lee A.J.C. and Ling R.S.M. (1974) A device to improve the extrusion of bone cement into the bone of the acetabulum in the replacement of the hip joint. *Biomed. Eng.* **9**, 1.

Lee A.J.C. and Ling R.S.M. (1984) Loosening. In Ling R.S.M. (ed.) *Complications of Total Hip Replacement*. Edinburgh, Churchill Livingstone, pp. 110–145.

Lee A.J.C. and Ling R.S.M. (1984) Stem breakage. In Ling R.S.M. (ed.) *Complications of Total Hip Replacement*. Edinburgh, Churchill Livingstone, pp. 146–171.

Lee A.J.C., Ling R.S.M. and Wrighton J.D. (1973) Some properties of polymethylmethacrylate with reference to its use in orthopaedic surgery. *Clin. Orthop.* **95**, 281.

Lee A.J.C., Perkins R.D. and Ling R.S.M. (1990) Time-dependent properties of polymethylmethacrylate bone cement. In Older M.J.W. (ed.) *Implant Bone Interface*. London, Springer-Verlag, pp. 85–90.

Lee A.J.C., Hooper R.M., Ling R.S.M., Brooks R., Gie G.A. and Hale D. (1993) Fretting as a source of particulate debris in total joint arthroplasty. In Turner-Smith A.R. (ed.) *Micromovement in Orthopaedics*. Oxford, Oxford University Press, vol. 12, pp. 82–98.

Lettin A.W.F., Ware H.S. and Morris R.W. (1991) Survivorship analysis and confidence intervals. *J. Bone Joint Surg.* **73B**, 729–731.

Lewis J.L., Askew M.J., Wixson R.L., Kramer G.M. and Tarr R.R. (1984) The influence of prosthetic stem stiffness and of a calcar collar on stresses in the proximal end of the femur with a cemented femoral component. *J. Bone Joint Surg.* **66A**, 280–286.

Linder L. (1977) The reaction of bone to the acute chemical trauma of bone cement. *J. Bone Joint Surg.* **59A**, 82.

Linder L. (1989) Osseointegration of metallic implants. 1. Light microscopy in the rabbit. *Acta Orthop. Scand.* **60**, 129–134.

Linder L. and Lundskog J. (1974) Incorporation of stainless steel titanium and vitalium in bone stock. *Injury* **6**, 277.

Linder L. and Hansson B.O. (1983) Ultrastructural aspects of the interface between bone and cement in man. *J. Bone Joint Surg.* **65B**, 646–649.

Linder L., Carlsson A., Marsal L., Bjursten L.M. and Branemark P.-I. (1988) Clinical aspects of osseointegration in joint replacement surgery. *J. Bone Joint Surg.* **70B**, 550–555.

Ling R.S.M. (1986) Observations on the fixation of implants to the bony skeleton. *Clin. Orthop. Rel. Res.* **210**, 80–96.

Ling R.S.M. (1991) Cementing technique in the femur. *Tech. Orthop.* **6**, 34–39.

Ling R.S.M. (1992) The use of a collar and pre-coating on cemented femoral stems is unnecessary and detrimental. *Clin. Orthop.* **285**, 73–83.

Lu Z, Ebramzadeh E., MacKellop H., Zahiri C. and Sarmiento A. (1992) The influence of stem–cement bonding strength on the cement stresses in total hip arthroplasty. *Transactions of the 38th Annual Meeting of the Orthopaedic Research Society* **17**, 377.

Markolf K.L. and Amstutz H.C. (1976) A comparative experimental study of stresses in femoral total hip replacement components: the effects of prosthesis orientation and acrylic fixation. *J. Biomech.* **9**, 73.

Markolf K.L., Amstutz H.C. and Hirschowitz M.D. (1980) The effect of calcar contact on femoral component micromovement. *J. Bone Joint Surg.* **62A**, 1315.

Marti R. and Besselaar P.P. (1981) Reconstruction of the acetabular roof and other bone grafts in total hip replacement and total hip revision. *J. Bone Joint Surg.* **63B**, 283.

McCarthy C.K., Steinberg G.G., Agren M., Leahey D., Wyman E. and Baran D.T. (1991) Quantifying bone loss from the proximal femur after total hip arthroplasty. *J. Bone Joint Surg.* **73B**, 774–778.

McCoy T.H., Salvati E.A., Ranawat C.S. and Wilson P.D. (1988) A 15 year follow-up study of 100 Charnley LFAs. *Orthop. Clin. N. Am.* **19**, 467–476.

McKee G.K. and Watson Farrar J. (1966) Replacement of arthritic hips by the McKee–Farrar prosthesis. *J. Bone Joint Surg.* **74B**, 245.

Malcolm A.J. (1990) Pathology of low-friction arthoplasties in autopsy specimens. In Older M.W.J. (ed.) *Implant Bone Interface*. London, Springer-Verlag, pp. 77–82.

Maloney W.J., Jasty M., Burke D.W. *et al.* (1989) Biomechanical and histological investigation of cemented total hip arthroplasties: the study of autopsy-retrieved femurs after 'in vivo' cycling. *Clin. Orthop. Rel. Res.* **249**, 129–140.

Maloney W.J., Jasty M., Rosenberg A. and Harris W.H. (1990) Bone lysis in well-fixed femoral components. *J. Bone Joint Surg.* **72B**, 966–970.

Mennem U. (1989) The use of clamp-on plates for forearm fractures. *Orthopaedics* **12**, 39–43.

Miles A.W., Clift S.E. and Bannister G.C. (1990) The effect of the surface finish of the femoral component in total hip replacement. *J. Bone Joint Surg.* **72B**, 736.

Miller J., Burke D.L., Stachiewicz J., Ahmed A. and Kelebay L.C. (1978a) Pathophysiology of loosening of femoral components in total hip arthroplasty. In *The Hip. Proceedings of the Sixth Open Scientific Meeting of the Hip Society.* St Louis, C.V. Mosby, p. 77.

Miller J., Tremblay G.R., Burke D.L., Ahmed A. and Kelebay L.C. (1978b) The injection of acrylic cement into cancellous bone as a method of the prevention of loosening of arthroplasty components. Paper read at the 24th Annual Meeting of the Orthopaedic Research Society, Dallas.

Mittlemeier T., Plitz W. and Russe W. (1986) The eccentric polythene acetabular cup: the role of cup wall thickness and design in implant loosening. In Kossovsky R. and Kossovsky N. (eds) *Materials Sciences and Implant Orthopaedic Surgery.* Dordrecht, pp. 223–232.

Mjoberg B. (1986) Loosening of the cemented hip prosthesis: the importance of heat injury. *Acta Orthop. Scand.* Suppl. 57.

Mjoberg B., Hansson L.I. and Selvik G. (1984) Instability, migration and laxity of total hip prostheses. A roentgen stereophotogrammetric study. *Acta Orthop. Scand.* **55**, 141–145.

Morrey B.F. and Ilstrup D. (1989) Size of the femoral head and acetabular revision in total hip replacement arthroplasty. *J. Bone Joint Surg.* **71A**, 50.

Morscher E. and Dick W. (1984) Cementless fixation of a polyethylene acetabular component. In Morscher E. (ed.) *The Cementless Fixation of Hip Endoprostheses.* Berlin, Springer-Verlag, pp. 200–204.

Morscher E. and Masar Z. (1988) Development and first experience with an uncemented press-fit cup. *Clin. Orthop.* **232**, 96.

Muller M. (1992) Lessons of thirty years of total hip arthroplasty. *Clin. Orthop.* **274**, 12–21.

Mulroy R.D. and Harris W.H. (1990a) The effect of improved cementing techniques on component loosening in total hip replacement. *J. Bone Joint Surg.* **72B**, 757–760.

Mulroy R.D. and Harris W.H. (1990b) Failure of acetabular autogenous grafts in total hip arthroplasty. *J. Bone Joint Surg.* **72A**, 1536–1540.

Munih M., Kralj A. and Bajd T. (1992) Bending moments in lower extremity bones for two standing postures. *J. Biomed Eng.* **14**, 293–302.

Murray D.W. (1992) Impingement and loosening of the long posterior wall acetabular implant. *J. Bone Joint Surg.* **74B**, 377–379.

Murray D.W. and Rushton N. (1992) Macrophages stimulate bone resorption when they phagocytose particles. *J. Bone Joint Surg.* **72B**, 988–992.

Neumann L., Freund K.G. and Sorenson K.H. (1994) Long-term results of Charnley total hip replacement. *J. Bone Joint Surg.* **76B**, 245–251.

O'Carroll P.F., Kim W.C., Kabo M. and Amstutz H.C. (1985) Membrane formation in response to acrylic and titanium in similar stress environment. *Transactions of the 31st Annual Meeting of the Orthopaedic Research Society* **10**, 89.

Oh I., Carlsson C.E., Tomford W.W. and Harris W.H. (1978) Improved fixation of femoral component after total hip replacement using a methacrylate intramedullary plug. *J. Bone Joint Surg.* **60A**, 608–618.

Oh I., Sander T.W. and Treharne R.W. (1985) Total hip acetabular cup flange design and its effect on cement fixation. *Clin. Orthop.* **195**, 304–309.

Older M.W.J. (1984) A ten to twelve year follow-up study of Charnley Arthroplasty of the hip. *J. Bone Joint Surg.* **66B**, 299–300.

Older M.J.W. (1986) Low-friction arthroplasty of the hip. A 10–12 year follow-up study. *Clin. Orthop.* **211**, 36–42.

Olerud S. and Karlstrom G. (1985) Recurrent dislocation after total hip replacement — treatment by fixing an additional sector to the acetabular component. *J. Bone Joint Surg.* **67B**, 402–405.

Park J.B., Malstrom C.S. and von Recum A.F. (1978) Intramedullary fixation of implants pre-coated with bone cement — a preliminary study. *Biomat. Med. Dev. Art. Org.* **6**(4), 361–373.

Parker-Williams J. and Vickers R. (1991) Major orthopaedic surgery on the leg and thromboembolism. Prophylatis now or negligence claims later. *Br. Med. J.* **303**, 531–532.

Patterson F.P. and Brown C.S. (1972) The McKee–Farrar total hip replacement. Preliminary results and complications of 368 operations performed in five general hospitals. *J. Bone Joint Surg.* **54A**, 257.

Paul J.P. (1976) Force actions transmitted by joints in the human body. *Proc. Roy. Soc. Lond.* **192**, 163–72.

Pavlov P.W. (1987) A fifteen year follow-up study of 512 consecutive Charnley–Muller total hip replacements. *J. Arthrop.* **2**, 151–156.

Pedersen D.R., Crowninshield R.D., Brand R.A. and Johnstone R.C. (1982) An axisymmetric model of acetabular components in total hip arthroplasty. *J. Biomech.* **15**, 305–315.

Pilliar R.M., Cameron H.U., Welsh R.P. and Binnington D.V.M. (1981) Radiographic and morphologic studies of load-bearing porous-surfaced structured implants. *Clin. Orthop. Rel. Res.* **156**, 249–257.

Pilliar R.M., Lee J.M. and Maniatopoulos C. (1988) Observations of the effect of movement on bone ingrowth into porous-surfaced implants. *Clin. Orthop. Rel. Res.* **208**, 108–113.

Radin E.L., Paul I.L. and Lowy M. (1970) A comparison of the dynamic force transmitting properties of subchondral bone and articular cartilage. *J. Bone Joint Surg.* **52A**, 444–456.

Ratliff A.H.C. (1984) Vascular and neurological complications. In Ling R.S.M. (ed.) *Complications of Total Hip Replacement.* Edinburgh, Churchill Livingstone, pp. 18–29.

Reckling F.W. and Dillon W.L. (1977) The bone–cement temperature during total joint replacement. *J. Bone Joint Surg.* **59A**, 80–82.

Reikeras O. (1982) Ten year follow-up of Muller hip replacements. *Acta Orthop. Scand.* **53**, 919–922.

Ritter M.A. and Sieber J.M. (1985) Prophylactic Indomethacin for the prevention of ectopic bone formation following total hip arthroplasty. *Clin. Orthop.* **196**, 217–225.

Ritter M.A., Keating E.M., Faris P.M. and Brugo G. (1990) Metal-backed acetabular cups in total hip arthroplasty. *J. Bone Joint Surg.* **72A**, 672–677.

Roberts D.W., Poss R. and Kelley K. (1986) Radiographic comparison of cementing techniques in total hip arthroplasty. *J. Arthroplasty* **1**, 241–247.

Rohlmann A., Mossner U., Bergmann G. and Kolbel R. (1982)

Finite-element-analysis and experimental investigation of stress in a femur. *J. Biomed. Eng.* **4**, 241.

Routledge P.A. and West R.R. (1992) Low molecular weight heparin. *Br. Med. J.* **305**, 906.

Rubash H.E. and Harris W.H. (1988) Revision of nonseptic, loose, cemented femoral components using modern cementing techniques. *J. Arthrop.* **3**, 241–248.

Ruff C.B. and Hayes W.C. (1982) Subperiosteal expansion and cortical remodelling of the human femur and tibia with aging. *Science* **217**, 945.

Rybicki E.F., Simonen F.A. and Weis E.B. (1972) The mathematical analysis of stress in the human femur. *J. Biomech.* **5**, 203.

Ryd L. (1992) Roentgen stereophotogrammetric analysis of prosthetic fixation in the hip and knee joint. *Clin. Orthop.* **276**, 56–65.

Rydell N. (1966) Forces acting on the femoral head prosthesis. *Acta Orthop. Scand.* Suppl. 86.

Saha S. and Pal S. (1984) Mechanical properties of bone cement: a review. *J. Biomed. Mat. Res.* **18**, 435–462.

Salvati E.A., Wilson P.D. Jr, Jolley M.N., Vakii F., Aglietti P. and Brown G.C. (1981) A ten-year follow-up study of our first one hundred consecutive Charnley total hip replacements. *J. Bone Joint Surg.* **63A**, 753–767.

Sarmiento A., Ebramzadeh E., Gogan W.J. and McKellop H.A. (1990) Cup containment and orientation in cemented total hip arthroplasties. *J. Bone Joint Surg.* **72B**, 996–1002.

Scheller A.D. and D'Errico J. (1982) Hip biomechanics and prosthetic design and selection in revision total hip replacement. In Turner R.H. and Scheller A.D. (eds) *Revision Total Hip Arthroplasty.* Grune and Stratton, New York, pp. 49–73.

Schmalzried T.P., Amstutz H.C. and Dorey F.J. (1990) Nerve palsy associated with total hip replacement. *J. Bone Joint Surg.* **73A**, 1074–1080.

Schmalzried T.P., Jasty M. and Harris W.H. (1992a) Periprosthetic bone loss in total hip arthroplasty. *J. Bone Joint Surg.* **74A**, 849–863.

Schmalzried T.P., Kwong L.M., Jasty M., Sedlacek R.C., Haire T.C., O'Connor D.O., Bragdon C.R., Kabo J.M., Malcolm A.J. and Harris W.H. (1992b) The mechanism of loosening of acetabular components in total hip arthroplasty. Analysis of specimens obtained at autopsy. *Clin. Orthop.* **274**, 60–78.

Schmidt S.A., Kjaersgaard-Andersen P., Pedersen N.W., Kristensen S.S., Pedersen P. and Nielsen J.B. (1988) The use of Indomethacin to prevent the formation of heterotopic bone after total hip replacement. A randomized, double-blind clinical trial. *J. Bone Joint Surg.* **70A**, 834.

Schreurs B.W., Huiskes R. and Slooff T.J.J.H. (1991) The initial stability of cemented and non-cemented stems, fixated with the bone grafting technique. *Orthop. Trans.* **15**, 439–440.

Selvik G. (1974) A roentgen stereophotogrammetric method for the study of the kinematics of the skeletal system. Thesis. Lund, A-V Centralen.

Sevitt S. (1981) Healing of medullary-nailed fractures. In *Bone Repair and Fracture Healing in Man.* Edinburgh, Churchill Livingstone, pp. 245–261.

Shelley P. and Wroblewski B.M. (1988) Socket design and cement pressurisation in the Charnley low friction arthroplasty. *J. Bone Joint Surg.* **70B**, 358–363.

Sherman R.P., Byrick R.J., Kay J.C., Sullivan T.R. and Waddell J.P. (1983) The role of lavage in preventing hemodynamic and blood gas changes during cemented arthroplasty. *J. Bone Joint Surg.* **65A**, 500–506.

Sloof T.J.J.H., Huskes R., van Horn J. and Lemmens A.J. (1984) Bone grafting in total hip replacement for acetabular protrusion. *Acta Orthop. Scand.* **55**, 593–596.

Soballe K., Brockstedt-Rasmussen H., Hansen E.S. and Bungar C. (1992) Hydroxyapatite coating modifies implant membrane formation. Controlled micromotion studied in dogs. *Acta Orthop. Scand.* **63**, 128–40.

Smith R.W. and Walker R.R. (1964) Femoral expansion in ageing women. *Science* **145**, 156.

Spector M., Shortkroff S., Hsu H.-P., Lane N., Sledge C.B. and Thornhill T.S. (1990) Tissue changes around loose prostheses: a canine model to investigate the effect of an anti-inflammatory agent. *Clin. Orthop. Rel. Res.* **261**, 140–152.

Stauffer R.N. (1982) Ten year follow-up study of total hip replacement. *J. Bone Joint Surg.* **64A**, 983–990.

St Clair Strange F.G. (1965) *The Hip.* William Heineman Medical Books, London.

Stone R.G., Weeks L.E., Hajdu M. and Stinchfield F.E. (1985) Evaluation of sciatic nerve compromise during total hip arthroplasty. *Clin. Orthop.* **201**, 26–31.

Sutherland C.J., Wilde A.H., Borden L. and Marks K.E. (1982) A ten year follow-up of one hundred consecutive Muller curved-stem total hip replacement arthroplasties. *J. Bone Joint Surg.* **64A**, 970–982.

Swanson S.A.V. (1977) Mechanical aspects of fixation. In Swanson S.A.V. and Freeman M.A.R. (eds) *The Scientific Basis of Joint Replacement.* London, Pitman Medical, pp. 130–157.

Tallroth K., Eskola A., Santavirta S., Konttinen Y.T. and Lindholm T.S. (1989) Aggressive granulomatous lesions after hip arthroplasty. *J. Bone Joint Surg.* **71B**, 571–575.

Thomas B.J., Salvati E.A. and Small R.D. (1986) The CAD hip arthroplasty. *J. Bone Joint Surg.* **68A**, 640–646.

Timperley A.J. and O'Dwyer K.J. (1993) Are comparisons comparable? The results of hip arthroplasty. Submitted for publication.

Timperley A.J., Ling R.S.M. and Jones P.R. (1992) The effect of surgical technique on the quality of hip arthroplasty. *J. Bone Joint Surg.* **74B**, Suppl. II, 139.

Timperley A.J., Gie G.A., Lee A.J.C. and Ling R.S.M. (1993) The femoral component as a taper in cemented total hip arthroplasty. *J. Bone Joint Surg.* **75B**, Suppl. I, 33.

Tonnis D. and Asai H. (1976) Untersuchungen uber die Locker-ungsraten verschiedener Hutfgelenksprothesen und under-schiedlicher Halslangen. *Arkiv. Orthop. Unfallchir.* **86**, 317.

Uhthoff H.K. (1973) Mechanical factors influencing the holding power of screws in compact bone. *J. Bone Joint Surg.* **55B**, 633–639.

Uhthoff H.K. and Germain J.-P. (1977) The reversal of tissue differentiation around screws. *Clin. Orthop.* **123**, 248.

Van Rens J.G. and Slooff T.J.J.H. (1984) The investigation of the painful total hip. In Ling R.S.M. (ed.) *Complications of Total Hip Replacement.* Edinburgh, Churchill Livingstone, pp. 231–241.

Vanderby R., Manley P.A., Kohles S.S., Belloli D.M. and McBeath A.A. (1989) A micromotion comparison of cemented and porous ingrowth total hip replacements in a canine model. *Orthop. Trans.* **13**, 456.

Vernon-Roberts B. and Freeman M.A.R. (1976) Morphological and analytic studies of the tissues adjacent to joint prostheses: investigations into the causes of loosening of prostheses. In Schaldach M. and Homan D. (eds) *Artificial Hip and Knee Joint Technology.* Berlin, Springer-Verlag, pp. 148–186.

Weber E.R., Daube J.R. and Coventry M.B. (1976) Peripheral neuropathies associated with total hip arthroplasty. *J. Bone Joint Surg.* **58A**, 66–69.

Wejkner B. and Stenport J. (1988) Charnley total hip arthroplasty: a 10–14 year follow-up study. *Clin. Orthop.* **231**, 113.

Wejkner B., Stenport J. and Wiege M. (1988) Ten-year results of the Charnley hip in arthrosis. *Acta Orthop. Scand.* **59**, 263.

Welch R.B., McGann W.A. and Picetti G.D. (1988) Charnley low-friction arthroplasty. A five to fifteen year study. *Orthop. Clin. N. Am.* **19**, 551–557.

Wiles P. (1988) The surgery of the osteo-arthritic hip. *Br. J. Surg.* **45**, 488.

Willert H. and Semlitsch M. (1976) Tissue reactions to plastic and metallic wear products of joint endoprostheses. In Gschwend N. and Debruner H.U. (eds) *Total Hip Prostheses*. Bern, Huber, p. 205.

Willert H.-G. and Semlitsch M. (1977) Reactions of the articular capsule to wear products of artificial joint prosthesis. *J. Biomed. Mat. Res.* **11**, 15.

Willert H.-G., Ludwig J. and Semlitsch M. (1974) Reaction of bone to methacrylate after hip arthroplasty. A long-term gross, light microscopic and scanning electron microscope study. *J. Bone Joint Surg.* **56A**, 1368–1372.

Wilson J.N. and Scales J.T. (1973) The Stanmore metal on metal total hip prosthesis using a three-pin type cup. *Clin. Orthop.* **95**, 239.

Wixson R.L. (1992) Do we need to vacuum mix or centrifuge cement? *Clin. Orthop.* **285**, 84–90.

Wiltse L.L., Hall R.H. and Stenehjem D.D.S. (1957) Experimental studies regarding the possible use of self-curing acrylic in orthopaedic surgery. *J. Bone Joint Surg.* **39A**, 961.

Wroblewski B.M. (1979) The mechanism of fracture of the femoral prosthesis. *International Orthop.* **3**, 137.

Wroblewski B.M. (1986) 15–20 year results of the Charnley low-friction arthroplasty. *Clin. Orthop.* **211**, 30–35.

Wroblewski B.M. and Siney P. (1992) Charnley low-friction arthroplasty in the young patient. *Clin. Orthop.* **285**, 45–47.

Wroblewski B.M. and van der Rijt. (1984) Intramedullary cancellous bone block to improve femoral stem fixation in Charnley low-friction arthroplasty. *J. Bone Joint Surg.* **66B**, 639–644.

Chapter 20.3
Cementless Total Hip Replacement

H. Phillips & J.K. Tucker

INTRODUCTION

There has been a revival of interest in cementless total hip replacement during the last decade. Published outcome studies demonstrating migration and subsidence of cemented components (Wroblewski, 1986; Pavlov, 1987) and a recognition of the technical difficulties of revising failed cemented joints were seen as good reasons for pursuing the cementless mode.

Meanwhile, improved cementing techniques with the use of lavage, intramedullary plugging, pressurization and an improved technique of mixing appear to have reduced the short-term loosening rate of cemented femoral components by a significant margin. Mulroy and Harris (1990) reported 3% aseptic loosening on the femoral side at 11 years, but 42% radiological loosening of the sockets. When evaluating the results of cementless systems, comparisons should only be made with such contemporary studies using modern cementing techniques.

Dobbs (1980) introduced the actuarial technique of survivorship analysis, which has been widely adopted for cemented hip replacements. The student of outcome, however, recognizes that there are no generally accepted criteria of failure other than the rather coarse marker of the need for revision. The measurement of pain eludes us and there are no absolute and accepted radiological features of failure in cemented or cementless hip replacements. Short-term results have been disappointing in some series of cementless replacements and there are no significant survivorship studies of the more recent cementless designs.

THE EARLY HISTORY OF CEMENTLESS DESIGNS

The earliest cementless designs were in the form of interposition arthroplasties. Sir Robert Jones allegedly used gold foil in 1902 and many other interposing materials followed: pigs bladder, muscle, fascia lata and skin. Hey Groves replaced the femoral head with ivory in 1921. Smith-Peterson (1948) experimented with many materials including glass, forms of plastic and finally, in 1939, vitallium alloy (Fig. 20.3.1). Wiles (1938) is usually accredited with having designed and used the first total hip replacement (Fig. 20.3.2). McKee of Norwich designed and used many implants for hip replacement from 1940 to 1960 (Fig. 20.3.3).

Kiaer (1951) introduced acrylic cement to orthopaedic surgeons and its subsequent use by Charnley and McKee detracted from further development in cementless design. Ring (1974) reported acceptable results with cementlesss replacements and Bryant (1991) found a cumulative survival rate of these implants of 60% after 21 years. Patterson (1987) drew attention to the fact that more than 80% of Ring replacements revised with cement were satisfactory 5 years after the second operation. He suggested that the absence of cement in the primary operation had improved the outcome of revision.

ANATOMICAL CONSIDERATIONS

The smooth transfer of load from the implant to bone with the generation of neither high nor low focal stress within bone is a function of the materials used, their elastic modulus and the efficiency of fixation. Bone cement as an adjuvent to fixation 'customizes' each implant and the composite makes allowances for the variation in geometry of the acetabulum and femur. On the contrary, the success of cementless designs depends on the creation of an optimum 'press-fit' which has to be achieved by careful machining of the bone, and accurate sizing and alignment of the prosthesis.

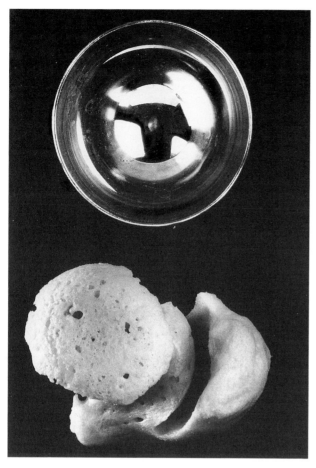

Fig. 20.3.1 A vitallium Smith-Peterson cup arthroplasty showing femoral head remodelling after 20 years.

THE PROXIMAL FEMUR

The anatomy of the proximal femur is very variable and indeed individualistic. The femoral head centre usually

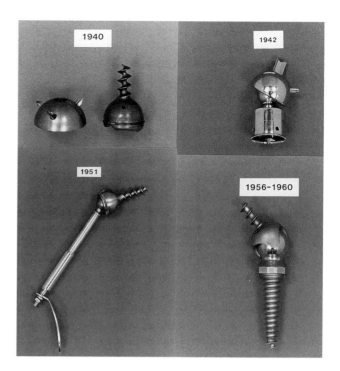

Fig. 20.3.3 The early designs of G.K. McKee of Norwich.

lies one diameter medial to and level with the tip of the greater trochanter when viewed in the coronal plane. As the neck-shaft angle increases, the centre of the femoral head will be increasingly proximal to the tip of the trochanter and at the same time approaches the axis of the shaft. With varus inclination of the femoral neck, the reverse is true. In the sagittal plane, the greater trochanter usually lies posterior to the proximal femoral shaft.

Noble *et al.* (1988) described the extremes of proximal femoral shape. In the 'stove pipe' femur the greater

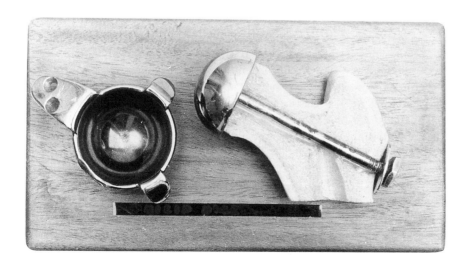

Fig. 20.3.2 The first total hip replacement by Philip Wiles. (Reproduced with permission from the British Orthopaedic Association.)

trochanter lies close to the axis of the shaft. The 'champagne glass' type of femur is wide proximally with the greater trochanter lying well lateral to the femoral axis (Fig. 20.3.4). The medullary canal is correspondingly narrow. Noble expressed these anatomical variations as an index—the canal flare index. In the elderly woman, the diameter of the endosteal cavity at the isthmus of the femoral shaft may approach that of the metaphysis. In contrast, men usually have a relatively narrow isthmus. When viewed from the side, the proximal femur is cranked. The metaphysis bows posteriorly to meet the anterior bow of the diaphysis. The recognition of these varying anatomical features of the proximal femur has major implications for the surgeon using cementless stems. Much can be learnt from pre-operative planning with transparent onlays but Phillips and Tucker (unpublished data) have found that plain radiographs are not accurate enough to choose the best shape and size of the femoral implant in an individual patient.

THE ACETABULUM

On the acetabular side, the congruence of the normal hip joint may be lost due to poor development or arthritis with secondary loss of bone. These acetabular defects have been classified by D'Antonio *et al.* (1988). Some may find this classification of the American Academy of Orthopaedic Surgeons comprehensive but cumbersome. For practical purposes a simple classification is all that is required (Table 20.3.1).

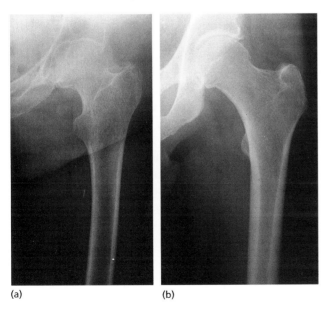

(a)　　　　　　　(b)

Fig. 20.3.4 (a) The 'stove pipe' type of femur; (b) the 'champagne glass' type of femur.

Table 20.3.1 Classification of acetabular bone loss

Rim
　Hip dysplasia
　Post-traumatic
　Osteoarthritic with superolateral migration
　Failed and migrated replacement

Medial wall
　Protrusio acetabuli
　Inflammatory arthritis
　Failed and migrated replacement

Universal
　Inflammatory arthritis
　Tumour
　Failed and migrated replacement

The presence of peripheral and medial osteophytes distorts the shape of the true acetabulum and reconstruction usually demands their removal.

Hip dysplasia is a frequent cause of early onset osteoarthritis. The superolateral defect is obvious, but less apparent is the absence of the anterior wall of the socket. The anteroposterior diameter of the anteverted dysplastic socket is quite small when compared with the mediolateral dimension. This asymmetry must be recognized when reaming the dysplastic socket during reconstruction.

FEMORAL COMPONENT DESIGN

When acrylic cement is used, even very ordinary surgical technique guarantees initial stability of the femoral component. Uncemented stems, however, introduce the problem of matching the shape of the implant and the shape of the bone. It is now recognized that a good press-fit where the whole of the implant surface is perfectly apposed to bone of good quality is difficult to attain. Complete endosteal contact can only be achieved by aggressive reaming and the use of very large femoral components. Paradoxically, large stiff implants, well-fixed distally, are associated with proximal stress shielding and bone resorption. Eng *et al.* (1987) considers that a tight press fit at the isthmus is the requirement for predictable fixation. The complex curvatures of the proximal femur preclude the use of a stem that completely apposes the endosteal cortex—such a stem could not be inserted. Straight-stem designs demand a recipient endosteal cavity within the proximal femur that is necessarily different from the original. Using straight instruments inserted proximally, posterior and lateral to the piriform fossa, alignment can be achieved in both planes in most femora. The stability of the implant depends on the presence of good cancellous bone but with straight stems there are always points of contact with endosteal cortex.

The obvious advantages of the straight stem concept are that the implant need not be 'handed' and, in general, straight instruments are more precise than curved ones.

Curved or 'anatomic' designs are necessarily handed and attempt to conform to the natural curves of the femur. There is no evidence that these implants appose better quality bone.

The proximo-distal mismatch of femoral shape and size has led to the development of modular designs. A two-part femoral stem system raises the concern of fretting corrosion at the metallic junction of the component parts, although this has not been evident in the short term.

Poss *et al.* (1988) have recommended computerized scanning as a technique to guide the manufacture of a femoral implant on an individual basis. The technique is flawed in that it does not take into consideration the quality of bone found at operation.

Mulier *et al.* (1988) described the intra-operative manufacture of the femoral component using laser scanning techniques on an exact elastomer mould of the prepared intramedullary canal. The benefits of this apparently precise technique are not supported by longer term results.

The protagonists of a collar in cementless stem designs argue their case on the basis of proximal loading of the femur. The authors' experience with one type of cementless stem with a committed collar and a precise neck cutting jig has not prevented stem subsidence but usually resulted in positive neck remodelling in the short term. The authors have not seen proximal stress shielding in a collared femoral design (Fig. 20.3.5). Whiteside and Easley (1989) support the use of a collar but in addition they emphasized the importance of a tight distal fit to prevent toggle of the stem.

The concept of osseointegration with smooth-surfaced implants may not be applicable to the hip and is probably unattainable. However, in spite of fibrous tissue anchorage uncemented smooth femoral implants often give a good short-term result (Fig. 20.3.5). The durability of this fixation is still an open question, particularly with respect to resistance to torsional forces.

ACETABULAR COMPONENT DESIGN

Cementless replacement of the socket has been the subject of much experiment in recent years. Polyethylene with and without metal backing in both hemispherical

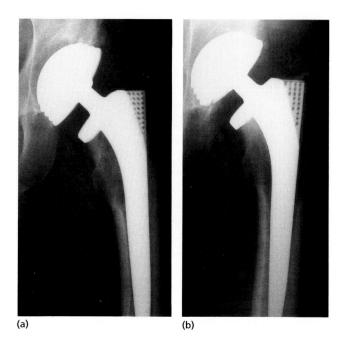

(a)   (b)

Fig. 20.3.5 A 55-year-old male with a cementless implant. Post-operative film (right). 4 years later (left) showing fibrous interface and the neocortex. There is good evidence of proximal loading. Note also migration of the threaded socket after 4 years.

and conical shape have been favoured by some. The concept of metallic threaded sockets with a polyethylene articulation and ceramic sockets of conical shape have also had their proponents.

Bertin *et al.* (1985) and Nunn (1988) reported encouraging early results of uncemented press-fit polyethylene sockets in direct contact with bone. Wilson-MacDonald *et al.* (1990), however, in reporting Morscher's cases, demonstrated the effect of polyethylene debris on the interface resulting in catastrophic loosening, massive granuloma formation and increasing revision rates after 6 years. Evidence of wear of the back of the acetabular component was the rule and a fibrous interface universal.

This study supports the thesis of Wroblewski (1979) that polyethylene should not come into contact with bone where there is the possibility of micro-movement. Ring (1983) and Andrew *et al.* (1985) have reported good results at up to 7 years with press-fit metal-backed polyethylene sockets.

SURFACE ENHANCEMENT OF IMPLANTS, BIOLOGICAL FIXATION AND POROUS INGROWTH OF BONE

During the last two decades, surgeons and engineers

have explored and tested the concept of biological attachment of implants directly to the skeleton. Much experience has been in the field of porous coated metal implants. Pilliar *et al.* (1975) showed that porous metal coatings will allow growth of bone into the pores. It is now accepted that a pore diameter of between 100 and 500 µm is critical for such ingrowth which includes a blood supply in addition to bone cells and matrix. Much larger pores will also allow ingrowth of bone but the process takes considerably longer. In the experimental model, bone appears in the pores of such implants within 2 weeks of implantation and reaches its maximum strength in 6–12 months. The quality and quantity of ingrown bone is superior in young animals and cortical ingrowth would appear to be much stronger than cancellous ingrowth.

Cameron *et al.* (1973) stated that micromotion of a coated implant within the recipient bone correlated with failure to achieve ingrowth. Initial stability is in practice vital and in the presence of excessive micromotion a fibrous interface develops. Such interfaces may be stable for years but their longer term outcome is unknown.

While porous metal surfaces of cobalt-chrome and titanium alloy have been popular in the clinical setting, other materials have been investigated. Ceramics are greatly hindered by their brittleness in the porous form but hydroxyapatite shows some early promise.

The manufacturing processes that have been applied to the surface of implants are summarized in Table 20.3.2. In practice, the strength of the bond between the coating and the implant itself has been variable and Buchert *et al.* (1986) reported separation of the coating. The implications of such separations are serious loss of stability, osteolysis due to particulate metal, and wear should the metal particles become intra-articular. Further, the use of the techniques of scintering and diffusion bonding at very high temperatures has resulted in a loss of compression fatigue strength and tensile

Table 20.3.2 Manufacturing processes applied to surfaces of implants

Grooves, slots and fins
  Machining

Cast surface
  Large beads casted on to the surfaces 1–2 mm in size

Layered coat
  Scintering or diffusion bonding under high temperatures

Surface coat
  Plasma spray technique in which only the powdered metal is heated

strength. Cook and Thomas (1991) have reported fracture of an acetabular component.

The retrieval of implants has allowed both qualitative and quantitative assessments of tissue ingrowth and the overall incidence of bone ingrowth has been disappointing. Cook *et al.* (1988) reported very little bone within the pores of retrieved sockets, the ingrowth being mainly fibrous. On the femoral side, they observed bone ingrowth but in very small amounts, and rarely saw ingrowth into metaphyseal bone. Eng *et al.* (1987) showed ingrowth at multiple points along a chrome-cobalt stem.

HYDROXYAPATITE COATING OF PROSTHESES

The search for materials that can form a long-term bond with the skeleton without fibrous tissue has led to the use of hydroxyapatite. This material is bioactive and has free calcium and phosphate at its surface which forms a chemical bond with bone. The transmission of tensile and shear forces is therefore a real possibility.

Geesink (1988) draws attention to the strength of the chemical fixation. Bonding hydroxyapatite onto a titanium femoral prosthesis using a plastic spraying technique has allowed Geesink to carry out chemical trials. He describes the development of an interface with high shear strength (30 MPa) within 3 months of implantation. His canine experiments show new bone and even Haversian systems at the surface of the coating. In this animal model fragmentation of the hydroxyapatite coating was described and there are reports of the failure of the metal/hydroxyapatite bond in humans. In the longer term, the success of hydroxyapatite as a biological coating will depend upon achieving optimum bonding to the metal substrate, optimum thickness and chemical purity of the material.

POROUS METAL-BACKED SOCKETS

Polyethylene sockets with porous metal backing have been fashionable in recent years. Chrome-cobalt and titanium alloy beads and titanium mesh have provided the metallic interface. Harris *et al.* (1983) demonstrated encouraging ingrowth in a canine model but the retrieval studies of Cook *et al.* (1988) showed only modest ingrowth of bone.

Whether press-fit sockets should be supplemented by screws, pegs or spikes to give initial stability and resist torque forces is controversial. Although Lachiewicz *et al.* (1989) claimed superiority for screw fixation in this regard, others including Freeman *et al.* (1983)

believe stability can be achieved without supplementary fixation even in the absence of bony ingrowth. The roentgenstereophotogrammetric studies of Baldursson *et al.* (1980) have shown the inevitability of early migration of almost all hip sockets and raises concern with regard to impingement and loosening of supplementary screws. In addition, fixation screws may represent a serious hazard to intra-pelvic neural and vascular structures. Wasielewski *et al.* (1990) have indicated that the 'safe' areas of the acetabulum which contain the best bone are posterior, superior and inferior. The medial wall must be avoided and the pubic bone entered with some caution. Eng *et al.* (1990) have reported that up to 6 years, porous metal-backed polyethylene cups are stable, but Callaghan *et al.* (1988) have, alarmingly, described bead loosening in more than one-third of his cases with one particular design.

THREADED ACETABULAR COMPONENTS

The early results of a variety of threaded socket designs using ceramic polymeric and metal shells were encouraging. Surgeons have experienced a very impressive feeling of stability and purchase on the recipient bone at the time of the operation. With longer follow-up, however, significant migration has been observed. Snorasson and Kärrholm (1990) applying roentgenstereophotogrammetry to threaded chrome-cobalt and titanium sockets showed medial migration of up to 2.5 mm proximally, and rotational migration of up to 5.7°. Eng *et al.* (1990) reported on 130 self-tapping metal threaded sockets at a mean of 3.9 years from insertion. 21% showed radiological signs of instability and 25% were said to be symptomatic as evidenced by buttock pain and an inability to straight-leg raise. Mahoney and Dimon (1991), using a ceramic threaded socket, also described a disappointing experience with migration, loss of fixation and lucencies in nearly one-third of patients followed to 4 years. Phillips and Tucker (unpublished data) have demonstrated a radiological migration rate in excess of 10% in a tapped threaded titanium socket at 3 years (Fig. 20.3.6). Huiskes *et al.* (1987), using finite element analysis, reported high stress on the leading thread of similar devices with evidence of stress shielding in the central and superior cancellous bone.

BONE RESORPTION AND REMODELLING SEEN WITH CEMENTLESS FEMORAL STEMS

The unreplaced proximal femur is externally loaded and

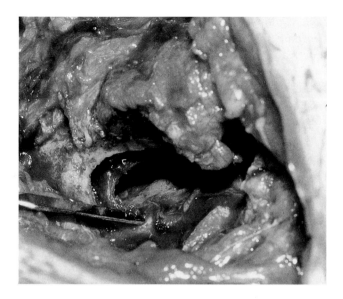

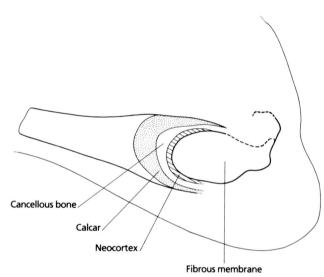

Cancellous bone
Calcar
Neocortex
Fibrous membrane

Fig. 20.3.6 The neocortex is very obvious at revision.

it is not surprising that an intramedullary stem, loading the femur from within, induces adaptive changes in femoral bone. Remodelling occurs according to the distribution of stress, which is dependent upon the geometry of the implant, its rigidity and its fixation.

Many patterns of remodelling have emerged. Distal fixation of the stem, easy to achieve by aggressive distal reaming, results in distal cortical thickening and density but at the same time there is a loss of proximal bone density. This proximal absorption of bone is attributed to stress shielding. Evidence for a collar taking load is seen by densification of the calcar (Fig. 20.3.5). Extensive radio-opaque line formation around the stem and parallel with it indicates the presence of a fibrous interface. The opaque line, which is in reality a sheath of new bone or 'neocortex' within the medullary canal, arises in response to micromotion (Fig. 20.3.5). The neocortex with its fibrous lining is very obvious at revision (Fig. 20.3.6). Cortical hypertrophy distally is not seen in the presence of a neocortex, suggesting perhaps a load carrying function for this new bone.

THE PROBLEM OF THIGH PAIN

Pain in the mid-thigh, which comes on with activity but is gradually eased by it, is a familiar symptom in failing cemented stems. Start-up pain and limp beginning soon after operation is unique to the cementless designs. Haddad *et al.* (1990) reported the incidence of thigh pain as being between 8 and 30%. Hedley *et al.* (1987) reported that the incidence of thigh pain decreased after the first year while Campbell *et al.* (1992) indicated that the symptom of thigh pain increased with time. Phillips and Tucker (unpublished data) have recorded an incidence of thigh pain of 14% and invariably the symptom has been progressive. The low incidence of thigh pain of 7% reported by Eng *et al.* (1987) is probably related to the rigid distal fixation achieved with his long chrome-cobalt implant. The literature fails to uniformly correlate pain with age and disease. The varying patterns of remodelling of the femur do not always precisely correlate with symptoms, neither does apparent fit and alignment universally match. The precise cause of thigh pain remains conjectural and Barrack

et al. (1992) imply that it might not be wholly related to stability and apparent bone ingrowth. Thigh pain is usually accompanied by an antalgic gait characterized by a lurch over the painful hip in the stance phase.

ENDOSTEAL EROSION IN CEMENTLESS REPLACEMENT

The generation of metallic and polyethylene wear debris is now recognized as a major problem in hip replacement irrespective of the type of fixation. Endosteal cortical erosions occur in loose and well-fixed cementless components (Fig. 20.3.7). Tanzer *et al.* (1992) showed in the presence of a stable femoral component that the erosions were usually distally placed and arose earlier than in a stable cemented femoral component as reported by Mahoney *et al.* (1990), and can occur as early as 2 years after operation. The erosions described were nearly always progressive. Histological examination of these granulomata have shown metallic and plastic debris or both. The metallic debris may arise from excessive wear of titanium heads and by crevice corrosion, or by abrasion of a loose metal implant against endosteum. Santavirta *et al.* (1990) reported aggressive granulomata around stable cementless stems which he considered were caused by high-density polyethylene wear products. The clinical implication of endosteal erosions in stable cementless implants is that such implants should be regularly followed up and observed, lest bone stock be seriously compromised by subsequent loosening. The

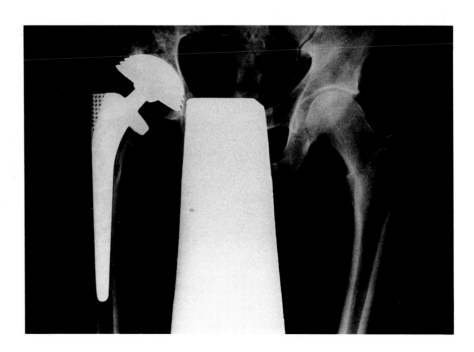

Fig. 20.3.7 Cementless stem 4 years after operation showing endosteal lysis in zone 3 of Gruen.

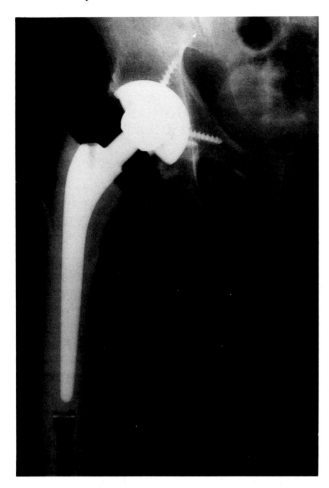

Fig. 20.3.8 The hybrid hip, cemented on the femoral side, with a press-fit uncemented socket.

outcome of presently used cementless designs may well be very dependent upon focal osteolysis and its progression.

THE CONCEPT OF THE HYBRID HIP

The short-term results of a variety of femoral components fixed without cement do not appear to have been as successful as those where cement has been used, yet cementless femoral designs are still recommended for the young. This paradox will be resolved by careful comparative and clinical studies in the longer term. For the time being, a cemented stem is likely to give the patient a good short-term result. On the contrary, cementless sockets with adjuvent fixation are producing results at least equal to those which use cement. Presently, a hybrid hip (Fig. 20.3.8) seems to be suitable for patients of any age.

REFERENCES

Andrew T.A., Berridge D., Thomas A. and Duke R.N.F. (1985) Long term review of Ring total arthroplasty. *Clin. Orthop.* **201**, 111–122.

Baldursson H., Hansson L.I., Olsson T.H. and Selvic G. (1980) Migration of the acetabular socket after total hip replacement determined by Roentgenstereophotogrammetry. *Acta. Orthop. Scand.* **51**, 535–540.

Barrack R.L., Jasty M., Bragdon C., Haire T. and Harris W.H. (1992) Thigh pain despite ingrowth into uncemented femoral stems. *J. Bone Joint Surg.* **74B**, 507–510.

Bertin K.C., Freeman M.A.R., Morscher E., Oeri A. and Ring P.A. (1985) Cementless acetabular replacement using a pegged polyethylene prosthesis. *Arch. Orthop. Trauma Surg.* **104**, 251–261.

Bryant M.J., Mollan R.A.B. and Nixon J.R. (1991) Survivorship analysis of the Ring Hip Arthroplasty. *J. Arthroplasty* **6**, 5.

Buchert P.K., Vaughn B.K., Mallory T.H., Eng C.A. and Bobyn J.D. (1986) Excessive metal release due to loosening and fretting of scintered particles on porous coated hip prostheses. *J. Bone Joint Surg.* **68A**, 606.

Callaghan J.J., Dysart S.H. and Savory C.G. (1988) The uncemented porous coated anatomic hip prosthesis. *J. Bone Joint Surg.* **70A** (3), 337–346.

Cameron H.U., Pilliar R.M. and MacNab J. (1973) The effect of movement on the bonding of porous metal to bone. *J. Biomed. Mat. Res.* **7**, 301.

Campbell A.C., Rorabeck C.H., Bourne R.B., Chess D. and Nott L. (1992) Thigh pain after cementless hip arthroplasty. *J. Bone Joint Surg.* **74B**, 63–66.

Cook S.D. and Thomas K.A. (1991) Fatigue failure of non cemented porous coated implants. A retrieval study. *J. Bone Joint Surg.* **73B**, 20–24.

Cook S.D., Barrack R.K., Thomas K.A. and Haddad R.J. (1988) Quantitative analysis of tissue ingrowth into human porous hip components. *J. Arthroplasty* **3**, 249.

D'Antonio R., Capello J.A., Borden W.N. *et al.* (1988) Classification and management of acetabular abnormalities in total hip arthroplasty. *Clin. Orthop.* **243**, 126.

Dobbs H.S. (1980) Survivorship of total hip replacements. *J. Bone Joint Surg.* **62B**, 168.

Eng C.A., Bobyn J.D. and Glassmann A.H. (1987) Porous coated hip replacement. The factors governing bone ingrowth, stress shielding and clinical results. *J. Bone Joint Surg.* **69B**, 45–55.

Eng C.A., Griffin W.L. and Marx C.L. (1990) Cementless acetabular components. *J. Bone Joint Surg.* **72B** (1), 53–59.

Freeman M.A.R., McLeod H.C. and Levai J-P. (1983) Cementless fixation of prosthetic components in total arthroplasty of the knee and hip. *Clin. Orthop.* **176**, 88–94.

Geesink R.G.T. (1988) Hydroxyapatite coated hip implants. Thesis, State University of Limburg, Maastricht, Netherlands.

Haddad R.J., Cook S.D. and Brinker M.R. (1990) A comparison of three varieties of non cemented porous coated hip replacements. *J. Bone Joint Surg.* **72B**, 2–7.

Harris W.H., White R.E. Jr, McCarthy J.C., Walker P.S. and Weinberg E.H. (1983) Bony ingrowth fixation of the acetabular component in canine hip joint arthroplasty. *Clin. Orthop.* **176**, 7–11.

Hedley A.K., Gruen T.A., Borden L.S., Hungerford D.S., Habermann E. and Kenna R.V. (1987) 2 year follow up of the P.C.A. non cemented total hip replacement. In *The Hip Proceed-*

ings of 14th Meeting of the Hip Society. St. Louis, C.V. Mosby, pp. 225–250.

Huiskes R., Peeters H. and Sloof T.J. (1987) Biomechanical analysis of load transfer in acetabular cup arthroplasty with cementless threaded sockets. *Transac. Orth. Res. Soc.* **12**, 508.

Kiaer M.S. (1951) Preliminary report on hip arthroplasty by use of acrylic head. *5th Congress Société Internationale de Chirugie Orthopédique et Traumatologie, Stockholm,* **5**, 33.

Lachiewicz P.F., Suh P.B. and Gilbert J.A. (1989) In vitro initial fixation of proous coated acetabular components. A biomechanical comparative study. *J. Arthroplasty* **4**, 3, 201.

Mahoney O.M. and Dimon J.H. (1991) Unsatisfactory results with a ceramic total hip prosthesis. *J. Bone Joint Surg.* **72A**, 663–671.

Mahoney W.J., Jasty M., Rosenberg A. and Harris W.H. (1990) Bone lysis in well fixed cemented femoral components. *J. Bone Joint Surg.* **72B**, 966–970.

Mulier J.C., Mulier M., Brady L.P., Stenhoudth H., Cauwe Y., Goosens M. and Elloy M.A. (1988) Intra-operative production of femoral prostheses. In Coombs (ed.) *Joint Replacement.* London, Orthotext, p. 163.

Mulroy R.D. and Harris W.H. (1990) The effect of improved cementing techniques on component loosening in total hip replacement. An 11 year radiographic review. *J. Bone Joint Surg.* **72B**, 757–760.

Noble P.C., Alexander J.W., Lindahl L.J. *et al.* (1988) The anatomic basis of femoral component design. *Clin. Orthop.* **235**, 148.

Nunn D. (1988) The Ring uncemented plastic on metal total hip replacement: 5 year results. *J. Bone Joint Surg.* **70B**, 40–44.

Patterson M. (1987) Ring uncemented hip replacements. The results of revision. *J. Bone Joint Surg.* **69B**, 374–380.

Pavlov P.W. (1987) A 15 year follow up study of 512 consecutive Charnley Müller total hip replacements. *J. Arthroplasty* **2**, 151.

Pilliar R.M., Cameron H.U. and MacNab J. (1975) Porous surface layered prosthetic devices. *Biomed. Eng.* **10**, 126.

Poss R., Walker P., Spector M., Reilly D., Robertson D.O. and

Sledge C.B. (1988) Strategies for improving fixation of femoral components. *Clin. Orthop.* **235**, 181–194.

Ring P.A. (1974) Total replacement of the hip joint—a review of 1000 operations. *J. Bone Joint Surg.* **56B**, 44–58.

Ring P.A. (1983) Ring U.P.M. total hip arthroplasty. *Clin. Orthop.* **176**, 115–123.

Santavirta S., Hoikka V., Eskola A., Konttinen V.T., Paavilainen T. and Tallroth K.A. (1990) Aggressive granulomatous lesions in cementless total hip arthroplasty. *J. Bone Joint Surg.* **72B**, 980–984.

Smith-Peterson M.N. (1948) Evolution of mould arthroplasty of the hip joint. *J. Bone Joint Surg.* **30B**, 59.

Snorrasson F. and Kärrholm J. (1990) Primary migration of fully threaded acetabular prosthesis. A Roentgenstereophotogrammetry analysis. *J. Bone Joint Surg.* **72B**, 647–652.

Tanzer M., Maloney W.J., Jasty M. and Harris W.H. (1992) The progression of femoral cortical osteolysis in association with total hip arthroplasty without cement. *J. Bone Joint Surg.* **74A**, 404–410.

Wasielewski R.C., Cooperstein L.A., Kniger M.P. and Rubash H.E. (1990) Acetabular anatomy and transacetabular fixation of screws in total hip arthroplasty. *J. Bone Joint Surg.* **72A**, 4, 501–508.

Whiteside L.A. and Easley J.C. (1989) The effect of collar and distal stem fixation on micromotion of the femoral stem in uncemented total hip arthroplasty. *Clin. Orthop.* **239**, 145.

Wiles P. (1938) The surgery of the osteoarthritic hip. *Br. J. Surg.* **45**, 488.

Wilson-MacDonald J., Morscher E. and Maser Z. (1990) Cementless uncoated polyethylene acetabular components in total hip replacement: 5–10 year results. *J. Bone Joint Surg.* **72B**, 423–430.

Wroblewski B.M. (1986) 15–21 year results of the Charnley Low Friction Arthroplasty. *Clin. Orthop.* **211**, 30.

Wroblewski B.M. (1979) Wear of high-density polyethylene on bone and cartilage. *J. Bone Joint Surg.* **61B** (4), 498–500.

Chapter 20.4
Total Knee Arthroplasty

J.N. Insall & G.R. Scuderi

INTRODUCTION

Cemented total knee arthroplasty (TKA) has evolved over the decades from simple surface replacement to highly technical designs, affording the orthopaedic surgeon the ability to correct deformities of the knee, maintain motion and relieve pain. The early prosthetic designs, introduced in the 1950s, were fully constrained, linked arthroplasties which placed high stress on the cement–bone interface resulting in loosening and failure. Other designs in the evolution were surface replacements with an insecure mechanical interlock between component and bone. Modern TKA has evolved to a condylar surface replacement, through the efforts of many investigators. At the Hospital for Special Surgery (HSS), New York, disappointing results with the unicondylar design led the authors towards the development of other total knee designs. Their initial duocondylar prosthesis had minimal bone resection and allowed for stability provided by the ligaments. Further design changes introduced the duopatellar prosthesis which had an anterior flange, allowing tricompartmental resurfacing and straight bone cuts. This was the direct forerunner of the total condylar knee prosthesis that was introduced in 1974 (Insall *et al.*, 1976, 1979, 1982, 1983a; Insall and Kelly, 1986; Vince and Insall, 1988).

The posterior stabilized (PS) knee prosthesis was introduced in 1978 as a modification of the already successful total condylar prosthesis (Insall *et al.*, 1982) (Fig. 20.4.1). Since the cruciate ligaments are sacrificed, the intercondylar spine of the tibial component and the transverse cam on the femoral component substitute for the posterior cruciate ligament. The interaction between the tibial spine and femoral cam as well as modifications in the centre of curvature of the prosthesis allows femoral rollback during flexion. Originally, the posterior stabilized tibial component was all polyethylene, but it has been demonstrated that metal-backed tibias transmit the load better to the underlying bone. In 1980, metal backing of the tibial implant was begun. Based on the success of the original posterior stabilized prosthesis, further modification to the Insall–Burstein posterior stabilized II prosthesis was performed in 1987 (Fig. 20.4.2). This is a completely modular system with the ability to modify the prosthesis at the time of surgery depending on individual needs. Available in this design are optional stems for both the femur and tibia, metal augmentations for the femur and metal wedges for the tibia. Polyethylene tibial inserts of various thicknesses are interchangeable on the metal tibial tray and have the capability of being either a standard posterior stabilized or a constrained condylar design. Further changes have included a wider range of component sizes to accommodate the individual patient and deepening of the patellar groove on the anterior flange of the femoral component to improve patellar tracking. The Insall–Burstein posterior stabilized II prosthesis has evolved to be the prosthesis of choice in the Knee Service at the Hospital for Special Surgery (Scuderi and Insall, 1989).

Controversy still exists regarding retention or sacrifice of the posterior cruciate ligament (PCL) (Dorr *et al.*, 1985, 1988; Alexiades *et al.*, 1989). Implant designs that retain the PCL have demonstrated excellent results (Hungerford, 1987; Ewald *et al.*, 1984) while PCL substituting prostheses have shown comparable results (Insall *et al.*, 1982; Scott *et al.*, 1988; Vince *et al.*, 1988; Scuderi and Insall, 1989). The PCL is usually contracted and shortened in fixed deformities of the knee and excision of the ligament affords easy correction of these fixed deformities. In designs that retain the PCL, it is necessary to partially release the PCL in order to correct fixed deformities. Exact tensing on the PCL so that the ligament is functional is often difficult. A tight PCL causes excessive rollback which results in a stiff and painful knee. If the preserved PCL is lax, the knee demonstrates a posterior lag and no evidence of rollback.

697

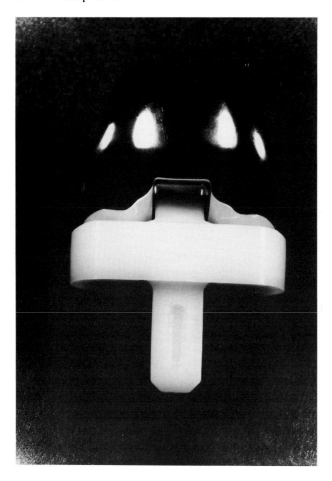

Fig. 20.4.1 The Insall—Burstein posterior stabilized knee prosthesis.

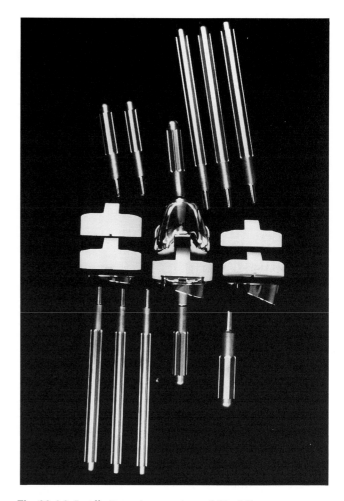

Fig. 20.4.2 Insall—Burstein posterior stabilized II.

Alexiades *et al.* (1989) have reported that the PCL in the arthritic knee is involved with the degenerative process. Histological evaluation has shown irregularity of the collagen architecture with loose myxoid and mucoid degeneration. The worse the deformity the more distortion to its microscopic architecture. Dorr *et al.* (1985) have reported that the arthritic PCL is not as strong as the normal ligament, but strong enough to sustain the anticipated loads of a patient with a total knee replacement. Biomechanical studies have shown that the ultimate load to failure of an arthritic PCL was 37% of normal while 54% less stiff (Dorr *et al.*, 1985). Dorr does, however, state that there have been no reported spontaneous ruptures of the PCL in a retaining design and there are numerous series of successful PCL prostheses (Ewald *et al.*, 1984; Hungerford, 1987).

INDICATIONS FOR TOTAL KNEE REPLACEMENT

In the presence of severe unremitting symptoms of degenerative joint disease, osteoarthritis and inflammatory arthritis which have failed medical management, total knee arthroplasty is indicated. After careful discussion with the patient concerning risks, benefits and alternative techniques such as tibial or femoral osteotomy, total knee replacement (TKR) is considered. Structural damage and knee joint deformity are indications for TKR especially in patients with rheumatoid arthritis and inflammatory arthritides. There may be an indication for TKR in post-traumatic arthritis. However, this is a special group of patients who tend to be younger and may place high demands upon their arthroplasty. In most cases patellofemoral arthritis can be treated with other techniques, but there may be cases with associated femorotibial changes or an occasional elderly patient with severe patellofemoral changes. Total knee replacement has been beneficial in this subgroup. When high tibial osteotomy has failed, TKR can be performed without difficulty (Windsor *et al.*, 1988). Total knee replacement in neuropathic joints is controversial and represents a technical challenge with respect to joint stability and bone loss (Soudry *et al.*, 1986a).

Contraindications to TKR include a sound painless knee arthrodesis in good position, genu recurvatum with associated quadriceps muscle weakness, a deficient quadriceps mechanism and active infection. There is controversy regarding TKR in patients with neuropathic joints.

OPERATIVE TECHNIQUE

An anterior midline approach allows full exposure of the distal femur and proximal tibia. Since the objective is to produce a knee that has approximately equal soft-tissue tension medially and laterally in flexion and extension, appropriate soft-tissue and ligament releases are performed before the bone cuts (Insall, 1981). For the varus deformity, ligament balance is achieved by progressively releasing the contracted medial soft tissues until they reach the length of the lateral ligamentous structures. The cruciate ligaments must be excised completely before starting the release because their presence will often inhibit correction. The medial release is performed by excising medial osteophytes from the femur and tibia and elevating a subperiosteal sleeve of soft tissue from the proximal medial tibia that includes the deep and superficial medial collateral ligament and the insertion of the pes anserinus tendon. Posteriorly the release is continuous with the semimembranosus insertion and the posterior capsule. Distally the release may include the deep fascia of the soleus and popliteus muscles. At the completion of the varus release, the limb is already aligned in the proper position; no further correction is needed and the bone cuts can be made in a standard manner (Fig. 20.4.3).

The principles for correction of a valgus deformity are similar to the varus release, but there are several differences due to anatomical variation. The lateral capsule is cut from the femoral condyle along with the lateral collateral ligament and popliteus tendon. There are occasions when the posterior capsule and lateral head of the gastrocnemius must be resected from the lateral femoral condyle. Similar to correction of a varus deformity, the corrected alignment should be checked each step of the way with the laminar spreaders. In severe valgus deformities associated with external rotation, the iliotibial band is contacted and must be released. It was originally described to transect this iliotibial band at the joint line, but recently the authors have begun to strip subperiosteally the iliotibial band from the lateral proximal tibia and Gerdy's tubercle (Fig. 20.4.4).

In fixed flexion contractures, the normal posterior

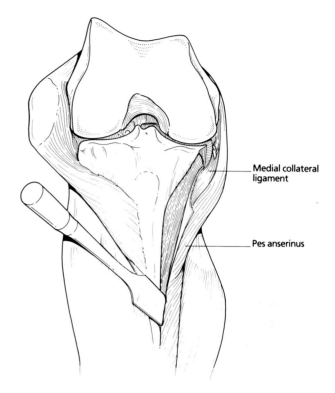

Fig. 20.4.3 The varus release.

Medial collateral ligament

Pes anserinus

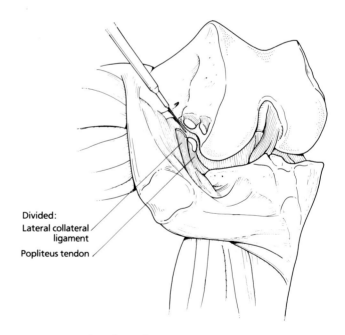

Fig. 20.4.4 The valgus release.

Divided:
Lateral collateral ligament
Popliteus tendon

recess and the capsule adherent to the femoral condyles are obliterated. For flexion contractures of 20° or less, more bone can be removed from the distal femur to compensate for the flexion contracture. For flexion contractures greater than 20°, however, a posterior release should be performed. With subperiosteal dissection along the posterior femoral condyles, the original recess can be re-established. The cruciate ligaments are excised releasing the fixed structures in the middle of the knee. The medial and lateral parts of the posterior capsule adjacent to the collateral ligaments are cut vertically to assist in their release. The medial and lateral posterior capsule is then cut transversely under direct vision to complete the capsular release (Fig. 20.4.5).

Once the soft tissues are balanced, the bone cuts are performed. The level of the tibial cut is constant and conservative at a level perpendicular to the long axis of the tibia. It should be 5 mm or less below the tibial plateau because tibial cancellous bone weakens rapidly as the distance from the articular surface increases (Hvid and Hansen, 1985). Contact between the tibial component and the peripheral cortical rim decreases stresses in the proximal tibia such that in sizing a tibial component it should extend to the cortices (Bourne and Finlay, 1986).

Resection of the femur follows tibial resection. The flexion gap produced should be rectangular in shape rather than trapezoidal. This can usually be achieved with adequate soft-tissue release. Occasionally, however, it may be necessary to actually rotate the femoral template until it becomes parallel to the cut tibial surface. This results in more bone resection from the posterior medial femoral condyle than the posterior lateral femoral condyle. At no time should the femoral template be internally rotated since this moves the patellofemoral groove of the femoral component medially, making it difficult for the laterally placed patella to capture the groove. Such malrotation of the femoral component may lead to patellar dislocation or subluxation. Once the correct amount of bone is resected and the soft tissue and ligaments are properly balanced, the size of the flexion and extension gaps should be equal.

Alignment is confirmed interoperatively with a rod and a limb line. The ideal limb alignment is 5–10° of valgus. The ideal placement of the tibial component is an angle of 90 ± 2° to the long axis of the tibial shaft on both the anteroposterior and lateral radiographs. The ideal placement of the femoral component is 7 ± 2° of valgus angulation on the anteroposterior radiograph and 0–10° of flexion on the lateral view (Scuderi and Insall, 1989).

The patella is routinely resurfaced and a uniform thickness of 10–14 mm preserved. The central fixation hole should be no larger than necessary and an all-polyethylene central dome patella is implanted. With the patellar component in place, the patella should track centrally in the femoral anterior flange without tilting to prevent patellar subluxation or, worse, patellar dislocation. Careful attention must be given to patellar tracking at the time of operation, and when necessary a lateral release or proximal realignment must be done. The authors perform their lateral release from the inside out, preserving the lateral superior genicular artery whenever possible, since sacrificing this vessel has been associated with an increase in patellar ischemia (Scuderi *et al.*, 1987). The most common cause of patellar dislocation in a review was error in operative technique (Merkow *et al.*, 1985). Internal rotation of the tibial component with respect to the tibia will cause external rotation of the tibia when the knee is reduced, resulting in lateral displacement of the tibial tubercle. This displacement increases the valgus vector and the tendency of the patella to sublux laterally. Correct rotational positioning of the tibial component is best achieved by aligning the intercondylar eminence of the tibial component with the tibial crest in the sagittal plane. Aligning the posterior margin of the plateau may not position the implant correctly with respect to the insertion of the patellar ligament.

Post-operatively, a soft compression dressing is used,

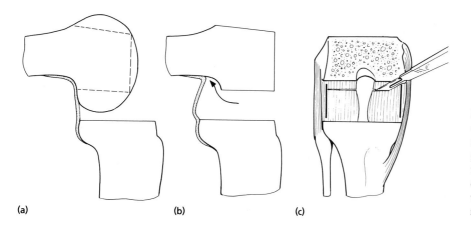

(a)   (b)   (c)

Fig. 20.4.5 Release of flexion contracture. (a) Standard femoral bone cuts; (b) subperioteal dissection along the posterior femoral condyles re-establishes the posterior recess; (c) the posterior capsule is cut transversely under direct vision to complete the posterior capsular release.

and since 1985, patients have been placed in continuous passive motion (CPM) machines immediately after surgery in the recovery room. Continuous passive motion is a useful adjunct to rehabilitation. Its use has reduced the time required to achieve 90° of flexion. A randomized prospective study revealed that CPM significantly improved early and late flexion of the knee, reduced the duration of stay in hospital and did not increase the incidence of superficial infection or problems with wound healing (Johnson, 1990). Reports have also demonstrated that CPM had no effect on long-term range of motion, knee rating scores and pain relief (Maloney *et al.*, 1990). Manipulation under general anaesthesia is used less frequently than previously reported to achieve flexion after total knee arthroplasty. Some patients are not willing to participate aggressively in their post-operative therapy and have difficulty obtaining 90° of flexion by the second to third post-operative week. The authors have found that manipulation is useful in this group of patients, with CPM a useful adjunct; however, this feeling is not accepted by all reviewers (Ritter *et al.*, 1989).

INSTRUMENTATION

Instrumentation in total knee arthroplasty has been refined since its early introduction. Most systems use extramedullary tibial guides because of the relative accessibility of the tibia. Intramedullary guides for the femur are popular and have been proven to be accurate, provided the femur is not excessively bowed or deformed and the centring hole is properly positioned. A radiograph of the entire femur is needed, so that when the intramedullary guide is used allowances can be made for bowing or deformity. The accuracy of the guide can be affected by the placement of the entry hole in the distal femur, and this can alter the distal femoral cut 2–3° in either direction. The accuracy of the extramedullary femoral guides depends on the precise location of the femoral head. Though this is relatively easy in the thin patient, it can be exceedingly difficult in the obese patient. However, extramedullary guides are beneficial in the presence of femoral shaft deformity, and the ideal system should include the option of intramedullary and extramedullary guides. The intramedullary guide can be misleading because of unusual femoral bowing and the rotational position of the femur. A variation of 2.5° was found between the positions of 20° internal rotation and 20° external rotation of the femur (Jiang and Insall, 1989). Intramedullary instrumentation provides sufficient accuracy when the femur has a normal anatomical shape. When an excessive degree of femoral bowing is

present, rotational attitudes can affect the roentgenographic measurements.

Cement technique

Cement technique and preparation have improved over the years. Fixation of methylmethacrylate to the cancellous bony surface is achieved by the irregular configuration of the bony interstices and the penetration of the cement into the microstructure of the cancellous bone. Bone preparation is critical to the intrusion of the methylmethacrylate into the cancellous bone. The cancellous bone is prepared with the use of pulsatile water lavage removing blood and debris from the bone interstices. After the bone is prepared in this fashion, manual pressure can give 3–4 mm of penetration. The difference in penetration between 1- and 3-min cement is not significant but drops appreciably after 4 min. Several investigators have studied the optimal depth of cement penetration into the cancellous bone for optimal strength of fixation and viability of bone (Krause *et al.*, 1982; Dorr *et al.*, 1984; Cheal *et al.*, 1985). Bone viability has been preserved when the methylmethacrylate is no thicker than 1 cm, but 1 cm of cement penetration is not needed for optimal fixation. Two to 5 mm of cement penetration is sufficient for optimal strength of the cement–bone composite. With soft rheumatoid bone, cement penetration may be deeper, and with hard sclerotic bone drill holes at least 6 mm should be prepared or else inadequate penetration will occur. Dorr *et al.* (1984) and Krause *et al.* (1982) have reported that cement failed within the cement column when the bone was strong and that the bone–cement interface failed when the bone was weak. Currently the authors believe that no more than 1–2 mm of cement penetration into bone is desirable. Excessive penetration of the cement into the bone at the time of primary arthroplasty causes excessive loss of bone stock during revision arthroplasty.

The results of total knee arthroplasty are closely aligned with surgical technique and are influenced by correct sizing, level of bone recession, level of the joint line, soft-tissue balance and most of all axial alignment. Based on these determinants, there are two schools of thought on the mechanism of loosening and failure of cement fixation. The first believes that the micromotion at the bone–cement interface grows even larger with accompanying loss of bone until the component is grossly loose. The other school argues that the mechanism of failure is due to subsidence, that is loosening because of bone overload. Overload occurs when the bone itself is very weak and osteoporotic, but most often it occurs because of uneven stress. Total knee replacements that loosen do so because of varus malalignment. Subsidence has nothing to do with the cement fixation or cement technique, although the level of tibial bone resection is important because cancellous bone is weaker further from the subchondral plate.

Cementless technique

In recent years, cementless designs have been popular. However, long-term results have yet to be reported. Rorabeck *et al.* (1988) compared cemented kinematic condylar and uncemented porous-coated anatomical (PCA) total knee replacements at 24 months and found higher knee scores with the cemented design. The revision rate for the cemented implant was 4% compared with 12% for the uncemented implant. Fixation of most cementless implants has been by fibrous tissue (Haddad *et al.*, 1987) and loosening of the porous coating has been identified in more than half of the patients. Rosenqvist *et al.* (1986) in a study of 34 PCA knees in patients with rheumatoid arthritis found more than one-half of the patients had radiographic evidence of loose beads as early as 3 months post-operatively, suggesting micromotion of the implants. In order to limit micro-motion and enhance fixation screws, stems and keels have been added to the implant designs but long-term follow-up has yet to be reported.

One final issue with porous-coated implants is metal corrosion, since with ingrowth designs the metallic surface area is substantially increased over that of cemented prostheses. High local metal ion concentrations have been reported in the soft tissue about the implant and consequences of these levels have yet to be determined.

Special problems

TIBIAL BONE LOSS

In primary total knee replacement, limited proximal tibial bone resection of 5 mm or less is recommended. However, with this limited bone resection in severe varus or valgus knees, a large defect may still remain. In those cases in which there is asymmetric bone loss from the upper tibia, the level of tibial resection should be at the usual level and not at the level of the defect. Resecting the proximal tibia at thicknesses greater than 5 mm places higher loads on the subchondral cancellous bone, possibly contributing to collapse of the cancellous bone and loosening of the cement–bone interface.

Autogenous bone grafting of tibial defects in total knee replacement permits a biocompatible and adaptable means of restoring the proximal tibial bone surface.

Dorr and Ranawat (1984) recommended that tibial bone grafting may be used for bone defects greater than 50% of the medial or lateral tibial plateau surface or a defect greater than 5 mm in height. It is contraindicated in Charcot joints or for defects that involve the entire medial or lateral tibial plateau. Several techniques have been described for bone grafting tibial defects in primary and revision total knee replacement using local autogenous bone (Dorr and Ranawat, 1984; Ranawat, 1985; Windsor *et al.*, 1986; Scuderi *et al.*, 1989b).

Our bone grafting technique utilizes a self-locking principle that obviates the need for permanent metal fixation (Scuderi *et al.*, 1989b). If there is a central tibial defect, the surgeon creates a trapezoidal defect, removing all sclerotic bone to expose the underlying cancellous bone. The trapezoidal shape allows a stable fit so that uniform compressive forces may be exerted over the entire graft recipient site. The bone taken from the intercondylar notch is suitable for grafting and is fashioned into a trapezoidal shape with a saw or burr. The bone block is tapped into place and should fit snugly into the defect in order to prevent cement from entering the crevices. Excess bone may be trimmed with a saw so that the graft fits flush with the tibial surface. A provisional prosthesis is placed to assure correct fit and alignment (Fig. 20.4.6).

For peripheral defects that involve the cortex, a trapezoidal defect is created with its widest base directed towards the centre of the tibia. The graft is temporarily secured with horizontally placed smooth Kirschner wires. They should remain in place until after excess bone is removed and the tibial component is cemented into place, preventing inadvertent dislodgement of the bone graft. It is important to position the base towards the centre of the tibia so that the graft will be locked in place. This technique allows only compressive forces to be exerted on the graft and prevents shear forces from dislodging the graft or compromising its incorporation.

Post-operatively, the routine is the same as that for standard total knee replacements except in cases where large defects have been grafted. In these situations partial weight-bearing with crutches is recommended for a period of 4–8 weeks until the bone graft is incorporated.

A review of 26 total knee replacements utilizing this technique demonstrated 22 (84.6%) excellent results, three (11.5%) good results and one (3.9%) fair result (Scuderi *et al.*, 1989). There were no poor results and the average post-operative Hospital for Special Surgery (HSS) knee score was 89 points. Radiographs demonstrated that all grafts were fully incorporated within the first year with cross trabeculation between the graft and proximal bone. Radiolucent lines were noted under the

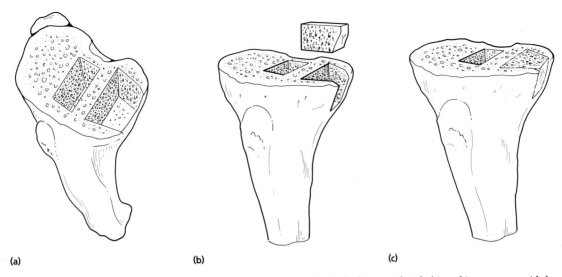

(a)   (b)   (c)

Fig. 20.4.6 Bone grafting technique. (a) The defect is shaped into a trapezoid; (b) the bone graft is fashioned into a trapezoid shape; (c) the bone graft is tapped into place and fits snugly.

medial tray of the tibial component in two knees, were less than 2 mm and were non-progressive. One medial bone graft was noted to have collapsed causing the radiolucency, but the tibial component did not change position at 56 months of follow-up. There has been no evidence of tibial component loosening and no arthroplasty has yet to be revised.

CUSTOM COMPONENTS

In primary total knee replacement for severe varus or valgus deformity, there may be severe bone loss requiring the use of custom components. Similar bone loss may also be found both on the femoral and tibial side during revision total knee replacement (Insall, 1986). Custom tibial prostheses incorporating metal wedges or separate metal wedges fixed beneath a metal-backed tibial tray have been implanted successfully and are biomechanically superior to cement alone (Urs *et al.*, 1988) (Fig. 20.4.7). In order to transmit the loads more efficiently, extended stems have been placed on these tibial trays. There is concern that intramedullary stems stress shield the proximal tibia and should be no longer than necessary to achieve fixation (Bourne and Finlay, 1986). Special consideration is required when utilizing tibial wedges since the shear stresses can be transmitted longitudinally into the tibial shaft with the intramedullary stem. In a similar fashion, when there is bone loss from the distal or posterior femoral condyles, metal augments may be put into the femoral component. Stemmed femoral components are utilized with these metal augmentations for better load distribution. The Insall–Burstein posterior stabilized II prosthesis with its modular components

allows the surgeon to adapt the prosthesis for individual needs at the time of surgery. Other implant designs also have the benefit of this modularity. These modular systems which have been successfully implanted obviate the need for custom-made implants.

In a recent review of treatment of non-unions about the knee utilizing custom total knee replacements with press-fit intramedullary stems, the results were successful (Kress *et al.*, 1990). The study included nine patients with non-unions about the knee who failed conservative or other operative treatment. There were four proximal tibial non-unions, two distal femoral non-unions and three supracondylar femur non-unions above previous total knee replacements. The six primary cases all had either associated post-traumatic or concurrent osteoarthritis in the affected knee. To facilitate healing, a press-fit intramedullary stem was incorporated into the total knee replacement. In an average follow-up of 6 years, the Hospital for Special Surgery knee score demonstrated four excellent, four good and one poor result.

CLINICAL EXPERIENCE

The posterior stabilized prosthesis is routinely used on the Knee Service at The Hospital for Special Surgery for all knees with competent collateral ligaments (Scuderi and Insall, 1989). In patients with significant bone loss, it may be necessary to utilize a custom prosthesis with metal augmentation and large intramedullary stems to transfer the load to cortical bone or to bone graft the bony defect (Urs *et al.*, 1988; Scuderi *et al.*, 1989). The constrained condylar prosthesis is used if there is loss of

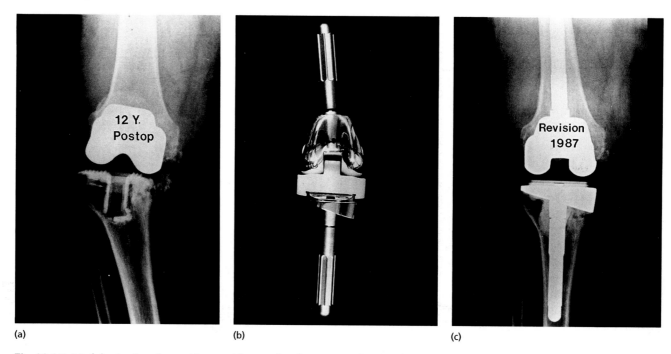

(a)   (b)   (c)

Fig. 20.4.7 Modular implant for revision total knee arthroplasty. (a) Radiograph of a failed total knee arthroplasty (TKA); (b) the assembled components prior to implantation; (c) the final radiograph.

the medial collateral ligament, severe valgus and flexion and combined deformities in which the posterior stabilized prosthesis would not suffice (Donaldson *et al.*, 1988).

At the time of introduction, there was concern that the increase in constraint with the posterior stabilized prosthesis would increase the rate of loosening. Clinically this has proven not to be the case. Stress analysis using finite element methods supports these clinical findings in that maximum tensile and compressive stresses under the plateau are no higher in the posterior stabilized prosthesis than in a prosthesis of similar geometry without the stabilizing cam (Bartel *et al.*, 1982). The records of the Knee Service at The Hospital for Special Surgery show that 1951 knee arthroplasties were performed between 1974 and 1985. The total condylar design was used in 326, of which six (1.8%) had tibial loosening. More recently, between 1978 and 1985, 1625 posterior stabilized prostheses were implanted, of which only three (0.18%) had tibial loosening (Insall, 1988).

A recent survivorship analysis of cemented primary total knee arthroplasties performed on the Knee Service at The Hospital for Special Surgery over a 15-year period demonstrated that the procedure was durable and predictable (Scuderi *et al.*, 1989). From 1974 to 1986, there were 1430 cemented primary total knee arthroplasties available for review. This includes 224 total condylar prostheses with a polyethylene tibial component (1974–1978), 289 posterior stabilized pros-

theses with an all-polyethylene tibial component (1978–1981) and 917 posterior stabilized prostheses with a metal-backed tibial component (1981–1986). There were 12 failures in the total condylar series, giving an average annual failure rate of 0.65% and a 15-year success rate of 90.56%. The posterior stabilized prosthesis with a polyethylene tibia showed an average annual failure rate of 0.27% and a 10-year success rate of 97.34% (Fig. 20.4.8). This prosthesis with a metal-backed tibial component gave an average annual failure rate of 0.19% and a 7-year success rate of 98.75% (Fig. 20.4.9). The overall survival rate was not influenced by sex or age, diagnosis or the percentage of ideal body weight. No metal-backed tibial components have yet been revised for loosening. The incidence of femoral loosening requiring revision was 0.89% in the total condylar group and 0.33% in the combined posterior stabilized group. The overall incidence of infection for all total knee replacements was 0.63%.

The Hospital for Special Surgery Knee Rating System is the most widely used for patient evaluation. Using this scale, a score of 85–100 points is termed an excellent result, 70–84 points good, 60–69 points fair and less than 60 points poor. An excellent result is close to normal function, taking into account such factors as age and the general state of the patient's health. Thus knees with an excellent rating are painless and stable, have at least 90° of flexion and do not in themselves restrict the activity of the patients. In the initial report on the

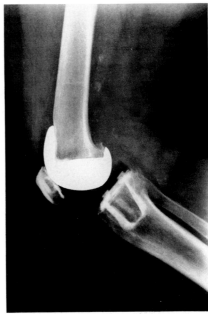

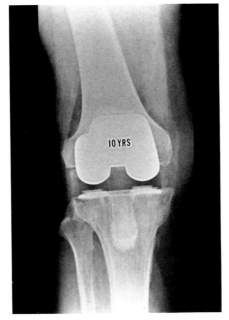

(a)

(b)

Fig. 20.4.8 Long-term radiograph of a posterior stabilized prosthesis with a polyethylene tibia. (a) Anteroposterior radiograph and (b) lateral radiograph.

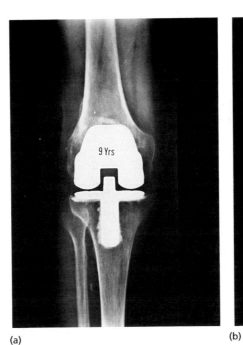

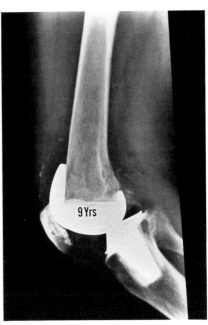

(a)

(b)

Fig. 20.4.9 Long-term radiograph of a posterior stabilized prosthesis with a metal-backed tibia. (a) Anteroposterior radiograph and (b) lateral radiograph.

posterior stabilized knee, 118 knees were followed for 2–4 years, 104 (88%) were rated excellent, 11 (9%) good or fair and three (3%) poor (Insall *et al.*, 1982). More recent follow-up of 96 knees followed for 8 years and longer revealed 76 (79.2%) excellent, 16 (16.7%) good, none fair and four (4.2%) poor (Vince *et al.*, 1988). This is a marked improvement in post-operative

function when compared with our results using other prostheses (Insall *et al.*, 1976, 1979).

Since the Hospital for Special Surgery system incorporates a functional component, the score tends to deteriorate as patients get older, although the knee remains unchanged. This led the American Knee Society to propose a new rating system which is simple, more exacting and more objective (Table 20.4.1). The rating is divided into separate knee and patient function scores. Increasing age or a medical condition will not affect the knee score (Insall *et al.*, 1989).

Several recent studies have demonstrated the successful application of cemented total knee arthroplasty in different conditions about the knee. The results of total knee arthroplasty using the posterior stabilized prosthesis in a small series of Charcot and Charcot-like joints have been good to excellent over an average of 3 years (Soudry *et al.*, 1986a). Pre-operatively, most patients in this study had demonstrated severe liga-

mentous laxity and bone loss. The posterior stabilized prosthesis had an added advantage in these cases through its inherent stability in flexion. In another series with post-traumatic arthritis, the posterior stabilized prosthesis had a 90% good to excellent result over an average of 4 years (Zelicof *et al.*, 1988). With Charcot joints, special attention must be given to ligamentous balancing and bone defects in the post-traumatic group. In yet another study, the use of the posterior stabilized knee for osteonecrosis yielded 86% excellent and good results at an average follow-up of 3.8 years (Stern *et al.*, 1988). In a recent study of total knee arthroplasty in gonarthrotic

Table 20.4.1 American Knee Society clinical rating system

	Points		Points
Patient category		*Deductions (minus)*	
A Unilateral or bilateral (opposite knee successfully replaced)		Flexion contracture	
		5°−10°	2
B Unilateral, other knee symptomatic		10°−15°	5
C Multiple arthritis or medical infirmity		16°−20°	10
		>20°	15
		Extension lag	
Pain		<10°	5
None	50	10−20°	10
Mild or occasional	45	>20°	15
Stairs only	40	Alignment	
Walking and stairs	30	5°−10°	0
Moderate		0°−4°	3 points each degree
Occasional	20	11°−15°	3 points each degree
Continual	10	Other	20
Severe	0	Total deductions	. . .
		Knee score	. . .
Range of motion		(If total is a minus number, score is 0.)	
(5° = 1 point)	25		
		Function	
Stability (maximum movement in any position)		Walking	50
		Unlimited	40
Anteroposterior		>10 blocks	30
<5 mm	10	5−10 blocks	20
5−10 mm	5	<5 blocks	10
10 mm	0	Housebound	0
Mediolateral		Unable	
<5°	15	Stairs	
6°−9°	10	Normal up and down	50
10°−14°	5	Normal up: down with rail	40
15°	0	Up and down with rail	30
Subtotal	. . .	Up with rail: unable down	15
		Unable	0
		Subtotal	. . .
		Deductions (minus)	
		Cane	5
		Two canes	10
		Crutches or walker	20
		Total deductions	. . .
		Function score	. . .

patients aged less than 55 years, there were 98% good and excellent results at an average follow-up of 5 years (Bowen *et al.*, 1990). When a subgroup of patients in this study, who may have been otherwise indicated for a high tibial osteotomy, were compared with long-term results of high tibial osteotomy, the clinical scoring was higher in the total knee arthroplasty group. There was no deterioration in the function of the prosthetic knees with time, as has been seen after high tibial osteotomy (Insall *et al.*, 1984; Windsor *et al.*, 1988).

Total knee arthroplasty in patients with rheumatoid arthritis has been successful and consistently relieves pain and improves function. Stuart and Rand (1988), in a recent study of total knee arthroplasty in young patients with rheumatoid arthritis, reported relief of pain and improvement in function. In patients with rheumatoid arthritis, however, the ability to walk is often limited by other joint involvement, including hips and feet. When comparing the Hospital for Special Surgery knee score in that study to the score obtained in a comparative study by Goldberg *et al.* (1988), the results were similar. Stuart and Rand (1988) reported an average post-operative score of 84, with 86% of patients achieving a good or excellent result. Goldberg *et al.* (1988) reported an average post-operative score of 85. However, Goldberg *et al.* (1988) did note that the functional ability deteriorated with longer follow-up. This loss of function was most often seen in the ageing patient who had difficulty climbing stairs unaided and walking distances. The knees with osteoarthritis had a higher final rate of failure (18%) and a lower average overall score (79 points) than those that were affected by rheumatoid arthritis (12% and 85 points, respectively). In a review and survivorship analysis of 112 knees, including 65 knees with rheumatoid arthritis and 47 with osteoarthritis with an average follow-up of 9.5 years, Ranawat and Boachie-Adjei (1988) found that the variables such as sex, age, diagnosis, thickness of the cement layer, level of tibial resection, and component alignment did not correlate with absence or presence of radiolucency. The only variable to influence the appearance of radiolucency was body weight. The clinical results were excellent to good in 92% of patients. Other reports have shown successful results with different types of implants (Trepte and Puhl, 1988). Laskin, in a review of 80 total condylar knee replacements in patients with rheumatoid arthritis followed for 10 years, showed a 24% failure rate with the major reasons for re-operation being loosening of the tibial component or late infection (Laskin, 1990).

Kjaersgaard-Andersen *et al.* (1990) have reported that total knee arthroplasty is an effective treatment for intractable chronic knee pain due to severe joint degeneration in haemophiliacs. Caution is necessary in HIV-positive patients because of the challenge to the patient's immune system, and the risk of transmitting the virus to the hospital staff.

Radiolucency

The appearance and development of radiolucencies do not seem to differ between the posterior stabilized and the total condylar prosthesis. The posterior stabilized prosthesis showed a 32% incidence of incomplete tibial radiolucent lines during the 2–4-year study (Insall *et al.*, 1982), whereas radiolucencies were observed in 36% of the total condylar implants at 5 years (Insall *et al.*, 1979). Although there may be concern that the incidence of radiolucent lines would increase with time, this does not appear to be the case. In a more recent and longer follow-up study of the posterior stabilized prosthesis, only one-third of the cases demonstrated radiolucencies at 8 years, which is similar to observations with the total condylar prosthesis at 10 years (Insall and Kelly, 1986; Vince *et al.*, 1988).

The American Knee Society Roentgenographic Evaluation System was developed for uniform reporting of radiographic results of total knee arthroplasty so comparisons could be made between different institutions and different implants. The system allows measurement of knee alignment, component position and has a numerical score for the prosthetic interface that assesses the quality of fixation (Ewald, 1989) (Fig. 20.4.10).

Mechanical failure

Mechanical failures in the authors' series were mainly attributable to error in operative technique and mechanical misalignment of the tibial component (Windsor *et al.*, 1989a). Post-operative varus tibiofemoral alignment, varus component positioning and excessive tibial bone resection may have predisposed knees to failure by tibial loosening. Though tibial loosening has been associated with overweight patients, there is no statistical correlation, and a recent review of total knee arthroplasties in obese patients failed to reveal this problem. No metal-backed posterior stabilized tibial component, however, has had to be revised for loosening. Femoral component loosening occurred much earlier than tibial component loosening, probably as a result of condylar osteoporosis and technical errors that are caused by overhang of the posterior aspect of the femoral component runners on the posterior femoral condyle or insufficient tibial component contact. In the long term a

ALIGNMENT: Recumbent ☐   Standing ☐

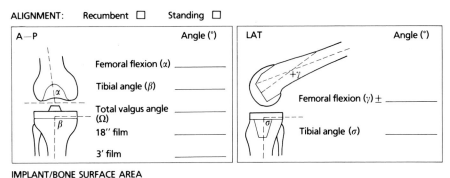

IMPLANT/BONE SURFACE AREA
   Percent area of tibial surface covered by implant

RADIOLUCENCIES: Indicate depth (mm) in each zone

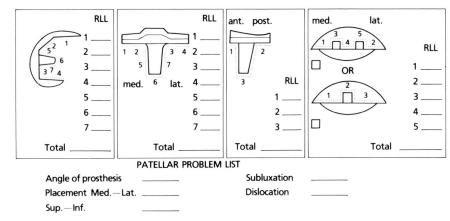

PATELLAR PROBLEM LIST

Angle of prosthesis	_____	Subluxation	_____
Placement Med.—Lat.	_____	Dislocation	_____
Sup.—Inf.	_____		

Fig. 20.4.10 The American Knee Society roentgenographic evaluation system.

well-aligned, cemented total knee arthroplasty with appropriate balanced ligaments will yield durable service with a low rate of mechanical failure at the femorotibial articulation.

Polyethylene wear characteristics

Recently polyethylene wear and breakage have been recognized. Debris from damage to the articular surface of polyethylene components of total knee arthroplasties have been shown to contribute to long-term problems such as loosening and infection. The biological response in the surrounding tissues by particles of polyethylene can cause endosteal resorption and deterioration of the bone implant interface (Bartel *et al.*, 1986). Contact between the metal femoral and polyethylene tibial components in total knee replacements results in a complex stress distribution on the surface and within the polyethylene. Perpendicular compressive stress is normal to the surface throughout the component. The maximum value occurs at the centre of the contact area. Near the edge of contact, the surface is stretched and tensile stresses occur in the polyethylene. Shearing and distortion of the polyethylene may occur by indentation of the

metal femoral component on the polyethylene tibial surface. The stresses on the polyethylene cause pitting and delamination of the articular surface with resultant debris. The contact between non-conforming articular surfaces in total knee arthroplasty results in significantly higher contact stresses on the polyethylene surface. The low conformity in posterior cruciate retaining designs increases polyethylene wear and results in edge loading of the components as well as instability. Total knee arthroplasty that is most conforming in the medial–lateral direction should be chosen to minimize the risk of surface damage. Maximum thickness of the polyethylene is recommended, in order to reduce stresses that lead to surface damage. Retrieved tibial components demonstrated that the most severe surface damage was to the flat tibial surfaces and thin polyethylene (4–6 mm) (Bartel *et al.*, 1986). A minimal thickness of polyethylene of 8 mm should be maintained whenever possible. The addition of carbon fibres to the polyethylene does not improve the resistance of polyethylene to surface damage (Wright *et al.*, 1988). This has been substantiated with experimental, analytical and clinical studies. Malalignment of components enhances polyethylene wear and will cause mechanical failure.

Patellar resurfacing

Patellar resurfacing is still a controversial issue (Soudry *et al.*, 1986b; Abraham *et al.*, 1988; Shoji *et al.*, 1989). It is the authors' belief, however, that the patella should be resurfaced in all arthroplasties. This has greatly reduced patellofemoral complaints after total knee arthroplasty in their experience. Now, they cement in place an all-polyethylene central dome patella. Metal-backed patellar prostheses are suspect due to the limited thickness of the polyethylene and associated wear and disassociation of the metal-backed patellar button. Hsu and Walker (1989) studied the wear and deformation of patellar components in total knee arthroplasty. They found that all plastic components suffer local deformation and underlying bone failure, whereas metal backing leads to eventual penetration of the metal on to the femoral flange owing to limited plastic thickness. Increased conformity of the patellar component on to the femoral flange increases the contact area and improves the situation. Care must be taken at the time of arthroplasty to maintain a centralized patella.

Patellar instability in the form of subluxation-dislocation after total knee replacement has been reported to range from 1 to 20% (Merkow *et al.*, 1985). Technical errors, surgical technique, trauma and prosthetic design have affected patellar tracking. Genu valgum or external rotational deformities of the tibia also predispose to lateral dislocation of the patella. Internal rotation of the tibial components with respect to the tibia causes external rotation of the tibia and lateral displacement of the tibial tuberosity in the reduced position. This displacement increases the valgus vector forces and the tendency of the patella to sublux laterally.

Proximal patellar realignment is an effective method of treatment for lateral dislocation of the patella after total knee replacement. The experience from the Knee Service at the Hospital for Special Surgery with this procedure reported all patients with good or excellent results without significant complications or redislocation (Merkow *et al.*, 1985).

If there is a severe malrotation of the tibial component in the horizontal plane, revision and repositioning of the tibial component to place a tuberosity in the correct sagittal plane is necessary. Traumatic disruption of the vastus medialis and medial retinaculum with patellar dislocation should be treated by early surgical repair and balancing of the extensor mechanism. The incidence of patellar fractures following total knee arthroplasty varies from 3% to 21%. This problem has been attributed to avascular necrosis of the patella secondary to the surgical approach, including medial arthrotomy and lateral release, patellar bone resection, thermal necrosis and anatomic variation. Management of patellar fractures may be conservative or surgical depending on the severity of the injury. Most fractures may be treated initially with cylinder cast immobilization for a period of 6 weeks, followed by active assisted exercises and isometric quadriceps strengthening. Surgical intervention is confined to these situations where there is a severely displaced transverse fracture of the patella or a comminuted fracture in which a large proximal pole is displaced to the point that the extension lag is severe and the patient's quadriceps function is poor. Fixation is often difficult and elaborate internal fixation should be avoided (Windsor *et al.*, 1989a).

A loose patellar button is also an indication for surgery, including removal of the patellar button and methylmethacrylate. If the bone stock is sufficient and the fracture healed, a new button can be reinserted; however, this case is rare (Windsor *et al.*, 1989).

A syndrome of patellofemoral dysfunction consisting of painful popping, catching or jumping of the patellar component can complicate total knee arthroplasty. Though the aetiology of this fibrous band is unclear, resolution of symptoms occurs after removal of the band (Thorpe *et al.*, 1990). With the original design of the posterior stabilized prosthesis, the patients were experiencing patellar 'catching' problems during flexion (Hozack *et al.*, 1989). This was attributed to the configuration of the anterior margin of the intercondylar notch and impingement of peripatellar soft tissue, particularly superiorly along the undersurface of the quadriceps tendon. In 1983, the posterior stabilized design was revised to incorporate a deeper patellar groove, allowing smoother tracking of the patella. Special attention is also given to excising the soft tissue and synovium from the superior peripatellar area (Scuderi and Insall, 1989).

Infection (see also Chapter 15)

Infection is the main cause of failure in total knee arthroplasty (Scuderi *et al.*, 1989a). Infections are usually described as early or late. Early infections usually result from contamination during operation but in rare instances may follow wound drainage or skin necrosis. A late infection is usually described as occurring 3 months after initial operation. The cause of late infection may be obscure. It may be due to transient bacteraemia from a site other than the knee. This would include dentition, ulcers, lungs, gastrointestinal tract and genitourinary tract. It may also be that late infection is the result of contamination at the time of the initial operation that has been dormant. Metastatic infections can be reduced by patient education, and prophylactic antibiotics should be taken to cover dental procedures and to treat obvious infections elsewhere in the body that may put the prosthesis at risk. The diagnosis of an infection is paramount. Early infections should be suspected when the patient's post-operative course demonstrates persistent fever and excessive swelling about the knee and pain beyond the first week. A sedimentation rate and white blood cell count may be helpful. When there is doubt, aspiration of the joint is indicated. The diagnosis of a late infection can be elusive. A painful total knee replacement without detectable mechanical cause should indicate infection until otherwise proven. The recommended procedure to establish the presence of infection is knee aspiration (Insall *et al.*, 1983b; Insall, 1986).

When the diagnosis of an early infection is made, particularly in the early post-operative course, incision, drainage and debridement are indicated leaving the components in place. The wound is closed over suction drains which are removed at 36 h. Appropriate intravenous antibiotic treatment is initiated. After 2 weeks the wound is inspected and reaspirated under strict aseptic conditions. If the wound is benign and the cultures are negative, antibiotic therapy is continued for an additional 4 weeks. If there is still evidence of infection with positive cultures, the components and cement are removed.

The treatment for a late infection is thorough debridement of the involved tissues and removal of the prosthesis and cement. Removal of the prosthesis may be difficult since the components may not be mechanically loose. Special instrumentation is recommended. The surgical procedure involves removal of the infected prosthesis and cement. The procedure is performed under tourniquet control but the limb is not exsanguinated with an Esmarch to minimize the risk of bacteraemia. The infected synovial membrane and pseudomembrane are thoroughly debrided. A sliding extraction hammer is useful for removal of the femoral and tibial components. The patellar prosthesis is removed using an oscillating saw to cut the stem and remove the button. All remaining cement is then removed. The wound is thoroughly irrigated with several litres of normal saline and antibiotic solution. Large-bore suction drains are left in the wound for 24−48 h. Irrigation in flow tubes is not used because of the risk of superinfection. All wounds are closed primarily and a bulky dressing with plaster splints is applied. The patient mobilizes non-weight-bearing, with a walker 4−7 days after operation (Insall, 1986).

All patients are given parenteral antibiotics for 6 weeks after removal of the prosthesis. The antimicrobial regimen is designed on the basis of quantitative *in vitro* sensitivity studies in which the minimum bactericidal concentration of a variety of antibiotics is determined for each infecting organism.

According to the patient's response to antibiotic therapy, future options are prolonged immobilization to produce painless pseudoarthrosis, arthrodesis and re-implantation of another prosthesis.

When the response to antibiotic therapy is successful, reimplantation is considered. Before reimplantation surgery, reaspiration of the knee may be performed. When the knee is exposed, Gram stains of the wound exudate are carried out and a tissue specimen is sent for frozen section. If any organisms are found, the wound is closed without reimplantation. Exposure for reimplantation can be difficult and care must be taken to avoid avulsing the tibial tubercle when the quadriceps is tight. A Coonse and Adams quadricepsplasty can be used if avulsion of the patellar tendon appears likely. Partial or complete skeletonization of the distal part of the femur or the proximal tibia may also be required. Usually a non-constrained resurfacing prosthesis can be used for reimplantation since a soft-tissue sleeve is preserved around the bones. The posterior stabilized prosthesis is recommended as a substitute for the posterior cruciate ligament. Occasionally the soft tissues are inadequate and a constrained condylar prosthesis will need to be utilized. The decision as to which prosthesis to use can be made at the time of implantation. The modular knee systems allow the surgeon a choice of implants. If there is bone loss from the distal femur or proximal tibia, metal augmentations can be utilized with associated intramedullary stems.

A recent study of two-stage reimplantation for the salvage of total knee arthroplasty complicated by infection demonstrated successful results with an average follow-up of 4 years. The results of this study suggested that the two-stage protocol for reimplantation, with a 6-week interval of intravenous antibiotic therapy is the procedure of choice. A patient who has polyarticular rheumatoid arthritis and in which the immunological system is suppressed may not be an ideal candidate for the protocol. Gram-negative bacterial infection may be treated with this protocol, provided the organism is sensitive to relatively non-toxic antibiotics. When the protocol cannot be followed, retention of a functioning arthroplasty has been unusual (Windsor *et al.*, 1990).

Wilson *et al.* (1990), in a review of 4171 total knee arthroplasties, reported an infection rate of 1.6%, predominantly of *Staphylococcus aureus*. The risk of infection was significantly increased in patients who had rheumatoid arthritis particularly men, in patients who had ulcers of the skin, and in patients who had a previous knee operation. Infection was also associated with obesity, recurrent urinary tract infections and oral use of steroids. The authors favoured a two-stage reimplantation, but in the presence of one or more of the risk factors, one-third of the infections recurred.

REFERENCES

Abraham W., Buchanan J.R., Daubert H., Greer R.B. III, and Keefer J.R.P.T. (1988) Should the patella be resurfaced in total knee arthroplasty? Efficacy of patellar resurfacing. *Clin. Orthop.* **236**, 128–134.

Alexiades M., Scuderi G., Vigorita V. and Scott W.N. (1989) A histologic study of the posterior cruciate ligament in the arthritic knee. *Am. J. Knee Surg.* 2(4), 153–159.

Bartel D.L., Burstein A.H., Santavicca E.A. and Insall J.N. (1982) Performance of the tibial component in total knee replacement. *J. Bone Joint Surg.* **64A**, 1026–1033.

Bartel D.L., Bicknell M.S. and Wright T.M. (1986) The effect of conformity, thickness, and material on stresses in ultra-high molecular weight components for total joint replacement. *J. Bone Joint Surg.* **68A**, 1041–1051.

Bourne R.B. and Finlay J.B. (1986) The influence of tibial component intramedullary stems and implant-cortex contact on the strain distribution of the proximal tibia following total knee arthroplasty. An in vitro study. *Clin. Orthop.* **208**, 95–99.

Bowen M.K., Stern S.H., Insall J.N. and Scuderi G.R. (1990) Total knee arthroplasty in gonarthrosis patients less than 55 years old. *Clin. Orthop.* **260**, 124–129.

Cheal E.J., Hayes W.C., Lee C.H., Snyder B.D. and Miller J. (1985) Stress analysis of a condylar knee tibial component: influence of metaphyseal shell properties and cement injection depth. *J. Orthop. Res.* **3**, 424–434.

Donaldson W.F., III, Sculco T.P., Insall J.N. and Ranawat C.S. (1988) Total condylar III knee prosthesis. Long-term follow-up study. *Clin. Orthop.* **226**, 21–28.

Dorr L.D. and Ranawat C.S. (1984) Bone grafts for tibial deficits in total knee arthroplasty. In Dorr L.D. (ed.) *Revision of Total Hip and Knee*. Baltimore, University Park Press, pp. 143–150.

Dorr L.D., Lindberg J.P., Claude-Faugere M. and Malluche H.H. (1984) Factors influencing the intrusion of methylmethacrylate into human tibiae. *Clin. Orthop.* **183**, 147–152.

Dorr L.D., Scott R.D. and Ranawat C.S. (1985) Controversies of total knee arthroplasty. A. Importance of retention of posterior cruciate ligament. In Ranawat C.R. (ed.) *Total-Condylar Knee Arthroplasty. Technique, Results and Complications.* New York, Springer-Verlag, pp. 197–202.

Dorr L.D., Ochsner J.L., Gronley J. and Perry J. (1988) Functional comparison of posterior cruciate-retained versus cruciate-sacrificed total knee arthroplasty. *Clin. Orthop.* **236**, 36–43.

Ewald F.C. (1989) The Knee Society total knee arthroplasty roentgenographic evaluation and scoring system. *Clin. Orthop.* **248**, 9–12.

Ewald F.C., Jacobs M.A., Miegel R.E., Walker P.S., Poss R. and Sledge C.B. (1984) Kinematic total knee replacement. *J. Bone Joint Surg.* **66A**, 1032–1040.

Goldberg V.M., Figgie M.P., Figgie H.E., III, Heiple K.G. and Sobel M. (1988) Use of a total condylar knee prosthesis for treatment of osteoarthritis and rheumatoid arthritis. *J. Bone Joint Surg.* **70A**, 802–811.

Haddad R.J., Jr., Cook S.D. and Thomas K.A. (1987) Current concepts review. Biological fixation of porous-coated implants. *J. Bone Joint Surg.* **69A**, 1459–1466.

Hozack W.J., Rothman R.H., Booth R.E., Jr. and Balderston R.A. (1989) The patellar clunk syndrome. A complication of posterior stabilized total knee arthroplasty. *Clin. Orthop.* **241**, 203–208.

Hsu H.-P. and Walker P.S. (1989) Wear and deformation of patellar components in total knee arthroplasty. *Clin. Orthop.* **246**, 260–265.

Hungerford D.S., Krackow K.A. and Kenna R.V. (1987) Two- to five-year experience with a cementless porous-coated total knee prosthesis. In Rand J.A. and Dorr L.D. (eds) *Total Arthroplasty of the Knee. Proceedings of the Knee Society, 1985–1986.* Rockville, Aspen Publishers Inc. pp. 215–235.

Hvid I. and Hansen S.L. (1985) Trabecular bone strength patterns at the proximal tibial epiphysis. *J. Orthop. Res.* **3**, 464–472.

Insall J.N. (1981) Technique of total knee replacement. In *Instructional Course Lectures, The American Academy of Orthopaedic Surgeons.* St Louis, C.V. Mosby, vol. 30, pp. 324–334.

Insall J.N. (1986a) Infection of total knee arthroplasty. In *Instructional Course Lectures, The American Academy of Orthopaedic Surgeons.* St Louis, C.V. Mosby, vol. 35, pp. 319–324.

Insall J.N. (1986b) Revision of total knee replacement. In *Instructional Course Lectures, The American Academy of Orthopaedic Surgeons.* St Louis, C.V. Mosby, vol. 35, pp. 290–296.

Insall J.N. (1988) Presidential address to the Knee Society. Choices and compromises in total knee arthroplasty. *Clin. Orthop.* **226**, 43–48.

Insall J.N. and Kelly M. (1986) The total condylar prosthesis. *Clin. Orthop.* **205**, 43–48.

Insall J.N., Ranawat C.S., Aglietti P. and Shine J. (1976) A comparison of four models of total knee-replacement prostheses. *J. Bone Joint Surg.* **58A**, 754–765.

Insall J., Scott W.N. and Ranawat C.S. (1979) The total condylar knee prosthesis. A report of two hundred and twenty cases. *J. Bone Joint Surg.* **61A**, 173–180.

Insall J.N., Lachiewicz P.F. and Burstein A.H. (1982) The posterior stabilized condylar prosthesis: a modification of the total condylar design. Two to four-year clinical experience. *J. Bone Joint Surg.* **64A**, 1317–1323.

Insall J.N., Hood R.W., Flawn L.B. and Sullivan D.J. (1983a) The total condylar knee prosthesis in gonarthrosis. *J. Bone Joint Surg.* **65A**, 619–628.

Insall J.N., Thompson F.M. and Brause B.D. (1983b) Two-stage reimplantation for the salvage of infected knee arthroplasty. *J. Bone Joint Surg.* **65A**, 1087–1098.

Insall J.N., Joseph D.M. and Msika C. (1984) High tibial osteotomy for varus gonarthrosis. A long-term follow-up study. *J. Bone Joint Surg.* **66A**, 1040–1048.

Insall J.N., Dorr L.D., Scott R.D. and Scott W.N. (1989) Rationale of the knee society clinical rating system. *Clin. Orthop.* **248**, 13–14.

Jiang C-C. and Insall J.N. (1989) Effect of rotation on the axial alignment of the femur. Pitfalls in the use of femoral intramedullary guides in total knee arthroplasty. *Clin. Orthop.* **248**, 50–56.

Johnson D.P. (1990) The effect of continuous passive motion on wound-healing and joint mobility after knee arthroplasty. *J. Bone Joint Surg.* **72A**, 421–426.

Kjaersgaard-Andersen P., Christiansen S.E., Ingerslev J. and

Sneppen O. (1990) Total knee arthroplasty in classic hemophilia. *Clin. Orthop.* **256**, 137–146.

Krause W.R., Krug W. and Miller J. (1982) Strength of the cement-bone interface. *Clin. Orthop.* **163**, 290–299.

Kress K.J., Scuderi G.R., Windsor R.E. and Insall J.N. (1993) Treatment of nonunions about the knee utilizing custom total knee replacements with press fit intramedullary stems. *J. Arthroplasty* **8** (1), 49–55.

Laskin R.S. (1990) Total condylar knee replacement in patients who have rheumatoid arthritis. A ten-year follow-up study. *J. Bone Joint Surg.* **72A**, 529–535.

Maloney W.J., Schurman D.J., Hangen D., Goodman S.B., Edworthy S. and Bloch D.A. (1990) The influence of continuous passive motion on outcome in total knee arthroplasty. *Clin. Orthop.* **256**, 162–168.

Merkow R.L., Soudry M. and Insall J.N. (1985) Patellar dislocation following total knee replacement. *J. Bone Joint Surg.* **67A**, 1321–1327.

Ranawat C.S. and Boachie-Adjei O. (1988) Survivorship analysis and results of total condylar knee arthroplasty. Eight- to 11-year follow-up period. *Clin. Orthop.* **226**, 6–13.

Ranawat C.S. (ed.) (1985) How to compensate for bone loss. In *Total-Condylar Knee Arthroplasty. Technique, Results and Complications.* New York, Springer-Verlag, pp. 95–104.

Ritter M.A., Gandolf V.S. and Holston K.S. (1989) Continuous passive motion versus physical therapy in total knee arthroplasty. *Clin. Orthop.* **244**, 239–243.

Rorabeck C.H., Bourne R.B. and Nott L. (1988) The cemented kinematic-II and the non-cemented porous-coated anatomic prostheses for total knee replacement. A prospective evaluation. *J. Bone Joint Surg.* **70A**, 483–490.

Rosenqvist R., Bylander B., Knutson K., Rydholm U., Rooser B., Egund N. and Lidgren L. (1986) Loosening of the porous coating of bicompartmental prostheses in patients with rheumatoid arthritis. *J. Bone Joint Surg.* **68A**, 538–542.

Scott W.N., Rubinstein M. and Scuderi G. (1988) Results after knee replacement with a posterior cruciate-substituting prosthesis. *J. Bone Joint Surg.* **70A**, 1163–1173.

Scuderi G.R. and Insall J.N. (1989) The posterior stabilized knee prosthesis. *Orthop. Clin. North Am.* **20**(1), 71–78.

Scuderi G., Scharf S.C., Meltzer L.P. and Scott W.N. (1987) The relationship of lateral releases to patella viability in total knee arthroplasty. *J. Arthroplasty* **2**(3), 209–214.

Scuderi G.R., Insall J.N., Windsor R.E. and Moran M.C. (1989a) Survivorship of cemented knee replacements. *J. Bone Joint Surg.* **71B**, 798–803.

Scuderi G.R., Insall J.N., Haas S.B., Becker-Fluegel M.W. and Windsor R.E. (1989b) Inlay autogeneic bone grafting of tibial defects in primary total knee arthroplasty. *Clin. Orthop.* **248**, 93–97.

Shoji H., Yoshino S. and Kajino A. (1989) Patellar replacement in bilateral total knee arthroplasty. A study of patients who had rheumatoid arthritis and no gross deformity of the patella. *J. Bone Joint Surg.* **71A**, 853–856.

Soudry M., Binazzi R., Johanson N.A., Bullough P.G. and Insall J.N. (1986a) Total knee arthroplasty in Charcot and Charcot-like joints. *Clin. Orthop.* **208**, 199–204.

Soudry M., Mestriner L.A., Binazzi R. and Insall J.N. (1986b) Total knee arthroplasty without patellar resurfacing. *Clin. Orthop.* **205**, 166–170.

Stern S.H., Insall J.N. and Windsor R.E. (1988) Total knee arthroplasty in osteonecrotic knees. *Orthop. Trans.* **12**, 722–723.

Stuart M.J. and Rand J.A. (1988) Total knee arthroplasty in young adults who have rheumatoid arthritis. *J. Bone Joint Surg.* **70A**, 84–87.

Thorpe C.D., Bocell J.R. and Tullos H.S. (1990) Intra-articular fibrous bands. Patellar complications after total knee replacement. *J. Bone Joint Surg.* **72A**, 811–814.

Trepte C.T. and Puhl W. (1988) Axial knee prostheses in patients with chronic polyarthritis. *Z. Rheumatol.* **47**, 213–218.

Urs W.K., Binazzi R., Insall J.N., Windsor R.E. and Padgett D. (1988) Custom total knee arthroplasty. *Orthop. Trans.* **12**, 711.

Vince K.G. and Insall J.N. (1988) Long-term results of cemented total knee arthroplasty. *Orthop. Clin. North. Am.* **19**(3), 575–580.

Vince K.G., Kelly M.A. and Insall J.N. (1988) Posterior stabilized knee prosthesis: follow up at five to eight years. *Orthop. Trans.* **12**, 157.

Wilson M.G., Kelley K. and Thornhill T.S. (1990) Infection as a complication of total knee-replacement arthroplasty. *J. Bone Joint Surg.* **72A**, 878–883.

Windsor R.E., Insall J.N. and Sculco T.P. (1986) Bone grafting of tibial defects in primary and revision total knee arthroplasty. *Clin. Orthop.* **205**, 132–137.

Windsor R.E., Insall J.N. and Vince K.G. (1988) Technical considerations of total knee arthroplasty after proximal tibial osteotomy. *J. Bone Joint Surg.* **70A**, 547–555.

Windsor R.E., Scuderi G.R. and Insall J.N. (1989a) Patellar fractures in total knee arthroplasty. *J. Arthroplasty Suppl.* **4**, 63–67.

Windsor R.E., Scuderi G.R., Moran M.C. and Insall J.N. (1989b) Mechanisms of failure of the femoral and tibial components in total knee arthroplasty. *Clin. Orthop.* **248**, 15–20.

Windsor R.E., Insall J.N., Urs W.K., Miller D.V. and Brause B.D. (1990) Two-stage reimplantation for the salvage of total knee arthroplasty complicated by infection. Further follow-up and refinement of indications. *J. Bone Joint Surg.* **72A**, 272–278.

Wright T.M., Astion D.J., Bansal M., Rimnac C.M., Green T., Insall J.N. and Robinson R.P. (1988) Failure of carbon fiber-reinforced polyethylene total knee-replacement components. A report of two cases. *J. Bone Joint Surg.* **70A**, 926–932.

Zelicof S.B., Scuderi G.R., Vince K.G., Urs W.K. and Insall J.N. (1988) Total knee arthroplasty in post-traumatic arthritis. *Orthop. Trans.* **12**, 547–548.

Chapter 21
The Cervical Spine

G. Bonney

INTRODUCTION

The cervical spine is a region of particular interest and importance to the orthopaedic surgeon because of its mobility, its liability to damage and its association with structures of vital importance, namely, the cervical part of the spinal cord, the cervical spinal nerves and the vertebral arteries. Pain in the neck with or without radiation to one or both upper limbs is a symptom very often encountered in the practice of medicine; the sequelae of injury to the neck are seen with increasing frequency. The causes of many of the pains so arising are ill-understood. The symptoms of disorder of the spinal cord or spinal nerves are less often encountered but when they are they demand thorough investigation and carefully planned treatment. The hazards of operating on the cervical spine must thoroughly be appreciated: this is no region for the attentions of the inexperienced or impatient surgeon.

ANATOMY OF THE CERVICAL SPINE

The cervical spine is made up of seven vertebrae, the uppermost two of which are of specialized form appropriate to their function. The atlas bears the weight of the skull and is in effect a ring of bone articulating above with the occiput by broad concave joints and below with the axis by broad flat joints. Its body has been fused with that of the axis to form the dens, which itself articulates with the back of the anterior arch of the atlas, retained by a transverse ligament.

The massive axis, its body prolonged cephalad by the dens, is in general plan like the five lower cervical vertebrae. The large lateral masses bear the upper and lower articular facets of the zygapophyseal joints. The strong pedicles meet at the lateral masses with the laminae, which join in the midline to form a bifid spine to which many of the muscles of the upper part of the

spinal column are attached. The transverse processes bear the foramina for the vertebral vessels, lying in a plane anterior to that of the zygapophyseal joints. The transverse (vertebrarterial) foramina of the atlas, morphologically different from those of the other cervical vertebrae, lie in a plane which cuts through the centre line of its upper articular facets (Fig. 21.1). Most of the rotation of the head on the trunk takes place at the atlanto-axial joint, while much of the flexion and extension occurs at the joints between the atlas and axis and between the axis and the third vertebra.

The third vertebra is much smaller and less massive than the axis; below it the vertebrae become progressively more massive until in the seventh the shape of the thoracic vertebra is foreshadowed, with well-developed pedicles, laminae and spine and with a large body. The laminae from the second down are imbricated, the upper lamina overlapping the lower.

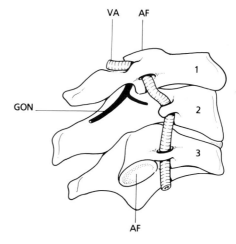

Fig. 21.1 The uppermost three cervical vertebrae, showing the relation of the vertebral artery to the atlanto-axial joint. AF: articular facet; GON: great occipital nerve; VA: vertebral artery. (After Frazer 1920.)

713

The intervertebral articulation is formed anteriorly by the anulus and nucleus of the intervertebral disc and by the neurocentral joints (Fig. 21.2). Posterolaterally it is formed by the zygapophyseal joints and their capsules (Fig. 21.2). The chief intervertebral ligaments are the ligamentum flavum between the laminae, the anterior and posterior longitudinal ligaments between the bodies, the inter-transverse and inter- and supra-spinal ligaments and the ligamentum nuchae.

The spinal canal is bounded by the bodies, pedicles and laminae, and between the bodies by the inter-vertebral discs and ligamenta flava. Bounded posteriorly by the zygapophyseal joints, above and below by adjacent pedicles and anteriorly by the bone and capsule of the neurocentral joints are the intervertebral canals for the passage of the spinal nerves in their dural sleeves (Fig. 21.2).

Contents of the spinal canal

Within the spinal canal lies the theca—the caudal continuation of the inner layer of the cranial dura mater—separated from the bony walls by a variable amount of fat and loose connective tissue. There is not, usually, much fat between the ligamenta flava and the dura mater. Within the dura is the filmy arachnoid mater, and within that the spinal cord floats in the spinal fluid, loosely connected to the bony wall on each side by the dentate ligaments. The cord's diameter is greatest at the sixth vertebral level, in relation to the origin and entry of the nerves of the brachial plexus.

Entering and leaving the cord are the cervical nerve roots—the multiple rootlets of the posterior system

entering the cord along the posterolateral sulcus and the fewer and thicker anterior roots leaving the anterolateral aspect of the cord. From the uppermost five segments spring on each side the roots of the spinal component of the accessory (eleventh cranial) nerve. These unite to pass cranially through the foramen magnum and so are lost to the orthopaedic surgeon until the nerve emerges again into the neck. The spinal nerve roots pass laterally and caudally in their sleeves of dura and arachnoid mater to enter the intervertebral canals. Here repose the posterior root ganglia, distal to which the roots unite to fuse with the epineurial prolongation of the dural sleeve and to emerge as the spinal nerves. These divide into anterior and posterior rami. The anterior rami go to form the cervical and brachial plexus; the posterior to innervate posterior cervical muscles and the skin of the back of the head and neck. The posterior ramus of the second nerve (the great occipital nerve) is large and important. Its ganglion is extradural; the nerve itself emerges between the posterior arch of the atlas and the lamina of the axis and passes cranially to innervate the skin of the back of the head, providing branches to supply the suboccipital muscles (Fig. 21.1).

The neural structures within the dura-arachnoid are very much more sensitive to trauma than are the peripheral nerves outside it. The spinal cord has, of course, the glial structure of supporting tissue characteristic of the central nervous system. At the transitional region (Berthold and Carlstedt, 1977) this gives way to the Schwann cell structure typical of the supporting tissue of the peripheral nerves, but the collagen content of the roots within the dura-arachnoid is far less than that of the peripheral nerves (Gamble, 1964). Handling which would not interfere with conduction along a peripheral nerve could result in permanent damage to a nerve root.

It is particularly important to note the increasing obliquity of the line of the nerve roots as we pass caudally down the cord. This is, of course, produced by the fact that the cord of the adult is markedly shorter than is the spinal canal. The angle subtended by the roots of the first thoracic nerve with the vertical line is no more than 20°. This disposition is of importance when the effects on nerve roots of space-occupying lesions within the canal are considered (Figs 21.3 and 21.4).

Vascular supply of the spinal cord

The cervical part of the spinal cord has a longitudinal and segmental blood supply. The studies of Chakravorty (1969) indicated:
1 that the contribution of the vertebral artery to the

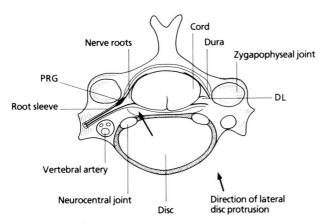

Fig. 21.2 Typical cervical vertebra, to show the relation of the root sleeve to the zygapophyseal and neurocentral joints and the direction of lateral disc protrusion (arrow). After MacNab (1983).

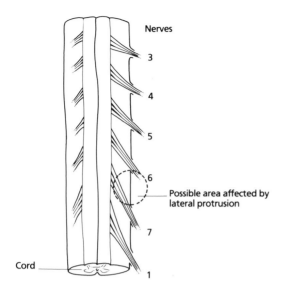

Fig. 21.3 The increasing obliquity of the cervical nerve roots and the relation of lateral disc protrusion to the cord and roots.

anterior spinal artery did not extend below the third cervical level; and

2 that radicular arteries maintained the blood supply below that level by contributing to the longitudinal anastomosis.

Radicular arteries of significant size commonly accompany one or more of the fourth to sixth cervical nerve roots.

The vertebral vessels

The vertebral arteries, arising from the first part of the subclavian arteries, enter the transverse processes of the sixth cervical vertebra and pass cephalad through the transverse processes of the next four vertebrae. They then traverse the transverse foramina of the atlas and wind posteriorly round the lateral masses to run for a short time in grooves in the upper surface on the posterior arch of the atlas (Fig. 21.1). Then, turning forward, they run alongside the uppermost part of the cord and medulla to pass through the foramen magnum and to join to form the basilar artery in front of the pons. Rarely, the vertebral arteries may enter the spinal canal between the atlas and the axis. With this anomaly, one or perhaps both arteries may be responsible for compression of the cervical cord. Satoh and colleagues (1993) describe such a case, in which the patient came with cervico-occipital pain. The vertebral veins accompany the arteries. Usually there are two on each side; one or both may pass through a foramen in the transverse process of the seventh vertebra.

The relationships of the cervical spine

Posteriorly and posterolaterally the cervical spine is covered by the mass of the spinal musculature, with the strong ligamentum nuchae in the midline. Laterally, muscles—notably the anterior and middle scalenes—take origin from, respectively, the anterior and posterior tubercles of the transverse processes. In the channels between these processes run the nerves of the brachial plexus. Anteriorly, the muscle cover (longus cervicis and longus capitis) is sparse and, in the midline, altogether absent. Here it gives place to the strong anterior

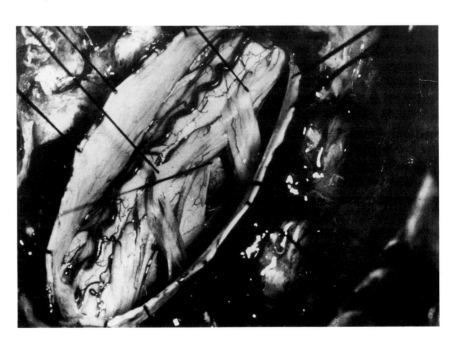

Fig. 21.4 The increasing obliquity of the cervical nerve roots as seen at operation. The cord has been rotated, at the time of taking the picture, by stays passed through the dentate ligaments.

longitudinal ligament. Directly in front lie the laryngo-pharynx and the tracheo-oesophagus, separated from the vertebral bodies by loose connective tissue. The cricoid cartilage usually lies at the level of the sixth vertebra. Lateral to the respiratory and alimentary tubes lie the carotid artery and internal jugular vein within the carotid sheath, the vagus (tenth cranial) nerve lying posteriorly between them. The recurrent laryngeal branch of the vagus passes on the left round the aortic arch and on the right round the brachio-cephalic (innominate) artery to lie laterally between the trachea and oesophagus. The cervical part of the sympathetic chain lies on each side on the anterior paravertebral muscles behind the carotid sheath.

SURGICAL APPROACHES TO THE CERVICAL SPINE

Operation on the cervical spine should not be undertaken by persons unfamiliar with its anatomy and relationships or imperfectly acquainted with operative techniques. The cervical spine is surrounded by important structures; it contains the vulnerable spinal cord and nerve roots and the vertebral vessels. The standard of anaesthesia must be high if unnecessary bleeding and consequent confusion are to be avoided. Even today both surgeon and anaesthetist must be acutely aware of the dangers of air embolism and of sudden loss of pressure within the theca. The patient must be carefully positioned. For anterior and anterolateral approaches the supine semi-sedentary position is admirable. For the posterior approach the prone head-up position is good; the forward-sitting position is excellent so long as proper precautions against air embolism and cerebral ischaemia are taken. In some circumstances, the lateral position is best. Apparatus should be on hand for stimulation of neural structures and recording of impulses. When hazard to the cord is apprehended, apparatus should be available for monitoring the cord's function by recording somatosensory impulses from the cortex. The value of such monitoring of the function of the cord has been shown by many workers (Engler *et al.*, 1978; Spielholz *et al.*, 1979; Landi *et al.*, 1980). It is, however, important to recall that the method is not and cannot be entirely reliable. Thus Spielholz and colleagues (1979) noted that there was no absolute correlation between main-tenance of potentials and preservation of clinical func-tion. Further, the use of the method in cases in which function of the cord is already compromised may be difficult.

Radiological facilities should be available in the oper-ation theatre so that levels may be verified and positions of grafts checked. Bipolar diathermy must be available for work so near conducting tissue. If the operation is likely to last for several hours special care must be taken to pad and protect bony parts, in particular the elbows, the sacrum and the knees. When the prone position is used, special care must be taken to protect the eyes.

The anterior approach

The direct anterior approach through the mouth and pharynx is applicable chiefly to operations on the upper-most part of the cervical spine and the base of the skull. With the mouth held open by a suitable 'gag', the tongue depressed and the soft palate retracted or divided, the posterior pharyngeal wall is exposed. The last is divided in the midline and the underlying vertebral bodies are cleared. By this route an exposure extending from the basi-occiput to the fifth vertebra can be made. It was first described by Southwick and Robinson (1957); later, Fang and Ong (1962) used it in the treatment of tuberculosis of the uppermost part of the spine. Its application was later extended by Bonney (1970), Thompson (1970) and Bonney and Williams (1985) in the UK and by others in the USA. There, Spetzler *et al.* (1979) refined the method by the use of the microscope, adding the further safeguard of monitoring the function of the spinal cord. Later Hadley *et al.* (1989) commented on this 'safe, efficacious approach for the treatment of selected patients with compressive pathology of the ventral brain stem and superior cervical cord'. Crockard and Bradford (1985) were bold enough successfully to extend the use of this approach to expose and remove a schwannoma anterior to the craniocervical junction. Crockard (1985) later indicated a further extension of the use of the approach in dealing with intracranial lesions. All who operate in this field owe a debt of gratitude to Crockard and his colleagues (1990) for their work in easing the performance of this operation and in smoothing the care of patients after it. Bonney and Williams (1985) indicated the restrictions on the use of bone grafts introduced through the mouth (Fig. 21.5). Initially, Crockard *et al.* (1985) preferred always to achieve stabilization by posterior fixation but Ashraf and Crockard (1990) later realized that in suitable cases the introduction of bone grafts through the mouth was permissible and successful. It is, however, important that the graft should:

1 be of iliac bone, with a large content of cancellous bone;
2 be well and firmly placed and locked into place;
3 be well covered by adequate suture of the overlying soft tissues.

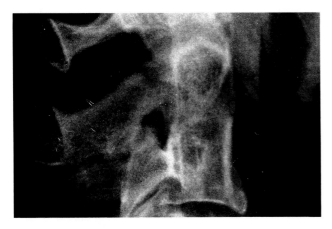

Fig. 21.5 A graft well placed between the second and third vertebral bodies by the transoral route, in a case of 'Hangman's fracture' of the axis. (Courtesy of Mr J.C. Strachan.)

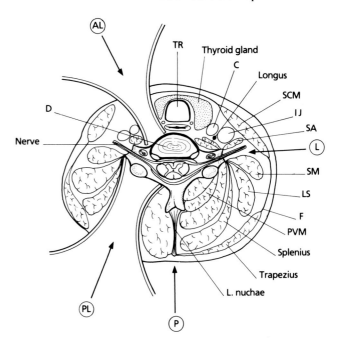

Fig. 21.6 The structures of the neck, showing four approaches: anterolateral (AL); posterior (P); posterolateral (PL) and lateral (L). PVM: paravetebral muscles; SA: scalenus anterior; SCM: sterno-cleido-mastoideus; SM: scalenus medius. (After Frazer 1920.)

If the graft becomes displaced, it may interfere with the healing of the overlying soft tissues and cause breakdown of the pharyngeal wound and consequent infection.

With improvement in operative and post-operative techniques, this operation now has an important place in the surgery of rheumatoid arthritis, neoplastic disease and other conditions in which the medulla and cord are distorted or compressed by agents anterior to them. Perhaps the gravest danger in its performance lies in the proximity of the vertebral arteries to the sides of the atlanto-axial articulations: a false move here can cause haemorrhage, which may be uncontrollable.

The anterolateral approach (Fig. 21.6)

Excellent exposure of the anterior aspect of the spine from the second cervical to the first thoracic vertebra is achieved by an approach made between, on the one hand, the laryngopharynx and the tracheo-oesophagus and, on the other, the carotid sheath (Robinson and Smith, 1955; Southwick and Robinson, 1957; Cloward, 1958). For further exposure of the lateral masses an alternative or additional approach may be made lateral to the carotid sheath. For ease of access in this more truly lateral approach (Verbiest, 1968) the surgeon must mobilize the sterno-cleido-mastoid muscle so that in the lower part of the neck entry can be made posterior to it. In the uppermost part of the neck the posterior inclination of the muscle allows the approach to be made anterior to it but in cases of special difficulty it may be detached from its upper insertion and retracted posteriorly. In these exposures the dissection follows natural tissue planes and little division of structures is necessary. Through the vertebral bodies and intervertebral discs

access is obtained to the spinal canal and to the root canals. The vertebral vessels are also easily accessible.

In the author's opinion, this operation is best done through a collar incision. The flaps are widely raised in the plane deep to the platysma and the medial border of the sterno-cleido-mastoid muscle is exposed. It is perhaps preferable, when no important contraindication exists, to make the approach to the left of the laryngopharynx because on this side the origin of the recurrent laryngeal nerve is more remote. The main drawback of the approach on the left side is that it carries, in difficult cases, the risk of damage to the thoracic duct. The supraclavicular nerves and—in the case of a high approach—the great auricular nerve are displayed and preserved, since troublesome hyperaesthesia can follow damage to them. It is important, too, to avoid damage to the mandibular branch of the facial nerve. The tendon of the omohyoid muscles is divided and the muscle bellies are retracted with slings. Entry is now made between the carotid sheath and the visceral tubes. No structures of importance have to be divided, but in the upper part of this dissection care has to be taken of the superior laryngeal and hypoglossal nerves. In the middle part it may be necessary to divide the middle thyroid vein and the inferior thyroid artery. In the lowest part of the dissection, when upper thoracic vertebrae are being approached, care has to be taken not to damage the recurrent laryngeal nerve.

In cases of great difficulty involving lesions at the cervicothoracic junction, a caudal extension of this approach can be achieved by the transclavicular approach described by Bonney (1977) — in fact, a revived and modified version of the approach of Fiolle and Delmas (1921). Birch *et al.* (1990) later described the further application of this method, in which the medial half of the clavicle and the upper lateral corner of the manubrium are elevated with the sternoclavicular joint on a pedicle of the sterno-cleido-mastoid muscle to expose the brachiocephalic (innominate) vessels and the uppermost part of the thoracic spine as far caudal as the fourth vertebra.

Once the spine is exposed the vertebral bodies are cleared of their ligaments and muscles and procedures are carried out as necessary. Closure — usually over a suction drain — should be done with meticulous care: omohyoid, fascia, platysma, skin. If the extended approach has been used, the manubrium and clavicle are replaced and fixed in position.

The important risk of this procedure, if carried out, for example, for the removal of an extensive tumour, is that of respiratory obstruction after operation. In such cases it is as well to retain the endotracheal tube until it is clear that there is no persistent obstruction. Careful observation of blood gases after removal of the tube is required. Tracheostomy is rarely necessary.

It is possible, though in the author's view very difficult, to expose the atlanto-axial joints and even the basi-occiput through the extension of the anterolateral approach described by Whitesides and Kelly (1966), used by MacNab (1967) and later developed by de Andrade and MacNab (1969) and Whitesides and McDonald (1978). This approach certainly retains the advantage of anterior approach to lesions placed anteriorly, while avoiding the disadvantages attached to, or thought to be attached to, the trans-oral approach. De Andrade and MacNab (1969) were indeed bold enough to suggest the use of this approach to gain access to lesions anterior to the brain stem. Riley (1973) extended and developed this approach to allow the whole of the cervical spine to be exposed by an antero-lateral route. The method is not recommended for use by surgeons of average or less than average skill.

The posterior approach

This was formerly the approach preferred. It is still preferred by some neurosurgeons. Certainly, it affords the best access to the contents of the theca in cases in which the lesion is lateral or posterior.

The midline vertical incision is deepened steadily through the ligamentum nuchae and the muscles are stripped as near to the bone as possible from the posterior vertebral elements. When access to the upper-most vertebrae is required, it is facilitated by stripping the muscles from the squamous part of the occipital bone. If extensive exposure of the occiput is required, a transverse component is added to the upper part of the incision to form a 'cross-bow'. The clearance is extended as far laterally as the lateral borders of the lateral masses. Care is necessary in exposing the posterior arch of the atlas and the atlanto-occipital membrane. The massive posterior elements of the axis serve as a reliable guide to levels. Bleeding should be controlled step by step, by diathermy, haemostatic material and retraction. It is unwise to start removing bone until satisfactory haemostasis has been achieved. Bleeding from cut bone surfaces should be checked by application of bone wax or similar haemostatic. The dura is exposed by removal of laminae and ligamenta flava.

It is very unwise to commence opening the dura be-fore haemostasis has been achieved. If possible, the dura should be opened without opening the arachnoid. The cut edges of the dura should be held up and apart by sutures to which light haemostats have been applied, in order to check the tendency to epidural bleeding manifested when pressure within the theca sinks because of escape of spinal fluid. Once the dura-arachnoid has been opened no sucker tip should intrude on the oper-ation field unprotected by a patty.

Closure of this incision is particularly important, for dehiscence may occur if it is not done with great care and in many layers. Modern suture materials have largely replaced black silk but sutures of the latter material act as good guides to depth if subsequent operations are necessary.

The posterolateral approach

In this approach, similar to that used for anterolateral decompression (lateral rhachotomy), the entry is made in the plane between the superficial and deep posterior cervical muscles (Alexander, 1946; Griffiths *et al.*, 1950; Capener, 1954). The former are detached from their midline attachments and retracted laterally; the para-spinal muscles are retracted medially and the medial and posterior scalene muscles and the splenius are detached from bone and retracted laterally. This incision is appropriate for the removal of a posterior remnant of a seventh cervical rib, in cases in which a further anterior approach might prove too hazardous. It affords good access to the lateral parts of the laminae, the zygapophyseal joints, the posterior aspects of the transverse processes and the proximal parts of the nerves of the brachial plexus.

Antibiotics

The tissues of the neck are in general very resistant to infection and if they are handled tenderly will continue to resist it well. When a large graft or foreign material is to be introduced, and in particular in transoral procedures, antibiotics should be used. At present the best for this purpose is cefuroxime, started before operation and continued for at least 72 hours.

External splinting of the neck

The introduction of the 'halo' splint (Thompson, 1962; Nickel *et al.*, 1968) was a decisive advance in the surgery of the cervical spine. Previous methods of 'splinting' by continuous skull traction or by fixation in a 'Minerva' plaster were to a varying degree unsatisfactory, though the former was made acceptable with the introduction of the 'Circolectric' bed. Indeed, it is still useful for patients with tetraparesis or tetraplegia and in particular for patients who have suffered serious injury to the cervical spine.

The 'halo' has the distinct advantages that it can be applied, with the jacket, before operation and that traction can be maintained through it during operation. At the conclusion of the procedure the two are united so that the spine is never unprotected. The material of which the halo apparatus is constructed can be varied so as to interfere as little as possible with magnetic resonance imaging (Ballock *et al.*, 1989). All orthopaedic surgeons working in this field, and all their patients, owe a debt of gratitude to the originators and developers of this method.

Splintage of lesser rigidity is afforded by moulded collars, by simple padded collars and by inflatable collars. It is unfortunately the fact that the better the fixation afforded, the less likely it is that the patient will tolerate the collar. It is a sad fact that many collars provided for many patients at considerable cost to the National Health Service rest unused for much of the time and are donned only for visits to the clinician. It is a sad fact, too, that many clinicians continue to believe that it is necessary to qualify the term 'collar' with the adjective 'cervical'*.

DIAGNOSIS OF CERVICAL SPINAL DISORDERS

Symptoms

The principal and most common symptom of cervical spinal disease is pain. The onset may be slow or acute; the level fluctuating; the occurrence episodic; the duration variable. The pain is usually felt in the neck; there may be radiation to both upper limbs and to the occiput or even to the frontal region. Occasionally, the pain is felt only in the limb or limbs. The orthopaedic surgeon is mistaken who thinks that every patient coming to him or her with cervicobrachial pain has a disorder of the cervical spine as a cause of the pain. Disease does not respect the subdivisions of medicine. Ischaemic heart disease may produce cervicobrachial pain, either in an acute episode of myocardial infarction or episodically in response to exertion. Conditions of soft tissues related to the cervical spine may cause pain, either in local disease or a part of a generalized process such as polyarteritis or polymyalgia rheumatica (Mackworth-Young and Hughes, 1990). In children, pain in the neck may be a symptom of meningeal infection or — more simply — of infection of the upper pharynx. Bland (1987) discusses possible causes of pain in the neck, and gives a good table of 'other potential causes'.

Discussing possible sources of pain arising from disorder of the intervertebral disc, MacNab (1971b) indicated (i) alteration in spinal mechanics; (ii) nerve root irritation; and (iii) pain derived from changes in the disc itself. The first might operate without important disorder of the disc and might involve principally the zygapophyseal joints, which are at least as liable to react to strain or injury as are the other synovial joints of the body. These joints are just as susceptible as are other synovial joints to involvement by the gouty process. Interference with a nerve root or rather with a root sleeve is primarily a mechanical matter: it is easy to visualize compression by nuclear protrusion medial to the neurocentral joint or lateral to it between the neurocentral and zygapophyseal joints. It may be, as MacNab (1971) has suggested, that it is necessary for the production of pain that the involved root sleeve must be

---

* My friend Dr Christopher Earl points out to me that one of the former editors of the *Quarterly Journal of Medicine* (probably Dr Denis Brinton) shared my view about 'cervical collars'. At the end of the article by R.A. Henson and M. Parsons (*Q. J. Med.* 1967, **36**, 205–222) there is a reference to 'tautologous collar'. Evidently, the editor deleted 'cervical' and noted 'tautologous'; the printer retained the 'tautologous' and the error was not picked up during the reading of the proofs.

'inflamed' or 'irritated' for this compression to produce pain. Observations in disorders of lumbar discs certainly suggest that an important degree of compression of a root sleeve is not necessarily associated with pain. It may of course be that the apparent hypersensitivity of 'inflamed' or 'irritated' tissues is caused by partial denervation. It is well known that partially denervated skin is often hyperaesthetic or dysaesthetic.

As to the third cause: pain may certainly arise from the disc itself, though whether this is due to increase of pressure or to accumulation within the disc of pain-producing polypeptides (Wall, 1971) is uncertain.

The confusion about the cause of pain due or thought to be due to disorder of cervical intervertebral joints is perhaps lightened by observations of the results of osteopathic treatment. Most clinicians have seen both acute and chronic cervical pain and stiffness resistant to the standard treatments of orthopaedics yet relieved instantly and lastingly by osteopathic manipulation. The author is indebted to his colleagues Richard Miller and Barrie Savory for an insight into the theory of their practice. Briefly, this depends on the proposal that the cause of pain is added strain placed on a weak cervical link by malposition in the upper part of the thoracic spine or at the cervicothoracic junction. Correction of that malposition removes the principal causative factor and leads to relief of pain. The results speak for themselves: osteopaths are entitled to use the famous phrase 'Eppur si muove'. This evidence points strongly to a mechanical element being prominent as a cause of pain: located probably in cervical zygapophyseal joints; intensified by manipulation of the joint itself, but relieved by removal of a precipitating factor in the uppermost part of the thoracic spine or at the cervicothoracic junction.

Persistently severe pain present night and day and not responding to simple treatment may indicate serious disease such as severe infection or new growth. Pain arising acutely from strain or injury and associated with paraesthesia, alteration of sensibility and weakness may indicate central protrusion or prolapse of the nucleus of a disc; the latter two symptoms may persist after subsidence of the pain. Radiation of pain to the head is often an indication of degenerative change in the cervical spine. It may be so severe as to partake of the qualities of migraine, and the term 'cervical migraine' was indeed accepted by Frykholm (1971). It is, however, important to remember that a cause of symptoms of this degree of severity and of this periodicity may be temporal arteritis.

PARAESTHESIAE

Paraesthesiae in the upper limbs may be associated with alteration of sensibility and paresis or paralysis. Clearly, these symptoms indicate affection of one or more spinal nerves. With affection of the cord there will be paraesthesiae and other sensory and motor symptoms in the lower limbs.

ISCHAEMIA

Disorder of the cervical spine may be expressed as symptoms of episodic ischaemia of the brain-stem caused by obstruction of one or both vertebral arteries. Persistent obstruction may lead to thrombosis of the basilar and posterior cerebellar arteries and to sudden death. The remarkable case histories related by Ford and Clark (1956) show that even in the healthy cervical spine rotation may cause such obstruction of healthy arteries with fatal consequences. Symptoms of visual impairment, of transient unconsciousness and of giddiness produced by movement of the head and neck on the trunk, should suggest the possibility of obstruction of vertebral arteries.

RESTRICTION

Pain is commonly associated with restriction of movement: with acute pain, the neck may be fixed in a position of deformity. In the case of infection all movements are severely limited, while with exacerbation of symptoms from degenerative disease extension is particularly painful. A significant degree of disc protrusion or prolapse is often compatible with the preservation of a good range of movement, though flexion to the side of the lesion is usually restricted. Deformity may accompany severe acute restriction or may develop slowly in the progression of spondylitis. Dysphagia may be associated with cervical spinal disease, usually with infection, though rarely from distortion of the oesophagus by large anterior osteophytes.

Very occasionally, the symptoms of a Claude Bernard-Horner syndrome form the presenting features of cervical spinal disease, the patient's first complaint being that of intermittent or progressive drooping of one eyelid. Other symptoms to be sought include those of affection of sphincter function.

Examination

The clinician should address the following questions when dealing with a patient complaining of cervico-brachial pain:
1 does the pain arise from the spinal column and related soft tissues?

2 does the pain arise from within the spinal canal?

3 is the process causing pain purely local, or is it a local manifestation of systemic disease.

Clearly, general examination and examination of the nervous system are required; it is as well too to examine joints for evidence of swelling and/or ligamentous laxity, and to examine the skin for abnormal laxity or tendency to bruise. Inspection of the pharynx should not be omitted in cases in which disease of the uppermost part of the cervical spine is suspected. The optic fundi should be examined and the neck should be auscultated when it is examined for posture, deformity, tenderness and range of movement. The significance of loss of the normal lordotic curve of the cervical spine has been well examined by Rechtman *et al.* (1961).

INVESTIGATION OF BLOOD

Probably the single most useful examination of blood is the measurement of erythrocyte sedimentation rate (ESR). Grievous errors have been avoided by the finding of abnormality in cases in which physical signs have been slight, absent or misleading. A raised ESR is a good though coarse indication of the presence of infection or of auto-immune disease. Clearly, other investigations are introduced as seems necessary. Their contribution is generally no more than confirmatory; taking of history and clinical examination make, or should make, the single largest contribution to diagnosis.

Imaging

The first step in imaging is by radiographic examination, which should include transoral views and views taken in anteroposterior, oblique and lateral projection. The radiographer should be careful to include all seven cervical vertebrae on the film taken in lateral projection, even if it is necessary to depress the patient's shoulders to ensure this inclusion. In cases of suspected instability, and especially in disorder of the atlanto-axial joints, views are taken with flexion and extension. It may be helpful to view the moving spine on the screen of the image-intensifier, but the danger of overexposure to radiation must be borne in mind. In former days, tomography was much used in the elucidation of problems in the cervical spine. It is still useful, but better images are now produced by computed tomography and by magnetic resonance imaging. The development of myelography with water-soluble contrast media greatly improved the quality of these images and reduced morbidity. In most cases the value of the information obtained far outweighs the inconveniences and risks,

but the investigation should never be recommended without clear indications for its performance, the chief of which is well-founded suspicion that there may be a lesion within the spinal canal.

EMISSION SCANNING

Emission scanning may be useful in cases of suspected infection, but the results with technetium are so non-specific as to be of limited value except in the very rare instance of osteoid osteoma. It may be the only means of investigation capable of showing this rare lesion. Scanning with indium-labelled white cells is more specific for infection but this investigation is only very occasionally indicated.

The introduction of computed tomography marked a great advance in imaging of the cervical spine, for with this technique it became possible clearly to detect abnormalities of soft tissues and to see the vertebrae and spinal canal in transverse section. It became possible to measure the extent of affection of the spinal cord and of the nerve roots (Marshall and de Silva, 1986). A few years after the introduction of computed tomography a new and wholly different technique of imaging emerged— namely, nuclear magnetic resonance. Although the method is intrinsically harmless, the presence of any metal objects in the body creates problems. Danger may arise from the exposure of such objects to the magnetic field in which the whole body is included; also, the presence of a metal object, say, in the head, may interfere with the imaging of any part of the body. The National Radiation Protection Board (1981) recommended certain precautions; more recently, Moseley (1994) summarized the dangers and difficulties.

Henderson (1983) outlined the history of the development of magnetic resonance imaging: since that time the technique has greatly been improved and with enhancement it has been possible clearly to show lesions within the brain and spinal cord (Miller *et al.*, 1988; Stack *et al.*, 1988; Valk, 1988; Parizel *et al.*, 1989). It may already be the case that magnetic resonance imaging has superseded all other methods of imaging of the cervical spine. Most clinicians, confronted with the choice of a single method of imaging, would now choose this; it is almost certain that with technical improvements its advantages will become decisive.

Particularly in the case of tumours involving the cervical spine it may be necessary to obtain evidence of extent by outlining the oesophagus (Fig. 21.7) or by visualizing the vertebral arteries by digital subtraction angiography. The former method has largely been superseded by the advance of magnetic resonance imaging,

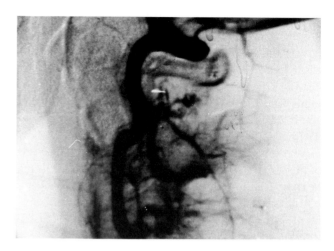

Fig. 21.8 Digital subtraction angiography, showing vertebral artery distorted by a rather invasive chondromyxoid fibroma of the third cervical vertebra. There is a 'blush' indicating the vascularity of the soft tissue extension of the tumour. (Courtesy of Dr D. Sutton.)

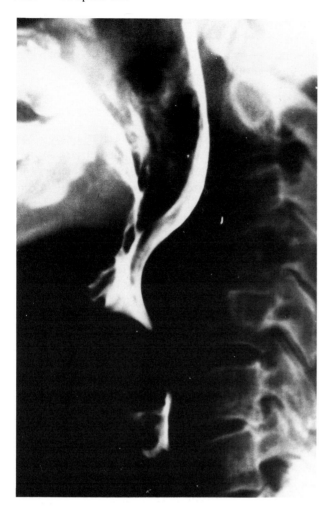

Fig. 21.7 Pharynx and oesophagus outlined by 'barium swallow' to show soft tissue extension of chordoma of the fourth vertebra.

but it is sometimes useful in difficult cases to know the course and state of the vertebral vessels (Fig. 21.8). The tumours themselves can often be visualized by angiography and useful information concerning their vascularity can be obtained. Further, it is likely that the incidence of damage to the vertebral vessels in cervical dislocation and fracture dislocation is underestimated. Lastly, one or both vertebral arteries may be affected by osteophytosis of the neurocentral joint: such affection may underlie the acute occlusion sometimes produced by manipulation of the neck.

It seemed that Nachemson (1989) had pronounced the obituary of discography as applied to the lumbar spine and that Sneider *et al.* (1964) had earlier done the same for the cervical spine, but later contributions seemed to indicate that the practice was still current (Osti *et al.*, 1990). Cervical discography was never widely used in the UK: it now seems that as a purely diagnostic investigation it has been superseded by magnetic resonance imaging. Simmons and Bhallia (1969) commented on the use of discography and 'discometry' as methods of determining the level or levels of origin of pain in degenerative disc disease. Certainly, it would be helpful in planning operative treatment if it were possible to rely on evidence from discography showing that the patient's pain arose from a particular level or levels. However, as long ago as 1971 Wickbom commented '. . . pains of a more or less similar distribution can be initiated from two or maybe even more discs. Furthermore, the distribution of the pains is not always the same if the injection is repeated'. Wickbom went on to comment on the risk of discitis following puncture. It may be that someone should pronounce for cervical discography the rites performed for its lumbar variant by Nachemson (1989).

Electrophysiological investigations

Dawson (1947) was the first to record from the scalp potentials evolved by stimulation of peripheral nerves. Bonney and Gilliatt (1958) were the first to record from nerves avulsed from the cord in cases of injury to the brachial plexus, and Jones (1979) and Landi *et al.* (1980) extended that work to observation of spinal evoked potentials in such cases. The diagnostic value of observations on evoked potentials was examined by Hattori *et al.* (1979) and their use during operation for correction of spinal deformity was described by Engler *et al.* (1978) and Spielholz *et al.* (1979). Since that time, monitoring of cord function during operation for correction of spinal deformity has become standard practice. The method of awakening the patient in order to test the integrity of conduction (Hall *et al.*, 1978) may be more reliable, but not all surgeons and anaesthetists are comfortable with this procedure. Examination of evoked potentials is useful in diagnosis of myelopathy, and electromyography may be helpful in separating peripheral lesions from those originating centrally.

PATHOLOGICAL CONDITIONS

It is hardly possible here to consider all the conditions that may affect the cervical spine. Instead, samples of conditions will be considered under the headings congenital; traumatic; degenerative; infective; autoimmune; metabolic; and neoplastic (benign and malignant, primary and secondary). Finally, some alternative methods for stabilizing the cervical spine will be considered.

Congenital malformations

Basilar impression

Primary basilar impression has been described as an upward movement of the base of the skull in the region of the foramen magnum (Raynor, 1983). Chamberlain (1939) described it as 'an unusual but important developmental abnormality of the occipital bone and upper cervical vertebrae'. The deformity consists of alteration towards the horizontal of the axis of the clivus, with shortening and thinning of the base-occiput. It is often associated with occipitalization of the axis; more importantly perhaps, it is often associated with Arnold-Chiari malformation (Cleland, 1883; Chiari, 1891; Schwalbe and Gredig, 1907). As a result, the dens intrudes into the foramen magnum. The extent of this intrusion can be estimated by observation of the relation of the dens to a line drawn from the posterior margin of the foramen magnum to the posterior margin of the hard palate (Chamberlain, 1939) or to a line drawn from the posterior margin of the hard palate (McGregor, 1948) (Fig. 21.9).

The consequence of the intrusion of the dens is to compress the medulla and the upper part of the spinal cord, with consequent tetraparesis. If an Arnold-Chiari malformation is also present, there may be signs of cerebellar dysfunction. In such circumstances, it may of course be difficult to separate the symptoms caused by external compression from those caused by the presence of a syrinx.

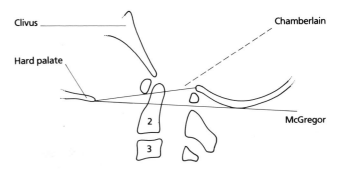

Fig. 21.9 Chamberlain's (1939) and McGregor's (1948) lines.

Diagnosis

Diagnosis depends principally on the radiological findings supplemented by the results of magnetic resonance imaging. The latter is of course helpful in determining the presence and extent of changes in the medulla and spinal cord. Treatment is necessarily by operative decompression. This may be by upper cervical laminectomy and removal of an appropriate amount of the squamous part of the occipital bone (Scoville and Sherman, 1951). When it is clear that the principal compression is exercised anteriorly by the intruding dens, transoral decompression is recommended. Derome *et al.* (1977), Delandsheer *et al.* (1977) and Pasztor *et al.* (1980) successfully used this approach. In the series of transoral interventions reported by Bonney and Williams (1985) there was one case of basilar impression (Fig. 21.10).

THE OS ODONTOIDEUM

The os odontoideum has been considered to be a separate dens whose fusion with the body of the axis has failed. However, the line of separation between dens and axis does not correspond with the line of the dens visible in the adult and the line of separation of the os does not run through the body of the axis (von Torklus and Gehle, 1972). The same workers suggest that the os is not an isolated dens but a bone existing apart from a hypoplastic dens (von Torklus and Gehle, 1968, 1969). With os odontoideum, the posterior arch of the atlas is often hypoplastic, while the anterior arch may be hypertrophic. The presence of an os odontoideum implies the possibility or even probability of atlanto-axial instability.

Differentiation from non-union of an initially unrecognized fracture of the dens is necessary; indeed, Fielding and Griffin (1974) considered that the origin of the os odontoideum was always such. The finding of an os odontoideum may be incidental, but symptoms associated

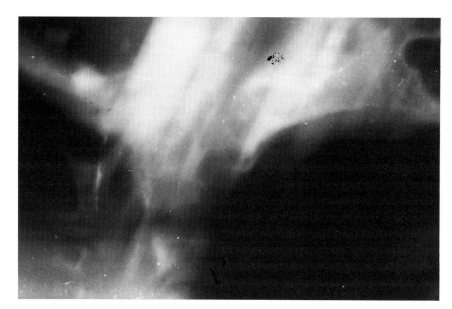

Fig. 21.10 Tomograph showing basilar impression in a youth of 13, with tetraparesis. Note the intrusion of the dens and the occipitalisation of the atlas.

with its presence range from episodic stiffness of the neck through transient tetraparesis to progressive myelopathy. The clinical finding of affection of the cord with associated evidence of atlanto-axial instability and of compression or distortion of the cord indicates stabilization (Greenberg, 1968; Greenberg *et al.*, 1968; Whitesides and McDonald, 1978).

KLIPPEL–FEIL SYNDROME (see also Chapter 8.1)

Klippel and Feil (1912) described a case of absence of cervical vertebrae with the thoracic cage going up to the base of the skull. In this case, necropsy showed complete fusion of all cervical vertebrae; the vertebral lesions were associated with pulmonary and renal disease. Nowadays, the term Klippel–Feil syndrome is used to describe persons with congenital fusion of cervical vertebrae; the presence of abnormality or disease of other systems is not necessarily implied, though a variety of conditions are in fact associated. The severity of the condition varies from affection of many vertebrae producing a short stiff neck and a low posterior hair-line to fusion at one level only. At this lowest end of the scale of affection, the finding of fusion may be incidental in a patient with pain in the neck after minor injury. The demonstration of Klippel–Feil syndrome should always alert the clinician to the possibility of disease or abnormality elsewhere in the spine and elsewhere in the body (Hensinger *et al.*, 1974). Its importance in the cervical spine lies in the possibility of development of instability above the fused segment at occipito-cervical level, or at an interval or intervals between fused segments. It is

likely, too, that the rigidity of the fused segments leads to the premature development of degenerative change in the residual mobile joints (Figs 21.11 and 21.12). Pain and radiculitis may arise from this. Stabilization by operation may be required for serious degrees of instability; decompression and stabilization may be required for persistent symptoms from degenerative change.

In certain inherited conditions such as Down's Syndrome, Morquio–Brailsford disease and osteogenesis imperfecta there may be significant instability at the atlanto-axial joint (Semine *et al.*, 1978). The more recent work of Stevens *et al.* (1991) has shown that in Morquio–Brailsford disease it is more the thickening anteriorly of the soft tissue than instability that causes affection of the spinal cord. In Ehlers–Danlos syndrome (Holton, 1987) in particular there is general joint laxity and instability of mobile vertebrae is seen. McKusick (1972) indicated that the major displacement principally seen was lumbosacral spondylolisthesis but the author has seen gross instability of the cervical spine in a patient referred by his colleague F. Horan. Serious instability of the cervical spine is seen in Larsen's syndrome (Micheli *et al.*, 1976). Secondary basilar impression in osteogenesis imperfecta was described by Pozo *et al.* (1984): they found the condition in three members of the same family, analysed the experience of others and stressed the hazard produced by compression of the medulla and cord at the level of the foramen magnum. Harkey *et al.* (1990) have reported the results of intervention for affection of the cord produced by basilar impression arising from osteogenesis imperfecta.

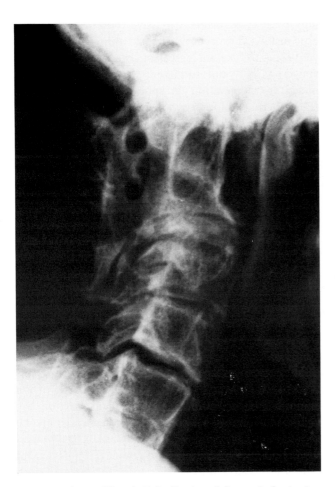

Fig. 21.11 Severe Klippel–Feil affection of the cervical spine in a man of 50, associated with other congenital malformations and causing intractable pain in the region of the ear.

Traumatic affections

Clearly, the consideration of fractures and fracture dislocations of the cervical spine has no place here. Three aspects will be considered: the 'acute stiff neck'; cervical disc protrusion and prolapse; and 'whiplash' injury.

THE 'ACUTE STIFF NECK'

Pain in the neck with stiffness and deformity is a common symptom in children and in adults. It may be a symptom of serious disease; it may be caused by processes that recede without revealing their nature. Evidently, the distinction between acute cervical pain and stiffness caused by transitory processes and similar symptoms caused by serious disease is of the greatest importance. In the cervical spine in particular, early diagnosis is important, because a dangerous process here may, if unrecognized, go on to produce irreversible changes in the cervical part of the spinal cord.

As has been indicated above, symptoms referred to the neck may have an origin outside this region; they may arise from the spinal column or from one of the contents of the spinal canal; they may arise in paravertebral structures; they may arise as part of a disease process affecting the whole body (Table 21.1).

In most cases of acute stiff neck the process is spontaneously reversible. Its nature has been debated at length, but little is in fact known about the reason why an otherwise healthy adult wakes with a stiff and painful neck or develops such a neck after exposure to a draught.

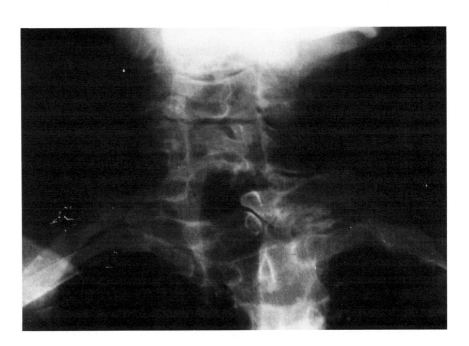

Fig. 21.12 Same patient as in Fig. 21.11. Note the degenerative changes in the 'mobile' joints.

Table 21.1 Some of the causes of acute pain in the neck, with or without stiffness.

Outside the neck
Myocardial infarction or ischaemia

Part of generalized disease
Auto-immune disease—polyarteritis; temporal arteritis
Gout
Polyarthritis
Acute rheumatism

In the neck, outside the spinal column
Acute pharyngeal infection
Acute paravertebral infection

In the spinal canal
Subarachnoid haemorrhage
Meningeal infection
Intradural tumour

In the spinal column
Acute disc protrusion or prolapse
Acute infection
Exacerbation of degenerative change
Tumour
Vertebral collapse
'Acute stiff neck'

Physical signs are confined to the neck; there are no signs of interference with the cord or with cervical nerves; there are no indications of generalized disease; radiographic examination shows no more than degenerative change in one or more of the joints of the lower part of the cervical spine; sedimentation rate is normal. In such cases, most treatments succeed: analgesics; protection with a collar; rest; local heat. Probably for the reasons advanced above, osteopaths are generally more successful with such cases than are the practitioners of so-called 'orthodox' medicine.

Fortunately, the distinction between 'orthodox' and 'unorthodox' (or perhaps better, anorthodox) practice has become blurred over the past 10 years, so that progressively more patients have been able to derive benefit from the methods of the practitioners of osteopathy and chiropractic. Very occasionally, the simple mode of screening indicated above fails, and the symptoms of incipient major nuclear prolapse go unrecognized. There are of course constant pointers to the graver diagnosis: severity of pain; complete failure to respond to treatment; deterioration under treatment; association with paraesthesiae in the limbs and trunk. Yet from time to time the distinction fails—chiefly, in the author's view, from failure of clinical sense. The

author has seen incipient massive central nuclear prolapse dismissed as 'acute stiff neck' although the patient was brought back with increasing severity of pain defying analgesics, rest and splintage; Pancoast tumour dismissed as 'imagination' in spite of the presence of a Claude Bernard-Horner syndrome; and persistence with manipulation in the face of increasing symptoms leading to damage to cord and spinal nerves in a case of lateral nuclear prolapse. All who treat patients with symptoms affecting the neck must at all times bear in mind the close proximity of vital conducting tissue.

The cause of acute stiff neck

It is perhaps most likely that the cause lies in a minor derangement of one or more interfacetal (zygapophyseal) or neurocentral joints on one or on both sides. Almost everyone has experienced a transient 'locking' of a joint—commonly, an elbow or a knee—associated with transient pain. It is not too far-fetched to surmise that the same may happen in the case of a posterolateral joint or joints in the cervical spine. The suggestion of precipitation by a derangement of the uppermost part of the thoracic spine or at the cervicothoracic junction has already been canvassed. It is hardly necessary to invoke derangement of an intervertebral disc as a cause or an association. Certainly, the acute synovitis of interfacetal joint or joints that must surely cause the acute stiff neck of gout produces symptoms and signs just like those of the 'acute stiff neck'.

CERVICAL INTERVERTEBRAL DISC PROTRUSION AND PROLAPSE

Almost certainly, protrusion and lateral prolapse of the nucleus of an intervertebral disc depends on increase of pressure within the anulus and in weakening of a part of it. Protrusion of nuclear material under a weakening annulus is followed by nuclear prolapse through the weakest part. That prolapse may be followed by migration (or sequestration) of the nuclear material. Protrusion and prolapse are usually posterior; in that situation they may be central or lateral.

Curiously, there is persistently a degree of confusion between pressure from soft protrusion or prolapse and pressure from osteophytes and degenerate disc material. This confusion may arise from the association of degenerative material with the hard osteophytes and with the associated fibrous hypertrophy of the annulus. Indeed, Wilson and Campbell (1977) considered that there had always to be a 'soft component' of a hard disc protrusion if symptoms of incapacitating severity were to be produced in cases of degenerative disease. This section considers solely the soft protrusion or prolapse of nuclear material in an otherwise healthy, or virtually healthy, cervical spine.

Lateral protrusion and prolapse

As MacNab (1983) has pointed out, the presence of the neurocentral joint exercises a decisive effect on the course of the protruding or prolapsing disc (Fig. 21.2). The nuclear material must pass medial to the joint, so that it cannot affect a single root in its sleeve in the intervertebral canal. It must affect the anterolateral aspect of the theca and the contained roots. As the size of the prolapsed material increases, the anterolateral aspect of the cord is affected. The levels commonly affected are those between the fifth and sixth and the sixth and seventh vertebrae. At these levels the nerves are descending obliquely so that a prolapse at one level is likely to affect adjacent sets of nerve roots: as many as three may be involved (Fig. 21.3). The patient comes with persistent pain and motor and sensory deficit, usually after an acute episode of pain associated with paraesthesia. Movement is limited: usually affected are lateral flexion to the side affected, and extension. There is alteration of sensibility and weakness in the territory of nerves affected. It is important to examine the trunk and lower limbs for evidence of affection of the cord. Radiographs will probably show some loss of intervertebral space at the affected level.

It is now likely that magnetic resonance imaging will wholly supersede myelography and computed tomography with enhancement as the investigation of choice in such cases. Certainly, when further investigation by myelography was deferred because of its invasive nature, many patients with symptoms and signs, such as those described, improved with the simplest of treatment — by rest and splintage with or without traction. Osteopathic treatment was successful in others. The supposed purpose of traction, intermittent or continuous, is to pull the vertebrae apart and, in the case of soft protrusion, to 'reduce' that protrusion. In the case of pain from degenerative change the purpose is, presumably, to pull the vertebrae apart and so to enlarge the root canal. Traction on the skull can certainly distract vertebrae, but it is doubtful whether continuous traction by halter or other similar method can do this and remain tolerable. The main role of 'closed' methods of continuous traction may be to enforce immobility.

Failure to improve or deterioration under treatment certainly indicates further investigation. In the author's view magnetic resonance imaging is the best choice, because of (i) the non-invasive character of the process and (ii) the superior image produced by the modern apparatus. The demonstration of nuclear material intruding into the canal combined with clinical evidence of failure to improve or deterioration under treatment is an indication for operation (Figs 21.13–21.15), though urgency is lacking if there is no element of interference with function of the cord. Indications for operation must be firm because of the serious commitment involved. Operation always involves proceedings very near a cord whose function may already be compromised, and even in the most skilled hands carries the risk of further damage.

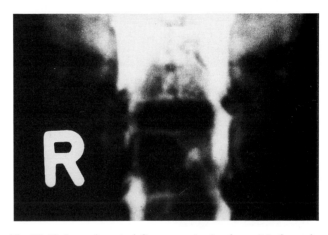

Fig. 21.13 Lateral cervical disc protrusion/prolapse. Myelograph shows lateral defect and obliteration of root sleeve on the right. Diagnosis confirmed at operation.

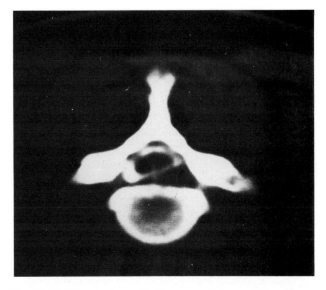

Fig. 21.14 CT scan shows displacement of theca and cord by anterolateral mass in the spinal canal. Diagnosis confirmed at operation.

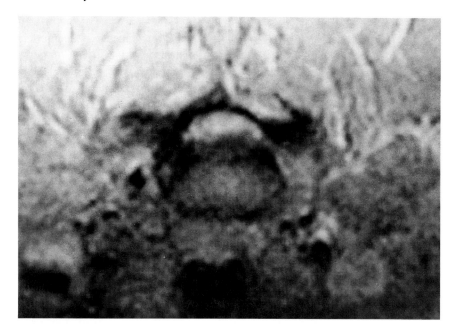

Fig. 21.15 Magnetic resonance imaging shows mass anterolaterally in the spinal canal displacing nerve root and cord. Signs of affection of upper motor neuron in ipsilateral lower limb and of lower motor neuron in ipsilateral upper limb.

The route chosen. Certainly, the posterior approach has always had the advantage that the surgeon is able to see theca and root sleeve, either through hemilaminectomy with partial facetectomy or through a more restricted exposure (Alexander, 1947). On the other hand, retraction of root sleeve and side of the theca is necessary for removal of the underlying prolapse or protrusion. Such retraction may, if pressed too hard or too long, damage permanently the contained conducting tissue (Fig. 21.16). Further, the option of concluding the process of decompression by intervertebral fusion is not easily available.

The author has for long preferred the anterior approach pioneered by Southwick and Robinson (1957) and later developed by Cloward (1958), Grote *et al.* (1991) and others. A further refinement aiding accuracy and lessening risk is afforded by the use of the microscope. The spine is exposed through the anterior approach and the level is identified on the X-ray screen; sufficient of the anterior part of the annulus is removed

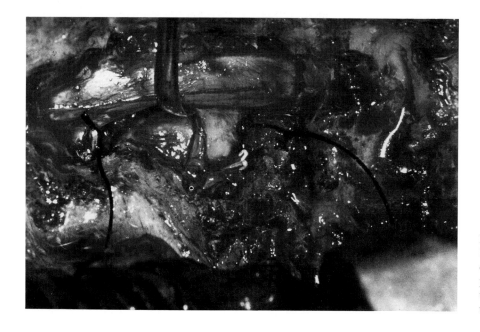

Fig. 21.16 Right lateral prolapse of disc between fifth and sixth vertebrae exposed by hemilaminectomy. Note the position of the prolapse and the elevator temporarily retracting the root sleeve and theca. (Courtesy of Dr H. Edwards.)

and the intervertebral space is entered. The space is opened out by the insertion of a suitable retractor and nuclear material is removed. Approaching the back of the space with care the operator is able to see and grasp the degenerate material as it enters the canal and to withdraw it (Fig. 21.17). The anterior dural face is then exposed and any other nuclear material herniated into the canal is withdrawn. Many neurosurgeons leave it at that, doubtless in the belief that the intervertebral joints are being preserved as happens in similar circumstances in the lumbar spine. Murphy and Gado (1972) found that when this procedure was followed, there was a high incidence of later spontaneous fusion, even though the cartilaginous end plates had not been removed. Martins (1976) was able to compare the results of removal of the disc with and without fusion. In the author's view little is lost and security is gained by combining fusion with removal of the disc. A rectangular graft is preferred to that of Cloward because of the superior degree of security offered. The end plates are removed centrally in the opposing vertebral bodies and the bone is undercut to receive the block graft from the ilium (Fig. 21.18).

Unnecessary and unsightly scarring is produced in the donor site by the use of curved incisions: a skin crease incision should be used over the ilium as in the neck. In most cases it is unnecessary to detach muscles from the crest since adequate exposure can be achieved by splitting them. After removal of a block of bone from the anterior buttress of the ilium the wound should be closed with care over a drain to minimize pain and stiffness after operation. With a well-fitting graft at one level and with intact posterior elements, splinting after operation is hardly necessary though the cautious use a simple collar is reassuring. After 6 weeks fusion is certainly secure enough to allow all splintings to be discarded. The results in such cases are excellent.

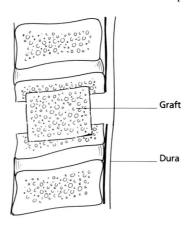

Fig. 21.18 Fusion after removal of disc. The end plates have been removed and the graft has been countersunk into adjacent vertebral bodies.

Central protrusion and prolapse

This serious event is, fortunately and unfortunately, rare. Fortunately, because its consequences can be very grave; unfortunately because its rarity may lead to failure of recognition. In one form acute stiff neck is associated with paraesthesiae which may affect all four limbs; symptoms persist and even increase in spite of rest, splintage and administration of analgesics. Bladder function is affected: the patient experiences impairment of bladder sensibility and difficulty in initiating micturition. The diagnosis must be made at this stage, preferably before it has been reached, though the signs of long tract affection may be slight. Brown and Crosby (1993) describe such a case, in which recognition came a little tardily, but in time. In the case of prolapse at a high level the long tracts to the upper limbs may be affected but more usually the signs in the upper limbs are mainly those of affection of the lower motor neurone. Time should not be lost waiting for magnetic resonance imaging, though if that investigation is available it is preferred. Myelography should give adequate information (Figs 21.19 and 21.20). Selladurai (1992) reports from Colombo on another mode of presentation. In 15 of his series of 26 patients below the age of 40 years seen and treated over a period of 10 years pain was not a feature; the progress of the affection of the cord was much slower than in the form described above. Selladurai rightly points to the importance of distinguishing this form of the condition from demyelinating disease.

It is likely that in the first instance the affection of the cord is purely mechanical and so, reversible; it is virtually certain that if pressure is continued the anterior spinal artery will be affected with disastrous consequences.

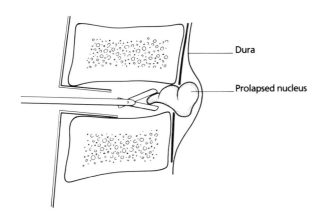

Fig. 21.17 Removal of sequestrated nucleus by anterior route.

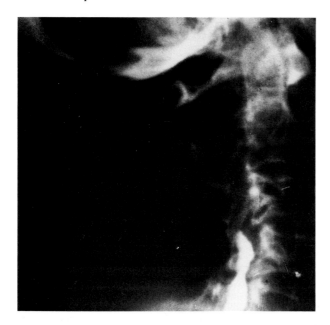

Fig. 21.19 Myelograph showing complete block to flow of contrast medium caused by central prolapse of disc between the third and fourth vertebrae. Diagnosis confirmed at operation by the posterior route. Complete recovery from tetraparesis.

Operation is a matter of urgency. Although formerly occasional successes were achieved with laminectomy and removal of the disc by the posterior approach, the common consequence of such a process was to confirm and deepen and perpetuate the paralysis. Operation should certainly be performed through the anterior route: the spine should be exposed, the intervertebral space marked and the disc opened widely. The prolapsed nucleus should then be withdrawn from the spinal canal and the anterior dura should be left fully exposed in the base of the bony excavation. There is a little doubt in such cases about the wisdom of fusion: the adjacent vertebrae should be fused once the canal has been cleared. The results of such interventions depend on the degree of damage suffered by the cord before operation and hence in the length of time between onset of symptoms and operation; they depend greatly on the operator's skill in avoiding further damage to the cord and on that of the anaesthetist in preventing hypoxia of the cord. In this connection, the author's observations on the behaviour of the cord after removal by the anterolateral route of a prolapsed thoracic nucleus are of interest (Chesterman and Bonney, 1964).

THE SEQUELAE OF 'WHIPLASH' INJURY

In a rear-end motor collision the unsupported head and neck are rapidly and violently extended until resistance is met. In the absence of a head restraint, the degree of extension is very great. With subsequent deceleration the neck is flexed until the chin meets the chest. The sequence of events is reversed in a true 'deceleration'

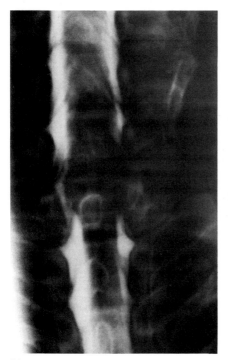

(a)

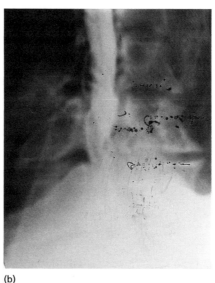

(b)

Fig. 21.20 (a) Almost complete block to flow of contrast medium in a case of massive prolapse of the disc between the sixth and seventh vertebrae of a 56-year-old woman. Diagnosis was delayed and tetraparesis persisted after operation (b).

injury when a car is stopped suddenly by collision. With the rather general introduction of head restraints the very severe damage to structures anterior to the cervical spine probably no longer occurs. In particular, the actual detachment of disc or discs from bone reported by MacNab (1964) probably takes place only when there is no head restraint or when the restraint is broken. However, damage still occurs at several levels and involves structures anterior and posterior to the vertebral bodies. As MacNab (1971(a)) remarks, 'disc herniation with root irritation and impairment of conduction rarely results from whiplash injury'.

Few will doubt that in cases of injury to the neck in which the damage is confined to the soft tissues, primary treatment should be by simple splintage after the possibility of fracture or dislocation has been excluded. Claims have been made regarding the superiority of the results of more active intervention, but it is doubtful whether they are justified (Pennie and Agambar, 1990). Probably, most patients so injured and so treated get better within 6 months. The problem remains of those patients who continue to get symptoms long after that term is up. Newman (1990) wisely remarks that 'In some, psychological factors and expectations of successful claims for compensation intermingle with the persisting symptoms'. However, he goes on to say that symptoms may persist after settlement of a claim and that persistence of symptoms is sometimes seen in patients who are not pursuing claims. Certainly, there is at about 7 years from injury an increased incidence of degenerative change in necks so injured. It is very rare for there to be in such cases any reliable evidence that localized degenerative change or disc protrusion is causing the persistent symptoms. Probably, operation is never indicated. Its injudicious performance often leads to increase of symptoms and consolidation of disability. The most important part of treatment consists of interest, reassurance and promotion of settlement. In time, most symptoms will subside, though the neck so damaged will remain liable to react with pain to strains that would not trouble a perfectly healthy cervical spine.

Curiously enough, in spite of the fact that damage to soft tissues is often severe, acceleration/deceleration injuries seem seldom to be associated with damage to the spinal cord. The author has under observation a patient in whom physical signs and appearances on magnetic resonance imaging could suggest such damage, but confirmation is not available. The whole situation may be different when the injured spine is not perfectly healthy but affected by degenerative change. It is of course well known that severe extension injury of the cervical spine in an elderly person may cause a deep lesion of the spinal cord. Initiation or exacerbation by 'whip-lash' injury of symptoms from a cervical spine already affected by degenerative change is well known; symptoms so produced are generally thought to be more severe and longer lasting than those arising from a cervical spine formerly healthy. The possibility is canvassed that such injury of a cervical spine already touched by degenerative change and of a spinal canal on which osteophytes have already encroached could initiate or precipitate myelopathy. The author has not seen such an event; great caution has to be used in such cases in interpreting the significance of findings or magnetic resonance imaging; in particular, it is necessary to avoid a *post hoc, propter hoc* argument. The encroachments on the spinal canal seen on magnetic resonance imaging after injury may well have been present for years. Here again, it is necessary to avoid confusion of thought between the soft protrusion of the acute event and the hard protrusion of the chronic change. At present, the last word is probably with Newman (1990): 'A large prospective study is needed ...'.

MYELOPATHY SECONDARY TO NON-UNION OF FRACTURE OF THE DENS

A proportion of fractures through the dens go undiagnosed; almost certainly some of these stay undiagnosed; others come to light with the appearance of symptoms of pain or of affection of the spinal cord through nonunion, pseudarthrosis and displacement. Nachemson (1960) was inclined to optimism concerning the outlook after fracture of the dens. However, it is probable that in about one-third of cases of undisplaced type II fracture treated by external immobilization there is non-union (Anderson and D'Alonzo, 1974). The incidence is higher in displaced fractures of this type so treated. Non-union and pseudarthrosis sometimes occur even after primary treatment by atlanto-axial fixation. In some instances of pseudarthrosis of the dens with displacement persistent pain and progressive myelopathy bring the lesion to attention. In former days it was considered enough to immobilize the atlanto-axial joint by posterior fusion; indeed, this procedure was successful in many cases, including, of course, those in which a mobile displacement was easily reducible by traction on the operation table.

Crockard *et al.* (1993) studied 16 patients with myelopathy secondary to non-union of fracture of the dens. They concluded that although persistent movement at the pseudarthrosis was clearly a factor in causing myelopathy, the persistent anterior compression inseparable from a fixed deformity also played an important part. It followed that in such cases removal of the anterior abnormality should supplement the fusion. This they did by combining transoral operation with stabilization, either in combination or as a staged procedure. Crockard and his colleagues were thus able to make the important observation that in no less than five cases the whole or part of the transverse ligament was trapped between the dens and its base. Important questions about the nature of the primary treatment in such cases are clearly raised by this observation.

Degenerative change

Degenerative change is common in the cervical spine, affecting most often the lower joints but occasionally affecting severely the atlanto-axial articulations. Its origins lie in the ageing process, in injury and, very occasionally, in disorder of metabolism (Harrold, 1956). The changes affect the zygapophyseal and neurocentral joints and the intervertebral discs. In the zygapophyseal and neurocentral joints the changes follow the common course of degeneration of articular cartilage with capsular thickening and later peripheral osteophytosis (Fig. 21.21). In the discs, the nuclei shrink and the annuli become hypertrophied; later, there is osteophytosis of the vertebral bodies. Sometimes degenerate nuclear material is extruded into the spinal canal. The vertebral changes may be associated with hypertrophy of the ligamenta flava. These changes and their effect on the neural tissues were well described by Holt and Yates (1966).

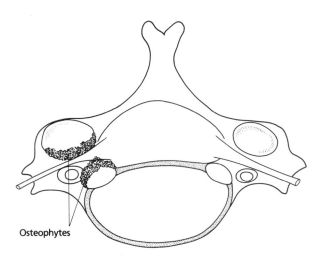

Osteophytes

Fig. 21.21 Osteophytosis of zygapophyseal and neurocentral joints threatening root sleeve and vertebral artery. After MacNab (1983).

The clinical consequences are pain, nerve root affection and affection of the spinal cord. Sometimes—more often perhaps than is suspected—one or both vertebral arteries may be affected. Pain probably arises from zygapophyseal and neurocentral joints as a result of synovitis and swelling. It is unlikely that it arises simply from osteophytic pressure on a root sleeve or root sleeves because under those circumstances it would surely be constant. All are familiar with the incidental finding of serious osteoarthritis with foraminal encroachment in radiographs of painless cervical spines. The possibility or even the probability of precipitation of symptoms by a cause lower down the spine has been discussed above. The pain, like that of osteoarthritis elsewhere, is typically episodic, induced by minor injury or exposure to cold, and is not associated with evidence of impairment of nerve function. It is local and radiated. It is not necessary to account for radiation of pain by invoking pressure on a root sleeve, for injection of hypertonic saline into intervertebral ligaments remote from the root sleeve will produce not only radiated pain but also peripheral 'tender spots' or 'fibrositic nodules'. As osteophytosis increases and as foramina are narrowed, the root sleeve and later the contained nerve roots are compressed.

For these reasons, operation is seldom indicated in the treatment of cervicobrachial pain from osteoarthritis without actual involvement of a root sleeve. White *et al.* (1973) concluded from examination of their series that they 'were unable to define what precisely constituted the operative indications'. They noted, however, that the best results were achieved in cases where there was: (i) clear evidence of radiculopathy; (ii) involvement of one level only; and (iii) a myelographic defect. It is often difficult to establish the level of origin of the pain; the condition often affects more than one level; there is little guarantee that neutralization of one or two levels will not be followed by production of pain at levels below or above that treated. The possibility of gout or of other generalized conditions should be excluded; treatment can nearly always be confined to simple splintage, simple analgesics and simple physiotherapy. Osteopathic treatment is regularly successful, though, as is the case with other treatments, it may have to be repeated. Manipulation is certainly best left to osteopaths. Clear hazards attach to manipulation under anaesthesia—in particular, to rotation during such proceedings. Injection of zygapophyseal joints with local analgesic and steroid under radiographic control is from time to time effective, as is the rather more hazardous cervical epidural injection. Only if the pain persists in spite of treatment and begins to mar the patient's life is it permissible to consider operation and then only if a reasonable certainty can be established concerning the level or levels of origin of pain. In the author's view, disc injection is an unreliable method of establishing the level of origin of pain. The guides have to be: (i) the distribution of the pain; (ii) the level or levels of tenderness; and (iii) the level or levels of affection and in particular of osteophytic encroachment on foramina as seen on radiographs. The operation proposed is necessarily intervertebral fusion, preferably by the anterior route at one or more levels. Patients must be warned that though such a fusion may for a time relieve pain, it is likely that symptoms are liable to recur through the development of changes at the levels below and above the fused segment.

Operation for intractable pain without objective evidence of radiculopathy is a much simpler business than that for radiculopathy or myelopathy. It is a simple matter of anterior approach to the cervical spine with fusion at one, two or three levels as seems indicated, without opening of the spinal canal or root canal. The most stable type of graft is rectangular and countersunk. The 'keystone' graft of Simmons and Bhallia (1969) is very stable. Perhaps unfortunately, these workers, in reporting a large series of operations, did not separate the results in patients with simple intractable pain from those in patients with pain associated with obvious neurological signs. There may subsequently have been some failure of clear thinking about the object of and indications for operation, about the type of operation required and about analysis of results.

Section of one or both great occipital nerves, either alone or in association with atlanto-axial fusion, has been used in the treatment of cervico-occipital pain. The rationale of this method is, in the author's view, far from being clearly defined. The author's best results in treatment of severe and persistent cervico-occipital pain caused by degenerative change in one or both atlanto-axial joints have been obtained by fusion; in one or two cases by fusion by the transoral route. An interesting sidelight is thrown on this subject by the recent publication of a further paper on the 'neck—tongue syndrome' (Orrell and Marsden, 1994). In this, cervico-occipital pain is associated with altered sensibility of the ipsilateral half of the tongue; sometimes with actual dysarthria, and on one occasion at least with pseudo-athetosis of the tongue. The association of lingual and cervico-occipital symptoms is traced to damage to lingual afferent fibres travelling in the hypoglossal nerve to second cervical spinal roots. It appears that the afferent fibres travelling in the hypoglossal nerve proper have only a proprioceptive function.

RADICULOPATHY

When a patient presents with pain associated with degenerative change and with objective evidence of affection of a nerve root or nerve roots, the question of decompression may have to be raised. It should be raised if pain is persistent in spite of treatment and if motor and sensory affection persists and increases. Level or levels of affection must be established by magnetic resonance imaging or by computed tomography (Fig. 21.22); the location of the neural lesion may further be identified by neurophysiological studies.

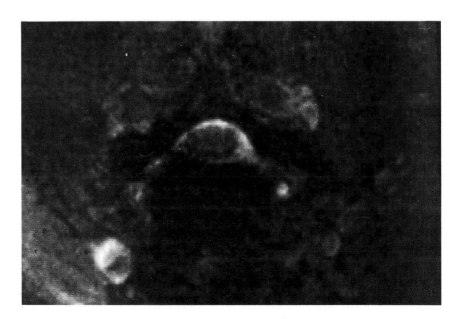

Fig. 21.22 Magnetic resonance imaging shows osteophytic encroachment on root canal at level C5/6.

The object of the operation is primarily to decompress the affected root sleeve or root sleeves. This may be done through a posterior approach, by hemilaminectomy with partial facetectomy. Here, the root sleeve is exposed and partly decompressed by the facetectomy; the bolder surgeon will go on to retract the root sleeve and to remove the osteophytes of the neurocentral joint lying anterior to it (Epstein *et al.*, 1969).

In the author's view, the preferred alternative in such cases is to approach the root sleeve from in front, through the disc and vertebral bodies, by way of an anterior approach. Here the microscope is very useful (Hankinson and Wilson, 1975). The vertebral bodies and discs are exposed and levels checked. Then the anterior anulus is removed and excavation of the adjacent vertebral bodies begins. The high-speed burr is the instrument of choice. As the back of the vertebral body and the posterior longitudinal ligament are approached, special care is necessary. Once a thin posterior shell of bone is left and the posterior longitudinal ligament is exposed, a very thin curved elevator can be placed to protect the anterior dura, though there should be no distortion of the membrane. The thin shell of bone can be removed with the burr and with very fine rongeurs any fragments of degenerate disc are removed. The anterior face of the dura is now exposed and it is possible to remove bone laterally from the anterior wall of the intervertebral foramen to expose the emerging root sleeve. The removal is continued until full decompression is achieved (Fig. 21.23).

Clearly, these proceedings have to be conducted with the utmost care, and the near presence of the cord has at all times to be borne in mind. The surgeon should always steady the working instrument with both hands; the assistant must not lose concentration and allow the protecting elevator to distort the theca or compress the cord. The Kerrison rongeurs are very good for removing bone in the depths of a wound, but in most situations in this approach to the spinal canal the foot of the instrument is liable to cause undesirable distortion of and pressure on the underlying dura. Bleeding from the vertebral body is well controlled with bone wax or with haemostatic paste; bleeding from epidural vessels is a more troublesome problem, but can usually be controlled with haemostatic sponge or with tiny patties. If the dura−arachnoid is punctured, there may be very troublesome bleeding from epidural vessels. This may best be controlled with stitches put through the dura and pulled forward so that the epidural space is closed. Holes in the dura should be closed; if they are left open a very troublesome leak may occur to form a huge pseudomeningocele in the front of the neck.

When foramina at adjacent levels are involved it is convenient to extend the bony excavation through the central vertebra. The depth of the excavation necessary to expose the dura will be shown first at one level, and this measure will serve as a useful guide at the next. A similar removal of osteophytes is carried out at the second level.

When the osteophytes have been removed at the level or levels involved, the vertebrae should be fused at one level if one level only has been opened; at two if two have been opened. It is best to use a block graft: with operation at a single level this graft unites adjacent vertebrae; with operation at two levels it traverses the channel in the middle vertebra and is firmly countersunk in the upper and lower vertebral bodies (Fig. 21.24). The easing of the graft into its bed is a matter for nice calculation and manipulation. As the graft is offered up, the anaesthetist gently and slowly extends the segment of neck by pressure from behind; the graft is placed in the lower or the upper vertebra and then eased and tapped down into the upper or lower vertebra. It is of the utmost importance that a ledge of bone should be left posteriorly on both vertebrae so that the graft cannot be punched back into the vertebral canal; the punch should be placed to overlap the edge of the graft so that when the latter goes home, the push of the punch will be arrested by impingement on the vertebral body.

With a graft well placed at a single level immobilization after operation is hardly necessary, but when a graft spans two or three levels it is sensible to protect the neck from sudden movement during the first 6 weeks after operation. Evidently, serial radiographic examin-

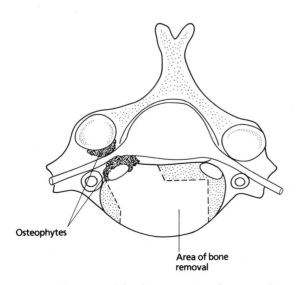

Osteophytes

Area of bone removal

Fig. 21.23 Bone removal for decompression of root canal.

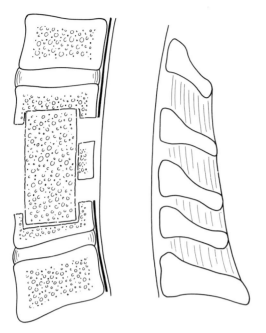

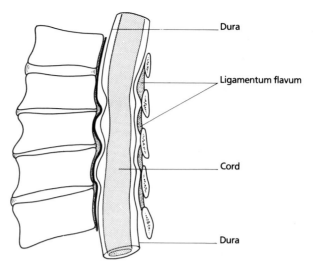

Fig. 21.25 Vertebral osteophytosis and hypertrophy of ligamenta flava cause compression of the theca and cord.

Fig. 21.24 Alternative method of fusion after decompression of root canals at two levels.

ations should be carried out to check the position of the graft and the process of incorporation. The complications are dealt with in the next section.

MYELOPATHY

When osteophytosis affects the posterior aspects of the vertebrae and is associated with a canal of small diameter and hypertrophy of the ligamenta flava (Stoltmann and Blackwood, 1964; Nurick, 1972), the theca is as it were gripped by a fist and the cord within it suffers (Fig. 21.25). Pallis *et al.* (1954) were among the first to study the condition and to relate symptoms and signs to the diameters of the cervical spinal canal. Taylor's (1964) and Chakravorty's (1969) studies drew attention to the role of the segmental arteries in the provision of nutrition to the spinal cord, but it is hardly possible to deny a role to the mechanical compression described or to the part played by that compression in compromising the blood supply of the cord. However, Adams and Logue (1971a,b) investigated the relation of the cord to the spinal canal on movement, and concluded that compression of the cord could not be the sole cause of this type of myelopathy. They made interesting suggestions about the role of traction and analysed closely the evidence then available from the studies of Pallis *et al.* (1954) and Stoltmann and Blackwood (1964). The ingenious experiments of Hakuda and Wilson (1972) indicated local ischaemia as a cause of myelopathy,

irreversibility being determined by disturbance in the blood supply from the systemic circulation through narrowing of vertebral, radicular and other arteries by arteriosclerosis and external pressure. A similar mechanism probably operates in myelopathy from ossification of the posterior longitudinal ligament (Leong *et al.*, 1988).

The clinical presentation of myelopathy is usually that of a patient in his or her forties or fifties with symptoms at first of fluctuating intensity indicating affection of the cord. Symptoms, generally bilateral, usually start in the lower limbs with dragging of the feet and numbness. Symptoms and signs in the upper limbs are usually caused by a mixture of myelopathy and radiculopathy: brisk reflexes accompanied by weakness and wasting. The posterior columns are often affected and Rombergism may be present. As time goes by symptoms become progressive and signs increasingly marked.

Diagnosis is based on evidence of compression of the cord as shown on magnetic resonance imaging (Fig. 21.26). The work of Nagata *et al.* (1990) has shown clearly the value of this method both in diagnosis and in observation after operation. Hattori *et al.* (1979) used spinal evoked potentials to measure the level and severity of the affection of the cord and to predict the results of operation. The distinction has to be made from other conditions causing disorder of the cord: new growth; subacute combined degeneration of the cord; syringomyelia; motor neuron disease; multiple sclerosis and various neuropathies. Pitt *et al.* (1990) described a remarkable case of tumour of the posterior elements of the axis producing symptoms simulating those of myelopathy from degenerative spinal disease.

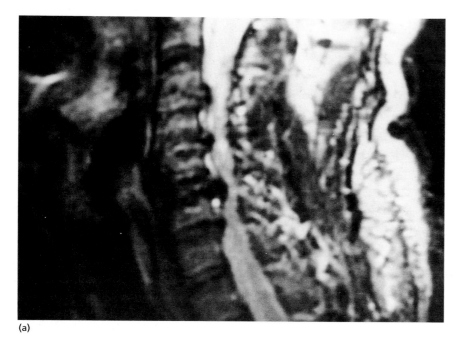

(a)

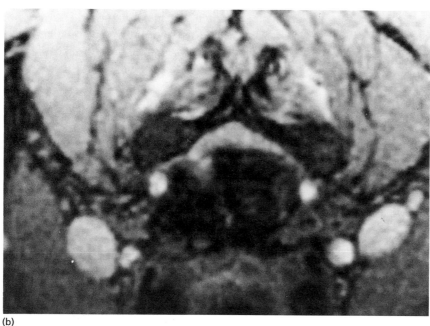

(b)

Fig. 21.26 Myelopathy from osteoarthritis with ossification of the posterior longitudinal ligament. Magnetic resonance imaging, showing affection of cord at four levels; maximal at the level C5/6. (a) Lateral projection, showing the levels affected. (b) Section at the level C5/6, showing extreme stenosis of the canal, with distortion of the cord. (Mr Nigel Harris' case; operation by Mr Rolfe Birch and the author, with early recovery.)

Treatment

Treatment is first attempted by 'immobilization' with a well-fitting collar, on the basis that the movement of the cord in relation to the bony walls of the canal during movement of the neck is thereby limited. It does indeed happen that in many cases the severity of affection diminishes with immobilization (Monro, 1984). At this stage, clearly, the changes are reversible. The timing of operation is a hard matter: on the one hand, it seems

sensible to intervene when the condition is in a reversible state; on the other, it seems perverse to subject a patient to a severe and possibly dangerous operation if his or her condition will be improved simply by wearing a collar. It seems sensible to intervene if:
1 there is no improvement with immobilization;
2 there is deterioration with immobilization;
3 improvement occurs to a point at which disability is still significant and seriously mars the patient's life.
It is clearly unwise to propose to operate in aged and

infirm patients. Further indications about the likelihood of success after operation can be gained from study of measurements of the diameter of the canal as shown by computed tomography (Fujiwara *et al.*, 1989). Shinomiya *et al.* (1990) indicated the role of measurement of evoked spinal cord potentials in differentiating local lesions with a good prognosis from extensive lesions with a poor prognosis.

Operation

The principal aims are to decompress the spinal cord and to improve its blood supply. Earlier attempts to do this were by the posterior approach, and that approach still has its adherents: laminectomy is performed over the affected segment of the cervical spine, usually from the third to the seventh cervical vertebrae. Ligamenta flava are removed. Although Clarke and Robinson (1956) reported disappointing results from this procedure, Knight (1964) advocated opening of the dura and division of the dentate ligaments to allow the cord to float back. Some have gone so far as to leave open the dura or to enlarge the tube by insertion of a homograft. Homografts of dura lyophilized or otherwise treated should no longer be used, because of the doubts raised about the transmission of Creutzfeld–Jakob disease (Martinez–Lage *et al.*, 1993). In these circumstances or in others in which it is necessary to repair a defect in the dura, it is best to use fascia lata or synthetic membrane.

Epstein *et al.* (1969) working through laminectomy were bold enough to remove osteophytes from in front of the cord but few have followed this example. The author indeed devised special instruments for this purpose and successfully followed Epstein's example, but soon abandoned the practice for the anterior approach. The proposal by Scoville (1961), Taylor (1964) and Epstein *et al.* (1978) to remove the medial part of the facet joints at appropriate levels in order to improve the segmental blood supply clearly received support from Chakravorty's (1969) findings. Hattori *et al.* (1980) devised an ingenious technique of laminoplasty designed to prevent the instability that commonly follows extensive laminectomy. Tsuji (1982), Kimura *et al.* (1984) and Tomita *et al.* (1988) reported on the results of similar procedures. Japanese workers have commented particularly on the high incidence of ossification of the posterior longitudinal ligament as a cause of myelopathy in their countrymen. The author's attempt to prevent instability by the preservation of the spines and interspinous ligaments during bone removal and by their replacement after decompression seems cumbersome in comparison with these methods.

Decompression of the theca in this manner can be expected to produce significant and significantly lasting improvement in about one-half of patients. The incidence of instability is uncertain; it is no doubt increased by combining hemifacetectomy with the laminectomy. Quite serious displacement may occur at one or two levels, making necessary external splintage by halo-jacket or internal fixation by anterior graft.

The anterior operation for myelopathy

Harris (1963) was among the first to propose and practise decompression of the cord by anterior operation. The proposal seems less attractive than that of posterior decompression in the case of the theca which conforms to the anterior curvature of the cervical spine and is compressed at several levels. Clearly, though, it is well conceived in the case of anterior compression at a single level either by purely degenerative changes or — more commonly — by deformity of the sequel of a previous subluxation.

In the case of affection at multiple levels the osteophytes can be removed at each level through a separate excavation. In this case, local grafting is not absolutely necessary, because fusion is likely to occur spontaneously. Alternatively, the central bone of the vertebral bodies can be removed throughout the length of the decompression and the gap can be bridged by a long graft (Fig. 21.27). By this procedure anterior decompression of the theca over a vertical extent of 3–7 cm

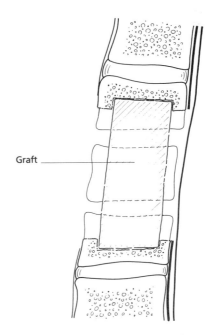

Graft

Fig. 21.27 Fusion at two levels after removal of bone and osteophytes.

and width of 10–12 mm can be achieved. After such a procedure, certainly, immobilization in a well-fitted collar is necessary. Hankinson and Wilson (1975) showed good results in a series of 51 patients in whom anterior decompression was performed at several levels. Yonenobu *et al.* (1985) preferred to reserve anterior operation for cases in which the cord was affected at three or fewer levels. For affection at more levels they recommended posterior operation.

Complications

Both anterior and posterior operations have their complications:

1 damage to conducting tissue;
2 damage to nearby structures;
3 general complications;
4 failure of fusion of graft.

Damage to conducting tissue. This complication is common to both methods of operation, though the liability is less with the posterior operation without opening of the dura. It must be remembered that in these cases the function of the cord is impaired and that a period of ischaemia or anoxia insufficient to damage a healthy cord may cause irreversible damage. If the dura is opened, the cord must be treated with extreme tenderness. It should not directly be retracted; rather, it should for short periods only, and only if absolutely necessary, be rotated or gently drawn aside by sutures placed in one or more dentate ligaments. It is clearly risky to remove osteophytes from in front of a cord approached through laminectomy.

The danger to the cord is greatest when the anterior approach is used. Errors or mishaps such as the penetration of the dura by an instrument or by a graft may be expected to cause damage, as may pressure exerted through the intact dura by the foot of a rongeur. If care is taken not to distort the theca, damage to the cord sufficient to produce clinical change can in general be avoided, but no patient before operation should be left in doubt about the hazards of proceedings within a few millimetres of this vital structure. Similar damage may be done in a similar manner to nerve roots; here too, great care must exercised.

When cord function is particularly poor or when particular danger is apprehended, it is wise to monitor function during operation, but that is sometimes difficult when function is already poor. The use of dexamethasone either as a prophylactic or for the event of damage to the cord has been commended (Delattre *et al.*, 1987). Contrary evidence relating to the use of methylpredni-

sone alone is provided by the work of Hitchon *et al.* (1989).

Damage to nearby structures. These complications too are chiefly those of the anterior route. The carotid vessel—perhaps atheromatous—may be damaged by overlong or overenthusiastic retraction; the recurrent laryngeal nerve may be stretched. When a high approach is used, the superior laryngeal nerve may be stretched and, higher still, the hypoglossal nerve may suffer. Assistants (and some surgeons) should constantly be reminded that they are dealing with living tissues which may cease to live if they are treated roughly.

If the dura-arachnoid is injured, there is the danger, in addition to that of immediate and troublesome bleeding, of a persistent leak of spinal fluid, with the formation of a large collection or even, very occasionally, of a fistula. It is important to be sure, before the gate is closed by the introduction of the graft, that there is no leak of spinal fluid. If there is doubt, it is as well to try the effect of jugular compression, though the additional bleeding that this may cause can obscure the field. Small wounds of the dura-arachnoid can usually be closed by suture; if suture is particularly difficult, or if there is a large gap or actual defect, a graft of fascia lata is effective. A small but persistent leak from a hole behind the bone can usually be sealed with a muscle graft reinforced by haemostatic sponge. In the case of formation of a large collection of fluid, re-forming in spite of treatment by aspiration and dehydration, it is necessary to re-explore, remove the graft and close the defect. In extreme cases a shunt may be necessary in order to ensure closure.

General complications. Air embolism and ischaemia of the brain and spinal cord are complications of the posterior approach to be avoided by careful techniques of positioning, anaesthesia and bandaging of the lower limbs and trunk. The particular complication of the anterior approach is, as has been said, oedema of the larynx and trachea leading to respiratory obstruction and anoxia.

Failure of fusion. Riley *et al.* (1969) indicated factors influencing the achievement of fusion, while Wilson and Campbell (1977) reviewed the results of 'discectomy' without the use of grafts. It remains the case that failure will be rare if:

1 the fusion involves one level only;
2 the graft is well and securely placed; and

3 (in cases of fusion at several levels) immobilization is adequate.

Infection in these well-vascularized tissues is rare.

Disorders of metabolism

The clinician has to consider:

1 disorders causing hyperostosis, such as osteitis deformans;

2 disorders causing demineralization through osteoporosis or osteomalacia, such as Cushing's syndrome; and

3 disorders causing arthropathy such as gout, pseudogout (articular chondrocalcinosis) (Ciricillo and Weinstein, 1989) and alkaptonuric ochronosis (Harrold, 1956; O'Brien *et al.*, 1963).

Paget's disease and Cushing's syndrome will be considered.

PAGET'S DISEASE

Osteitis deformans is the commonest 'metabolic' disease of bone. The combined processes of osteoclasis and osteogenesis usually produce enlargement of bone. The vascularity of the bone is much increased in the active phase of the disease. The combination of bone resorption and bone formation may lead to deformity (Fig. 21.28). Wyllie (1923) reported two cases in which the cord was affected by involvement of the thoracic spine, and Sadar *et al.* (1972) reported specifically on neurological involvement in Paget's disease of the vertebral column. Their principal observation was of compression of the cord by the stenosis of the spinal canal produced by hyperostosis but they drew attention to the interesting fact of cord involvement in the absence of myelographic block. In those days treatment was necessarily by operation for decompression, but in 1981 Douglas *et al.* indicated good relief of cord compression by treatment with calcitonin or diphosphonates. In one of their cases there was actual collapse of the fifth cervical vertebral body—an occurrence in some ways similar to that shown in Fig. 21.28. The cervical spine was involved in only one of Lander and Hadjipavlou's (1991) series of 84 patients. Bull *et al.* (1959) reported on the effects of secondary basilar impression caused by Paget's disease of the skull.

CUSHING'S SYNDROME

Cushing (1932) described the condition produced by hyperplasia of the adrenal cortex secondary to overproduction of adrenocorticotrophic hormone by an

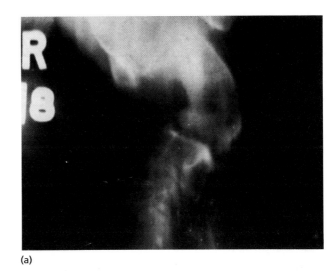

(a)

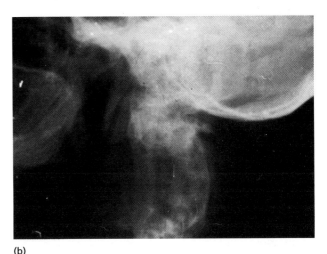

(b)

Fig. 21.28 Osteitis deformans of the uppermost part of the cervical spine causing progressive tetraparesis. Early improvement after positive decompression, later recurrence. Improvement after partial correction of deformity and anterior (trans-oral) fusion. (Courtesy of Mr Bernard Harries.)

adenoma of the pituitary gland. Since that time it has been recognized that similar hyperplasia could be produced by a primary adrenocortical adenoma or by a secreting tumour elsewhere than in the pituitary gland. Jeffcoate (1988) reviewed the choices for and results of treatment in Cushing's disease; Carpenter (1986) discussed principally the validity of diagnostic methods.

In the later stages the clinical features are easily recognizable: obesity; wasting of muscle; easy bruising; thin skin; abdominal striae; demineralization and deproteinization. The main diagnostic thrust comes from history and physical signs; confirmation by cortisol suppression by dexamethasone is clearly necessary.

Imaging by computed tomography is likely to show enlargement of adrenal glands or tumour of an adrenal gland. Occasionally, radiographic examination will show evidence of pituitary adenoma (Fig. 21.29).

In such cases, the weakening of the bones may persist after specific treatment by hypophysectomy or adenomectomy and by affection of the cervical spine may cause myelopathy. Stabilization with or without decompression may be required (Figs 21.30 and 21.31). In this situation, as in others in which several levels of the cervical spine are affected, it is as well to use a graft or grafts of cortical bone taken from the tibia. The objections to removing cortical bone from a tibia already wasted by osteoporosis have perhaps been overstated. In these situations, two cortical grafts, curved if necessary, are inserted into a trough formed anteriorly in the vertebral bodies and firmly jammed at each end into a vertebral body. This technique has been very helpful in dealing with extensive vertebral disease from all causes. It is important that the grafts should be well placed and well fitting and introduced so that after operation they will be under compression.

Auto-immune disease

The particular aspect of auto-immune disease with which this section is concerned is of course that of arthropathy, but, as has been said, other manifestations may mimic those of the bones and joints of the neck. It is with the effects of *rheumatoid arthritis* that the orthopaedic surgeon is chiefly concerned. The effect of the progressive disorder is to disorganize the joints of the cervical spine

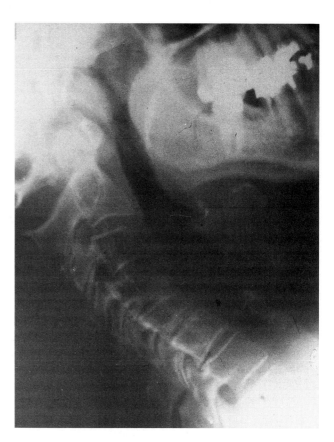

Fig. 21.30 Osteoporosis, subluxation and collapse in Cushing's disease leading later to tetraparesis (Courtesy of Prof. W.I. McDonald.)

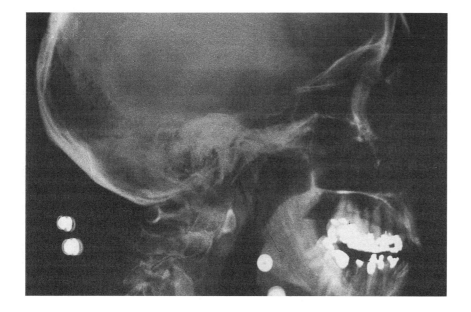

Fig. 21.29 Erosion and enlargement of the pituitary fossa produced by basophil adenoma in a case of Cushing's disease. Diagnosis confirmed at operation. (Courtesy of Prof. W.I. McDonald.)

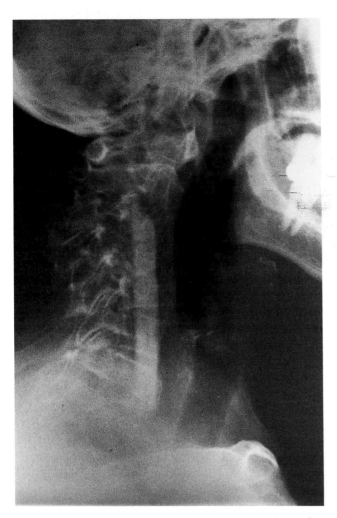

Fig. 21.31 Same patient as in Fig. 21.30, after correction and grafting. Recovery from tetraparesis. (Courtesy of Prof. W.I. McDonald.)

affected than any lower joint. There are three components of the affection of the atlanto-axial joint: forward subluxation of the atlas and skull on the axis (Fig. 21.32); upward migration of the dens so that it intrudes into the foramen magnum (Fig. 21.33); and formation of pannus in the articulation between the dens and the atlas, with destruction of the transverse ligaments (Fig. 21.34). The first and second components may coexist; intrusion of the dens can hardly take place without a degree of forward subluxation of the atlas, but subluxation without intrusion is of course possible. Posterior dislocation of the atlas on the axis is possible only if the dens has been badly eroded or broken, but rotary dislocation can occur (Sherk, 1978). It may be significant that 16 of the 19 patients in Crellin's (1970) series had had prolonged treatment with steroids. A more recent review of the subject, with a 10-year follow-up, is provided by Santavirta *et al.* (1991).

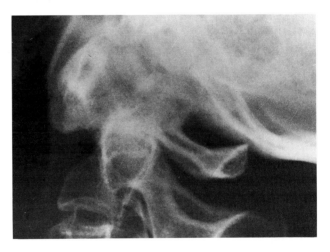

Fig. 21.32 Rheumatoid arthritis of the atlanto-axial joint. Subluxation with erosion of dens. (Courtesy of Mr Rolfe Birch.)

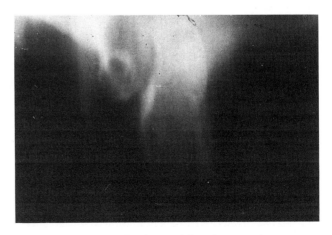

Fig. 21.33 Rheumatoid arthritis of the atlanto-axial joint. Intrusion of dens (tomograph).

at one or more levels so as to lead to instability (Conlon *et al.*, 1966). This instability may, in the mobile cervical spine, increase to the point of causing distortion of the spinal canal and interfering with the function of the cord and cervical nerves. That interference may be compounded by pressure from the growth of the pannus associated with the disease. It may be acting on a cord and nerves already influenced by neuropathy associated with the disease; as Hauge (1961) demonstrated, there may be an associated inflammatory arachnoiditis. One or both vertebral arteries may be at risk because of the distortion of the line of the transverse foramina. The level most commonly affected is that between the atlas and axis, but more than one level may be involved in any one patient (Conlon *et al.*, 1966; Crellin *et al.*, 1970). In the series of 19 patients reported by Crellin *et al.* (1970) two or more levels were affected in five cases, and the atlanto-axial joint was far more often

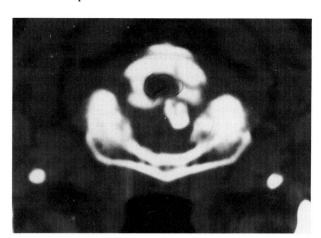

Fig. 21.34 Rheumatoid arthritis of the atlanto-axial joint. CT scan with enhancement shows dens separated from axis by pannus. The dens impinges on the cord. (Courtesy of Mr Rolfe Birch.)

SYMPTOMS

Pain is common, but is by no means a constant symptom. Particularly at the atlanto-axial joint pain may be slight, or may perhaps be masked by pain from a peripheral joint or joints. In these circumstances the first symptoms may be those of affection of the spinal cord, with alteration of sensibility and paraesthesia, and later with disturbance of motor function. Affection of the brainstem by intrusion of the dens may lead to oculomotor symptoms and difficulty in swallowing. As in all types of disorder of the spinal cord, disturbance of sphincter function is an important warning symptom. The careful examiner may from time to time detect evidence of affection of the descending nucleus of the trigeminal (fifth cranial) nerve, in alteration of corneal sensibility. There is clearly a range of findings in clinical examination, from normal sensory and motor function to spastic tetraparesis.

Whereas atlanto-axial instability may exist in rheumatoid arthritis without evidence of affection of the spinal cord, such affection is likely to develop in one-third to one-half of such cases (Mathews, 1969). In a few cases, there may be symptoms of interference with the flow through the vertebral arteries: dizziness with flexion of the neck or disturbance of vision. Very occasionally, such interference is the cause of sudden death.

Imaging (see also Chapter 30)

The preferred method of examination is by magnetic resonance imaging. This allows the situation of the bones and the shape of the spinal canal to be seen and in addition shows the cord and the extent of the pannus. In the absence of this facility, computed tomography gives useful information (see Figs 21.24–21.26), but plain radiographic examination is often misleading in dealing with the atlanto-axial joint.

Digital subtraction angiography is indicated when symptoms clearly suggest obstruction of a vertebral artery or of vertebral arteries. It may be necessary, in order to show distortion or obstruction, to take films with the neck in a position approximating that at which symptoms are caused.

Treatment

When instability exists without affection of the spinal cord, simple external splintage is adequate, though if pain is severe and is not controlled by splintage, thoughts will turn to stabilization by operation. Clark *et al.* (1989) take a bolder line, reminding us of the catastrophic consequences of sudden neural involvement from a sudden increase of instability. Unfortunately, stabilization at one level in the middle or lower part of the cervical spine may well be followed by the development of instability at another level or at other levels. Crellin *et al.* (1970) confined operation to patients in whom instability was associated with affection of the cord. It may be that evidence of affection of vertebral arteries by itself may be an adequate indication for operation, though usually such interference is associated with evidence of disorder of the spinal cord.

Simple forward subluxation of the atlas on the axis is probably best treated by posterior atlanto-axial stabilization with graft and wires. At the time of operation the vertebrae — the displacement is almost always readily reducible — held in reduction by traction on the 'halo' which at the end of the procedure is united to the jacket. A firm fixation can be achieved in this way, but if the patient is so seriously affected as to be unable to tolerate a halo-jacket, more elaborate methods may be used in order to avoid the need for external splintage (Cregan, 1966; Crockard *et al.*, 1990). The interlaminar clamp described by Moskovich and Crockard (1992) used with an interposed graft, may come to supersede wiring. It is in any case important to ensure that conducting tissue is not damaged when wires are passed under laminae. For reasons not wholly clear, Newman and Sweetnam (1969) advocated occipitocervical fusion in all cases of atlanto-axial instability in which operation was recommended (Fig. 21.35). Their well-argued advocacy was not and has not yet been sufficient to convince this author: he prefers the more precise indications given by Hamblen (1967).

Intrusion of the dens is best treated by transoral removal combined with fusion. Pannus is, of course, removed at the same time. Bonney and Williams (1985) set out the factors inimical to success after transoral introduction of a bone graft, and 5 years later these indications were appreciated by Ashraf and Crockard (1990). When the patient is receiving steroids, stabilization is best carried out by the posterior route, as suggested by Crockard *et al.* (1985). It is not difficult to achieve secure fusion in appropriate cases with an anterior graft: it is quite well achieved by other methods in patients in whom transoral grafting is inappropriate. In a recent communication Crockard *et al.* (1990) indicated a move away from bone grafting in association with posterior fixation with metal and wires, adducing as reasons frequent failure and poor general condition of some patients. It remains to be seen whether metallic internal fixation alone will suffice to maintain position for sufficiently long: the results described seem to indicate that whenever possible bony fusion should be sought.

It is doubtful if there is any longer any indication for the wide posterior decompression formerly used in cases of intrusion of the dens. Such wide decompression

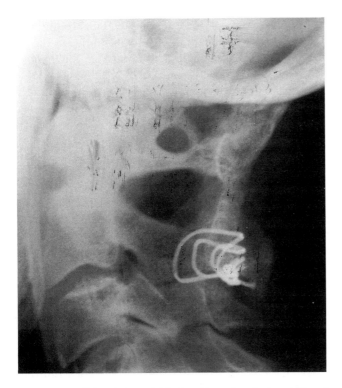

Fig. 21.35 Solid occipito-axial fusion. Operation for instability of the atlanto-axial joint produced by fracture through the base of the dens.

involved a difficult subsequent fusion from the second vertebra or lower vertebrae to the occiput: a formidable proceeding in a patient already seriously ill and probably subject to the side-effects of treatment with steroids. In some patients in this category, affection of the temporo-mandibular joints may make it difficult sufficiently to open the mouth to gain access to the pharynx; that may lead to difficulty in intubation. Section of the mandible may even be required. There may already be formidable difficulties in intubation because of stiffness of the neck. Sometimes, retrograde intubation through tracheotomy may be necessary. The grave decision for operation in such cases has to be taken on the basis that without operation the patient is likely or indeed certain to slide into severe spastic tetraparesis, with all its distressing and probably mortal consequences. Very high standards of anaesthesia, operative surgery and post-operative care are required.

Lower fusions

When instability at a lower level is complicated by affection of the spinal cord or vertebral arteries, stabilization is best achieved by the anterior operation with the insertion of some type of locking or countersunk graft. Such stabilization may later have to be extended, but it is doubtful whether 'prophylactic' stabilization at levels above and below the unstable segment is justifiable. It is important before operation to measure the extent of pannus within the spinal canal. If formation of pannus appears to be compromising the theca, it may be necessary to enter the spinal canal and remove it before inserting the graft. If it is a matter simply of instability of one vertebra or another, it is sufficient to confine operation to simple fusion without entering the canal. Fusion is readily achieved but it is important thereafter to keep the spine under observation in case of subluxation at another level.

LATE DEFORMITY IN ANKYLOSING SPONDYLITIS

The causes and methods of treatment of ankylosing spondylitis have been canvassed over several years and with increasing knowledge and attention the incidence of late deformity has perhaps been lessened. However, patients still present with stiffness and deformity so severe that they cannot lift their gaze from the ground. Such patients ask for the opportunity at least to be able to look straight forward and even to lift their line of vision above the horizontal. In some cases still, the deformity has become so extreme that the chin has come to rest on the chest. In all such cases, the difficulties and dangers of correction by operation are serious: there is often difficulty with intubation and the restricted movement of the thoracic cage increases the liability to pulmonary complications. Nevertheless, correction is possible and safe if care is taken throughout. Acting on the basis that lesions of the cauda equina are more likely to be recoverable than are lesions of the cord, and that a lesion of the cauda is a less catastrophic event than is one of the cord, Smith-Petersen *et al.* (1945) and Adams (1952) chose to correct the deformity by acting upon the lumbar spine. Adams indeed later carried this work to a high pitch of perfection. The disadvantage in the male of the occasional occurrence of sterility through intra-vesical ejaculation produced by damage to the lumbar sympathetic outflow was outweighed by the advantages accruing from correction of deformity.

Urist (1958) was sufficiently bold and skilful successfully to correct extreme deformity by osteotomy through the lowest part of the cervical spine, removing posterior elements widely and extending the resection laterally to the transverse processes. Most of the procedure was done with local analgesia, supplemented at the time of fracture of the spine by nitrous oxide and oxygen. Correction was done slowly, while the conscious patient was able to respond to tests for the integrity of cord function. In this case indeed, lumbar osteotomy would have conferred but small benefit, for deformity had gone so far that the patient's chin had come to rest on the manubrium. Simmons (1972) was similarly successful using a similar technique at the cervicothoracic junction. Clearly, there is a place for cervical spinal osteotomy when deformity is so great that the chin has come to or near to the manubrium, and when lumbar osteotomy would not produce adequate correction of the line of vision without gross distortion of the lumbar spinal canal. Continuous monitoring of cord function is essential: either through the use of local anaesthesia, through 'wake-up' testing at the time of correction, or through constant monitoring of cortical evoked potentials. It is important, too, adequately to remove posterior and lateral elements so that (i) correction can readily be achieved by fracture through anterior elements and (ii) there is no pinching of the theca by posterior elements when the gap is closed after correction. The actual process of correction should be slow, accompanied by constant monitoring of cord function. Correction is best maintained with a halo-jacket. It is an agreeable feature in such cases and a reward for the daring of surgeon and patient that the fractured spine is remarkably stable and that rapid union is the rule. The malady that originally produced the fixed deformity here becomes the ally and friend of the patient and surgeon.

The surgeon must, however, bear in mind that ankylosing spondylitis is almost always associated with restriction of movement of the thoracic cage. The possibility of respiratory complications has to be kept in mind and appropriate steps have to be taken to prevent them. An even more dangerous complication is introduced by the possibility of cardiac affection. Ansell *et al.* (1958) were probably the first to describe the affection of the aortic valve associated with ankylosing spondylitis: they found a very low incidence of this lesion. Takkunen *et al.* (1970) found a much higher incidence of cardiac affection: they found evidence of cardiomyopathy in 35 of 55 patients with 'rheumatic spondylitis', though only in a minority of these cases was it possible to assign a cause. It is clearly important that the condition of the heart should be investigated fully before operation. Even when that has been done, a cardiomyopathy not fully revealed by investigation may lead to complications after operation.

Infection

TUBERCULOSIS (see also Chapter 15)

In former days in the UK, infection of bone meant for most clinicians, tuberculous infection. The rise in living standards in the 1950s, 1960s and 1970s, together with improvements in diet, housing and preventive medicine, largely removed tuberculosis of bone from the indigenous population. It was indeed still seen in first-generation immigrants from Africa, Asia and the Caribbean, but it was by then treatable with specific drugs; additionally, the proportion of the population composed of first-generation immigrants decreased. It remains to be seen whether the increase of deprivation in the late 1980s will be associated with a rise in the incidence of tuberculosis generally and of bone tuberculosis in particular. There has already been a suggestion of such an increase (Sennett, 1991).

The bone is the primary site of tuberculous infection of the cervical spine: the body rather than the lateral or posterior elements. As the disease proceeds, it affects other vertebral bodies through the disc or by subperiosteal spread. As destruction proceeds an abscess is formed from granulation tissue, necrotic material and caseous matter. With destruction of bone comes deformity. The pattern of affection of the uppermost part of the cervical spine is rather different from that obtaining elsewhere—the difference is perhaps dictated by the different anatomical arrangements. Thus, the affection is more truly one of the atlanto-axial joints with destruction of those joints and consequent instability.

Neural affection

Griffiths *et al.* (1956a) defined the two broad types of neural affection associated with spinal tuberculosis: affection associated with the acute stages of the disease and affection associated with late deformity. The spread of 'early onset' affection is of course wide, and in this group there are several variations. Of particular importance are those cases in which the onset of neural affection is the first symptom, in some of whom the onset resembles that of a spinal tumour. The steady advance of recognition, improved methods of treatment and decline in the incidence of the disease have now made uncommon the myelopathy caused by deformity late in the disease process.

Presentation

Cervical spinal tuberculosis may present with pain and stiffness, and in its early stages in the UK of the 1990s may present serious difficulties in diagnosis. It may present with signs of tetraparesis, especially when the uppermost joints are involved. Radiological changes in the bone may be slow to develop, but the soft tissue shadow of an abscess may be apparent early. The more advanced methods of imaging will evidently be helpful to the establishment of a diagnosis of infection, but the cause of that infection may not be revealed until material is available for examination. Distinction has to be made from other types of infection, from eosinophilic granuloma, from tumour and in the case of the atlanto-axial joints, from rheumatoid disease (Fig. 21.36).

Treatment

The work of Wilkinson (1950) and later that of Hodgson and Stock (1960) provided a much-needed impetus for the advance of treatment of spinal tuberculosis. They showed that results could be improved and the incidence of deformity lessened by operation combined with specific drug therapy. The aim of operation was and is, to remove necrotic tissue and to promote fusion by grafting of bone. A little later, Fang and Ong (1962) opened the way to the development of the transoral operation for disease of the uppermost part of the spine. The objectives of operation in spinal tuberculosis are:
1 diagnostic;
2 drainage of abscess and removal of necrotic material;

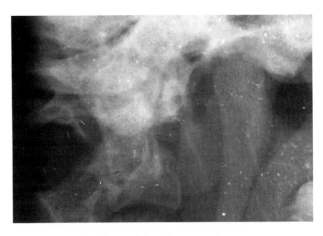

Fig. 21.36 Tuberculosis of the atlanto-axial joint in a young Asian woman. Tetraparesis before operation; recovery after transoral debridement and graft and specific therapy. (Courtesy of Dr Harold Edwards.)

3 (in case of tetraparesis) extra-thecal decompression of the cord; and
4 stabilization.

Clearly, operation sets the scene for successful long-term anti-tuberculous therapy by a combination of isoniazid, rifampicin and pyrazinamide over the first 2 months, with a much longer phase of treatment with isoniazid and rifampicin. The neurotoxicity of streptomycin is now well known, and ethambutol may produce visual disturbances. These indications and precautions are well set out in the British National Formulary (1990).

The series of Griffiths *et al.* (1956c) contained only five cases of paraplegia in cervical spinal disease. They noted that Roaf had, in a case too recent to be included, succeeded in decompressing the cord at the sixth and seventh cervical level by an anterolateral trans-vertebral approach. It was of course shortly after the publication of *Pott's Paraplegia* that Southwick and Robinson (1957) described the approach to the cervical spine that has since become the standard method. Undertaken before the disease has advanced to produce myelopathy, the operation can be confined to drainage, debridement and bone grafting. External protection will be required in most cases for a period of 2 or 3 months. When there is compression of the cord, operation has to include decompression with actual opening of the spinal canal in order to ensure that there is no residual pressure on the theca and the contained cord.

The atlanto-axial joint

It may be possible (Fang and Ong, 1962; Bonney and

Williams, 1985) to achieve both debridement and stabilization by transoral operation, but as Hsu and Yau (1983) have indicated, the lack of substance of the anterior elements caused by the ravages of the disease 'makes grafting an unrewarding proposition'. In such circumstances, it is better to limit the transoral procedure to debridement and to secure stability by posterior operation. Serious splintage, by halo-jacket, is needed unless secure internal fixation can be achieved. Fang and Ong (1962) warned particularly about the dangerous proximity of the vertebral arteries when the transoral operation is performed for tuberculous infection with destruction of bone.

Deformity after tuberculous infection

It is rare nowadays for deformity to develop after tuberculous infection sufficient so to distort the spinal canal as to interfere with the function of the cord. In such cases the impairment of function of the cord is at first due to mechanical compression; later, to permanent occlusion of vessels. It is unlikely in such cases that there will be any evidence of active disease. A serious decision confronts the patient and the surgeon: whether to embark on an operation that may prove curative or may precipitate tetra- or paraplegia, or to leave the condition to shade gradually and inevitably into paralysis. Certainly, 'decompressive laminectomy' should not be considered in such cases: the concept of the procedure is faulty and the practice commonly precipitates tetraplegia even when there has apparently been no new interference with the cord. The operation to be proposed is the difficult and delicate one of removing the obstructing kyphus formed by the vertebral bodies from in front by opening up the spinal canal and burring away bone until the theca is exposed throughout the length of the excavation. The utmost care must be taken to avoid increasing pressure on the theca by the insertion of any but the thinnest instrument between bone and theca. In the presence of very severe angulation, this will be extremely difficult. Once the theca has been decompressed, the levels are stabilized by the insertion of a graft. This is one of the situations in which grafts of cortical bone may be appropriate. This operation, the equivalent in the cervical spine of thoracic 'anterolateral decompression' (Alexander, 1946; Dott, 1947; Capener, 1954; Griffiths *et al.*, 1956) produces good results if it is carried out before irreversible changes have been produced in the cord and if it is done by one with extensive experience armed with all resources for gauging depth and monitoring function.

Pyogenic infection (see also Chapter 15)

Pyogenic infection, often acute but sometimes shading into chronicity, may arise *de novo*, or secondarily after needling of an intervertebral disc or discs. In its secondary form it may in the early stages be difficult to distinguish from the non-specific 'discitis' that occurs after injection of fluid or contrast medium into the nucleus. The organism commonly concerned is staphylococcus: in primary infection *Staphylococcus aureus*; in secondary infection *Staphylococcus albus*. The infection usually involves anterior elements, and most frequently involves the vertebral end-plate and disc. As it progresses, the nucleus is destroyed and an abscess forms. Later, bone is destroyed and other levels are involved. The formation of an epidural abscess may lead to affection of the cord.

Neither primary nor secondary pyogenic infection of the cervical spine (vertebral osteomyelitis) is too easily recognizable. When a disc has been infected, the operator is reluctant to believe that symptoms of pain and stiffness can be due to infection produced by his or her aseptic proceedings. When the patient presents *de novo* with acute cervical pain and stiffness, the condition is too often attributed to a 'slipped disc'. Even the development of dysphagia from formation of a retropharyngeal abscess may fail to strike a chord, and it may only be the onset of symptoms of tetraparesis that brings the realization of the cause (Fig. 21.37). The routine taking of temperature has now, regrettably, fallen into desuetude in many hospitals and consulting rooms; if this were not so, many cases might earlier be recognized. The erythrocyte sedimentation rate and blood count are very often revealing, the former rising to high levels as the infection proceeds. This rise is often accompanied by a neutrophil leucocytosis. Blood culture may be positive, but the delay imposed by this investigation means that its results are of little help in determining whether to start treatment. The results if positive can provide a useful guide in the choice of antibiotic. The experience of Kemp *et al.* (1973a) seemed to indicate that estimation of levels of anti-alpha-haemolysin was of no great help in diagnosis. Dealing apparently entirely with lesions in the thoracic and lumbar spine, they proposed early operation in all or nearly all cases for: (i) establishing diagnosis; (ii) clearing out infected tissue; and (iii) stabilization. It is unwise to expect that in the early stages radiographic examination will show more than the signs of abscess formation. The next indication is that of diminution of intervertebral space; evidence of destruction of bone follows but diagnosis should be made before such a sign

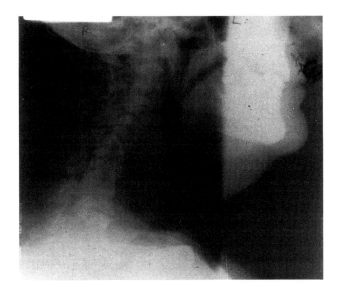

Fig. 21.37 Radiograph showing soft tissue shadow of large prevertebral abscess in a case of staphylococcal infection at the level C5/6. Diagnosis confirmed at operation.

is visible. Computed tomography and magnetic resonance imaging make possible a very exact diagnosis of the site and extent of the disease, but confirmation is only possible by examination of pus.

Epidural abscess

Epidural abscess in the cervical region commonly arises in connection with vertebral osteomyelitis (Heusner, 1948). It is, of course, the principal cause of the affection of the cord associated with the infection, although, as Baker *et al.* (1975) noted, 'the lesions in the cord may be more extensive than can be accounted for by mechanical effects of compression alone'. It may be the sparsity of epidural fat in the cervical region that makes epidural abscess without osteomyelitis less common here than it is in the thoracic and lumbar regions. The association with osteomyelitis, which usually affects the vertebral bodies, favours the development anteriorly of the abscess. It is rare for the infection to penetrate the dura mater: it appears that in the series of Baker *et al.* (1975) no penetration of the dura was found, and there was none in Hutton's (1956) single case. On the other hand, Hulme and Dott (1954) indicated a liability to penetration of the dura in the cervical region, because of the adherence anteriorly of the dura. Even without penetration of the dura there are changes in the spinal fluid: elevation of the protein level and of the white cell count.

Treatment

There is, in the author's view, a good case for giving a broad spectrum antibiotic such as cefuroxime if pain perists at a high level 24 h after needling of a cervical disc or discs. It is objectionable, particularly to microbiologists, to use a powerful drug in the absence of knowledge of the nature of the infecting organism, but the consequences of delay are too serious to allow such nice considerations to influence decision. Microbiologists are not, in any case, required to confront patients with severe and intractable pain after a surgical procedure. The antibiotic can be stopped if there is subsidence of pain without elevation of the erythrocyte sedimentation rate and without progressive radiological changes. Osti *et al.* (1990) dealing in general and experimentally with infective discitis after discography, indicated an incidence of 1–4%, commended the prophylactic use of a single dose of cephazolin and showed that this drug penetrated to the nucleus.

In the case of primary infection, operation is required if:

1 there is an abscess;
2 the cord is affected;
3 pain fails to respond to adequte treatment with antibiotics; and
4 there is persistent doubt about diagnosis.

With these indications, operation will no doubt be recommended in most cases, though the case reported by Mendelson *et al.* (1993) shows that even when nerve roots are affected antibiotics alone may bring resolution. In this case *Staphylococcus aureus* was found on blood culture. Since in most cases anterior elements are affected, the anterior route is commonly chosen for drainage of the abscess and removal of nuclear debris from the intervertebral space or spaces. Epidural abscesses are best drained by this route when they are situated principally anterior to the theca. It is of prime importance to take adequate amounts of pus and debris for examination, culture and testing of sensitivity. Whereas a broad-spectrum antibiotic can be used before operation in the absence of exact knowledge of the infecting organism, the choice can and should be made more exact once the nature and sensitivity of the infecting organism is known. Sterility on culture should not inhibit the administration of antibiotics if (i) cocci have been seen on the film of the material or (ii) clinical and radiological evidence and findings at operation strongly suggest a pyogenic infection.

Since fusion is very likely to occur through natural process, the function of bone grafting is mainly in the prevention or mitigation of deformity. In this respect the views of Kemp *et al.* (1973b) and of Stone *et al.* (1989) command respect.

Neoplasms

INTRADURAL TUMOURS

The orthopaedic surgeon cannot expect to be spared seeing one or more patients who present with symptoms caused by the presence of intradural tumours. Indeed, such tumours may produce symptoms that bring the patient past the general practitioner into the orthopaedic clinic. Such symptoms are more commonly produced by tumours within the thoracic or lumbar theca, but a cervical intradural tumour may bring a patient with pain in and stiffness of the neck and with symptoms and signs of affection of nerve root or roots. Extramedullary tumours account for three out of four intradural tumours and are more likely than are intramedullary tumours to cause symptoms thought to fit a patient for the orthopaedic clinic. Most extramedullary intradural tumours are meningiomas or neurofibromas or schwannomas. Of these, meningiomas may cause no more than a slight erosion of a pedicle, while the others may produce enlargement of an intervertebral foramen. Diagnosis has to be sought by myelography or, better, by computed tomography or magnetic resonance imaging. The removal of these tumours is best left to those with experience of intradural work (Fig. 21.38).

Tumours of the cervical spine are primary and secondary; benign and malignant.

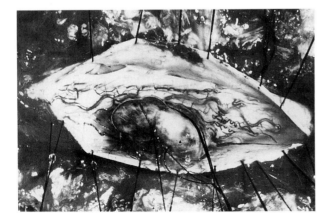

Fig. 21.38 Meningioma at the seventh cervical level causing first cervicobrachial pain and later tetraparesis. (Courtesy of Dr Harold Edwards.)

PRIMARY BENIGN TUMOURS

The common benign tumours are aneurysmal bone cyst and its variants; osteoblastoma; chondromyxoid fibroma and osteochondroma. Osteoid osteoma is rare. It is more likely to affect a pedicle or lamina than a body. Solitary plasmocytoma and solitary eosinophilic granuloma might be included. As the causation of new growth is increasingly canvassed and the field of causes is widened, it may be perverse to seek such differentiation. In their discussion of the relationships of eosinophilic granuloma of bone, Schajowicz and Slullitel (1973) mentioned five 'vertebral' cases, but did not identify the vertebrae affected. These benign tumours are more common than are primary malignant growths; they affect broadly the same age groups. It is the vertebral body that is usually affected but the tumours may spread to involve lateral and posterior elements or may affect primarily only one of these. Pitt *et al.* (1990) showed a remarkable case in which an osteochondroma of the arch of the axis was responsible for tetraplegia. In this case, removal of the arch and tumour combined with stabilization was followed by an excellent recovery.

The cervical spine may be affected in neurofibromatosis, but vertebral deformity and scalloping of vertebral bodies are not necessarily associated with neurofibromatous growths (Figs 21.39 and 21.40). On the other hand, the 'dumb-bell' neurofibroma, part of which lies in the spinal canal and part is para- or intravertebral, is well recognized. There is, of course, a definite incidence of malignant change in neurofibromatosis which has been put as high as 10%. Curtis *et al.* (1969) reported on the incidence of tumours in 32 reported cases and eight of their own cases of paraplegia associated with neurofibromatosis. Tumours, including three meningiomas, were found in 17 cases. The incidence of tumours in the series reported by Winter *et al.* (1979) was much the same: eight tumours in 16 patients with compression of the cord or cauda equina. In the remaining cases the compression was caused by angulation of the spinal canal. Craig and Govender (1992) reviewed eight cases of neurofibromatosis involving the cervical spine: in five of these there was neurological deficit, and in four a mass. The presence of neural defect was not necessarily connected with the presence of a mass. In one case—that of a 54-year-old man—the mass was malignant.

Some of these tumours, neurofibroma and osteoblastoma in particular, may behave in a manner that suggests local malignancy, and become locally invasive. In one case of osteoblastoma (Figs 21.41 and 21.42) tumour tissue was found in the lumen of the left brachio-

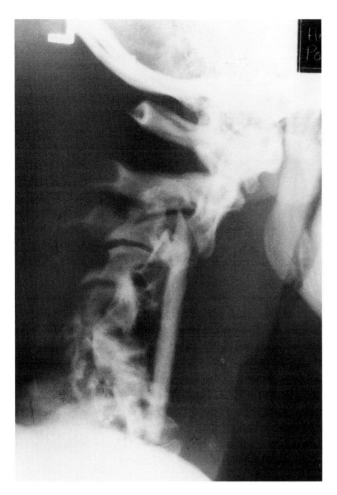

Fig. 21.39 Neurofibromatosis. Deformity without vertebral tumour, causing pain and tetraparesis. Radiograph taken soon after operation.

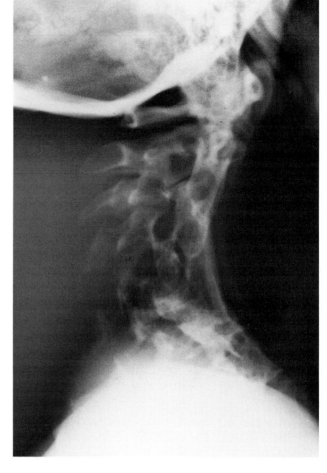

Fig. 21.40 Same case as in Fig. 21.39, 3 years later. Solid fusion. Relief of pain and tetraparesis.

cephalic (innominate) vein. Another growth verging on malignancy is the desmoid tumour (desmoplastic fibroma; musculo-aponeurotic fibromatosis). These growths seem to affect the cervical spine in two ways: either as tumours within the vertebrae (Scheer and Kuhlman, 1963; Rabhan and Rosai, 1968) or as tumours extrinsic to the vertebral column (Fig. 21.43). These tumours do not metastasize, but are locally so invasive that complete removal may necessitate the removal of important structures.

Presentation and diagnosis

Benign tumour of the cervical spine may declare itself with local and radiated pain of gradual onset, or may come to light with acute symptoms of affection of the cord or of spinal nerve roots or of both. Often enough, initial removal of the tumour will have been followed by

recurrence and extension. The presentation of osteoid osteoma is characteristically and misleadingly with chronic pain with few, if any, detectable physical signs. Commonly enough, when no cause for pain can be demonstrated, such patients are referred to psychiatrists. Fortunately, most psychiatrists refer them back, but the proliferation in the UK of 'Pain Clinics' or 'Pain Relief Clinics' offers a new peril for those patients. These clinics were formerly conceived as places for the palliative treatment of patients with intractable pain from incurable malignant disease. In the hands of clinicians such as Lipton *et al.* (1973) they provided both relief from pain and admirable insights into the mechanisms of pain. In other such clinics the study of pain was pursued and important advances were made. With improvement in the treatment of malignant disease, the original reason for the establishment of such clinics largely disappeared, but many have persisted, to provide

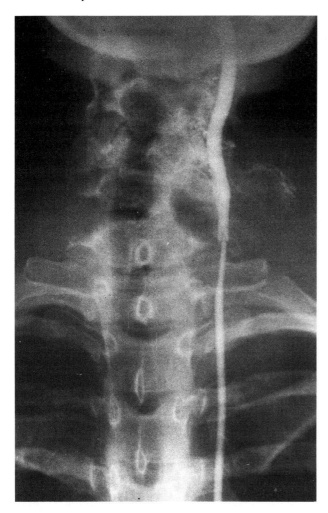

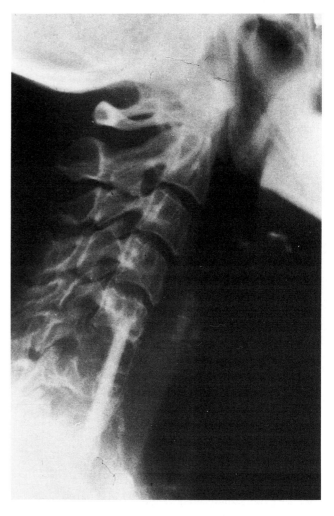

Fig. 21.41 Invasive osteoblastoma of the sixth and seventh vertebrae, with affection of cord and nerve roots. Radiograph showing destructive vertebral lesion with soft tissue extension.

Fig. 21.42 Same case as in Fig. 21.41, after removal and stabilisation. Later radiotherapy (Dr J.N. Godlee). Full recovery at 10-year follow-up.

a convenient home for patients with pain of undetermined origin. Some of the results of this transfer of responsibility have been in the highest degree unfavourable both to the patients and to the referring clinicians. Orthopaedic surgeons in particular should remember that it is their responsibility to determine the cause of pain and that every orthopaedic clinic is or should be, a 'Pain Clinic' (McCain, 1985).

In the absence of a previous history of intervention, the diagnosis of tumour is usually raised as a result of radiographic examination showing an osteolytic lesion (Fig. 21.44). Further information is sought by computed tomography or magnetic resonance imaging and by examination of blood for exclusion of myelomatosis. Diagnosis is of course easier when there are cutaneous and other manifestations of neurofibromatosis. Osteoid osteoma may be revealed by emission scanning. Very

often confirmation will have to be obtained from biopsy. Needle biopsy can be used when the tumour is in the vertebral body; it must be performed with exceptional care when the tumour is in the posterior or lateral elements. Often, the results of such biopsy are inconclusive because of the paucity of material obtained.

Operations

Open biopsy is often best performed as the first stage of operative removal of the tumour. The results of examination of frozen sections are not of course so reliable as those of examination of fixed and prepared specimens but the grosser errors can be avoided by using this method.

The extent of operation varies according to the extent of the tumour, but the aim in all cases should be the

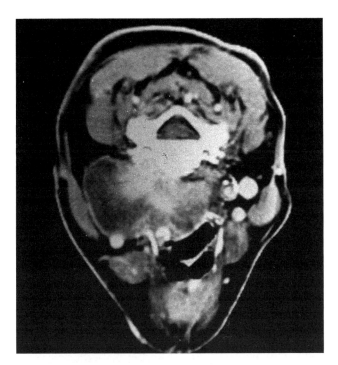

Fig. 21.43 Magnetic resonance imaging shows a large extravertebral tumour. (Mr K.J.H. Mallett's case. Tumour removed by Mr Rolfe Birch and the author.)

complete eradication of neoplastic material. In cases in which the vertebral body alone is involved, the lesion can be removed with the curette and sucker and marginal bone with the high-speed burr. The defect is then repaired with a graft of iliac bone well set into the vertebral

bodies above and below the site of the tumour. When the tumour is more extensive, more elaborate procedures are necessary for its eradication. These will be considered with operations for primary and secondary malignant disease. The procedures are well described by Verbiest (1965) and by Fielding *et al.* (1979).

PRIMARY MALIGNANT TUMOURS

The principal primary malignant tumours are chordoma, osteoclastoma, chondrosarcoma, osteosarcoma and Ewing's sarcoma. Evidently, neurofibroma with malignant change has to be included. Myelomatosis may be considered. The presentation is with pain, with or without symptoms of involvement of the spinal cord and nerve roots. The diagnosis can be adumbrated on the basis of radiological findings and further information may be obtained by magnetic resonance imaging, but confirmation has usually to be obtained by biopsy.

The place of operation in the treatment of these tumours has been debated. It has three objectives:
1 the radical removal of tumour and of tumour-bearing bone;
2 the relief of pressure on the spinal cord and nerve roots; and
3 the stabilization of the affected levels after removal of bone and tumour.
Whereas the first objective can often be achieved in dealing with malignant tumours of the limbs and trunk, it is far less likely to be achieved in the cervical spine, where the proximity of vital structures inhibits or

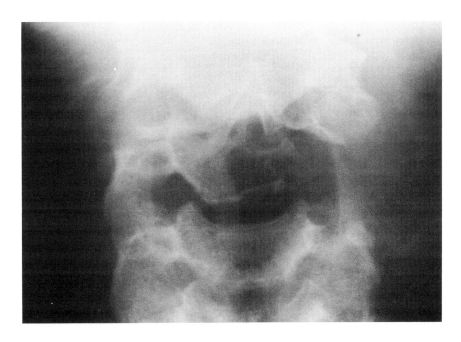

Fig. 21.44 Chondromyxoid fibroma of third vertebra, with extensive destruction of body, lateral mass and pedicle. Diagnosis confirmed at operation.

prevents a truly radical removal. However, Fielding *et al.* (1979) showed that it could be done. Verbiest (1983) has indeed described 'complete corporectomy'. The author has on occasion gone far in this direction and has succeeded in restoring conduction along the cord. He ventures to suggest 'somectomy' as preferable to 'corporectomy'. It is likely that the place of such radical operation in these conditions is to set the stage for specific cytotoxic therapy and radiotherapy.

It is certain that radical operation has a place in the treatment of particular tumours: chordoma; chondrosarcoma; desmoid tumour; neurofibroma (Harwick and Miller, 1979; Eriksson *et al.*, 1981). It has a clear place in these and other tumours when function of the cord is compromised. The effect of the tumours upon the cord is at first, without doubt, simply deformation and local ischaemia through pressure. Later, the condition becomes irreversible through permanent vascular occlusion. The initial reaction of the tumour to cytotoxic therapy or to radiotherapy may be by swelling. That swelling compromises still further the function of the cord and may determine irreversibility of the lesion. It is almost certainly a sound plan, if no contraindication exists, to operate to relieve pressure on the cord as a preliminary to specific treatment.

Operation

Operation for malignant tumours or invasive primary tumours of the cervical spine has to be planned and executed with very great care. The site and extent of the tumour in the bone must be determined by magnetic resonance imaging; the course and relations of the vertebral vessels should be defined by digital subtraction angiography. Clearly, general examination and investigation should have established the state of the patient's general health and should so far as possible have given any information on the nature of the tumour. It should, for instance, have been possible to recognize by appropriate examinations the presence of multiple myelomatosis or of secondary malignant disease, either in the vertebra or from the vertebra. If it is expected that extensive resection will be necessary and will lead to instability, the halo should be fitted before operation.

In most cases the primary approach will be anterolateral to the vertebral body, on the side of greater extent of the tumour or of greater affection of cord or cervical nerves. If it is expected that a lateral approach will be necessary, the sterno-cleido-mastoid muscle and the carotid sheath should be mobilized to permit an approach behind them. If there is caudal extension of the tumours, access should be ensured by using the transclavicular approach with elevation of a pedicle of sterno-cleido-mastoid muscle, half of the manubrium, the sternoclavicular joint and the medial half of the clavicle (Bonney, 1977; Birch *et al.*, 1990). This approach has the advantage of mobilization of the sterno-cleido-mastoideus at the same time, so opening the way to a lateral approach. The brachiocephalic and subclavian vessels are isolated and the origin of the vertebral artery is defined. The dome of the pleura is depressed or separated from the tumour mass. It is as well, on the right side, to see the recurrent laryngeal nerve as it approaches the laryngopharynx. The phrenic nerve and cervical ganglionated chain may have to be sacrificed. The proximal part of the brachial plexus is defined and its relation to the tumour is determined. The laryngopharynx and tracheo-oesophagus are mobilized. The surgeon should be in a position broadly to define the anterior and lateral aspects of the tumour and to gauge its superior and inferior extent. The surgeon should also be able to feel its posterolateral aspect.

It is now necessary to work away with the rongeurs, the burr and the sucker removing the tumour from the bone and mobilizing the superficial part of the tumour from the soft tissues. In the course of these proceedings the theca and root sleeves may be exposed over a varying extent; the vertebral vessels are likely to be exposed running in front of the line of the plexus. The dissection may take the surgeon to the front, side and even the posterolateral aspect of the theca. The resection of bone may involve most of the vertebral body, an intervertebral disc or discs, the anterior and posterior tubercles and the rest of the transverse process, and even part or all of the lateral mass bearing the facets. The chief sources of bleeding are the tumour, the epidural veins and the vertebral vessels. If the vertebral artery is wounded or divided it should be repaired. Haemostasis is secured with ligatures, clips, bone wax, haemostatic sponge and the bipolar diathermy. The nerves of the brachial plexus should if possible be spared, but it may be inevitable that they come in for more severe handling than would in other circumstances be advisable.

At the conclusion of this removal the surgeon is confronted by a gap in the cervical spine, continuity sometimes being maintained by no more than the contralateral zygapophyseal joint and the interlaminar and interspinous ligaments with the theca crossing the gap. Sufficient stability for the present and good stability for the future can be secured by the insertion of cortical grafts well fitted into the bodies of the vertebrae above and below the field of resection (Fig. 21.45). Usually these are enough, with the intact posterior and contralateral posterolateral elements, to produce a degree of

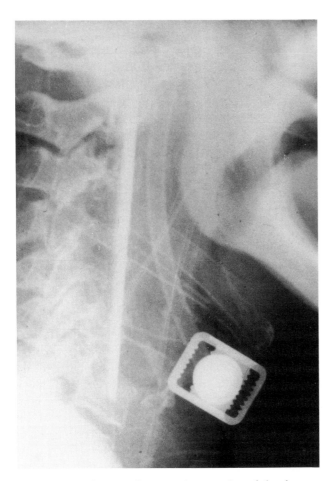

Fig. 21.45 Stabilization after extensive resection of chordoma.

stability adequate for transfer of the patient into the halo-jacket. In cases of very extensive removal, when the introduction of tibial grafts does not seem to produce adequate stability, posterior wiring may be added. The wound is very carefully closed over drains and the clavicle, sternoclavicular joint and manubrium are replaced. The place of tracheostomy in such cases has been discussed. Halo-jacket fixation will be required. It may be inconvenient in operations in the middle or lower cervical spine to have the patient in a jacket during operation.

It has been said, but it bears repeating, that operation is to be regarded in appropriate cases as a proceeding preliminary to treatment with cytotoxic drugs or by radiotherapy. Osteoclastoma is generally sensitive to irradiation, while chordoma is resistant. The latter tumour is likely to recur and to become increasingly invasive after apparently successful primary removal and stabilization. Verbiest (1983) reserved the suspect term 'vertebrectomy' for excision of the whole vertebra — a procedure that entails a two-stage removal of body and lateral processes, and at the same time or later, of the posterior elements.

DUMB-BELL TUMOURS

Among these rare tumours neurofibromas and schwannomas predominate. The neurofibromas are always potentially malignant; the schwannomas are sometimes primarily malignant. The problem of removal has recently been addressed by Clavel (1988), Sharma *et al.* (1989), and Viard *et al.* (1989). Sen and Sekhar (1990) have dealt more particularly with the problem of removing tumours lying in front of the theca and cord, but their experience with an 'extreme lateral approach' is relevant to the problem posed by dumb-bell tumours.

When they affect the neck, dumb-bell tumours may present as a mass (Clavel, 1988) or with symptoms of affection of the spinal cord (Sharma *et al.*, 1989). The object is to remove the tumour at a single operation, through one approach. That approach is lateral and anterolateral, with exposure of the extracanalicular part of the tumour, the vertebral bodies, the transverse processes, the lateral masses and the vertebral artery.

Once the 'root' of the tumour entering the spinal canal has been identified, its extracanalicular part can be removed in order to facilitate access to the appropriate intervertebral foramen. The foramen is likely to be much enlarged by the presence of the tumour, but the surgeon is fortunate who finds that the access so provided is sufficient to permit withdrawal of the intraspinal part of the tumour. Depending on the situation of that part of the tumour in relation to the spinal cord and on its longitudinal extent, access is gained by anterolateral removal of body and transverse process or by enlargement of the foramen by removal of the lateral mass or masses bearing the facets. The vertebral artery must, of course, be identified, liberated and guarded. If the tumour is intradural, the dura is opened and it is separated from the front of the cord in the plane of the arachnoid mater. Sen and Sekhar (1990) use the ultrasonic aspirator to 'debulk' the tumour before removal, so as to avoid any manipulation of the cord. After such proceedings, there will almost certainly be difficulty in obtaining closure of the dura. Reservations have already been expressed about the use of lyophilized dura for closing a defect; instead, fascia lata or synthetic membrane should be used. It may be enough to close the overlying soft tissues very securely. Removal is much simpler when the intracanalicular part of the tumour is extradural. When a malignant schwannoma is inextricably associated with the nerve roots, the latter must be sacrificed. Since in most such cases there is already marked interference with conduction, the additional loss of function may be slight. In cases of great difficulty it may be impossible to remove both components of the tumour through a single approach. It is then necessary to combine a lateral and anterolateral approach with a posterior approach, either in one session or as two separate operations. It seems safer to first remove the intraspinal tumour, through a posterior approach in such cases.

SECONDARY TUMOURS

Secondary deposit in bone occurs most commonly from tumours of the breast, lung, thyroid gland, kidney and prostate gland, though of course other primary sites may be the origin of such metastasis. In the case of metastasis from breast cancer, the primary disease has commonly declared itself, so that the occurrence of spread to bone is recognized as such either by routine observations or at the onset of pain. In the case of metastasis from pulmonary and renal cancer, the first symptom of disease may arise from the deposit in bone. Constans *et al.* (1983) were able to report their findings in a series of no less than 600 cases. The principal presenting symptom is pain, but this may soon be followed by symptoms of interference with the function of the spinal cord or spinal nerves.

Operation may be indicated when pain is very severe and intractable through instability produced by extensive destruction of bone. It may be indicated when there is evidence of interference with the function of the spinal cord. Clearly, decision in these cases is extremely difficult: the patient may be seriously ill; the tumour may well be susceptible to hormonal, cytotoxic or radiotherapy; only in the case of secondary deposit from a renal tumour is there any good possibility of cure. The author rejects the proposition that in all cases of secondary deposit in the cervical spine primary treatment should be by cytotoxic, hormonal or radiotherapy. When there is extreme instability, with or without evidence of affection of the spinal cord, there is a case for operation: (i) to remove tumour; (ii) to restore stability; and (iii) to relieve pressure on the spinal cord. The argument that in such cases the affection of the cord is irreversible, from occlusion of vessels, is shown by experience to be incorrect. The contrary argument, that with the initiation of specific therapy there may be swelling of the tumour with consequent increase in the depth of cord affection, is also shown by experience to be correct. Clearly, there is no case for intervening in cases in which the depth of paralysis indicates an irreversible condition of the cord. On the other hand, many patients with para- or tetra-paresis from spinal secondary deposit may be afforded by operation months or years of life made tolerable by relief of the neural affection or instability. In the UK of the 1990s the question of the 'cost-effectiveness' of such interventions has been canvassed, though comparison of the relative costs of intervention and non-intervention would be difficult to the point of impossibility. Clearly, the most cost-effective course would be that of hastening the patient's death or of permitting the patient to die without any attempt at treatment. Many clinicians will hope that such arguments will not readily be accepted.

The procedure for removal of secondary deposit in the cervical spine differs little from that described for the removal of primary malignant tumours. Evidently the resection may be less extensive, for the main thrust of curative treatment must come from specific methods (Fig. 21.46). The theca should be decompressed and affected levels stabilized. In the case of some secondary renal growths in which the primary tumour is revealed only after examination of material removed at the time of operation on the spine, and in which there is no other metastasis, later removal of the renal tumour with the kidney may be indicated (Fig. 21.47). Special difficulty is encountered with Pancoast tumours, in which the bony lesion represents perhaps a simple extension of the apical pulmonary growth (Fig. 21.48). These tumours are intensely invasive, rather sclerotic, completely without capsule and extremely difficult to remove. Complete removal is impossible, but in appropriate cases it is possible to remove enough to secure decompression of the cord and to allow local stabilization.

MALIGNANCY IN THE AXIS

It is convenient here to consider the treatment of secondary deposit in the axis together with that of primary malignant tumour. At this level in the cervical spine destruction of bone produces instability so severe as to cause the most severe and intractable pain. The author has seen three patients so affected who literally had constantly to hold their heads on (Fig. 21.49). With extension of the tumour there may be interference with the spinal cord, but in general the call is for stabilization.

Operation

In this site, unlike other sites, adequate biopsy can be obtained without compromising the performance of any later operation. It can be done simply and quickly by the transoral route, so long, of course, as the tumour occupies the body of the bone (Hastings *et al.*, 1968).

When the tumour is in the body of the bone, it is best

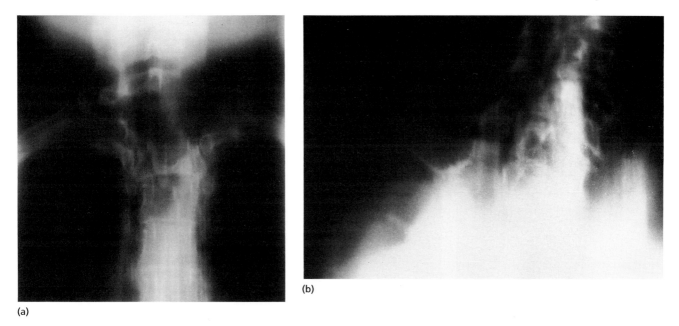

(a)

(b)

Fig. 21.46 Tomographs showing secondary thyroid tumour at the cervicothoracic junction, causing severe paraparesis. (a) Extensive destruction of bone. (b) After removal and stabilization.

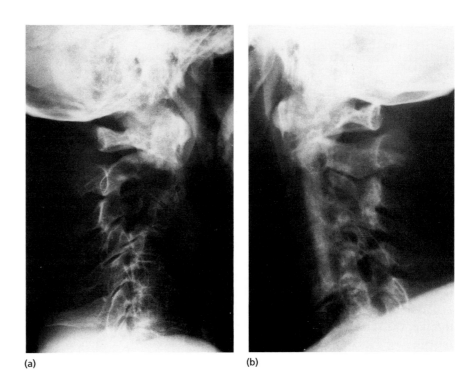

Fig. 21.47 Secondary renal carcinoma. (a) Destructive lesions of second, third and fourth vertebrae. (b) After resection and stabilization.

(a)

(b)

removed by the transoral route. Access is very good, and extensive removal of tumour is possible. If the patient is not receiving steroids, the level can be stabilized by an anterior graft. In other cases, posterior stabilization can be done. An early instance of such proceeding was reported by Laurence and Bonney (1969).

PARAVERTEBRAL TUMOURS

Very occasionally, the orthopaedic surgeon is confronted by a ganglioneuroma in the neck. These benign tumours, which occur in the sites favoured by phaeochromocytomas, contain ganglion cells and some Schwann-like

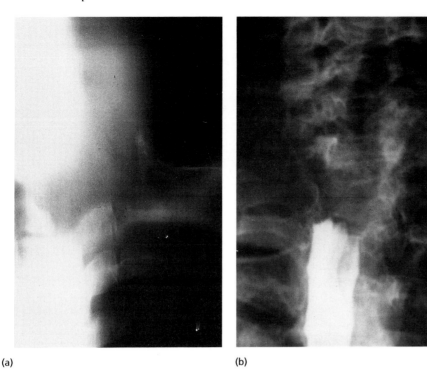

(a)   (b)

Fig. 21.48 Pancoast tumour.
(a) Tomograph showing extensive
destruction at the cervicothoracic
junction. (b) Myelograph shows block to
flow of contrast medium. Paraparesis
partly relieved by decompression and
stabilization.

cells (Gruhn and Gould, 1990). They are peculiar in
that, though electronmicroscopy shows them to contain
neurosecretory granules, and though they have been
shown to produce neuropeptide hormones, few are
associated with symptoms of hormonal disorder. They
may be very extensive, running from the base of the
skull to the pleural apex. They are, however, well
encapsulated and can be removed fully by wide exposure
and careful dissection.

Other methods of stabilization of the cervical spine

It may occur that stabilization becomes necessary but
that it cannot be attempted by the anterior route. In
other cases it may seem sensible to secure stabilization
by the posterior route after extensive laminectomy. The
method most commonly used is that of wire fixation:
through the spines or through the laminae or beneath
the laminae; with or without interposed grafts of cancellous bone. Wires may also be placed across the zygapophyseal joints after erasion of the articular surfaces;
again, grafts of cancellous bone may be added. It is of
particular importance that if, while holes are being
drilled for the passage of interlaminar or transfacetal
wires, spinal fluid appears, the significance of this should
be appreciated. It is preferable to pass the wire or wires
under vision, while the dura is slightly depressed with a
very thin elevator, than to pass a wire or wires through

conducting tissue, even if the former process is rather
more time consuming. The cervical spine is not the best
situation for the posterior introduction of plates and
bolts, because the posterior elements are so fragile. On
the other hand, bent metal rods or frames or various
description can well be used to hold the posterior
elements by wires (Cregan, 1966; Crockard *et al.*, 1990).
The use of such frames may of course be supplemented
by the addition of grafts. Some have relied on the
superior strength of the lateral masses to use screws
passed across the interfacetal joints (Hanson *et al.*, 1991).
This principle has been extended to the use of plates
fixed by such screws to the back of the lateral masses.

Knight (1964) proposed and practised the insertion
posteriorly of moulds of methylmethacrylate for stabilization of the cervical spine in cases of intractable pain
from degenerative disease. The method is applicable in
certain cases, though nowadays it finds its main application in stabilization by introduction anteriorly after
removal of vertebral bodies.

Methods for anterior stabilization

With the proliferation of devices for insertion in order to
replace joints, there has been a considerable increase in
the number of implants offered for stabilization of the
spine. Böhler and Gaudernak (1980) used plates for
anterior stabilization of fracture-dislocations of the

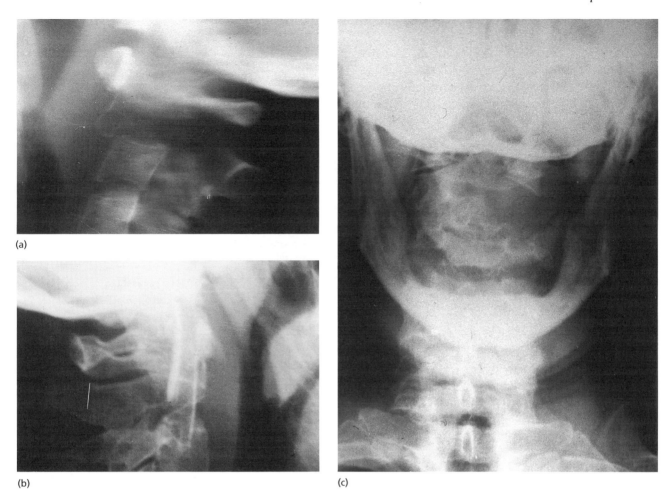

Fig. 21.49 Malignancy in the axis. (a, b) Secondary carcinoma. (a) Transoral view shows destruction of the body of the axis. (b) After transoral removal and stabilization. (c) Osteoclastoma of the axis.

lower cervical spine. Since that time many others have recorded their experience of this and of other methods (Bremer and Nguyen, 1983; Tippets and Apfelbaum, 1988; Caspar *et al.*, 1989; Garvey *et al.*, 1992). Difficulties with plates secured by screws that engage the posterior cortex of the body have to some extent been overcome by the use of special plates secured by hollow screws (Morscher *et al.*, 1986; Suh *et al.*, 1990). Reservations must remain concerning the placing of foreign material in so close a relation with the back of the pharynx and oesophagus, but the use of slim plates of titanium has reduced that potential disadvantage. The claims of methylmethacrylate as a material for filling defects and promoting stabilization after extensive removal of bone should not be disregarded, though the introduction of such large amounts of foreign material may add to the risk of infection (Dunn, 1977). The block of methylmetnacrylate is introduced when it is in a malleable plastic state. It must be cooled as it hardens

by continuous spraying with cold saline. It is anchored to adjacent vertebrae by wire or screw. Metallic implants secured by acrylic cement have been used for the same purpose (Ono and Tada, 1975). The advantages to all concerned of a firm metallic internal fixation during the process of stabilization of a graft are very great. Most series seem to be concerned chiefly with problems of instability in the thoracic and lumbar regions (Flatley *et al.*, 1984; Siegal *et al.*, 1985), but Turner *et al.* (1988) seem to indicate some experience with stabilization of the cervical spine. In their early cases they used bone grafts, but later came to rely on plates and screws and on Zielke or slot rods. Recent experiences with devices to secure extensive fusion in cases of rheumatoid arthritis are narrated by Hukuda and Katsuura (1994).

The use of Kiel bone, formerly much promoted, seems to have fallen into desuetude, though the anterior elements of the cervical spine form an excellent location for this material. A block of Kiel bone well placed and countersunk between vertebral bodies can be expected to remain in place and to become incorporated. Best of all materials, no doubt, is vascularized bone. Freidberg *et al.* (1989) described the successful use of a vascularized fibular graft in replacing three cervical vertebral bodies. The time-consuming nature of this admirable procedure may limit its application.

Stabilization for paralysis

Sometimes the orthopaedic surgeon is called upon simply to act as an operative mason and to straighten and stabilize the spine of a patient whose head has drooped forwards ineluctably because of established or progressive paralytic disease. In such cases a fixation that will be permanent through incorporation is required; it is unwise to rely on internal splintage by prostheses, which will become loose. The author's experience with very long cortical grafts has been disappointing: even with stabilization from the second cervical to the first thoracic vertebra, deformity has recurred at levels above and below the fixed segment. It may be that in such cases the even more extensive stabilization by the posterior route is more successful (Perry and Nickel, 1959). Many methods are now available for posterior and posterolateral instrumentation, including screw plates and plates secured by transfacetal screws (Nazarian and Louis, 1991).

ACKNOWLEDGEMENTS

The author wishes to express his gratitude and sense of obligation to former nursing and medical colleagues at St Mary's Hospital and other hospitals who assisted and guided him in the clinical work and care of patients that form the basis of this monograph, and in particular to Mrs M. Taggart, formerly nursing sister in charge of patients, records and medical staff at St Mary's Hospital, to Dr Jennifer Jones, anaesthetist, in charge of the Intensive Care Unit of the same hospital, to Mr Rolfe Birch, orthopaedic surgeon, to Dr David Sutton, radiologist, and to Dr J.N. Godlee, oncologist and radiotherapist. The author is also grateful to colleagues from other hospitals who entrusted to him the care of many of the patients whose cases are illustrated here, and to the patients who endured and in most cases survived. He recalls to the young men and women who follow him the words of Paré 'I treated him; God cured him'; and more particularly the words of Sherlock Holmes 'It has all been done before'.

REFERENCES

Adams C.B.T. and Logue V. (1971a) Studies in cervical spondylotic myelopathy. I: Movements of the cervical roots, dura and cord and their relation to the course of the extrathecal roots. *Brain* **94**, 557–568.

Adams C.B.T. and Logue V. (1971b) Studies in cervical spondylotic myelopathy. II: The movement and contour of the spine in relation to the neural complications of cervical spondylosis. *Brain* **94**, 569–586.

Adams J.C. (1952) Technique, diagnosis and safeguards in osteotomy of the spine. *J. Bone Joint Surg.* **34B**, 226–232.

Alexander G.L. (1946) Neurological complications of spinal tuberculosis. *Proc. R. Soc. Med.* **39**, 730–734.

Alexander G.L. (1947) Prolapsed intervertebral disc. *Edinburgh Med. J.* **54**, 14–29.

Anderson L.D. and D'Alonzo R.T. (1974) Fractures of the odontoid process of the axis. *J. Bone Joint Surg.* **56A**, 1663–1674.

Andrade J.R. de and MacNab I. (1969) Anterior occipito-cervical fusion using an extra-pharyngeal approach. *J. Bone Joint Surg.* **51A**, 1621–1626.

Ansell B.M., Bywaters E.G.L. and Doniach I. (1958) The aortic lesion of ankylosing spondylitis. *Br. Heart J.* **20**, 507–515.

Ashraf T. and Crockard H.A. (1990) Transoral fusion for high cervical fractures. *J. Bone Joint Surg.* **72B**, 76–77.

Baker A.S., Ojemann R.G., Swartz M.N. and Richardson E.P. (1975) Spinal epidural abscess. *N. Engl. J. Med.* **293**, 463–468.

Ballock R.T., Hajek P.C., Byrne T.P. and Garfon S.R. (1989) The quality of magnetic resonance imaging, as affected by the composition of the halo orthosis. *J. Bone Joint Surg.* **71A**, 431–432.

Berthold E.A. and Carlstedt T. (1977) Observations on the morphology at the transition between the peripheral and the central nervous system in the cat. *Acta Physiol. Scand.* Supplement **446**, 23–42.

Birch R., Bonney G. and Marshall R.W. (1990) A surgical approach to the cervical spine. *J. Bone Joint Surg.* **72B**, 904–907.

Bland J.H. (1987) *Disorders of the Cervical Spine.* Philadelphia, W.B. Saunders, pp. 6 and 7.

Böhler J. and Gaudernak T. (1980) Anterior plate stabilisation for fracture-dislocations of the lower cervical spine. *J. Trauma* **20**, 203–205.

Bonney G. (1970) Stabilisation of the upper cervical spine by the transpharyngeal route. *Proc. R. Soc. Med.* **63**, 896–897.

Bonney G. (1977) Some lesions of the brachial plexus. *Ann. R. Coll. Surg. Engl.* **59**, 298–386.

Bonney G. and Gilliatt R. (1958) Sensory nerve conduction after traction lesion of the brachial plexus. *Proc. R. Soc. Med.* **51**, 365–367.

Bonney G. and Williams J.P.R. (1985) Trans-oral approach to the upper cervical spine. *J. Bone Joint Surg.* **67B**, 691–698.

Bremer A.M. and Nguyen T.Q. (1983) Internal metal plate fixation combined with anterior interbody fusion in cases of cervical spine injury. *Neurosurgery* **12**, 649–653.

British National Formulary (1990) British Medical Association and the Pharmaceutical Press, vol. 19, p. 229.

Brown J.N. and Crosby A.C. (1993) Acute soft tissue injuries of the cervical spine. *Br. Med. J.* **307**, 439–440.

Bull J., Nixon W., Pratt R. and Robinson P. (1959) Paget's disease of the skull and secondary basilar impression. *Brain* **82**, 10–22.

Capener N. (1954) The evolution of lateral rhachotomy. *J. Bone Joint Surg.* 36B, 173–179.

Carpenter P.C. (1986) Cushing's syndrome: update of diagnosis and management. *Mayo Clin. Proc.* 61, 49–58.

Caspar W., Burbier D.D. and Klare P.M. (1989) Anterior cervical fusion and Caspar plate fixation for cervical trauma. *Neurosurgery* 25, 491–502.

Chakravorty B.G. (1969) Arterial supply of the cervical spinal cord and its relation to the cervical myelopathy in spondylosis. *Ann. R. Coll. Surg. Engl.* 45, 232–251.

Chamberlain W.E. (1939) Basilar impression (platybasia). *Yale J. Biol. Med.* 11, 487–496.

Chesterman P. and Bonney G. (1964) Spastic paraplegia caused by sequestrated thoracic intervertebral disc. *Proc. R. Soc. Med.* 57, 87–88.

Chiari H. (1891) Ueber Veränderungen des Kleinhirns unfolge von hydrocephalie des Grosshirns. *Deutsche Med. Wochenschr.* 17, 1172–1175.

Ciricillo S.F. and Weinstein P.R. (1989) Foramen magnum syndrome from pseudogout of the atlanto-occipital ligament. *J. Neurosurg.* 71, 141–143.

Clark C.R., Goetz D.D. and Menezes A.M. (1989) Arthrodesis of the cervical spine in rheumatoid arthritis. *J. Bone Joint Surg.* 71A(3), 381–392.

Clarke E. and Robinson P.K. (1956) Cervical myelopathy: a complication of cervical spondylosis. *Brain* 79, 483–510.

Clavel M. (1988) C2 Neurofibroma. A Case Report. *Spine* 13, 589–591.

Cleland J. (1883) Contribution to the study of spina bifida, encephalocele and anencephalus. *J. Anat. Physiol.* 17, 257–292.

Cloward R.B. (1958) The anterior approach for removal of ruptured cervical disks. *J. Neurosurg.* 15, 602–617.

Conlon P.W., Isdale I.C. and Rose B.S. (1966) Rheumatoid arthritis of the cervical spine. *Ann. Rheum. Dis.* 25, 120–126.

Constans J.P., de Divitiis E., Donzelli R., Spaziante R., Meder J.F. and Haye C. (1983) Spinal metastases with neurological manifestations. *J. Neurosurg.* 59, 111–118.

Craig J.B. and Govender S. (1992) Neurofibromatosis of the cervical spine. *J. Bone Joint Surg.* 74B, 575–578.

Cregan J.C.F. (1966) Internal fixation of the unstable rheumatoid cervical spine. *Ann. Rheum. Dis.* 25, 242–252.

Crellin R.Q., Maccabe J.J. and Hamilton E.B.D. (1970) Severe subluxation of the spine in rheumatoid arthritis. *J. Bone Joint Surg.* 52B, 244–251.

Crockard H.A. (1985) The transoral approach to the base of the brain and the upper cervical cord. *Ann. R. Coll. Surg. Engl.* 67, 321–325.

Crockard H.A. and Bradford R. (1985) Transoral transclival removal of a schwannoma anterior to the cranio-cervical junction. *J. Neurosurg.* 62, 293–295.

Crockard H.A., Pozo J.L., Ransford A.O. and Hutton P.A.N. (1985) One-stage trans-oral anterior decompression and posterior stabilisation in cervical myelopathy complicating rheumatoid arthritis. *J. Bone Joint Surg.* 67B, 498–499.

Crockard H.A., Calder I. and Ransford A.O. (1990) One-stage trans-oral decompression and posterior fixation in rheumatoid atlanto-axial subluxation. *J. Bone Joint Surg.* 72B, 682–685.

Crockard H.A., Heilman A.E. and Stevens J.H. (1993) Progressive myelopathy secondary to odontoid fractures: clinical, radiological and surgical features. *J. Neurosurg.* 78, 579–586.

Curtis B.M., Fisher R.L., Butterfield W.L. and Saunders F.P.

(1969) Neurofibromatosis with paraplegia. *J. Bone Joint Surg.* 51A, 843–861.

Cushing H. (1932) The basophil adenomas of the pituitary body and their clinical manifestations (pituitary basophilism). *Bull. Johns Hopkins Hosp.* 50, 137–195.

Dawson G.D. (1947) Cerebral responses to electrical stimulation of peripheral nerve in man. *J. Neurol. Neurosurg. Psych.* 10, 134–140.

Delandsheer J.M., Caron J.P. and Jomin M. (1977) Voie trans-bucco-pharyngée et malformations de la charniére cervico-occipitale. *Neurochirurg.* 23(4), 276–281.

Delattre J.Y., Arbit E., Thaler M.T., Rosenblum M.K. and Posner J.B. (1987) A dose-response study of dexamethasone in a model of spinal cord compression caused by epidural tumour. *J. Neurosurg.* 70, 920–925.

Derome P., Caron J.P. and Hurth M. (1977) Indications de la voie trans-bucco-pharyngee et malformations de la charniere cranio-vertébrale. *Neurochirurg.* 23, 282–285.

Dott N.M. (1947) Skeletal traction and anterior decompression in the management of Pott's paraplegia. *Edinburgh Med. J.* 54, 620–627.

Douglas D.L., Duckworth T., Kanis J.A., Jefferson A.A., Martin T.J. and Russell R.G.G. (1981) Spinal cord dysfunction in Paget's disease of bone. *J. Bone Joint Surg.* 63B, 495–503.

Dunn E.J. (1977) The role of methylmethacrylate in the stabilisation and replacement of tumours of the cervical spine. *Spine* 2(1), 15–24.

Engler G.L., Spielholz N.I., Bernhard W.N., Danziger F., Merkin H. and Wolff E.E. (1978) Somatosensory evoked potentials during instrumentation for scoliosis. *J. Bone Joint Surg.* 60A, 528–532.

Epstein J.A., Carras R., Lavine L.S. and Epstein B.S. (1969) The importance of removing osteophytes as part of the surgical treatment of myelo-radiculopathy in cervical spondylosis. *J. Neurosurg.* 30, 219–226.

Epstein J.A., Epstein B.S., Lavine L.S., Carras R. and Rosenthal A.D. (1978) Cervical myeloradiculopathy caused by arthrotic hypertrophy of the posterior facets and laminae. *J. Neurosurg.* 49, 387–392.

Eriksson B., Gunterberg B. and Kindblom L.-G. (1981) Chordoma: a clinico-pathologic and prognostic study of a Swedish national series. *Acta Orthop. Scand.* 52, 49–58.

Fang H.S.Y. and Ong G.B. (1962) Direct anterior approach to the upper cervical spine. *J. Bone Joint Surg.* 44A, 1588–1604.

Fielding W.J. and Griffin P.P. (1974) Os odontoideum: an acquired lesion. *J. Bone Joint Surg.* 56A, 187–190.

Fielding J.W., Pyle R.N. and Fietti V.G. (1979) Anterior cervical vertebral body resection and bone-grafting for benign and malignant tumours. *J. Bone Joint Surg.* 61A, 251–253.

Fiolle J. and Delmas J. (1921) (Translated and edited by C.G. Cumston) *The Surgical Exposure of Deep-seated Blood Vessels.* London, W. Heinemann, pp. 61–67.

Flatley T.J., Anderson M.H. and Anast G.T. (1984) Spinal instability due to malignant disease. *J. Bone Joint Surg.* 66A, 17–52.

Ford F.R. and Clark D. (1956) Thrombosis of the basilar artery with softenings in the cerebellum and brain stem due to manipulation of the neck. *Bull. Johns Hopkins Hosp.* 98, 37–42.

Frazer J.E. (1920) *The Anatomy of the Human Skeleton.* London, J & A Churchill.

Freidberg S.R., Gumley G.J., Pfeifer B.A. and Hybels R.L. (1989) Vascularized fibular graft to replace resected cervical vertebral bodies. *J. Neurosurg.* 71, 283–286.

Frykholm R. (1971) The clinical picture. In Hirsch C. and Zotterman Y. (eds) *Cervical Pain*. Pergamon Press, pp. 5−16.

Fujiwara K., Yonenobu K., Ebara S., Yamashita K. and Ono K. (1989) The prognosis of surgery for cervical compression myelopathy. *J. Bone Joint Surg.* **71B**(3), 393−398.

Gamble H.J. (1964) Comparative electron-miscroscopic observations on the connective tissues of a peripheral nerve and a spinal nerve root in a rat. *J. Anat.* **98**, 17−25.

Garvey T.A., Eismont F.J. and Roberti L.J. (1992) Anterior decompression, structural bone grafting and Caspar plate stabilisation for unstable cervical spine fractures and/or dislocations. *Spine* **17**, S431−S435.

Greenberg A.D. (1968) Atlanto-axial dislocations. *Brain* **91**, 655−634.

Greenberg A.D., Scoville W.B. and Davy L.M. (1968) Trans-oral decompression of atlanto-axial dislocation due to odontoid hypoplasia. Report of two cases. *J. Neurosurg.* **20**, 266−269.

Griffiths D.L.I., Seddon H.J. and Roaf R. (1956a) *Pott's Paraplegia*. Oxford, Oxford University Press, pp. 1−21.

Griffiths D.L., Seddon H.J. and Roaf R. (1956b) *Pott's Paraplegia*. Oxford, Oxford University Press, pp. 50−73.

Grote W., Kalff R. and Roosen K. (1991) Die operative Behandlung zervikaler Bandscheibenvorfälle. *Zentralblatt für Neurochirurgie* **52**, 101−108.

Gruhn J.G. and Gould V.E. (1990) In Kissan J.M. (ed.) *Anderson's Pathology*. St Louis, C.V. Mosby, vol. 33, p. 1613.

Hadley M.M., Spetzler R.F. and Sonntag V.K.H. (1989) The transoral approach to the upper cervical spine. *J. Neurosurg.* **71**, 16−23.

Hakuda S. and Wilson C.B. (1972) Experimental cervical myelopathy. *J. Neurosurg.* **37**, 631−652.

Hall J.E., Levine C.R. and Sudhir K.G. (1978) Intra-operative awakening to monitor spinal cord function during Harrington instrumentation and spine fusion. *J. Bone Joint Surg.* **60A**, 533−536.

Hamblen D.L. (1967) Occipito-cervical fusion; indications, technique and results. *J. Bone Joint Surg.* **49B**, 33−45.

Hankinson H.L. and Wilson C.B. (1975) Use of the operating microscope in anterior cervical discectomy without fusion. *J. Neurosurg.* **43**, 452−456.

Hanson P.B., Montesano P.X., Sharkey N.A. and Rauschning W. (1991) Anatomic and biomechanical assessment of transarticular screw fixation for atlanto-axial instability. *Spine* **16**, 1141−1145.

Harkey H.L., Crockard H.A., Stevens J.M., Smith R. and Ransford A.O. (1990) The operative management of basilar impression in osteogenesis imperfecta. *Neurosurgery* **27**, 782−786.

Harris P. (1963) The anterior approach to excision of cervical discs. *Proc. R. Soc. Med.* **56**, 807−808.

Harrold A.J. (1956) Alkaptonuric arthritis. *J. Bone Joint Surg.* **38B**, 537−538.

Harwick R.D. and Miller A.S. (1979) Craniocervical chordomas. *Am. J. Surg.* **138**, 512−516.

Hastings D.E., MacNab I. and Lawson V. (1968) Neoplasms of the axis and atlas. *Can. J. Surg.* **11**, 290−296.

Hattori S., Saiki K. and Kawai S. (1979) Diagnosis of the level and severity of cord lesion in cervical spondylotic myelopathy. *Spine* **4**(6), 478−485.

Hattori S., Miyamoto T. and Kawai S. (1980) Choice of the surgical treatment for cervical myelopathy with multiple spondylotic protrusions. *Eighth Annual Meeting of the Cervical Spine Research Society*.

Hauge T. (1961) Chronic rheumatoid polyarthritis and spondylarthritis associated with neurological symptoms and signs occasionally simulating an intraspinal expansive process. *Acta Chirurg. Scand.* **120**, 395−401.

Henderson R.G. (1983) Nuclear magnetic resonance imaging: a review. *J. R. Soc. Med.* **76**, 206−212.

Hensinger R.N., Lang J.E. and MacEwen G.D. (1974) Klippel−Feil syndrome: a constellation of associated anomalies. *J. Bone Joint Surg.* **56A**, 1246−1253.

Heusner A.P. (1948) Nontuberculous spinal epidural abscess. *N. Engl. J. Med.* **239**, 845−854.

Hitchon P.W., McKay T.C., Wilkinson T.T., Girton R.A., Hanson T. and Dyste G.N. (1989) Methylprednisolone in spinal cord compression. *Spine* **14**(1), 16−22.

Hodgson A.R. and Stock F.E. (1960) Anterior spine fusion for the treatment of tuberculosis of the spine *J. Bone Joint Surg.* **42A**, 295−310.

Holt S. and Yates P.O. (1966) Cervical spondylosis and nerve root lesions. *J. Bone Joint Surg.* **48B**, 407−423.

Holton J.B. (1987) *The Inherited Metabolic Diseases*. Edinburgh, Churchill Livingstone, pp. 313−317.

Hsu L.C.S. and Yau A.C.M.C. (1983) In Baily R.W. (ed.) *The Cervical Spine*. Philadelphia, J.B. Lippincott, p. 342.

Hukuda S. and Katsuura A. (1994) Operations for subluxation of the cervical spine in patients with rheumatoid arthritis: a transition from short fusion to long fusion. *Orthopaedics* **2**, 118−124.

Hulme A. and Dott N.M. (1954) Spinal epidural abscess. *Br. Med. J.* **i**, 64−68.

Hutton P.W. (1956) Acute osteomyelitis of the cervical spine with epidural abscess. *Br. Med. J.* **i**, 153−154.

Jeffcoate W.J. (1988) Treating Cushing's Disease. *Br. Med. J.* **298**, 227−228.

Jones S.J. (1979) Investigation of brachial plexus traction lesions by peripheral nerve and spinal somatosensory evoked potentials. *J. Neurol. Neurosurg. Psych.* **42**, 107−116.

Kemp H.B.S., Jackson J.W., Jeremiah J.B. and Hall A.J. (1973a) Pyogenic infections of bone occurring primarily in intervertebral discs. *J. Bone Joint Surg.* **55B**, 698−714.

Kemp H.B.S., Jackson J.W., Jeremiah J.B. and Cook J. (1973b) Anterior fusion of the spine for infective lesions in adults. *J. Bone Joint Surg.* **55B**, 715−734.

Kimura I., Oh-Hama M. and Shingu H. (1984) Cervical myelopathy treated by canal-expansive laminaplasty. *J. Bone Joint Surg.* **66A**(6), 914−920.

Klippel M. and Feil A. (1912) Un cas d'absence des vertébres cervicales avec cage thoracique remontant jusqu' à la base du craine. *Nouvelle Iconographie de la Salpétrière* **25**, 223−250.

Knight G.C. (1964) Neurosurgical treatment of cervical spondylosis. *Proc. R. Soc. Med.* **57**, 7−10.

Lander P. and Hadjipavlou A. (1991) Intradiscal invasion of Paget's Disease of the spine. *Spine* **16**, 46−51.

Landi A., Copeland S.A., Wynn Parry C.B. and Jones S.J. (1980) The role of somatosensory evoked potentials and nerve conduction studies in the surgical management of brachial plexus injuries. *J. Bone Joint Surg.* **62B**, 492−496.

Laurence M. and Bonney G. (1969) Malignant destruction of the axis—two-year survival. *Proc. R. Soc. Med.* **62**, 2−3.

Leong J.C.Y., Fang D., Woo E., Huang C.Y. and Lau H.K. (1988) Cervical myelopathy due to ossification of the posterior longitudinal ligament. *Brain* **111**, 769−793.

Lipton S. (1973) Pain control and the management of advanced malignant disease. *Proc. R. Soc. Med.* **66**, 607–609.

McCain M.A. (1985) Chordoma in a chronic pain patient. *Arch. Phys. Med. Rehabil.* **66**(7), 457–458.

McKusick V.A. (1972) *Heritable Disorders of Connective Tissue*, 4th edn. St Louis, C.V. Mosby, pp. 292–371.

McGregor M. (1948) The significance of certain measurements of the skull in the diagnosis of basilar impression. *Br. J. Radiol.* **21**, 171–181.

Mackworth-Young C.G. and Hughes G.R.V. (1990) Complications of rheumatic and connective tissue disease. In Swash M. and Oxbury J. (eds) *Clinical Neurology*. Edinburgh, Churchill Livingstone, pp. 1678–1694.

MacNab I. (1964) Acceleration injuries of the cervical spine. *J. Bone Joint Surg.* **46A**, 1797–1799.

MacNab I. (1967) Anterior occipito-cervical fusion. *J. Bone Joint Surg.* **49A**, 1010–1011.

MacNab I. (1971a) The 'Whiplash Syndrome'. *Orthop. Clin. North Am.* **2**(2), 389–403.

MacNab I. (1971b) The mechanism of spondylogenic pain. In Hirsch C. and Zofferman Y. (eds). *Cervical Pain*. Pergamon Press, pp. 89–95.

MacNab I. (1983) Symptoms in cervical disc degeneration. In Bailey R.W. (ed.). *The Cervical Spine*. Philadelphia, J.B. Lippincott, pp. 388–394.

Marshall R.W. and de Silva R.D.D. (1986) Computerised axial tomography in traction lesions of the brachial plexus. *J. Bone Joint Surg.* **57A**, 938–948.

Martinez-Lage J.F., Sola J., Poza M. and Esteban J.A. (1993) Pediatric Creutzfeld–Jakob disease: probable transmission by a dural graft. *Child's Nervous System* **9**, 239–242.

Martins A.N. (1976) Anterior cervical discectomy with and without interbody bone graft. *J. Neurosurg.* **44**, 290–295.

Mathews J.A. (1969) Atlanto-axial subluxation in rheumatoid arthritis. *Ann. Rheum. Dis.* **28**, 260–266.

Mendelson G.M., Hunt J.B. and Baron J.H. (1993) Cervical osteomyelitis and magnetic resonance imaging. *J. Roy. Soc. Med.* **86**, 298–299.

Micheli L.J., Hall J.E. and Watts H.G. (1976) Spinal instability in Larsen's syndrome. *J. Bone Joint Surg.* **58A**, 562–565.

Miller D.M., Rudge P., Johnson G., Kendall B.E., MacManus D.G., Moseley I.F., Barnes D. and McDonald W.I. (1988b) Serial gadolinum enhanced magnetic resonance imaging in multiple sclerosis. *Brain* **111**, 927–939.

Monro P. (1984) What has surgery to offer in cervical spondylosis? In Warlow C. and Garfield J.S. (eds) *Dilemmas in the Management of the Neurological Patient*. Edinburgh, Churchill Livingstone, pp. 168–187.

Morscher E., Sutter F., Jennis M. and Olerud S. (1986) Die vordere Verplattung der Halswirbelsaule mit dem Hohlschrauben-plattensystem. *Der Chirurg.* **57**, 702–707.

Moseley I. (1994) Safety and magnetic resonance imaging. *Br. Med. J.* **308**, 1181–1182.

Moskovich R. and Crockard H.A. (1992) Atlanto-axial arthrodesis using interlaminar clamps. *Spine* **17**, 261–267.

Murphy M.G. and Gado M. (1972) Anterior cervical discectomy without interbody bone graft. *J. Neurosurg.* **37**, 71–74.

Nachemson A. (1960) Fracture of the odontoid process of the axis. A clinical study based on 26 cases. *Acta Orthopaed. Scand.* **29**, 185–217.

Nachemson A. (1989) Lumbar discography – where are we today? *Spine* **14**, 555–557.

Nagata K., Kiyenaga K., Okashi T., Sugara M., Miyazaki S. and Inoue A. (1990) Clinical value of magnetic resonance imaging for cervical myelopathy. *Spine* **15**, 1088–1096.

National Radiation Protection Board (1981) Exposure to nuclear magnetic resonance clinical imaging. *Radiography* **47**, 258–260.

Nazarian S.M. and Louis R.P. (1991) Posterior internal fixation with screw plates in traumatic lesions of the cervical spine. *Spine* **16**, S64–S71.

Newman P.K. (1990) Whiplash injury. *Br. Med. J.* **301**, 395.

Newman P. and Sweetnam R. (1969) Occipito-cervical fusion. *J. Bone Joint Surg.* **51B**, 423–431.

Nickel V.L., Perry J., Garrett A. and Heppenstall M. (1968) The halo: a spinal skeletal traction fixation device. *J. Bone Joint Surg.* **50A**, 1400–1409.

Nurick S. (1972) The pathogenesis of the spinal cord disorder associated with cervical spondylosis. *Brain* **95**, 87–100.

O'Brien W.M., La Du B.N. and Bunim J.J. (1963) Biochemical pathologic and clinical aspects of alcaptonuria, ochronosis and ochronotic arthropathy: review of world literature (1584–1962). *Am. J. Med.* **34**, 813–838.

Ono K. and Tada K. (1975) Metal prosthesis of the cervical vertebra. *J. Neurosurg.* 562–566.

Orrell R.W. and Marsden C.D. (1994) The neck-tongue syndrome. *J. Neurol. Neurosurg. Psych.* **57**, 348–352.

Osti O.L., Fraser R.D. and Vernon Roberts B. (1990) Discitis after discography. *J. Bone Joint Surg.* **72B**, 271–276.

Pallis C., Jones A.M. and Spillane A.D. (1954) Cervical spondylosis: incidence and implications. *Brain* **77**, 274–289.

Parizel P.M., Baleriaux D., Rodesch G. *et al.* (1989) DTPA enhanced MR imaging of spinal tumours. *Am. J. Roentgenol.* **152**, 1087–1096.

Pasztor E., Vajda J., Piffko P. and Horvath M. (1980) Transoral surgery for basilar impression. *Surg. Neurol.* **14**, 473–476.

Pennie B.H. and Agambar L.J. (1990) Whiplash injuries. *J. Bone Joint Surg.* **72B**, 277–279.

Perry J. and Nickel V.L. (1959) Total cervical spine fusion for neck paralysis. *J. Bone Joint Surg.* **41A**, 37–60.

Pitt M.C., Monro P.S. and Uttley D. (1990) Numb, clumsy hands may indicate a surgically treatable cause of myelopathy in the elderly. *J. R. Soc. Med.* **63**, 119–120.

Pozo J.L., Crockard H.A. and Ransford A.O. (1984) Basilar impression in osteogenesis imperfecta. *J. Bone Joint Surg.* **66B**, 233–238.

Rabhan W.N. and Rosai J. (1968) Desmo-plastic fibroma. *J. Bone Joint Surg.* **50A**, 487–502.

Raynor R.B. (1983) Congenital malformations of the base of the skull. In Bailey R.W. (ed.) *The Cervical Spine*. Philadelphia, J.B. Lippincott, vol. 5, pp. 147–155.

Rechtman A.M., Borden A.G.B. and Gershon-Cohen J. (1961) The lordotic curve of the cervical spine. *Clin. Orthop.* **20**, 208–216.

Riley L.H. (1973) Surgical approaches to the anterior structures of the cervical spine. *Clin. Orthop.* **91**, 16–20.

Riley L.H., Robinson R.A., Johnson K.A., Walker A.E. (1969) The results of anterior interbody fusion of the cervical spine. *J. Neurosurg.* **30**, 127–133.

Robinson R.A. and Smith G.W. (1955) Anterolateral cervical disc removal and interbody fusion for cervical disc syndrome. *Bull. Johns Hopkins Hosp.* **96**, 223–224.

Sadar E.S., Walton R.J. and Gossman H.H. (1972) Neurological dysfunction in Paget's disease of the vertebral column. *J. Neurosurg.* **37**, 661–665.

Santavirta S., Kontinnen Y.T., Laasonen E., Honkann V., Antiipoika I. and Kauppi V. (1991) Ten-year results of operations for rheumatoid cervical spine disorders. *J. Bone Joint Surg.* **73B**, 116–120.

Satoh S., Yamamoto N., Kitagawa Y., Umemori T., Susaki T. and Iida T. (1993) Cervical cord compression by the anomalous vertebral artery presenting with neuralgic pain. *J. Neurosurg.* **79**, 283–285.

Schajowicz F. and Slullitel J. (1973) Eosinophilic granuloma of bone and its relationship to Hand–Schuller–Christian and Letterer–Siwe syndromes. *J. Bone Joint Surg.* **55B**, 545–565.

Scheer G.E. and Kuhlman R.E. (1963) Vertebral involvement by a desmoplastic fibroma. *JAMA* **185**(2), 669–670.

Schwalbe E. and Gredig M. (1907) Uber Entwicklungstörungen der Kleinhirns Hirnstamms und Halsmarkes bei spina bifida (Arnold'sche und Chiari'sche Missbildung). *Beiträge zur Pathologischen Anatomie und zur allgemeinen Pathologie* **40**, 132–194.

Scoville W.B. (1961) Cervical spondylosis treated by bilateral facetectomy and laminectomy. *J. Neurosurg.* **18**, 423–428.

Scoville W.B. and Sherman I.J. (1951) Platybasia. *Ann. Surg.* **133**, 486–502.

Selladurai B.M. (1992) Cervical myelopathy due to nuclear herniations in young adults: clinical and radiological profile, results of microdiscectomy without interbody fusion. *J. Neurol., Neurosurg. Psych.* **55**, 604–608.

Semine A.A., Ertel A.N., Godberg M.J. and Bull M.J. (1978) Cervical spine instability in children with Down syndrome (trisomy 21). *J. Bone Joint Surg.* **60A**, 649–642.

Sen C.N. and Sekhar L.N. (1990) An extreme lateral approach to intradural lesions of the cervical spine and foramen magnum. *Neurosurg.* **27**, 197–204.

Sennett K. (1991) *Independent* 12 February 1991, p. 7.

Sharma B.S., Banerjee A.K. and Kak V.K. (1989) Malignant schwannoma of brachial plexus presenting as spinal cord compression. *Neurochirurg.* **32**, 189–191.

Sherk H.H. (1978) Atlanto-axial instability and acquired basilar invagination in rheumatoid arthritis. *Orthop. Clin. North Am.* **9**(4), 1053–1063.

Shinomiya K., Okamito A., Komori H., Matsuoka Y., Yoshida H., Muto N. and Furya K. (1990) Prognosticating study for cervical myelopathy using spinal cord potentials. *Spine* **15**, 1053–1057.

Siegal T., Tiqva P. and Siegal T. (1985) Vertebral body resection for epidural compression by malignant tumours. *J. Bone Joint Surg.* **67A**, 375–382.

Simmons E.H. (1972) The surgical correction of flexion deformity of the cervical spine in ankylosing spondylitis. *Clin. Orthop.* **86**, 132–143.

Simmons S. and Bhallia S.K. (1969) Anterior cervical discectomy and fusion. A clinical and biomechanical study with eight year follow-up. *J. Bone Joint Surg.* **51B**, 220–237.

Smith-Petersen N.M., Larsen C.B. and Aufranc O.E. (1945) Osteotomy of the spine for correction of deformity in rheumatoid arthritis. *J. Bone Joint Surg.* **27**, 1–11.

Sneider S.E., Winslow O.P. and Pryor T.H. (1964) Cervical diskography: is it relevant? *JAMA* **188**(2), 163–165.

Southwick W.O. and Robinson R.A. (1957) Surgical approaches to the vertebral bodies in the cervical and lumbar regions. *J. Bone Joint Surg.* **39B**, 631–644.

Spetzler R.F., Selman W.R., Nash C.L. and Brown R.H. (1979) Transoral microsurgical odontoid resection and spinal cord monitoring. *Spine* **4**, 506–510.

Spielholz N.I., Benjamin N.V., Engler G.L. and Ransohoff J. (1979) Somatosensory evoked potentials during decompression and stabilisation of the spine. *Spine* **4**, 500–505.

Stack J.P., Antouin N.M., Jenkins J.P.R., Metcalfe R. and Isherwood I. (1988) Gadolinum DTPA as a contrast agent in magnetic resonance imaging of the brain. *Neuroradiol.* **30**, 145–154.

Stevens J.M., Kendall B.E., Crockard H.A. and Ransford A. (1991) The odontoid process in Morquio-Brailsford's disease. *J. Bone Joint Surg.* **73B**, 851–858.

Stoltmann H.F. and Blackwood W. (1964) The role of the ligamenta flava in the pathogenesis of myelopathy in cervical spondylosis. *Brain* **87**, 45–50.

Stone J.L., Cybulski G.R., Rodriguez J., Gryfinski M.E. and Kant R. (1989) Anterior cervical debridement and strut-grafting for osteomyelitis of the cervical pine. *J. Neurosurg.* **70**, 879–883.

Suh P.B., Kostuik J.P. and Esses S.I. (1990) Anterior cervical plate fixation with the titanium hollow screw plate system. *Spine* **15**, 1079–1081.

Takkunen J., Vuopala U. and Somaki H.I. (1970) Cardiomyopathy in ankylosing spondylitis. *Ann. Clin. Res.* **2**, 106–112.

Taylor A.R. (1964) Vascular factors in the myelopathy associated with cervical spondylosis. *Neurology* **14**, 62–68.

Taylor L.J. (1984) Multifocal avascular necrosis after short-term high-dose steroid therapy. *J. Bone Joint Surg.* **66B**, 431–433.

Thompson H. (1962) The 'halo' traction apparatus: a method of external splinting of the cervical spine after injury. *J. Bone Joint Surg.* **44B**, 655–661.

Thompson H. (1970) Transpharyngeal fusion of the upper cervical spine. *Proc. R. Soc. Med.* **63**, 893–896.

Tippets R.H. and Apfelbaum R.I. (1988) Anterior cervical fusion with the Caspar instrumentation system. *Neurosurgery* **22**, 1008–1013.

Tomita K., Nomura S., Umeda S. and Baba H. (1988) Cervical laminoplasty to enlarge the spinal canal in multilevel ossification of the posterior longitudinal ligament with myelopathy. *Arch. Orthop. Traum. Surg.* **107**, 148–153.

Torklus D. von and Gehle W. (1968) Das os odontoideum als okzipital-wirbelmanifestation. *Radiologia Clinica et Biologica* **37**, 321.

Torklus D. von and Gehle W. (1969) Neue Perspektiven der Entwicklungstörungen der oberen Halswirbelsäule. *Zeitschr. Orthop. Grenzgebiete* **105**, 78.

Torklus D. von and Gehle W. (1972) *The Upper Cervical Spine.* Stuttgart, George Thieme, p. 45.

Tsuji H. (1982) Laminoplasty for patients with compressive myelopathy due to so-called spinal canal stenosis in cervical and thoracic regions. *Spine* **7**(1), 28–34.

Turner P.L., Prince H.G., Webb J.K. and Sokal M.P.J.W. (1988) Surgery for malignant extradural tumours of the spine. *J. Bone Joint Surg.* **70B**, 451–456.

Urist M. (1958) Osteotomy of the cervical spine. *J. Bone and Joint Surg.* **40A**, 833–843.

Valk J. (1988) Gd-DTPA in the MR of spinal lesions. *Am. J. Roentgenol.* **150**, 1163–1168.

Verbiest H. (1965) Giant cell tumours and aneurysmal bone cysts of the spine. *J. Bone Joint Surg.* **47B**, 699–713.

Verbiest H. (1968) A lateral approach to the cervical spine: technique and indications. *J. Neurosurg.* **28**, 191–203.

Verbiest H. (1983) Tumours involving the cervical spine. In Bailey R.W. (ed.) *The Cervical Spine*. Philadelphia, J.B. Lippincott, pp. 439, 440.

Viard H., Sautreaux J.-L., Haas O., Bernard A., Goudet P. and Barry P. (1989) Tumeurs nerveuses en sablier. *Chirurgie* **115**, 521–525.

Wall P.D. (1971) The mechanisms of pain associated with cervical vertebral disease. In Hirsch C. and Zotterman Y. (eds) *Cervical Pain*. Oxford, Pergamon Press, p. 203.

White A.A., Southwick W.O., Deponte R.J., Gainor J.W. and Hardy R. (1973) Relief of pain by anterior cervical spine fusion for spondylosis. *J. Bone Joint Surg.* **55A**(3), 525–534.

Whitesides T.E. and Kelly R.P. (1966) Lateral approach to the upper cervical spine for fusion. *Southern Med. J.* **59**, 879–883.

Whitesides T.E. and McDonald A.P. (1978) Lateral retropharyngeal approach to the upper cervical spine. *Orthop. Clin. North Am.* **9**(4), 1115–1127.

Wickbom I. (1971) X-ray methods for presenting changes in the cervical spine and discs. In Hirsch C. and Zotterman Y. (eds) *Cervical Pain*. Oxford, Pergamon Press.

Wilkinson M.C. (1950) Curettage of tuberculous disease in the treatment of spinal caries. *Proc. R. Soc. Med.* **43**, 114–115.

Wilson D.H. and Campbell D.D. (1977) Anterior cervical discectomy without bone graft. *J. Neurosurg.* **47**, 551–555.

Winter R.B., Moe J.H., Bradford D.S., Lonstein J.E., Pedrus C.V. and Weber A.M. (1979) Spine deformity in neurofibromatosis. *J. Bone Joint Surg.* **61A**, 677–694.

Wyllie W.G. (1923) The occurrence in osteitis deformans of lesions of the central nervous system with a report of four cases. *Brain* **46**, 336–351.

Yonenobu K., Fuji T., Ono K., Okada V., Yamamoto T. and Harada N. (1985) Choice of surgical treatment for multisegmental cervical spondylotic myelopathy. *Spine* **10**, 710–716.

Chapter 22
Low Back Pain

J.R. Johnson

INTRODUCTION

Four out of five people suffer from low back pain at some time in their life. However, 80–95% of patients having an acute attack recover within 3 months. In the majority of patients presenting to a doctor with back pain, no objective cause of the pain can be found even after a thorough examination. One study in the USA found that back pain was the most frequent cause of limitation of activity in people under the age of 45 years and ranked only third after heart disease and arthritis in the 46–65-year-old age group.

The prognosis for patients whose back pain persists for longer than 6 months is poor. Many never return to work and the problem seems to be increasing. Back ache has become one of the commonest causes of disability in the UK. Twelve million days are lost by 300 000 people every year. Roughly one million patients consult their GP for back pain every year. Of these, some 300 000 are referred to hospital, 30 000 are eventually admitted to hospital for one reason or another and 5000 require an operation on the back. The number of permanently disabled back sufferers in the UK is estimated at around 80 000. Disability associated with back ache appears to be on the increase. In the USA, in the 1970s and 1980s, the number of people registered disabled with back pain increased by 168%, while the population only increased by 12.5%. There has certainly been a change in attitude over the past 50 years with more patients complaining of a back injury rather than back ache, perhaps with compensation in mind. Although back ache reaches a peak in the middle years, degenerative changes continue throughout life. It has been shown that there is no obvious relationship between degenerative changes and low back pain (Fig. 22.1). Indeed low back pain seems to occur with about the same frequency in patients in sedentary occupations as those doing heavy labour. Many believe that almost all low back pain is caused by

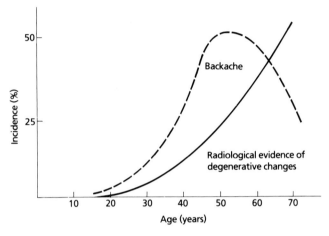

Fig. 22.1 Although radiological changes progress relentlessly with age, the incidence of back ache peaks in the fifties and there is therefore no good relationship between radiography and patient symptoms.

poor sitting posture and much work is now being done in the field of ergonomics to try to improve posture at home and in the workplace to reduce the time lost through episodes of back pain.

This chapter will consider the common clinical syndromes causing back pain with reference to the appropriate investigations and management of these problems. When examining a patient, possible differential diagnoses should never be forgotten. Pain referred to the spine is common in many non-orthopaedic conditions, e.g. vascular, renal, gastrointestinal and gynaecological. Normally there are other symptoms in these related areas which help make the diagnosis, but this is not always so.

DIAGNOSIS

As in other areas of medicine, the diagnosis of spinal

765

conditions depends largely on the history and physical examination.

History

Often the only symptom is pain and it may be extremely difficult to identify the location of the pain because it is often non-specific. It is important to try to describe the character of the pain, for example, whether it is dull or sharp.

The site of the pain is important. This can be demonstrated by the patient in the form of a pain drawing (Fig. 22.2) which is useful in showing the site and distribution of the pain, and in psychological evaluation (Ransford *et al.*, 1976). Patients are usually happy to record their pain on a drawing and this can then be put in the patient records.

An important aspect of the history-taking is to elicit what factors make the pain better or worse. Back pain is normally related to activity and patients should be specifically asked whether they are better or worse standing, sitting, walking or resting. For example, continuous pain which extends through the night, suggests a spinal tumour. A patient with an acute disc may find sitting

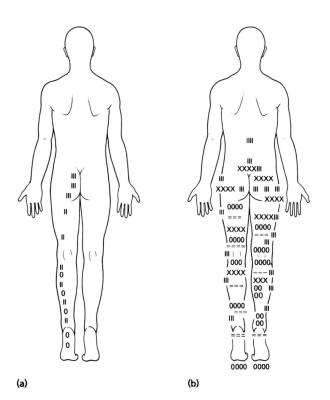

(a)   **(b)**

Fig. 22.2 Pain. (a) Patient describing the physical pattern of an S1 sciatica from a disc prolapse; (b) patient with simple back ache is communicating distress. (From Ransford *et al.*, 1976).

difficult and be better getting up and walking around, whereas a patient with spinal stenosis may not be able to walk far and will be relieved by sitting. It is useful to know how the pain started, whether there is a history of injury, and whether the pain is getting better or worse. The most accurate way to measure pain is by asking the patient to use a visual analogue scale from 0 to 10.

Another useful technique is to try to assess the degree of disability of the patient in everyday life. There are various pain and disability questionnaires available, which can be useful in assessing patients who have chronic pain.

Psychological assessment

Psychological factors can obviously affect the way patients experience and express their pain. In most cases, it is not necessary to undertake a formal psychological assessment of patients with back pain. These techniques, however, have been shown to be useful in patients with chronic pain, patients involved in litigation and patients who are clearly emotionally distressed (see below).

The examination

It should be remembered that a clinical examination is really a snapshot of a particular patient's impairment at a particular time on the day they are examined. Many of the tests described are subjective observations by an examiner. Recording in the notes is often vague and variations between examiners are common. There have been numerous attempts over the past few years to improve and standardize examination techniques. The aim is to ensure reproducibility between examiners and to have specific objective tests of lumbar impairment. This applies mainly to examination of the back itself. There is usually much less dispute over findings in the associated neurological examination. A suggested detailed examination technique is given in Appendix 2, p. 782.

Computer-aided diagnosis

There have been several recent studies made of the diagnostic performance of clinicians against that of a computer. With the advent of new computer programs, using artificial intelligence techniques, there have been studies to suggest that the computer can often outperform the clinician in the assessment of low back disorders (Mathew *et al.*, 1988).

Trunk-strength testing

There are now commercially available machines which test flexion/extension and to assess isometric, isotonic or isokinetic trunk strength in the sagittal and axial planes. These methods are useful in training patients to use their trunk muscles and in the assessment of patients with chronic low back pain. They have also been used to identify malingerers who are not putting their full effort into their spinal movement (see below). Waddell (1982) has shown that pain disability and impairment are all closely interrelated (Fig. 22.3) and to get an accurate assessment of the degree of severity of an impairment, all these elements have to be taken together.

DEGENERATIVE BACK DISEASE

Most low back disorders are caused by degeneration of one form or another, either in the disc itself or in the facet joints. There are three stages of the degenerative process. First, there is an initial phase of damage to the disc which is followed by an unstable phase where most of the problems arise. With time, further degeneration leads to a period of stabilization and any pain or discomfort disappears. The exception to this occurs when the degenerative change causes root involvement.

The degenerative process starts quite early in life with loss of some of the water content, and therefore hydrostatic pressure, within the nucleus of the disc. This, combined with minor repetitive injuries to the disc, causes secondary changes in the posterior facet joints.

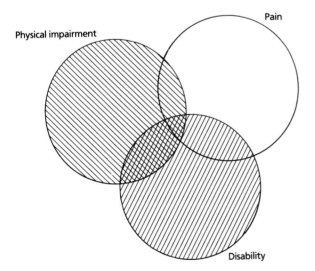

Fig. 22.3 The relationship between pain, disability and impairment showing the correlation and overlap between them. (From Waddell, 1982.)

While these progressive changes occur in everybody, not all patients suffer from back pain and it is probably the addition of more severe injuries that cause the clinical syndromes.

Mechanism of injury

There are two mechanisms involved in injury: rotational strains and compressive forces. Rotation mainly affects L4 and L5 and above, whereas L5 and S1 are more commonly affected by compressive forces which affect the disc first. This explains why the L4 and L5 joints are more susceptible to facet damage and degenerative changes.

Rotational strains of the disc initially cause circumferential tears but, later, radial tears occur from the edge of the annulus to the nucleus pulposus. It is down these radial tears that the nucleus can herniate to cause a prolapsed intervertebral disc.

There are three common clinical syndromes associated with degenerative changes in the lumbar spine.
1 The prolapsed intervertebral disc. This usually affects the young adult patient.
2 Lumbago. This syndrome causes severe back pain usually without sciatic or root symptoms and affects the middle-aged population.
3 Lateral canal stenosis (spinal stenosis). This is a syndrome causing root symptoms in the older patient.

The prolapsed intervertebral disc

Disc problems usually occur in patients in their twenties and forties although they can occur even into the sixties and seventies on occasion. At the other end of the spectrum is the adolescent disc which may occur between the ages of about 14 and 17 years.

Herniation of a disc can occur at any level but by far the commonest levels are L4 and L5, and L5 and S1. They therefore affect the root passing to the sciatic nerve and give rise to the main symptom of sciatica.

CLINICAL FEATURES

Patients with an acute prolapse intervertebral disc usually present with a variable amount of low back pain and sciatica. Often sciatica is the predominant symptom and is usually the more severe of the two symptoms. Sciatica should be defined as pain extending down the line of the sciatic nerve beyond the knee into the calf, as referred pain from the back or even from the hip can extend as far as the knee. Unlike referred pain, sciatic pain is normally associated with other neurological symptoms such as numbness, tingling, pins and needles or weakness. There is often a history of trauma and previous attacks of back pain without sciatica. Generally, the pain is made worse by sitting, especially driving, or standing for too long but is eased by getting up and walking around. The pain may be exacerbated by straining, for example coughing or sneezing. Lying down or resting relieves the pain.

On examination, there is a loss of the normal lumbar lordosis and patients often have a sciatic tilt of the spine to one side or the other. This is often called a 'scoliosis' but is distinguished from true scoliosis by the fact that there is no rotation of the spine. Flexion is usually very limited and increases the leg pain. Straight leg raising is usually grossly reduced on the side of the disc lesion and there is a positive sciatic stretch test. Pain on the affected side caused by lifting the unaffected leg is called 'crossed leg pain' and is almost pathognomonic of a prolapsed intervertebral disc. In addition there may be objective neurological signs such as an absent ankle jerk, weakness of the foot muscles or numbness in the L5 or S1 distribution.

INVESTIGATION (see Chapter 30)

Magnetic resonance imaging scanning, with its increasing availability, is the investigation of choice for the acute disc lesion in the younger patient. This investigation avoids radiation, is non-invasive and will clearly show a prolapsed intervertebral disc. It is often possible to distinguish between the contained disc and a sequestrated fragment which may be useful in helping to decide the best form of management (Fig. 22.4).

Computed tomography scanning, without contrast, is usually adequate for the young patient with an acute prolapsed intervertebral disc, if magnetic resonance imaging scanning is not available. In fact, in the lumbar spine generally, computed tomography scanning alone can show a prolapsed intervertebral disc without adding contrast. In the older patient, because of the associated degenerative changes, it may be difficult to identify the level of compression unless contrast medium is added to the investigation.

Radiculography alone will show the acute disc lesion as an impression in the dye column and under or non-filling of the nerve root on the affected side; however, this is an invasive procedure which is not without complications, and has been largely superseded by magnetic resonance imaging and computed tomography scanning.

MANAGEMENT

The majority of young patients presenting with the clinical syndrome of an acute prolapsed intervertebral disc will settle, with conservative management, over a period of 6–8 weeks. At the time of the initial severe episode of back pain and sciatica, a period of bed-rest, up to a week, may be helpful, especially if combined with anti-inflammatory drugs, pain killers and possibly a muscle relaxant. This period of bed-rest need not be in hospital, provided the facilities for full rest exist at home. After this, treatment by physiotherapy or other alternative methods may help, although it is difficult to know whether this actually shortens the period of natural healing.

INDICATIONS FOR SURGERY

The only absolute indication for surgery is the patient with an acute cauda equina syndrome with severe back pain, often bilateral sciatica and with bladder involvement. This requires immediate investigation and, if a central disc protrusion is shown, urgent surgery. Other indications for surgery are:
1 A patient with a progressive neurological deficit.
2 Patients who are not progressing and still have sciatic symptoms and signs after a period of bed-rest and physiotherapy. It is usually impossible to identify these patients within 3–6 weeks of treatment.
3 The patient with severe neurological symptoms when first seen, i.e. foot drop or quadriceps weakness, indicating a high disc.

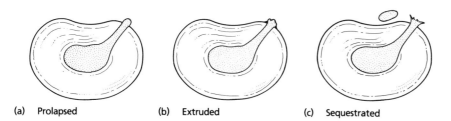

(a) Prolapsed   (b) Extruded   (c) Sequestrated

Fig. 22.4 Types of disc herniations. In all disc herniations the annular fibres are disrupted. In the prolapsed disc, the nucleus is confined by the outer fibre of the annulus. In the extruded disc, the nucleus breaks through and comes to lie under the posterior longitudinal ligament. In the sequestrated disc a free fragment of nuclear material comes to lie in the spinal canal.

4 The patient in whom the attack is not the first and has had recurrent attacks of severe back pain and sciatica over many months.

Surgery, by whatever method, is mainly directed towards removal of the protruding disc material and is therefore successful if the main symptom is sciatica. An assessment should be made of the ratio between low back pain and sciatica and surgery only offered if sciatica is the major symptom.

OPERATIVE TREATMENT

There is now quite a wide choice of procedure for the simple prolapsed intervertebral disc that has not responded to conservative measures. Minimally invasive techniques for removal of the disc have been developed, starting with microdiscectomy in the mid-1970s. More recently, various percutaneous techniques have been developed and even the use of the laser is being explored.

The aim of all these techniques is to relieve the sciatic pain and thus restore the patient's quality of life. With so many techniques now available it is difficult to make comparisons; it is probably true to say, however, that there are slight differences in the indications for the use of the various methods.

PERCUTANEOUS TECHNIQUES

Chemonucleolysis

The use of chymopapain to dissolve the nucleus of the disc was first suggested by Lyman Smith (1963) in the 1970s. There is a general consensus of opinion that this technique has a success rate of about 70%. The failure rate, in almost all cases, is due to the fact that percutaneous techniques cannot work in cases where there is a sequestrated disc protrusion or where there is lack of communication between the disc protrusion and the centre of the disc. Even with good magnetic resonance imaging scanning, it is sometimes impossible to be sure whether the disc is contained or not. Obviously, this technique should not be used in patients where there is clear evidence of sequestration or in patients over the age of 40 years, where there may be an element of facet joint degeneration contributing to the cause of root irritation. The best results have been obtained in younger patients with a typical acute prolapsed intervertebral disc. There have now been 10-year follow-up studies on the use of chymopapain, showing that these patients are not distinguishable from patients treated by surgery, except that there is a slight trend for surgical patients to have a higher incidence of repeat operation.

The procedure is carried out under local anaesthesia but with the anaesthetist present in case there is any anaphylactic reaction. The recorded rate of anaphylactic shock in a large series in Europe is 0.14%. It is advisable to have an intravenous infusion running and adrenaline ready in case it should be needed. Some centres give antihistamines and a small dose of steroid with the pre-medication.

Percutaneous discectomy (Fig. 22.5)

This approach was started by Hijikata in Japan in 1975. In this technique, a small (5 mm) cannula is inserted under image-intensifier control using the percutaneous route. This procedure is technically difficult at the L5 – S1 level because of the brim of the pelvis. Initially, a manual technique was developed and, in both Europe and America, specially developed arthroscopes have been used to view the disc so that disc material can be removed under direct vision.

In 1985, Onik reported a series of patients in which an automated aspiration probe (nucleotome) had been used to automatically cut and suck nuclear tissue again through the percutaneous route. This technique uses a 2-mm aspiration probe, again under image-intensifier control.

At about the same time, Asscher in Austria and others in America started to use a laser fibre placed under fluoroscopic control. Various lasers have been tried, e.g. neodymium: YAG, KTP, argon and ultraviolet. All these wavelengths appear to be suitable for use in the lumbar spine. There is no objective evidence, as yet, as to

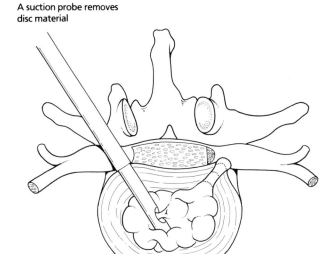

A suction probe removes disc material

Fig. 22.5 Percutaneous discectomy.

whether these techniques will be any advance over the ordinary percutaneous discectomy or chymopapain.

The percutaneous methods and the laser appear to give success rates of around 60–70%. As with chymopapain, the main reason for failure appears to lie in failing to recognize the sequestrated disc fragment. As for chymopapain, the indication should be the younger patient with the symptoms and signs of a unilateral acute prolapsed intervertebral disc with appropriate findings on imaging. The advantages of these techniques are the short hospital stay (day-case or overnight stay at the most) and the low overall complication rate. It is too early to tell whether these patients will have a higher recurrence rate compared with surgery and chymopapain in the long term. Certainly, the results of percutaneous discectomy are not as predictable as those of open discectomy.

Microdiscectomy (Fig. 22.6)

This technique was described in the mid-1970s, simultaneously by Williams in the USA and Yasargil and Caspar in Europe. After identification of the level, using the image intensifier in the operating room, a 2-cm skin incision is used, the ligamentum flavum is incised and the disc removed using the operating microscope. Several studies have shown that this procedure allows a more rapid convalescence with a shorter in-patient hospital stay and a more rapid return to work. The success rate is similar to that for standard disc surgery at around 90%. However, several groups have found that the hospital stay has been halved from 7 to 3–4 days. The com-

plication rate is similar to that of conventional disc surgery although there is probably a higher incidence of operating at the wrong level or missing pathology such as a sequestrated disc. Whether there is a higher rate of disc space infection (discitis) or a higher incidence of recurrent disc prolapse has not been proven and further longer-term studies are required.

Laminotomy (Fig. 22.7)

This technique involves removing a small amount of the lamina of the vertebra above the disc together with the ligamentum flavum on the side of the disc protrusion. Usually the muscles are only stripped on the symptomatic side. Using this technique, a protruding or sequestrated disc can be removed and the disc space cleared out.

Laminectomy (Fig. 22.8)

Laminectomy may be either hemi or total. Hemilaminectomy is sometimes useful for the exploration of two discs on the same side and a total laminectomy is occasionally used for removal of a large central disc lesion or to give better exposure, when there has been a complication, such as a dural tear. It may be necessary in order to adequately decompress a spinal stenosis (see below).

Foramenotomy/partial facetectomy (Fig. 22.9)

These techniques are used to enlarge the foramen through which the nerve root leaves the spinal canal.

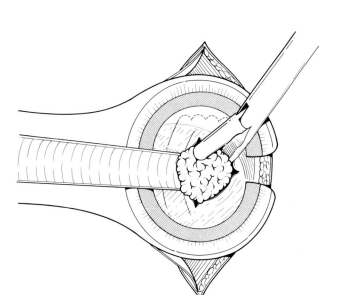

Fig. 22.6 Microdiscectomy.

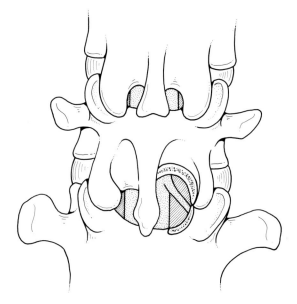

Fig. 22.7 Laminotomy.

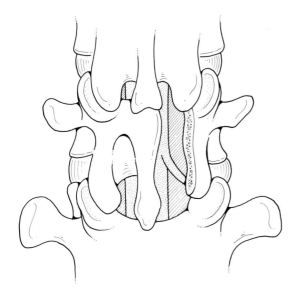

Fig. 22.8 Laminectomy.

This normally involves removing some of the superior facet of the vertebra below the disc and is a useful technique for dealing with lateral disc prolapses or lateral canal stenosis (see below).

Lumbago (back pain without sciatica)

This syndrome is characterized by back pain without sciatica. Patients often complain of a long history of low back pain which is intermittent. This is associated with more severe attacks which are often set off by some minor incident such as lifting or turning. The pain is associated with stiffness and often the patients find they are unable to get out of bed the day after the injury. The pain seems to be worse in the mornings and is often associated with stiffness which gradually subsides through the day. The acute attack usually subsides after 3–7 days and the patient gradually returns to normal over the ensuing 4–5 weeks. Often patients are woken at night, as they turn, as this sets off the pain and this suggests that some of the pain arises in the facet joints as well as in the disc.

The pain is in the lower lumbar area and may radiate into the buttocks. However, there is never any true sciatica with pain beyond the knee nor are there any associated neurological symptoms such as numbness or tingling. The pain is generally worse standing for prolonged periods or getting up from the sitting position, and by bending.

On examination there is often a loss of the lumbar lordosis caused by back spasm. All spinal movements are limited but particularly flexion. Straight-leg raising is normally fairly unrestricted although there is sometimes some pain in the back as the hamstrings are tightened. There is no neurological deficit on examination.

INVESTIGATIONS (see Chapter 30)

Plain radiography may show some degree of disc space narrowing but the investigation of choice is the magnetic resonance imaging scan which will show the degenerative disc or discs. The degenerate disc may be associated with a central disc bulge. This is differentiated from a prolapsed intervertebral disc by the fact that it is central, contained and usually not bulging to any severe degree.

MANAGEMENT

The degenerate disc is probably the commonest cause of back ache in the middle-aged group of patients. Having excluded any non-spondylogenic cause for the pain (e.g. malignancy), the patient can be reassured that this is just 'wear and tear' in their back and that the overall prognosis is good. As the disc continues to degenerate, the vertebrae sink closer together and the 'instability' resolves.

Usually, these patients respond well to advice from the physiotherapist on back-strengthening exercises and the back school with advice on how to lift and avoid exacerbating the problem. Wearing a corset during periods of prolonged standing or sitting may also help.

Acute attacks of lumbago usually respond to a period

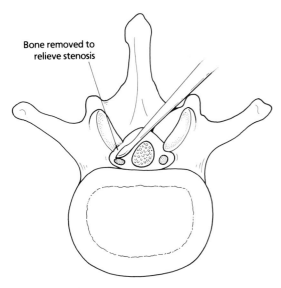

Bone removed to relieve stenosis

Fig. 22.9 Partial facetectomy.

of bed-rest together with the use of anti-inflammatory drugs, pain killers and if necessary a muscle relaxant.

Indications

There are no absolute indications for surgery in this condition. However, surgery may be advised in the younger patient with disc degeneration confined to one or at the most two discs. The main indication is pain following unsuccessful conservative management of the condition. The aim is to do the minimum to stabilize the affected segment but, before doing this, it is important to know that the discs on either side of the affected level are normal. Magnetic resonance imaging scanning will indicate which discs have a normal signal and if necessary provocative discography can also be carried out. This involves putting a needle into the lower lumbar discs, injecting some dye to see if the discs are normal, at the same time assessing whether the injection causes the sort of pain that the patient normally suffers.

Technique

Fusion may be carried out anteriorly using a trans-abdominal or retroperitoneal approach or more usually posteriorly, with bone graft placed between the transverse processes (Fig. 22.10). The latter approach may be combined with the use of some form of internal fixation. The current trend is to use pedicular screws combined with rods or plates to provide an immediate stable fixation of the diseased segment. The patient may then be mobilized quickly without a corset; however, there is no good evidence that these patients do any better in the long term than patients fused with bone graft alone.

Recently, a new technique has been described in which pedicle screws above and below the degenerate disc are connected with polyester bands. These pull the facet joints into extension and cause increased pressure on the posterior half of the disc. This technique is claimed to avoid the main disadvantage of fusion which is to put excessive strains on the normal discs above. At the same time, the 'instability' at the degenerate level is controlled. In the short term, this technique appears to work but longer-term studies are needed. Work is also progressing on an artificial disc. There is already one artificial disc commercially available and others are being evaluated. Again, long-term studies would be needed to show if these are an effective method of treatment for this type of problem.

Perhaps more important than the technique of fusion

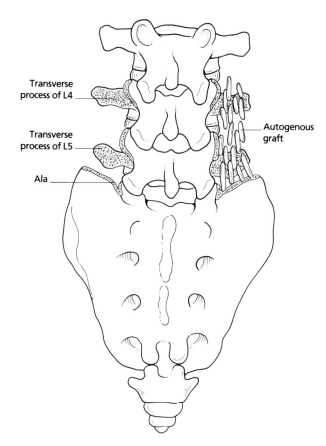

Fig. 22.10 Lateral mass or intertransverse fusion. (From Wiltse, 1968.)

is the selection of the patient and there is no doubt that the young patient with one level disc disease is likely to do better than the middle-aged patient with generalized degeneration and who is making a claim for an accident at work (see below).

Lateral canal stenosis (spinal stenosis) (Fig. 22.11)

This condition tends to affect the middle-aged-to-elderly patient and is characterized by intermittent claudication, i.e. pain on walking, relieved by rest. There is often a long history of low back pain before the leg symptoms start. The leg pain is characterized by pain on walking or standing; the walking is usually worse on inclines or going upstairs and is relieved by sitting or leaning forward. There is often a feeling of heaviness in the legs but usually not the typical numbness or tingling associated with a disc protrusion. Although lying down normally relieves all mechanical back pain, these patients are often unable to lie flat because the increased lordosis causes further pressure on the nerves.

On examination, the patient often stands with the

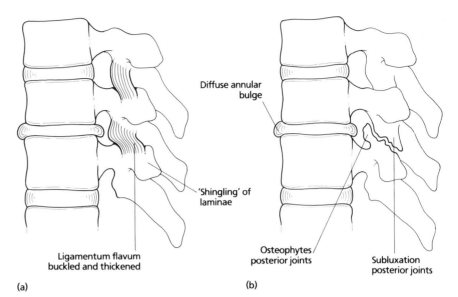

Fig. 22.11 In degenerative spinal stenosis, the spinal canal is narrowed by shingling of the laminae and by buckling of the ligamentum flavum. The arthritic posterior joints may hypertrophy and also encroach on the midline giving rise to further compression of the cauda equina. The emerging nerve roots are commonly compressed as they course through the narrow subarticular gutter.

(a) Ligamentum flavum buckled and thickened

(b) Diffuse annular bulge · 'Shingling' of laminae · Osteophytes posterior joints · Subluxation posterior joints

back flexed and walks with a slight stoop forwards. Flexion is normally full but extension is reduced and painful. Straight leg raising is often normal and it is quite common for there to be no objective neurological signs, although there may be a patchy sensory disturbance or absent reflexes.

The main differential diagnosis is vascular intermittent claudication. Distinction may be difficult. Patients with back pain suffer from vascular disease and may not have normal pulses. In the absence of a history of arterial disease and with normal pulses the condition is likely to be neurogenic in origin. One simple test is the bicycle test, whence cycling tolerance of the patient will be relatively unlimited if the condition is caused by neurogenic claudication. This is despite the fact that the patient may not be able to walk very far. If on the other hand there is vascular claudication, then the exercise tolerance is the same, whether the patient is walking or cycling.

INVESTIGATION

Magnetic resonance imaging scanning will show the areas of narrowing, but if there is more than one level involved, it may be difficult to see exactly which nerve roots are affected, with the current quality of scanning. With better quality scanners becoming available, this may not be so much of a problem in the future. Similarly computed tomography scanning alone tends to over-diagnose the number of levels of degeneration and does not show the nerve roots clearly. As far as surgical planning is concerned, the investigation of choice is still the radiculogram with or without associated computed tomography scanning. It is useful to have a dynamic study which allows the spine to be viewed in flexion and extension so that nerve root filling can be assessed accurately. Often, despite the fact that several levels are involved, only one level is causing the symptoms and it may be that only one level needs to be decompressed.

MANAGEMENT

Many patients can be managed with conservative measures, either by keeping within their exercise tolerance or by wearing a corset which will often reduce the lordosis enough to relieve symptoms. There may be a place for epidural injections and root-sleeve injections of local anaesthetic and steroid which can often work for a considerable length of time. Often deterioration is slow and for this reason conservative measures may be very successful.

SURGERY

Indications

The main indication for surgery is to relieve the symptoms of pain on walking and enable the patients to increase their walking distance and ability. Accurate pre-operative planning with a radiculogram and or scanning is important, so that the minimum amount of tissue is removed in order to achieve an adequate decompression.

Technique

The old technique of total laminectomy has now been

largely superseded by more limited focal decompressions of the individual nerve roots. The midline sections of a computed tomography or magnetic resonance imaging scan show no compression in the midline and therefore it is unnecessary to remove the midline structures. The aim is to reduce the size of the facet joints which are pressing on the nerve roots by a partial facetectomy or removal of the medial half of the facet joint releasing the nerve roots out to the foramen on each side (Fig. 22.9) (Getty *et al.*, 1981). If adjoining levels have to be decompressed, a thin bar of lamina can be left to support the dorsal spine and midline structures.

In some patients the narrowing is associated with a degenerative spondylolisthesis; this occurs particularly at L4 and L5 and a fusion may need to be added to the decompression, at this level, in patients in whom the disc space is still well preserved. If the affected disc is already narrow, then decompression alone is usually satisfactory, as no further slip will occur.

Failed back syndrome (post-laminectomy syndrome)

Not all patients do well after spinal surgery. Probably the most important reason for failure is the inappropriate selection of patients for surgery. Even with a good selection of patients, however, there may be failures either early or late.

In the case of disc surgery, early failures may be due to operation at the wrong level or on the wrong side, failure to find a sequestrated disc fragment, or damage to the nerve root or cauda equina. Late failures of disc surgery are usually due either to a recurrent disc, which may occur in up to 5% of patients, or to post-operative scarring.

In the case of degenerative disc disease, early failures may be due to failure of the fusion mass, i.e. pseudo-arthrosis or technical problems with internal fixation. Late failures may be due to degeneration at the disc above the fusion.

With spinal stenosis, early failures may be due to inadequate decompression or to technical complications with damage to nerve roots. Late failures may be due to recurrent disease or disease affecting another level, causing similar symptoms.

It is generally true that each successive operation to salvage a previous operation will be less successful. However, this may not be true if a specific new problem is identified pre-operatively and is found at operation.

Success with failed back patients therefore depends on good quality investigations. Plain radiographs may be useful in showing how much bone has been removed at a previous operation and in checking that the correct level and side has been operated upon. Up to now, the other investigations such as radiculograms, computed tomography scans and venograms have been relatively unhelpful because of their inability to distinguish between scar tissue (epidural fibrosis) and recurrent disc problems. They may, however, still be useful in identifying pathology if it is occurring at another level.

The main advance in any investigation of the problem back has been with the improvements in magnetic resonance imaging scanning. Using specific sequences it is now possible to differentiate between scar tissue and recurrent disc.

Therefore if there is a recurrent disc or other pathology at a different level or a previous inadequate decompression, then second or even third time surgery may be successful. If, on the other hand, the problem is due to scar tissue, then further surgery is unlikely to help. In the later case caudal epidural injections may help in dividing adhesions.

If surgery is not possible, an indirect approach by control of pain may be helpful and a combined approach with the use of the local pain clinic may be indicated.

Psychological factors may play a big part in the failed back syndrome and it is for this reason that the selection of patients pre-operatively is so important (see below). Often these problem patients are not diagnosed correctly until they have had several operations, by which time salvage is difficult.

Complications of spinal surgery

It should not be forgotten that spinal surgery carries with it a mortality rate. In two recent series there was a mortality rate of about 0.1%. Cauda equina lesions have been reported in 0.2% and dural lacerations in 2–4% of cases (Simmons and Wilber, 1978). Obviously, a dural laceration does not normally cause any problem unless a secondary meningocoele develops. The treatment of a dural laceration depends on its size. If it is very small or very large it may be left, otherwise the dura should be sutured or sealed with fibrin clot glue. Nerve root lesions occur in about 0.5% of cases. The result may be a foot drop or sphincter problem or areas of anaesthesia in the leg or perineum. Infection is rare but discitis or inflammation of the disc space may occur in about 0.1% of cases. Patients with discitis present with severe back pain and a raised erythrocyte sedimentation rate. Treatment should be with bed-rest or a plaster jacket, antibiotics and the patient will normally recover without further intervention. Deep infection is rare and it is treated by further exploration and curettage of the disc space.

BEHAVIOURAL SYNDROMES (PSYCHOGENIC BACK PAIN)

These patients develop an abnormal response to what starts as a genuine attack of back pain. Patients develop a lack of ability to cope with daily activities and subconsciously exaggerate their symptoms and disability. While it would clearly be impracticable to subject every patient arriving in the clinic to a full battery of psychological tests, there are some simple tests that can be added to the routine examination and if the level of suspicion is raised, further assessments can be carried out (see Appendix 2).

History

As already stated, mechanical back pain is normally associated with increased pain on activity, relieved by rest. Obviously patients who do not fit into this category either have a more sinister cause for their pain, which is non-spondylogenic, or may have a psychological cause for the pain. Pain affecting the arm and leg on one side, pain affecting the whole body, or glove and stocking numbness of the whole limb should be regarded with suspicion.

Before examination it may be useful to ask the patient to complete a pain drawing (Fig. 22.2) (Ransford *et al.*, 1976).

Examination (see Appendix 2)

On examination various inappropriate signs have been described (Waddell *et al.*, 1980), e.g. axial loading of the head, rotation of the body, apparent limitation of straight leg raising when lying but not when sitting and cog-wheel weakness of the foot have all been described. Waddell (1980) has shown quite clearly that patients in whom the inappropriate symptoms and signs are positive do not do as well following surgery, even if there is a demonstrable pathology shown on investigation or at operation.

Litigation

It is quite common for patients involved in litigation to develop the behavioural neuroses described above. These patients usually present themselves for examination for a medical report on behalf of their solicitors. The injury, which has always occurred at work, is usually over a year old. Despite the time factor, the patient can always remember the exact date of the incident and the exact details. The severity of the injury is usually out of all proportion to the apparent disability of the patient when seen for examination some years later. The patient has usually never returned to work from the date of the accident. The patient often brings a partner with them to help them dress and undress and walks with one or two sticks or even is brought in in a wheelchair. On examination, there is usually gross exaggeration of the limitation of spinal movements with added sound affects, e.g. grunts and groans. The inappropriate signs described above are all positive. The main point about the physical signs is that they are often inconsistent between different examinations and different examiners. Confrontation with the patient does not seem to help and they usually just become aggressive. This is because the behavioural syndrome has become subconscious and the patient does not believe that he or she is malingering. There is research being carried out using trunk-strength testing machines which can pick up inconsistencies in the effort required to flex and extend against resistance.

In addition to this group, there is a small number of definite malingerers who are trying to make a financial gain from a minor accident at work. These have been caught in the past by using private investigators and video cameras to provide evidence of them walking normally to and from the doctors' surgery or even doing manual work.

SPONDYLOLISTHESIS

Spondylolisthesis is the slipping of one vertebra from another. This can be partial or even complete. The term was described by Kilian in 1854 and later classified first by Newman and then by the International Society for the Study of the Lumbar Spine. The classification is as follows (Fig. 22.12):

1 Congenital.

Type A dysplastic. In this case, the articular facets are orientated axially and are often combined with spina bifida. This together with a rounded top to the sacrum, allows the L5 vertebrae to slip.

Type B. This has a sagittal orientation allowing an unstable junction between L5 and S1.

Type C. Other congenital abnormalities such as congenital kyphosis.

2 Isthmic. In these cases the lesion is in the pars intra-articularis.

(a) Lytic. In this type there is a stress fracture of the pars.

(b) Elongated. This has a elongated but intact pars which may be secondary to an old healed stress fracture.

3 Degenerative. This is due to long-standing instability

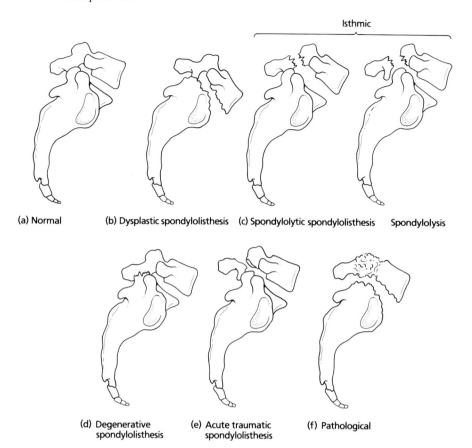

Isthmic

(a) Normal   (b) Dysplastic spondylolisthesis   (c) Spondylolytic spondylolisthesis   Spondylolysis

(d) Degenerative spondylolisthesis   (e) Acute traumatic spondylolisthesis   (f) Pathological

Fig. 22.12 Classification of lumbospondylolisthesis. (After Wiltse *et al.*, 1976.)

with a degenerative disc; it usually occurs at L4–L5 and is described further under the heading of lateral canal stenosis (see above, p. 772).

4 Post-traumatic. This results from acute fractures in the areas of the bony hook other than the pars itself.

5 Pathological. This type results from generalized or localized bone disease. With destruction of the posterior elements, the vertebrae can slip on the one below.

6 Post-surgical or iatrogenic. This is due to loss of the posterior bony support secondary to wide surgical decompression.

There is a strong genetic element to both the dysplastic and isthmic types of spondylolisthesis. This was shown in a study by Wynn-Davies and Scott who often noted an association with spina bifida occulta at L5 or S1 or both. The incidence of spondylolisthesis is around 5% although it is never seen in children below the age of 5 years. The suggestion therefore, is, that there is a combination of a congenital abnormality and stress of the pars caused by trauma. In these patients, there is a congenital risk for fracture at the pars and also for a slip of the dysplastic type, caused by hypoplasia of the posterior arches of L5 or S1 or both.

The other type of isthmic spondylolisthesis seen commonly occurs in young adults engaged in strenuous training. The incidence of pars defects in young female gymnasts is nearly four times the average of normal. The incidence of spondylolisthesis is clearly larger than the number of patients who complain of low back pain. Studies of the natural history of types 1 and 2 have been carried out. From these, it would appear that isthmic spondylolisthesis with a slip of up to 10% carries no higher risk of low back pain than a patient with no slip. For a slip between 10% and 25% there may be some increase in the instance of back pain and sciatica. Beyond 25% is almost certain that patients are predisposed to symptoms.

The slipping in types 1 and 2 appears to occur soon after puberty. At this stage, patients may present either with pain and or spasm in the spinal muscles and in particular the hamstrings. On examination, there is usually a sciatic scoliosis in the lumbar spine and reduction of straight leg raising. Neurological signs are very uncommon.

If there is a sudden slip, patients can present acutely with the so-called 'lumbar crisis'; these patients present tilted forward into flexion with much spasm and the hamstrings are so tight they cannot stand up straight. This gives them a rather bizarre posture and gait.

Management

In view of the natural history of the condition, the management of spondylolisthesis should be conservative if possible. Indeed, in several series, patients treated conservatively with low-grade spondylolisthesis have done rather better in the long term than patients who have had surgery.

Conservative management

Initially, patients usually present with pain with or without spasm and an abnormal gait. These patients should be stopped from any sporting activities, given a lumbosacral support, analgesia as required and then monitored on a regular basis with yearly radiography to ensure that the displacement does not increase. Young patients presenting with a lumbar crisis may require an initial period of bed-rest and if this does not settle, may require surgery.

In the skeletally mature patient, the treatment is by conservative measures, for example analgesia, corset and physiotherapy.

Surgery

Children with type 1 and type 2 spondylolisthesis may require surgery if they (i) present with a lumbar crisis, (ii) present with a displacement which is already more than 50% and (iii) continue to progress, despite regular observation and conservative management. These patients do very well with a fusion *in situ*, without decompression, using the lateral spinal approach described by Wiltse (1968) (Fig. 22.10). They get up after a few days and do not usually require a corset or brace. If there is a large slip with rotation of the L5 vertebrae, then the fusion should be carried up to the level of L4. Attempts have been made to reduce and fuse severe slips; however, there is a danger of neurological complications and long-term follow-up studies have shown that fusion *in situ* is perfectly satisfactory.

Type 2 isthmic spondylolisthesis

These are often stress fractures in young athletes, e.g. fast bowlers in cricket. In the acute stages, it may be difficult to see the fracture and this may only be shown as a crack revealed by a hot spot on a bone scan.

Oblique films reveal the classic 'Scottie dog' silhouette. If the pars defect occurs at L5 in an adult, the situation is stable and no slip is likely. However, at L4 and above, later degenerative changes in the disc may cause the situation to deteriorate and spondylolisthesis to increase.

Treatment

Again, the acute pars fracture can be treated conservatively with rest and a plaster jacket. Normally these will heal quite satisfactorily within 3–6 months. Even if the fracture does not heal, patients are often asymptomatic and able to resume their sporting activities.

If the patient is young and there is no slip, the pars intra-articularis can be fused or repaired. The earliest technique was described by Buck (1970) who passed a screw through the pars interarticularis with or without bone graft. Nicol and Scott (1986) advocated passing wires around the base of the transverse processes and winding them around the spinous process. Morscher *et al.* (1984) has described a hook which goes around the loose lamina and screws into the lateral mass. Although these work in the young patient the question is whether they would be asymptomatic if treated conservatively in any case. Over the age of 25 years, simple repair may not work because of degenerative changes in the associated disc.

In the older patient, in whom there is continuing pain and failed conservative management, an intertransverse fusion, by the Wiltse technique, is very successful at the L5–S1 level (Fig. 22.10) At levels above this, treatment depends on whether the disc space is of a normal height and whether the patients have neurological symptoms. In the older patient, with a spondylolisthesis and sciatica, decompression alone with resection of the whole lamina (Gill's operation) is often successful especially at L5–S1. At levels above this, however, further slipping may occur as the disc degenerates. Therefore, at these levels, fusion is used for patients with back pain only and decompression and fusion used for patients with sciatic symptoms. With the advent of good methods of internal fixation using pedicle screws, fusion above the level of L5 is normally performed by combining internal fixation with lateral mass bone graft.

CONGENITAL ABNORMALITIES AFFECTING THE LUMBAR SPINE

Spina bifida

Minor degrees of spina bifida are common but as stated above are quite commonly associated with other lesions such as spondylolisthesis. Spina bifida occulta is of no importance and the incidence of back pain in these patients is no higher than in the normal population.

Severe spina bifida is less common with pre-natal assessment and diagnosis and unselective closure of the defect is no longer practised.

Segmental abnormalities

Abnormalities of segmentation are common with either lumbarization of S1 or sacralization of L5 but, again, there is no evidence that these abnormalities cause an increased incidence of back pain. The incidence of some form of segmental anomaly is probably in the region of 15%.

Dysraphism

These patients have a bifurcation or splitting of the spinal cord often associated with a bony spike in the midline between the halves.

Patients often present with back pain with variable neurological symptoms and signs. They may need surgical treatment to free the tethered spinal cord and excise any midline bone.

OTHER CONDITIONS AFFECTING THE LUMBAR SPINE

Trauma

Fractured spines occur in young adults, often as a result of a fall from a height. This may be a suicide attempt or a fall off a building site. Patients with fractures of the calcaneum should always be assessed carefully for spinal fractures. Management of these fractures may be conservative or operative following careful assessment. If there is a complete paraplegia patients are usually transferred to a spinal injuries unit. With no paraplegia or partial paraplegia there may be an indication for surgery if computed tomography scanning shows encroachment of the spinal canal at the level of the fracture. These fractures normally occur in the thoracolumbar region and if there is a significant kyphosis or burst fracture, patients may require reduction and stabilization with internal fixation.

In the elderly woman spontaneous fractures may occur in the lumbar spine due to osteoporosis; these are normally treated conservatively with bed-rest and analgesia. Secondary malignancy has to be excluded

in these patients by clinical examination and bone scanning.

Infection (see Chapter 15)

Infected lesions normally attack the disc and then involve the vertebral bodies on either side (Fig. 22.13). Radiographic changes may not develop for 6–8 weeks after the acute infection starts. Infective agents are commonly *Staphylococcus* or tuberculosis, although increasingly, other rare organisms, e.g. *Salmonella*, are seen in the spine.

A more localized inflammation of the disc or discitis may occur after surgery. These patients present with acute severe low back pain with much muscle spasm.

INVESTIGATION

Investigation may include radioactive bone scans together with needle biopsy under radiographic control so that the appropriate antibiotics can be used.

TREATMENT

Most infections can be treated with conservative management although the occasional case of tuberculosis has to be opened and drained. Collapsed vertebrae can then be filled with bone graft.

A good approach for the infected spine, which is usually only over one level, is the costotransversectomy with an extra-peritoneal approach into the infected area.

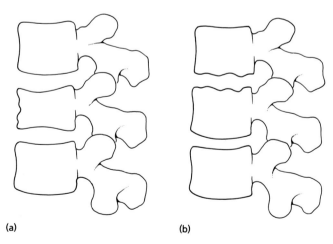

(a)   (b)

Fig. 22.13 The radiological differentiation between tumours and infection. (a) A typical tumour affecting the vertebral body initially; (b) a spinal infection which affects the disc first and then the bodies subsequently.

TUMOURS

Primary tumours of the lumbar spine are rare, accounting for about 0.4% of all tumours. They are often missed because they present with the universal complaint of low back pain, but unlike mechanical pain, the pain tends to be constant. There should always be a high index of suspicion in patients who have symptoms of back pain at night or pain at rest. Radicular pain or neurological signs are often a late presentation. It is not unusual for the interval from onset of symptoms for the diagnosis to be prolonged, particularly with benign lesions.

Benign tumours

The most common benign spinal lesions are hae-mangiomas, osteoid osteomas and osteoblastomas. Giant-cell tumours and aneurysmal bone cysts also occur in the lumbar spine. Diagnosis is normally by computed tomography scanning, magnetic resonance imaging scanning and or a bone scan.

Malignant tumours

Malignant tumours tend to arise from the main vertebral body with its subsequent collapse and this is the main differentiation between a likely tumour and infection that affects the disc space. The mean age at diagnosis is higher for patients with malignant tumours than those with benign tumours, and the commonest neoplasms are secondary deposits from another primary.

Patients with primary malignant tumours more commonly have associated neurological symptoms and signs.

The most common malignant neoplasm is myeloma but other primary malignant tumours have been seen in the spine, e.g. chordoma, chondrosarcoma, Ewing's sarcoma and osteosarcoma.

Metastatic tumours

Two-thirds of cancer cases develop metastases and the skeletal system is the third most common site. The most common primary tumours that metastasize to bone are breast and prostate followed by thyroid, lung and kidney. The spine is the most common site of the skeletal metastases irrespective of the primary tumours. Spinal metastases are often asymptomatic being dis-covered by routine bone scans as part of follow-up treatment.

Treatment may be operative or non-operative. If there is no neurological impairment, the patients are normally irradiated or given chemotherapy, depending on the primary tumour. If there is a neurological deficit which is slowly progressive, again radiation often works well. Depending on the tumour and the prognosis, however, surgery may be the treatment of choice in patients who are becoming paraplegic. The current approach to tumours, because they tend to involve the vertebral bodies, is an anterior approach with decompression of the tumour and stabilization using internal fixation together with bone graft, a bone substitute or metallic strut or device.

GROWTH DISORDERS

Osteochondritis (Calvé's disease)

This is an extremely rare cause of back pain. Treatment is with conservative measures and the vertebra normally returns back to its normal shape. The differential diag-nosis is from solitary eosinophilic granuloma which has similar radiographic appearances.

Scheuermann's disease

Although classically this affects the dorsal spine causing kyphosis, it may cause anterior irregularity and lipping in the lumbar spine though these are often radiographic findings and are of little clinical significance.

Lumbar scoliosis (see Chapter 4)

Lumbar scoliosis may occur in adults, either because of inadequate treatment of adolescent scoliosis or because of subsequent osteoporosis. Patients may develop sciatic symptoms with lateral canal stenosis caused by osteo-arthritic changes developing in the facet joints. Recently, attempts have been made to correct adult scoliosis. There has, however, been a high complication rate and normally patients are treated on their symptoms with localized decompressions of spinal stenosis as and where necessary.

Arthropathies

Ankylosing spondylitis classically affects young men (see also Chapter 17). As well as back pain, there is associated stiffness of the spine and a good clue to the diagnosis is that patients often experience aches and pains of a rheumatic nature in other joints in the body. These patients may also suffer night pain.

On examination, stiffness of the spine is found, but

usually no limitation of movements of the lower limbs or neurological signs. Classically, a restricted chest expansion may be found although this is not always so. Radiography may show early changes in the sacro-iliac joints but often they are normal. Blood tests may show seropositivity. Technetium bone scans may be helpful in showing areas of increased uptake in the sacro-iliac joints and in the spine itself. Eventually, the sacro-iliac joints ossify followed by the lumbar spine and occasionally the hips. Without treatment, increasing kyphosis develops until patients can no longer see where they are walking. The apex of the kyphosis is often in the upper thoracic region. Untreated disease like this is increasingly rare as it is possible to prevent this complication occurring with early postural treatment and physiotherapy. The modern treatment is with anti-inflammatory drugs together with at least 20 min of physiotherapy daily.

If ankylosis of the hips occur, a total hip replacement may be valuable in correcting fixed flexion deformities. Although the kyphosis occurs in the upper thoracic spine, it is safer to correct the spine in the upper lumbar region and this can be done by a wedge osteotomy combined with internal fixation.

METABOLIC DISORDERS (see also Chapter 14)

Osteoporosis

Osteoporosis is normally asymptomatic unless a pathological fracture occurs (see trauma above, p. 778).

Fractures may cause severe pain and may require inpatient bed-rest followed by physiotherapy and analgesia. By the time fractures occur, it is usually rather late to treat the osteoporosis, particularly as the only effective treatment is probably hormone replacement therapy. Premature osteoporosis may occur in younger patients on steroids or with other hormonal abnormalities.

Osteomalacia

Back pain may occur with this condition which is due to lack of vitamin D. This may occur in patients who are vegetarian or in patients who have had radical gastric surgery or renal disease. Back pain may occur but there is normally generalized skeletal pain and often fractures in the peripheral skeleton.

APPENDIX 1 ANATOMY OF THE LUMBAR SPINE: THE VERTEBRA

Vertebral body

The body of the vertebra consists of a thin cylinder of cortical bone filled with soft cancellous bone. As the bone ages, it loses calcium and strength and then becomes vulnerable to compression, resulting in the fracture seen in osteoporotic elderly patients.

The upper lumbar vertebrae are cylindrical in shape with slight flattening posteriorly; however, the lower lumbar vertebra becomes progressively more kidney-

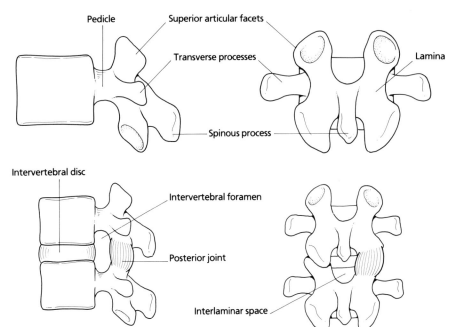

Fig. 22.14 The skin-marking technique of measuring lumbar flexion.

shaped and this affects the stresses that are brought to bear on the intervertebral disc.

Vertebral arch

The vertebral arch consists of dense cortical bone and starts with the pedicle which projects from the upper part of the body. The superior facet projects from the upper end and from the lower end the lamina and the inferior facet hang down over the disc below. The part between the two facet joints is called the pars intra-articularis which is an area subject to developmental failure and trauma (Fig. 22.14).

The transverse processes project laterally and are equivalent to the ribs of the thoracic region. The fifth transverse process may be attached to the sacrum on one or other sides in about 5% of patients.

The spinus processes in the lumbar spine are large and square and may be absent at L5 and below.

The facet joints have an important variation in alignment. Throughout the lumbar spine at L3−L4, they lie in the sagittal plain and allow little or no rotation, at L4−L5 and at the lumbosacral level, the joints lie more obliquely and allow some rotation. The lower facet joints may also be asymmetrical and there is a suggestion that this affects the disc at the L4−L5 and lumbosacral levels and may cause degeneration.

The spinal canal (Porter *et al.*, 1980) is oval proximally and becomes triangular in shape as one progresses distally. The capacity of the canal tends to reach a narrow point at L4−L5 and then starts to enlarge again towards the sacrum.

The L4−L5 level therefore tends to be the most vulnerable segment both because of the narrow spinal canal and because of facet joint hypertrophy. This results in the L4−L5 level being the commonest site for degenerative spondylolisthesis and for spinal stenosis.

Facet pain tends to refer in to the buttock and back of the thighs. It does not radiate beyond the knee. There are usually no sensory or motor disturbances. The pain is often worse in extension.

Intervertebral disc

The intervertebral disc consists of an outer annulus fibrosus of strong fibres arranged in radial ply configuration and softer nucleus which takes the forces of compression. The disc is separated from the vertebral body by the cartilaginous end plate which rests on a thin layer of cortical bone (Hickey *et al.*, 1980). In the lower kidney-shaped discs, the stresses tend to be concentrated at the areas of maximum convexity, i.e. at the two poles of the disc. The disc itself is reinforced anteriorly and posteriorly by the anterior and posterior longitudinal ligaments. Disc damage is thought to arise because of compression plus rotation which tends to occur at the lower disc levels.

The nucleus pulposus consists of a proteoglycan complex which retains water and acts as a shock absorber by distributing the stresses of compression to the surrounding annulus. At birth the nucleus has a water content of 88% which drops to about 80% by the age of 12 years. With increasing age, the nucleus continues to dry out and changes from a gelatinous structure. Nachemson (1981) has shown that pressure within the nucleus varies with posture, being highest when sitting with the back unsupported and lowest when lying supine. Lifting and bending can therefore cause sudden fluctuations in disc pressure.

The disc is relatively avascular and therefore has a limited capacity to heal. The nerve supply is mainly peripheral and discogenic pain is therefore deep aching-type pain.

Muscles and ligaments

These structures play a vital role in supporting and controlling the vertebral column. Pain arising in these structures has the same character and distribution as pain arising in the vertebral bodies and discs, with varying acuteness depending on the mechanism of injury.

The pain from a sprained ligament is aggravated by passive stretching. The pain in a damaged muscle is aggravated by active contraction of the damaged muscle. Both are relieved by relaxing the damaged tissue.

The ligaments of the sacro-iliac joints are often singled out for special attention. The diagnosis of chronic sacro-iliac strain is no longer fashionable but undoubtedly does occur later in pregnancy and in the early puerperium. It can also occur in association with certain sports, in particular Association Football, where chronic laxity in the sacro-iliac ligaments can occur. This results in pain both in the region of the sacro-iliac joints and in the symphysis pubis. Confirmation of this instability can be obtained by taking anteroposterior radiographs of the pelvis with the patient standing on one leg at a time when the level of the pubic rami will be noted to change (Harris and Murray, 1974).

Spinal cord and lumbar nerve roots

The spinal cord ends opposite either the first or second lumbar vertebra in the adult and more distal in the infant. Below this level, the dural tube contains the lumbar and spinal roots, the cauda equina. At the upper levels of the lumbar spine, the roots pass more horizontally and laterally and lie above the related disc space.

The lower roots lie more vertically so that a disc lesion in the conventional posterolateral situation will tend to involve the root passing to the vertebra below but, if large or with a lateral extension, can involve the root at the same level. For instance, a disc lesion at the L4−L5 level involves the L5 root and only the L4 root if there is a significant portion laterally. Similarly, the disc lesion at the lumbosacral level most commonly involves the first sacral root.

Distribution of the nerve roots

Segmental variations are common and it is therefore difficult to pinpoint the level of a lesion clinically. Where it is necessary to know the level accurately, i.e. when surgery is planned, precise localization is made with radiological investigations such as magnetic resonance imaging scanning.

Sensation

Published dermatomes are a reasonable guide with L4 being distributed down the medial side of the calf, L5 down the outer side of the calves and S1 on the sole and up the back of the legs.

Motor

Each movement of joint in the leg is controlled by two spinal segments (Last, 1963) which progress steadily caudally and are generally adequate for clinical assessment. Hip flexion is controlled by L2 and L3, hip extension by L4 and L5, knee extension by L3 and L4, and knee flexion by L5 and S1. Dorsiflexion of the ankle is controlled by L4 and L5 and plantar flexion by S1 and S2. Extensor hallucis longus is normally controlled by L5 and flexor hallucis longus by S1.

Root irritation

In acute disc lesions and true inflammatory conditions, the root is irritated and inflamed and responds to the slightest contact with pain radiating down the distribution of root. This pain is sharp, well defined and sometimes excruciating to the extent that the accompanying numbness or tingling is submerged. The related muscles go into protective spasm producing limited movement and the adoption of a posture which minimizes the contact with the inflamed nerve root.

When the sciatic roots are involved, the normal lordosis is obliterated and a sciatic scoliosis may develop. The direction of the scoliosis is unrelated to the side of the disc prolapse and depends more on the relationship of the disc to the nerve root. Limitation of forward flexion and straight leg raising is normally accompanied by a positive sciatic stretch test (see Appendix 2).

Root compression

When the root is actually compressed, pain as above may occur but in extreme instances pain disappears leaving areas of depressed sensation or even anaesthesia, motor weakness and depression of reflexes. On relief of this compression, within a reasonable period, sensation and motor power recover but the reflexes seldom return to normal. If compression is maintained too long, recovery of sensation and motor power may not occur. Large central disc prolapses are particularly notorious for causing permanent paralysis of bladder and bowel.

Root entrapment

Degenerative changes with or without pre-existing congenital stenosis can result in narrowing of the spinal and neural canals leading to the roots being trapped in rigid bony canals which they exactly fit.

At rest, the patient is free of symptoms and apart from the expected degree of loss of motion for a patient of that age, no abnormality can be found on clinical examination. If the patient stands or walks for any length of time, pain with or without radiation into one or both legs develops. It is ill-defined and is accompanied by various sensory symptoms and motor phenomena. The patient has difficulty in describing these and they can include various paraesthesiae with cramp-like pain in the muscles, or a feeling of the muscles being leaden or wooden or simply that the muscles will not act.

This pattern is similar to that of intermittent claudication due to muscle ischaemia and is aggravated by walking up hill and climbing stairs. Unlike intermittent vascular claudication, neurogenic claudication is not relieved by standing and relief is only gained from sitting or bending forwards. Patients with neurogenic claudication have normal pulses and often find they can ride a bicycle although they cannot walk.

Patients with neurogenic claudication are often ignored because so little is found on clinical examination. If the patient is exercised, however, sensory and motor changes may be noted.

Unfortunately, spinal stenosis and vascular intermittent claudication tend to affect the same age group of

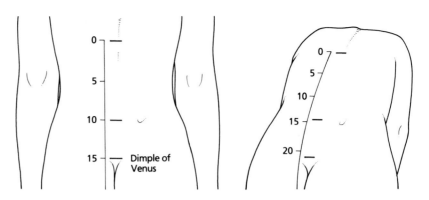

Fig. 22.15 The components of a lumbar vertebra: the body, the superior and inferior facets, the transverse and spinous processes, and the intervertebral foramen and its relationship to the intervertebral disc and the posterior joint.

patients and indeed may occur in the same individual which may make diagnosis difficult.

Vascular supply

The arterial supply to the neural elements in the lumbar spine is not so critical as in the cervical and dorsal regions (Domisse, 1974). The veins are in direct communication with the abdominal and pelvic veins without any valvular control between the two systems. When operating on the spine, it is therefore essential to position the patient so that there is no compression of the abdomen, otherwise venous bleeding may be disastrous.

The intimate relationship between the spinal and pelvic veins also explains the risk of spread of infection to the lumbar spine from the lower renal tract, bladder and prostate (Crock *et al.*, 1973).

The veins on the anterior wall of the spinal canal form a ladder-like pattern and it is possible to visualize these veins by lumbar venography. This technique has been used to demonstrate disc protrusions. It is a technically difficult procedure however, and is not helpful in patients who have had previous surgery. This technique has rather been superseded by good radiculography and more recently magnetic resonance imaging scanning.

APPENDIX 2 EXAMINATION OF THE SPINE

Clinical examination is really an assessment of patient impairment at a particular time. Many parts of the examination are subjective and therefore recording is vague and variations between examiners are often widespread. It is normal with any examination of the back to start with the patient standing. In order to avoid confusion between back movement and hip movement or hamstring tightness, the skin-marking technique is useful (Fig. 22.15) Skin marks are made in the back and when the patient bends forward, the increase in distance between the upper and lower marks are taken as a measure of lumbar flexion; alternatively, a goniometer can be used.

Pain, on extending from the flexed position, often suggests problems in the facet joints, such as lateral canal stenosis or segmental instability. A sciatic tilt on forward flexion suggests a prolapsed intervertebral disc. Although lateral flexion and rotation are often measured, these tests have little clinical significance.

Patient prone on the couch

With the patient prone on the couch, palpation down the length of the spine may reveal areas of tenderness. Again, however, this is of variable reliability. While the patient is prone, it is useful to carry out the femoral stretch test with lifting of the thigh and then flexion of the knee (Fig. 22.16). If this causes pain down the front of the thigh, the femoral stretch test is positive. Finally, it is often much easier to test the ankle jerks by flexing the knee to 90° and carrying out the ankle reflex in the prone position.

Patient supine on the couch

With the patient supine on the couch, straight leg raising tests can be performed, followed by the Lasegue test and bow-string sign. Restriction of straight leg raising suggests root irritation. Pain in the opposite leg, i.e. cross-leg pain, is highly suggestive of a prolapsed intervertebral disc. Increased tension can be put on the sciatic root by dorsiflexion of the ankle which aggravates the pain in the back. Tension can be removed by flexing the knee and flexing the hip. If the knee is extended from this position and causes pain, Lasegue's test is positive.

The best test for sciatic tension is the bow-string test (Fig. 22.17). The hip is flexed to 90° and the knee extended as far as the patient will tolerate and then

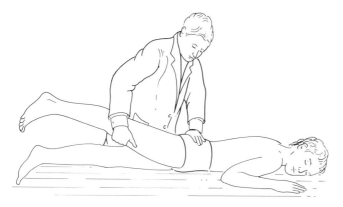

Fig. 22.16 The femoral stretch test with the compression of L4. The patient experiences pain down the front of the thigh. This pain is aggravated if the hip is extended and then the knee flexed.

pressure is applied with the thumb to the hamstrings. This will immediately cause pain if the test is positive.

Nerve compression signs

A standard neurological examination is then performed. Usually, any sensory, motor or reflex deficit will be confined to a single root origin and therefore the finding of whole leg pain or whole leg weakness or indeed stocking anaesthesia suggests a non-organic cause.

NON-ORGANIC SIGNS

Waddell (1980) described five tests to perform during the routine back examination:
1 Superficial or non-anatomical tenderness. In this test, the skin is lightly pinched (the pinch test) over a wide area of lumbar skin. If this causes pain, the test is positive.
2 Axial loading of the skull. If the patient complains of low back pain on vertical loading of the skull, by the examiner's hand, this test is regarded as positive. Similarly, rotation of the shoulders and pelvis in the same plane should not cause back pain.
3 Distraction. A commonly used test is that of distraction during straight leg raising, i.e. if the patient is made to sit up on the couch with the legs extended in front and there is no pain as the legs are lifted with the patient sitting, this is clearly an inappropriate response. In the USA, this is called the 'flip test'.
4 Regional disturbances. These are motor or sensory deficits that do not coincide with normal anatomical pathways, e.g. cog-wheel weakness of the foot or apparent weakness of the foot when the patient can heal-and-toe walk when standing.

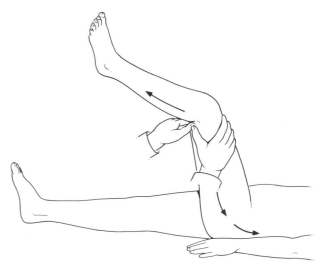

Fig. 22.17 The bow-string test. When eliciting the Bow-string test the patient's foot should be allowed to rest on the examiner's shoulder with the knee flexed slightly at the limit of straight leg raising. Firm pressure is then applied by the examiner's thumbs in the popliteal fossa and reproduction of leg pain indicates root tension.

5 Overreaction, e.g. muscle spasms, tremor, collapsing while being examined.
Normally examination of the patient is followed up with plain radiographs of the lumbar spine with a coned lateral view of the lumbosacral level. A full blood count and erythrocyte sedimentation rate may also be performed together with biochemistry if indicated.

SPINAL INVESTIGATIONS
See Chapter 30.

REFERENCES

Buck J.E. (1970) Direct repair of the defect in spondylolisthesis. *J. Bone Joint Surg.* **52B**, 432−437.
Caspar W. (1977) A new surgical procedure for lumbar disc herniation causing less tissue damage through a microsurgical approach. *Adv. Neurosurg.* **4**, 74−79.
Crock H.V., Yoshwizawa H. and Kane S.K. (1973) Observations on the venous drainage of the human vertebral body. *J. Bone Joint Surg.* **55B**, 528−533.
Domisse G.F. (1974) The blood supply of the spinal cord. A factor in spinal surgery. *J. Bone Joint Surg.* **56B**, 225−235.
Getty C.J.M., Johnson J.R., Kirwan E.O'G. and Sullivan M.F. (1981) Partial undercutting facetectomy for bony entrapment of the lumbar nerve root. *J. Bone Joint Surg.* **63B**, 330−335.
Gill G.G. (1955) Surgical treatment of spondylolisthesis without spinal fusion. *J. Bone Joint Surg.* **37A**, 493−520.
Harris N.H. and Murray R.O. (1974) Lesions of the symphysis in athletes. *Br. Med. J.* **4**, 211.

Hickey D.S. and Hinkins D.W.L. (1980) Relation between the structure of avascular fibrosis and the function and failure of the intervertebral disc. *Spine* 5, 106−116.

Hijikata S.A. (1975) A method of percutaneous nuclear extraction. *J. Toden. Hosp.* 5, 39−46.

Last R.J. (1963) *Anatomy. Regional and Applied*, 3rd edn. Edinburgh, Churchill, p. 39.

Mathew B., Norris D., Hendry D. and Waddell G. (1988) Artificial intelligence in the diagnosis of low back pain and sciatica. *Spine* 13, 168.

Morscher E., Gerber B. and Fasel J. (1984) Surgical treatment of spondylolisthesis by bone grafting and direct stabilisation of spondylolysis by means of a hook. *Arch. Orthop. Trauma Surg.* 103. 175−178.

Nachemson A.L. (1981) Disc pressure measurements. *Spine* 6, 93.

Newman P.H. (1963) The etiology of spondylolisthesis. *J. Bone Joint Surg.* 45B, 39−59.

Nicol R.O. and Scott J.H.S. (1986) Lytic spondylolysis-repair by wiring. *Spine* 11, 1027−1030.

Onik G., Helms C., Ginsberg L., Hoaglund I.T. and Morris J. (1985) Percutaneous lumbar discectomy using a new aspiration probe. *AJNR* 6, 290−293.

Porter R.W., Hibbert C. and Wilman P. (1980) Backache and the lumbar canal. *Spine* 5, 99−105.

Ransford A.O., Cairns D. and Moonly V. (1976) The pain drawing as an aid to the psychological evaluation of patients with low back pain. *Spine* 1, 127−134.

Simmons E.H. and Wilber I.G. (1978) Complications of spinal surgery for discogenic disease and spondylolisthesis. In Epps C. (ed.) *Complications of Orthopaedic Surgery*. Philadelphia, J.B. Lippincott, pp. 1181−1214.

Smith L., Garvin P.J. and Jennings R.B. (1963) Enzyme dissolution of the intervertebral disc. *Nature* 198, 1398.

Waddell G., McCulloch J., Kummel G. and Venner R. (1980) Nonorganic physical signs in low back pain. *Spine* 5, 117.

Wilkie R. and Beetham R. (1980) Transfemoral lumbar epidural venography. *Spine* 5, 424−431.

Williams R. (1978) Micro-lumbar discectomy. A conservative surgical approach to the virgin herniated lumbar disc. *Spine*, 3, 175−182.

Wiltse L.L., Bateman J.G., Hutchinson R.H. and Welson W.E. (1968) The paraspinal sacrospinalis-splitting approach to lumbar spine. *J. Bone Joint Surg.* 50A, 919−926.

Wiltse L.L., Newman P.H. and MacNab I. *et al.* (1976) Classification of spondylolisthesis. *Clin. Orthop.* 117, 23−29.

Yasargil M.G. (1977) Microsurgical operations for herniated lumbar disc. *Adv. in Neurosurg.* 4, 81−82.

Chapter 23
The Shoulder

I.G. Kelly

INTRODUCTION

Until recently, those interested in problems of the shoulder often referred to it as the 'forgotten joint'. The upsurge in interest during the last decade has resulted in this term becoming outmoded but it may be worth remembering for its inaccuracy. The 'shoulder' is a complex of joints and forgetting this fact can make the orthopaedic surgeon's task impossible. The glenohumeral, acromioclavicular, sternoclavicular, scapulothoracic and subacromial joints are moved by their associated muscles to position and stabilize the upper limb for function.

The shoulder joint complex has an enormous range of motion and this is achieved by the sacrifice of intrinsic bony stability at the glenohumeral joint together with motion at the other joints in the complex. This results in large stresses upon the soft tissues which may predispose to degenerative conditions as the individual ages and makes the glenohumeral joint highly susceptible to dislocation. The most common presenting symptoms of shoulder disease, therefore, are pain and instability.

SURGICAL ANATOMY

It is not the intention here to present a comprehensive overview of shoulder anatomy but the surgeon must be aware of certain facts if the pathogenesis and treatment of shoulder conditions are to be understood.

The shoulder girdle straddles the apex of the rib cage with the sternoclavicular joint as its only secure articulation with the axial skeleton. The scapula is supported by muscles on the posterior chest wall and the glenoid thus comes to face anteriorly and inferiorly and is matched by the 35° retroversion of the humeral head on its shaft — a feature that produces overlap of the images of the humeral head and glenoid on anteroposterior projections of the 'shoulder'.

The humeral head is larger than the glenoid face and has a much smaller radius of curvature. This last fact is partially compensated for by the presence of the glenoid labrum. This structure resembles the menisci in the knee but is constructed of fibrous tissue rather than fibrocartilage (Gardner, 1963). Its existence has been challenged by Moseley (1969) but most authors regard it as an extension of the inferior glenohumeral ligament (Bigliani, 1989).

The glenohumeral ligaments (Fig. 23.1) are thickenings in the anterior capsule of the glenohumeral joint and, although not easily appreciated at open operations, are well seen through the arthroscope. They undoubtedly play a role in stabilizing the joint but are not alone in this. Three ligaments are described: superior, middle and inferior. De Palma (1983) regards the superior to be the superior margin of the subscapularis bursa and not a real entity. The middle ligament arises deep to the inferior insertion of the subscapularis into the lesser tuberosity and extends superiorly behind the tendon to insert into the neck of the scapula just beyond the glenoid rim. It may extend as high as the 1 or 2 o'clock position on the glenoid face. The inferior glenohumeral ligament arises distal to the articular margin of the humeral head and crosses to the glenoid where it gains attachment via the labrum.

The acromioclavicular joint is highly variable in its shape and orientation. By contrast with the glenohumeral joint it possesses considerable stability which it derives from its strong superior ligament together with its intra-articular disc and capsule — preventing anteroposterior displacement — and the two coracoclavicular ligaments which limit superior motion.

The sternoclavicular joint is the most stable in the complex by virtue of strong anterior and posterior capsular ligaments augmented by the interclavicular ligament and the costoclavicular ligament to the first rib. A strong articular disc also makes an important

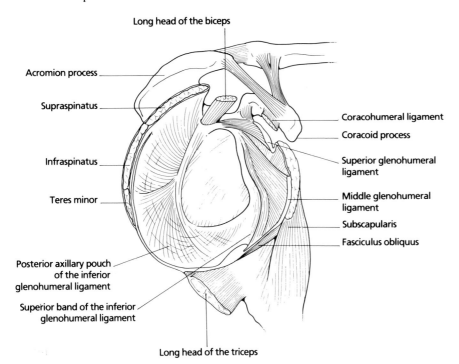

Fig. 23.1 The anatomy of the glenohumeral ligaments.

contribution. Traumatic dislocation of this joint is unusual and requires considerable violence.

The subacromial joint is not a true anatomical joint but is a common site of pathology and merits separate consideration. It comprises the undersurface of the acromion together with the coracoacromial ligament and the coracoid which articulate with the greater tuberosity of the humerus and the insertion of the supraspinatus tendon with the subacromial or subdeltoid bursa acting as the joint cavity. Pathological changes in any of these components are capable of producing symptoms.

The joints of the shoulder complex interact during motion of the upper limb. Because of the orientation of the humeral head and the glenoid, the humerus must rotate externally during elevation if conflict between the greater tuberosity and the acromion is to be avoided. At the same time the clavicle must rotate and differential movement between the clavicle and the acromion begins at about 90° of flexion. It thus follows that a patient who lacks external rotation will be unable to elevate the arm fully and that painful pathology in the acromioclavicular joint will manifest itself at and beyond 90° of flexion.

Elevation of the upper limb is also accompanied by movement of the scapula around the chest wall and the relationship between this movement and that of the humerus is in a ratio of about 2:1 (Wallace, 1982). This produces the clinically recognizable scapulohumeral

rhythm which will be disturbed by almost any pathology within the shoulder girdle.

The muscles that power the shoulder joints can be considered in three groups—deltoid, the rotator cuff and those muscles that stabilize the scapula.

The deltoid is the largest and most powerful muscle at the shoulder and in humans its power has been enhanced over that in other species by the enlarged acromion and the distal insertion into the humerus. It behaves as three units, the anterior and posterior of which are unipennate with the middle portion being multipennate allowing it to maintain power through a large range of motion even when its origin is brought close to its insertion. The anterior deltoid is at risk in many of the standard approaches to the shoulder and must be treated with respect since its loss imposes considerable disability in the form of reduced ability to elevate the arm. The deltoid receives its innervation from the large circumflex nerve which arises from the posterior cord of the brachial plexus and passes over the anterior aspect of the subscapularis muscle to join the posterior humeral circumflex artery as it winds around the neck of the humerus in contact with the bone. It is prudent to locate this nerve if operating on or near the subscapularis and if using a deltoid splitting approach the split should be limited to 5 cm from the acromion since the nerve runs on the deep surface of the deltoid muscle approximately 6 cm distal to the acromial margin.

The rotator cuff muscles comprise supraspinatus,

infraspinatus, teres minor and subscapularis. The supraspinatus and subscapularis have generous tendinous insertions but teres minor and infraspinatus have only limited tendinous areas making repair of a rupture more difficult. Subscapularis is innervated by two nerves arising from the posterior cord of the brachial plexus and entering the muscle on its anterior surface. This permits this muscle to be mobilized off the scapula without risk—a procedure often required during cuff repair or glenohumeral arthroplasty. The supraspinatus and infraspinatus muscles are innervated by the suprascapular nerve which arises high in the neck and passes down through the suprascapular notch (where it may be compressed beneath the transverse ligament) and along the base of the scapular spine. It is at risk during attempts to mobilize the supraspinatus muscle from the scapula.

The rotator cuff muscles stabilize the humeral head and facilitate the initiation of movements. Their tendons are at risk from attrition as they pass beneath the coracoacromial arch during motion.

The muscles that stabilize the scapula are the serratus anterior, the trapezius, the rhomboids and the levator scapulae. The last two muscles pull the scapula towards the thoracic vertebrae. The serratus anterior and the trapezius act to control the rotation of the scapula on the chest wall and paralysis of either will result in winging of the scapula.

The tendon of the long head of biceps runs an intra-articular course and may be involved in a variety of pathological processes. It probably acts as a depressor and stabilizer of the humeral head. Rupture of the tendon is easily recognized clinically but should alert the surgeon to the possibility of an associated rupture of the rotator cuff since it emerges from the capsule and through the rotator cuff tendons in the area most liable to damage.

Finally, this brief overview must consider the musculocutaneous nerve. This nerve passes through the substance of the coracobrachialis at a variable distance below the coracoid process. (Richards *et al.*, 1987). It is particularly at risk when the coracoid is detached as part of the approach to the shoulder and is best palpated before any bony section is made and protected from traction thereafter. Fortunately, it is possible to perform most shoulder operations without detaching the coracoid process.

IMAGING

Although the majority of problems afflicting the shoulder involve the soft tissues, good radiology is essential to highlight or exclude associated bony pathology.

The glenohumeral joint lies at approximately 30° to the coronal plane and it is therefore essential to rotate the patient to obtain an image that demonstrates the joint space (Fig. 23.2). A second view should always be obtained and the author's preference is for the axillary projection (Fig. 23.3) which has the added advantage that it also provides an image of the acromioclavicular joint. If the range of abduction is limited, however, this projection can be difficult or impossible to obtain and in this situation the author uses an apical oblique projection (Fig. 23.4) (Wallace and Hellier, 1983; Garth *et al.*, 1984). In the acute situation, the routine use of such a second 'lateral' projection will prevent posterior dislocation of the glenohumeral joint from being overlooked. This is a surprisingly common occurrence and results in costly litigation for the surgeon as well as suffering for the patient.

The author routinely examines the acromioclavicular joint using an anteroposterior projection with the beam angled 15° cephalad (Fig. 23.5). Internally and externally rotated anteroposterior projections can be helpful in demonstrating calcified deposits and the outlet view or transcapular lateral projection allows the acromion to be visualized. The sternoclavicular joint is difficult to visualize using plain radiography but the serendipity view (Rockwood, 1984) can sometimes provide useful images.

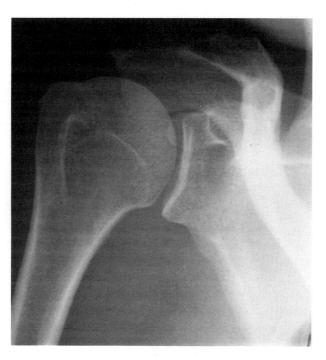

Fig. 23.2 Anteroposterior projection of the glenohumeral joints showing the joint space.

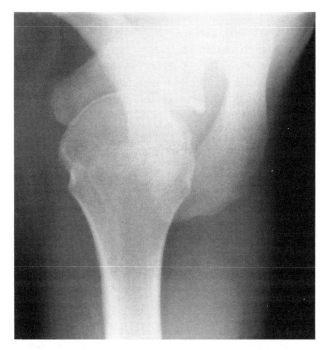

Fig. 23.3 An axillary projection of the shoulder. Note that the acromioclavicular joint space can be seen through the image of the humeral head.

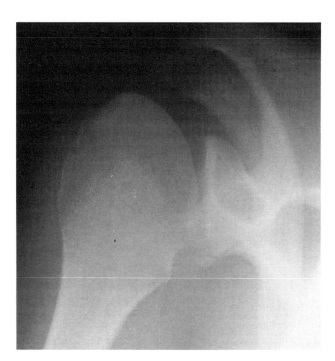

Fig. 23.4 An apical/oblique projection which can be performed without moving the arm from the side. This is a particularly useful projection in patients with shoulder instability.

Arthrography, especially double-contrast arthrography, of the glenohumeral joint is of value in investigating possible ruptures of the rotator cuff or the state of the capsule in the 'frozen shoulder'. It does not, however, provide any information about the size or location of a tear. Computed tomography double-contrast arthrography provides very useful information about the intraglenohumeral joint structures and has a place in the investigation of glenohumeral instability.

Magnetic resonance imaging is now a well-established

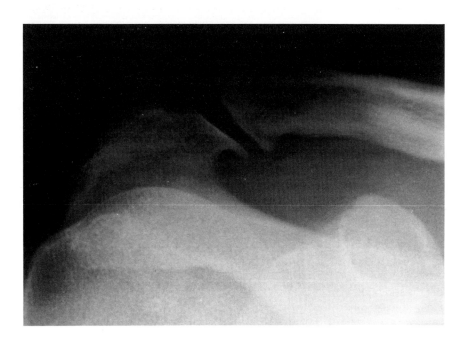

Fig. 23.5 A cephalic tilt view to show the acromioclavicular joints. Note the inferior osteophytes in this illustration.

method of investigation and reports suggest that it is of particular value in the assessment of the rotator cuff in impingement syndromes. It appears to be a little inferior to computed tomographic–arthrography in the investigation of instability.

Ultrasonography can provide a useful non-invasive method of investigating the rotator cuff and in skilled hands (Mack *et al.*, 1985) has proved valuable in demonstrating rotator cuff pathology.

ARTHROSCOPY

The glenohumeral joint and the subacromial joint are amenable to arthroscopic examination and, indeed, this approach has done much to improve our understanding of shoulder anatomy and function. Arthroscopy can be used both diagnostically and therapeutically but, as at the knee, the surgeon should be thoroughly familiar with diagnostic arthroscopy before attempting any operative procedures. There is a wide range of normal variation at the shoulder and this can be the cause of considerable confusion. A wide experience is therefore essential. Operative procedures are limited and their role has not yet been proven. Long-term results are awaited.

Indications

Arthroscopy must only be performed for specific reasons and it is not acceptable to use it as a substitute for proper clinical assessment. The vast majority of shoulder problems can be diagnosed using clinical means together with one or more of the imaging methods described above. The major indications for arthroscopy are as follows.

1 To provide information regarding shoulder instability either in place of, or as an addition to, radiographic methods.
2 To assess the rotator cuff from both the glenohumeral and subacromial sides. This can be very valuable in identifying the presence, size and location of tears.
3 To investigate the cause of pain or other symptoms arising from the glenohumeral joint when other investigative methods have proved unhelpful.
4 To obtain biopsy specimens under direct vision.
5 To perform arthroscopic surgery.

Diagnostic arthroscopy

Under general anaesthesia, the patient is positioned in the lateral position with the affected shoulder uppermost. The beach chair position frequently used for many forms of shoulder surgery can also be used. It is necessary to be able to apply traction to the limb and this can be done by an assistant — a tiring task — or by the use of a mechanical system. Several commercial systems are available but a paediatric skin traction kit applied to the forearm and connected to a weight and pulley system is usually adequate. Traction is not applied until after the joint has been entered.

After draping the shoulder with the arm free on a gutter rest, the posterior portal is selected. This allows good visualization of the glenohumeral joint and is also the easiest way of entering the joint. The point of skin entry lies 1.5 cm distal and 1 cm medial to the posterior angle of the acromion and corresponds to a fibrous septum between the fibres of the posterior and middle deltoid. An arthroscopic cannula or an intravenous cannula is then directed from this point towards the coracoid process anteriorly. Entry into the joint is usually easily appreciated but can be difficult in obese patients. Once the cannula is in place the trochar is removed and the joint is inflated using a 50 ml syringe of saline. Copeland and Barrett (1990) have described a useful sign confirming placement of the cannula within the joint and preventing extravasation of saline into the soft tissues which may make subsequent examination difficult or impossible. As the saline is injected, the arm will rise from its rest internally rotating and abducting only if the cannula is within the joint cavity.

After the joint is inflated, a short incision is made with a number 11 blade and a standard 4 mm diameter arthroscope with its blunt obturator is inserted in the same way as the cannula. Once the joint is entered, the traction system is set up with the arm in 45° of flexion and up to 45° of abduction. This range reduces the stresses on the brachial plexus while permitting good visibility (Klein *et al.*, 1987). The arm can be rotated to facilitate viewing of the various parts of the joint. This can sometimes also involve contortions on the part of the surgeon since the arthroscope has to be moved through a wide range of positions. Fortunately, the development of solid-state video cameras has overcome this and has been of considerable benefit to shoulder arthroscopy.

The surgeon must have a system for examining the joint and it is usual to commence with the tendon of the long head of biceps which is easily identifiable. Its insertion to the superior glenoid margin is the key landmark and a place to return to if one loses one's way. Above the tendon is the undersurface of the supraspinatus tendon and below it lies the glenoid face with its labral margin. The labrum can be inspected around the circumference of the glenoid and is variable in width. The superior, posterior and inferior glenoid recesses can also be examined at this time and may be the site of loose bodies. By rotating the head externally, the bare area on the posterior aspect can be seen and must be distinguished from the humeral head defect commonly seen in unstable shoulders. This latter defect involves the articular surface.

If traction is applied, the anterior part of the joint can be reached and a prominent finding is the superior margin of the subscapularis tendon and the opening into the subscapularis recess. The glenohumeral ligaments (see above) can be seen with the middle ligament being particularly prominent.

Further examination requires the use of a probe or hook and this should be inserted through an anterior portal. To avoid damage to the musculocutaneous nerve, the site of this portal must be carefully chosen. From within the joint it is the space bounded by the biceps tendon, the superior border of the subscapularis and the anterior glenoid rim. Placing the arthroscope against this area will illuminate the skin and indicate the site which must be lateral to the coracoid process. Confirmation of the site is gained by passing a needle before inserting the probe.

Other portals are often required for arthroscopic surgery. For example, the subacromial region may be better visualized using an entry portal lateral to the acromion. The reader is referred to specialist works on operative arthroscopy for fuller details (Ellman, 1988; Bunker and Wallace, 1991).

Operative arthroscopy

Various operative procedures have been performed arthroscopically at the shoulder and mention will be made of these in the appropriate sections of this chapter.

SHOULDER PAIN

The innervation of the shoulder is such that pain is mediated through the supraclavicular nerves (mainly C4 but also C3), the circumflex nerve with its cutaneous distribution at the deltoid insertion (C5) and the suprascapular nerve which has no significant cutaneous branches. The shoulder thus shares innervation with the phrenic nerve and pain arising in the pleura, diaphragm or gall bladder may be felt in the shoulder (Fig. 23.6). Similarly, by means of the interconnections in the sympathetic trunk, pain arising in the cervical discs or facets may be referred to the shoulder and is a common cause of diagnostic confusion. It is therefore important to remember that pain in the shoulder may be extrinsic

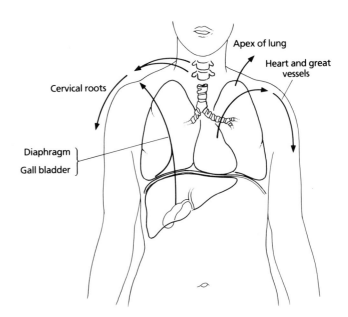

Fig. 23.6 Diagrammatic representation of the extrinsic sources of shoulder pain. (Reproduced with permission from Churchill Livingstone.)

in origin. Extrinsic shoulder pain does not usually worsen with shoulder movement but may do so particularly if the cervical spine is involved. Intrinsic shoulder pain is almost always aggravated by shoulder movement.

The innervation of the shoulder tends to produce patterns of pain that can be of help in reaching a diagnosis. Thus, pain localized to the region of the acromioclavicular joint by the patient usually indicates pathology in that joint which can be confirmed by physical signs and other tests. Subacromial pathology results in less precisely localized pain, usually felt over the point of the shoulder radiating to the area of the deltoid insertion. The patient may present clutching the upper arm with the opposite hand. The glenohumeral joint gives rise to anterior or, less commonly, posterior pain associated with radiation to the deltoid insertion. Unfortunately, the patient's description of the pain is not always so clear-cut and, as will be seen later, in patients with polyarthritis there can be difficulties in interpretation.

The author has no wish to present a method of examining the shoulder but it should be noted here that the presence of painful arcs (in flexion or abduction) can localize the site of the pain and pathology (Fig. 23.7). The well-known subacromial arc is from approximately 80° to 120° of abduction resulting in the pattern no pain−pain−no pain. A high painful arc will be present with acromioclavicular pathology and is a terminal arc in flexion or abduction. On occasion it will be present along with the subacromial arc.

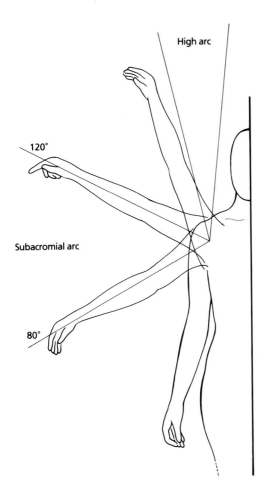

Fig. 23.7 Painful arcs of abduction can be useful in determining the site of shoulder pain. The high arc represents impingement beneath the acromioclavicular joint. (Reproduced with permission from Churchill Livingstone.)

Most of the conditions affecting the shoulder complex produce pain and they will be dealt with in the following sections.

DEGENERATIVE CONDITIONS

Osteoarthritis of the glenohumeral joint (Fig. 23.8) is uncommon and is usually secondary to trauma or avascular necrosis. Rarely, it can appear in individuals who subject their shoulders to large stresses over long periods (Kessel and Bayley, 1986). The patient presents with typical glenohumeral pain and limitation of movement, particularly rotations. The radiological appearances are typical with loss of glenohumeral joint space and tear-drop osteophytes on the inferior aspect of both the humeral head and the glenoid. If the symptoms are severe, treatment is by arthroplasty.

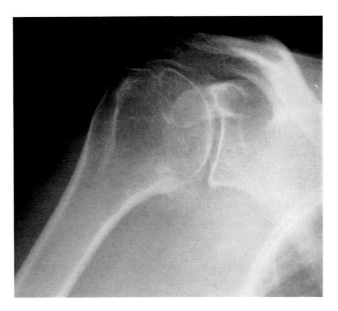

Fig. 23.8 Osteoarthritis of the glenohumeral joint. Note the inferior osteophyte on the humeral head.

The acromioclavicular joint is much more commonly involved by osteoarthritic change and this may be post-traumatic—following subluxation or dislocation or as a consequence of an intra-articular fracture of the outer end of the clavicle—or occupational resulting from repeated elevation of the arm or working with the arms overhead. The patient can frequently localize the pain to the joint and adducting the arm across the trunk or behind the back will reproduce the pain in the joint. A high painful arc may also be present as long as elevation past 90° is possible. Radiographs show narrowing of the joint space with superior, anterior and inferior osteophytes. These latter may compress the rotator cuff tendon causing a subacromial type of painful arc or even rupture of the cuff (see later). This condition is overlooked with surprising frequency, attention usually being directed more towards the subacromial joint. The diagnosis can be confirmed by injecting a small amount (1 ml) of local anaesthetic into the joint and abolishing the pain. Local treatment by physiotherapy or steroid injection may be effective but failing this excision of the outer 1–1.5 cm of the clavicle is necessary. It should be noted that this interferes with the integrity of the shoulder girdle and reduces its strength such that a patient engaged in heavy labouring work may not be able to return to such an occupation.

IMPINGEMENT SYNDROMES

The subacromial joint is also frequently involved in degenerative disease but at this site the condition is not usually called osteoarthritis but 'refractory painful arc syndrome' or, more internationally, 'impingement syndrome'. The subacromial impingement syndrome is only one of several impingement syndromes and all will be discussed here.

Watson (1991) has defined the impingement syndromes as 'clinical conditions where pain occurs during part of the excursion of the glenohumeral joint due to compression of an element of the rotator cuff against an element of its immediate relations'. The rotator cuff elements are the tendons of its muscles plus that of the long head of biceps and the relations are the components of the coracoacromial arch. The changes that ageing produces in the rotator cuff together with the accumulated effects of repeated minor trauma mean that these conditions are most often seen in patients over the age of 40 years.

In some patients the typical pain with a demonstrable subacromial arc occurs after a bout of intense activity such as trimming a hedge or playing tennis. It is hypothesized that this repetitive trauma injures the cuff producing an inflammatory response with swelling of the tendon and the overlying bursa. Any attempt at flexion or abduction then brings this area into conflict with the overhanging acromion and results in pain. This acute form usually responds well to rest or local measures such as ice or ultrasonography. Occasionally steroid injection may be of value but the site of the pain should always be confirmed by the prior injection of local anaesthetic. Neer (1972) advocates the instillation of 10 ml of local anaesthetic into the subacromial space in his 'impingement test' but the author favours using no more than 1 ml which allows for greater specificity and can permit the differentiation of different types of impingement syndrome. Very occasionally, surgical decompression of the subacromial space is necessary.

The chronic form of impingement is that most commonly seen in orthopaedic clinics. There is not usually a history of intense activity but more a gradual onset of pain during elevation of the arm. It is felt that thickening of the tendon and the loss of tone in the cuff muscles with ageing associated with repetitive minor trauma results in impingement with the coracoacromial arch which in turn stimulates bursa formation. Over a long period of time, the bursa thickens and becomes a space-occupying lesion perpetuating the impingement. Reactive osteophyte formation occurs along the anterior margin of the acromion and along the line of the coracoacromial ligament further compromising the rotator cuff tendon. This may ultimately result in rupture of the cuff.

Variations in shoulder anatomy are well known and Bigliani *et al.* (1986) have described three types of acromion (Fig. 23.9). In a study of 140 cadaveric shoulders, the acromion was flat (Type I) in 17%, curved (Type II) in 43% and hooked (Type III) in 40%. Of the 71 cadavers, 58% had the same pattern on each side. Of the 33% of rotator cuffs that had full thickness tears, 73% had Type III acromions, 24% Type II and 3% Type I. In an extension of this study, Morrison and Bigliani (1987) observed the morphology of the acromion on the lateral scapular views of 200 patients with shoulder problems. Of those with rotator cuff rupture, 80% had hooked acromions and 20% had curved. However, those patients with impingement syndromes without cuff tears had a normal distribution of acromial types. It is difficult to establish whether the hooked acromion is the cause or the result of cuff tear — the osteophytes that form along the anterior margin of the acromion can produce this effect. Nevertheless, these observations lend some support to the rationale of anterior acromioplasty in attempting to convert all acromia to the shape of Type I.

The osteophytes that form on the underside of the degenerative acromioclavicular joint can also impinge against the rotator cuff and in these patients the typical subacromial type of painful arc is accompanied by a terminal arc often producing pain from 90° to 180° of abduction. Some patients have no evidence of any changes in the subacromial region or the acromioclavi-

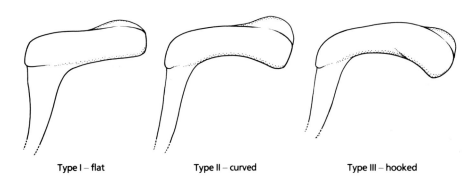

Type I – flat   Type II – curved   Type III – hooked

Fig. 23.9 Diagram to show the three acromial types described by Bigliani *et al.* (1986).

cular joint and injection studies can locate the impingement to the coracoacromial ligament. The remaining element of the coracoacromial arch, the coracoid process, can also contribute to impingement and this unusual condition was first reported by Gerber *et al.* (1985). Pain is provoked by internally rotating the flexed or abducted arm. Pain is felt anteriorly and commonly radiates to the arm and sometimes to the proximal forearm. Three types are recognized: (i) idiopathic, usually associated with anatomical variations in the shape of the coracoid; (ii) iatrogenic, often following surgery involving coracoid osteotomy and/or transfer; and (iii) traumatic, after proximal humeral or coracoid fractures. The diagnosis, once suspected, can be confirmed by abolition of the symptoms using a subcoracoid injection of local anaesthetic.

Impingement may also result from any condition that allows upward migration of the humeral head, e.g. rotator cuff rupture or suprascapular nerve palsy. It is also important to realize that joint laxity can be associated with impingement and glenohumeral stability should always be assessed when examining a patient presenting with the symptoms of impingement, particularly if they are below the age of 40 years.

Management

In its mild form, chronic impingement may respond to a change in the way the limb is used for work or recreation. For example, it may be possible to eliminate overhead working. Physiotherapy comprising local measures to reduce pain and rotator cuff muscle and deltoid strengthening can be very helpful and a short course of a non-steroidal anti-inflammatory agent may facilitate this.

The place of local steroid injections and, more particularly, their number is confused. There is no doubt that these injections can be helpful and, in some patients, they can settle the problem completely. The injection, however, must be given to the site of the pathology and that is not always the site of maximal tenderness or even the site suggested by the history and examination! Beware the patient who attends the clinic with the history of having had numerous injections, none of which has had any effect. It is likely that none was placed appropriately. It is the author's practice to localize the site of the impingement using small injections (1 ml) of 1% lignocaine and this, together with the clinical features, confirms the diagnosis of impingement. Thereafter, the author injects a suitable steroid preparation, often with a long-acting local anaesthetic, into the same site. If there is no response over a 3 week period, there is no repeat of the injection but other, usually surgical,

methods of treatment are considered. If there is an incomplete or short-lasting response the author will consider repeating the injection on one occasion only. Failure to obtain a lasting response indicates the need for other measures. This approach avoids the risk of multiple injections which, as Watson (1985) has shown, results in softening of the rotator cuff.

Failure to respond to any of the above measures results in the need to consider surgical treatment and anterior acromioplasty as described by Neer (1972) provides the means of achieving decompression of the rotator cuff in the majority of cases. The procedure may be performed open or arthroscopically (Ellman, 1988). Radical acromionectomy has no place in the management of shoulder pain and, by removing the origin of the deltoid muscle and promoting scarring between the deltoid and the rotator cuff, it can significantly worsen the patients symptoms and function. Salvage is virtually impossible.

In the open operation, the patient is positioned in the so-called beach-chair position with the head elevated to approximately 60° (Fig. 23.10). Arthroscopy of the glenohumeral joint can be carried out first to exclude any intra-articular lesions. A short incision is made commencing in front of, or over, the acromioclavicular joint and extended distally and slightly laterally parallel to the line of the axillary crease (Fig. 23.11a). The incision is deepened to expose the insertion of the deltoid into the clavicle and this muscle is detached by incising

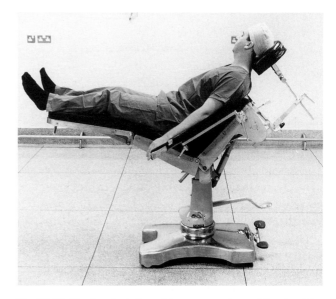

Fig. 23.10 The beach-chair position commonly used for shoulder surgery. If a neurosurgical head rest is not available a head ring can be used on a standard table.

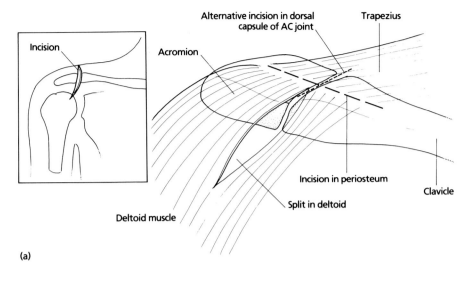

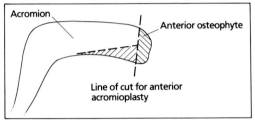

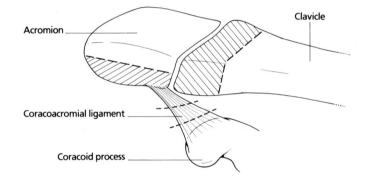

Fig. 23.11 (a) Diagram to show the approaches used for acromioplasty. The periosteum over the acromion and clavicle can be opened in the line of the clavicle or an incision can be made through the dorsal capsule of the acromioclavicular joint. In either case, the split in the fibres of deltoid should not extend 5 cm beyond the acromion in order to protect the axillary nerve. (b) Structures resected when decompressing the rotator cuff. Note the angle of the acromial resection.

the short tendon of insertion and the clavicular periosteum in the line of the clavicle in such a way as to permit secure re-attachment at the conclusion of the operation. The deltoid fibres are split from the clavicle for a distance of no greater than 5 cm to avoid damage to the circumflex nerve on the deep surface of the muscle, thus creating two flaps which can be retracted. An alternative approach is to incise the dorsal capsule of the acromioclavicular joint in line with the split in deltoid and then to elevate the medial and lateral flaps off the underlying bone (Fig. 23.11a). This allows for an easier repair but can create difficulties if the periosteum is too thin.

The exposed acromion is inspected and any overhanging anterior osteophytes are removed. The anterior

two-thirds of the undersurface are then removed using an oblique osteotomy and any remaining deep projections are removed (Fig. 23.11b). Osteophytes projecting down from the acromioclavicular joint can also be removed at this stage after first resecting the coracoacromial ligament—beware of the acromial branch of the thoracoacromial artery running along the posterior margin of the ligament. The outer end of the clavicle can be removed at this time if the acromioclavicular joint is significantly involved. At least 1 cm of the outer clavicle should be removed with more being resected posteriorly than anteriorly.

The usually thickened subacromial bursa can be removed exposing the surface of the rotator cuff for inspection. Any tears can be repaired through this approach.

Closure requires firm re-attachment of the deltoid muscle through drill holes in the bone if necessary. Passive motion commences immediately post-operatively and active motion is not commenced until a full passive range has been achieved.

It is important to be aware of the results of this procedure and of the need for skilled and often prolonged physiotherapy treatment. Moderate pain may persist for as long as 4–5 weeks and patients should be warned to expect this or their will to cooperate with their rehabilitation may be compromised. Neer (1972) reported satisfactory results in 15 of 16 patients in his initial series, but Thorling *et al.* (1985) obtained good-to-excellent results in only 33 of 51 patients in his series. Post and Cohen (1986) reported that 11% of their series continued to have significant pain after acromioplasty; 56% of those with weakness prior to surgery complained of weakness post-operatively and 29% with pre-operative limitation of motion remained restricted. In athletes, Tibone and his associates (1985) found that only 43% returned to their previous level of sport and 20% continued to have moderate-to-severe pain.

Ellman (1988) introduced the arthroscopic technique for rotator cuff decompression. The arthroscope is introduced through the posterior approach and the suction burr is passed through the anterior portal to perform the acromioplasty. Ellman recommends the use of two needles to identify the position of the acromioclavicular joint and the coracoacromial ligament. If this ligament is to be divided, either a knife or electrocautery can be used. If the latter is chosen, the irrigation fluid must be substituted with distilled water or electrocautery will not take place. Bleeding from the acromial branch of the thoracoacromial artery can cause visibility problems.

The reasons for failure in all methods include poor patient selection, inadequate decompression, advanced rotator cuff pathology and failure of rehabilitation. The acromioclavicular joint is frequently overlooked as a source of pathology/pain and five of the failures in Post and Cohen (1986) were attributed to this. Careful use of local anaesthetic test injections can minimize this problem. It is important to ensure that the subacromial region is adequately decompressed by inserting a finger while an assistant applies traction to the arm. Any residual bony prominences or osteophytes should be removed. When performing an arthroscopic decompression (Ellman, 1988) it can be very difficult to judge the amount of acromion resected and too little or too much may be removed. Advanced rotator cuff disease with deep surface tears is very difficult to recognize unless using an arthroscopic approach and will militate against a good result by allowing upward migration of the humeral head. Finally, prolonged immobilization of the shoulder following acromioplasty predisposes to adhesion formation and the development of a stiff and painful shoulder. Passive mobilization — to protect the deltoid re-attachment — should commence on the first post-operative day and a supervised structured rehabilitation programme should be followed thereafter.

ROTATOR CUFF RUPTURE

Neer (1972) proposed that impingement could lead to rotator cuff failure and reported that 95% of cuff tears were associated with impingement. However, Codman (1934) described what he termed 'rim rents' in which the deep surface of the rotator cuff was torn at its insertion to the greater tuberosity and he argued that these were the origin of cuff tears. DePalma (1983) described tearing away of the innermost fibres of the cuff from their insertion beginning in the fifth decade and Petterson (1942) indicated that these tears increased in size over the next three decades. Uhthoff *et al.* (1986) observed that partial thickness tears were almost always found on the deep surface of the cuff tendon. These observations do not seem to accord with Neer's suggestion that impingement results in cuff rupture.

Most cuff tears occur in patients over the age of 40 years, increasing in frequency over the ensuing three decades, suggesting that age-related changes may be important in their aetiology. Many tears occur without a history of injury in patients with sedentary occupations and bilateral tears are not uncommon — trauma alone therefore cannot be the cause.

Mack *et al.* (1985) have suggested that the likely pathogenesis is progressive fibre failure in an ageing cuff which distorts the vascular supply, thus prejudicing healing, and weakens the cuff permitting upward migration of the humeral head. This migration produces additional damage and provokes the development of subacromial or acromioclavicular spurs which have been described in association with cuff tears (Peterson *et al.*, 1983). The cuff may totally fail by attrition or may succumb to minor trauma. Neer's finding of the high association of cuff tears with impingement can be explained in this way, which also accords with the observations of many other researchers.

Patients with cuff ruptures usually give a history of previous shoulder pain often with crepitus on movement. Some may describe a specific incident but many give no such history. Most complain of weakness of elevation with pain. It should be noted here that patients over 50 years and who sustain a traumatic dislocation have a high risk of sustaining a cuff rupture and that this is frequently misdiagnosed as an axillary nerve palsy.

The clinical findings are diagnostic but care must be taken in eliciting them. In the acute presentation there will be no muscle wasting but this quickly develops and will involve the supraspinatus, infraspinatus or both spinati. Some patients cannot initiate elevation or abduction at all and all will have difficulty in carrying out these movements against resistance. Elevation is usually accompanied by a shrugging motion produced by the overworking deltoid. The passive range of motion is nearly always preserved. In a thin patient, a gap can sometimes be felt in the cuff by extending the shoulder and palpating anterior to the acromion.

The most important tests of cuff function involve assessing the strength of the rotator muscles. Supraspinatus is tested by asking the patient to abduct the arm from the side of the trunk against resistance and the examiner palpates the body of the muscle during the test. Infraspinatus function is assessed by holding the patient's elbow to the side and testing the power of external rotation against the examiner's resisting hand. Comparison with the opposite side is essential and it is important to note that weakness may only be detected in one of these muscles. The reduction in power may be subtle especially if there is pain and great care must be taken to perform these tests properly. Abolition of the pain using a subacromial injection of local anaesthetic can facilitate the test. Brems (1987) found an association between the power of external rotation and the size of the cuff tear.

Although a cuff tear can be diagnosed easily from the history and clinical signs in most cases, this is not always the case and it is worth obtaining confirmation whenever the diagnosis is suspected. This is best achieved using double-contrast arthrography or ultrasonography although the latter is highly operator-dependent. Magnetic resonance imaging may be of value and is undergoing evaluation at present. Neither arthrography nor magnetic resonance imaging give a good indication of the size or location of the tear while ultrasonography, in experienced hands, can be very useful in this regard. Many surgeons carry out arthroscopy immediately before repair in order to establish the size and location of the tear.

Treatment

Not all rotator cuff tears require operative treatment and, indeed, many are not symptomatic. If symptoms are present, treatment must be directed towards pain relief and the restoration of function.

Non-operative treatment can be considered in those patients with pain but little functional impairment and those with limited demands upon their shoulders—these tend to be older patients. Subacromial steroid injection can be of value in relieving pain but the effects are usually limited and unless a firm decision has been taken not to proceed to surgery under any circumstances, it should probably not be repeated. Watson (1985) has demonstrated the deleterious effects of steroid upon the strength of the rotator cuff and thus on the quality of the surgical repair. Non-steroidal agents can be of value and physiotherapy aimed at strengthening the remaining rotator cuff muscles and the deltoid can be helpful. Such exercises must be gentle and involve a gradual increase in intensity or they will exacerbate any pain. They must also be continued for at least 6 weeks before any improvement is seen.

Rotator cuffs do not heal spontaneously, probably because of the presence of synovial fluid, but Takagishi (1978) reported good results in 44% of those patients treated non-operatively.

Operative treatment is indicated if the tear is sufficiently symptomatic to interfere with the patient's lifestyle. In practice, this means most full-thickness tears in patients younger than 70 years of age. The approach to the cuff is the same as that used for management of the impingement syndromes and the decompression of the cuff is necessary for both a good result and to improve the exposure. Kessel and Watson (1977) described a transacromial approach for cuff repair but, although this can provide excellent exposure, this author has found an unacceptable incidence of morbidity following its use. Repair should be carried out as soon as possible after diagnosis and within 3 weeks of an acute tear if at all possible to avoid the problems of cuff retraction and tendon edge degeneration. Unfortunately, acute cuff tears are frequently overlooked in casualty departments and presentation is late in the majority of cases.

Small tears of the cuff usually involve supraspinatus and can be closed easily by side-to-side suture. The author prefers to use a slowly absorbed suture such as PDS (Ethicon) but non-absorbable material can also be used. The margins of the tear should be trimmed prior to closure. Neer (1990) emphasizes that it is not necessary to trim away all scar tissue or abnormal tendon.

Larger tears nearly always involve avulsion of the cuff from its lateral insertion and are often L-shaped. Repair involves mobilization of the tendons with elevation of the subscapularis from the front of the scapula and the supraspinatus from the spine of the scapula taking care to avoid injury to the suprascapular nerve. Division of the capsule around the margin of the glenoid can also be helpful. Mobilization can be time-consuming but is nearly always rewarding. Repair of the tendon to the tuberosity can be accomplished by suturing it to bone through a trough cut just lateral to the articular surface. The residual part of the tear can then be repaired in side-to-side fashion. The repair should be carried out with the arm by the side. This permits the early mobilization essential to a good result. The use of abduction splints has been described and they can be of benefit in protecting repairs. However, they are unlikely to contribute to a good result when the tendon has been repaired in abduction.

Occasionally, the tear is massive and closure is impossible despite extensive mobilization. A variety of methods have been described for managing this situation including transfer of part of the tendon of subscapularis (Cofield, 1982), latissimus dorsi transfer (Gerber *et al.*, 1988), posterior deltoid transfer (Takagishi *et al.*, 1975), and debridement of the cuff (Apoil *et al.*, 1977). Synthetic or fascial grafts have not proved successful but Wallace (1990) has described the use of a Dacron hood in association with a humeral head replacement with encouraging initial results.

The results of rotator cuff repair in the literature are usually from centres with a special interest in the problem and the occasional shoulder surgeon should bear this in mind when advising the patient. Rotator cuff repair can be extremely difficult and good results depend upon attention to detail in patient assessment, surgical technique and post-operative rehabilitation. Neer *et al.* (1988) reported 77% excellent results and 14% satisfactory in 233 repairs with an average follow-up of 4.6 years. Cofield (1985) amalgamated many of the results in the literature and concluded that pain relief occurred in 87% and the patient was satisfied in 77% of cases. Comparison of the results of cuff repair, however, is limited by the lack of a uniform method of describing the type and size of the tear, the quality of the cuff tissue and the quality of the result.

CALCIFYING TENDONITIS

This is a common condition in which calcium is deposited in the rotator cuff tendon. It must be appreciated that the process of deposition and the continuing presence of calcium in the cuff is painless. However, resorption of the calcium often causes intense pain. Although there have been many theories for the aetiology of this condition, at present it appears appropriate to consider it to be degenerative in nature.

The calcium is deposited in the rotator cuff tendon and not the bursa. The supraspinatus tendon is most frequently involved and, in common with other pathology in this tendon, the lesion occurs in the area just medial to its insertion — the 'critical zone' of Moseley and Goldie (1963). This zone appears to be hypovascular and it is hypothesized that its few vessels are compressed against the coracoacromial arch in abduction or flexion further emphasizing the poor vascularity. There appears to be a diminution in the vascularity of the entire tendon with age and Brewer (1972) has suggested that this is the main reason for degeneration. It is hypothesized that this loss of vascularity will result in fibre necrosis in the already vascularly compromised 'critical zone' followed by dystrophic calcification. Some support for this theory is provided by the observation that calcification is rarely seen in patients under the age of 30 years, although Uhthoff and his colleagues (1976) argue against a degenerative cause in view of the healing of the tendon after the calcium has been resorbed.

Clinical features

Calcifying tendonitis has its peak incidence in the fifth decade, involves the dominant and non-dominant shoulders with equal frequency, and is unusual in manual workers.

It is most important to realize that in its formative and resting phases, calcifying tendonitis is not painful. The patient may complain of an aching in the shoulder as a result of the associated condition but the deposit does not cause pain. In this phase, radiographs demonstrate the calcium clearly (Fig. 23.12) and the unwary surgeon must guard against incriminating it in a patient presenting with a painful shoulder. Unusually the deposit can be so large as to cause subacromial impingement with a painful arc but this should be diagnosed specifically.

Once resorption of the deposit occurs, the patient may present with severe pain of acute onset sometimes requiring opiates for relief. Associated with the pain is restriction of all shoulder movements and septic arthritis must be considered as a differential diagnosis. Radiographs at this stage will usually show a 'fluffy' opacity. Although this is the only episode in many patients, some experience recurrent episodes of acute pain with local discomfort and tenderness between them.

Treatment

Unless there is impingement due to the calcium deposit, patients are asymptomatic in the resting phase and no therapy is necessary.

In the acute phase, the symptoms demand immediate action and, in the majority of patients, injection of local anaesthetic into the subacromial region is helpful. The addition of depot steroid may be of value but Murnaghan

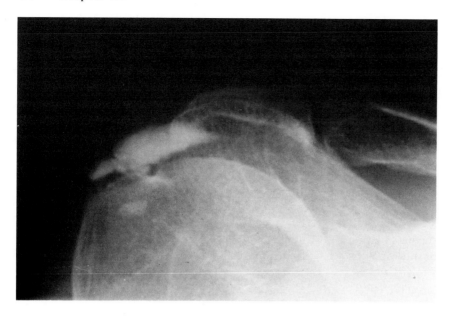

Fig. 23.12 A large calcified deposit in the supraspinatus tendon. Calcification in the resting phase is not painful but a deposit as large as that shown may be associated with subacromial impingement.

and Mackintosh (1955) could find no difference between local anaesthetic and steroid in a controlled trial. Needling of the deposit with lavage has been advocated by DePalma and Kruper (1961). The needle is introduced into the area of maximum tenderness and local anaesthetic is used for the lavage.

If the foregoing measures prove to be unsuccessful, surgical removal of the deposit(s) may be required.

FROZEN SHOULDER

This term is a much abused description of the shoulder with adhesive capsulitis. Its evocative nature has led to it being used inappropriately for any stiff and painful shoulder and, in the author's experience, occasionally for any painful shoulder (Keating and Kelly, 1990). Such lax usage of the diagnosis can make the interpretation of the literature difficult.

Like much else connected with the shoulder, the term is attributed to Codman (1934) but other terms have been, and are still, used. The most common are periarthritis and capsulitis. Neviaser (1945) described the pathological changes in 'frozen shoulder' as 'adhesive capsulitis' and this term is also sometimes used synonymously. Lundberg (1969) proposed that the stiff and painful shoulder was considered to be primary or secondary frozen shoulder with the latter group comprising those with a post-traumatic stiff shoulder.

The pathological changes described by Neviaser (1945) comprise contraction of the capsule which, as a result, adheres to the humeral head. He also found thickening of the subacromial bursa.

Many theories have been proposed for its aetiology but none has proved to be entirely satisfactory. There appears to be a definite association with lack of activity (Johnstone, 1959; Lundberg, 1969) and immunological factors have also been implicated (Macnab, 1973; Bruckner and Nye, Bulgen *et al.* 1982, 1981).

Clinical features

Primary frozen shoulder occurs most commonly between the ages of 40 and 70 years with equal sex incidence. The non-dominant shoulder is most frequently affected and recurrence of the condition in the same shoulder is rare. The condition is unusual in manual workers. There is an increased incidence of the condition in insulin-dependent diabetics and bilateral involvement is seen more commonly in this group.

Onset is spontaneous with no prior history of trauma and the development of symptoms is gradual. Pain is the initial feature and may be poorly localized. It increases in severity over the first few weeks and is associated with a progressive loss of motion at the shoulder. By about 4 months, the rest pain disappears and sharp pain on attempted movement persists. Glenohumeral movements are almost totally absent and this is sometimes called the 'frozen phase' (DePalma, 1983). In an untreated patient there will be a gradual recovery in the range of motion over the next 6–18 months—the 'thawing phase'—although some patients fail to recover fully.

The important finding on examination in any phase is the restriction of glenohumeral motion which is best seen in the rotations. Any patient who does not have some restriction of external rotation does not have a frozen shoulder.

The diagnosis can usually be made clinically but confirmation can be obtained by performing a shoulder arthrogram (Fig. 23.13). This will show obliteration of the inferior capsular recess with a tight glenohumeral joint space and variable filling of the sheath of the tendon of the long head of biceps.

Treatment

The aim of treatment is to relieve discomfort and promote the return of motion and many approaches have been described. In the initial or 'freezing' phase support for the shoulder with gentle mobilization associated with the use of ice or other local measures at physiotherapy can be helpful. Non-steroidal anti-inflammatory agents may also be effective.

Once the pain has settled, mobilization and strengthening exercises are the treatment of choice but controversy surrounds the use of additional methods.

Steroid injections have been advocated in this condition, often in the form of paired injections into the glenohumeral joint and the subacromial bursa. In a

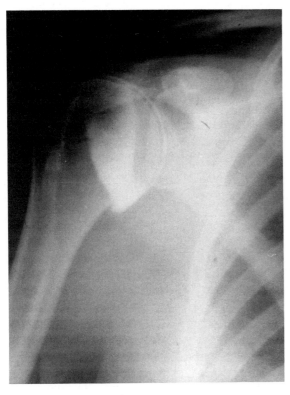

Fig. 23.13 Typical appearances of an arthrogram in adhesive capsulitis. The inferior capsular recess has been obliterated and contrast can be seen in the tendon sheath of the long head of biceps.

controlled study Bulgen *et al.* (1984) failed to show any difference between paired injections and analgesics with exercises. Hollingsworth (1983), in a controlled crossover trial, showed that 26% of a small group of patients gained more benefit from intra-articular steroid injection than injections into tender points. The case for steroid injection remains to be established.

Manipulation under anaesthetic has also provoked much controversy with condemnation on the grounds of damage to the rotator cuff tendons (DePalma, 1952). Lundberg (1969) showed that manipulation increased the rate of return of shoulder motion but that it did not shorten the duration of the condition. There are no well-controlled studies of its use and the published results show a variable success rate. The author has found it to be useful in those patients with well-established stiffness who are not responding to physiotherapy.

The procedure must be performed under general anaesthetic and the patient must have been previously informed of the need to cooperate with a physiotherapy programme after the manipulation. It does not produce a dramatic cure! The arm is held close to the shoulder and the author prefers to begin by gently stretching the shoulder into flexion thereby stressing and ultimately rupturing the inferior capsule. This is facilitated by placing the other hand on the spine of the scapula to stabilize it. Rupture of the capsule is easily appreciated by the tearing sensation it produces. Only after full flexion is possible will the author proceed to gently develop rotation and it is occasionally not possible to achieve much improvement. Repeated manipulations can be used if thought to be indicated. Intra-articular steroid along with the manipulation has been advocated by some authors. Post-operatively, immediate physiotherapy is essential. In the past the author treated these patients as day cases but has found that they respond better if detained overnight or until they can cooperate fully with a mobilization programme.

Andren and Lunberg (1965) demonstrated that capsular rupture could be achieved by distension at arthrography and their results are similar to those reported for manipulation. Ogilvie-Harris and Wiley (1986) have reported the favourable results of arthroscopic release in a large group of patients but the author feels that the results may be the result of the capsular distension required for arthroscopy to take place.

Rarely, surgical intervention will be necessary and Neer (1990) has described the technique of open release including division of the coracohumeral ligament.

Despite its extensive literature frozen shoulder remains, in the words of Codman (1934) 'difficult to define, difficult to treat and difficult to explain ...'.

RHEUMATOID ARTHRITIS

The shoulder complex is commonly affected by rheumatoid arthritis but, even in this condition, the glenohumeral joint appears to be involved less often than the other joints of the shoulder girdle.

It has been reported that 80% of all hospitalized rheumatoid patients have shoulder involvement (Petersson, 1986) and it has been estimated that two-thirds of all adult patients with rheumatoid arthritis complain of shoulder pain (Gschwend, 1980). The author's own studies (Kelly, 1990) have indicated that the acromioclavicular joint and the subacromial joint are the site of pain in 60% of rheumatoid patients with painful shoulders and this should be borne in mind when assessing these patients.

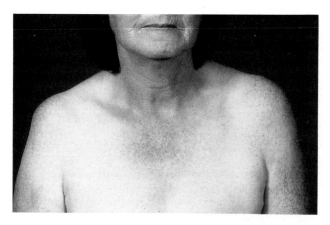

Fig. 23.14 This patient with rheumatoid arthritis shows the typical appearance of medialization in her right shoulder. This is a result of loss of bone and joint space and not merely muscle wasting.

CLINICAL FEATURES

It has already been indicated that shoulder pain is common in this group of patients. It may be part of a flare in disease activity when, if it settles as the flare subsides, it will not attract the patient's attention. Recurrent episodes are associated with a gradual loss of motion, especially external rotation, secondary to the patient resting the painful limb across the trunk, and by the time the patient presents with 'shoulder problems' motion may be severely restricted and the radiological changes may be advanced. Sometimes the shoulder is involved in isolation and the patient presents early with mild radiological changes and reversibly restricted motion.

The location of the pain is frequently of little diagnostic assistance in identifying the site of the pain and radiographs are of limited value in this regard (Kelly, 1990). It is usually felt anteriorly and over the point of the shoulder radiating towards the deltoid insertion.

Motion is lost gradually with limitation of elevation and restriction of rotation if the glenohumeral joint is involved. Muscle wasting is almost invariable and is often as much a reflection of the disease itself as the shoulder involvement. With increasing destruction, the glenohumeral joint becomes medialized giving a characteristic appearance (Fig. 23.14) which, when bilateral, was likened to a Bordeaux wine bottle by Neer (1990), and suggesting more severe muscle wasting than has actually occurred.

Several radiographic grading systems have been proposed for the rheumatoid shoulder but that which is most widely used by surgeons and rheumatologists is the system of Larsen *et al.* (1977) which has versions for both the acromioclavicular and glenohumeral joints

(Fig. 23.15a,b). It should be noted that the acromioclavicular joint expands as the degree of involvement increases.

MANAGEMENT

When assessing the rheumatoid patient with shoulder pain the first priority is to identify the source of the pain so that treatment can be directed appropriately. The author has found the use of 1 ml injections of 1% lignocaine into the components of the shoulder joint complex to be of particular value in this regard (Fig. 23.16). The glenohumeral joint is always injected last and is frequently not injected if pain has been relieved by injections to extra-glenohumeral sites (Kelly, 1990). If the patient is referred at a very early stage and has only mild limitation of movement and function, it may be prudent to delay such injection testing until the effects of drug manipulation together with physiotherapy and/or hydrotherapy have been evaluated. These last measures are usually all that is required by many patients in the early stages.

If injection testing has been used, it is useful to follow the local anaesthetic with a steroid preparation to the site of the pain and to review the patient after 3–4 weeks. Steroids are often successful but if they have no effect after a successful local anaesthetic injection surgery is likely to be required. The harmful effects of steroid injection have already been alluded to and this approach avoids the overuse of steroid by placing it at the site of the pain. If it has no effect there is no logic in repeating the injection.

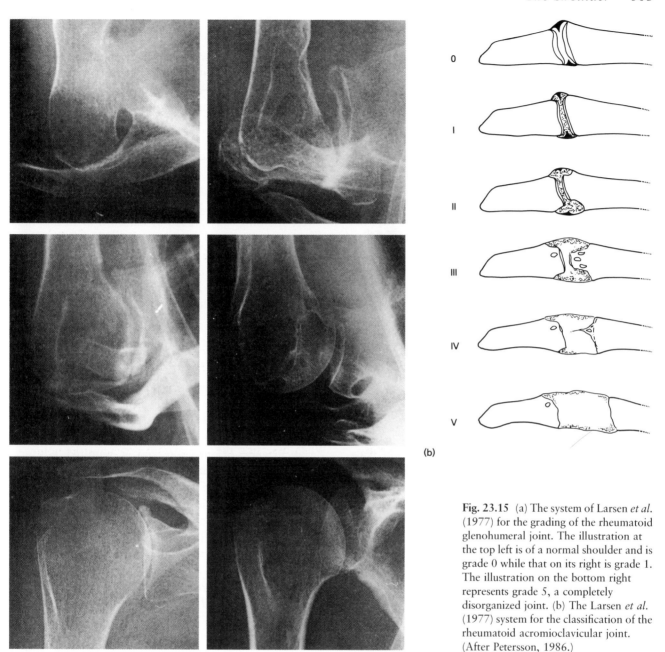

(b)

(a)

Fig. 23.15 (a) The system of Larsen *et al.* (1977) for the grading of the rheumatoid glenohumeral joint. The illustration at the top left is of a normal shoulder and is grade 0 while that on its right is grade 1. The illustration on the bottom right represents grade 5, a completely disorganized joint. (b) The Larsen *et al.* (1977) system for the classification of the rheumatoid acromioclavicular joint. (After Petersson, 1986.)

SURGICAL MANAGEMENT

The surgical management of rheumatoid arthritis of the shoulder varies with the joint that is involved. Of the surgical procedures commonly used in the management of arthritic joints arthrodesis is the least used because of the actual or potential involvement of associated joints. Synovectomy remains popular in continental Europe but is not commonly used in the UK. Excision arthroplasty of the subacromial and acromioclavicular joints can be very useful and replacement arthroplasty of the glenohumeral joint is now well established. In this section only on synovectomy and the extraglenohumeral arthroplasties will be discussed. Arthrodesis and glenohumeral arthroplasty will be discussed in the following sections.

The author's indication for surgical intervention is the failure of medical therapy, including appropriately placed steroid injections, in a patient with severe pain and limitation of function and the type of surgery is determined by the results of the injection test.

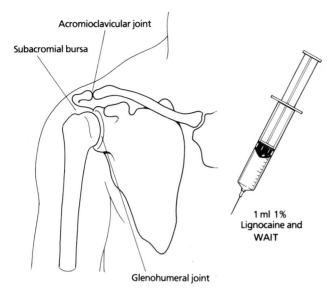

Acromioclavicular joint

Subacromial bursa

1 ml 1%
Lignocaine and
WAIT

Glenohumeral joint

Fig. 23.16 Injection testing of the shoulder joint complex.

Subacromial region

Visible or palpable subacromial bursae causing sub-acromial pain should be removed as a matter of some urgency since it has been the author's experience that they are frequently associated with rotator cuff tears which are often small and multiple. It is the author's practice to perform an anterior acromioplasty and divide the coracoacromial ligament at the same time and this is also the procedure of choice when there is subacromial pain without the enlarged bursa.

The procedure is performed in exactly the same way as described for the impingement syndromes.

Acromioclavicular joint

Although, this joint can be involved in isolation, it is more usually affected along with the subacromial region. Management is by excision of the outer 1–1.5 cm of the clavicle accompanied by anterior acromioplasty and division of the coracoacromial ligament when the sub-acromial region is also involved.

Petersson (1986) has reported good results for excision arthroplasty of the acromioclavicular joint in this group of patients and, in a group of 24 shoulders followed from 18 months to 5 years, the author has also found excellent pain relief, good recovery of motion and excellent return of function in all but one case, using a combination of anterior acromioplasty and excision of the acromioclavicular joint.

Glenohumeral joint

If the injection tests indicate the glenohumeral joint as the main site of pain and the sphericity of the humeral head is maintained—an unusual combination in the author's experience—synovectomy is preferable to arthroplasty.

In a group of 54 shoulders (48 patients) undergoing synovectomy, Pahle and Kvarnes (1985) reported that all but 10 had an increased range of motion and improved function at a mean follow-up of 10 years (range 1–16 years). Most of these glenohumeral joints were radiologically graded as Larsen II or III and none was more advanced. The authors indicated that it was not always possible to make a firm decision regarding synovectomy until after the arthrotomy because radiographic signs are late. If the sphericity of the humeral head was lost, they performed a replacement arthroplasty.

GLENOHUMERAL ARTHROPLASTY

When Péan replaced the shoulder and proximal humerus of a Parisian baker suffering from tuberculous osteomyelitis in 1891 it was the first example of the replacement of any joint. However, Péan's surgery failed due to a recurrence of infection and it required advances in surgical and anaesthetic technology before Neer was able to introduce a successful humeral head replacement in the 1950s. Glenohumeral joint replacement has progressed from that time with a variety of implants being described. These can be considered in three groups—unconstrained, partially constrained and constrained.

1 *Unconstrained.* Prostheses in this group copy the normal anatomy and therefore depend upon the integrity of the rotator cuff and deltoid muscles for stability. They are typified by the Neer prosthesis (Fig. 23.17) which comprises a stemmed humeral component with a head which is a section of a sphere with 40-mm radius of curvature and a matching glenoid component.

Cup arthroplasties have been described by Steffee and Moore (1984), Jonsson *et al.* (1986) and Copeland (1990). This type of unconstrained arthroplasty involves the placing of a metal cup over the shaped humeral head remnant.

2 *Partially constrained.* Any of the unconstrained prostheses can be converted to partially constrained types by increasing the amount of cover provided for the head by the glenoid component, usually by the provision of an extended upper lip. These prostheses are more

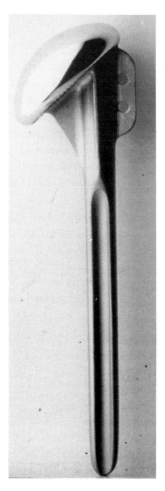

Fig. 23.17 The Neer II humeral prosthesis.

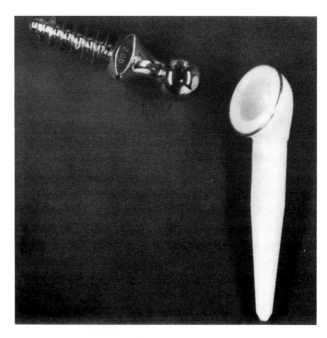

Fig. 23.18 The Kessel shoulder arthroplasty.

stable but transfer more stress to the glenoid bone and make closure of the rotator cuff difficult or impossible. **3** *Constrained.* Constrained arthroplasties have a linked scapulohumeral articulation permitting rotation but preventing translation of the humeral head on the glenoid. Its intrinsic stability means that it does not need a rotator cuff to function but also leads to considerable loads on the fixation of the implant.

Several designs have been described but they fall into two groups—those with the ball of the joint on the humeral side and those with it on the glenoid. The advantage of the latter is that the centre of rotation of the joint is lateralized and this helps to avoid impingement of the humerus against the acromion. An example of this type is the Kessel prosthesis (Kessel and Bayley, 1979) (Fig. 23.18) and the other group is exemplified by the Stanmore prosthesis (Fig. 23.19) (Lettin and Scales, 1972).

Indications

Any condition that affects the glenohumeral joint and results in pain and loss of function provides an indication for arthroplasty. As indicated above it is essential to ensure that the glenohumeral joint is indeed the source of the pain, especially in conditions such as rheumatoid arthritis. Some conditions, such as avascular necrosis of the humeral head, may involve only the humeral head and in this situation only the head will need to be replaced.

Glenohumeral arthroplasty is contraindicated if there is active or recent infection, if there is a Charcot joint or if there is paralysis of *both* the deltoid and the rotator cuff muscles. Severe loss of bone stock may also make arthroplasty impossible. In most of these situations arthrodesis becomes the method of choice.

The choice of constrained or unconstrained prostheses depends largely upon the quality of the rotator cuff. In the early days of shoulder arthroplasty it was believed that cuff rupture was common but Neer *et al.* (1982) reported a 5% incidence of cuff tears in osteoarthritis and 42% in patients with rheumatoid arthritis. Cofield (1983) found cuff tears in 19% of his osteoarthritic patients and 24% of his rheumatoid patients. In the author's own group of 180 rheumatoid shoulders, there were 28 cuff tears but it should be noted that the cuff was thin but intact in 80%. In his group of 176 shoulders with differing diagnoses, Cofield (1983) reported that of

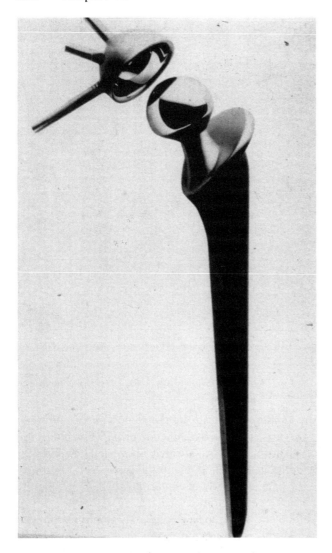

Fig. 23.19 The Stanmore shoulder replacement.

48 cuff tears, 27 were smaller than 5 cm and 21 were larger. The majority could be repaired by simple suture and all but six were amenable to repair. Thus about 90% of all shoulders have, or can be provided with a functional rotator cuff and can therefore be considered for treatment with an unconstrained prosthesis.

Post *et al.* consider constrained arthroplasty to be a salvage procedure for the relief of pain when gleno-humeral motion is desired and other methods such as arthrodesis are felt to be inappropriate. Thus it can be used when the rotator cuff is irreparable but the surgeon must be familiar with the results of each prosthesis.

Results

Comparison of the results of shoulder arthroplasty in the literature is made difficult by the lack of a common assessment system and the failure to separate diagnostic groups. Different pathologies present different problems and must be considered separately.

Pain relief is good or excellent in 90% of patients in all diagnostic groups in all series reporting the use of unconstrained arthroplasties (Neer *et al.*, 1982; Cofield, 1984; Pahle and Kvarnes, 1985; Kelly *et al.*, 1987). The results for constrained prostheses are more difficult to assess because of a high incidence of painful complications in many series. It would appear that pain relief is satisfactory in between 85 and 90% of the uncomplicated cases.

Ranges of motion and functional results are highly dependent upon the diagnostic group. For example, in Neer's series of 273 arthroplasties (Neer *et al.*, 1982) 40 with osteoarthritis gained an average of 77° of elevation, 43 with rheumatoid arthritis gained 57° degrees and 35 performed for old trauma gained only 33°. Similar figures were reported by Cofield (1984). Useful rotation is usually regained but again the diagnosis has a major bearing on this. The range of elevation achieved is closely linked to the state of the rotator cuff (Cofield, 1983). Barrett and his colleagues (1987) noted that all patients who had an intact cuff pre-operatively could attain at least 90° of elevation but three shoulders with minor or moderate cuff tears averaged 87° and six shoulders with massive tears averaged only 37°. This need not seriously interfere with function, however, since most activities of daily living are performed below shoulder level and are more related to rotational movements. Motion after constrained arthroplasty appears to be as good as that after unconstrained but results are difficult to compare because of differing methods of presentation.

The functional results are also extremely difficult to compare. Details of the function after arthroplasty for osteoarthritis are rarely given but it appears that the ability to work at, or above, shoulder level is reduced in all groups. Indeed, the difference in functional results between the diagnostic groups is not as great as the differences in the ranges of movements obtained. For the constrained prostheses, function is either not considered or merely recorded as being 'improved'.

Complications

The complications following unconstrained arthroplasty are post-operative rotator cuff failure, instability, fracture of the humerus, infection and neurovascular injury and the last three are shared by constrained prostheses together with loosening. Radiographic lucency around the glenoid component is common in unconstrained arthroplasties often approaching 80% (Amstutz *et al.*, 1981; Cofield, 1984; Kelly *et al.*, 1987; Kelly, 1990). However, clinical loosening of the glenoid component in unconstrained arthroplasties is uncommon amounting to fewer than 2%. Kelly (1990) has reported that no lucent line showed progression beyond two years in a group of 69 rheumatoid shoulders followed for a minimum of 3 years and an average of 5.5 years.

Post-operative rotator cuff tear has been reported in between 3 and 15% of patients and although it is associated with severe limitation of movements against gravity, the majority of patients regain useful function.

Instability of the joint in the form of anterior or posterior dislocation or subluxation is uncommon, occurring in approximately 2% of reported shoulders.

Intra-operative fracture usually involves the humerus and is more commonly encountered when the bone is osteoporotic as in rheumatoid arthritis. It is unusual but if recognized it is easily managed by the use of a long-stemmed component.

Neurovascular injury is rare but is well described and usually involves the circumflex nerve or the lateral cord of the brachial plexus (Wilde *et al.*, 1984; Sledge *et al.*, 1989).

The incidence of infection is extremely low with Neer reporting only one infection in his series of 193 shoulders and there being no early infections and one late infection (16 months) in the author's own group of 180 shoulders.

Although loosening of unconstrained prostheses is rare, constrained devices are more prone to this as a result of the increased load transferred to the bone−prosthesis interface. Lettin and Scales reported 10 loose glenoids in their series of 50 Stanmore shoulders and Kessel and Bayley (1979) reported two in his group of 24 shoulders.

Summary

Glenohumeral arthroplasty is now a well-established procedure. Most patients can be managed using an unconstrained prosthesis and the results show a very low complication rate with a useful return of motion and function. As with all joint replacements, pain relief is very good. The results obtained depend upon the state of the rotator cuff tendon and the extent to which the local anatomy is distorted.

ARTHRODESIS

Arthrodesis of the glenohumeral joint is not commonly performed but provides an alternative when arthroplasty is contraindicated and may be useful in the salvage of failed arthroplasties (Neer and Kirby, 1982; Kelly *et al.*, 1987). It provides a permanent solution but at the price of losing the rotational movements so essential for normal function and in rheumatoid patients it may be accompanied by the loss of motion at other joints in the upper limb secondary to immobilization.

The published results vary particularly with regard to the patient's ability to attend to their perineal care or to feed themselves (Cofield and Briggs, 1979; Rybka *et al.*, 1979). It appears likely that this is a result of the position used for the fusion. The majority of the suggested positions involve placing the hand to the mouth or forehead at the time of surgery and this can obviously be accomplished using a range of elbow and shoulder positions (Barr *et al.*, 1942; Rybka *et al.*, 1979; Raunio, 1981). The position of the arthrodesis must allow personal hygiene, must allow the arm to lie comfortably by the side with minimal scapular winging and must provide maximum strength for lifting, pulling and pushing (Rowe, 1974).

Part of the difficulty in deciding what is the optimum position is the different methods of measurement used with either the vertebral border of the scapula, the side of the trunk or the midline of the trunk being adopted as the datum. Another source of problems is the often quoted paper from Barr and his colleagues on a working committee of the American Orthopaedic Association (Barr *et al.*, 1942) which made recommendations for position based upon a study of 101 young patients with poliomyelitis. The needs of these patients are such that more abduction is required for good function and the position recommended by Barr is not suitable for non-paralysed patients. Work by Rowe (1974) and Jonsson (1988) suggests that a position of 20° of abduction measured from the side of the trunk, 20−30° of forward flexion measured from the sagittal plane and 20−40° of internal rotation measured from the sagittal plane with the arm by the side is the most appropriate. Both DePalma (1983) and Post (1989) are in agreement with this. Achieving this position at operation remains a problem and large positioning errors have been reported (Cofield and Briggs, 1979; Jonsson, 1988). Jonsson (1988) has developed a jig to facilitate positioning but most surgeons must rely on avoiding excessive abduction or flexion at operation.

Many methods of achieving glenohumeral fusion have been described. The aim is to achieve and maintain contact between the cancellous bone of the head of the humerus and the glenoid to enable bony union to occur in the desired position. The methods described can be classified as intra-articular (Watson-Jones, 1933; Carrol, 1957), extra-articular (Gill, 1931; Putti, 1933; Brittain,

1952), combined intra- and extra-articular (Moseley, 1961; Beltran *et al.*, 1975) and methods using compression (Charnley and Houston, 1964; Hawkins and Neer, 1987). The extra-articular methods were designed for the management of infected joints, especially tuberculosis. Most current procedures involve a combination of intra-articular and extra-articular methods and the use of internal fixation. The author's own preference is to use the method of Gill (1931) in which the surfaces of the joint are denuded of articular cartilage and subchondral bone and the decorticated acromion is fractured at its base and turned down into a slot cut in the head of the humerus (Fig. 23.20). Once the desired position has been obtained it is fixed using two AO screws passed across the glenohumeral joint into the scapular neck. Excision of the outer end of the clavicle can give a poor cosmetic result and Hawkins and Neer (1987) found that it had little, if any, effect upon the range of elevation which it is intended to improve.

INSTABILITY

This section considers the problems posed by recurrent dislocation or subluxation of the glenohumeral joint. The instability can be unidirectional when it is most usually anterior in direction but is sometimes posterior. Instability can also be multidirectional. It is important to distinguish *multidirectional instability* when the patient is symptomatic from *multidirectional laxity* when there are no symptoms and to realize that it is possible for a patient with multidirectional laxity to suffer from unidirectional instability.

Classification

Glenohumeral instability can be classified under several headings. There may be *complete dislocation* when spontaneous relocation does not occur or *subluxation* when complete separation of the articular surfaces does not occur. Dislocations or subluxations may be *atraumatic* or *traumatic*, *anterior*, *posterior* or *inferior* and *acute* or *recurrent* although only the last will be considered here. If the patient is thought to intentionally contribute to the dislocation or subluxation the term *voluntary* is used. The majority of dislocations are, however, *involuntary*.

The crucial distinction to make when considering a recurrently unstable shoulder is whether the instability is traumatic or atraumatic. Rowe (1956), in a study of 500 dislocations, found that 96% were traumatic and 4% atraumatic. Traumatic instability is usually unilateral, is frequently associated with a Bankart lesion and usually requires surgical treatment—the so-called *TUBS shoulder*. Atraumatic instability, on the other hand, is often multidirectional and is said to be frequently bilateral. It usually responds well to a rehabilitation programme but if surgery is required an inferior capsular shift type of procedure should be used—this is the *AMBRI shoulder*. Although bilateral laxity is very common in this type of shoulder, the author has found bilateral instability to be rare.

Factors contributing to recurrent instability

Rowe and Sakellarides (1961) and Simonet and Cofield (1984) have demonstrated the importance of age in determining the risk of recurrent dislocation following a single episode of anterior dislocation. In Rowe's series, the incidence of recurrence in patients in their second decade was 94%, the third decade 79% and the fourth decade 50%. Thereafter the incidence fell sharply. In Cofield's study, 65% of patients under 20 years suffered recurrence of dislocation but a further 19% had symptoms of instability. Between 20 and 40 years, 40% suffered recurrence with 9% experiencing instability symptoms and over 40 years there were no recurrences but 10% had symptoms of instability. In a study of factors contributing to recurrent instability Rowe and Sakellarides (1961) found that the age of the patient was the most significant factor determining the incidence of recurrence. Other factors have been identified including length of immobilization and the degree of violence

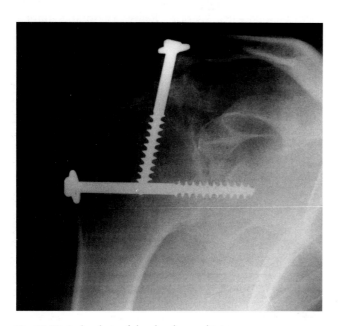

Fig. 23.20 Arthrodesis of the glenohumeral joint.

involved. However, in a study of athletes, Henry and Genung (1982) showed no significant difference in the incidence of recurrent dislocation between those immobilized and those not. Similarly, Hovelius and his colleagues (1983) showed no difference in the recurrence rates of two groups of patients under 40 years of age immobilized for 3 weeks or mobilized in a sling from day one. Despite these reports most authors recommend immobilization for 3–6 weeks in patients under 40 years! The author's recommendation is to rest the arm in a shoulder immobilizer for one week, thereafter mobilizing the joint according to the degree of pain. The degree of violence is difficult to estimate and the presence of an associated fracture is no reflection of this but a consequence of the changing properties of the tissues of the shoulder with age.

Clinical features

In the majority of patients there is no difficulty in reaching the diagnosis of recurrent dislocation since the glenohumeral joint dislocates during activities involving flexion/abduction and external rotation and frequently requires hospital relocation providing radiographic confirmation of the injury. The patient who suffers from recurrent subluxation, however, can present many problems and a high index of suspicion is required. This type of patient usually complains of the shoulder 'going out' but always manages to relocate the joint alone or with assistance. Occasionally, the patient may complain of the arm 'going dead' during the wind-up phase of a throwing activity or when preparing to serve at tennis. Between episodes, both types of patient are usually symptom-free but may alter their lifestyle to avoid situations which provoke instability.

Examination must try to confirm the presence of instability and its direction. This involves the use of provocative tests. The presence of an anterior apprehension sign is a sensitive indicator of anterior instability. This is performed by grasping the affected shoulder with one hand so that the thumb lies posterior to the humeral head and the fingers lie anterior. The other hand is then used to abduct and extend the arm. In a positive test, the patient will stop the examiner — verbally or physically — because of the sensation of impending dislocation.

It is more difficult to identify posterior instability. It is best to have the patient supine on a couch and the arm is then passively elevated to 90° in flexion. A hand is then placed under the scapula and the other hand grasps the elbow pushing the humeral head posteriorly. Posterior subluxation may be felt but this is frequently not the case and it is only by extending the arm to 90° of

abduction while maintaining the longitudinal pressure that the clunk of relocation is recognized.

Inferior instability or laxity can be demonstrated by longitudinal traction on the arm as it lies by the patient's side. In a positive test a sulcus appears below the acromion (Fig. 23.21). Anterior and posterior instability or laxity can be demonstrated by grasping the humeral head between the finger and thumb of one hand and attempting to move it anteriorly and posteriorly against the glenoid while stabilizing the scapula with the other hand.

By using these tests and obtaining a good history it is nearly always possible to decide upon the presence and direction of instability.

Radiographic assessment

Good quality radiographs must be obtained and these must include at least two views of the joint. The author's practice is to obtain an anteroposterior projection of the glenohumeral joint together with an axillary projection. In the acute situation, an apical oblique projection (Garth *et al.*, 1984; Richardson *et al.*, 1988) avoids moving the arm from the side to obtain the 'lateral projection'. These projections are useful for demonstrating Hill–Sachs lesions (1940) or fractures of the glenoid margin and facilitate the identification of posterior dislocations (Fig. 23.22).

Most of the lesions associated with shoulder instability involve soft-tissue structures and require to be demonstrated by contrast studies, magnetic resonance imaging or arthroscopy. The most useful contrast study in this group of patients is the double-contrast computed

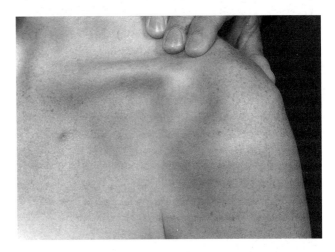

Fig. 23.21 Positive sulcus sign. Longitudinal traction has been applied to the patient's arm.

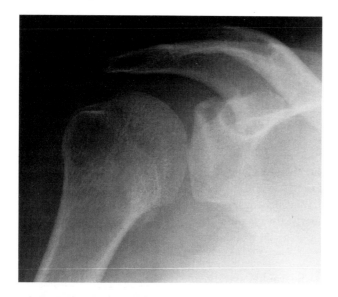

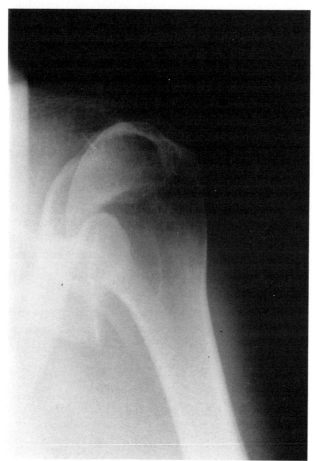

tomography arthrogram (Resch *et al.* 1990). This investigation does not provide the diagnosis of instability but it is useful to demonstrate the associated pathology. It can provide useful confirmation in those few cases where the diagnosis is in doubt and it allows the surgeon to plan the surgical repair. Bankhart lesions, capsular laxity, glenoid abnormalities and Hill–Sachs lesions can all be shown using this technique (Fig. 23.23). Magnetic resonance imaging (Resch *et al.* 1990) has so far proven inferior to computed tomography–arthrography in the investigation of instability but developments in both hardware and software may improve its efficacy.

Arthroscopy

Like computed tomography–arthrography, arthroscopy can be useful in demonstrating pathology within the glenohumeral joint and providing evidence for the direction of the instability.

Treatment

While recurrent dislocation will require surgical repair if it is occurring frequently enough to cause the patient problems, recurrent subluxation often responds to a course of rotator cuff strengthening exercises performed over a period of at least 6 months. This involves isometric

Fig. 23.22 (a) Anteroposterior projection of a posterior fracture dislocation of the shoulder. Unfortunately this injury is commonly overlooked in Accident & Emergency departments. A second radiological projection must always be performed. (b) An apical/oblique projection of the same shoulder shown in (a). This clearly demonstrates the posterior fracture dislocation of the glenohumeral joint.

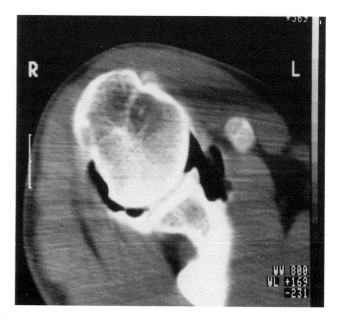

Fig. 23.23 A double contrast computed tomography arthrogram of the glenohumeral joint demonstrating detachment of the anterior labrum and a Hill–Sachs lesion in the posterior aspect of the humeral head.

exercises below shoulder level. Surgery is indicated if this regimen fails.

In the most common situation of unidirectional anterior dislocation a large number of procedures have been described. These involve soft-tissue repair of the labrum or capsule, tightening of the anterior capsule, transfer of the coracoid process, the use of an anterior bone block or de-rotation osteotomy. The results of the many published series are difficult to interpret because of differences in presentation with some authors including post-operative subluxation with the failures and some not considering it.

The most commonly used and best documented procedure is the Bankart operation which has been elegantly described by Rowe *et al.* (1978). Avulsion of the glenoid labrum represents avulsion of the inferior glenohumeral ligament from the glenoid and its re-attachment appears to be the logical treatment. It can be a difficult operation, involving the refixation of the labrum using sutures passed through holes in the glenoid margin. These holes can be difficult to drill and pose the risk of fracture of the glenoid rim greatly increasing the complexity of the repair. The recent introduction of suture anchors placed into drill holes in the glenoid neck have helped to simplify the procedure.

The shoulder is approached through the deltopectoral groove and the deltoid is reflected off the underlying fascia. The subscapularis is divided approximately 3 cm medial to its insertion — midway along the length of the tendon — and is then elevated off the underlying capsule. The arm is fully externally rotated and the capsule is divided at the level of the glenoid rim allowing inspection of the interior of the joint. The Bankart lesion is identified and the glenoid neck is cleared of soft tissue. The bone underlying the avulsed labrum or capsular remnants is roughened using an awl and drill holes are made through the glenoid rim for the passage of sutures or into the glenoid margin for the use of suture anchors. The capsule is re-attached to the glenoid rim and the labrum or its remnants is sutured over this. Subscapularis is then repaired without shortening.

If a Bankart lesion is not present the anterior capsule — if lax — can be plicated as described by Osmond-Clarke (1948) in the Putti–Platt procedure. Care must be taken to avoid overtightening since this will result in a disabling loss of external rotation. This can be avoided by ensuring that at least 30° of external rotation is possible during surgery.

Transfer of the coracoid process to the glenoid neck as in the Bristow procedure is popular in continental Europe and can give good results in experienced hands (Gazielly and Godeneche, 1991). Technical consider-ations are paramount and accurate placement of the coracoid is essential. This procedure causes extensive scarring which can make revision extremely difficult.

Arthroscopic repair

Arthroscopic repair of the Bankart lesion is now well established and two approaches have been described. The first uses sutures passed through the neck of the glenoid which anchor the anterior capsule and are tied together against the posterior glenoid (Morgan and Bodenstab, 1978). The second, more popular procedure involves the placing of one or more staples to re-attach the labrum to the glenoid rim (Johnson, 1986). These are demanding procedures and preliminary results from experts (Caspari *et al.*, 1990; Maki, 1990) have only yielded success rates of 80%. Their use is popular in sportsmen but it should be noted that the healing of the Bankart lesion is no quicker using this method and return to sporting activities is no earlier than with the open operation.

Posterior instability

Recurrent traumatic posterior instability is not common but is well recognized. Even in the traumatic cases there is often increased joint laxity and it is worth treating the patient with a 6-month course of rotator cuff strengthening before embarking on operative treatment.

In most cases posterior capsular plication is used but if there is excessive glenoid retroversion (recognized from the computed tomography — arthrogram or special radiographic projections) a posterior opening wedge glenoid osteotomy is used in addition (Kretzer and Scott, 1982). The success rate is not as high as for anterior instability.

Multidirectional instability

It is important to recognize this condition since the use of anterior capsular plication procedures will not be successful and may convert a predominantly anteriorly dislocating joint into a posteriorly unstable joint. Computed tomography — arthrography and arthroscopy can help to avoid this mistake.

If rotator cuff strengthening exercises fail to work over a period of 6–12 months, surgery has to be considered. This must achieve tightening of all parts of the capsule and several procedures have been described. The inferior capsular shift procedure of Neer and Foster (1980) is one of the most widely used but it is difficult to perform and attention to detail is essential. This is not an operation for the occasional shoulder surgeon. It is technically difficult, there is a moderately high risk of injuring the axillary nerve and rehabilitation is demanding of both the therapist and patient. There are few published results of this procedure. Neer's small series reports good results but Wallace (personal communication) reports 50% recurrence of instability in his series. In the author's own group of 12 patients only one has minor symptoms of 'instability' but this is a soft-tissue procedure in patients with lax soft tissue and it may well be that recurrence is merely a matter of time.

SUMMARY

The shoulder is a complex of joints which act in concert to facilitate the placing of the upper limb. The design and interaction of these joints is such that pathology occurs mainly in the soft-tissue elements in the form of degeneration and failure. While imaging can be of great value, it remains limited and the mainstay of shoulder assessment is the eliciting of a good history and the performance of a careful examination. By combining this information with a knowledge of the applied anatomy of the shoulder and the pathogenesis of shoulder problems accurate diagnoses can be made and appropriate therapies devised.

REFERENCES

Amstutz H.C., Sew Hoy A.L. and Clarke I.C. (1981) UCLA anatomic total shoulder. *Clin. Orthop.* **155**, 7–20.

Andren L. and Lundberg B.J. (1965) Treatment of rigid shoulders by joint distension during arthrography. *Acta Orthop. Scand.* **36**, 45–53.

Apoil A., Dautry P., Moinet P.H. and Kochlin, P.H. (1977) Le syndrome dit de rupture de la coiffe des rotateurs de l'epaule. Apropos de 70 interventions. *Rev. Chir. Orthop.*, Suppl. II, 63.

Barr J.S., Freiberg J.A., Colonna P.C. and Pemberton B.A. (1942) A survey of end results on stabilisation of the paralytic shoulder. *J. Bone Joint Surg.* **24A**, 699–707.

Barrete W.P., Franklin J.L., Jakins S.E. *et al.* (1987) Total shoulder arthroplasty. *J. Bone Joint Surg.* **69A**, 865–872.

Beltran J.E., Trilla J.C. and Barjan, R. (1975) A simplified compression arthrodesis of the shoulder. *J. Bone Joint Surg.* **57A**, 538–541.

Bigliani L.U. (1989) Anterior and posterior capsular shift for multidirectional instability. *Tech. Orthop. B*, 36–45.

Bigliani L.U., Morrison D. and April E.W. (1986) The morphology of the acromion and its relationship to rotator cuff tears. *Orthop. Trans.* **10**, 228.

Brems J.J. (1987) *Digital Muscle Strength Measurement in Rotator Cuff Tears.* Paper presented at the American Shoulder and Elbow Surgeons' Third Open Meeting, San Francisco.

Brewer B.J. (1979) Aging of the rotator cuff. *Am. J. Sports Med.* **7**, 102–110.

Brittain H.A. (1952) *Architectural Principles of Arthrodesis*, 3rd edn. Edinburgh, E. and L. Livingstone.

Brucner F.E. and Nye C.J.S. (1981) A prospective study of adhesive capsulitis of the shoulder in a high risk population. *Q. J. Med.* **198**, 191–204.

Bulgen D.Y., Binder A., Hazleman B.L. *et al.* (1984) Frozen shoulder: prospective clinical study with an evaluation of three treatment regimens. *Ann. Rheum. Dis.* **43**, 353–360.

Bulgen D.Y., Binder A., Hazleman B.L. and Park J.P. (1982) Immunological studies in frozen shoulders. *J. Rheumatol.* **9**, 893–898.

Bunker T.D. and Wallace W.A. (1991) *Shoulder Arthroscopy.* London, Martin Dunitz.

Carrol R.E. (1957) Wire loop arthrodesis of the shoulder. *Clin. Orthop.* **9**, 185–189.

Casparai R.B., Savoie F.H. and Myers J.F. (1990) Arthroscopic reconstruction of anterior shoulder instability. In Post M., Morrey B. and Hawkins R.J. (eds) *Surgery of the shoulder*, St Louis, Mosby Year Book.

Charnley J. and Houston J.K. (1964) Compression arthrodesis of the shoulder. *J. Bone Joint Surg.* **46B**, 614–620.

Codman E.A. (1934) *The Shoulder.* Boston, Thomas Todd.

Cofield R.H. (1982) Subscapular muscle transposition for repair of chronic rotator cuff tears. *Surg. Gynaecol. Obstet.* **154**, 667–672.

Cofield R.H. (1983) Unconstrained shoulder arthroplasty. *Clin. Orthop.* **173**, 97–108.

Cofield, R.H. (1984) Total shoulder arthroplasty with the Neer prosthesis. *J. Bone Joint Surg.* **66A**, 899–906.

Cofield R.H. (1985) Current concepts review: rotator cuff disease of the shoulder. *J. Bone Joint Surg.* **67A**, 974–979.

Cofield R.H. and Briggs B.T. (1979) Glenohumeral arthrodesis. Operative and long term functional results. *J. Bone Joint Surg.* **61A**, 668–677.

Copeland S. (1990) *Cementless total shoulder replacement.* In Surgery of the Shoulder. Post M., Morrey B.F., Hawkins R.J. (eds.) St. Louis, Mosby Year Book.

Copeland S. and Barrett D. (1990) A new physical sign in shoulder arthroscopy. *J. Bone Joint Surg.* **71B**, 860.

DePalma A.F. (1952) Loss of scapulohumeral motion (frozen shoulder). *Ann. Surg.* **135**, 193–204.

DePalma A.F. (1983) *Surgery of the Shoulder*, 3rd edn. Philadelphia, J.B. Lippincott.

DePalma A.F. and Kruper J.S. (1961) Long term study of shoulder joints afflicted with and treated for calcific tendonitis. *Clin. Orthop.* **20**, 61.

Ellman H. (1988) *Arthroscopic Subacromial Decompression: One to Three Year Follow-up Study.* Instructional Course Lectures, American Academy of Orthopaedic Surgeons, Atlanta, Georgia.

Gardner E. (1963) Prenatal development of the human shoulder joint. *Surg. Clin. N. Am.* **43**, 1465–1470.

Garth W.P., Slappey C.E. and Ochs T.W. (1984) Roentgenographic demonstration on instability of the shoulder. The apical oblique projection. A technical note. *J. Bone Joint Surg.* **66A**, 1450–1453.

Gazielly D.F. and Godeneche J.L. (1991) The use of coracoid transfer for recurrent anterior glenohumeral instability. In Watson M.S. (ed.) *Surgical Disorders of the Shoulder.* Edinburgh, Churchill Livingstone, pp. 355–362.

Gerber G., Ternier G. and Ganz R. (1985) The role of the coracoid process in the chronic impingement syndrome. *J. Bone Joint Surg.* **67B**, 703–708.

Gerber C., Vinh T.S., Hurtel R. *et al.* (1988) Latissimus dorsi transfer for the treatment of massive tears of the rotator cuff. *Clin. Orthop.* 232, 51–61.

Gill A.B. (1931) New operation for arthrodesis of the shoulder. *J. Bone Joint Surg.* 13A, 287–295.

Grey R.J. (1978) The natural history of idiopathic frozen shoulder. *J. Bone Joint Surg.* 60, 564.

Gschwend N. (1980) *Surgical Treatment of Rheumatoid Arthritis*. Philadelphia, W.B. Saunders.

Hawkins R.J. and Neer C.S. (1987) Functional analysis of shoulder fusion. *Clin. Orthop.* 223, 65–76.

Henry J.H. and Genung J.A. (1982) Natural history of gleno-humeral dislocation revisited. *Am. J. Sports Med.* 10, 135–137.

Hill H.A. and Sachs N.D. (1940) The grooved defect of the humeral head. A frequently unrecognised complication of dislocations of the shoulder joint radiology 35, 690–700.

Hollingsworth G.R. (1983) Comparison of injection techniques for shoulder pain. *Br. Med. J.* 287, 1339–1341.

Hovelius L., Eriksson K., Fredin H. *et al.* (1983) Recurrences after initial dislocation of the shoulder: results of a prospective study of treatments. *J. Bone Joint Surg.* 65A, 343–349.

Johnson L.L. (1986) Shoulder arthroscopy. In Johnson L.L. (ed.) *Arthroscopic Surgery, Principles and Practice* St. Louis, C.V. Mosby, pp. 1301–1445.

Jonsson E. (1988) Surgery of the Shoulder. Thesis, University of Lund, Sweden.

Jonsson E., Egund N., Kelly I.G. *et al.* (1986) Cup arthroplasty of the rheumatoid shoulder. *Acta Orthop. Scand.* 57, 542–546.

Johnstone J.T.H. (1959) Frozen shoulder in patients with pulmonary tuberculosis. *J. Bone Joint Surg.* 41, 877–882.

Keating J.F. and Kelly I.G. (1990) Frozen shoulder: a retrospective analysis of 56 patients. *J. Orthop. Rheumatol.* 3, 11–14.

Kelly I.G. (1990) *Shoulder replacement in rheumatoid arthritis*. In Post M., Morrey B.F. and Hawkins R.J. (eds) *Surgery of the Shoulder*. St. Louis, Mosby Year Book , pp. 305–307.

Kelly I.G. (1990) Surgical management of the rheumatoid shoulder. The surgical management of rheumatoid arthritis. *Ann. Rheum. Dis.* 49 (Suppl. 2), Heberden Papers, 824–829.

Kelly I.G., Foster R.S. and Fisher W.D. (1987) Neer total shoulder replacement in rheumatoid arthritis. *J. Bone Joint Surg.* 69B, 723–736.

Kessel L. and Watson M.S. (1977) The transacromial approach to the shoulder for ruptures of the rotator cuff. *Int. Orthop.* 1, 153–154.

Kessel L. and Bayley I. (1979) Prosthetic replacement of the shoulder: preliminary communication. *J. Roy. Soc. Med.* 72, 748–752.

Kessell L. and Bayley I. (1986) *Clinical Disorders of the Shoulder*, 2nd edn. Edinburgh, Churchill Livingstone.

Klein A.H., France J.C., Mutschler T.A. and Frew F.H. (1987) Measurement of brachial plexus strain in arthroscopy of the shoulder. *Arthroscopy* 3, 45–52.

Kretzler H. and Scott D.J. (1982) Posterior glenoid osteotomy for posterior dislocation of the shoulder. In Bayley I. and Kessel L. (eds). *The Shoulder*. Berlin, Springer-Verlag, pp. 95–97.

Larsen A., Dale K. and Eek M. (1977) Radiographic evaluation rheumatoid arthritis in related conditions by standard reference films. *Acta Radiol. (Diag.)* 18, 481–491.

Lettin A.W.F. and Scales J. (1972) Total replacement of the shoulder joint. *Proc. Roy. Soc. Med.* 65, 373–374.

Lundberg B.J. (1969) The frozen shoulder. *Acta Orthop. Scand.* (Suppl.) 119, 1–59.

Mack L.A., Matsen F.A., Kilcoyne R.F. *et al.* (1985) Evaluation of the rotator cuff. *Radiology* 157, 205–209.

Macnab I. (1973) Rotator cuff tendonitis. *Ann. Roy. Coll. Surg.* (Engl.) 53, 271–287.

Maki N.J. (1990) Arthroscopic stabilization for recurrent shoulder instability. In Post M., Morrey B. and Hawkins R.J. (eds) *Surgery of the Shoulder*. St Louis, Mosby Year Book.

Morgan C.D. and Bodenstab A.B. (1978) Arthroscopic suture repair: techniques and early results. *Arthroscopy* 3, 111–122.

Morrison D.S. and Bigliani L.U. (1987) *The Clinical Significance of Variations in Acromial Morphology*. Paper presented at the American Shoulder and Elbow Surgeons' Third Open Meeting, San Francisco.

Moseley H.F. (1961) Arthrodesis of the shoulder in the adult. *Clin. Orthop.* 20, 156–162.

Moseley H.F. (1969) *Shoulder Lesions*, 3rd edn. Baltimore, Williams & Wilkins.

Moseley H.F. and Goldie I. (1963) The arterial pattern of the rotator cuff of the shoulder. *J. Bone Joint Surg.* 45B, 780–789.

Murnaghan G.F. and MacIntosh D. (1955) Hydrocortisone in painful shoulders controlled trial. *Lancet* 21, 798–800.

Neer C.S. (1972) Anterior acromioplasty for the chronic impingement syndrome in the shoulder. A preliminary report. *J. Bone Joint Surg.* 54A, 41–50.

Neer C.S. (1990) *Shoulder Reconstruction*. Philadelphia, W.B. Saunders.

Neer C.S. and Foster C.R. (1980) Inferior capsular shift for involuntary inferior and multi-directional instability of the shoulder. *J. Bone Joint Surg.* 62A, 897–908.

Neer C.S. and Kirby R.M. (1982) Revision of humeral head and total shoulder arthroplasties. *Clin. Orthop.* 170, 189–195.

Neer C.S., Watson K.C. and Stanton F.J. (1982) Recent experience in total shoulder arthroplasty. *J. Bone Joint Surg.* 64A, 319–337.

Neer C.S., Flatow E.L. and Lech O. (1988) *Tears of the Rotator Cuff: Long Term Results of Anterior Acromioplasty and Repair*. Presented at the American Shoulder and Elbow Surgeons' Fourth Meeting, Atlanta, Georgia, February.

Neviaser J.S. (1945) Adhesive capsulitis of the shoulder. *J. Bone Joint Surg.* 27A, 211–222.

Ogilvie-Harris D.J. and Wiley A. (1986) Arthroscopic surgery of the shoulder. *J. Bone Joint Surg.* 68B, 201–207.

Osmond-Clarke H. (1948) Habitual dislocation of the shoulder. The Putti–Platt operation. *J. Bone Joint Surg.* 30B, 19–25.

Pahle J.A. and Kvarnes L. (1985) Shoulder synovectomy. *Ann. Chirurg. Gynaecol.* 74 (Suppl. 198), 37–39.

Pahle J.A. and Kvarnes L. (1985) Shoulder replacement arthroplasty. *Ann. Chirurg. Gynaecol.* 74 (Suppl. 198), 85–89.

Peterson J. and Gentfed C.F. (1983) Ruptures of the supraspinatus tendon—The significance of distally pointing acromioclavicular osteophytes. *Clin. Orthop.* 174, 143.

Petterson G. (1942) Rupture of the tendon aponeurosis of the shoulder joint in anterior/inferior dislocation. *Chirurg. Scand.* (Suppl.) 77, 1–184.

Petersson C.J. (1986) Painful shoulders in patients with rheumatoid arthritis. *Scand. J. Rheumatol.* 15, 275–279.

Post M. (1989) *The Shoulder—Surgical and Non-Surgical Management*, 2nd edn. Philadelphia, Lea & Febiger.

Post M. and Cohen J. (1986) Impingement syndrome. *Clin. Orthop.* 207, 126–132.

Post M., Haskell S.S. and Jablon M. (1980) Total shoulder replacement with a constrained prosthesis. *J. Bone Joint Surg.* 62A, 237–335.

Putti V. (1933) Arthrodesis for tuberculosis of the knee and of the shoulder. *Chir. Orgaani. di Movimento* **18**, 217.

Raunio P. (1981) Arthrodesis of the shoulder joint in rheumatoid arthritis. *Reconstruct. Surg. Traumatol.* **18**, 48–54.

Resch H., Furtschegger A., Medden D. *et al.* (1990) The value of different screening methods in the diagnosis of shoulder lesions: ultrasonography, arthrography, CT, MR imaging, arthroscopy, bursoscopy. In Post M., Morrey B.F. and Hawkins R.J. (eds) *Surgery of the Shoulder.* St. Louis, Mosby Year Book, pp. 22–26.

Richards R.R., Hudson A.R., Bertoia J.T. *et al.* (1987) Injury to the brachial plexus during Putti–Platt and Bristow procedures. A report of eight cases. *Am. J. Sports Med.* **15**, 374–380.

Richardson J.B., Ramsay A., Davidson J.K. and Kelly I.G. (1988) Radiographs in shoulder trauma. *J. Bone Joint Surg.* **70B**, 457–460.

Rockwood C.A. (1984) Subluxation and dislocations about the shoulder. In Rockwood Jnr. C.A. and Green D.P. (eds) *Fractures in Adults.* Philadelphia, J.R. Lippincott.

Rowe C.R. (1956) Prognosis of dislocations of the shoulder. *J. Bone Joint Surg.* **38A**, 957–977.

Rowe C.R. (1974) Re-evaluation of the position of the arm in arthrodesis of the shoulder in the adult. *J. Bone Joint Surg.* **56A**, 913–922.

Rowe C.R. and Sakellarides H.T. (1961) Factors related to recurrences of anterior dislocations of the shoulder. *Clin. Orthop.* **20**, 40–48.

Rowe C.R., Patel D. and Southmead W.W. (1978) The Bankhart procedure—long term end result study. *J. Bone Joint Surg.* **60A**, 1–16.

Rybka V., Raunio P. and Vainio K. (1979) Arthrodesis of the shoulder in rheumatoid arthritis. A review of 41 cases. *J. Bone Joint Surg.* **61B**, 155–158.

Simonet W.T. and Cofield R.H. (1984) Prognosis in anterior shoulder dislocation. *Am. J. Sports Med.* **12**, 19–24.

Sledge C.B., Kozinn S.C., Thornhill T.S. and Barrett W.P. (1989) Total shoulder arthroplasty in rheumatoid arthritis in rheumatoid arthritis surgery of the shoulder. In Lettin S.W.F. and Petersson C. (eds) *Rheumatology,* vol. 12, Basel, Karger, pp. 95–102.

Steffe A.D. and Moore R.W. (1984) Hemiresurfacing arthrosplasty of the shoulder. *Contemp. Orthop.* **9**, 51–59.

Takagishi N. (1978) Conservative treatment of the ruptures of the rotator cuff. *J. Jap. Orthop. Ass.* **52**, 781–787.

Takagishi N., Okabe Y., Latseuzaki N. *et al.* (1975) Treatment of the rotator cuff tear. *J. Jap. Orthop. Ass.* **49**, 698.

Thorling J., Bjerneld H., Hallin G. *et al.* (1985) Acromioplasty for impingement syndrome. *Acta Orthop. Scand.* **56**, 147–148.

Tibone J.E., Jobe F.W., Kirwan R.K. *et al.* (1985) Shoulder impingement syndrome in athletes treated by anterior acromioplasty. *Clin. Orthop.* **198**, 134–140.

Uhthoff H.K., Sarkar K. and Maynard J.A. (1976) Calcifying tendonitis. *Clin. Orthop.* **118**, 164–168.

Uhthoff H.K., Loehr, J. and Sarkar K. (1986) The pathogenesis of rotator cuff tears. In *Proceedings of the Third International Conference on Surgery of the Shoulder, Fukuora, Japan.*

Wallace W.A. (1982) The dynamic study of shoulder movement. In Bayley I. and Kessel L. (eds) *Shoulder Surgery.* Berlin, Springer-Verlag.

Wallace W.A. (1990) The Nottingham dacron hood reinforcement for unconstrained shoulder replacement. In Post M., Morrey B.F. and Hawkins R.J. (eds) *Surgery of the Shoulder.* St. Louis, Mosby Year Book, 277–281.

Wallace W.A. and Hellier M. (1983) Improving radiographs of the injured shoulder. *Radiography* **49**, 229–233.

Watson M.S. (1985) Major ruptures of the rotator cuff: The results of surgical repair in 89 patients. *J. Bone Joint Surg.* **67B**, 618–624.

Watson M.S. (1991) *Surgical Disorders of the Shoulder.* Watson M.S. (ed.). Edinburgh, Churchill Livingstone.

Watson-Jones R. (1933) Extra-articular arthrodesis of the shoulder. *J. Bone Joint Surg.* **15B**, 862–871.

Wilde A.H., Borden L.S. and Brems J.J. (1984) Experience with the Neer total shoulder replacement. In Bateman J.E. and Welsh R.P. (eds) *Surgery of the Shoulder.* St. Louis, C.V. Mosby, pp. 224–228.

Chapter 24

The Hand, Wrist and Elbow

T.G. Wadsworth

EXAMINATION

The upper limb consists of a series of levers interposed by joints, extending from the shoulder to the tips of the digits: this mechanical chain is controlled not only by muscle action but by stabilizing features of the capsulo-ligamentous structures at the various joints as well as the shape of the articular surfaces (Fig. 24.1). The function of the upper limb is as follows. Firstly, the shoulder is used to position the hand while elbow movement provides appropriate length for the required task; rotation of the forearm then places the hand in position and thereafter the digits and wrist are appropriately used. Grip is reinforced by appropriate muscle stabilization of the upper limb proximally and of the body. Any deficiency in the linkage system will cause impairment of overall function so it is important to make full assessment of the upper limb in the clinical examination.

Normal stance of the thumb and fingers is much influenced by complex muscle action, especially the balancing role of the intrinsic musculotendonous units in relation to the extrinsic finger flexor and extensor tendons: this important role is exemplified by clawing of the ring and little fingers in advanced ulnar neuropathy (Fig. 24.2).

The hand and upper limb should first be visually inspected, taking into account any general medical features, including rheumatoid disease, psoriasis, gout and pulmonary disease (Fig. 24.3).

Examination of the nails can sometimes be suggestive of various medical conditions: splinter haemorrhages in the longitudinal axis of the nail may occur with subacute bacterial endocarditis while spoon-shaped nails, termed koilonychia, can be seen in anaemia.

Beau's lines are transverse in the nail and an indicator of periods of severe illness. Grooving and elevation of the nails, the latter known as onycholysis, is typical of psoriasis and the skin rash is usually obvious. Clubbing of the fingers with overhang of the nail is typical of heart and lung disease producing cyanosis, but it can also be idiopathic and familial in nature. Overhang of the nail can, of course, on occasion be due to traumatic damage to the digit.

Rarely, a melanoma is seen in the nail-bed, 75% of such cases involve the thumb or great toe and account for 2–3% of all melanomas in white people, a higher proportion in dark-skinned individuals: the usually brown to black discoloration in the nailbed is typically situated proximally. Pigment involvement of the posterior nail-fold is said to be ominous and indicating an

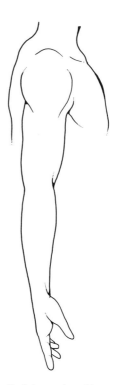

Fig. 24.1 The upper limb is a series of levers, interposed by joints, extending from the digital tips to the shoulder.

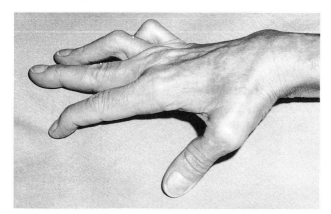

Fig. 24.2 Complex musculotendonous action accounts for the normal stance of the hand. This is an example of imbalance with respect to ulnar neuropathy with clawing of the ring and little fingers.

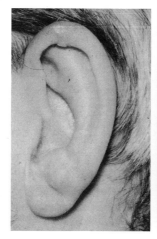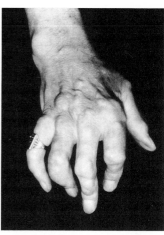

Fig. 24.3 Typical changes of gout in the ear and hand. General medical features should be considered such as rheumatoid disease, psoriasis, gout and pulmonary osteoarthropathy in evaluating the hand and upper limb.

advanced stage, this being known as Hutchinson's sign. The condition occurs with equal frequency in men and women, most often aged 55–65 years.

Fungal infections and paronychia are important conditions seen in the area of the nail. Painful elevation of the nail can result from a subungual exostosis arising dorsally from the distal phalanx.

The digits have an important involvement in systemic lupus erythematosus and in Raynaud's syndrome. Severe cases of frostbite result in gangrene of the digits and embolus from a proximal arterial plaque may have the same result. Acrocyanosis can be seen typically in young women without any apparent important underlying cause. The Allen test is useful in evaluating vascularity of the hand (Fig. 24.4).

Where a finger has been amputated, usually for trauma, loss of length should be measured after placing the palms of both hands accurately together with the other fingers terminally in line. Stability of the three joints of the finger should be assessed and in the case of the metacarpophalangeal joint it is important to test this in full flexion where normally the collateral ligaments on either side of the joint are at full stretch (Fig. 24.5).

From a functional point of view, it is important to assess whether the pulps of the fingers reach the palmar skin and, if not, the short-fall in distance should be appropriately measured. Extension and flexion are easily measured and it is important also to assess abduction and adduction, together with range of motion of the interphalangeal and metacarpophalangeal joints (Fig. 24.6).

Digital angular and rotatory deformity should be noted, as should limitation of normal span between the thumb and index finger with loss of normal abduction of the thumb.

Where there is web-space contracture, limitation of abduction of the thumb should be measured and compared with that of the other hand; stability of the joints of the thumb should be assessed, particularly the metacarpophalangeal joint. This disability is seen in the rheumatoid patient and psoriatic arthritic patients and after trauma, especially to the ulnar collateral ligament (Fig. 24.7).

Arthritis at the basal thumb joint is likely to be accompanied by easily visible and palpable swelling, and here the 'grind' test is useful in locating the area of painful disability at the trapeziometacarpal articulation, the examiner grasping the thumb and rotating the digit while it is compressed. However, similar osteoarthritic change can be pan-trapezial or isolated to the trapezio-scaphoid articulation.

Grip of the hand is, of course, of paramount importance in use of the upper limb. Pinch grip varies in type with the thumb engaged against the finger in pulp, key, precision and chuck grip. Where there is painful disability of the index finger key grip can be substituted by the thumb engaging the middle or ring finger.

With regard to examining grasp of the hand as a whole, this varies between hook, span and power grip; palm push is concerned with pressing on the palm to elevate the body or to compress objects. Considerable physical use of the hand in manual work activities is typically exhibited by calluses on the palm.

Grip and pinch strength should be assessed with an appropriate meter for each and the test should be

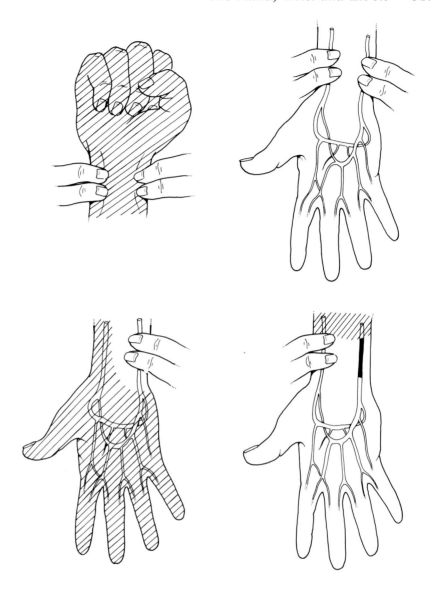

Fig. 24.4 The Allen test for patency of the radial and ulnar arteries. Firstly, both are occluded by the examiner while the fist is clenched. The radial and ulnar arteries are then sequentially released after the digits are extended by the patient. The blanched hand returns to a normal colour when pressure is relieved at either artery unless obstruction is present.

repeated on three occasions to see if a consistent value is given (Fig. 24.8).

Scars and contractures are commonly seen in the palm of the hand and in the digits: many are due to traumatic lesions, these sometimes being accompanied by digital shortening, and there may be proximally referred tenderness by percussing amputation neuromata.

Dupuytren's disease is characterized by pitting of the palmar skin and nodularity and relative immobility of the skin, and in many cases there are obvious bands involving the digits, often producing contractures. In some, there is an accompanying lesion of the plantar fascia rarely causing varus deformity of the great toe and more rarely the penis, this being termed Peyronie's disease.

Various deformities may be seen in the rheumatoid patient such as flexion of the interphalangeal joints,

boutonnière, swan-neck and angular abnormality of the interphalangeal joints while ulnar drift is a common problem.

In rheumatoid disease there may also be deformity of the thumb with prominence of the basal joint and either severe flexion deformity of the metacarpophalangeal joint with matching hyperextension of the interphalangeal joint or the opposite deformity in others. There is frequently obvious synovitis, most easily seen on the dorsum of the wrist in the active stage of the disease and also in the digital joints, less often in the flexor sheaths.

Rupture of the extensor pollicis longus tendon results in the stance of the thumb being across the palm of the hand with inability to extend: this not only occurs in the rheumatoid arthritic patient but also after a Colles' fracture, usually in the post-healing stage of the fracture.

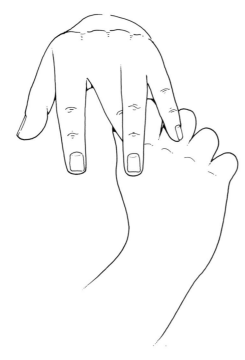

Fig. 24.5 Testing for stability of the finger collateral ligaments at the metacarpophalangeal joint, normally stable in maximum flexion.

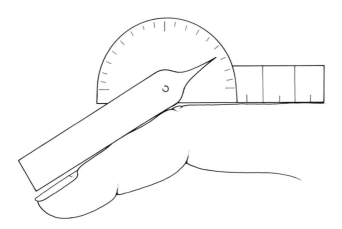

Fig. 24.6 A goniometer should be used to measure accurately digital joint motion; it is also functionally important to assess whether or not the finger pulp impacts into the palm on flexion.

This is typically an attrition lesion occurring in the third compartment of the extensor retinaculum at Lister's tubercle.

In the psoriatic patient, there may be spectacular shortening of the fingers with collapse of the interphalangeal joints in particular and also in the metacarpophalangeal and interphalangeal joints of the thumb with considerable loss of function.

It is useful to assess whether the palmaris longus

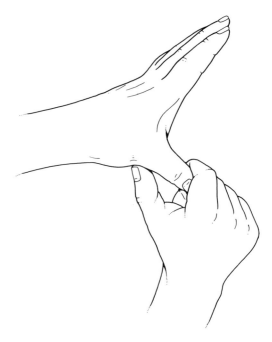

Fig. 24.7 Testing for stability of the ulnar collateral ligament at the metacarpophalangeal joint of the thumb.

tendon is present if a tendon graft procedure is required in a particular individual: here, the thumb should be opposed to the little finger and then the wrist palmar-flexed when the tendon comes easily into relief and can be readily seen (Fig. 24.9).

Testing for the deep-finger flexor tendons is achieved simply by the examiner anchoring the middle phalanx and asking the individual to bend the distal phalanx. With regard to the superficialis tendon, it is necessary to anchor the other three fingers in extension, with the knowledge that the deep flexor tendons are intimately bound at the wrist, and then it is easy to assess action in isolation of the superficialis tendon in a particular finger (Fig. 24.10).

In the caput ulnae syndrome of the rheumatoid arthritic patient, the head of the ulna is prominent, the wrist displaced volarly and there may be rupture of the digital extensor tendon mechanism. Most typically the ring and little fingers are then held in flexion with the inability to fully extend and there is likely to be some restriction of forearm rotation.

Severe digital contracture with tapering of the fingers and shininess of the skin is typical of the late stage of reflex sympathetic dystrophy, often also known as algo dystrophy and Sudeck's atrophy.

Range of motion of the wrist should be compared on both sides: dorsiflexion is best estimated with the palms together and palmar-flexion with the backs of the hands

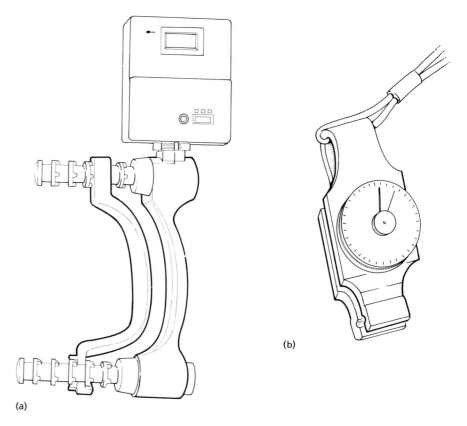

Fig. 24.8 Grip (a) and pinch (b) meters. Normal grip strength in the adult dominant hand averages 47.6 kg in the male and 24.6 kg in the female, the value depending on age and occupation, while minor hand strength is 45 kg and 22.4 kg respectively. Lateral pinch grip averages 7.5 kg and 4.9 kg in the adult dominant male and female hand respectively; average strength in the minor hand is 7.1 kg and 4.7 kg respectively.

(a)

(b)

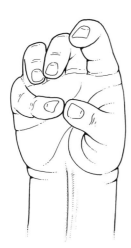

Fig. 24.9 Testing for the presence of a palmaris longus tendon, present in 85% of individuals. The tendon is seen in relief on opposition of the thumb to the little finger with the wrist palmar-flexed.

similarly held, a goniometer being used in mensuration while, additionally, radial and ulnar deviation movement needs to be estimated (Fig. 24.11).

In examining the elbow, the shape should firstly be observed: most often normally valgus, especially in females after puberty; rectus, i.e. straight; or varus. The elbow is best seen when the patient stands with the elbow in extension and the forearm supinated, inspection being made both from the front and the back. Exaggerated valgus may be a result of trauma or sex-chromosome abnormality, e.g. Turner's syndrome. Likewise varus deformity, always abnormal, can result from supracondylar fracture of the humerus in childhood, typically associated with rotational deformity and accompanying limitation of motion or, again, sex-chromosome anomalies (Fig. 24.12). Olecranon bursitis is characterized by soft-tissue swelling at the point of the elbow, this sometimes being accompanied by an olecranon spur observed on the lateral radiograph.

Range of elbow motion is calculated from the extended to the flexed position, commencing at 0° and appropriate comparison of the other side is made: on occasions, there is normally hyperextension of the joint, e.g. +10°. It is easiest to measure forearm rotation by anchoring the elbows at the side of the body at 90° of flexion: from the position of zero rotation, supination and then pronation are readily calculated (Fig. 24.13).

Neurological assessment of the hand and upper limb should be carefully accomplished, firstly in regard to sensory loss. Sensory deficit in radial nerve lesions is confined to the dorsilateral aspect of the hand. Sensory deficit in ulnar nerve lesions proximal to the dorsal

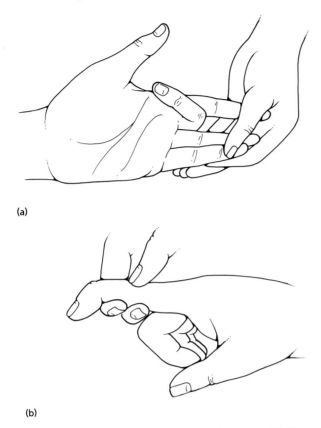

(a)

(b)

Fig. 24.10 Demonstrating function of the finger superficialis (a) and deep flexor tendons (b).

cutaneous branch result in sensory loss of the dorsi-medial aspect of the hand and wrist as well as the ring and little fingers. With nerve compression within Guyon's canal at the wrist, sensory loss is confined to the ring and little fingers and sensation is intact if compression is at the pisohamate hiatus or in the palm of the hand, e.g. compression by a simple ganglion. With median nerve compression within the carpal tunnel,

sensory loss is hardly ever profound and is typically best seen in the middle finger; compression of the nerve at the pronator teres muscle results in more extensive sensory loss with the superficial palmar branch being involved.

The much less common condition of anterior interosseous nerve compression results in weakness of the long flexor of the thumb and the deep flexors of the index and middle fingers: an interesting diagnostic feature is collapse into extension of the interphalangeal joint of the thumb and the distal interphalangeal joint of the index finger on pulp pinch of these two digits (Fig. 24.14).

Sensory loss can be particularly difficult to assess in a small child, particularly after a painful lacerating injury to the palm or digit. The ninhydrin sweat test can be used with fingerprints being taken on the sprayed filter paper, the colour test depending on lack of sweating 30 minutes after division of a digital nerve.

Sensation should be tested for carefully, avoiding concern and anxiety in the patient: firstly, a wisp of cotton wool should be used then judicious use of a fine pin and greater specificity can be sought by the two-point discrimination test.

Stereognosis can also be an important feature of neurological examination of the hand, asking the individual to recognize, with the eyes closed, common objects such as a coin.

Motor deficit of the median nerve at the carpal tunnel is readily diagnosed by observing thenar wasting and weakness of opposition of the thumb to the little finger; nerve compression at the pronator teres muscle if severe is additionally exhibited by weakness of the deep flexor muscles to the index and middle fingers and also of the long flexor of the thumb.

Advanced ulnar nerve deficit is easily seen by appro-

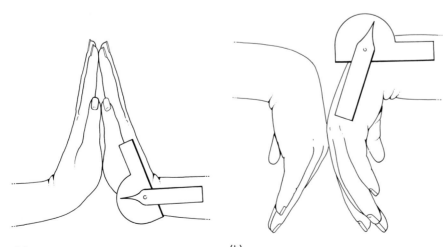

(a)   (b)

Fig. 24.11 Mensuration of wrist motion.

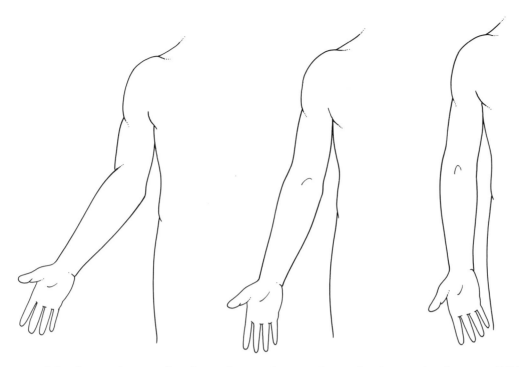

Fig. 24.12 Variants of the elbow angle: normally valgus and greater in post-pubescent females, occasionally rectus. Childhood supracondylar fracture may result in cubitus varus, while lateral condylar fractures in the child may readily result in abnormal valgus; interestingly, sex-chromosome anomalies can influence elbow shape.

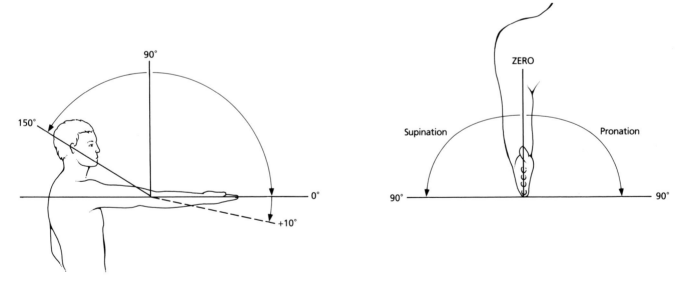

Fig. 24.13 Mensuration of elbow and forearm rotation motion.

priate intrinsic muscle wasting of the hand and, in proximal lesions, of the flexor carpi ulnaris and there is also diminished function of the deep flexor muscles of the ring and little fingers.

Weakness of abduction of the fingers from each other and of adduction as well as of adduction of the thumb into the palm of the hand are additional features, while Froment's sign is typical of the advanced case of ulnar neuropathy—the thumb is pressed palm down on a surface, the metacarpophalangeal joint becomes extended

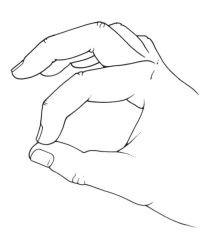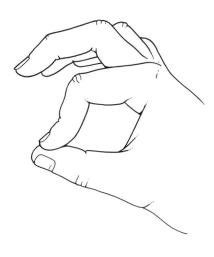

Fig. 24.14 Pathological stance from the normal, on pulp pinch of the thumb and index finger, in anterior interosseous compression neuropathy.

and the interphalangeal joint flexed as a consequence of severe weakness of the thumb adductor and the deep head of the flexor pollicis brevis muscles.

Radial nerve motor loss involves the extensors of the wrist and of the digits while posterior interosseous nerve compression, typically at the level of the Arcade of Frohse of the supinator muscle, results in digital extensor weakness.

There are two volume-reduction tests for nerve compression lesions in the upper limb, the ulnar nerve within the cubital tunnel and the median nerve at the carpal tunnel.

1 The Wadsworth elbow flexion test depends on the anatomical features of tautness of the arcuate ligament, forming the roof of the cubital tunnel, during elbow flexion and bulging superficially of the medial ligament when the elbow is in this position.

The elbow is kept fully flexed with the wrist in neutral position to avoid confusion with the Phalen test and it is important to avoid surface compression of the elbow. A positive result is signalled by initiation or aggravation of numbness and/or paraesthesiae in the ulnar nerve distribution at the hand, a positive result being found most often within 2 minutes (Fig. 24.15).

2 The Phalen test depends on the fact that the volume of the carpal tunnel is least in palmar flexion: the wrist is held in this position for 1–2 minutes, a positive result being signalled by initiation or aggravation of numbness and/or paraesthesiae in the median nerve distribution (Fig. 24.16).

Radiographic examination may be required and standard views of the hand, wrist, elbow and radio-ulnar joints may be supplemented by special views when necessary—the cubital tunnel of the elbow is well visualized with accurate delineation of the skeletal structures in the radiographic view described by the author (1977) (Fig. 24.17).

Consideration of radioisotope and computerized tomography scanning may be given in appropriate cases. It has been found that magnetic resonance imaging can be most useful at the elbow, while arthrography has its place in appropriate cases in examination of the wrist, elbow and the radio-ulnar joints. Arthroscopy is increasingly being used to visualize the complex articular structure of the wrist, especially useful in determining subtle instability, and also of the elbow and proximal radio-ulnar joints.

TREATMENT PRINCIPLES

Conservative and surgical management of hand, wrist and elbow problems often demand special skills, essentially learned by expert example and supervision.

Particularly concerning the hand, enthusiastic co-operation of the patient is mandatory and the help of an experienced therapist is also essential in the rehabilitation programme. Certain cases also require appropriate splintage.

Hand surgery is necessarily precise and is most often performed under pneumatic tourniquet control: the time scale here should be no more than 90 minutes in general, certainly no longer than 120 minutes. If a procedure takes longer, the tourniquet requires release for 10 minutes and reinflation for a further limited period of time. It is possible to prolong tourniquet time by appropriate freezing of the hand and upper limb.

The tourniquet should be placed high on the arm reaching to the axilla and should be appropriately padded, particularly around the edges, by wool. After application of the tourniquet, the limb should be elevated

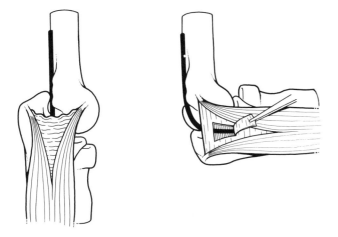

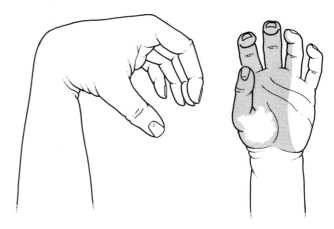

Fig. 24.16 The Phalen *wrist flexion test* for compression neuropathy of the median nerve at the carpal tunnel.

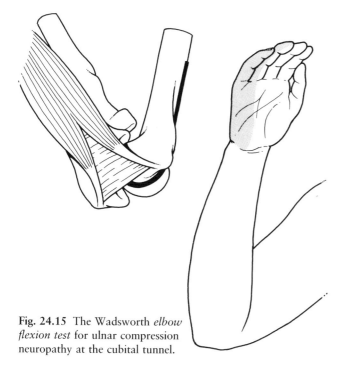

Fig. 24.15 The Wadsworth *elbow flexion test* for ulnar compression neuropathy at the cubital tunnel.

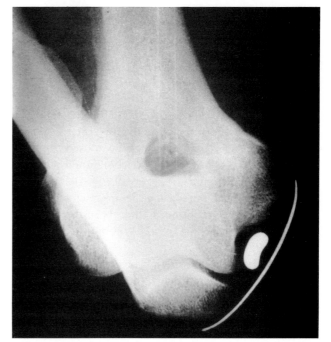

Fig. 24.17 The author's radiographic view of the elbow which defines the skeletal anatomy of the cubital tunnel: with the patient sitting at the side of the table, the elbow is fully flexed and the arm externally rotated, the tube being aligned appropriately. The roof of the cubital tunnel and the ulnar nerve are here superimposed.

and then decongested either by applying an Esmarch bandage from the tip of the digits upwards to the tourniquet or, more simply, an exsanguinator. The tourniquet should be elevated to no more than 250 mmHg in a normotensive adult.

Anaesthesia for hand and upper limb surgery should be general anaesthesia or blockage of the brachial plexus. Bier's and digital anaesthetic block are not without hazard and therefore are not recommended, but on occasion isolated blockage of the ulnar nerve within the cubital tunnel, the median nerve at the wrist and the superficial radial nerve dorsilaterally at the wrist can be performed. However, a tourniquet cannot be comfort-

ably tolerated under these circumstances for longer than 30 minutes.

It should be mentioned that haematoma block within several hours of injury is an excellent form of anaesthesia for manipulation of certain wrist fractures, particularly for Colles' fracture.

Surgical technique can be aided in appropriate cases by the use of a magnifying loop or the dissecting micro-

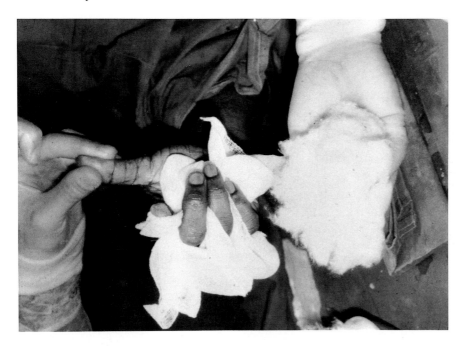

Fig. 24.18 Dressing regime for the hand.

scope. After appropriate suturing, plastic spray should be applied to the surgical wound and it is important that dressings be loosely applied. Teased-up wool should be placed in the palm of the hand (Fig. 24.18).

It is important that dressings be loosely applied, including between the fingers, and wool should be placed around the fingers and the remainder of the hand, the thumb if necessary, but leaving the tips open for inspection. The wool is continued into the upper forearm and then a dorsal splint, p.o.p. or plastic is applied (Fig. 24.19).

The ideal splintage position is of slight dorsiflexion of the wrist and, very importantly, the metacarpophalangeal joints of the fingers should be flexed to over 70° when the collateral ligaments are at maximum stretch and so extension contracture of these joints is avoided. Likewise, the interphalangeal joints are flexed no more than 10° when the collateral ligament system is at greatest stretch. The thumb should be kept well out of the palm with an appropriate pad of wool in order to avoid adduction contracture which can severely limit future hand function.

After trauma or a surgical procedure, there is the frequent complication of oedema: in this circumstance the collateral ligaments of the fingers may very well become fixed in the immobilized position. If the digits are splinted appropriately, no subsequent restriction of motion will occur, but there will be significant and most often permanent loss of motion if this dictum is not adhered to. It is usual after severe trauma or surgery to elevate the hand and upper limb at the side of the bed

for at least 48 hours in a Bradford sling (Fig. 24.20); whatever digital movement is possible should be encouraged and appropriate circulatory observation is made.

For the best results, an informed, co-operative and enthusiastic patient is ideal: those few patients who exhibit a different attitude are doomed to worst results however expert the surgical procedure and subsequent management by the clinician.

The therapist should assess the hand prior to appropriate rehabilitation measures. This includes assessment of swelling and restriction of motion, and the various modalities to assess sensation, including light touch with cotton wool, proprioception, two-point of discrimination and stereogenosis, as well as abnormal sensory patterns, e.g. hypersensitivity and paraesthesiae. Psychosocial assessment is also a necessary part of the therapists evaluation in many cases as well as the patient's goals in terms of activities of daily living, work and social and leisure pursuits.

Appropriate therapy includes an active and passive regime and the use of silicone baths in earlier stages, then perhaps paraffin wax as well as ultrasound. Furthermore, splintage is often an important feature of the rehabilitation programme as well as appropriate exercises to encourage the patient to grip and improve function of the hand and wrist and upper limb (Fig. 24.21).

With regard to the forearm and elbow, the therapist should concentrate on an active exercise programme rather than intermittent passive movements which can, quite often, prove counter-productive with increasing stiffness and decreasing function. It is best to achieve

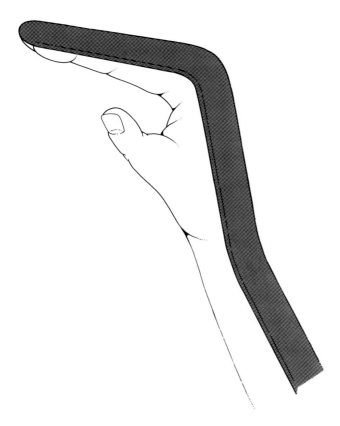

Fig. 24.19 Proper stance of the hand and wrist when splinted: finger metacarpophalangeal joints flexed greater than 70°, the interphalangeal joints almost straight, the thumb abducted from the palm and the wrist moderately dorsiflexed.

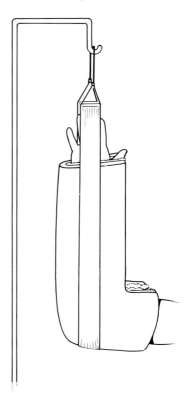

Fig. 24.20 Elevation of the upper limb is usual for 48 hours after hand surgery.

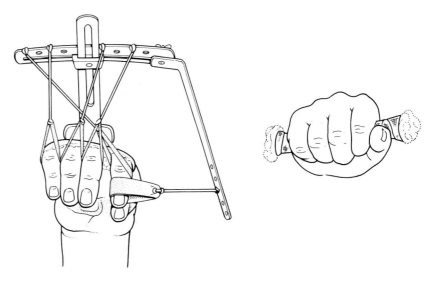

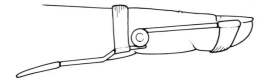

Fig. 24.21 Various modalities of rehabilitation treatment after hand surgery are often required, including silicone and paraffin wax baths as well as an active and passive exercise programme. Here, two examples of splints and an exerciser are demonstrated.

increase in forearm rotation by keeping the elbow locked into the body and at right angles.

Rehabilitation of the post-traumatic stiff elbow can be carried out by continuous passive motion on an appropriate machine. This is usually after surgical arthrolysis, but on occasion surgery can be avoided.

SURGICAL APPROACHES

Whenever possible, surgical incisions in the hand should follow dermal cleavage lines. Of course, care must be taken to avoid damage, particularly to neurological and vascular structures. It should be remembered that the main venous drainage of the hand proceeds dorsally and venous interference here as well as with lymphatics can result in disabling chronic swelling of the hand with consequent limitation of function.

It is probably best to use longitudinal linear incisions at the dorsum of the digits and in the remainder of the hand so that adequate exposure can be accomplished without causing neurological or venous damage; however, in such simple operations as resection of a ganglion on the dorsum of the wrist, it is best to use a transverse incision, with appropriate care, as this will heal with the least cosmetic disability (Fig. 24.22).

Midlateral incisions at the fingers and thumb are safe, provided that the surgical approach is posterior to the line of the neurovascular structures.

Palmar incisions should follow the natural creases.

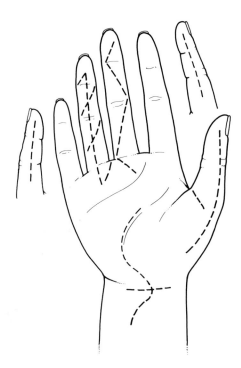

Fig. 24.23 Volar incisions at the hand and wrist, including the commonly used Bruner approach on the palmar surface of the middle finger and Z-plasty of the ring finger.

Proximally, they should be located to the inner side of the thenar crease, so avoiding damage to the superficial palmar branch of the median nerve; if a palmar incision has to be extended proximally to the lower forearm, for example flexor synovectomy, then there should be an appropriate curve at the wrist flexion crease (Fig. 24.23). The best incision for draining the pulp of the finger is a transverse distal approach.

The Bruner approach for the fingers, with extension into the palm where necessary, is a favoured incision. The midlateral approach to the index finger and the similar medial incision for the little finger can be particularly useful. Z-plasty sometimes has to be performed in order to lengthen, in particular, the palmar skin: this is most often necessary in certain cases of Dupuytren's disease and post-traumatic wound scarring. It is very important that the limbs be of equal length and that the angles be 60°: this technique can also be useful in thenar contracture (Fig. 24.24). A skin graft may be required for the recurrent case of Dupuytren's contracture.

When skin grafting is required in the hand, then a full-thickness graft can be taken from the inner aspect of the arm above the elbow, the front of the elbow or wrist and the groin (Fig. 24.25). A split skin graft is best taken from the thigh. In other cases, more sophisticated plastic procedures may be required, e.g. a cross-finger or neurovascular flap.

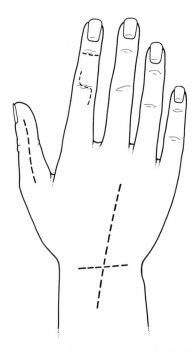

Fig. 24.22 Surgical incisions on the dorsum of the hand and wrist.

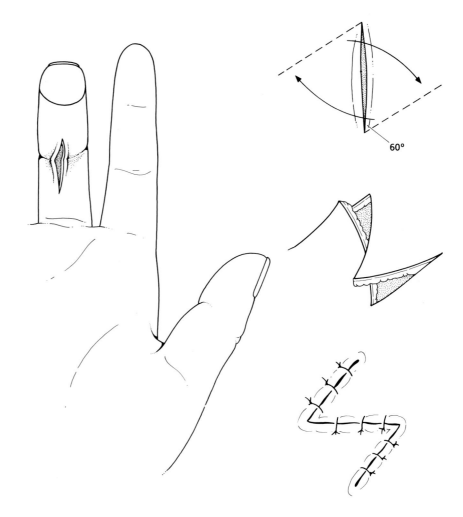

Fig. 24.24 Technique of Z-plasty for skin contracture of the finger.

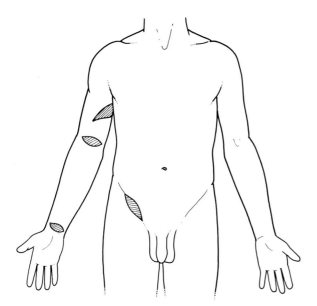

Fig. 24.25 Full-thickness free skin grafts can readily be taken from the inner aspect of the arm, the front of the elbow and wrist and the groin.

A number of surgical approaches are available for the elbow: anterior, medial, lateral and posterior, some of these having specific indications (Fig. 24.26). The short, oblique, posterior approach is ideal for resection and replacement of the radial head. The more extensive posterior approaches involve longitudinal splitting of the triceps tendon; construction of a tongue of this tendon, distally based; or elevating the muscle from the medial side of the lower humeral shaft; the Boyd technique being most useful in surgical treatment of the Monteggia injury. The lateral, medial and anterior incisions are also well established approaches to the elbow.

CLINICAL PROBLEMS

The nail

Traumatic subungual haematoma can be a very painful condition. Symptoms are relieved by simple trephining:

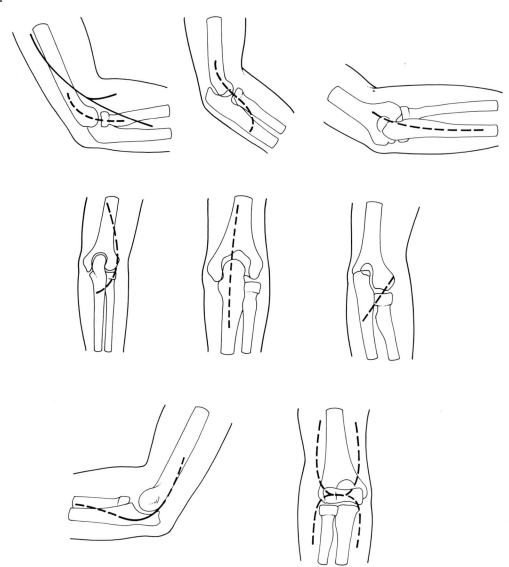

Fig. 24.26 Surgical approaches to the elbow: lateral, posterior, medial and anterior. Care has to be taken to avoid damage to the radial and posterior interosseous nerves in laterally approaching the elbow. The short oblique posterior approach is useful for radial head resection while the proximally extended posterior approach at the ulna is particularly useful in reconstructive surgery for the Monteggia injury. Other approaches at the back of the joint involve either splitting the triceps tendon, construction of a distally based tongue of the tendon or medial peeling of the triceps muscle from the humerus.

this can be accomplished by using the heated end of a paper clip, cautery or a hypodermic needle. Otherwise, a segment of the nail may have to be removed.

Nail bed lacerations, simple or stellate, can be carefully cleaned up and sewn with colourless absorbable sutures: the avulsed nail, after careful cleaning, can be replaced and sutured in position using non-absorbable 4/0 sutures. It is important to achieve continuous contact of the nail with its bed. Typically, the replaced nail will remain in position for 2 months until the proximal part of the new nail forms.

Lacerating injuries of the nail fold can be difficult and an ungual flap may have to be constructed to gain appropriate access.

Complex injuries of the nail bed often involve fracture of the distal phalanx and, under such circumstances, the fracture should be accurately reduced and fixed with a longitudinal Kirschner wire while the nail bed laceration is carefully sewn together.

Replacement of avulsed nail bed is important and if the nail remains attached to the nail bed then this should be preserved; irretrievable loss of a segment of the nail bed can be dealt with by a split skin graft, although this is often unsuccessful with regard to the new nail properly bedding down.

Germinal matrix should, of course, always be preserved, and if displaced should be replaced appropriately. If no nail bed is available then consideration can be given to using that of a toe.

Claw nails can be functionally and cosmetically unacceptable: the nail bed can be recessed in position over the distal phalanx using an appropriate flap, so that the distal pulp can be reconstructed. Alternatively, the nail bed can be resected down to the lunula while a lateral neurovascular flap is constructed, this being placed distally at the open pulp. The nail is stabilized by a Kirschner wire longitudinally through the pulp and into the distal phalanx, while the defect caused by taking the flap is covered by a split thickness skin graft.

Paronychia is a common infection of the periungual area of the digit: treatment by a short course of antibiotics is usually effective before abscess formation. Thereafter, the abscess should be drained and the proximal segment of the nail resected: resistant cases may be due to fungal infection, in which case appropriate antifungal ointment can be regularly applied for a period of time. Chronic paronychia can sometimes be treated successfully by several applications of short-wave diathermy in the physiotherapy department.

The digital pulp

Simple lacerations usually produce no serious long-term effect. However, loss of tissue can be a problem, especially if distal amputation is involved at the terminal phalanx, with bone exposed in the wound.

Where the bone and subcutaneous tissue is intact, creeping epitheliazation can effectively restore proper function, provided that the wound area is 1 cm^2 or less, with especially good results being obtained in children. Larger defects of similar depth can be readily treated by split thickness skin grafting.

A particular problem arises in wounds of greater depth with involvement of the terminal phalanx; the bone should be appropriately smoothed out and skin cover obtained.

If it is possible to advance a palmar flap it is best to use the V−Y technique. On the other hand, a thenar or cross-finger pedicle flap may also be used, the secondary defect being covered with a split thickness skin graft.

Terminalization is a simple technique in appropriate cases, involving partial resection of the distal phalanx to provide ease of cover, using the remaining pulp skin.

Digital neuromata can be troublesome in terms of tenderness, with proximal pain radiation after traumatic amputation: this is a difficult problem to deal with, particularly in the severe case. Various surgical options are available including silastic capping of the end of the nerve. However, often the best solution is to transpose the nerve onto the dorsum of the finger, where it is less subject to external trauma.

A felon is a term given to deep infection in the pulp of the digit. Pus needs to be drained off and this is easily accomplished by a unilateral linear incision, with appropriate insertion of a drain for a period of about 48 hours. Radiographs should be taken pre-operatively and if osteomyelitis is present (typically not seen on X-ray under 10 days), then appropriate bony débridement is required.

Digital joint injuries

Mallet deformity of the finger is common, resulting from traumatic rupture of the lateral bands at their insertion into the distal phalanx, this sometimes being accompanied by an avulsed fragment of bone. Depending on elasticity of capsuloligamentous structures, there is a tendency for hyperextension deformity at the proximal interphalangeal joint because of overpull of the central skin mechanism at the middle phalanx. The wearing of a plastic mallet splint for 6 weeks usually produces an excellent result; if there is a large avulsed fragment of bone this is best secured percutaneously with a Kirschner wire, this being removed in 4−6 weeks (Fig. 24.27). Consideration can be given to rebalancing the finger in a chronic case by percutaneous tenotomy of the central slip, although this tends to be more effective in the rheumatoid arthritic patient.

The opposite, and much less common, deformity is that produced by traumatic rupture of the central slip mechanism and here the lateral bands tend to sublux in a volar direction to increase direct pull on the distal phalanx so that flexion deformity of the proximal interphalangeal joint is accompanied by hyperextension at the distal interphalangeal joint, known as the boutonnière deformity.

Treatment of the acute case is by immobilization of the interphalangeal joints by a straight padded splint on the dorsal surface, importantly not including the metacarpophalangeal joint and this should be kept in position for 6 weeks (Fig. 24.28). With the chronic case, consideration can be given to percutaneous tenotomy of the distal insertion of the lateral bands, but again, as in mallet deformity, this is more often effective in the rheumatoid patient. Otherwise, reconstruction of the central slip mechanism can be accomplished in a number

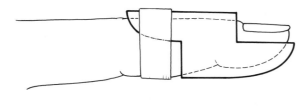

(a)

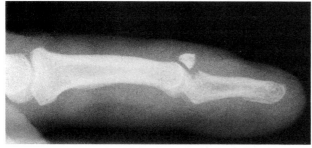

(b)

Fig. 24.27 The plastic splint (a) commonly used for traumatic mallet deformity of the finger; also illustrated (b) is the unusual case where a large fragment of bone has been avulsed dorsally from the base of the terminal phalanx.

of ways, e.g. by inserting a small palmaris longus graft with its surrounding fascia or dividing the lateral bands, then crossing them over in an X-stance and appropriately suturing the tendon together.

In the acute case of a large bony fragment off the dorsum of the base of the middle phalanx, this requires securing percutaneously with a Kirschner wire for 6 weeks.

Dislocation of the digital joints is not a common injury, usually easily treated by closed manipulation and appropriate temporary splintage, following which an active exercise programme should be instituted. However, metacarpophalangeal dislocation, particularly in the thumb, can be impossible to reduce closed because of button-holing of the head of the metacarpal through the soft tissues and in these cases open reduction through a judicious palmar incision may have to be performed.

Strain of ligamentous structures should be considered, particularly so at the metacarpophalangeal joints. In the case of the finger, it is important to test for this by flexing the joint maximally until the lateral ligament mechanism is at full stretch and then to deviate the finger radially and ulnarward so that there is appropriate painful discomfort when the damaged ligament is stretched as well as local tenderness. A Bedford soft splint immobilizing the affected digit to its neighbour is useful in treatment over a period of several weeks and this may be supplemented by steroid and local anaesthetic injection into the damaged ligament as well as by physiotherapy measures such as ultrasound, laser and interferential treatment.

With regard to the thumb, it is the ulnar collateral ligament of the metacarpophalangeal joint that is most often affected. Trauma without ligamentous instability is easily treated by immobilization in a scaphoid cast for several weeks, alternatively by steroid and local anaesthetic injection and physiotherapy as indicated for the finger.

A more serious injury is rupture of the ulnar collateral ligament, often with an avulsed fragment emanating from the base of the proximal phalanx. Surgical repair is required and immobilization in a scaphoid-type cast for 6 weeks, after which a rehabilitation programme is commenced (Fig. 24.29).

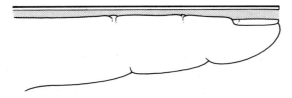

Fig. 24.28 A straight splint, immobilizing both interphalangeal joints, for traumatic boutonnière deformity of the finger.

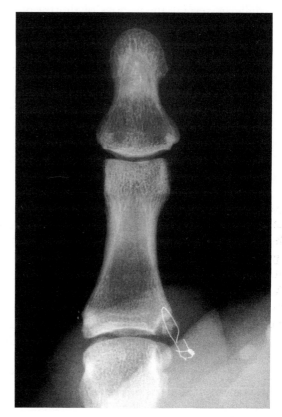

Fig. 24.29 Method of repair for rupture of the ulnar collateral ligament of the metacarpophalangeal joint of the thumb.

Unfortunately, this injury is often 'missed' and it is not unusual for the case to eventually be referred for expert treatment several months after the causative incident. Of course, it is then difficult to treat: a new ligament can be reconstructed using fascia, a palmaris longus tendon graft or a synthetic ligament; alternatively the elongated scar tissue can be divided and then overlapped with acceptable results in most cases. For particularly chronic and painful disability it may be necessary to arthrodese the metacarpophalangeal joint of the thumb in slight flexion.

Angular and/or rotatory deformity of the finger can follow from metacarpal or phalangeal fractures resulting in impairment of grip and, in some, overlapping of the affected digit with the adjacent finger on gripping. Corrective osteotomy can be considered in such cases, particularly when warranted by functional disability in a particular individual.

It is rare for such rotatory deformity to be a problem in the thumb. However, there may be significant deformity at the trapeziometacarpal joint at the base of the thumb in case of missed or maltreated Bennett's fracture. The fact of the matter is that such individuals with this problem unusually have significant disability, but in the case of painful symptoms at the base of the thumb causing limitation of use of the hand then arthrodesis of the trapeziometacarpal joint is the easy surgical option.

Unfortunately, fracture-subluxation of the proximal interphalangeal joint of the finger is often missed or its nature not properly appreciated. Flexion deformity and painful limitation of motion can be a disabling feature of such injury and an attempt at surgical reconstruction should be made. Even up to 6 months post-injury, the displaced palmar fragment at the base of the middle phalanx can sometimes be elevated into position and secured with a wire suture after reduction of the displaced joint (Fig. 24.30).

When reconstruction of the base of the phalanx and reduction of subluxation has been satisfactorily accomplished then for several weeks the finger should be immobilized with a Kirschner wire along its length as far as the base of the proximal phalanx in the flexor sheath.

If this proves impossible, resection of the joint and the insertion of a Swanson silastic prosthesis, with or without grommets, can often be satisfactorily accomplished with pleasing restoration of adequate function (Fig. 24.31). Following such surgery and similarly after bony and soft-tissue repair, an appropriate rehabilitation programme is mandatory, including the temporary use of a spring brace.

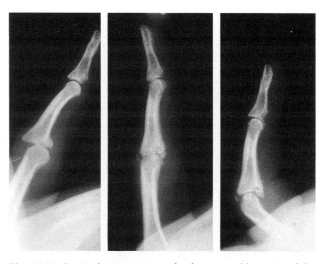

Fig. 24.30 Surgical reconstruction for fracture-subluxation of the proximal interphalangeal joint of the finger: the fracture fragment has been reduced and fixed with a wire suture.

Soft-tissue lesions

Distally placed soft-tissue lesions in the finger are likely to be xanthomata. Rarely, lipomata are seen in the hand and may occupy the palm and/or the digit, particularly on the palmar surface and can extend to the lateral or medial border.

Even less frequently, soft-tissue swelling of the finger or thumb can rarely be due to villonodular synovitis. Synovitis produces swelling in the digit, this usually in rheumatoid disease and is similarly seen in the palm and carpal tunnel.

The simple ganglion is most commonly seen on the dorsum of the wrist, although it is more likely to cause functional disability with pain on gripping when it is seen as a small, tense, pea-like structure lying to either side of the finger on the palmar surface at its base. These lesions are caused by soft-tissue mucoid degeneration, typically of the dorsal capsule at the wrist joint.

Important functional disability can occur due to neurological compression by a ganglion, e.g. the ulnar nerve at the cubital tunnel of the elbow, at the wrist, the piso-hamate hiatus and in the palm of the hand. Similarly, the median nerve may be compromised by a ganglion within the carpal tunnel.

If sufficiently large, and not multilocular, the lesion may be aspirated and hydrocortisone with local anaesthetic injected into the sac effectively, particularly ganglia on the dorsum of the wrist. Otherwise, surgical resection, when appropriate, is the best form of treatment; however, there is a significant recurrence rate which should be explained to the patient prior to surgery.

An inclusion dermoid resulting from injury and a

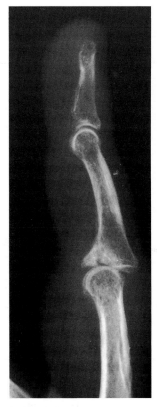
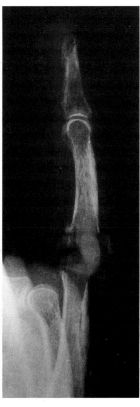

Fig. 24.31 Joint resection and insertion of a Swanson silastic prosthesis for chronic fracture-subluxation of the finger proximal interphalangeal joint.

This is a degenerative process at the entrance of the fibrous flexor sheath with accompanying local flexor synovitis. The result is periodic stiffening of the digit and, in the more advanced cases, actual locking, usually in flexion, which is painful and disabling.

In the early case, injection of steroid and local anaesthetic within the entrance of the fibrous flexor sheath often may be curative and can be repeated for recurrence on two further occasions. If unsuccessful, surgical decompression of the proximal fibrous flexor sheath is required (Fig. 24.32).

Rarely, the condition in the thumb can be congenital, with the infant exhibiting inability to move the thumb out of the palm. It is mandatory in these cases for surgery to be performed or else there is risk of improper growth and function of the thumb, the procedure probably best being performed at 12 months of age.

Occasionally, a nodule may form in the deep flexor tendon and locking can then occur between the tendonous slips of the superficial flexor. Reduction of accompanying synovitis by steroid and local anaesthetic injection can sometimes be helpful, otherwise resection of a single slip of the superficial flexor will have to be performed.

Flexor synovitis can effect any or all of the digits of the hand and also the carpal tunnel. Well-known causes are rheumatoid disease and repetitive use of the hand and wrist in certain manual workers. Tuberculosis,

cause of painful swelling of the digit can sometimes even be found within a phalanx.

A glomus tumour is an unusual condition producing tenderness at the nail fold.

A mucous cyst is not infrequently seen in the area of an interphalangeal joint, which may be osteoarthritic, and sometimes at the base of the nail.

Aneurysm at the hand and wrist can be a result of traumatic injury while haemangiomata may sometimes be quite extensive in the hand.

A neurilemmoma is an unusual lesion and, when present at the hand and wrist, most often emanates from the median nerve.

A pyogenic granuloma is occasionally seen in the digit, usually distally, this abnormal tissue being much prone to bleeding. The lesion should be curetted by a hot cautery.

Flexor tendon triggering of the fingers and thumb is not uncommon in individuals beyond middle age and can be traumatic in origin, including younger individuals. Of the fingers, the middle is most often involved, but sometimes several digits may be affected sequentially or at the same time.

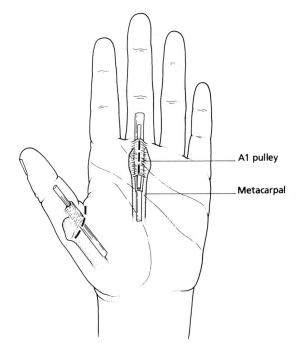

Fig. 24.32 Surgical release for triggering of the thumb and finger.

although rare nowadays, should be borne in mind in the chronic case.

If trauma is the cause, cessation of repetitive work activity should result in resolution of the problem in the course of time. In others, consideration should be given to appropriate steroid and local anaesthetic injection while intermittent splintage can also be useful.

Where the condition is chronic and unresolved by conservative measures, especially where carpal tunnel syndrome is present, then surgical synovectomy becomes necessary.

Suppurative tenosynovitis can have serious consequences and the patient requires hospitalization. With flexor tendon sheath involvement there tends to be a history of penetrating trauma although this may not be obvious.

There is very painful and tender swelling of the digit, particularly along the flexor tendon sheath and there is accompanying erythema. The digit is moderately flexed and, typically, passive extension of the interphalangeal joints of the finger causes pain.

Drainage through a lateral incision is made and a drain may be inserted, the tendon sheath being irrigated with sterile saline; a catheter may be left in place for postoperative irrigation. It is mandatory that an appropriate intravenous antibiotic regime be set up in the beginning.

Infection may occur in the mid-palmar and thenar spaces. Incision and drainage is required and antibiotics are given appropriately.

A penetrating wound from a tooth may occur into the metacarpophalangeal joint of a digit during an assault. Infection here can be serious indeed and surgical exploration, drainage and debridement of necrotic tissue is required and the wound should be initially left open and a drain inserted. Non-traumatic infective arthropathy can also occur, even gonococcal infection, typically associated with urethral discharge: here the joint should be aspirated and an appropriate antibiotic regime instituted after identification of the causative organism, including intravenous administration.

Tuberculosis is now uncommon in this country and such infective arthropathy in the hand and wrist is rarely seen; the condition may rarely follow a puncture wound. The disease can be diagnosed by culture and histological examination. Appropriate antituberculous drugs are usually effective for treatment, although resistant cases are now being seen.

Herpes infection is unusual but is most likely to be seen in those with exposure to oral contact such as dental and medical personnel. The vesicle is typically seen in the vicinity of the nail and pulp. The condition may be helped by acyclovir in the form of ointment and oral medication.

De Quervain's syndrome

This was first described in 1895, women being affected more often than men and, typically, the condition affects those of middle age and over. There is often a repetitive traumatic basis for this condition.

The complaint is of radial wrist pain particularly on gripping and sometimes discrete swelling is noticed by the patient. There is a tender firm swelling laterally at the wrist overlying the radial styloid, best seen when the wrist is viewed in profile from the radial side.

Resisted extension of the thumb is painful and the Finkelstein test, described in 1930, is useful: the fingers are gently clenched over the thumb which is held adducted and flexed across the palm of the hand and the examiner then passively moves the wrist into ulnar deviation, this being accompanied by radial wrist pain (Fig. 24.33).

Pathologically, there is thickening of the soft tissue at the fibro-osseous sheath at the radial styloid which contains the extensor pollicis brevis and abductor pollicis longus tendons. It must be said that aberrant tendons are known to sometimes run across the radial styloid process and these may also be involved.

Most often symptoms are relieved by steroid and local anaesthetic injection into the thickened tissue over the involved tendons and such injection may be repeated on no more than two further occasions for recurrence.

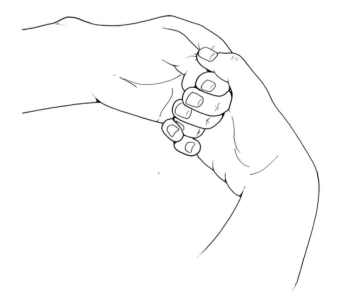

Fig. 24.33 The Finkelstein test for de Quervain's tenosynovitis stenosans.

It is unusual for surgical decompression to be required: this is easily accomplished through a longitudinal incision. It is essential to avoid damage to the terminal branch of the radial nerve or else a painful and tender neuroma will certainly result, symptoms then being worse than the initial problem (Fig. 24.34).

The enclosed tendons should be decompressed and search should be made for any aberrant tendon which should also be similarly treated.

The unusual condition of flexor carpi radialis indicis tendonitis is said to be degenerative in nature, the tendon lying in a tunnel on the medial side of the trapezium within the fibres of the flexor retinaculum. Tenderness is located over the anterior aspect of the radial side of the carpus and resisted pronation of the forearm tends to worsen painful disability. In the early stages appropriate steroid and local anaesthetic injection may be helpful, otherwise the roof of the tunnel requires surgical decompression.

Olecranon bursitis, when infective in nature, requires antibiotic treatment and aspiration of fluid, sometimes surgical drainage; other cases can be traumatic in origin or associated with arthropathy. It is unwise, generally speaking, to resect the protective bursal sac over the point of the elbow.

Typically, rheumatoid nodules occur on the extensor surfaces of the upper forearm and resection of these is for cosmetic or biopsy reasons only.

It is highly unusual to see rupture of the distal biceps tendon, typically preceded by degenerative change. There is antecubital swelling and also a bulbous lesion in the arm when active elbow flexion is attempted and supination of the forearm is weak. The proximal end of the ruptured tendon can be anastomosed to the brachialis near its insertion, less often direct suture of the tendon can be accomplished.

Dupuytren's disease

Dupuytren described permanent contraction of the fingers due to a disease of the palmar aponeurosis in his lecture at the Hotel-Dieu Hospital in Paris in December 1831, subsequently reported in 1832 and 1834.

However, the condition appears to have been first described by Felix Plater of Basel in 1614 and there were subsequent descriptions of this disease prior to Dupuytren's lecture: by Henry Cline in 1778 and Sir Astley Cooper in 1822.

The palmar fascia extends from an apex proximally in the palm in a triangular fashion: the proximal extent being contiguous with the palmaris tendon which is present in 85% of individuals. Septal partitions in the palm are most obviously developed distally and here merge with the transverse metacarpal ligament.

The palmar fascia contains numerous bands of fibrous tissue and distally in the palm there are well-defined transverse fibres which limit the span of abduction of the fingers, the so-called natatory ligaments. The corresponding ligament in the thenar cleft is called the distal commissural ligament (Fig. 24.35).

Distal extensions of the palmar fascia insert into the fibrous flexor sheath of the fingers. The pretendinous bands to each finger lie so that they proceed from the level of the metacarpophalangeal joint at either side of the digit.

In the space between the natatory ligament, the pretendinous bands and the superficial transverse ligament of the palm lie the neurovascular bundles to the fingers; this space also contains fat.

Deep palmar extensions of the fascia divide the palm into intermetacarpal and metacarpal spaces, the former containing the flexor tendons and lumbrical muscles and the latter the interosseous muscles and neurovascular bundles.

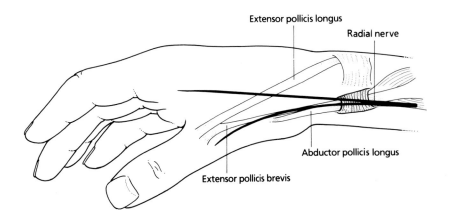

Extensor pollicis longus

Radial nerve

Abductor pollicis longus

Extensor pollicis brevis

Fig. 24.34 Surgical release of de Quervain's tenosynovitis stensosans: care should be taken to avoid damaging the terminal radial nerve.

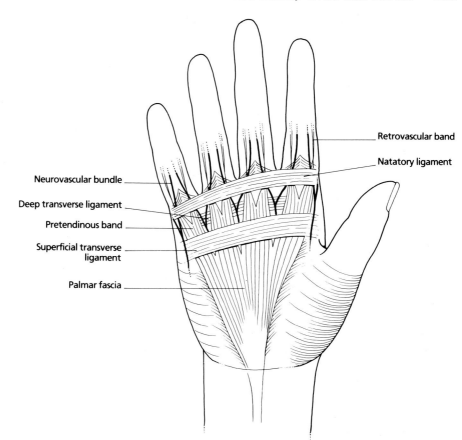

Retrovascular band

Natatory ligament

Neurovascular bundle

Deep transverse ligament

Pretendinous band

Superficial transverse ligament

Palmar fascia

Fig. 24.35 Anatomical features of the palmar fascia.

Research continues into the cause of Dupuytren's disease and there is known to be a relatively high level of hyaluronate in normal palmar fascia while high levels of glycosaminoglycans have been found in the tissue of Dupuytren's disease, more so in cellular bands and nodules than dense fibrous cords. Proliferation of fibrous collagen is a major biochemical factor in Dupuytren's disease.

Dupuytren's disease is rarely seen before the age of 40 and is mainly a disease of older white males. The male/female ratio in those aged 50–64 is 8:1 and over age 75 is 2:1.

The condition is rare in black people, Chinese and Asians but is particularly common in diabetic and epileptic individuals and those with a strong family history of the condition. There is also a high incidence of Dupuytren's disease in those suffering from tuberculosis. There is an association in some individuals with swelling in the plantar fascia, Lederhose nodules, and Peyronie's disease—the corpora cavernosa of the penis being involved in the latter.

The prognosis is worse if there is a high alcohol intake with liver impairment and in epileptic individuals on long-term phenobarbitone medication. Also, the pres-

ence of nodularity on the dorsum of the interphalangeal joints of the fingers, so-called knuckle pads, first described by Garrod in 1904, can also be a poor prognostic feature.

Where there is a strong Dupuytren's diathesis, it may be that trauma can provoke the condition and some believe that long-term administration of phenobarbitone, such as to an epileptic individual, can actually cause Dupuytren's disease.

In the early stages, there is nodular formation in the palm of the hand, particularly within the palmar fat between the dermis and the palmar fascia at the level of the metacarpophalangeal joints, typically accompanied by adhesion and dimpling of the skin. The nodules consist of dense active cellular fibrous tissue and there is typically hypertrophy of the epidermis overlying the prominent nodules in the palm.

In the more advanced case, there is thickening and contracture of the pretendinous bands as well as the vertical partitions of the palmar fascia deep in the palm.

Lack of proper abduction of the affected digits and, importantly, flexion contracture of the metacarpophalangeal and interphalangeal joints of the fingers can readily occur. Fortunately, the anatomical fact that the collateral ligament system of the metacarpophalangeal joint is maximally stretched at 70° and beyond easily allows for correction of the flexion deformity of the knuckle joint with appropriate surgical management.

Thickening and contracture of the retrovascular digital bands causes contracture of both the metacarpophalangeal and proximal interphalangeal joints. The fact that the collateral ligament system of the proximal interphalangeal joint is lax in flexion means that it can be difficult to undo flexion contracture of this joint with the collateral ligaments effectively shortened and fixed.

Involvement of Landsmeer's ligament, the oblique retinacular ligament, causes limitation of extension of the distal interphalangeal joint as well as flexion contracture of the proximal interphalangeal joint, producing the so-called boutonnière deformity.

On occasions, a 'phalangeal band' exists in apparent isolation, producing flexion contracture of the proximal interphalangeal joint. Such a band in the little finger may arise at its base from the tendon of abductor digiti minimi.

The ring and little fingers are the most commonly affected digits in Dupuytren's disease. In the most severe cases, all the digits, including the thumb, may be involved (Fig. 24.36).

It is impossible to forecast the course of the disease with any accuracy in a particular individual. However, it is possible to predict speed of progress in certain individuals, especially so in the presence of alcoholism, epilepsy treated with phenobarbitone, where there is a strong family history and the presence of knuckle pads overlying the proximal interphalangeal joints of the fingers, while onset at an early age is likely to signal a particularly aggressive form of the disease.

Where digital contracture is mild or absent, the patient should be instructed to passively extend the digits frequently and to sit on the hand from time to time with the palm downwards. Ideally, the patient should be checked every 6 months for progress of the disease. It is useful for the individual to massage the skin over the Dupuytren's tissue in order to keep the skin as soft as possible, warm olive oil being particularly useful.

Dupuytren's contracture is an unpredictable condition and so are the results of surgical management. It is important that the patient is appropriately made aware of this prior to any surgical treatment.

Fasciotomy was first openly performed by Dupuytren in 1831 and percutaneous fasciotomy by Sir Astley Cooper in 1822, this supplemented by use of a splint to maintain the involved finger in the straight position. Fasciotomy may occasionally be useful, but should only be performed as proximally as possible in the palm in

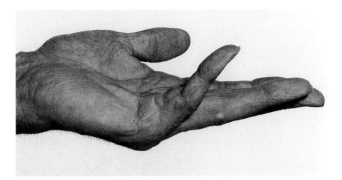

Fig. 24.36 A case of Dupuytren's contracture.

order to avoid neurovascular damage. It is best to use a small tenotome for the percutaneous method. Fasciotomy can sometimes be useful in the beginning of the procedure for limited fasciectomy, particularly to partially overcome severe flexion deformity of the digit so that the skin incision may be more easily extended distally.

Timing of surgical treatment can be difficult and should be limited to overcoming digital contracture; there is less urgency in regard to flexion contracture of the metacarpophalangeal joint than that of the proximal interphalangeal joint and in the latter it is best to operate early for flexion contracture of 30° or beyond.

Limited fasciectomy is the treatment of choice for digital contracture in Dupuytren's disease. There are numerous incisions available, but it is usual to either make a longitudinal straight incision over the digit and into the palm using the Z-plasty technique for closure or the zig-zig incision of Bruner.

In the case of the index and little fingers, mid-lateral and midmedial longitudinal incisions respectively can be usefully made with an extension transversely at the level of the distal palmar crease and then proximally from there. It is unwise to surgically treat more than two digital rays at a time.

Deep dissection should commence proximally where the neurovascular structures are most deeply placed and, after their identification, such dissection should carefully proceed distally with minimal undermining of the skin flaps. The more distal the dissection, the greater the hazard to neurovascular structures that are frequently surrounded by Dupuytren's tissue in the distal palm and within the finger.

In fact, there can be considerable distortion within the digit of these structures. Dupuytren's tissue has to be dissected off the fibrous flexor sheath of the digit and contracted deep septa of the palmar fascia that are affected should be resected. There is typically no difficulty after appropriate fasciectomy in fully releasing contracture of the metacarpophalangeal joint. The same cannot be said about advanced contracture of the proximal interphalangeal joint. However, gentle sustained manipulation of the joint on the operating table after limited fasciectomy can often satisfactorily result in elimination of even quite severe flexion deformity: when unsuccessful, surgical division of the palmar capsule and partial release of the collateral ligaments should be attempted.

Of course, appropriate splintage and a rehabilitation programme is necessary here. In some severe cases, consideration can be given to arthrodesis of the proximal interphalangeal joint in less severe flexion, dorsal wedge osteotomy of the proximal phalanx or replacement of the joint by a Swanson silastic implant.

It is important to release the tourniquet and to secure haemostasis for skin closure; a drain, either corrugated or suction, inserted into the palmar wound should be removed after 48 hours. Plastic skin spray is applied to the wound and then loose dressings; teased-up wool is applied to the palmar surface of the hand and then Velband, this extending into the wrist, while the tips of the digits should remain exposed. The bandage should be loosely applied and the limb kept elevated for 48 hours and an active exercise programme commenced.

Within several days of surgery, the hand can be readily immersed in a silicone bath and after healing of the skin wound this can be changed to paraffin wax baths. The rehabilitation programme should include an active and passive regime and, particularly in the case of the proximal interphalangeal joint, intermittent use of a spring base.

Skin grafting is sometimes required, particularly in the recurrent case. When sufficiently severe, skin contracture can often be dealt with at primary or secondary surgery by appropriate Z-plasty of the skin.

When there has been recurrence, dermofasciectomy has to be considered, combined with appropriate skin grafting (Fig. 24.37). Application of a full-thickness skin graft requires a satisfactory bed, including an intact fibrous flexor tendon sheath. It is convenient to take the full-thickness graft from the anterior fold of the elbow.

The open-palm technique was first described by McCash in 1964, particularly for elderly patients. A transverse distal palmar crease incision is used with appropriate exposure of contracted fasia, selective fasciectomy then being performed. The open palmar wound is covered with vaseline gauze, appropriate dressings and the application of wool and a bandage. The dressing is replaced on the fifth day, this regime being repeated until the wound has appropriately epithelialized and an active and passive exercise programme has to be instituted.

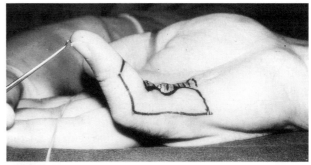

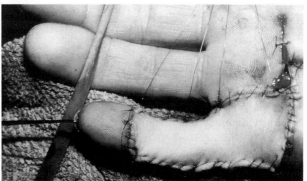

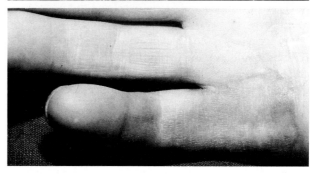

Fig. 24.37 Limited fasciectomy and skin grafting for Dupuytren's disease. (Courtesy of Andrew M. Logan.)

Volkmann's ischaemic contracture

This is an example of compartment syndrome involving the forearm. A common aetiological factor is external compression at the anterior aspect of the elbow and upper forearm, the notorious example being a supracondylar fracture in childhood. However, compression from an overtight cast for other traumatic lesions as well as penetrating and blunt trauma are responsible for other cases to which should be added arterial injury from cardiac catheterization and injection for drug addiction.

The early warning symptom is deep unrelenting pain in the forearm which may be accompanied by distal pallor and coolness as well as paraesthesiae.

The fascial compartment in the anterior aspect of the forearm has either increased by the volume of its contents or there is decrease in its size. Blood flow ceases if the tissue pressure exceeds the critical closing pressure of Burton (1951). Interruption of arterial and venous flow can result in decreased tissue perfusion and increased exudation following increased capillary permeability, another cause of increase in compartmental pressure; decreased tissue perfusion can result in death of muscle and nerve.

The end result can be an infarct, particularly of the deep forearm musculature, i.e. the deep flexors of the fingers and the long flexor of the thumb.

The diagnosis of impending ischaemic contracture should be urgently made on clinical evidence: this can be supplemented by estimating intracompartmental pressure with needling, use of a Doppler stethoscope, and arteriography.

Urgent treatment is mandatory: the constricting cast should be immediately removed and prompt relief of compartmental pressure in the antecubital fossa and forearm may be accomplished by fasciotomy, this including wide opening of the skin and subcutaneous tissues, the lacertus fibrosis and fascia overlying the muscles of the forearm.

It is necessary to completely restore vascular continuity, this being accomplished in some by fasciotomy alone; in others, there appears to be spasm of the brachial artery and this can be appropriately 'milked' so that blood flow occurs. In other cases, surgery on the brachial artery is required: either in the form of resection and primary end-to-end anastomosis or in more extensive damage the interposition of a reversed lower limb vein graft. At the time of surgery, a supracondylar fracture requires internal fixation to produce stability.

Median nerve damage due to vascular impairment may occur, less frequently neuropathy of the ulnar and radial nerves.

In the late case, there is unsightly and highly disabling flexion contracture of the digits and of the wrist with adduction deformity of the thumb and intrinsic plus deformity of the fingers.

The milder chronic case may be surgically rehabilitated by distally sliding the common flexor origin at the inner aspect of the elbow as well as off the ulna, interosseous membrane and the radius, the ulnar nerve being transposed anteriorly to lie next to the median nerve. The digits and wrist need to be immobilized in extension for 3 weeks, except that the finger metacarpophalangeal joints should be flexed, and a rehabilitation programme is mandatory.

In more advanced cases, progressive deformity in the early months may be aborted by resecting the fibrotic mass in the volar aspect of the forearm, the ideal time being between 4 and 6 months post-injury.

In the late case, adduction contracture of the thumb may have to be released by stripping the adductor muscle from its origin at the middle finger metacarpal. Intrinsic tendon release is required when there has been ischaemic contracture of the intrinsic musculature producing swan-neck deformity of the fingers.

In the less severe chronic case, neurological impairment may well reasonably improve, but in the more severe case consideration may have to be given to cable-grafting of the irretrievably damaged segment of the median nerve in particular.

Reflex sympathetic dystrophy

This unusual condition, also known as Sudeck's atrophy and algo-dystrophy, is disabling and worrisome to both patient and clinician. The cause remains a mystery, although it is well known to typically follow such surgical procedures as resection of a ganglion at the hand or wrist, limited fasciectomy for Dupuytren's disease and Colles' fracture; psychological factors may play a part.

The early features are complaints of unusually troublesome pain, soft-tissue swelling and exquisite tenderness in the hand with circulatory changes in the skin that may appear purple and cold; excess perspiration may also occur.

With this persistent painful condition, there is a predisposition to the diathesis and an abnormal sympathetic reflex. The normal sympathetic reflex does not shut off at the appropriate time after it normally initially causes vasoconstriction to prevent excessive blood loss or swelling, after which there is gradual vasodilatation as it is necessary for the body to repair the damaged tissue. Because of intensive vasoconstriction, localized ischaemia is produced and this in turn produces 'pain reflex'. The four cardinal signs of reflex sympathetic dystrophy are pain, swelling, stiffness and discoloration.

Initially there is hyperhydrosis and later dryness of the skin and there are osseous changes of demineralization, pseudomotor and temperature changes, atrophy, vasomotor instability and palmar fibromatosis. Diagnostic confirmation can be gained if there is a definite degree of relief resulting from interruption of the sympathetic reflex.

Eventually, tapering deformity of the fingers may develop with extreme stiffness of the digits and wrist as well as flexion deformity of the fingers and thumb; in some, the forearm, elbow and shoulder may be involved and the classic radiographic features are of mottled decalcification and osteoporosis.

Reasonable return of function may be obtained in many of these patients by active and passive exercise conducted with the help of a therapist: paraffin wax baths are useful.

Guanethidine sympathetic blockage can be useful as may be a short course of prednisolone 5 mg three times a day over 6 weeks. A combination of small doses of diazepam may also help. It is often best to admit the patient to hospital for such treatment and for the arm to be kept elevated much of the time; fitting of spring braces to the fingers to undo flexion deformity of the proximal interphalangeal joints should also be part of the rehabilitation programme.

Although the metacarpophalangeal joints may exhibit limited flexion, the temptation to perform capsulotomy should be avoided in individuals who appear to over-react to a serious extent and the likelihood is that the condition could be worsened with further surgical insult.

Arm–hand vibration syndrome

Use of tools causing vibration dates from 1883, with reports of associated symptoms in the hand in the early 1900s. In order to establish the diagnosis, there has to be a history of exposure to vibration and exclusion of other possible causes of symptoms.

Vibration white finger has been a prescribed disease since 1985 and its occurrence in association with certain occupations may give rise to compensation by the government; workers may also sue their employers in the civil courts.

Furthermore, the Health and Safety at Work Act 1974 requires employers to do all that is reasonably practicable to safeguard their employees' health. Since the beginning of 1993, management of health and safety regulations further specify that the employer makes suitable and sufficient assessments of hazards and risk in the workplace and ensures that appropriate health surveillance is carried out and no doubt this will be expanded with regard to the European Community Directive on physical hazards in the workplace. It is nowadays thought that the syndrome is more than Raynaud's phenomenon due to vibration and there are neurological changes that can be even more important: clinical assessment should be followed by appropriate investigations of vascular and neurological function, while the cold provocation test, including measurement of the systolic blood pressure in the finger, is of some value.

Of course, neurophysiological tests can be of particular importance in detecting the presence of entrapment neuropathies and other neuropathies unrelated to work activity. All is not known about this condition but when suspected, it is obviously prudent to alter the workstyle of the patient.

Repetitive strain injury

Characteristically, arm pain in those individuals with this diagnosis does not conform to any identifiable anatomical or pathological pattern: such individuals more often than not have jobs involving highly repetitive activities. Curiously, despite subsequent avoidance of possible pain-inducing activities, many of these individuals report non-improvement, even deterioration, and eventually litigate. There are two related conditions recognized as 'prescribed disorders': cramp of the hand or forearm in people with an occupation maintaining long periods of handwriting, typing or other repetitive movements, and traumatic inflammation of the tendons of the hand and forearm and associated tendon sheaths in any occupation entailing manual labour or frequent or repeated movements of the hand or wrist. Occasionally, definitive and well-known lesions *can* without question be caused by highly repetitive use of the hand and upper limb in less than ideal conditions, such as carpal tunnel syndrome, de Quervain's tenosynovitis stenosans and lateral and medial epicondylitis at the elbow.

It has been suggested that repetitive strain injury syndrome is referred pain from the neck; on the other hand, it has been estimated that one-tenth of the population at some time has pain in the neck and arm or both, quite often associated with degenerative osteo-arthritic change in the neck.

It must be said that there is presently insufficient conclusive evidence to prove repetitive strain injury is causative of anything other than the specifically described conditions already mentioned.

A whole host of other descriptive terms have been used for so-called repetitive strain injury. Occupational overuse syndrome (OOS), overuse syndrome, muscle overuse syndrome, occupational cervicobrachial disorder (OCD), cumulative trauma disorder (CTD), regional pain syndrome, localized fibrositis or fibromyalgia syndrome, chronic upper limb pain syndrome, occupational neuralgia, cramp, palsy, work-related upper limb disorder, refractory cervicobrachial pain (RCBP) and static stress syndrome.

In the 19th century, writers were called scriveners and scriveners palsy was described in 1864. This affected those in occupations where writing was incessant and the pain was said to be burning or aching in character and accompanied by a feeling of cold and fatigue and numbness in the fingers, as well as cramp, to the extent that writing had to cease. The term writer's cramp has also been used.

On the other hand, occupational neurosis has also been a diagnosis for such individuals, described as long ago as 1911 by W.E. Paul, a Boston neurologist.

It is not unusual with individuals diagnosed as suffering repetitive strain injury to have an apparent psychological disorder in regard to overanxiety and to seek blame for their condition. The question is whether the diagnosed condition affects their personalities or such conditions tend to occur in this particular type of individual. The concept of mass hysteria should also be mentioned, particularly in the context of the 'Australian epidemic' where certain features were said to come into play: a stressful life; everyday aches and pains which may be as bad as usual at the end of the day in a keyboard worker; a strongly held belief in the symptomatic individual that repetitive movement *can* injure the hand and upper limb; reinforcement from fellow workers, Trade Unions, the press and other peer groups; medical diagnosis and certification from work in the absence of physical signs; easy access to workers compensation scheme and a favourable sociopolitical milieu for acceptance of repetitive strain injury as a compensatable condition. Sadly, individuals exhibiting symptoms which some would regard as repetitive strain injury, have overanxious personalities and it seems seldom indeed that such individuals are given adequate appropriate reassurance, although counselling and physiotherapy measures are typical treatment modalities.

Extensor tendon damage

Occasionally, a non-rheumatoid, elderly individual may exhibit medial translocation of the extensor tendon mechanism which, when severe, can cause significant disability because the finger cannot be extended at the metacarpophalangeal joint. The realignment of the extensor tendon mechanism can usually be performed by overlap procedure on the dorsilateral aspect of the extensor hood (Fig. 24.38).

Closed rupture of the extensor pollicis longus tendon is well known to occur in the rheumatoid arthritic patient and after the healing stage of a Colles' fracture. Disability is profound with inability to elevate the thumb from the palm in order to grasp objects. Typically, this is an attrition lesion in the third compartment of the extensor retinaculum as the tendon courses round Lister's tubercle.

A number of surgical techniques are available for restoration of extension to the thumb, the most popular being transfer of the extensor indicis tendon which requires two surgical incisions and does lead to some weakness of extension of the index finger. Among other techniques, an intercalated tendon graft can be considered.

A useful alternative is to use the extensor carpi radialis

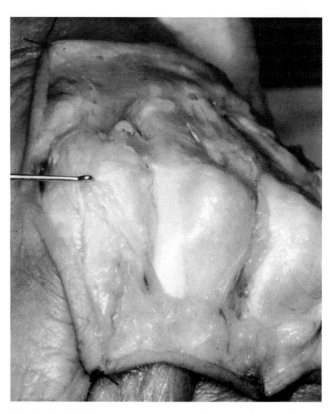

Fig. 24.38 Medial translocation of the finger extensor tendons, resulting in flexion deformity of the metacarpophalangeal joints: this can be corrected by centralization of the tendons by a lateral overlapping procedure of the extensor hood.

longus tendon: maximum length of the tendon transfer is required when it is released from the base of the index metacarpal (Fig. 24.39). The transposed tendon is similar in girth to the extensor pollicis longus and is normally anatomically adjacent while only a single incision is required. This technique has proven to be a highly successful procedure, described by the author in 1986.

Lacerating injuries of the extensor tendons to the digits proximal to the knuckles are usually easily repaired with excellent functional results. It is important, as in flexor tendon injuries, to immobilize the metacarpophalangeal joint in flexion beyond 70° and the interphalangeal joints just short of full extension for a period of 3–4 weeks in a splint.

When there is soft-tissue crushing of the dorsum of the hand and wrist, apart from lacerating injury, it is necessary on occassion to perform, after soft-tissue healing, the two-stage procedure of silastic rodding and secondary tendon grafting.

In regard to the unusual and interesting condition of snapping or dislocation of the extensor carpi ulnaris tendon, when symptomatically disabling, surgical stabilization can be considered. In the normal anatomy, this

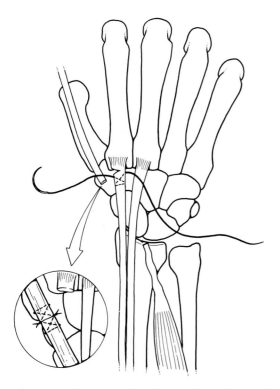

Fig. 24.39 The author's simple technique of transferring the extensor carpi radialis longus tendon from the base of the index metacarpal to the distal segment of the ruptured extensor pollicis longus tendon.

tendon is angular in its course as it proceeds distally to its insertion when the forearm is fully supinated: it is in this stance of the forearm that trauma can occur and typically there is acute onset of pain with a mild sensation of snapping. In the acute case, application of a cast with the forearm in pronation and the wrist dorsiflexed with slight radial deviation for several weeks is curative. However, the chronic disabling case can be surgically treated in the manner of Spinner and Kaplan. This procedure involves raising a flap of extensor retinaculum in the neighbourhood of Lister's tubercle of the radius, the base being maintained at the inner aspect of the extensor digiti minimi. This flap is passed under the displaced extensor carpi ulnaris tendon from the radial side, the free end of the flap then being sutured onto itself and adjacent soft-tissue and ulnar periosteum after which the forearm is immobilized for 3 weeks and then a removable wrist splint for 2 further weeks.

Flexor tendon division

The flexor tendons in the lower forearm and palm receive nutrition by vascular perfusion via the longitudinally orientated vessels from the surrounding paratenon.

Within the fibrous flexor sheath, there is diffusion from the synovial fluid and also vascular perfusion from the vincular system.

Longitudinally running vessels in the deep flexor tendon interconnect at the level of the digital joints, the intra-tendonous vasculature being fed by a longitudinal vessel on the dorsal surface of the tendon, this being continued with vessels on the short vinculum distally and the long vinculum proximally. Between the vinculae there is a zone of potential ischaemia within the tendon (Fig. 24.40).

The dorsal vessel is reinforced by branches of vessels supplying the superficialis insertion, these running along each limb of the insertion of this tendon, converging in the decussation to form a dorsal vessel similar to that of profundus. Intratendonous patterns within the superficialis tendon are similar to those in the profundus.

In assessing potential difficulty of surgical treatment, it is useful to use the zone system and consider the anatomical construction of the fibrous flexor sheath into annular (A) and cruciform (C) pulleys, the former being thicker and preventing bow-stringing of the tendon (Fig. 24.41). The particularly difficult problem here is where both flexor tendons have been divided in zones one and two, this commencing proximally at the level of the metacarpal neck. The A1 and oblique pulleys are of great importance in the thumb.

Closed flexor tendon rupture is unusual and is seen more often in the rheumatoid patient. In rheumatoid disease, the deep flexor tendons to the digits may often be ruptured in the carpal tunnel, particularly where there is carpal bone erosion and severe synovitis.

In non-rheumatoid cases, closed rupture is usually traumatic in origin with the level of the lesion being situated at the distal insertion of the deep flexor tendon; radiographs are necessary as in some cases a segment of bone has been avulsed from the distal phalanx. In the acute case, appropriate repair can usually be readily made, but disability in the average individual may not be great and surgery is not always mandatory, certainly not for the little finger.

It is rarely necessary to consider sophisticated, often two-stage surgery in the rheumatoid individual with closed tendon rupture affecting only one or two digits and even such a lesion of the long flexor tendon of the thumb often does not lead to important loss of function.

Lacerating injuries of the flexor tendon mechanism in the digits can present problems in surgical management, rehabilitation and long-term disability.

It is important to assess fully neurological, vascular and tendonous damage with lacerating wounds of the palmar surface of the hand and wrist. As a general

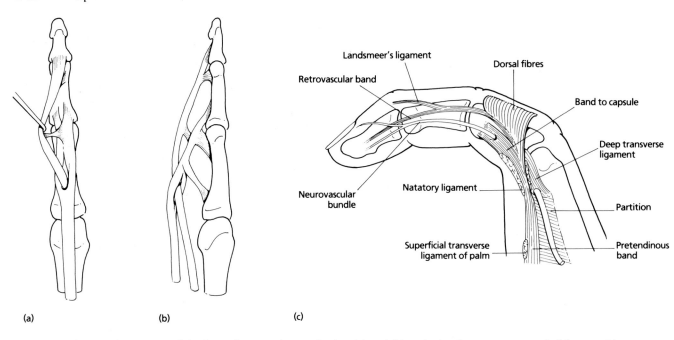

(a)   (b)   (c)

Fig. 24.40 The vincular systems of the finger flexor tendon mechanism (a) and (b) and other important anatomical features (c).

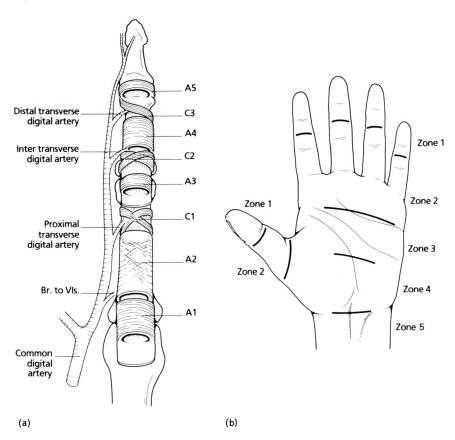

(a)   (b)

Fig. 24.41 (a) The finger flexor pulley system. (b) Zoning in the hand is useful in considering surgical treatment of flexor tendon injuries.

principle, such damage should be dealt with primarily unless the wound is heavily contaminated.

It is, of course, necessary that surgery for tendonous, neurological and vascular damage is performed in an expert manner, with pneumatic tourniquet control ideally and under brachial block or general anaesthesia with a hand table and proper instrumentation being available. There is seldom difficulty in surgically primarily anastamosing divided flexor tendons proximal to the distal palmar crease.

Likewise, isolated division of the deep flexor tendon distal to the sublimis slips should be dealt with by primary suture. However, this technique is unlikely to be successful if delayed beyond 2 or 3 weeks post-injury, the problem then being retrieval of the proximal segment of the tendon. If the injury is in the chronic stage, a definite option is to leave well alone, certainly where a single digit is concerned, particularly so the little finger. A 'sublimis finger' can be functionally useful and the distal interphalangeal joint can be arthrodesed in 30° of flexion if necessary.

Surgical reconstruction of the deep finger flexor tendon mechanism in the chronic stage involves a two-stage procedure in most cases, firstly by silastic rodding and then tendon grafting, but the end result often does not justify this time-consuming treatment.

Division of both flexor tendons within the fibrous flexor sheath of the finger provides a difficult surgical challenge, particularly so in regard to ensuring proper tendon glide. Such damage caused by a simple lacerating injury may be repaired in one of two ways: either by tendon grafting or by primary direct suture. Primary or delayed primary repair is now regarded as the treatment of choice.

On the other hand, tendon damage associated with a crushing and lacerating injury cannot be so treated. The damaged skin should first be attended to appropriately, sometimes involving a skin-grafting procedure. Here, after the skin has healed, a silastic rod should be inserted temporarily, extending from the retained distal stump of the deep flexor tendon and brought proximally either into the palm or lower forearm where it is attached to the appropriate tendon, the flexor tendon mechanism otherwise being resected. It is frequently necessary in these cases to construct pulleys in the digit, at least one at the level of the centre of the middle phalanx and the other at the base of the finger using resected tendon and the damaged fibrous flexor sheath should be resected (Fig. 24.42). It is, of course, necessary that passive motion of the digital joints is maintained by a proper rehabilitation regime.

Provided all goes well with the healing of the soft tissues, the permanent tendon graft is then rail-roaded along the pseudo-sheath that has formed. It is, of course, mandatory to very carefully handle the damaged tendon tissue so as to minimize subsequent fibrous scarring.

If it is decided to go for flexor tendon grafting the wound should simply be cleaned up and sutured. Once skin healing has occurred satisfactorily, some weeks after the accident, then the flexor tendon graft procedure

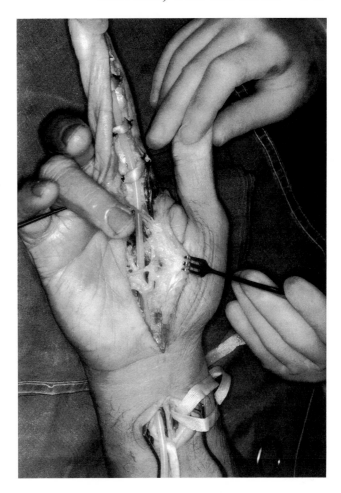

Fig. 24.42 First-stage finger flexor tendon reconstruction, using a silastic rod which results is the formation of a smooth endothelial-lined channel through which the tendon graft can subsequently glide; new pulleys have been formed in the finger, using resected tendon. This two-stage technique can be used in the lacerated and contused finger and after failed previous flexor tendon surgery.

can be performed. If neurological damage has had to be repaired, appropriate splintage will have to be maintained for at least 3 weeks.

Prior to tendon grafting, full passive range of motion of the affected digit is essential and this exercise programme should be clearly explained to the patient.

The ideal donor tendon for grafting is the palmaris longus, present in 85% of individuals; if absent on the side of injury it may be present at the opposite forearm and wrist. If both palmaris longus tendons are absent then the long extensor tendon to the fourth toe should be used. Appropriate use of a tendon stripper minimizes skin scarring; the peritendonous sheath of the donor graft should be preserved and the tendon tissue, of course, has to be handled gently.

In the absence of the palmaris longus tendon and where more than one digit has to be treated, the extensor tendons of the middle three toes are useful for tendon grafts; a further alternative is the extensor indicis proprius. The plantaris tendon gives a long, thin tendon graft and is said to be present in 80% of individuals but its presence cannot be clinically predicted.

On occasion, the superficial flexor tendon can be transposed from one digit to its neighbour; it is also occasionally useful to transpose the ring or middle finger superficialis tendon to the thumb with complicated lacerating injury to the flexor pollicis longus tendon. It is useful to use the Bruner incision for the ring and middle fingers: the alternative for the index and little fingers is a midlateral or medial incision respectively which is appropriately extended into the palm.

The damaged superficial deep and flexor tendons of the finger are resected into the palm, a distal profundus stump being left for subsequent anastomosis; included in the surgical technique is identification and appropriate preservation of the neurovascular structures. Where the proximal interphalangeal joint is hyperextensible, it is often best to leave one tail of the sublimis at its distal attachment and to suture the proximal end into the flexor sheath proximal to the joint.

Pulleys of the fibrous flexor sheath should be preserved over at least the middle of the middle phalanx and at the base of the proximal phalanx; if the sheath has been severely damaged it may have to be resected *in toto* and pulleys constructed from resected tendon tissue. It is essential to retain an adequate pulley mechanism to avoid bow-stringing deformity of the tendon graft (Fig. 24.43).

The tendon graft should firstly be sutured to the profundus stump at the distal phalanx: either the Bunnell criss-cross suture or the Kessler technique can be used (Fig. 24.44); alternatively, the distal end of the tendon graft can be sutured into bone, the suture being brought through the pulp and tied over a button.

The tendon graft is then taken through the pulley mechanism and sewn into the proximal profundus stump distal to the origin of the lumbrical muscle. An oblique split should be made in the profundus tendon and the graft threaded through this prior to suture. It is important to bury the tendon stump to avoid encouraging development of dense local adhesion formation. It is essential to have a proper stance of the digit at the moment of proximal suture of the graft; it is useful here to obtain skin closure of the digit prior to this to allow for tension within the finger.

Improper flexion deformity of the finger can result from the anastamosis being too short and also there is

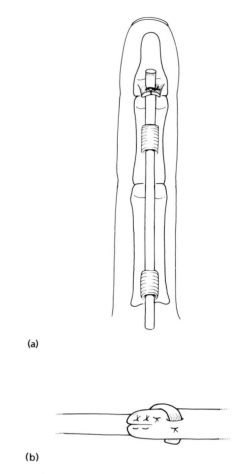

(a)

(b)

Fig. 24.43 (a) Flexor tendon grafting for division of both flexor tendons in the finger: either as a delayed primary procedure or after silastic rodding. (b) Proximal anastomosis.

the risk of overpull of the lumbrical muscle with swan-neck deformity and this might have to be in due course corrected by surgical release of the intrinsic tendon at the base of the finger.

With regard to the crushed and lacerated finger where a silastic tendon rod has been inserted, the tendon graft should be rail-roaded. The tendon graft is first temporarily sutured to the distal end of the silastic rod, then the old incision on the volar surface of the wrist or palm is opened and the rod carefully pulled proximally, the tendon graft following. The proximal end of the tendon graft is then sutured appropriately, as already described, to the profundus tendon in the lower forearm or palm, care being taken to obtain proper stance of the affected finger.

Primary repair of the flexor tendon mechanism can be considered in the fibrous flexor sheath of the finger associated with a relatively clean and simple lacerating wound, particularly in the younger adult and in the child.

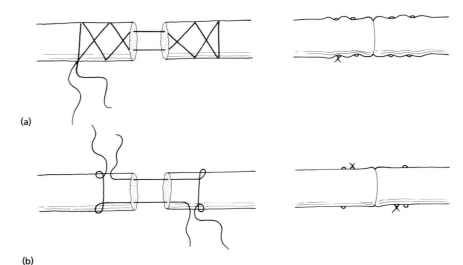

Fig. 24.44 The Bunnell (a) and Kessler (b) techniques of tendon suture.

Usually, the wound will require extending proximally and distally; the fibrous flexor sheath is then resected carefully to an appropriate extent at the level of tendon damaged.

Apposition of the tendon ends is facilitated by passive flexion of the digit and wrist.

The ends of the divided tendon should be very carefully handled; on occasion, the palm has to be opened in order to retrieve the proximal stump.

Tendon anastamosis should be carefully accomplished, the best results being obtained when the synovial sheath of the tendon can be brought over the anastamosis site and sutured in position with absorbable fine catgut sutures. It is best, certainly in the adult, to repair only the deep flexor tendon, the sublimis being sacrificed within the digit. In the child, both tendons can sometimes be anastomosed provided the technique is particularly fine and expert.

Whether the technique of reconstruction of the flexor tendon mechanism is by primary repair or secondary tendon grafting, a posterior well-padded splint should be applied with the metacarpophalangeal joints of the fingers flexed at least 70° and the interphalangeal joints just short of extension while the thumb should be held well abducted from the palm, the wrist being at neutral. Very early active movement of the digits of the hand should be encouraged within the protective splint and it is helpful to use the Kleinert technique by attaching a rubber spring to the nail by an adhesive technique or placing a wire suture distal to the nailbed (Fig. 24.45).

After three weeks, a dorsal splint should be used intermittently and kept on through the night while the daily rehabilitation programme proceeds with an active and passive regime, supervised by a therapist, and it can

also be helpful to use silicone and paraffin wax baths for a period of time.

Sometimes the result of even expert surgical management is disappointing and tenolysis can be considered for some individuals 6–12 months after tendon surgery to improve tendon glide, this to be followed by a reasonably aggressive rehabilitation programme.

There can be particular difficulty in rehabilitating children under 5 years of age, but in the long-term such young patients tend to do well.

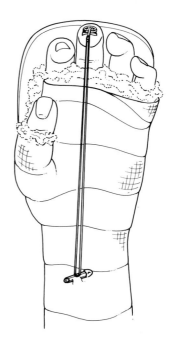

Fig. 24.45 The Kleinert technique for rehabilitation after finger flexor tendon reconstruction.

The wrist

CARPAL INSTABILITY

The anatomy of the wrist joint is complex and consists of capsuloligamentous structures together with the articular surface of the carpometacarpal, intercarpal and radiocarpal articulations together with the triangular fibrocartilage at the ulna.

It is best to consider the carpus as three vertical columns, where both dynamic and static instability can occur:

1 between the lateral column consisting of the scaphoid, trapezium and trapezoid and the central column composing the lunate and capitate;
2 between the medial column, the triquetrum, and the central column of the lunate or hamate;
3 proximally between the single unit of the entire carpus and the articular surface of the radius and the triangular articular disc, frequently resulting from changes at the lower radius.

Loss of scapholunate integrity can result in dorsiflexion of the lunate at the radiocarpal articulation: the normal alignment of radius, lunate and capitate is lost, this being termed dorsal intercalated segmental integrity, or DISI.

By contrast, and less frequently, loss of triquetral control on the lunate can result in its flexion together with the scaphoid at the radiocarpal articulation, this being termed volar intercalated segmental instability, or VISI.

Dorsal subluxation of the carpus at the radiocarpal articulation is typically seen in malunited Colles' fracture; midcarpal instability may also be seen in this injury. Of course, early diagnosis of sprains and subluxation or dislocation of the carpus is mandatory for proper treatment. In the case of a sprain, it is usually sufficient to immobilize the wrist in slight palmar flexion in a cast for several weeks. Capsuloligamentous tearing can be repaired, sometimes arthroscopically, after reduction of any displacement. However, in the late case it is more likely that limited carpal fusion will give the best result.

Nowadays, there are recognized subdivisions of the main types of traumatic carpal instability. Scapholunate dissociation is relatively commonly seen, the clinical diagnosis depending on the examiner pressing the thumb on the distal pole of the scaphoid with the forearm fully pronated and the wrist in ulnar deviation. The wrist is then radially deviated while pressure is maintained, the proximal pole of the scaphoid then subluxing dorsally. The typical radiographic finding is of a pathological gap between the lunate and the scaphoid, commonly known as the 'Terry Thomas' sign (Fig. 24.46). Sometimes, there is the opportunity for capsuloligamentous stabilization of the replaced scaphoid, but more often than not arthrodesis is required, either of the scaphoid to the lunate or to the trapezium. Stabilization can sometimes be accomplished arthroscopically (Fig. 24.47). In the chronic case that has degenerated into osteoarthritic change, consideration can be given to surgical resection of the scaphoid and its replacement with a silastic or titanium implant together with limited carpal arthrodesis, e.g. lunocapitate. It should be said that there have been occasional reports of wrist synovitis with silastic carpal implants.

Symptomatic midcarpal instability following Colles' fracture can be sometimes relieved by effective osteotomy of the lower radius, usually in those under age 60 who have adequate pre-operative range of wrist motion; in other cases, appropriate limited arthrodesis can be considered.

Injury can result in lunotriquetral sprain, greater violence sometimes resulting in palmar flexion instability with rotational force being an important factor in the production of this condition. Diagnosis can be difficult

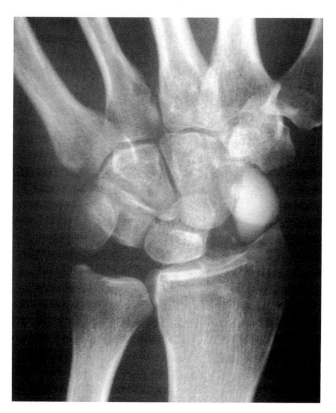

Fig. 24.46 The 'Terry Thomas' radiographic sign of scapholunate dissociation, demonstrating the pathological gap between the two bones.

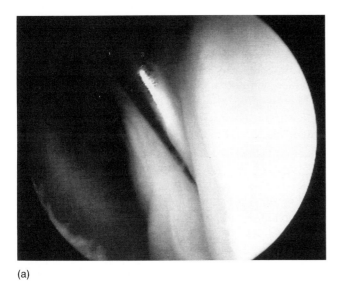

(a)

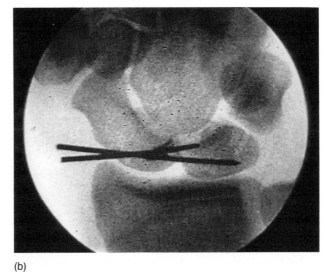

(b)

Fig. 24.47 Arthroscopic stabilization of scapholunate dissociation: firstly, the probe is seen in the scapholunate interval prior to reduction (a), after which pins are used for fixation (b). (Courtesy of A. Lee Osterman.)

and often the only sign is localized tenderness at the inner aspect of the carpus. In the acute case, the wrist should be immobilized in an above-elbow cast for at least 6 weeks, the wrist being ulnar deviated and dorsiflexed with the cast moulded at the pisiform. Symptoms are usually satisfactorily resolved in this way but if there is chronic disability then triquetrolunate arthrodesis can be considered.

The rare condition of triquetrohamate instability can sometimes be effectively treated by immobilizing the wrist in an above-elbow cast with the forearm supinated and the wrist at neutral. In others, with persistent disability, treatment may be successfully accomplished by surgical fusion of this articulation but, in the long-term, it may be better to consider combined arthrodesis of the lunate, capitate, triquetrum and hamate. Soft-tissue reconstruction can also be considered. The diagnosis is suggested by painful snapping produced by bringing the hand into and out of ulnar deviation while the forearm is pronated, with the examiner longitudinally compressing the wrist.

The unusual major injury of trans-scaphoid perilunate dislocation results in considerable dorsal deformity of the carpus and stiffness, sometimes also median compression neuropathy.

In the acute case it is often possible to perform satisfactory closed reduction, although screw fixation of the scaphoid fracture may often be required: appropriate cast immobilization for at least 6 weeks is necessary. In the chronic unrecognized case, then open reduction, sometimes arthrodesis, of the wrist, is then required.

While many carpal injuries are readily diagnosed clinically and radiographically, there are other more subtle conditions of instability that can be difficult to diagnose and to treat. Arthrographic and arthroscopic examination as well as cineradiography can be useful in these cases.

Of course, displacement of carpal joints requires reduction, either closed or operative as the case may be and additional measures such as capsuloligamentous reconstruction or arthrodesis can be additionally necessary.

Ulnar-plus deformity with painful medial wrist disability and impingement can sometimes be satisfactorily relieved by appropriate steroid and local anaesthetic injection. The ulnocarpal impingement syndrome can occur in childhood as a result of premature closure of the lower radial epiphysis arrest following trauma.

Adults with this condition, without radio-ulnar arthrosis, when sufficiently symptomatic can be dealt with by ulnar recession osteotomy. Others, exhibiting arthritic change can be suitably treated by ulnar head resection or, preferably, by lower ulnar shaft cuff resection, combined with arthrodesis of the inferior radio-ulnar joint in the manner of Suavé–Kapandji (Fig. 24.48), this procedure typically produces a near-normal appearance of the wrist, ulnar translocation of the carpus is obviated and uncomfortable disability of the resected end of the ulnar shaft, sometimes a feature with ulnar head resection, is avoided.

Ulnocarpal impingement syndrome can vary from simple wear to involvement of the lunate and ulna with

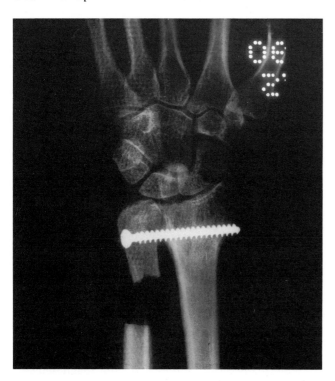

Fig. 24.48 The Sauvé–Kapendj procedure. This can be a useful operation for symptomatic instability of the inferior radio-ulnar joint as well as for restricted forearm rotation.

chondromalacia and in others there is perforation of the triangular fibrocartilage which may also be accompanied by ligamentous damage and, in the final stages, ulno-carpal osteoarthritis.

Attenuation or tearing of the volar aspect of the triangular fibrocartilage can lead to dorsal displacement of the ulna in pronation as the ulnocarpal ligaments are relaxed in this position. On the other hand, similar pathology at the dorsal margin of the cartilage allows for volar subluxation of the ulnar head. The osseous shape of the convexity of the ulnar articular surface and the margins of the sigmoid notch are also of importance in rotational stability.

Trauma to the triangular fibrocartilage may result in central perforation while avulsion in other cases may be medial or lateral; the medial and lateral cases can be accompanied by fracture.

Clinical suspicion of derangement of the triangular fibrocartilage can be confirmed by arthrography and arthroscopic examination.

Non-disabling symptoms can often be dealt with by the wearing of a removable splint on the wrist for several weeks, perhaps combined with physiotherapy treatment and steroid and local anaesthetic injection.

In other cases, where there is important disability,

consideration then has to be given to repair of the triangular fibrocartilage while limited debridement in other cases can be performed arthroscopically. In some, ulna recession osteotomy may have to be performed to produce symptomatic relief.

In other cases a small fracture fragment off the ulnar articular surface may need to be resected, while larger fragments should be repositioned and internally fixed.

KEINBOCK'S DISEASE

This is sometimes known as lunate malacia: the precise cause remains unknown, although a number of theories are available.

However, it is known that the condition is typically accompanied by a somewhat medially placed lunate compared with the normal subject and there can be uneven compression between the radius and ulnocarpal complex with typically relative shortening of the ulna.

The radiographic changes progress from increased density and normal shape of the lunate and the development of cystic changes then collapse and fragmentation, the final stage demonstrating perilunate osteoarthritic change.

Conservative treatment consists of a removable splint, which can relieve painful symptoms in these relatively young patients.

There is a considerable variety of surgical procedures available: revascularization by inserting into the lunate a segment of radius kept attached to the pronator quadratus, bone grafting, proximal carpectomy, partial or total arthrodesis of the wrist and resection of the lunate and its replacement with a silastic or titanium implant (Fig. 24.49).

On the other hand, 'joint levelling' has become popular at the proximal side of the wrist joint, particularly so in the earlier stages of the condition before significant collapse of the lunate has occurred; one method is to lengthen the distal ulnar shaft.

Radial shortening is perhaps preferable, best performed with a longitudinal volar–radial incision, and a segment of distal radius is resected sufficient to equalize the level of the distal radius and ulna, internal fixation being required either by plate and screws or appropriately thick Kirschner wires and a plaster cast should be worn for 6 weeks (Fig. 24.50).

MALUNION OF LOWER RADIAL FRACTURES

In the case of malunion of lower radial fractures at the wrist, particularly Colles' fracture, the wrist is working at a mechanical disadvantage with hand and wrist

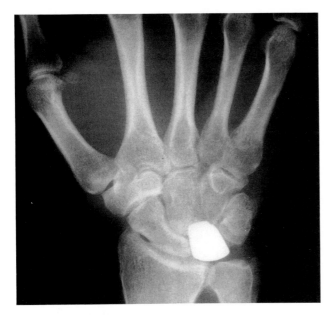

Fig. 24.49 The Swanson titanium implant for Keinbock's disease.

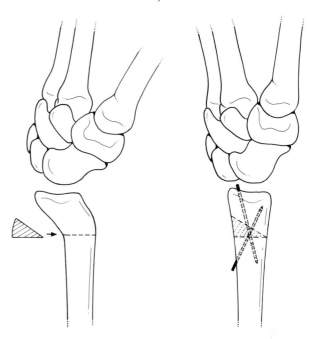

Fig. 24.51 Lower radial osteotomy for malunion of a Colles' fracture: indicated for chronic uncomfortable malfunction, rarely performed in those over 60 years old.

function being limited quite apart from embarrassing cosmetic deformity. Also, in the case of malunion in Colles' fracture, uncomfortable midcarpal instability may be a continuing problem.

For corrective lower radial osteotomy, a longitudinal volar–radial approach to the radius is best, centred along the flexor carpi radialis indicis tendon; a dorsal approach may also be used.

Usually, an open wedge osteotomy is performed (Fig. 24.51). A motorized saw can readily be used but completion of the osteotomy is safest by judicious use of the osteotome at the dorsal and radial cortex to avoid tendon damage. Bone is harvested from the iliac crest of the pelvis and internal fixation is required either by plate

and screws, securing the osteotomy on either side, or by Kirschner wires. Particularly where there is painful ulnar head deformity as a result of a Colles' fracture, consideration may have to be given to realigning the ulna by recession osteotomy of the lower shaft of this bone or by the Sauvé–Kapendji procedure, either at the same time as the lower radial osteotomy or at a second procedure.

In general, corrective lower radial osteotomy should be confined to those under age 60, particularly in women with osteoporotic change; there should be at least a

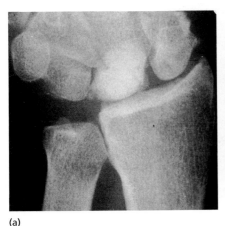

(a)

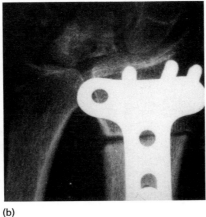

(b)

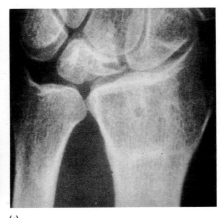

(c)

Fig. 24.50 Radial recession osteotomy for Keinbock's disease: particularly indicated in the earlier stages of the disease, in the presence of relative shortening of the ulna. (a) Pre-operative. (b) The osteotomy with internal fixation. (c) Appearance at follow-up.

preoperative range of wrist motion of 50% of normal without degenerative osteoarthritic change at the radiocarpal joint.

Muscle and tendon transfers

Rupture of the finger extensor tendons in rheumatoid disease is part of the caput ulnae syndrome and most often affects the ring and little fingers and here, after appropriate synovectomy and resection of the ulnar head, possibly its prosthetic replacement, then simple cross-over anastomosis of the distal ends of the ruptured tendons to the intact extensors of the index and middle fingers is readily accomplished.

Where the middle finger and rarely the index finger are also involved then tendon transfer is required and a good result can be expected by transferring the superficial flexor tendon from either the middle or ring finger through a constructed window in the interosseous membrane of the forearm, the end of the tendon transfer then being threaded through the distal ruptured extensor tendon segments (Fig. 24.52).

In the case of permanent paralysis of the abductor and short flexor muscles of the thumb with loss of opposition, opponensplasty should be considered in the appropriate case: a useful method is to transpose the superficial flexor tendon of the middle or ring finger. The tendon is released through a palmar digital incision and brought through a pulley fashioned from part of the flexor carpi ulnaris tendon, the main insertion being kept intact through the volar−medial approach at the wrist. A short lateral incision is made at the thumb and the finger

flexor tendon is pulled through subcutaneously to be sewn into the tendonous insertion of the short abductor tendon (Fig. 24.53).

In the case of permanent clawing of the ring and little fingers from an ulnar nerve lesion, a useful procedure is that described by Zancolli where the released superficial flexor is brought back on itself over the A1 pulley at the base of the finger and is sutured with the metacarpophalangeal joint in the straight position, this being known as the dynamic Zancolli operation (Fig. 24.54).

This surgeon also devised, for similar anatomical reasons, the static procedure of proximal advancement of the volar capsule of the metacarpophalangeal joint, both procedures being performed through a transverse distal palmar incision.

Irreparable paralysis from a posterior interosseous nerve lesion can be dealt with by transferring the superficial flexor tendons of the middle and ring fingers through a window in the interosseous membrane to provide power for the extensor tendons of the fingers and the long thumb extensor and in this operation the flexor carpi radialis indicis tendon is transferred to the abductor pollicis longus and extensor pollicis brevis.

If the radial nerve has been irreparably damaged the operation described should be supplemented by transference of the pronator teres into the radial carpal extensors.

Muscle transfers around the elbow usually apply to flaccid paralysis resulting from anterior poliomyelitis, traction lesions of the brachial plexus and, occasionally, in those patients suffering from muscular dystrophy and arthrogryposis.

In such cases, careful functional assessment is manda-

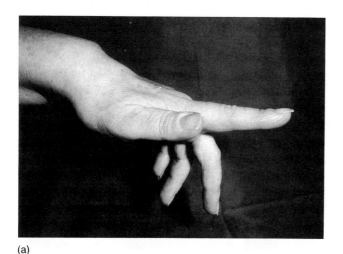

(a)

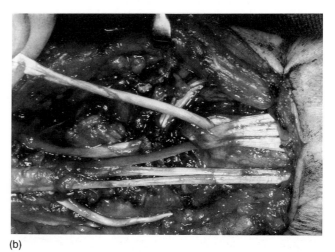

(b)

Fig. 24.52 Flexor superficialis transfer, from either the middle or ring finger, for closed rupture of the middle finger, ring and little fingers in the rheumatoid caput ulnae syndrome (a). The ulnar head has been resected and replaced with a silastic implant and the forward-displaced extensor carpi ulnaris tendon replaced and stabilized (b).

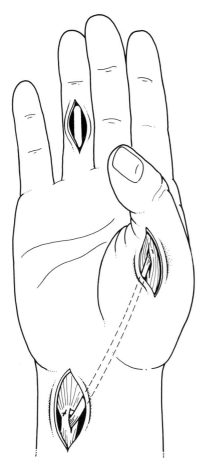

Fig. 24.53 Opponensplasty, using the middle or ring finger superficialis tendon.

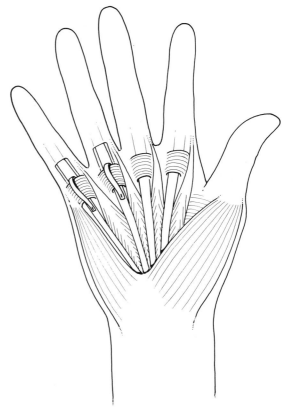

Fig. 24.54 The dynamic Zancolli procedure for chronic clawing of the ring and little fingers as a result of ulnar neuropathy.

tory and it can be difficult to select the appropriate operation in an individual case; accurate muscle charting is important and the strength of the proposed muscle to be transferred should not be overestimated. So far, no effective muscle transfer has yet been devised to restore active extension of the elbow.

Pectoralis major transfer to restore active elbow flexion can be effective if good scapula control and glenohumeral stability are present. If the shoulder joint is weak, arthrodesis of the shoulder maybe additionally required.

The Steindler procedure is particularly useful in patients with a traction lesion involving the upper trunk of the brachial plexus only. The common flexor origin is divided and then button holed through the intermuscular septum approximately 2.5 cm above the medial epicondyle. With the elbow still held at right angles, the common extensor origin is then divided, mobilized and transposed 1 cm proximal to its usual attachment, being sutured into the lateral intermuscular septum.

Clark's pectoral transfer involves freeing the pectoralis major with its overlying fascia from the sixth rib, a strip of muscle 7.5 cm wide is mobilized proximally to the interspace between the third and fourth ribs, the nerve supply being carefully preserved at this level.

A second L-shaped incision is made in the lower third of the arm and the transverse component is at the anterior elbow crease; the distal biceps tendon is exposed and a subcutaneous tunnel is fashioned, connecting the two incisions; the free end of the pectoral muscle is then withdrawn down the arm. The fascial origin is then anastomosed to the distal biceps tendon with the elbow at the right angle (Fig. 24.55).

The elbow should be immobilized in a posterior splint at the right angles for about 3 weeks after which an active exercise programme is instituted. This particular transfer is probably the first choice for restoration of elbow flexion.

The Brookes–Seddon pectoral transfer involves detaching the tendon of insertion of pectoralis major at the bicipital groove and then anastomosing this to the detached tendon of the extensor carpi radialis longus,

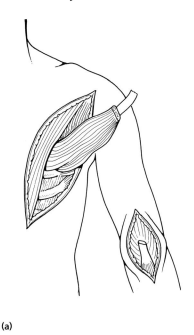

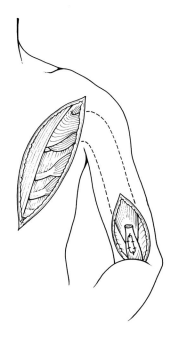

(a)   (b)

Fig. 24.55 (a, b) The Clark pectoral transfer is one of several operative procedures to restore active flexion to the elbow as well as conferring an element of active supination. This operation is particularly indicated for those with an isolated lesion of the upper trunk of the brachial plexus which has failed to recover.

which is firstly button-holed through and sewn into the distal biceps tendon.

d'Aubigne and Postel modified the Clark pectoral transfer. Here the detached insertion of the pectoralis major from the bicipital groove is attached to the coracoid process with a good line of action being provided.

The triceps transfer should be avoided when possible in view of possible serious consequences from loss of active extension of the elbow, the chief indication being for traction lesions of the brachial plexus.

In this procedure, the incision extends from the middle of the arm distally and posteromedially, following the line of the ulnar nerve, then proceeding to the subcutaneous border of the ulna.

The triceps muscle and tendon are detached from their insertion into the olecranon and also freed from the posterior aspect of the medial intermuscular septum above the elbow: the medial intermuscular septum has to be resected, the triceps tendon being button-holed into the musculotendonous junction of the biceps with tension being such that there is no undue force on the transferred muscle with the elbow held at the right angle.

Latissimus dorsi transfer was first described by Hovnanian in 1956; the whole of the muscle is detached from its origin and swung around on its neurovascular pedicle and then passed distally and attached either to the tubercle of the radius or the olecranon.

Zancolli modified this technique in 1973 and he has made the point that in certain appropriate cases arthro-

desis of the glenohumeral articulation of the shoulder provides improved flexion power of the elbow.

In the Zancolli modification, part of the thoracolumbar fascia is taken from its distal origin for subsequent attachment of the transplant to the biceps tendon. This is a fairly involved procedure during which a tunnel is made within the pectoralis major muscle after identifying the coracoid process. This allows attachment of the proximal end of the latissimus dorsi muscle to the corocoid process. The brachial fascia is incised to allow room for the muscle belly of latissimus dorsi to be passed down to the distal incision and it is necessary here to exercise great care to avoid kinking of the neurovascular pedicle.

Surgery for spasticity

It is sometimes possible to significantly improve function in those individuals seriously afflicted by serious flexion deformity of the hand and wrist and of the elbow by appropriate surgical measures, an expert rehabilitation programme being essential. Such individuals usually have a history of severe head injury, cerebral palsy or stroke.

It is, of course, mandatory to assess fully such individuals, particularly as to whether extensive surgery and prolonged rehabilitation could produce any significant reward in terms of function; this should include proper assessment of sensory modalities, including stereognosis.

With regard to elbow flexion deformity, it is best

improved by distal sliding of the common flexor musculature; the anterior capsule may also have to be surgically divided.

Severe flexion deformity of the fingers and wrist may be satisfactorily dealt with by transfer of the distally divided superficialis tendons at the wrist to the proximally divided deep flexor tendons. Z-lengthening of the long thumb and wrist flexors should also be performed and the digits brought into the straight position with the wrist at 15° of dorsiflexion. Of course, appropriate splinting and intensive rehabilitation is required.

Adduction deformity of the thumb in spastic conditions can sometimes be satisfactorily relieved by release of the adductor muscle from the middle finger metacarpal through a palmar incision.

Epicondylitis

Medial epicondylitis is sometimes called golfer's elbow: characteristically, there is tenderness at the common flexor origin and accentuation of painful disability by full passive extension of the elbow with the forearm supinated and the wrist dorsiflexed.

Usually, effective treatment is steroid and local anaesthetic injection which may be repeated on no more than two further occasions as there is a distinct risk of subcutaneous fat necrosis and dimpling of the skin as well as depigmentation, particularly so in black people. Alternative management is physiotherapy in the form of ultrasound, laser and interferential treatment. In those unusual cases refractory to such measures, surgical release of the common flexor origin at the medial epicondyle can be considered.

By far the more common condition is lateral epicondylitis, so-called tennis elbow, and here the lesion involves the proximal tendon of extensor carpi radialis brevis. Local tenderness laterally at the elbow is typical of the condition while painful disability is aggravated by passive extension of the elbow with the forearm fully pronated and the wrist palmar-flexed.

Resisted radial deviation and dorsiflexion of the wrist often similarly aggravates painful disability. Another test is to elicit lateral elbow pain by resisted dorsiflexion of the middle finger, no doubt explained by the distal tendonous insertion of extensor carpi radialis brevis into the middle finger metacarpal. This test is also positive in the unusual condition of posterior interosseous nerve compression at the supinator muscle which can sometimes mimic lateral epicondylitis, it is said, because of a cutaneous branch of this nerve radiating to the lateral aspect of the elbow.

There are other causes of lateral elbow pain apart from lateral epicondylitis and it is important to take appropriate X-ray films to eliminate the possibility of radiohumeral arthritis and the rare condition of soft-tissue ectopic calcification.

In the vast majority of cases, lateral epicondylitis is successfully treated by steroid and local anaesthetic injection, repeated on no more than two further occasions for recurrence. Physiotherapy treatment as for medial epicondylitis can sometimes be effective as well as immobilizing the limb in a sling, sometimes supplemented by a posterior splint with the elbow at right angles over a period of several weeks.

However, about 10% of individuals are unrelieved conservatively and here surgical treatment can be considered with several well-known operative procedures being available. Most popular is the modified Bosworth operation where the common extensor tendon is released and the proximal half of the annular ligament resected, since the lateral ligament of the elbow is connected to the common extensor origin as well as to this ligament (Fig. 24.56).

Percutaneous tenotomy of the common extensor tendon can also be performed while some prefer to curette the damaged area of tendon and to repair it into bone. Another procedure is to Z-lengthen the distal tendon of extensor carpi radialis brevis in order to reduce tension in this musculotendonous unit.

In the chronic case of lateral epicondylitis, an attractive alternative to surgery is to manipulate the elbow under general anaesthesia. Chronic painful disability appears to be associated with adhesion formation beneath the

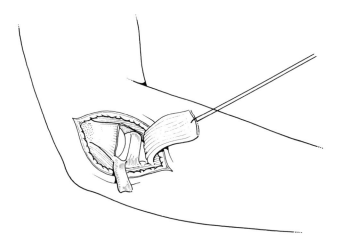

Fig. 24.56 The modified Bosworth lateral release procedure for chronic lateral epicondylitis: other surgical treatment options are percutaneous tenotomy of the common extensor tendon, repair of this tendon and elongation of the distal tendon of the extensor carpi radialis brevis.

damaged tendon and satisfactory break-down of these adhesions most often results in cure. Importantly, this technique is only usually effective under general anaesthesia: before the manipulation, steroid and local anaesthetic should be injected into the proximal tendon of extensor carpi radialis brevis at the lateral humeral epicondyle. The patient is supine on the operating table and the elbow is forcefully, but carefully, fully extended from the fully flexed position with the forearm in pronation and the wrist palmar-flexed. Typically, there is an audible snap and there is usually immediate relief of painful disability (Fig. 24.57).

In cases of resistant medial epicondylitis, manipulative treatment under general anaesthesia with the addition of steroid and local anaesthetic injection at the common flexor origin can also be considered. The elbow is forcefully and gently manipulated from being fully flexed into the extended position, with the forearm fully supinated and the wrist dorsiflexed (Fig. 24.58). The alternative treatment for the chronic case is tenotomy of the common flexor tendon at the medial humeral epicondyle, care being taken to avoid damage to the ulnar nerve, particularly when it is hypermobile.

In all cases of enthesopathy of the elbow, strain on the upper limb should be avoided, particularly in sports activities and provoking physical work, for at least 3 months and this applies to cases where surgery or manipulation has been performed for epicondylitis.

It is highly unusual in the author's experience to find posterior interosseous nerve compression causing lateral elbow pain. When present, it is usually associated with a well-formed arcade of Frohse. A sometimes helpful clinical sign is pain on resisted supination of the forearm, with the elbow held in extension thus eliminating the biceps action. Surgical release is easily performed through an anterior incision with a section of the fibrous arcade being resected.

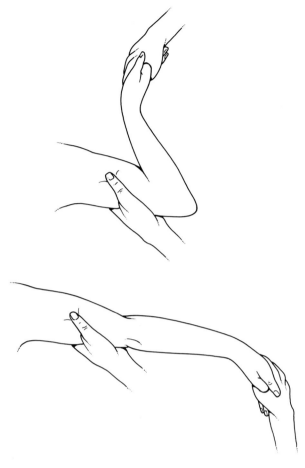

Fig. 24.58 Chronic medial epicondylitis may be treated by manipulation under general anaesthesia and injection of steroid and local anaesthetic.

Habitual dislocation of the elbow

This unusual condition typically commences in childhood and adolescence and it seems that failure of the postero-lateral capsular and ligamentous structures to heal in reasonable position after trauma is a probable cause in

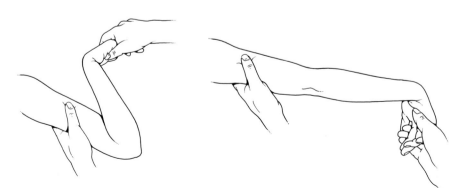

Fig. 24.57 An attractive and most often successful method of treatment for chronic lateral epicondylitis is manipulation under general anaesthesia. At the same time, steroid and local anaesthetic is injected into the common extensor tendon to minimize build-up of further adhesions. Strain on the hand and upper limb should subsequently be avoided for three months.

most while there may be congenital laxity of the capsule in others.

The several operative procedures available are as follows: bone grafting to improve the coronoid process; translocation of the detached biceps tendon into a constructed hole in the ulna; anterior translocation of a strip of triceps aponeurosis and similarly a length of biceps tendon posteriorly, both through a hole constructed in the olecranon fossa; another procedure is to re-attach the damaged posterolateral capsule and lateral ligament to roughened bone laterally at the lower humerus.

The abnormal carrying angle

Normally there is a valgus angle that is symmetrical and on average greater in the female than the male after puberty. Some individuals normally exhibit cubitus rectus, with no angle. Mention has been made of the pathological alteration of the shape of the elbow with sex-chromosome anomalies, usually not requiring surgical correction (Fig. 24.12).

Supracondylar fracture in childhood can typically cause varus, or gunstock, deformity and in these cases there is also rotational deformity of the lower humerus. This deformity can sometimes produce awkward disability of the upper limb and corrective osteotomy should be considered at skeletal maturity if the deformity is 20° or more.

It is easiest to perform a lateral wedge osteotomy (Lloyd-Roberts 1978), either through a lateral or posterior surgical approach, but leaving the inner cortex of the humerus intact. The osteotomy can be secured either with two screws placed laterally and brought together with a wire or else with an appropriate plate and screws. Another method is to construct a lateral proximal flange of humerus and to insert this into the distal fragment; security is obtained by a screw transgressing this tongue and proceeding from the lateral to medial cortex.

Moderate valgus deformity may be a long-term consequence of radial head fractures, particularly where the radial head has been resected. More significant valgus can occur after the common injury of lateral condylar fracture in childhood: this can occur because of malunion, premature epiphysial fusion or non-union. Essentially there is deficiency or absence of the lateral lip of the trochlea, allowing the ulna to migrate laterally (Fig. 24.59).

The important consequence is approximation of the arcuate ligament of the cubital tunnel to the floor with risk of compression neuropathy of the ulnar nerve. Unlike cubitus varus, the altered shape of the elbow in

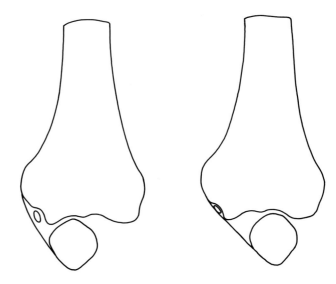

Fig. 24.59 Childhood lateral condylar fracture can lead to deficiency of the lateral lip of the trochlea: the ulna slides laterally, producing cubitus valgus, and the roof of the cubital tunnel consequently approaches the floor. There is long-term risk of compression ulnar neuropathy.

the form of cubitus valgus does not in itself usually produce important functional disability and corrective osteotomy is rarely indicated. It should be pointed out that such surgical correction could not influence the altered state of affairs within the cubital tunnel.

Surgical arthrolysis of the post-traumatic stiff elbow

Significant flexion deformity and stiffness of the elbow can result in considerable functional disability in use of the hand and upper limb. Such loss of motion typically is a result of intra-articular fracture, particularly of the lower humerus. However, injudicious and lengthy immobilization in a cast for simple injuries such as undisplaced radial head fracture can also result in this important disability.

In some cases, bony incongruity is a major factor and in all there is considerable thickening of the anterior capsule in particular as well as adhesion formation.

While an active exercise programme can sometimes be effective in gaining elbow movement, intermittent passive stretching by a therapist is most often counter-productive with eventual deterioration of elbow movement.

Surgical arthrolysis can often produce a pleasing result, but no guarantee can be given and it is important to establish with the patient that there is a small risk of damage to important neurovascular structures around the elbow which could result in sensory deficit, wasting and weakness in the hand.

Probably the best overall surgical approach is lateral and this can be supplemented by a medial incision, especially where there is particular concern over the ulnar nerve (Fig. 24.60). Surgery is best performed under general anaesthesia and a pneumatic tourniquet placed high on the arm. A straight lateral incision gives adequate access to both the anterior and posterior aspects of the elbow.

It is important to firstly identify the anterior capsule and to carefully separate this from the overlying brachialis muscle and to put a dissector in place for further surgery. Adhesions within the joint anteriorly and beneath the capsule are appropriately divided and the capsule elevated from the humerus. The anterior capsule is carefully partially resected. Any adhesion formation posteriorly at the elbow can also be dealt with through this approach.

Bony incongruity causing limited motion should be resected and the bleeding bed sealed with Horsley's bone wax. Where restriction of forearm rotation is also a feature of the case, adhesions can be dealt with at the proximal radio-ulnar joint and if there is considerable disabling bony deformity of the radial head this can be resected and consideration given to its replacement with a silastic or titanium prosthesis.

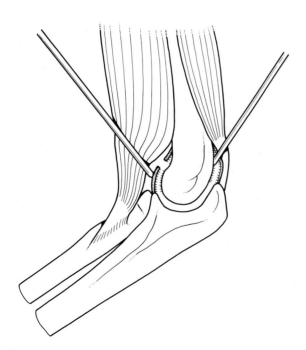

Fig. 24.60 The lateral surgical approach for post-traumatic stiffness: both the anterior and posterior aspects of the elbow are easily reached.

Rehabilitation is, of course, crucial to obtain the best result: at this time, continuous passive motion is favoured, certainly for the case where extensive surgery has been required for removal of bone as well as soft-tissue release.

The continuous passive motion machine is used day and night, and appropriate medication is administered when necessary, over a period of at least 2 weeks: thereafter, an active exercise programme for the elbow and forearm should be maintained with the help of physiotherapy supervision and intermittent use of an anterior splint in maximum extension of the elbow, sometimes also a flexion splint.

Elbow stiffness may be associated with ectopic bone within the brachialis muscle: this can result from even minor trauma while stretch injury of the brachialis from overvigorous physiotherapy by passive exercising could be a significant factor in some and it can also be seen after head injury. Growth of the lesion is progressive and usually ceases after 6 months.

It is best to operate in these cases in the area of myositis ossificans when this is mature, assessment being made by radio-isotope scanning and the radiographic appearance. In this type of lesion, the best surgical approach is anterior, either that of Henry or Fiolle and Delmas, but a lateral approach can also be used.

Arthritis of the elbow and proximal radio-ulnar joints

The majority of patients presenting with arthritis are suffering from rheumatoid disease: osteoarthritis is less frequently seen and is either secondary to intra-articular skeletal damage with other cases being of unknown aetiology. Other causes of arthritis are distinctly uncommon at this joint.

Unfortunately, moderate to severe rheumatoid disease of the elbow is often accompanied by similar changes at the glenohumeral articulation of the shoulder. Restriction of shoulder movement, particularly of rotation, results in further force being applied to the elbow in activities of daily living, this no doubt, at least in part, being responsible for loosening of constrained elbow prostheses within bone.

Of course, in the severe rheumatoid case, there are inevitably important questions as to priority of treatment of the hand, wrist, elbow and shoulder. It is certainly the case that, somewhat more frequently nowadays, shoulder and elbow prostheses are being inserted in the ipsilateral limb in order to improve overall function. With arthritis of the hips and knees requiring crutch-walking, it is best to reserve reconstructive procedures on the hand and upper limb until appropriate lower limb treatment is accomplished and there is improved walking ability when crutches can be discarded.

Treatment options for the severely disabling case of rheumatoid elbow arthritis include the following: synovectomy, sometimes combined with radial head resection; resectional arthroplasty, with or without an interpositional material; and total prosthetic replacement of the elbow joint, such prostheses being non-, semi- or unconstrained in type (Fig. 24.61). Arthrodesis is a rarely chosen procedure.

In actual fact, the opportunity rarely arises for synovectomy that is entirely suitable for the elbow where the articular surfaces are more or less intact, the procedure being performed prophylactically to attempt to guard against deterioration of the joint.

Interestingly, cases are seen where the disease is most evident laterally with accompanying erosion of the radial head and it is here that synovectomy combined with radial head resection is sometimes useful. Synovectomy usually has to be performed through at least two surgical incisions.

Replacement of the radial head can be considered, either by a silastic or metallic prosthesis, in order to avoid valgus deformity and shortening of the radius. The former resulting in risk of compression neuropathy of the ulnar nerve within the cubital tunnel and the latter possibly leading to symptomatic instability at the inferior radio-ulnar articulation.

Total prosthetic replacement has to be considered in the case of moderate to severe rheumatoid change in the elbow causing unacceptable painful disability in particular. However, there has been something of a 'graveyard' of prostheses over the years and, even now, such surgery is not entirely out of the province of clinical trial.

It is best to restrict the amount of bone resected and to preserve capsuloligamentous structures as far as possible. It is well known that fully constrained prostheses have in the past had an unacceptably high failure rate, which has been due to the amount of bone resected as well as additional forces on the elbow joint from accompanying shoulder disability.

Unfortunately, it has not been uncommon to find a windscreen wiper effect with the tip of the stem of the prosthesis eroding through cortical bone, usually of the ulna, and considerable disability has led to removal of the prosthesis and grave risk of a flail upper limb. On occasion, this can be reduced by a bone graft set in between the lower humeral pillars with resection arthroplasty being the salvage procedure.

Semiconstrained prostheses have been designed to allow a certain amount of global mobility at the elbow while guarding against subluxation of the prosthetic

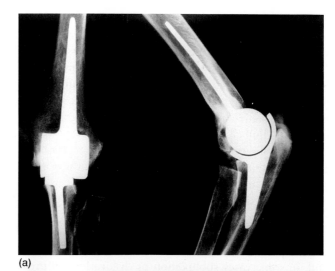

(a)

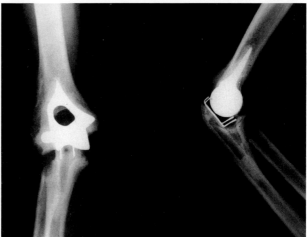

(b)

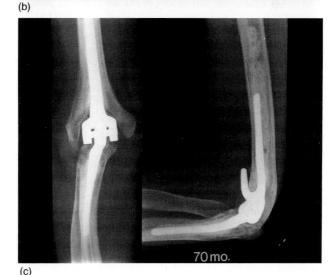

(c)

Fig. 24.61 The Wadsworth 2 elbow prosthesis (a) is unconstrained, the articular surfaces being simple concavo-convex in contrast to the Souter prosthesis where there is an anatomical articular surface (b). The Coonrad–Morrey prosthesis is semiconstrained and is particularly suitable for certain cases of revision surgery (c).

articular surfaces: however, in effect some of these prostheses have acted as fully constrained prostheses with the risks already mentioned.

It is thought by many that an unconstrained prosthesis is best, but there have been design problems, such prostheses having a more or less anatomical configuration or a simple concavoconvex articulating surface linking the humeral and ulnar components. Here, there is the possibility of minimal bone resection, but the components need to be set in bone in such a way that there is not undue laxity and, likewise, the capsulo-ligamentous structures should be preserved as far as possible.

Unfortunately, failure even with this type of prosthesis can be spectacular, e.g. after infection and/or loosening and, in some cases subluxation or dislocation, so providing a distinct challenge for further reconstruction of the joint.

It must be said that the indication for prosthetic replacement of the elbow joint is severe painful disability causing unacceptable loss of use of the upper limb, restriction of motion being very much a secondary consideration.

The situation may be so difficult after failed elbow prosthetic surgery that arthrodesis of the joint has to be considered. Unfortunately, there is simply no 'good' position for the stiff elbow for all activities of daily living and a very severe compromise has to be accepted, in these circumstances, by the patient—the best position perhaps being that of 90° of flexion.

In other cases, the last resort is for an external brace, preferably made of plastic, and this needs to extend high up into the arm and into the forearm and even then can be a difficult contraption for the patient to cope with.

Osteoarthritis of the elbow is typically not only accompanied by stiffness but episodes of locking because of the frequent presence of loose bodies. If the latter is a particular problem, these objects can be removed, often with good result, either by arthrotomy or by arthroscopic measures.

In the well-chosen case, the procedure of lower humeral fenestration arthroplasty in the manner of Outerbridge and Kashiwagi can give an excellent result (Fig. 24.62). A window is constructed, through a posterior triceps-splitting incision, in the lower humerus; osteophytes can be resected and loose bodies can even be removed from the front of the joint through the constructed aperture. There is the opportunity for greater motion in extension with the tip of the olecranon proceeding into the opening in the lower humerus.

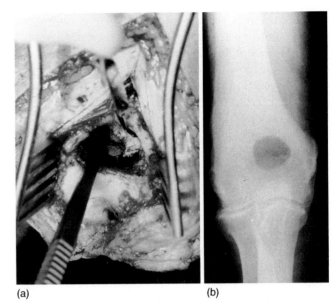

(a)   (b)

Fig. 24.62 (a, b) Lower humeral fenestration arthroplasty. This can be a useful procedure in the well-chosen case of osteoarthritis of the elbow; loose bodies may be removed through the constructed aperture.

Arthrodesis of the elbow

This should be a last-resort procedure in as much that there is no particular position of arthrodesis that allows for other than limited use of the upper limb.

Most often, this unusual procedure is performed after failed prosthetic replacement of the elbow and when there has been considerable bone loss from trauma.

Several methods of arthrodesis are available, a bone graft usually being taken from the iliac crest of the pelvis. Angled plate and screw fixation of the humerus and ulna is typically performed. The usual position for arthrodesis is at the right angle, forearm rotation being preserved whenever possible.

Congenital anomalies

These encompass difficult and sometimes untreatable conditions, mainly dealt with in Chapter 8.1.

The bony septum between the olecranon and coronoid fossae is occasionally absent when a supracondylar foramen is said to be present.

A supracondylar process is rarely present, extending from the anterior aspect of the lower humeral shaft from which the ligament of Struthers proceeds to be inserted into the medial humeral epicondyle. The arch so-formed contains the brachial artery and the median nerve while the ulnar nerve courses around the base of the abnormal bone.

The stage is set for possible development of the supra-condylar process syndrome with compression neuropathy of the median nerve which may result in considerable neurological deficit, a negative Phalen test and involvement of the pronator teres, the latter differentiating this particular syndrome from the case of compression of the median nerve within this muscle.

Other congenital anomalies of the elbow, sometimes causing diagnostic confusion, are antecubital, para-trochlear and accessory coronoid bones and the patella cubiti.

Variation in the elbow carrying angle can be indicators of congenital and developmental abnormalities.

Baughman *et al.* (1973) first reported that those chromosome anomalies that decrease vertical height tend to increase the carrying angle, while those increasing vertical height decrease or invert the carrying angle. There is a spectrum of elbow abnormalities with maximal cubitus valgus in XO phenotype, decreasing valgus in XX and XY while one X or Y supernumerary cases tend to produce a varus carrying angle accompanied by radio-ulnar synostosis and radial head dislocation in the presence of multiple supernumerary sex chromosomes. A well-known example of cubitus valgus is Turner's syndrome, 45XO phenotype.

Congenital proximal radioulnar synostosis is unusually seen and is a random developmental defect, the radius and ulna usually being normal in length: this may be incidentally found and also in other congenital deficiency of the upper limb, e.g. upper limb partial hemimelia and in acheira and adactylia.

In a bilateral case, said to be present in 60%, it can sometimes be useful to position the forearm of the non-dominant upper limb into supination with the palm upward so that the individual has adequate bipalmar prehension in activities of daily living, this particularly so where both forearms are locked in the position of pronation; it should be mentioned that rotatory wrist motion can usefully compensate for lack of proper forearm rotation, especially in youngsters.

Congenital dislocation of the radial head is rarely seen and may be positioned anteriorly, posterior or laterally, this condition being usually relatively asymptomatic except to say that there may be modest restriction of flexion and extension at the elbow and also of forearm rotation. Radial head displacement can also occur as a result of unrecognized trauma, accompanied by fracture of the ulnar. It is unusual for surgery to be required for congenital dislocation of the radial head.

Radial club hand is associated with longitudinal absence of the radius, often associated with other anomalies, most cases being bilateral; additionally, the thumb is typically rudimentary and there may be extension deformity of the elbow as well as impairment of index finger and middle finger function.

In cleft hand deformity the deficiency can simply be soft tissue in nature between the middle and ring fingers while there may be absence of the middle ray and a combination of syndactyly of the remaining digits.

Apert's and Poland's syndromes include the non-hereditary form of symphalangism, i.e. stiffness of the digital joints, especially of the proximal interphalangeal articulation of the finger, as well as syndactyly. The hereditary form of symphalangism is a dominant trait. In appropriate cases, the only treatment to consider is arthrodesis of the proximal interphalangeal joint at the best angle for function.

Syndactyly can be total with the involved digits entirely united together or incomplete. On the other hand, the condition can be complex and there is bony union of the digits together. The distal segments of the involved digits are fused with proximal fenestration between them in the very unusual condition of acrosyndactyly. With syndactyly, separation of the digits can be performed between 6 and 12 months of age, urgency depending upon discrepancy of length.

Polydactyly most often involves the radial aspect of the hand: there may be no skeletal structure present, normal phalanges may be articulated with a bifid metacarpal, or the extra digit simply contains a metacarpal bone. Where the phalanges articulate with the bifid metacarpal, there is typically associated syndactyly. On the other hand, with an extra thumb, there may be an additional skeletal unit. In many cases, the supernumerary digit is readily resected, the situation, of course, being more difficult in the more complicated case.

Camptodactyly is a commonly seen flexion deformity, typically of the little finger and occurring at the proximal interphalangeal joint. This deformity involves all the tissues of the digit but without important functional deficit, surgical management being seldom if ever indicated.

Clinodactyly is an angular deformity of the digit located at the middle phalanx with appropriate deformity at the articular surface of the involved interphalangeal joint. There is severe skeletal deformity in delta phalanx which also produces angular deformity. In these cases, it is sometimes possible to form an open-wedge osteotomy with bone grafting in order to lengthen and correct the shape of the digit, but it must be said that the result is not always entirely satisfactory.

Congenital triggering of the thumb, affecting the interphalangeal joint often remains unrecognized until some months after birth, passive extension typically being accomplished with a click, but in other cases the digit is locked in flexion. Surgical release should be performed at 12 months of age, certainly no longer than 4 years old, 30% of cases spontaneously resolving within the first 12 months after birth.

Clasp thumb exhibits flexion deformity of the metacarpophalangeal and interphalangeal joints. Many of these cases resolve with the thumb being splinted in extension for 3–6 months while others go on to require tendon transfer for the deficient extensor tendon mechanism in the more severe case as well as release of the flexion contracture.

Constriction rings of the digits are typically non-hereditary and can be simple or complicated by distal deformity or joint fusion. Spontaneous amputation is sometimes an inevitable result and early surgical release is required, e.g. by Z-plasty.

Hypoplasia of the thumb ranges from a minor disorder to the floating thumb which is vestigial and attached proximally to the metacarpophalangeal joint area of the index finger.

Hereditary stiffness of the digital joints is more common on the ulnar side of the hand, typically with shortening of the middle phalanx, and there is little that can be effectively done to improve function apart from maintaining available function by appropriate use of the hand.

Digital overgrowth is a non-hereditary condition and is termed macrodactyly, most often unilateral. The condition may be static and seen at birth, with enlargement keeping pace with normal growth. However, the progressive type is not typically apparent until 2 years of age and is more aggressive in nature, growth being accelerated compared with the normal digits. There may be associated digital tip ulceration due to neuro-vascular impairment and it is important in these cases to eliminate the additional problem of a haemangioma.

Such conditions can be very difficult to treat surgically, with reduction often resulting in a poor result; furthermore, osteotomy may have to be considered in order to correct length and shape of the involved digit.

The question of surgery in adults presenting with congenital anomalies should be carefully weighed: it must be said that many such individuals manage reasonably well in activities of daily living and have accommodated satisfactorily to their long-standing deficit with regard to normal function. Most of these individuals are best left alone, e.g. syndactyly of all four fingers with an intact thumb is an instance where an individual may cope adequately during a lengthy lifespan (Fig. 24.63).

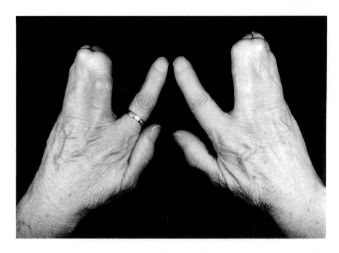

Fig. 24.63 Example of useful function of both hands with severe syndactyly.

Tumours

An enchondroma in the phalanx or metacarpal may require curettage and bone-grafting to give stability to the bone in order to avoid the possibility of pathological fracture.

While the dyschondroplastic lesions of Ollier's disease appear to be rather unsightly, it is unusual for them to undergo malignant change in the hand but this is more likely in the similar skeletal lesion in Maffucci's syndrome, associated with multiple haemangiomata. Resection of the lesion, sometimes digital amputation, is required, particularly so with suspicion of malignant change.

Malignant tumours, including skeletal metastases, are indeed rare at the hand and wrist. When seen in the hand, osteo- and chondrosarcomas can be surgically treated by amputation of the involved finger or the whole of the appropriate digital ray when the metacarpal is the site of the lesion (Fig. 24.64). Appropriate chemotherapy should be given for an osteosarcoma.

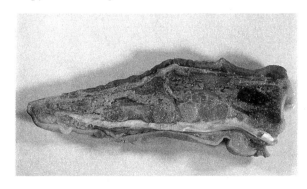

Fig. 24.64 An example of a low-grade chondrosarcoma of the right index finger in a young male adult, treated by amputation through the distal metacarpal shaft.

Malignant primary skeletal lesions proximal to the hand most often require amputation of the limb, although on occasion surgical resection may be accomplished.

FURTHER READING

Ashbell G.R. and Lipscomb P.R. (1967) The changing treatment of Volkmann's ischaemic contracture from 1955 to 1965 at the Mayo Clinic. *Clin. Orhop.* **50**, 215–223.

Barton N.J., Hooper G., Noble J. and Steel W.M. (1992) Occupational causes of disorders in the upper limb. *Br. Med. J.* **304**, 309–311.

Baughman F.A. Jr, Wadsworth T.G., Demaray M.J. and Higgins J.V. (1973) The carrying angle in sex chromosome anomalies. *Fourth International Conference on Birth Defects*. Vienna, Austria.

Baughman F.A. Jr, Higgins J.V., Wadsworth T.G. and Demaray M.J. (1974) The carrying angle in sex chromosome anomalies. *J. Am. Med. Assoc.* **230**, 718–720.

Bell D.S. (1989) 'Repetition strain injury': an iatrogenic epidemic of simulated injury. *Med. J. Aust.* **151**, 280–284.

Bogumill G.P. and Fleegler E.J. (1993) *Tumors of the Hand and Upper Limb*. Edinburgh, Churchill Livingstone.

Boyd H.B. (1940) Surgical exposure of the ulna and proximal third of the radius through one incision. *Surg. Gynaecol. Obstet.* **71**, 86–88.

Braun R.M., Vise G.T. and Roper B. (1974) Superficialis to profundus tendon transfer. *J. Bone Joint Surg.* **56A**, 466–472.

Browne C.D., Nolan B.M. and Faithfull D.K. (1984) Occupational repetition strain injuries. Guidelines for diagnosis and management. *Med. J. Aust.* **140**, 329–332.

Buckle P. (1987) Musculoskeletal disorders of the upper extremities: The use of epidemiologic approaches in industrial settings. *J. Hand Surg.* **12A**, 885–889.

Bunnell S. (1953) Ischaemic contracture in the hand. *J. Bone Joint Surg.* **35A**, 88–101.

Burton A.C. (1951) On the physical equilibrium of small blood vessels. *Am. J. Physiol.* **164**, 319–329.

Campbell W.C. (1932) Incision for exposure of the elbow joint. *Am. J. Surg.* **15**, 65–67.

Campbell Semple J. (1991) Tenosynovitis, repetitive strain injury, cumulative trauma disorder, and overuse syndrome, et cetera. *J. Bone Joint Surg.* **73B**, 536–538.

Cassebaum W.H. (1952) Operative treatment of T and Y fractures of the lower end of the humerus. *Am. J. Surg.* **83**, 265–270.

Chigot P.-L. (1974) Foreword. In Hueston J.T. and Tubiana R. (eds) *Dupuytren's Disease*. Edinburgh, Churchill Livingstone.

Cohen M.L., Arroyo J.F., Champion G.D. and Browne C.D. (1992) In search of the pathogenesis of refractory cervicobrachial pain syndrome. *Med. J. Aust.* **156**, 432–436.

Eaton R.G. and Green W.T. (1975) Volkmann's ischaemia. A volar compartment syndrome of the forearm. *Clin. Orthop.* **113**, 58–64.

Evans D.M. (1992) *Skin Cover in the Injured Hand*. Edinburgh, Churchill Livingstone.

Ferguson D.A. (1987) 'RSI': putting the epidemic to rest. *Med. J. Aust.* **147**, 213–214.

Finkelstein H. (1930) Stenosing tenovaginitis at the radial styloid process. *J. Bone Joint Surg.* **12**, 509–540.

Fitton J.M., Shea F.W. and Goldie W. (1968) Lesions of the flexor carpi radialis tendon and sheath causing pain at the wrist. *J. Bone Joint Surg.* **50B**, 359–363.

Fisk G.R. (1970) Carpal instability and the fractured scaphoid. *Ann. Roy Coll. Surg. Eng.* **46**, 63–76.

French P.R. (1959) Varus deformity of the elbow following supracondylar fractures of the humerus in children. *Lancet* ii, 439–441.

Fry H.J.H. (1986) Overuse syndrome of the upper limb in musicians. *Med. J. Aust.* **144**, 182–185.

Green D.P. (1988) *Operative Hand Surgery*, 2nd edn. Edinburgh, Churchill Livingstone.

Hadler N.M. (1992) Arm pain in the workplace. A small area analysis. *J. Occup. Med.* **34**, 113–119.

Harrison J. (1993) Hand transmitted vibration. *Br. Med. J.* **307**, 79–80.

Henry A.K. (1973) *Extensile Exposure*, 2nd edn. Edinburgh, Churchill Livingstone.

Holden C.E.A. (1979) The pathology and prevention of Volkmann's ischaemic contracture. *J. Bone Joint Surg.* **61B**, 296–300.

Hooper G. (1990) *Colour Atlas of Hand Disorders*. Edinburgh, Churchill Livingstone.

Horwich M. and Wadsworth T.G. (1955) Post traumatic inoculation tuberculosis. *Br. Med. J.* **2**, 1060–1062.

Hueston J.T. (1961) Limited fasciectomy for Dupuytren's contracture. *Plast. Reconstr. Surg.* **27**, 569–585.

Hueston J.T. (1963) *Dupuytren's Contracture*. Edinburgh, E. and S. Livingstone.

Hueston J.T. (1969) The control of recurrent Dupuytren's contracture by skin replacement. *Br. J. Plast. Surg.* **22**, 152–156.

Hunter J.M. and Salisbury R.E. (1971) Flexor-tendon reconstruction in severely damaged hands. *J. Bone Joint Surg.* **53A**, 829–858.

Hunter J.M., Mackin E.J. and Callahan A.D. (1995) *Rehabilitation of the Hand: Surgery and Therapy*, 4th edn. St. Louis, C.V. Mosby.

Huskisson E.C. (1992) *Repetitive Strain Injury*. London, Charterhouse Conference and Communications Ltd.

Hutchinson J. (1857) Melanotic disease of the great toe, following a whitlow of the nail. *Trans. Path. Soc. Lond.* **8**, 404.

Kasdan M.L., Amadio P.C. and Bowers W.H. (1994) *Technical Tips for Hand Surgery*. Philadelphia, Hanley & Belfus, Inc.

Kashiwagi D. (1985) *Elbow Joint, Proceedings of the International Seminar, Kobe*, Japan. Amsterdam, Elsevier Science.

Lister G. (1993) *The Hand*, 3rd edn. Edinburgh, Churchill Livingstone.

Lloyd-Roberts G.C. (1978) A technique of supracondylar osteotomy to correct cubitus varus. Personal communication.

Mattson R.H., Cramer J.A., McCutchen C.B. and the Veterans Administrations Epilepsy Co-operative Study Group (1989) Barbiturate-related connective tissue disorders. *Arch. Intern. Med.* **149**, 911–914.

McAuliffe J.A., Burkhalter W.E., Ouellette E.A. and Carneiro R.S. (1992) Compression plate arthrodesis of the elbow. *J. Bone Joint Surg.* **74B**, 300–304.

McFarlane R.M., McGrouther D.A. and Flint M.H. (1990) *Dupuytren's Disease*. Edinburgh, Churchill Livingstone.

Mekosha H. and Jakubowicz A. (1991) Repetition strain injury: The rise and fall of an 'Australian' disease. *Crit. Social Pol.* **11**, 18–37.

Milch H. (1936) Bilateral recurrent dislocation of the ulna at the elbow. *J. Bone Joint Surg.* **18**, 777–780.

Milford L. (1987) The hand. In Crenshaw A.H. (ed.) *Campbell's Operative Orthopaedics*, 7th edn. St Louis, C.V. Mosby.

Mital, M.A. (1979) Lengthening of the elbow flexors in cerebral palsy. *J. Bone Joint Surg.* **61A**, 515–522.

Molesworth W.H.L. (1930) Operation for complete exposure of the elbow joint. *Br. J. Surg.* **18**, 303–307.

Morrey B.F. (1993) *The Elbow and its Disorders*, 2nd edn. Philadelphia, W.B. Saunders.

Mouchet A. (1898) *These de Docteur*, Paris.

O'Neill O.R., Morrey B.F., Tanaka S. and An K.-N. (1992) Compensatory Motion in the Upper Extremity after Elbow Arthrodesis. *Clin. Orthop.* **281**, 89–96.

Osborne G.V. and Cotterill P. (1966) Recurrent dislocation of the elbow. *J. Bone Joint Surg.* **48B**, 340–346.

Panas J. (1878) Sur une cause peu connue de paralysie due nerf cunital. *Arch. Gen. Med.* (Paris) **2**, 5–22.

Phalen G.F. (1966) Carpal tunnel syndrome 17 years experience in diagnosis and treatment of 654 hands. *J. Bone Joint Surg.* **48A**, 211–228.

Quintner J. (1991) The RSI syndrome in historical perspective. *Int. Disabil. Stud.* **13**, 99–104.

Rayan G.M. (1983) Recurrent dislocation of the extensor carpi ulnaris in athletes. *Am. J. Sports Med.* **11**, 183–184.

Razeman J.P. and Fisk G.R. (1988) *The Wrist*. Edinburgh, Churchill Livingstone.

Reichenheim P.P. (1947) Transplantation of the biceps tendon as a treatment for recurrent dislocation of the elbow. *Br. J. Surg.* **35**, 201–204.

Roles N.C. and Maudsley R.H. (1972) Radial tunnel syndrome. *J. Bone Joint Surg.* **54B**, 499–508.

Skoog T. (1948) Dupuytren's contracture. *Acta Chirug. Scand.* **96** (Suppl), 139.

Sledge C.B. and Weissmann B.N. (1986) *Orthopaedic Radiology*. Philadelphia, W.B. Saunders.

Spence S.H. (1989) Cognitive-behaviour therapy in the management of chronic occupational pain of the upper limbs. *Behav. Res. Ther.* **27**, 435–446.

Spinner M. and Kaplan E.B. (1970) Extensor Carpi ulnaris. Its relationship to stability of the distal radio-ulnar joint. *Clin. Orthop.* **68**, 124–129.

Struthers J. (1849) On a peculiarity of the humerus and humeral artery. *Mon. J. Med. Sci.* **9**, 264–267.

Swanson A.B. (1973) *Flexible implant resection arthroplasty in the hand and extremities*. St Louis, C.V. Mosby.

Swanson A.B., Goran-Hagert C. and Swanson G. de Groot (1987) Evaluation of impairment in the upper extremity. *J. Hand Surg.* **12A**, 896–926.

Symeonides P.P. (1972) The humerus supracondylar process syndrome. *Clin. Orthop.* **82**, 141–143.

Taleisnik J. (1980) Post-traumatic carpal instability. *Clin. Orthop.* **149**, 73–82.

Taleisnik J. (1985) *The Wrist*. Edinburgh, Churchill Livingstone.

Van Gorder G.W. (1940) Surgical approach in supracondylar 'T' fractures of the humerus requiring open reduction. *J. Bone Joint Surg.* **22**, 278–298.

Verdan C. (1960) Primary repair of the flexor tendons. *J. Bone Joint Surg.* **42A**, 647–657.

Wadsworth T.G. (1964) Premature epiphysial fusion after injury of the capitulum. *J. Bone Joint Surg.* **46B**, 46–49.

Wadsworth T.G. (1972) Injuries of the capitular (lateral humeral condylar) epiphysis. *Clin. Orthop.* **85**, 127–142.

Wadsworth T.G. (1977) The external compression syndrome of the ulnar nerve at the cubital tunnel. *Clin. Orthop.* **124**, 189.

Wadsworth T.G. (1979) A modified postero-lateral approach to the elbow and proximal radio-ulnar joints. *Clin. Orthop.* **144**, 151–153.

Wadsworth T.G. (1982; Spanish edn. 1986) *The Elbow*. Edinburgh, Churchill Livingstone.

Wadsworth T.G. (1986) Extensor carpi radialis longus transfer for rupture of the extensor pollicis longus tendon. In Boswick J.A., Jr (ed.) *Advances in Upper Extremity Surgery and Rehabilitation*. Rockville, Maryland, Aspen.

Wadsworth T.G. (1987) Tennis elbow: conservative, surgical and manipulative treatment. *Br. Med. J.* **294**, 621–624.

Wadsworth T.G. (1990) The elbow. In Foy M.A. and Fagg P.S. (eds) *Medicolegal Reporting in Orthopaedic Trauma*. Edinburgh, Churchill Livingstone.

Wadsworth T.G. (1990) Colles' fracture. *Br. Med. J.* **301**, 192–194.

Wadsworth T.G., Broome G.H.H. and Tustin J.E. (1992) Surgical arthrolysis of the post-traumatic stiff elbow. Orthopaedic proceedings. *J. Bone Joint Surg.* **74B**, 150–151.

Wadsworth T.G. (1993) Prosthetic replacement of the arthritic elbow. *Curr. Opin. Rheumatol.* **5**, 322–328.

Whipple T.L. (1992) *Arthroscopic Surgery of the Wrist* Philadelphia, J.B. Lippincott.

Zancolli E.A. (1957) Clawhand caused by paralysis of the intrinsic muscles, a simple surgical procedure for its correction. *J. Bone Joint Surg.* **39A**, 1076–1080.

Zancolli E.A. and Mitri H. (1973) Latissimus dorsi transfer to restore elbow flexion. *J. Bone Joint Surg.* **55A**, 1265–1275.

Zancolli E.A. (1979) *Structural and Dynamic Bases of Hand Surgery*, 2nd edn. Philadelphia, J.B. Lippincott.

Chapter 25
The Knee

W.N. Scott, M.S. McMahon, S.M. Craig & J.N. Insall

SURGICAL ANATOMY

The knee, exposed to forces in excess of five times body weight per step, consists of three articulations: (i) the patellofemoral; (ii) the tibiofemoral; and (iii) the tibiofibular (Kettelkamp and Jacobs, 1972). The basic characteristics of the human knee can be traced back almost 300 million yaers (Heller and Langman, 1964). The knee of Erypos, the common ancestor of all living reptiles, birds and mammals, had a bicondylar femur articulating with a relatively flat tibia and a rudimentary femoral fibular articulation (Drachman and Sokoloff, 1966; Dye, 1987; Ferkel *et al.*, 1989). Embryologically, the knee joint arises from the blastemal interzone.

The blood supply to the skin around the knee is random, sustained by both an intrinsic and extrinsic source. The intrinsic contributors to the blood supply of skin overlying the knee are the perforating branches of the superior and inferior genicular systems. The extrinsic blood supply originates from three sources: (i) the descending genicular branch of the superficial femoral artery; (ii) the recurrent branch of the anterior tibial artery; and (iii) the descending branch of the lateral femoral circumflex artery.

The blood supply of the skin overlying the knee is such that a transverse incision combined with a straight midline longitudinal incision is the most favourable combination of incisions. As the incisions approach parallel, their bases and consequently the origin of their blood supplies become increasingly narrower, jeopardizing the points of intersection of combined incisions. Parallel incisions depend for their blood supply on vessels coming from the superior and inferior intact segments of skin. The survival of skin under these circumstances is unpredictable and is dependent on the width of the superior and inferior pedicles (Craig, 1987) (Fig. 25.1).

Bony anatomy

The femur, the tibia and the patella are the three bones that define the knee joint. The articulation is described in terms of three distinct compartments: (i) medial; (ii) lateral; and (iii) patellofemoral. The significant extra-articular landmarks about the knee are: (i) Gerdy's tubercle, which corresponds to the insertion of the iliotibial band and is located 1–2 cm lateral to the tibial tubercle; (ii) the proximal tibiofibular joint, located in the posterolateral aspect of the tibia; and (iii) the adductor tubercle, which is just proximal to the medial epicondyle.

Imbedded within the quadriceps tendon, the patella is the largest sesamoid bone in the body. It is triangular at its superficial surface and more oval appearing on its articulating surface. The widened proximal portion tapers inferiorly at the origin of the patellar ligament (tendon). The blood supply originates from as many as

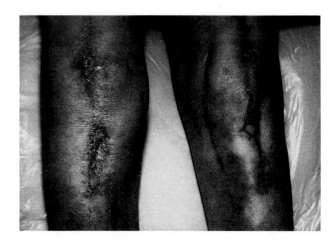

Fig. 25.1 The lateral or medial parapatellar incision, even when very long can safely coexist with the midline approach to the knee joint. (Reproduced by permission from Scott, 1987.)

12 nutrient arteries at the inferior pole and which run upwards on the anterior surface in a series of furrows (Scapinelli, 1968; Insall, 1984a). The articular surface of the patella is divided into seven facets (Insall, 1984). The medial and lateral facets are divided into equal thirds, superiorly and inferiorly, with the seventh facet being the most medial portion called the 'odd facet'. Wiberg (1941) and Warren and Marshall (1979) identified three shapes based on the position of the vertical ridge.

The patellofemoral joint is the most incongruous joint in the body and it is this lack of conformity which contributes to many of the problems noted in patellar tracking. Maximum patellofemoral contact occurs at 45° (Aglietti *et al.*, 1975; Goodfellow *et al.*, 1976). In full extension, the lower-most portion of the patella is in contact, and it progresses proximally as the knee is flexed.

The term 'sulcus' or 'trochlear groove' refers to the anterior distal surface of the femur that articulates with the patella. The lateral condyle has a greater anterior–posterior length and medial–lateral width than the medial condyle. The origins of both cruciate ligaments, ligamentum mucosum and ligaments of Humphrey and Wrisberg are located in the intercondylar notch. The anterior cruciate ligament originates on the postero-medial aspect of the lateral femoral condyle, while the posterior cruciate arises from the lateral aspect of the medial femoral condyle. The ligamentum mucosum originates from the most superior aspect of the notch.

The distal femur is in contact with the proximal tibia at all times throughout the range of motion of the knee. The addition of menisci converts this non-conforming geometry into a joint capable of sustaining significant functional loading (Insall, 1984a). The tibial plateau is sloped in an anterior-to-posterior direction from 7° to 10° and contains a greater surface area on the medial plateau which is almost flat compared with the convex lateral plateau. While the interspinous area corresponds to the midportion of the plateau, it is not necessarily the centre of the axis of rotation. The true axis of rotation lies between the tibial tubercle (10–15° external rotation) and the midportion of the tibial plateau.

Menisci

The semicircular medial and lateral menisci are fibrocartilagenous in consistency and are joined to each other anteriorly by the transverse ligament. They increase femoral–tibial congruity throughout the range of motion of the knee. The medial meniscus is wider posteriorly than anteriorly and its overall length measures approximately 3.5 cm. Posteriorly, it is attached to the medial capsule or deep medial collateral ligament. The lateral meniscus is more circular than the medial meniscus. The posterior attachment of the lateral meniscus has two variable ligamentous structures which run anterior (ligament of Humphrey) and posterior (ligament of Wrisberg) to the posterior cruciate ligament (Heller and Langman, 1964; Morrison, 1967; Insall, 1984; Rosenberg and Kolowich, 1990). The blood supply for the medial and lateral menisci arises from the medial and lateral genicular arteries. Vessels enter the menisci both from a superior and inferior position and develop from a series of peri-meniscal capillaries that are present in the synovial and capsular tissues (Arnoczky and Warren, 1982).

Anterior compartment

The quadriceps muscle group and corresponding structures occupy the anterior compartment and allow for extension of the knee. Traversing both the hip and knee joints, the quadriceps is composed of the rectus femoris, vasti lateralis, medialis and intermedius (Fig. 25.2). The rectus femoris inserts into the superficial border of the patella as the most superficial layer of the trilaminar tendon. The vastus lateralis inserts into the lateral aspect of the patella and extends distally as the lateral retinaculum. The vastus medialis has two components, the vastus medialis longus and its most distal and obliquely oriented fibres, the vastus medialis obliquis, which inserts into the medial border of the patella. The combination of the vastus medialis and lateralis insertion is the middle layer of the trilaminar quadriceps tendon. The vastus intermedius is the deepest layer of the quadriceps tendon, inserting into the superior aspect of the patella. The articularis genus muscle consists of a few muscle fibres running beneath the vastus intermedius and inserting into the suprapatellar capsule.

At approximately 8 cm proximal to the superior pole of the patella the quadriceps muscle tapers to form the trilaminar quadriceps tendon. While very thin superiorly, the tendon increases in width as it approaches the patella. The most superficial part of the tendon then continues distally in an expansion over the most superficial aspect of the patella as it condenses inferiorly to coalesce with the patellar ligament (tendon). As the quadriceps tendon inserts into the superior pole of the patella, there is an intimate relationship with the medial and lateral retinaculum. The retinaculum parallels the quadriceps and patella tendon, coalescing with the capsule which inserts into the respective sides of the patella and tibial plateau. The blood supply of the quadriceps

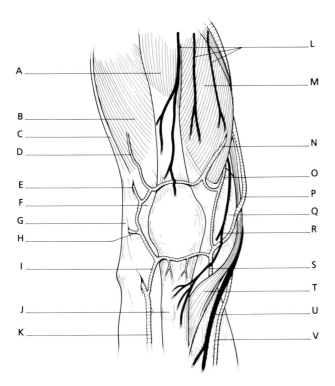

Fig. 25.2 The vasculature on the anterior aspect of the knee.
(A) Rectus femoris, (B) vastus lateralis, (C) iliotibial tract,
(D) descending branch of the lateral femoral circumflex artery,
(E) superior lateral genicular artery, (F) lateral patellar
retinaculum, (G) biceps femoris tendon, (H) inferior lateral
genicular artery, (I) anterior tibial recurrent artery, (J) patellar
ligament, (K) anterior tibial artery, (L) cutaneous nerve of the
thigh, (M) vastus medialis, (N) articular branch of the descending
genicular artery, (O) superior medial genicular artery,
(P) saphenous branch of the descending genicular artery,
(Q) medial patellar retinaculum, (R) infrapatellar branch of the
saphenous nerve, (S) inferior medial genicular artery,
(T) sartorius, (U) saphenous nerve, (V) greater saphenous vein.
(Redrawn by permission from Scott, 1991.)

tendon, patella and patellar tendon arises from both an
extrinsic and intrinsic source.

Medial compartment

Warren and Marshall (1979) have divided the medial
side of the knee into three layers. Layer 1, which includes
the crural fascia, is superficial to the superficial medial
collateral ligament (Fig. 25.3a). Layer 2 is the layer of
the superficial medial collateral ligament, considered the
primary static stabilizer to valgus stress (Fig. 25.3b).
Layer 3, the true capsule of the joint, is the most
intimate connection with the synovium (Fig. 25.3c).
While very thin anteriorly, there is a thickening of layer

3 deep to the superficial medial collateral ligament,
identified as the deep medial collateral ligament.

The sartorius, gracilis and semitendinosus tendons
each insert into the pes anserinus on the anteromedial
aspect of the proximal tibia. Innervated by the sciatic
nerve, supplied from the profunda femoris and popliteal
arteries, the semimembranosus has the same innervation
and blood supply as the semitendinosus, but inserts
more superficially and posteriorly on the medial condyle
of the tibia. The gracilis is supplied through an anterior
branch of the obturator nerve, while the sartorius is
supplied by branches of the femoral nerve.

Lateral compartment

Several authors have described the lateral side of the
knee as consisting of three layers (Kaplan, 1962;
Hollinshead, 1974; Johnson, 1979; Insall, 1984a;
Schultz *et al.*, 1984; Main and Scott, 1991). Layer 1
includes the iliotibial tract and the superficial portion of
the biceps femoris (Fig. 25.4a). The iliotibial band
inserts into Gerdy's tubercle on the lateral aspect of the
tibial tubercle. The biceps femoris muscle inserts into
the fibular head. Layer 2 contains the quadriceps retinaculum anteriorly and the patellofemoral ligaments
(Fig. 25.4b). Layer 2 also includes the lateral collateral
ligament which originates on the lateral epicondyle of
the femur and inserts into the head of the fibula. Layer
3, defined as the joint capsule, incorporates the arcuate
and fabellofibular ligaments (Fig. 25.4c). The arcuate
ligament is in the posterolateral aspect of the knee just
behind the lateral collateral ligament. The primary function of the popliteus muscle is internal rotation of the
knee, 'unlocking the knee' being accomplished by virtue
of the contour of the articulation and retracting the
posterior aspect of the lateral meniscus (Gray, 1959;
Hollinshead, 1974; Insall, 1984a; Main and Scott,
1991).

Posterior compartment

The posterior compartment of the knee contains the
joint capsule, the medial and lateral portion of the
gastrocnemius muscle and the plantaris muscle. Both the
medial and lateral heads of the gastrocnemius arise from
the respective posterior condyles of the femur and capsule of the knee joint. The plantaris muscle originates on
the lateral supracondylar line of the femur and the
oblique popliteal ligament of the knee joint. The floor of
the popliteal fossa is composed of the posterior surface
of the femur, posterior capsule, oblique popliteal ligament and the popliteus muscle. More superficially are

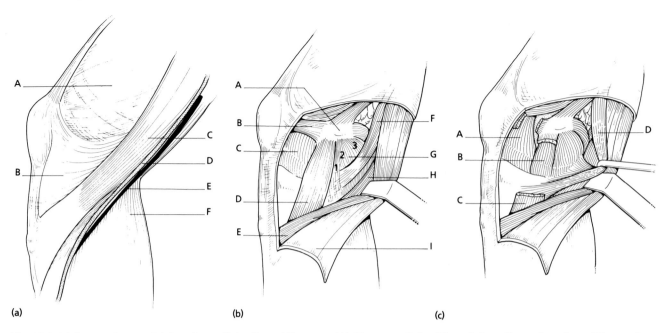

Fig. 25.3 (a) Layer 1 is superficial to the medial collateral ligament. (A) Vastus medialis, (B) medial patellar retinaculum, (C) sartorius, (D) greater saphenous vein, (E) saphenous nerve, (F) medial head of the gastrocnemius muscle. (b) Layer 2 includes the medial collateral ligament. (A) Adductor tubercle, (B) patellar-femoral ligament, (C) anterior joint capsule, (D) superficial medial collateral ligament, (E) gracilis, (F) semimembranosus, (G) posterior oblique ligament, (H) semitendinosus, (I) sartorius (cut). (c) Layer 3 is the capsular layer. (A) Anterior joint capsule, (B) deep medial collateral ligament, (C) superficial medial collateral ligament (cut), (D) semimembranosus. (Redrawn by permission from Scott, 1991.)

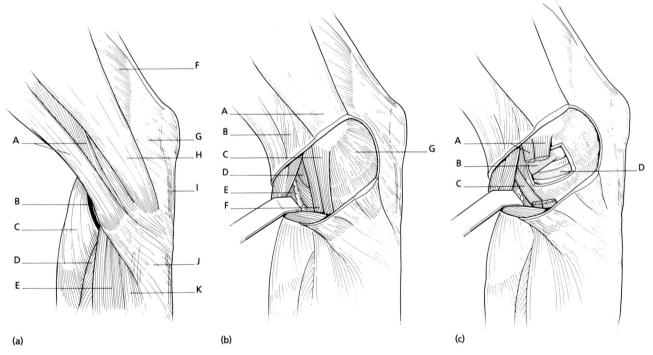

Fig. 25.4 (a) Layer 1 of the lateral side includes the iliotibial tract and the superficial portion of the biceps femoris. (A) Biceps femoris, (B) common peroneal nerve, (C) lateral head of the gastrocnemius muscle, (D) soleus muscle, (E) peroneus longus, (F) vastus lateralis, (G) lateral patellar retinaculum, (H) iliotibial band, (I) patellar ligament, (J) tibialis anterior, (K) extensor digitorum longus. (b) Layer 2 contains the lateral retinaculum and patellar–femoral ligaments. (A) Iliotibial band (cut), (B) biceps femoris, (C) fibular collateral ligament, (D) posterolateral joint capsule, (E) arcuate ligament, (F) fabellofibular ligament, (G) anterolateral joint capsule. (c) Layer 3 is the joint capsule and includes the arcuate and fabellofibular ligament. (A) Cut fabellofibular and fibular collateral ligaments, (B) popliteus tendon, (C) arcuate ligament, (D) lateral meniscus. (Redrawn by permission from Scott, 1991.)

the popliteal vessels, tibial and common peroneal nerves, saphenous vein, posterior femoral cutaneous nerve and the articular branch of the obturator nerve (Fig. 25.5).

Neurovascular supply

Virtually the entire blood suppy of the knee arises from the geniculate circulation (Scapinelli, 1968; Reider *et al.*, 1981). The arteries that supply the anastomotic ring include the supreme (descending) genicular, medial and lateral superior genicular, medial and lateral inferior genicular and anterior tibial recurrent arteries. The cruciate ligaments are supplied by the middle genicular artery, a direct branch of the popliteal artery which traverses the posterior joint capsule at the level of the

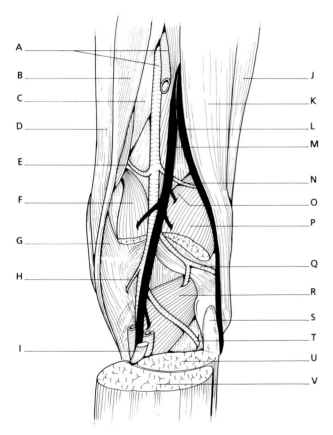

Fig. 25.5 Popliteal anatomy. (A) Popliteal artery and vein, (B) semitendinosus, (C) adductor magnus, (D) semimembranosus, (E) superior medial genicular artery, (F) medial head of the grastrocnemius muscle, (G) semimembranosus, (H) inferior medial genicular artery, (I) plantaris tendon, (J) iliotibial tract, (K) biceps femoris, (L) common peroneal nerve, (M) tibial nerve, (N) superior lateral genicular artery, (O) plantaris, (P) lateral head of the gastrocnemius muscle, (Q) inferior lateral genicular artery, (R) popliteus, (S) fibula, (T) anterior tibial artery, (U) soleus muscle, (V) gastrocnemius muscle. (Redrawn by permission from Scott, 1991.)

intercondylar notch. The patella itself is supplied by the midpatellar vessels penetrating the middle third of the anterior surface and the inferior pole vessels which anastomose at the inferior pole of the patella.

The obturator (L2 to L4), femoral (L2 to L4) and sciatic (L4, L5, S1, S2) trunks each contribute to the innervation to the knee joint. At the level of the knee, Kennedy *et al.* (1982) have demonstrated two distinct groups of nerves innervating the joint: (i) the posterior group, which includes the obturator and posterior articular branch of the posterior tibial nerve; and (ii) the anterior group, composed of articular branches of the femoral, common peroneal and saphenous nerves.

Cruciate ligaments

Composed of multiple collagen fascicles, the anterior cruciate ligament is approximately 38 mm in length and 1 cm in width. Microscopically, the interlacing fibrils (150–250 nm in diameter) are grouped into fibres (1–20 µm in diameter) and then a subfascicular unit (100–250 µm in diameter) (Arnoczky, 1983, 1991). The anterior cruciate ligament has a synovial membrane envelope and is described as being intra-articular but extra-synovial. This synovium is richly endowed with vessels from the middle genicular artery. The anterior cruciate ligament receives its neurological innervation from the tibial nerve, infiltrating the capsule posteriorly. The ligament arises from the posterolateral corner of the medial aspect of the lateral femoral condyle in the intercondylar notch (Fig. 25.6a,b). The tibial attachment is in a fossa in front of and lateral to the anterior tibial spine.

The posterior cruciate ligament arises from the lateral aspect of the medial femoral condyle in the vicinity of the intercondylar notch (Fig. 25.6a,b). While it is somewhat wider (13 mm), its length (38 mm) approximates that of the anterior cruciate ligament. The tibial attachment is not intraarticular, but over the back of the tibial plateau, approximately 1 cm distal to the joint line.

EXTENSOR MECHANISM INJURIES

The extensor mechanism includes the quadriceps muscles, quadriceps tendon, medial and lateral retinaculum, patellar tendon (ligament) and the tibial tubercle. Since this anatomical complex occupies the most superficial aspect of the knee, it is the most commonly injured. The forces traversing the quadriceps tendon, patella and patellar ligament often exceed five times body weight. As the level of activity increases, these forces are often eccentrically applied and may

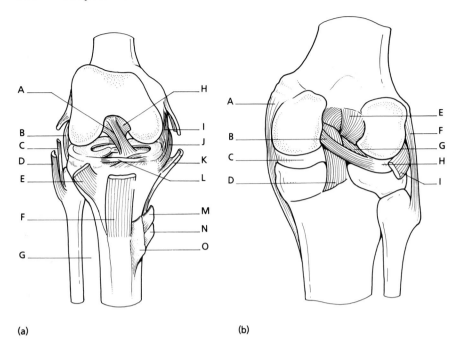

(a)   (b)

Fig. 25.6 The relationship of the intercondylar structures in the flexed knee.
(a) (A) Anterior cruciate ligament, (B) popliteus tendon, (C) fibular collateral ligament, (D) biceps femoris tendon, (E) iliotibial tract, (F) patellar ligament, (G) interosseus membrane, (H) posterior cruciate ligament, (I) deep medial collateral ligament, (J) semimembranosus, (K) superficial medial collateral ligament, (L) transverse ligament, (M) gracilis, (N) semitendinosus, (O) sartorius.
(b) (A) Superficial medial collateral ligament, (B) ligament of Wrisberg, (C) medial meniscus, (D) posterior cruciate ligament, (E) anterior cruciate ligament, (F) fibular collateral ligament, (G) ligament of Humphrey, (H) lateral meniscus, (I) popliteus tendon. (Redrawn by permission from Scott, 1991.)

result in tendon ruptures, articular cartilage impaction, and/or patella dislocations. Extensor mechanism muscular strength is derived from the quadriceps group (Figs 25.2 and 25.7). The line of pull of the quadriceps is always in a valgus orientation, measuring 12° in men and 15° in women. The synovial cavity has several embryological invaginations called 'plica' that persist into adult life. These have often been associated with anterior knee symptoms and can be acutely ruptured (Fig. 25.8). Tendon ruptures are very rare in young individuals with muscle tears predominating. The combination of extensor mechanism contraction and a concurrent applied stretching usually result in either muscle or tendon disruption. In almost all situations, these ligament and tendon ruptures must be repaired surgically.

Quadriceps tendon rupture

Quadriceps tendon rupture is more common in the sixth or seventh decade and is most likely a consequence of decreased vasculature. The tear can involve either a portion of the trilaminar tendon or its entirety. Its level usually corresponds to the amount of flexion at the time of injury. It is imperative that the repair be of sufficient quality to allow motion as early as possible.

Unlike the Achilles' tendon rupture, the quadriceps disruption is often associated with intense pain and the

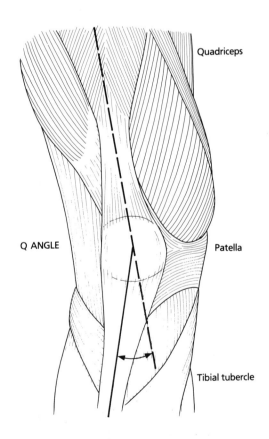

Fig. 25.7 The Q (quadriceps) angle as measured from the anterior superior iliac spine, through the central portion of the patella and to the tibial tubercle. (Redrawn by permission from Insall, 1984e.)

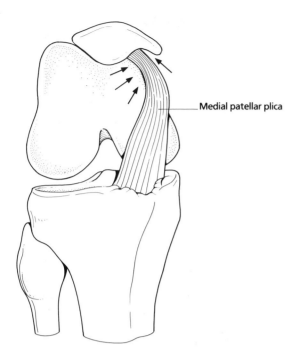

Fig. 25.8 The occasional abrasive rubbing which can be seen with a medial plica syndrome. (Redrawn by permission from Insall, 1984e.)

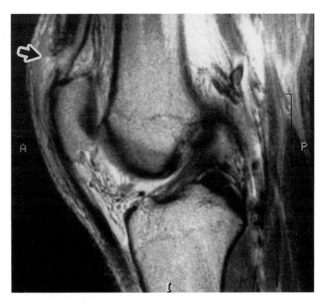

Fig. 25.9 Sagittal view of the knee through the patellar ligaments. The arrow points to rupture of the quadriceps tendon near its attachment to the patella. There is increased signal through the tendon as well as loss of continuity of the fibres. In addition, there is oedema in the surrounding soft tissue.

patient is usually unable to walk without assistance. While this would appear to be an easily diagnosed injury, in a series of 17 cases, seven were initially misdiagnosed (Ramsey and Miller, 1970). After subsidence of the initial discomfort, symptoms might dissipate especially if either the medial or lateral retinaculum is still intact. Physical findings include a palpable defect and an obvious swelling secondary to a haemarthrosis. The knee cannot be extended if the quadriceps tendon is completely ruptured. If a delay in diagnosis and treatment is encountered, the patient is often able to ambulate, but will do so with a stiff knee. Radiographs will often reveal a patella situated lower than its normal position. Magnetic resonance imaging is quite helpful in delineating quadriceps tendon ruptures (Fig. 25.9).

Incomplete tears of the quadriceps tendon should be immobilized in full extension. This should be continued for a period ranging from 4 to 6 weeks with a subsequent progressive discontinuation of immobilization using a protected programme. Unless it can be completely ascertained that the quadriceps injury is partial, surgical intervention is mandatory. Exposure of the tear is most easily performed through a straight midline incision. The authors prefer debriding the ragged ends and, if the situation is favourable, using a direct end-to-end suturing reinforced with a Bunnell-type suture from the proximal portion of the tendon to the distal portion and/or the proximal pole of the patella. Each layer does not have to be approximated separately, but must be included in the confluent re-approximation of the entire tendon. The sutures should be placed with the knee in full extension and, if it appears somewhat tenuous, it is wise to reinforce the repair site with a proximal portion of the quadriceps tendon as recommended by Scuderi (1958), Larson (1984) and Scott (1991). It is also prudent to protect the suture line using either a pull-out wire, or a strong non-absorbable suture.

Reconstruction of a chronic quadriceps tendon rupture is usually carried out with a great deal of difficulty. When the quadriceps tendon has to be lengthened, several approaches can be used depending on the defect. Incomplete portions of the proximal tendon can be turned down to bridge the gap, or the tendon can be lengthened with autogenous or synthetic materials. It is imperative not to allow the extensor mechanism to be in a position of relative patella baja as this will jeopardize subsequent knee motion.

Post-operative range of motion should be permitted as soon as possible. In the acute setting, it is possible to begin range of motion within 4–6 weeks if the ideal circumstances have been achieved. The patient should be able to straight leg raise with the cast or Velcro immobilizer in full extension for 10 days prior to commencement of range of motion exercises. Ideally it would be helpful to have the patient realize 90° of flexion within a month after beginning the motion stage of the therapy. Coincident with this is the continuance of the quadriceps exercise, achieving quadriceps strength sufficient to lift at least 10% of the body weight. When the patient is able to sustain resistance equal to 5% body weight, it is usually a good sign for discontinuing protected ambulation with crutches (approximately 6–8 weeks) and progressing to a sleeve-type brace with medial and lateral hinges. Therapy must be continued until quadriceps parity between the affected and non-affected leg is achieved. In the acute repair this will usually take 6 months. For late reconstructions, the principle of post-operative treatment is the same, but the course is usually longer. Prognostically, in patients sustaining an acute repair the quadriceps strength has been returned to normal, yet in those undergoing late reconstructions, a persistent extensor deficit may persist.

Patellar tendon rupture

Disruption of the patellar tendon is relatively rare, occurring only one-third as frequently as quadriceps tendon rupture. The mechanism of injury is similar to that noted with the quadriceps tendon, i.e. a forceful contraction of the quadriceps muscle interrupted by a passive stretching. Patellar tendon rupture usually occurs in those under 40 years and is often associated with a previous history of tendonitis and steroid injections. These injuries are associated with marked pain and are secondary to significant trauma. A palpable defect is usually present, although significant swelling can mask this sign. Patella alta is frequently seen on radiographs. Magnetic resonance imaging is even more specific (Fig. 25.10).

An incomplete disruption of the patellar tendon should be immobilized from 3 to 6 weeks in full extension. Complete tears require surgical intervention. Midsubstance tears which are less frequent than proximal disruptions can be re-approximated by direct suturing after debriding of ragged edges. Tension-relieving measures such as a proximal or distal pull-out non-absorbable suture should be undertaken. The inferior pole of the patella or tibial tubercle may be drilled for re-attachment of avulsions. Delayed reconstruction of the patellar tendon is difficult because of tissue loss that has ensued and contraction of the extensor mechanism. Kelikian *et al.* (1957), Larson (1984) and Scott (1991) use the semitendinosus, while Scuderi (1958), Larson (1984) and Scott (1991) have suggested using a flap of quadriceps tendon that has been turned down to cover the defect.

Post-operative treatment should consist of 6 weeks of

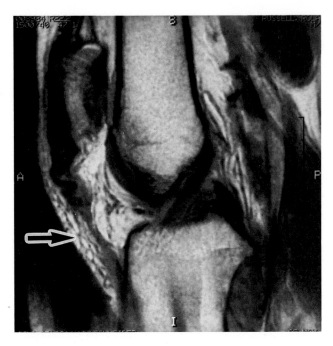

Fig. 25.10 Sagittal view of the knee through the patellar ligaments. Arrows point to loss of the low signal of the inferior patellar ligament as well as waviness of the ligament consistent with a sprain or partial tear. Note that the fibres of the ligament are thinned and there is increased signal in the inferior patellar ligament. (Courtesy of Dr. Morton Schneider.)

immobilization with Velcro-type splints and protected weight-bearing. Thereafter, motion should be gradually instituted with concurrent quadriceps strengthening. The best results are in those ruptures that are repaired early. Patella baja is a major complication of patellar tendon repair.

DISORDERS OF THE PATELLA

Non-operative and operative treatment choices must include an understanding of the radiological evaluation of the patellofemoral joint, chondromalacia, osteoarthritis, osteochondral fractures, malalignment syndromes, synovial plicae, bursitis, overuse syndromes and dislocations. The patella is subject to potential imbalance between the medial and lateral aspects of the quadriceps muscle group (Fig. 25.3). It is this dynamic activity that causes a great deal of variation between static evaluations of patellofemoral motion and the dynamics of this particular articulation. It is this differential that often explains why a patient with a normal Q angle and relatively normal radiographic values is still susceptible to patellar subluxation. The most significant abnormal force on the patellofemoral joint is a result of the lateral pull on the patella, from the vastus lateralis and the lateral retinaculum, with contributions from the iliotibial band.

The patella is frequently impacted with a resultant adverse effect — traumatic chondromalacia. In addition, virtually any rotational force to the knee can result in a similar patellar injury. Hyperextension of the knee causes a direct impact on the patella, usually affecting the inferior pole. Abnormal anatomy exposes the patient to similar situations with less violent injuries. The authors prefer the classification of patellar disorders proposed by Insall (1984) which is based on the appearance of cartilage damage: (i) usually normal cartilage: (ii) variable cartilage damage; and (iii) significant cartilage damage.

Usually normal cartilage

The four causes of patellar disorders with usually normal cartilage are: (i) peri-patellar causes (bursitis and tendonitis); (ii) overuse syndromes; (iii) sympathetic dystrophy; and (iv) patellar anomalies. There are four bursa around the knee and these are susceptible to an inflammatory response, the pre-patellar (most commonly affected), the infrapatellar, the deep patellar and the anserine. Inflammation of the bursa is self-limiting and can be treated with the usual non-operative modalities such as ice and rest. As aspiration of these bursa, especially the pre-patellar bursa, can result in persistent drainage and even infection, caution should be exercised.

Tendonitis of the extensor mechanism may occur anywhere along the course of the quadriceps or patellar tendons. When calcification is present at the inferior pole of the patella, it is termed Sinding–Larson–Johanssen syndrome, whereas calcification or tenderness along its insertion into the tibial tubercle is identified as Osgood–Schlatter's disease (Sinding–Larson, 1921; Insall, 1984a; Larson, 1984; Scott, 1991). None of these entities usually requires operative treatment, but they respond to non-operative treatment that must include quadriceps stretching and strengthening exercises. Injuries of the infrapatellar fat pad are usually diagnosed only by clinical examination. Increasing recreational demands have resulted in more frequent diagnosis of knee overuse syndromes.

Disproportionate extensor mechanism pain, whether a result of trauma or surgery, must raise the suspicion of sympathetic dystrophy (DeTakats, 1965; Ficat and Hungerford, 1977). Manifestations of this entity are diffuse but usually characterized by intense disproportionate pain, stiffness, skin discoloration and decreased skin temperature. Patella symptoms with a normal appearing articular cartilage can also be secondary to

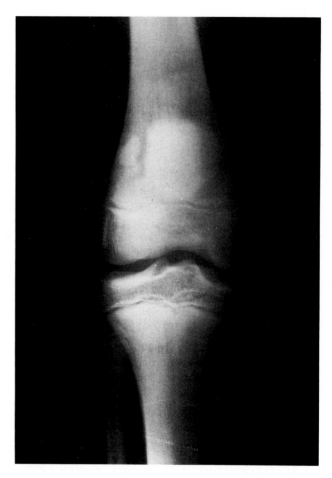

Fig. 25.11 Anteroposterior radiogram revealing a tripartite patella.

developmental abnormalities, such as bipartite and tripartite patella (Fig. 25.11). In those individuals with persistent discomfort, the non-fused piece of bone can be removed without jeopardizing the function of the extensor mechanism (Scott, 1991).

Variable cartilage damage

Both synovial plicae and malalignment syndromes can produce variable cartilage damage. Patellar subluxation and dislocation are often grouped together in discussing malalignment syndromes. Cartilage damage has often been described with dislocating patellae and, in fact, small fracture chips may often be seen on axial radiograms. The diagnosis of patellar malalignment is often made by abnormal clinical values or radiographic indices. Patella alta is another malalignment that can similarly result in a subluxation and often dislocation. Understanding the mechanism of pain in patients with a malalignment syndrome is difficult since articular cartilage has no nerve endings. Theoretically, pain might be secondary to an overload on the subchondral bone due to a softening of the articular cartilage or an associated synovitis. It is interesting to note that in two series (Insall *et al.*, 1976; Scuderi *et al.*, 1988) pain and articular cartilage changes did not have a direct correlation.

Significant cartilage damage

Chondromalacia, osteoarthritis, osteochondral fractures and osteochondritis are among the disorders of the patella which cause significant cartilage damage. Budinger (1906) has been given credit as the first person to describe chondromalacia. Outerbridge (1961) described four stages of chondromalacia: Stage I—swelling and softening of the cartilage (Fig. 25.12); Stage II—fissuring within the softened areas (Fig. 25.13); Stage III—fasciculations or breakdown of the articular cartilage almost to the level of the subchondral bone (Fig. 25.14); and Stage IV—destruction of the articular cartilage with the subchondral bone exposed (Fig. 25.15) (Rand, 1990). Histologically, Stage IV is virtually indistinguishable from osteoarthritis.

Pathological changes can occur on either one or both surfaces of the patellofemoral joint. The aetiology of chondromalacia has been attributed to surface degeneration, age-related degeneration, abnormal ridges of the patella, malalignment, direct trauma, patellar shape, biochemical alteration and loss of bone compliance. Immobilization has been observed to be a contributing cause. The biochemical and histological analysis of cartilage taken from both chondromalacia and osteoarthritic patella do indeed suggest that this is a continuum in a disease process. The clinical correlation, however, is difficult since the osteoarthritic patient is usually older and usually does not give a long history of chronic knee discomfort.

Chondromalacia is often the result of direct trauma to the patella. These chondral fractures often result in loose bodies that will perpetuate a synovial reaction and chronic effusion. Osteochondritis dissecans of the patella, a rare entity, is usually central in origin. Excision of the loose fragment is usually required and unfortunately, often encompasses more than 25% of the articular surface.

Radiological evaluation of the patellofemoral joint

Routine radiographic evaluation of the knee includes an anteroposterior, lateral, tunnel and axial view. The anteroposterior view, in addition to assessing femoral–tibial angle and medial- and lateral-joint space altera-

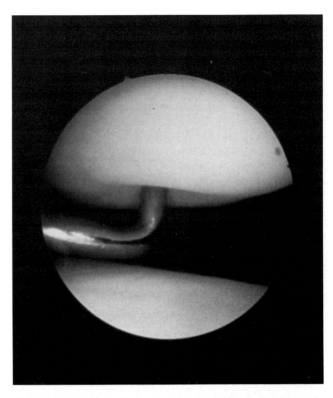

Fig. 25.12 Softening of patellar articular cartilage, Stage I chondromalacia, Outerbridge classification.

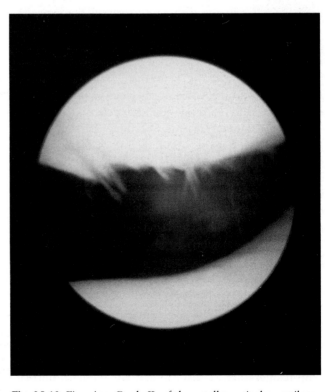

Fig. 25.13 Fissuring, Grade II, of the patellar articular cartilage.

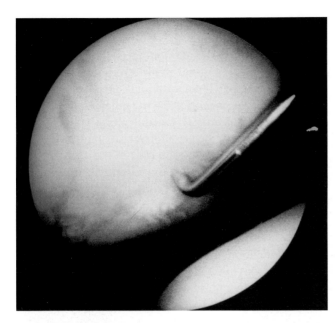

Fig. 25.14 Arthroscopic demonstration of Grade III chondral changes on the patella.

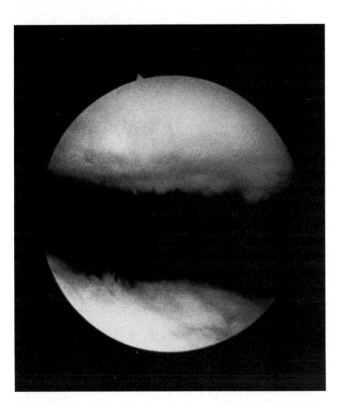

Fig. 25.15 Grade IV chondromalacia or oesteoarthritis of both the patella and trochlea.

tions, will show the size, position and integrity of the patella. Bipartite patellar (Fig. 25.11) fractures and osteochondritis dissecans can very often be identified in this particular view. The lateral view is helpful in esti-

mating the height of the patella in relationship to the joint line. Essentially, there have been four methods of measuring whether a patient has patella alta or infera: Boon-Itt (1930), Blumensaat (1938), Insall and Salvati (1971) and Blackburne and Peel (1977). Blumensaat's measurement is based on a lateral view taken with the knee flexed 30°. In this projection, the lower pole of the patella should lie on a line projected anteriorly from the intercondylar notch (Blumensaat's line) (Fig. 25.16). The Insall and Salvati method describes a normal patellar height in relationship to the patellar tendon. The patellar tendon should not have an increased dimension of more than 20% of the patellar height (Fig. 25.17). Blackburne and Peel utilize a ratio between the perpendicular distance from the lower articular margin of the patella to the tibial plateau and the length of the articular surface of the patella.

An axial view of the knee is indispensable in assessing patellofemoral alignment (Jaroschy, 1924; Hughston, 1969, 1972; Ficat, 1970; Jacobson and Bertheussen, 1974; Laurin *et al.*, 1979). Merchant and Mercer (1974), Merchant (1987) and Merchant *et al.* (1974) use a technique in which the radiographic beam is positioned proximally and the cassette below the knee. The knees are flexed 45° over the end of the table (Fig. 25.18). The

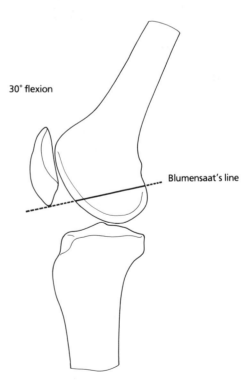

Fig. 25.16 Blumensaat's line projects the intercondylar line of the femur to the lower pole of the patella. (Reproduced by permission from Insall, 1984e.)

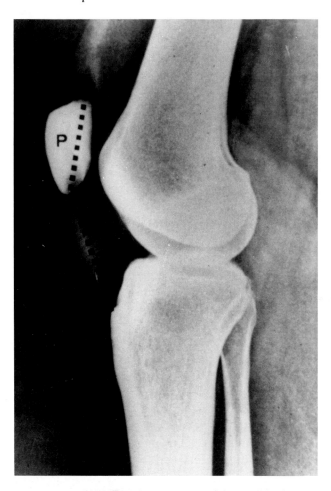

Fig. 25.17 Radiographic demonstration of the Insall–Salvati technique. (Reproduced by permission from Insall, 1984.)

sulcus angle is measured to establish a zero reference line (Fig. 25.19). A second line is projected from the apex of the sulcus angle to the lowest point of the articular ridge of the patella. The angle between these two lines is the congruence angle. If the apex of the patellar articular ridge is lateral to the zero line, the congruence angle is designated positive, whereas if it is medial, the congruence angle is negative (Fig. 25.20).

Methods of treatment

All patients with patellofemoral pain, with the possible exception of an acute dislocation of a malaligned patellofemoral articulation, should undergo an initial conservative therapeutic regimen. This approach should include an education so that they might understand the diagnosis, a restriction or refinement in activities, a strengthening programme, bracing and possibly orthotics.

While walking and running are beneficial to cardiovascular conditioning, they elevate patellofemoral contact pressure. A conditioning programme should entail strengthening of the quadriceps muscles to alleviate stress at the patellofemoral joint. Hyperextension of the knee during quadriceps strengthening should be avoided as it accentuates patellofemoral compression. Immobilization of the patellofemoral joint should be very brief (less than 48 h) and only in the acute setting. Further immobilization encourages muscle atrophy and subsequent increased stress at the patellofemoral joint. Bracing of the patellofemoral joint is usually achieved by means of pads placed to stress relieve the patella while restricting motion. Medication for the treatment of patellofemoral problems should be used sparingly. While there was initially some speculation that salicylates protected against fibrillation, this study, based on a small series, has not been corroborated. Icing the knee immediately after activities is probably as effective as analgesics. Orthotics decrease the impact load of the joints of the lower extremity including the knee. The quality of footwear today is such that running shoes probably obviate the need for orthotics.

Surgery is certainly an option for the patient whose symptoms of extensor mechanism dysfunction have not responded to a conservative therapeutic regimen. The types of surgical procedures range from those affecting the articular cartilage (shaving, drilling) to re-alignments and biomechanical enhancements (tibial tubercle elevation). In patients with no malalignment, arthroscopic debridements and shaving will sometimes alleviate symptoms. Although drilling of subchondral bone to stimulate fibrocartilagenous ingrowth has had unpredictable success, there have been many reports of patient's symptoms being accentuated by this procedure.

Re-alignment procedures have included lateral retinacular releases and those which extend into the vastus lateralis, as well as proximal re-alignments and distal re-alignments. Lateral releases are performed to decrease the lateral vector on patella tracking throughout its range of motion. Clinical relief of symptoms has been realized in upwards of 75% of patients with recurrent subluxation undergoing lateral release. It has been suggested that formal re-alignment procedures be reserved for those patients with histories of documented dislocations (Jacobson and Bertheussen, 1974; Scuderi *et al.*, 1988; Scott, 1991). Immediate reconstruction of the disrupted retinaculum after acute dislocations should be considered in patients who have obvious clinical and radiologic malalignment and are active. Post-operative results with proximal re-alignment procedures have been encouraging. With increased understanding of joint

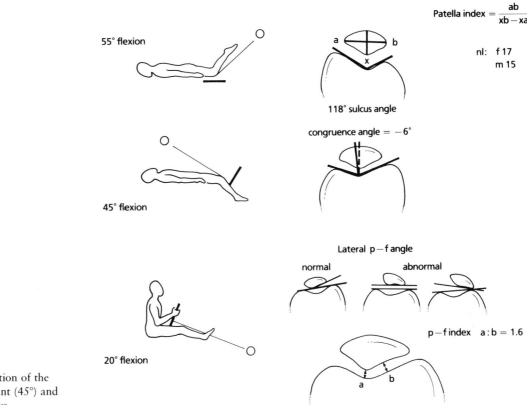

Fig. 25.18 A representation of the Hughston (55°), Merchant (45°) and Laurin (20°) patella views.

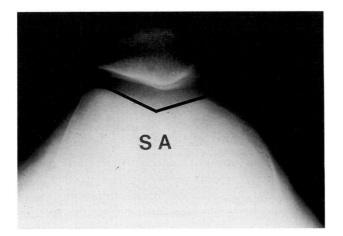

Fig. 25.19 The sulcus angle.

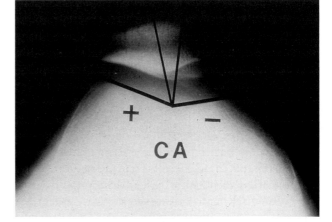

Fig. 25.20 Assessment of the congruence angle.

physiology, the best operative treatment is now facilitated by commencing range of motion on the first postoperative day. Using this protocol, most patients achieve full range of motion by 3 weeks post-operatively.

The Elmslie–Trillat and Hauser techniques have frequently been performed. In the Elmslie–Trillat method, the tibial tubercle is displaced medially up to 1 cm, pivoting on a distal base (Trillat *et al.*, 1964; Elmslie,

1978). Unfortunately, multiple series have reported late osteoarthritis (Cox, 1945; Heywood, 1961; Hampson and Hill, 1975; Hughston and Walsh, 1979) with distal transfers. Patellofemoral joint pressure can be minimized if the effective lever arm of the patella is increased. This concept is the basis for the tibial tubercle elevation, i.e. Maquet procedure (Fig. 25.21) (Maquet, 1974) (see Chapter 19). Maquet calculated that elevating the tibial

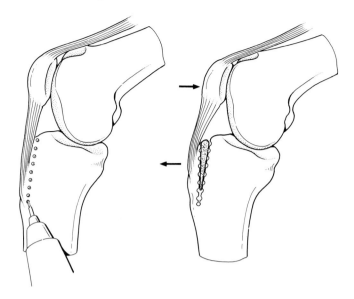

Fig. 25.21 In the Maquet procedure the tubercle is elevated, increasing the lever arm of the patella and theoretically decreasing contact pressure. (Redrawn by permission from Scott, 1991.)

tubercle by 2 cm reduced patellofemoral forces by 50%. This procedure has had moderate success, but is associated with marked complications, primarily skin problems due to the tubercle elevation and subsequent skin tension. In the patient with recalcitrant patellofemoral pain, patellectomies have been used but the basic problem has been the marked reduction in quadriceps strength.

CHONDRAL AND OSTEOCHONDRAL INJURIES

Arthroscopy has greatly aided clinical delineation of chondral injuries. Demonstration of articular cartilage involvement in knee injuries has elucidated many of the complaints and cause for persistent discomfort in the symptomatic patient. An excellent description of gross and histological characteristics of articular cartilage has been presented by Rand (1990). To the naked eye, the articular cartilage appears as a smooth covering of the joint surface. This is, of course, deceptive since articular cartilage, composed of cells (chondrocytes) in an extracellular matrix, is a highly complex anatomical structure. Under 5% of tissue volume in articular cartilage is composed of cells, less than any other tissue in the body. Articular cartilage is also unique in that there is no vascular, neural or lymphatic contribution involved with its maintenance. Subsequently, nourishment is dependent on a diffusion of nutrients (Andren and Wehlin, 1960; Mankin, 1970, 1974). In addition to diffusion of

nutrients, anaerobic pathways are well developed in chondrocytes to allow for synthesis of the extracellular matrix. The thickness of the articular cartilage is between 3 and 5 mm throughout the knee (Hall and Wyshak, 1980; Hoshino and Wallace, 1987; Rand, 1990).

Questions have persisted concerning the ability of articular cartilage to heal defects. The avascularity of articular cartilage prevents a vascular response when there is cartilage injury alone. When the subchondral bone is also injured, then a vascular response might ensue. While human studies suggest that articular cartilage is not ordinarily repaired (Collins, 1949; Paget, 1969; Redfern, 1969; Stockwell and Meachim, 1973; Rand, 1990), animal studies suggest that articular cartilage injuries are capable of healing by intrinsic repair (Calendruccio and Gilmer, 1962). It appears that superficial cartilage lacerations will not heal by an intrinsic response but they do not seem to lead to osteoarthritic changes.

When bone is injured, it forms a fibrin clot which is subsequently replaced by granulation tissue and then fibrous tissue (DePalma *et al.*, 1966; Mankin, 1974, 1982). The reparative tissue is almost always fibrocartilaginous although some animal species have displayed healing of full-thickness defects with hyaline cartilage. The fibrocartilage, mostly type I, does not seem to be very durable (Covery *et al.*, 1972; Mitchell and Shepherd, 1976; Cheung *et al.*, 1978; Furukawa *et al.*, 1980). A review of osteochondral fractures in humans reveals that the subchondral bone healing was with fibrous tissue only and articular chondrocytes seem to contribute significantly to the repair response (Milgram, 1986; Rand, 1990).

Clinical considerations

Both endogenous and exogenous sources inflict acute and repetitive trauma upon articular cartilage. An abnormal motion can result in a shearing type of force which can injure the superficial zone of the articular cartilage. Bauer and Jackson (1988) identified six different types of lesions of the articular cartilage. In their series they found that rotational forces in direct trauma were the most common cause of injury. In most of their cases the lesions were in the weight-bearing area of the articular cartilage and usually in the medial compartment. The most commonly associated lesion was a tear of the meniscus. The six types of changes were identified as linear crack, stellate fracture, flap, crater, fibrillation and degrading (Fig. 25.22).

Chondral injuries are frequently difficult to diagnose in so far as they can mimic meniscal and synovial

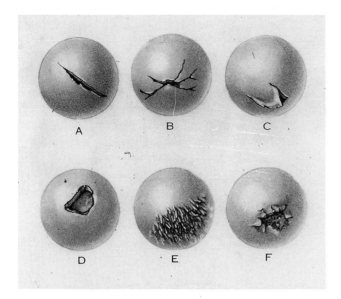

Fig. 25.22 Articular cartilage changes as described by Bauer and Jackson. (A) Linear, (B) stellate, (C) flap, (D) crater, (E) fibrillation, (F) degrading. (Reproduced by permission from Scott, 1991.)

injuries. Symptoms are somewhat non-specific, often associated with an effusion. Pain can be either localized or diffuse. Intermittent locking, recurrent effusions, crepitus and persistent pain may all be associated with chondral injuries; this can be a diagnostic dilemma since extensor mechanism dysfunction and meniscal injuries can present similarly. When the chondral injury is associated with subchondral bone involvement, the subsequent radiopaque loose body will be readily apparent on standard radiograms. The tunnel view is particularly important in the under 18 age group, who are susceptible to osteochondritis dissecans. This lesion is most often seen on the lateral aspect of the medial femoral condyle and is usually unilateral (74%) and twice as common in males (Aichroth, 1971, 1977). Arthrography has been used in the past to delineate large osteochondritis lesions, but has not been helpful in small lesions. Magnetic resonance imaging seems insensitive for detecting defects of less than 3 mm (Gylys-Morin *et al.*, 1987). Arthroscopy certainly remains the most accurate method of detailing the chondral defect.

Fragments of articular cartilage greater than 5 mm in diameter should be removed. Smaller pieces of articular cartilage will often imbed in the synovium and become asymptomatic. Arthroscopy allows for identification of the site of origin, delineating the extent of the chondral fracture. Trimming of the localized lesions has been beneficial in most series (Hubbard, 1987; Kelly, 1990). Debridement by itself, however, which is usually con-

fined to the arthritic population is less predictable alleviating symptoms for 75% of patients in short-term follow-up (Shahriaree, 1986). Any reparative process would be dependent on stimulating the subchrondral bone via drill holes to subsequent formation of fibrin clots as outlined above. Open reduction and internal fixation of ostoechondral fractures have been attempted with Kirschner wires and screws. Long-term results with these treatments do not favour either technique and, in fact, several large series report good results after removal of the osteochondral fragment (Rosenberg, 1964; Ahstrom, 1965; Kennedy *et al.*, 1966; Paget, 1969; Smillie, 1971; Bauer and Jackson, 1988). In general, small fragments need not be replaced, but when dealing with large fragments comprising at least 25% of the joint surface area consideration must be given to replacing the fracture fragment. Post-operatively, there should be no joint immobilization as range of motion is encouraged. To date, there has been no evidence to favour non-weight-bearing for more than 6 weeks. Cartilage transplantation with autografts or allografts is becoming more of an accepted procedure, albeit associated with significant problems.

THE MENISCUS

The meniscal blood supply is limited to the periphery, with the internal and intermediate regions being primarily avascular (Arnoczky and Warren, 1982; Insall, 1984c; Hosea *et al.*, 1991). The blood supply to the menisci originates from the lateral and medial superior and inferior genicular arteries. Unlike articular cartilage, the meniscus contains sensory nerve endings within its substance. Their course is similar to the blood supply and essentially supplies the outer third of the meniscus (Rosenberg and Kolowich, 1990). These semilunar cartilages are functional extensions of the tibial articulation of the knee. Without the menisci the tibial articulation is incongruous with the femur.

The medial meniscus is crescentic in shape. The posterior fibres of the anterior horn connect through the transverse ligament which runs across the medial aspect of the tibial plateau to connect with the lateral meniscus. The mid-aspect of the medial meniscus is firmly attached to the deep medial collateral ligament. Posteriorly, the medial meniscus is anchored to the posterior intercondylar area (Fig. 25.6). The lateral meniscus is much more of a closed circle with a wider surface area anteriorly. Posteriorly it is attached in the intercondylar area to the posterior cruciate ligaments from the ligaments of Humphrey (the anterior meniscal–femoral ligament) and Wrisberg (the posterior meniscal–femoral ligament). The circumferential arrangement of the collagen fibres, thought to be in response to the predominantly circumferential forces on the meniscus, is the dominant pattern, although there are a few radial fibres.

In the young individual without a previous knee injury, meniscal tear is normally a consequence of a twisting motion. This can be in association with a collateral or cruciate ligament injury, or it may be isolated. In the acute setting there is usually a delayed swelling due to synovial reaction after 6 hours. Joint line tenderness is usually present and is probably one of the most distinctive clinical findings. Swelling and tenderness associated with locking has also been considered for some time as a hallmark of meniscal tears. Numerous manoeuvres have been suggested to localize the site of the meniscal tear. They include the Steinmann test (Fig. 25.23), Apley test (Fig. 25.24) and McMurray test (Fig. 25.25). These tests, by manipulating the joint, attempt to elicit tenderness at the specific site of the tear.

As with other conditions of the knee, routine radiographs should be performed. For years the gold standard of diagnostic testing for meniscal tears was arthrography. There has been scepticism regarding its efficacy and interpretation of cruciate and collateral ligament disruptions (Ireland *et al.*, 1980; Selesnick *et al.*, 1985; Savory *et al.*, 1987). The advent of magnetic resonance imaging and arthroscopy has made the role of arthrography diminish significantly. Many retrospective studies have suggested an accuracy of greater than 90% in interpretation of both meniscal and cruciate ligament disruption. Meniscal tears are identified by a disruption of the low intensity signal within the meniscus as viewed on a magnetic resonance imaging scan. A Grade I tear is identified by a small disruption of the homogeneous signal (Fig. 25.26a,b). In Grade II tears, the disruption is more pronounced, but does not extend through either the superior or inferior surface. Arthroscopically, a Grade I or II tear cannot be visualized. The Grade III tear, disruption of the homogeneous signal with extension to either the superior or inferior surface is a clinically significant tear (Fig. 25.27).

Methods of treatment

The present trend of minimizing the resection of meniscal tears, and in certain circumstances re-attaching the menisci, has resulted from the noted Fairbank's changes seen post-meniscectomy (squaring, ridging and narrowing of the joint spaces). These changes are consistent with the function of menisci demonstrated to sustain 40–50% of the total load transmitted across the knee

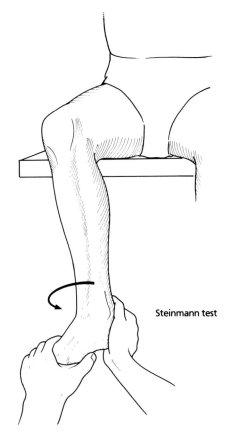

Fig. 25.23 In the Steinmann test, the patient is sitting with the leg bent over the table approximately 90°. To assess the medial side, the foot is externally rotated alerting the physician to discomfort arising from the medial aspect of the joint. (Redrawn by permission from Insall, 1984e.)

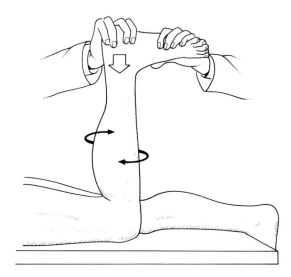

Fig. 25.24 In the Apley–Grind test, the prone patient flexes the knee 90°. The examiner compresses the joint while simultaneously rotating it. Meniscal pain is often discovered, yet this test is by no means pathognomonic of a meniscal tear.

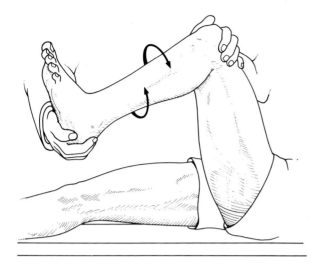

Fig. 25.25 The McMurray test is performed with the knee flexed 90° and slowly extended with an external rotation force. It might be positive for a posterior peripheral medial meniscus tear. (Redrawn by permission from Insall, 1984e.)

joint (Ricklin *et al.*, 1971; Seedham *et al.*, 1974; Shrive, 1974; Walker and Erkman, 1975). Arthroscopy has certainly enhanced our understanding and treatment of meniscal as well as ligament injuries.

The types of meniscal tears include bucket-handle, flap, horizontal, radial, degenerative and double-radial tear of a discoid meniscus (Savory *et al.*, 1987; Rosenberg and Kolowich, 1990). More common in younger patients and frequently associated with anterior cruciate disruption, bucket-handle tears are vertical and longitudi-

nal in orientation. The bucket-handle tears are three times as common in the medial as compared to the lateral meniscus and can displace into the knee with development of the classic locked knee (Fig. 25.28). Arthroscopically, these tears are removed in the classical triangular approach. In this setting, three portals are used when resection of the displaced fragment is indicated.

Radial tears are more frequently found on the medial aspect of the lateral meniscus. Operative treatment of the radial tear is local excision with the remaining rim contoured and stabilized. The flap tear is one of the most common meniscal tears and is believed to propagate from either the radial or bucket-handle tear. The horizontal cleavage tear produces a ragged appearance and has been identified as the most common tear. Similar to the radial tear, the horizontal tear is most often found in association with a meniscal cyst. Surgical excision is similar to that of a radial tear in which the disrupted segment is excised back to its base. Chronic tears, degenerative in nature, often have a combination of the patterns described. These areas of disruption are often associated with degenerative articular changes, and it becomes questionable at times which is more symptomatic, the articular cartilage disruption or the meniscus pathology. In general, the basic principle of minimal meniscal excision applies once again to this type of tear pattern. The diagnosis of an asymptomatic discoid lateral meniscus by itself does not require surgical intervention. At surgery, the meniscus is trimmed back to a stable rim which resembles in shape a normal meniscus.

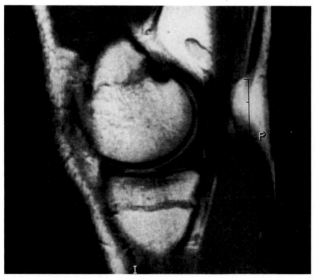

(a)

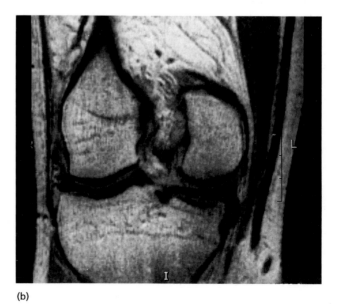

(b)

Fig. 25.26 Sagittal (a) and coronal (b) sections of a normal meniscus, which demonstrate a normal low-intensity signal and contour. (Courtesy of Dr Morton Schneider.)

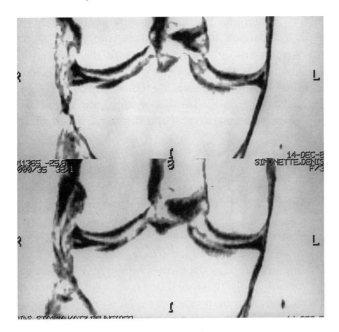

Fig. 25.27 Coronal image demonstrates a linear area of increased signal in the body of the lateral meniscus. This does not reach a meniscal surface, and therefore, would be consistent with a Grade II degeneration. (Courtesy of Dr Morton Schneider.)

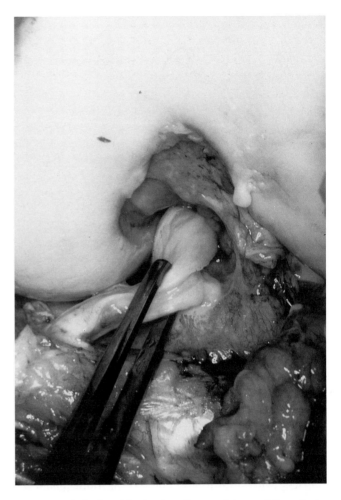

Fig. 25.28 A displaced bucket-handle tear of the medial meniscus as seen at arthrotomy.

Arnoczky's studies on the peripheral blood supply of menisci has encouraged many investigators to repair the meniscus in its vascular zone (Scapinelli, 1968; Cabaud *et al.*, 1981; Wirth, 1981; Arnoczky and Warren, 1982; 1983; DeHaven, 1985; Graf *et al.*, 1987; Savory *et al.*, 1987; Henning *et al.*, 1988; Rosenberg *et al.*, 1988; Glashow *et al.* 1989). Many short-term studies have suggested a high rate of healing, approaching 98% in one series (Morgan and Casscells, 1986; Henning *et al.*, 1988). Three basic techniques have been described (DeHaven, 1985; Graf *et al.*, 1987): (i) open repair; (ii) inside-out technique (Barber and Stone, 1985; DeHaven, 1985; Morgan and Casscells, 1986; Rosenberg *et al.*, 1986; Scott *et al.*, 1986); and (iii) outside-in technique. Meniscal repair should be performed on non-degenerative longitudinal tears in the vascular zone and which are less than 3 cm in length. In general, an unstable knee is not one in which meniscal repairs should be considered. There is some controversy as to this concept, but most studies suggest that ligament instability is a relative contraindication for meniscal repair.

At present, open complete meniscectomy is contraindicated under all circumstances. Post-operatively, the uncomplicated partial meniscal resection in a knee with minimal or no disruption of the articular cartilage may be treated aggressively. Restriction of weight-bearing should be only on a symptomatic basis and the patient should be encouraged to begin strengthening exercises the night of surgery. Range-of-motion exercises should be initiated the following morning. Return-to-normal activities are dependent on the patient regaining full strength in the muscle groups surrounding the knee. In patients undergoing meniscal repair, the present approach is to restrict weight-bearing for 4–6 weeks. Range of motion may be initiated and strengthening is encouraged.

The patient can easily perform quadriceps exercises at home. Fifty repetitions per 24-h period, simultaneously or interspersed, seems to be effective. Progression to resistance with ankle weights has also been quite helpful. The rule of thumb has been to increase resistance between 4.5 and 12 kg per week to approximately 10% of the patient's body weight. Return to activity can be initiated when the strength of the operative leg equals that of the non-operative extremity. It is important that patients do not strengthen either the quadriceps or hamstring group by exceeding full extension or flexion beyond 90°. Exceeding these limits, hyperextension or flexion beyond 90°, will often cause patellofemoral symptoms, particularly in the immediate post-operative period.

Major complications of arthroscopic surgery are infection, vascular and nerve injury, synovitis and persistent drainage. Although these complications can occur, they are certainly very rare (Insall, 1984; Scott, 1990). Popliteal artery disruption has been reported, albeit infrequently, with arthroscopic surgery. The prognosis of operative treatment of meniscal tears is fully dependent on technical ability and associated intra-articular pathology. There have been some groups, however, identified as not doing as well post-operatively and these include those with associated pathology, primarily degenerative changes or ligament insufficiency. The question that still remains to be answered concerns the long-term effect of partial meniscectomies on osteo-arthritic changes.

COLLATERAL LIGAMENTS

A conservative approach towards isolated collateral ligament injuries has been advocated for Grade I and II sprains, but remains somewhat controversial for Grade III injuries. Typically, an injury to the medial collateral ligament may very well involve any or all of the structures from layers 1 to 3: the crural fascia, the deep medial collateral ligament and the superficial medial collateral ligament. The posterior extension of the medial collateral ligament, the posteromedial capsule, includes the posterior oblique ligament described by Hughston (Hughston and Eilers, 1973; Hughston *et al.*, 1980; Reider, 1991). The posteromedial corner also has an intimate relationship with the semimembranosus tendon and it has been conjectured that there is a dynamic relationship with this tendon and the posteromedial corner. Similarly, the origin of the superficial medial collateral ligament (layer 3) is believed to be reinforced by a contribution from the vastus medialis obliquis.

The medial capsular layers provide stability to valgus stress. Selective cutting studies on cadavers have been conducted by Grood *et al.* (1981), Warren *et al.* (1974) and Inove *et al.* (1987). The medial collateral ligament is the primary medial stabilizer at 30° of flexion whereas it is a secondary contributor at full extension. In full extension, the anterior cruciate ligament is a primary stabilizer with a contribution from the posteromedial capsule.

The quadruple complex has been described by Kaplan (1962) as providing functional stability to varus stresses. This complex includes the iliotibial band, biceps muscle and tendon, lateral collateral ligament and popliteus. The posterior third of the lateral supporting structures is known as the 'arcuate complex'. It includes the lateral collateral ligament, arcuate ligament and an extension of the popliteus muscle. The posterior third of the lateral ligamentous complex is reinforced by the biceps, popliteus and lateral head of the gastrocnemius. The extracapsular lateral collateral ligament originates from the lateral epicondyle and attaches to the fibular head. According to Grood *et al.* (1981), the lateral collateral ligament is a primary restraint to varus stress at both 5° and 25° of flexion. The lateral capsule and arcuate ligament make a minor contribution to varus restraint. The iliotibial band and popliteus tendon biomechanically play a very insignificant role in restricting varus stress statically; however, there is undoubtedly a significant dynamic stabilizing role.

Many joints throughout the body are constrained by ligaments, tendons, capsule and/or menisci. Sprains are injuries that produce some degree of increased elongation or rupture of either single or multiple collagen fibres. Clinically testing for a degree of injury is based on three grades with Grade 0 being considered normal. Grade 1 (mild) is less than 0.5 cm opening of the joint. Grade 2 (moderate) is a 0.5−1 cm opening and Grade 3 (severe) is greater than 1 cm of opening. An alternative nomenclature is as follows: zero is normal, 1+ is a translation of 0.5 cm, 2+ is 0.5−1 cm and 3+ is 1−1.5 cm. Throughout the literature a Grade 4 terminology has developed indicating greater than 1.5 cm.

Clinical considerations

Collateral ligament injuries about the knee are the result of either direct or rotational injuries. With an injury to the medial side of the knee, for instance, the force is almost always applied on the lateral aspect of the knee. The combination of a torsional and valgus moment much more typically causes an injury to both the medial collateral and anterior cruciate ligaments (Hughston and Barrett, 1983; Indelicato, 1983; Mont, 1990). The magnitude of the valgus injury will sequentially cause disruption of the primary medial stabilizer (medial collateral ligament), and possibly the secondary stabilizer, the anterior cruciate ligament. Injuries to the lateral stabilizing ligaments of the knee result from a medially directed force which almost always involves a rotational component applied to the tibia. Compared to the valgus injuries, medial direct forces to the knee are rather infrequent. The cruciate ligaments can also be involved, once again depending on the magnitude of the forces applied.

While a patient with an isolated Grade 1 (up to one-third of the ligament torn) or Grade 2 (one-third to two-thirds of the ligament torn) injury may immediately return to a sporting event, rarely will a patient do so with a Grade 3 (greater than two-thirds torn) sprain, which is typically associated with an anterior cruciate disruption. The patients often feel a ripping sensation, with discreet tenderness apparent to the examiner. The patient will frequently prefer some sort of protection whether it be an ace bandage, immobilizer or crutches as the knee feels insecure with weight-bearing. Pain can almost always be duplicated upon appropriate stressing of either the affected medial or lateral ligamentous complex. The degree of injury will be manifested by the degree of opening of the knee. With an isolated collateral ligament injury, swelling is not always an absolute feature. Swelling, if it does occur, will be noted within several hours, suggestive of blood-vessel disruption rather than of a synovial reaction. The absence of swelling may be indicative of a significant injury which has disrupted the capsule allowing blood to dissect down the calf and thus not be apparent intra-articularly.

When testing for instability, the medial collateral ligament should be stressed at both 0° and 30° of flexion. The medial collateral ligament is reinforced at 0° of flexion by the secondary restraint, the anterior cruciate ligament. At 30° of flexion, however, the testing is specific for the medial collateral ligament. In addition to instability, pain will usually be experienced by the patient, especially with Grade 1 and Grade 2 injuries. For lateral instability, a varus force is gently applied.

The routine radiographic analysis of the knee will not disclose an injury to the collateral ligaments unless there has been a bony avulsion. In the chronic injury, however, it is very common to see evidence of calcification at the origin of the medial collateral ligament (Pellegrini—Stieda phenomenon) (Noyes *et al.*, 1974). Stress films have been recommended in the past and are certainly helpful when more specific testing is not possible (Fig. 25.29). In addition to the previously discussed advantages of magnetic resonance imaging in identifying meniscal lesions, this procedure has been quite helpful in delineating the site of disruption of the collateral complexes (Fig. 25.30). The tears can usually be seen by a decreased signal intensity along the course of the collateral ligaments.

Methods of treatment

Grade 1 and 2 collateral ligament injuries should be

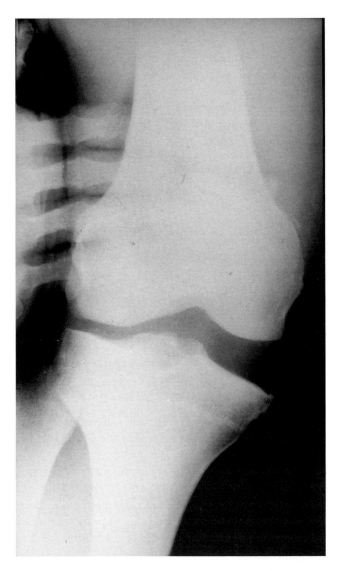

Fig. 25.29 Valgus stress test performed with standard radiograms will often reveal a Grade III tear of the medial collateral ligament.

treated non-operatively as long as the anterior cruciate ligament has not also been disrupted. It is, however, rather unusual for the anterior cruciate to be damaged with a Grade 1 or 2 injury. The non-operative approach consists of three phases: Phase I — pain and inflammation control; Phase II — strengthening; and Phase III — return to functional levels (Rettig, 1991). Immobilization can be discontinued within 5 days. Quadriceps strengthening exercises should be commenced initially. Protection in the form of a cane or sleeve brace is recommended for the first week. A sleeve-type brace with a hinge should be used throughout Phase I and II and even in Phase III which is a return to more functional activities such as running and cutting. In Grade 3 collateral ligament injuries in which it has been ascertained

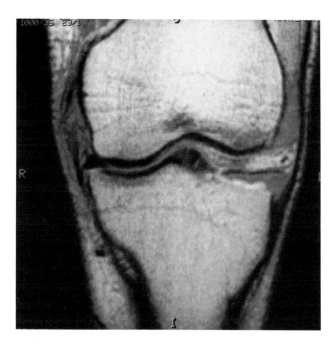

Fig. 25.30 A magnetic resonance imaging coronal view of the knee through the medial collateral ligament. There is blood and oedema involving the subcutaneous tissues. Note that the iliotibial band in comparison is a continuous dark signal. (Courtesy of Dr Morton Schneider.)

be too tight. Medial collateral ligament injuries can be approached through direct medial incision over the collateral structure preferably localized to the area of maximum tenderness and disruption. With tears of the medial collateral ligament and posterior oblique ligament, Hughston advocates a careful dissection of re-attachment of the posterior oblique ligament. For lateral instability, the more popular procedures include the Losee 'sling-and-reef' technique for lateral extra-articular instability (Fig. 25.31) and the Andrews lateral tenodesis of the iliotibial band (Fig. 25.32) or the Hey Groves fascia lata technique (Fig. 25.33). As a rule, most patients can return to a full sporting life with the isolated Grade 1 to 3 ligament injuries between 6 and 12 weeks. It is thus the authors' protocol to keep them in a sleeve-type brace with medial and lateral metal reinforcement for approximately 1 year after the injury. Isolated injuries to the collateral ligaments when treated conservatively are not associated with future instability or meniscal lesions. Indeed, meniscal lesions are rare, occurring less than 4% of the time with Grade 1 and 2 injuries and in the range 0−13% in Grade 3 injuries (Macey, 1939; Derscheid and Garrick, 1981; Ritter *et al.*, 1983; Rettig, 1991).

CRUCIATE LIGAMENTS

Individuals who were first credited with repairs of the anterior cruciate included Battle (1900), Goetjes (1913), Hey Groves (1919), Campbell (1936) and Smith (Snook, 1936). The approach towards cruciate ligament injuries is one of the most controversial areas in orthopaedic surgery. The posterior cruciate ligament is injured much less commonly than the anterior cruciate ligament. The primary function of the posterior cruciate ligament is to

that the anterior and posterior cruciate ligaments are not involved, non-operative treatment is also the preferred method of treatment (Indelicato, 1983).

Operative treatment of collateral ligaments usually occurs only in the setting of a concomitant cruciate disruption. Surgically, a direct end-to-end suture is permissible but an interlacing Bunnell-type repair is more advisable. Stiffness can be a major problem in collateral ligament repair and thus the repair should not

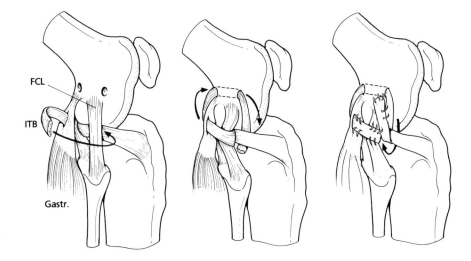

Fig. 25.31 Losee 'sling-and-reef' technique for lateral extra-articular instability. (Redrawn by permission from Scott, 1991.)

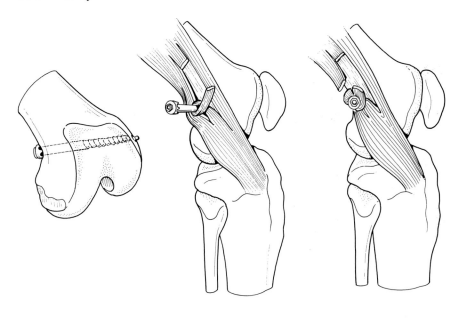

Fig. 25.32 The Andrews lateral tenodesis of the iliotibial band. (Redrawn by permission from Scott, 1991.)

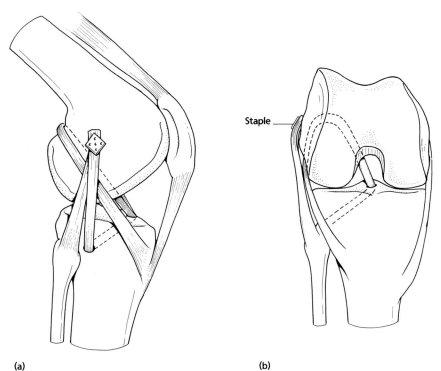

Staple

(a)   (b)

Fig. 25.33 The Hey Groves fascia lata technique for lateral reconstruction. (Redrawn by permission from Insall, 1984e.)

prevent posterior displacement of the tibia on the femur. This ligament accounts for 95% of the restraining force for such displacement (Meyers *et al.*, 1975).

In the most publicized Instrom testing of the anterior cruciate ligament and certain substitutes, Noyes *et al.* (1978) reported that the anterior cruciate ligament bone complex is able to withstand approximately 1730 N (400 lb) before complete rupture. During daily activities, it was shown that the anterior cruciate ligament is

subjected to only 454 N (100 lb) and that ligaments in young adults can stretch 25% without failure. Increasing age, however, is associated with a definite decrease in the load-bearing characteristics of the anterior cruciate ligament. In trying to assess the relative strength of cruciate substitutes, Noyes *et al.* (1978) performed Instrom tests on several preparations including patellar tendon with its associated retinaculum, a patellar tendon bone preparation, iliotibial band and the semitendinosus tendon. The biomechanical data on anterior and posterior cruciate ligament substitutes is complicated by the question of whether 'dynamic' reconstructions exist. Insall (1984e), in describing the intra-articular transfer of the iliotibial band, felt that the anatomy suggested this procedure could be both a static and dynamic reconstruction.

In general, ligaments can elongate 10–25% of their resting length (Scott, 1991). Cruciate ligament injuries can, like collateral ligament injuries, be partial. An anterior cruciate ligament injury usually involves a twisting manoeuvre associated with sudden deceleration, abduction/external rotation, hyperextension, or rarely a varus and internal rotation movement. Posterior cruciate disruption is normally caused by a posteriorly directed force on the proximal tibia. Hyperextension and abduction/external rotation movements have also been described in the production of posterior cruciate ligament injuries.

The diagnosis of a torn anterior cruciate ligament is often suggested by the circumstances of the injury. The twisting deceleration type of injury, with or without contact, is often associated with a 'pop' and swelling present within a few hours. While swelling is a characteristic to look for, complacency should be avoided if swelling is not apparent since capsular tears allow the fluid to extravasate from the joint. It is important to remember that the presence of an acute haemarthrosis is usually indicative of a cruciate ligament injury although it may also be associated with chondral fracture, patellar dislocation, peripheral meniscal tear or intraarticular fracture. An examination within minutes of injury is probably the most productive examination. It is very difficult thereafter for most patients to relax enough to perform the diagnostic tests.

Classification of instability

The American Orthopedic Society for Sports Medicine (AOSSM) Research and Education Committee (1976) has formulated a classification system that combines clinical and operative findings. This system includes knee instabilities which are best classified as either straight (non-rotatory or one plane), rotatory (simple or two plane), or combined. While this system has been generally accepted, it should be noted that there are significant objections to its use. Noyes *et al.* (1974) and Daniel (1988) believe that an infinite number of different combinations of instability can exist when injuries occur in more than one plane.

A rating of zero instability implies normal laxity, 1+ is an anterior translation of less than 0.5 cm, 2+ is

between 0.5 and 1 cm, and 3+ is between 1 and 1.5 cm. Grade 4, a colloquial rating, indicates a translation of greater than 1.5 cm. The rotatory instabilities include anteromedial, posteromedial, anterolateral, posterolateral and combined. In anteromedial instability, the anteromedial aspect of the tibial plateau pivots abnormally allowing increased anterior translation. Anteromedial rotatory instability (AMRI) is defined as tibial abduction, external rotation and anterior translation. Depending on the magnitude of forces, AMRI indicates a ruptured anterior cruciate ligament, disruption of the posteromedial corner and the medial collateral ligament. The rotatory instabilities described are the final positions of the knee at the time of the examination as a result of the specific injuries. Abnormal translation should be assessed after examination of the non-affected extremity. Anterolateral rotatory instability (ALRI) corresponds to rupture of the lateral capsular ligament, lateral collateral ligament and anterior cruciate ligament. Varus injury and internal rotation is the usual mechanism of injury. Stability can be detected by the pivot shift manoeuvre, MacIntosh test, jerk test, ALRI test and Losee test.

In posteromedial rotatory instability (PMRI), the medial tibial plateau is able to displace posteromedially. This suggests an injury usually by hyperextension and valgus forces affecting the medial collateral ligament, medial capsular ligament, posterior oblique ligament and anterior cruciate ligament. The posterior cruciate ligament must be intact thus providing the axis of rotation for both posteromedial and posterolateral displacement. Posterolateral rotatory instability produces a reverse pivot shift and involves the posterolateral capsule, primarily arcuate complex and anterior cruciate ligament. There have been multiple attempts at developing mechanical ligament testing devices. Presently, there are three such devices that are most commonly used, the KT-1000 Arthrometer, the Stryker Knee Laxity Tester and the Genucom.

Tests for instability

Numerous clinical tests can be used to assess various ligamentous injuries in the knee. The Lachman test (Fig. 25.34) is probably the most sensitive manoeuvre for eliciting anterior cruciate disruption, particularly in the acute setting where considerable motion of the patient's knee is too painful to be tolerated (Kennedy *et al.*, 1974). This test (Norwood *et al.*, 1977) has been described with the knee comfortably flexed between 15 and 30°. The anterior drawer test is performed with the patient in the supine position and the knee flexed 90° (Figs 25.35 and 25.36). The examiner should be certain

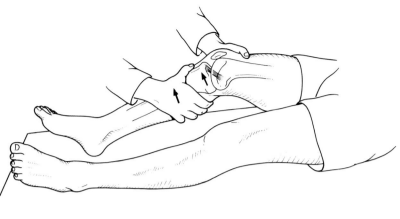

Fig. 25.34 The Lachman test is performed with the knee flexed between 15° and 30°. (Redrawn by permission from W.N. Scott, *Ligament and Extensor Mechanism Injuries of the Knee: Diagnosis and Treatment*, 1991, C.V. Mosby.)

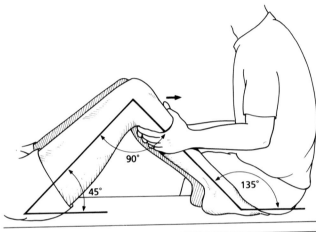

Fig. 25.35 The anterior drawer test is performed with the patient supine and the effected knee bent 90°. The examiner then exerts an anterior force to detect any asymmetry between the two legs. (Redrawn by permission from J.N. Insall, *Surgery of the Knee*, 1984, Churchill Livingstone.)

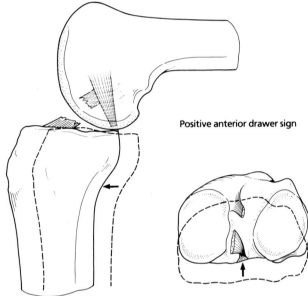

Positive anterior drawer sign

Fig. 25.36 A positive anterior drawer test, with the knee in neutral position, signifies a torn anterior cruciate ligament. (Redrawn by permission from J.N. Insall, *Surgery of the Knee*, 1984, Churchill Livingstone.)

that the foot points forward without any rotatory movement, and the patient is relaxed. With the foot stabilized and each hand enveloping the proximal tibia, a forward pull is made. The examiner can elicit anteromedial or anterolateral instability by performing the drawer test with the foot in external rotation (anteromedial) (Fig. 25.37) or internal rotation (anterolateral) (Fig. 25.38). Sometimes there may be a discrepency between the Lachman test and the drawer test; this has been attributed to a differential injury to the anteromedial and posterolateral bundles of the anterior cruciate ligament. A negative Lachman indicates an intact posterolateral bundle, while a positive anterior drawer indicates a disrupted anteromedial bundle. The posterior drawer test is done in a similar fashion with the examiner trying to displace the tibia posteriorly rather than anteriorly (Figs 25.39 and 25.40).

A patient's description of the knee 'going out' is described as the 'pivot shift phenomenon' (MacIntosh and Galway, 1972; Galway and MacIntosh, 1980). The MacIntosh test (MacIntosh and Galway, 1972) (Fig. 25.41) is performed with the knee extended and valgus stress applied to the proximal tibia with the foot internally rotated. As the knee is flexed, the lateral tibial plateau will subluxate forward until 20–40° of flexion when the tibia is reduced by the iliotibial tract moving posteriorly. The 'jerk' test begins with the knee in a flexed position (Fig. 25.42) as contrasted to the extended position of the MacIntosh manoeuvre (Fig. 25.43). Thus, the tibia is starting out in a reduced position and there will be a sudden 'jerk' between 20 and 40° of flexion as

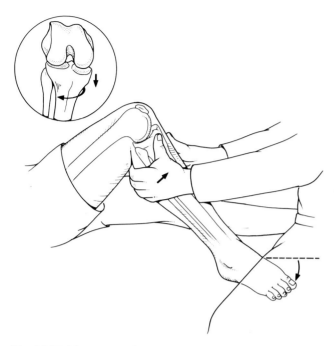

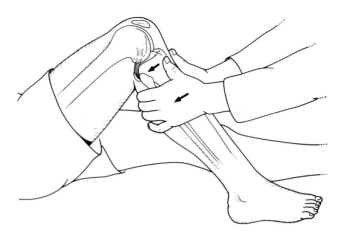

Fig. 25.39 The posterior test is performed in the same fashion as the anterior drawer (Fig. 25.38) except that the examiner exerts a posterior force. (Redrawn by permission from W.N. Scott, *Ligament and Extensor Mechanism Injuries of the Knee: Diagnosis and Treatment*, 1991, C.V. Mosby.)

Fig. 25.37 The anterior drawer test with the knee in 15° of external rotation (Slocum) illustrates posteromedial capsule and usually anterior cruciate ligament disruption. (Redrawn by permission from W.N. Scott, *Ligament and Extensor Mechanism Injuries of the Knee: Diagnosis and Treatment*, 1991, C.V. Mosby.)

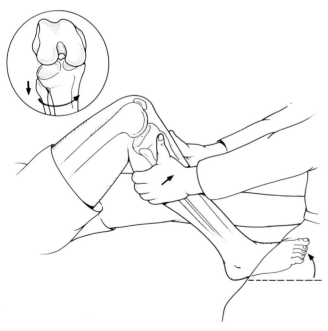

Fig. 25.38 Anterior drawer with the knee in 30° of internal rotation illustrates posterolateral capsule and anterior cruciate ligament disruption. (Redrawn by permission from W.N. Scott, *Ligament and Extensor Mechanism Injuries of the Knee: Diagnosis and Treatment*, 1991, C.V. Mosby.)

the knee extends. This phenomenon is a subluxation of the lateral tibial plateau anteriorly.

To diagnose posterolateral rotatory instability, use can be made of the external rotation and recurvatum test, the posterolateral drawer test and the reverse pivot shift (Hughston *et al.*, 1976; Hughston and Norwood, 1980; Jacob *et al.*, 1981; Reider, 1991). In the external rotation recurvatum test, the affected extremity is held by the toes with the leg in extension. The posterolateral drawer test is done with the knee flexed between 60° and 90° and the foot externally rotated. When a posterior drawer test is performed, the lateral tibial plateau will displace posteriorly. A reverse pivot shift manoeuvre is performed by providing a valgus stress to a flexed knee with the foot in external rotation. As the knee is extended, the lateral tibial plateau will be reduced from its posterolateral position, a movement visible at the moment of reduction (Fig. 25.43).

Arthroscopic examination is the best method of assessing the condition of the anterior cruciate ligament. Observation of the posterior cruciate ligament, however, is more difficult arthroscopically, and it is probably not as reliable as magnetic resonance imaging which has been a major help in evaluating the integrity of the anterior and posterior cruciate ligaments. A normal anterior cruciate ligament will present as a homogeneous dark ligamentous structure extending from the lateral femoral condyle to the tibial plateau (Fig. 25.44). While magnetic resonance imaging diagnosis of complete tears of the anterior cruciate ligament has reached the 90% accuracy range, partial tears remain difficult to assess. During arthroscopy, the insertion of the anterior cruciate

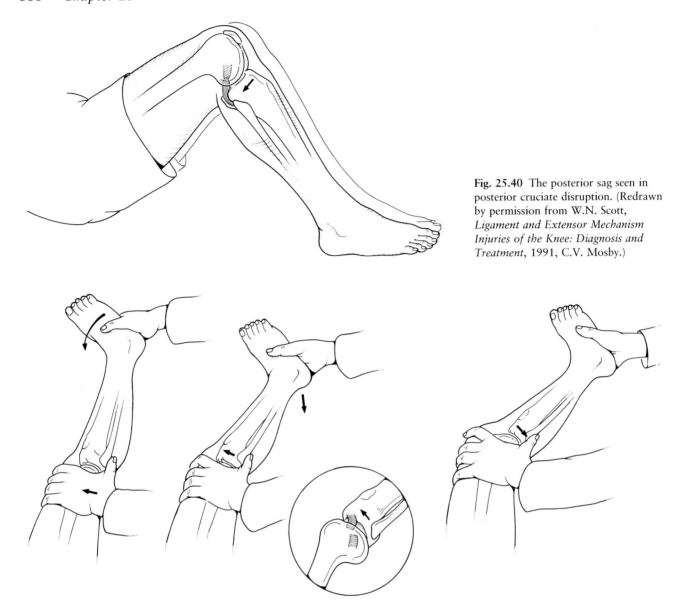

Fig. 25.40 The posterior sag seen in posterior cruciate disruption. (Redrawn by permission from W.N. Scott, *Ligament and Extensor Mechanism Injuries of the Knee: Diagnosis and Treatment*, 1991, C.V. Mosby.)

Fig. 25.41 In the pivot shift of Galway and MacIntosh, the test is done with the knee in full extension while applying a valgus and internal rotation stress. The 'clunk' of reduction is felt in the first 20−30° of flexion. (Redrawn by permission from W.N. Scott, *Ligament and Extensor Mechanism Injuries of the Knee: Diagnosis and Treatment*, 1991, C.V. Mosby.)

ligament on the tibial plateau can appear relatively normal, only to find a disruption in the proximal 20% of the ligament (Fig. 25.45). The origin of the posterior cruciate ligament can usually be assessed through a standard anterolateral portal. It is often necessary to use an anteromedial portal to see the midsubstance of the posterior cruciate ligament. To fully assess its insertion on the back of the tibia, a posterior medial puncture site is required with the probe usually entering through an anteromedial portal.

Methods of treatment

Even the proponents of non-operative treatment agree that the untreated anterior cruciate ligament 'leads to anterior laxity, rotatory instabilities, and meniscal tears, and there is a definite increase in roentgenographic changes of joint space narrowing and osteoarthritis' (McDaniel and Dameron, 1983). Approximately one-third of patients with an isolated anterior cruciate ligament injury will probably not develop functional

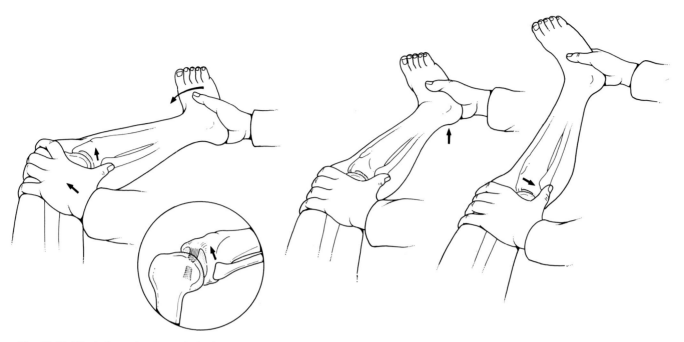

Fig. 25.42 The jerk test begins with the knee in flexion while applying a valgus and internal rotation force. The thumb pushes the tibia forward and the clunk of reduction is felt as the knee approaches full extension. (Redrawn by permission from W.N. Scott, *Ligament and Extensor Mechanism Injuries of the Knee: Diagnosis and Treatment*, 1991, C.V. Mosby.)

instability. Two-thirds, however, will have some functional instability (Noyes *et al.*, 1983). Development of osteoarthritis at a later time certainly seems to occur with a higher incidence although no unequivocal data have been presented (McDaniel and Dameron, 1983). Similarly, it is important to understand that at this stage there are no long-term cruciate reconstruction or repair studies that unequivocally prove operative treatment will prevent the development of arthritic changes. The risk:benefit ratio must include assessment of the patient's lifestyle, willingness to comply with rehabilitation and long-term conditioning. Associated ligament injuries certainly might compel the surgeon to be more aggressive in suggesting operative treatment although, once again, the natural history of multiple ligamentous injuries about the knee is not truly known. It is, however, logical to assume that the non-operative treatment in this situation has less of a chance of success than in the isolated anterior cruciate ligament injury.

Non-operative therapy can begin soon after treating any associated meniscal or articular cartilage injuries. Considering the function of the anterior cruciate ligament, resisting anterior displacement, it is important to rehabilitate the hamstring muscle group and maintain strength in the quadriceps and proximal muscle groups. Stress-relieving strengthening methods are begun almost immediately and include swimming and non-weight-bearing strengthening modalities such as hamstring

strengthening in a flexed position and bicycle riding. Once the patient's strength has reached acceptable standards as determined by various testing modalities, the patient should be braced and may commence activities (Saraniti *et al.*, 1991).

Much controversy exists as to whether bracing of the ligamentously injured knee is beneficial (Bach, 1991). While it was somewhat tempting to 'prophylactically brace' football players to minimize career-threatening ligament injuries, the data associated with these studies have been inconclusive. A functional knee brace is designed for the unstable knee (Bach *et al.*, 1988) (see Chapter 34). While these braces have been designed to control pathological laxity in the anterior cruciate-deficient knee, clinical and biochemical studies have refuted these claims (Markolf *et al.*, 1976; Butler *et al.*, 1980; Fukubayashi *et al.*, 1982; Hanten and Pace, 1987; Branch *et al.*, 1988).

The physician should first review all the operative and non-operative alternatives with the patient. If it is decided that surgery is the best treatment, the physician has three options: (i) primary repair; (ii) intra-articular reconstruction; and (iii) combined intra- and extra-articular reconstruction. A successful reconstruction should allow the knee to develop the following: (i) functional motion; (ii) stability; (iii) limit long-term development of osteoarthritic changes; (iv) reinnervation of the joint; (v) reproducibility; and (vi) minimization of the potential

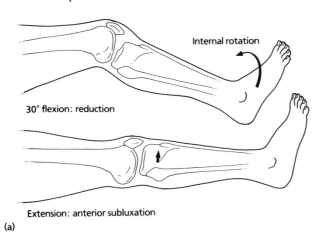

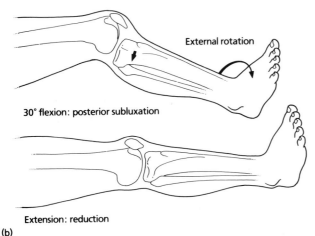

Fig. 25.43 In the pivot shift test, while the foot is internally rotated, the tibia will sublux forward with knee extension (a) In the reverse pivot shift test (b) the tibia will sublux posteriorly with flexion. (Redrawn by permission from J.N. Insall, *Surgery of the Knee*, 1984, Churchill Livingstone.)

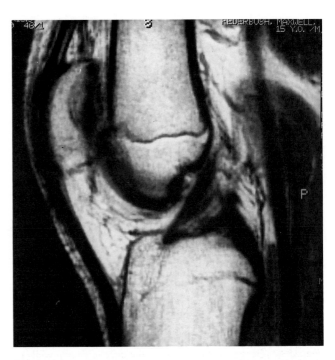

Fig. 25.44 Thin section sagittal and coronal views demonstrate a normal low-intensity signal, forming the anterior cruciate ligament at 3 mm (A) slices. (Courtesy of Dr. Morton Schneider.)

for complications. It is important to try to return the static stability as close as possible to the normal extremity. While no difference is ideal, a 1+ grade is almost always functionally acceptable to the patient. The repaired or reconstructed ligament must be adequately protected during revascularization and subsequent recollagenization. The cruciate substitute should be of adequate strength. It is important for the patient to achieve a range of motion from 10° to 110° quickly and thus minimize patellofemoral complications. Primary repair of the anterior cruciate ligament, while initially encouraging, has had poor 5-year evaluations. In reviews by Sherman and Bonamo (1988) and Wickiewicz (1987) the isolated repairs have shown a steady erosion of the early good results.

The four types of intra-articular reconstructions are: (i) static; (ii) static and dynamic; (iii) allografts; and (iv) prosthetic. The most commonly used static reconstructions are the intra-articular semitendinosus transfer, patellar tendon transfer and its variations (of which the most common today is bone−patella tendon−bone preparation), the gracilis and proximally based iliotibial band reconstructions.

The tendon of the semitendinosus has been utilized as either a free graft or a partially attached transfer. It maintains either its origin or insertion and may sometimes be augmented with gracilis tendons. Multiple authors have suggested the use of the semitendinosus as a static intra-articular stabilizer passed through a drill hole in the proximal tibia and re-routed over the top of the lateral femoral condyle (Bianchi, 1983). Improvements in arthroscopic techniques have allowed the semitendinosus to be used in this fashion with screw, washer or double-staple fixation. Arthroscopic advancements have encouraged the use of tibial and femoral tunnels although some over-the-top procedures are still performed. The unitunnel technique advocated by Hendler *et al.* (1988) certainly is quite amenable to arthroscopic performance. While clinical success has been quite rewarding in multiple series, the lack of a bone-to-bone fixation in either the femoral or tibial tunnel has remained as an unattractive feature. The contraindication is damage to the semitendinosus tendon itself. A relative contra-its initial strength. Clancy (1988a) suggests that the revascularization is much quicker because Arnoczky's study did not take into account femoral and tibial bone tunnels and their input to the revascularization. This procedure has gained widespread clinical acceptance and the early results seem promising.

Approximately one-third of the width of the patellar tendon is harvested with a patellar and tibial bone block attached to the tendon. The harvesting incision can be extended to the medial placement of the tibial drill hole. Arthroscopic assistance is of utmost importance in locating and preparing the intercondylar notch and the drill hole at the posteromedial aspect of the lateral femoral condyle. Fixation of the structure has been through the use of an interference fit screw, malleolar screw, or when brought in the over-the-top fashion without a proximal bone graft with the use of a staple or screw and washer techniques (Clancy, 1988a; Wang and Hewson, 1988; Reider, 1991). Rehabilitation based on clinical experience has been reported to be 6 months.

Intra-articular transfer of the iliotibial muscle tendon unit as described by Insall is the most commonly utilized static and dynamic reconstruction for anterior cruciate insufficiency. The iliotibial band has probably accounted for more intra- and extra-articular cruciate reconstructions than any other supporting structure about the knee (Nicholas and Minkoff, 1978; Insall *et al.*, 1981; Scott and Schosheim, 1983; Insall, 1984b, e; Scott *et al.*, 1985). The proximally based intra-articular procedure has been described independently by two separate authors, Insall (1981) and Nicholas and Minkoff (1978). In the Insall technique, the anterior portion of the iliotibial band and its continuous relationship with the lateral retinaculum, its proximal connection to the fascia overlying the vastus lateralis and its interstitial attachment to the lateral intermuscular septum, were maintained and tubed to increase the cross-sectional area and subsequent strength. While initially performed in 1976, several modifications have improved the static stability of this procedure (Fig. 25.46). The largest published series to date has shown a direct correlation with improved static stability and limited dissection (Scott *et al.*, 1985; Scott, 1991). The advantages of this technique are that it allows immediate range of motion and full weight-bearing within 3–4 weeks.

Intra-articular transfer of the iliotibial band is successful in almost 85% of patients (Scott *et al.*, 1985; Scott, 1991). Unlike all other cruciate reconstructions, parity of hamstring muscle strength is usually achieved at 6–8 weeks post-operatively with the iliotibial transfer. Quadriceps strength, however, takes longer and would be a limiting factor in the patient's return to vigorous athletic

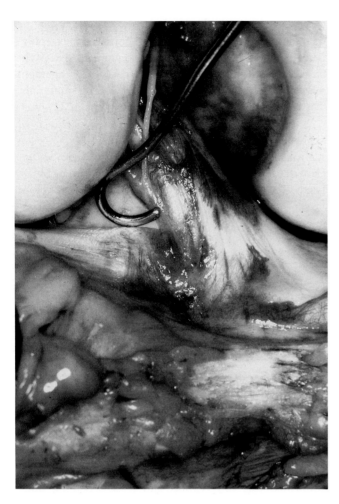

Fig. 25.45 The inferior portion of the anterior cruciate appears normal at arthrotomy yet proximal portion (above the hook) manifests the disruption of the fibres.

indication would be a concurrent medial capsular and ligamentous complex injury.

Arthroscopic-assisted cruciate reconstruction with a bone–patellar tendon–bone graft is a commonly performed procedure. This particular preparation of patellar tendon is now the most commonly used method. Clinical results with the bone–patellar tendon–bone preparation have been quite encouraging, and in fact, as early as 1983, Clancy (1988a) stated that 'none of the fifty patients had an episode of instability after operation'. The procedure has undergone modifications including the use of a vascularized fat-pad pedicle, although subsequent studies have shown it to be ineffective (Reider, 1991). The healing properties of this free graft have been shown by Arnoczky *et al.* (1982) to take 2–6 months to revascularize and at least another 6–8 weeks to recollagenize. Their studies also show that one year after implantation the preparation only has one-half of

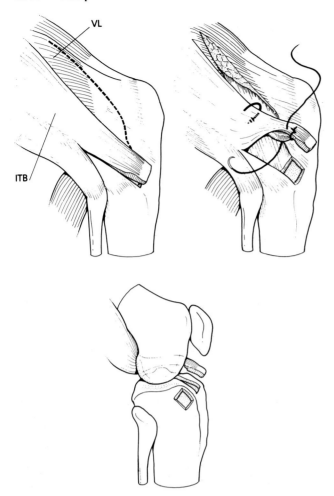

Fig. 25.46 Several of the modifications of the Insall intra-articular transfer of the iliotibial band include the limited posterior dissection which maintains the attachment to the lateral intermuscular septum. (Redrawn by permission from W.N. Scott, *Ligament and Extensor Mechanism Injuries of the Knee: Diagnosis and Treatment*, 1991, C.V. Mosby.)

activities. Once there is symmetrical extensor strength, the patient is then returned to sporting endeavour. This procedure is contraindicated in the presence of an acute lateral capsular ligamentous injury.

The third type of intra-articular reconstruction of the anterior cruciate-deficient knee utilizes allografts. The most commonly used allograft now is the bone−patellar tendon−bone preparation and in the last few years has seen a limited application. Early results are controversial and relate to the method of preservation and preparation of the allograft.

Synthetic material was first used as a substitute for knee ligaments in 1906. In the 1990s, there are four general categories of prosthetic ligaments: (i) permanent; (ii) stent; (iii) augmentation; and (iv) ingrowth or scaffold. The permanent prosthetic ligaments include

Gore-Tex (polytetrafluoroethylene), Xenotech (bovine ligament, Stryker Dacron velour graft, Proflex (polyethylene) and Dacron-hytrel fibre ligament. The stent type of prosthetic implants are Proplast, LAD (ligament augmentation device) and various Dacron materials. The only augmentation type of device is the LAD which is a braided polyproplyene. The fourth category of artificial ligaments are those materials that act as a scaffold while theoretically promoting ligamentous ingrowth. The representative ligaments are carbon fibres, Leeds-Keio (a Dacron open weave), a Dacron-velour fascia lata composite, high-strength Dacron, ABC ligament (a carbon and Dacron composite) and allografts. The Gore-Tex experience, for instance, has shown a steady decline from two- to five-year evaluations, with one-third of all patients complaining of buckling at the five-year evaluation (DuToit, 1967; Ahlfeld *et al.*, 1987; Scott, 1991). On the other hand, the addition of a LAD to a patella tendon autograft has resulted in improved stability (Ahfeld *et al.*, 1987).

Numerous authors have advocated combined intra- and extra-articular reconstructions as a treatment for anterior cruciate deficiency. In the report by Yost *et al.* (1981) it did not seem to make any difference as to whether any extra-articular procedure was performed or whether an acute repair of either collateral ligament was performed at the time of cruciate reconstruction. Subsequent authors (Sherman and Bonamo, 1988) have confirmed this observation and it is becoming quite common not to address collateral ligament injuries at the time of cruciate substitution nor to try and 'reinforce' the cruciate reconstruction with extra-articular procedures. In chronic instability, however, the chance for repair of the collateral structures is not present and it is often necessary to combine an extra-articular procedure to resist the secondary instabilities that might have appeared.

Since there is no surgical technique in which it has been unequivocally proven that intervention has either delayed or eliminated the development of degenerative joint disease, we strongly believe that no patient should have an anterior cruciate reconstruction solely for the purpose of 'not developing arthritis'. Thus, in non-aggressive or non-athletic individuals, a non-operative approach might be best.

Treatment of posterior cruciate injury

Treatment options for posterior cruciate ligament tears are predicated on the severity of the injury (partial or complete) and whether there has been an avulsion (Fig. 25.47) or an interstitial tear (Fig. 25.48). In numerous

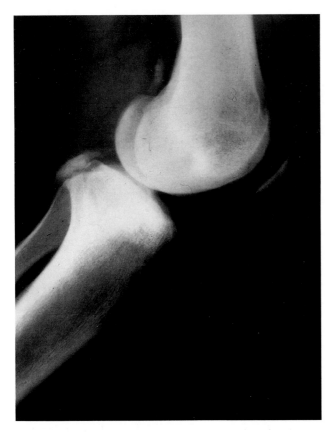

Fig. 25.47 Obvious avulsion of the posterior cruciate ligament which inserts on the posterior portion of the tibia. (Reproduced by permission from W.N. Scott, *Ligament and Extensor Mechanism Injuries of the Knee: Diagnosis and Treatment*, 1991, C.V. Mosby.)

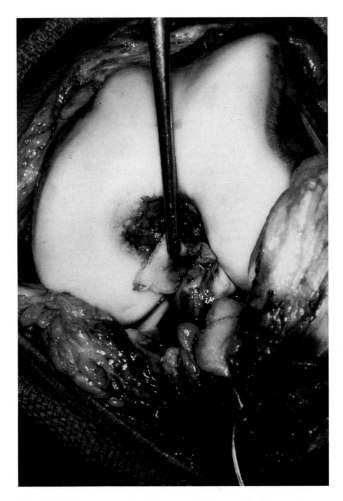

Fig. 25.48 Intraoperative photograph of an avulsed posterior cruciate ligament. (Reproduced by permission from W.N. Scott, *Ligament and Extensor Mechanism Injuries of the Knee: Diagnosis and Treatment*, 1991, C.V. Mosby.)

articles (Kennedy, 1967; Kennedy and Galpin, 1982; Clancy *et al.*, 1983; Cross and Powell, 1984; Parolic and Bergfeld, 1986; Clancy, 1988b) the suggestion is rather obvious that surgical treatment of acute injuries seems to have the best prognosis. In addition, most posterior cruciate ligament injuries are usually associated with other major ligamentous disruption throughout the knee whether it be anterior or collateral capsular ligament disruption.

Meyers' evaluation of 14 avulsion injuries showed that the use of a long leg cast for 8 weeks resulted in non-union in four of five minimally displaced fractures with eventual 'significant functional disability' (Meyers *et al.*, 1975). Similarly, in that same series the operative repair of these avulsions gave excellent results in almost 90% of cases. With avulsions, re-attachment of the avulsed fragment is the treatment of choice. The most commonly utilized approach is that of Abbott and Carpenter (1944) which directly visualizes the insertion of the posterior cruciate on the tibia allowing re-approximation.

Dandy and Poosey (1982) reported that subjective and objective results were not related when a non-operative approach was used with acute interstitial injuries. The patients seem to tolerate instability and did not want to undergo the rigors of a surgical reconstruction. Treatment of these interstitial injuries consists of a brief period of immobilization which gives relief of symptomatic complaints and an aggressive quadriceps rehabilitation programme. Direct surgical repair of acutely injured interstitial posterior cruciate ligament injuries has had minimal success (Bianchi, 1983; Clancy, 1988b; Scott, 1991). Several approaches have been used for reconstructing this ligament including substitution by the popliteus tendon, semitendinosus and gracilis, lateral meniscus, semimembranosus, medial head of the gastrocnemius and the patellar tendon (Elmslie, 1978; Insall and Hood, 1982; Kennedy and Galpin, 1982; Scott, 1991).

Clancy *et al.* (1983) and Clancy (1988b) reported 90% good-to-excellent static results for 'the past ten years with utilization of repair and a patellar tendon graft for the treatment of acute PCL [posterior cruciate ligament] injuries'. They suggest a vertical tibial tunnel to allow for ease of retrograde passage of the bony portion of the patellar tendon graft. This procedure has recently been used augmenting the patellar tendon with a ligament augmentation device with some improved static stability. In an acutely injured posterior cruciate ligament it is the authors' belief that operative treatment probably has the greatest potential for success. The authors have observed that incorporation of the ligament augmentation device with a patella tendon graft has resulted in a decrease in the post-operative posterior sag sign (Fig. 25.40).

The authors utilize the medial head of the gastrocnemius when the patellar tendon has been previously used. Substituting the medial head of the gastrocnemius muscle with a bone block attachment is potentially both a static and dynamic reconstruction. Results with this procedure have been reported by Hughston *et al.* (1980), Kennedy (1982) and Insall (1982, 1984), and the conclusions are that while static stability is often not improved the subjective feeling is acceptable (Scott, 1991) (Fig. 25.49).

The complications of anterior or posterior cruciate reconstruction include infection, haematoma, skin necrosis, knee stiffness, prolonged effusion, tendonitis, extensor mechanism discomfort, patellar fracture, muscle hernia, sympathetic dystrophy, vascular injury and neurological injury. Arthroscopic surgical techniques are believed to minimize patellofemoral complications. It is fair to say that early mobilization is the most important contributing factor to minimize extensor mechanism discomfort as evidenced by the authors' own review of arthrotomy procedures. With the patellar tendon graft gaining popularity in both anterior and posterior cruciate reconstructions, attention must be focused on the complications that can occur using this structure. Tendonitis, infrapatellar contracture syndrome, rupture of the patellar tendon and patellar fracture have all been reported (Insall *et al.*, 1972).

DISLOCATIONS OF THE KNEE

Knee dislocation occurs rarely with the average orthopaedist observing one or two throughout an entire career (Fig. 25.50). In the Mayo Clinic only 14 knee dislocations were recorded during an interval of two million admissions (Montgomery, 1987).

The popliteal artery courses through a fibrous tunnel

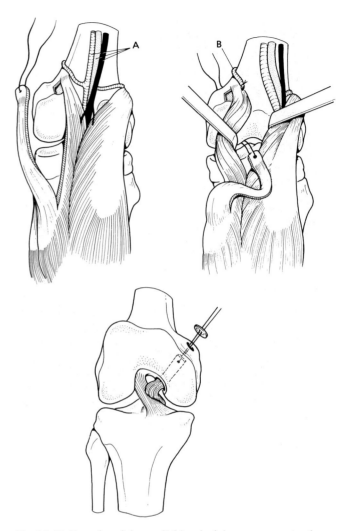

Fig. 25.49 Transfer of the medial head of the gastrocnemius for posterior cruciate insufficiency. (A) Popliteal artery, vein, nerve, (B) medial superior genicular artery. (Redrawn by permission from W.N. Scott, *Ligament and Extensor Mechanism Injuries of the Knee: Diagnosis and Treatment*, 1991, C.V. Mosby.)

at the level of the adductor hiatus. After it gives off the five genicular branches at the level of the knee joint, it passes deep to the soleus where it traverses another fibrous tunnel. The fixation of the artery in these tunnels causes a proximal and distal tethering, particularly at the time of a knee dislocation.

The five types of knee dislocations are anterior, posterior, medial, lateral and rotatory (usually posterolateral). These dislocations are always described with the tibia in relation to the femur, i.e. an anterior dislocation implies that the tibia is displaced anterior to the femur. An anterior dislocation is usually a result of a hyperextension in excess of 30° (Siliski, 1991). In these injuries the posterior cruciate and possibly the anterior cruciate are torn, and depending on the magnitude of

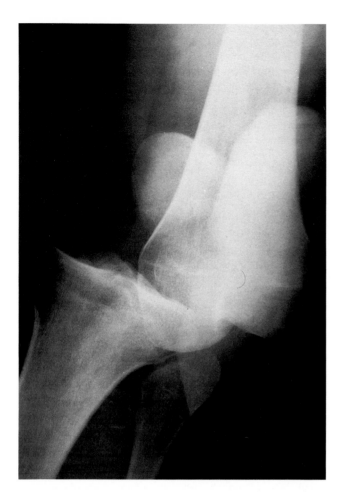

Fig. 25.50 Radiographic demonstration of a dislocated knee. (Reproduced by permission from W.N. Scott, *Ligament and Extensor Mechanism Injuries of the Knee: Diagnosis and Treatment*, 1991, C.V. Mosby.)

the injury, the popliteal artery may be lacerated. In a posterior dislocation, the tibia is translated posteriorly with disruption of both cruciate ligaments, and once again, depending on the magnitude of displacement, the popliteal artery. In a series by Green, involving 245 cases, 31% were anterior dislocations, 25% posterior, 13% lateral, 4% rotatory, 3% medial and 20% unspecified (Green and Allen, 1977).

The clinical presentation of a dislocated knee is of such gross distortion as to make the diagnosis apparent. It is most important not to take radiographs in the displaced position as an immediate reduction should be attempted. The mechanism of injury always involves a significant force whether it be an automobile accident or a sporting injury. The first concern is the arterial supply and the presence of a distal pulse does not exclude significant arterial injury. Similarly, peroneal nerve injury must be immediately assessed especially in the posterior

and posterolateral dislocations. Ligament injury with a traumatic dislocation of the knee is predictable as long as the displacement exceeds 10–25% of the ligament's resting length. Gross instability is readily apparent after reduction.

An angiogram should be performed after all knee dislocations. If there is disruption of the popliteal artery, then a vein graft is the preferred method of treatment. Most authors recommend the use of a contralateral saphenous vein interposition graft since ipsilateral popliteal vein injury is common. If the limb ischaemia exceeds 6 h, then a fasciotomy should be performed at the time of vascular repair. Peroneal nerve injury has been reported in 35% of cases (Shields *et al.*, 1969; Sisto and Warren, 1985; Siliski, 1991). The decision to operate on the nerve injury is controversial since no treatment modality has been irrefutably effective (Sisto and Warren, 1985; Siliski, 1991). Management of the ligamentous injuries has also remained controversial. A review by Sisto and Warren (1985) found that stiffness was more of a problem than instability. Meyers and Kennedy (1963) concluded that open repair of all ligaments has a greater prediction of success. In view of the problem with stiffness it seems reasonable to advocate open repair in all situations where vascular anastomosis has been re-established or in active patients. If there is no vascular contraindication to repairing the disrupted ligament structures at the time of the arterial surgery, then ligament repair should be done simultaneously. Neurolysis or direct anastomosis of disrupted nerves still is debatable in the authors' opinion. It would seem that immediate surgery might only be indicated in situations where this can be done microscopically, and the vasculature is intact. Post-operative treatment is aimed at establishing an early range of motion as quickly as possible while ascertaining that no neurovascular damage is being done. Range of motion should be completed within 4–6 weeks, with strengthening begun accordingly.

REFERENCES

Abbott L.C., Saunders J.B., Bosh F.C. and Anderson C.E. (1994) Injuries to the ligaments of the knee joint. *J. Bone Joint Surg.* **16**, 503–521.

Aglietti P., Insall J., Walker P.S. and Trent P. (1975) A new patella prosthesis. *Clin. Orthop.* **107**, 175–187.

Aglietti P., Insall J. and Cerulli G. (1983) Patellar pain and incongruence. I. Measurements of incongruence. *Clin. Orthop.* **176**, 217.

Ahstrom J.P. (1965) Osteochondral fracture in the knee joint associated with hypermobility and dislocation of the patella. *J. Bone Joint Surg.* **47A**, 1491–1502.

Ahlfeld S.K., Larson R.L. and Collins H.R. (1987) Anterior cruciate ligament reconstruction in the chronically unstable knee using an expanded PTFE prosthetic ligament. *Am. J. Sports Med.* **15**, 326–330.

Aichroth P. (1971) Osteochondritis dissecans of the knee. *J. Bone Joint Surg.* **53B**, 440.

Aichroth P.M. (1977) Osteochondral fracture and osteochondritis dissecans in sportsmen's knee injuries. *J. Bone Joint Surg.* **59B**, 108.

American Orthopedic Society for Sports Medicine Research and Education Committee, 1976.

Andren L. and Wehlin L. (1960) Double-contrast arthrography of the knee with horizontal roentgen ray beam. *Acta Orthop. Scand.* **29**, 307.

Arnoczky S.P. (1983) Anatomy of the anterior cruciate ligament. *Clin Orthop.* **172**, 19–25.

Arnoczky S.P. (1991) Physiological principles of ligament injuries and healing. In Scott W.N. (ed.) *Ligament and Extensor Mechanism Injuries of the Knee: Diagnosis and Treatment.* St. Louis, C.V. Mosby.

Arnoczky S.P. and Warren R.F. (1982) Micro-vasculature of the human meniscus. *Am. J. Sports Med.* **10**, 90.

Arnoczky S.P. and Warren R.F. (1983) The micro-vasculature of the meniscus and its response to injury: an experimental study in the dog. *Am. J. Sports Med.* **11**(3), 131–141.

Arnoczky S.P., Tarvin G.B. and Marshall J.L. (1982) Anterior cruciate ligament replacement using the patella tendon: an evaluation of graft revascularization in the dog. *J. Bone Joint Surg.* **64**, 217.

Bach B. (1991) Ligament testing devices and bracing. In Scott W.N. (ed.) *Ligament and Extensor Mechanism Injuries of the Knee: Diagnosis and Treatment.* St. Louis, C.V. Mosby.

Bach B.R. Jr., Flynn W., Warren R.F. and Wickiewicz T.L. (1988) KT 1000 arthrometer evaluation of normal, acute, and chronic anterior cruciate ligament patients. *Orthop. Trans.* **12**, 194.

Bach B.R. Jr., Warren R.F., Flynn W. *et al.* Generalized ligamentous laxity and its affect on KT 1000 evaluation of normal and ACL deficient knees. (In preparation.)

Bach B.R. Jr., Wang C.W., Du L.R. and Hager C.A. A comparative study of the anterior drawer, Lachman, and pivot shift tests and the KT 1000 knee ligament arthrometer in the clinical diagnosis of ACL insufficiencies. (Submitted for publication.)

Barber F.A. and Stone R.G. (1985) Meniscal repair: an arthroscopic technique. *J. Bone Joint Surg.* **67B**(1), 39–41.

Battle W.H. (1900) A case after open section of the knee joint for irreversible traumatic dislocation. *Clin. Soc. Lond. Trans.* **33**, 232.

Bauer M. and Jackson R.W. (1988) Chondral lesions of the femoral condyles: a system of arthroscopic classification. *J. Arthroscop. Rel. Surg.* **4**(2), 97–102.

Bianchi M. (1983) Acute tears of the posterior cruciate ligament: clinical study and results of operative treatment in twenty-seven cases. *Am. J. Sports Med.* **11**, 308.

Blackburne J.S. and Peel T.E. (1977) A new method of measuring patella height. *J. Bone Joint Surg.* **59B**, 241.

Blumensaat C. (1938) Die Lageabweichungen und Verrenkungen der Kniescheibe. *Ergeb. Cir. Orthop.* **31**, 149.

Boon-Itt S.B. (1930) The normal position of the patella. *J. Roentgen Soc.* **24**, 389.

Branch T., Hunter R. and Reynolds P. (1988) Controlling anterior tibial displacement under static load: a comparison of two braces. *Orthopaedics* **11**, 1249–1252.

Brattstrom H. (1970) Patella alta in non-dislocating knee joints. *Acta Orthop. Scand.* **41**, 578–588.

Budinger K. (1906) Ueber Ablosung von Gelenktulen und ver-

wandte Prozesse. *Dtch. Z. Chir.* **84**, 311.

Butler D.L., Noyes F.R. and Grood E.S. (1980) Ligamentous restraints to anterior–posterior drawer in the human knee. *J. Bone Joint Surg.* **62A**, 259–270.

Cabaud H.E., Rodkey W.G. and Fitzwater J.E. (1981) Medial meniscus repairs: an experimental and morphological study. *Am. J. Sports Med.* **9**(3), 129–134.

Calendruccio R.A. and Gilmer W.S. (1962) Proliferation, regeneration, and repair of articular cartilage of immature animals. *J. Bone Joint Surg.* **44A**(3), 431–455.

Campbell W.C. (1936) Repair of the ligaments of the knee. *Surg. Gynec. Obstet.* **62**, 964.

Cheung M.S., Cottrell W.H., Stephenson K. and Nimni M.E. (1978) *In vitro* collagen biosynthesis in healing and normal rabbit articular cartilage. *J. Bone Joint Surg.* **60A**, 1076–1081.

Clancy W.G. (1988a) Arthroscopic anterior cruciate ligament reconstruction with patella tendon. *Tech. Orthop.* **2**, 4.

Clancy W.G. (1988b) Repair and reconstruction of the posterior cruciate ligament. *Operat. Orthoped.* **3**, 1656.

Clancy W.G., Shelbourne K.D., Zoeller G.B. *et al.* (1983) Treatment of knee joint instability secondary to rupture of the posterior cruciate ligament. *J. Bone Joint Surg.* **65A**, 310–322.

Collins D.H. (1949) *The Pathology of Articular and Spinal Diseases.* London, Edward Arnold.

Covery F.R., Akeson, W.H. and Keowin G.H. (1972) The repair of large osteochondral defects. *Clin. Orthop.* **82**, 253–262.

Cox F.J. (1945) Traumatic osteochondritis of the patella. *Surgery* **17**, 93.

Craig S.M. (1987) Soft tissue considerations. In Scott, W.N. (ed.) *Total Knee Revision Arthroplasty.* London, Grune Stratton.

Cross M.J. and Powell J.F. (1984) Long-term follow-up of posterior cruciate ligament rupture: a study of 116 cases. *Am. J. Sports Med.* **12**, 191–297.

Dandy D. and Poosey R. (1982) Long-term results of unrepaired tears of the posterior cruciate ligament. *J. Bone Joint Surg.* **64B**, 92–94.

Daniel D.M. (1988) Diagnosis of knee ligament injury: tests and measurements of joint laxity. In Feagan J.A. (ed.) *The Cruciate Ligament.* New York, Churchill Livingstone.

DeHaven K.E. (1985) Meniscus repair in the athlete. *Clin. Orthop.* **198**, 31–35.

DePalma A.F., McKeever C.D. and Subin D.K. (1966) Process of repair of articular cartilage demonstrated by histology and autoradiography with tritiated thymidine. *Clin. Orthop.* **48**, 229–242.

Derscheid G.L. and Garrick J.G. (1981) Medial collateral ligament injuries in football: non-operative management of Grade I and Grade II sprains. *Am. J. Sports Med.* **9**, 365–368.

DeTakats G. (1965) Sympathetic reflex dystrophy. *Med. Clin. N. Am.* **49**, 117.

Drachman D.B. and Sokoloff L. (1966) The role of movement in embryonic joint development. *Dev. Biol.* **14**, 401.

DuToit G.T. (1967) Knee joint cruciate ligament substitution: the Lindmann (Heidelberg) operation. *S. Africa J. Surg.* **5**, 25.

Dye S.F. (1987) An evolutionary perspective of the knee. *J. Bone Joint Surg.* **69A**(7), 976.

Elmslie R.C. (1978) Unpublished work at St. Bartholomew's Hospital, London, 1912–1932. In Smillie I.S. (ed.) *Diseases of the Knee Joint.* Edinburgh, Churchill Livingstone.

Ferkel R.D., Fox J.M., Wood D., DelPizzo W., Friedman M.J. and Snyder S.J. (1989) Arthroscopic second look at the Gore-Tex ligament. *Am. J. Sports Med.* **17**(2), 147–153.

Ficat P. (1970) *Patholozie Femora-Patellaire.* Paris, Masson.

Ficat P. and Hungerford D.S. (1977) *Disorders of the Patello-Femoral Joint*. Baltimore, Williams & Wilkins.

Fukubayashi T., Torzilli P.A., Sherman M.F. and Warren R.F. (1982) An *in vitro* biomechanical evaluation of anterior—posterior motion of the knee. *J. Bone Joint Surg.* **64A**, 258—264.

Furukawa T., Eyre D.R., Koide S. and Glimcher M.J. (1980) Biochemical studies on repair cartilage resurfacing experimental defects in the rabbit knee. *J. Bone Joint Surg.* **62A**, 79—89.

Galway H.R. and MacIntosh D.L. (1980) The lateral pivot shift: a symptom and sign of anterior cruciate ligament insufficiency. *Clin. Orthop.* **147**, 45.

Glashow J.L., Katz R., Schneider M. and Scott W.N. (1989) Double-blind assessment of the value of magnetic resonance imaging in the diagnosis of anterior cruciate and meniscal lesion. *J. Bone Joint Surg.* **71A**, 113—119.

Goetgis H. (1913) Über Verletzungen der Ligamenta cruciata des Kniegelenks. *Dtch. Z. Chir.* **123**, 221.

Goodfellow J., Hungerford D.S. and Zindel M. (1976) Patellofemoral joint mechanics and pathoogy. *J. Bone Joint Surg.* **58B**, 287—290.

Graf B., Doctor T. and Clancy W. Jr. (1987) Arthroscopic meniscal repair. *Clin. Sports Med.* **6**(3), 525—536.

Gray H. (1959) *Gray's Anatomy of the Human Body*, Goss, C.M. (ed.) Philadelphia, Lea & Febiger.

Green N.E. and Allen B.L. (1977) Vascular injuries associated with dislocation of the knee. *J. Bone Joint Surg.* **59A**, 236—239.

Grood E.S., Noyes F.R., Butler D.L. and Suntay W.T. (1981) Ligamentous and capsular restraints preventing straight medial and lateral laxity in intact human cadavera knees. *J. Bone Joint Surg.* **63A**, 1257—1269.

Gylys-Morin V.M., Hajek P.C., Sartoris D.J. and Resnick D. (1987) Articular cartilage defects: detectability in cadavera knees with MRI. *Am. J. Roentgen.* **148**, 1153—1157.

Hall F.M. and Wyshak G. (1980) Thickness of articular cartilage in the normal knee. *J. Bone Joint Surg.* **62A**, 408—413.

Hampson W.G.J. and Hill P. (1975) Late results of transfer of the tibial tubercle for recurrent dislocation of the patella. *J. Bone Joint Surg.* **57B**, 209.

Hanten W.P. and Pace M.B. (1987) Reliability of measuring anterior laxity of the knee joint using a knee ligament arthrometer. *Phys. Ther.* **67**, 357—359.

Heller L. and Langman J. (1964) The menisco-femoral ligaments of the human knee. *J. Bone Joint Surg.* **46B**, 307.

Hendler R.C. (1991) Intra-articular semitendinosus anterior cruciate ligament reconstruction. In Scott W.N. (ed.) *Ligament and Extensor Mechanism Injuries of the Knee: Diagnosis and Treatment*. St. Louis, C.V. Mosby.

Henning C.E., Clark J.R., Lynch M.A., Stallbaumer R., Yearout K.M. and Vequist S.W. (1988) Arthroscopic meniscus repair with a posterior incision. *Am. Acad. Orthop. Surg. Instruct. Course Lect.* **37**, 209—221.

Hey-Groves E.W. (1919) The crucial ligaments of the knee joint: their function, rupture, and the operative treatment of the same. *J. Surg. (Br.)* **7**, 674—675.

Heywood A.W.B. (1961) Recurrent dislocation of the patella. *J. Bone Joint Surg.* **43B**, 508.

Hollinshead W.H. (1974) *Textbook of Anatomy*. Hagerstown, Harper & Row.

Hosea T.M., Tria A.J. and Bechler J.R. (1991) Embryology of the knee. In Scott W.N. (ed.) *Ligament and Extensor Mechanism Injuries of the Knee: Diagnosis and Treatment*. St. Louis, C.V. Mosby.

Hoshino A. and Wallace W.A. (1987) Impact-absorbing properties of the human knee. *J. Bone Joint Surg.* **69B**, 807—811.

Hubbard M.J.S. (1987) Arthroscopic surgery for chondral flaps in the knee. *J. Bone Joint Surg.* **69B**, 794—796.

Hughston J.C. (1969) Subluxation of the patella in athletes. In *American Academy of Orthopaedic Surgeons Symposium on Sports Medicine*. St. Louis, C.V. Mosby.

Hughston J.C. (1972) Reconstruction of the extensor mechanism for subluxating patella. *J. Sports Med.* **1**, 6—13.

Hughston J.C. and Eilers A.F. (1973) The role of the posterior oblique ligament in repair of acute medial (collateral) ligament tears of the knee. *J. Bone Joint Surg.* **55A**, 923—940.

Hughston J.C. and Walsh W.M. (1979) Proximal and distal reconstruction of the extensor mechanism for patella subluxation. *Clin. Orthop.* **144**, 36.

Hughston J.C. and Norwood L.A. (1980) The postero-lateral drawer test and external rotational recurvatum test for postero-lateral rotatory instability of the knee. *Clin. Orthop.* **147**, 82.

Hughston J.C. and Barrett G.R. (1983) Acute antero-medial rotary instability: long-term result of surgical repair. *J. Bone Joint Surg.* **65A**, 145—153.

Hughston J.C., Andrews J.R., Cross M.J. and Moschi A. (1976) Classification of knee ligament instabilities. Part I. The medial compartment and cruciate ligament. *J. Bone Joint Surg.* **58A**, 159—172.

Hughston J.C., Bowden J.A., Andrews J.R. *et al.* (1980) Acute tears of the posterior cruciate ligament. *Clin. Orthop.* **164**, 59—77.

Indelicato P.A. (1983) Non-operative treatment of complete tears of the medial collateral ligament of the knee. *J. Bone Joint Surg.* **65A**, 323—329.

Inove M., McGurk-Burleson E., Hollis J.M. *et al.* (1987) Treatment of the medial collateral ligament injury. I. The importance of anterior cruciate ligament on the varus—valgus knee laxity. *Am. J. Sports Med.* **15**, 15—21.

Insall J.N. (1984a) Anatomy of the knee. In Insall J.N. (ed.) *Surgery of the Knee*. New York, Churchill Livingstone.

Insall J.N. (1984b) Chronic instability of the knee. In Insall J.N. (ed.) *Surgery of the Knee*. New York, Churchill Livingstone.

Insall J.N. (1984c) Meniscectomy. In Insall J.N. (ed.) *Surgery of the Knee*. New York, Churchill Livingstone.

Insall J.N. (1984d) The menisci of the knee. In Insall J.N. (ed.) *Surgery of the Knee*. New York, Churchill Livingstone.

Insall J.N. (1984e) *Surgery of the Knee*. New York, Churchill Livingstone.

Insall J.N., Falvo K.A. and Wise D.W. (1975) Chondromalacia patellae: a prospective study. *J. Bone Joint Surg.* **58A**, 1—8.

Insall J.N. and Salvati E. (1971) Patella position in the normal knee joint. *Radiology* **101**, 101.

Insall J.N. and Hood R.W. (1982) Bone-block transfer of the medial head of the gastrocnemius for posterior cruciate insufficiency. *J. Bone Joint Surg.* **64A**, 691—699.

Insall J.N., Goldberg V. and Salvati E. (1972) Recurrent dislocation and the high-riding patella. *Clin. Orthop.* **88**, 67—69.

Insall J.N., Joseph D.M., Aglietti P. and Campbell R.D. Jr. (1981) Bone-block iliotibial-band transfer for anterior cruciate insufficiency. *J. Bone Joint Surg.* **63A**, 560—569.

Ireland J., Trickey E.C. and Stoker D.J. (1980) Arthroscopy and arthrography of the knee: a critical review. *J. Bone Joint Surg.* **62B**(1), 3—6.

Jacob R.P., Hassler H. and Strarubli H.U. (1981) Instability of the lateral compartment of the knee. *Acta Orthop. Scand. (Suppl.)* **191**.

Jacobson K. and Bertheussen K. (1974) The vertical location of the patella. *Acta Orthop. Scand.* **45**, 436.

Jaroschy W. (1924) Die diagnostische Verwerbarkeit der Patellaraufnahemen. *Fortschr. Roentgenstr.* **31**, 781.

Johnson L.L. (1979) Lateral capsular ligament complex: anatomical and surgical considerations. *Am. J. Sports Med.* **7**, 156–160.

Kaplan E.G. (1962) Some aspects of functional anatomy of the human knee joint. *Clin Orthop.* **23**, 18–29.

Kelikian H., Riashi E. and Gleason J. (1957) Restoration of quadriceps function in neglected tear of the patella tendon. *Surg. Gynecol. Obstet.* **104**, 200–204.

Kelly M. (1990) Arthroscopy: loose bodies. In Scott, W.N. (ed.) *Arthroscopy of the Knee.* Philadelphia, W.B. Saunders.

Kennedy J.C. (1963) Complete dislocation of the knee joint. *J. Bone Joint Surg.* **45A**, 889–904.

Kennedy J.C. (1967) The posterior cruciate ligament. *J. Trauma* **7**, 367.

Kennedy J.C. and Galpin R.D. (1982) The use of the medial head of the grastrocnemius muscle in the posterior cruciate-deficient knee: indications, technique, and results. *Am. J. Sports Med.* **10**, 63–74.

Kennedy J.C., Grainger R.W. and McGraw R.W. (1966) Osteochondral fractures of the femoral condyles. *J. Bone Joint Surg.* **48B**, 437–440.

Kennedy J.C., Weinberg H.W. and Wilson A.S. (1974) The anatomy and function of the anterior cruciate ligament. *J. Bone Joint Surg.* **56A**, 223–237.

Kennedy J.C., Alexander I.J. and Hayes K.C. (1982) Nerve supply of the human knee and its functional importance. *Am. J. Sports Med.* **10**, 329–335.

Kettelkamp D.B. and Jacobs A.W. (1972) Tibio-femoral contact area: determination and implications. *J. Bone Joint Surg.* **54A**, 343–356.

Larson R. (1984) Fractures and dislocations of the knee. In Rockwood C.A. and Green D.P. (eds) *Fractures in Adults.* Philadelphia, J.B. Lippincott.

Laurin C.A., Dussault R. and Levesque H.P. (1979) The tangential X-ray investigation of the patello-femoral joint: X-ray technique, diagnostic criteria and their interpretation. *Clin. Orthop.* **144**, 16.

Macey H.B. (1939) A new operative procedure for repair of ruptured cruciate ligaments of the knee joint. *Surg. Gynecol. Obstet.* **69**, 108.

MacIntosh D.L. and Galway H.R. (1972) The lateral pivot shift: a symptomatic and clinical sign of anterior cruciate insufficiency. Read at the Annual Meeting of the American Orthopedic Association, Tucker's Town, Bermuda.

MacNab I. (1964) Recurrent dislocation of the patella. *J. Bone Joint Surg.* **46B**, 498.

Main W.K. and Scott W.N. (1991) Knee anatomy. In Scott W.N. (ed.) *Ligament and Extensor Mechanism Injuries of the Knee: Diagnosis and Treatment.* C.V. Mosby.

Mankin H.J. (1970) The articular cartilage: a review. *Am. Acad. Orthop. Surg. Instruct. Course Lect.* **19**, 204–224.

Mankin H.J. (1974) The reaction of articular cartilage to injury and osteoarthritis. I. *N. Engl. J. Med.* **291**, 1285–1291.

Mankin H.J. (1982) Current concept review: the response of articular cartilage to mechanical injury. *J. Bone Joint Surg.* **64A**, 460–465.

Maquet P. (1974) Biomechanische Aspekte der Femur–Patella Beziehungen. *Z. Orthop.* **112**, 620.

Markolf K.L., Mensch J.S. and Amstutz H.C. (1976) Stiffness and laxity of the knee—the contribution of the supporting structures. A quantitative *in vitro* study. *J. Bone Joint Surg.* **58A**(5), 583–593.

McDaniel W.J. and Dameron T.B. (1983) The untreated anterior cruciate ligament rupture. *Clin. Orthop.* **172**, 158–163.

Meachim G. (1963) The effect of scarification on articular cartilage in the rabbit. *J. Bone Joint Surg.* **45B**, 150–161.

Merchant A.C. (1987) Patella–femoral disorders. In Crenshaw A.H. (ed.) *Campbell's Operative Orthopedics.* St. Louis, C.V. Mosby.

Merchant A.C. and Mercer R.L. (1974) Lateral release of the patella: a preliminary report. *Clin. Orthop.* **103**, 140–145.

Merchant A.C., Mercer R.L., Jacobsen R.H. *et al.* (1974) Roentgenographic analysis of patello-femoral congruence. *J. Bone Joint Surg.* **56A**, 1391.

Meyers M.H., Moore T.M. and Harvey J.P. (1975) Follow-up notes on articles previously published in the *Journal.* Traumatic dislocation of the knee joint. *J. Bone Joint Surg.* **57A**, 665–672.

Milgram J.W. (1986) Injury to articular cartilage joint surfaces. II. Displaced fractures of underlying bone. *Clin. Orthop.* **206**, 236–247.

Mitchell N. and Shepherd N. (1976) The resurfacing of adult rabbit articular cartilage by multiple perforations through the subchondral bone. *J. Bone Joint Surg.* **58A**, 230–233.

Mont M.A. (1990) Classification of ligament injuries. In Scott W.N. (ed.) *Ligament and Extensor Mechanism Injuries of the Knee.* St. Louis, C.V. Mosby.

Montgomery J.B. (1987) Dislocation of the knee. *Orthop. Clin. N. Am.* **18**, 149.

Morgan C.D. and Casscells S.W. (1986) Arthroscopic meniscus repair: a soft approach to the posterior horns. *Arthroscopy* **2**(1), 3–12.

Morrisson J.B. (1967) The Forces Transmitted to the Human Knee Joint During Activity. PhD thesis, University of Strathclyde.

Nicholas J.A. and Minkoff J. (1978) Iliotibial band transfer through the intercondylar notch for combined anterior instability (ITPT procedure). *Am. J. Sports Med.* **6**, 341–353.

Norwood L.A., Shields C.L., Russo J., Kerlan R.K., Jobe F.W., Carter V.S., Blazina M.E., Lombardo S.J. and Del Pizzo W. (1977) Arthroscopy of the lateral meniscus in knees with normal arthrograms. *Am. J. Sports Med.* **5**, 271–274.

Noyes F.R., DeLucas J.L. and Torvik P.J. (1974) Biomechanics of anterior cruciate failure: an analysis of strain-rate sensitivity and mechanism of failure in primates. *J. Bone Joint Surg.* **56A**, 236–253.

Noyes F.R., Butler D.L., Grood E.S., Basses H.R.W. and Hosea T. (1978) Clinical parodoxies of anterior cruciate instability and a new test to detect its instability. *Orthop. Trans.* **2**, 36.

Noyes F.R., Butler D.L., Paulos L.E. and Grood E.S. (1983) Intra-articular cruciate reconstruction. I. Perspective on graft strength, vascularization, and immediate motion after replacement. *Clin. Orthop.* **172**, 71–79.

Outerbridge R.E. (1961) The aetiology of chondromalacia patellae. *J. Bone Joint Surg.* **43B**, 752.

Paget J. (1969) Healing of cartilage. *Clin. Orthop.* **64**, 7–8.

Parolic J.M. and Bergfeld J.A. (1986) Long-term results of non-operative treatment of isolated posterior cruciate ligament injuries in the athlete. *Am. J. Sports Med.* **14**, 35.

Sixth International Symposium on Prosthetic Ligament Reconstruction of the Knee. March 3–5, 1989, Los Angeles.

Ramsey R.H. and Miller G.E. (1970) Quadriceps tendon ruptures: a diagnostic trap. *Clin. Orthop.* **70**, 161–164.

Rand J.A. (1990) Arthroscopic diagnosis and management of

articular cartilage pathology. In Scott W.N. (ed.) *Arthroscopy of the Knee.* New York, W.B. Saunders.

Redfern P. (1969) On the healing wounds in articular cartilage. *Clin. Orthop.* 64, 4–6.

Reider B. (1991) Arthroscopic anterior cruciate ligament reconstruction with patella tendon combinations. In Scott W.N. (ed.) *Ligament and Extensor Mechanism Injuries of the Knee: Diagnosis and Treatment.* St. Louis, C.V. Mosby.

Reider B., Marshall J.L. and Warren R.F. (1981) Persistent vertical septum in the human knee joint. *J. Bone Joint Surg.* 63A, 1185–1187.

Rettig A.C. (1991) Medial and lateral ligament injuries. In Scott W.N. (ed.) *Ligament and Extensor Mechanism Injuries of the Knee: Diagnosis and Treatment.* St. Louis, C.V. Mosby.

Ricklin P., Ruttiman A. and delBuone M.S. (1971) Meniscus lesions. In *Practical Problems of Clinical Diagnosis, Arthrography, and Therapy.* New York, Grune & Stratton.

Ritter M.A, McCarroll J., Wilson F.D. and Carlson S.R. (1983) Ambulatory care of medial collateral ligament tears. *Phys. Sports Med.* 11, 47.

Rosenberg N.J. (1964) Osteochondral fracture of the lateral femoral condyle. *J. Bone Joint Surg.* 46A, 1013–1026.

Rosenberg T.D. and Kolowich P.A. (1990) Arthroscopic diagnosis and treatment of meniscal disorders. In Scott W.N. (ed.) *Arthroscopy of the Knee.* New York, W.B. Saunders.

Rosenberg T.D., Paulos L.E., Parker R.D., Harner C.D. and Kolowich P.A. (1988) The well leg support. *Arthroscopy* 4(1), 41–44.

Rosenberg T.D., Scott S.M., Coward D.B. *et al.* (1986) Arthroscopic meniscal repair evaluated with repeat arthroscopy. *Arthroscopy* 2(1), 14–20.

Saraniti A., Sweitzer D. and Sweitzer R. (1991) Rehabilitation for extensor mechanism and ligament injuries. In Scott W.N. (ed.) *Ligament and Extensor Mechanism Injuries of the Knee: Diagnosis and Treatment.* St. Louis, C.V. Mosby.

Savory C.G., Polly D.W., Sikes R.A. *et al.* (1987) A prospective comparison study of magnetic resonance imaging and arthroscopy of the knee. (Abstract.) *Am. J. Sports Med.* 15, 389.

Scapinelli R. (1968) Studies on the vasculature of the human knee joint. *Acta Anat.* 70, 305–331.

Scott G.A., Jolly B.L. and Henning C.E. (1986) Combined posterior incision and arthroscopic intra-articular repair of meniscus. *J. Bone Joint Surg.* 68A, 847–861.

Scott W.N. (1990) *Arthroscopy of the Knee.* New York, W.B. Saunders.

Scott W.N. (1991) *Ligament and Extensor Mechanism Injuries of the Knee: Diagnosis and Treatment.* St. Louis, C.V. Mosby.

Scott W.N. and Schosheim P.M. (1983) Intra-articular transfer of the iliotibial band muscle tendon unit. *Clin. Orthop.* 172, 97–101.

Scott W.N., Ferriter P. and Marino M. (1985) Intra-articular transfer of the iliotibial tract. *J. Bone Joint Surg.* 67A, 532–538.

Schultz R.A., Miller D.C., Kerr C.S. and Micheli L. (1984) Mechanoreceptors in human cruciate ligaments. *J. Bone Joint Surg.* 66A, 1072–1076.

Scuderi C. (1958) Ruptures of quadriceps tendon: study of twenty tendon ruptures. *Am. J. Surg.* 95, 626–635.

Scuderi G., Cuomo F. and Scott W.N. (1988) Lateral release and proximal realignment for patellar subluxation and dislocation. A long term follow-up. *J. Bone Joint Surg.* 70A, 856–861.

Seedham B.B., Dowson D. and Wright V. (1974) The functions of the menisci: a preliminary study. *J. Bone Joint Surg.* 56B, 381.

Selesnick F.H., Nole H.B., Bachman D.C. and Steinberg F.L. (1985) Internal derangement of the knee: diagnosis by arthrotomy. *Clin. Orthop.* 198, 26–30.

Shahriaree H. (1986) Chondromalacia. In Whipple T.L. (ed.) *Arthroscopic Surgery Desk Reference.* Redondo Beach, California, Bobit Publishing.

Sherman M.F. and Bonamo J.R. (1988) Primary repair of the anterior cruciate ligament. *Clin. Sports Med.* 7(4), 739–750.

Shields L., Mitral M. and Cave E.F. (1969) Complete dislocation of the knee: experience at the Massachusetts General Hospital. *J. Trauma.* 9, 192–215.

Shrive N. (1974) The weight bearing mode of the menisci of the knee. *J. Bone Joint Surg.* 56B, 381.

Siliski J.M. (1991) Traumatic dislocations of the knee. In Scott W.N. (ed.) *Ligament and Extensor Mechanism Injuries of the Knee: Diagnosis and Treatment.* St. Louis, C.V. Mosby.

Siliski J.M. and Plancher K. (1989) Dislocation of the knee. American Association of Orthopedic Surgery Meeting.

Sinding-Larson C. (1921) A hitherto unknown affection of the patella in children. *Acta Radiol.* 1, 171.

Sisto D.J. and Warren R.F. (1985) Complete knee dislocation. *Clin. Orthop.* 198, 94–101.

Smillie I.S. (1971) *Injuries of the Knee Joint.* Baltimore, Williams & Wilkins.

Snook G.A. (1983) A short history of the anterior cruciate ligament and the treatment of tears. *Clin. Orthop.* 172, 11–13.

Stockwell R.A. and Meachim G. (1973) The chondrocytes. In Freeman M.A.R. (ed.) *Adult Articular Cartilage.* New York, Grune & Stratton.

Trillat A., Dejour H. and Couette A. (1964) Diagnostic et traitement des subluxations recidivantes de la rotule. *Rev. Chir. Orthop.* 50, 813.

Walker P.S. and Erkman M.J. (1975) The role of the menisci in force transmission across the knee. *Clin. Orthop.* 109, 184.

Wang J.B. and Hewson G.F. (1988) Anterior cruciate ligament reconstruction using the lateral one-third of the patella tendon. *Tech. Orthop.* 2, 4.

Warren L.F. and Marshall J.L. (1979) The supporting structures and layers on the medial side of the knee. *J. Bone Joint Surg.* 61A, 56–62.

Warren L.F., Marshall J.L. and Girgis F. (1974) The prime static stabilizer of the medial side of the knee. *J. Bone Joint Surg.* 56A, 665–674.

Wiberg G. (1941) Roentgenographic and anatomic studies on the femoro-patellar joint. *Acta Orthop. Scand.* 12, 319–410.

Wickiewicz T.L., Kaplan N. and Warren R.F. (1992) Primary surgical treatment of anterior cruciate ligament ruptures: a long term follow-up study.

Wirth C.R. (1981) Meniscus repair. *Clin. Orthop.* 157, 153–160.

Yost J.G., Chekofsky K., Schosheim P. and Scott W.N. (1981) Intra-articular iliotibial band reconstruction for anterior cruciate ligament insufficiency. *Am. J. Sports Med.* 9, 220–224.

Chapter 26
The Ankle and Foot

N.H. Harris

INTRODUCTION

Although this chapter will give an account of conditions presenting in the adult, it should be recognized that many of them are residual deformities which were first noticed at birth or during the early years of life (see Chapter 7). Rheumatoid arthritis is excluded as it is discussed elsewhere (see Chapter 18.2).

Many of the patients presenting with foot complaints are elderly and it is essential to routinely assess the peripheral circulation, not only because pain in the foot may be vascular in origin, but also because it will influence the type of treatment offered. Assessment of a foot problem is incomplete unless the examination is conducted with the patient standing and walking. Finally, the shoes should always be carefully inspected as these will frequently reveal the cause of the pain.

COMBINED DEFORMITIES AFFECTING THE ANKLE AND FOOT

Untreated or relapsed talipes equinovarus

The essential deformity is a variable degree of fixed equinus at the ankle joint, varus (inversion) at the subtaloid joint and varus, adduction and plantar flexion (plantaris) at the midtarsal joint. The most common cause is an incompletely corrected or relapsed congenital talipes equinovarus in childhood. A similar deformity may be associated with other conditions that first manifest themselves in infancy and childhood, namely cerebral palsy, malformations resulting from abnormal splitting of the notochord (spinal dysraphism) including spina bifida, occulta and cystica, myelodysplasia and poliomyelitis. The underlying cause in all these conditions is a weakness of the dorsiflexors and peronei in the presence of normal or strong and spastic calf and tibialis posterior muscles.

Conditions that usually first manifest in the adult include spinocerebellar degeneration (peroneal muscular atrophy, Friedreich's ataxia), multiple sclerosis, traumatic paraplegia and cerebral vascular disease and trauma which may result in hemiplegia. All of the above-mentioned conditions may of course present with other deformities, e.g. pes equinus and pes cavus, depending on the muscle groups most severely affected. It follows that some of the common combined ankle and foot deformities in adults are simply a manifestation of serious neurological disease which may or may not be progressive; unless this is borne in mind, operative treatment could end in disaster.

SYMPTOMS AND SIGNS

The patient presents with a foot deformity that is painful. In addition, footwear poses a considerable problem. It is not difficult to establish if the deformity started in childhood. The pain when walking, especially in shoes, is the patient's main concern; it is principally the result of abnormal pressure on the outer border of the foot where callosities develop, and the excessive strain on capsular ligaments of the affected joint (Fig. 26.1). The patient's gait should be observed and this will explain the symptoms. In addition to the deformity, the affected joints are relatively stiff, particularly if the aetiology is congenital talipes, previous surgery has been undertaken, spasticity is present with secondary capsular and ligamentous contractures (Fig. 26.2) or secondary osteoarthritis has developed. The degree of passive correction must be assessed as this will have a bearing on treatment. The following associated features may be present: upper or lower motor neurone signs, limb shortening, a small foot, muscle wasting, and trophic skin changes, which may be due to sensory loss as in spinal dysraphism (Fig. 26.3). The lumbar spine should be carefully examined both clinically and radiologically to exclude the last

901

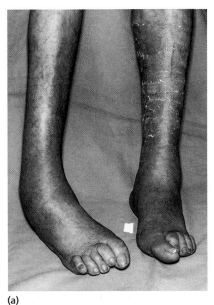

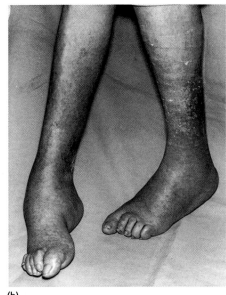

(a)   (b)

Fig. 26.1 (a,b) Relapsed congenital talipes equinovarus. Note the inversion, high varus heel and medial cavus. Excess load is taken on the outer border of the foot.

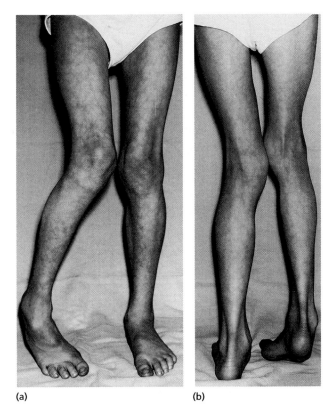

(a)   (b)

Fig. 26.2 (a,b) Spastic diplegia. Note the typical posture of the legs and severe equinovarus deformity of the right foot.

condition. A neurological opinion is always advisable in order to exclude progressive disease. Radiographs of the foot and ankle will indicate the presence of osteoarthritis.

TREATMENT

Symptomatic relief may be obtained in some patients by a combination of specially made shoes with appropriate insoles, chiropody and occasionally a calliper. Such therapy is best reserved for patients with progressive neurological disease and the elderly who may have associated vascular disease or other serious medical problems. In all other instances the object must be to obtain a plantigrade, balanced foot which sometimes has the added bonus of avoiding the need for surgical shoes. If full passive correction is possible, as it is sometimes in poliomyelitis for example, transfer of the tendon of the tibialis anterior to the lateral side of the foot may be sufficient. In some patients this operation will be combined with a soft-tissue release including elongation of the Achilles' tendon and division of the posterior capsule of the ankle joint. If the soft-tissue contracture is severe or if secondary osteoarthritic changes are present, these operations are contra-indicated. In these and in other very severe deformities, the problem is best dealt with by either a triple arthrodesis or a wedge tarsectomy if the deformity is principally in the midtarsal region.

If it is thought that equinus is a major feature of the deformity then a Lambrinudi type of triple arthrodesis will be indicated. The principle of this operation (Fig. 26.4) is as follows:

1 A wedge of bone is removed from the talus and calcaneus.

2 The calcaneocuboid joint and the lower part of the navicular are also excised.

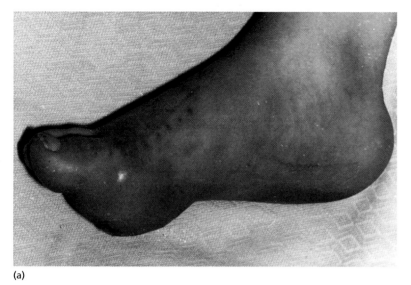 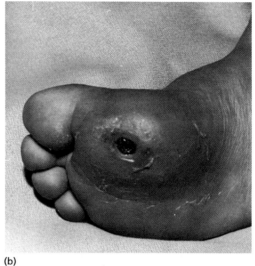

(a) (b)

Fig. 26.3 (a,b) This patient had a myelomeningocoele repaired in infancy. Pes cavus developed, followed by a trophic ulcer under the first metatarsal head; the medial sesamoid sequestrated. Correction of the depressed first metatarsal was attempted by means of a Robert Jones tendon transplant.

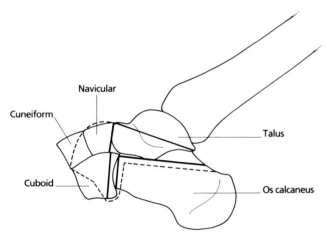

Fig. 26.4 The principle of Lambrinudi's triple arthrodesis. The solid line indicates the excision for the standard procedure, and the broken line that which is used for severe deformity.

3 The remainder of the talus is inserted between the navicular and cuboid bone.

4 If the deformity is very severe, full correction will only be possible if a large wedge is removed, and the naviscular and the superior part of the cuboid are excised, and with wide resection of the calcaneocuboid joint.

5 The lower half of the cuneiform is excised so as to fit on the remaining beak of the talus.

The operation is more successful if done for deformity rather than pain and for fixed deformity rather than a passively correctable one. Some residual equinus can easily be compensated for by raising the heel. It should be remembered that residual equinus may be beneficial to compensate for a short leg.

A note of caution should be sounded with regard to cerebral palsy. A transfer of the tendon of tibialis anterior may produce an overcorrection and a severe calcaneovalgus deformity will follow. The problem can largely be avoided by splitting the tendon and transferring half to the lateral side. Arthrodesis of the ankle should seldom be necessary but occasionally has to be done in order to restore stability; sometimes it will be combined with triple arthrodesis so as to avoid the need for a calliper.

Pes calcaneus

This deformity consists of a dorsiflexed foot at the ankle and is usually fixed, though some degree of passive correction may be possible in the young adult. When the patient stands or walks, the point of the heel is generally the only part of the foot that comes into contact with the ground and painful callosities develop in this area. The deformity results from paralysis of the calf muscles as seen in poliomyelitis.

TREATMENT

Restoration of muscle balance is normally reserved for children although a muscle transplant such as transfer of the long extensors to the calf, which may be combined with a bone operation, is sometimes indicated in the adult. Cholmeley (1953) described Elmslie's two-stage procedure which consists of a removal of a wedge from the posterior part of the subtaloid joint and a dorsal wedge tarsectomy to correct plantaris deformity.

Pes equinus and plantaris

A fixed plantarflexion deformity at the ankle (equinus) is usually the result of a condition that first presents in childhood; examples are cerebral palsy, spina bifida, poliomyelitis and compensation for leg shortening. If it presents for the first time in an adult, some of the more common causes are lateral popliteal nerve palsy, peripheral neuritis (e.g. diabetic neuropathy), hemiplegia and paraplegia. It not infrequently follows a tibial fracture, and there are two possible factors involved. The leg may be incorrectly encased in plaster with the foot in equinus or there is development of a compartment syndrome in which there is impairment of the arterial circulation with later development of a calf contracture. The latter sequence of events is often missed because the examining doctor does not think of the possibility when the patient complains of increasing pain and numbness in the toes.

A flexion deformity at the midtarsal joint is referred to as plantaris. This is sometimes clinically mistaken for ankle equinus with which it may coexist (Fig. 26.5). The author is aware of instances where the mistaken diagnosis has led to correction by ankle arthrodesis with disastrous consequences. The aetiology is similar to equinus deformity.

TREATMENT

Equinus

A mobile deformity may be controlled by one of the many forms of foot drop device. The patient may prefer the alternative, namely a muscle transplant. The most effective is to transfer the tendon of tibialis posterior through the interosseous membrane to the dorsum of the foot. If shortening is present, some degree of fixed equinus is a useful compensatory mechanism and should not be disturbed.

A calf contracture may be improved by elongation of the Achilles' tendon, and if necessary division of the posterior capsule of the ankle joint. It is important to remember that in some patients with paralytic equinus there is a need for the deformity to maintain stability. Careful assessment is required in these patients because elongation of the Achilles' tendon, which inevitably weakens the calf, may make it more difficult to walk. With these patients, and also those who are unlikely to

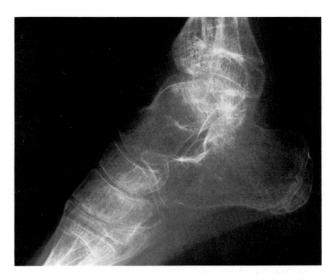

Fig. 26.5 Plantaris deformity at the midtarsal joint. Clinically it may be confused with ankle equinus.

gain adequate correction by soft tissue release alone, the Lambrinudi type of triple arthrodesis is appropriate (see p. 902).

Plantaris

In order to produce a plantigrade foot, the most effective operation is a dorsal wedge tarsectomy.

CONDITIONS PRINCIPALLY AFFECTING THE ANKLE JOINT AND ADJACENT STRUCTURES

The unstable ankle

The stability of the ankle joint depends on the anatomical configuration of the talus and mortice, the ligaments and muscle balance of the foot. Direction of muscle action and gravity combine to encourage forward displacement of the leg but it is resisted by the direction of the collateral ligaments and by the fact that the body of the talus is wedge-shaped, the broader end being anterior. It follows that the most unstable position of the joint is when the foot is plantar-flexed, for in this position the narrow end of the wedge-shaped body of the talus is only loosely engaged by the malleoli.

Instability is usually the result of rupture of one or more parts of the lateral ligament of the ankle joint, though a developmental type is recognized, in which case both ankles are generally affected. An important predisposing factor is weakness of the peroneal muscles. The mechanism of injury has been described by Glasgow *et al.* (1980). They have shown that following an inversion strain with the foot plantar-flexed, the anterior talofibular ligament ruptures. The result of this injury is that forward subluxation of the talus in the mortice occurs but it is stable to a varus stress. If the rupture extends posteriorly to involve the calcaneofibular ligament and medially to involve the anterior capsule, a marked tilt of the talus with varus stress and anterior subluxation can be produced with the foot plantigrade or in equinus. An isolated calcaneofibular rupture produces a minor degree of varus instability with the foot plantigrade and there is no anterior subluxation.

SYMPTOMS

The patient complains of pain and swelling on the anterolateral aspect of the joint. In addition, the joint gives way especially when walking on uneven surfaces. In the acute stage a diagnosis of a sprained ankle is made, simple strapping is applied and very occasionally the possibility of a complete ligament rupture is considered. Even if such a diagnosis is made and it is treated by immobilization in a cast, subsequent instability may follow later. The past history of injury is obtained in most chronic problems.

SIGNS

Invariably it is possible to elicit tenderness over the attachment of the affected ligament; there may or may not be some swelling. If the instability is severe, it may be possible to detect the tilt or anterior subluxation of the talus. The strength of the peronei should be tested and lateral popliteal nerve palsy excluded.

RADIOLOGY

The varus tilting of the talus is demonstrated by an anteroposterior radiograph while stressing the joint (Fig. 26.6a). Sometimes a compression defect may be noted on the medial aspect of the talus and it represents an osteochondral fracture produced by impingement of the medial malleolus during forced inversion (Fig. 26.6b). Failure to demonstrate the tilt does not exclude instability because anterior subluxation may be the cause, and indeed both types may coexist, depending upon the degree of damage to the lateral ligament complex. Anterior subluxation is most easily demonstrated by lying the patient prone with the feet over the end of the table; downward pressure is applied to the heel while a lateral radiograph is taken.

TREATMENT

Conservative measures are seldom effective; they consist of strengthening the peroneal muscles and alterations to the heel of the shoe. For women, lowering and broadening the heel and for men floating out the heel on the lateral side are the available techniques.

Operative treatment has a high success rate, and it is

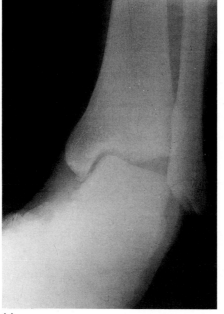 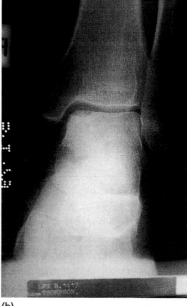

Fig. 26.6 Varus tilting of the talus. (a) Note the significant talar tilt. (b) Note the compression defect (osteochondral fracture) on the medial part of the superior articular surface of the talus.

(a)　　　　　(b)

usually possible for the patient to resume sporting activities. The principle of the operation is to produce a tenodesis effect by using the tendon of peroneous brevis.

The Watson-Jones (1976) procedure has been largely replaced by a similar one which is just as effective, described by Evans (1953). The tendon is divided 2–3 cm proximal to the lateral malleolus, re-routed through the latter and then sutured to itself under moderate tension (Fig. 26.7). The short-term functional results are excellent; however, it seems that functional stability deteriorates after about 14 years (Karlsson *et al.*, 1989). The probable reason is that the tenodesis does not effectively control the anterior subluxation which results from rupture of the anterior talofibular ligament, especially when the foot is in equinus.

An alternative procedure which gives 94% excellent or good results at 10 years is reported by Snook *et al.* (1985). The Chrisman–Snook operation uses half the peroneus brevis tendon to replace both the talofibular and calcaneofibular ligaments (Fig. 26.8).

Osteochondritis dissecans of the talus

This lesion is an example of the localized ischaemic necrosis of the subarticular bone. The condition usually occurs after epiphyseal closure. It is essentially a sequestrum with overlying healthy articular cartilage and there is a plane of cleavage separating dead from surrounding healthy bone. The cause is obstruction to the blood supply, probably of traumatic origin. If the fragment remains undisplaced, spontaneous healing is likely. Alternatively, a fragment may separate into the joint to become a loose body. Secondary osteoarthritis may follow later.

The talus is the second most common site of this type of lesion. It affects the medial side of the superior convex articular surface (Fig. 26.9). The history of pain and swelling is the usual presentation and locking will occur if the fragment is loose. The condition may settle down after rest in a plaster. In the long term, the lesion does not progress, and secondary osteoarthritis seldom, if ever, occurs. If symptoms persist, the joint should be explored and a decision can then be made as to whether the fragment should be removed or replaced after drilling the subchondral bone.

Recurrent dislocation of the peroneal tendons

In this condition, the peroneal tendons sublux anteriorly over the lateral malleolus as the foot is actively dorsiflexed and return with plantar-flexion. It occurs spontaneously or is the result of trauma. The patient presents

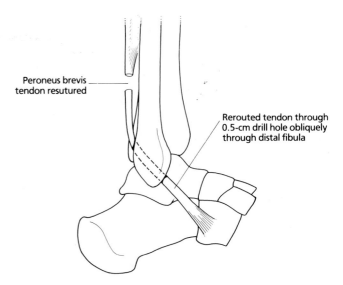

Fig. 26.7 Diagrammatic representation of Evans' peroneal tenodesis operation for instability of the ankle following rupture of the lateral ligament.

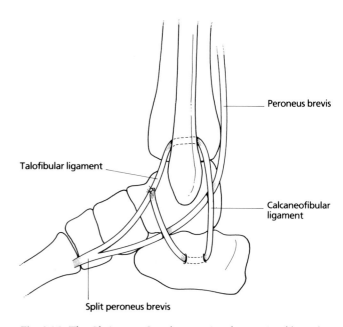

Fig. 26.8 The Chrisman–Snook operation for repair of lateral ligament of the ankle. Note the split peroneus brevis tendon passing through the fibula to replace the anterior talofibular ligament. It then passes through a tunnel in the calcaneum to form the calcaneofibular ligament.

with pain, clicking or a feeling of giving way. Treatment is surgical and consists of turning down an osteoperiosteal flap from the lateral malleolus over the tendon.

Tarsal tunnel syndrome

This syndrome is caused by compression of the posterior tibial nerve as it passes deep to the flexor retinaculum

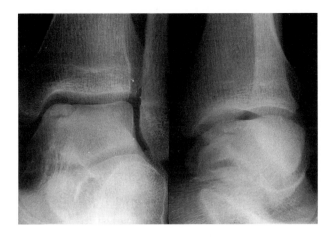

Fig. 26.9 Osteochondritis dissecans of the talus. Note the large osteochondral fragment on the superomedial aspect of the articular surface. (Reproduced by kind permission of the X-ray Museum, Royal National Orthopaedic Hospital.)

behind the medial malleolus. The patient complains of a burning sensation on the medial side of the sole of the foot. The pain is aggravated by exercise and the patient is usually woken at night. Positive Tinel's sign may be elicited over the nerve at the site of compression, and altered sensation may be present in the skin supplied by the nerve. Peripheral vascular disease is excluded by the presence of normal peripheral pulses as is a neurological lesion by the presence of normal reflexes and the absence of motor weakness. The diagnosis is confirmed by nerve-conduction studies which will show a delay at the level of compression. Treatment is operative and consists of decompression of the posterior tibial nerve by dividing the flexor retinaculum.

Tendovaginitis of the tibialis posterior tendon

This lesion is most commonly a non-specific inflammatory swelling of the synovial sheath surrounding the tendon of tibialis posterior; rheumatoid arthritis is sometimes the cause. The tendon itself is not infrequently much enlarged though its appearance to the naked eye is otherwise normal. The patient presents with pain and swelling of gradual onset on the inner side of the ankle. Examination reveals a rather diffuse swelling in the line of the tendon and localized tenderness. Inversion of the foot is restricted and painful. Treatment may be conservative at first. A hydrocortisone injection into the sheath while carefully avoiding the tendon with or without a walking cast are the usual methods. A more certain cure can be obtained by complete division of the tendon sheath, a portion of which should always be sent for biopsy and synovectomy if appropriate.

Bursitis at the Achilles' tendon insertion

An adventitious bursa lies superficial to, and the calcaneal bursa is deep to, the insertion of the Achilles' tendon. Inflammatory swelling of the deep bursa may be non-specific or it may be the first manifestation of rheumatoid arthritis, Reiter's disease or ankylosing spondylitis. Relief of symptoms is obtained by raising the heel, avoiding local pressure from the shoe, and if these measures fail a carefully planned injection of hydrocortisone may be tried. Inflammation and swelling of the superficial bursa are most commonly seen in women athletes who have an enlarged posterosuperior angle of the os calcis. The swelling is on the posterolateral aspect of the heel (Fig. 26.10). It may be quite large and is impinged upon by the back of the shoe. The symptoms are worse in the winter months and are often associated with chilblains. The only effective treatment is wide excision of the prominent bone from the os calcis (Fig. 26.11) taking care not to significantly disrupt the insertion of the Achilles' tendon. If this is unavoidable, then it is wise to apply a walking cast about 3 weeks after the operation. Pressure with the finger over the lower end of the tendon should easily displace it forwards if sufficient bone has been removed.

Some athletes wear trainers with a large posterior tongue which may cause pressure on the Achilles' tendon insertion producing pain and swelling and it is as well to inspect the footwear if this is suspected.

Peritendonitis (paratenonitis) of the Achilles' tendon

This condition is most frequently seen in athletes, particularly long-distance runners. In its acute form the paratenon is inflamed and the sheath is distended with fluid. It often progresses to become a chronic lesion (Kvist and Kvist, 1980). The paratenon is thickened with fibrous adhesions between the tendon and surrounding structures; nodules may be present in the sheath or tendon and they possibly represent the effects of partial rupture of degenerative fibres in the Achilles' tendon.

SYMPTOMS AND SIGNS

In the acute or chronic stage, the patient complains of pain and swelling that is aggravated by exercise and their functional ability is inevitably impaired. In the acute stage, the distal part of the tendon is thickened and tender; crepitus is present in the acute stage only. Thickening of the adjacent tissues is a feature of the chronic condition.

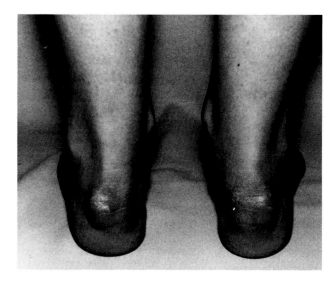

Fig. 26.10 Note the prominent heel swelling which is mainly the result of a chronically inflamed superficial bursa.

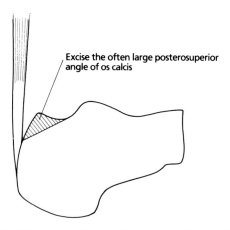

Excise the often large posterosuperior angle of os calcis

Fig. 26.11 Diagram to illustrate the portion of bone which is excised for 'heel bumps'; partial release of the Achilles' tendon insertion is sometimes necessary.

A useful diagnostic test is the appearance on a lateral radiograph of the tendon with the opposite normal side for comparison. In the chronic condition, the normal dark triangular shadow representing the tendon is either obscured or irregular.

TREATMENT

It is generally agreed that treatment for the chronic forms of disease is unsatisfactory. The usual measures are rest from physical activity, physiotherapy, raising the heel of the shoe and steroid injections into the tendon sheath. Unless great care is taken, the latter may precipitate tendon rupture. Operation is indicated if the relatively short period of conservative treatment fails. It consists of extensive stripping of the thickened paratenon, division of the crural fascia which is left open, complete freeing of the Achilles' tendon and immediate post-operative mobilization.

Rupture of the Achilles' tendon

Complete rupture most commonly presents with a sudden onset during the course of an unaccustomed form of exercise, such as squash or tennis. The rupture occurs at about 3 cm proximal to the insertion which is often the site of degenerative changes in later life.

SYMPTOMS AND SIGNS

The principal symptom is pain in the calf accompanied by an audible snap. The patient can walk but not with a normal heel−toe gait. In the acute stage, a gap will be felt at the site of rupture and it will be tender; bruising may be visible. Plantar-flexion is present but is of much reduced power. If the patient kneels on a chair and the calf is gently squeezed, plantar-flexion of the foot does not occur if the tendon is ruptured. The latter test is useful in patients who present not uncommonly weeks or months after the injury; in such patients the gap at the site of rupture is impalpable because it is filled with organizing tissue.

TREATMENT

In the early stages some surgeons advocate conservative treatment which consists of immobilization in a cast for 8 weeks with the foot in some degree of equinus, followed by wearing a raised heel for a few weeks with physiotherapy. The period of recovery may take many months and there is a 10% risk of repeat rupture. Operative treatment is favoured by most surgeons; it ensures that the tendon unites with the correct length, weight-bearing is safe after 2 weeks, the period of immobilization is 6 weeks and total recovery time much less than with conservative treatment. For the patient who presents late, surgery is obligatory. The tendon will have united with lengthening and therefore the scar filling the gap must be excised; the defect is closed by using two strips of calf muscle aponeurosis about 1-cm wide, attached distally and turned down and threaded through the distal stump of the tendon (Fig. 26.12).

In the author's experience, the results of late repair are most rewarding, though full recovery may take several months. It is strongly advised that absorbable suture material should be used in all these procedures and so avoid infection and a persistent sinus.

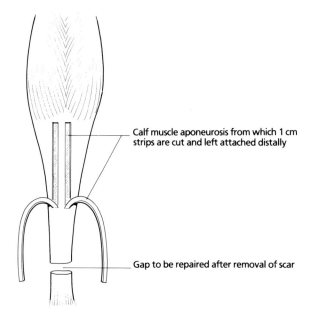

Fig. 26.12 Diagram to show a method of repair for late rupture of the Achilles' tendon.

Calf muscle aponeurosis from which 1 cm strips are cut and left attached distally

Gap to be repaired after removal of scar

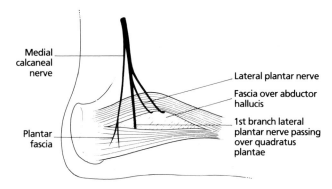

Medial calcaneal nerve

Plantar fascia

Lateral plantar nerve

Fascia over abductor hallucis

1st branch lateral plantar nerve passing over quadratus plantae

Fig. 26.13 Diagram to show the medial calcaneal nerve and the branch of the lateral plantar nerve which may be compressed.

THE FOOT

Chronic heel pain

The commonest site of pain is at the attachment of the thickened central part of the plantar aponeurosis and the intrinsic muscles to the medial calcaneal tuberosity. The aperneurosis is attached distally to the flexor tendon sheaths, plantar plates of the metatarsophalangeal joints and base of proximal phalanges. During walking, as the toes dorsiflex, the aporneurosis is tightened and raises the longitudinal arch.

It is likely that over a period of years in some patients who are overweight or have a particular occupation, for example, repetitive stress occurs at the attachment of the aponeurosis and associated flexor brevis muscles. An inflammatory reaction is set up, and sometimes a periosteal reaction develops leading to spur formation. A stress fracture of the medial calcaneal tuberosity has been reported. The condition is generally referred to as plantar fascilitis. When considering treatment, it is noteworthy that a spur is a secondary phenomenon and it is not likely to be the cause of symptoms.

Unless well recognized, a relatively common cause of pain is entrapment of the first branch of the lateral plantar nerve as it passes horizontally between the deep fascia of abductor hallucis and quadratus plantae muscles (Fig. 26.13).

Some other conditions that have to be excluded as the cause of pain are gout, Reiter's disease, ankylosing spondylitis and first sacral nerve root compression.

SYMPTOMS AND SIGNS

The chronic stress lesion characteristically causes pain at the inferomedial aspect of the heel which is worse when first rising from bed in the morning; local tenderness will be found and frequently a spur will be noticed on radiography. Nerve entrapment causes pain and paraesthesiae in the distribution of the nerve, associated with local tenderness.

TREATMENT

Heel pain for whatever cause usually responds to conservative measures such as a Rose's modified valgus insole, ultrasonic or laser therapy, and occasionally a steroid injection.

Surgery has a high morbidity and unless great care is taken, the calcaneal nerves will be damaged producing an unpleasant painful area on the weight-bearing aspect of the heel. Surgery should not be contemplated until conservative therapy has been given at least a 6 months' trial. It is in any event best reserved for nerve entrapment. An oblique incision is likely to avoid the calcaneal sensory nerves (Fig. 26.14), which should be proximal to the incision, and the deep fascia of the abductor hallucis muscle is divided.

Pes planovalgus

AETIOLOGY

A number of conditions that are first seen in childhood are the cause of a variable degree of valgus deformity in

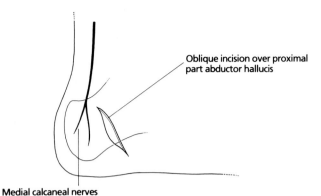

Oblique incision over proximal
part abductor hallucis

Medial calcaneal nerves

Fig. 26.14 Oblique medial heel incision to expose first branch lateral plantar nerve, avoiding the more proximal calcaneal nerves.

the adult. Some of the more common problems will be discussed.

CONGENITAL

The most familiar problem is tarsal coalition, a condition that has been reviewed by Mosier and Asher (1984). It is a fibrous, cartilagenous or osseous union between two tarsal bones, most commonly calcaneonavicular or talocalcaneal.

In about half the patients, the condition is bilateral. They present with symptoms in the second decade, usually pain in the midfoot, worse with activity and eased by rest. A notable feature is severe peroneal muscle spasm and valgus deformity (Fig. 26.15). Attempting passive inversion produces severe pain and increases the spasm. Radiography confirms the diagnosis (Fig. 26.16),

but it should be stressed that not all patients with peroneal spasm have a tarsal coalition; equally, a tarsal coalition may be symptomless.

By the time an adult presents with symptoms, there is a significant possibility that secondary osteoarthritic changes will be present, particularly in the talonavicular joint, and this influences the choice of treatment.

If symptoms are minimal, appropriate supports with or without surgical shoes are likely to be successful. A short period in a walking cast may be helpful when symptoms are more severe. Failed conservative measures is the principal indication for operation. It is most unlikely that resection of the coalition tissue could be as successful as it is in the adolescent. If it is to be done, the patient should be warned accordingly. The most reliable procedure for persistent symptoms is a triple arthrodesis.

ANATOMICAL

Anatomical causes include rotational abnormalities of the femur and tibia (see Chapter 10), genu valgum and supination of the forefoot in which there is an elevated first metatarsal. The deformity is often not recognized because the foot is incorrectly examined. The patient should lie prone with the heel held in neutral position, and it will be noted that the first metatarsal head is higher than others (forefoot supination). In order to walk with a plantigrade foot, the patient compensates by pronating the foot.

POSTURAL

Patients who are obese and stand for long periods at work often associated with poor footwear will develop a

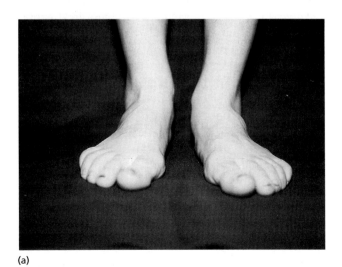

(a)

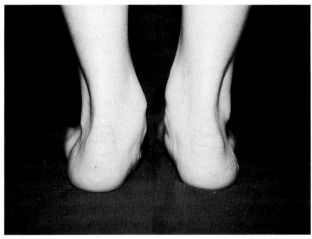

(b)

Fig. 26.15 (a,b) Bilateral peroneal spastic flat feet. Note the typical valgus deformity caused by peroneal muscle spasm.

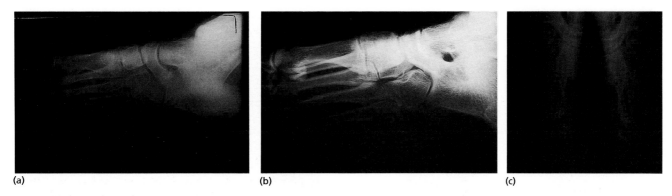

(a)   (b)   (c)

Fig. 26.16 (a–c) Tarsal coalition. Note the calcaneonavicular bar.

postural valgus deformity. Poor muscle tone after a long illness may also be a factor.

NEUROLOGICAL

Paralysis of the inverters from whatever cause allows the foot to roll into valgus (Fig. 26.17). In cerebral palsy, aductor spasm combined with overaction of the evertors similarly produces a valgus foot.

INFLAMMATORY

The most frequently seen example is rheumatoid arthritis. The subtaloid joint is invariably involved and this will produce a secondary peroneal spasm similar to that seen in adolescent spasmodic flat foot (see p. 910). Additional factors are destruction of ligaments and in some instances there has been a spontaneous rupture of the tendon of the tibialis posterior.

SYMPTOMS AND SIGNS

The most common complaint in the adult is pain, usually aching, which is worse at the end of the day and may be accompanied by swelling. A valgus foot may be associated with hallux valgus, retracted toes and meta-tarsalgia, any one of which may be the patient's principal complaint.

The patient is asked to stand and walk and any rotational abnormalities are noted. The foot is examined for mobility of the tarsal joints, the presence of forefoot deformities, intrinsic muscle function and local tenderness. Finally, shoes should be inspected for signs of abnormal wear and suitability.

TREATMENT

Whatever the cause, most patients should benefit from muscle-strengthening exercises, especially the intrinsics. Advice on suitable footwear is imperative but, as with weight reduction, it is often not accepted by the patient. Suitable insoles (see Chapter 34) offer good palliation especially in the elderly, and if they are to be effective, comfortable surgical shoes may have to be provided. Some patients with a severe mobile flat foot (e.g. in cerebral palsy and poliomyelitis) do not respond satis-factorily to conservative measures which may include instrinsic exercises, insoles or a calliper—usually an outside iron and inside T-strap. In such instances, Dwyer (1961) recommends operative treatment to tilt the heel into varus so that it can effectively support the head of the talus; he advises an opening wedge osteotomy on the outer side of the os calcis and insertion of bone which thus increases its height. The effect is to direct the line of action of the Achilles' tendon to the medial side and so balance either overacting evertors or weak inverters. Lengthening of the Achilles' tendon may be done at the same time or preferably left until later.

Where patients have associated forefoot deformities, these are dealt with as necessary. If secondary osteo-arthritic changes or rheumatoid arthritis have produced a painful rigid pronated foot, relief of symptoms can be obtained by a triple arthrodesis if conservative measures fail.

Pes cavus

The deformity usually presents in childhood and is discussed in detail elsewhere (see Chapter 7). However, adults do sometimes present with an established deform-ity which has not been treated, or alternative treatment in childhood has not been entirely successful. The essen-tial features (Fig. 26.18) vary in degree in individual patients, and consist of progressive varus deformity of the heel which shifts the line of action of the Achilles' tendon medially, thus allowing it to act as an invertor,

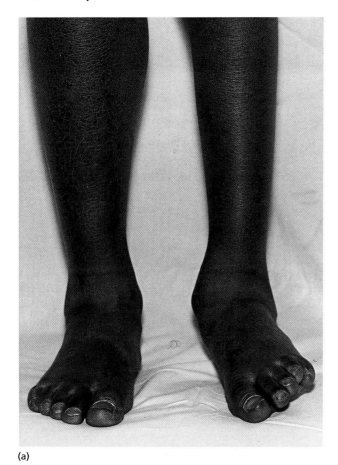

(a)

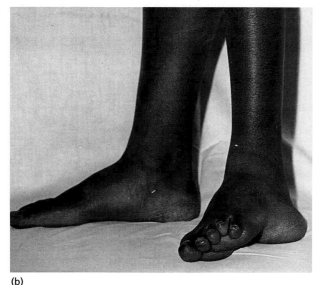

(b)

Fig. 26.17 (a,b) Paralytic valgus deformity. The patient had poliomyelitis in childhood; note the atrophied/left calf and a severe valgus deformity.

not only on the heel itself but also on the plantar fascia which becomes contracted. Equinus of the forefoot (plantaris) occurs at the midtarsal joint and all the toes

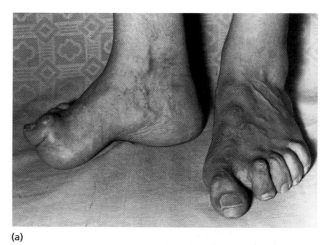

(a)

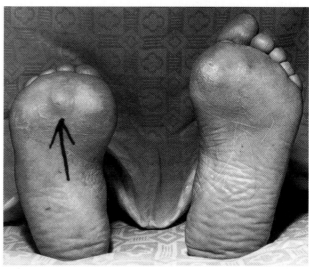

(b)

Fig. 26.18 (a,b) Pes cavus. Note the claw toes, prominent metatarsal heads, and the plantaris and medial cavus of the smaller right foot. Although not well shown, the right heel is inverted.

become retracted, with hyperextension at the metatarso-phalangeal joint and flexion at the interphalangeal joints. The latter deformity is mobile at first and by the time of presentation in the adult it is visually a fixed contracture. The toe deformities are associated with impaired intrinsic muscle function and therefore the patient can no longer flex the toes at the metatarsophalangeal joint. It follows that abnormal stress falls on the metatarsal heads in the push-off phase of walking.

SYMPTOMS AND SIGNS

There may be no symptoms in the relatively mild deformities especially if care is taken with footwear. At some time the patient is likely to complain of difficulty in obtaining suitable shoes, which rapidly become deformed. Painful callosities develop along the outer border of the foot, on the plantar aspect of the metatarsal heads and on the dorsum on the proximal interphalangeal joints. If secondary osteoarthritic changes are present then general aching and stiffness will be an additional complaint.

Characteristic deformities are unmistakable (Fig. 26.18). It is important to exclude a neurological basis for the deformity, and if one is found to decide whether or not it is progressive. The site of callosities is noted and the degree of passive correction of the affected joints is ascertained. Weight-bearing radiographs will confirm the clinical findings and indicate the presence of osteoarthritic change.

TREATMENT

It is occasionally possible to give relief of symptoms with a moulded cavus insole made from a cast and incorporated into surgical shoes. Failure to obtain relief by these means, or if the patient declines surgical footwear, is an indication for surgical treatment. The patient should be told a deformity is progressive and therefore in the young adult it would be reasonable to advise surgical correction which is likely to prevent more serious problems in later life.

It is unlikely that a soft-tissue release will be of significant benefit in the adult. In the young adult with relatively mobile joints, a good correction of the varus heel is obtained by a calcaneal osteotomy (Dwyer, 1959). The principle is to remove a large laterally based wedge from the outer aspect and place the heel into slight valgus. Following the operation, the high medial arch will flatten under the stress of weight-bearing and the deformed toes will gradually straighten. If the toes do not straighten or the forefoot deformity is severe or fixed, then in addition a dorsal wedge tarsectomy at the tarsometatarsal level should be undertaken. Procedures so far mentioned will preserve motion of the subtaloid and midtarsal joints. If secondary osteoarthritic changes are judged to be largely responsible for the symptoms, a triple arthrodesis will be necessary.

The toe deformities require separate consideration. For mobile clawing of the lesser toes, the flexor-to-extensor transplant is recommended. It was first performed by Girdlestone (1947) and the technique and results have been described by Taylor (1951) and Pyper (1958). The object of the operation is to transfer the long flexor tendon into the dorsal expansion to enable them to replace the function of the intrinsic muscles. It is not necessary to splint the toes afterwards as this can be achieved by a suitable plaster. For the halux, a re-commended operation is a fusion of the interphalangeal joint and transfer of the long extensor into the neck of the first metatarsal.

If there is a fixed deformity of the lesser toes arthrodesis of the interphalangeal joints and internal fixation with intramedullary Kirschner wires is advised. It may be necessary to perform an extensor tendon tenotomy and dorsal capsulotomy of the metatarsophalangeal joints at the same time. The principle of the operation (Lambrinudi, 1938) is to produce a dynamic redistribution of power so that the long flexors exert all their action on the metatarsophalangeal joints.

CONDITIONS PRINCIPALLY AFFECTING THE FOREFOOT

There are a number of conditions that are due to or associated with poor intrinsic muscle function, and they have in common a claw toe deformity. Numerous other conditions are due to a specific local pathological process and include, for example, halux valgus and rigidus, hammer toes and digital neuroma.

Claw toes

Most commonly the deformity is due to intrinsic muscle deficiency for which there is no obvious cause, and when this is so it is most often seen in women who have worn inappropriate footwear, e.g. shoes which can only be held in place by flexion of the toes. The deficiency may sometimes be age-related even when sensible shoes are worn.

There are a number of specific conditions with which the muscle deficiency is associated, e.g. halux valgus, pes cavus (idiopathic and neurogenic), neurological conditions such as poliomyelitis and peroneal muscular atrophy, following a compartment syndrome (e.g. after a tibial fracture) and in association with reflex sympathetic dystrophy. Two common medical conditions affect muscle control of the toes, i.e. rheumatoid arthritis and diabetes.

The effect of the deficiency is to produce retraction of the toes or a claw deformity; the metatarsophalangeal joints are all hyperextended and the interphalangeal joints flexed (Fig. 26.19). At first the deformity is mobile and passively correctable; later it is fixed. In the later stages, pressure on the dorsum of the fixed claw deformity depresses the metatarsal heads which will take an increasing load causing a severe metatarsalgia.

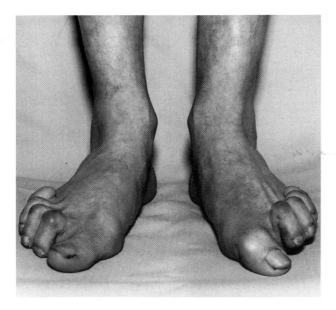

Fig. 26.19 Claw toes.

TREATMENT

Clearly, if there is an association deformity such as a pes cavus (see p. 911) treatment will be directed at this as well as the toes, if appropriate.

In the early stages an attempt should be made to correct the intrinsic deficiency and correct footwear inadequacies. A suitable orthotoic to reduce pressure from the forefoot is often helpful.

Surgical correction should only be considered after several months' trial of the preceding measures. It is the author's experience that when the patient first presents, very often only one toe — the second — is symptomatic. Careful examination will often reveal some deformity in the third and fourth toes also. Furthermore, if only the second toe is corrected, the patient soon presents again with third and fourth toe metatarsal head pain. It is probably wise therefore to advise the patient (and the reason for so doing) that the second, third and possibly fourth toes should be corrected at the same time.

For the mild deformities, a soft-tissue release may be all that is necessary; at the metatarsophalangeal joints, extensor tenotomy and dorsal capsulotomy, and if necessary release of the collateral ligaments, are useful procedures. At the proximal interphalangeal joint, division of the flexor tendons should be considered. In some patients with mobile claw toes — in pes cavus or from some neurological disorder, for example — the Girdlestone tendon transplant is appropriate; if there is a fixed deformity at the interphalangeal joint, joint fusion is appropriate (see p. 913).

More severe deformity at the metatarsophalangeal joint amounting to subluxation or dislocation is unlikely to respond to soft-tissue procedures. The recommended operation is a Helal osteotomy (Helal, 1975) in the coronal plane of the metatarsal neck, the object of which is to relax the soft tissues and elevate the metatarsal heads. The operation gives consistently good results, and is more reliable than either excision of the base of the proximal phalanx or excision of the metatarsal head, both of which produce excessive shortening of the toe which often becomes functionless. An alternative method for elevating the metatarsal heads is a dorsal-based wedge osteotomy at the metatarsal base (Thomas, 1974).

Hallux valgus

Valgus displacement of the hallux is often one feature of the numerous structural changes in the forefoot (Fig. 26.20). The essential deformity is a medial subluxation of the first metatarsal head out of the joint cavity; the sesamoids are left behind so there is an apparent rather than a true lateral displacement of these bones. The base of the proximal phalanx is tethered by the deep transverse ligaments and the adductor and flexor brevis which are attached to the plantar aspect of the base of the proximal phalanx; it follows that the hallux will rotate as well as deviate laterally. As the hallux displaces, so the long extensor tendon will bow-string across the joint and will act as a deforming force. The medial capsule of the metatarsophalangeal joint stretches, the tendon of the abductor hallucis displaces onto the plantar aspect, and the lateral capsule contracts. The medial aspect of the articular surface of the metatarsal head becomes exposed and a vertical groove develops between the functional articular surface and the medial prominence (exostosis).

Degenerative changes subsequently develop in the joint. The swelling (bunion) on the medial aspect of the first metatarsal head consists of a callosity, a subcutaneous bursa and the medial head prominence; the bursa sometimes becomes inflamed and an infected sinus may occasionally develop. The first metatarsal is almost invariably deviated from the second toe to a variable degree (metatarsus primus varus) (Fig. 26.21). The foot is frequently pronated and the forefoot splayed, particularly in older patients. The function of the intrinsic muscles is compromised and clawing or retraction of the toes soon follows; the toes are often cramped together and relatively functionless. Painful callosities develop to the metatarsal heads due to excessive stress. The second toe may be compressed from the dorsum or elevated

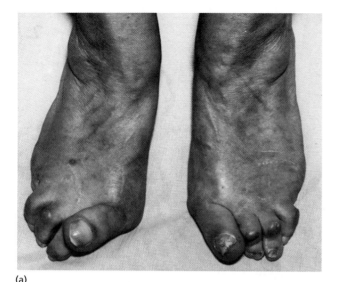

(a)

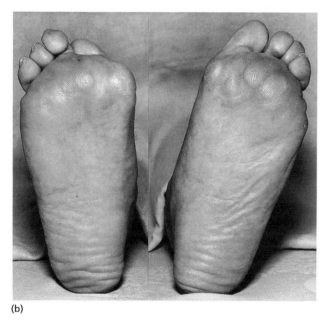

(b)

Fig. 26.20 Hallux valgus (a) Note the subluxed and rotated hallux, overlapping of the second toe on right foot, hammer deformity of the second and third toes on the left foot and (b) callosities under the prominent metatarsal heads.

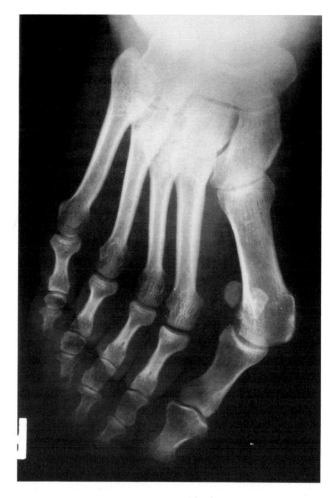

Fig. 26.21 Weight-bearing radiograph to show adduction of the first metatarsal which exposes the tethered lateral sesamoid. Note the medial head prominence ('exostosis') and lateral subluxation of the proximal phalanx at the first metatarsophalangeal joint (Piggott's subluxated type of hallux valgus).

from the plantar aspect by the deviated hallux (Figs 26.20a and 26.22). The second toe and its metatarsal head are subjected to greater stress than normal from weight-bearing and the result is a flexion deformity at the proximal interphalangeal joint and retraction or subluxation at the metatarsophalangeal joint (hammer toe deformity) (Fig. 26.20a).

AETIOLOGY

Controversy on this matter is unresolved. Some of the more fashionable theories will be discussed briefly because they have a bearing on treatment.

About 60% of patients give a family history of the condition and they will present earlier with symptoms (Bonney and MacNab, 1952). Although 90% of patients who come to surgery are female, there is in fact very little difference in incidence between the sexes.

Varus displacement on the first metatarsal is thought by many to be a primary aetiological factor. There may be an inherent weakness in those structures which hold the first metatarsal in position. Hardy and Clapham (1952) do not accept this theory and they believe that displacement of the hallux precedes that of the metatarsal. Piggott (1960) after considering the available

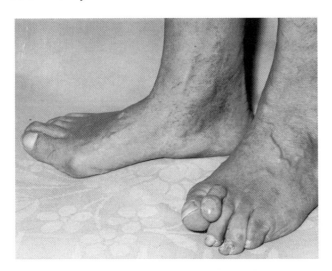

Fig. 26.22 Hallux valgus. Note that the second toe on the left foot has been elevated by the laterally deviated hallux.

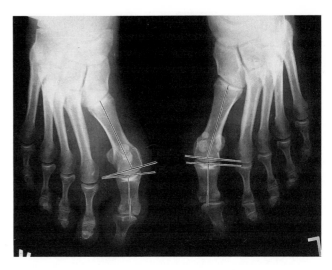

Fig. 26.23 Hallux valgus. (a,b) Note on the left that the articular surfaces of the great toe are congruous but are set more obliquely to the long axis of the shaft. On the right the articular surfaces are not congruous (Piggott's deviated type) and there is increased valgus.

evidence, suggests that medial deviation of the first metatarsal is secondary to lateral displacement of the proximal phalanx. Shoes are certainly not a primary aetiological factor; however, the greater incidence of women presenting for surgery is possibly explained by the wearing of high heels. Normally there is some degree of spreading of the metatarsals, and they will spread further in the take-off phase of walking. If there was an inherent weakness in the structures that stabilize the first metatarsal or there is excessive stress from wearing high heels, there would be a tendency to further spreading of the metatarsals.

NATURAL HISTORY

The deformity usually starts in adolescence and a knowledge of the natural history would therefore be helpful if guidance on prevention is to be given to the patients. Piggott (1960) has studied the problem. He states that measurements of the hallux valgus angle from standing weight-bearing radiographs indicated that the first metatarsophalangeal joint may be congruous as in a normal joint. He considers it is an exaggeration of the normal tilting of the articular surface of the base of the proximal phalanx and the metatarsal head (Fig. 26.23a) and that it does not progress and is therefore not a pathological condition. Pathological hallux valgus may be classified as either deviated or subluxed (Figs 26.21 and 26.23b); these two types represent different stages of the lateral displacement at the proximal phalanx. If the joint is subluxed, progression is likely; if it is deviated, some (but by no means all) will progress.

SYMPTOMS

The adolescent seeks advice for cosmetic reasons and to some extent because of difficulty in obtaining comfortable shoes. Mothers who have a similar deformity usually bring their child along early before there are significant symptoms. The older patient complains of pain which may be confined to the bunion or the subluxed second toe. In severe deformities, metatarsal head pain is an additional complaint. Shoe problems are an equally common complaint.

SIGNS

A clinical estimate of the amount of hallux valgus is made with the patient standing. The presence of rotation, deformity of the lateral toes and plantar callosities are noted. The range of motion of the great toe joint is estimated. The degree of stiffness, indicating the presence of osteoarthritis, is an important factor which determines the most appropriate treatment.

Radiographs of the weight-bearing foot will allow the angle of valgus, its type and the intermetatarsal angle to be measured. The presence of degenerative changes in the joint of the great toe may be demonstrable.

TREATMENT

Chiropody gives considerable palliative relief from pain. In addition, some chiropodists are sufficiently well trained to give advice as to what constitutes a sensible shoe, and such advice is clearly most important for the adolescent. Surgical footwear, with or without suitable insoles, is an alternative to operation. This should always be considered as a primary method of treatment for the elderly person with a severe forefoot deformity involving the hallux and lateral toes, in any patient who has a poor peripheral circulation and in those patients with rheumatoid arthritis on whom operative treatment is not contemplated.

When surgery is considered, it is a good principle to avoid operation until after skeletal maturity. The indications for operation and the type of operation will vary according to the age of the patient.

YOUNG ADULTS

The indication for operation is progressive deformity, and useful guidance for making a judgement is provided by Piggott's radiological criteria (Piggott 1960); thus if the joint is subluxed or if a previously deviated joint has progressed to subluxation, operation is indicated. Persistent symptoms unrelieved by conservative measures are also an indication for operative treatment. In many of these patients the symptoms are minimal, but the patient may be anxious to know if the condition will deteriorate. If this is the surgeon's opinion then it is entirely reasonable to recommend a prophylactic operation. It is important to note that in this age group the available operations are curative as opposed to palliative and it is probably unwise to recommend this type of operation in someone over the age of about 40 years. This is a factor that should be taken into account when discussing with the patient the need for an operation and how soon it should be performed.

There is no single operation of choice, but it should be unequivocally stated that there is no place for an arthroplasty in this age group. The operation of choice is a metatarsal osteotomy; it is a curative operation in the sense that it is designed to correct the underlying deformity. A variety of operations have been described. Osteotomy at the base of the first metatarsal to correct the varus is the author's preference (Fig. 26.24). It is based on a procedure described by Golden (1961); the principal modifications are to use a 2.8-mm screw for internal fixation and to perform a soft-tissue release of the metatarsophalangeal joint (division of the adductor hallucis and lateral capsulotomy). Weight-bearing in a cast starts about 10 days after the operation and is continued for a further 2 weeks. In a review of the results in 41 patients (66 feet) with an age range of 17–60 years followed-up for 1–6 years, 93% had no pain in the metatarsophalangeal joint, 95% did not have a shoe problem, 80% had a range of dorsiflexion to ≥40° and 69% had ≥40° of plantar flexion (Fig. 26.25).

An oblique osteotomy of the metatarsal shaft has been described by Wilson (1963) (Fig. 26.26). The operation has many advocates but one criticism is that significant shortening of the hallux results which, if it does not impair function, will be cosmetically unacceptable for some patients and may be followed by lateral toe metatarsalgia, though this is more likely to occur if the distal fragment were displaced dorsally. The success rate, as with most osteotomies, is in the region of 90% (Helal, 1981). Distal osteotomy is a common procedure, but there are many variations on the original operation established by Hohmann (1925). Modifications were devised by Peabody (1931), Hawkins *et al.* (1945) and Mitchell *et al.* (1958). The Mitchell operation is generally accepted as a satisfactory procedure. A different modification was recommended by Thomasen and the results were reported by Mygind (1952) and Gibson and Piggott (1962). A further modification is recommended by Adams (1976).

The principle of all these operations is similar, namely to displace the metatarsal head laterally, and the vari-

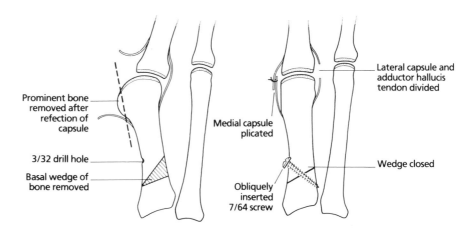

Fig. 26.24 Diagrammatic representation of the author's technique (modified Golden operation) of basal osteotomy for correction of hallux valgus with varus of the first metatarsal.

Prominent bone removed after refection of capsule

3/32 drill hole

Basal wedge of bone removed

Lateral capsule and adductor hallucis tendon divided

Medial capsule plicated

Obliquely inserted 7/64 screw

Wedge closed

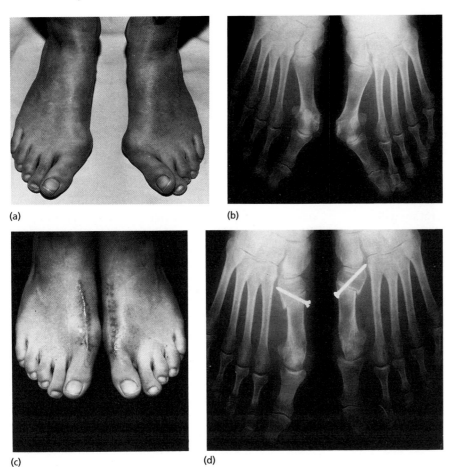

(a)   (b)

(c)   (d)

Fig. 26.25 (a) Bilateral hallux valgus in a 20-year-old female. Note the rotation of the hallux on the left and overlapping of the second toe. (b) Weight-bearing radiograph. Note the varus of the first metatarsal. (c) Following basal osteotomy the deformity has been corrected. (d) Radiograph to show the osteotomy and screw fixation.

ations have been devised to improve stability (Fig. 26.27). The success rate is in the region of 90% and the failures are usually the result of recurrence of deformity, lateral toe metatarsalgia (from dorsal angulation of the distal fragment and/or excessive shortening of the hallux) and stiffness of the metatarsophalangeal joint.

THE OLDER PATIENT

There is no doubt that the basal osteotomy described gives satisfactory results in patients over 40 years of age. However, it is probably best reserved for those patients who do not have significant osteoarthritis of the metatarsophalangeal joint and in the absence of deformity of the lateral toes with metatarsalgia; the same criteria apply to other types of osteotomy that have been described.

Arthrodesis

It is impossible to be precise about the indications for arthrodesis. In general it should be considered when the deformity is severe and secondary osteoarthritic

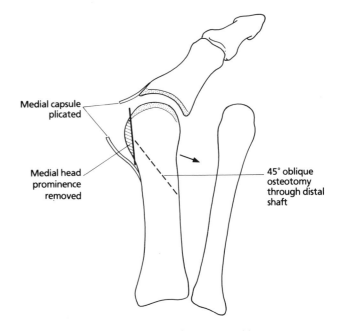

Fig. 26.26 Wilson's osteotomy. After the 45° oblique osteotomy, the distal fragment is displaced medially by half the width of the bone, and some plantar displacement. The medial capsule is plicated.

Medial capsule plicated

Medial head prominence removed

45° oblique osteotomy through distal shaft

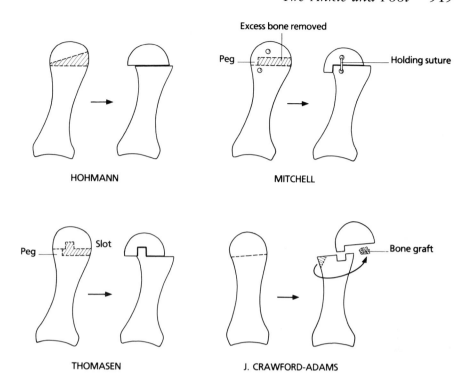

Fig. 26.27 Some examples of distal first metatarsal osteotomy for correction of hallux valgus.

changes are present with significant stiffness of the metatarsophalangeal joint. In such patients it is likely that additional procedures will have to be undertaken for deformities of the lateral toes and metatarsalgia (Raymakers and Waugh, 1971). The technique varies and it is probably of little consequence provided attention is paid to certain details, particularly the position of arthrodesis—a residual valgus of 20–30°, 20° of dorsiflexion (less in men) and neutral rotation. Fixation of the correct angle of dorsiflexion is of critical importance and is best achieved by dorsiflexing the foot to 90° and measuring the angle between the hallux and the plantar surface of the foot. The principal complications are malposition of the arthrodesis, interphalangeal joint osteoarthritis and failure of fusion. Fitzgerald (1969) has reviewed the long-term results.

Arthroplasty

Keller's operation (Keller, 1912) is a palliative operation that has stood the test of time, but the long-term results remain controversial (Rogers and Joplin, 1947; Jordan and Brodski, 1951; Bonney and MacNab, 1952). Following operation, the great toe bears weight in about 40% of patients and loading of the first metatarsal head is increased.

It is generally accepted that attention to certain factors is of considerable importance if poor results are to be avoided. Selection of patients is a major factor; the operation should be avoided if the metatarsophalangeal joint is affected by significant osteoarthritic change and in very active patients who are on their feet all day; the exception is those feet severely affected by rheumatoid arthritis or on which a Keller's procedure is part of the forefoot arthroplasty. It is best avoided in patients under 60 years of age and significant pain under the second and third metatarsal heads is a relative contraindication; in such instances, an osteotomy is likely to be more successful. In patients with >40° of hallux valgus and/or significant varus of the first metatarsal, resection of the proximal phalanx would need to be excessive resulting in a short functionless toe; in such instances, arthrodesis is probably the operation of choice.

No operation is likely to be successful unless sensible, well-fitting shoes are worn. Undoubtedly some of the failures are due to poor technique following operation by inexperienced surgeons; either too little or too much of the proximal phalanx is removed, the tight extensor hallucis longus is not corrected and inadequate soft-tissue repair is undertaken. Correct bandaging and splinting of the toe after operation are extremely important and teaching the patient to flex the toes and walk with a plantigrade foot is essential.

A significant improvement in the anatomical and functional results is obtained by maintaining distraction of the toe with an intramedullary Kirschner wire or a staple (Thomas, 1962). The author has attempted to obtain the same effect by using a Swanson silastic toe prostheses. Thomas's technique is probably more universally applicable particularly in the very severe deformities and in feet affected by rheumatoid arthritis.

The Mayo arthroplasty in which the first metatarsal head is excised and a capsular flap is used to separate the bone ends, fell into disfavour about 30 years ago, mainly because it was thought that excision of the metatarsal head would increase the incidence of metatarsalgia. However, results at least as good (and some would claim better) than those following Keller's procedure can be obtained (Bonney and McNab, 1952; Rix, 1986); Rix introduced a number of small modifications that have probably improved the success rate of the operation.

Failed Keller's arthroplasty

Generally, the operation fails because of poor patient selection and operative technique. The hallux may be excessively short and functionless, clawed or is fixed in a position of dorsiflexion. Active motion is much reduced and metatarsalgia may be severe. If a salvage operation is to be considered, then the choice is between insertion of a silastic spacer and arthrodesis. Each patient presents with a combination of numerous complicating factors; a decision regarding further operation (or surgical footwear) and the type of operation must be left to detailed discussion with each patient.

Excision of the medial head prominence ('exostectomy')

Simple excision of the prominent bone and careful resuturing and tightening of the medial capsule are best reserved for those elderly patients whose bunion is the only problem with its characteristic pain and/or repeated inflammation, causing difficulty in fitting shoes and the resultant loss of independence. There is a high risk of increasing valgus deformity after this operation and it should not be performed except in special circumstances, an example of which has been described above.

Hallux rigidus

This condition signifies a painful limitation of dorsiflexion of the hallux, initially with a normal range of plantar flexion. Later, those movements are restricted in association with osteoarthritic changes in the joint. The patient may present as an adolescent (usually female), or as an adult when the male is more common.

AETIOLOGY

Osteochondritis dissecans of the first metatarsal head is thought to be a primary factor (Goodfellow, 1966). Repeated minor trauma may cause the osteochondritis or by itself may be responsible for a synovitis, muscle spasm and contracture of the capsule. Others consider that the primary cause is congenital elevation of the first metatarsal (Lambrinudi, 1939; Kessel and Bonney, 1958). The majority opinion, however, is that the latter is secondary to the flexion deformity which results from the painful flexor spasm affecting the joint. Hallux rigidus may be secondary to rheumatoid arthritis or gout.

SYMPTOMS AND SIGNS

At first the pain is intermittent and is aggravated by walking, even in bare feet. The pain is significantly worse when wearing high-heeled shoes. Later, in the older patient when osteoarthritis is established, pain becomes continuous and may wake the patient at night. A dorsomedial prominence is often troublesome (Fig. 26.28). Stiffness may be an additional complaint.

In the early acute stages, the first metatarsophalangeal joint may be slightly enlarged from an effusion and is tender; dorsiflexion will be restricted and painful. In later stages, the joint is enlarged and in particular a tender dorsomedial osteophyte and bursa (bunion) is present. Dorsiflexion is markedly restricted and so to a lesser extent is plantar flexion. Sometimes the toe is held in flexion by muscle spasm. Inspection of the plantar aspect of the foot and the shoe will indicate that most of

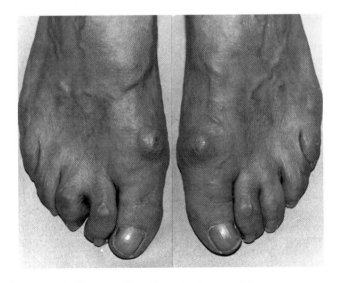

Fig. 26.28 Hallux rigidus. Note the dorsomedial prominence.

the weight-bearing load is being taken on the lateral side. Radiographs may be normal or show evidence of osteochondritis dissecans or various stages of joint degeneration may be visible (Fig. 26.29).

TREATMENT

It is worth trying the fitting of a concealed metatarsal rocker bar to the shoe. If this fails, or is unacceptable to the patient, then surgery is advised.

In the rare instances when persistent severe pain makes operation necessary in the adolescent the procedure of choice is an osteotomy of the base of the proximal phalanx (Bonney and MacNab, 1952), the short-term results of which are excellent and were reviewed by Kessle and Bonney (1958). Essential prerequisites for the success of the operation are 30% of pre-operative plantar flexion and a normal or near normal radiograph. The essential features of the operation are excision of a dorsally based wedge from the base of the proximal phalanx, and closure of the gap so that some of the residual plantar flexion range is converted into functional dorsiflexion. The operation undoubtedly confirms long-lasting benefit (Citron and Neil, 1987).

In the adult, a similar operation can be employed provided degenerative changes are not demonstrable. When there is considerable pain and stiffness associated with osteoarthritis, many surgeons will recommend arthrodesis. The results have been reviewed by Moynihan (1967) and Wilson (1967) who described the CONE arthrodesis, and by Fitzgerald (1969). The disadvantages are that decreased weight is taken under the first metatarsal head and increased weight under the second and third metatarsal head. The result is the onset of, or aggravation of, metatarsalgia; compensatory osteoarthritis of the interphalangeal joint is common and non-union occurs in about 40% of patients, but not all have symptoms. The type of footwear is severely restricted.

Keller's arthroplasty still has its advocates but probably should be reserved for the elderly. The disadvantages are that the toe is often significantly shortened and weight transfer to the lateral side causes or aggravates metatarsalgia as occurs after arthrodesis; fixed hyperextension sometimes occurs, and the cosmetic result is often poor.

The author's recommendation is an arthroplasty using the Swanson silastic prosthesis (Swanson *et al.*, 1979) to replace the excised base of the proximal phalanx (Fig. 26.29) and the operation is usually applicable to all adult age groups. The implant seems to last indefinitely, pain relief and restoration of function are remarkably consistent and recovery is rapid. Very occasionally infection is the only significant complication and if this unfortunately occurs, then removal of the implant leaves a remarkably good pseudarthrosis. The operation should

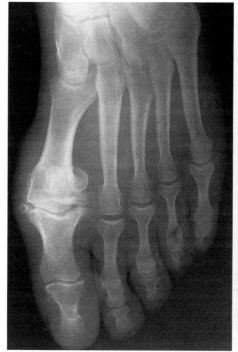 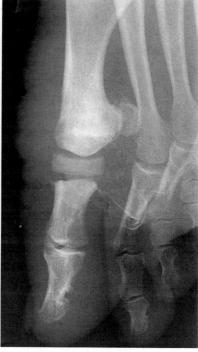

Fig. 26.29 Radiography to show advanced osteroarthritis of great toe joint treated by excision and insertion of a silastic prothesis.

(a) (b)

certainly be considered before an arthrodesis which has a much longer recovery period and not insignificant complications. For those who advocate the Keller's arthroplasty, the insertion of a silastic implant at the same time undoubtedly adds to the quality of the functional and anatomical result.

Hammer toes

This deformity most commonly affects the second toe, but the third and fourth are also sometimes involved. It is commonly congenital.

The deformity is a fixed contracture producing hyperextension at the metatarsophalangeal joint and flexion at the interphalangeal joint; the distal joint is extended but frequently it is an isolated condition with no associated abnormalities in the forefoot. The deformity not infrequently accompanies a hallux valgus. Pain occurs on the plantar aspect of the metatarsal head where the joint is often subluxed and there is usually a painful corn on the dorsum of the proximal joint.

A mallet toe is a fixed flexion deformity of the terminal joint; the nail is commonly deformed and an apical callosity is usually present.

TREATMENT

Chiropody may give useful but temporary relief, otherwise operative treatment is advised. For the proximal joint alone, arthrodesis is recommended and the most reliable and convenient technique is excision of the joint and fixation with a Kirschner wire. The same technique is applicable if both interphalangeal joints are to be fused or a mallet deformity only is to be corrected. For the latter, it may be preferable to amputate the terminal phalanx, particularly if the nail is deformed or painful. If there is a subluxation of the metatarsophalangeal joint, then extensor tendon tenotomy and dorsal capsulotomy may be sufficient to correct a mild deformity. In most instances it would be necessary to elevate the metatarsal head by means of Helal's osteotomy of the metatarsal neck as previously described (p. 914).

The fifth toe

Isolated pressure symptoms arise either as a result of a congenital dorsal displacement (Fig. 26.30) or from prominence of the metatarsal head with an inflamed bursa associated with varus displacement of the toe (Fig. 26.31). The latter is often present in the foot with hallux valgus and varus displacement of the other toes.

Dorsal displacement is best treated by a dorsal V—Y-

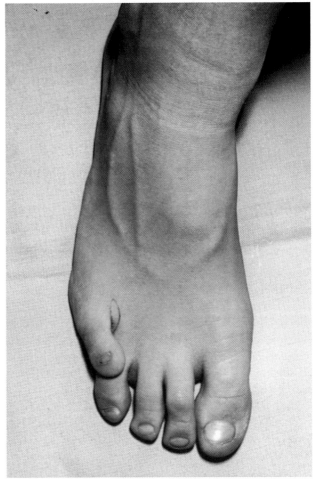

(a)

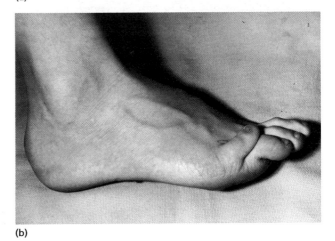

(b)

Fig. 26.30 (a,b) Congenital dorsal displacement of the fifth toes.

plasty, lengthening of the extensor tendon and dorsal capsulotomy of the metatarsophalangeal joint. The toe must be held in the correct position for 3 weeks, either with strapping or by use of a Kirschner wire.

Prominent metatarsal head is best treated by an

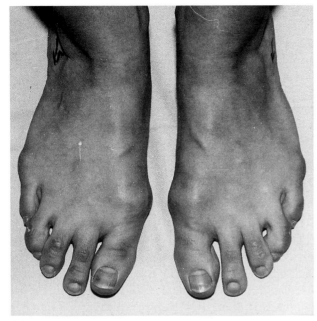

(a)

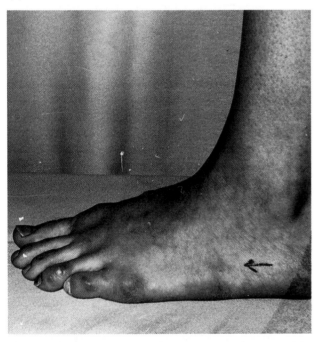

(b)

Fig. 26.31 (a,b) Note the varus displacement of the fifth toe associated with a prominent metatarsal head and callosity.

oblique osteotomy in the sagittal plane, displacing the head medially and proximally.

Soft corns

These are usually found in the fourth cleft. They are commonly caused by pressure between the lateral con-dyle of the proximal phalanx of the fourth toe and the medial aspect of the fifth toe where the corn is generally found. Relief may be given by a domed metatarsal insole that separates the fourth and fifth toe. If an operation is needed, the excision of the bony prominence is the most appropriate procedure.

Digital neuroma (Morton's metatarsalgia)

This lesion is a degenerative change in a plantar nerve immediately proximal to its bifurcation and adjacent to the distal part of the transverse intermetatarsal ligament. The affected part of the nerve develops a fusiform swelling which is not a true neuroma, and it contains degenerating and regenerating axons. It is likely that ischaemia is the underlying aetiological factor (Nissen, 1948). Any cleft may be affected but it is more commonly seen between the third and fourth toes. Women are affected more commonly than men.

SYMPTOMS AND SIGNS

Acute pain is felt on the plantar aspect of the forefoot often spreading to one or more toes; it may be accom-panied by paraesthesiae. Pain is related to weight-bearing, is relieved to some extent by removing the shoe and is aggravated by a shoe with a high heel. Night pain occurs occasionally.

The single most important physical sign is acute tenderness when pressure is exerted by the finger on the affected nerve in the web space on the plantar aspect. Rolling the finger from side to side while exerting pressure sometimes produces a painful click as the neuroma is displaced.

TREATMENT

Attention must be paid to the suitability of the shoes. A domed metatarsal insole sometimes gives temporary relief. Excision of the neuroma is usually required if permanent relief is to be obtained. The surgical approach is through an adequate plantar incision and the resection of the nerve must be sufficiently proximal to prevent the later development of a painful neuroma on the proximal end of the nerve.

Intermetatarsophalangeal bursitis

The bursa is situated dorsal to the transverse metatarsal ligament and adjacent to the joint capsule between the second and third and the third and fourth metatarsal heads. Bursitis may be non-specific or a manifestation of rheumatoid arthritis. Sometimes the swelling is large enough to be visible and cause the toes to spread apart (Fig. 26.32). The pain is indistinguishable from that caused by a digital neuroma. The treatment of choice is excision.

Rheumatoid arthritis

In addition to swelling from joint involvement (Fig. 26.33) or a bursitis it may be due to synovial protrusion from a tendon sheath or an isolated cyst in the sub-

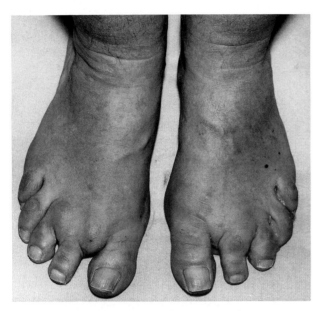

Fig. 26.32 Intermetatarsophalangeal bursitis. Note the bilateral bursa in the first and second cleft causing separation of the toes.

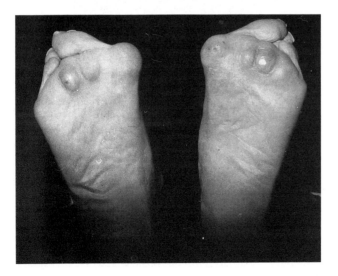

Fig. 26.33 Rheumatoid arthritis. Note the 'cystic' lesions from involvement of the metatarsophalangeal joints, and note also the typical severely retracted toes.

cutaneous tissues (Fig. 26.34). The presence of such a lesion usually means that conservative treatment will fail. The whole subject of rheumatoid arthritis is discussed in Chapter 18.2.

OTHER CYSTIC SWELLINGS

All these lesions may cause pain and include a ganglion, epidermoid cyst (inclusion dermoid) and an adventitious bursa on the plantar aspect of the great toe sesamoid. The lesions are treated by surgical excision.

Plantar warts

This lesion is caused by a virus which probably enters the skin through a small unrecognized breach in the epidermis. The common site is on the plantar aspect of the metatarsal heads and it presents as one or more painful round or oval lesions which are commonly mistaken for callosities (Fig. 26.35). Sometimes multiple lesions coalesce to form a mosaic which is very resistant to treatment.

Callosities occur only on pressure areas; warts may not occur at these sites. Tenderness to pressure is much less with a callosity, and lateral squeezing produces much more pain in a wart. Epithelial skin ridges are interrupted by a wart but not by a callosity. Punctate bleeding occurs as a wart is pared down.

TREATMENT

Single warts are best treated by curettage followed by

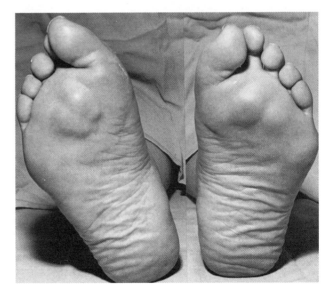

Fig. 26.34 Rheumatoid arthritis. Note the large rheumatoid subcutaneous cysts.

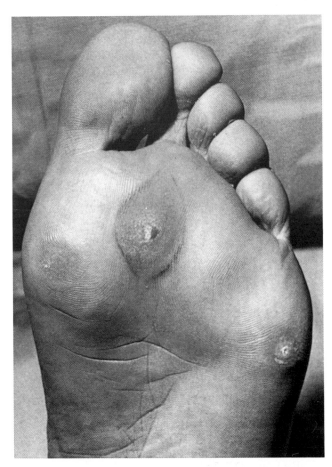

Fig. 26.35 Verruca. Note the typical appearance of the two lesions, in particular the interruption of the epithelial skin ridges.

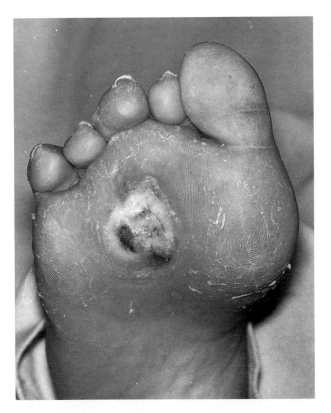

Fig. 26.36 An infected ulcer which followed treatment for a callosity over the prominent second metatarsal head.

cauterization of the cavity wall. A mosaic-type lesion should be treated with 30–40% salicylic acid. Occasionally, it may be necessary to resort to wide excision leaving the area open to heal spontaneously.

Penetrating ulcer

This lesion is more appropriately considered later in respect of the diabetic foot (p. 928). Sometimes non-specific ulceration occurs as a result of inappropriate chiropody for a metatarsal head callosity or simply from neglect. Secondary infection invariably follows (Fig. 26.36).

Metatarsal stress fracture (March fracture)

The different varieties of stress fracture have been fully described by Devas (1975). Usually it affects the second or third metatarsal shaft (Fig. 26.37) but one or all may be involved. The fourth or fifth metatarsal may be affected by a transverse basal fracture (Fig. 26.38).

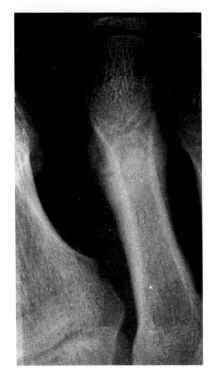

Fig. 26.37 March fracture. Note the periosteal new bone around the neck of the metatarsal. (Reproduced by kind permission of the X-ray Museum, Royal National Orthopaedic Hospital.)

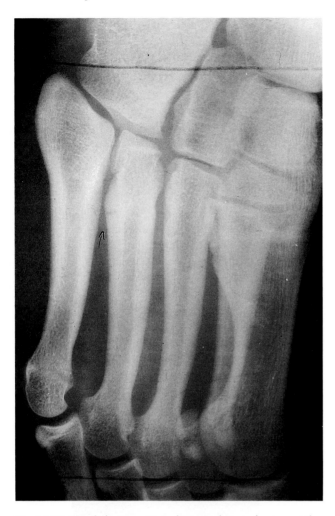

Fig. 26.38 March fracture. Note the typical stress fracture at the base of the fourth metatarsal.

SYMPTOMS AND SIGNS

Classically, the patient complains of pain in the foot after exercise and later on during exercise, and the pain is usually associated with a certain degree of swelling. If there is a long history there may even be pain at rest.

Local tenderness and swelling are the usual findings. In the early stages, the radiographs are negative but after about 3 weeks, an area of callus will be visible and sometimes a transverse or an oblique fracture line affecting one cortex will be noted. An isotope scan is a useful diagnostic aid in the early stages.

TREATMENT

Rest from physical activity is the most important aspect of treatment and this applies particularly to athletes; it may be supplemented by strapping or a cast for 3–4 weeks.

Freiberg's infraction (osteochondritis)

This condition starts in adolescence but may not present until early adult life or later. The natural history has been described by Smillie (1967).

Usually it is the second metatarsal head that is affected. The cause is ischaemic necrosis of the epiphysis, starting as a fissure fracture and passing through various stages of softening, fragmentation and absorption. Spontaneous healing with minimal head distortion does occur, but sometimes in the adult considerable distortion has taken place and secondary osteoarthritis is likely to intervene later.

SYMPTOMS AND SIGNS

Pain under the affected metatarsal head with exercise is the only significant complaint, usually associated with swelling. The metatarsal head is obviously enlarged and tender. Radiography will confirm the diagnosis (Fig. 26.39).

TREATMENT

When the condition presents in the adult, irreversible changes have generally taken place so that Smillie's bone grafting procedure is inappropriate. For those patients, if relief is not obtained by a metatarsal insole, permanent relief can be obtained either by excision of the head alone or replacement with a Swanson silastic hinge prosthesis.

The great toe sesamoids

Patients sometimes present with quite acute pain in the

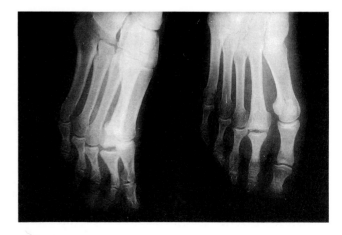

Fig. 26.39 Freiberg's osteochondritis of the second metatarsal head. Note that the articular surface is irregular and the enlarged head has collapsed.

region of the sesamoids, almost always on weight-bearing. Well-localized tenderness is demonstrable over one or other sesamoid. An axial radiological projection will demonstrate the sesamoids which may well have normal appearance. Sometimes the bones are multipartite and a fracture is diagnosed, but this appearance is also found in symptomless feet; in other instances, the bone is dense or stippled and the diagnosis of sesamoiditis is made; again the apparent abnormality is consistent with a symptomless foot. Very little is known about the cause of the pain but, despite our ignorance, it is relieved by excision of the bone which is thought to be the source of trouble. A detailed study of the sesamoids has been made by Gallocher (1967). The joint between the metatarsal head and the sesamoid is affected by degenerative changes (rheumatoid arthritis and osteoarthritis), usually associated with similar changes affecting the metatarsophalangeal joint with or without a hallux valgus.

Generally, it is thought to be unwise to remove both sesamoids because the loss of the flexor hallucis tendon insertion will cause clawing of the great toe.

THE NAILS

Ingrowing toe nail (onychryptosis)

This is an example of a very common, relatively minor condition which causes considerable disability, but generally will receive poor treatment.

The nail plate penetrates the lateral nail fold; inflammation quickly follows and granulation is formed (Fig. 26.40). One or both nail folds may be affected. The aetiology is the result of lateral pressure from ill-fitting shoes with or without appropriate nail cutting.

TREATMENT

In the early stages before a significant degree of infection has occurred, the condition should be treated by a chiropodist who will often cure the condition. When infection is clinically obvious, it is wise to undertake a two-stage procedure, i.e. avulsion of the nail to allow the sepsis to be eliminated, followed later by a definitive operation to cure the problem. All too frequently, however, the patient is given no further advice following the first stage and the condition recurs.

There are two techniques which, if properly executed, will effect a cure. Unless the nail is grossly deformed or chronic infection (which may be fungal) has supervened, a wedge resection is indicated. In other instances, the nail and the bed must be oblated and the operation of choice is a procedure recommended by Zadik (Townsend and Scott, 1966). The principal complication is recurrence of a spike of nail and this is invariably due to the fact that there has been inadequate removal of the nail bed.

Onychogryphosis

In this condition, the nail is grossly thickened and deformed (Fig. 26.41) usually as a result of tight shoes and trauma. It is most frequently seen in the elderly. Palliative treatment from a chiropodist should be advised in the elderly, but in all other instances oblation of the nail bed will be necessary to effect a cure.

Subungual exostosis

This condition usually presents as pain and swelling at

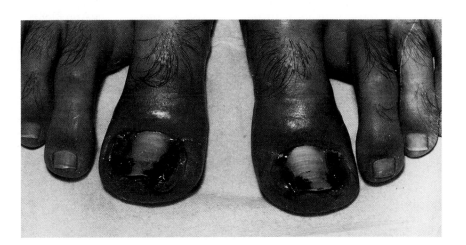

Fig. 26.40 Chronically infected ingrowing toe nails.

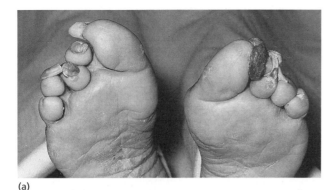

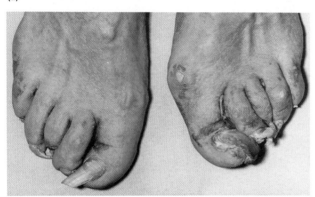

(a)

(b)

Fig. 26.41 (a,b) Onychogryphosis.

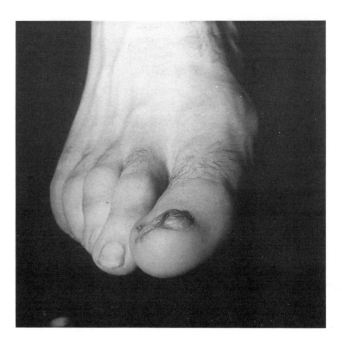

Fig. 26.42 Subungual exostosis of the great toe. Note the elevated nail.

the end of a toe. Obvious nail elevation is seen (Fig. 26.42). The exostosis arising from the terminal phalanx is easily removed after first avulsing the nail.

THE DIABETIC FOOT

Despite improved management of diabetes, the incidence of foot problems remains high. Complications affecting the foot are responsible for about 20% of diabetic admissions. Correct management depends on an accurate diagnosis of the underlying aetiological factors, and identifying those patients particularly at risk so that appropriate preventative measures can be taken.

AETIOLOGY

The lesions have been classified by Oakley *et al.* (1956) as septic, neuropathic, ischaemic and any combination of these. Usually more than one factor is involved though one is usually dominant in most patients. The neuropathic changes may affect soft tissues, joint or both.

SEPSIS

This is seldom a primary event and is nearly always superimposed on a neuropathic or vascular lesion, often after minor trauma. Unless recognized early and effectively treated, infection may prejudice the outcome for survival of the limb.

NEUROPATHY

This is usually a chronic condition of gradual onset due to a lesion in the peripheral nerves resulting from a metabolic disorder associated with the diabetes. A progressive polyneuropathy is the most common pattern. The soft tissues and joints are affected in varying degree. Control of the diabetes is more important than its duration when considering the incidence of neuropathy. Abnormalities of nerve conduction occur; the sensory neuropathy is the most common and manifests itself as early loss of pain and temperature sensation, and later loss of touch sensibility in a stocking distribution, distal impairment or loss of vibration sense and early loss of the ankle jerk. Loss of autonomic function leads to trophic skin changes such as hyperkeratosis; infection may enter through the cracks that develop in the brittle skin; the nails are often deformed and thickened. An intrinsic muscle palsy is the first manifestation of a motor neuropathy and leads to mobile and later fixed clawing of the toes (Fig. 25.43). It follows that excessive load will be taken on the metatarsal heads; callosities develop through which infection may enter, but due to the loss of pain sensibility the patient will be unaware

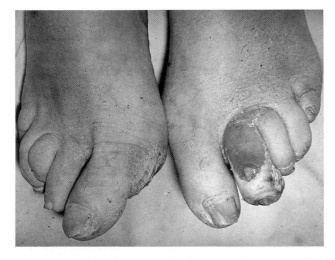

Fig. 26.43 Diabetic foot. Note the claw toes and gangrene of left second toe. (Reproduced by kind permission of Dr. Bob Elkeles.)

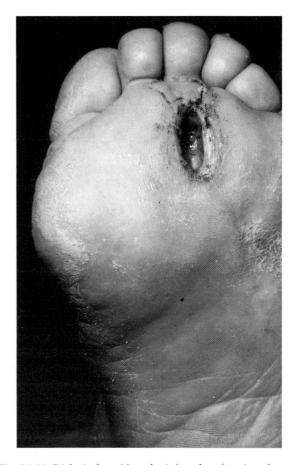

Fig. 26.44 Diabetic foot. Note the infected perforating ulcer. (Reproduced by kind permission of Dr. Bob Elkeles.)

that anything is wrong. Later, ulcers occur which rapidly extend to involve the bone or joints (Fig. 26.44). Charcot joints occur in patients with chronic disease, particularly if there have been periods of poor control of the diabetes. Load distribution under the feet of diabetics has been critically examined by Stokes *et al.* (1975), and their findings are important both with regard to the aetiology of the lesion and its management. Plantar pressure measurements have shown that most neuropathic ulcers can be correlated with areas of high pressure (Duckworth *et al.*, 1985).

VASCULAR CHANGES

Large- and small-vessel disease occurs, although the former is more common. Atherosclerosis is possibly more common in diabetics than in patients of the same age and the general population, but there is no proof that this is so. What is not in doubt is the fact that ischaemia of the foot is common in diabetics and peripheral gangrene of one or more toes may develop, usually as a result of the combined effects of neuropathy and sepsis (Fig. 26.45). Large-vessel disease is responsible for ischaemic ulceration in the majority of patients. The onset is usually a blister on the dorsum of the toes, side of the foot or the heel. Ulceration with surrounding erythema follows, and it fails to heal. If sepsis intervenes, the ulcer enlarges with surrounding cellulitis and swelling, and gangrene will follow in many cases.

DIAGNOSIS

It is of considerable importance to distinguish between

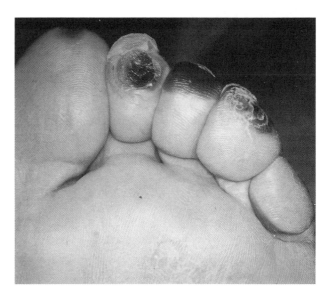

Fig. 26.45 Diabetic foot. Note the gangrene involving the terminal part of the toes. (Reproduced by kind permission of Dr. Bob Elkeles.)

ischaemic gangrene of the toe and a neuropathic lesion that is essentially a pressure sore; the former may lead to radical local ablation or a below-knee amputation whereas the latter will be amenable to some form of relatively simple local surgery.

The absence of pain in the presence of an infected ulcer or gangrene of the toe suggests a neuropathic lesion and would be confirmed by neurological examination. A typical neuropathic ulcer is painless and surrounded by greatly thickened epidermis. Deformity at the site of the ulcer is usually seen. Excess vascular granulation tissue is present in the floor of the ulcer. Rigid clawing of the toe suggests intrinsic muscle palsy. Ischaemia will be suggested by a painful ulcer which fails to heal and there may be a history of claudication. This will be detected by careful examination of the skin for the absence of hairs and the presence otherwise of the peripheral pulses with the help of Doppler ultrasound; the presence of sepsis will also be noted. It should always be borne in mind that an apparently superficial lesion is often a manifestation of extensive deep infection and necrosis of soft tissues, bone and joint structure.

INVESTIGATIONS

Radiography is of considerable assistance. Rarefaction of bone, periostisis and sequestrum formation suggest sepsis (Fig. 26.46). Neuropathic arthropathy is suggested by hypertropic bone destruction of joints. The midtarsal region is most frequently affected and results in either a rocker-bottom foot or valgus of the forefoot. Arteriography is only of value if disease of the proximal arterial vessels is suspected. The Doppler test will confirm the presence and extent of an ischaemic lesion and may therefore be of prognostic value. An isolated penetrating ulcer in the sole of the foot should not present a diagnostic problem if a complete history and examination are made. An alternative cause for such a lesion is any condition that produces a sensory deficit in the foot, e.g. leprosy (see p. 15) and a myelomeningocoele (Fig. 26.47).

TREATMENT

In general, a diabetic foot should be managed by a combination of medical, orthopaedic and chiropodial expertise.

PROPHYLACTIC

Patients should always be warned of the dangers of inadequate control of the diabetes. They must also

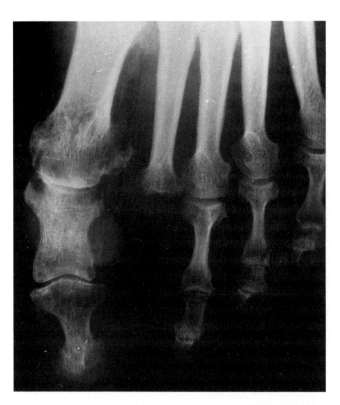

Fig. 26.46 Radiograph of diabetic foot. The second toe had been removed but a chronic discharging sinus developed. Note the erosions affecting the great toe joint and the second metatarsal head indicating chronic infection. The patient had a sensory neuropathy and developed gangrene of the hallux.

receive instruction in the regular washing of the feet, avoidance of minor trauma by not walking in bare feet, cutting toe nails correctly, wearing appropriate socks and shoes which should be made of wool. Surgical footwear with a moulded insole may be necessary, particularly if deformity is present. Excessive heat and cold must be avoided. Many patients are elderly, and have poor vision; their feet must receive regular attention from a chiropodist. If a patient is confined to bed for any reason the heels are prone to the rapid onset of pressure sores. The feet must be protected from the weight of the bed clothes, and the heel protected by suspending the legs in padded slings which must allow the patient to move freely in the bed.

CONSERVATIVE MEASURES

If infection is suspected, it must be treated vigorously with bed-rest, elevation and antibiotics. Infection with ischaemia is a dangerous combination; conservative treatment and infection may result in amputation and in such instances adequate surgical drainage must be undertaken. Ischaemic symptoms such as rest pain, especially

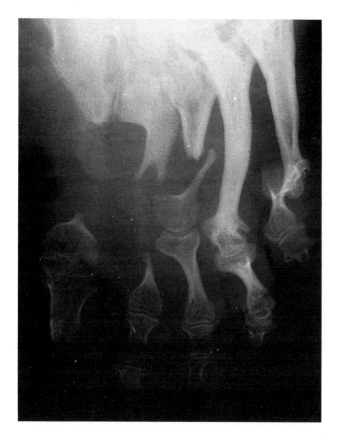

Fig. 26.47 Radiograph of foot of patient with myelo-meningocoele. Note the extensive bone destruction which is typical of the changes associated with neuropathy and secondary infection.

at night, may be controlled by analgesics, keeping the foot cool at night and a bed-time alcoholic drink. If pain is not relieved by these simple measures, amputation should be recommended without delay.

A neuropathic lesion will heal following application of simple measures to keep the affected part clean and dry; it is, of course, imperative to exclude deep infection which significantly alters the prognosis. Attention must be paid to the shoes so as to avoid pressure and, if necessary, special shoes will have to be made.

Mobile claw toes can be helped by incorporating a metatarsal insole in the shoes; rigid clawing is best managed either by surgical shoes or by a metatarsal rocker-bar.

OPERATIVE MEASURES

Adequate pre-operative care is essential and may permit less radical surgery than was first contemplated. Control of the diabetes is clearly essential and, in addition, reduction of oedema by elevation and control of infection

by antibiotics are important prerequisites. It is advisable to avoid using a tourniquet and suturing of wounds is not recommended unless tension is totally eliminated and it is certain that infection has been fully controlled.

Neuropathy plus infection

For lesions confined to a single toe, amputation through a metatarsophalangeal joint is recommended; if several toes are involved, a less troublesome foot will result from ablation of all the toes. Following this latter procedure, balance is surprisingly good and the insertion of a toe block permits the patient to wear normal shoes. If the metatarsal is involved, it must be excised with the toe and the skin flaps allowed to fall together; in some instances more than one ray has to be excised. For these patients, consideration should be given to advising amputation of the remaining uninvolved toes so as to avoid the inevitable later development of deformity. If limited amputation and drainage procedures fail to control the infection, a below-knee amputation should be advised. However, it must always be remembered that in the absence of ischaemia, a radical amputation can be deferred for a long time because healing will occur in most instances even if it is slow, provided there is careful attention to detail and the patient cooperates fully with the programme of management.

THE ISCHAEMIC FOOT

In the early stages, either bed-rest or crutches non-weight-bearing for a time combined with antibiotics, local debridement and good footwear are appropriate measures. Suitable insoles will relieve pressure on the ulcer. Control of deformity such as claw and hammer toes with prominent metatarsal heads, equinus or cavus may be necessary before the ulcer will heal.

In more advanced cases, toe amputation or ray resection may be necessary.

It should be borne in mind that the patient may have a treatable atherosclerotic lesion and a vascular surgeon should always be consulted.

The problem in the ischaemic foot is no different from the non-diabetic ischaemic foot; however, reconstructive arterial surgery is less likely to be successful in a patient with diabetes because, generally, the atherosclerosis is widespread and more often peripheral. Almost all these patients will come to an amputation below or through the knee.

Ischaemia with infection

In this condition, the usual presentation is a foot with one or more gangrenous toes. It has a poor prognosis and the sudden deterioration and loss of diabetic control are not uncommon. If a single toe is involved it is worth attempting a local amputation but the patient must be told there is only about a 30% chance of success, namely primary healing and saving the foot. In the majority, and if more than one toe is involved, a below-knee amputation is the procedure of choice.

REFERENCES

Adams J.C. (1976) *Standard Orthopaedic Operations.* Edinburgh, Churchill Livingstone.

Bonney G. and MacNab (1952) Critical survey of operative results. *J. Bone Joint Surg.* **34B**, 366.

Chomeley J.A. (1953) Elmslie's operation for calcaneus foot. *J. Bone Joint Surg.* **34B**, 46.

Citron N. and Neil M. (1987) Dorsal wedge osteotomy of the proximal phalanx for hallux rigidus. *J. Bone Joint Surg.* **69B**, 835.

Devas M. (1975) *Stress Fractures.* Edinburgh, Churchill Livingstone.

Duckworth T., Boulton A.J.M., Betts A.P. *et al.* (1985) Plantar pressure measurements and the prevention of ulceration in the diabetic foot.

Dwyer F.C. (1959) Osteotomy of the calcaneum for pes cavus. *J. Bone Joint Surg.* **41B**, 80–86.

Dwyer F.C. (1961) Osteotomy of the calcaneum in the treatment of grossly everted feet with special reference to cerebral palsy. *Huitième Congrès Internationale de Chirurgie Orthopédique et de Traumatologie*, p. 892.

Dwyer F.C. (1964) The relationship of variations in size and inclination of the calcaneus to the shape and function of the whole foot. *Ann. Roy. Coll. Surg.* **34**, 120.

Evan D.L. (1953) Recurrent instability of the ankle—a method of surgical treatment. *Proc. Roy. Soc. Med.* **46**, 343.

Fitzgerald J.A.W. (1969) A review of long-term results of arthrodesis of the first metatarsophalangeal joint. *J. Bone Joint Surg.* **51B**, 488.

Gallocher J. (1967) A study of the sesamoid bones and related structures in the first metatarsophalangeal joint of the foot. *Chiropodist* **22** (12).

Gibson J. and Piggott H. (1962) Osteotomy of the neck of the first metatarsal in the treatment of hallux valgus. *J. Bone Joint Surg.* **44B**, 349.

Girdlestone G.R. (1974) Physiotherapy for hand and foot. *J. Chartered Soc. Physiother.* **32**, 167.

Glasgow M., Jackson A. and Jamieson A.M. (1980) Instability of the ankle after injury to the lateral ligament. *J. Bone Joint Surg.* **62B**, 196.

Golden G.N. (1961) Hallux valgus, the osteotomy operation. *Br. Med. J.* **1**, 1361.

Goodfellow J. (1966) Aetiology of hallux rigidus. *Proc. Roy. Soc. Med.* **59**, 821.

Hardy R.H. and Clapham T.C.R. (1952) Hallux valgus—predisposing anatomical causes. *Lancet* **1**, 1180.

Hawkins F.B., Mitchell C.L. and Hendrick D.W. (1945) Correction of hallux valgus. *J. Bone Joint Surg.* **44B**, 349.

Helal B. (1975) Metatarsal osteotomy for metatarsalgia. *J. Bone Joint Surg.* **57B**, 187.

Helal B. (1981) Surgery for adolescent hallux valgus. *Clin. Orthopaed.* **157**, 50–63.

Hohmann G. (1925) Der Hallux Valgus und die übrigen Zehenverkrummingen. *Ergeb. Chir. Orthop.* **18**, 308.

Jordan M.H. and Brodski A.E. (1951) Keller's operation for hallux valgus and hallux rigidus. *Arch. Surg.* **62**, 586.

Karlsson J., Bergsten T., Lansinger O. *et al.* (1989) Lateral instability of the ankle treated by Evans' procedure. *J. Bone Joint Surg.* **70B**, 476.

Keller W.L. (1912) Further observations on the surgical treatment of hallux valgus and bunions. *NY Med. J.* **95**, 696.

Kessel L. and Bonney G. (1958) Hallux rigidus in the adolescent. *J. Bone Joint Surg.* **40B**, 668.

Kvist H. and Kvist M. (1980) The operative treatment of chronic calcaneal paratenonitis. *J. Bone Joint Surg.* **62B**, 353.

Lambrinudi C. (1938) Metatarsus primus elevatus. *Proc. R. Soc. Med.* **31**, 1273.

Mann R.A. and Clanton T.O. (1988) Hallux rigidus: treatment by cheilectomy. *J. Bone Joint Surg.* **70A**, 400.

Mitchell C.L., Flemming J.L., Allen R. *et al.* (1958) Osteotomy—bunionectomy for hallux valgus. *J. Bone Joint Surg.* **40A**, 41.

Mosier K.M. and Asher M. (1984) Tarsal coalition in peroneal spastic flat foot. *J. Bone Joint Surg.* **66A**, 976.

Moynihan F.J. (1967) Arthrodesis of the metatarsophalangeal joint of the great toe. *J. Bone Joint Surg.* **49B**, 544.

Mygind J.B. (1952) Operation for hallux valgus. Report of Danish Orthopaedic Association. *J. Bone Joint Surg.* **34B**, 529.

Nissen K.I. (1948) Plantar digital neuritis: Morton's metatarsalgia. *J. Bone Joint Surg.* **30B**, 84.

Oakley W., Catterall R.C.F. and Martin H.M. (1956) Aetiology and management of lesions of the foot in diabetes. *Br. Med. J.* **2**, 953.

Peabody C.W. (1931) The surgical cure of hallux valgus. *J. Bone Joint Surg.* **13**, 273.

Piggott H. (1960) Natural history of hallux valgus in adolescence and early adult life. *J. Bone Joint Surg.* **42B**, 749.

Pyper J.B. (1958) The flexor—extensor tendon transplant operation for claw toes. *J. Bone Joint Surg.* **40B**, 528.

Raymakers R. and Waugh W. (1971) The treatment of metatarsalgia with hallux valgus. *J. Bone Joint Surg.* **53B**, 684.

Rix R.R. (1968) Modified Mayo operation for hallux valgus and bunion—a comparison with the Keller procedure. *J. Bone Joint Surg.* **50A**, 1368.

Rogers W.A. and Joplin R.J. (1947) Hallux valgus weak foot and Keller's operation—An end-result study. *Surg. Clin. North Am.* **27**, 1295.

Smillie I.S. (1967) Treatment of Freiberg's infraction. *Proc. Roy. Soc. Med.* **60**, 29.

Snook G.A., Chrisman D. and Wilson T.C. (1985) Long-term results of the Chrisman—Snook operation for reconstruction of the lateral ligament of the ankle. *J. Bone Joint Surg.* **67A**, 1.

Stokes I.A.E., Faris I.B. and Hutton W.C. (1975) The neuropathic ulcer and loads on the foot in diabetic patients. *Acta Orthop. Scand.* **41**, 839.

Swanson A.B., Lumsden R.M. and Swanson G.D. (1979) Silicone implant arthroplasty of the great toe. *Clin. Orthop.* **142**, 30.

Taylor R.G. (1951) The treatment of claw toes by multiple transfer of flexor into extensor tendons. *J. Bone Joint Surg.* **33B**, 539.

Thomas F.B. (1962) Keller's arthroplasty modified. *J. Bone Joint Surg.* **44B**, 356.

Thomas F.B. (1974) Levelling the tread. *J. Bone Joint Surg.* **56A**, 314.

Townsend A.C. and Scott P.J. (1966) Ingrowing toe nails and onychogryphosis *J. Bone Joint Surg.* **48B**, 354.

Watson-Jones R. (1976) *Fracture and Joint Injuries*, 5th edn. Edinburgh, Churchill Livingstone, p. 115.

Wilson J.N. (1963) Oblique displacement osteotomy for hallux valgus. *J. Bone Joint Surg.* **45B**, 552.

Wilson J.N. (1967) Cone-arthrodesis of the first metatarsophalangeal joint. *J. Bone Joint Surg.* **49B**, 98.

Chapter 27

Surgical Disorders of Peripheral Nerves

R. Birch

INTRODUCTION

Function of the musculoskeletal system is dependent upon the peripheral nerves and this chapter outlines their structure, function and some disorders of function.

STRUCTURE AND FUNCTION

The peripheral nerves consist of bundles of nerve fibres with connective tissues and their vascular supply. The conducting elements of peripheral nerves are the axons, which are extensions of cells within the dorsal root ganglion (the somatic afferent), in the ventral horn of the spinal cord (somatic efferent) or in the autonomic ganglia (the sympathetic and parasympathetic). The axon with its sheath of satellite cells, the Schwann cells, form the nerve fibre. Nerve fibres are enveloped by the endoneurial sheath or tube, a condensation of the endoneurium and of the cell membrane of the Schwann cells. The diameter of axons ranges from less than 1 μm to 20 μm. The smallest axons are embraced by continuous columns of Schwann cell processes. They are called 'non-myelinated nerve fibres'. Larger axons are surrounded by a lamellar envelope of myelin, and are called 'myelinated nerve fibres'. Myelin is formed by the Schwann cells and forms a cylinder along the axon which narrows at the nodes of Ranvier (Fig. 27.1a−c).

Axons transmit information by means of the action potential, a self-propagating constant amplitude impulse caused by the exchange of sodium and potassium ions across voltage-sensitive channels or pores within the membranes of the axons. In non-myelinated fibres this process occurs along the length of the axolemma and occurs at the rate of about 1 m/sec. In myelinated nerve fibres, ion exchange is restricted to the axon where it is relatively exposed at the node of Ranvier. This saltatory (jumping) conduction allows much higher speed of trans-

mission of the axon potential, up to 70 m/sec for the largest diameter axons.

In addition to transmitting information by means of axon potentials, the axons also afford chemical transmission of organelles and substances within their cytoplasm. Chemical transport occurs both centrifugally and centripetally. Slow systems of transmission of 0.1−2 mm/day and fast systems up to 400 mm/day have been recognized.

The fast centrifugal transport system conveys transmitter agents, lipids, glycoproteins, amino acids and polypeptides. The slow centrifugal system conveys materials for the maintenance of the membrane and the cytoskeleton, such as the constituent proteins of microtubules, neurofilaments and microfilaments. The fast centripetal system is of increasing clinical interest, for it conveys the neuronotrophic factors important for cell survival.

The connective tissues

Nerve fibres are embedded within the endoneurium, a connective-tissue space of collagen fluid fibroblasts and capillaries. The perineurium is the best delineated of the connective-tissue envelopes of peripheral nerve. It is formed from lamellae of flattened cells which are derived from fibroblasts. Up to 15 layers of these cells define collections of nerve fibres into bundles or fascicles. The perineurium is the major source of the tensile strength of a peripheral nerve. It is a diffusion barrier. The contents of the bundle within the perineurium are under pressure. Experimental 'windowing' of the perineurium leads to herniation of the contents and to local demyelination. The epineurium is a condensation of areolar connective tissue surrounding numbers of nerve bundles. It contains collagen, fat, fibroblasts and other cell types. The extrinsic vascular system of longitudinal vessels runs within

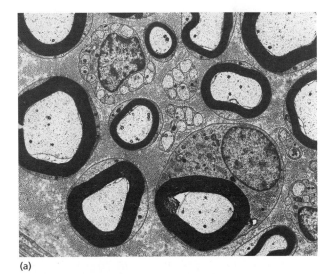

(a)

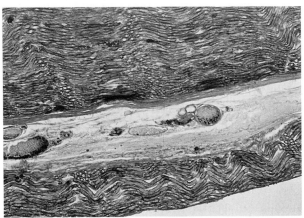

(b)

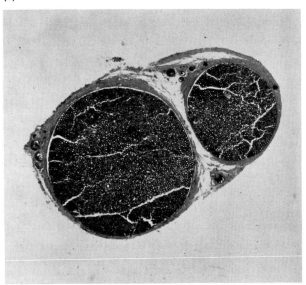

(c)

the epineurium supplied at essentially constant intervals by pedicles entering from adjacent vascular axes. The epineurial system communicates with the intrinsic vascular system passing between the bundles and within the endoneurium.

The epineurium forms the greater proportion of the cross-sectional area of a nerve trunk. Sunderland (1978) has shown that the epineurium constitutes 30−75% of the cross-sectional area of a nerve trunk, that the proportion of epineurium is greater in multifascicular nerves, and that it is greater where nerves traverse joints. He also noted that fat within the epineurium was prominent in the human sciatic nerve in the buttock and at the hip. The epineurium is responsible for protection against compression, and to a lesser extent against tension. It certainly allows a nerve trunk to glide independently of adjacent tissues, notably at joints. When it is scarred it becomes adherent to adjacent tissue. Pain and loss of function follow.

A functional classification of nerve fibres

The nerve action potential is characterized by a series of peaks. Matching these with nerve fibre diameter allows a broad classification of function (Table 27.1). The largest nerve fibres, α-fibres, conducting at rates between 70 and 130 m/sec control skeletal muscle fibre and convey impulses for proprioception. A-β fibres are responsible for sensations of touch and of pressure. A-δ fibres carry impulses for pain, touch and temperature. Less is known about the large numbers of C fibres, which are non-myelinated but these include the postganglionic sympathetic fibres and are responsible for some types of pain sensation, characterized by a burning and rather unpleasant quality.

This considerable oversimplification leads to the question, what is the real function of such specialized sensory receptors as Meissner or Paccinian corpuscles? Are such organelles responsible for specific perceptions such as

Fig. 27.1 (a) Mouse sciatic nerve (× 4250). Clusters of non-myelinated nerve fibres embedded within Schwann cell cytoplasm. A large myelinated nerve fibre surrounded by Schwann cell cytoplasm containing numerous organelles lies close to a Schwann nucleus. (b) Longitudinal section of rat sciatic nerve (Weigert−Pal technique × 100). Wavy-form dark-staining nerve fibres are surrounded by a well-defined perineurium. The epineurium contains numerous blood vessels. (c) Transverse section of rat sciatic nerve (Weigert−Pal technique × 40). Myelinated nerve fibres organized in two clearly defined bundles.

Table 27.1 Nerve action potentials and fibre diameter in relation to function

Diameter (μm)*	Conduction velocity (m/sec)	Function
A-α MNF (12−20)	70−130	Extrafusal muscle fibres, proprioception
A-β MNF (5−12)	30−70	Touch, pressure
A-γ MNF (3−6)	15−30	Intrafusal muscle fibre
A-δ MNF (2−5)	10−30	Pain, touch, temperature
B MNF (1.5−3)	3−15	Pre-ganglionic sympathetic fibres
C NMNF (<2.0)	0.5−2	Pain, post-ganglionic sympathetic fibres

* MNF, myelinated nerve fibre; NMNF, non-myelinated nerve fibre.

touch, vibration, pressure or stretching? Iggo (1977, 1986) in two important reviews, has shown that they do. The morphology of sensory receptors in the skin has been defined by electron microscopy, and their physiological characteristics by quantitive electrophysiological investigations. Correlation of morphology and physiology followed combining percutaneous microelectrostimulation and recording from individual nerve fibres and their sensory receptors in conscious subjects and matching these responses with the evoked sensory perceptions (Ochoa and Torebjork, 1983). This work confirms that there are four groups of sensory receptors with large myelinated axons in glabrous skin; Paccinian corpuscles, Meissner corpuscles, Merkel discs and Ruffini endings. There are two kinds of thermoreceptor with fine-myelinated or non-myelinated axons. Rapidly adapting afferent units have Meissner corpuscles as receptors and electrical stimulation of these produces a sensation of non-painful tapping. Increasing the frequency of stimulation caused changes in sensation from tapping to flutter vibration. The sensation was consistent, there was no quality of pressure, tickling, heat or cold, or pain whatever the frequency or pattern of stimulation. The sensation of sustained pressure is conveyed by slowly adapting units that have Merkel discs as their receptors. Stimulation of Paccinian corpuscle units cause sensations of tickling or vibration.

Table 27.2 shows the proven functions of different sensory receptors. Again, this is a considerable oversimplification. Iggo emphasizes the modulatory effect of the central nervous system on the trains of impulses reaching it through peripheral nerves. Wynn-Parry (1986) emphasized that the sensory function of the hand in discriminating between objects and textures is based upon the stimulation of many thousands of sensory receptors and a central interpretation of the volleys of impulses.

Some surgical implications

The blood supply to the peripheral nerve trunks is rich and it is very difficult to produce ischaemia within a nerve by ligation of pedicles entering into the epineurium. However, compression or stretching of a nerve will induce ischaemia, by inducing venous stasis. Lundborg (1988) has persuasively argued that the perineurium forms the sheath around a bundle or fascicle of nerve fibres which constitutes a compartment and that manipulation of a nerve may induce an increased intracom-

Table 27.2 Some skin sensory units

Receptor	Physiological name	Morphological receptor	Stimulus	Nerve fibre	Sensation evoked
Low-threshold mechanoreceptors	Slow adapting, SA1	Merkel cell	Maintained skin displacement	A-β	Sustained pressure
	Rapid adapting, RA	Meissner corpuscle	Transient skin displacement	A-β	Tapping
	Rapid adapting	Paccinian corpuscle	Transient skin displacement	A-β	Buzzing, flutter
Thermoreceptors	Cooling	Cold receptor		A-δ and C	Cooling
	Warming	Warm receptor		C	Warming
Nocioceptors	Myelinated nocioceptor	Unmyelinated fibre Schwann cell complex in basal epidermis	Harmful skin deformation	A-β and A-δ	Sharp pain
	C polymodal nocioceptor	?	Harmful heat, chemicals	C	Burning pain

partmental pressure with associated oedema and ischaemia. It is also clear that interference with the perineurium in the course of an operation is harmful. The perineurium should not be breached. For these reasons the surgeon will always exercise great care in operations of decompression or transposition. So-called 'internal' neurolysis is reserved only for cases of partial transection of a nerve where intact bundles are preserved, resecting only those which have formed a neuroma.

Acute compression in the unconscious patient causes severe disturbance of function. Lack of care in positioning the anaesthetized patient may result in neuropathy of the brachial plexus, of the ulnar nerve at the elbow, or of the common peroneal nerve at the neck of the fibula. As Wadsworth (1977) pointed out the iatrogenic cubital tunnel syndrome has a poor prognosis, and full recovery is exceptional. The earliest symptoms of compartment syndrome, following fracture or operation, reflect disturbance of peripheral nerve function, and are evidence of external compression of that nerve trunk. These include pain, disturbance of sensation, and progressive weakness. Neglect of these symptoms will lead to ischaemic contracture or worse. Larger sensory and motor myelinated nerve fibres are more susceptible to pressure than the non-myelinated variety; sweating, vasomotor control and touch are commonly spared in simple conduction block. Conversely the smallest fibres, A-δ and C are the first to be blocked by local anaesthesia and severe pain suggests an irritative lesion of a nerve, from an encircling suture or from haematoma compression.

SOME CAUSES OF NERVE INJURIES
(Table 27.3)

Open wounds

It is useful to distinguish between open- and closed-nerve lesions although the mechanisms of injury may overlap. The special report from the Medical Research Council (1954) is a work of unparalleled exactitude and range. The experience of war wounds dictated a policy of delayed nerve suture. Seddon (1975) advised primary nerve repair in particularly favourable cases, of an uncontaminated wound, if a surgeon of skill and experience was available with requisite facilities. Rank *et al.* (1973) introduced a very useful concept of the tidy and the untidy wound in their discussion of the timing of repair of nerves and of tendons. Most open wounds in civilian practice would come into their category of the tidy wound and in these, granted Seddon's requirements, primary repair is preferred. Delay is still the wisest

Table 27.3 Causes of nerve injuries

Lesion	Characteristic	Agent
Open	Tidy	Knife, glass, scalpel
	Untidy	Missile, burn, open fracture — dislocation
Closed	Compression — ischaemia	Pressure neuropathy in the anaesthetized patient. Compartment syndrome
	Traction — ischaemia	Fracture dislocation
	Thermal	Acrylic cement, electrical burn
	Irradiation	Irradiation neuritis
	Injection	Regional anaesthetic block, intravenous or intra-arterial catheterization

course when there is a real risk of infection. Obvious examples include the gunshot or missile injury, the thermal injury, and the complex open fracture with heavy contamination of muscle and other tissues.

Compression and traction

Both compression and traction upon a nerve induce ischaemia. Of the two, traction is the more harmful. Lundborg and Rydevik (1973) showed that venous flow was blocked when a nerve was stretched 8% beyond resting length and that complete ischaemia was induced when the nerve was stretched to 15%. Kwan and Woo (1991) showed that conduction was significantly disturbed when a nerve trunk was stretched to as little as 6%. Rupture is the extreme form of traction lesion and is commonly associated with fractures or dislocations. It is increasingly clear that the sciatic nerve at the hip is particularly vulnerable to traction during operations for fracture or replacement arthroplasty. Arthroplasty for congenital dislocation of the hip carries a 5% risk of compromising sciatic nerve function (Schmalzreid and Amstutz, 1991).

Thermal injuries

Cold injuries to nerves have been well described. Denny Brown *et al.* (1945) showed severe cold caused Wallerian degeneration but there was no disruption of the connective-tissue sheaths of the nerves so that regeneration was possible. Less has been written about heat injuries. Dale (1954) and DeVicenti *et al.* (1969) described electrical burns showing how serious these were because of extensive muscle necrosis. Wilkinson and Clarke (1992) described two cases of burns of the brachial plexus in unconscious patients. The skin injury was full thickness and there was very little recovery from the burn of the underlying nerve. Birch *et al.* (1992) described a case where the sciatic nerve was virtually destroyed by extruded cement and went on to show the nerve was damaged to a margin of about 5 mm from the cement (Fig. 27.2a–c). Care to remove extraneous cement is obviously important but when such an accident occurs it does seem reasonable to resect the damaged segment of the nerve and to graft it.

Irradiation neuritis (IN)

Although pain and loss of function in a limb following radiotherapy to the axilla or the pelvis for cancer may indicate recurrent disease, direct injury to the brachial or lumbosacral plexus by irradiation is an important differential diagnosis. No distinct clinical features indicate a certain diagnosis of IN. Kori *et al.* (1981) reported that lesions of the upper trunk with associated lymphoedema suggested IN, whereas severe pain with involvement of the lower trunk with a Bernard–Horner syndrome indicated recurrence. However, IN may cause the most intense pain and it may affect all or any part of the plexus. Vautrin (1954) reported on IN in five patients with different primary cancers. There was progressive and irreversible progression of the lesion. Speiss (1972) demonstrated the changes in the axon and in the myelin sheath following irradiation and concluded that these

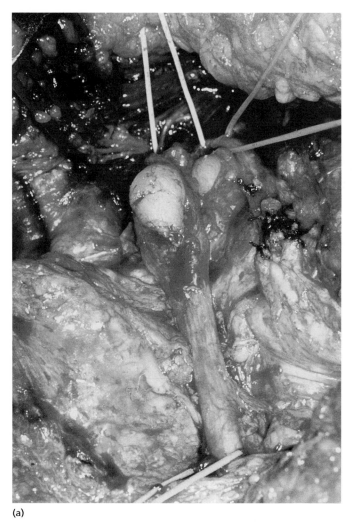

(a)

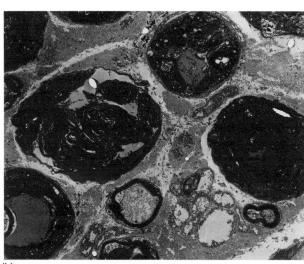

(b)

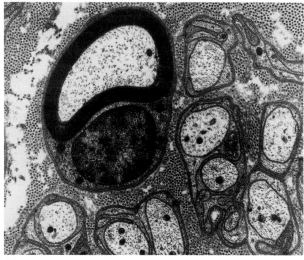

(c)

Fig. 27.2 (a) Sciatic nerve stretched over extruded cement from total hip arthroplasty. (b) Biopsy from the nerve adjacent to cement showing necrosis (× 3600). (c) Biopsy of the nerve 2 cm from the cement. The appearances are normal (× 10 800).

changes together with vasculitis led to progressive endo-neurial fibrosis. The late development of malignant peripheral nerve-sheath tumours after irradiation is now clearly established (Sordillo *et al.*, 1981; Ducatman and Scheithauer, 1983).

Findings at operation suggest that there is often an element of external compression from fibrosis of adjacent muscles. Such underlying anatomical abnormalities as a cervical rib may contribute to the problem. In some cases, intense thickening of fascial sheath and of the epineurium is evident, with obliteration of the longit-udinal blood vessels. Examination of biopsies shows intense endoneurial fibrosis and demyelination. Associ-ated thrombosis of the subclavian artery can occur.

Narakas *et al.* (1989) described the evolution of the lesion in 126 patients in whom operation had been performed. They found that symptoms commenced at between 6 months and 18 years after treatment but they also refer to patients in whom recurrence of breast carcinoma became apparent 17 years after initial pre-sentation. A typical presentation for IN is when the patient notes pins and needles in the thumb and index finger between 18 months 3 years after treatment. A diagnosis of carpal tunnel syndrome is made although close examination shows impairment of lateral cord function with weakness of elbow and wrist flexors.

Investigations are of limited value, although Albers *et al.* (1981) have described rhythmic voluntary muscle contraction in some patients and suggest that there is a typical electromyographic pattern in IN, termed 'myokymia'. Computed tomography scans may be useful in demonstrating fibrosis with narrowing of the sub-clavian vein and also in demonstrating metastases (Cooke *et al.*, 1988).

Drug treatment is probably valueless and two types of operations have been described. The first is where the brachial plexus is decompressed by excision of adjacent scar tissue. Pain is relieved and deterioration halted in about 50% of cases (Narakas, 1989). The author has performed this operation in 35 patients, finding recur-rence of malignant disease in five cases. Significant pain relief occurred in 18 patients; serious complications included failure of wound healing, deterioration in neurological function and thrombosis of the axillary artery.

Other operations go further and attempt to improve the blood supply to the damaged nerves combining neurolysis with a free transfer of a vascularized flap of omentum. Brunelli *et al.* performed this in 63 patients and achieved substantial pain relief in pain in 55 cases (Narakas, 1989). There was much less improvement in function. IN is underdiagnosed. It is progressive and it is

painful and in about one-third of patients, all function is lost and pain becomes so severe that operation within the spinal cord may prove necessary. The reader is referred to the excellent recent review of Thomas and Holdorff (1993) who discuss radiation-induced neuro-pathy as well as other neuropathies caused by physical agents.

Injection

Injection injuries to nerves should be no more than a matter of historical interest, unfortunately this is not the case. The sciatic nerve, the brachial plexus, the nerves to the shoulder and the nerves in front of the elbow are particularly at risk from injection for therapeutic pur-poses, from cannulation of adjacent vessels for contrast studies or parenteral feeding and from regional anaes-thesia. Seddon (1975) has described 24 cases. Pain was often severe and recovery often limited. He demonstrated intense intraneural fibrosis often extending far within a nerve. Hudson (1993) confirmed that damage to the nerve was related not only to the chemical nature of the offending agent but also whether this was injected within the nerve or merely adjacent to it. In an experimental series he showed that such commonly used agents as lignocaine, procaine, hydrocortisone and triamcinolone produced extensive degeneration and fibrosis when injected into the rat sciatic nerve.

A grasp of the anatomy of the neurovascular axis of limbs should abolish these injuries. When a conscious patient complains immediately of very severe pain in the distribution of a nerve during the course of an injection, it must be assumed that the needle is in a nerve and although there is still controversy about the role of operation in this condition, the author believes that it is wise to expose the nerve, to incise the epineurium but not the perineurium, and to irrigate the nerve trunk with physiological Ringer's solution.

A CLASSIFICATION OF NERVE INJURIES

A classification of nerve injuries is only useful if it can be readily applied in clinical diagnosis. Two systems are in general use, the physiological described by Seddon and the anatomical of Sunderland. The author prefers Seddon's classification although Sunderland's scheme does help in the understanding of traction lesions. Table 27.4 outlines the two systems.

Table 27.4 Classification of nerve injuries

Seddon	Sunderland	Functional loss	Anatomical lesion	Neurophysiological
Neurapraxia (non-degenerative)	Grade I	Muscle power, gnosis	Axon and nerve fibre sheath intact	Distal conduction maintained — no fibrillation
Axonotmesis (degenerative)	Grade II, III	All modalities	Interruption and distal Wallerian degeneration of axon	Conduction lost, fibrillation
Neurotmesis (degenerative)	Grade IV, V	All modalities	Interruption of the nerve trunk, Wallerin degeneration	Conduction lost, fibrillation

Neurapraxia

This is a conduction block. There is no interruption of the axon or of the nerve fibre. Power and discriminatory sensation are lost, and pressure sense and sympathetic function are maintained. The prognosis is excellent assuming that the causal lesion has been removed. True neurapraxia is not common in clinical practice. One example is the loss of conduction seen in a nerve trunk exposed at operation with a proximal suprasystolic cuff. The muscle twitch, from stimulation of the nerve, weakens and disappears at about 30 minutes and is rapidly restored to normal when the cuff is removed. This transient conduction block is clearly ischaemic. Prolonged conduction block is sometimes seen after such mishaps as overlong use of a tourniquet cuff or after an unduly high cuff pressure has been used. Ochoa *et al.* (1972) showed that there was a morphological change in the nerve fibre with a characteristic deformity of the nodes of Ranvier which are displaced away from the compressed segment of the nerve. There is distortion and fracturing of the paranodal myelin. Gilliatt's (1980) excellent review of acute conduction block clearly analyses this form of the lesion and it is one of particular clinical significance. Birch and St. Clair Strange (1990) went so far as to coin the term 'neuramanosis', in a description of three patients where decompression of a nerve trunk which had not been working for many months was followed by rapid recovery. The report has merit in drawing attention to this lesion although the authors were probably not justified in introducing another term.

Pain is not an important feature in neurapraxia. Electrical conduction in the distal nerve trunk persists and as there is no denervation of muscle fibrillation potentials are not seen. Neurapraxia, or worse, neuro-praxia is commonly used to describe lesions of nerves which are plainly degenerative. A surgeon who considers the diagnosis for a nerve which is not working where there is a wound over the course of the nerve is surely unwise.

Axonotmesis

The axons are interrupted, Wallerian degeneration follows, but the connective-tissue envelopes of the nerve and the nerve fibre sheaths are intact. If the cause of the lesion is removed then spontaneous recovery occurs. A typical example is the radial nerve palsy following closed fracture of the shaft of the humerus, where over 70% recover.

Neurotmesis

The nerve trunk is divided. It is the commonest finding in open wounds but also occurs in traction lesions.

The clinical features of axonotmesis and neurotmesis are identical. All function is lost. After Wallerian degeneration has occurred, there is no distal conduction in the nerve trunk, and fibrillation potentials appear within the denervated muscle at about three weeks from the injury. Clinical diagnosis of nerve lesions is simplified by asking whether this is a non-degenerative lesion (nerve conduction block, neurapraxia) or is it a degenerative lesion (axonotmesis, neurotmesis) (Thomas and Ochoa, 1993). The one consistently reliable physical sign for a degenerative lesion of a mixed nerve trunk or a cutaneous nerve is loss of sudo- and vasomotor function of the post-ganglionic sympathetic fibres. The affected part is red and dry. Neurapraxia cannot be considered as a diagnosis with this evidence.

The next question for the clinician is to distinguish

between the two types of degenerative lesion: those which will recover spontaneously and those where recovery can only be expected after the nerve has been repaired. Neurotmesis is the most likely diagnosis where there is a wound over the course of the nerve and this includes surgical wounds (Fig. 27.3). Axonotmesis is more likely in closed fractures and dislocations, in many traction lesions and in ischaemic injury but overlap between these categories is common so that exploration of the nerve may be necessary to assess the extent of the injury. Traction lesions are particularly difficult, especially in the infraclavicular brachial plexus and in the obstetric brachial plexus palsy. A frequent finding in such cases is apparent continuity of the nerve trunk although this is stretched and may become so coiled as to resemble a twisted barley sugar. There may be no recovery in these cases because the conducting elements, the Schwann tubes and the perineurium have been disrupted over a long segment of the nerve.

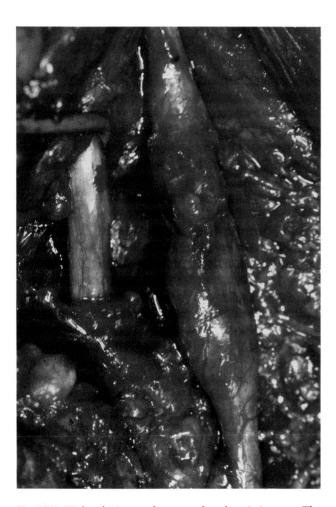

Fig. 27.3 High-velocity gunshot wound to the sciatic nerve. The tibial nerve recovered — axonotmesis. The common peroneal nerve was disrupted — neurotmesis.

Two investigations are particularly useful in distinguishing between the degenerative lesion of favourable prognosis from that where spontaneous recovery cannot be expected. The first is clinical. Tinel (1919) described how percussion along the course of a peripheral nerve, from distal to proximal induced intense paraesthesia within the territory of that nerve when the examining finger came to a neuroma. If Tinel's sign advances down the limb, at the predicted rate of regeneration for a degenerative lesion, which is roughly 1 mm a day or 1 inch a month, then recovery can be expected. If Tinel's sign remains firmly fixed at the level of the injury to the nerve, then it must be assumed that the nerve has been transected. Electromyography is the second useful investigation. This may show early re-innervation of muscles still apparently paralysed.

DEGENERATION AND REGENERATION

When a nerve trunk is cut, Wallerian degeneration occurs in the distal trunk with early disintegration of the axon cylinder and then more slowly, breakdown of the myelin sheath. There is a great increase in cell population of Schwann cells, fibroblasts and macrophages. Schwann cells form essentially orderly columns, the bands of Bungner, and synthesize neuronotrophic factors such as nerve growth factor. This intense biological response prepares an environment favourable to the reception and guidance of regenerating axons. Proximally, axons throw out sprouts, the growth cones (Fig. 27.4a,b). In favourable situations, the growth cones enter the bands of Bungner. If there has been no repair, the growth cones meander into connective tissue or other foreign tissue to form a neuroma. There is increasing awareness of the significance of central changes. Axotomy in the neonatal animal leads to extensive death within a population of parent neurones, particularly within the spinal cord. Although central cell death is less marked in adult animals, it is significant particularly in proximal and severe injuries of nerves such as the traction rupture or avulsion of brachial plexus. Bonney (personal communication, 1975) noted atrophy of the ipsilateral spinal cord during operations of hemilaminectomy to establish the diagnosis in injuries of the brachial plexus. Dyck *et al.* (1984) showed a marked reduction in the ventral motor neurone pool in the spinal cord of patients who had had previous amputation of the lower limb.

There is growing appreciation of the role of neuronotrophic factors (NTF) in regeneration. The reader is referred to the important review of Richardson (1991). It is now known that nerve growth factor is essential

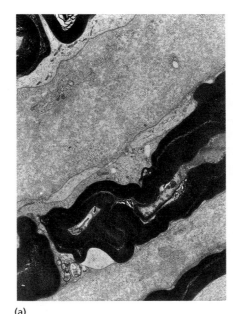

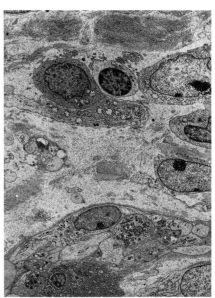

Fig. 27.4 (a) Human ulnar nerve (× 2000). Distal stump 3 weeks after division. The axons have collapsed; there is disruption of the myelin sheath. (b) The proximal stump (× 1600). Numbers of axon sprouts and Schwann cell extensions are seen. There is intense nuclear activity.

(a)

(b)

in the maintenance of sympathetic and some sensory neurones. Ciliary neuronotrophic factor prevents the death of motor neurones in the facial nerve nucleus of the rat. Further studies of NTF in the regeneration of human peripheral nerves is already clinically significant. Anand *et al.* (1991) described the first recognized clinical example of deprivation of sensory nerve growth factor presenting as an autonomic and sensory neuropathy. More recently Anand *et al.* (1993) have shown that the NTF levels are reduced in injured nerve stumps biopsied during operations for repair of the brachial plexus and they suggest that local administration of NTF may be indicated.

It is now clear that NTF are substances influencing the survival and growth of nerve cells, and are of great importance in regeneration after repair of a nerve. NTF are synthesized not only by target organs but also by the cell population within the distal stump. How do the new nerve fibres find their way to their proper target? The modern view follows the work of Cajal and Ramon (1928) who saw chemotropism and contact guidance as complementary rather than conflicting processes. Diffusible proteins synthesized as in a distal nerve segment do exert a neurotropic influence on axon sprouts and Lundborg (1988) has proven that the distal nerve segment is essential for axonal growth and guidance.

Some knowledge of this classical and contemporary work is an essential basis of the biological approach to nerve repair. A surgeon should aim to assist the process of regeneration, not interfere with it.

Prognosis after nerve repair

Factors governing prognosis after nerve repair are well known and only some of the more obvious ones will be discussed here. It is convenient to separate those relating to the injury and the patient, which we may call the inevitable, from those that are in control of the surgeon.

AGE

McEwan (1962) reviewed a large series of repairs of median and ulnar nerves showing that children under 15 years did much better than older patients. Other series suggest that there is an inexorable decline in the quality of results with increasing age (Birch and Raji, 1991). Pain seems to be a more severe problem in the older patients. Severe nerve injuries in infancy are perhaps an exception to this general rule. The prognosis for the severe obstetric brachial plexus palsy is poor. Shortening of the limb and trophic disturbance are striking consequences of lesions of major trunk nerves in early childhood.

THE WOUND

The prognosis is worse in more destructive wounds, and three features stand out: destruction of the nerve, destruction of tissues and above all ischaemia mitigate against a good result.

THE NERVE

Results after nerve repair of such predominantly motor nerves as the musculocutaneous and posterior interosseous are almost always better than for such mixed nerve trunks as the sciatic, the median and the ulnar nerve. This may be explained by impaired, imperfect return of sensation. No adult regains truly normal sensation after a repair of a mixed or a cutaneous nerve and this is clearly important for the median nerve.

LEVEL

The more proximal the lesion, the poorer the outlook, and the results after suture of ulnar and median nerves progressively decline with more proximal levels of injury. It is unusual to see functional recovery in the small muscles of the hand when either of these nerves has been damaged above the elbow. It is also unusual to see return of gnosis.

DELAY

Delay in treatment is one of two factors which are under the surgeon's control. Delay is the most important factor in poor prognosis. Zachary (1954) described critical intervals after which repair was not worthwhile, suggesting that this interval was 9 months for the ulnar nerve injured above the elbow. This lesson, drawn from war-time experience, has been repeatedly confirmed in larger published series describing outcome after repair of median and ulnar nerves, nerves in the lower limb and the brachial plexus. Why is delay so important? It is known that the central changes, including cell death, are progressive. The biological milieu of the distal stump also becomes progressively unfavourable. There are progressive and ultimately irreversible changes in target organs including the skin, the sensory receptors, the skeletal muscle and sweat glands (Fig. 27.5). Morphological studies suggest that skeletal muscle cannot be expected to work if denervation exceeds 2 years although protective sensation may be restored after longer intervals than this. An added complication of delay is progressive secondary deformity. Most notable are the equinus deformity of common peroneal nerve palsy, internal rotation and adduction contracture of the shoulder after injuries of the brachial plexus and fixed extension deformity of metacarpophalangeal joints with flexion deformity of the proximal interphalangeal joints after median and ulnar nerve injuries. In one respect, trophic changes are most severe in children. Shortening of the limb seen in severe obstetric brachial plexus palsy is as much as 15–20% and similar length discrepancies

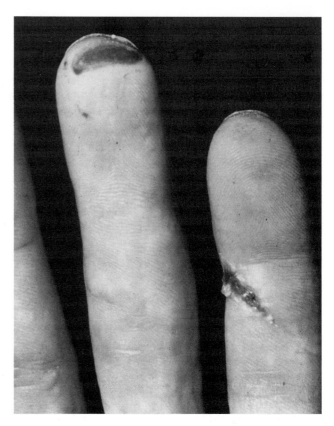

Fig. 27.5 Atrophy of the skin with scars from unnoted wounds 18 months after section of median nerve.

follow severe injection injuries to the sciatic nerve in infancy. The shortening is very much more marked after injury to a major nerve trunk than it is following poliomyelitis.

TECHNICAL ASPECTS

Technical aspects are also, of course, under the surgeon's control. Operations of nerve suture, grafting and transfer are fully described elsewhere (Birch, 1991). The principles of these operations follow those governing the treatment of wounds and include wound excision to prevent sepsis and urgent restoration of the circulation and of tissue perfusion. The skeleton must be stabilized, preferably by a technique that allows early movement. Muscle and tendons are carefully repaired. Repair of the synovium over individual tendons is important. Healthy full-thickness skin cover must be achieved, if need be by rotation or free flaps. Repair of blood vessels is of outstanding importance, and not only of the major axial vessels essential for the survival of the limb (Fig. 27.6a, b). Recovery after repair of ulnar, tibial and of digital sensory nerves is significantly better if the adjacent artery is repaired. Swelling and compression must be

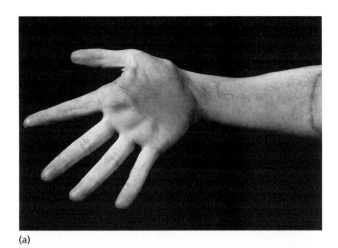

(a)

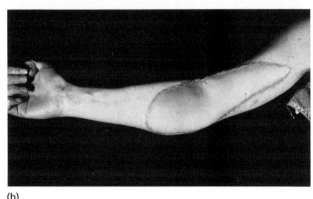

(b)

Fig. 27.6 (a,b) Missile injury destroyed the median nerve and brachial artery in this patient. Function was restored by combining grafting of the nerve, reversed vein graft of the artery, a free latissimus dorsi myocutaneous flap and high median transfer.

prevented, by open decompression and by meticulous attention to the posture of the splinting of the limb. Mobilization is planned and progressive and the aim is to return to normal activities as soon as possible. Urgent recognition and treatment of two serious complications, ischaemia and pain, is essential for a worthwhile result. The availability and the skill to use the appropriate instruments and sutures with magnification either by loupes or the operating microscope are prerequisites. In delayed or neglected cases, nerve repair must follow abolition of sepsis, skeletal stability, excision of scar with replacement by full thickness skin, and correction of fixed deformity.

SUTURE, GRAFTING AND OTHER METHODS OF NERVE REPAIR

Primary suture of nerves is best. This is possible in most clean lacerations in civilian practice. Direct suture may be practised in some late cases, when the prepared nerve

ends can be drawn comfortably together with, say, a 6-0 nylon suture, without flexion of the adjacent joints. The necessary post-operative flexion of joints should not be extreme, the elbow at no more than 70° and the wrist no more than 30°. The huge sciatic nerve is something of an exception, because so little autogenous graft is available and worthwhile results can be achieved if the suture line is protected from tension by mobilizing the hip in extension and the knee in 90° of flexion. Turnbuckle plasters or hinged splints allow progressive mobilization of the joints. Seddon (1963) set out the principles underlying nerve grafting and Millesi and coworkers (1968, 1972) have presented overwhelming evidence showing that tension impairs, or even prevents, regeneration. Merle and De Medinacelli (1991) carefully emphasized the technical details—notably delicacy of touch.

The importance of blood supply to a nerve graft was recognized by St. Clair Strange (1947) who developed the operation of ulnar nerve pedicle graft in repair of seemingly hopeless injuries to the median nerve. The free vascularized cutaneous nerve graft is a time-consuming operation providing one or two strands of vascularized graft. Jamieson's team extended the pedicle operation in repair of severe lesions of the brachial plexus, using the redundant ulnar nerve as a free vascularized graft. An analysis of 63 of these operations showed that useful elbow flexion was restored in two-thirds of patients but return of hand function was rare (Birch *et al.*, 1988). This was disappointing. It must be admitted that the free vascularized nerve graft has a limited application where there is a densely scarred bed or some severe traction lesions of the brachial plexus when the prognosis for the ulnar nerve is hopeless.

Nerve transfer is another useful technique in other seemingly irretrievable situations. Transfer of a normal hypoglossal nerve into the distal stump of a damaged facial nerve was well established before nerve grafting. Seddon (1963) described the first cases of restoration of elbow flexion by transfer of intercostal nerves to the musculocutaneous nerve. The chief indication for the operation is in otherwise irreparable lesions of the brachial plexus and Nagano *et al.* (1989) report on their results of intercostal transfer to musculocutaneous nerve in 179 patients. Over 80% of their cases regained functional flexion at the elbow. The subject has been extensively reviewed by Narakas (1987a) and Birch (1992).

Alternatives to nerve grafts

Glasby *et al.* (1992) have described the frozen muscle graft in repair of peripheral nerves and more recently have extended this to the repair of spinal nerves injured within the spinal canal. Although the technique remains unproven in the repair of major trunk nerves, and although the known deficiencies of the technique include fragmentation during preparation of the muscle and diminished calibre of regenerating nerve fibres as they pass through the graft, none the less the technique is promising and it is now the author's preferred method for the treatment of painful sensory neuromas. The idea of providing a suitable biological environment for nerve regeneration has recently been extended by Lundborg (1991) who reports a case of recovery of an ulnar nerve through a tissue chamber. These two strands of recent work are potentially of great significance for they emphasize the importance of the supporting cellular elements, Schwann cells and fibroblasts and neuronotrophic factors.

NERVE INJURIES IN FRACTURES AND DISLOCATIONS

This is a particularly difficult problem for the orthopaedic surgeon because of the difficulty in diagnosis of nerve lesions. In over half of simple closed fractures, the nerve will recover spontaneously. Operation for diagnosis and repair is often indicated when bone fragments are widely displaced after high-energy injury, after dislocations and in open fractures. Fractures of the pelvis and of the hip present difficulties in distinguishing between injuries to the lumbosacral plexus and to the sciatic nerve. Associated vascular injuries are frequent, and they are commonly neglected, a matter which is particularly disheartening at a time when techniques of vascular repair have become so consistently reliable. De Bakey and Simeone (1955) analysed outcome of vascular injuries from the Second World War treated, as was the practice then, by ligation of injured arteries. Table 27.5 shows the rate of amputation following ligation of major trunk vessels. The reader's attention is drawn to the aftermath of failure to repair the subclavian, the

Table 27.5 Limb loss after ligation of damaged major vessels during the Second World War (from De Bakey and Simeone, 1955)

Vessel	Incidence (%)
Subclavian	28.6
Axillary	43.2
Common brachial	55.7
Brachial	25.8
External iliac	46.7
Common femoral	81.1
Superficial femoral	54.8
Popliteal	72.5

axillary, the common brachial, the femoral and the popliteal arteries. This changed dramatically after a policy of repair using a reversed vein graft was introduced in later conflicts. Further impetus followed microvascular surgical techniques developed for re-implantation and free vascularized tissue-transfer work (Birch, 1987). Bonney (1963), in reporting a case of rupture of the common femoral artery from closed fracture of the femoral shaft wrote, 'Surgeons treating fractures of long bones must be prepared to treat associated vascular injury'. The author follows this view. The reader is urged to study the outstanding review from Barros d' Sa (1992) who refers to experience drawn from missile injury to the lower limb in Northern Ireland and describes the success of a closely coordinated approach between vascular and orthopaedic surgeons to these difficult injuries.

Seddon (1975) has set out some principles in the treatment of nerves injured in closed fractures: 146 from 212 of his cases of nerves injured in fractures or dislocations within the upper limb spontaneously recovered to near normal levels. Less than one-half of his 57 cases of nerve lesions after skeletal injury in the lower limb recovered to normal or near normal levels. He pointed out that nerves are at risk from rupture or entrapment after dislocations, and that they were more at risk from transection in open fractures. He suggested that the nerve could be treated expectantly if a reasonable reduction could be achieved, implying no interposition of soft tissues and if there was no hint at all of vascular injury. He recommended that palsy of the sciatic nerve from closed fracture of the shaft of the femur was an indication for urgent exploration of the nerve. Four areas seemed to present particular difficulties for the fracture surgeon and these are the pelvis and hip, the knee, the elbow, and the shoulder.

Pelvis and hip

The lumbosacral plexus is at risk in more severe fracture dislocations of the pelvis (Fig. 27.7a). Life-threatening multiple injuries demand first priority in treatment but the chance to improve function by nerve repair is granted the surgeon more frequently now, such that more such patients survive. The diagnosis is evident from clinical examination for sensory loss extends well beyond the territory of the sciatic nerve (Fig. 27.7b); the flexors of the hip and extensors of the knee are weak or paralysed, and there may be sphincter dysfunction. The injury is a traction lesion and rupture within the spinal canal is frequent (Fig. 27.7c,d).

The sciatic nerve is at risk in fracture dislocations of

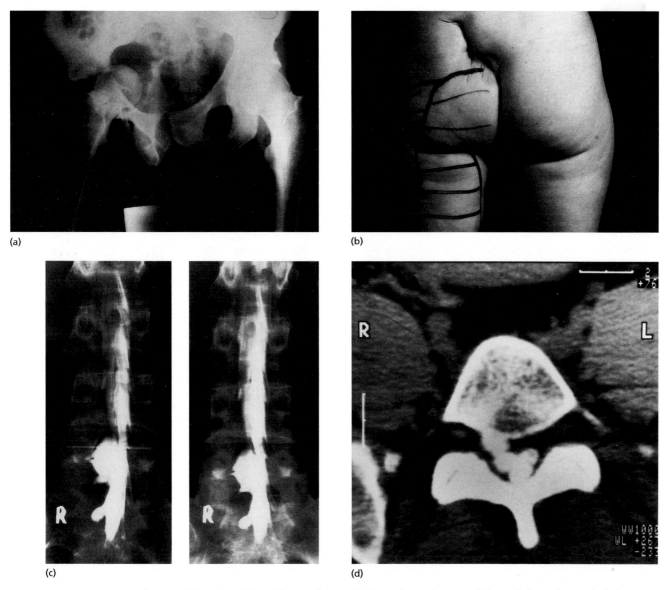

Fig. 27.7 (a) A severe open fracture dislocation of hip with nerve injury. (b) Loss of sensation extends beyond the territory of sciatic nerve. (c,d) Myelogram scan and computed tomography confirmed injury to L5 and S1 spinal nerves within the spinal canal.

the hip and the incidence is highest in posterior column fractures. Epstein (1980), in his review of 830 cases seen personally, identified 68 nerve injuries, an incidence of 8%. Good recovery occurred in 43% but a poor result followed in 32%. Letournel and Judet (1981) recorded 57 nerve injuries in 469 patients treated by reduction and internal fixation, a pre-operative incidence of 12%. This rose to 17.4% in the posterior column group. They emphasized the need for careful examination of the patients before operation, acknowledging that 16 of their cases had not been 'properly examined'. This series suggests that early reduction and fixation of the pelvis is helpful to the nerve, for in 36 cases of nerve injury

where there was early intervention, recovery was good in 21; it was poor in 13. They emphasized the real risk to the sciatic nerve during operation. 30 of their cases developed sciatic palsy after intervention and recovery was poor in 13 of these. They described how meticulous care for the nerve, and a combination of femoral traction with flexion of the knee, reduced the incidence of intra-operative injury from 18% to 9%.

The conclusions drawn from this meticulous study of a very large series commands respect. It is important to distinguish, by clinical examination, between injury to the lumbosacral plexus and injury to the sciatic nerve. Sciatic nerve lesions in displaced fracture dislocations of the hip demand urgent reduction. If open reduction is performed, then the nerve should be displayed, removing loose bony fragments which may compress or impale it. It must be acknowledged that there is a significant risk to the sciatic nerve in operations for open reduction and internal fixation and that the prognosis for recovery of such lesions is not at all good.

The knee

There are two common patterns of injury to nerves at the knee: vascular injury from dislocation or fracture dislocation.

The popliteal artery is ruptured in about 3% of supracondylar fractures of the femur and in at least 30% of dislocations of the knee (Fig. 27.8a,b). The artery, or more commonly, the major branches, are ruptured in about 10% of displaced fractures of the proximal tibia. Treatment of a vascular injury determines outcome for the leg as well as for the nerve because the nerve lesion is usually secondary to compression and ischaemia. De Bakey and Simeone (1955) reported that 364 of 502 legs were amputated after ligation of the popliteal artery. After a policy of repair of the vessel adopted in the Korean and Vietnam Wars, the ampu-

tation rate decreased from 73 to 32% (Rich *et al.*, 1969).

The foot may be plainly ischaemic from the outset but secondary thrombosis may occur hours or even days after injury to the intima of the vessels. Doppler flow studies may mislead and while angiography is always useful in confirming diagnosis and in localizing the arterial injury, it must not delay operation. Unless the arterial flow is restored within 6 hours at the most, preferably less than this, the limb is irretrievably marred (Fig. 27.9a,b).

Barros d' Sa and Moorhead (1989) have shown how intraluminal shunts have simplified treatment of these difficult injuries, particularly when wound contamination and fracture comminution prevent the simple technique outlined above. Coordination of orthopaedic and vascular surgeons begins with the planning of the incision and restoring flow by shunts, which then allows a careful and unhurried skeletal fixation. Finally, the arterial repair can be performed without risk of disruption by bone fragments.

THE COMMON PERONEAL NERVE

Platt (1928) described lesions of the common peroneal

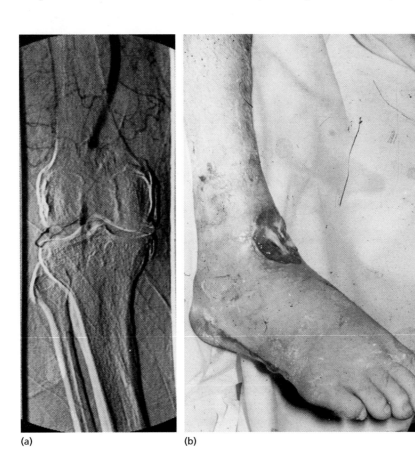

(a)   (b)

Fig. 27.8 (a) Dislocation of knee causing rupture of popliteal artery. The artery was not repaired. (b) The appearance of the foot on removal of the plaster cylinder.

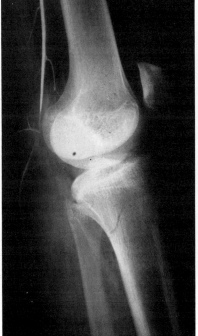

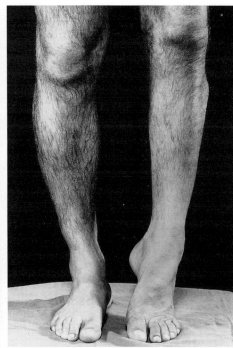

Fig. 27.9 (a) False aneurysm of popliteal artery following arthroscopic meniscectomy. (b) The appearance of the leg. Diagnosis was delayed for 3 weeks.   (a)   (b)

nerve from adduction injuries of the extended knee. These are severe injuries. Force that is sufficient to rupture the lateral structures of the knee joint may extend to injure both cruciate ligaments. In cases where the tibial nerve and popliteal vessels are involved, the outlook for the leg is poor. Seddon (1975) in discussing traction injuries of the common peroneal nerve referred to 11 cases where both divisions of the sciatic nerve had been injured in lateral dislocation of the knee. Of 26 patients where the neural lesion was confined to the common peroneal nerve, he found that 18 had functional recovery spontaneously. Partial recovery occurred in two of three nerves sutured. The author has grafted 17 ruptures of the common peroneal nerve caused by adduction injuries of the knee. Functional dorsiflexion of the foot was achieved in eight patients, and worthwhile eversion of the foot in three others. Wide retraction of stumps was found in all of these cases and the gap, after preparation of the nerve faces, ranged from 8 to 18 cm. No recovery occurred in any case where the repair was performed at over 6 months from injury. The author believes that the ruptured nerve should be grafted at the first operation, at the same time as the operation for ligament repair. At the very least, the operation for repair of lateral ligaments should include exposure of the nerve, and if this has been ruptured then the ends should be gently approximated.

The elbow

Wilkins (1991) reviewed 61 series including over 7000 cases of supracondylar fracture. He found an incidence of nerve injury in 7%, the radial being most commonly affected and it seemed that more than half of all these went on to full spontaneous recovery. Ottolenghi (1960) reviewed 830 cases and found arterial compromise in 5% (Fig. 27.10). Ischaemic contracture occurred in less than 1% suggesting that early recognition and treatment had been effective in the great majority of cases. Hallett (1981) reported a series of median nerves trapped within the joint after reduction of a dislocation. This was a valuable contribution, giving some indications for exploration of the nerve.

It is useful to restate some guidelines for treatment. If there is no hint of vascular compromise, and if the fracture or dislocation has been well reduced then it is reasonable to observe the nerves. If arterial injury is suspected then this should be explored urgently and the injured nerve exposed at the same time. If reduction is imperfect and if the nerve injury is a complete degenerative one, with loss of sudo- and vasomotor function, then this is a relatively strong indication for early exploration.

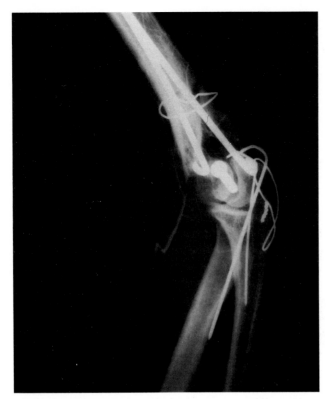

Fig. 27.10 Rupture of brachial artery with fracture of distal humerus. The artery was not repaired, and the fracture was fixed internally. The entire flexor compartment of the forearm necrosed.

Shoulder

Lesions of nerves following injuries to the shoulder range from isolated circumflex palsy to very complex and severe injuries to the whole of plexus. The severe infraclavicular lesion will be discussed later (p. 955). The axillary artery is at risk particularly in older patients, and it is one of the most common vascular injuries in civilian practice (Fig. 27.11a–c). Bigliani *et al.* (1991) record that ruptures of the axillary artery secondary to fractures or dislocations of the shoulder account for 6% of all arterial injuries. Stableforth (1984) recorded an incidence of 5% of arterial lesions in his series of fractures of the proximal humerus. An associated injury to the rotator cuff is not uncommon, particularly in the elderly. Functional recovery in three of the author's cases after repair of rupture of suprascapular and axillary nerves was very poor despite return of muscle bulk, and only later did we diagnose the rotator cuff rupture which explained this. The integrity of the cuff is easily assessed by arthroscopy in the urgent case and either by computed tomography scan with contrast enhancement or magnetic resonance imaging scan in later cases. It is

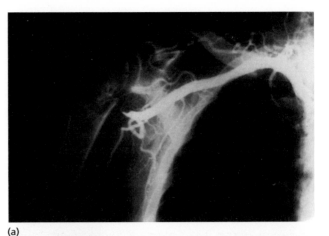

(a)

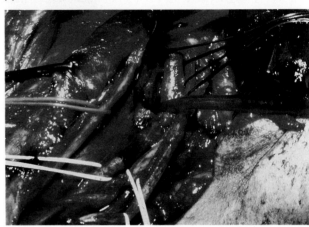

(b)

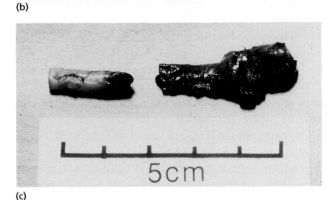

(c)

Fig. 27.11 (a) Fracture dislocation of shoulder in a 63-year-old man with rupture of the axillary artery. (b) The artery exposed. Note the segment of thrombus at the site of rupture of intima. Repair by vein graft. (c) The resected calcified vessel.

now the author's policy to exclude lesions of the rotator cuff before going on to exploration of the nerves to the shoulder.

Published work on the incidence and the natural history of the nerve lesion is surprisingly limited. Stableforth (1984) found an incidence of 6% of nerve lesions in a series of 81 fractures of the proximal humerus. Leffert and Seddon (1965) and Seddon (1975) took an optimistic view, suggesting that the great majority of nerve injuries recovered spontaneously. However, Seddon (1975) found full recovery in only 14 of his 27 axillary nerve lesions. It is likely that the axillary nerve is only partially injured in the majority of cases. Blom and Dahlback (1970) described 24 cases of isolated circumflex nerve lesions; all of these went on to full recovery but their electromyographic examination showed that the injury was incomplete in 15. Nunley and Gable (1991) recommend that the axillary nerve should be explored if there is no clinical or electromyographic evidence of recovery at between 2 and 3 months after injury and the author agrees with this view. Results from grafting of the axillary nerve, when that is done within 6 months of injury, are good. Petrucci *et al.* (1982), Millesi (1980) and Narakas (1989) considered that 80% of their results were good or excellent from a total of 45 repairs.

One particularly uncomfortable question for orthopaedic surgeons is the relation between nerve injury and the timing and technique of reduction of a dislocation of shoulder. Of course, reduction is an emergency. The risk to the brachial plexus increases by the hour as it lies tightly stretched over the head of the humerus while remaining compressed deep to the subscapularis. Flaubert (1827) described the tragic consequences from an attempt at closed reduction which led to rupture of the axillary artery and avulsion of the whole of the plexus from the spinal cord. Nerves may be damaged after successful relocation by compression from haematoma and increasing paralysis, and loss of sensation over the course of 24–48 hours after relocation is a strong indication that the axillary artery or vein has been ruptured. The author is inclined to the view that persisting severe pain with loss of function through the cords of the plexus even after successful relocation of the simple low-energy dislocation of the shoulder is a strong indication for exploration and decompression. It is rare to find frank rupture of nerve trunks. The medial cord, in particular, appears stretched and oedematous. In some cases pain relief has been remarkable.

IATROGENIC INJURIES

Irradiation neuritis and injection injuries to nerves have been mentioned earlier (p. 939). Turning to accidental injuries to nerves caused by the surgeon, it is perhaps logical to consider these under three headings. First are those which follow neglect to detect risk factors; next are those which occur during the operation either from a faulty positioning or from faulty operating technique; and lastly, the recognition and treatment of the injury.

Pre-operative

The surgeon should recognize factors which put a patient at risk and these include endocrine disorders, notably diabetes and thyroid disease, which predispose to neuropathy. The risks from anaemia, hypertension, ischaemic heart disease and malignant disease are well known but not all orthopaedic surgeons are aware of the very real hazard of using a tourniquet in the lower limb after arterial reconstruction. A tourniquet should not be used for lower-limb work after femoral popliteal bypass grafting. To do so carries a very real risk of losing the leg (Mansfield, 1992). Hereditary sensory motor neuropathy and hereditary compression neuropathy are uncommon conditions but should perhaps be considered in the differential diagnosis of patients presenting with seemingly commonplace nerve-entrapment syndromes.

Intra-operative

Cooper (1991) reviewed compression neuropathies from faulty positioning of patients on the operating table and in recovery wards. The sciatic and common peroneal nerves are particularly at risk in lithotomy, the brachial plexus from the Trendelenberg position and the ulnar and lateral femoral cutaneous nerves in the prone position. Hypovolaemia, hypotension, and cold, particularly in patients with anaemia or coagulopathy, are significant factors in causation of compression neuropathy. A permanent deficit after compression lesion of the brachial plexus was found in between 5 and 22% of patients, and for between 10 and 27% of patients in common peroneal nerve palsies. Wadsworth and Williams (1973) emphasized the danger of permanent dysfunction from compression of the ulnar nerve in the anaesthetized patient. The surgeon has a difficult but unavoidable duty to attend to the positioning of the patient during anaesthesia and to attend to the protection of the vulnerable trunk nerves such as the brachial plexus, the ulnar nerve and the common peroneal nerve. The head should be positioned in the midline avoiding undue extension or lateral flexion. The shoulder should not be abducted beyond 90° and care should be taken to prevent accidental extension of the shoulder particularly when combined with extension of the elbow. Padding at the elbow and knee should be standard practice in all of our operating theatres. The surgeon must be cautious in use of the tourniquet, to avoid it wherever possible, to ensure that adequate checks are made of the pressure recording equipment, that the cuff is not too narrow, and that the cuff is inflated for as short a time as possible. Cuff pressure should not exceed 200 mmHg in the arm and 300 mmHg in the leg. Ischaemic time should neither exceed 90 min in the upper limb nor 2 h in the leg and preferably the period of ischaemia should be less than this.

Table 27.6 shows the number of trunk nerves divided or otherwise irreparably damaged during the course of operation seen in the author's unit. It excludes accidental injuries to sensory nerves such as superficial radial, medial cutaneous nerve of forearm, sural and saphenous and palmar digital nerves. Nerve injuries during arthroplasties of the hip are discussed later (p. 954). Orthopaedic surgeons were responsible for about one-half of these cases. The accident occurred during emergency operations for treatment of a fracture or vascular problems in one-third of cases. Delay in diagnosis was a striking feature exceeding 6 months in nearly one-half of these cases. Some of the worst cases occurred when operations had been performed as day cases under local anaesthetic. Several of these, involving nerves within the posterior triangle of the neck, were diagnosed by the family practitioner as the surgeon had neither seen the patient after the operation nor had arrangements been made for them to attend for follow-up.

Table 27.6 Intraoperative injuries of trunk nerves*

Nerve	Number of cases
The neck	
Accessory nerve	18
Long thoracic nerve	4
Brachial plexus	22
The upper limb	
Musculocutaneous	4
Radial	15
Posterior interosseous	5
Median	5
Anterior interosseous	3
Ulnar	9
The lower limb	
Femoral	3
Sciatic	1
Common peroneal nerve	15
Tibial	3
Total	91

* Excludes damage to sensory nerves and to femoral and sciatic nerves in hip arthroplasty.

Nerves at risk

The accessory nerve is extremely vulnerable in its course across the posterior triangle of the neck. In most of our cases, the operation performed was for lymph-node biopsies. All of these patients experienced significant pain and disability, so much so that some were dismissed as hysterical. Paralysis of the upper fibres of the trapezius muscle leads to lack of support of the upper limb and a secondary traction upon the brachial plexus and this is probably the source of the severe pain (Fig. 27.12). Good or excellent results followed repair of the nerve if it were performed within 6 months of the accident. The upper trunk of the brachial plexus is surprisingly superficial and this too is at risk of injury during operations for lymph-node biopsy (Fig. 27.13a). The lower trunk of the brachial plexus and the long thoracic nerve is vulnerable during operations for thoracic outlet syndrome or cervical sympathectomy (Fig. 27.13b). The femoral nerve is at risk from operations in the inguinal region (Fig. 27.14a,b). The common peroneal nerve is superficial as it winds around the neck of the fibula and in most of these cases it is ligated or avulsed through short incisions used for the treatment of varicose veins (Fig. 27.15).

Plainly, prevention is the best course. Strachan and Ellis (1971) described an exposure to minimize risks to the posterior interosseous nerve. Adams (1964) described an approach to minimize risk to the sciatic nerve during ischiofemoral arthrodesis. The surgeon must be familiar with the anatomy of the nerves in the field of operation

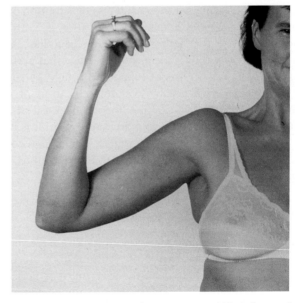

Fig. 27.12 Iatrogenic section of accessory nerve. Note the wasting of trapezius and impaired glenohumeral movement.

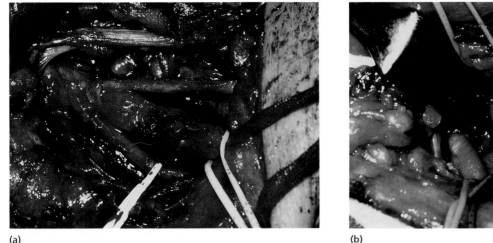
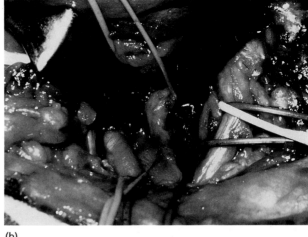

(a) (b)

Fig. 27.13 (a) Damage to the posterior division of the upper trunk in operation for biopsy of swelling. The operation was performed in a day-care theatre. The diagnosis was made by the general practitioner 6 weeks later. (b) Section of the lower trunk of the brachial plexus in operation for excision of first rib.

and long incisions are best to expose structures at risk, particularly when normal anatomy has been distorted by scar. The practice of removing 'ganglions' or 'synovial cysts' through small incisions which give no glimpse of important axial structures is to be deprecated. The stimulator should be available in all operations performed in the vicinity of major nerves, particularly when

pathology or scarring from previous operations distorts the normal planes. The unexpected finding of an intra-neural tumour is best resolved either by enucleation of a benign schwannoma or desisting from interference altogether.

The delay in diagnosis in many of these cases seems inexplicable. When a patient awakes from an operation

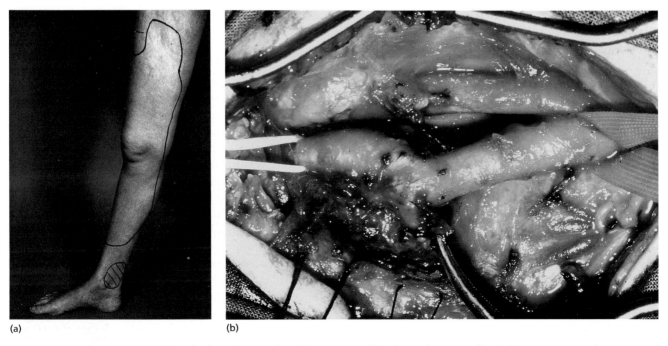

(a) (b)

Fig. 27.14 (a) This patient complained of numbness and inability to extend her knee after inguinal node biopsy. Her complaints were ignored for 8 months. (b) The appearance of the femoral nerve when this was exposed. On review, the original biopsy plainly contained large numbers of myelinated nerve fibres.

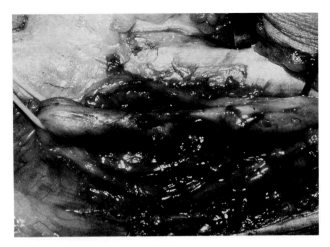

Fig. 27.15 The common peroneal nerve is at risk in operations for varicose veins.

with signs of a lesion within a nerve in the field of that operation, it must be assumed that the nerve is divided and the diagnosis of 'neurapraxia' or conduction block is unwise. Bonney (1986) commented, 'if there is an incision over the line of a main nerve and if, after operation, there is complete paralysis including vasomotor and sudomotor paralysis in the distribution of that nerve, speculation is unnecessary; the nerve has been cut and there will be no recovery until the nerve is explored and repaired'. Severe pain is a feature of partial or irritative lesions of nerves caused by persistent pressure or by accidental ligation and these complaints should not be dismissed.

Sensory nerves

Accidental injury to a palmar digital nerve during the course of a difficult operation for Dupuytren's contracture is understandable and remarkably few patients are unduly troubled. Injury to other sensory nerves, however, may bring about disabling pain, seemingly out of proportion to the nerve which has been damaged. Two nerves, in particular, stand out as being troublesome: the superficial radial nerve at the wrist and the medial cutaneous nerve of the forearm at the elbow. Injury to the terminal branches of the sural nerve and of the long saphenous nerve may also lead to severe pain. Regrettably many of these injuries occur during so-called trivial operations for release of stenosing tenovaginitis or golfers elbow. The best treatment here is prevention, by careful placing of the incision and by careful dissection. A wide range of treatments has been recommended for the painful sensory neuroma—none of them is entirely satisfactory. It seems illogical to treat a painful cut nerve by cutting more proximally although excision of a subcutaneous neuroma and burying the proximal nerve stump more deeply is often effective. It is more logical to restore continuity of the divided nerve and it is in this particular situation that frozen muscle graft is proving so promising.

The nerves at the hip

A nerve palsy after a successful hip arthroplasty is a most unpleasant occurrence for both the patient and the surgeon. Information on incidence and causation has been sparse until relatively recently. Ratcliffe (1984) conducted a survey amongst orthopaedic surgeons in the UK and collected 50 cases. Traction seemed to be the most important feature in the 16 femoral nerve palsies which usually followed an anterolateral approach to the hip. There was no clear relation between the adopted approach and the sciatic nerve palsy. Some instances of direct injury to the nerve were described, including accidental division by the knife or compression by wire or suture. Haematoma, compressing the nerve, or bleeding within the nerve did occur in patients on anticoagulant therapy. He recommended that steps be taken to exclude a lesion within the spinal canal, and commented on the rarity of a true common peroneal nerve injury at the knee. He described several cases where urgent reexploration improved the situation by relieving the nerve from compression by haematoma, or strangulation by wire or suture.

Schmalzreid and Amstutz (1991) reviewed over 3000 consecutive hip arthroplasties at the University of California, Los Angeles (UCLA). They found a 1% incidence of nerve palsies after primary hip replacements; this rose to 2–3% after revision arthroplasty. Patients with a primary diagnosis of congenital dislocation of the hip were at particular risk, with an incidence of 5.8% of lesions. They found that femoral and obturator nerve palsies were most often associated with extrusion of methyl methacrylate cement. A lateral transtrochanteric approach was used in the majority of their cases and in a cadaveric study they demonstrated that the sciatic nerve was at risk from being compressed between the posterior edge of the osteotomized trochanter and the ischium after dislocation, flexion and internal rotation of the hip (Fig. 27.16). They found that those patients who did well recovered within 6 months, and that those with severe pain did badly; 24% of their patients were left with severe disability.

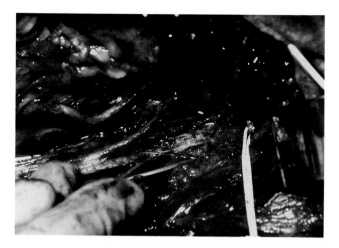

Fig. 27.16 Complete and painful palsy of sciatic nerve after a difficult total hip arthroplasty. The appearance of the nerve suggests a combination of compression and traction; there is obliteration of the longitudinal epineurial vessels and surrounding fibrosis.

Table 27.7 Nerve injuries at hip arthroplasty

Mode	Agent	Femoral	Sciatic	Total
Direct	Knife			
	Suture wire	2	2	4
	Cement	1	4	5
		1	2	3
Indirect	Haematoma			
	Ischaemia	1	3	4
	Traction–compression	1	1	2
		3	16	19
Total		9	28	37

The authors make several recommendations. The patient should be warned of the risk of injury. Particular care is taken to support the limb during the operation, and the sciatic nerve is exposed during revision arthroplasty. In high-risk cases, neurophysiological monitoring of the sciatic nerve is performed, recording from the nerve just distal to the sciatic notch. Since adopting this protocol their incidence of nerve palsy in primary cases has been reduced to 0.6%, and in revisions to 1.8%.

The author has seen 37 cases of injury to femoral or sciatic nerves and Table 27.7 shows the cause of these. There is no clear relation between the approach and the nerve injury. No case of isolated injury to the common peroneal nerve was found, and where that diagnosis had been considered clinical examination, supplemented by electromyography, confirmed weakness of the lateral hamstrings. All of these nerves were injured at the hip. Direct injuries were found in 12 cases, and in four more cases the nerve was compressed by haematoma or there had been an intraneural bleed. In two cases, nerves were injured indirectly from ischaemia from accidental injury to the iliac or femoral arteries.

A combination of traction and compression appeared to be the most common cause of all. Exploration in these cases showed the nerve entrapped and tethered within scar tissue to a varying degree, with a thickened epineurium and obliteration of longitudinal blood vessels. In some, a degree of conduction block was demonstrable.

External neurolysis of the nerve was usually followed by some improvement in pain and sensation in this group of patients. In four patients, colleagues had performed urgent re-exploration before referral, finding one case of transection of the sciatic nerve, one case of strangulation by suture and two cases of compression by haematoma. Relief of pain and recovery of a nerve was good in three of these four, and certainly better than equivalent cases where no such prompt action had been taken.

Perhaps now it is right to offer some guidelines for this difficult complication. It seems inescapable that patients must be warned of the risks of nerve damage. Particular care should be taken in high risk cases and the recommendations from UCLA that the sciatic nerve be seen and protected throughout the operation does appear reasonable. The value of intraoperative monitoring of the nerve remains unclear; its use reflects particularly high standards of care and it does not give immunity to the nerve. If a patient awakes with a severe pain or with a complete lesion of either femoral or sciatic nerve, then the surgeon is best advised to re-explore that nerve urgently. A remedial cause may be found, of extruded cement, strangulation, or tight compression of the nerve trunk from haematoma. It is very much less clear what to do when the injury is partial and there is little pain. The risk of leaving a potentially treatable condition alone is to be balanced against the risk of subjecting patients who may be elderly or otherwise infirm to a second anaesthetic, and an operation that carries with it a risk of introducing sepsis into the field.

THE BRACHIAL PLEXUS

Serious injuries of the brachial plexus are the most complex and difficult of peripheral nerve lesions. One of the reasons for this is that the central nervous system is so frequently involved, by avulsion of spinal nerves directly from the spinal cord. The great majority follow closed traction injury. The last 25 years has seen very significant changes in approaches to diagnosis and to treatment. It is convenient to separate those occurring at birth from those occurring later.

Traction and open lesions of the brachial plexus

In the Medical Research Council's special report on peripheral nerve injuries (1954), Brooks concluded that operative repair was usually valueless after reviewing 170 cases of open wounds from Second World War casualties. This view was endorsed at the Sicot meeting in Paris in the 1960s when interested surgeons concluded that no operations for repair in traction and gunshot injuries of the brachial plexus were fruitless. Many patients in the UK with complete lesions of the brachial plexus were treated by early amputation, arthrodesis of the shoulder and a prosthesis but many patients did not use them. Bonney (1959) in a meticulous study of the natural history of the condition in 25 patients noted that 12 remained in severe pain several years after their injury and Wynn-Parry *et al.* (1987) showed that 112 out of 122 patients with pre-ganglionic injury continue in severe pain at 3–30 years after the accident.

It is perhaps strange that such a pessimistic approach was so widespread. Patients with complete lesions of the brachial plexus were left with a useless arm or an amputation and about two-thirds of them continued to experience severe pain. Yet the principles for diagnosis and repair had already been clearly defined, mostly by work in the UK. The foundation of diagnosis was Bonney's (1954) introduction of the concept of pre- and post-ganglionic injuries. The work of Bonney and Gilliatt (1958) is the basis of all modern neurophysiological investigation. The usefulness of myelography in diagnosis had been established by Davis and Bligh in 1966. Seddon (1963) had already given grafting respectability and he described several cases of successful intercostal nerve transfer. Vascularized nerve grafts had been developed by St. Clair Strange (1947) and Young and Medawar (1940) had reported on sutureless repair of nerves with fibrin glue.

Narakas and Verdan (1969) and Millesi (1968) recommenced surgical endeavour using microsurgical technique and their early results encouraged others to a more creative approach.

Epidemiology

It is very difficult to find accurate information of the incidence, causation and social implications of these severe injuries. There are about 350 cases of complete or partial supraclavicular traction injuries every year in the UK (Goldie and Coates, 1992) and about 150 of severe infraclavicular lesions. Iatrogenic injuries to the brachial plexus have already been discussed. The incidence of open wounds from knife or gunshot increases every year and now forms about 10% of the total of patients referred to the author's unit. Rosson (1988) reviewed over 200 patients injured in motor cycle accidents, finding that 90% were under 25 years, that nearly one-half held only a provisional licence and that the motor cycle had an engine capacity of 125 cc or less in over one-third. He established that the dominant limb was injured in over 60%, and that there were severe injuries to the head, the chest, the viscera or to other limbs in 50%. More than one-third of his patients remained unemployed at more than one year after the accident.

Management rests on the following: (i) prompt and accurate diagnosis of level and extent of the lesion; (ii) operation for re-innervation of the limb or for appropriate muscle transfer; and (iii) a closely supervised scheme of rehabilitation which has, as its central aim, return to normal work and normal life as soon as possible. A multidisciplinary retraining programme with provision of specialized splinting and the recognition and treatment of pain is essential.

Diagnosis

The extent of neural injury is obvious to clinical examination and can be made by any orthopaedic surgeon with the assistance of the MRC's *Aids to the Examination of Peripheral Nerves*. The level of injury may be more difficult. Is the injury intradural, have spinal nerves been torn directly from the spinal cord (pre-ganglionic), or is there a rupture in the posterior triangle of the neck or below the clavicle (post-ganglionic)? Some clinical features are helpful in this. Weakness of trapezius, and serratus anterior, loss of sensation above the clavicle and paralysis of the ipsilateral hemidiaphragm indicate avulsion of the upper roots of the brachial plexus (Fig. 27.17a–c). A Bernard–Horner syndrome with pain points to avulsion of C8 and T1 and fracture or dislocation of the first rib or the transverse process of C7 supports this diagnosis. In the worst cases, swelling and deep bruising in the posterior triangle points to complete avulsion of all five spinal nerves. The radiographs may show that the cervical spine has been tilted away from

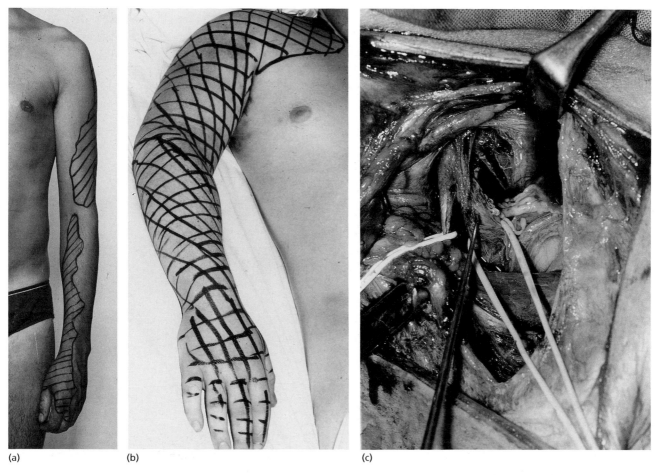

Fig. 27.17 (a) The loss of sensation from injury to C5 and C6 nerves. (b) Loss of sensation extending above the collar bone, indicating injury to the cervical plexus, is associated with the worst injuries to the brachial plexus. (c) Exploration revealed dorsal root ganglia and spinal nerve rootlets of C5 and C6.

the side of impact or the upper limb may appear distracted from the chest.

PHYSIOLOGICAL INVESTIGATION

These are based on the fact that Wallerian degeneration *does not occur* in the sensory afferent nerve fibres passing to the dorsal root ganglion in those cases where the injury is between the dorsal root ganglion and the spinal cord. They are useful at about 3 weeks, when Wallerian degeneration will have taken place in post-ganglionic ruptures and in the efferent motor fibres. Injection of histamine into normal skin induces a flair, mediated by the axon reflex. In pre-ganglionic injuries, the afferent axons remain myelinated and a normal flair is seen. In post-ganglionic injuries, all nerve fibres degenerate and the flair disappears. The sensory action potentials in the trunk nerves of the upper limb persist in patients with

pre-ganglionic injury. Intraoperative neurophysiological studies, by stimulating the exposed brachial plexus and recording from electrodes over the scalp or over the skin of the neck must now be regarded as an essential step in diagnosis. They may be misleading and they are not quantitative but they are extremely valuable (Fig. 27.18).

Imaging

Yeoman (1968) compared myelography with findings at operation confirming the investigation as a useful one (Fig. 27.19a). Marshall and De Silva (1986) showed that a computed tomography scan with contrast enhancement was more accurate than myelography particularly for C5 and C6. It is reasonable to predict that magnetic resonance imaging will soon replace the invasive investigations (Fig. 27.19b).

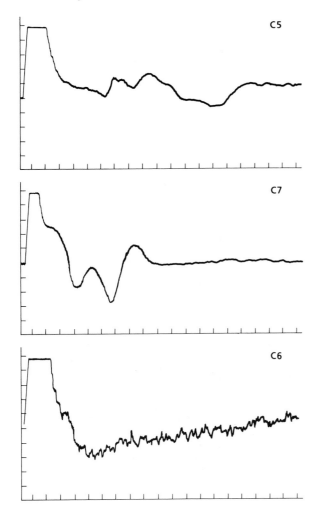

Fig. 27.18 Sensory evoked potentials recorded during exploration of the brachial plexus. The individual spinal nerves were stimulated and records made from electrodes attached to the skin of the scalp. Good traces were recorded from C7 and from C5 but none for C6 (top right) confirming pre-ganglionic injury to this nerve.

INDICATIONS FOR OPERATION

The purpose of operation is to establish diagnosis, and the prognosis, and to improve that prognosis wherever possible by nerve repair or transfer. We should acknowledge that advances in anaesthesia now allow for long and delicate work to be done in confidence that the circulation and ventilation are maintained. The discriminating use of neuromuscular blocking agents allows sensitive neurophysiological investigations during the exploration.

Given adequate skill and facilities, open wounds of the plexus from knife or glass should be treated according to the principles governing such injuries—by primary repair. The same cannot be said for the closed traction

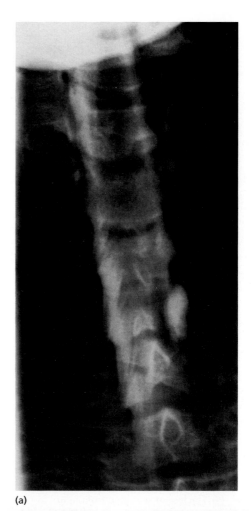

(a)

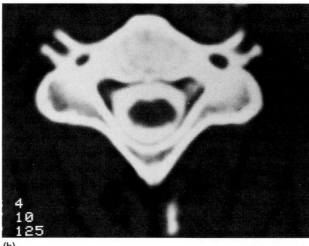

(b)

Fig. 27.19 (a) Myelogram showing pseudomeningocoele C7, obliteration of root shadow at C6. (b) Computed tomograph/myelogram in this case confirmed pre-ganglionic injury of C5.

lesions. A history of high-energy injury, together with the clinical features already outlined, may permit urgent exploration of the plexus and this is the author's policy in selected patients. However, life-threatening injuries to the head, of the chest and the viscera must take priority and it must be emphasized that urgent exploration demands a versatility of skill in dealing with unexpected injury to the great vessels. It also carries risk from air embolism and coming from a sudden leak of cerebrospinal fluid. There is no doubt that results of repair within a few days of injury are better than when repair is performed later and results decline progressively with the interval from injury to repair. It must be emphasized, however, that this is not work for the occasional operator and can only be performed in adequately equipped hospitals. Intraoperative neurophysiological investigation is essential in urgent operations.

Surgical pathology (Tables 27.8 and 27.9)

Arterial injury is common, occurring in over 10% of cases of supraclavicular injury and in over 30% of the infraclavicular lesions (Fig. 27.20a,b). The incidence of pre-ganglionic injury is high. Injury to the spinal column is not uncommon in complete lesions. A Brown-Séquard syndrome is found in about 10% of such cases. Repair of the first or second parts of the subclavian artery is desirable but not always essential, as sufficient collateral supply may ensure a living arm, but this is certainly not the case for rupture of the axillary artery in infra-clavicular lesions. Prognosis is determined by urgent restoration of the circulation and if this is delayed by

Table 27.9 Pre-ganglionic injury to spinal nerves confirmed at exploration

C4	C5	C6	C7	C8	T1	Total
NR	50	118	151	162	152	633 in 229 patients (Narakas, 1987)
3	52	58	57	51	50	270 in 100 consecutive explorations (Birch, 1992)

NR, not recorded.

more than 6 hours, irretrievable ischaemia of muscle and nerve trunks dooms the limb.

Ruptures of nerve trunks may be repaired by conventional grafting using cutaneous sensory nerves or, in severe cases, with proof of hopeless injury to the C8 and

Table 27.8 Operations for traction lesion of brachial plexus, St. Mary's Hospital–Royal National Orthopaedic Hospital, 1977–1991

Lesion	n
Supraclavicular	
Complete pre-ganglionic – no repair	80
Mixed and incomplete lesion – no repair	135
Repair	
graft	185
vascularized ulnar nerve graft	63
accessory and/or intercostal transfer	277
others	15
Total	755
Rupture of subclavian artery in:	88
Infraclavicular	164
Rupture of subclavian or axillary artery in:	70

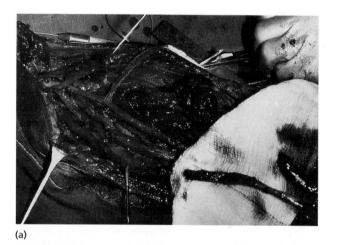

(a)

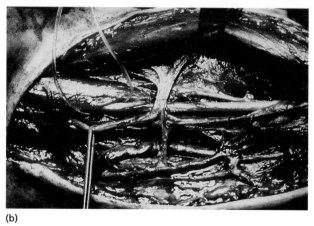

(b)

Fig. 27.20 (a) Infraclavicular lesion of brachial plexus, rupture of radial and median nerves, fracture of humerus. Case of Mr G.L.W. Bonney. (b) Rupture of musculocutaneous and ulnar nerves. The axillary artery was ruptured at the level of the coracoid.

T1 nerves by strands of free vascularized ulnar nerve. Direct repair is not possible in pre-ganglionic injury and two types of nerve transfer are proving most useful. These include transfer of the accessory nerve to the suprascapular nerve and transfer of three or four intercostal nerves to the musculocutaneous nerve or lateral cord. It is now possible to give a reasonable indication of the results of these different operations.

1 Repair of ruptures in the posterior triangle achieves worthwhile function at shoulder and in elbow in about two-thirds of cases. Vascularized ulnar nerve graft is perhaps a little better.

2 Nerve transfer has radically improved the outlook for shoulder and elbow in patients with pre-ganglionic injury of C5, C6 and C7 (Fig. 27.21). If it is possible to combine this with conventional repair, useful return of hand function can be anticipated in children and in some adults.

3 Reinnervation of the limb secures significant pain relief in many patients and we have seen some example of surprising and gratifying mitigation of pain following intercostal transfer (Fig. 27.22a,b).

4 Delay in repair is harmful—the earlier repair is performed the better. In repairs after 6 months, failure is the rule.

5 Results after primary grafting of nerves, at the same time as urgent repair of ruptured axillary and subclavian vessels, are better than where nerve repair is delayed.

Rehabilitation

The timing of recovery after nerve repair is prolonged and the extent of that recovery uncertain. After operation the patients are advised to expect recovery over years rather than months and a multidisciplinary approach is necessary to help them adjust to their disability and return to normal life. Wynn-Parry established the Rehabilitation Unit at the Royal National Orthopaedic Hospital, London, and a brief description of the approach used there will be given. Patients are admitted for short periods of 1 or 2 weeks, and they work with a coordinated team towards clearly defined ends. Physiotherapy and occupational therapy should be for short but intensive periods. We have had patients saying they have not returned to work because they have continued to attend for treatment for two or three times a week for many months to their local Physiotherapy Department. The ward is a low-dependency unit. It is run by experienced nurses who are in a good position to recognize psychological and social problems. Sister in Charge coordinates the multidisciplinary team and nursing staff are responsible for making serial plaster of Paris splints for correc-

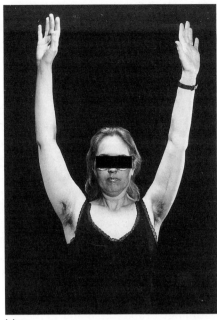

(a)

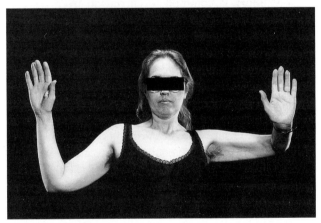

(b)

Fig. 27.21 (a,b) The result following repair by graft of rupture C5, C6 and C7. The operation was performed within 48 h of injury.

tion of deformity. Physiotherapists work to overcome deformity, to develop strength and coordination and are also responsible for transcutaneous nerve stimulation for pain. Occupational therapists continue functional training within a Department which is equipped with many of the features found in the workplace. They assess the need for special instruments or adaptations. They are responsible for fitting and training in orthoses. Psychologists and speech therapists contribute in the treatment of those recovering from associated head injuries, some 10% of our patients, and the Disablement Resettlement Officer is a valuable link with employers, assisting resettlement in previous work or retraining.

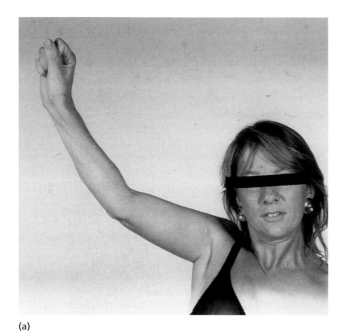

(a)

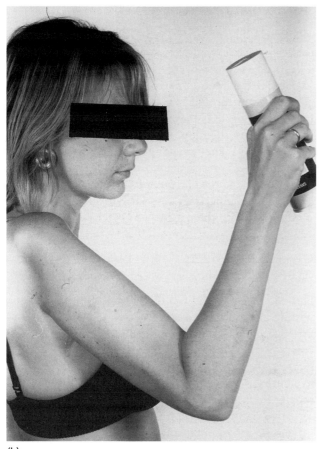

(b)

Fig. 27.22 (a,b) This patient suffered pre-ganglionic injury of C5 and C6. She had a great deal of pain. Six weeks after injury the accessory nerve was transferred to the suprascapular nerve and intercostal nerve to the musculocutaneous nerves. The result at one year is shown. Her pain was abolished.

Pain

Severe pain is usual in patients after pre-ganglionic injury. The description of pain is typical: constant, crushing or burning pain in the anaesthetic hand, with lightning shoots of pain of great severity passing down the whole of the limb. It interferes with concentration and with sleep in most patients; it commences on the day of injury in about one-half. If no repair is performed there is some improvement of pain in perhaps one-half of patients but if it persists for 3 years then it will be permanent. The majority of patients find that distraction at work or play eases pain, a very strong argument for insisting (and indeed firmly encouraging) return to some form of occupation. Drugs are of limited use, although anti-epileptic drugs, e.g. carbamazepine, sometimes relieve the shooting pains. Tricyclic anti-depressants are sometimes helpful in older patients with long-established pain. Transcutaneous nerve stimulation is useful. Wynn-Parry and colleagues (1987) reviewed 52 patients finding substantial diminution in pain in 26 cases. It is important that patients are carefully trained in the use of this equipment; a short out-patient trial is useless.

OPERATIONS FOR PAIN

Surgeons with considerable experience find that successful regeneration eases pain. There is a significant difference between patients who have had an operation of repair with some limited recovery from those who have had no operation at all or those where there has been no recovery. The easing of pain is unpredictable even after the most extensive nerve repair and indeed, a few patients have had new increasing pain during regeneration. There have been quite dramatic examples of pain relief following successful intercostal nerve transfer and this coincides with clinical evidence of recovery of the reinnervated muscles at about 10–12 months after the operation. Having exhausted all other modes of treatment there remain a group of patients who remain utterly demoralized by extreme pain and for these a direct approach to the central nervous system is a last resort; stimulating or ablating central afferent pathways may prove necessary. Thomas (1987, 1988) and Bruxelle *et al.* (1988) have carefully reviewed their experience with the DREZ (dorsal root entry zone) lesion and found it helpful in about one-half of patients. Complications from injury to the spinal cord are severe, occurring in about 10%, and the operation can only be considered as a last resort. The reintroduction of dorsal column stimulation has yielded to some promising early results but its role is not yet established.

Palliative operations

Palliative or reconstructive operations are useful in some cases. They should be integrated within the overall plan for rehabilitation and advised only when there is a clearly defined need and an equally clear solution. Results from standard muscle or tendon transfer are disappointing after severe injuries of the brachial plexus perhaps because of the widespread disturbance of sensation and loss of power. Ross and Birch (1991) reviewed operations about the shoulder finding that glenohumeral arthrodesis was indicated only for well-adjusted patients who had returned to work, with irreparable lesions of C5 and C6. Alnot and Abols (1984) and Marshall and colleagues (1988) have reviewed the results of operation for restoration of elbow flexion. Both concluded that triceps-to-biceps transfer was the most successful, but this operation costs the patients most in loss of function. The results are far inferior, in range of motion and in power, to those following successful repair of the musculocutaneous nerve. The standard flexor to extensor transfer, so reliable for injuries of the radial nerve is much less so in patients with C5/6/7 lesions because there is no motor for wrist extension and sensation in thumb and index is lost (Fig. 27.23).

Amputation has a definite place in patients with complete lesions of the brachial plexus. The largest series is Fletcher's (1981) and his criteria for recommending the operation were strict. Most of his patients were pleased that they had gone on to amputation and they also found some use for the prosthesis. He emphasized that serious pain was a contraindication to the operation and was best reserved for those already back at work and otherwise reintegrated. The author follows these recommendations, restricting amputation for those patients back at work and whose useless limb is a hazard from unnoted injury or infection. Careful explanation must be given that amputation cannot relieve residual pain from the nerve injury.

Work

Loss of function in the dominant upper limb in the young manual worker is a very severe handicap. Some patients totally bypass the rehabilitation process. They use their own initiative, returning to work within weeks of the accident, and decline offers of splints or further operations. Most patients are unable to do this. Seventy patients with complete lesions of the brachial plexus were referred to the rehabilitation unit of the Royal National Orthopaedic Hospital for retraining for work. After follow-up of at least 3 years, 80% of these were at work, 35 with their original firms, 25 in different trades (Wynn-Parry *et al.*, 1987). Petry and Merle (1989) discuss experience from the rehabilitation unit in Nancy. Forty-nine patients were retrained for work between 1980 and 1984 and, after 3 years, one-third had returned to their previous employer, some in a different capacity; a further one-third were retrained into other occupations. Rehabilitation may be impeded by process for compensation through the courts. The author has had patients saying that they have been advised not to go back to work because it might interfere with their compensation. The surgeon, therefore, has a duty to give a clear and precise diagnosis and prognosis as early on as possible to the patient and their legal advisor. It is also clear that the chief responsibility for the rehabilitation rests with the patient.

OBSTETRIC BRACHIAL PLEXUS PALSY (OBPP)

Platt (1973) described OBPP as a 'vanishing condition', writing at a time when incidence was diminishing, but this no longer seems to be the case. While OBPP is common in countries with poorly developed obstetric services, the incidence is still as high as 0.4 in every 1000 live births in Western Europe. Enthusiasm for operative repair (Kennedy, 1903) was followed by a more conservative approach and it has been assumed that the prognosis for spontaneous recovery is good. More detailed analysis of the natural history of the condition and dissatisfaction with the results of palliative operations of muscle transfers has stimulated a more active approach. It became evident that a baby who had not fully recovered by 3 months would have a permanent defect in the afflicted limb and that children with a

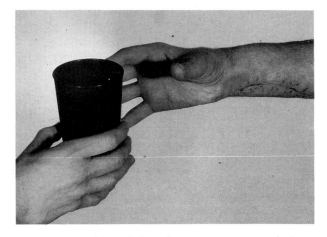

Fig. 27.23 A useful result from flexor to extensor transfer in a patient with irreparable injury C5, C6, C7.

persisting complete lesion at 3 months have a poor prospect for return of function.

Danyou (1851) confirmed at post-mortem that OBPP was caused during birth and Duchenne (1861) described four cases of C5 and C6 paralysis of a condition later termed Erb's palsy. Sever (1925) reported from over 1000 cases, showing that recovery was on the whole good with appropriate and careful conservative treatment. In the early 1980s, some surgeons with very considerable experience in the treatment of adult lesions of the brachial plexus turned their attention to the birth lesion (Morelli, 1984; Narakas, 1987b). Gilbert (1989) now has the largest series of operated cases, some 280 between 1977 and 1989.

Risk factors

Two groups of infants are particularly at risk and the larger group includes the heavy baby with shoulder dystocia. A smaller proportion of babies are born by breech, often very small; these have the most severe and complete lesion. Analysis of 200 consecutive babies seen in the author's unit shows a substantially higher mean birth weight than the UK national average. It seems that the mothers tended to be shorter and heavier than average and that they tended to gain more weight than usual during the pregnancy. In three cases, OBPP was found after caesarian section. In one case, an ultrasound scan showed the cord to be wrapped around the neck of the fetus 2 weeks before delivery and it seems that this is a true example of intrauterine causation. In two babies, Brown-Séquard syndrome was evident. In several others, neonatal hypoxia caused damage to the central nervous system and in these cerebral palsy and OBPP coexisted.

Clinical course

In many instances, recovery occurs within a few days where the injury is a conduction block. If paralysis persists to 3 weeks then the nerve injury is degenerate and prognosis less certain. A widely used classification for these children is useful as a guide to prognosis (Table 27.10).

Table 27.10 Classification of obstetric brachial plexus palsy

Group 1	C5–6	Paralysis shoulder, biceps
Group 2	C5, 6, 7	Paralysis shoulder, arm, wrist extension
Group 3	C5-T1	Complete paralysis
Group 4	C5-T1	Complete paralysis and Bernard–Horner syndrome

Comparing the outcomes in this series (Table 27.10) with others that have been published it is clear that the outlook for full recovery for Group 1 is good; about 90% of children make complete spontaneous recovery. Over one-half of the children in Group 2 are left with some permanent loss at the shoulder (Fig. 27.24) but in both Groups 1 and 2 function in the hand can be considered normal. Few children in Group 3 go on to full spontaneous recovery (Fig. 27.25) and none at all in Group 4.

Early treatment

Treatment commences within days of birth and it is directed towards maintaining a full range of passive movements throughout the limb, particularly at the shoulder where internal rotation and adduction contractures occur so rapidly. A skilful physiotherapist advises the parents. These exercises need to be performed several times every day. Splints are not used. Electromyography is useful at about 10 weeks in those babies with persisting complete paralysis or where there is no clinical evidence

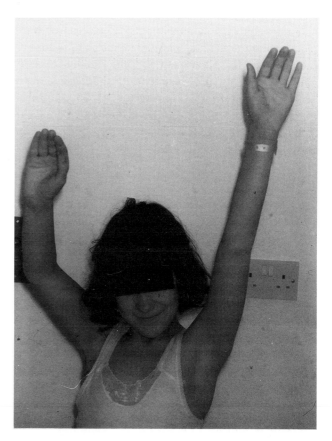

Fig. 27.24 Obstetric brachial plexus palsy, Group 2. There is notable impairment of shoulder function; the hand is smaller.

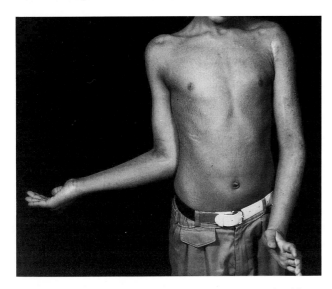

Fig. 27.25 Obstetric brachial plexus palsy, Group 3. Shoulder and elbow flexors remain virtually paralysed.

of recovery into the deltoid and into the biceps. This may reveal one of three things: first, and most favourable, is evidence of reinnervation of the paralysed muscles, with many polyphasic units; next, partial innervation may be demonstrated, with some muscle fibres showing voluntary contraction but without evidence of additional reinnervation; last, and most unfavourable, is that of extensive fibrillation potentials with no evidence of reinnervation at all. An absent or diminished nerve action potential from median or ulnar nerves confirms a degenerative lesion. A normal median or ulnar nerve action potential in a limb which is completely paralysed suggests that the lesion is a most serious one, and it is intradural or pre-ganglionic. Operations for diagnosis and repair is recommended to the parents in Group 1 and in Group 2 babies if there has been no clinical evidence of recovery to the biceps and the deltoid within 3 months, unless electromyography shows strong reinnervation. This recommendation may be made somewhat earlier in Group 3 and 4 babies. Gilbert (1989) uses myelography pre-operatively. The author does not, but a magnetic resonance imaging scan under light sedation is increasingly promising.

Findings at operation

The operation requires meticulous haemostasis and a most thorough knowledge of the normal anatomy of the neck and its variations by the surgeon. An obvious neuroma within the upper trunk is a common finding, indicating rupture of C5, C6 and sometimes of C7 but rather atrophic nerves without neuroma, which respond

little to stimulation point to intradural injury (Fig. 27.26). We rely heavily on intraoperative neurophysiological studies, stimulating the exposed spinal nerve and recording from electrodes attached to the skin of the scalp and of the neck (Fig. 27.27). This investigation, when taken with histological examination of biopsies and the post-operative course suggest that the incidence of pre-ganglionic injury is high (Table 27.11).

Gilbert (1989) describes results of 178 repairs with a minimum follow-up of 3 years: 124 infants fell into Group 1 and Group 2 and pre-ganglionic injury to at least one spinal nerve was found in 29 cases. Normal or good function at the shoulder and elbow was restored in 80%. Predictably results were not as good in the 54 babies in Group 3 and in Group 4. In Group 4, Gilbert confirms that all spinal nerves have been damaged, with pre-ganglionic injury in some and post-ganglionic rupture of others. Of the 54 babies in Groups 3 and 4, good shoulder function was achieved in 35% and was considered useful in 50%. In the hand, the long flexors of the digits regained functional power in 75% and function was gained in the intrinsic muscles in 50%.

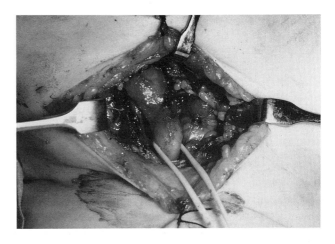

Fig. 27.26 Rupture of the upper trunk in a 3-month-old baby. Obstetric brachial plexus palsy, Group 1.

Table 27.11 Obstetric brachial plexus palsy. Findings in 62 explorations—310 spinal nerves*

Level	Intact	LIC	Rupture	Pre-ganglionic
C5	0	11	40	9
C6	0	12	38	10
C7	8	30	4	18
C8	32	11	0	17
T1	32	9	2	17

* 73 avulsions (25%).

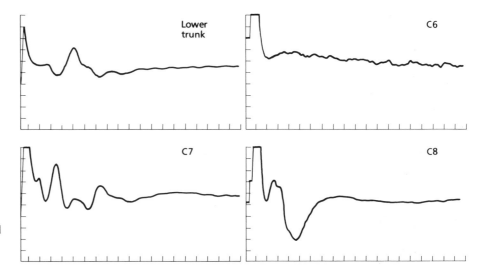

Fig. 27.27 Evoked potentials recorded during exploration. These confirm intradural injury to C6.

Deformity and palliative operations

Palliative operations are useful in mitigating disability by releasing contracture and by muscle transfer. On the whole, the results of muscle or tendon transfer are unpredictable and are inferior to equivalent operations in poliomyelitis or for simple peripheral nerve injuries. The reasons for this include impaired recovery in muscles available for transfer, loss of sensation and co-contraction of antagonistic muscles. In severe lesions, the limb is excluded from fine function altogether and is used as a helper only, and in these cases, interference with deformity might lose what little function there is. Fixed elbow flexion assists bringing the hand to the face and a functional ankylosis between the scapula and humerus afford a stable platform of motion within limited range. Reinnervation of the limb is the basis of function and physiotherapy supplements this in three ways. First, and most important, is the prevention of deformity. Next, assiduous exercises assist the development of the new functional patterns after muscle and tendon transfer and finally, use of the limb is encouraged during nerve regeneration. Formal physiotherapy is reserved for short and intensive periods. The bulk of the work must be done by the parents and the child should be encouraged to enter into all play and sporting activities. There is a risk of enhancing disability by overzealous attendance at therapy departments or by interference in daily activity in play or in school by those caring for the child.

Later operations

Improvement after muscle or tendon transfers is limited and these operations should only be recommended when the functional deficit, and the means of overcoming it, are clearly defined. Assessment by an experienced occupational therapist can be very useful, particularly before any proposed work in the forearm and hand.

Fixed internal rotation at the glenohumeral joint is perhaps the most common and significant deformity. It may proceed to posterior subluxation or dislocation of the head of the humerus (Fig. 27.28). Loss of 40° of passive external rotation, which does not respond to stretching, is best treated by the operation of subscapularis recession performed at between 12 and 18 months. The arm is immobilized in a plaster of Paris spica for a period of 6 weeks, in full abduction and external rotation at the shoulder. A significant and even dramatic improvement in function for the whole of the upper limb is usual. Muscle transfers to restore active movements of the shoulder are less satisfactory.

Indications for operations in the elbow and hand

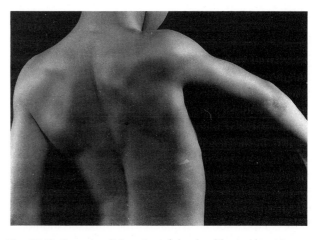

Fig. 27.28 Posterior dislocation of the shoulder in obstetric brachial plexus palsy, Group 2.

remain unclear. Fixed supination or pronation contraction, often with dislocation of the head of the radius, disables the hand and is perhaps best treated by rotation osteotomy of the radius with realignment of the biceps tendon. Flexor-to-extensor tendon transfer, if successful, is beneficial but it can prove a most difficult transfer to retrain. Tendon transfers within the hand require much caution for the gain may be outweighed by loss of an adapted function but it is worthwhile improving the posture of the thumb in relation to the digits.

COMPRESSION AND ENTRAPMENT NEUROPATHY

We have already seen that compression of a nerve causes distortion of the myelin sheath and later, demyelination (Gilliatt, 1980). It is also known that relatively low external pressure of 20–30 mmHg blocks the venous flow through the affected segment of the nerve and it also impedes external transport. Higher pressures of 130–150 mmHg cause acute blocks of conduction in peripheral nerves. Large-diameter fibres are more sensitive, both to compression and to ischaemia, than smaller fibres. If the cause of compression is not relieved, Wallerian degeneration with loss of axons occurs. Neurophysiological investigations are invaluable in the diagnosis of these conditions and also in predicting outcome. Focal demyelination causes slowing or blocking of conduction across the affected segment of the nerve but conduction distally is maintained. There is no denervation of muscle. Prognosis after release of the compression is, on the whole, good. Axonal loss leads to mild slowing of conduction but a diminution of nerve action potential and sensory action potential. Electromyography showing fibrillation of potentials within the muscles confirms denervation and the prognosis here is worse.

A local compression syndrome (carpal tunnel syndrome, ulnar neuropathy) may be the first sign of an underlying generalized neuropathy or of systemic disease. Nerves in patients with diabetic neuropathy are particularly at risk from compression. Patents recovering from Guillain–Barré syndrome are prone to peroneal nerve palsy and a lesion of the ulnar nerve at the elbow may be the first clinical evidence of leprosy. There is a rare familial disorder of inherited pressure-sensitive neuropathy. Dissociated loss of pain and temperature in the lower limbs is a feature of Type 1 hereditary sensory motor neuropathy. Before making a sure diagnosis of local compression neuropathy, the surgeon should at least consider the possibility of an underlying disorder and should be prepared to exclude diabetes, renal disease, thyroid disease and rheumatoid arthritis. An erythrocyte sedimentation rate is a simple enough screening test. The possibility of the space-occupying lesion should also be considered, of a tumour within or adjacent to a nerve at the elbow or at the root of the limb. Pain and sensory disturbance in the hand may be the first indication of Pancoast's tumour involving the brachial plexus. Diagnosis of carpal tunnel syndrome in irradiation neuritis is a common error. There may be more central compression of a spinal nerve from intervertebral disc lesion or from osteoarthritis. Rarely, abnormalities in the hand or leg point to a lesion within the spinal cord; wasting of the small muscles of the hand may be taken as evidence of compression of the ulnar nerve to cursory examination when the underlying diagnosis is syringomyelia.

Many compression syndromes and numerous causes have been described but there are a number of common features. Pain is the most common complaint, and there is usually disturbances of sensation within the territory of the affected nerve. Muscle weakness is less common. Patients are almost always able to outline the areas of abnormal sensation and this corresponds with the cutaneous territory of the afflicted nerve. Pain is often much less precisely localized and may be experienced in other parts of the limb. The course of the nerve should be examined, seeking abnormality in adjacent joints or other structures may be compressing the nerve. The MRC volume, *Aids to the Examination of the Peripheral Nervous System* (1976), is always useful.

Carpal tunnel syndrome

This is the commonest of the compression syndromes. Sepsis, crushing injuries and fractures of the wrist may cause acute compression of the nerve. Carpal fractures, tenosynovitis, anomalous muscles and tumours are other occasional causes but usually there is no obvious aetiology. The patient experiences pain and abnormal sensations in the hand, often extending beyond the territory of the median nerve. Symptoms are usually worse at night and may be eased by elevation or shaking of the hand. Sensory disturbance will be found in over 50% of patients and weakness of the thenar muscles in about one-quarter. In mild cases, a resting splint may help and this is useful for many patients whose symptoms arise during pregnancy. If symptoms persist, however, open decompression is indicated. This should be a simple and reliable operation but damage to the palmar cutaneous branch, the thenar motor branch, and the superficial palmar arch will leave the patient a good deal worse off than before. The safest approach is by a longitudinal incision on the ulnar side of the thenar crease. On occasion the nerve is adherent to the flexor retinaculum. The author does not agree that internal neurolysis is necessary, and is not persuaded of the value of endoscopic decompression.

Compression of the ulnar nerve at the elbow

The ulnar nerve runs in a tunnel behind the medial condyle of the elbow (the cubital tunnel). The floor of the tunnel is formed by the humerus and the medial ligament of the elbow, the roof by the aponeurosis between the humeral and ulnar heads of flexor carpi-ulnaris. The nerve is at risk from entrapment in valgus deformity of the elbow, from osteoarthritis in the floor of the tunnel, from synovial cysts or benign tumours.

Patients experience pain and abnormal sensation in the territory of the ulnar nerve, there may be no clinical weakness of the intrinsic muscles of the hand but electromyography will demonstrate denervation in many cases. Tenderness and swelling of the ulnar nerve at the entrance to the tunnel is usual, percussion here causing paraesthesia in the territory of the nerve. A light padded splint should be recommended for early or mild cases. The complications of poorly conducted decompressions or transpositions are severe, and may lead to an intractable pain state. Open decompression is best done through a posterior incision avoiding branches of the medial cutaneous nerve of the forearm and if there is no obvious abnormality of the joint or in the tunnel, then local decompression by division of the roof of the tunnel (Osborne, 1970) is adequate. Deep transposition of the ulnar nerve is indicated when the elbow is deformed or when there is marked osteoarthritis involving the tunnel. The operation is a difficult one. The nerve must pass smoothly to lie next to the median nerve on brachialis and the medial intermuscular septum should be widely resected to prevent angulation. Ideally, the longitudinal blood vessels passing with the nerve are preserved. Haematoma is a serious complication and best treated by urgent decompression.

Thoracic outlet syndromes

These are some of the most confusing and controversial of all disorders of peripheral nerves. They are considered rare by some authorities, common by others. Perhaps the term is too broad, for it includes the dangerous occlusion of the subclavian artery without any involvement of the brachial plexus at all, and on the other hand the true neurogenic lesion without any vascular involvement. These are clearly defined entities and they are both uncommon. The majority of patients present with symptoms indicating impairment of blood flow and impairment of nerve conduction. Wilbourne (1993) in an extensive review of thoracic outlet syndromes proposed a simple classification into subgroups, which is very helpful. Before considering these we should turn now to the anatomy of the thoracic outlet.

The subclavian vessels and the brachial plexus arch over the first rib which forms the base of a narrow triangle, the other boundaries being scalenus anterior and scalenus medius. This may be distorted by accessory ribs, accessory muscles, or a fibrous band passing from the transverse process of C7 to the first rib. The area may be distorted after fracture of first rib or of clavicle. Space-occupying lesions, such as tumours, cause compression particularly of the subclavian vein and brachial plexus.

ARTERIAL THORACIC OUTLET SYNDROME

The first endarterectomy was performed by Dos Santos in 1946 for obstruction of the subclavian artery deep to the scalenus anterior muscles. Rob and Standeven (1958) described the dangerous vascular complications of this condition. It is rare, almost always unilateral, and the usual cause is a fully formed cervical rib. Post-stenotic dilatation and then an aneurysm forms distal to the compression site. Thrombus forms within the aneurysm, throwing off emboli; proximal thrombosis may occur. Increasingly severe ischaemia occurs within the limb with frank claudication pain, hand pallor after exercise and loss of distal pulses. Symonds (1927) described nine cases of embolism in the right common carotid artery, and six of his patients were left with permanent left hemiplegia with irreversible ischaemia of the right arm. The orthopaedic surgeon should be on the alert for this rare but extremely dangerous variation of thoracic outlet syndrome. Urgent investigation including Doppler flow studies and digital subtraction angiography are necessary, before proceeding to decompression and reconstruction of the artery. The reader is referred to the outstanding review of Parry and Eastcott (1992).

TRUE NEUROGENIC THORACIC OUTLET SYNDROME

This rare condition was clearly defined by Gilliatt and his colleagues in 1970. Before their work, many patients with neurological disturbance in the hand were diagnosed as thoracic outlet syndrome when in fact they had carpal tunnel syndrome. The lower trunk of the brachial plexus is stretched over a taut band arising from a small cervical rib or an elongated transverse process of C7 to the first rib. Weakness and wasting of the small muscles of the hand is constant, and these patients experience pain and paraesthesia along the medial aspect of the forearm and the medial two fingers. Radiographs of the neck confirm the bony abnormality, and neurophysiological investigations are diagnostic, confirming denervation of the intrinsic muscles of the hand and lower amplitudes for the median motor and ulnar sensory patentials. Decompression by excision of the band relieves pain but is very rarely followed by improvement in strength.

COMBINED VASCULAR AND NEUROLOGICAL THORACIC OUTLET SYNDROME

This is more common and it is the most difficult to diagnose and to treat. Patients complain of pain, often in the scapular region and sometimes worse at night. There is weakness of grip but rarely wasting; there is disturbance of sensation which may extend to the whole of the hand but which may be confined to the median or to the ulnar territories. Minor vascular symptoms are common. Hand pallor after exercise or elevation of the limb, followed by engorgement and cyanosis is a frequent complaint. Exacerbation of symptoms on elevation of the arm is typical. Obliteration of the radial pulse on elevation of the arm is often taken as an important diagnostic feature but of course this occurs in many healthy subjects. Greater significance should be attached to two findings. First, there is obvious prominence and tenderness of the plexus in the posterior triangle of the neck as it passes over the accessory rib or band and next, there is a bruit from the subclavian artery. The surgeon should be extremely cautious before recommending operation unless these two physical signs are found. Nerve-conduction studies are usually normal and the most useful supporting investigation is digital subtraction angiography confirming stenosis and sometimes post-stenotic dilatation of the subclavian artery. The purpose of the operation is to confirm and relieve the cause of the disturbance and exposure of both the brachial plexus and the subclavian artery is necessary. A nerve stimulator is essential. The first thoracic nerve may be stretched to a web of tissue over an anomalous band or bone. The first rib usually requires excision.

PAIN

Pain is the chief reason that drives patients to see doctors and it is for doctors to define the cause. The patient's own description often points to diagnosis; all too frequently that description is ignored or dismissed.

The trend to referring patients to a 'pain clinic' before attempting to establish diagnosis to relieve the cause is thoroughly bad practice. Sympathetic block, in one form or another, is undoubtedly valuable in the treatment of certain types of injury to peripheral nerves, but it must be acknowledged that such blocks are regularly applied on empirical grounds alone. It is nonsensical to use these techniques in many patients with neurological disease. Some examples that are of particular relevance to the orthopaedic surgeon include the intense bursting pain of compartment syndrome or ischaemia, the often agonizing pain following partial transection of a major nerve trunk or irritation of that trunk by an encircling suture, the boring pain with bizarre sensory disturbance from compression of the spinal cord or syringomyelia and the burning pain of certain types of neuropathy. Pain following pre-ganglionic injury to the brachial plexus is characteristic and it indicates the involvement of the central nervous system. There is a deep, constant, crushing or burning pain felt in the anaesthetic hand; superimposed upon this are the lightening pains so severe as to double the patient up. The first indicates de-afferentation of the limb, the second points to abnormal hyperactivity of the neurones within the substantia gelatinosa and the dorsal horn. It may be useful to define the terms now in common use: *allodynia* is a normally non-painful stimulus, such as light touch, experienced as pain; *hyperpathia* or *hyperalgesia*, is an exaggerated response to a painful stimulus. A combination of symptoms allows definition of two particular pain states.

Physiological mechanisms

The perception of pain is mediated through two groups of nerve fibres. The A-δ group are small myelinated axons, $3-6\,\mu m$ in diameter, and conduct at the rate of about 20 m/sec. These are mechanoreceptors and are responsible for the perception of sharp or pricking pain which is well localized, classically termed 'epicritic pain'. The unmyelinated C afferent fibres are polymodal nociceptors and respond to potentially harmful thermal, mechanical and chemical stimuli. These are responsible for burning, delayed, dull, poorly localized pain, classically termed 'protopathic'. Intraneural microstimulation of the fascicles within a mixed nerve trunk show that some pass solely to skin or to muscle. Microstimulation of skin nerve fascicles causes either the protopathic (C-fibre) type of pain or the sharp (A-δ) epicritic pain. Localization is accurate whereas stimulation of muscle nerve fascicles causes a characteristic cramping pain, poorly localized, and sometimes referred to remote parts.

The C-fibres are particularly sensitive to changes in their local environment, from ischaemia and electrolyte imbalance, and it is not unreasonable to imagine that the local changes in circulation in the swollen hand or foot excite these nerves.

The afferent fibres pass to their cell bodies in the dorsal root ganglion, and from there they enter the dorsal spinal horn. Most C-fibres pass to their synapse in Layer 2 of the dorsal horn, the substantia gelatinosa. A-δ fibres synapse in Layers 1 and 5. Classically, two projecting pathways for transmission for nociceptor activity have been described. The spinothalamic tract lying in the anterolateral cord projects contralaterally to the posterolateral thalamus, ending in the thalamo-corticol neurones. The projection from here is to the somatosensory cortex. It has been said that this pathway is responsible for the localization and the intensity of pain. The second pathway, the spinoreticulothalamic, is polysynaptic and lies more ventrally in the spinal cord. It projects to the medullary and midbrain reticular formation, from there by ill-defined pathways to the cerebral cortex.

The behaviour of the central neurone and their projecting pathways is profoundly altered after injury to a peripheral nerve. Nearly all of these observations come from experimental work in animals and their clinical relevance is not always clear. Nerve fibres at the site of damage in the nerve trunk become more excitable, and there is increased activity within the neurones of the dorsal horn. The receptive areas of neurones in the dorsal column nuclei, in the thalamus and in the somato-sensory cortex increase after peripheral nerve injury and they become more active. The establishment of the abnormal central patterns of function may be part of the explanation for that fearful situation of the chronic pain state which is resistant to local distal intervention at the site of the original injury to the peripheral nerve. The prognosis for function after repair of the nerve deteriorates with time. The prognosis for relief of pain after an injury to a peripheral nerve trunk similarly deteriorates with delay. Infusion of local anaesthetic into incisions or wounds, or adequate use of opiates after operation, demonstrates that prevention is better than cure.

What is prejoratively termed 'anecdotal' evidence of the importance of the higher centres should not be dismissed too lightly for there is a key to the understanding of pain in General Paget not knowing that he had lost his leg at the Battle of Waterloo until his Commander in Chief had advised him of this mishap. Beecher (1956) described his experience with the war wounded at the Battle of Anzio. Three-quarters of his patients required no analgesia at all and he explained this because for them the wound was relief from war and the threat of death. The orthopaedic surgeon will ponder on the harm done to patients by process for compensation after injury. Journals are full of papers that describe how the outcome is worse in 'workmen's compensation' cases, an unpalatable fact for any surgeon attempting to rectify the consequences of iatrogenic nerve injury. A particularly tragic example of the possible relevance of CNS endogenous opiates is the sight of an intravenous drug addict who cannot be relieved of somatic pain by conventional therapeutic doses of morphine.

Causalgia

This term was introduced by Mitchell from his experience in the American Civil War (1872). Causalgia means burning pain and the best definition comes from the MRC Report of 1954. Causalgia follows injury to a major nerve trunk. It is severe, spontaneous, persistent and it usually has a burning quality. It may spread beyond the territory of the injured nerve and it is characteristically aggravated by physical and emotional stimuli. True causalgia is rare. It was recognized after high-velocity missile injuries to nerve trunks in war and such injuries are not common in civil practice (Fig. 27.29). The nearest equivalent is the intense pain following injury to the brachial plexus or proximal median and ulnar nerves in the upper limb or to the sciatic or tibial nerves in the lower limb. Unfortunately, many of these are iatrogenic. The afflicted part is intolerant of examination and stimulation and there is usually excessive sweating and vasomotor instability. Trophic changes which include atrophy of the skin, stiffness of

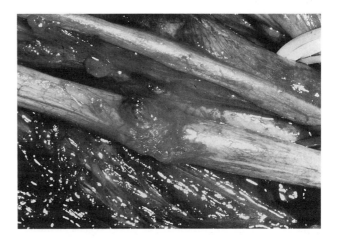

Fig. 27.29 Causalgia after a gunshot wound partially transecting median nerve. The pain was abolished by cervical sympathectomy.

the joints and osteoporosis of the skeleton may progress so far as to render the limb useless.

Reflex sympathetic dystrophy (RSD)

This has been defined by the International Association for the Study of Pain and it is characterized by continuous pain associated with sympathetic overactivity in the distal portion of the limb often after mild injury without a direct injury to a major nerve. There is continuous burning pain which is made worse by movement, stimulation of skin, or stress. Early on, the hand or foot is red, warm and swollen and there is usually excess sweating. Later the part becomes cold and blue and there is marked atrophy of the soft tissues with joint stiffness and loss of hair. Hannington-Kiff (1974) showed that this pain may be abolished by the intravenous injection of guanethidine, or by other agents which deplete neurotransmitters in adrenergic sympathetic endings. RSD loses credibility as a diagnosis when it is used as a catch-all phrase for any swollen or painful hand after a fracture or other injury, and Thomas and Ochoa (1993) described several syndromes that fulfil the criteria for RSD which cannot be explained on the basis of excess sympathetic activity nor on the sensitization of nociceptors to catecholamine neurotransmitters. The author believes that many examples of so-called RSD, notably in the hand, are the result of inadequate treatment of a fracture or a crush injury. The elementary principles of elevation, and early mobilization to prevent swelling, have been neglected. Splints or bandages improperly applied worsen the swelling (Fig. 27.30a). There are published series reporting that RSD is a common complication of treatment of a Colles fracture; perhaps those authors should consider whether their own protocol of treatment has not in fact contributed to this seeming high incidence. Adams (1978) introduced a policy of treatment for patients with these fractures which is based on the early restoration of function and, having followed this technique, the author has been impressed by how rarely RSD occurs. Adams stipulated that the fracture must be reduced and held in position with an incomplete dorsal plaster of Paris splint. The patient attends the fracture clinic every day in the first week after injury, elevation and active movements of the fingers are encouraged there, and the splint is rebandaged to allow for change in swelling. The plaster is completed on the seventh day after injury. Adams' insistence on daily attendance for rebandaging and exercises enables doctors concerned to detect the earliest evidence that things are not going well, that there is undue pain, abnormal swelling and stiffness requiring appropriate

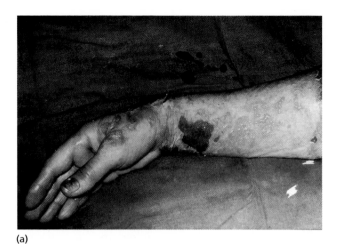

(a)

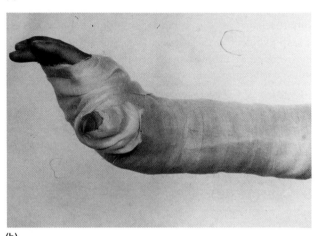

(b)

Fig. 27.30 (a) Reflex sympathetic dystrophy after incorrect splinting of a fracture of wrist. Note blisters and skin loss from overzealous bandaging. (b) The hand splinted after operation of tendon transfer. Note that it is in position of function. The plaster slab is incomplete; it is not compressing the limb; only those joints which must be immobilized are protected.

treatment. RSD should be regarded as a preventable complication, not as an inevitable consequence of certain types of injury. The surgeon should think very carefully before imputing psychological instability to the patient for this largely iatrogenic complication.

A surgical response to post-operative pain

Severe post-operative pain indicates that something has gone wrong. The patient's description of the pain of ischaemia or compression, of partial transection of a nerve trunk or of irritation by a foreign body is so characteristic as to be diagnostic. The surgeon must consider alternative diagnoses, such as bleeding into the spinal canal or an unrecognized peripheral neuropathy. Two particular iatrogenic nerve injuries cause severe pain that is not easily explained. Section of the accessory nerve high in the posterior triangle of the neck or injury to the long thoracic nerve usually causes severe and debilitating pain afflicting the whole of the upper limb and the shoulder girdle. A possible explanation for this is that the limb is no longer supported adequately and there is a traction upon the brachial plexus. Neuralgic amyotrophy may be a diagnosis in these cases but it must be one of exclusion and if these two motor nerves stop working after an incision over their course, then only re-exploration can establish that they have not been accidentally damaged.

The cutaneous neuroma

Neuroma formation is an inevitable consequence of section of any nerve. Injury to certain nerves of sensation may cause pain seemingly beyond all proportion. These include the superficial radial nerve of forearm, the medial cutaneous nerve of forearm, the sural and the long saphenous nerve. It is remarkable that these nerves which are often used in grafting are so prone to pain states after injury to their distal branches. A number of operations have been described, and none of them is wholly satisfactory. The subject is fully reviewed by Herndon and Hess (1991). Most studies of operative treatment are illogical for they ignore two inevitable factors: (i) a neuroma is a normal biological response to section of a nerve, and neuroma formation cannot be prevented; (ii) if a cut nerve causes pain, then cutting that same nerve more proximally cannot be expected to abolish pain. The long history of ablative operations in the spinal cord or even more proximally for pain relief shows that relief is usually transient, and that pain returns more severely. The most logical solution is to restore continuity of the nerve but using another cutaneous nerve as a graft risks inducing a second painful neuroma and adds to sensory loss. The frozen muscle graft (Glasby *et al.*, 1992) is a potentially promising solution for this problem. Stirrat *et al.* (1991) reported on a series of freeze−thawed muscle graft (FTMG) in repair of damaged cutaneous nerves in the upper limb. Pain was improved in over 70% of the upper-limb neuromas; results for the lower limb were very much worse.

The chronic pain state

After reasonable and appropriate treatment there are still despairing and depressed patients who remain in pain. These induce a sense of despair and depression in the attending surgeon. The surgeon should try not to pass the burden to other colleagues and should at least do what he or she can to establish the cause, the underlying cause of this state, and to remember that appropriate earlier intervention might have prevented its development. Some lessons are worth repeating. The single most effective way of alleviating the pain of severe traction lesion of the brachial plexus is to reinnervate the limb. This should be done early. Timely and skilful use of sympathetic blockade, when performed early, is successful in many cases of causalgia and of reflex sympathetic dystrophy. Dobyns (1991) outlines a holistic approach to this problem. He deprecates reliance on sympathetic overactivity as the explanation, and emphasizes the need to establish cause. He refers to the importance of recognition of psychological and social factors which may bear on the continuation of severe chronic pain. Dobyns emphasizes early recognition and treatment and the need for one doctor to be in overall charge of the patient.

Treatment of the common pain state follows two paths. These are complementary and they are not mutually exclusive. The first is an attempt to restore order to cerebral interpretation of afferent stimuli from the periphery. On the whole, ablative operations in the central nervous system will fail although some results of the DREZ lesion are promising for patients with malignant infiltration of peripheral nerves and, to a lesser extent, in patients with severe pain from pre-ganglionic injury to the brachial plexus. The reintroduction of implanted stimulators adjacent to the peripheral nerves or spinal cord is promising. Cooney (1991) described 25 cases of implants adjacent to peripheral nerve trunks. The majority were helped. Tai (personal communication) has obtained strikingly promising results in severe cases of pain following traction lesion of brachial and the lumbosacral plexus.

The second mode relies on drugs. Two types are potentially useful. The first suppresses abnormal hyperactivity in central neurones. The anticonvulsant agents, carbamazepine or phenytoin, first applied for trigeminal neuralgia, have a role in treating the convulsive pain of avulsion lesion. The second group, the tricyclic antidepressants, block the re-uptake of monoamine transmitters. Willner and Low (1993) reviewed the indications for these agents, and emphasized the severity and the danger of their side-effects. This impressive review concludes by emphasizing the role of the nerve microenvironment, the need to develop agents that will stabilize the peripheral nerve membrane without central effects and the need for rigorously designed clinical studies.

PERIPHERAL NERVE TUMOURS

Peripheral nerve tumours present problems in clinical diagnosis, in classification and in treatment. Avoidable damage to major nerve trunks is seen far too often after operations on benign tumours. In neurofibromatosis, the involvement of other systems may be more significant than the lump within the nerve and careful judgement is necessary in deciding which tumours should be removed and which can be left. Patients with this condition should be advised about risks of malignant transformation of a benign tumour and the risks of transmission of the disease to children. The prognosis for malignant nerve tumours is poor and the indications for excision, compartmentectomy and amputation remain unclear.

Origin and classification of nerve tumours

Until relatively recently, large published series of benign tumours did not distinguish clearly between schwannoma and neurofibroma. Major early studies suggested that malignant nerve tumours were the most common of sarcomas. The confusion about histogenesis has been clarified by electron microscopy and by immunohistochemical studies. Urich (1993) has comprehensively reviewed the pathology of peripheral nerve tumours. He points out that the Schwann cell expresses the S-100 protein and the LEU-7 membrane antigen. Perineurial cells are S-100 negative but are positive for the epithelial membrane antigen. Fibroblasts express vimentin and produce fibronectin. Electron microscopy has confirmed that schwannomas are formed from Schwann cells, and that neurofibromas arise from varying proportions of Schwann cells, perineurial cells and fibroblasts. The long-standing debate about the origin of the perineurial cell has been decisively settled in favour of the fibroblast.

Although most peripheral nerve tumours are easily recognizable by their clinical features, diagnosis in the larger tumours, of those within the body cavities and of the malignant tumours, requires a study of clinical, histological and ultrastructural and immunohistochemical features. A large schwannoma arising within the lumbosacral plexus or femoral nerve may be taken for a soft-tissue sarcoma, such as a leiomyosarcoma. Presence of the S-100 protein indicates that the tumour is in fact a benign schwannoma. This finding will deter the surgeon from an unnecessary and crippling wide excision.

Table 27.12 shows a classification of nerve tumours, and the numbers of cases seen by the author are shown in Tables 27.13 and 27.14.

Table 27.13 Number of cases based on type of tumour

Tumour type	Non-neurofibromatosis	Neurofibromatosis
Schwannoma	81	⎫
Solitary neurofibroma	16	⎬ 30
MPNST*	15	5
PNET†	3	2

* Malignant peripheral nerve sheath tumour.
† Peripheral (primitive) neurectodermal tumour.

Table 27.14 Other benign tumours or tumour-like conditions (32 cases); see also Table 27.13

Intraneural ganglion	6
Angioma	4
Lipoma	3
Amyloid	1
Focal hypertrophic neuropathy	4
Extra-abdominal fibromatosis (dermoid)	7
Fibro-fatty infiltration (lipohamartoma of the median nerve)	7

Table 27.12 Classification of peripheral nerve tumours

Tumour	Benign	Malignant
Nerve sheath tumours	Schwannoma (neurilemmoma), solitary neurofibroma, plexiform neurofibroma (in neurofibromatosis)	Malignant peripheral nerve sheath tumour (MPNST) includes malignant schwannoma, neurofibrosarcoma, nerve sheath fibrosarcoma
		Peripheral or primitive neurectodermal tumour (PNET) includes neuroepithelioma, peripheral neuroblastoma, extra-osseous Ewing's sarcoma
Neuronal tumours	Ganglioneuroma	Ganglioneuroblastoma, neuroblastoma

The solitary benign schwannoma (neurilemmoma, neurinoma)

The schwannoma can be removed from its nerve of origin without loss of function. Sex distribution is equal and the peak incidence is between the third and sixth decade. The most common site is the head and neck, including the brachial plexus and spinal nerves, followed by the upper and lower limbs. Slow-growing deep-seated tumours in the mediastinum and retroperitoneum may grow to such a size as to be mistaken for soft-tissue sarcomas.

The usual presentation is a painful lump. The swelling is mobile from side to side but not in the vertical axis of the limb and the single most useful physical sign is irradiating painful paraesthesia in the territory of the nerve on percussion, similar to Tinel's sign. The epineurium forms a capsule about the tumour which lies eccentrically within the nerve trunk (Fig. 27.31a). Large tumours develop cysts and show degenerative changes of haemorrhage, calcification and hyalinization. Engorged and tortuous epineurial vessels course over the capsule of the tumour. The cut surface is yellowish in larger tumours, cystic and it may be blood-stained. The diagnostic histological features are the organization of Schwann cells either into areas of compact bundles (Antonin type A tissue) or in a less-orderly arrangement of spindle-shaped or oval cells in a loose matrix (Antoni type B tissue). Diagnosis is confirmed by specific immunohistochemical and ultrastructural features. Schwannomas strongly express the S-100 protein and electron microscopy shows Schwann cells forming layers and stacks of long cytoplasmic extensions surrounded by a basement membrane.

Schwannomas are treated by removing the tumour without damaging the nerve (Fig. 27.31b). The diagnosis should be apparent before operation or at least at exposure. No less than 18 patients in this series suffered irreparable damage from unnecessary resection of parts of the brachial or lumbosacral plexus of the femoral and sciatic nerves and other major mixed nerve trunks.

The solitary neurofibroma

The typical neurofibroma arising in a major nerve trunk is easily recognizable. Enzinger and Weiss (1988) point out that neurofibromas occur in younger patients, that cutaneous nerves are most commonly involved and that degenerative changes are unusual. Neurofibromas do not possess a true capsule and staining for S-100 protein is less intense and less uniform than in the schwannoma. These are uniformly grey-white, translucent, rubbery

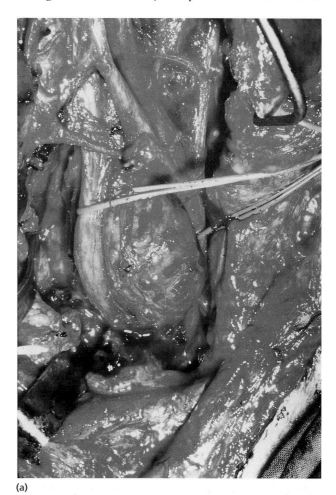

(a)

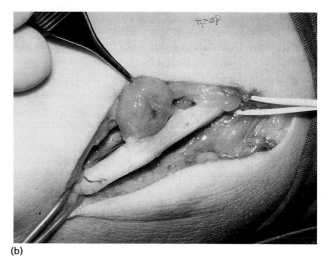

(b)

Fig. 27.31 (a) A schwannoma arising in C5. Note the displacement of the conducting elements. (b) Enucleation of a schwannoma from the ulnar nerve at the elbow. The nerve is intact.

and fibrous tumours. They are less vascular than the schwannomas. Enneking (1983) described two features helpful in diagnosis: 'a large vascular non-reactive oval fusiform mass in intimate proximity to a displaced vascular bundle is very suggestive of a neurofibroma'. The second feature is multiple nodules within the mass. Neurofibromas are clinically important for four major reasons. First, they may grow to a very large size causing pressure on adjacent structures (Fig. 27.32a—c). Next, a neurofibroma of a spinal cord may extend into the spinal canal, the dumbell tumour which is more common in neurofibromas than in schwannomas (Fig. 27.33). Thirdly, the neurofibroma of a trunk nerve is inseparable from nerve bundles which become intimately involved within it so that enucleation is not possible. Fourthly, there is a slight but definite risk of malignant transformation at about 1%.

Neurofibromatosis

There have been recent major advances from studies of prevalence, inheritance, molecular genetics and the natural history of this condition (see Chapter 1). The reader is referred to the excellent review of Riccardi (1990). Two studies in south-east Wales by Huson and her colleagues (1989a,b) found a prevalence of 1 in 4950 of the population; 41 of their 135 cases were new mutations. They give clear guidelines on genetic counselling. The features of the two main syndromes, neurofibromatosis type 1 (NF1) or Von Recklinghausen's disease, and type 2 neurofibromatosis (NF2) or central neurofibromatosis are shown in Table 27.15. There are mixed forms and also localized variants.

Neurofibromatosis type 1 is a disorder of the central and peripheral nervous systems, the skeleton and vessels. It is protean and there are four major causes of death: (i) massive plexiform neurofibroma in the mediastinum involving the airways; (ii) astrocytomas of optic chiasma, brainstem or cerebellum; (iii) cervical paraspinal neurofibromas; (iv) malignant peripheral nerve sheath tumour (MPNST). Phaeochromocytoma is a rare cause of death. The chief sources of morbidity include plexiform neurofibroma, gigantism, intracranial astrocytoma, congenital glaucoma, tibial pseudarthrosis and spinal deformity, renovascular hypertension and speech and learning defects.

Less than one-half of the patients presenting in this series with neurofibromatosis type 1 knew of their condition. Only a few of those who did know were aware of the implications of the diagnosis. The surgeon may be the first to make the diagnosis and should work closely with the clinical geneticist so that the patient and

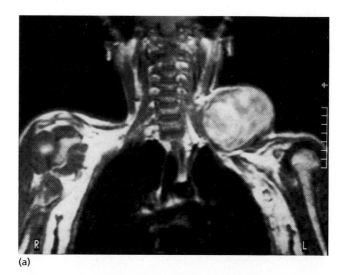

(a)

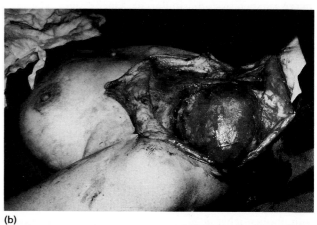

(b)

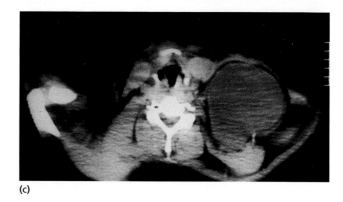

(c)

Fig. 27.32 (a) Massive solitary neurofibroma in posterior triangle of the neck. (b) The tumour exposed by the transclavicular approach. There was no loss of neurological function. (c) Computed tomography scan of large solitary neurofibroma in the posterior triangle of the neck. The capsule appears well defined.

family are adequately advised. The support group LINK have produced excellent fact sheets on neurofibromatosis types 1 and 2. A reasonable estimate of the risk of MPNST in a patient with neurofibromatosis type 1 is

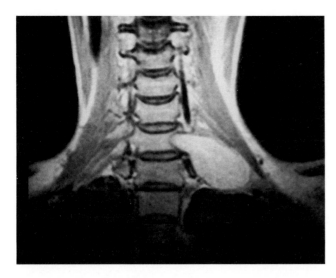

Fig. 27.33 Magnetic resonance imaging scan of schwannoma in C8 nerve with intraspinal extension. Successfully removed by combined anterior and posterior approach. Mr R. Bradford's case.

about 3%. These tumours present most commonly in adolescence or early adult life and they are characterized by pain, increase in size of a pre-existing neurofibroma and loss of neural function.

Table 27.15 Neurofibromatosis

Characteristic	Peripheral neurofibromatosis (NF1)	Central neurofibromatosis (NF2)
Incidence	60 per 100 000	0.1 per 100 000
Inheritance	Autosomal dominant — gene locus on the proximal long arm of chromosome 17	Autosomal dominant. Gene locus on the distal long arm of chromosome 22
Diagnostic features	Six or more café au lait patches. Axillary or inguinal freckling. Two or more neurofibromas, or one plexiform neurofibroma, optic glioma. Two or more Lisch nodules. Pseudarthrosis, sphenoid dysplasia	Bilateral VIII nerve tumours. Two or more of neurofibroma, meningioma, glioma, schwannoma, juvenile posterior subcapsular lenticular opacity. A unilateral VIII nerve tumour with a first degree relative who has established NF2

Surgical considerations

Operations are necessary to establish the diagnosis, to relieve pain, and to remove pressure on adjacent structures including the spinal cord. Severe pain, progressive loss of nerve function, and a tender mass were obvious in all patents with MPNST in this series. We have already seen that there is a danger of unnecessary injury to major nerve trunks in the treatment of benign nerve tumours. Biopsy in MPNST must be performed properly to avoid local dissemination of tumour but also to obtain adequate tissue for study in these often very pleomorphic tumours. A tumour of a peripheral nerve may be the first sign of neurofibromatosis; a thorough physical examination and family history will confirm this. Both computed tomography and magnetic resonance imaging scans provide invaluable information about the size and nature of the tumours within body cavities or in the limbs, and are essential in analysis of extension into the spinal canal (Fig. 27.34). Digital subtraction angiography (see Chapter 30.2) is useful in demonstrating the relation of the tumour to axial vessels.

OPERATION

Neuromuscular blocking agents should be avoided to allow intraoperative nerve stimulation. Magnification by loupes or operating microscope should be available. In large tumours, the surgeon may have to excise and repair major vessels, stabilize the spinal column and repair nerves. Frozen sections are sometimes helpful in MPNST particularly by showing that the proposed limit

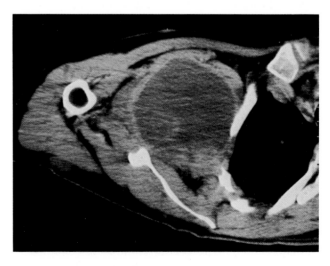

Fig. 27.34 Transverse computed tomography scan of highly malignant peripheral nerve sheath tumour in axilla extending into the posterior triangle. There is no capsule.

of resection is adequate. Incisions must allow adequate exposure of axial structures. Some of the worst iatrogenic cases that we have seen followed small incisions made by inexperienced surgeons in the day care theatre. Bonney's transclavicular approach (Bonney *et al.*, 1990) is invaluable in difficult cases of tumour in the brachial plexus. Crockard and Bradford (1985) successfully removed a schwannoma anterior to the craniovertebral junction by the transoral–transclival route. Tumours arising in the neck or at the cervicothoracic junction demand an approach that allows adequate exposure of the spinal nerves, the vertebral bodies and the vertebral arteries.

In a benign schwannoma, or in a benign tumour arising from a nerve which is still conducting, the incision is made in the capsule remote from conducting elements which are usually visible from nerve bundles stretched tightly over the tumour. An intracapsular resection is performed in a benign schwannoma, using a fine dissector to develop the plane between the tumour and its capsule. In most neurofibromas, partial excision of the tumour allows preservation of conducting bundles. In others in which conduction has been lost, the normal architecture of the nerve is obliterated.

Malignant peripheral nerve sheath tumours

The schwannoma may be malignant from the outset, neurofibromas are always potentially so. MPNSTs will develop in between 3 and 5% of patients with neurofibromatosis type 1. They are also a late complication of radiotherapy. A review of the literature describing over 700 cases of MPNST (Birch, 1993) suggests there are two populations. One-third of these tumours occur in patients with neurofibromatosis. These patients are younger, with a peak decade of incidence at 20–30 years. Malignant tumours in NF arise more centrally and the prognosis is very much worse than for the solitary MPNST (Fig. 27.35). In these, the peak incidence is in the fourth, fifth and sixth decades and the tumours arise more peripherally. The head, neck and upper limbs account for 40%; the lower limb is the site of approximately one-third. The remainder occur within the trunk, usually arising from spinal nerves in close relation to the spinal column.

Pain is the cardinal symptom, and there is almost always clinical evidence of loss of nerve function. A tender enlarging mass is found in all but the most deeply seated tumours. The clinical features and findings at operation are more important in the diagnosis of MPNST than are histological characteristics, most of all in the low-grade malignant neurofibroma. The smaller

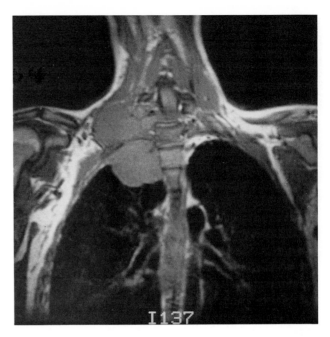

Fig. 27.35 Extra-osseous Ewing's sarcoma, arising from the sympathetic chain.

tumours appear as fusiform swellings within a nerve trunk; they are hard and the nerve is surrounded by vascular adhesions. Oedema of the adjacent tissues is a significant finding. In larger tumours the diagnosis is obvious. The tumour may have burst out of the epineurium extending into muscle or bone. Some large tumours develop as multilobular masses, there may be cystic changes with haemorrhage, and in the most rapidly growing tumours there is extensive necrosis. The most common histological appearance is similar to fibrosarcoma, with masses of spindle-shaped cells organized into sweeping bundles or lamellae. Metaplastic differentiation occurs in over 20% of MPNST, bone, cartilage and muscle being the most common tissues found. Epithelioid differentiation into glandular or squamous tissue is less common.

There is little evidence that radiation or chemotherapy improves survival although there may be a temporary response in metastases. It may be possible to excise the nerve of origin sufficiently widely to effect cure and compartmentectomy is reasonable in occasional cases involving a dispensable nerve. Amputation is indicated for recurrence after local incision, when the tumour has burst through the epineurium, or when a previous poorly planned biopsy has contaminated the field. Amputation cannot cure cases with proximal spread within the nerves or when there are already metastases. The particular difficulties of treating tumours of their brachial plexus are set out in two excellent series, Lusk *et al.* (1987) and Sedel *et al.* (1989). The prognosis is very poor. Forequarter amputation is advised for most cases but this is impractical when tumour has extended to the spinal column or canal.

The peripheral neurectodermal tumours, a group which includes neuroepithelioma, the peripheral neuroblastoma, and perhaps some cases of extraosseous Ewing's sarcoma, are rare. These tumours are radiosensitive and do respond to appropriate chemotherapy.

PROGNOSIS

The prognosis for MPNST is poor. Unfavourable features include a proximal or central origin, large size and neurofibromatosis. Five-year survival and disease-free intervals of about 50% have been reported for a solitary MPNST. In neurofibromatosis, reported figures for 5-year survival range from 16 to 30%.

ACKNOWLEDGEMENTS

I should like to thank Mr Stephen Gshmeissner of the Royal College of Surgeons for preparation of electron micrographs 27.1(a,b), Oota Boundy of the Institute of Orthopaedics for preparation of the other photographs and Mrs Margaret Taggart for collation of records and preparation of manuscript.

REFERENCES

Adams J.C. (1964) Vulnerability of the sciatic nerve in closed ischiofemoral arthrodesis by nail and graft. *J. Bone Joint Surg.* **46B**, 748–763.

Adams J.C. (1978) *Outline of Fractures*, 7th edn. Edinburgh, Churchill Livingstone, pp. 159–169.

Albers J.W., Allen A.A., Bastron J.A. and Daube J.R. (1981) Limb myokymia. *Muscle Nerve* **4**, 494–504.

Alnot J.Y. and Abols Y. (1984) Réanimation de la flexion du coude pars transferts tendineaux dans les paralysies traumatique du plaxus brachial de l'adulte. *Rev. Chir. Orthop.* **70**, 313–323.

Anand P., Birch R., Foley P., Sincropi D.V. and Peroutka S.J. (1993) Nerve growth factor in injured human peripheral nerve: indications for nerve repair. *J. Neurol. Neurosurg. Psych.* In press.

Anand P., Rudge P., Mathias C.J. *et al.* (1991) New autonomic and sensory neuropathy with loss of adrenergic sympathetic function and sensory neuropeptides. *Lancet* **337**, 1253–1254.

Barros d'Sa, A. (1992) Arterial injury. In Eastcott H.H.G. (ed.) *Arterial Surgery.* Edinburgh, Churchill Livingstone, pp. 355–414.

Barros d'Sa, A. and Moorhead R.J. (1989) Combined arterial and venous intraluminal shunting in major trauma of the lower limb. *Eur. J. Vasc. Surg.* **3**, 577–581.

Beecher H.K. (1956) Relationship of significance of wound to the pain experienced. *J. Am. Med. Ass.* **161**, 1609.

Bigliani L.U., Craig E.V. and Butters K.P. (1991) Fractures of the shoulder. In Rockwood C.A., Green D.P. and Bucholz R.W. (eds) *Fractures in Adults.* 3rd edn. Philadelphia, Lippincott, pp. 871–1020.

Birch R. (1987) The place of microsurgery in orthopaedics. In Catterall A. (ed.) *Recent Advances in Orthopaedics 5.* Edinburgh, Churchill Livingstone, pp. 165–186.

Birch R. (1991) The repair of peripheral nerves. In Bentley G. and Greer R.B. (eds) *Rob & Smith's Operative Surgery, Orthopaedics.* Part I, 4th edn. London, Butterworth Heinemann, pp. 24–38.

Birch R. (1992) Advances in diagnosis and treatment in the closed traction lesion of the supraclavicular brachial plexus. In Catterall A. (ed.) *Recent Advances in Orthopaedics.* Edinburgh, Churchill Livingstone, pp. 65–76.

Birch R. (1993) Peripheral nerve tumours. In Dyke P.J. and Thomas P.K. (eds) *Peripheral Neuropathy*, 3rd edn. Philadelphia, W.B. Saunders, pp. 1623–1640.

Birch R. and St. Clair Strange F.G. (1990) A new type of peripheral nerve lesion. *J. Bone Joint Surg.* **72B**, 312–313.

Birch R. and Raji A.R.M. (1991) Repair of median and ulnar nerves. *J. Bone Joint Surg.* **73B**, 154–157.

Birch R., Dunkerton M., Bonney G. and Jamieson A.M. (1988) Experience with the free vascularised ulnar nerve graft in repair of supraclavicular lesions of the brachial plexus. *Clin. Orthop. Rel. Res.* **237**, 96–104.

Birch R., Bonney G., Dowell J. and Hollingdale J. (1991) Iatrogenic injuries of peripheral nerves. *J. Bone Joint Surg.* **73B**, 280–282.

Birch R., Wilkinson M.C.P., Vijayan K.P. and Gschmeissner S. (1992) Cement burn of the sciatic nerve. *J. Bone Joint Surg.* **74B**, 731–733.

Blom S. and Dahlback L.O. (1970) Nerve injuries in dislocations of the shoulder joint and fractures of the neck of the humerus. *Acta Chir. Scand.* **136**, 461–466.

Bonney G. (1954) The value of axon responses in determining the site of lesion in traction lesions of the brachial plexus. *Brain* **77**, 588–609.

Bonney G. (1959) Prognosis in traction lesions of the brachial plexus. *J. Bone Joint Surg.* **41B**, 4.

Bonney G. (1963) Thrombosis of the femoral artery complicating fracture of the femur. *J. Bone Joint Surg.* **45B**, 344–345.

Bonney G. (1986) Iatrogenic injuries of nerves. *J. Bone Joint Surg.* **68B**, 9–13.

Bonney G. and Gilliatt R.W. (1958) Sensory nerve conduction after traction lesion of the brachial plexus. *Proc. R. Soc. Med.* **51**, 365–367.

Bonney G., Birch R. and Marshall R.W. (1990) An approach to the cervicothoracic spine. *J. Bone Joint Surg.* **72B**, 904–907.

Bruxelle J., Travers V. and Thiebaut J.B. (1988) Occurrence and treatment of pain after brachial plexus injury. *Clin. Orthop. Rel. Res.* **237**, 87–95.

Cajal S. and Ramon Y. (1928) *Degeneration and Regeneration of the Nervous System.* London, Millford.

Cooke C.J., Powell S. and Parsons C. (1988) The diagnosis by computer tomography of brachial plexus lesion following radiotherapy for carcinoma of the breast. *Clin. Rad.* **39**, 602–606.

Cooney W.P. (1991) Chronic pain treatment with direct electrical nerve stimulation. In Gelberman R.H. (ed.) *Operative Nerve Repair and Reconstruction.* Philadelphia, Lippincott, pp. 1551–1562.

Cooper D.E. (1991) Nerve injury associated with patient positioning in the operating room. In Gelberman R.H. (ed.) *Operative
Nerve Repair and Reconstruction.* Philadelphia, Lippincott,
pp. 1231–1242.

Crockard H.A. and Bradford R. (1985) Transoral–transclival
removal of a schwannoma anterior to the craniovertebral junction. *J. Neurosurg.* **62**, 293.

Dale R.H. (1954) Electrical accidents: a discussion with illustrative
cases. *Br. J. Plas. Surg.* 44–66.

Danyou M. (1851) Paralysie du membre supérieur chez le
nouveau–né *Bull. Soc. Chir.* **2**, 148.

Davis E.R. and Bligh A.S. (1966) Myelography in brachial plexus
injury. *Br J. Radiol.* **39**, 362–371.

De Bakey M.E. and Simeone F.A. (1955) Acute battle-incurred
arterial injuries. Surgery in World War II. Vascular surgery.
Medical Department, US Army, Washington, US Government
Printing Office, pp. 60–148.

Denny Brown D.E., Adams R.D., Brenner C. and Docherty M.M.
(1945) The pathology of injury to nerve induced by cold. *J.
Neuropath. Exp. Neurol.* **4**, 305–323.

DeVincenti F.C., Moncreif J.A. and Pruitt E.A. (1969) Electrical
injuries: overview of 65 cases. *J. Trauma* **9**, 497–507.

Dobyns J.H. (1991) Pain dysfunction syndrome. In Gelberman
R.H. (ed.) *Operative Nerve Repair and Reconstruction.*
Philadelphia, Lippincott, pp. 1489–1496.

Ducatman B.S. and Scheithauer B.W. (1983) Post-irradiation
neurofibrosarcoma. *Cancer* **51**, 1028–1033.

Duchenne G.B.A. (1861) *De l'Éléctrisation Localisée et de son
Application à la Pathologie et à la Thérapeutique,* 2nd edn.
Paris, J.B. Baillière, p. 353.

Dyck P.J., Nukada H., Lais C.A. and Karnes J. (1984) Permanent
axotomy. A model of chronic neuronal degeneration preceded
by axonal atrophy, myelin remodelling and degeneration. In
Dyck P.J., Thomas P.K., Lambert E.H. and Bunge R. (eds)
Peripheral Neuropathy, 2nd edn. Philadelphia, W.B. Saunders,
pp. 660–690.

Enneking W.E. (1983) *Musculo-skeletal Tumour Surgery.* New
York, Churchill Livingstone.

Enzinger F.M. and Weiss F.W. (1988) *Soft Tissue Tumours,* 2nd
edn. St. Louis, C.V. Mosby.

Epstein H. (1980) *Traumatic Dislocation of the Hip.* Baltimore,
Williams & Wilkins.

Flaubert M. (1827) Mémoire sur plusieurs cas de luxation dans
lesquels les efforts pur le réduction ont été suivis d'accidents
graves. *Répert. Gén. d'Anat. Physiol. Pathol.* **3**, 55–69.

Fletcher (1981) Amputation of the upper limb. In Wynn-Parry
C.B. (ed.) *Rehabilitation of the Hand,* 4th edn. London,
Butterworth.

Gilbert A. (1989) Indications et résultats de la chirurgie du plexus
brachial dans le paralysie obstétricale. In Alnot J.Y. and Narakas
A.O. (eds) *Les Paralysies du Plexus Brachial.* Monographies du
groupe d'Étude de la Main, No. 15. Paris, Expansion Scientifique
Française, pp. 228–239.

Gilliatt R.W. (1980) Acute compression block. In Sumner A.J.
(ed.) *The Physiology of Peripheral Nerve Disease.* Philadelphia,
W.B. Saunders, pp. 287–315.

Gilliatt R.W., Lequesne P.M., Logue V. and Sumner A.J. (1970)
Wasting of the hand associated with the cervical rib or band. *J.
Neurol. Neurosurg. Psych.* **33**, 615.

Glasby M.A., Carrick M.J. and Hems T.E.J. (1992) Freeze thawed
skeletal muscle autografts used for brachial plexus repair in the
non-human primate. *J. Hand Surg.* **17B**, 526–535.

Goldie B.S. and Coates C.J. (1992) Brachial plexus injury: a
survey of incidence and referral pattern. *J. Hand Surg. (Br.)*
17B, 86–88.

Hallett J. (1981) Entrapment of the median nerve after dislocation
of the elbow. *J. Bone Joint Surg.* **63B**, 408–412.

Hannington-Kiff J.G. (1974) Intravenous regional sympathetic
block with guanethidine. *Lancet* **1**, 1019–1020.

Harkin J.C. and Reid R.J. (1969) Tumours of the peripheral
nervous system. In *Atlas of Tumour Pathology,* 2nd Series,
Classical 3. Washington, Armed Forces Institute of Pathology.

Herndon J.H. and Hess A.V. (1991) Neromas. In Gelberman R.H.
(ed.) *Operative Nerve Repair and Reconstruction.* Philadelphia,
Lippincott, pp. 1525–1540.

Hudson A.R. (1993) Peripheral nerve surgery. In Dyke P.J.
and Thomas P.K. (eds) *Peripheral Neuropathy,* 3rd edn.
Philadelphia, W.B. Saunders, pp. 1674–1690.

Huson S.M., Compston D.A.S., Clark P. and Harper P.S. (1989a)
A genetic study of von Recklinghausen neurofibromatosis in
south-east Wales. Part 1. *J. Med. Gen.* **26**, 704–711.

Huson S.M., Compston D.A.S. and Harper P.S. (1989b) A genetic
study of von Recklinghausen neurofibromatosis in south-east
Wales. Part 2. Guidelines for genetic counselling. *J. Med. Gen.*
26, 712–721.

Iggo A. (1977) Cutaneous and subcutaneous sense organs. *Br.
Med. Bull.* **33**, 97–102.

Iggo A. (1986) Cutaneous sensory mechanisms. *J. Bone Joint
Surg.* **68B**, 19–20.

Kennedy R. (1903) Suture of the brachial plexus in birth paralysis
of the upper extremity. *Br. Med. J.* **1**, 298–301.

Kori S.H., Foley K.M. and Posner J.B. (1981) Brachial plexus
lesions in patients with cancer: 100 cases. *Neurology* **31**,
45–50.

Kwan M.K. and Woo S.L.Y. (1991) Biomechanical properties
of peripheral nerves. In Gelberman R.H. (ed.) *Operative
Nerve Repair and Reconstruction.* Philadelphia, Lippincott,
pp. 47–54.

Leffert R.D. and Seddon H.J. (1965) Infraclavicular brachial
plexus injuries. *J. Bone Joint Surg.* **47B**, 9.

Letournel E. and Judet R. (1981) *Fractures of the Acetabulum.*
Berlin, Springer Verlag.

Lundborg G. (1988) *Nerve Injury and Repair.* Edinburgh,
Churchill Livingstone.

Lundborg G. (1991) Neurotropism, frozen muscle grafts and
other conduits. *J. Hand Surg.* **16B**, 473–476.

Lundborg G. and Rydevik B. (1973) Effects of stretching the tibial
nerve of the rabbit: preliminary study of the intraneural circulation and the barrier function of the perineurium. *J. Bone Joint
Surg.* **55B**, 390–401.

Lusk M.D., Klein D.G. and Garcia C.A. (1987) Tumour of the
brachial plexus. *Neurosurgery* **21**, 439.

Mansfield A.O. (1992) Personal communication. Hazards of TED
stockings. London, Vascular Society Meeting, St. Mary's
Hospital.

Marshall R.W. and de Silva R.D. (1986) Computerized axial
tomography in traction injuries of the brachial plexus. *J. Bone
Joint Surg.* **68B**, 734–738.

Marshall R.W., Williams D.M., Birch R. and Bonney G. (1988)
Operations to restore elbow flexion after brachial plexus injuries.
J. Bone Joint Surg. **70B**, 577–582.

McEwan L.E. (1962) Median and ulnar nerve injuries. *Austral.
NZ J Surg.* **32**, 89–104.

Medical Research Council Special Report Series No. 282 (1954)

Peripheral Nerve Injuries, Seddon H.J. (ed.). London, HMSO.

Medical Research Council, (1976) *Aids to the Examination of the Peripheral Nervous System*. Memorandum No. 45. London, HMSO.

Merle M. and De Medinacelli L. (1991) Applying cell surgery to nerve repair: a preliminary report on the first ten human cases. *J. Hand Surg.* **16B**, 499–504.

Millesi H. (1968) Zum Problem de Überbruckung von Defecten peripherer Nerven. *Wien Med. Wochenschr.* **118**, 182–187.

Millesi H. (1980) Nerve grafts: indications, techniques and prognosis. In *Management of Peripheral Nerve Problems*. Philadelphia, W.B. Saunders, pp. 425–426.

Millesi H., Meissl G. and Berger A. (1972) The interfasicular nerve grafting of the median and ulnar nerves. *J. Bone Joint Surg.* **54A**, 727–750.

Mitchell S.W. (1872) *Injuries of Nerves and their Consequences*. Philadelphia, Lippincott.

Morelli E., Raimondi P.L. and Saporiti E. (1984) Il loro trattamento precoce. In Pipino F. (ed.) *Le Paralisi Ostetriche*. Bologna, Aulo Gaggi, pp. 57–76.

Nagano A., Tsuyama M., Ochiai N., Hara T. and Takahashi M. (1989) Direct nerve crossing with the intercostal nerve to treat avulsion injuries of the brachial plexus. *J. Hand Surg.* **14A**, 980–985.

Narakas A.O. (1987a) Traumatic brachial plexus injuries. In Lamb D.W. (ed.) *The Paralysed Hand*. Edinburgh, Churchill Livingstone, pp. 100–115.

Narakas A.O. (1987b) Obstetrical brachial plexus injuries. In Lamb D.W. (ed.) *The Paralysed Hand*. Edinburgh, Churchill Livingstone, pp. 116–135.

Narakas A.O. and Verdan C. (1969) Les greffes nerveuses. *Z. Unfall Berufskr.* **3**, 137–152.

Narakas A.O., Brunelli G., Clodius L. and Merle M. (1989) In Alnot J.Y. and Narakas A.O. (eds) *Traitement Chirurgical des Plexopathies Postactinique 1989 Les Paralysies du Plexus Brachial*. Monographies du Groupe d'Études de la Main, No. 15. Paris, Expansion Scientifique Française, pp. 240–249.

Nunley J.A. and Gabel G. (1991) The axillary nerve. In Gelberman R.H. (ed.) *Operative Nerve Repair and Reconstruction*. Philadelphia, Lippincott, pp. 437–444.

Ochoa J. and Torebjork E. (1983) Sensations evoked by intraneural microstimulation of single mechano-receptor units innovating the human hand. *J. Physiol.* **342**, 633–654.

Ochoa J., Fowler T.J. and Gilliatt R.W. (1972) Anatomical changes in peripheral nerves compressed by a pneumatic tourniquet. *J. Anat.* **113**, 433–455.

Osborne G.V. (1970) Compression neuritis ulnar nerve at the elbow. *The Hand*, 2–10.

Ottolenghi C.E. (1960) Acute ischaemic syndrome, its treatment, prophylaxis of Volkman's syndrome. *Am. J. Orthop.* **2**, 312–316.

Parry E.W. and Eastcott H.H.G. (1992) Cervical rib and thoracic outlet syndrome. In Eastcott H.H. (ed.) *Arterial Surgery*, 3rd edn. Edinburgh, Churchill Livingstone, pp. 333–354.

Petrucci F.S., Morelli A. and Raimondi P.L. (1982) Axillary nerve injuries: twenty-one cases treated by nerve graft and neurolysis. *J Hand Surg.* **7**, 271–278.

Petry D. and Merle M. (1989) Le réinsertion sociale des blessés atteints de paralysie traumatique du plexus brachial. In Alnot J.Y. and Narakas A.O. (eds) *Le Paralysies du Plexus Brachial*. Monographies du Groupe l'Étude de la Main, No. 15. Paris, Masson, pp. 224–227.

Platt H. (1928) On the peripheral nerve complications of certain fractures. *J. Bone Joint Surg.* **10**, 403.

Platt H. (1973) Obstetrical Paralysis: a vanishing chapter in orthopaedic surgery. *Bull Hosp Joint Dis.* **34**, 4–21.

Rank B.K., Wakefield A.R. and Hueston J.T. (1973) *Surgery of Repair as Applied to Hand Injuries*, 4th edn. Edinburgh, Churchill Livingstone.

Ratcliffe A.H.C. (1984) Vascular and neurological complications. In Ling R.S.M. (ed.) *Complications of Total Hip Replacement* (*Current Problems in Orthopaedics*). Edinburgh, Churchill Livingstone, pp. 18–29.

Riccardi V.M. (1990) Neurofibromatosis. In Kennard C. (ed.) *Recent Advances in Clinical Neurology*, No. 6. Edinburgh, Churchill Livingstone, pp. 187–208.

Rich N.M., Bauch J.H. and Hughes C.W. (1969) Popliteal artery injuries in Vietnam. *Am. J. Surg.* **118**, 53–134.

Richardson P.M. (1991) Neurotrophic factors in regeneration. *Curr. Opin. Neurobiol.* **1**, 401–406.

Rob C.G. and Standeven A. (1958) Arterial occlusion complicating thoracic outlet syndrome. *Br. Med. J.* **2**, 709–712.

Ross A. and Birch R. (1991) Reconstruction of the paralysed shoulder after brachial plexus injuries. In Tubiana R. (ed.) *The Hand*, Vol. 4. Philadelphia, W.B. Saunders.

Rosson J.W. (1988) Closed traction lesions of the brachial plexus: an epidemic among young motorcyclists. *Injury*, **19**, 4–6.

Schmalzreid T.P. and Amstutz H.C. (1991) Nerve injury and total hip arthroplasty. In Gelberman R.H. (ed.) *Operative Nerve Repair and Reconstruction*. Philadelphia, Lippincott, pp. 1245–1254.

Seddon H.J. (1963) Nerve grafting: Fourth Watson-Jones Lecture of the Royal College of Surgeons of England. *J. Bone Joint Surg.* **45B**, 447–461.

Seddon H.J. (1975) *Surgical Disorders of the Peripheral Nerves*, 2nd edn. Edinburgh, Churchill Livingstone.

Sedel L., Alnot J.Y., Raimondi P.L. *et al.* (1989) Les tumeurs de plexus brachial. In Alnot J.Y. and Narakas A. (eds) *Les Paralysies du Plexus Brachiale*. Monographies du Groupe pour l'Étude de la Main, No. 15. Paris, Expansion Scientifique Française.

Sever J.W. (1925) Obstetrical paralysis. Report of eleven hundred cases. *J. Am. Med. Ass.* **85**, 1862–1865.

Sordillo P.P., Helson L., Hajdu S.L. *et al.* Malignant schwannoma, clinical characteristics, survival and response to therapy. *Cancer* **47**, 2503–2509.

Speiss H. (1972) Schädigungen am peripheren Nervensystem durch Ionisierende Strahlen. In *Schriften reihe Neurologie*, Neurology Series, Bd. 10. New York, Springer Verlag.

Stableforth P.G. (1984) Four-part fractures of the neck of the humerus. *J. Bone Joint Surg.* **66B**, 104–108.

St. Clair Strange F.G. (1947) An operation for nerve pedicle grafting preliminary communication. *Br. J. Surg.* **34**, 423–425.

Stirrat A.N., Birch R. and Glasby M.A. (1991) Applications of muscle autograft in peripheral nerve injury. *J. Bone Joint Surg.* **73B** (suppl. 2), 166–167.

Strachan J.C.H. and Ellis B.W. (1971) Vulnerability of the posterior interosseous nerve during radial head resection. *J. Bone Joint Surg.* **53B**, 320.

Sunderland S. (1978) *Nerves and Nerve Injuries*, 2nd edn. Edinburgh, Churchill Livingstone.

Sunderland S. (1991) *Nerve Injuries and Their Repair. A Critical Appraisal*. Edinburgh, Churchill Livingstone.

Symonds C.P. (1927) Cervical rib: Thrombosis of the subclavian artery. Contralateral hemiplegia, probably embolic. *Proc. R. Soc. Med.* **20**, 1244–1245.

Tai M. (1992) Personal communication. Implanted cervical cord stimulators for intractable pain. The West Midlands Experience, Fracture Symposium, Royal National Orthopaedic Hospital, London.

Thomas D.G.T. (1987) Dorsal root entry zone thermocoagulation. *Adv. Tech. Stand. Neurosurg.* **15**, 99–114.

Thomas D.G.T. (1988) Dorsal root entry zone thermocoagulation. In Schmidek H.H. and Sureet W.G. (eds) *Operative Neurosurgical Techniques*, 2nd edn. Philadelphia, W.B. Saunders, pp. 1169–1176.

Thomas P.K. and Holdorff V. (1993) Neuropathy due to physical agents. In Dyke P.J. and Thomas P.K. (eds) *Peripheral Neuropathy*, 3rd edn. Philadelphia, W.B. Saunders, pp. 990–1014.

Thomas P.K. and Ochoa J. (1993) Clinical features and differential diagnosis. In Dyke P.J. and Thomas P.K. (eds) *Peripheral Neuropathy*, 3rd edn. Philadelphia, W.B. Saunders, pp. 749–774.

Tinel J. (1919) Les paresthésies précoces après suture ou greffe nerveuse. *Rev. Neurol.* **26**, 521.

Urich H. (1993) Pathology of tumours of cranial nerves, spinal nerve roots and peripheral nerves. In Dyke P.J. and Thomas P.K. (eds) *Peripheral Neuropathy*, 3rd edn. Philadelphia W.B. Saunders, pp. 1641–1672.

Vautrin C. (1954) Déficit moteur du membre supérieur après radiothérapie cervico-axillaire à dose elévée. *Memoir d'Électro-Radiologie*, 40, Institute du Radium, Universite de Paris.

Wadsworth T.G. (1977) The external compression syndrome of the ulnar nerve at the cubital tunnel. *Clin. Othop. Rel. Res.* **124**, 189.

Wadsworth T.G. (1982) *The Elbow.* Edinburgh, Churchill Livingstone.

Wadsworth T.G., Williams J.R. (1973) Cubital tunnel external compression syndrome. *Br. Med. J.* **1**, 662.

Wilbourn A.J. (1993) Brachial plexus disorders. In Dyke P.J. and Thomas P.K. (eds) *Peripheral Neuropathy*, 3rd edn., Vol. 2. Philadelphia, W.B. Saunders, pp. 911–950.

Wilkins K.E. (1991) Fractures and dislocations of the elbow. In Rockwood C.A., Wilkins K.E. and King R.E. (eds) *Fractures in Children*, 3rd edn. Philadelphia, Lippincott, pp. 509–820.

Wilkinson M.C.P. and Clarke J.A. (1992) Burns to the brachial plexus. *Injury* **23**, 342–343.

Willner C. and Low P.A. (1993) Pharmacological approaches to neuropathic pain. In Dyke P.J. and Thomas P.K. (eds) *Peripheral Neuropathy*, 3rd edn. Philadelphia, W.B. Saunders, pp. 1709–1720.

Wynn-Parry C.B. (1986) Sensation. *J. Bone Joint Surg.* **68B**, 15–19.

Wynn-Parry C.B., Frampton V. and Monteith, A. (1987) Rehabilitation of patients following traction lesions of the brachial plexus. In Terzis, J.K. (ed.) *Microreconstruction of Nerve Injuries*. Philadelphia, W.B. Saunders, pp. 483–495.

Yeoman P.M. (1968) Cervical myelography in traction injuries of the brachial plexus. *J. Bone Joint Surg.* **50B**, 253–260.

Young J.Z. and Medawar P.B. (1940) Fibrin suture of peripheral nerves. *Lancet*, **2**, 126.

Zachary R.B. (1954) *Results of Nerve Suture.* Medical Research Council Special Report Series, No. 282. London, HMSO, pp. 354–388.

Chapter 28

Cysts and Tumours of the Musculoskeletal System

H.B.S. Kemp, J.A.S. Pringle & D.J. Stoker

INTRODUCTION

The occurrence of cysts and benign tumours of bone is extremely rare. Such lesions represent 24% of all tumours of bone (Dahlin and Unni, 1986). Primary malignant bone tumours are also relatively uncommon and yet, nevertheless, they account for a significant proportion of tumours occurring in childhood and adolescence. This is instanced by the study of Kramer *et al.* (1983) among white children up to the age of 14 years in the USA where malignant tumours of bone are the seventh commonest tumour of childhood, an incidence of 6.3 per 1 000 000. After the age of 14, the proportion rises because of the fall in the rate of occurrence of neuroblastoma and Wilms' tumours (Birch *et al.*, 1980). The age and sex incidence of osteosarcoma among white children in the USA shows a preponderance of approximately 9:5 in relation to Ewing's sarcoma with a slight male preponderance which becomes more marked for both tumours in males, particularly in late adolescence. Although the incidence of tumours in the UK is approximately the same as that reported in the USA, in all probability some 20% of all patients are not formally recorded.

There have been numerous studies of adolescent bone tumours to determine the relationship of tumours to skeletal growth (Price, 1955, 1958; Weinfeld and Dudley, 1962). Osteosarcoma of the upper limb usually occurs earlier than tumours of the lower limb, possibly due to the earlier phase of accelerated growth of the humerus in adolescent development. In various studies of limb growth, the distribution of height of children with the two common primary conditions shows a small but significant difference in the height of patients with these tumours over control children (Fraumeni, 1967; Poldenak 1985a,b). Further, the relative risk of these tumours is related to the skeletal growth of the individual, particularly in those above the 97th percentile, especially in

boys during a period of maximal growth acceleration between the ages of 12 and 17 years. Other work has shown a peak incidence for girls from 12 to 14 years as against boys, who peak from 13 to 17 years (Miller, 1976). There is evidence to suggest that there is a higher mortality in boys over the age of 13 years. There is also a definite indication that the incidence of bone sarcoma is directly related to growth rate and bone turnover. There is a racial difference in the occurrence of bone tumours, and the most striking difference is the extreme rarity of Ewing's sarcoma in blacks as against whites regardless of the ethnic background of blacks (Glass and Fraumeni, 1970; Jensen and Drake, 1970; Huvos *et al.*, 1983b). Chinese children have an equally low incidence of Ewing's sarcoma (Li *et al.*, 1980). There is considerable unpublished data concerning ethnic variations in the incidence of tumours in various racial groups and for which there is no logical explanation. Genetics and familial disease have a significant role in governing the manifestation of bone tumours (Aurias *et al.*, 1983; Turc-Carel *et al.*, 1983). Obviously, retinoblastoma treated by irradiation would exhibit a high incidence of post-radiation sarcoma as these are essentially iatrogenic and the incidence has fallen in direct relation to the dose of radiation (Sagerman *et al.*, 1969; Jensen and Miller, 1971; Kitchin, 1976; Francois, 1977; Friend *et al.*, 1986). Patients who have been treated for retinoblastomas, however, and who have survived exhibit a higher incidence of remote sarcoma and carcinoma and irradiation does not necessarily promote this manifestation of tumours. The gene responsible has been localized to the G14 band on the long-arm of chromosome 13 (13G14). Mutations affecting this gene can be inherited or arise somatically (Sparkes *et al.*, 1980; Ward *et al.*, 1984). More recently, Porter *et al.* (1992) have established that a higher proportion of patients with osteosarcoma are from pedigrees that fulfil the strict criteria necessary for the diagnosis of the Li–Fraumeni cancer family syndrome. Bone tumours may arise in relation to other inherited diseases which may affect or involve bones such as adamantinoma in fibrous dysplasia and Ollier's disease (multiple enchondromatosis). It is also recognized in Maffucci's syndrome (Schwartz and Alpert, 1964; Unni and Dahlin, 1979; Goodman *et al.*, 1984). Malignant tumours can and do arise in patients who have previously been treated for other forms of cancer and sarcoma by radiotherapy or by the ingestion of radioactive material (Martland, 1929; Cahan *et al.*, 1948; Strong *et al.*, 1979; Huvos *et al.*, 1985). Irradiation intentionally or accidentally produces bone death and subsequent bone necrosis. However, at the margin of the area of radiation it stimulates an area of intense and active bone repair and it is in this reactive zone at an interval of approximately a median of 6 years that post-radiation sarcoma occurs (Hatcher, 1945; Arlen *et al.*, 1971; Weatherby *et al.*, 1981). Today, the use of radio-therapy has become more sophisticated. In consequence, the area treated is subjected to the use of multi-angle application or progressively-diminishing windows, reducing the risk of creating a hyperactive zone of bone turnover.

The incidence of primary sarcoma of bone falls between the ages of 20 and 40 years and then reputedly rises due to Paget's disease and, as mentioned, post-radiation sarcoma (Price and Goldie, 1969). It has, in consequence, been suggested that sarcoma of bone therefore has its highest incidence between the ages of 60 and 80 years. There is no doubt, however, that sarcoma arising in Paget's disease is a consequence upon the increased turnover of bone that occurs in this condition, but the increase in incidence is relatively small due to this disease (Wick *et al.*, 1981; Greditzer *et al.*, 1983; Haibach *et al.*, 1985) and many workers consider that the major cause of the increase in sarcoma in this age group is in consequence of the extensive use of radiotherapy. Though there are no epidemiological studies to support this observation, it is of interest to note that the incidence of Paget's disease among patients in the older age group referred to the Supra-regional Bone Tumour Centres in the UK is extremely low. The aetiology of Paget's disease remains unknown but current work suggests that it could be the sequel to contracting a slow-acting virus from domestic animals in childhood (O'Driscoll and Anderson, 1985; Gordon *et al.*, 1991). The results of treatment of Paget's sarcoma are singularly disappointing. The survival rate is a median of 8 months and a 2-year survival is no more than 17%.

Although our knowledge of the aetiology of bone tumours is progressively increasing and current research is suggesting that patients with bone tumours have an identifiable chromosomal defect, as with all forms of cancer, multiple factors are probably necessary for the stimulus of oncogenesis, the development of a tumour and subsequent uncontrolled malignant growth.

RADIOLOGICAL DIAGNOSIS

Without the assistance of radiology, to the orthopaedic surgeon a bone tumour essentially is a painful swelling. With the availability of a plain radiograph the elements of a coherent differential diagnosis begin to appear. Other information—clinical, haematological, bio-chemical, etc.—may need to be added, but imaging methods remain, short of biopsy, the most important factors in diagnosis and management.

Despite the introduction of new sophisticated imaging techniques, the plain film remains pre-eminent in the primary diagnostic evaluation of any solitary bone lesion. The radiograph is the best imaging method for the demonstration of the pattern of bony destruction, permeation and the zone of transition, basic internal architecture and periosteal reaction. For the foreseeable future, if one includes a digitalized system, the plain radiograph will remain the main method for radiological diagnosis of musculoskeletal neoplasm. The newer techniques—radionuclide scintigraphy, computed tomography and magnetic resonance imaging—have extended the overall capabilities of radiology. Their value lies more in the staging and management of such tumours, an equally important role. Serious errors in diagnosis most commonly occur when films are inadequate or of poor quality. Constant vigilance is required in control of the radiographic quality to ensure the greatest possible resolution of cortical and trabecular detail, together with the demonstration of soft-tissue shadows. It is a necessary truism to say that the whole of the relevant region must be depicted; so often a misdiagnosis occurs when part of a tumour or even a second lesion lies just off the edge of the radiograph. Equally, as not all regions are depicted adequately on standard views, it is important to discuss the radiological investigation with the interested radiologist at an early stage. Once adequate films are available, diagnosis and further investigation must be achieved through a methodical and analytic radiological approach.

The plain radiograph in diagnosis

Poor radiographs are commonly accepted and used as an excuse to proceed to computed tomography examination, only to provide evidence that competent radiography would have shown. Worse, plain radiography is sometimes bypassed altogether on the false assumption that new technology is better, whereas the new information is different and supplementary.

Under certain limited circumstances, the plain radiograph alone is sufficient to establish the diagnosis of a benign and self-limiting tumour or tumour-like lesion. Examples of such lesions (Fig. 28.1), which often do not require intervention, include simple cartilage-capped exostoses, non-ossifying fibromas, sometimes a simple bone cyst (Fig. 28.2), post-traumatic ossification, fibrous dysplasia or a stress fracture. In the majority of symptomatic bone tumours, however, biopsy is essential in order to reach a definitive diagnosis. The radiologist usually can indicate the site most likely to provide adequate representative material for a histological diagnosis. Often, also, a needle or trephine biopsy performed by the radiologist will be the best means of providing histological material without interfering with future management.

The radiologist does not work in isolation. The diagnosis and management of bone tumours depends on teamwork. The responsibility for the final diagnosis, or indeed, the inability to make a diagnosis, rests with the histopathologist. In many cases, the radiological diagnosis will be confirmed by the pathologist. In others, the radiologist's differential diagnosis will include the primary diagnosis offered by the pathologist, and this will prove acceptable to the radiologist. Occasionally, the diagnosis offered by the pathologist will be unacceptable or even bizarre in the light of the radiological features; the radiologist must then challenge its validity. Such

diagnostic irreconcilability usually stems from examination of a small or unrepresentative biopsy, which can contain necrotic or reactive tissue; indeed, sometimes only the pseudocapsule of the tumour has been sampled. The radiological information, moreover, reflects gross pathological anatomy not otherwise available to the pathologist. Reappraisal of various radiological and pathological features will often result in a working diagnosis for the surgeon.

General principles of radiological diagnosis

Orthodox radiology only provides a two-dimensional image of a three-dimensional structure. The relative absence of contrast between muscle and most tumours makes the plain radiograph almost valueless in the diagnosis of a tumour originating in the soft tissues. With bone, the situation is very different. Its well-defined structure and the contrast produced by the presence of fat within the medulla and around the periosteum and muscle bundles enables the form of any destructive process to be depicted and categorized.

AGE OF THE PATIENT

This is a major consideration in the diagnosis of bone tumours. Many neoplasms show a predominant incidence confined to perhaps two decades and a range of common and acceptable incidence beyond which it is unwise to make the diagnosis unless the features are unmistakable.

Carcinomatous metastases are the most common

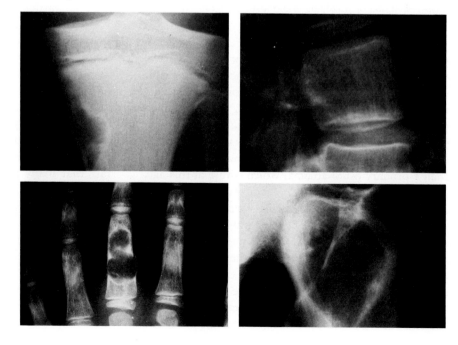

Fig. 28.1 'Leave-me alone' lesions. Certain lesions of bone can be diagnosed as benign or latent conditions not generally requiring biopsy. The examples here are a non-ossifying fibroma (top left), a haemangioma of vertebral body (top right), an enchondroma with pathological fracture (bottom left) and long-standing fibrous dysplasia of the intertrochanteric region (bottom right).

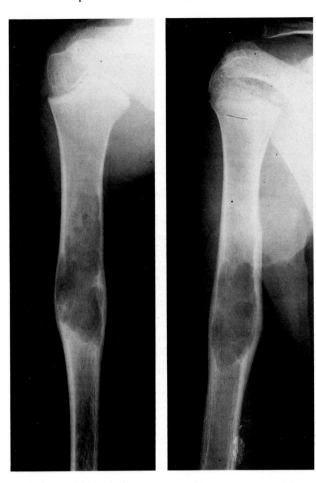

Fig. 28.2 Solitary bone cyst. This lesion normally begins in the proximal shaft of the humerus of a child and is left behind as growth occurs, so that it appears to migrate distally. The proximal shaft of the humerus is the commonest site for this lesion which shows expansion or scalloping of the cortex and a moderately well-defined margin.

malignancies of bone in patients over the age of 50 years. An atypical metastasis will be encountered in this age group more often than even the most radiologically typical primary bone neoplasm. Thus, a sclerotic neoplasm of bone with spiculated periosteal reaction and a soft-tissue mass in a man of 70 years is very much more likely to be a metastasis from carcinoma of the prostate than a primary osteosarcoma, which is rare at this age.

The commoner primary bone neoplasms of childhood — osteosarcoma and Ewing's tumour — are uncommon under the age of 5 years and excessively rare under the age of 2 years. Osteosarcoma is the predominant primary neoplasm of bone in the second decade of life, and Ewing's sarcoma cannot really be diagnosed with any confidence over the age of 30 years. Giant-cell tumour of bone is uncommon in children and the older adult; about 85% of these tumours are found between the ages of 18 and 45 years. The likelihood of a neoplasm being a giant-cell tumour in a patient with unfused epiphyses at the metaphyseal location of the lesion is very low. In an older patient, the radiological appearance suggestive of a giant-cell tumour in a typical subarticular location is more likely to be due to a metastasis. The common primary malignant tumour of bone in the middle-aged or elderly patient is the chondrosarcoma.

LOCATION OF THE TUMOUR

While some tumours can arise almost anywhere in the skeleton, certain predilections exist and have to be taken into account.

Primary malignant neoplasms of bone, with the exception of myeloma, are rare in the vertebral column. Thus, any lesion in the axial skeleton in the middle-aged and elderly should suggest a metastasis from carcinoma, or myelomatosis; the presence of similar lesions should therefore be sought in other parts of the skeleton as each of these disorders tends to produce multiple lesions. The most common tumour metastasizing to bone in the first decade of life is neuroblastoma. Because the red marrow has not disappeared from the appendicular skeleton, such lesions are often widespread. Histioreticuloses such as eosinophilic granuloma (Langerhans cell histiocytosis) and primary histiocytic lymphoma tend also to occur in sites of residual red marrow. In contrast, most primary bone tumours tend to occur in areas of rapid growth, particularly affecting the distal femur, proximal tibia and proximal humerus. Exceptions to this tendency abound, particularly in tumours that present after childhood, and include chordoma with its predilection for involving either end of the spine, chondrosarcoma, predominantly affecting the pelvis and femur and adamantinoma with a peculiar propensity for involvement of the tibial shaft.

Johnson's metabolic field theory states that 'a tumour of a given cell type usually arises in that metabolic field where the homologous normal cells are most active' (Johnson, 1953). This statement is supported by the fact that many primary tumours of bone arise in the metaphysis.

Within the bone, while most neoplasms are centred on the medulla, a parosteal osteosarcoma, as its name indicates, is related to the subperiosteal cortex.

Benign bone tumours also are often associated with characteristic sites. A non-ossified fibroma is usually located subcortically in the diametaphysis of a long bone in the lower limb. A giant-cell tumour almost invariably is subarticular by the time it is clinically and radiologically apparent but sometimes will involve the site of an earlier apophysis (Fig. 28.3). More than 80% of solitary bone cysts occur in the proximal third of the humerus (Fig. 28.2) or the proximal third of the femur. It must be recalled that not all tumour-like appearances are caused by neoplasms. Eosinophilic granuloma may mimic a tumour or infection (Fig. 28.4).

Radiographic demonstration of purely medullary lesions is relatively insensitive as a lesion cannot be identified until 40–50% of the bone mass has been removed. In contrast, even a small area of erosion of cortical bone will become evident on the plain film.

In most cases, the destruction of bone associated with tumours is not a direct effect of the neoplastic cells. It is mediated through resorption by osteoclasts, direct pressure by the tumour mass, by associated hyperaemia or by an alteration in the physiology of the bone (Madewell *et al.*, 1981).

As it enlarges, a neoplasm of bone causes a modification of host bone at its interface with the tumour. This is mediated mainly by the activity of the osteoclasts and

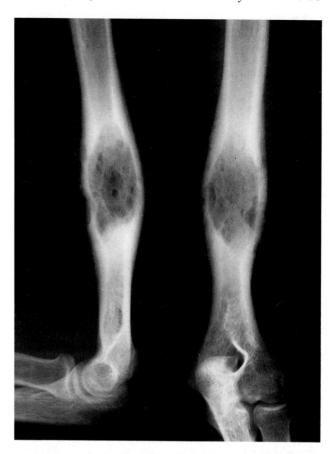

Fig. 28.4 Eosinophilic granuloma. This lesion of unknown aetiology often appears quite aggressive and, in this case, has caused considerable expansion of the bone, mimicking a benign bone tumour. Although the progress is generally benign, biopsy is often required to establish the diagnosis.

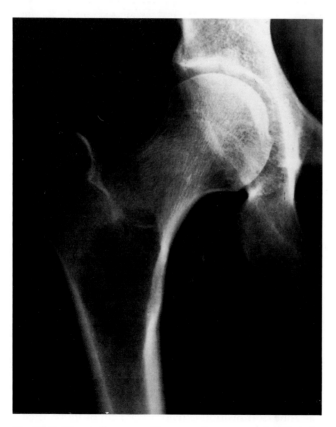

Fig. 28.3 Giant-cell tumour. These tumours commonly affect the ends of bones in young adults and are therefore subarticular in location. The relationship probably owes more to the site of a previous growth plate as apophyses can also be involved. In this woman in her thirties, pathological avulsion of the lesser trochanter has occurred as a result of the tumour.

osteoblasts of the host bone. The patterns produced reflect the rate of growth of the tumour (Lodwick, 1971), thus:

Grade I—geographical pattern (slow growth).
Grade II—moth-eaten pattern (intermediate growth).
Grade III—permeative pattern (rapid growth).

Grade I pattern

There is slow erosion of the cortex with sharp margination; destructive change in the medulla will not produce a geographic appearance unless it also produces sclerosis.

Grade I has been divided further into three subtypes—IA, IB and IC.

Type IA. A geographical lesion with sclerosis of its margin. This exemplifies the typical benign bone lesion such as a solitary bone cyst (Fig. 28.2), quiescent enchondroma, chondromyxoid fibroma, monostotic fibrous dysplasia and Brodie's abscess.

Type IB. A geographical lesion with no sclerosis of its margin. Type IB lesions often appear 'punched-out' (Fig. 28.5). They do have some medullary sclerotic reaction in that it is the minimal sclerosis of the margin that makes them visible, but this is not an obtrusive feature. However, when the cortex is involved to even a small degree, the lesion becomes visible without the need for cortical sclerosis. This radiological appearance is rather more active than in type IA lesions and especially in benign chondroid neoplasms and more slowly growing giant-cell tumours.

Type IC. A geographical lesion with ill-defined margins. This amounts to a locally infiltrative process, short of a Grade II appearance. Neoplasms showing this degree of biological activity include giant-cell tumours (Fig. 28.3), actively growing chondromas, low-grade chondrosarcomas, certain metastases and low-grade osteosarcomas.

Grade III pattern

At its least detectable stage radiologically, this pattern involves partial lysis of the cancellous bone of the medulla. Potential penetration of the cortex must be assumed (Fig. 28.6). When destruction of the cortex first becomes visible it is ill-defined, but nevertheless enables the lesion to be identified radiologically. A more reactive medullary lesion, such as a Brodie's abscess, becomes visible not because of cortical involvement but on account of subtle sclerosis of its medullary margins. This explanation of the difference between geographic and permeating lesions runs counter to that proposed by some authors (Madewell *et al.*, 1981).

Grade II pattern

This pattern lies intermediately between the other two grades and may be difficult to distinguish at times from a coarsely permeating pattern; it probably constitutes the most difficult area of assessment in this classification. It has been suggested that accuracy in grading can be maintained by modifying the categories (Lodwick *et al.*, 1980). In this modification, Grade III can include moth-eaten and/or permeating patterns but with no geographical components; Grade II can include a similar mixture but with geographical components.

Determination of what constitutes one of these patterns necessitates the introduction of the concept of the zone

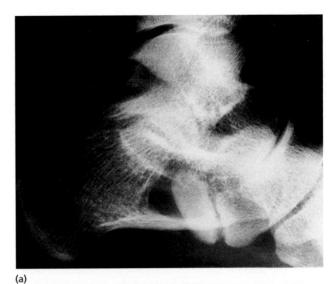

(a)

(b)

Fig. 28.5 Aneurysmal bone cyst. (a) In this moderately well-defined lesion of the calcaneus, the differential diagnosis from the commonly occurring simple cyst in this location may be difficult. On the computed tomography scan (b) the lesion is shown to be quite large with thinning of the cortex and expansion.

of transition between normal and abnormal bone. The radiologist has to decide at what point, at the edge of the tumour, the bone is clearly abnormal and where it is entirely normal. A region will remain where it is not possible to say categorically whether the bone is either normal or abnormal—this is the zone of transition. When the zone measures only a few millimetres, the edge is sharp (geographical); when it is indistinct and the zone of transition extends over 1 cm or more, then a more permeating lesion is present. A moth-eaten lesion essentially is a permeating lesion that is composed of larger, often elliptical or irregular, lytic areas, probably resulting from patchy erosion of the cortex (Fig. 28.4); usually, the zone of transition is less than 1 cm.

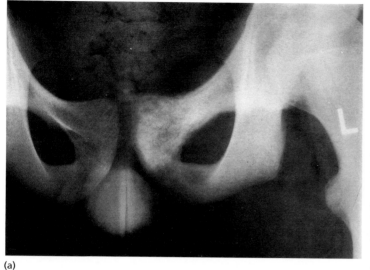

(a)

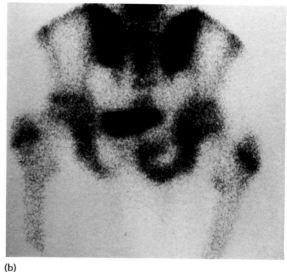

(b)

Fig. 28.6 Ewing's sarcoma. (a) In this 14-year-old boy, a permeating lesion with some reactive bony sclerosis is shown. The cortex is almost certainly breached and a soft tissue extension is suggested above the pubic ramus. (b) Bone scintigraphy shows the extent of the increase in uptake to lie far beyond the region suggested on the plain film. Not all of this activity is necessarily due to tumour as non-malignant reactive vascularity can also produce a similar response.

In addition to the pattern of bony destruction, the reaction of the tissues of the host must also be assessed. Slow growth permits time for the host bone to surround the tumour with reactive new bone. In the medulla this takes the form of an enveloping endosteal sclerosis, while the outer cortex (periosteum) responds by producing a shell of new bone of variable thickness. An increase in the rate of growth subsequently will reduce the thickness of this reactive bone.

Sometimes the margin of the lesion varies in its definition. Although occasionally the radiographic technique can alter the appearance, it cannot make an ill-defined lesion better defined; so it is most probable that the best defined region reflects the true activity of the neoplasm. This must not be accepted if the change is from a relatively slowly extending margin on one side to an overtly aggressive one on another. In this circumstance, the possibility that the lesion has changed its grade of malignancy (dedifferentiation) has to be considered. Thus a chondrosarcoma may dedifferentiate into a fibrosarcoma or malignant fibrous histiocytoma, or a lower grade of osteosarcoma may change to an orthodox and highly malignant variety. Malignant transformation of benign disorders also may occur; chondrosarcomatous transformation may affect an osteochondroma, and Paget's disease or radiation osteitis may be complicated by sarcomatous change.

The most important diagnostic feature in determining malignancy, or at least local aggressive behaviour, of a neoplasm is the presence of extension into the soft tissues. Sometimes the periosteum is visualized by the formation of a thin shell of new bone that demonstrates that the tumour is likely to lie within the bony envelope (Fig. 28.5b). On other occasions, a large, well-defined tumour mass is clearly extra-osseous, and this implies malignancy (Fig. 28.7).

Most initial periosteal reactions are non-specific and linear. Multilaminar reactions indicate a periodicity of the tumoral extension. Such an appearance is classically attributed to Ewing's sarcoma, but it is rare even in the presence of that tumour. The formation of parosteal new bone perpendicular to the cortical margin is usually reactive in nature because such bony spicules follow the lines of the prominent Sharpey's fibres, which bind the periosteum to the cortex until the force elevating it stretches or ruptures them. Although classically associated with osteosarcoma, when the reactive spiculation may be supplemented by the presence of tumoral bone, such a 'sunburst' reaction is by no means confined to that tumour. More delicate perpendicular spicules are to be found in the presence of Ewing's sarcoma, and a sunburst reaction is not uncommon in low-grade chronic cellulitis.

Skeletal scintigraphy

This method of imaging is highly sensitive but non-specific, and hence is rarely diagnostic in the field of

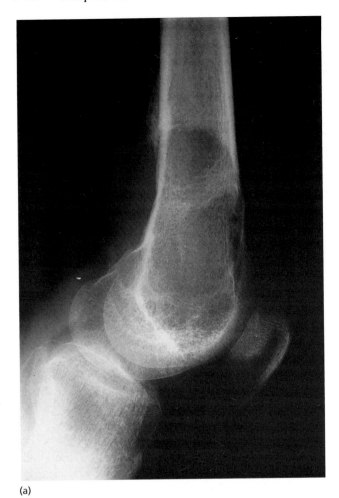

(a)

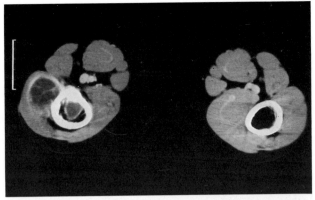

(b)

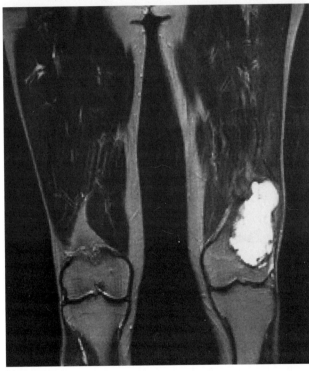

(c)

bone tumours. Probably its most valuable function is in the demonstration or exclusion of multiple metastatic lesions. Lytic metastases may not be visible on a plain film for several months after their demonstration on a bone scan. It is therefore always important to confirm that a lesion in a middle-aged patient is solitary as, if multiple lesions are evident at scintigraphy, the chances of a primary neoplasm being present diminish markedly. Similarly, certain malignant tumours have a propensity for producing 'skip' lesions in a more proximal location.

In respect of solitary bone tumours, scintigraphy can provide some element of differential diagnosis. Uptake of the phosphorus−technetium complex relates to both the vascular supply and the metabolic activity of the bony lesion. Demonstration of such activity is of great value where the lesion is small or not clearly identifiable on the radiograph (Fig. 28.8). Many highly malignant tumours such as osteosarcoma produce scans with intense activity and irregular outlines (Murray, 1980), often overestimating the extent of the tumoral involvement as the surrounding reactive tissues also take up the

Fig. 28.7 Osteosarcoma. A destructive lesion affects the distal shaft of the femur in this young adult. On the plain film (a) there is very little evidence of the formation of tumour bone which might establish the diagnosis radiologically. The cortex has almost certainly been breached with a posterior tumour extension with reactive periosteal triangles at the margins. Anteriorly, the cortex is thinned by permeation. (b) On the computed tomography scan in this patient, not only is the medullary involvement by the tumour demonstrated but a clear indication of the formation of periosteal new bone and soft-tissue extension of the lesion is apparent. Within the soft-tissue extension of lower attenuation, mineralization is shown, suggesting the diagnosis. (c) Magnetic resonance imaging. On this sequence the extremely bright intensity of the signal of the tumour demarcates it sharply from the bone and surrounding soft tissue. The soft-tissue extension is well shown and would be more clearly defined by reference to the adjoining slices.

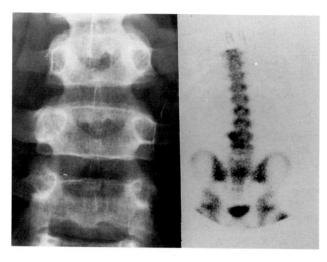

Fig. 28.8 Osteoid osteoma of the right side of a lumbar vertebra. The pedicle on the right is enlarged and sclerotic, indicating the activity of the tumour and the bony overgrowth in response. The activity is confirmed by the radionuclide bone scan, which shows increased uptake in the region of the pedicle.

radionuclide. The marrow permeation of a Ewing's sarcoma often leads to a lesser activity but may show activity along the length of the bone far beyond any abnormality detected on the radiograph (Fig. 28.6b).

Variation in the uptake of a tumour may reflect its vascular pattern with peripheral uptake in a tumour, such as an aneurysmal bone cyst (Gunterberg *et al.*, 1977); other tumours may outstrip their blood supply and undergo central necrosis or haemorrhage, reflected in reduced central photon activity on a bone scan.

Nevertheless, in terms of staging, radionuclide scans do tend to indicate the extent of the combined neoplastic defect of bone and the surrounding reactive tissue changes and oedema.

Arteriography (see also Chapter 30.2)

As it is an invasive procedure, the value of arteriography in the diagnosis and management of bone tumours has always been in dispute. Its value has been stressed in the past (Voegeli and Uehlinger, 1976). In the opinion of one of the authors (D.J.S.) it has never had an important or necessary place in the diagnosis of such lesions. Its value in the delineation of a soft-tissue extension has been removed by the introduction of computed tomography and even more so by magnetic resonance imaging, the value of both being extended by contrast media. None of these methods is, however, infallible, as magnetic resonance imaging produces false positives caused by peritumoral oedema involving the region of the main vessels.

In two areas, arteriography still seems to have a place. Firstly, it remains valuable in the demonstration of tumours of vascular origin, benign or malignant. Secondly, in the embolization of large vascularized tumours that might otherwise be unsuitable for more than palliative therapy, prior diagnostic angiography is essential. Together, these applications relate to only a small percentage of tumours seen by orthopaedic surgeons.

STAGING OF TUMOURS

Staging—defining the extent of the lesion

One of the radiological differences between the extension of a malignant neoplasm and an infection from the bone into the soft tissues is that the margin of the malignant tumour is defined better than the infective mass. Differentiation of such changes requires good soft-tissue radiography; nevertheless, the observation is extremely valuable. Greater accuracy in staging can be obtained by adding the information obtained from the more recently available imaging modalities—computed tomography (CT) and magnetic resonance imaging (MRI). The objective of staging is the prediction of the degree of risk of local recurrence or distant metastasis and the implication of this on surgical and chemotherapeutic management. The system for the staging of musculoskeletal sarcomas adopted by the Musculoskeletal Tumor Society (Enneking *et al.*, 1980) and subsequently by the American Joint Committee for Cancer Staging and End Results Reporting (Enneking, 1986) depends greatly upon radiological information. Not only does staging specifically relate to the radiographic grade, radionuclide scintigraphy, angiography and CT, but many so-called clinical elements of grading, site and distant spread are based primarily on radiological information.

Computed tomography (see also Chapter 30.1)

Although it does not play a major part in the primary radiological diagnosis, CT is superior to the plain radiograph in a number of areas of interest. It is of most use in:

1 Determining the intramedullary extension of the tumour (Fig. 28.7b) on serial transverse axial slices.
2 Determining the presence and extent of extraosseous extension of the neoplasm (Fig. 28.7b).
3 Demonstrating the relationship between the tumour and important adjoining structures, in particular the involvement by tumour of major vessels perhaps even

following their demonstration by intravascular injection of contrast medium.

4 Demonstrating certain characteristics of the tumour, such as mineralization of the matrix, which may be important in the diagnosis (Fig. 28.7b).

5 Contributing to staging of the disease by demonstrating certain local anatomical relationships and the presence or absence of pulmonary or nodal metastases.

In terms of superficial lesions, it is usually possible to determine if a parosteal lesion originating in soft tissue is involving the cortex itself or simply stimulating periosteal reaction.

CT was the first imaging technique to assess, with any degree of accuracy, the extent of medullary involvement by a primary neoplasm of bone (Fig. 28.5b). Measurement of the attenuation value within a representative volume of medulla is more accurate than a visual impression and can be compared with the result either of the normal medulla, away from the tumour site, or with the other limb. Similarly, when a tumour is essentially fatty in nature, for example on the plain film, CT can almost always distinguish a benign lipoma with a value equivalent to fat (about −95 Hounsfield units (HU)) from a liposarcoma with a value usually between −70 and +50 Hu (Halldorsdottir *et al.*, 1982).

The radiological grading already referred to on examination of the plain radiograph has its counterpart in the CT scan, although this is probably a less reliable and vastly more expensive method of obtaining such information. Thus, CT features signifying geographical and permeating involvement of bone can be shown (Brown *et al.*, 1986). CT has less value in showing local recurrences following the use of metallic prostheses, as artefacts reduce the quality and accuracy of the examination.

As mentioned above, the most sensitive screening method of detecting metastases, or early involvement of bone by a primary neoplasm, is radionuclide scintigraphy. Radiographic skeletal surveys are much less sensitive and entail greater radiation dose to the patient. A unified approach, logically combining the two imaging modalities, will reduce the number of inappropriate examinations (Mall *et al.*, 1976). In the small but significant number of patients with positive scintigraphic examination and negative radiographs, CT may play an important role. Providing radiographs of good quality are studied to exclude the presence of abnormalities which are clearly non-neoplastic, asymmetry in medullary density may indicate metastatic involvement due to cellular replacement of marrow fat. It has been suggested that a difference of medullary CT number of greater than 20 Hu between limbs is abnormal (Helms *et al.*, 1981).

CT is superior to conventional tomography in the demonstration of pulmonary metastases. In 1978, Muhm *et al.* demonstrated that in 35% of their patients more nodules were revealed by CT. In 15.6% of this group, CT revealed nodules where none was shown by whole-lung tomography; in the remainder, CT simply identified more pulmonary nodules in each case. CT has evolved technically since that date and, in a series of 32 patients with osteosarcoma (Vanel *et al.*, 1984), lung tomography demonstrated only half the metastases shown by a third generation CT scanner. It is probable that the main benefit of CT lies in its identification of subpleural nodules, which accounted for about half the metastases.

Magnetic resonance imaging (MRI)
(see also Chapter 30.1)

MRI offers a number of advantages that can be used in the evaluation of musculoskeletal tumours. It involves no ionizing radiation, the resolution of contrast is excellent and continues to improve, and the ability to scan directly in the coronal and sagittal planes offers advantages for staging and the planning of treatment.

The total magnetic resonance image depends on a number of factors, including proton density, relaxation times (T1 and T2) and flow within vessels. Manipulation of the pulse sequences can alter the relative contribution of each of these elements, although the relative intensities of most musculoskeletal tissues are constant through most combinations of repitition time (TR) and echo delay time (TE) in common clinical usage.

Heavily calcified structures, such as cortical bone, contain only a small number of protons. Hence magnetic resonance produces a poor signal from cortical bone and has little value in the direct evaluation of its structure. As a consequence, MRI has little place in the initial diagnosis of a neoplasm of bone. Fortunately, however, fat in the bone marrow and the extra-osseous soft tissues produces a high signal intensity with most combinations; hence the cortical bone is identified by default, lying between the marrow and the periosseous fat. Air, ligaments, tendon and fibrocartilage also show a very low signal intensity, while muscle and hyaline cartilage show an intermediate intensity of signal. A significantly different behaviour is shown by fluid-filled structures, oedematous tissue, neoplasia and haematoma. All of these tend to produce elevated values of T1 and T2 and hence show low signal intensity on T1-weighted sequences and higher intensity on T2-weighted sequences. It should be noted that, just as in CT, a haematoma changes its signal with age. The T1 and T2 constants tend to decrease progressively so that they show high intensity with T2-weighted sequences as well as T1-weighted sequences after a number of days (Swensen *et al.*, 1985).

MRI cannot, of itself, accurately differentiate between a malignant and a benign neoplasm of bone, although there is some evidence to support this in the case of soft-tissue tumours. Of more importance is the ability provided for specific demonstration of pathological changes in the bone marrow and the extra-osseous tissues. It is into these regions that the spread of neoplasms occurs, and MRI can therefore supply information about the extent and staging of either a tumour arising in bone or of metastatic spread to bone. MRI is now the most sensitive single method of assessing medullary involvement by tumour (Zimmer *et al.*, 1985). It is also able to demonstrate penetration of cortical bone and involvement of an articular surface; hence it is the most valuable imaging method for staging of musculoskeletal neoplasms (Fig. 28.7c). Evidence that the use of short-time inversion recovery (STIR) sequences make the extent of the lesion more conspicuous (Golfieri *et al.*, 1989).

Early expectations that MRI would be able to identify specific tumour matrix and thus predict the histology have not been realized, except in the case of fluid-filled structures and possibly lipomas. Lipomas can be differentiated from liposarcomas, as with CT (Dooms *et al.*, 1985). The content of a lipoma is normal fat, so that with spin-echo imaging a high-intensity image is shown that is maintained at most pulse sequences. Brightness of this degree is, however, not confined to fat, and difficulty may initially be experienced in distinguishing the signal from a lipoma from that of a soft-tissue haematoma (Sundaram *et al.*, 1987). Fluid-filled structures appear of relatively low intensity on a T1-weighted sequence and brighten considerably when the sequence is more T2-weighted. The future use of intravenous contrast agents in MRI promises to improve the ability to recognize various types of neoplastic tissue.

Both CT and MRI can demonstrate the presence of extra-osseous soft-tissue extension (Aisen *et al.*, 1986). When the soft-tissue encroachment is bounded by a thin egg-shell of residual bone, and hence may be merely an aggressive benign lesion such as an aneurysmal bone cyst contained by the periosteum, MRI will often not detect the bony rim of the lesion. In this specific circumstance, CT may offer an advantage over both plain radiography and MRI. In other circumstances, the evidence indicates that MRI is superior to CT in differentiating tumour from the adjoining muscle (Aisen *et al.*, 1986; Bohndorf *et al.*, 1986). T2-weighted images are most valuable in the definition of extra-osseous

tumour from peritumoral oedema and surrounding normal tissue. However, it must be stated that, in high-grade malignant tumours, differentiation of neoplastic tissue from peripheral oedema is not always possible (Bohndorf *et al.*, 1986). Improved resolution over CT is particularly evident in coronal and sagittal MRI scans, which are vastly superior to the reformatted images obtained with CT. MRI produces superior images, particularly in the extremities, where the presence of thick cortical bone may result in significant CT streak artefacts (Richardson *et al.*, 1986). Prosthetic implants or metallic clips may produce local field defects with MRI, but these interfere with the scan to a much lesser degree than do the severe artefacts of CT.

Present evidence indicates that MRI is more valuable than CT in the pre-operative assessment of musculoskeletal neoplasms. It is, moreover, important to reflect that in terms of its potential development and exploitation, MRI technology is at a relatively primitive stage.

MRI is likely to offer considerable advantages in the assessment of response to treatment with radiotherapy and chemotherapy. Successful response to treatment is shown by reduction in extra-osseous tumoral mass and perhaps reduction in the intensity of the previous MRI signal (Cohen *et al.*, 1984), especially in T2-weighted sequences (Holscher *et al.*, 1990). The precise cause for the latter is not yet clear, but is likely to be multifactorial.

THE PLACE OF NEEDLE BIOPSY IN THE DIAGNOSIS OF BONE TUMOURS

In the investigation of tumours of the musculoskeletal system, the diagnosis ultimately depends upon the histological examination of a representative sample of lesional tissue; biopsy is therefore the most crucial procedure in the diagnosis of many musculoskeletal neoplasms. Biopsy must be an elective procedure, planned as part of the investigative process in which all members of the team—the surgeon, radiologist and pathologist—have a role to play. Initially, the radiologist may be able to identify a non-neoplastic lesion, which does not require biopsy. Such lesions include traumatic lesions such as stress fractures and myositis ossificans, infection, metabolic and degenerative conditions as well as tumour-like disorders such as fibrous dysplasia. If a true neoplasm cannot be excluded, biopsy is mandatory. In the older patient, a radionuclide bone scan will be required to confirm or exclude multiple metastases, not only for diagnostic purposes, but because a choice of site for biopsy may be provided.

Open biopsy enables the surgeon to obtain a large amount of tissue, which is likely therefore to be representative, but is accompanied by a considerable complication rate. Problems relating to subsequent management of the patient as a consequence of inappropriate technique occur in 20% of cases; infection occurs in an additional 20%. The performance of open biopsy adversely affects prognosis and successful limb salvage in a further group of patients (Mankin *et al.*, 1982).

Although the problems of needle biopsy of bone are similar, they are of much lesser magnitude, with a reported complication of only 0.2% even in spinal cases (Moore *et al.*, 1979). Despite this advantage, considerable controversy still persists over the use of needle techniques for the biopsy of musculoskeletal lesions. In the authors' unit, it is the policy to obtain tissue whenever possible by a percutaneous method (Stoker *et al.*, 1991). Percutaneous biopsy has a particular attraction in inaccessible sites, such as the spine. In a personal series of 135 vertebral biopsies (Stoker and Kissin, 1985), tissue adequate for diagnosis was obtained in 93.4% of patients, with complications, all of a minor nature, in only three patients. These biopsies were undertaken under fluoroscopic control; CT guidance is often unnecessary but in certain situations is invaluable for localization of the tumour. Ultrasonographic guidance is only of real value when a large soft-tissue extension or a cortical window to the tumour is present.

Most percutaneous biopsies can be undertaken under local anaesthesia with sedation by intravenous benzodiazepines; an overnight stay in hospital is rarely required on the basis of the biopsy alone. In cases of thoracic vertebral biopsy, it may be considered advisable to obtain a chest radiograph within the first 12–24 hours, although, in the author's series, no single pneumothorax was produced.

In lesions of flat bones, such as the pelvis, it is advisable to obtain a CT scan to define the anatomy, even if biopsy is not to be CT-directed; such information is useful in locating any soft-tissue extension and in defining a 'window' in the cortex made by the neoplasm.

Operative treatment is almost always affected by biopsy, certainly in converting an intracompartmental lesion into an extracompartmental one, but the effect of the planned needle biopsy is less. The track of the needle can be excised completely at the definitive operation and the biopsy scar will not affect the definitive surgical procedure when, as is preferable, the biopsy is performed at the referral centre.

Needle or trephine biopsy therefore offers advantages to the surgeon and to the patient. To the histopathologist, however, at first sight, it offers little but tribulation. Instead of a large amount of tissue from an incisional biopsy, only small cores of tissue are provided. A trephine with an inside core of ⩾2 mm has been shown to minimize histological distortion (Fyfe *et al.*, 1983), while the larger the diameter of the trephine, the greater the complications. The Jamshidi needle (Jamshidi and Swaim, 1971) is favoured for routine use; its non-serrated cutting edge causes minimal damage to surrounding tissues, including neurovascular structures. The needle used has an external diameter of 3 mm and as a consequence of its tapered tip being smaller than its barrel diameter, it causes little or no crush artefact. The histopathologist receives the whole specimen apart from material sent for culture. Fresh imprint preparations are made on microscope slides by the operator; these can be stained immediately on receipt, so that a working diagnosis may be possible prior to the decalcification of the main specimen, which is preserved in formol–saline. In addition, the imprint preparations are available for the pathologist to undertake immunohistochemical staining techniques for more accurate identification of the pathological process; such procedures replace the frozen section.

Solitary cysts of bone do not require biopsy as such. Puncture by two needles under fluoroscopic control permits the fluid to be flushed out and contrast medium injected to confirm the nature of the lesion. It is general practice to encourage healing by then making an intralesional injection of corticosteroid.

PATHOLOGY — THE CLASSIFICATION OF BONE TUMOURS

With the introduction of new techniques, the histopathologist plays an increasingly important role in the management of primary bone tumours. Frozen-tissue sections are now rarely used to establish a diagnosis as they are difficult to prepare and interpret and, at times, they can be grossly misleading. The use of touch imprints can often confirm or even establish a diagnosis. They are made by obtaining a core biopsy with a Jamshidi or Trucut needle or a small quantity of tumour obtained at open biopsy is divided with a scalpel to produce a fresh surface. Excess blood is carefully removed with a clean dry swab and the material is then placed on a clean, dry glass slide, and it is then carefully lifted off. This technique is continued repeatedly to form a circular group of imprints on each slide. Approximately six contacts should be made with the central area of each slide, which is then air-dried. Preferably three of four slides should be prepared in this way. Subsequently, the slides may be stored or examined immediately. While one slide is examined using conventional stains, the remainder are usually reserved for enzyme, histochemical and immunochemical examination. This technique can frequently give an accurate diagnosis, particularly where the histopathologist is able to consider the clinical findings with the surgeon and review the radiological investigations with a radiologist. When it is not possible to give an immediate diagnosis based on an imprint, biopsy material for accurate assessment requires careful fixation and equally careful decalcification if a satisfactory histological assessment is to be made. It is for this reason that patients with a suspected bone lesion should preferably be referred to a centre specializing in the management of bone tumours so that the histological material is not only correctly processed but can be examined by all the modern histological techniques that are available.

Bone is comprised of specialized connective tissue that has the ability to evolve into different matrices, namely osteoid, bone, cartilage and collagen. Tumours arising in bone are traditionally classified according to their pattern of differentiation. Within any one group of lesions there is a variation in manifestation from the benign to the overtly malignant. Primary tumours may arise in bone but which are not peculiar to bone in that they are derived from supporting tissues and, as such, may have a vascular, neurological or adipose origin. Myeloma and lymphoma may be confined to bone when they originally present. A small number of tumours arise from cell rests. Further, there is one group of bone tumours, the malignant round-cell tumours, which includes Ewing's sarcoma, which were until recently of unknown histogenesis.

Tumours arising from osteoblastic cells (Table 28.1)

OSTEOID OSTEOMA AND BENIGN OSTEOBLASTOMA

Histologically indistinguishable, these two are quite dissimilar clinically and radiologically and in their gross pathological presentation, which is quite disparate (Schajowicz and Lemos, 1970). Occurring generally in childhood and young adults, they consist of fine trabeculae of osteoid in a highly vascular matrix of osteoblasts and osteoclasts. Traditionally, osteoid osteomas measure less than 1 cm (Byers, 1968) and, unlike the benign osteoblastoma, are surrounded by a dense matrix of woven bone. Very occasionally, osteoblastoma can be locally aggressive (Jackson, 1978), particularly when they are not adequately excised, and they may occasionally undergo malignant transformation and metastasize (Schajowicz and Lemos, 1976; Merryweather *et al.*, 1980).

OSTEOSARCOMA

Osteosarcoma are the commonest primary malignant bone tumours arising in the metaphysis of long bones in juxtaposition to the diaphyseal growth plate. The tumours occur most frequently in those regions of long bones exhibiting the maximum growth potential. Thus, in order of frequency they affect the distal femur, the proximal tibia, the proximal femur and the proximal humerus, though rarely they can occur in relation to any growth plate. Arising in medullary tissue, the tumour permeates and destroys surrounding cortical bone. The periosteum acts as a barrier to the expanding tumour. However, it is elevated by the distending mass and osteoid is laid down at right angles to the cortex in relation to the subperiosteal blood vessels and Sharpey's fibres forming the characteristic sunray spicules, while at the extremity of the tumour a margin of pathological callus forms the so-called Codman's triangle. When ultimately the tumour ruptures through the periosteum, tumour growth is unrestricted and, in consequence, the

Table 28.1 Bone-forming tumours

| Benign | Intermediate | Malignant | |
		Low-grade	High-grade
Osteoma*	Aggressive osteoblastoma*	Low-grade central osteosarcoma*	High-grade central osteosarcoma
Parosteal osteoma*		Osteoblastoma-like osteosarcoma*	High-grade juxtacortical osteosarcoma*
Osteoid osteoma		Parosteal osteosarcoma*	Multicentric osteosarcoma*
Benign osteoblastoma		Periosteal osteosarcoma*	Histological subtypes of osteosarcoma
			common mixed
			chondroblastic
			fibroblastic
			osteoblastic
			osteoclast-rich
			telangiectatic
			small cell

* Rare.

pattern of tumour bone formation becomes totally irregular. Although most osteosarcomas have a classical radiological appearance, on occasion the picture is so atypical that the definitive diagnosis is entirely dependent on the histological findings. Although it was originally believed that it was necessary to demonstrate the presence of osteoid or bone formation by the tumour cells in order to confirm the diagnosis, it is now accepted that specific staining for alkaline phosphatase, demonstrating its presence in tumour cells, is diagnostically conclusive (Sanerkin, 1980). Most high-grade osteosarcomas show a mixed histological pattern, though occasionally they present a dominant cellular picture (see Table 28.1).

PAROSTEAL OSTEOSARCOMA

This rare tumour (Unni *et al.*, 1976a), probably representing no more than 2% of all osteosarcomas, has a peak occurrence in the third and fourth decade. Occurring, as they do, well beyond the florid growth of youth, their growth is slow and organized, and they are often misdiagnosed clinically in the initial stage as a myositis ossificans or even osteochondroma. Accurate histological diagnosis is essential in order to plan adequate wide surgical resection (Kavanagh *et al.*, 1990) and, on occasion, to consider the role of chemotherapy in management. Unless this is done, then like other slow-growing tumours, these lesions have a singular tendency to recur. The commonest site for these tumours is the distal femur in the popliteal fossa. The characteristic histological feature of these tumours is a collagenous spindle-celled stroma interspersed with well-defined trabecular bone formation. The absence of osteoblasts on the bone surface differentiates them from reactive callus formation and other lesions such as myositis ossificans. At a late stage in the elaboration of these tumours, they may permeate the underlying cortex, encroaching on the medullary cavity, and it is at this phase that pulmonary metastases may occur. Further, at this advanced state of development these tumours may differentiate into high-grade sarcomas (Wold *et al.*, 1984). When this takes place, then the subsequent management is the same as that instigated in the treatment of osteosarcomas.

PERIOSTEAL OSTEOSARCOMA

This is an even rarer tumour (Unni *et al.*, 1976b) that has a predilection for the proximal tibia, occurring in the young to the middle-aged. Matching the radiological appearance histologically, this lesion is predominantly a chondroid tumour. The peripheral zone contains cells of a high-grade pleomorphic tumour adjacent to thin-walled vascular spaces and scattered areas of lace-like osteoid. Imprints are positive for intracellular alkaline phosphatase. Establishing the histological differentiation is important in planning treatment as these tumours are particularly sensitive to chemotherapy, showing a marked response in terms of mineralization and trabecular maturation, thus enhancing the indications for conservative management.

Tumours arising from chondroblastic cells (Table 28.2)

In particular, in assessing such tumours, it is essential to be aware of the patient's age, the site of the lesion and, more importantly, whether the lesion is symptomatic. Though possibly of lesser significance is whether there is overall radiological evidence of active expansion of the lesion. For instance, a lesion in a child, such as an enchondroma, even though it is showing some cellular activity, could be safely regarded as benign on the basis of cartilage growth; in an adult, this would justifiably warrant a diagnosis of a malignant chondrosarcoma if it was demonstrating a similar histological pattern of behaviour.

CHONDROMA (ENCHONDROMA, OLLIER'S DISEASE)

Enchondroma in the growing skeleton may be single or multiple. They are relatively cellular and evidence of comparative growth is seen in relation to the number of binucleate cells that are present. In Ollier's disease, the appearance may be of concern to the pathologist, particularly as these lesions may continue to grow after skeletal maturation. It is the responsibility of the clinician to monitor such patients critically as a small percentage do become malignant. Fortunately, these patients do not exhibit familial disease.

OSTEOCHONDROMA (ECCHONDROMA, DIAPHYSEAL ACLASIA)

Pedunculated or sessile, these lesions communicate with the underlying medullary cavity; they constitute areas of discongruate aberrant development of the diaphyseal growth plate. Consisting of both bone and cartilage, it is the cartilage cap which predominates. Clinically, whereas a smooth cartilage cap is usually indicative of a benign lesion, the presence of a soft friable 'cauliflower-like' covering is generally associated with a potential risk of recurrence and also of subsequent malignant change.

Table 28.2 Cartilage tumours

Benign	Intermediate	Malignant
Enchondroma (chondroma) solitary or multiple Osteochondroma (cartilage capped exostosis) solitary or multiple Chondromyxoid fibroma Benign chondroblastoma	A group of cartilage tumours with evidence of active growth after skeletal maturity is reached Locally-recurring non-metastasizing	Chondrosarcoma, Grades I, II and III (sometimes subdivided into primary and secondary chondrosarcomas, the latter arising in a pre-existing benign lesion) Clear-cell chondrosarcoma Mesenchymal chondrosarcoma Dedifferentiated chondrosarcoma

CHONDROMYXOID FIBROMA

These are extremely rare tumours affecting adolescents and young adults. The characteristic radiological appearance is of a lesion that approaches but never embraces the articular surface of the tibia or humerus with the propinquity of the giant-cell tumour. Histologically, it consists of pseudolobules of myxoid chondroid tissue, the areas between the lobules consisting of highly vascular fibroblastic tissue. The presence of numerous osteoclasts may be confusing to the inexperienced pathologist. Further, many cells may appear pleomorphic and inexperience may lead the pathologist to misdiagnose myxoid chondrosarcoma as chondromyxoid fibroma, leading to inadequate surgical clearance and subsequent tumour recurrence.

BENIGN CHONDROBLASTOMA

This tumour invariably arises in relation to the diaphyseal growth plate of the immature skeleton and only rarely in relationship to the growth plate of the epiphysis. Occasionally, the differentiation between giant-cell tumours and chondroblastomas may prove difficult. However, the presence of islands of chondroid differentiation, the uniformly rounded appearance of the mononuclear cells and the occasional presence of delicate pericellular calcification ('chicken wire' calcification) are important features in establishing the diagnosis of chondroblastoma. Although local recurrences may occur following incomplete removal, it is remarkable that in such difficult surgically-approachable sites the recurrence rate is not considerably higher.

CHONDROSARCOMAS

These tumours are invariably the slowest-growing tumours that occur as primary malignant bone tumours. They are, therefore, underestimated not only by the surgeon but also by the pathologist. They are not sensitive to chemotherapy or radiotherapy. If they are not treated on the first occasion by radical surgical clearance then, if they recur, almost invariably each successive recurrence shows an increase in the histological stage of malignancy. Like their counterpart in tumours of osteoblastic origin, the parosteal osteosarcoma, the other slow-growing tumour, unless their initial extirpation is carefully planned local recurrence and ultimate metastatic spread results in the death of the patient. Unfortunately chondrosarcomas are all too frequently referred to a supraregional centre after inadequate resection, penetration of the periosteum or pathological fracture has taken place. Chondrosarcoma of the pelvis and axial skeleton, in general, have a poor prognosis, not because they tend to have an initially higher grade of malignancy, but because they present later clinically and adequate resection is technically more difficult.

The histological grade of these particular tumours is closely related to the prognosis. *Grade I chondrosarcomas* are similar in appearance to benign cartilage, though occasional binucleate forms are present, confirming active growth. If biopsy material shows the permeation of intertrabecular spaces, this is sufficient to regard the lesion as malignant. *Grade II chondrosarcomas*, in addition to being softer and more friable, exhibit a more myxoid histological appearance with a more pleomorphic cellular pattern while the matrix is less defined. *Grade III chondrosarcomas* may consist of gelatinous pools of matrix, areas of necrosis and little solid tumour tissue. Histologically, there are extensive areas of mucoid material, degeneration and necrosis. Further, there is markedly increased cellularity, cellular atypia, bipolar forms and mitoses.

Dedifferentiated chondrosarcoma

The term 'dedifferentiated chondrosarcoma' refers to the coexistence of Grade I chondrosarcoma with a high-grade component usually of the malignant fibrous histiocytoma type, though occasionally it may be an osteosarcoma. This is seen in 10% of cases (Dahlin and Beabout, 1971; McFarland *et al.*, 1977). In addition, inadequately treated low-grade chondrosarcomas which recur locally repeatedly over a period of time due to inadequate resection gradually become higher in grade and may ultimately dedifferentiate.

Clear-cell chondrosarcoma

This rare tumour (Unni *et al.*, 1976b) tends to occur in the proximal humerus. There is expansion of the bone with endosteal erosion and thinning of the cortex. Histologically, there is a mixture of strikingly clear cells, delicate benign trabecular bone, osteoclast giant cells and a variable amount of chondroid matrix. The clear cell areas may be difficult to distinguish from metastatic clear-cell carcinoma of the kidney. However, the clear-cell chondrosarcomas are S-100 positive and cytokeratin negative in contrast to renal carcinomas, which give the inverse reaction.

Mesenchymal chondrosarcoma

A rare highly-malignant tumour (Bertoni *et al.*, 1983; Huvos *et al.*, 1983c), it shows a predilection for the jaw and the ribs. Histologically distinctive, it consists of islands of chondroid tissue surrounded by primitive mesenchymal tumour cells, occasionally with a distinctive haemangiopericytoma-like pattern.

Tumours arising from fibroblastic cells (Table 28.3)

NON-OSSIFYING FIBROMA

Classical non-ossifying fibroma are usually small and asymptomatic and radiologically typified by bearing a close relationship to cortical bone in both the antero-posterior and lateral radiographs. Believed to be most frequently observed in relationship to the distal femur and proximal tibia, this may be a reflection on the incidence of the number of radiographs as a routine of the knee joint. Essentially, a 'leave alone' lesion, when biopsied they consist of spindle-cell fibroblasts arranged in a storiform pattern with foci of foamy histiocytes

and scattered osteoclasts. They are self-limiting and occasionally heal. Histologically similar to benign fibrous histiocytoma, their site of occurrence does not usually correspond with that of malignant histiocytoma. A small number continue to progress in the adult skeleton and require surgical management. This group is referred to as benign fibrous histiocytoma.

DESMOPLASTIC FIBROMA

Histologically resembling fibromatosis of soft tissue, these lesions are slowly progressive and permeative, and it is this infiltrative pattern of the margin that helps to distinguish them histologically. They do not metastasize.

MALIGNANT FIBROUS HISTIOCYTOMA

These uncommon tumours occur in the mature skeleton. Originally classified with fibrosarcoma, in general it was subsequently recognized that a tumour similar to malignant fibrous histiocytoma of the soft tissue can also occur in bone (O'Brien and Stout, 1964; Capanna *et al.*, 1984; Ros *et al.*, 1984; Huvos *et al.*, 1985a; Boland and Huvos, 1986). Histological features are similar. The cells are predominantly spindle shaped and arranged in a storiform pattern. They produce varying amounts of collagen. The tumour cells exhibit marked pleomorphism. Scattered through the field are tumour giant cells and osteoclast giant cells. A proportion of malignant fibrous histiocytomas are associated with a previous infarct (Mirra *et al.*, 1974) or fracture or areas of abnormal bone such as Paget's disease. Unlike their soft-tissue counterpart, malignant fibrous histiocytoma of bone respond to chemotherapy (Earl *et al.*, 1993).

FIBROSARCOMA

Now that malignant fibrous histiocytoma has become established as an entity, true fibrosarcoma are recognised as extremely rare. They only occur in the mature skeleton, though they are occasionally misdiagnosed in earlier age groups when they are, in fact, fibroblastic osteosarcoma. Histologically, these tumours have a typical pattern of spindle cells or elongated oval cells

Table 28.3 Fibrous tumours

Benign	Intermediate	Malignant
Non-ossifying fibroma	Desmoplastic fibroma	Malignant fibrous histiocytoma
Osteofibrous dysplasia		Fibrosarcoma
Benign fibrous histiocytoma		

arranged in a herring-bone pattern of interdigitating bundles. The tumour cells elaborate a various amount of collagen.

Tumours containing osteoclast giant cells (Table 28.4)

GIANT-CELL TUMOURS (OSTEOCLASTOMAS)

Giant-cell tumours (Jaffe *et al.*, 1940) account for 5–10% of primary bone tumours. It is now accepted that they almost invariably arise in the mature skeleton at the site of an epiphyseal, diaphyseal or apophyseal growth plate. Like malignant tumours, the order of frequency of the sites of occurrence are the distal femur, the proximal tibia, the proximal femur, the proximal humerus and, an uncommon site for malignant tumours, the distal radius. Classical giant-cell tumours are in an intermediate category in that they cannot be regarded as truly benign or as malignant in that they have a metastatic potential. However, these metastases when they do occur in less than 0.5% (Rock *et al.*, 1984) exhibit an unusual feature in that they do not infiltrate the host area. They implant and then mimic the primary tumour, elaborating an egg-shell of bone around the periphery. The primary tumour is always intimately related to an angle between the articular surface and the cortical bone, and they have, in addition, an endosteal margin, which is moderately well defined. Ultimately, the tumour becomes expansile, but always remains surrounded by a thin egg-shell of cortex. Only when a pathological fracture occurs or when there has been injudicious surgery does the tumour break outward into the surrounding soft tissue, where it can rapidly extend between muscle planes. The gross histological appearance is of a soft friable haemorrhagic material which is a reddish-brown, yellow or occasionally grey, resembling raw liver. The histological picture is one of mononuclear 'stromal' cells containing a variable number of normal mitotic figures. Distributed throughout this tissue are large numbers of 'reactive' multinucleate osteoclast giant cells that have inadvertently given the tumour its name. It is thought that the primary cell in the tumour is similar to the inactive osteoblast, the bone lining cell, whose role in normal bone turnover is to prepare the bone for resorption and to recruit and activate the osteoclast. It seems probable that resting osteoblasts remaining at the site of a fused growth plate may give rise to a giant-cell tumour. With the development of the tumour, osteoclasts progressively migrate into its substance. Grading of these tumours is unsatisfactory in that selective sampling is heterogeneous, and the rare event of a metastasis may even occur in a Grade I tumour.

Tumours arising from extra-osseous medullary tissues

Commonly referred to as 'malignant round-cell tumours of bone', this group includes Ewing's sarcoma, atypical Ewing's, Askin tumour and a group of tumours exhibiting neural features, the primitive neuroectodermal (PNET) tumour and metastatic neuroblastoma. In an older age group, small-cell carcinoma of the bronchus may need to be excluded by positive reactions to cytokeratin markers. The old classification included so-called 'reticulin cell sarcoma' which occurred in an older age group. In contrast to Ewing's tumour, the cells did not contain glycogen though they produced copious reticulin fibres. With the advent of immunohistochemistry, it has been shown that reticulin cell sarcomas are lymphoma presenting in bone. The majority are high-grade non-Hodgkin B-cell lymphomas. They may present as an isolated focus or be part of a more generalized process. They respond well to both chemotherapy and radiotherapy and rarely require surgical resection except where there is a pathological fracture.

EWING'S SARCOMA

Until recently of unknown histogenesis, it is now regarded as a poorly differentiated tumour of neural origin (Triche and Cavazzana, 1988). It is rarely seen over the age of 25 years. Generally affecting the diaphysis of long bones, it may affect the bones of the pelvis and the ribs. A similar tumour occurs in the soft tissues. It is highly malignant and the worst feature of the tumour is

Table 28.4 Lesions containing osteoclast giant cells

Non-neoplastic	Benign	Intermediate	Malignant
Brown tumour (hyperparathyroidism)	Non-ossifying fibroma	Giant-cell tumour	Malignant fibrous histiocytoma
Pigmented villonodular synovitis involving bone	Aneurysmal bone cyst	Aggressive osteoblastoma	Osteoclast-rich osteosarcoma
	Benign chondroblastoma		Clear-cell chondrosarcoma
	Chondromyxoid fibroma		
	Benign fibrous histiocytoma		

its permeative facility, rapidly invading the marrow cavity of the medulla, the vascular spaces of the cortex, the periosteum and surrounding soft tissues. Previously, characteristic layerings of appositional new bone has been described as 'onion skin layering'. Seen only in rare slow-growing tumours, the majority show only minimal radiological elevation of the periosteum by new bone as the associated vessels are rapidly infarcted by tumour cells and, in the majority of patients, lysis of this new bone is frequently seen, leaving occasionally only indeterminate Codman's triangles. Radiologically, particularly in the pelvis, large soft-tissue masses are observed. Tumour cells are small, uniform and round, and although in many instances mitotic figures are relatively few, the tumours are consistently of a high-grade of malignancy. It is currently believed that these sarcomas are poorly differentiated neuroectodermal tumours (Mierau, 1985; Dehner, 1986). Because of the rapid tumour growth and associated necrosis in some instances, there may be a systemic response, occasionally the patient exhibiting a pyrexia, anorexia and weight loss. Open biopsy reveals so-called 'pus formation', and a mistaken diagnosis of osteomyelitis is occasionally made. Histologically, the classic Ewing's sarcoma cells contain intracytoplasmic glycogen, while production of reticulin fibres is sparse. Although Ewing's sarcoma contain glycogen, it is easily depleted by inappropriate fixation. However, it is well preserved in imprint preparations. Below the age of 5 years, it is particularly important to exclude the alternative diagnosis of neuroblastoma. A large panel of antibodies is required to establish the diagnosis of malignant round cell tumours of bone. Chemotherapy and radiography may appear clinically to have a dramatic effect on both the intraosseous tumour and soft-tissue extensions (MacVicar *et al.*, 1992). However, surgical resection is indicated where this is feasible as scattered microfoci of tumour are found in the majority of resected specimens in bone and/or soft tissue. These microfoci are sufficient to lead to late local relapse if they are not resected. Currently, it is the practice to exhibit chemotherapy with subsequent resection of the skeletal lesion. Then, depending on the histological examination of the extremities of the resection, radiotherapy is judiciously introduced.

Tumours arising in abnormal bone

The association of malignant fibrous histiocytoma with pre-existing bone infarction is well recognized. A variety of sarcomas may occur in bone affected by Paget's disease. Rarely, malignant changes may occur in fibrous dysplasia or fibrocartilaginous mesenchymoma. Sarcomas also arise in irradiated bone.

Tumours arising in cell rests

CHORDOMA

Arising in notochordal remnants, these affect essentially the upper cervical spine and sacrococcygeal regions. Commonly, they occur in the middle-aged. Death is due to extension and local attrition, though metastases occur in 10%. Macroscopically, the tumour consists of soft translucent mucinous material. Histologically, the cells are filled with vacuoles of mucin and are referred to as 'physaliferous cells'. Positive reaction for cytokeratin distinguishes the tumour from myxoid chondrosarcoma.

ADAMANTINOMA

This is a rare tumour of long bones with a predilection for the tibia (90%). It is occasionally multiple in the tibia or it may be multifocal involving the tibia, fibula and os calcis. There is an association with pre-existing osteofibrous dysplasia. The classical site is the junction of the upper and middle third of the tibia on the subcutaneous surface. Radiologically, there is a typical soap-bubble appearance, whereas pre-existing fibrous dysplasia usually produces an associated 'ground glass' effect. Histologically, the lesions resemble fibrous dysplasia but with clefts and spaces lined by epithelial cells which may have a squamous- or basal-cell appearance. A similar tumour occurs in the jaw where it is referred to as an ameloblastoma (Eve's disease). Although electron microscope studies have confirmed the epithelial nature of the cells (Rosai, 1969), Huvos and Marcove (1975) noted the similarity of the epithelial cells to proliferating angioblasts and suggested a vascular origin. However, immunohistochemistry has demonstrated conclusively an epithelial rather than a vascular origin. Concern should be exercised before making a diagnosis of adamantinoma in an unusual site and the possibility of metastatic squamous-cell carcinoma should be considered.

SURGERY OF BONE DEFECTS AND SOLID BENIGN BONE LESIONS

Lesions such as enchondromas may require removal in that they occasionally cause deformities or pathological fractures, particularly when they affect the small bones of the hands. They should be widely resected and only grafted when the continuity of the bone is at risk.

Sessile and pedunculated osteochondromas should be treated conservatively except when they restrict joint function or interfere with the individual's normal activities. If they are excised, the base should be generously saucerized into the medullary bone in order to prevent local recurrence. Although it is uncommon, these lesions have a tendency to recur, and if they do, the recurrence often exhibits a higher potential towards malignant change.

Simple bone cysts are often responsible for pathological fractures in childhood and adolescence. It is a common though erroneous belief that following fracture such lesions are usually filled by new bone formation, an occurrence which is exceptional. Campanacci *et al.* (1986) have claimed considerable success, treating such lesions by irrigation and then by injecting with steroids. Others using this technique have been less successful. Many authors have suggested that with skeletal maturity, simple bone cysts undergo involution. This is not necessarily true, though such lesions are less likely to fracture in adult life. Aneurysmal bone cysts are variable in their behaviour. They may be relatively quiescent. When they are, they may respond to the Campanacci method of treatment. Equally, they can be locally aggressive, expanding the bone and causing collapse of the epiphyseal plates when they are in juxtaposition to articular surfaces. When this occurs, they should be treated according to the site of occurrence. In the distal radius, the bone is fenestrated and a wide clearance obtained by curettage. Unlike giant-cell tumours, they rarely destroy the subarticular bone but, because expanded cortical bone at this site is so fragile, they are generally grafted with autogenous bone.

Solid benign tumours of bone are most suitably treated by curettage. In order to do so, however, as Sim *et al.* (1983) states, adequate exposure is essential. In consequence, the fenestration of the cortical bone must equal the extent of the lesion if the tumour is to be completely visualized. Once the content of the cavity has been cleared, the subsequent management is debatable. In this country, the two major centres take considerable care in removing the wall of the tumour, either by removing the margin of the lesion by the use of a burr or removing it systematically, gouging away the abnormal bone until normal cortical or medullary bone is seen (Kemp, 1987). Other centres have used suction curettage (Conrad *et al.*, 1985). The cavity is then cleared using pulsatile lavage. Sim *et al.* (1983) then used phenol to sterilize the cavity. Johnston (1985) employed hydrogen peroxide. Cryosurgery has been advocated as a successful technique (Marcove *et al.*, 1978; Jacobs and Clemency, 1983; Malawer and Zielinski, 1983), but there is a high incidence of soft-tissue morbidity coupled with subsequent iatrogenic fractures using this method.

Osteoid osteoma are unusual lesions occurring predominantly in the pedicles of the spine and in the lower limbs. They account for 11% of benign bone lesions (Dahlin and Unni, 1986). Presenting with pain particularly at night, the pain is frequently but not always relieved by aspirin. The lesions are usually identified by their typical radiological presentation and are confirmed by technetium and computed tomography scanning. They are, in general, easily removed if visualized at operation with an image intensifier and an appropriate core cutter is employed. However, it is essential that the material is examined by a histopathologist in order to confirm that resection is complete. If any part of the lesion has been left behind, early re-exploration is recommended in that late overt recurrences are notoriously difficult to localize because these recurrences are invariably sclerotic (Marsh *et al.*, 1975).

Osteoblastoma, though not differing histologically, are usually larger than osteoid osteoma. They are often painful but not to the same exquisite degree as that produced by an osteoid osteoma, which elaborate prostaglandins, stimulating response by the host bone. Sometimes the symptomatology elucidated by these lesions can be extremely bizarre when they are identified accidentally, particularly when the patient is being assessed radiologically for some other condition. These two lesions are essentially the only two benign bone tumour lesions occurring in the posterior elements of the immature spine, and when they occur they invariably cause a painful scoliosis, a manifestation which in itself is virtually diagnostic.

Osteochondroma are the commonest benign bone tumours and represent 40% of all benign lesions (Dahlin and Unni, 1986). Treated expectantly, they only need to be removed if they are symptomatic and exhibiting evidence of growth or causing mechanical limitation of function. Chondroblastoma occur in relationship to the growth plates of immature bone, extending primarily into the epiphysis or the metaphysis. Generally treated by curettage, it is surprising how rarely they recur in that the approach to such lesions is frequently difficult and the clearance is usually unsatisfactory (Dahlin and Ivins, 1972; Huvos and Marcove, 1973).

Despite claims made by various workers that their particular method of treatment is the most efficacious, the recurrence rate of many of the benign tumours still remains depressingly high in the region of 25% in terms of the appendicular skeleton and as much as 50% in the axial skeleton. This applies particularly to giant-cell tumours, which have a close affinity with the subchondral surface of the affected joint. Despite the care that may be taken in removing the bony wall of the cavity left after curettage, it is rarely possible to remove the isolated bone spicules containing tumour cells from the subarticular cartilage without disturbing the continuity of the joint surface. Curettage alone is reported to have a recurrence rate approaching 50% (Campanacci *et al.*, 1975; Marsh *et al.*, 1975; Willert and Enderle, 1983; Campanacci *et al.*, 1986; Sim *et al.*, 1987). It has been a traditional and compulsive practice of orthopaedic surgeons to use autograft, allograft or xenograft to fill the bone defect left after the removal of benign lesions. Autograft medullary bone is generally well incorporated, but cortical autograft is only remodelled slowly. Further, harvesting autogenous bone is not without problems of morbidity. Despite claims to the contrary, allografts do elicit an antibody response by the recipient. The only allografts of any virtue are medullary slivers used in spinal fusion where they appear to provide a transitory scaffold for osteogenesis. Xenografts are, on occasion, associated with secondary osteomyelitis. They are never incorporated into the host bone, though paradoxically, however, they may rarely stimulate a brisk allergic response on the part of the host which, by walling off the graft by depositing bone, provides additional support to the affected areas. The xenograft is treated by the host as foreign material and is gradually eroded over an infinite period of time, frequently in excess of 20 years. As an alternative to bone grafts, bone cement has been widely advocated (Wouters, 1974; Persson and Wouters, 1976; Willert and Enderle, 1983; Persson *et al.*, 1984; Conrad *et al.*, 1985; Johnston, 1985). Thought by some to kill tumour cells during polymerization, it is responsible for masking tumour recurrence and causes the recurrence to expand centrifugally. Long-term studies by Willert (1985) suggest that the cement damages the articular cartilage and, as a result, 38% of his patients clinically manifested osteoarthritis prematurely. The two major centres in the UK rarely ever use bone grafts for management of defects. The rationale for avoiding grafts is that there is no morbidity in harvesting grafts; there is considerable clinical evidence to suggest that grafts interfere and even inhibit the potential of the host to regenerate bone to fill the deficit, and possibly, even more importantly, the presence of graft material masks the radiological manifestation of tumour recurrence.

Malignant bone tumours

The two principle tumours occurring in the immature or young adult skeleton are osteosarcoma and Ewing's sarcoma. The highest incidence of osteosarcomas occurs in the adolescent during the growth spurt and the commonest site is directly related to those areas where growth potential is at a maximum, generally affecting the juxtaepiphyseal metaphysis. Ewing's sarcoma, while commonly affecting the same age group, is more diffuse

in the site of occurrence, affecting the axial skeleton more commonly and, when involving long bones, not necessarily showing a predilection of site.

Prior to the introduction of chemotherapy by Rosen *et al.* (1982), the only available treatment for malignant tumours was amputation and radiotherapy, and the two were occasionally used in conjunction (Cade, 1955). The survival rate varied between 10 and 20% (Carter, 1980). Today, the combination of conservative surgery, chemotherapy and, in some instances, radiotherapy has increased the survival rate to 65% in some centres (Rosen *et al.*, 1983). Conservative surgery is interpreted variously in different countries. The current practice in terms of management is to treat the patient with chemotherapy and to allow a window between the third and fourth course of therapy for surgical treatment. Only rarely is it possible to resect a malignant tumour without interfering with the continuity of a long bone, though if a wide margin can be obtained, then this is justifiable. However, it is possible to resect part of the pelvic ring with such a margin and to replace the deficit with suitable bone grafts or, when the hip joint is involved, by endoprosthetic replacement (Steel, 1978; Enneking and Dunham, 1978).

Since the majority of bone tumours essentially affect the appendicular skeleton and most frequently the bones of the lower limb, the principles of conservative management will be discussed in relation to the knee and hip joint and to a lesser extent the shoulder. When deciding on proposed management, however, treatment should always be discussed with the patient, and if the patient is a minor, in conjunction with the parents, and their wishes and expectations must be taken into consideration. Further, judgement may be influenced by social, ethnical and economic factors.

Even today, as already mentioned, patients are referred to the supraregional units with tumours that are so advanced that it would not be possible to obtain an adequte clearance to permit replacement surgery, while others are so grossly infected due to previous open biopsy that this precludes conservative treatment (Mankin *et al.*, 1982). With few exceptions, the majority of such patients can only be treated by amputation or disarticulation coupled with adjuvant chemotherapy. Further, the vast majority of these patients will already have secondary pulmonary deposits and, therefore, have a poor prognosis. The principle behind conservative surgery is that the tumour should be widely excised (Enneking *et al.*, 1980; Enneking, 1986). Although a logical concept, it cannot be followed in practice in that at the knee, for instance, a wide excision would mean resection of a neurovascular bundle and the overlying

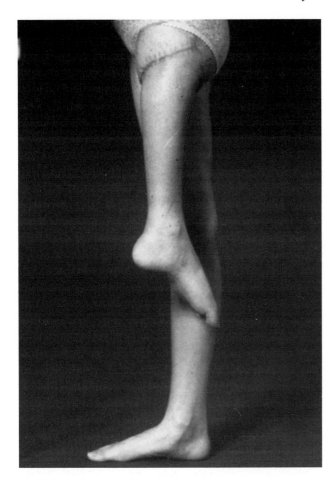

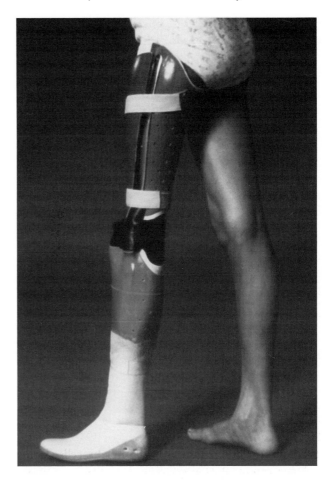

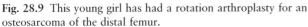

Fig. 28.9 This young girl has had a rotation arthroplasty for an osteosarcoma of the distal femur.

Fig. 28.10 The girl (see Fig. 28.9) is able to walk in a custom-built orthosis using her own ankle to flex the knee.

skin. Fortunately, in that in the majority of cases the periosteum is acting as an anatomical barrier to tumour spread, more modified surgery can be performed. Various methods of replacing the deficit at the knee after resection have been advocated. One of the earliest methods employed intramedullary nailing and sliding grafts (Merle d'Aubigne and Dejournay, 1958). Although a logical concept, this deprived the patient of knee movement and, further, graft incorporation took an extremely long time. A method favoured in Germany and Holland (Van Nes, 1950; Winkelmann, 1983; Winkler *et al.*, 1986) is to resect the tumour and then to approximate the residual bone and arthrodese this to the unaffected bone after rotating the distal portion of the limb through 180° (rotational arthroplasty). The ankle joint will then function within its limited range of movement as a proxy knee joint (Figs 28.9 and 28.10). In the USA and in Russia (Lexer, 1925; Volkov, 1970; Parrish, 1973; Mankin *et al.*, 1976), the use of allografts

has been popularized. While sound in principle, there are many disadvantages. First, it is becoming increasingly difficult to obtain allografts that can be guaranteed to be free from HIV and other infections. Second, as McKibbin (1971) has shown, allografts of bone induce a slow immune response by the host, and although initially the host vessels enter the allograft through the cut surface in particular, ultimately vascular invasion ceases and lymphocytic islands are laid down around these vessels. Consequently, the vast proportion of the donor bone remains avascular and ultimately stress microfractures cause gradual collapse. In the UK, as a sequel to the work of Professor Scales and his successor, Professor Walker, and the Department of Biomedical Engineering at Stanmore, the use of extensive endoprosthetics has developed over the past 40 years (Burrows, 1968; Burrows *et al.*, 1975; Scales, 1983; Sweetnam, 1983; Bradish *et al.*, 1987; Ross *et al.*, 1987). Present-day prostheses consist of cobalt chrome molybdenum

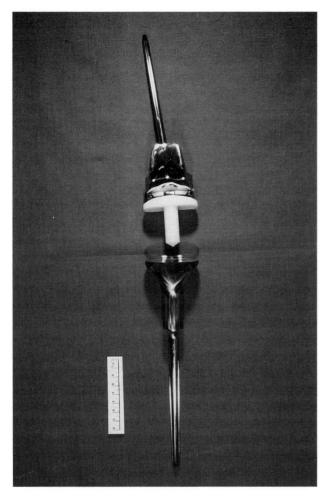

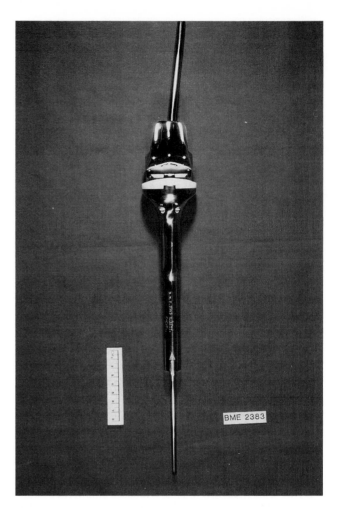

Fig. 28.11 The SMILES prosthesis is a hinged prosthesis. It has an interlink that permits rotation to occur at the knee joint. This particular prosthesis was made for a patient with a giant-cell tumour of the proximal tibia.

Fig. 28.12 A more extensive prosthesis is required for the replacement of malignant tumours occurring at this site.

bearings coupled with titanium alloy shafts and intra-medullary pins in order to achieve lightness of the prosthesis, while the bushes of the prosthesis consist of RCH-1000. Such extended joints, necessarily in the earlier stage of prosthetic development, were dependent on captive or hinged joints. These have now been modified to allow 10° of internal and external rotation of the knee when flexed. This advance occurred as a sequel to the introduction of a linked joint by the Department of Biomedical Engineering at Stanmore. It is known as the SMILES prosthesis (Figs 28.11 and 28.12). Technically, in the long-term, replacements of the distal femur have presented relatively few problems. However, replacements of the proximal tibia have not been as successful due to a number of local problems. First, re-attachment of the quadriceps tendon to the tibial component is not always successful as the use of

Terylene tape in the past has produced a soft-tissue reaction and, on occasion, tissue breakdown. Various methods of extending the tendon so that it can be directly attached to the tibial component are now being employed. Oxidation of the titanium alloy has resulted in tissue staining and pigmentation and, on occasion, sterile abscess formation.

To avoid these problems, a number of modifications have been introduced. At surgery, the medial head of the gastrocnemius is mobilized and brought anteriorly to cover the prosthesis in its subcutaneous aspect and the prosthesis is now sculptured to accommodate this. Further, it is possible with these modifications to approximate the deep fascia on either side of the tendon so that the prosthesis is almost entirely covered. Finally, in order to prevent oxidization, the prosthesis is now subjected to a chemical process which produces a surface layer of titanium nitrite so that oxidization no longer occurs.

Replacements of the hip joint are, in general, extremely successful, though when the resection is extensive the insertion of the abductors into the greater trochanter is lost. The abductors can be attached to the fascia lata or to a fenestrated shaft of the prosthesis. The latter technique is relatively successful for, although such an attachment is not necessarily permanent, it allows scarring by fibrous tissue to achieve a more efficient function of the abductors. Approximately 50% of these patients with hip replacements will walk without a Trendelenberg gait.

Giant-cell tumours occasionally occur in the femoral head and neck. These lesions at this site can never be adequately curetted because of the difficulties of the surgical approach, and it is preferable to perform a prosthetic replacement as a primary procedure in these cases. Tumours affecting the diaphysis of long bones such as the tibia and femur can be treated either by the use of a medullary prosthesis or by the use of a fibular graft or a vascularized fibular graft. Sometimes the latter is coupled with internal plating. These techniques are, in general, successful in that the graft ultimately hypertrophies. On occasion, when a tumour of the shaft is well circumscribed, it is possible to resect the lesion and then to treat the patient by using bone transport.

Tumours may occasionally involve the proximal fibula. Contrary to current belief, such tumours can be resected with impunity as the resection does not disturb function of the knee joint. Tumours of the distal tibia are rare. They have previously been treated by resection and grafting either with fibular or ilial bone. Currently, they are being managed by the insertion of prostheses, though these procedures are essentially experimental at this stage.

Lesions of the pelvis are treated by wide excision of the tumour. Those affecting the pubic rami and the ischial rami can often be treated by resection alone. If the lesion encroaches on the acetabulum, it is necessary to resect the hip joint. Depending on the nature of the tumour, the patient can be left with the so-called 'hanging hip' or, preferably, with a custom-built prosthesis made in the Department of Biomedical Engineering, Stanmore, and which can be attached directly to the residual ilial wing. The main problem arising with surgery of this nature at this site is that there will be an imbalance of muscle function which may necessitate intensive postoperative physiotherapy. Tumours arising more posteriorly, particularly those involving the ilial wing, are most suitably managed by wide resection of the lesion and the insertion of fibular grafts to restore continuity,

for failure to reconstruct the pelvic ring at this site inevitably leads to a collapse of the pelvic ring.

Tumours of the sacrum almost invariably present major problems. Whereas partial resections may not produce gross neurological deficits, total sacral resection deprives the patient of bladder and bowel control and, if the S1 root cannot be preserved, it seriously affects lower limb function. Total sacrectomy is only justified as a life-preserving procedure. Reconstruction after resection is dependent on internal fixation augmented with bone grafts.

Tumours of the upper limb essentially affect the proximal humerus. Prosthetic replacement of such lesions has the added disadvantage that part of the rotator cuff is inevitably lost. Attempts at reconstruction, even when the surgery is relatively conservative because of the nature of the tumour, are not necessarily successful (Ross *et al.*, 1987). This is in part due to the fibrosis which inevitably follows the resection, though in part it is due to the inability to re-attach the rotator cuff to the prosthesis satisfactorily. Nevertheless, it preserves glenohumeral stability and facilitates normal elbow and hand function. Elbow joint replacement usually permits an adequate range of movement providing that the integrity of the proximal radio-ulnar joint can be reconstituted. However, the occurrence of tumours at this site is extremely uncommon. Tumours of the distal radius are equally uncommon. To date, prosthetic replacements have been unsuccessful. Curettage and grafting is used in the management of most benign lesions. Occasionally, particularly in the case of giant-cell tumours that have destroyed the articular surface, the distal radius is resected and replaced with a free graft of the proximal fibula which is plated. In those rare instances where the tumour is malignant, the lesion is widely excised and the distal ulna is arthrodesed to the carpal bones.

In general, it is an infrequent occurrence for a tumour to involve the whole of the medullary cavity of a long bone. However, when this occurs in either the humerus or the femur, it has been possible to replace the whole bone and the associated joints.

Extending prostheses (Fig. 28.13)

Tumours of growing bone present an additional problem in terms of management, particularly when they involve actively-growing epiphyses. A standard replacement would leave the young patient with a short limb. To overcome this difficulty, an extending prosthesis was designed by the Department of Biomedical Engineering, Stanmore (Sneath *et al.*, 1984). There are two components. The passive component replacing the bone

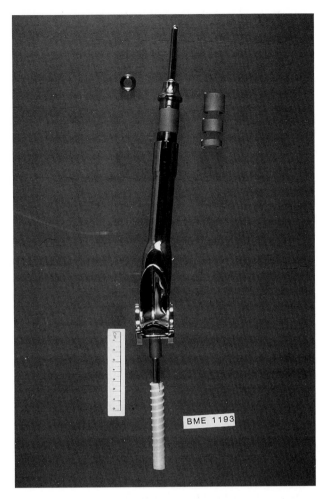

Fig. 28.13 Extending prostheses are required for the immature skeleton. In this prosthesis used to replace the distal femur, the femoral component is periodically extended by the use of 'C' clips inserted surgically. In the unaffected tibia, a polyethylene sleeve is inserted into the medullary canal. It sheaths the piston, which is attached to the floating tibial table, which allows the piston to be extended as growth takes place.

deficit consists of a barrel with an extrudible piston. The initial system consisted of a worm-screw mechanism. Subsequently, extension was achieved by inserting tungsten carbide ball bearings through a port in the side of the barrel. Another method which is presently used is achieved by fitting C-rings after the prosthesis has been physically extended at operation. These procedures can all be repeated at regular intervals during growth. Occasionally, it may even be necessary to replace part or whole of the component in order to maintain length. The active component consists of an RCH-1000 sleeve which is sunk into the medullary canal beyond the growth plate. A close-fitting medullary rod carries the component of the joint on the epiphyseal side of the growth plate. As growth occurs at the plate, the rod is extruded and normal elongation of the bone takes place. In the majority of patients with a growth potential, by using these methods it has been possible to extend the limb so that leg equalization is maintained.

Tumours of the spine

Tumours of the vertebral bodies present particular problems to the surgeon. If they are to be resected then careful planning is required to ensure that complete resection can be achieved, preferably at one procedure. Soft tissue, particularly nerve roots, may need to be sacrificed. Following resection, it is essential to obtain spinal stability using the most appropriate form of internal fixation.

Surgery of bone tumours and of the associated soft tissues present a constant challenge to the oncological orthopaedic surgeon in that these problems are never routine. Surgeons can no longer approach these cases in isolation. To be successful in terms of management, not only are they dependent on their radiological colleagues and the histopathologist, they also rely on the support of the paramedical team consisting of trained nursing staff, cancer counsellors, physiotherapists and occupational therapists in addition to junior staff.

REFERENCES

Aisen A.M., Martel W., Braunstein E.M. *et al.* (1986) MRI and CT evaluation of primary bone and soft-tissue tumors. *Am. J. Roentgen.* **146**, 749–756.

Arlen M., Higinbotham N.L., Huvos A.G. *et al.* (1971) Radiation-induced sarcomas of bone. *Cancer* **28**, 1087–1099.

Aurias A., Rimbaut C., Buffe D., Dubousset J. and Mazabraud A. (1983) Chromosomal translocations in Ewing's sarcoma. *New Eng. J. Med.* **309**, 496–497.

Bertoni F., Picci P. and Bacchini P. (1983) Mesenchymal chondrosarcoma of bone and soft tissue. *Cancer* **52**, 533–541.

Birch J.M., Marsden H.B. and Swindell R. (1980) Incidence of malignant disease in childhood: a 24 year review of the Manchester Children's Tumour Registry data. *Br. J. Cancer* **42**, 215–223.

Bohndorf K., Reiser M., Lochner B., Feaux de Lacroix W. and Steinbrich W. (1986) Magnetic resonance imaging of primary tumours and tumour-like lesions of bone. *Skel. Radiol.* **15**, 511–517.

Boland P.J. and Huvos A.G. (1986) Malignant fibrous histiocytoma of bone. *Clin. Orthop. Rel. Res.* **204**, 130–134.

Bradish C.F., Kemp H.B.S., Scales J.J. and Wilson J.N. (1987) Distal femoral replacement—the long term results using the custom made Stanmore hinged total knee replacement. *J. Bone Joint Surg* **69B**, 276–284.

Brown K.T., Kattapuram S.V. and Rosenthal D.L. (1986) Computed tomographic analysis of bone tumors; patterns of cortical destruction and soft tissue extension. *Skel. Radiol.* **15**, 448–451.

Burrows H.J. (1968) Major prosthetic replacement of bone: lessons learnt in seventeen years. *J. Bone Joint Surg.* **50B**, 225–226.

Burrows H.J., Wilson J.N. and Scales J.T. (1975) Excision of tumour of humerus and femur, with restoration by internal prostheses. *J. Bone Joint Surg.* **57B**, 148–159.

Byers P.D. (1968) Solitary benign osteoblastic lesions of bone: osteoid osteoma and benign osteoblastoma. *Cancer* **22**, 43–57.

Cade S. (1955) Osteogenic sarcoma: a study based on 133 patients. *J. Roy. Coll. Surg. Edin.* **1**, 79–111.

Cahan W.G., Woodard H.Q., Higinbotham N.L. *et al.* (1948) Sarcoma arising in irradiated bone: report of eleven cases. *Cancer* **1**, 3–29.

Campanacci M. (1979) Malignant degeneration in fibrous dysplasia. *Ital. J. Orthop. Traumatol.* **5**, 373–381.

Campanacci M., Guinti A. and Olmi R. (1975) Giant-cell tumours of bone: a study of 209 cases with long-term follow-up in 130. *Ital. J. Orthop. Traumatol.* **1**, 249–277.

Campanacci M., Capanna R. and Picci P. (1986) Unicameral and aneurysmal bone cysts. *Clin. Orthop. Rel. Res.* **204**, 25–36.

Capanna R., Bertoni F. and Bacchini P. (1984) Malignant fibrous histiocytoma of bone. The experience at the Rizzoli Institute: report of ninety cases. *Cancer* **54**, 177–187.

Carter S.K. (1980) The dilemma of adjuvant chemotherapy for osteogenic sarcoma. *Cancer Clin. Trials* **3**, 29–36.

Cohen M.D., Klatte E.C., Baehner R. *et al.* (1984) Magnetic resonance imaging of bone marrow disease in children. *Radiology* **151**, 715–718.

Conrad E.U., Enneking W.F. and Springfield D.S. (1985) Giant cell tumor treatment with curettage and cementation. In Enneking W.F. (Chairman) *Abstracts of the International Symposium on Limb Salvage in Musculoskeletal Oncology, Orlando, Florida, October 2–5, 1985.* Bristol-Myers/Zimmer Orthopaedic Symposium in cooperation with the Orthopaedic Research and Education Foundation. American Orthopaedic Association.

Dahlin D.C. and Beabout J.W. (1971) Dedifferentiation of low-grade chondrosarcomas. *Cancer* **28**, 461–466.

Dahlin D.C. and Ivins J.C. (1972) Benign chondroblastoma: a study of 125 cases. *Cancer* **30**, 401–413.

Dahlin D.C. and Unni K.K. (1986) *Bone Tumors: General Aspects and Data on 8542 Cases*, 4th edn. Springfield, Charles C. Thomas.

Dehner L.P. (1986) Peripheral and central primitive neuroecto-dermal tumors: a nosological concept seeking a consensus. *Arch. Pathol. Lab. Med.* **110**, 997–1006.

Dooms G.C., Hricak H., Sollitto R.A. and Higgins C.B. (1985) Lipomatous tumors and tumors with fatty component: MR imaging potential and comparison of MR and CT results. *Radiology* **157**, 479–483.

Earl H.M., Pringle J., Kemp H.B.S., Morrittu L., Miles D. and Souhami R. (1993) Chemotherapy of malignant fibrous histio-cytoma of bone. *Ann. Oncol.* **4**, 409–415.

Enneking W.F. (1986) A system of staging musculoskeletal neo-plasms. *Clin. Orthop. Rel. Res.* **204**, 9–24.

Enneking W.F. and Dunham W.K. (1978) Resection and recon-struction of primary neoplasms involving the innominate bone. *J. Bone Joint Surg.* **60A**, 731–746.

Enneking W.F., Spanier S.S. and Goodman M.A. (1980) A system for the surgical staging of musculoskeletal sarcoma. *Clin.*

Orthop. Rel. Res. **153**, 106–120.

Francois J. (1977) Retinoblastoma and osteogenic sarcoma. *Ophthalmologica* **175**, 185–191.

Fraumeni J.F. (1967) Stature and malignant tumours of bone in childhood and adolescence. *Cancer* **20**, 967–973.

Friend S.H., Bernards R., Rogel, J.S. *et al.* (1986) A human DNA segment with properties of the gene that predisposes to retino-blastoma and osteosarcoma. *Nature* **323**, 643–646.

Fyfe I.S., Henry A.P.J. and Mulholland R.C. (1983) Closed vertebral biopsy. *J. Bone Joint Surg.* **65B**, 140–143.

Glass A.C. and Fraumeni J.F. (1970) Epidemiology of bone cancer in children. *J. Nat. Cancer Inst.* **44**, 187–190.

Golfieri R., Baddeley H., Pringle J. and Souhami R. (1989) The role of the STIR sequence in magnetic resonance imaging exam-ination of bone tumours. *Br. J. Radiol.* **63**, 251–256.

Goodman S.B., Bell R.S., Fornasier V.L., de Demeter D. and Bateman J.E. (1984) Ollier's disease with multiple sarcomatous transformations. *Hum. Pathol.* **15**, 91–93.

Gordon M.T., Anderson D.C. and Sharp P.T. (1991) Canine distemper virus localised in bone cells of patients with Paget's disease. *Bone* **12**, 195–201.

Greditzer H.G., McLeod R.A., Unni K.K. *et al.* (1983) Bone sarcomas in Paget's disease. *Radiology* **146**, 327–333.

Gunterberg B., Kindblom L-G. and Laurin S. (1977) Giant-cell tumour of bone and aneurysmal bone cyst—a correlated histo-logic and angiographic study. *Skel. Radiol.* **2**, 65–74.

Haibach H., Carrell C. and Dittrich F.J. (1985) Neoplasms arising in Paget's disease of bone: a study of 82 cases. *Am. J. Clin. Pathol.* **83**, 594–600.

Halldorsdottir A., Ekelund L. and Rydholm A. (1982) CT diag-nosis of lipomatous tumors of the soft tissues. *Arch. Orthop. Traum. Surg.* **100**, 211–216.

Hatcher C.H. (1945) The development of sarcoma in bone sub-jected to roentgen or radium irradiation. *J. Bone Joint Surg.* **27**, 179–195.

Helms C.A., Cann C.E., Brunelle F.O. *et al.* (1981) Detection of bone marrow metastases using quantitative computed tomo-graphy. *Radiology* **140**, 745–750.

Holscher H.C., Bloem J.L, Nooy M.A., Taminian A.H.M., Eulderink F. and Hermans J. (1990) The value of MR imaging in monitoring the effect of chemotherapy on bone sarcomas. *Am. J. Roentgen.* **154**, 763–769.

Huvos A.G. and Marcove R.C. (1973) Chondroblastoma of bone: a critical review. *Clin. Orthop. Rel. Res.* **95**, 300–312.

Huvos A.G. and Marcove R. (1975) Adamantinoma of the long bones. A clinicopathological study of fourteen cases with vascu-lar origin suggested. *J. Bone Joint Surg.* **57A**, 148–154.

Huvos A.G., Butler A. and Bretsky S.S. (1983a) Osteogenic sar-coma associated with Paget's disease of bone. A clinicopatho-logic study of 65 patients. *Cancer* **52**, 1489–1495.

Huvos A.G., Butler A. and Bretsky S.S. (1983b) Osteogenic sar-coma in the American black. *Cancer* **52**, 1959–1965.

Huvos A.G., Rosen G. and Dabska M. (1983c) Mesenchymal chondrosarcoma. A clinicopathological analysis of thirty-five patients with emphasis on treatment. *Cancer* **51**, 1230–1237.

Huvos A.G., Heiweil M. and Bretsky S.S. (1985a) The pathology of malignant fibrous histiocytoma of bone. A study of 130 patients. *Am. J. Surg. Pathol.* **9**, 853–871.

Huvos A.G., Woodard H.Q., Cahan W.G. *et al.* (1985b) Post-radiation osteogenic sarcoma of bone and soft tissues: a clinico-pathologic study of 66 patients. *Cancer* **55**, 1244–1255.

Jackson R.P. (1978) Recurrent osteoblastoma: a review. *Clin.*

Orthop. Rel. Res. **131**, 229–233.

Jacobs P.A. and Clemency R.E. Jr. (1983) Closed cryosurgical treatment of giant cell tumor, aneurysmal bone cyst and other lesions of bone (Abstract). *Orthop. Transact.* **7**, 195–196.

Jaffe H.L., Lichtenstein L. and Portis R.B. (1940) Giant cell tumour of bone: its pathological appearance, grading, supposed variants and treatment. *Arch. Pathol.* **30**, 993–1031.

Jamshidi K. and Swaim W.R. (1971) Bone marrow biopsy with unaltered architecture: a new biopsy device. *J. Lab. Clin. Med.* **77**, 335–342.

Jensen R.D. and Drake R.M. (1970) Rarity of Ewing's sarcoma in Negroes. *Lancet* **1**, 777–779.

Jensen R.D. and Miller R.W. (1971) Retinoblastoma: epidemiologic characteristics. *New Engl. J. Med.* **285**, 307–311.

Johnson L.C. (1953) A general theory of bone tumours. *Bull. N.Y. Acad. Med.* **29**, 164–171.

Johnston J. (1985) Treatment of giant cell tumour of bone by aggressive curettement and packing with bone cement. In Enneking W.F. (Chairman) *Abstracts of the International Symposium on Limb Salvage in Musculoskeletal Oncology, Orlando, Florida, October 2–5, 1985*, pp. vi–13 (Bristol-Myers/Zimmer Orthopaedic Symposium in cooperation with the Orthopaedic Research and Education Foundation). American Orthopaedic Association.

Kavanagh T.G., Cannon S.R., Pringle J., Stoker D.J. and Kemp H.B.S. (1990) Parosteal osteosarcoma — Treatment by wide resection and prosthetic replacement. *J. Bone Joint Surg.* **72B**, 959–965.

Kemp H.B.S. (1987) Limb conservation surgery for osteosarcoma and other primary bone tumours. *Baillière's Clin. Oncol.* **1(1)**, 111–136.

Kitchin F.D. (1976) Genetics of retinoblastoma. In Rees A.E. (ed.) *Tumors of the Eye*, pp. 90–132. Hagerstown, MA, Harper and Row.

Kramer S., Meadows A.I., Jarrett P. and Evans A.E. (1983) Incidence of childhood cancer: experience of a decade in a population-based registry. *J. Nat. Cancer Inst.* **70**, 49–55.

Lexer E. (1925) Joint transplantations and arthroplasty. *Surg. Gynaecol. Obstet.* **40**, 782–809.

Li F.P., Fraumeni J.R. Jr., Mulvihill J.J. *et al.* (1988) A cancer family syndrome in twenty four kindreds. *Cancer Res.* **48**, 5358–5362.

Li F.P., Tu J., Liu F. and Shiang E. (1980) Rarity of Ewing's sarcoma in China. *Lancet* **1**, 1255–1257.

Lodwick G.S. (1971) *The Bones and Joints.* Chicago, Year Book.

Lodwick G.S., Wilson A.J., Farrell C. *et al.* (1980) Estimating rate of growth in bone lesions: observer performance and error. *Radiology* **134**, 585–590.

MacVicar A.D., Olliff J.F.C., Pringle J., Ross Pinkerton C. and Husband J. (1992) Ewing's sarcoma — imaging of chemotherapy-induced changes with histologic correlation. *Radiology* **184**, 859–864.

McFarland G.B. Jr., McKinley L.M. and Reed R.J. (1977) Dedifferentiation of low grade chondrosarcoma. *Clin. Orthop. Rel. Res.* **122**, 157–164.

Madewell J.E., Ragsdale B.D. and Sweet D.G. (1981) Radiologic and pathologic analysis of solitary bone lesions. Part I. Internal margins. *Radiol. Clin. North Am.* **19**, 715–748.

Malawer M.M. and Zielkinski C.J. (1983) Giant cell tumor of bone: cryosurgery and 'en-bloc' resection, current concepts and recommendations for treatment. *Orthop. Transac.* **7** (Abstract), 492.

Mall J.C., Bekerman C., Hoffer P.B. and Gottschalk A. (1976) A unified radiological approach to the detection of skeletal metastases. *Radiology* **118**, 323–328.

Mankin H.J., Fogelson F.S., Thrasher A.Z. and Jaffer F. (1976) Massive resection and allograft transplantation in the treatment of malignant bone tumours. *New Engl. J. Med.* **294**, 1247–1255.

Mankin H.J., Lange T.A. and Spanier S.S. (1982) The hazards of biopsy in patients with malignant primary bone and soft tissue tumors. *J. Bone Joint Surg.* **64A**, 1121–1127.

Marcove R.C., Weiss L.D., Vaghaiwalla M.R. and Pearson R. (1978) Cryosurgery in the treatment of giant cell tumors of bone: a report of 52 consecutive cases. *Clin. Orthop. Rel. Res.* **134**, 275–289.

Marsh B.W., Bonfiglio M., Brady L.P. and Enneking W.F. (1975) Benign osteoblastoma: range of manifestations. *J. Bone Joint Surg.* **57A**, 1–9.

Martland H.S. (1929) Occupational poisoning in manufacture of luminous watch dials. *J. Am. Med. Ass.* **92**, 466–473.

McKibbin B. (1971) Immature joint cartilage and homograft reaction. *J. Bone Joint Surg.* **53B**, 123–135.

Merle d'Aubigne R. and Dejournay J.P. (1958) Diaphyso-epiphyseal reconstruction for bone tumours at the knee. *J. Bone Joint Surg.* **40B**, 385–395.

Merryweather R., Middlemass J.H. and Sanerkin N.G. (1980) Malignant transformation of osteoblastoma. *J. Bone Joint Surg.* **62A**, 381–384.

Mierau G.W. (1985) Extraskeletal Ewing's sarcoma (peripheral neuroepithelioma). *Ultrastruct. Pathol.* **9**, 91–98.

Miller R.W. (1976) Aetiology of childhood bone cancer: epidemiologic observations. *Recent Results Cancer Res.* **54**, 50–62.

Mirra J.M., Bullough P.M. and Marcove R.C. (1974) Malignant fibrous histiocytoma and osteosarcoma in association with bone infarcts. Report of four cases, two in caisson workers. *J. Bone Joint Surg.* **56A**, 932–940.

Moore T.M., Meyers M.H., Patzakis M.J., Terry R. and Harvey J.P. (1979) Closed biopsy of musculoskeletal lesions. *J. Bone Joint Surg.* **61A**, 375–379.

Muhm J.R., Brown L.R., Crowe J.K. *et al.* (1978) Comparison of whole lung tomography and computed tomography for detecting pulmonary nodules. *Am. J. Roentgen.* **131**, 981–984.

Murray I.P.C. (1980) Bone scanning in the child and young adult. Part I. *Skel. Radiol.* **5**, 1–14.

Neifeld J.P., Michaelis L.L. and Doppman J.L. (1977) Suspected pulmonary metastases: correlation of chest X-ray, whole lung tomograms and operative findings. *Cancer* **39**, 383–387.

O'Brien J.E. and Stout A.P. (1964) Malignant fibrous xanthoma. *Cancer* **17**, 1445–1455.

O'Driscoll J.B. and Anderson D.C. (1985) Past pets and Paget's disease. *Lancet* **ii**, 919–921.

Parrish F.F. (1973) Allograft replacement of all or a part of the end of a long bone following excision of a tumour. *J. Bone Joint Surg.* **55A**, 1–22.

Persson B.M. and Wouters H.W. (1976) Curettage and acrylic cementation in surgery of giant cell tumors of bone. *Clin. Orthop. Rel. Res.* **120**, 125–133.

Persson B.M., Ekelund L., Lövdahl R. and Gunterberg B. (1984) Favourable results of acrylic cementation for giant cell tumors. *Acta Orthop. Scand.* **55**, 209–214.

Polednak A.P. (1985a) Primary bone cancer incidence in blacks and whites in New York State. *Cancer* **55**, 2883–2890.

Polednak A.P. (1985b) Human biology and epidemiology of

childhood bone cancers: a review. *Hum. Biol.* **57**, 1–26.

Porter D.E., Holden S.T., Steel C.M. *et al.* (1992) Patients with osteosarcoma may belong to Li–Fraumeni cancer families. *J. Bone Joint Surg.* **74B**, 883–886.

Price C.H.G. (1955) Osteogenic sarcoma: an analysis of the age and sex incidence. *Br. J. Cancer* **9**, 558–574.

Price C.H.G. (1958) Primary bone-forming tumours and their relationship and skeletal growth. *J. Bone Joint Surg.* **40B**, 574–593.

Price C.H.G., and Goldie W. (1969) Paget's sarcoma of bone. A study of 80 cases from the Bristol and Leeds Bone Tumour Registries. *J. Bone Joint Surg.* **51B**, 205–224.

Revell P.A. and Scholtz C.L. (1979) Aggressive osteoblastoma. *J. Pathol.* **127**, 195–198.

Richardson M.L., Kilcoyne R.F., Gillespy III T., Helms C.A. and Genant H.K. (1986) Magnetic resonance of musculoskeletal neoplasms. *Radiol. Clin. North Am.* **24**, 259–267.

Rock M.G., Pritchard D.J. and Unni K.K. (1984) Metastases from histologically benign giant-cell tumor of bone. *J. Bone Joint Surg.* **66A** 269–274.

Ros P.R., Viamonte M. Jr. and Rywlin A.M. (1984) Malignant fibrous histiocytoma. Mesenchymal tumour of ubiquitous origin. *Am. J. Radiol.* **142**, 753–759.

Rosai J. (1969) Adamantinoma of the tibia: electron microscopic evidence of its epithelial origin. *Am. J. Clin. Pathol.* **51**, 786–792.

Rosen G., Caparros B., Huvos A.G. *et al.* (1982) Pre-operative chemotherapy for osteogenic sarcoma; selection of post-operative adjuvant chemotherapy based on the response of the primary tumour to pre-operative chemotherapy. *Cancer* **49**, 891–895.

Rosen G., Marcove R.C., Huvos A.G. *et al.* (1983) Primary osteosarcoma: eight year experience with adjuvant chemotherapy *J. Cancer Res. Clin. Oncol.* **106** (Suppl.), 55–67.

Ross A.C., Wilson J.N. and Scales J.T. (1987) Endoprosthetic replacement of the proximal humerus. *J. Bone Joint Surg.* **69B**, 656–661.

Sagerman R.H., Cassady J.W., Tretter P. and Ellsworth R.M. (1969) Radiation induced neoplasia following external beam therapy for children with retinoblastoma. *Am. J. Roentgen.* **105**, 529–535.

Sanerkin N.G. (1980) Definitions of osteosarcoma, chondrosarcoma and fibrosarcoma of bone. *Cancer* **46**, 178–185.

Scales J.T. (1983) Bone and joint replacement for the preservation of limbs. *Br. J. Hosp. Med.* **29**, 220–232.

Schajowicz F. and Lemos C. (1970) Osteoid osteoma and osteoblastoma. Closely related entities of osteoblastic derivation. *Acta Orthop. Scand.* **41**, 272–291.

Schajowicz F. and Lemos C. (1976) Malignant osteoblastoma. *J. Bone Joint Surg.* (Br.) **58B**, 202–211.

Schwartz D.T. and Alpert H.R. (1964) The malignant transformation of fibrous dysplasia. *Am. J. Med. Sci.* **247**, 1–20.

Sim F.H. (ed.) (1983) Principles of surgical treatment. In *Diagnosis and Treatment of Bone Tumors: A Team Approach*, pp. 23–25. Thorofare, NJ, Slack.

Sim F.H., Beauchamp C.P. and Chao E.Y.S. (1987) Reconstruction of musculoskeletal defects about the knee of tumor. *Clin. Orthop. Rel. Res.* **221**, 188–201.

Sneath R.S., Scales J.T. and Wright K.W.J. (1984) *The Use of 'Growing' Endoprostheses to Induce or Accommodate Lengthening of the Limb in the Child or the Adult*, p. 48. Abstracts of the 16th SICOT Congress, London.

Sparkes R.S., Sparkes M.C., Wilson M.G. *et al.* (1980) Regional assessment of genes for human esterase D and retinoblastoma to chromosome band 13q14. *Science* **208**, 1042–1044.

Steel H.H. (1978) Partial or complete resection of the hemipelvis. *J. Bone Joint Surg.* **60A**, 719–730.

Stoker D.J. and Kissin C.M. (1985) Percutaneous vertebral biopsy: a review of 135 cases. *Clin. Radiol.* **36**, 569–577.

Stoker D.J., Cobb J.P. and Pringle J.A.S. (1991) Needle biopsy of musculoskeletal lesions. A review of 208 procedures. *J. Bone Joint Surg.* **73B**, 498–500.

Strong L.C., Henderson J., Osbourne B.M. and Sutow W.W. (1979) Risk of radiation-related subsequent malignant tumours in survivors of Ewing's sarcoma. *J. Nat. Cancer Inst.* **62**, 1401–1405.

Sundaram M., McGuire M.H. and Herbold D.R. (1987) Magnetic resonance imaging of osteosarcoma. *Skel. Radiol.* **16**, 23–29.

Sweetnam R.D. (1983) Limb preservation in the treatment of bone tumours. *Ann. Roy. Coll. Surg. Engl.* **65**, 3–7.

Swensen S.J., Keller P.L., Berquist T.H., McLeod P.A. and Stephens D.H. (1985) Magnetic resonance imaging of hemorrhage. *Am. J. Roentgen.* **145**, 921–927.

Triche T., Cavazzana A. (1988) Round cell tumours of bone. In Krishnan Unni, K. (ed.) *Bone Tumours*, pp. 199–224. Churchill Livingstone, New York.

Ture-Carel C., Philip I., Berger M-P. *et al.* (1983) Chromosomal translocations in Ewing's sarcoma. *New Engl. J. Med.* **309**, 497–498.

Unni K.K., Dahlin D.C. and Beabout J.W. (1976a) Parosteal osteogenic sarcoma. *Cancer* **37**, 2644–2675.

Unni K.K., Dahlin D.C. and Beabout J.W. (1976b) Periosteal osteogenic sarcoma. *Cancer* **37**, 2476–2485.

Unni K.K. & Dahlin D.C. (1979) Premalignant tumours and conditions of bone. *Am. J. Surg. Pathol.* **3**, 47–58.

Vanel D., Henry-Amar M., Lumbroso J. *et al.* (1984) Pulmonary evaluation of patients with osteosarcoma: roles of standard radiography, tomography, CT, scintigraphy and tomoscintigraphy. *Am. J. Roentgen.* **143**, 519–523.

Van Nes C.P. (1950) Rotation-plasty for congenital defects of the femur. *J. Bone Joint Surg.* **32B**, 12–16.

Voegeli E. and Uehlinger E. (1976) Arteriography in bone tumours. *Skel. Radiol.* **1**, 3–14.

Volkov M. (1970) Allotransplantation of joints. *J. Bone Joint Surg.* **52B**, 49–53.

Ward P.S., Packman P.S., Loughman W. *et al.* (1984) Location of the retinoblastoma susceptibility gene(s) and the human esterase D locus. *J. Med. Genet.* **21**, 92–95.

Weatherby R.P., Dahlin D.C. and Ivins, J.C. (1981) Post-radiation sarcoma of bone: review of 78 Mayo Clinic cases. *Mayo Clin. Proc.* **56**, 294–306.

Weinfeld M.S. and Dudley H.R. (1962) Osteogenic sarcoma. *J. Bone Joint Surg.* **44A**, 269–276.

Wick M.R., McLeod R.A., Siegal G.P. *et al.* (1981) Sarcomas of bone complicating osteitis deformans (Paget's disease): fifty years experience. *Am. J. Surg. Pathol.* **5**, 47–59.

Willert H.G. (1985) Clinical results of the temporary acrylic bone cement plug in the treatment of bone tumors: a multicentric study. In Enneking W.F. (Chairman) *Abstracts of the International Symposium on Limb Salvage in Musculoskeletal Oncology, Orlando, Florida, October 2–5, 1985* (Bristol-Myers/Zimmer Orthopaedic Symposium in cooperation with the Orthopaedic Research and Education Foundation). American Orthopaedic Association.

Willert H.G. and Enderle A. (1983) Temporary bone cement plug: an alternative treatment of large cystic tumorous bone lesions near the joint. In Kotz R. (ed.) *Proceedings of the 2nd International Workshop on the Design and Application of Tumor Prostheses for Bone and Joint Reconstruction*, pp. 69−72. Vienna, Egerman.

Winkelmann W. (1983) Die Umdrehplastik bei malignem proximalen Femurtumoren. *Z. Orthopädie* **121**, 547−549.

Winkler K., Beron G., Kotz R. *et al.* (1986) Einfluss des lokalchirurgischen Vorgehens auf die Inzidenz von Metastasen nach neoadjuvanter Chemotherapie des Osteosarcoms. *Z. Orthopädie* **124**, 22−29.

Wold L.E., Unni K.K. and Beabout J.W. (1984) Dedifferentiated parosteal osteosarcoma. *J. Bone Joint Surg.* **66A**, 53−59.

Wouters H.W. (1974) Tumeur à cellules géantes de l'extrémité distale du fémur avec fracture intra-articulaire de genou: traitée par excochléation et remplissage avec du ciment osseux. *Rev. Chir. orthopéd. Réparat. l'Appareil Moteur* **60** (supplement 2), 316.

Zimmer W.D., Berquist T.H., McLeod R.A. *et al.* (1985) Bone tumours: magnetic resonance imaging versus computed tomography. *Radiology* **155**, 709−718.

Chapter 29

Chemotherapy and Radiotherapy in the Treatment of Primary Malignant Bone Tumours

R.L. Souhami & A. Cassoni

INTRODUCTION

In the last 20 years there have been considerable advances in the treatment of primary bone tumours. These advances have resulted in an improved cure rate and a lower risk of amputation. A better understanding of the interplay between chemotherapy, radiation and surgery has led to an increased awareness that the management of primary bone tumours can no longer be undertaken in centres where such cases are rarely seen. All primary bone tumours are rare and it is now clearly essential for them to be managed in specialized units. Increasingly, referral to such specialist centres is being undertaken even before the diagnosis is made. Management begins with an accurate diagnosis, and bone tumour pathology is difficult as well as being uncommon. Inaccurately and poorly placed open biopsies seriously compromise the possibility of conservative limb surgery and accurate diagnosis can often be made by needle biopsy. Response to treatment is also assessed histopathologically and detailed examination of the resection specimen can be helpful in determining prognosis.

Future progress will undoubtedly involve intensification of treatment and refining of the surgical procedures. The planning and execution of surgery in the middle of intensive chemotherapy is a difficult task. The radiation therapist has also to be fully conversant with the problems of irradiation being given at the same time as chemotherapy and in an area which has either been the site of a resection or where a resection may subsequently be carried out.

PRINCIPLES OF CHEMOTHERAPY

Cytotoxic chemotherapy damages the reproductive integrity of cells. Nuclear DNA appears to be the main target for the lethal effects of many drugs. It is of great interest that the sensitivity of tumour types varies widely but is in roughly the same ranking order for drugs of widely differing classes. Thus lymphoma of bone is sensitive to most cytotoxic drugs, whatever their chemical structure, and chondrosarcoma is resistant. Ewing's sarcoma is a relatively sensitive tumour and osteosarcoma less so.

The main classes of agents used in bone sarcomas are:
1 *Alkylating agents*, e.g. cyclophosphamide and ifosfamide. The latter has been shown to be very active in Ewing's sarcoma but the renal and CNS toxicity is considerable and great care is needed in its administration.
2 *Anthracyclines*, e.g. doxorubicin. These intercalate between the DNA strands and alter the configuration of the helix. Doxorubicin is myelosuppressive, vesicant and causes hair loss. It is highly active in osteosarcoma, Ewing's sarcoma and lymphoma.
3 *Vinca alkaloids* of which the most widely used is vincristine. This is active in bone lymphoma and Ewing's sarcoma. It is not myelosuppressive but causes peripheral neuropathy and is vesicant.
4 *Platinum drugs*, e.g. cisplatin. This is an active drug in osteosarcoma but less is known of its use in Ewing's sarcoma. It is nephrotoxic and is extreme in inducing nausea. The newer analogue carboplatin causes less nausea and nephrotoxicity but does cause more bone marrow suppression. Little is known yet of its activity in Ewing's sarcoma or osteosarcoma.
5 *Antitumour antibiotics*, e.g. actinomycin D which has activity in Ewing's sarcoma. Although used in some protocols for osteosarcoma, its activity is not well substantiated.

Chemotherapy of malignant bone tumours is a task for oncologists and not for surgeons! Intensive combination chemotherapy is dangerous, time-consuming and requires great attention to detail. In inexpert hands the toxicity increases and inappropriate dose reductions lead to worse results. The combination of chemotherapy and radiotherapy is especially dangerous (see below).

The dovetailing of chemotherapy, surgery and radiation means careful, collaborative treatment planning for each patient.

The long-term sequelae of chemotherapy in childhood and early adult life are matters of concern and will undoubtedly lead to modification of treatments in the years ahead. The most important complications are:

1 *Growth delay in childhood and adolescence.* This is due in part to a direct effect on pulsatile pituitary growth hormone release. Measurement of growth velocity must be made during follow-up of all children treated with cytotoxic chemotherapy.

2 *Cardiac toxicity.* This is a major long-term complication of doxorubicin administration and is related to total dose and schedule of administration. Subclinical defects of left-ventricular function are common and the long-term sequelae of these are not yet known.

3 *Renal toxicity.* Both cisplatin and ifosfamide are nephrotoxic causing impaired glomerular filtration and tubular damage. Long-term effects can be minimized by careful attention to dose, schedule and details of drugs administration.

4 *Infertility.* This is an almost universal problem for males treated with large doses of alkylating agents. It appears to be less severe with drugs such as cisplatin and doxorubicin. The period of reproductive life may be shortened in women. Pelvic irradiation involving the ovaries leads to complete cessation of ovarian function.

5 *Second cancers.* Alkylating agents (especially melphalan and chlorambucil) are associated with an increased risk of leukaemia. Doxorubicin appears to decrease the latent period before radiation-induced bone sarcoma appears.

PRINCIPLES OF RADIOTHERAPY

Ionizing radiation has been used to destroy malignant tissue since early this century. At therapeutic doses, cell death is due to damage to DNA, resulting in loss of genetic material. Death of the damaged cell occurs after subsequent mitosis. Both malignant and normal tissues will sustain this damage, but, by administering the radiation in a number of small doses rather than one large dose, it is possible to eradicate tumour while maintaining the integrity of the tumour-bearing normal tissue. Fractionation of radiotherapy over several weeks is the basis of the currently accepted therapeutic ratio between tumour destruction and normal tissue tolerance.

The effectiveness of radiation in treating any tumour depends on the natural history of the disease. Effective local control has limited impact on survival if the risk of metastases is high. Like surgery, it is a local treatment and its usefulness is in local tumour destruction where surgery is not possible or morbidity unacceptable. Various factors influence the efficacy of radiation in producing tumour sterilization. Tumour bulk is an important prognostic factor as the level of cell kill is exponentially related to dose. The chances, therefore, of eliminating all cells are greater the smaller the number there are to start with.

Some tumours are more radiosensitive than others. Among bone tumours, lymphoma and Ewing's sarcoma are relatively sensitive, while osteosarcoma and chondrosarcoma are amongst the most resistant. The intrinsic cellular sensitivity varies with tissue type, but differences in tumour population kinetics, as well as elements of the tumour environment such as hypoxia, also affect tumour control.

Radioresponsiveness, as judged by regression of detectable masses, while related to tumour control, does not necessarily predict control. Where clonogenic cells proliferative slowly, radiation-induced cell death may occur long after the radiation has been inflicted. Regression of masses of soft-tissue sarcoma or infiltrative fibromatosis, for example, may occur over many months or even years. Where a considerable proportion of the tumour is composed of non-cellular elements such as osteoid, chondroid or fibrous tissue, persistent tumour bulk may not reflect the degree of clonogenic cell kill.

Acute effects of radiotherapy

Normal tissues will experience both acute and late side-effects to a degree and severity that will depend on the radiation dose, the nature and volume of normal tissue included in the volume. Inclusion of a large amount of the gastrointestinal tract will produce side-effects during and immediately after the course of therapy. Nausea, sore mouth and diarrhoea may occur depending on the precise site treated. The inclusion of bone marrow, in large vertebral or pelvic fields, for example, while uncommonly producing marrow depression alone, may further depress or maintain depression produced by chemotherapy.

Late effects of radiotherapy

Should acute morbidity prove unacceptably severe, treatment may be interrupted or modified. However, some tissues only exhibit damage months or years after radiation. The late morbidities most relevant to bone tumours are those affecting limb function. Radiation of active epiphyses will stop growth and, where possible, these are excluded from the field. Where vertebrae must be irradiated the full width should be included to prevent scoliosis. Soft tissues, when treated to doses necessary to control sarcomas, will become firmer and stiffer. This may be marked where joint capsules are radiated. With careful radiotherapy technique and an active prophylactic physiotherapy programme, these effects can be minimized and ankylosis avoided.

The spinal cord is able to tolerate lower doses than other tissue and damage will not be manifest for months or even years. Where the cord cannot be excluded from the high dose volume the risk can be minimized by using smaller doses in each fraction. Peripheral nerves are rarely damaged by doses of 50–60 Gy but higher doses, especially to the brachial plexus, may produce painful neuropathy.

Second malignancy

The carcinogenic and leukaemogenic potential of ionizing radiation and certain cytotoxic agents are well described. The level of risk and factors affecting it in patients treated for cancer are, however, complex. The familial form of retinoblastoma is associated with greatly increased risks of osteosarcoma at any site and this risk is even greater in the irradiated field. A young age at radiation increases the risk of radiation-induced cancer. Radiation quality and total dose also affect risk in ways not yet entirely clear.

Radiation-induced bone sarcomas have been reported by many authors and have been extensively studied. A relative risk of 649 in those treated for Ewing's was found by Tucker *et al.* (1987) with a cumulative risk of approximately 5% at 20 years for a group of patients treated for a variety of tumours. These were predominantly osteosarcomas and chondrosarcomas, and the majority were within or close to the radiation field. The risk of developing bone sarcomas is less for cancers of adult life but radiation-induced bone sarcomas do occur and the prognosis is poor since the tumours are aggressive (Huvos, 1986).

Total body radiation

This may be used as part of intensive chemotherapy regimens that require bone marrow transplantation. This approach has been used in relapsed Ewing's sarcoma but must still be considered experimental. The whole body is radiated at continuous low dose rate over 6–8 h to 10 Gy or in 6–8 fractions over 3–4 days to 12–14 Gy.

Radiotherapy for palliation

Radiotherapy may be very effective in palliation in several circumstances. It is most effective in the more sensitive tumours such as Ewing's sarcoma but may produce rapid relief from bone pain even in the more resistant tumours. Such treatment may be given in a few high-dose fractions. Where symptoms are due to compression, however, high doses are required in osteosarcoma and high-grade spindle-cell sarcomas. Multiple sites of metastases in sensitive tumours may respond to a single hemibody radiation or to intravenous radioactive strontium.

OSTEOSARCOMA

Chemotherapy

Studies of chemosensitivity of osteosarcoma have usually been carried out in patients who have had previous cytotoxic chemotherapy and who have pulmonary metastases. In this setting metastatic osteosarcoma has not shown itself to be a tumour that is sensitive to many cytotoxic agents. Clinical trials of this kind, however, underestimate the effectiveness of chemotherapy since drug resistance is usually present and the sensitivity of established metastases may be different from that of micrometastases which are assumed to be present when chemotherapy is used as an adjuvant to surgery in patients who do not have visible metastatic disease.

A list of the most active agents is shown in Table 29.1. Methotrexate (MTX) was one of the first agents to be used in osteosarcoma and has typically been used in high-dose MTX. High-dose MTX can be given safely provided that great care is taken over drug administration and the details of folic acid rescue. Jaffe *et al.* (1973)

Table 29.1 Approximate response rates to single chemotherapeutic agents in metastatic osteosarcoma. Data taken from Bramwell (1987) and Pratt (1979)

Drug	Response (%)*
Cyclophosphamide	14
Actinomycin D	10
Melphalan	15
Doxorubicin	20
Cisplatin	20
High-dose methotrexate	25
Ifosfamide	25

* Most responses are partial. Includes both previously treated and untreated cases.

and Isacoff *et al.* (1978) showed that partial remissions could be achieved in metastatic disease using doses of 50 mg/kg or more. Overall the response rate to high dose methotrexate as a single agent is probably of the order of 25–35%. There has been no conclusive evidence that, as a single agent, high-dose MTX has an advantage over lower doses of methotrexate. Although this drug schedule is being incorporated into clinical practice without a firm basis it seems probable that this is the most effective use of the drug. The controversies over high-dose MTX are well reviewed by Grem *et al.* (1988).

Doxorubicin (Adriamycin) produces regression in approximately 25% of tumours (Cortes *et al.*, 1972; Pratt and Shanks, 1974; Pratt, 1979). The optimum dose and schedule for doxorubicin has not been evaluated. Most regimens use doxorubicin in divided doses over 2–3 days. There is some evidence that cardiotoxicity, which is a considerable problem with doxorubicin therapy, is less if very high peak plasma values are not achieved and a divided or infusion regimen may help to lower the incidence of this complication. Cisplatin is an active agent (Rosen *et al.*, 1980; Gasparini *et al.*, 1985; Pratt *et al.*, 1985). Response rates of 15–27% are recorded in previously treated patients which places the drug with the same range of activity as high-dose MTX and doxorubicin. Ifosfamide has been introduced into chemotherapy of osteosarcoma and responses of 25% are recorded in previously treated patients (Brade *et al.*, 1985; Klegar *et al.*, 1986). Other agents such as cyclophosphamide and melphalan appear to have lower activity—perhaps of the order of 10–20% (see review by Bramwell, 1987).

Intra-arterial chemotherapy has been intensively studied but no firm evidence has been produced for its improved efficacy over chemotherapy by the intravenous route. Although intra-arterial chemotherapy would be attractive if it allowed a greater proportion of patients to undergo conservative, limb salvage, surgery, it must not be forgotten that the main aim of chemotherapy is to treat metastasis and limb perfusion has not been developed for this purpose. The drug most commonly used in limb perfusion is cisplatin (Mavligit, 1981; Jaffe *et al.*, 1989). Responses occur in over 70% of patients as judged histologically by tumour necrosis. Jaffe *et al.* (1989) showed that healing of the tumour may be so dramatic that soft-tissue masses may disappear and pathological fractures can heal. Doxorubicin has been used intra-arterially (Stephens *et al.*, 1987) and so has high-dose MTX (Jaffe *et al.*, 1983). High-dose MTX, however, achieves very high blood levels when given intravenously and doxorubicin can only be given safely in a large artery. These considerations restrict the use of both drugs intra-arterially. The COSS group in West Germany are conducting a randomization between intra-arterial and intravenous cisplatin in the context of a combination chemotherapy adjuvant study. In this situation it may be difficult to show whether one route has an advantage over the other but this is the realistic setting for intra-arterial treatment.

Each of these agents is accompanied by significant short-term and long-term toxicity. High-dose MTX has to be very carefully handled since prolonged excretion can lead to dangerous myelosuppression, mucositis and renal damage. The drug is extremely expensive, and so is the folinic acid rescue needed for its safe use. Transient elevation of liver transaminases are almost always observed. Cisplatin is the agent most disliked by patients since it causes severe nausea and vomiting. In recent years this has been partially mitigated by the use of 5-HT$_3$ antagonists but the complication is still severe. There is both short-term and long-term alteration of renal function. In the short term, elevations of blood urea and serum creatinine are frequent and tubular disorders with loss of calcium and magnesium may give rise to clinical tetany. In the longer term, peripheral neuropathy and progressive renal impairment may be seen. The peripheral neuropathy, usually subclinical, has become more prominent as experience with high-dose platinum has been gained. Doxorubicin causes myocardial damage. This is not usually clinically apparent unless doses greater than 450 mg/m^2 are given. Nevertheless it has to be borne in mind that patients with osteosarcoma are young and considerable subclinical left-ventricular damage may occur which may only be apparent in later adult life as coronary artery disease develops. Ifosfamide is now recognized as being severely nephrotoxic, causing renal tubular defects with loss of amino acids, phosphate and calcium. These renal tubular defects may be long lasting and biochemical osteomalacia, and even clinical rickets, may develop. For these reasons there is considerable attention being paid to ways of minimizing long-term toxicity in patients with osteosarcoma. It may be possible to identify patients at low risk of metastasis who may be treated with less intensive chemotherapy programmes. At the present time, however, the long-term results (see below) are not sufficiently encouraging to justify reduction of the amount of chemotherapy for all patients.

Combination chemotherapy is generally associated with a higher response rate in metastatic osteosarcoma, although again the problems of previous treatment lead to an underestimation of the effects of drug treatment. Examples of response rates with various combinations

Table 29.2 Response rates to combination chemotherapy in metastatic osteosarcoma

Drug	Response (%)*
CP, HDMTX, VCR	30–40
CP, DOX	25–45
CY, VCR, DOX, ACT	25
CY, VCR, DOX, DTIC	25
B, CY, ACT	35

* Responses are complete and partial, and are composites of small-scale studies. They are therefore approximations. CP, cisplatin; HDMTX, high-dose methotrexate; VCR, vincristine; DOX, doxorubicin; ACT, actinomycin D; B, bleomycin.

Table 29.3 Some non-randomized trials of adjuvant chemotherapy in operable osteogenic sarcoma (trial size greater than 50 patients)

Trial	Protocol†	n	Relapse-free survival (%)
Rosen *et al.* (1979, 1982)	T4, T5	52	48
	T7	54	80
	T10	79	92*
Pratt *et al.* (1984)	HDMTX DOX, CP	51	51†
Eckhardt *et al.* (1985)	DOX, VCR, HDMTX	57	62‡
Ryan *et al.* (1990)	CY, VCR, DOX	58	40 (10-year follow-up
Cortes *et al.* (1981)	DOX	88	48 (6-year follow-up)

* Follow-up only 22 months.
† Follow-up only 30 months.
‡ Follow-up only 32 months.
HDMTX, high-dose methotrexate; DOX, doxorubicin; CP, cisplatin; VCR, vincristine; CY, cyclophosphamide; DTIC, dicarbazine.

are shown in Table 29.2. From this it can be seen that the combinations using cisplatin, high-dose MTX and doxorubicin are among the most active. Response duration is usually short in metastatic disease.

ADJUVANT CHEMOTHERAPY

This was introduced in the early 1970s. Among the first studies were those carried out by Jaffe *et al.* (1974) and Rosen *et al.* (1974). These studies were uncontrolled. The early results of Jaffe *et al.* (1974) were greeted with great enthusiasm but attempts to repeat the comparison of the use of adjuvant high-dose methotrexate with historical controls led to less impressive results (Rosenberg *et al.*, 1979). Rosen and his colleagues at the Memorial Sloan–Kettering Hospital carried out a series of uncontrolled studies of combination chemotherapy as an adjuvant to surgery (Rosen *et al.*, 1974, 1978, 1982; Rosen, 1985). These regimens were based on high-dose methotrexate, doxorubicin and a drug combination of bleomycin, cyclophosphamide and actinomycin D (Table 29.2). In the later studies chemotherapy was given before definitive surgery and if there was a poor histological response in the resection specimen, platinum and doxorubicin were used post-operatively.

The early results of the most complex of these programmes—the so-called T10 protocol—were impressive with two-year survival rates in excess of 80% (Rosen *et al.*, 1982). Interpretation of this seemingly dramatic improvement in survival was made difficult by the very short follow-up period, the lack of any prospective control, the alteration in selection criteria which had occurred during the 1970s with the introduction of computed tomography scanning and the fact that the results were being reported from a single centre, making comparisons with multicentre studies difficult. Taylor

et al. (1985) suggested that survival of patients being treated with adjuvant chemotherapy was improving without chemotherapy as a result of case selection and other factors. Edmondson *et al.* (1984) showed, in a very small study where high-dose methotrexate was randomized to no treatment, that there was no difference in survival. Representative results of these uncontrolled adjuvant therapy studies are shown in Table 29.3.

There was therefore considerable controversy at this time about the role of adjuvant chemotherapy. Although most investigators felt that some progress was being achieved by the use of chemotherapy, it was not clear to what extent the reported improved results were due to the chemotherapy alone, and whether the undoubted toxicity and expense of chemotherapy justified the effort (Lange and Levine, 1982). The publication of two studies comparing chemotherapy with a control group has resolved some of this difficulty but not all. In 1986 Link *et al.* (1986) reported on behalf of the multi-institutional osteosarcoma study. This study was a comparison of immediate T10-based chemotherapy versus no chemotherapy until disease became evident on relapse. The study was difficult to perform since many patients refused randomization. In the small number (36) who agreed to be randomized there was a clear difference in relapse-free survival in favour of chemotherapy given at diagnosis. This difference was also apparent in those patients who refused to be randomized but who elected either for or against chemotherapy. At the time of the report (1986), however, there was no difference in overall survival between the two policies. A long-term follow up of this study is awaited. Eckhardt and co-workers (1985) from the University of California, Los Angeles carried out a study of somewhat different design in which, after initial intra-arterial doxorubicin and tumour irradiation, 27 patients received no further chemotherapy following surgery and 32 patients received post-operative treatment with high-dose methotrexate and vincristine, doxorubicin and BCD (bleomycin, cyclophosphamide, dactinomycin; see Table 29.2). There was a significant improvement in relapse-free survival and overall survival in patients who received adjuvant chemotherapy post-operatively.

There are many major questions still to be determined about adjuvant chemotherapy for osteosarcoma. Firstly, what is the long-term outlook at the present time for patients treated with combination chemotherapy programmes? We do not have many long-term follow-up data on patients treated with intensive combination chemotherapy. In a report on the long-term follow-up from the South West Oncology Group on patients treated with CY-VADIC (see Table 29.2), the survival curve showed relapse continuing after chemotherapy to 10 years (Ryan *et al.*, 1990). Although 65% of patients were alive at 3 years, and 55% at 5 years, by 10 years only 40% of patients had not died. A recent report from the Memorial Sloan–Kettering Hospital (Meyers *et al.*, 1992) describes the long-term survival of 279 patients treated with adjuvant chemotherapy. The T10 protocol produced a 75% 5-year survival from this single centre. Adverse prognostic factors were increased age, Afro-American origin, and a poor histological response to chemotherapy in the resection specimen.

Many oncologists are now becoming increasingly familiar with late relapse following chemotherapy. Although late pulmonary metastasis can occasionally be salvaged by thoracotomy (see below), some of these late relapses are of high-grade aggressive osteosarcoma and many patients die. It seems likely, from long-term follow up in European studies, that at the present time about 55–60% of patients will be cured with the use of adjuvant chemotherapy. This compares favourably with series reported in the early 1970s when either no chemotherapy or low-dose chemotherapy was used and survival was approximately 25–35% (MRC, 1986).

The second question is whether chemotherapy of the T10 type using multiple agents and lasting 44 weeks is necessary to produce optimum results. In the recent European Osteosarcoma Intergroup (EOI) study results

comparable to T10 have been achieved with only 17 weeks therapy using doxorubicin and cisplatin in full dose (Bramwell *et al.*, 1988). This group is undertaking a formal randomized comparison between a T10-based programme and this two drug regimen. The trial has now been closed with 400 patients randomized. If the results are equal this will allow development of programmes which are of higher intensity but shorter duration.

Increasing intensity of treatment may prove difficult since current regimens are already severely myelo-suppressive and nephrotoxic. The use of haemopoietic growth factors may allow a modest increase in the amount of drug delivered but it is likely that other toxicities than myelosuppression will then prove dose limiting. The EOI is exploring more intensive regimens of treatment in patients with metastasis, for example a dose-intensive combination chemotherapy programme using doxorubicin, cisplatin, ifosfamide and high-dose methotrexate. It seems, at the present time, that the main obstacle to progress lies in incompletely effective chemotherapy in approximately 45% of patients. In other patients, where there is a low risk of metastasis (small tumours, low alkaline phosphatase, no inflammatory signs around the tumour), it may be possible to reduce chemotherapy, particularly doxorubicin, in view of the long-term toxic effects. It is still not clear, however, whether such patients can be accurately defined before chemotherapy begins.

It is now the usual practice to give chemotherapy before surgery. This practice was introduced by Rosen *et al.* (1979) who advanced several reasons for it being a logical development. The most important of these were that the use of chemotherapy allowed response to cytotoxic drugs to be assessed both clinically and histopathologically. The second major reason was that it left time for planning of definitive surgery, particularly conservative surgery. If a response to chemotherapy was achieved then conservative surgery might be technically possible in patients who, at the outset, had only borderline operable tumours. It was also suggested by Rosen *et al.* (1982) that the histopathological response could be used as a guide to selecting post-operative chemotherapy. This argument seems flawed since it has not been the experience in this cancer, or indeed in other tumours, that tumours which are resistant to multiple agents of one kind will nevertheless retain useful sensitivity to other drugs. Some degree of cross-resistance between cytotoxic drugs is usually observed. Experience from the West German Coss-82 studies (1988) suggests that it is an unwise policy to leave out effective agents (particularly cisplatin and doxorubicin) and reserve these for patients who are not responding subsequently.

Pre-operative ('neo-adjuvant') chemotherapy has thus become a fairly accepted practice in the management of osteosarcoma. There are, however, several clinical problems with its use. Firstly, if patients do not respond to chemotherapy significantly, this allows metastases to occur which might not otherwise have taken place. Secondly, poorly or non-responsive tumours may grow, making conservative surgery less possible after treatment than it was at the time of diagnosis. Thirdly, chemotherapy response may lead to conservative surgery being carried out under circumstances which are not altogether wise. Thus diffuse muscle infiltration, pathological fractures, and a large soft-tissue mass are all pointers towards a high risk of local recurrence. Even if there is a response to chemotherapy this may not eradicate all microscopic disease at the site of the surgery and local recurrence rates may rise. Finally, there is now a tendency to imply to patients that conservative surgery is the aim of treatment and to create a pressure for chemotherapy even under circumstances where amputation is clearly the only possible surgical procedure. It should be remembered that many patients lead an acceptable and well-adjusted life after amputation and that the object of treatment is to save the patient's life and prevent untreatable local recurrence. Clinicians must avoid being 'boxed into a corner' by appearing to promise limb preservation under circumstances where it is ill-advised.

Response assessment therefore becomes of critical importance. At the present time this is judged clinically in most cases, but computed tomography scanning can help by showing reduction in soft-tissue mass. Other techniques that have been used include serial quantitative isotope scanning and magnetic resonance imaging scanning but these are not yet either well validated or generally available.

A further problem with the use of pre-operative chemotherapy is that, with intensive myelosuppression, the timing and the performance of the surgery become a matter of considerable expertise. It is unwise to allow long delays in chemotherapy both before and after surgery and the coordination between oncologist and surgeon has to be finely adjusted. This is a further reason why the management of these highly specialized problems are best carried out in centres with particular experience.

Radiotherapy in osteosarcoma

Radiotherapy does not usually play a role in the primary management of this reputedly radioresistant tumour. Useful responses may, however, be achieved although

high doses are required. Complete necrosis may be produced in 30% of those irradiated to 60–70 Gy (Cade, 1955) and in up to 80% when given with chemotherapy (Caceres *et al.*, 1984). Experience with radiotherapy as an adjuvant to surgery, where margins are limited by anatomical constraints, suggests that microscopic disease may be controlled. Improved survival compared with surgically treated historical controls has been suggested in mandibular and maxillary osteosarcoma following post-operative radiotherapy alone (Chamber and Mahoney, 1970) or with chemotherapy (De Fries *et al.*, 1970; Akbiyik and Alexander, 1981).

These observations indicate that osteosarcoma is not totally radioresistant and may have a role where there is residual microscopic disease. Marked regression of bulky tumours, however, is unusual. High doses are necessary even for palliation and attempts to palliate large, painful limb primaries may be fruitless, particularly if most of a limb circumference must be treated.

Prophylactic pulmonary radiation

Adjuvant lung irradiation has been studied, primarily in osteosarcoma, with varying results. Two studies, one randomized, using doses of 20 Gy report improved survival rates (Breur *et al.*, 1978; Newton *et al.*, 1978) while others, using lower doses with or without concomitant chemotherapy, reported no benefit (Rab *et al.*, 1976; Caceres *et al.*, 1978).

Overall, prophylactic pulmonary radiation has no demonstrated value in current intensive combined modality protocols. It may, however, have a role in those with established pulmonary disease, following excision and this is the subject of clinical investigation at present. Increased pulmonary toxicity may occur after exposure to cytotoxics with actinomycin or bleomycin, especially. Mediastinal radiation may carry the risk of subsequent cardiomyopathy in those who have received maximal doses of antracyclines. Doses of 20 Gy in 12–15 fractions are well tolerated although they may produce subclinical changes in pulmonary function. Higher doses to smaller areas of particular risk may be given in addition.

Treatment of special problems in osteosarcoma

SMALL-CELL OSTEOSARCOMA

This variant of osteosarcoma was first reported by Sim *et al.* in 1979. The tumour is composed of small cells and resembles Ewing's sarcoma or lymphoma. It is distinguished from Ewing's sarcoma if the cells can be shown to produce alkaline phosphatase. It is distinguishable from lymphoma by the fact that the cells do not stain for common leucocyte antigen. According to Ayala *et al.* (1989), the tumour cells may contain intracytoplasmic glycogen. In that series the prognosis seemed poor with 50% of patients dead in 2 years and a poor response of distant metastases to chemotherapeutic treatment.

TELANGIECTATIC OSTEOSARCOMA

These large destructive tumours constitute about 10% of all cases of osteosarcoma (Huvos *et al.*, 1982). In this series, where patients were given adjuvant chemotherapy, the prognosis did not appear to be worse than for conventional osteosarcoma. Chemoresponsiveness was also reported by Chawla *et al.* (1985) who showed responses in five of eight patients treated with intra-arterial cisplatin and intravenous doxorubicin and DTIC. Subsequently, Rosen *et al.* (1986) reported histopathological response in 11 of 16 patients who had pre-operative chemotherapy of the T10 type.

PAROSTEAL OSTEOSARCOMA

This tumour is of relatively low grade malignancy with a much lower risk of metastasis. Occasionally, metastases do occur and dedifferentiation of the tumour to a high-grade osteosarcoma is also recorded (Wold *et al.*, 1984). Adjuvant chemotherapy is not given for typical parosteal osteosarcoma but is usually administered if there are major areas of high-grade tumour within the primary resection specimen, or if metastases or dedifferentiation occur.

PERIOSTEAL OSTEOSARCOMA

Periosteal osteosarcoma is of relatively high grade (Unni *et al.*, 1976) but with a lower risk of metastasis than in conventional central osteosarcoma. It is not known if adjuvant chemotherapy will affect the relatively low rate of metastasis. It should be given if there is extensive local infiltration or if metastases occur. It is our current practice to treat all these patients with adjuvant chemotherapy for 9 weeks both pre- and post-operatively.

OSTEOSARCOMA DURING PREGNANCY

Huvos *et al.* (1985) could find no evidence that pregnancy worsens the prognosis of osteosarcoma but the necessity for early chemotherapy means that termination is advised if the patient is in the first trimester. If the patient is in the third trimester early delivery is undertaken (Simon *et al.*, 1984).

POST-RADIATION AND PAGET'S OSTEOSARCOMA

These tumours are usually of high grade histologically and appearances may not always be of classical osteosarcoma. In Paget's disease malignant fibrous histiocytoma and lymphoma may also develop and post-radiation sarcomas may also have a marked spindle-celled component similar to malignant fibrous histiocytoma (Haibach *et al.*, 1985). The tumours often arise in the axial skeleton, and, when they do surgery may be extremely difficult particularly if the patient is elderly. Nevertheless surgical resection has to be the mainstay of treatment and the sensitivity of these tumours to chemotherapy is largely unexplored. Huvos *et al.* (1986) found a very poor prognosis for both radiation and Paget's sarcoma.

OSTEOSARCOMA IN OLD AGE

In the elderly osteosarcoma often arises in an area of Paget's disease or at an irradiated site but about 40% of cases arise in an otherwise normal bone. Huvos *et al.* (1986) found that fibrohistiocytomatous forms were the most frequent with osteoblastic histology being the second most common type. The tumours are more commonly axial skeletal than the classical osteosarcoma of childhood and adolescence. As in Paget's sarcomas and radiation sarcomas, the mainstay of treatment is surgical but there are serious problems due to the tumour location. Chemotherapy of the intensity of that given to young patients is seldom possible. The overall survival is poor with only 4% surviving 5 years when associated with Paget's disease but with 30% 5-year survival for those arising in an otherwise normal bone.

Conclusions

There is no doubt that chemotherapy has improved the survival of osteosarcoma. Figure 29.1 shows the survival curves for children with osteosarcoma diagnosed in the UK between the years 1971 and 1985. It can be seen that in each 2-year period there has been a steady improvement in survival but the most dramatic increase has come following 1983 at a time when national intensive programmes for chemotherapy were first introduced. These survival curves represent the true state of affairs in a single country for children below the age of 16 years. Nevertheless 50% of patients are not cured and

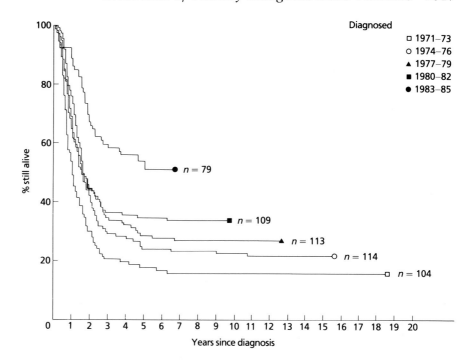

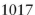

Fig. 29.1 Survival for all UK children with osteosarcoma under the age of 16 in the period 1971–1985. (From Stiller and Bunch, 1990, with permission.)

future advances will come from improving chemotherapy and from diminishing toxicity.

A major obstacle in showing that results are improving lies in the fact that even improvements in survival of 10–15% (all that realistically can be expected from a new chemotherapy programme) requires trials of 500 patients or more. In such a rare disease this is only possible by national and international collaboration and this must surely be the aim.

EWING'S SARCOMA

Single-agent chemotherapy

Unlike osteosarcoma, Ewing's sarcoma shows a much higher response rate to cytotoxic drug administration. The most useful drugs are alkylating agents, doxorubicin, actinomycin and vincristine.

Alkylating agents were among the first drugs to be used in Ewing's sarcoma. Sutow and Sullivan (1962) showed that cyclophosphamide was active in metastatic disease and these findings were confirmed by Samuels and Howell (1967). Cyclophosphamide has been the standard alkylating agent used in the disease although other drugs such as mustine and chlorambucil are also active. In recent years there has been considerable interest in the use of ifosfamide which differs from cyclophosphamide in the position of one of the chloroethyl groups. Ifosfamide is a highly effective agent in Ewing's sarcoma with response rates approaching 40%

even in patients previously treated with chemotherapy (Magrath *et al.*, 1986). The activity of ifosfamide has led to its incorporation in many recent programmes of chemotherapy treatment in the disease. The sensitivity of Ewing's sarcoma to alkylating agents has led to the use of very high-dose melphalan as a treatment in relapsed disease. Although responses are frequently seen (Graham-Pole *et al.*, 1984) such responses are usually short lived and high-dose alkylating chemotherapy is not an established treatment.

Vincristine was shown to be active by Selawry *et al.* (1968) and has been incorporated into most programmes of treatment, as has actinomycin. Doxorubicin was introduced by Wang *et al.* (1971) and by Oldham and Pomeroy (1972). The importance of doxorubicin in current programmes was emphasized by a multi-institutional randomized trial, IESS-1 (Nesbit *et al.*, 1981), which showed that the addition of doxorubicin to vincristine, actinomycin and cyclophosphamide significantly improved the disease free survival at 2 years and subsequently (Nesbit *et al.*, 1990). Other drugs with useful activity are etoposide and BCNU (Palma *et al.*, 1972). The latter is limited in its use by the prolonged myelosuppression which nitrosureas produce.

There seems little doubt that the major determinant of prognosis in Ewing's sarcoma is the volume of the tumour at the time of presentation. Both Hayes *et al.* (1989) and Jürgens *et al.* (1988) have shown that tumour volume is the most important determinant and probably accounts for the difference in prognosis which is always observed between limb Ewing's sarcoma and axial skel-etal (particularly pelvic) Ewing's sarcoma. Tumours in the pelvis often grow to enormous size before diagnosis is made. Almost all published series show that pelvic primaries carry a particularly poor prognosis. In assess-ing the results of combination chemotherapy pro-grammes it is important to keep in mind that different proportions of patients with different size tumours will almost certainly account for substantial differences in long-term results. Only randomized trials are capable of distinguishing the value of one treatment with another. Such randomized comparisons have seldom been made in Ewing's sarcoma and accounts for the uncertainty which surrounds the details of many of the current treatment programmes.

It seems probable that the small, round-cell tumour of bone with neuroendocrine features histologically (primitive neuroectodermal tumours: PNET), have a worse prognosis than classical Ewing's sarcoma. PNETs often occur in the chest wall and tend to be more common in young men. There may also be an increased tendency to metastasis generally, and to sites unusual for classical Ewing's sarcoma, such as lymph nodes and brain. Several reports (Hartman *et al.*, 1991; Schmidt *et al.*, 1991) have indicated a rather adverse outcome.

The report of Hayes *et al.* (1989) from St. Jude's Hospital indicated that 3-year survivals in excess of 70% could be obtained with combination chemotherapy using relatively low-dose cyclophosphamide and doxo-rubicin. The drugs were given in a sequential manner. These data require independent confirmation and com-parison with other regimens. The second intergroup Ewing's sarcoma study is evaluating more intensive chemotherapy based largely on cyclophosphamide and doxorubicin but long-term results are not yet available. At the Memorial Sloan–Kettering Hospital, Rosen has reported a series of studies in Ewing's sarcoma (Rosen *et al.*, 1981; Rosen, 1982). These programmes (called T2, T6 and T9) have used multi-agent chemotherapy including vincristine, doxorubicin, actinomycin D and cyclophosphamide, initially over a period of 18 months. Subsequently bleomycin, BCNU and low-dose metho-trexate were added but the drug programme was con-tinued for 9 months. In the latest publication (Rosen, 1982), disease free survival rates of 65%, 76% and 90% were reported for axial skeletal lesions, lesions in the proximal long bones and distal bones respectively. These are outstanding results from a single institution and have not been independently confirmed.

In the UK, the UKCCSG used vincristine, doxorubicin, actinomycin and cyclophosphamide with an overall sur-vival of 39% over 4 years. This study included many

patients with poor prognosis and a later follow-up than is usually reported in most of the previous studies. In the current MRC/UKCCSG programme, intensive chemo-therapy with ifosfamide, vincristine and doxorubicin is used as induction treatment with actinomycin substi-tuted for doxorubicin after the primary tumour has been treated with either surgery or radiotherapy at 12 weeks. Current results (unpublished) indicate that there is prob-ably an improved outlook compared with the results of the previous study although comparisons with historical data are always suspect. A very similar approach to the UK group has been adopted by the Cooperative Ewing's Sarcoma studies in West Germany. In a 5-year follow-up report (Jürgens *et al.*, 1988) a disease free survival of 51% was reported.

Figure 29.2 shows the overall survival for all children below the age of 16 years with Ewing's sarcoma diag-nosed between 1971 and 1985 in the UK (Stiller and Bunch, 1990). It can be seen that, contrary to the results in osteosarcoma, there appears to have been little change in survival during this period. It should be noted, how-ever, that the more intensive programmes of treatment have only recently been introduced.

One of the outstanding problems in the management of Ewing's sarcoma is the optimum management of the local tumour. Although Ewing's sarcoma is radiosen-sitive (in comparison with osteosarcoma), the long sur-vival now being achieved with chemotherapy means that late relapse at the local site has been fairly frequently observed (Gasparini *et al.*, 1981). This, again, is related to tumour bulk (Jürgens *et al.*, 1988). Late relapse is particularly likely to occur in pelvic primaries even with high doses of radiation. Surgical excision of the tumour may help to reduce the risk of local recurrence but, of course, surgical excision is easier with small tumours than with large ones, and the problem of local control is less pressing with small lesions.

Radiotherapy in Ewing's sarcoma

Debate continues over the roles of radiotherapy and surgery in the management of primary Ewing's sarcoma, as advances in surgical techniques allow conservative techniques for increasing numbers of patients. Direct comparison of surgery and radiotherapy must be inter-preted with caution because of the effect of bulk on case selection, local control and survival. Ewing's sarcoma is radiosensitive as judged both by tumour shrinkage and long-term control. Control rates of 50–70% are reported for radiotherapy alone, increasing to 70–90% when used with effective combination chemotherapy (Perez *et al.*, 1977). Nevertheless, there are several concerns

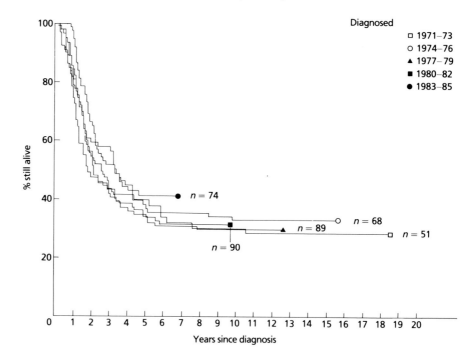

Fig. 29.2 Survival for all UK children with Ewing's sarcoma under the age of 16 in the period 1971–1985. (From Stiller and Bunch, 1990, with permission.)

regarding its use. The local control rates reported may be overoptimistic. Currently, survival is 40–50%, most relapse occurring within 3 years. A series of patients treated at the National Cancer Institute demonstrated persistent, residual tumour at the primary site in 13 out of 20 autopsies despite the absence of suspicious clinical or radiological features (Telles *et al.*, 1978). If survival is improved by more effective chemotherapy, more patients may be at risk of local relapse.

As more patients survive, the problems of treatment-induced second malignancies become apparent. That associated with radiation in Ewing's sarcoma is osteosarcoma within the radiation field. The incidence varies between institutions and, critically, on length of follow-up. Four out of 24 Ewing's patients were reported from the M.D. Anderson (Strong *et al.*, 1979) while only 3 of 251 from the IESS-I study developed osteosarcoma (Perez *et al.*, 1981). Dose and radiation quality may also be relevant; the M.D. Anderson series were treated to higher doses, and some with orthovoltage.

The third issue relates to morbidity. Sufficient reporting of morbidity is rarely provided to allow assessment of the long-term consequences of local treatment. Radiotherapy should be avoided for primaries of the foot and hand or where a growing epiphysis would be included. Current practice in the UK is to offer surgery wherever possible. Radiation is added if there is residual microscopic disease at the edge of the resection specimen.

Both the dose and volume required have been changed by the development of effective cytotoxic regimens. It is

no longer considered necessary to irradiate the whole length of the bone. Sparing of the epiphyses distant to the tumour does not compromise control (MacIntosh *et al.*, 1975; Suit, 1975). There is also a suggestion that local relapse rate associated with inadequate radiation fields is reduced with more effective cytotoxic regimens (Perez *et al.*, 1981). Attempts to reduce dose to 30–35 Gy following actinomycin and cyclophosphamide induction resulted in an increased relapse rate (Hayes *et al.*, 1983; Thomas *et al.*, 1984). There is, however, no demonstrable dose response beyond 45–50 Gy with intensive chemotherapy (Thomas *et al.*, 1984; Jürgens *et al.*, 1988). Complications have a clear dose response. Current recommendations are to treat a wide volume to 40–45 Gy with a further 10–15 Gy to the site of the primary. The volume is based on the prechemotherapy extent with a margin of 5 cm where possible.

Principles of radiotherapy planning and treatment

The nature of the radiotherapy affects both local control and morbidity. The CESS study in Ewing's showed a fall in local relapse when radiotherapy was planned centrally (Jürgens *et al.*, 1988). Skeletal problems in irradiated children are less severe in patients currently treated than in those between 1940 to 1970 as a result of more sophisticated approaches (Butler *et al.*, 1990).

The first step is the definition of the target volume, using similar considerations to those used to plan a surgical resection. The full width of the tumour-bearing bone must be included, with a reasonable margin, defined around the pre-chemotherapy volume and taking into consideration the surgical procedure and findings. A minimum margin of 5 cm is used where possible. It is usual to reduce the field for the final third of treatment, giving the highest dose to the area of greatest risk. Various measures may be taken to reduce tissue morbidity. Small bowel may be excluded by positioning the patient prone for treatment of posterior tumours, treating with the bladder full, or by the surgical implantation of a spacer such as a gel filled breast prosthesis (Ball *et al.*, 1990). Limb morbidity may be minimized by several measures, most important of which is to leave unirradiated a strip of skin and subcutaneous tissue to allow lymphatic drainage of the distal limb. Where possible epiphyses and joint spaces are excluded from the field. Long-term effects are minimized by using small doses per fraction. Radical doses of the order of 45–60 Gy are given in 2 Gy fractions. Optimum dose distribution within the target volume should be achieved using custom made beam shaping blocks, wedge modification of beams and compensators where necessary. To reduce errors and allow volumes to be kept as small as possible immobilization devices should be produced for each patient. Of great importance to the eventual functional result is the continual emphasis on the maintenance of mobility during therapy and the subsequent year. Post-irradiation fibrosis continues to develop over years, but the major effects are seen by 2 years.

Long bones radiated to doses required for sarcoma are at risk of fracture. This is related to the degree of weakness produced by the tumour itself. The risk can be minimized by avoiding irradiation of the entire circumference of bone, where possible within the volume and, where the distal limb is radiated, by excluding one long bone from the high-dose volume.

Combined radiotherapy and chemotherapy

These agents may be used together in the management of certain tumours (Steel and Peckham, 1979). Ewing's sarcoma is the most common bone tumour where this approach is used . Lymphoma and inoperable osteosarcoma may also require treatment with both modalities. The basis of this approach is that of spatial cooperation and additive cell kill. There are, however, several problems in using these two modalities together. Prolongation of radiotherapy over a longer time than usual, or administered as several split courses, is known at other sites to be less effective than a continuous course over 5 to 6 weeks, due to proliferation of surviving tumour cells (Maciejewscki *et al.*, 1983). Similarly, an interval of 6 to

8 weeks in cytotoxic therapy, leaving disease outside the radiation field untreated, is also not ideal. Administration of radiation and chemotherapy at the same time, however, will increase the incidence and severity of both acute and late side-effects.

Various alternatives have been explored, such as postponing radiation to the end of chemotherapy, continuing low-dose chemotherapy during radiation, using agents least likely to enhance radiation damage and new methods of changing the sequence of radiation and chemotherapy and changes in fractionation. At present there is no demonstrated advantage for any new approach.

While survival continues to be limited by metastatic disease rather than local relapse, priority should, perhaps, be given to optimum systemic treatment. Nevertheless, morbidity and quality of life will be influenced greatly by the quality of the radiotherapy and any enhancement in morbidity by sequencing drugs or changing fractionation to allow continuation of chemotherapy, must be monitored carefully.

There is, therefore, a considerable dilemma about the local treatment in Ewing's sarcoma. The outcome of local surgery and endoprosthetic replacement in young adults and in children is very uncertain. The resection margins may be involved, in which case radiation will have to be added to the local excision; the life of endoprostheses is by no means certain; the functional results of endoprosthetic replacement in some sites (for example the upper humerus) is often only mediocre. On the other hand, radiation treatment carries the unavoidable risk of the late induction of radiation sarcoma with a life time of follow-up (Newton *et al.*, 1991). The balancing of these uncertainties is at present almost impossible. Only long-term follow-up of carefully controlled studies, where patients have been treated in a uniform manner, would indicate the correct local treatment for each individual site of the sarcoma. In the meantime current practice is tending to favour surgery, wherever this can be done safely and without mutilation, and keeping radiotherapy to a minimum, unless the tumour margins are incompletely excised.

Future directions in the therapy of Ewing's sarcoma

Undoubtedly chemotherapy will need to be intensified in high-risk cases since it is quite clear that the major problem is failure to control systemic disease. New agents such as etoposide, new strategies such as high-dose chemotherapy with autologous bone marrow transplantation (Simon *et al.*, 1984), and new adjuncts to chemotherapy such as haemopoietic growth factors, may all help to increase the efficacy of chemotherapy.

Local control is still a problem and in the pelvis and for very large proximal primaries combinations of surgery and radiation may be necessary to improve results. Finally, national and international collaboration will be necessary in order to conduct randomized trials where one form of treatment can be systematically compared with another. As with osteosarcoma even improvements as large as 15% in treatment outcome can only be observed in trials containing several hundred patients. For a tumour as rare as Ewing's sarcoma it is inescapable that international collaboration will be necessary.

MALIGNANT FIBROUS HISTIOCYTOMA OF BONE (MFHB)

This is a recently described entity which accounts for approximately 5% of all primary malignant bone tumours. The cell of origin is not known but the tumour is characterized by spindle cells producing collagen, marked pleomorphism and the cells being arranged in a 'storiform' pattern.

Several series have described the prognosis of MFHB treated with surgery alone. In the large series of 48 patients from the Rizzoli Institute Capanna *et al.* (1984) reported a 32% 3-year survival and 25% 10-year survival. Similar results were reported in 28 patients by Dahlin *et al.* (1977) with 33% of patients relapse-free at 5 years. Pooling all patients, 30% of patients were long-term survivors out of 133 patients in six reported series (Earl *et al.*, 1987). These rather poor results have led several groups to explore the use of chemotherapy in recent years. A variety of agents have been used, usually in combination. Chemosensitivity of the tumour has been reported by Rosen *et al.* (Rosen, 1982; Urban *et al.*, 1983; Weiner *et al.*, 1983; Den Heete *et al.*, 1985). All these groups have shown that the tumours respond clinically to combination chemotherapy and that histopathological necrosis of the tumour is frequently observed. In our own group (Earl *et al.*, 1993) 16 patients have been treated with primary chemotherapy, including ifosfamide, doxorubicin and high-dose methotrexate and over 95% of necrosis of the tumour has been found at resection in 10 cases.

With such a rare tumour it is difficult to be sure whether chemotherapy will improve long-term survival. Randomized studies in this and other high-grade spindle-cell sarcomas of bone are extremely difficult due to the rarity. The European Osteosarcoma Intergroup, which includes the Medical Research Council Bone Sarcoma Working Party, has started a non-randomized trial of doxorubicin and cisplatin as a neo-adjuvant and adjuvant chemotherapy programme in surgically resectable

MFHB. Long-term results of patients treated with chemotherapy may give some indication that survival is being improved. At the present time, such patients should be entered into well-defined programmes of treatment so that we can add to our store of knowledge (the protocol of the MRC/EOI is currently accepting patients with this diagnosis).

PRIMARY NON-HODGKIN'S LYMPHOMA OF BONE (NHLB)

This disease is uncommon. The definition is that it is a lymphoma arising primarily in bone without evidence of nodal disease ante-dating the onset of the tumour. It is common for non-Hodgkin's lymphoma to involve bone marrow, but the distinction between bone-marrow involvement in the context of generalized non-Hodgkin's lymphoma and primary NHLB is usually straightforward. Typically the tumour involves the femur or humerus, and produces a lytic lesion which may fracture. Histologically, there may be confusion with round-cell tumours of bone, such as Ewing's sarcoma, but the use of leucocyte−common antigen to stain the infiltrating lymphocytes usually makes the diagnosis clear (Dosoretz *et al.*, 1982).

For truly stage IE disease, the mainstay of treatment has been radiotherapy. Local control with doses of 45−50 Gy is nearly always achieved (Dosoretz *et al.*, 1983). It is difficult to be certain of the true stage of the tumour, however, and although for some patients local treatment alone may be adequate (Mendenhall *et al.*, 1987) in the last 15 years patients have usually been treated with chemotherapy as well as radiation. This seems particularly important when there is evidence of involvement of the adjacent nodal sites. In the report of Bacci *et al.* (1986) 26 patients were treated with radiotherapy and chemotherapy and only three of these had relapsed at the time of the report. In several of these series the late sequel of second, radiation-induced cancers of bone have been recorded in a few patients. It is not clear whether, in localized NHLB, local control can be achieved with chemotherapy alone. It will be very difficult to assess this point since the tumour is so rare and the results of treatment of early stage disease are excellent.

Patients with more widespread disease (with dissemination beyond the first lymph node site or into bone marrow and liver) are in a worse category. There is difficulty in assessing the results of treatment since Stage 4 disease is difficult to interpret as the bone lesion may be secondary to a lymphoma arising at another site. Intensive combination chemotherapy programmes have been used to treat these patients (Reimer *et al.*, 1977; Koziner *et al.*, 1982). Long-term survival is obtained in approximately 40% of patients (Earl *et al.*, 1987).

CHONDROSARCOMA

Even when high-grade or metastatic, most forms of chondrosarcomas appear resistant to chemotherapy, although systematic exploration of the value of drug treatment has not been undertaken. Occasional responses have been reported to methotrexate and alkylating agents but the clinical value of the response is usually minimal. An exception is mesenchymal chondrosarcoma where responses to osteosarcoma-type chemotherapy have been reported. There is also evidence that the small cell component of mesenchymal chondrosarcoma is relatively radiosensitive (Harwood *et al.*, 1980).

Chondrosarcomas are generally radioresistant but occasional long-term survivors are reported and tumour regression noted in those treated with radiotherapy alone. High doses of 50–60 Gy are required. Harwood reports disease-free survival in six of 12 patients with well- or moderately differentiated tumours followed up for 3–16 years after treatment with radiotherapy alone (Harwood *et al.*, 1980). Thirty-eight patients at Princess Margaret Hospital, Toronto, treated with chemotherapy and radiotherapy to 40 Gy had an actuarial survival of 41%, and 36% at 5 and 10 years with 55% local control (Krochak *et al.*, 1983). The M.D. Anderson experience suggests a possible benefit for neutrons. Of patients local control was achieved by radiation in 70%, all the failures having been treated with photons only (McNaney *et al.*, 1982). Dedifferentiated and mesenchymal variants have a poor prognosis mainly because of metastatic spread, but radiation may be effective in controlling local disease during the patient's lifetime.

REFERENCES

Akbiyik N. and Alexander L.L. (1981) Osteosarcoma of the maxilla treated with radiation therapy and surgery. *J. Nat. Med. Assoc.* 73, 355–356.

Ayala A.G., Ro J.Y., Raymond A.K. *et al.* (1989) Small cell osteosarcoma: A clinicopathologic study of 27 cases. *Cancer* 64, 2162–2173.

Bacci G., Jaffe N., Emiliani *et al.* (1986) Therapy for primary non-Hodgkin's lymphoma of bone: a comparison of results with Ewing's sarcoma. Ten years experience at the Instituto Ortopedico Rizzoli. *Cancer* 57, 1468–1472.

Ball A.B., Cassoni A., Watkins R.M. *et al.* (1990) Silicone implant to prevent visceral damage during adjuvant radiotherapy for retroperitoneal sarcoma. *Br. J. Radiol.* 63, 346–348.

Brade W.P., Herdrich K. and Varini M. (1985) Ifosfamide –

pharmacology, safety and therapeutic potential. *Cancer Treat. Rev.* 12, 1–47.

Bramwell V.H.C. (1987) Chemotherapy of operable osteosarcoma in bone tumours. In Souhami R.L. (ed.) *Baillière's Clin. Oncol.* 1(1), 175–203.

Bramwell V., Burgers M., Sneath R. *et al.* (1988) Preliminary report of the first European Osteosarcoma Intergroup Study. *Am. Ass. Clin. Oncol.* Abstract.

Breur K., Cohen P., Scheisguth O. *et al.* (1978) Irradiation of the lungs as an adjuvant therapy in the treatment of osteosarcoma of the limbs. An EORTC randomised study. *Eur. J. Cancer* 14, 461–471.

Butler M.S., Robertson W.W., Rate W., D'Angio G.J. and Drummond D.S. (1990) Skeletal sequelae of radiation therapy for malignant childhood tumours. *Clin. Orthop.* 251, 235–240.

Caceres E., Zaharia M., Moran M. *et al.* (1978) Adjuvant whole lung radiation with or without Adriamycin treatment in osteogenic sarcoma. *Cancer Treat. Rep.* 62, 297–299.

Caceres E., Zaharia M., Valdivia *et al.* (1984) Local control of osteogenic sarcoma by radiation and chemotherapy. *Int. J. Rad. Oncol. Biol. Phys.* 10, 35–39.

Cade S. (1955) Osteogenic sarcoma: at study based on 133 patients. *J. Roy. Coll. Surg.* (Edin.) 1, 79.

Capanna R., Bertoni F., Bacchini P. *et al.* (1984) Malignant fibrous histiocytoma of bone. The experience of the Rizzoli Institute: report of 90 cases. *Cancer* 54, 177–187.

Chambers R.G. and Mahoney W.D. (1970) Osteogenic sarcoma of the mandible: current management. *Am. Surg.* 46, 463–471.

Chawla S.P., Raymond A.K., Carrasco C.H. *et al.* (1985) High rates of complete remission limb salvage and prolonged survival in telangiectatic osteosarcoma after pre-operative chemotherapy with intra-arterial cisplatinum and systemic Adriamycin. *Proc. Am. Soc. Clin. Oncol.* 4, 152.

Cortes E.P. and Holland J.F. (1981) Adjuvant chemotherapy for primary osteogenic sarcoma. *Surg. Clin. N. Am.* 61, 1391–1404.

Cortes E.P., Holland, J.F., Wang J.J. and Sinks L.F. (1972) Doxorubicin in disseminated osteosarcoma. *JAMA* 221, 1132–1138.

Dahlin D.C., Unni K.K. and Matsuno T. (1977) Malignant (fibrous) histiocytoma of bone: fact or fancy? *Cancer* 39, 1508–1516.

de Fries H.O., Perlin E. and Leibl S.A. (1970) Treatment of osteogenic sarcoma of the mandible. *Arch. Otolaryngol.* 105, 358–359.

den Heete G.J., Schraffordt-Koops H., Kamps W.A. *et al.* (1985) Treatment of malignant fibrous histiocytoma of bone: A plea for primary chemotherapy. *Cancer* 56, 37–40.

Dosoretz D.E., Raymond A.K., Murphy G.F. *et al.* (1982) Primary lymphoma of bone. The relationship of morphologic diversity to clinical behaviour. *Cancer* 50, 1009–1014.

Dosoretz, D.E., Murphy G.F., Raymond K. *et al.* (1983) Radiation therapy for primary lymphoma of bone. *Cancer* 51, 44–46.

Earl H.M. (1987) Chemotherapy of rare malignant bone tumours. *Baillière's Clin. Oncol.* 1(1), 223–239.

Earl H.M., Pringle J., Kemp H. *et al.* (1993) Chemotherapy of malignant fibrous histiocytoma of bone. *Ann. Oncol.* 4, 409–415.

Eckhardt J.J., Eilber F.R., Grant T.T. *et al.* (1985) Management of stage IIB osteogenic sarcoma: experience at the University of California, Los Angeles Cancer Treatment Symposia 3, 117–130.

Edmondson J.H., Green S.J., Ivins J.C. *et al.* (1984) A controlled pilot study of high dose methotrexate as post-surgical adjuvant treatment for primary osteosarcoma. *J. Clin. Oncol.* 2, 152–156.

Gasparini M., Lombardi F., Gianni C. and Fossati-Belani F. (1981) Localised Ewing's sarcoma: results of integrated therapy and analysis of failures. *Eur. J. Cancer Clin. Oncol.* 17, 1205–1209.

Gasparini M., Rouessé J., Van Oosterom A. *et al.* (1985) Phase II study of cisplatin in advanced osteogenic sarcoma. *Cancer Treat. Rep.* 69, 211–213.

Graham-Pole J., Lazarus H.M., Herzig R.H. *et al.* (1984) High dose melphalan therapy for the treatment of children with refractory neuroblastoma and Ewing's sarcoma. *Am. J. Pediat. Hemat. Oncol.* 6, 17–26.

Grem J.L., King S.A., Wittes R.E. and Leyland-Jones B. (1988) The role of methotrexate in osteosarcoma. *J. Nat. Cancer Inst.* 80, 626–656.

Haibach H., Carrell C. and Dittrich F.J. (1985) Neoplasms arising in Paget's disease of bone: a study of 82 cases. *Am. J. Clin. Pathol.* 83, 594–600.

Hartman K.R., Triche T.J., Kinsella T.J. and Miser J.S. (1991) Prognostic value of histopathology in Ewing's sarcoma. Long-term follow-up of distal extremity primary tumours. *Cancer* 67, 163–171.

Harwood A.R., Krajbich J.I. and Fornasier V.L. (1980) Radiotherapy of chondrosarcoma of bone. *Cancer* 45, 2749–2777.

Hayes F.A., Thompson E.I., Sustu H.O. *et al.* (1983) The response of Ewing's sarcoma to sequential cyclophosphamide and Adriamycin induction therapy. *J. Clin. Oncol.* 1. 45–51.

Hayes F.A., Thompson E., Meyer W. *et al.* (1989) Therapy for localised Ewing's sarcoma of bone. *J. Clin. Oncol.* 7, 208–213.

Huvos A.G. (1986) Osteogenic sarcoma of bones and soft tissues in older persons. A clinicopathologic analysis of 117 patients older than 60 years. *Cancer* 57, 1442–1449.

Huvos A.G., Rosen G., Betsky S.S. *et al.* (1982) Telangiectatic osteosarcoma: a clinico-pathologic study of 124 cases. *Cancer*, 49, 1679–1689.

Huvos A.G., Butler A. and Betsky S.S. (1985) Osteogenic sarcoma in pregnant women. Prognosis, therapeutic implications and literature review. *Cancer* 56, 2326–2331.

Isacoff W.H., Eilber F., Tabbarah H. *et al.* (1978) Phase II clinical trial with high dose methotrexate therapy and citrovorum factor rescue. *Cancer Treat. Rep.* 62, 1295–1304.

Jaffe N., Farber S., Traggis D. *et al.* (1973) Favorable response of osteogenic sarcoma to high dose methotrexate with citrovorum rescue and radiation therapy. *Cancer* 31, 1367–1373.

Jaffe N., Frei E., Traggis D. and Bishop Y. (1974) Adjuvant methotrexate and citrovorum factor treatment of osteogenic sarcoma. *New Engl. J. Med.* 291, 994–997.

Jaffe N., Purdich J., Knapp J. *et al.* (1983) Treatment of primary osteosarcoma with intra-arterial and intravenous high dose methotrexate. *J. Clin. Oncol.* 1, 428–431.

Jaffe N., Raymond K., Ayala A. *et al.* (1989) Effect of cumulative courses of intra-arterial *cis*-diamminedichloroplatin-II on the primary tumour in osteosarcoma. *Cancer* 63, 63–67.

Jürgens H., Exner U., Gadner H. *et al.* (1988) Multidisciplinary treatment of primary Ewing's sarcoma of bone. A 6-year experience of a European Cooperative trial. *Cancer* 61, 23–32.

Klegar K., Ryan L., Elias A.D. *et al.* (1986) Ifosfamide (IFF) for advanced previously treated sarcomas: phase II. *Proc. Am. Soc. Clin. Oncol.* 5, 132.

Koziner B., Little C., Passe S. *et al.* (1982) Treatment of advanced histiocytic lymphoma. An analysis of prognostic variables. *Cancer* 49, 1571–1579.

Krochak R., Harwood A.R., Cummings B.J. *et al.* (1983) Results of radical radiation for chondrosarcoma of bone. *Radiother. Oncol.* 1, 109–115.

Lange B. and Levine A.S. (1982) Is it ethical not to conduct a prospectively controlled trial of adjuvant chemotherapy in osteosarcoma? *Cancer Treat. Rep.* 66, 1699–1704.

Link M.P., Goorin A.M., Miser A.W. *et al.* (1986) The effect of adjuvant chemotherapy on relapse-free survival in patients with osteosarcoma of the extremity. *New Engl. J. Med.* 134, 1600–1606.

Maciejewski B., Preuss-Bayer G. and Trott K.R. (1983) The influence of the number of fractions and the overall treatment time on local control make complication rate in squamous cell carcinoma of the larynx. *Int. J. Radiat. Oncol. Biol. Phys.* 9, 321–328.

MacIntosh D.J., Price C.H.G. and Jeffree J.M. (1975) Ewing's tumour: a study of behaviour and treatment in forty-seven cases. *J. Bone Joint Surg.* 57, 331–340.

Magrath I., Sandlund J., Raynor A. *et al.* (1986) A phase II study of ifosfamide in the treatment of recurrent sarcomas in young people. *Cancer Chemother. Pharmacol.* 18 (suppl. 2), S25–28.

Mavligit G.M. (1981) Intra-arterial cisplatin for patients with inoperable skeletal tumors. *Cancer* 48, 1.

McNaney D., Lindberg R.D., Ayala A.G. *et al.* (1982) Fifteen-year radiotherapy experience with chondrosarcoma of bone. *Int. J. Radiat. Oncol. Biol. Phys.* 8, 187–190.

Medical Research Council (MRC) (1986) A trial of chemotherapy in patients with osteosarcoma (a report to the Medical Research Council by their working party on bone sarcoma). *Br. J. Cancer* 53, 513–518.

Mendenhall N.D., Jones J.J., Kramer B.S. *et al.* (1987) The management of primary lymphoma of bone. *Radiother. Oncol.* 9, 137–145.

Meyers P.A., Heller G., Healey J. *et al.* (1992) Chemotherapy for nonmetastatic osteogenic sarcoma: The Memorial Sloan–Kettering experience. *J. Clin. Oncol.* 10, 5–15.

Nesbit M.E., Perez C.A., Tefft M. *et al.* (1981) Multimodal therapy for the management of primary non-metastatic Ewing's sarcoma of bone: an Intergroup Study. *Nat. Cancer Inst. Monogr.* 56, 255–262.

Nesbit M.E., Gehan E.A., Burgert E.O. *et al.* (1990) Multimodal therapy for the management of primary, non-metastatic Ewing's sarcoma of bone: A long term follow up of the first Intergroup Study. *J. Clin. Oncol.* 8, 1664–1674.

Newton K.A. and Barrett A. (1978) Prophylactic lung irradiation in the treatment of osteogenic sarcoma. *Clin. Radiol.* 29, 493–496.

Newton W.A., Meadows A.T., Shimada H. *et al.* (1991) Bone sarcomas as second malignant neoplasms following childhood cancer. *Cancer* 67, 193–201.

Oldham R.K. and Pomeroy R.C. (1972) Treatment of Ewing's sarcoma with Adriamycin (NSC-123127). *Cancer Chemother. Rep.* 56, 635–639.

Palma J., Gailani S., Freeman A. *et al.* (1972) Treatment of metastatic Ewing's sarcoma with BCNU. *Cancer* 30, 909–913.

Perez C.A., Razek A.A., Tefft M. *et al.* (1977) Analysis of local control in Ewing's sarcoma. *Cancer* 40, 2864–2873.

Perez C.A., Tefft M., Nesbit M.E. *et al.* (1981) The role of radiation therapy in the management of non-metastatic Ewing's sarcoma of bone. Report of the Intergroup Ewing's Sarcoma Study. *Int. J. Radiat. Oncol. Biol. Phys.* 7, 141–149.

Pratt D.B. (1979) Chemotherapy of osteosarcoma — an overview. In Van Oosterom A.T. *et al.* (eds) *Therapeutic Progress in Ovarian Cancer, Testicular Cancer and the Sarcomas*, pp. 329–347. The Hague, Martinus Nijhoff.

Pratt C.B. and Shanks E.C. (1974) Doxorubicin in treatment of malignant solid tumours in children. *Am. J. Dis. Child.* 127, 534–536.

Pratt C.B., Green A.A., Fleming I.D. *et al.* (1984) Results of adjuvant chemotherapy for 77 patients with osteosarcoma of an extremity 1973–1981. *Proc. Am. Soc. Clin. Oncol.* 3, A257.

Pratt C.B., Champion J.E., Senzer N. *et al.* (1985) Treatment of unresectable or metastatic osteosarcoma with cisplatin or cisplatin–doxorubicin. *Cancer* 56, 1930–1933.

Rab G., Ivins J., Childs D. *et al.* (1976) Elective whole lung irradiation in the treatment of osteogenic sarcoma. *Cancer* 38, 939–942.

Reimer R.R., Chabner B.A., Young R.C. *et al.* (1977) Lymphoma presenting in bone. Results of histopathology, staging and therapy. *Ann. Intern. Med.* 87, 50–55.

Rosen G. (1982a) Current management of Ewing's sarcoma. *Progr. Clin. Cancer* 8, 267–282.

Rosen G. (1982b) Sarcomas of the soft tissue and bone. In De Vita V.T. *et al.* (eds) *Cancer. Principles and Practice of Oncology*, p. 1072. Philadelphia, Lippincott.

Rosen G. (1985) Preoperative (neoadjuvant) chemotherapy for osteogenic sarcoma: a ten year experience. *Orthopaedics* 8, 659–664.

Rosen G., Suwansirikul S., Kwon C. *et al.* (1974) High dose methotrexate with citrovorum factor rescue and Adriamycin in childhood osteogenic sarcoma. *Cancer* 33, 1151–1163.

Rosen G., Huvos A.G., Mosende C. *et al.* (1978) Chemotherapy and thoracotomy for metastatic osteogenic sarcoma: a model for adjuvant chemotherapy and the rationale for the timing of thoracic surgery. *Cancer* 41, 841–849.

Rosen G., Marcove R.C., Caparros B. *et al.* (1979) Primary osteogenic sarcoma. The rationale for preoperative chemotherapy and delayed surgery. *Cancer* 43, 2163–2177.

Rosen G., Nirenberg A. and Caparros B. (1980) Cisplatin in metastatic osteogenic sarcoma. In Prestayko A.W. *et al.* (eds) *Cisplatinum: Current Status and New Developments*, pp. 465–475. New York, Academic Press.

Rosen G., Caparros B., Nirenberg A. *et al.* (1981) Ewing's sarcoma: ten-year experience with adjuvant chemotherapy. *Cancer* 46, 2204–2213.

Rosen G., Caparros B., Huvos A.G. *et al.* (1982) Preoperative chemotherapy for osteogenic sarcoma: selection of postoperative adjuvant chemotherapy based on the response of the primary tumor to preoperative chemotherapy. *Cancer* 49, 1221–1230.

Rosen G., Huvos A.G., Marcove R. and Nirenberg A. (1986) Telangiectatic osteogenic sarcoma. *Clin. Orthop.* 207, 164–173.

Rosenberg S.A., Chabner B.A., Young R.C. *et al.* (1979) Treatment of osteogenic sarcoma. I. Effect of adjuvant high-dose methotrexate after amputation. *Cancer Treat. Rep.* 63, 739–751.

Ryan J., Baker L., Benjamin R. *et al.* (1990) Long term follow up in the cure of osteogenic sarcoma. *Chir. Organi. Mov.* 75 (suppl. 1), 48–49.

Samuels M.L. and Howe C.D. (1967) Cyclophosphamide in the management of Ewing's sarcoma. *Cancer* 20, 961–966.

Schmidt D., Herrmann C., Jürgens H. and Harms D. (1991) Malignant peripheral neuroectodermal tumor and its necessary distinction from Ewing's sarcoma. *Cancer* 68, 2251–2259.

Selawry O.S., Holland J.F. and Wolman I.J. (1968) Effect of vincristine on malignant solid tumors in children. *Cancer Chemother. Rep.* 53, 497–500.

Sim F.H., Unni K.K., Beabout J.W. and Dahlin D.C. (1979) Osteosarcoma with small cells simulating Ewing's tumor. *J Bone Joint Surg.* 61A, 207–215.

Simon M.A., Phillips W.A. and Bonfiglio M. (1984) Pregnancy and aggressive or malignant bone tumors. *Cancer* 53, 2564–2569.

Steel G.G. and Peckham M.J. (1979) Exploitable mechanisms in combined radiotherapy–chemotherapy: the concept of additivity. *Int. J. Radiat. Oncol. Biol. Phys.* 5, 85–91.

Stephens F.O., Tattersall M.H.N., Marsden W. *et al.* (1987) Regional chemotherapy with the use of cisplatin and doxorubicin as primary treatment for advanced sarcomas in shoulder, pelvis and thigh. *Cancer* 60, 724–735.

Stiller C.A. and Bunch K.J. (1990) Trends in survival for childhood cancer in Britain diagnosed 1971–85. *Br. J. Cancer* 62, 806–815.

Strong L.C., Herson J., Osborne B.M. *et al.* (1979) Risk of radiation related subsequent malignant tumours in survivors of Ewing's sarcoma. *J. Nat. Cancer Inst.* 62, 1401–1406.

Suit H.D. (1975) Role of therapeutic radiology in cancer of the bone. *Cancer* 35 (Suppl. 3), 930–935.

Sutow W.W. and Sullivan M.P. (1962) Cyclophosphamide therapy in children with Ewing's sarcoma. *Cancer Chemother. Rep.* 23, 55–60.

Taylor W.F., Ivins J.C., Pritchard D.J. *et al.* (1985) Trends and variability in survival among patients with osteosarcoma: a 7 year update. *Mayo Clin. Proc.* 60, 91–104.

Telles N.C., Rabson A.S. and Pomeroy T.C. Ewing's sarcoma: an autopsy study. *Cancer* 41, 2321–2399.

Thomas P.R., Perez C.A., Meff J.R. *et al.* (1984) The management of Ewing's sarcoma: role of radiotherapy in local tumour control. *Cancer Treat. Rep.* 68, 703–710.

Tucker M.A., Dangio J.G., Boice J.E. *et al.* (1987) Bone sarcoma linked to chemotherapy and radiotherapy in children. *New Engl. J. Med.* 315, 588–593.

Unni K.K., Dahlin D.C. and Beabout J.W. (1976) Periosteal osteogenic sarcoma. *Cancer* 37, 2476–2485.

Urban C., Rosen C., Huvos A.G. *et al.* (1983) Chemotherapy of malignant fibrous histiocytoma of bone. A report of five cases. *Cancer* 51, 795–802.

Wang J.J., Cortes E., Sinks L. and Holland J.F. (1971) Therapeutic effect and toxicity of Adriamycin in patients with neoplastic disease. *Cancer* 28, 837–843.

Weiner M., Sedlis M., Johnston A.D. *et al.* (1983) Adjuvant chemotherapy of malignant fibrous histiocytoma of bone. *Cancer* 51, 25–29.

Winkler K., Beron G., Delling G. *et al.* (1988) Neoadjuvant chemotherapy of osteosarcoma: results of a randomized co-operative trial (Coss-82) with salvage chemotherapy based on histological tumour response. *J. Clin. Oncol.* 6, 329–337.

Wold L.E., Unni K.K. and Beabout J.W. (1984) Dedifferentiated parosteal osteosarcoma. *J. Bone Joint Surg.* 66A, 53–59.

Section 3
Special Topics

Chapter 30

Radiological Investigations: Modern Investigative Procedures

Chapter 30.1

Spine: Myelography, Computed Tomography and Magnetic Resonance Imaging

B.E. Kendall & J.M. Stevens

INTRODUCTION

The purpose of this chapter is to discuss the applications of radiographic computed tomography (CT), magnetic resonance imaging (MRI) and myelography to the elucidation of conditions affecting the spine. Emphasis is placed on advantages and disadvantages of each of these modalities for demonstrating aspects of spinal anatomy and pathology with the aim of facilitating rational judgement on the choice of test and clear communication to a department of clinical imaging.

COMPUTED IMAGING TECHNIQUES

Computed imaging techniques involve the computed reconstruction of images from sets of linear projection data (Brooks and Di Chiro, 1976). The object is divided into a series of cubical or rectangular volume elements (voxels), characteristics of which are measured so that their intensity can be represented by a number and/or displayed using an appropriate grey scale or occasionally a colour code as a picture element (pixel) to constitute an image. Pixels are rarely smaller than approximately 0.3 mm; this is far larger than the size of silver halide granules in conventional radiographic film emulsion, so that computed images are often classified as relatively low-resolution images. Digital acquisition is a major advantage: (i) images are suitable for direct transmission to storage sites or other destinations; (ii) the display can be manipulated to accentuate contrasts within specified numerical ranges (window settings); (iii) linear, area and volume measurements of known accuracy can be made electronically; (iv) reconstructions may be made using different computational algorithms to accentuate or more accurately define boundaries between various tissues; and (v) the data can be reformatted in multiple planes. Advanced image-processing techniques are becoming increasingly accessible including various types of surface display resulting in images with three-dimensional effects. These have great potential for detailed study of complex skeletal features, but tend to be slow with the computing power usually available and have found limited clinical application.

Image quality depends upon both spatial and contrast resolution. Unfortunately, these are linked to energy input and any option which increases one usually reduces the other. Spatial resolution is dependent on the size of the field of view, the size of the computational matrix, and the selected slice thickness in multiplanar imaging. Contrast resolution is dependent on the signal-to-noise ratio (SNR) and is increased by increasing the size of the volume elements in the image. In the spine, the natural tissue contrasts between bone, fat and cerebrospinal fluid (CSF) are high. Within the spinal theca, however, contrast between neural tissue and CSF is considerably less.

Radiographic computed tomography

Computed tomography is a planar data-acquisition technique. The numerical value of each picture element is expressed in Hounsfield units (HU) and represents the radiographic attenuation coefficient of the volume element measured relative to that of water at body temperature. Perception of bone detail is increased by reducing the pixel size, and reducing the slice thickness. Both of these strategies reduce soft-tissue contrast and compromises are usually chosen. Multiplanar reformatting is only of value when voxel size is relatively small, and when planning to use this facility, slice thicknesses need to be narrow. This prolongs significantly the examination time during which the patient must be still to avoid artefacts, which may be inappropriate or impossible for some patients. It also increases radiation exposure which must be considered in younger patients, particularly when radiosensitive organs such as the thyroid gland and gonads are included in the measuring field. Metal implants cause serious and unavoidable degradation of the images. Metal-induced artefacts can occasionally be avoided by modifying the angulation of the slice although this is seldom possible; they are minimized by using the thinnest possible slices and maximizing the radiographic exposure factors. Multiplanar imaging is more difficult in the presence of spinal curvatures, both from the point of view of patient positioning within the field of view and also in interpretation of the images. Many currently available machines do not have sufficiently advanced post-processing facilities to electronically correct for spinal curvatures.

The major advantage of computed tomography (CT) over plain radiography is greatly improved tissue contrast; high spatial resolution alone is not of value if tissue contrast is poor. Secondly, CT is a tomographic modality which facilitates localization to specific regions. Thirdly, CT provides axial images of the spinal canal which greatly aids the evaluation of pathological processes and planning surgical strategies. It has rendered conventional focal plane radiographic tomography obsolete in virtually all clinical situations.

The major disadvantage of CT is limited ability to demonstrate longitudinal views of the spine. Such views can be generated directly only in very special circumstances, but even then positioning is difficult and usually not entirely satisfactory. The usual way to generate longitudinal images is by multiplanar reformatting and rarely more than five vertebral segments can be included in a single block of images. Particularly if multiplanar reformatting is planned, acquisition times can be as much as 40 min and patient movement within this period can ruin attempts at useful multiplanar reformatting from the reconstructed slices. This drawback has been largely overcome by the introduction of spiral CT. This modality will allow 2 mm thick contiguous sections suitable for reformatting to be made over a length of 15 cm in approximately 1 minute. The CT gantry has an aperture of limited width which may restrict a study in special circumstances such as severe scoliosis, very obese individuals, and when there is a large amount of life-support material required as in a severely injured patient.

SPECIAL TECHNIQUES WITH COMPUTED TOMOGRAPHY

Intravenous contrast enhancement

Intravenous contrast enhancement is usually unnecessary in spinal CT because: (i) natural tissue contrast usually is sufficient to demonstrate normal and pathological anatomy; (ii) in most of the common extradural pathologies such as herniated disc fragments enhancement is slight or absent; (iii) normal intradural structures do not enhance so that visualization of roots and spinal cord is not improved; and (iv) intravenous contrast enhancement is not totally innocuous (deaths from their use are recorded in the UK every year, and there is no means of identifying reliably patients at risk).

Computed myelography

The term 'intrathecal contrast enhancement' is best avoided because it can lead to confusion within an imaging department; myelography and CT are performed on different pieces of equipment often in widely separated locations. It is the authors' opinion that, other than in exceptional circumstances, this should be preceded by a conventional myelogram. The myelogram is particularly useful when significant pathology is present in unexpected sites enabling the CT study to be focused on the regions of principal interest; moreover, the information necessary for diagnosis and treatment planning may be clearly apparent on the myelogram so that a following CT becomes redundant.

The advantages of CT after myelography are that: (i) extradural pathology not visible on a myelogram may be demonstrated; (ii) bone destruction, which can be of considerable help in differential diagnosis, is shown more clearly and at an earlier stage; (iii) anatomical location of a lesion, in relation to the dura and the spinal cord is more exact; (iv) contrast penetration may outline cysts; (v) the severity of spinal cord compression can be more accurately assessed; and (vi) electronic measurements may be applied to this and other variables.

Computed discography, epidurography, epidural venography

Epidural opacification techniques such as epidural myelography where water soluble contrast medium is injected intentionally under pressure into the extradural space, and epidural venography, are now obsolete. The value of discography as a provocative test is controversial. The clinical value of demonstrating morphological changes, in particular radial tears of the annulus fibrosis, by discography is virtually non-existent and the addition of CT to this procedure is considered by the authors to be pointless.

CT-guided biopsy and injection

Computed tomography is useful as an aid to accurate

placement of needles or trocars for diagnostic biopsy and injections for pain relief into joints or close to nerve roots. Sections made during the insertion help in ensuring that the needle does not pass through potentially harmful regions such as the pleura, spinal canal or aorta. A CT image made with the needle in place confirms that the pathological region has been biopsied.

Magnetic resonance imaging

Protons carry a positive charge and they spin around their own axis at high speed so that when they are placed in a strong magnetic field they behave like small magnets, aligning with the field and gyrating around its axis in an angular motion termed 'precession'. The rate of precession is in the radiofrequency range; it depends on a characteristic property of the nucleus, termed the 'gyro-magnetic ratio', and the strength of the magnetic field. If radiofrequency energy at the same rate as the precession is applied at right angles to the magnetic field, it produces two effects: (i) it augments the angle of precession and thus increases the energy of the system; (ii) it brings the precessing protons into phase or resonance. When the radiofrequency pulse is terminated the resonating excited protons return the radiofrequency signal and the numerical value of the voxel in MRI indicates the intensity of this signal at the time of recording. The initial intensity depends on the number or density of protons within the voxel and the amount of energy which could be added to them. The latter depends on two main factors. The first is a characteristic property of the particular tissue itself termed the 'T1 relaxation time'. This is in the region of $200-900$ msec for the solid tissues of the nervous system but considerably longer for liquids like CSF. The second factor is the time allowed for the tissue to relax between radiofrequency stimulating pulses. If such pulses are applied at intervals of $300-500$ msec the tissues having longer relaxation times will have incompletely recovered their equilibrium state and will absorb a lesser proportion of the radio-frequency energy than those with the shorter T1 which are more relaxed. A relatively short interval between the radiofrequency pulses (TR) will thus allow distinction between tissues having short and long T1 values. A longer TR ($2000-2500$ msec), on the other hand, will allow time for all tissues to return to equilibrium and for the protons within them to absorb similar amounts of radiofrequency energy which will thus be proportional to the number of protons or proton density and relatively uninfluenced by the T1 value. The proton density varies little between most soft tissues but the low signal reflected from gases such as air, heavy calcification and dense cortical bone is due to their low proton content. The protons synchronized by the radiofrequency pulse dephase rapidly due to the influence of charged particles causing magnetic inhomogeneities in their immediate environment. This dephasing causes rapid loss of signal and it is characterized by a relaxation time (T2) which is much shorter than T1, rarely more than 150 msec and also much less dependent on field strength. Images influenced mainly by T2 are made on a long TR series after sufficient time for dephasing has been allowed, usually after an interval of about 80 msec.

Images can thus be produced in which the signal reflected from the voxels is dominated or weighted by proton density, T1 or T2 effects.

There are several other factors that influence signal return. The most important of these are flow, magnetic susceptibility and paramagnetic contrast agents.

The protons from each section transmit at a given frequency to which the receiver coil is tuned. Signals at other frequencies are not recorded, so that if protons are carried into a section in flowing blood, pulsating CSF or diffusing fluids, the lack of signal from them may be reflected as a dark region or signal void. Similar changes in signal occur when flow is taking place across a slice due to changes relative to the phase or frequency encoding magnetic field gradients. It is possible to compensate for the effects of flow by using special pulse sequences and also to specifically record flow effects, which is the basis of magnetic resonance angiography.

Ferric iron in large molecules, or when contained within cells as in haemosiderin-containing macrophages, or desoxyhaemoglobin within red blood cells, possesses magnetic effects that can result in local alterations of the magnetic field and thus cause localized increase in the rate of dephasing of protons and hence low signal on T2-weighted sequences, an effect which is proportionate to the strength of the magnetic field. This effect is seen normally in the central nuclei of the brain beginning after childhood and increasing with age and in certain pathological conditions. It does not occur normally in the spine but is a feature of abnormal conditions, particularly when breakdown products of haemoglobin are present following haemorrhage and it is an important cause of artefact from ferromagnetic implants. Even tiny fragments separated from a drill bit during surgery can be an important source of artefact (Fig. 30.1.1).

Certain paramagnetic substances facilitate T1 relaxation and thus increase signal on T1-weighted sequences. Naturally occurring substances in this category include methaemoglobin and melanin. Methaemoglobin is an oxidation product of haemoglobin occurring in subacute haematomas and it causes a characteristic high signal,

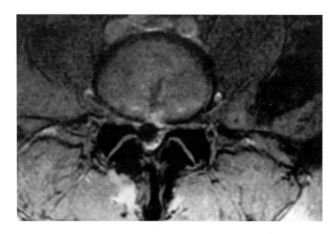

Fig. 30.1.1 Axial MRI of the lumbar spine at the level of L5 (T2-weighted image, from a multiplanar gradient related echo sequence known as MPGR). The cerebrospinal fluid yields high signal and appears white, creating a myelographic effect. However, the rounded filling defect within the theca (arrow) was not seen on T1-weighted images, and was a susceptibility artefact presumed to be from iron shavings left after a previous laminectomy. Such shavings are seldom visible on plain radiography or CT, but gradient recalled echo acquisitions are particularly sensitive to magnetic materials. Such artefacts fortunately are uncommon.

facilitating the diagnosis of such lesions which may be difficult using all other imaging modalities. Melanoma deposits may be suspected for similar reasons though such deposits are also notably prone to intratumoral haemorrhage.

Magnetic resonance possesses many advantages. These include:

1 Absence of any ionizing radiation. At field strengths currently in use, magnetic resonance has no known biological hazards. MRI may therefore be repeated as necessary to obtain multiple parameters and planes of imaging and for follow-up studies, which is of particular importance in young patients presenting for example with dysraphic lesions.

2 Since images are constituted from radiowaves, they can be produced with similar resolution in any plane. This is of particular advantage in the examination of a longitudinal structure such as the spinal column and cord especially in the rather common situations where the precise level from which symptoms are originating cannot be determined on clinical grounds.

3 Magnetic resonance is free of bone induced artefacts, which detract from the value of CT. This is an important factor in favour of high-quality magnetic resonance for demonstration of the spinal cord and subarachnoid space for which it can replace myelography and computed myelography in almost all circumstances.

4 Marked sensitivity to pathological changes. Each of

the parameters which influence signal intensity can be made the dominant factor producing contrast discrimination in a particular image sequence. Many lesions which are not visible on CT are routinely shown by magnetic resonance. These include degree of hydration of the nucleus pulposus, composition of bone marrow and red—yellow marrow conversion, early evidence of cellular infiltration of fatty marrow, many plaques of demyelination, various myelopathies, cord cysts and neoplasms, particularly those of low grade.

5 The anatomical relationship of lesions to adjacent structures, particularly the spinal cord, vertebrae and blood vessels is almost always adequate for determination of surgical approach.

6 Low toxicity-enhancing agents are available. These have proved of particular value for (i) surveys for intrathecal metastases from primary CNS neoplasms or in conditions in which multiple neoplasms are commonly present as in neurofibromatosis and Von Hippel—Lindau syndrome and (ii) assessment for recurrent disease after surgery, particularly in distinction of additional disc prolapse or of inflammatory disease in the presence of fibrosis.

Contraindications and limitations include certain implanted magnetic materials, which may be induced to move. These include:

1 Certain aneurysm clips and metallic foreign bodies related to the spinal cord, eye or ear.

2 Cardiac pacemakers and other devices susceptible to radiofrequency changes.

3 Up to 5% of patients are claustrophobic and are unable to remain within the machine for the duration of the procedure. Many children are frightened by the appearance of the machine or the noise of the gradient coils and require either heavy sedation or anaesthesia.

4 Life-support apparatus is more difficult to monitor within the magnetic field although this is largely overcome by more specialized equipment.

5 Occasionally, patients are unable to fit into the magnet either due to gross obesity or skeletal deformities.

6 Currently patients are not examined during the first trimester of pregnancy though there is no evidence that the procedure is in fact harmful at this time.

7 Patient movement, even slight, can result in suboptimal images, as can minor malfunctions of the machine. In a proportion of cases image quality is disappointing.

SPECIAL TECHNIQUES WITH MRI

Spinal imaging is routinely performed using surface coils to achieve maximum signal-to-noise ratio and exclude artefacts arising in deeper structures. Imaging is usually performed segmentally, but phased array coils are available which allow simultaneous whole spine imaging.

Intravenous contrast enhancement

Paramagnetic contrast agents, cause local reduction in T1 and thus increase the signal on T1 weighted sequences when given intravenously, they are retained within the normal blood−brain barrier but penetrate many pathological tissues. The chief among them in current use is gadolinium detoxified by chelation with DPTA (diethylene triaminepenta-acetic acid). This is a very safe but not totally innocuous agent which is injected in small dosages, its effects being apparent in extremely low concentration. Blood−brain barrier changes can be detected with much greater sensitivity using gadolinium plus MRI than with iodine contrast media utilizing CT, although the same general principles apply to each.

Fast-imaging methods and whole-volume acquisition

Fast-imaging techniques usually employ reversing magnetic field gradients to re-establish resonance (GRE), and imaging times can be reduced to a few seconds per slice on most modern equipment. The trade-off is overall increase in noise and characteristic artefacts (due to motion, magnetic susceptibility differences and chemical shift) generated or accentuated by the gradient acquisition (Fig. 30.1). These may significantly exaggerate the size of osteophytes or degree of cord or root compression (Czervionke and Daniels, 1988) though this can be at least partly overcome by modification of rephasing gradients. Volume acquisition reduces this problem, and permits generation of ⩾64 slices at thicknesses down to 1 mm in reasonably short times (<10 min), and these then can be presented in different formats (Tsuruda *et al.*, 1989).

MYELOGRAPHY

Myelography involves the intrathecal injection of potentially irritant and neurotoxic contrast agents. Although serious side effects are rare when modern non-ionic contrast media are used, for most patients myelography is an unpleasant experience which should be imposed only when strictly necessary. As alternative diagnostic methods, in particular MRI, become more widely available and realistically priced the ethical position of myelography will become increasingly questionable.

Myelography in experienced hands remains the most consistently reliable way of demonstrating the contents of the entire spinal canal from foramen magnum to sacrum, or the presence of obstruction of the spinal theca. This is true for relatively uncooperative patients and for a wide range of body habitus and spinal curvatures. Clinical localization is not invariably reliable, so that inclusion of, for example, the thoracic region when images of the lumbar theca have failed to provide an unequivocal explanation for all the clinical features may be crucial. The term 'radiculogram' was appropriate at the time when water-soluble contrast media were too toxic for demonstration of the spinal cord, but unfortunately it has persisted. To restrict a myelogram to examination of the lumbar thecal sac when evaluating patients with back pain and sciatica removes its major advantage over CT.

Myelography remains the most sensitive method of demonstrating the intradural roots and rootlets, showing minimal but significant intradural abnormalities such as small neurofibromas, and for distinguishing normal and abnormal intradural vessels, crucial to the diagnosis of most spinal arteriovenous malformations.

The disadvantages of myelography are that it outlines only the thecal sac and its contents which occupy only part of the spinal canal. It is considerably less sensitive than CT or MRI at demonstrating epidural disease and the internal structure of the spinal cord.

Complications

Headache is very frequent after myelography, and is usually maximal several hours later. It seldom lasts more than 24 hours but can last several days. Also, although a clinically obvious confusional state is rare, minor changes in mentation are not uncommon. The appearance of or exacerbation of leg or arm pain shortly after the myelogram occurs in about 6% of studies, and it may persist for several hours. Very occasional complications, which occur in less than 0.1%, include cranial nerve palsies, paralysis, seizures and even death. A cause of major neurological morbidity in cervical myelography has been intramedullary injection of contrast medium when lateral C1−C2 punctures were performed (Robertson and Smith, 1990). Now that more benign contrast media are available this entry point is appropriate only when the study cannot be satisfactorily accomplished from lumbar injection. Complications of lumbar puncture such as intraspinal haemorrhage are exceptionally rare, and occur more often in elderly subjects, and those with coagulation defects and/or hypertension (Fig. 30.1.2).

Despite this list, outpatient myelography, to avoid the expense and inconvenience of hospital admission, is an

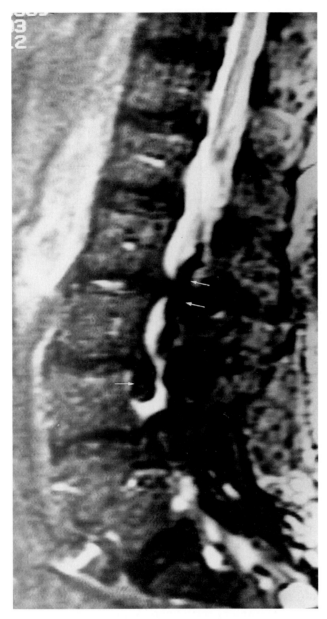

Fig. 30.1.2 Rapid T2-weighted sagittal MRI of the lumbar spine, acquired on a coarse matrix to reduce imaging time. Despite low resolution, an epidural haematoma is shown (arrows) which became symptomatic 40 min after the myelogram and required surgical removal. A large disc herniation is also shown (single arrow).

acceptable technique for the majority of patients (Vezina *et al.*, 1984), with the proviso that good community care is available and there are immediate re-admission facilities.

There are no absolute contraindications to myelography, but relative contraindications include known sensitivity to iodine or radiographic contrast media and major clotting defects. Controlled epilepsy is not a contraindication.

Situations in which a myelogram may still be necessary

These situations include:
1 inadequate availability of computed imaging facilities, or unacceptability by the patient for any reason;
2 equivocal findings on CT or MRI;
3 multiple levels of abnormality of similar severity are shown by CT or MRI, when focal clinical features are present relating to a single root;
4 suspected spinal arteriovenous malformation with negative MRI when spinal angiography is contemplated.

ANATOMICAL ASPECTS

The spinal cord

The normal spinal cord usually cannot be seen on plain CT in the thoracic and lower cervical regions. It is well shown on conventional myelography, but its cross-sectional contour is visible only on computed myelography. Both longitudinal and cross-sectional images of the spinal cord are available on MRI, and good quality machines can consistently show the anterior and posterior horns of the grey matter and also reveal signal differences between parts of the white matter columns (Fig. 30.1.3).

The midsagittal diameter of the spinal cord in the cervical region varies little from level to level, and is between 8 and 10 mm as measured from an average conventional myelogram, and approximately 7–8 mm on CT or MRI. The transverse diameter on the other hand is broader in the lower cervical region. The cross-sectional shape of the spinal cord is ovoid in the mid- and lower cervical regions and tends to be more round in the thoracic, lumbar and upper cervical regions. The

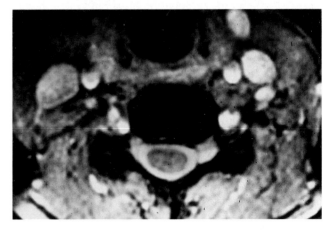

Fig. 30.1.3 Axial MRI of the cervical spine at C5–C6 (T2-weighted image from a multiplanar gradient recalled echo sequence). Internal structure of the spinal cord is shown.

anterior median sulcus varies in width especially in the cervical region. The spinal cord normally terminates at the lower border of L1 but this can vary by one segment and still be normal. The cross-sectional area of the spinal cord in the cervical region is approximately 70–90 mm. It should be emphasized that errors in measurements on images are usually of the order of 10–15% and can be higher.

Intradural spinal roots and cerebrospinal fluid

Intradural portions of the spinal nerves are not shown by plain CT. They are shown best by myelography and computed myelography, and usually can be shown well by modern MRI. Intradural roots are not necessarily shown well on routine MRI protocols, so if there is a particular interest in the intradural roots such as in the diagnosis of arachnoiditis, special pulse sequences may be necessary (Fig. 30.1.4). In myelography and computed myelography, water-soluble contrast medium is often of sufficient density to exceed the specific gravity of the

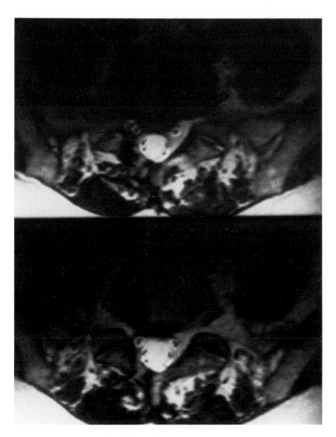

Fig. 30.1.4 Axial MRI of the lumbar spine. This is a T2-weighted image from a fast spin echo sequence with all available movement compensatory strategies applied. The individual roots of the cauda equina are consistently well shown using such a technique.

spinal cord and roots which therefore tend to float in dense contrast medium.

In the cervical region the posterior rootlets appear larger than the anterior, and in the lumbar region the anterior and posterior roots appear approximately equal in size. Intradural roots are usually invisible in the thoracic region on any imaging modality. At the level of L1, the conus medullaris is usually shown as a central small round structure from which the anterior and posterior roots of the cauda equina radiate in four curved linear aggregations, two on each side. Between L2 and L4 the roots aggregate symmetrically in clusters on either side of the midline, often appearing on MRI as a crescentic posterior conglomerate mass in which individual roots can be resolved. At the level of L4, the roots are fewer and more peripheral in location, and symmetry may not be present; however, individual anterior and posterior roots are usually distinguishable, and although they may seem in contact with the lateral aspect of the theca they should be identifiable as rounded individually distinct structures. The roots usually lie peripherally within the theca as they cross the intervertebral disc above their dural ostia, but in the case of S1 the dural ostia usually lie just above the L5–S1 disc.

ROOT SHEATHS

The root sheaths terminate proximal to the dorsal root ganglia; root cysts arising from the region of the termination are relatively frequent. The spinal theca is tethered to the spinal nerves at this point, and the root sheath is also usually relatively loosely attached to the margins of the intervertebral canal. The root sheaths vary in size and length. The root sheaths of C1 and C2 are small and usually invisible, and the root sheaths between T2 and T12 usually are inconspicuous. In the cervical region C8 is usually has largest root sheath. In the lumbar region the root sheaths are longest from L5 to S2, and are relatively short between L1 and L2; the S1 root sheath is usually the largest of all and often diverges from the theca at the level of the upper border of the L5–S1 disc whereas the other lumbar root sheaths diverge from the theca below the lower border of the intervertebral disc (Fig. 30.1.5). Root sheath cysts are often large on S2 roots and often erode the sacral canals.

The root sheaths are not always distributed symmetrically, and sometimes adjacent root sheaths exit very close together and may even be conjoined. This occurs most commonly at L5 and L4 vertebral levels (Fig. 30.1.6). There is usually no associated skeletal anomaly save that the lateral recess at the level of the conjoining is relatively wide. The importance of this

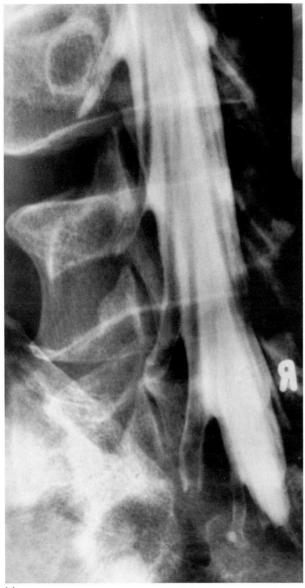

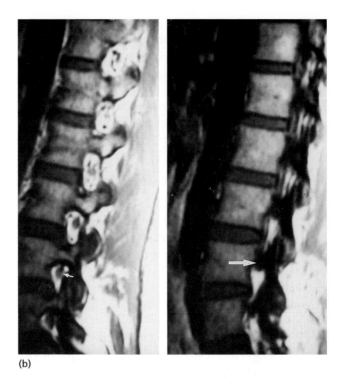

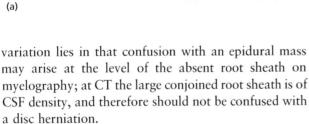

(a)

(b)

Fig. 30.1.5 (a) Water-soluble myelogram, lumbar region, showing the relationship of the roots and root sheaths to the pedicles, apophyseal joints and intervertebral discs.
(b) Parasagittal T1-weighted MRI of the lumbar spine showing, on the left, the infrapedicular parts of the nerve root canals (intervertebral foramen) containing the dorsal root ganglia (arrow), and on the right, the subarticular parts of the nerve root canals (the lateral recesses) containing the medial openings of the subarachnoid sheaths of the spinal nerves just below each disc (arrow).

variation lies in that confusion with an epidural mass may arise at the level of the absent root sheath on myelography; at CT the large conjoined root sheath is of CSF density, and therefore should not be confused with a disc herniation.

CEREBROSPINAL FLUID

Signal from CSF on MRI is modulated significantly by cardiosynchronous longitudinal to and fro movement which becomes progressively damped with increasing distance from the foramen magnum. Areas of stagnant or turbulent flow in wide CSF spaces, such as the cervical part of the cisterna magna and often the posterior subarachnoid space in the thoracic region, can

result in appearances that on occasions have been misinterpreted as significant pathology.

Epidural soft tissues

Visible structures in epidural soft tissues are fat and veins, and the dorsal root ganglia which, together with radicular veins, lie mainly in the intervertebral canals. The dura is in contact with the posterior longitudinal ligament and medial aspect of the pedicles, and usually also is loosely attached to the base of the spinous processes. Epidural fat surrounds the theca except in these situations; it occupies the intervertebral canals and lies anterior to the posterior longitudinal ligament at the level of the vertebral bodies (Schellinger *et al.*, 1990).

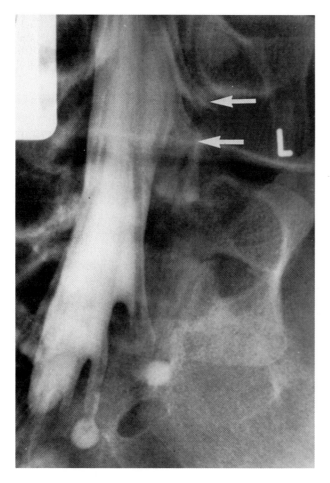

Fig. 30.1.6 Myelogram showing the L4 and L5 spinal roots on the left piercing the dura immediately adjacent to each other though not strictly conjoined (arrows).

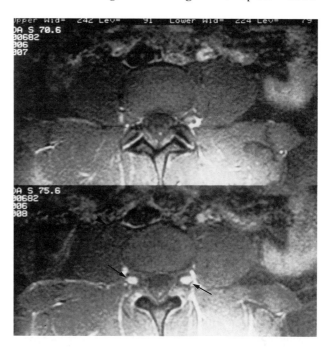

Fig. 30.1.7 Axial T-weighted image of the lumbar spine at L4–L5, made after intravenous gadolinium–DTPA, and a special radiofrequency pulse has been applied to relatively suppress signal from fat which appears dark in this image. The arrows indicate the L4 dorsal root ganglia.

Epidural fat in the thoracic region frequently interposes between the spinous processes and theca from T2 and T10, where it may be as thick as 6 mm and occupy more than half of the sagittal diameter of the thoracic spinal canal. In the thoracic and cervical regions, fat often interposes between the theca, root sheaths and pedicles.

Most visible epidural veins lie anteriorly in the spinal theca and also occupy the inferior parts of the root canals below the spinal nerves. The dorsal root ganglia are large conspicuous structures in the lumbar region on both CT and MRI lying in the intervertebral foramina. In the cervical region only MRI is capable of showing them, and they appear as fusiform structures occupying much of the volume of the intervertebral canals. The ganglia yield a relatively high signal on T2 and most gradient recalled (fast) imaging sequences, though generally lower than the CSF in adjacent root sheaths. An important feature of dorsal root ganglia is that they enhance diffusely and strongly after intravenous gadolinium–DTPA (Fig. 30.1.7).

Skeletal elements and intervertebral discs

The vertebrae are best shown by CT, especially when performed on high-resolution modes. Multiplanar reformatting in the parasagittal or oblique parasagittal planes can be helpful in accurately defining the anatomy of the intervertebral canals and the apophyseal joints. Skeletal structures are reasonably well shown by MRI, and the state of the bone marrow can best be assessed by MRI (Yuh *et al.*, 1989). In children and young adults the axial skeleton contains predominantly red marrow. This is partly replaced by fatty marrow with advancing years and the replacement may be a diffuse or patchy process. The latter results in discrete foci of high signal on T1-weighted sequences which should not be mistaken for a disease process. The fatty marrow reflects high signal on T1- and lower signal on T2-weighted sequences. Highly cellular marrow reflects low signal on T1- and higher on T2-weighted sequences, whether the cells be normal haematogenous or neoplastic or inflammatory in nature.

The paravertebral soft tissues are shown best by MRI but are also reasonably shown by plain CT and by computed myelography. Conventional radiographs are relatively insensitive for recognizing bone destruction, over 50% of bone mass having to be absent before it will be clearly recognizable.

The appearance of intervertebral discs has been the subject of extensive study. The posterior surface of a normal intervertebral disc is slightly concave on axial section except L5–S1 where it is either straight or slightly convex. Internal structure appears of uniform low signal on T1-weighted MRI but is visible on T2-weighted MRI (Fig. 30.1.8). In a normal young adult, the central tissue composed of type II collagen and proteoglycans is clearly distinguishable on T2-weighted sections as a region of higher signal from the dense type I collagenous structure of the outer layers of the annulus fibrosus and hyaline cartilage lining the vertebral end plate, yielding low signal. The compact collagenous horizontal equatorial nuclear lamina appears in adolescence as a low signal structure partly dividing the disc into upper and lower halves on T2-weighted images. It becomes complete in many adults (Yu *et al.*, 1989a). Normal ageing is associated with dehydration and fibrosis of the nucleus which causes signal loss on T2-weighted sequences. This process is not accompanied by annulus bulging or loss of disc height, which may indeed be increased by development of concavity of the vertebral end plates.

Loss of disc space height, usually accompanied by reduced signal from a central part of the disc, either alone or in combination with bulging of the annulus fibrosis >2.5 mm beyond the posterior margin of the vertebral body, is associated with radial tears of the annulus fibrosus; these features are regarded as signs of degeneration to be distinguished from normal maturation (Fugiwara *et al.*, 1989; Yu *et al.*, 1989b) (Fig. 30.1.8).

The intervertebral foramina in the lumbar region can be divided into superior and inferior recesses, the lower recess containing veins and fat, the upper mainly the dorsal root ganglion. The intervertebral disc forms the anterior margin of the inferior recess. The lateral recess of the spinal canal lies medial to the pedicle under cover mainly of the superior articular process and pars inter-articularis of the same vertebra. It contains the spinal theca and medial part of the spinal root sheath. The lateral recess normally contains little or no epidural fat. In the cervical region, the intervertebral canals are bounded anteriorly by the uncovertebral joints and posteriorly by the posterior joints.

ABNORMALITIES OF THE SPINAL CORD

Chronic and acute compression

Chronic spinal cord compression results in deformity of the cross-sectional shape of the spinal cord congruous with the shape of the deforming agent. Considerable

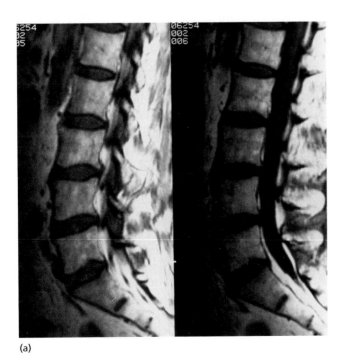

(a)

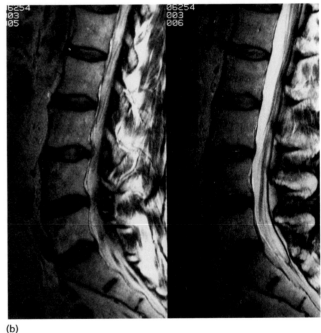

(b)

Fig. 30.1.8 Sagittal MRI of the lumbar spine, to show the normal structure of mid and upper lumbar discs and degeneration in the L4–L5 and L5–S1 discs. Left image is T1-weighted, and the right T2-weighted. The intradural roots are well shown on the T2-weighted images.

deformation of the spinal cord is possible without any pathological change being detectable in its substance, but when the midsagittal diameter or cross-sectional area are reduced by over 50%, pathological changes usually are present. Slow compression produces mainly areas of demyelination with little or no obvious axonal disruption. Rapid compression produces variable amounts of swelling and central necrosis even when deformation is relatively slight. In diseases such as cervical spondylotic myelopathy, both types of cord damage are frequently present.

Autopsy studies have shown that there is reasonable correlation between pathological changes in cord substance and the nature and severity of clinical disability. Correlation of clinical features with alteration in the external contour of the spinal cord is poor, however, and only becomes demonstrable at all when the spinal cord deformity is in excess of 50%. Unfortunately, it has been shown that when the cross-sectional area of the spinal cord is reduced to ≤30 mm, or by more than 50%, associated clinical features usually persist despite decompressive surgery (Fugiwara *et al.*, 1989). A '50% rule' therefore can be defined. When compressive cord deformity is <50%, it is not possible to decide whether or not compression alone is responsible for clinical disability; when >50%, a direct causal relationship becomes more likely but pari passu is less likely to be reversible. While this discouraging rule generally is true for spinal cord compression due to cervical spondylosis and other processes such as subluxations from rheumatoid arthritis, clinical features from even severe spinal cord compression due to slowly growing tumours such as meningiomas often recover: demyelination is reversible, but necrosis which may result from even minor traumatic episodes is not.

Plain CT is of limited value in assessing the severity of spinal cord compression. Myelography usually accurately represents the severity of spinal cord compression and its longitudinal extent. However, errors can arise when the compression is eccentric, central with marked anterior concavity of the spinal cord surface, or when a lateral film of a myelogram is oblique. The cross-sectional images provided by computed myelography are more reliable for indicating the severity of spinal cord compression. The patient is in the supine position when scanned, however, and the neck mildly flexed, a position in which the spinal cord often will not be in contact with anterior osteophytes. Fortunately, the spinal cord has a limited capacity for elastic recoil and usually retains its deformed shape long after compression has been removed (Stevens *et al.*, 1987).

Acute traumatic compression may result in fusiform swelling of the spinal cord. This may be shown by myelography, computed myelography or MRI. In addition, as well as revealing any osseous, disc or ligamentous damage and significant encroachment on the spinal or intravertebral canals, MRI frequently shows signal changes within the substance of the spinal cord which are usually maximal at the site of spinal cord compression and uncommonly extend more than one or two segments beyond. The most frequent change is increased signal on T2-weighted images which may be due to reversible oedema and is not necessarily of poor prognostic significance for eventual recovery; changes consisting of low signal on T1 and high signal on T2 are likely to represent more severe damage such as myelomalacia (necrosis), which is associated with poor functional recovery. A central area of high signal on T1-weighted and low signal within a larger area of high signal on T2-weighted images indicates haematomyelia, and usually is a poor prognostic sign (Ramananskas *et al.*, 1989; Stevens, 1990).

Chronic post-traumatic myelopathy usually is accompanied by cystic change in the region of the spinal cord injury. Most often this is localized to the site of injury, but can be extensive and may involve the whole spinal cord which frequently becomes distended. Clinical correlation with an ascending or progressive myelopathy is not as close as was suggested in the past. Although post-traumatic cysts may be shown by plain CT it is not a reliable or recommended mode of study. Myelography may demonstrate enlargement, thinning, flattening or irregularity of the spinal cord, or it may appear normal. Occasionally contrast medium can be seen entering the cord through a tear in the region of the injury where frequently there is a complete or partial myelographic block. Computed myelography more sensitively demonstrates contrast penetration into the spinal cord. This occurs at a variable rate and may not appear for 6–24 hours after the myelogram, necessitating delayed post-myelography CT for demonstration. Contrast medium may be retained in intramedullary cavities for many hours or even days. MRI demonstrates intramedullary cysts as well-circumscribed areas of homogeneous signal change, low on T1- and high on T2-weighted images. Pulsatile CSF movements within cysts may result in low signal on T2-weighted images and when present confirms conclusively the fluid nature of the cyst contents. MRI also frequently shows extensive high signal throughout the remaining substance of the spinal cord on T2-weighted images, a finding that correlates poorly with the level of clinical myelopathy.

Localized, mainly central, necrosis of the spinal cord usually is referred to as 'myelomalacia'. This can extend into otherwise non-contused spinal cord substance for many segments as fusiform columns or spindles of necrotic tissue. Such changes are identifiable on delayed post-myelography CT as areas of abnormal accumulation of contrast medium within spinal cord substance, and on MRI as areas of low signal on T1-weighted and uniformly high signal on T2-weighted images (Mehalic *et al.*, 1990). This process is difficult to distinguish with certainty from cysts containing drainable fluid.

Neoplasms

The main intramedullary neoplasms encountered are gliomas (astrocytomas and ependymomas), haemangioblastomas and very occasionally metastases. The former usually are diffuse, and the latter two localized; all are commonly associated with intramedullary cyst formation which may be extensive. Plain CT may demonstrate intramedullary cysts as areas of lower attenuation. Myelography, however, is necessary to demonstrate the extent of cord expansion, which usually is fusiform over several segments. Sometimes the entire spinal cord is enlarged. Enlarged vessels on the surface of the swollen cord increase the probability of haemangioblastoma though some ependymomas are highly vascular and occasionally cord swelling occurs with intramedullary arteriovenous malformations. Computed myelography usually will distinguish solid from cystic areas provided early and delayed imaging is performed.

MRI is the preferred method of assessing intramedullary neoplasms. Solid and cystic areas can usually be distinguished, and most intramedullary neoplasms show enhancement with intravenous gadolinium–DTPA. In clinical practice, MRI can distinguish reliably idiopathic syringomyelia from most intrinsic neoplasms associated with syrinx, whether or not gadolinium is administered. Post-contrast MRI is usually necessary to demonstrate the very focal nature of haemangioblastomas. Gliomas frequently are relatively well circumscribed within cord substance but usually extend over many cord segments.

Syringomyelia

Syringomyelia is usually associated with mild-to-moderate descent of the cerebellar hemispheres into the upper part of the spinal canal, referred to as cerebellar ectopia or Chiari type I malformation. A small proportion are due to post-traumatic or post-inflammatory myelopathy and some are associated with spinal cord tumours. In about up to 20% of cases, however, no cause can be found. A major role of imaging is to demonstrate any causative lesion and to elucidate the anatomy to determine therapeutic strategy.

Though plain CT may show low attenuation within a spinal cord cyst, a normal study does not exclude one and CT is usually unhelpful. On myelography, the spinal cord appears enlarged in about 80% of cases, small in about 10% and normal in about 10%; size may vary with posture. Enlargement is diffuse and usually involves many segments, but occasionally is localized. Contrast medium rarely is discernible within the cyst in non-traumatic syringomyelia. Computed myelography demonstrates concentric enlargement of the cross-section of the spinal cord. Contrast medium probably enters the cyst from the subarachnoid space in all cases, though this often is most clearly apparent 6–24 hours after the myelogram (Fig. 30.1.9). MRI is the best modality for demonstrating the extent and nature of intramedullary cysts. In idiopathic cases without cerebellar ectopia, administration of intravenous gadolinium–DTPA may be necessary to further exclude an intrinsic tumour. Signal from intramedullary cysts is low on T1-weighted images but varies on T2-weighted image due to the variable mobility of the fluid within the cyst. Signal change is rarely seen in uninvolved cord substance in Chiari-associated and idiopathic syringomyelia.

Inflammatory conditions

The most frequent inflammatory condition is multiple sclerosis in adults and acute disseminated encephalomyelitis in children; acute infections are commonly due to enteroviruses and Echo viruses, and bacterial causes include *Borrelia*. More chronic lesions, which include HIV-I infections and AIDS and inflammatory sequelae, are increasingly frequent. Also intramedullary granulomas are occasionally encountered due either to tuberculosis or sarcoidosis.

Plain CT is of no value in these conditions. Myelography may show focal enlargement of the spinal cord usually involving only a few segments, or eventually may show atrophy which is sometimes profound. Computed myelography is expected to show concentric enlargement of the spinal cord cross-section or in chronic cases shrinkage and distortion. Intramedullary cysts may form which can become extensive and indistinguishable from syringomyelia of other aetiology; early and delayed contrast penetration of these cysts may be observed on computed myelography.

MRI is the most sensitive modality for detecting this type of pathology, but even so, in acutely presenting multiple sclerosis clinically isolated to the spinal cord,

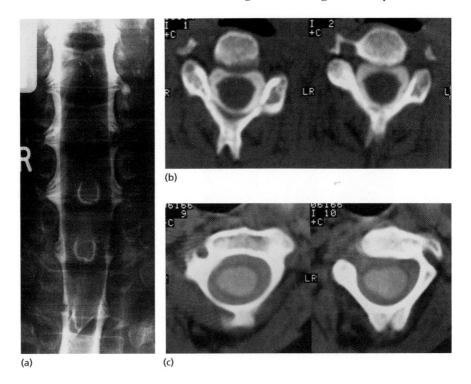

Fig. 30.1.9 Syringomyelia. (a) Myelogram; (b) immediate post-myelography CT; (c) delayed post-myelography CT (see text for description).

(a)

(b)

(c)

it may be positive in little more than 50% of cases (Fig. 30.1.10). In approximately 50% of patients with clinically isolated spinal multiple sclerosis, MRI will show lesions in the brain. These may occur in other types of encephalomyelitis also. Necrosis may be apparent as areas of more circumscribed low signal on T1-weighted images and high signal on T2-weighted images, and some enhancement may occur on T1-weighted images after the administration of intravenous gadolinium–DTPA. Syringomyelia may develop as described on p. 1040. In granulomas, meningeal involvement may also be apparent with irregularity and partial obliteration of the subarachnoid space, which also may be shown by myelography, and sometimes meningeal enhancement after gadolonium–DTPA.

Congenital abnormalities

The commonest congenital abnormalities are the lipomyelomeningodysplasias, which can present early or in adult life with or without external evidence of spinal dysraphism. The lumbosacral segments almost invariably are involved. Some lipomas are entirely intra-medullary, being enclosed by an intact dura and spinal canal which frequently is focally expanded at the site of the lesion. The fatty nature of components are shown by plain CT, but precise localization usually requires myelography of the whole spine and foramen magnum and full anatomical display of the affected region (Vezina *et al.*, 1984) is then provided by subsequent CT. MRI fulfils all functions and is the diagnostic modality of choice (Fig. 30.1.11).

Diastematomyelia is often suggested by plain film which shows focal enlargement of the spinal canal without erosion sometimes with partial vertebral fusion and or sagittal osseous spur. While plain CT may permit recognition of the abnormality, particularly if there is a split dural tube or spinal canal, definitive evaluation and confirmation of a split cord usually requires myelography and even better computed myelography. MRI demonstrates the lesion well.

Congenital cystic lesions involving the spinal cord are usually developmental and include ependymal, dermoid, or enterogenous cysts. Much less commonly they may be a consequence of vascular occlusion or traumatic labour. Plain CT may demonstrate associated bony anomalies such as butterfly vertebra and may reveal fatty components of a dermoid, but usually myelography is required to localize the lesion. The spinal cord typically shows abrupt localized expansion which may also involve the spinal canal, and following CT may demonstrate the lesion to be of relatively low density. MRI is the diagnostic test of choice showing all features that are visible on either CT or myelography.

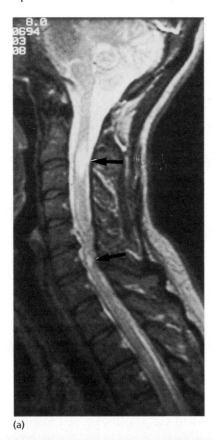

(a)

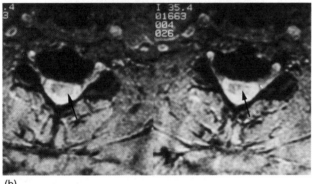

(b)

Fig. 30.1.10 MRI of the cervical spinal cord. (a) T2-weighted sagittal images. (b) Volume gradient recalled axial images. Several plaques of multiple sclerosis are shown (arrows). Spondylosis is probably irrelevant.

Vascular abnormalities

INFARCTION

Acute spinal cord infarction usually results in little or no radiologically demonstrable changes, although signal abnormalities have been shown in presumed acute cases on MRI. The late effects of infarction producing spinal cord atrophy can be shown by myelography and post-

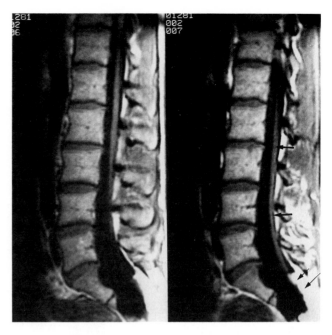

Fig. 30.1.11 MRI of lipomyelomeningodysplasia in the lumbar region. T1-weighted sagittal image. Single arrows, spinal cord; double arrows, transdural lipoma.

myelography CT, as well as MRI by small size of the spinal cord and signal changes within it. These appearances, however, are rarely specific enough for the radiological appearances in isolation to suggest the correct diagnosis.

VASCULAR MALFORMATIONS

Most spinal 'angiomas' are dural arteriovenous fistulae with intradural drainage. True intramedullary lesions are either arteriovenous malformations of variable size and/or localized arteriovenous fistulae. All these arteriovenous shunts distend and enlarge intradural veins, and cause variable alterations in cord substance related to ischaemia and/or congestion, which can be very extensive. Intramedullary malformations may show localized spinal cord swelling. They may be complicated by haemorrhage into the spinal cord and which could be shown but not excluded by plain CT. CT, therefore, has no role in diagnosis. MRI is most sensitive at detecting the presence of intramedullary haemorrhage, either past or present, and often shows enlarged vessels, but myelography is more sensitive than MRI at detecting enlarged intradural veins. Cases undergoing therapeutic evaluation require spinal angiography.

Non-shunting vascular malformations which are not usually revealed by spinal angiography include capillary, cavernous and telangiectatic angiomas; these also may be associated with intramedullary haemorrhage. The spinal cord may be mildly expanded at the site of the lesion but often it has a normal external contour. The diagnosis of these low flow lesions usually requires MRI; plain CT, myelography and computed myelography are often normal or at best non-specific, and spinal angiography also is usually normal (Fig. 30.1.12).

INTRADURAL ABNORMALITIES

Neoplasms

Although a wide variety of tumours can occur in the intradural space, the vast majority are neurofibromas, meningiomas or metastases.

Plain spine radiographs or CT may show clear evidence of a neurofibroma as an extraspinal mass, with erosion of the margins of an adjacent intervertebral foramen and/or the spinal canal, but definitive evaluation usually requires myelography, preferably followed by CT, or MRI (Figs 30.1.13 and 30.1.14).

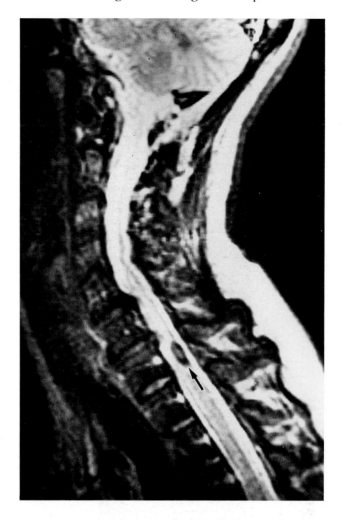

Fig. 30.1.12 (*Right*) MRI cervical spine, T2-weighted sagittal image, made 4 days after a whiplash injury. A circumscribed area of low intensity is shown in the dorsal columns of the spinal cord (arrow) presumed to represent blood products in relation to an incidental intramedullary angioma. The patient complained of neck and right shoulder pain, and this lesion lay at C7. Further angiomas are present at the craniocervical junction.

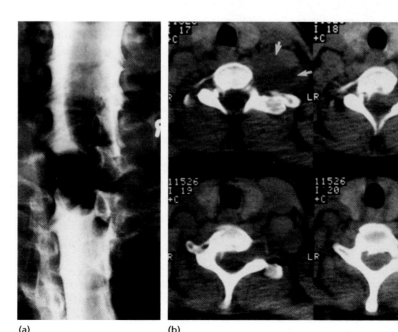

Fig. 30.1.13 Neurofibroma at C7 on the left. (a) Myelogram. (b) Immediate post-myelogram CT at C7. Contrast is almost completely excluded from the subarachnoid space. The lesion has a large extraspinal component (arrows).

(a)

(b)

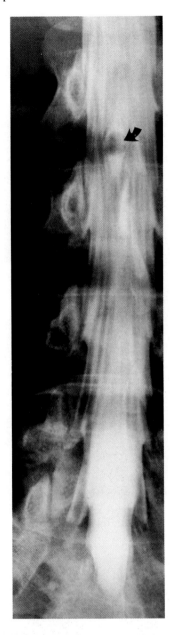

Fig. 30.1.14 Myelogram showing a small neurofibroma (arrow). A small lesion like this is unlikely to be shown by a routine MRI performed for back pain or radiculopathy.

Meningiomas generally occur in the thoracic region and affect older women, but they can involve the cervical region and foramen magnum in both men and women. They very occasionally produce recognizable changes in skeletal tissues, and rarely have extradural components of significant size. They are uncommonly shown by heavy calcification within the tumour, but generally myelography or MRI is essential for the diagnosis of intraspinal meningioma, and CT may be necessary after myelography to provide definitive evidence of its extramedullary location (Fig. 30.1.15).

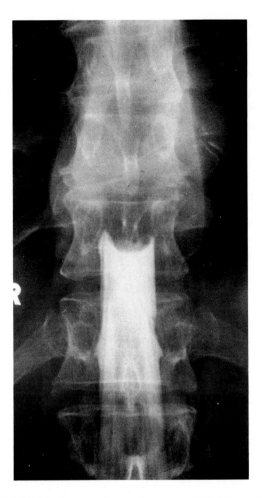

Fig. 30.1.15 Myelogram of a meningioma at T11. The typical appearance of obstruction of the subarachnoid space by an intradural mass is well shown.

Intradural metastases are most sensitively detected by myelography whether or not followed by CT. They produce either nodular masses or diffuse thickening of roots. This can be difficult to recognize on MRI, although intravenous gadolinium−DTPA improves detectability and approaches the sensitivity of myelography for detection of such masses. Both myelography and MRI, with and without gadolinium enhancement, however, are usually negative in patients with clinical and cytological evidence of intradural metastatic involvement (Yousem *et al.*, 1990).

Inflammation

Arachnoiditis may occur in a wide variety of contexts. Most arachnoiditis encountered in clinical practice probably arises iatrogenically as a result of substances injected either intentionally or unintentionally into the spinal theca. Arachnoiditis can also accompany predominantly epidural inflammation and fibrosis. Arachnoiditis results in adhesion of the intradural nerve roots to each other and to the theca itself. Extensive adhesions may result in loculation of the subarachnoid space, and may be accompanied by secondary changes in the spinal cord such as myelomalacia and cyst formation. Plain CT has no role in primary diagnosis, although it may show evidence of the causative agents such as iophendylate (Myodil or Pantopaque) or Thorotrast, and very occasionally extensive calcification occurs in the dura which may be recognizable on plain radiographs or CT.

Myelography has been the definitive test and probably remains the most sensitive for diagnosing minimal changes. Good-quality MRI is just about as sensitive as myelography or post-myelography CT (Delamarker *et al.*, 1990) (Fig. 30.1.16), and has the additional advantage of demonstrating parts of the spinal canal which may be rendered inaccessible to myelographic contrast medium by intradural adhesions. Changes in the spinal cord are also most sensitively shown by MRI. MRI is useful in the search for other types of pathology, and in particular recurrent disc herniation when arachnoiditis is present, but not necessarily the cause of non-specific symptoms.

Arachnoiditis may arise from spinal infections, of which tuberculosis is a leading cause particularly in some underdeveloped countries. It may also result from cystercercosis, and in this condition mobile intradural bladders may be visible on myelography or MRI.

EXTRADURAL ABNORMALITIES

Degenerative conditions

INTERVERTEBRAL DISCS

The distinction between normal maturation which is a diffuse process and degeneration which generally is more focal has been noted; both processes are, however, usually present together in the elderly. Recent studies have indicated that degeneration of the nuclear matrix invariably is associated with radial tears of the annulus fibrosis of variable severity and extent in addition to the concentric tears which are a feature of normal ageing (Yu *et al.*, 1989a). Bulging of the outer layers of the annulus fibrosis >2.5 mm beyond the margins of the vertebral bodies implies the presence of radial tears of the annulus fibrosis (Yu *et al.*, 1989a).

The earliest changes of degeneration are shown by MRI, and consist of reduction in signal from the central parts of the disc on T2-weighted images, signifying decrease in hydration. Penetration of the outer layers of the annulus fibrosis by relatively hyperintense nuclear material on T2-weighted images gives direct evidence of radial tears; it is commonly shown in moderately advanced, but only occasionally on routine, imaging in early degeneration. Granulation tissue in radial tears is also demonstrable in T1-weighted images made after the intravenous injection of gadolinium−DPTA. In advanced degeneration, the nucleus is replaced by fibrous tissue (T1- and T2-weighted low signal) which may develop cystic spaces containing fluid (T2-weighted high signal) or gas (T1- and T2-weighted low signal).

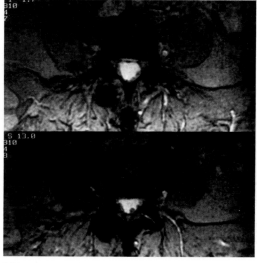
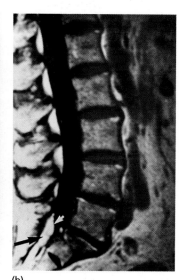

Fig. 30.1.16 (a) Axial MRI at L5 level, T2-weighted (gradient echo image). Intradural roots are adherent to the dura. Adhesion needs to be distinguished from normal peripheral location of roots, usual below L4, where the individual roots remain visible, although their distribution may not be precisely asymmetrical. (b) Sagittal T1-weighted MRI image of the lumbar spine showing the characteristic high signal of residual Myodil in the caudal thecal sac (arrows). (a)   (b)

Nuclear protrusions are shown as posterolateral, smooth but eccentric bulges of the annulus fibrosis. Nuclear herniations are definite intraspinal masses usually extending above or below the intervertebral disc, but in fact they nearly always are *contained* by the posterior longitudinal ligament which constitutes the posterior boundary of the anterior epidural space (Schellinger *et al.*, 1990). Sequestered fragments have lost contact with the disc of origin, and can lie anywhere in the spinal canal including posteriorly. Imaging can be unreliable in making the distinction between sequestrations and true herniations and those contained by the posterior longitudinal ligament or its lateral extensions (Schellinger *et al.*, 1990); this may be particularly significant when percutaneous discectomy or chemonucleolysis is contemplated. Plain CT and MRI usually are adequate to demonstrate these lesions and their effects on extradural roots and thecal sac (Figs 30.1.17–30.1.20).

A definite diagnosis can be made when continuity with the disc of origin is apparent, and the density of the fragment is similar to that of disc material, although on MRI the T2-related signal is often slightly higher. If image quality is inadequate to provide a definitive diagnosis, which is much less likely with MRI than CT, myelography may be required. Myelography may also be indicated when clinico-radiological correlation is poor and the possibility of an alternative diagnosis to intervertebral disc disease or spinal degeneration is suspected on clinical grounds.

Sclerotic bone reaction is usual in the parts of the vertebral bodies adjacent to degenerate discs. On MRI it returns low signal on both T1- and T2-weighted sequences. Reactive granulation tissue occurs less frequently and causes low signal on T1- and high on T2-weighted sequences, enhancing with gadolinium-DTPA which may also involve the disc. Red bone

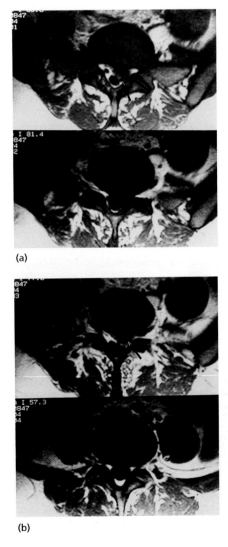

(a)

(b)

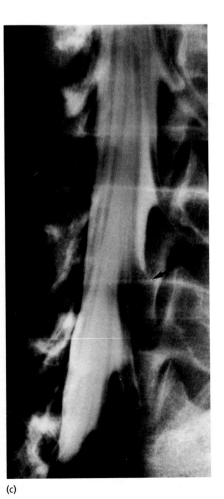

(c)

Fig. 30.1.17 (a) Axial MRI (T1-weighted image) showing a large extended fragment entrapping the left S1 root (arrow). (b) Axial MRI (T1-weighted image) showing a small protrusion (arrow) not causing definite root entrapment. (c) Myelogram showing compression of the left L5 root by a focal L4–L5 disc protrusion. The root is compressed in the subarticular part of the root canal (lateral recess) (arrow).

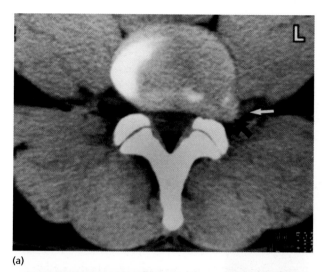

(a)

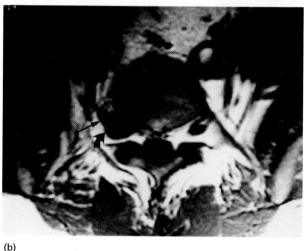

(b)

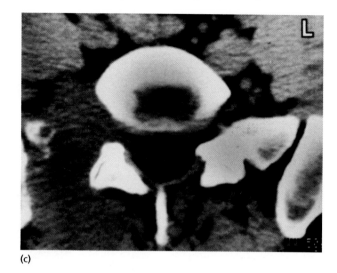

(c)

Fig. 30.1.18 Far lateral disc protrusions shown on (a) CT and (b) MRI. These lesions are not visible on myelography and compress the root leaving the spinal canal beneath the pedicle of the vertebra above. The small arrows indicate the compressed dorsal root ganglia. (b) Shows how sometimes these lesions are confused with a neurofibroma. (c) Axial plain CT, showing a large destructive mass arising in the lateral mass of L5 and invading the L5 intervertebral foramen on the right. This sarcoma was not shown by myelography; even this degree of bone destruction was difficult to recognize on the myelogram.

marrow may be replaced by fatty marrow adjacent to the disc which gives high signal on T1-weighted and normal signal on T2-weighted sequences. None of these changes appears to have clinical significance.

OSTEOARTHROSIS

Osteoarthrosis in the posterior joints, combined with ligament thickening and diffuse bulging of the annulus fibrosis associated with degeneration of the intervertebral disc often accompanied by subluxation, is the usual cause of degenerative canal stenosis. These changes are well shown by axial imaging techniques, particularly plain CT and MRI (Modic *et al.*, 1988) (Fig. 30.1.21). Myelography is seldom indicated for further elucidation of these conditions in the lumbar spine, but is more useful in the cervical spine where it will show the severity of spinal cord compression. Good-quality MRI

is just as effective, however, at showing spinal cord compression and has the additional advantage of revealing internal cord damage.

Reparative processes associated with ligament degeneration may result in intraspinal masses which histologically can resemble mucoid cysts or fibrocartilaginous material simulating nuclear protrusions. These may occur anywhere in the spinal canal and arise from the posterior longitudinal ligament, transverse ligament of the atlas, ligamenta flava (Fig. 30.1.22) or the synovium of the posterior joints themselves (Fig. 30.1.23). Sometimes the degenerate ligaments and reparative masses become heavily calcified or ossified and involve many segments of the spine; extensive ossification in the posterior longitudinal ligament in the cervical spine possibly should be classified here. Local masses may superficially simulate meningioma, from which they are distinguished by recognition of their extradural origin.

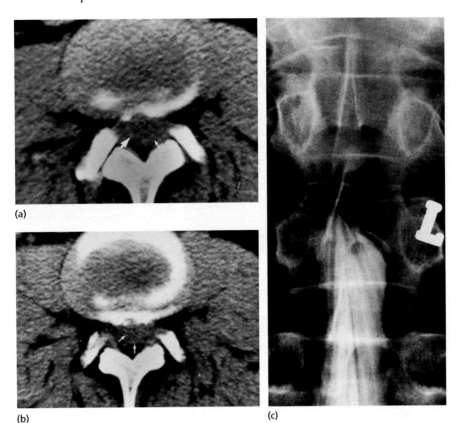

(a)

(b)

(c)

Fig. 30.1.19 Large lumbar disc protrusion. (a) and (b) are images from a plain CT at L3–L4. A very large disc protrusion is evident, but is difficult to recognize because it occupies most of the spinal canal. The arrows indicate its outline. It was missed on this study, but shown unequivocally on the myelogram (c), performed 2 days later. The patient had clinically severe cauda equina compression.

The extensive lesions may cause diffuse narrowing of the spinal canal requiring wide decompression. (Yamashita *et al.*, 1990).

These conditions are shown well by plain CT especially when ossified or calcified and also by MRI. Where MRI is not available myelography may be required to demonstrate more precisely the effects on neural structures in the cervical and thoracic regions.

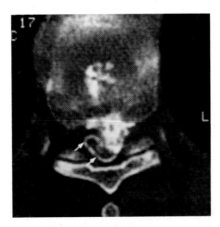

Fig. 30.1.20 A large calcified thoracic disc protrusion shown on a computed myelogram. The spinal cord is indicated by arrows. Thoracic disc herniations commonly calcify like this.

THE POST-OPERATIVE SPINE

Surgery on the spinal canal usually results in conspicuous epidural scar tissue. This tends to contract over time, and may exert traction with distortion of the spinal theca. Scar tissue generally shows as a poorly demarcated region in which there is either obliteration or diminution of the amount of epidural fat and it can make interpretation of computed images more difficult. CT or MRI should be avoided in the very early post-operative period, because oedema and haematoma often obliterate anatomical features to such an extent that interpretation becomes unreliable. Residual or recurrent nuclear herniation is more likely to appear as a focal mass deforming the theca or roots by pressure rather than by traction. Plain CT may permit confident recognition of scar tissue from recurrent or associated nuclear protrusion, but its accuracy is only about 80%. Intravenous contrast usually results in detectable enhancement of epidural scar tissue less than 2 years old, but some enhancement may occur around recurrent disc herniations, and scar tissue more than 2 years old may not show enhancement. MRI usually plus gadolinium-enhanced MRI is the definitive method of recognizing scar tissue from recurrent or residual disc herniation,

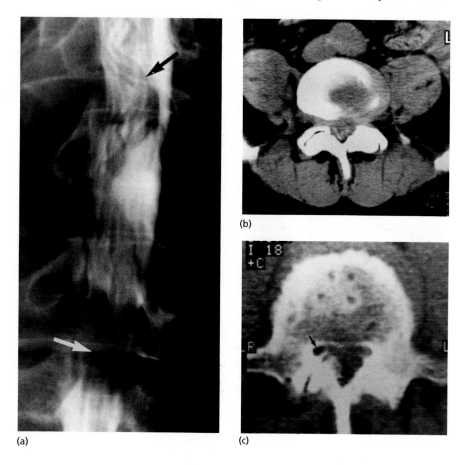

Fig. 30.1.21 Lower lumbar canal stenosis. (a) Myelogram showing a compressed subarachnoid space at L4—L5 (white arrow) with redundant sinuosity of the elongated roots above (black arrow). (b) A following CT showing a diffusely bulging intervertebral disc and osteoarthritic changes in the posterior joints. (c) Plain CT in another patient with a severe localized canal stenosis due to osteophytes. A stenotic later recess is indicated by the arrow.

(a)   (c)

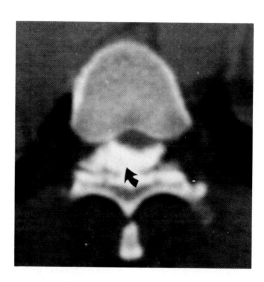

Fig. 30.1.22 Axial plain CT at T11 showing an ossified mass in the position of the ligamentum flavum (arrow).

whether alone or, as is more usual, in combination (Hueftle *et al.*, 1988) (Fig. 30.1.24). Persistent pain a few weeks or months after back surgery may be associated with infection either in the disc itself or in the surgical wound; MRI is the most sensitive technique for suggesting this and sometimes will indicate an abscess which would benefit from surgical drainage (Fig. 30.1.25).

In the cervical region, failure to respond to surgery or recurrent symptoms of myelopathy or radiculopathy may be due to persistent spinal cord compression due to inadequate decompression at the time of the original surgery. Although it is sometimes stated that posterior osteophytes resorb after adequate spinal fusion, in practice this process, if it occurs at all, is generally too slow or insufficient. Also, persistent spinal cord compression due to residual osteophytes is shown in up to 60% of patients with persistent or recurrent symptoms (Clifton *et al.*, 1990). Plain CT may show that the spinal canal is still significantly narrowed, but additional imaging is advisable in case there are soft disc protrusions at other levels which the plain CT may fail to

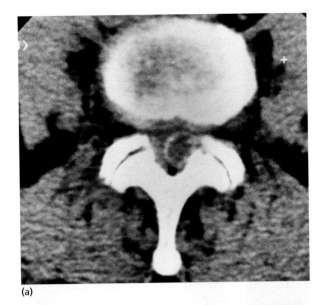

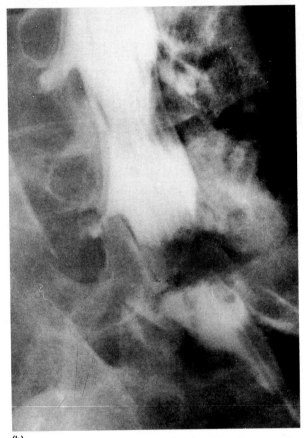

Fig. 30.1.23 (a) Plain CT at the L4–L5 disc level showing a cyst-like mass attached to the apophyseal joint and protruding into the spinal canal. (b) Myelogram of the same case. Synovial cyst.

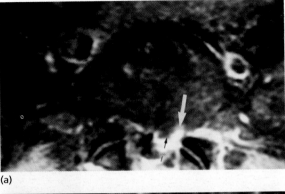

(a)

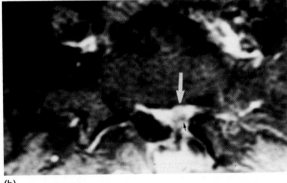

(b)

Fig. 30.1.24 (a,b) Axial T1-weighted MRI images at L5–S1. Fat suppression has been applied, and gadolinium–DTPA administered intravenously. The brightly enhancing intraspinal tissue (white arrow) is mainly post-operative scar tissue; within the scar, however, a small residual disc fragment is visible (black arrow).

show (Fig. 30.1.26). MRI should show both features adequately and when available should remove the necessity for myelography.

IMAGING FOR BACK PAIN, SCIATICA AND BRACHALGIA

These are the commonest clinical contexts for which spinal imaging is requested. The aims of imaging are to exclude causes such as neoplasia and infection, in which plain radiography has a very limited role, and to identify various types of spondyloarthrosis in which plain radiography is obsolete.

Back pain and sciatica

Myelography should only be considered as an initial investigation when there are strong clinical grounds for suspecting disease of roots within the thecal sac or involving spinal cord. Plain CT of the lower three disc

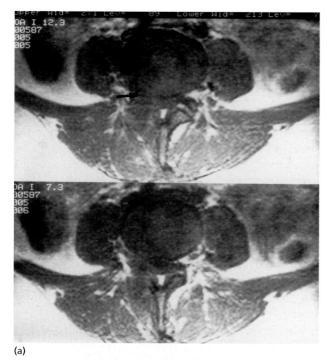

(a)

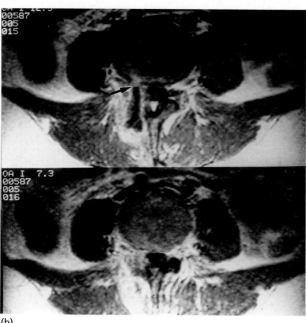

(b)

Fig. 30.1.25 Axial T1-weighted MRI before (a) and after (b) intravenous gadolinium–DTPA. Large abscess cavity is shown in the extraspinal soft tissues extending into the intervertebral disc (arrows).

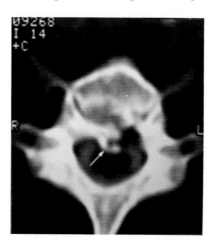

Fig. 30.1.26 Axial image from a post-myelography CT at C6. Persistent spinal cord compression is shown due to an incompletely removed osteophyte (arrow). An anterior fusion and osteophytectomy had been performed 3 years earlier; the fusion was successful, but much of the osteophyte remains.

gadolinium–DTPA is given when indicated, and the pathological regions included. In the context of isolated back pain and non-specific leg or buttock pain, plain CT has a little more to offer over plain radiography in assisting in the exclusion of causes other than spondylo-arthrosis. Spondylolisthesis can be equally well shown by appropriately angled or reformatted CT or by MRI and both congenital and degenerative canal stenosis are revealed by either modality.

Discography still is advocated by some to identify a specific pain provocative level when multiple discs are shown to be abnormal by MRI (Yu *et al.*, 1989b). The idea, however, that discography can definitively indicate and localize a discogenic origin for back or leg pain in the absence of root compression, and that having done so the pain necessarily will be cured by discectomy or fusion at that level, has never been adequately substantiated; unless this happens, the value of discography will remain controversial.

Brachalgia

The cervical root canals are difficult to image, and the probability of an extra-spinal site of neural entrapment is higher than for sciatica. Imaging has yet to prove of value in demonstrating nerve entrapment in peripheral sites such as thoracic inlet, elbow and carpal tunnel. Peripheral nerve conduction studies are a necessary adjunct to imaging, but results can be unreliable. Plain radiography, including oblique views, are valueless in accurately defining the degree of stenosis of cervical root canals. Plain CT is better, but clinicoradiological

levels is an appropriate first investigation for sciatica. MRI is even better, because in addition to showing all the relevant articulations it will also replace myelography for detection of intradural disease and spinal cord involvement when appropriate pulse sequences are used, correlation remains poor and there may not be enough soft-tissue contrast to identify extruded disc material or deformation of root sheaths or thecal sac. Myelography remains a reliable test to demonstrate compression of cervical root sheaths and thecal sac, and both sensitivity and specificity are improved by adding CT. In theory, modern high-resolution MRI should be the investigation of choice, but results can be inconsistent even on the best equipment. Various strategies have been devised such as imaging in the plane of the root canals, and whole-volume techniques which can generate thin slices. Thin slices reduce susceptibility effects which may render location of boundaries uncertain within limits of 1–2.5 mm, not very satisfactory when imaging a structure as narrow as a cervical root canal (Fig. 30.1.27).

Trauma

Plain radiography remains the examination of choice for localizing fractures and dislocations of the spine. Plain CT is far more sensitive than plain radiography at demonstrating the extent of the disruption, and therefore the likelihood of instability and the state of the spinal canal (Figs 30.1.28 and 30.1.29). Plain CT, however, may not detect fractures, particularly if they are not displaced and the fracture line runs approximately in the plane of the CT section, unless thin sections are acquired (≤3 mm) for reformatting in coronal, sagittal or oblique planes as necessary. This is essential if laminar, lateral mass and dens fractures are to be recognized with adequate sensitivity. Plain CT is generally inadequate to demonstrate the state of the spinal cord and other soft tissues within the spinal canal and if MRI is not available, myelography may be indicated in spinal trauma if clinical disability is thought to be due to acute disc herniation, usually in the absence of major fractures.

MRI of good quality is the diagnostic test of choice if neurological disability is present in that it may demonstrate changes within the spinal cord as well as epidural tissues and paraspinal tissues, including compressing subdural and extradural haematomas. Usually it is adequate to demonstrate bony, disc and ligamentous injuries.

MRI has shown traumatic disc herniation to be relatively frequent particularly in the cervical region. Ligament disruption is recognized by discontinuity of the low-signal fibrous bands, often with intervening high-signal haemorrhagic fluid on T1-weighted sequences. In

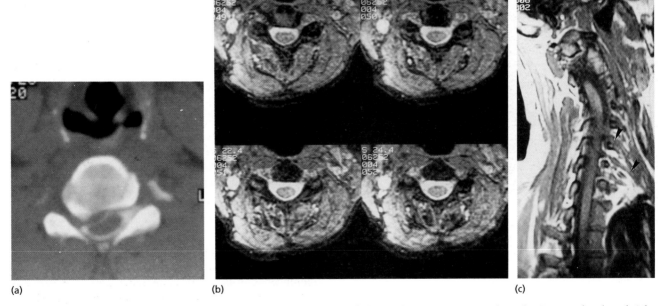

(a)   (b)   (c)

Fig. 30.1.27 (a) Axial image from a computed myelogram at C5–C6. Soft disc is shown compressing the right C6 root sheath and right side of the spinal cord. Such lesions are easily shown by myelography, and generally correlate well with clinical features. More lateralized lesions create greater diagnostic difficulty. (b) A set of images from a volume MRI study of the cervical spine using a gradient echo technique. Sections are 2 mm thick. Several images of each intervertebral canal are generated using this method, which probably has the best chance of diagnosing entrapment of cervical roots confined to the root canals and lateral to the theca. This case is normal. (c) Oblique T1-weighted MRI of the cervical spine in the plane of the left C5–C8 spinal root canals, showing the roots and parts of the trunks of the bronchial plexus (arrows).

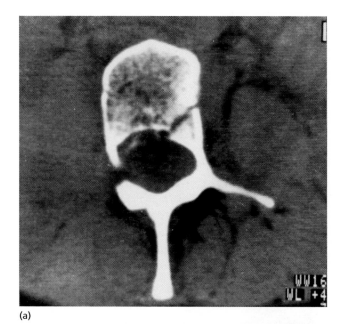

(a)

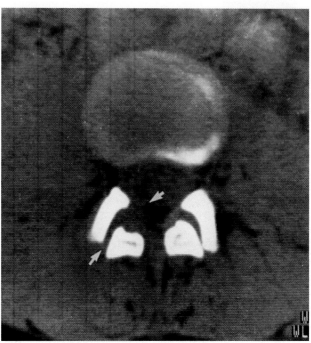

(b)

Fig. 30.1.28 Axial CT of the lumbar spine at L2 and the L2–L3 disc space. Fractures of the body of L2 were shown on plain radiography. CT showed involvement of posterior aspects of the L2 body, and disruption of the apophyseal joints especially the right with capsular swelling (arrows).

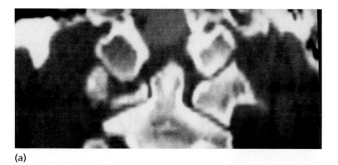

(a)

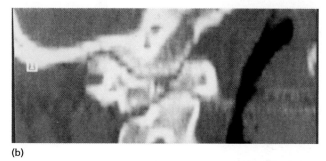

(b)

Fig. 30.1.29 Coronal (a) and oblique parasagittal (b) reformatted image of the craniovertebral junction generated from a stack of 1.5 mm axial slices on plain CT. Fracture of the right lateral mass of C1 is well shown.

the case of penetrating injuries, the possibility of inducing cord damage by movement of ferromagnetic fragments should be considered and preliminary plain films are essential.

Defects in the interarticular parts of the neural arches of the lumbar and rarely cervical vertebrae can be associated with instability. Occasionally these are clearly congenital in origin, because of the presence of other dysplastic features. Most, however, represent chronic ununited fractures. On CT they typically appear as irregular defects, sometimes with small detached bony fragments, and accompanied by sclerosis. Some displacement is usual but not invariable, which requires reformatting for adequate evaluation. On MRI, the defects usually are accompanied by low signal on T1- and T2-weighted images due to sclerosis and fibrosis, and displacement is shown in sagittal and parasagittal images. In practice, it can be difficult to distinguish spondylolisthesis due to traumatic pars interarticularis defects from that due to severe osteoarthritis in the apophyseal joints.

Traumatic brachial or lumbosacral plexopathies are often pre-ganglionic avulsion injuries. Avulsion occurs either at the spinal cord or intervertebral foramen, the latter occurring most commonly in the lumbar region. In each case, the relevant root sheaths are usually damaged, and pseudomeningocoeles may develop though they are not invariable (Fig. 30.1.30). Myelography probably remains the most reliable method of confirming avulsion of intradural rootlets from the cervical cord; following CT will best demonstrate the presence and extent of

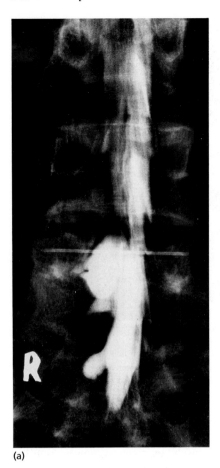

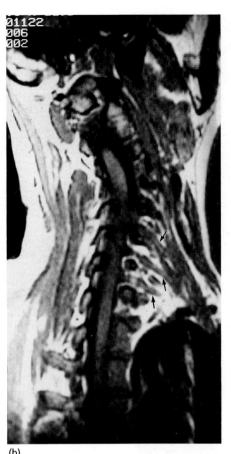

(a)   (b)

Fig. 30.1.30 (a) Myelogram showing avulsion injuries of multiple lumbosacral roots of the left side. (b) Oblique MRI of the cervical region, T1-weighted. Normal case. The roots and lower trunks of the left brachial plexus (arrows) are well shown by images of this sort of quality and may remove the need for myelography in many cases of traumatic brachial plexopathy.

associated meningocoeles, though these usually are not of relevance even when large or having extensive intraspinal components. Good-quality MRI should be as reliable as computed myelography in the cervical region, and may be at least as good and possibly even better than myelography and CT in the lumbosacral region when avulsion may have occurred at the intervertebral foramen (Fig. 30.1.29b).

Whiplash mechanism injuries may result in fractures, fracture dislocations, acute disc herniations and spinal cord contusion, which may be shown readily by the various imaging modalities. In the common post-whiplash syndromes, however, which consist mainly of pain, typically there are no specific abnormalities on plain radiography, CT or myelography. MRI shows evidence of focal or multifocal cervical disc or other type of degenerative canal stenosis in about 70% of such cases, but again specificity is lacking. Very occasionally unexpected and formerly unrecognized pathology is uncovered such as syringomyelia, spinal cord tumour or angioma (see Fig. 30.1.11).

Inflammatory conditions

INFECTIONS

Spinal osteomyelitis usually manifests as a destructive discovertebral lesion. CT is far more sensitive than plain radiography at demonstrating bone destruction which characteristically has a moth-eaten appearance adjacent to the disc space (Figs 30.1.31 and 30.1.32). MRI is the most sensitive and specific diagnostic test for diagnosing infectious lesions involving an intervertebral disc and adjacent bone. Abnormalities precede changes on radionuclide studies and the latter are not specific. Specific features are a relatively high signal on T2-weighted sequences from a narrow intervertebral disc with loss of the normal dark line representing the vertebral end plate, and changes in the adjacent vertebral bodies consisting of low signal on T1- and high signal on T2-weighted images which replace the entire vertebral end plate. Such changes in the vertebral bodies on MRI need to be distinguished from reactive changes secondary to degenerative intervertebral disc disease which do not extend across the entire and usually intact end-plate. An

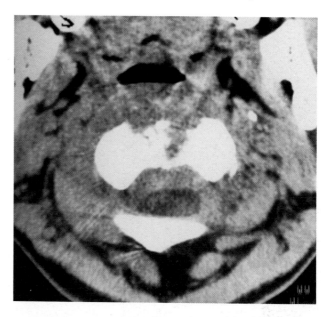

Fig. 30.1.32 Axial CT through the upper part of the body of C2 showing ragged bone destruction anteriorly and diffuse soft-tissue swelling also involving the extradural intraspinal tissues. The thecal sac is compressed. Pyogenic retropharyngeal abscess with involvement of C1 and C2.

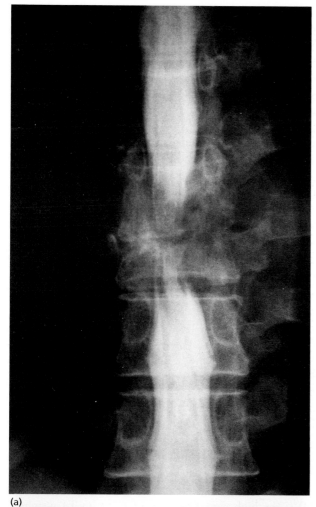

(a)

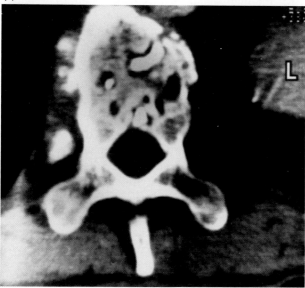

(b)

Fig. 30.1.31 Tuberculous spondylitis. (a) Myelogram showing extradural compression of the thecal sac and spinal cord, loss of the T6–T7 disc space, and paravertebral mass. (b) Axial CT showing typical bone destruction, and also, in this case dense sequestrata.

adjacent abscess within the spinal canal or paravertebral tissues may be evident. Primary epidural abscess is usually an extensive lesion lying posteriorly and laterally; it also can be recognized on MRI which is the ideal method for exclusion of an underlying adjacent focus of osteomyelitis.

Non-pyogenic infections such as tuberculosis affecting vertebral bodies or apophyseal joints may present less-typical appearances. On MRI the resemblance to metastatic disease may be close. Extensive spread beneath the longitudinal ligaments with epidural and extra-spinal abscess formation is a helpful distinguishing diagnostic feature.

OTHER TYPES OF INFLAMMATION

Destructive discovertebral lesions can occur in rheumatoid arthritis and the seronegative arthropathies (Fig. 30.1.33). They can also occur in some of the crystal deposition diseases such as pseudogout, and in chronic dialysis patients.

Rheumatoid arthritis most frequently affects the cervical spine, particularly the atlanto-axial articulations. Such typical cervical spine findings are subluxations, erosions and inflammatory soft-tissue masses. Plain CT shows erosions, and also may show inflammatory soft-tissue masses, particularly when these contain calcification. Rotations and subluxations also are

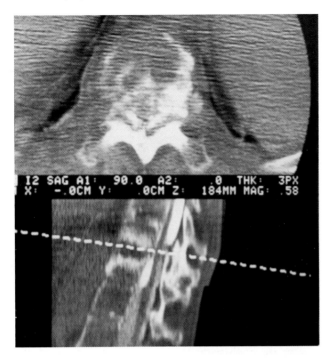

Fig. 30.1.33 Andersson-type lesion in ankylosing spondylitis, shown by post-myelography CT. The axial image (above) has been prescribed from the mid-sagittal reformatted image (below).

shown by plain CT although thin-section imaging for reformatting particularly in the sagittal and coronal planes may be necessary to demonstrate them well. Flexion and extension studies can be done on CT to evaluate the dynamics. Accurate demonstration of inflammatory soft-tissue masses and compression of the spinal cord and subarachnoid space usually is necessary when surgery is contemplated, and this requires myelography followed by CT (Fig. 30.1.34). MRI shows all these features and also may show intrinsic spinal cord

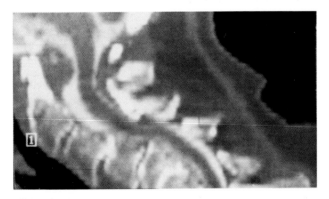

Fig. 30.1.34 Rheumatoid arthritis of the cervical spine shown by post-myelography CT. There are subaxial subluxations, concentric erosion of the dens and an inflammatory retrodental soft-tissue mass. This image was made in extension, the flexion image showed anterior atlanto-axial subluxation.

damage. In most circumstances MRI should replace the need for myelography and CT in these difficult cases, which often need repeated assessment on both conservative treatment and after surgery. The composition of inflammatory soft-tissue masses in rheumatoid arthritis, sometimes referred to as pannus, is related to disease activity. Florid pannus, in distinction to mature fibrous tissue, enhances with gadolinium–DTPA and is capable of rapid resorption after fixation of the affected mobile segment. Both florid pannus and synovial effusions are generally of high signal on T2-weighted images, and usually being associated with mobile subluxations, tend to change in position relative to the bones and ligaments with flexion extension. Fibrous pannus tends to reflect low signal on T2-weighted images and usually is associated with relatively fixed subluxation and itself tends to be immobile.

Neoplasms

Most extradural neoplasms are metastases or other disseminated malignancies, including multiple myeloma, lymphoma and leukaemia. A major feature usually is the presence of bone destruction which may be combined with sclerosis. The neural arch is often involved and a local paravertebral extension is usual. These features are demonstrated more effectively by CT than by isotope scans or plain radiography (Fig. 30.1.35), and are often recognizable on good-quality MRI (Fig. 30.1.36). Diffuse or focal infiltration of marrow is usually evident on MRI, the high signal of fatty marrow on T1-weighted sequences being replaced by low-signal tissue. MRI also distinguishes neoplastic collapse of the vertebral body from a chronic fracture (Yuh *et al.*, 1989). High signal on T1-weighted sequences does not occur with neoplastic collapse unless dexamethasone has been given and the neoplastic cells have been replaced by fat. So, intense signal on all sequences is much more frequent in osteopenic and post-traumatic collapse, but it can occur with neoplastic collapse. Vertebral haemangiomas reflecting high signal on T1-weighted and often patchy low signal on T2-weighted sequences are also inactive lesions requiring no treatment.

CT- or MRI-guided biopsy of suspected metastatic lesions of the spine will provide confirmatory histology in 70–80% of cases when decompression is not indicated (Murphy *et al.*, 1988).

Primary bone tumours are usually localized by plain radiography. CT demonstrates bone destruction and a large soft-tissue mass, or localized textural change usually with expansion of bone. In the spine, most large lesions such as osteoblastoma, giant-cell tumour and many aneurysmal bone cysts are indistinguishable. Some aneurysmal bone cysts, however, produce a characteristic appearance on CT and more frequently on MRI, consisting of multiple cysts of variable density or signal, sometimes with evidence of gravitational layering within them; a thin rim of bone remaining around the periphery is also a very suggestive feature. Osteoid osteomas can also be characteristic on CT when central ossification within a low-density nidus is evident, surrounded by sclerotic bone reaction. When MRI is not available, evaluation of the state of neural structures will usually require myelography and this is a good time to perform CT for full assessment.

Skeletal dysplasias

Skeletal dysplasias involving the spine may cause dwarfism and abnormal curvatures, and also may result in compression of neural structures directly. This is usually due to (i) spinal canal stenosis as in achondroplasia, (ii) soft-tissue thickening as in some of the mucopolysaccharidoses, and/or (iii) ligamentous laxity with subluxation as in mucopolysaccharidoses, Down's syndrome and multiple epiphyseal dysplasia. Most subluxations occur at the craniovertebral junction, where they are often associated with os odontoideum.

Clinical features may identify the likelihood of cord compression and plain radiography is usually necessary to locate deformities and subluxations. CT provides information about cross-sectional configuration and actual size of the spinal canal, and also more reliably demonstrates anomalies such as fusions and os odontoideum; thin-section imaging adequate for multiplanar reformatting is necessary (Fig. 30.1.37). When there are neurological abnormalities, MRI, when available, will evaluate the effects of skeletal and soft-tissue abnormalities upon neural structures; otherwise myelography plus CT is usually indicated.

GENERAL CONCLUSION

It is the authors' opinion that in the interest of avoiding unnecessary investigations *the first line investigation* should be MRI for most painful conditions of the spine and conditions in which there is suspected or definite neural involvement. When MRI is not available, CT and/or myelography may need to be considered. Suspicion of spinal cord or cervical root lesion indicate myelography in the first instance, most other situations plain CT. CT, however, has little to offer in the context of non-specific back pain. We cannot overemphasize that the ethical position of myelography as an initial

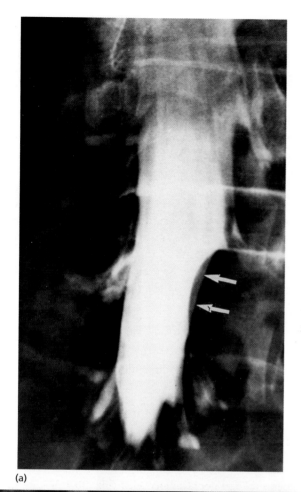

(a)

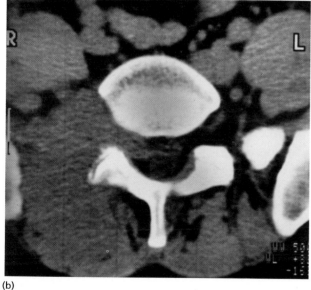

(b)

Fig. 30.1.35 Sarcoma of sacrum. (a) Myelogram showing a right-sided impression on the lower theca (arrows); no definite bone destruction was visible. (b) Plain CT at L5 in the same case showing a huge soft-tissue mass and destruction of the right lateral mass.

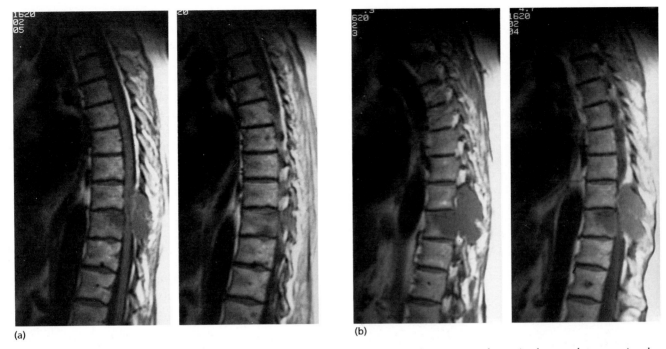

(a)

(b)

Fig. 30.1.36 (a,b) Sagittal T1-weighted MRI of the thoracic region, showing a large soft-tissue mass destroying bone and compressing the spinal cord. Metastatic carcinoma of the breast.

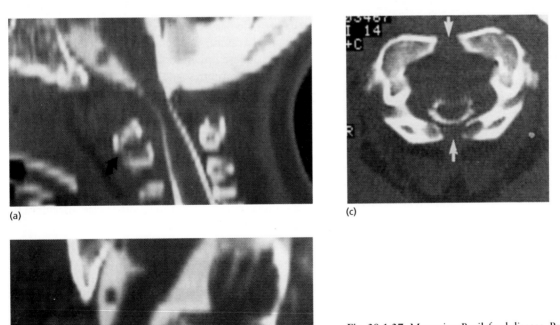

(a)

(b)

(c)

Fig. 30.1.37 Morquio–Brailsford disease. Post-myelography CT. (a) and (b) are mid-sagittal reformatted images in flexion and extension, and (c) is an axial image through C1. The spinal cord is markedly compressed by an anterior soft-tissue mass in both flexion and extension. The subdental synchondrosis is indicated by the black arrow. The cranial part of the dens is not ossified, and there are defects in the anterior and posterior arches of the atlas. All of these structures will ossify if movement is prevented by craniocervical fusion.

investigation for back pain and sciatica is growing increasingly doubtful.

REFERENCES

Avrahami E., Tudmore R. and Dally O. (1989) Early MR demonstration of spinal metastases in patients with normal radiographs and CT and radionuclide bone scans. *J. Comput. Assist. Tomogr.* **13**, 598–602.

Brooks R.A. and Di Chiro G. (1976) Principles of computer assisted tomography. *Phys. Med. Biol.* **21**, 689–705.

Clifton A., Stevens J.M., Whitear P. and Kendall B.E. (1990) Identifiable causes of poor outcome in surgery for cervical spondylosis. *Neuroradiology* **32**, 450–455.

Czervionke L.F. and Daniels D.L. (1988) Cervical spine anatomy and pathological processes: application of new MR imaging techniques. *Radiol. Clin. N. Am.* **26**, 921–948.

Delamarker R.B., Ross J.S., Masaryk T.J., Modic M.T. and Bohlman H. (1990) Diagnosis of lumbar arachnoiditis by magnetic resonance imaging. *Spine* **15**, 304–310.

Fugiwara K., Yonenobu K., Ebara S., Yamashita K. and Ono K. (1989) The prognosis of surgery for cervical compression myelopathy—an analysis of factors involved. *J. Bone Joint Surg.* **71B**, 393–398.

Hueftle M.G., Modic M.T., Ross J.S. *et al.* (1988) Lumbar spine: post-operative MR imaging with Gd-DTPA. *Radiology* **167**, 817–824.

Mehalic T.F., Pezzuti R.T. and Applebaum B.I. (1990) Magnetic resonance imaging and cervical spondylotic myelopathy. *Neurosurgery* **26**, 217–227.

Modic M.T., Maaryk T.J., Ross J.S. and Carter J.R. (1988) Imaging of degenerative disc disease. *Radiology* **168**, 177–186.

Murphy W.A. and Destouch J.M. (1988) Percutaneous biopsy of the spine. In Kricun M.E. (ed.) *Imaging Modalities in Spinal Disorders.* London, W.B. Saunders, pp. 643–662.

Ramananskas W.I., Wilner H.I., Meter J.J., Lazo A. and Kelly J.K. (1989) MR imaging of compressive myelomalacia. *J. Comput. Assist. Tomogr.* **13**, 399–404.

Robertson H.J. and Smith R.D. (1990) Cervical myelography. Survey of modes of practice and major complications. *Radiology* **174**, 79–83.

Schellinger D., Manz H.J., Vidic B. *et al.* (1990) Disc fragment migration. *Radiology* **175**, 831–836.

Stevens J.M. (1990) The spine and spinal cord. *Curr. Opin. Neurol. Neurosurg.* **3**, 894–901.

Stevens J.M., O'Driscoll D., Yu L. and Ananthapavan A. (1987) Some dynamic factors in compressive deformity of the cervical spinal cord. *Neuroradiology* **29**, 136–142.

Tsuruda J.S., Norman D., Dillon W., Newton T.H. and Mills D.G. (1989) Three-dimensional gradient-recalled MR imaging as a screening tool for diagnosis of cervical radiculopathy. *Am. J. Neuroradiol.* **10**, 1263–1271.

Vezina J.L., Fontaine S. and Laperviere J. (1984) Outpatient myelography with fine-needle technique—an appraisal. *Am. J. Neuroradiol.* **10**, 615–617.

Yamashita Y., Takahashi M., Matsumo Y. *et al.* (1990) Spinal cord compression due to ossification of ligaments. MR imaging. *Radiology* **175**, 843–848.

Yousem D.M., Patrone P.M. and Grossman R.I. (1990) Leptomeningeal metastases: MR evaluation. *J. Comput. Assist. Tomogr.* **14**, 255–261.

Yu S., Haughton V.M., Sether L.A., Ho K.C. and Wagner M. (1989a) Criteria for classifying normal and degenerated lumbar intervertebral discs. *Radiology* **170**, 523–526.

Yu S.W., Haughton V.M., Sether L.A. and Wagner M. (1989b) Compression of MR and discography in detecting radial tears of the annulus. A postmortem study. *Am. J. Neuroradiol.* **10**, 1077–1082.

Yuh W.T.L., Zachar C.K., Barloon T.J., Sata Y. Sickels W.J. and Hawes D.R. (1989) Vertebral compression fractures; distinction between benign and malignant causes with MR imaging. *Radiology* **172**, 215–218.

Chapter 30.2
Angiography in Orthopaedics

A. Al-Kutoubi

ARTERIOGRAPHY

Arteriography is not a commonly used radiological modality in orthopaedic surgery but it has a significant role in the appropriate clinical setting.

Conventional angiography necessitates a puncture of an artery and the introduction of a catheter as close as possible to the area of interest. The femoral artery is commonly used but puncture of the axillary or brachial arteries is sometimes undertaken. The advent of digital subtraction angiography (DSA) has made it easier to obtain adequate images. The technique is based on the use of electronic detectors linked to the radiographic equipment. The detectors receive the radiation and store the data in digital form. These data can then be manipulated to produce a clear image which is then printed on a film. The detectors are considerably more sensitive than the radiographic films, therefore excellent images can be obtained using a much lower dose of contrast. Another advantage is that the images can be viewed 'live' during the procedure and further images obtained in different positions if necessary without delay and without moving the patient. This is invaluable in trauma patients and in cases where therapeutic procedures prove necessary.

The sensitivity of the electronic detectors made it possible for reasonable images of the major arteries to be aquired without direct arterial puncture. Intravenous DSA is performed by injecting contrast in a peripheral, or more commonly, central vein and images of the arterial phase are then obtained. Intravenous injections require a larger dose of contrast but this is not usually a problem with the new low-osmolar and non-ionic contrast media. The major advantage of intravenous DSA is that it can be performed on an out-patient basis and avoids the complications of direct arterial puncture such as haematoma formation, dissection and thrombosis. Imaging of the peripheral arteries of the limbs, however, still requires intra-arterial approach.

Indications

TRAUMA

Vascular injury is a fairly common association in severe trauma. Peripheral arterial injury is usually obvious clinically but the extent of damage is often difficult to assess without angiography particularly if arterial reconstruction proves necessary. Intimal tears, thrombosis and transection of the arteries reflect the severity of the injury. A common site for intimal tears is across the shoulder and knee joints which are liable to severe dislocation, but disruption of the arterial supply can occur at any site where the bones are in close contact with the vessels (Figs 30.2.1–30.2.4). Injury to the spine and pelvis may be associated with damage to intra-abdominal organs and their vascular supply. The presence of damage to the renal arteries, for instance, may change the order of priorities in the management of trauma patients (Fig. 30.2.5).

Arteriovenous fistulae and false aneurysm formation are commonly seen in penetrating and bullet injuries (Figs 30.2.6 and 30.2.7). These can be treated by transcatheter embolization with a good measure of success.

Vascular trauma may be missed at the time of injury but manifests later. The classic example of this is the traumatic aneurysm of the distal arch of the aorta due to deceleration injury to the chest (Fig. 30.2.8). Injury to the first and second ribs is associated with a high incidence of vascular trauma.

Thrombosis, false aneurysm and arteriovenous fistula formation may happen as a result of surgical procedures and manipulation (Fig. 30.2.9). Angiography will demonstrate the extent of damage and assess the possibility of transcatheter treatment.

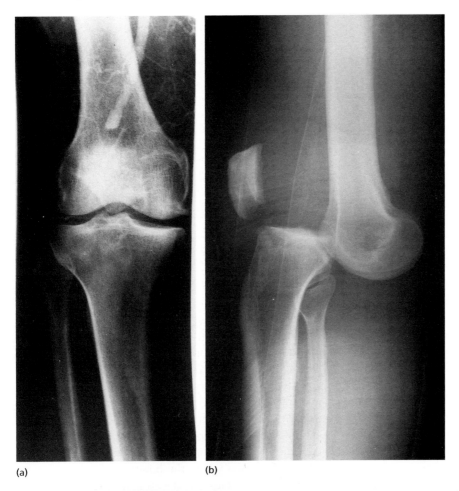

(a)   (b)

Fig. 30.2.1 (a) Complete disruption and occlusion of popliteal artery following knee dislocation. (b) Lateral view of the knee.

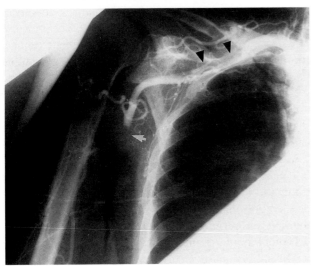

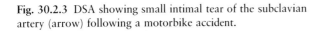

Fig. 30.2.2 Occlusion of axillary artery secondary to dissection after shoulder dislocation (arrow). The dissection flap extends medially into the subclavian artery (arrowheads).

Fig. 30.2.3 DSA showing small intimal tear of the subclavian artery (arrow) following a motorbike accident.

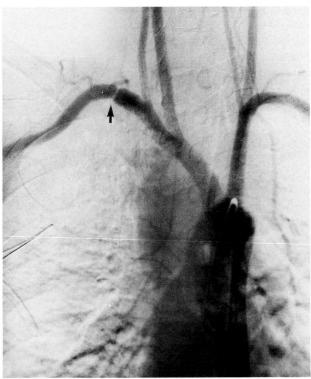

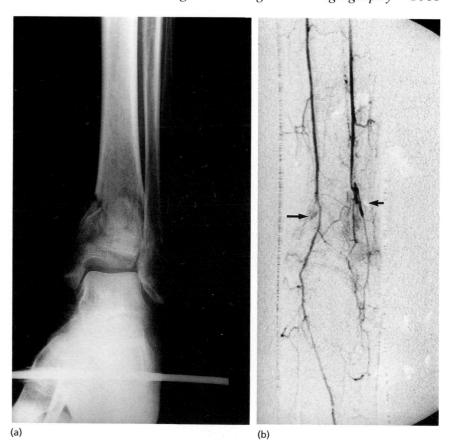

Fig. 30.2.4 (a) Comminuted fracture of the ankle. (b) DSA showing interruption of the anterior tibial artery (short arrow) and disruption of the posterior tibial artery (long arrow).

(a)

(b)

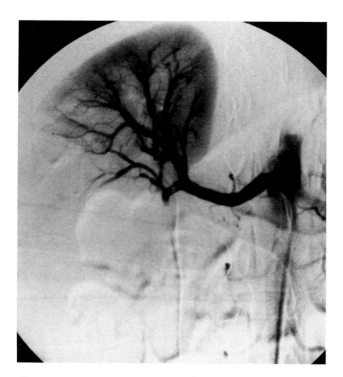

Fig. 30.2.5 Traumatic transection of the renal artery. Only the upper half of the kidney is perfused.

TUMOURS

The modern imaging techniques including computed tomography and magnetic resonance imaging scanning provide most of the required information in bone and soft-tissue tumours prior to surgery but occasionally the extent of vascular involvement needs to be assessed in detail so that the surgical approach may be planned. The angiographic pattern may provide some prognostic information as vascular tumours tend to be more aggressive but it is not possible to predict the histological diagnosis from the angiographic features. The extent of the tumour and intraosseous involvement are depicted by angiography. Neovascularity, pooling of contrast and invasion of the vessels are features suggestive of malignancy (Figs 30.2.10–30.2.12). It is not always possible, however, to distinguish between benign and malignant tumours nor is it easy to differentiate tumour from infection. The only exception is in the case of haemangiomata and congenital arteriovenous malformations where the angiographic pattern is often specific (Figs 30.2.13 and 30.2.14) and treatment is primarily by the transcatheter route. Glomus tumours are rare but occur commonly in

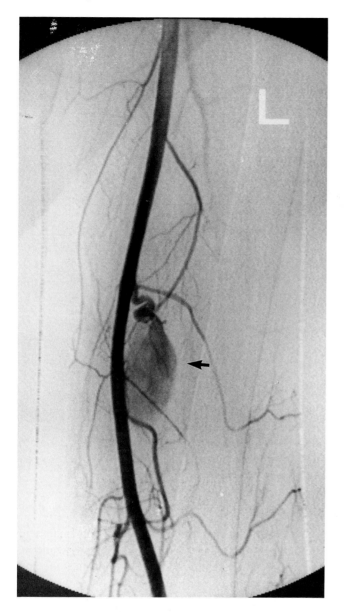

Fig. 30.2.6 False aneurysm of the superficial femoral artery (arrow) from penetrating injury.

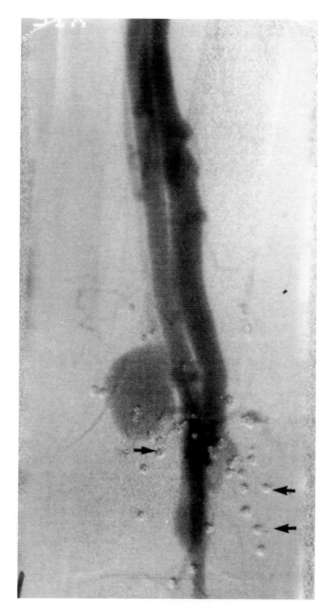

Fig. 30.2.7 Traumatic arteriovenous fistula of the popliteal artery. Shrapnels are visible in the soft tissues (arrows).

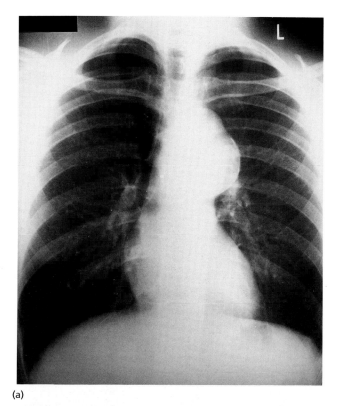

(a)

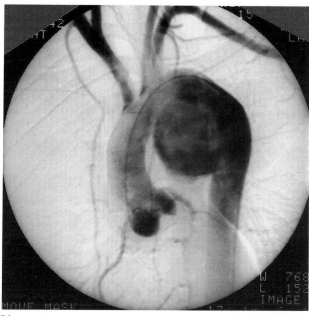

(b)

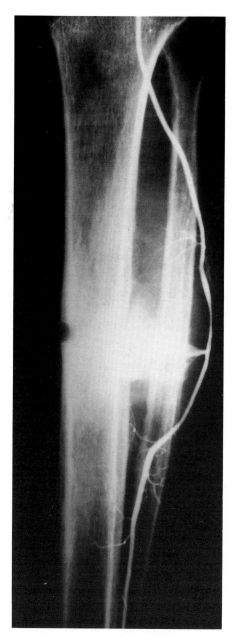

Fig. 30.2.9 Traumatic perforation of anterior tibial artery with false aneurysm formation following bone biopsy. (Courtesy of Mr J.R. Kenyon.)

Fig. 30.2.8 (a) Chest radiograph showing a mass related to the aortic arch with a calcified margin. (b) DSA shows a large aneurysm of the distal arch due to deceleration injury 15 years earlier.

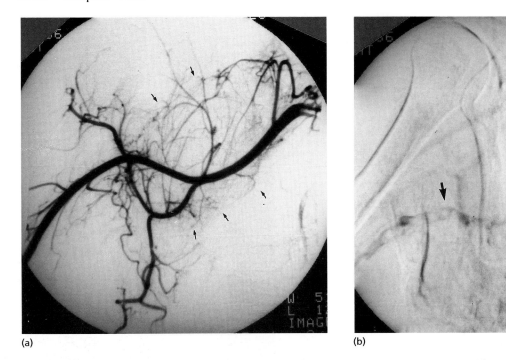

(a)

(b)

Fig. 30.2.10 (a) Neurofibrosarcoma (arrows) receiving supply from the displaced axillary artery. (b) Venous phase showing invasion and obstruction of the axillary veins (arrow).

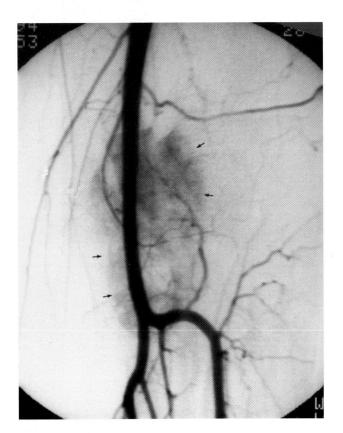

Fig. 30.2.11 Histiocytoma in upper tibia (arrows) receiving supply from genicular branches of popliteal and anterior tibial arteries.

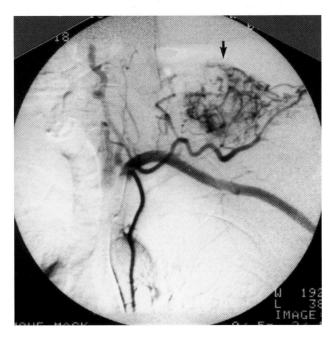

Fig. 30.2.12 Haemangiosarcoma in shoulder (arrow). The supply comes from the costocervical trunk.

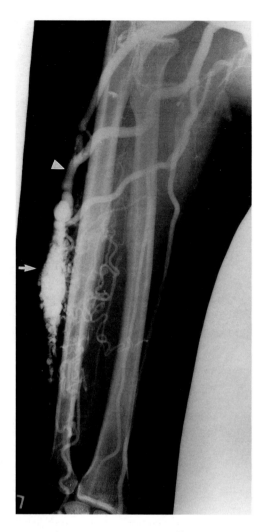

Fig. 30.2.13 Soft-tissue arteriovenous malformation (arrow) in the forearm. Early filling of the draining veins is noted (arrowhead).

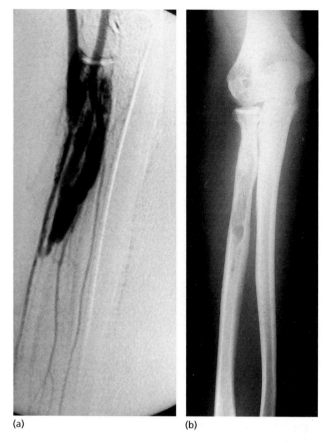

(a)   (b)

Fig. 30.2.14 (a,b) Arteriovenous malformation arising within the proximal radius. Large channels are seen in the cortex of the radius due to the enlarged vessels.

the hands and feet and present as an area of exquisite pain over the tumour. Angiography is the definitive imaging modality in these lesions and may be the only imaging technique that confirms the diagnosis (Fig. 30.2.15).

ARTERIAL DISEASE

Arteriography by the intra-arterial or intravenous method is the main investigation in primary arterial disease which occasionally mimics orthopaedic conditions (Fig. 30.2.16). Popliteal aneurysms may be confused for Baker's cysts. Entrapment of the popliteal artery (Fig. 30.2.17) is a condition seen primarily in young athletic men who are often seen by the orthopaedic surgeon before the vascular specialist. Assessment of the arterial and venous involvement in the thoracic inlet syndrome

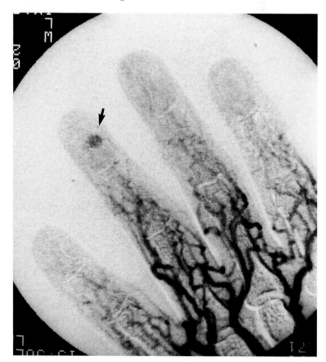

Fig. 30.2.15 Glomus tumour in the ring finger (arrow).

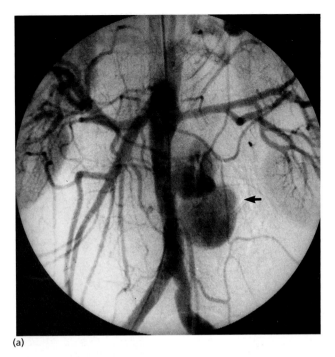
(a)

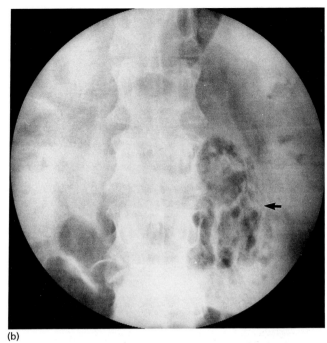
(b)

Fig. 30.2.16 (a) Mycotic aneurysm of aorta (arrow) due to *Salmonella* infection in a patient who presented with acute back pain. (b) Air (arrow) is seen in the region of the aneurysm.

forms a significant part of the investigation in this complex and difficult condition (Figs 30.2.18 and 30.2.19).

Raynaud's phenomenon may be a manifestation of some of the rheumatological disorders such as sclero-

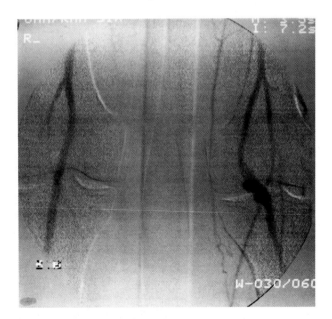

Fig. 30.2.17 Medial deviation of the popliteal arteries on both sides due to entrapment. There is aneurysmal dilatation on the left side.

derma and rheumatoid arthritis (Fig. 30.2.20). The extent and severity of the disease may be assessed by arteriography before treatment with prostaglandins and other agents. The diagnosis of polyarteritis nodosa is often confirmed by the demonstration by arteriography of micro-aneurysms in the renal or mesenteric circulation.

MISCELLANEOUS CONDITIONS

Severe cases of frostbite are associated with significant arterial damage. The decision whether or not to amputate may be influenced by the angiographic demonstration of patent arteries in the foot or toes. Gas gangrene secondary to trauma or in drug addiction may be associated with arterial or venous damage which will require angiographic assessment (Fig. 30.2.21). Avascular necrosis of the femoral head can be diagnosed by selective angiography but this is much more easily demonstrated by magnetic resonance imaging scanning and angiography is only reserved for the occasional atypical or inconclusive case.

THERAPEUTIC PROCEDURES

Congenital arteriovenous malformations can be arterial, capillary or venous. Transcatheter embolization is the treatment of choice for the arterial and capillary varieties

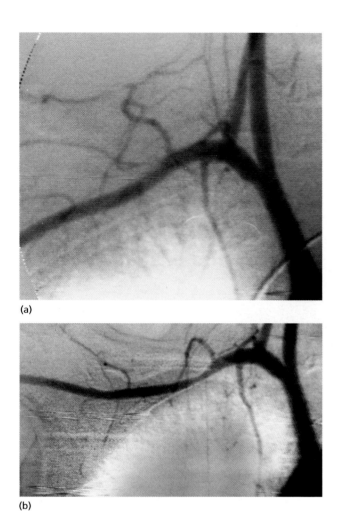

(a)

(b)

Fig. 30.2.18 Views of the subclavian artery in neutral position (a) and in abduction (b) showing moderately severe narrowing on abduction at the level of the first rib.

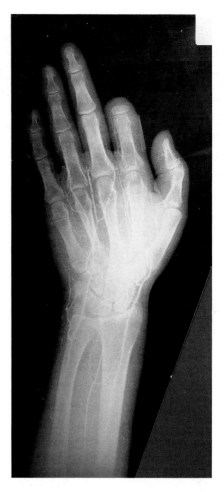

Fig. 30.2.20 Scleroderma. Occlusion of most digital branches and soft-tissue loss.

Fig. 30.2.19 DSA study in neutral position and in abduction. There is complete obstruction of the left subclavian artery on abduction (small arrow). Severe narrowing of the subclavian vein is also demonstrated (large arrow).

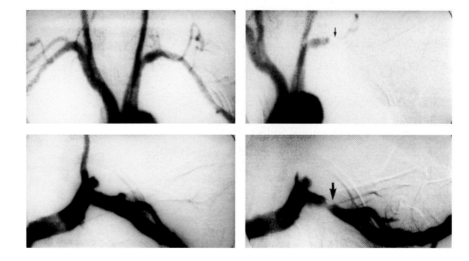

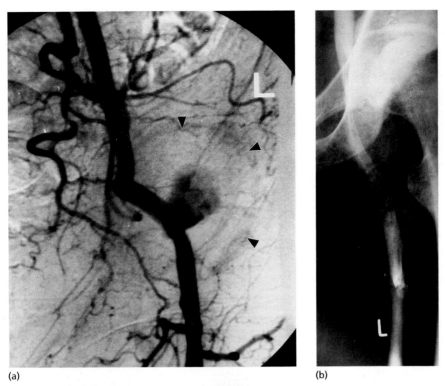

(a)

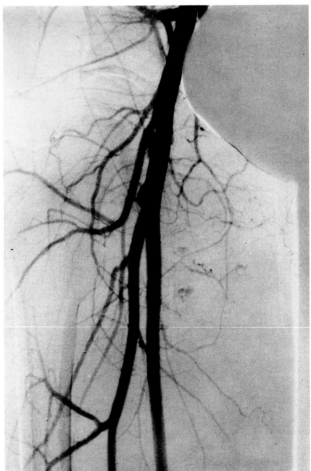

(b)

Fig. 30.2.21 (a) False aneurysm in femoral artery (arrowheads) in a drug addict. (b) Venogram showing compression of the femoral vein and gas in the tissues.

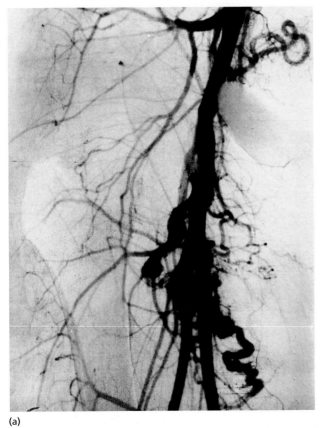

(a)

Fig. 30.2.22 (a) Arteriovenous malformation in the buttock and upper thigh. (b) After transcatheter embolization, the appearances are normal.

(b)

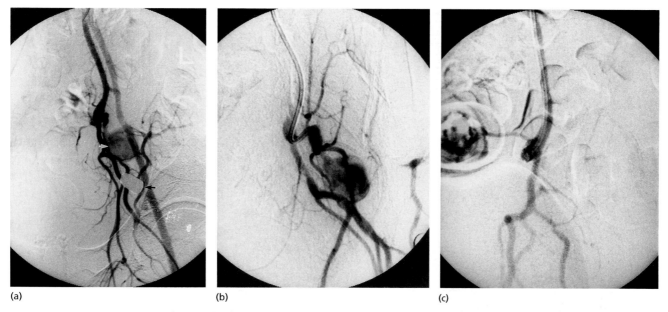

(a)   (b)   (c)

Fig. 30.2.23 (a) False aneurysm of a branch of the internal iliac artery (white arrow) from a bullet (black arrow) injury. The patient had had the external iliac artery repaired at the initial presentation but represented with symptoms of nerve compression in the pelvis. (b) Catheter selectively positioned in the injured artery. (c) Total occlusion of the aneurysm after embolization.

as surgical intervention often results in enlargement of the lesion and the formation of new feeders. The delivery of the embolization particles selectively to the bed of the malformation can result in total cure. Two or three embolization procedures are often required to achieve a satisfactory result (Fig. 30.2.22).

Traumatic false aneurysms and arteriovenous fistulae can be similarly treated with embolization particularly if the condition of the patient does not permit surgery or the lesion is difficult to treat surgically (Fig. 30.2.23).

Thrombolytic therapy for acute arterial or venous occlusion is seldom used in the orthopaedic practice. Thrombolysis of acute subclavian vein thrombosis in the thoracic inlet syndrome, for instance, is effective and will result in quick relief of the acute symptoms (Fig. 30.2.24).

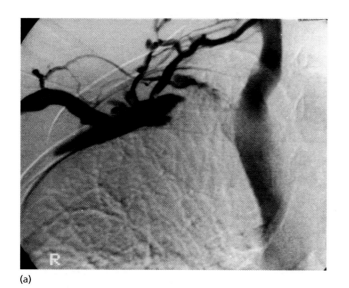
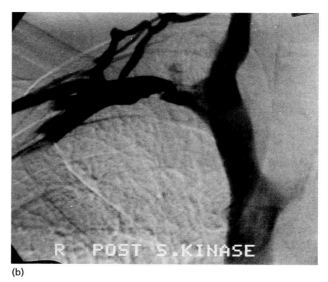

(a)   (b)

Fig. 30.2.24 (a) Total thrombosis of the subclavian vein. (b) After thrombolysis, the vein is now patent. The acute symptoms subsided completely.

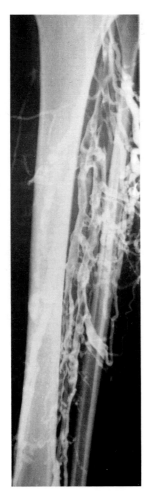

Fig. 30.2.25 Extensive deep-vein thrombosis in calf veins following hip surgery.

VENOGRAPHY

Deep-vein thrombosis of the calf is a common medical problem as an acute presentation which may mimic orthopaedic conditions or as a complication of orthopaedic surgical procedures (Fig. 30.2.25). Venography is the best method in diagnosing and demonstrating the extent of the thrombosis, particularly the presence of fresh or loose clot in the femoral or iliac veins. Surgical extraction or the insertion of a caval filter may then follow. Occasionally the demonstration of venous com-pression due to extrinsic causes or after surgical pro-cedures will require detailed venography of the upper or lower limbs.

SUMMARY

Digital subtraction angiography plays a useful role in orthopaedic surgery. Intravenous DSA can be performed on an out-patient basis and is sufficient for visualization of the major arteries but intra-arterial studies are required for detailed assessment of the small peripheral arteries and if transcatheter therapeutic procedures are planned.

FURTHER READING

Adler J. and Hooshmand I. (1973) The angiographic spectrum of the thoracic outlet syndrome with emphasis on mural thrombosis and emboli and congenital vascular anomalies. *Clin. Radiol.* **24**, 35.

Bloem J.L., Tamianou A.H.M., Euldrink F., Hermans J. and Pauwels E.K.J. (1988) Radiologic staging of primary bone sarcoma: MR imaging, scintigraphy, angiography and CT cor-related with pathological examination. *Radiology* **169**, 805.

Carrasco C.J., Charanasangavej C., Raymond A.K. *et al.* (1989) Osteosarcoma: Angiographic assessment of response to pre-operative chemotherapy. *Radiology* **170**, 839.

Carroll R.E. and Berman A.F. (1972) Glomus tumours of the hand: Review of the literature and report of 28 cases. *J. Bone Joint Surg.* **54**, 691.

Hudson J.M., Enneking W.F. and Hawkins I.F. (1981) The value of angiography in planning surgical treatment of bone tumours. *Radiology* **138**, 283.

Klatte E.C., Becker G.J., Holden R.E. and Yune H.Y. (1986) Fibrinolytic therapy. *Radiology* **159**, 619.

Mistretta C.A., Crummy A.B., Strother C.M. (eds) (1982) *Digital Subtraction Angiography. An Application of Computerized Fluoroscopy.* Chicago, Year Book Medical Publishers.

Rose S.C. and Moore E.E. (1987) Angiography in patients with arterial trauma: Correlation between angiographic abnormalities, operative findings and clinical outcome. *Am. J. Roentgen.* **149**, 613.

Scalfani S.J.A., Cooper R., Shaftan G.W., Goldstein A.S., Glanz S. and Gordon D.H. (1986) Arterial trauma: Diagnostic and thera-peutic angiography. *Radiology* **161**, 165.

Stamatakis J.D., Kakkar V.V., Sagar S., Lawrence D., Nairn D. and Bentley P.G. (1977) Femoral vein thrombosis and total hip replacement. *Br. Med. J.* **2**, 223.

Yakes F.W., Haas D.K., Parker S.H. *et al.* (1989) Symptomatic vascular malformations. Ethanol embolotherapy. *Radiology* **170**, 1059.

Chapter 31

Biomechanics of Joints and Joint Replacements

A.A. Amis

INTRODUCTION

This chapter does not deal with the properties of the natural tissues which make up human joints, since such data are already available (Nordin and Frankel, 1989). It concentrates, instead, on the functional aspects of joint mechanics—the movements of the joints and the forces acting on them during normal activities. It is primarily an understanding of the forces acting on the joints which allows the surgeon to understand why the bones have their particular load-bearing architecture, why certain fractures are difficult to keep reduced, or why prosthetic joints have been designed to a certain pattern. This, then, is fundamental in helping surgeons to anticipate what will befall their work after the operation.

THE HIP

Hip motion

The spherical geometry allows rotation about all three axes of flexion–extension, abduction–adduction and internal–external rotation. Ellis and Stowe (1982) noted that motion varies greatly between subjects, so the normal limb should be taken as a reference for loss of motion. The most frequent motion is that required for walking, which Murray *et al.* (1964) showed to be from approximately 30° flexion to 10° extension, accompanied by some 8° pelvic rotation (Fig. 31.1).

Forces on the hip—static analysis

Various authors have presented simplified analyses of hip joint forces for one- and two-legged stance. Maquet (1985) noted that the hips take equal shares of the weight of head, trunk and upper limbs if the subject stands symmetrically, leading to a hip load of 0.31 BW

(BW = body weight). This is likely to be a considerable underestimate, however, because it neglects the postural muscle actions which maintain the body on top of the femora. Williams and Svensson (1968), in a three-dimensional analysis of single leg stance, showed that allowing for the postural muscle equilibrium raised the joint force by 1.5 BW. This was because the centre of gravity is posterior to the centres of the hips when standing erect, necessitating tensions in the ilio-psoas muscle and ilio-femoral ligament to prevent hip hyperextension. These tensions add to the hip force.

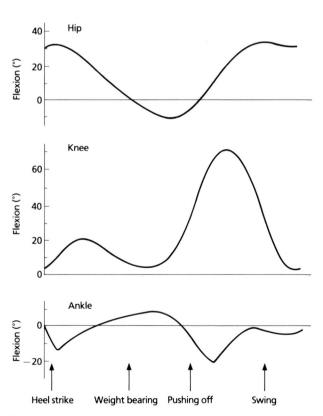

Fig. 31.1 Flexion–extension of hip, knee and ankle when walking. (From Murray *et al.*, 1964.)

1073

In one-legged stance, the centre of gravity of the parts of the body acting onto the supporting hip (head, trunk, upper limbs and opposite leg) is located on the far side of the lumbar spine. This weight causes the pelvis to tend to drop, rotating about the centre of the hip (Fig. 31.2). The abductor muscle tensions that prevent the pelvis dropping may be found in a simplified two-dimensional analysis by examining rotational equilibrium about an anterior–posterior axis. To maintain equilibrium, the abductor muscles must impose an equal and opposite turning moment about the hip. Thus $W \times a = M \times b$, where a is the moment arm of the partial body weight W (0.81 BW; Maquet, 1985) about the centre of the hip, and b is the moment arm of the estimated mean line of action of the abductors about the hip centre. This gives an abductor muscle force

$$M = \frac{W \times a}{b}$$

or

$$M = \frac{0.81\,\text{BW} \times 110}{47}$$

so

$$M = 1.9\,\text{BW}$$

The 'moment arm' is the perpendicular distance of the line of action of the force away from the pivot point at the centre of the hip. Dimensions a and b can be found from radiographs, using a wire plumbline aligned to the supporting foot to locate the line of action of the centre of gravity for dimension a. Note that the calculated abductor muscle force, $M = 1.9\,\text{BW}$, is the minimum possible, since it neglects the effects of antagonistic muscle actions that maintain posture.

The downward actions of gravity acting on the body, and of the abductors pulling on the ilium, must be opposed by the equal and opposite reaction force of the femoral head pressing upwards into the acetabulum. This hip joint reaction force can be found graphically. Since the free part of the body, i.e. that part supported by the femoral head, can be assumed to have only three forces acting on it (W, M, H; Fig. 31.2a), a force vector triangle can be drawn to scale, with the lengths of the sides of the triangle proportional to the magnitudes of the forces, and with the correct directions taken from the radiograph (Fig. 31.2b). Since the magnitude and direction of both W and M are known, the third side of the triangle is easily obtained. If the three force vectors did not close the triangle, it would signify that an unbalanced force resultant existed, and the body would not be in equilibrium. The magnitude and direction of the hip-joint reaction force H can be measured directly from the diagram: $H = 2.64\,\text{BW}$, acting at 21° to the vertical.

The hip-joint force can also be calculated directly from the data available, knowing that it is equal and opposite to the forces acting on the joint. This is most easily done by resolving the forces into vertical and horizontal components and considering them separately. Thus the vertical component $H_V = W + M\cos 30°$, where 30° is the angle of the abductor muscles from vertical (Fig. 31.2b).

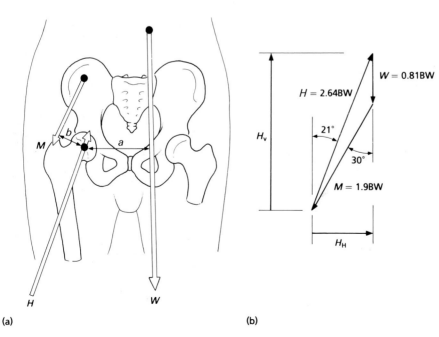

(a) (b)

Fig. 31.2 (a) Static analysis of single leg stance forces on the hip. The abductor muscles impose an equal and opposite turning moment about the hip to that caused by the body weight. (b) The hip-joint force can be derived by constructing a force vector triangle, knowing the magnitude and direction of W and M, to find H. The mathematical derivation uses the vertical and horizontal components of the forces separately to find H_H and H_V, from which H can be calculated.

Using values found above,

$$H_V = 0.81\,BW + 1.9\,BW \times 0.866$$

so

$$H_V = 2.46\,BW$$

Similarly, for horizontal equilibrium,

$$H_H = M \sin 30° = 1.9\,BW \times 0.5$$

so

$$H_H = 0.95\,BW$$

The combined effect of these horizontal and vertical force components can be calculated:
Hip force,

$$H = H_V^2 + H_H^2$$

so

$$H = (2.46\,BW^2 + 0.95\,BW^2) = 2.64\,BW$$

This force is acting at angle *a* from the vertical and

$$\tan a = \frac{H_H}{H_V} = \frac{0.95}{2.46}$$

Thus $a = \tan^{-1} 0.39 = 21°$.

Note, in Fig. 31.2b, how the mathematical derivations of H_V and H_H correspond to the parts of the force vectors drawn — it is simply another way to do the same thing. The mathematical method is always used in more complex analyses.

The above analysis for one-legged stance did not allow for all aspects of static equilibrium, since only the muscle force components controlling rotation about an anterior–posterior axis were considered. Consideration of flexion–extension and internal–external rotation would take such an analysis nearer the true joint force, which would be higher. Williams and Svensson (1968), for example, then predicted 6 BW for the hip force.

Dynamic loading of the hip

The major load-bearing activity is locomotion, a situation which requires more complex dynamic analysis. The underlying reason is revealed by stroboscopic or slow-motion cinephotography: the centre of gravity of the body undulates up and down, and also sways from side to side, as a person walks (Murray *et al.*, 1964). In the single-legged stance phase of walking, the centre of gravity is high, while the free leg swings past. The centre of gravity then falls as the heel approaches and strikes the ground. In order to arrest the fall, the reaction forces acting through the joints of the legs must oppose the

dynamic inertial load as well as the static body weight, leading to a higher force. During walking there is a period of overlap in the gait cycle when both feet are on the ground — as load is taken by the heel strike of the leading foot, then the body weight is accelerated upwards by plantarflexion of the trailing foot, leading to toe-off.

The best-known analysis of this action (Paul, 1967) showed hip joint forces of 4 BW after heel strike and 7 BW before toe-off. In order to make this prediction, Paul measured the forces acting between the foot and the ground, by means of a force plate. This was effectively a floor tile mounted on force transducers, which were linked to amplifiers and recorders. The force data could be synchronized to cine film of the subject, allowing the inertial effects of thigh and shank accelerations to be added. This led to data on forces and moments acting on and about the hip at different points in the walking cycle. To complete the analysis, Paul had to allow for the moments acting about the hip, by adding muscle forces to counteract them. This was done in the same manner as in the simple single leg-stance analysis described above. The many muscles crossing the hip had to be grouped together in terms of their functions, to simplify the analysis, in the same way that the actions of gluteus medius, gluteus minimus and tensor fascia lata were grouped together as an idealized 'abductor' described above. The muscles were taken as being relaxed or active on the basis of electromyography linked to the gait cycle.

Although the prediction of hip force from such an analysis depends on many assumptions concerning the line of action or intensity of particular muscle actions, the basic double-peaked hip joint force waveform (Fig. 31.3) found by Paul (1967) has been reproduced by other studies. An interesting comparison was provided by Rydell (1966), who implanted strain gauged hip prostheses into patients, then monitored the forces. Rydell found lower peak forces than Paul, but higher values during the swing phase.

Although there have been many simplified analyses of hip forces in the coronal plane the anterior–posterior forces cannot be ignored. Examination of Paul's results shows that there is a considerable anterior–posterior force acting onto the femoral head shortly before toe-off. Figure 31.3, from Berme and Paul (1979), shows a posteriorly-acting force of 1.7 kN at 50% of the gait cycle, at the same time as a vertical force of 1.8 kN acts downwards onto the femoral head. This arises from the actions of the gluteal muscles pulling around the trochanteric region to extend the hip. Thus, as well as bending the neck in the coronal plane, the neck also bends posteriorly, setting up a torsion load on the

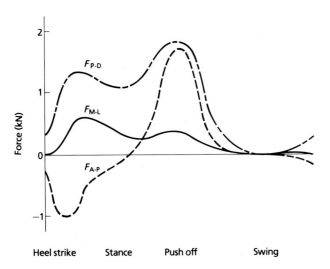

Fig. 31.3 Variation of hip-joint force during one cycle of walking gait. The force components F_{A-P}, F_{M-L} and F_{P-D} act on the anterior, medial and proximal aspects of the femoral head, respectively. (From Berme and Paul, 1979.) Large-force components act simultaneously on the proximal and anterior aspects of the hip during the push-off phase of the gait cycle. A−P = anterior−posterior; M−L= medial−lateral; P−D = proximal−distal.

proximal femoral shaft (Fig. 31.4). Appreciation of this load action, which can be much higher when climbing stairs or rising from a chair, has led to the introduction of prosthetic stems which allow retention of the femoral neck, thus aiding rotational stability (Nunn *et al.*, 1989).

The importance of hip-joint force analysis arises from

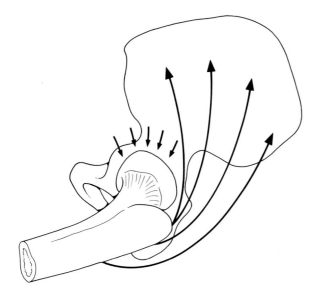

Fig. 31.4 In the stance phase of walking, or when rising from a chair, the gluteal muscles pull the femoral head anteriorly against the acetabulum, causing a tortion load on the proximal femur.

the use of the results in the design of implants, both joint replacements and fracture fixators such as nail plates. Large cyclic loads can lead to fatigue failures, in either the porotic bone of the femoral neck, or the metallic stem of an implant.

Femoral neck stresses

The stresses in the neck of the femur, arising from the joint loading predicted above, are represented in Fig. 31.5. With a normal neck-shaft angle of 125°, the neck of femur is approximately 50° from the vertical. This means that the joint force, approximately 20° from vertical in the coronal plane illustrated, imposes a bending load on the neck of the femur. Because of the angle at which the force acts on the femoral head, it is most convenient to analyse its effects by splitting the force into axial and transverse components. The axial component induces an axial compressive stress throughout the cross-section of the femoral neck. The transverse component, acting through the centre of the head, tends to shear the neck, or displace the head transversely. However, because it has a moment arm between its line of action and the femoral neck section being analysed, it also imposes a moment on the femoral neck. This bending moment causes tensile stresses on the superior aspect of the neck, and compressive stresses on the inferior aspect. The tensile stresses are partly offset by the axial compressive stress, but the resultant obtained by super-imposing the stress fields arising from the axial and transverse forces is a small tensile stess and a larger compressive stress, as shown in Fig. 31.5. Radiographs show arrays of trabeculae orientated to these loads.

It is well known that the femoral neck weakens with ageing, as bone mass is resorbed. Eventually the tensile stresses increase (because the joint loads act on a diminishing area of bone) to the point where the tensile fatigue strength of the bone is exceeded, and transcervical fracture occurs. Such fractures are usually treated with a telescoping lag screw−bone plate assembly (Fig. 31.6). These devices are available in a range of neck−shaft angles, the 135° model being most popular. Unfortunately, this is not aligned with the joint force even in the coronal plane, which means that a bending load is imposed on the shank of the screw, and the shank is then more likely to bind, rather than slide, in the barrel. Although it is more difficult to drill through the trochanteric femur at an acute angle, a 150° screw−plate assembly will be less inclined to fail by screw bending and more likely to allow efficient fracture-line impaction, as the device will then telescope in line with the forces imposed (Amis *et al.*, 1987).

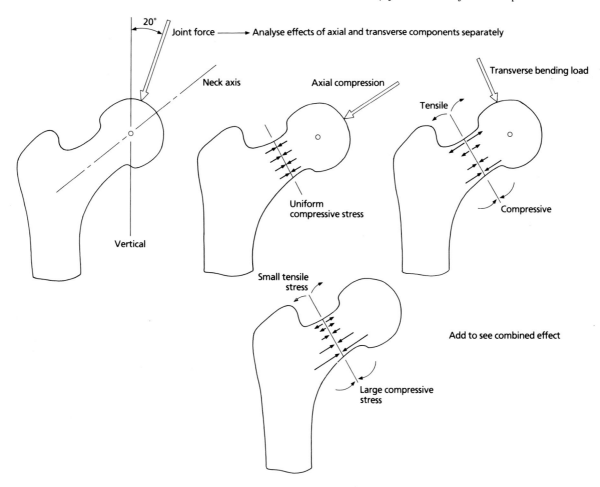

Fig. 31.5 Stresses acting on the neck of the femur can be derived by adding the effects of the compressive and bending components of the load, leaving a tensile stress in the superior aspect and a larger compressive stress in the inferior aspect.

Hip-joint prostheses

The evolution of hip replacements has been guided primarily by attempts to allow for the joint forces described above, since these cause looosening and prosthesis breakage. Interest in hip replacement was stimulated by Judet and Judet (1950), who used a short-stemmed femoral head replacement made of the acrylic polymer methyl methacrylate (Fig. 31.7a). The implant stem was inserted along the neck, towards the lateral cortex. Although chemically the same as the polymethyl methacrylate bone cement used commonly, moulded components have far superior mechanical properties when cured at elevated temperature and pressure, when they take on the characteristics best known as Perspex (or Plexiglass in the US). The hip forces, however, caused fatigue failures of the acrylic stems, so the design soon incorporated a stainless-steel stem reinforcement. The basic problem, though, was that the joint forces had to be carried by a small area of the endosteal surface of the femoral neck, causing implant migration into varus. A further problem was excessive wear of the acrylic, leading to tissue reactions to the debris.

Longer intramedullary stems were introduced by Moore (1952) (Fig. 31.7b) and Thompson (1952), which obtained stability in the medullary canal of the femoral shaft and soon proved superior to the Judet-type fixation. This pattern remains the basis for most hip prostheses. The hip forces, acting only 20° from vertical in the coronal plane, wedge the long stem into the medulla. The length of these stems allows bending loads to be opposed by relatively small forces spaced well apart on the medial calcar and the lateral diaphysis. The Moore and Thompson implants were hemi-arthroplasties and were not satisfactory if the acetabulum was deficient. Total hip replacements overcame this problem by providing an acetabular 'cup' component; McKee and Watson-Farrar (1966) described a total hip prosthesis using the Thompson stem and Ring (1968) used the Moore stem.

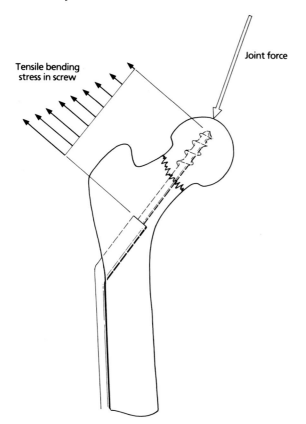

Fig. 31.6 Typical lag screw–bone plate assembly for treatment of femoral neck fracture, with a 135° neck–shaft angle. Because the hip-joint force acts at 20° to the vertical, a bending load is imposed on the screw, which may fail to slide or fracture where it enters the barrel.

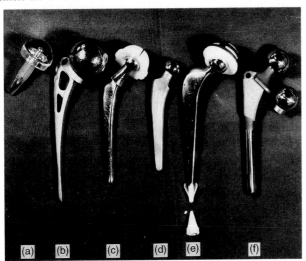

Fig. 31.7 Evolution of hip prostheses. (a) Judet acrylic hemi-arthroplasty; (b) Moore hemi-arthroplasty; (c) Charnley total replacement, with stainless-steel stem and polyethylene cup; (d) computer-aided design (CAD) straight stem; (e) collarless Exeter polished stem, with cement restrictor and stem tip centralizer; (f) VSP stem, with modular neck length, proximal ingrowth fixation zone with collar, and polished stem tip. (e) and (f) use a metal-backed cup.

At this time, in the mid-1960s, Charnley (1967) introduced cold-curing acrylic resin ('bone cement') for prosthetic fixation. The McKee–Watson-Farrar cup was cemented, although the Ring cup was screwed into the bone. Bone cement had several advantages over the previous press-fit stem fixation. The principal attraction was that bone cement could fill the medullary cavity of an osteoporotic femur, as expected in elderly patients. Thus there was no need to rasp away within a pathologically thin cortex, while simultaneously providing load transfer over a large surface area, reducing the shear stress on the interface. In contrast, press-fit stems imposed high stresses on the localized areas of prosthesis–cortex contact. Charnley and Kettlewell (1965) did various experiments on this matter, and showed that the use of cement caused a significant reduction in prosthesis–bone movement under load. Since bone cement works as a grouting agent, rather than as an adhesive, early practice recommended that a layer of cancellous bone trabeculae be left within the cortex to allow interdigitation of the cement. Stem loosening, however, has been linked to the presence of a cancellous layer where the stem rested on the medial cortex of the femoral neck. This is not surprising when the relative strengths of cancellous and cortical bone are known — 5 MPa and 150 MPa (N/mm^2) ultimate compressive strength, respectively. More recent practice has therefore involved removal of the cancellous interlayer. As well as loosening, tenuous support for the proximal stem after calcar resorption had occurred predisposed it to fatigue failure. This was compounded by the Charnley stems being relatively slender (Fig. 31.7c), hence having low bending resistance, and also being made of stainless steel with relatively low fatigue strength. In order to understand why fatigue fracture secondary to calcar resorption happens, the phenomenon of 'stress shielding' must be understood.

If the materials behave elastically, they deform in proportion to the load applied. The imposed strain e (deformation per unit length) is proportional to the stress s (load per unit area) and inversely proportional to the inherent stiffness of the material, often the Young's modulus E, so $e = s \div 1/E$. Thus for the prosthesis, which has a very high stiffness, the strain deformation caused by a given load will be very much smaller than the amount that the bone would be deformed by that load. Referring to Fig. 31.8, the whole of load W is taken by the metal implant at level A, and by the bone at level B. The load passes from metal to bone between these sections, via the bone cement. The load on the implant stem at A causes it to deform in response to the stress. If the stem has a cross-section of $150\,mm^2$,

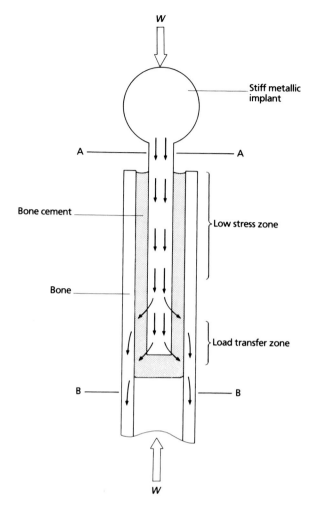

Fig. 31.8 Simplified model of stem fixation. The load is taken entirely by the metal at A–A and by bone at B–B. 'Stress shielding' causes the load to transfer near the stem tip, by-passing the proximal bone.

the stress = W/150. For a joint load $W = 1750\,N$ (ca. 2.5 BW), the stress is 11.67 MPa (N/mm²). Thus, with stainless steel having a Young's modulus of 193 GPa, this stress will impose a strain of:

$$\frac{11.67 \times 10^6}{193 \times 10^9} = 60 \times 10^{-6}$$

This means that a steel stem carrying 1750 N along its length of 130 mm will shorten by $130 \times 60 \times 10^{-6}$, or 0.008 mm. In practice, there is usually an interlayer of fibrous tissue between cement and bone, and also between prosthesis and cement (unless the cement has bonded to an adherent polymethyl methacrylate 'precoat' surface on the metal). Thus, if the fibrous tissue layers have a thickness of 0.1 mm, the stem could deform elastically without transferring axial load to the surrounding femoral neck at all if it is anchored securely at

its tip. Even with perfect bonding, the neck of femur will only be deformed as far as the metal it contains. In this case, assume that the bone strain will also be 60×10^{-6}. Cortical bone has an axial Young's modulus of 14 GPa (Burstein *et al.*, 1976), so the induced stress due to the strain deformation will be 0.22 MPa. If the outer diameter of the femur is 25 mm, and the cortex 4-mm thick, the stress of 0.22 MPa acting over 164 mm² cross-section corresponds to a force of 36 N in the bone, i.e. 2% of the load. The result of this is that the majority of the load is carried by the metal, and the bone is by-passed. There must then be a zone of concentrated load transfer at the tip of the stem. Although this is a greatly simplified analysis, it shows how stress shielding causes disuse atrophy of the proximal femur and endosteal hypertrophy at the stem tip. The result is a stem gripped firmly at its tip but relatively unsupported against bending loads proximally. It is not surprising to find a history of femoral stem fatigue fractures near the midstem region — Charnley reported one in 1971, six in 1973, and by 1979 Wroblewski had a personal series of 40 fractured stem revisions.

The manufacturers then tried to reduce the bending load in the coronal plane and relatively straight stems with a small head–stem offset were introduced around 1980 (Fig. 31.7d). Unfortunately, although this reduced or even eliminated the moment arm of the joint force vector about the midstem section in the coronal plane, this manoeuvre also brought the femur closer to the centreline of the body. Thus the hip abductors had their moment arm about the centre of the hip reduced, necessitating much larger muscle — and hence joint — forces in order to maintain equilibrium of the body on the femoral head as in Fig. 31.2(a). This caused larger anterior–posterior bending loads on the stems, thus predisposing them to fail in a different direction (Brown *et al.*, 1984). The subsequent introduction of forged and cold-worked alloys with enhanced fatigue strengths has eliminated the stem failure problem and allowed a return to a more normal head–shaft relationship.

A different strategy utilizes a polished stem with a smooth taper (Fig. 31.7e). This allows it to wedge into place, raising the femoral hoop (i.e. transverse 'bursting') stress proximally, reducing calcar resorption. This has led to good clinical results (Fowler *et al.*, 1988), partly because the stem can migrate, settling within the cement, without disrupting the cement–bone interface.

Stress shielding has led to the evolution of more sophisticated implants intended for bone ingrowth fixation, interlocking directly with the proximal bone after being forced into close apposition. This requires accurate cavity formation and a tapered prosthesis shape that wedges in. The surfaces may consist of multiple small beads, cast integrally with the core ('Madreporique' finish; Lord *et al.*, 1979), or else sintered-on several layers deep (Turner *et al.*, 1986). Alternatives include wire meshes bonded to the surface or a hydroxyapatite coating. These studies have again shown cortical hypertrophy at the distal stem, suggesting stress-shielding, when the coating completely covered the stems. More recent designs (Fig. 31.7f) localize the ingrowth fixation material to the calcar region, while the distal stem is left as a polished rod. Thus the axial load transfers from metal to bone proximally, while the distal intramedullary stem locates laterally to resist bending loads by a cantilever action. Thus, two distinct implant stem types have emerged, with or without a collar or other means to ensure proximal load transfer. Both types have produced good clinical results and have mechanical arguments to support their use (Kwong, 1990), so it is likely that both will continue alongside each other. It must be remembered, though, that it will require a lot of clinical experience to show superiority over the long-term results achieved with earlier cemented prostheses (Rothman and Cohn, 1990) particularly since Mulroy and Harris (1990) have shown a significant reduction in the loosening rate of hip stems when more modern cement injection and pressurization techniques are used.

A more conservative approach to the femur was tried in several centres in the 1970s, with the development of 'double-cup' arthroplasties. These implants used a thin metallic shell to resurface the femoral head after it had been formed into a spigot, articulating within a thin-walled acetabular cup (Goldie *et al.*, 1979). This appeared very desirable because it preserved the femoral neck, and it was argued that failure would allow easy revision to a conventional design. Unfortunately, the short-term failure rate was unacceptable (Jolley *et al.*, 1982). The femoral shell migrated off of the femoral head into varus, and this was linked to high fixation stresses and bone necrosis arising from damage to the blood supply on the superior aspect of the femoral neck (Crock, 1980).

Acetabular components have also evolved through several stages, requiring hemispherical or conical bone cavities. The original cast cobalt–chrome alloy cups, such as with the McKee–Watson–Farrar hip (McKee and Watson–Farrar, 1966), became unpopular on two grounds. Firstly, it is usual for there to be a high coefficient of friction when two components of the same metal rub together. This was implicated in causing a high friction torque, leading to loosening. A second reason was 'metallosis'—the tissue reaction to metallic wear debris. This led to Charnley's second main contri-

bution in hip replacement, a metal-on-polymer bearing with a lower coefficient of friction. After an abortive start with polytetrafluoroethylene, Charnley chanced upon ultra-high molecular-weight polyethylene. In order to reduce the friction torque to a minimum, Charnley reduced the radius of the femoral head at which it acted. This allowed a thick-walled socket within the acetabulum. However, although a mean wear rate of only 0.07 mm per year was reported, this applied to an elderly group of patients. As the indications widened, cases of severe penetration of the cup were seen. This acceleration was sometimes caused by entrapment of abrasive bone cement debris, but creep deformation (a cold-flow phenomenon under load) also acted. The result was excessive superomedial head migration, which then allowed the side of the femoral neck to impinge on the rim of the cup, leading to loosening (Fig. 31.9). In response to this, most manufacturers settled on a larger head size, of approximately 32-mm diameter.

The fixation of acetabular sockets is often regarded as more critical than that of the femoral stem (Mulroy and Harris, 1990), with a greater likelihood of at least partial radiolucent zones at the bone–cement interface. This probably arises because the pelvic girdle is a relatively thin structure that deforms significantly under load. Stress analysis has shown that the highest stresses arise superiorly from the acetabulum, as expected. The upward force in the acetabulum counteracts the forces of the abductors arising from the ilium, and the sacro-iliac joint force. The bone structure is well adapted to resist deformation in bending, being essentially a 'sandwich' of two cortical surfaces separated by a cancellous core (Jacob *et al.*, 1976). Thus it is analogous to modern yacht construction, in which fibre-reinforced plastics sheath a light foam core. This arrangement optimises the bending strength-to-weight ratio. Despite this, a superiorly-directed load will deform the bone in that direction, tending to pull the inferior margins of an acetabular cup away from the bone. It thus became standard practice to drill large cement 'keying' holes through the subchondral plate in diverging directions, in order to maintain a gross interlock with the bone, even if the cement were separated from it by a thin fibrous layer. The addition of wide flanges around acetabular cups aids cement entrapment and hence allows a higher pressure to be exerted on insertion, causing better cement/bone interdigitation (Oh *et al.*, 1985). Following the publication of several stress analyses of acetabular cup–bone interactions, which suggested that a rigid cup would impose lower stresses (Vasu *et al.*, 1982; Harris, 1984) 'metal-backed' components have become popular. These sometimes take the form of a truncated cone with

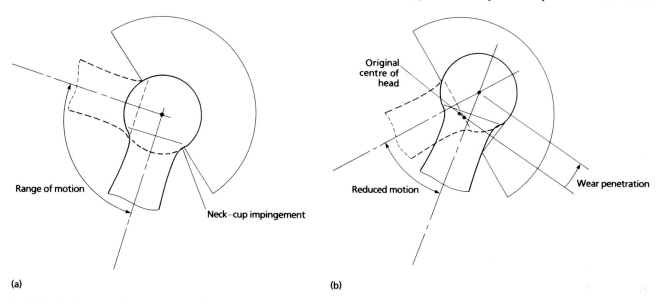

Range of motion

Neck–cup impingement

(a)

Original
centre of
head

Reduced motion

Wear penetration

(b)

Fig. 31.9 Mechanism of impingement of femoral neck with reduced range of motion after wear penetration, leading to cup loosening.

an interrupted coarse thread on the exterior surface, for cement-free fixation. A claimed advantage is that such designs will allow the polyethylene liner to be replaced if it wears out. Meanwhile, Ritter *et al.* (1990) have reported significantly worse survival rates for metal-backed cups compared with polyethylene cups of the same prosthesis type. Rothman and Cohn (1990) have noted that although acetabular cups may have radiolucent zones, several large series have reported nearly 100% survival rates for both Charnley and metal-backed cups at ten years.

THE KNEE

Although it is the largest joint in the body, the form and function of the knee predisposes it to mechanical problems. The joint surfaces are adapted to a large range of flexion–extension motion, not as a stable 'roller-in-trough' configuration, but as a 'roller on a flat plate', since the former would obliterate the freedom for axial rotation between femur and tibia that is a necessary part of lower limb function. The result is an inherently unstable joint that must rely on ligaments and muscles for kinematic control. Injury to these soft tissues is not unexpected, since the joint carries the large forces of locomotion at the intersection of the longest bony 'levers' in the body.

Knee motion

The main function of the knee is the flexion action which allows the foot to be raised from, or the body

lowered towards, the ground. This is obviously needed when negotiating steps, but it is a fundamental part of normal locomotion. It is possible to walk without knees, but a stiff-legged gait means that the centre of gravity of the body must rise and then fall in a trajectory that is an arc centred at the ankle, as the hip passes over the fixed foot in the stance phase of gait. This raising and lowering is wasteful of energy, and hence tiring, and is avoided in normal walking by knee flexion in the midstance phase, allowing the centre of gravity to remain at a relatively constant height. Thus the normal pattern of motion (Murray *et al.*, 1964) is that of Fig. 31.1, with the knee extended as the foot reaches forwards for heel strike, flexion in stance, then extension before the leg pushes off from the toes. Because the load-bearing knee flexes at midstance, there is not enough ground clearance for the swinging leg to avoid the toes dragging unless that knee is then flexed 70°.

While tibiofemoral motion approximates to a hinge, flexion does not take place about a fixed axis. Because the tibial plateau is relatively flat, the femur tends to roll backwards and forwards in flexion and extension. This is controlled towards the limits of motion, principally by muscle actions and the cruciate ligaments, and also by the need to 'climb uphill' over the horns of the menisci. The situation is analogous to the driving wheel of a car, tethered to the ground by a rope attached near to its axle. The wheel is driven round, but the rope prevents progress, so the tyre slips and a relative motion occurs between it and the ground. Because of this, the surfaces of the femoral condyles are constrained to undergo a mixture of rolling and sliding in relation to the tibia.

The menisci must move posteriorly and anteriorly with flexion and extension, particularly on the lateral side, to follow the moving areas of contact of the condyles on the tibial plateau.

If tibiofemoral motion or equilibrium is to be analysed, the axis about which rotation occurs must be identified. In the sagittal plane, the femoral condyles do not have a constant radius. The posterior aspect is approximately circular, and this blends into a larger radius anteriorly. At each particular angle of flexion, the femur would rotate about a point at the centre of the contact radius if the tibiofemoral motion consisted solely of sliding. However, the mixture of rolling and sliding induced by the cruciates causes the centre of rotation to move towards the joint line. It can be located by means of the Reuleaux method of double-exposure radiographs (Fig. 31.10) at any angle of flexion. This double-position technique is generally applicable to the discovery of the centre of rotation of one body relative to another, being useful in complex situations such as the wrist. An approximate method for the knee is to locate the intersection of the cruciates in the sagittal plane. This follows from the definition of the 'instant centre of rotation'—all other points on the body are instantaneously rotating around that point, neither approaching nor receding from it. This includes the cruciate origins on the femur, so the centre of rotation must be at the ligaments' intersection if they are not changing length.

Tibial rotation may be caused actively through a range of approximately 60° when the knee is flexed 90°, but is inhibited progressively as the knee extends. This is caused by tightening of the ligaments and posterior capsular and popliteal tissues. The posterior tissues have slanting fibre orientations that can resist tibial rotation. As the knee extends, the tibia is controlled so that it rotates externally—the 'screw home' mechanism, which has been measured in gait by Levens *et al.* (1948).

Static analysis of tibiofemoral joint force

A 'static' analysis can be used in situations where movement is slow, because errors arising from inertial effects will be negligible. A typical heavily-loaded situation occurs when a subject rises from a chair without the aid of the arms. In this activity, the knee is flexed beyond 90°, the ankle is dorsiflexed, and the hip flexed, so that the centre of mass of the body is brought towards a vertical line through the contact area between feet and ground (Fig. 31.11a). The body weight (BW) tends to flex the knees, and it can be assumed that they share this equally. So for each knee the flexion effect is a moment of force BW/2 multiplied by the perpendicular distance

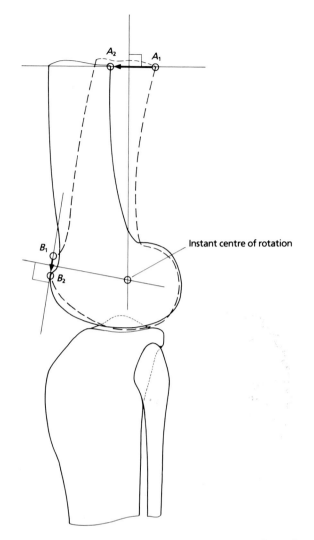

Fig. 31.10 The Reuleaux double-exposure technique allows the centre of rotation to be found, since all points on the femur rotate about it. This uses two points identifiable on a radiograph, with a small arc of movement between two exposures. The path of any point is centred at the axis, so a perpendicular to the path gives a circle radius. The intersection of two radii must be the centre of the circle, at the instant centre of rotation.

between the line of action of the force and the instant centre of rotation of the knee. To be in equilibrium, the knee must be acted on by an equal and opposite extension moment arising from the patellar tendon tension (PT). Thus, from Fig. 31.11(a), $BW/2 \times d = PT \times e$. Thus the patellar tendon tension, $PT = BW/2 \times d/e$. If $BW = 700\,N$, $d = 200\,mm$ and $e = 35\,mm$, $PT = 2000\,N$, or 2.9 BW.

The tibiofemoral joint force (TF) may now be calculated. Figure 31.11(a) shows the forces acting on the limb distal to the joint line. Lesser forces, such as the weight of the shank, have been omitted for clarity.

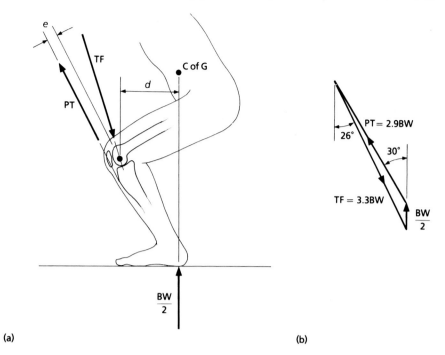

Fig. 31.11 (a) Forces when rising from a chair: the centre of mass of the body is above the foot–floor contact, giving a moment arm *d*. For equilibrium, the patellar tendon must exert a moment equal and opposite to that caused by the body weight, so $BW/2 \times d = PT \times e$. (b) The tibiofemoral joint force can be found by constructing the force vector triangle, knowing both the magnitude and direction of BW/2 and PT.

(a)

(b)

Knowing the magnitude and direction of PT and BW/2, TF may be found by solving the force vector triangle shown in Fig. 31.11(b), giving TF = 3.34 BW, acting at 26° from the vertical. Thus the tibiofemoral joint force of 3.34 BW is caused mainly by the patellar tendon tension, 2.9 BW, rather than direct compression arising from the body weight. The tendon tension depends primarily on the distance of the line of action of the body weight from the rotation axis. An extreme situation arises when rising from a squatting position, when the moment arm may reach 0.35 m and both patellar ten-

dons may reach tensions of 5 BW. It has been calculated that weight lifters can exert 16 BW!

The patellofemoral joint

The main function of the patella is to lift the line of action of the extensor mechanism away from the surface of the distal femur. This increases the moment arm of the patellar tendon about the centre of rotation of the knee and thus decreases the tendon tension needed to resist knee flexion moments. Figure 31.12 demonstrates

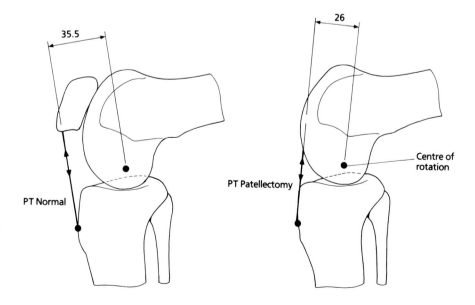

Fig. 31.12 Patellectomy reduces the moment arm of the patellar tendon about the centre of rotation, requiring 36% greater tension in the patellar tendon to produce the same extension moment, since $35.5 = 1.36 \times 26$.

that a patellectomy would require an increase in patellar tendon tension of 36% in order to produce the same knee extension effect, a muscle force increase beyond the capacity of many patients, leading to difficulty with daily activities such as stair climbing. Since the musculotendinous complex now takes a shorter path around the end of the femur, there is excess length in the soft tissues. This causes 'extensor lag' when walking, in which knee extension does not follow the accustomed relationship to muscle shortening in gait.

It was shown above that tibiofemoral joint forces rose as the knee was flexed, mainly due to the increased moment arm of the line of body weight from the knee. This is repeated at the patellofemoral joint, but the phenomenon is magnified here. Firstly, the patellar tendon tension must rise as the knee flexes because the flexion moment caused by body weight is increasing. Secondly, there is a geometrical effect which compounds this, as the tendon and muscle tensions change direction in flexion. With the knee extended as in Fig. 31.13(a), the patellofemoral joint force (PF) is seen to be approximately a half of the patellar tendon tension (PT). The diagram was constructed by drawing in the lines of action of the patellar and quadriceps tendons, then adding the joint force PF. As seen in Fig. 31.13, the three forces must intersect at a point if the patella is to be in equilibrium. Furthermore, the line of action of PF should pass through the patellofemoral contact area, and should

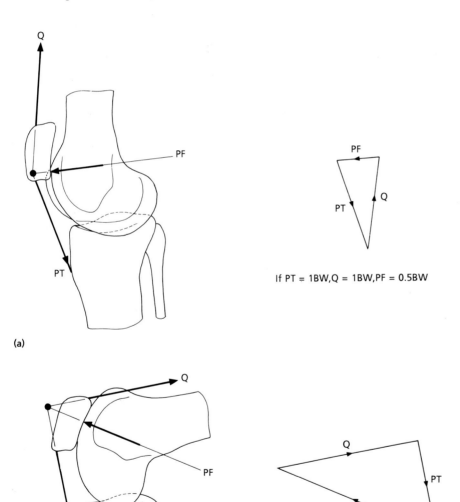

If PT = 1BW, Q = 1BW, PF = 0.5BW

(a)

If PT = 1BW, Q = 1.6BW, PF = 1.9BW

(b)

Fig. 31.13 (a) Patellofemoral joint force constructions near full extension and at 90° flexion. Note how the joint force rises with flexion for a constant patellar tendon tension, and how the quadriceps tension is greater than the patellar tendon tension in flexion.

be approximately normal to the joint surfaces, since the friction coefficient is low in human joints. Thus the diagram gives the directions of the three force vectors, which can then be drawn as a force vector triangle, from which their relative magnitudes can be measured. If this procedure is repeated for the knee at 90° flexion, as in Fig. 31.13(b), it is seen that the line of action of the quadriceps tension has rotated with the femur, while the patellar tendon has scarcely moved, leading to the force vector construction shown. The patellofemoral contact force has increased in relation to the patellar tendon tension by a factor of nearly four times that seen in Fig. 31.13(a). This is why patellofemoral pain usually manifests itself when the knee is flexed.

The force vector construction of Fig. 13.13(b) indicates a quadriceps tension 1.6 times that of the patellar tendon. Various publications have given the erroneous impression that patellar tendon tension is equal to quadriceps tension because of the low friction in the patellofemoral joint. Such a statement can only be correct if the joint force vector bisects the angle between their lines of action, as in Fig. 31.13(a). The situation is clearer if an analogous situation is considered, as in Fig. 31.14. The truck represents the patella, pulled by strings PT and Q. If it is in left–right equilibrium, the horizontal component of tension Q must be equal and opposite to PT, so Q is obviously larger than PT.

As the knee flexes, the patella slides into the trochlear groove, maintaining a constant distance from the tibial tuberosity. The patellofemoral contact is initially near the distal pole of the patella (Fig. 31.13a), where this small contact area has relatively low forces applied to it. With increasing flexion, the contact area moves prox-

imally (Fig. 31.13b), until there is a band of contact across the widest part of the patella, in order to resist the larger patellofemoral force in this posture. In extreme flexion, the patella bridges across the intercondylar notch, with two contact areas on the anterior part of the condyles. It is because the patella passes onto the condylar bearing surfaces that partial knee replacements of the patellofemoral type have not been introduced widely, since they would either interfere with the tibiofemoral articulation, or else cause the patella to pass off of the femoral component.

The patellofemoral force analysis above was a two-dimensional approximation to a three-dimensional situation. When viewed in coronal projection, it is seen that the patella is pulled laterally (Fig. 31.15), due to the valgus angulation (sometimes known as the Q angle) between the quadriceps mechanism and the patellar tendon. This is no problem normally, because the prominent lateral facet of the patellar groove keeps the patella stable. This can be shown by considering a transverse section through the contact area with the knee near full extension (Fig. 31.16). In this diagram, the anterior–posterior force component of PF is that found in Fig.

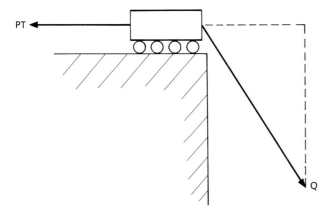

Fig. 31.14 Representation of the extensor mechanism with the knee flexed. The truck represents the patella, pulled by strings PT and Q. If it is in left–right equilibrium, the horizontal component of tension Q must be equal and opposite to PT, so Q is obviously larger than PT.

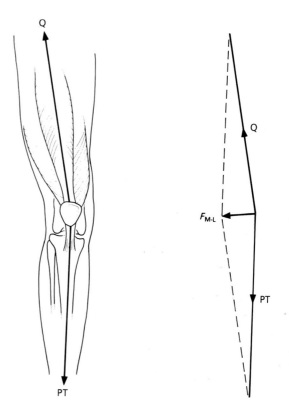

Fig. 31.15 The patella is pulled laterally, due to the valgus angulation (sometimes known as the Q angle) between the quadriceps mechanism and the patellar tendon.

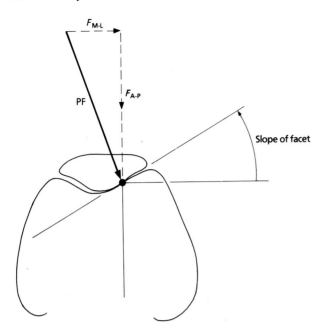

Fig. 31.16 Transverse section through the patellofemoral contact near full extension, showing how the anterior–posterior (AP) and medial–lateral (ML) force components derived in Figs 31.15(a) and 31.17 maintain the patella in a stable position against the slope of the lateral facet of the groove, as long as the slope of the facet is greater than $\tan^{-1}$ ML/AP.

31.13(a), while the medial–lateral component of the same force is that found in Fig. 31.15. The situation is stable if PF deviates from the sagittal plane less than the slope angle of the lateral facet of the patellar groove. So, for stability, tan (slope angle) > medial–lateral/anterior–posterior components of PF. This shows that the patella can be stabilized in the groove by reducing the medial–lateral component (such as by medialization of the tibial tuberosity), or by increasing the anterior–posterior component (as happens during flexion). Osteotomy to increase the slope of the lateral facet has also been described for cases where the trochlear groove is abnormally shallow.

The patella can also be re-aligned by anterior elevation of the tibial tuberosity. This increases the moment arm of the patellar tendon about the centre of rotation, and tilts the patella because it is anchored in a different direction. The tuberosity is usually elevated 20 mm (Maquet, 1984), moving the contact area superiorly, perhaps away from existing lesions, while the increase in moment arm reduces the patellofemoral contact forces near full extension, relieving pain when walking.

Dynamic analysis of knee forces

Although the static force analysis above has shown how

loads are caused at the knee, the majority of joint loading occurs during dynamic ambulatory activities. The classic work examining forces on the knee during walking, and other activities such as ascending ramps or descending stairs, was that of Morrison (1968, 1969). Figure 31.17 shows the external forces and moments acting on and about the knee when walking. The force components graph shows that the predominant force is axial compression F_{axial}, with small anterior–posterior forces $F_{A–P}$ that would cause cruciate tensions. The double-peaked waveform shows that load is greatest soon after heel-strike, when the foot arrests the body's descent, and also approaching toe-off, as the foot pushes the body upwards and forwards. The $F_{A–P}$ curve goes

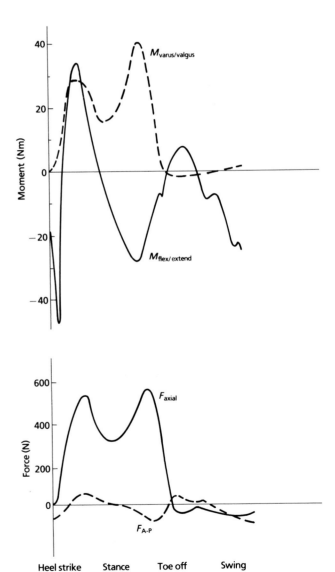

Fig. 31.17 Forces and moments acting on the knee when walking. (Morrison, 1968.)

positive and negative, which means that the tibia is pushed anteriorly and posteriorly, necessitating actions in both cruciates sequentially if the muscles do not provide stability. The joint moments tend to cause angulation of the knee. $M_{\text{flex/extend}}$ acts about the flexion–extension axis: the sharp negative peak at heel-strike shows that the impact force tends to extend the knee, so hamstrings action is needed. The moment then becomes positive, flexing the knee-after-heel strike, so this is when quadriceps acts to arrest the body's descent. Towards toe-off, the moment becomes negative again, so gastrocnemius acts, both to control knee extension and to plantarflex the foot to push off from the ground. Perhaps unexpectedly, the $M_{\text{varus/valgus}}$ curve is strongly positive, showing that the knee is subjected to strong varus actions during load-bearing. This arises because the line of action of the ground reaction forces passes medially to the knee during the stance phase (Fig. 31.18). Knee and hip stability are thus controlled simultaneously by tension in the iliotibial tract during stance phase. It follows that the majority of the compressive load on the knee is taken by the medial condyle (Fig. 31.18). This finding appears initially not to conform to static loading analysis in the coronal plane, when it has been emphasized that the centres of hip, knee and ankle should be in a straight line on load-bearing anterior–posterior radiographs, but this configuration does not mean that static loads need to pass up the centre of the tibia to the knee. Denham and Bishop (1978) showed that the line of action could move 8 cm mediolaterally with trunk leaning in static one-legged stance, while Harrington (1974) found 4-cm movement when walking. The important point of the hip–knee–ankle line is that small angulations of knee prostheses, or joint deformity arising from cartilage loss in one compartment, cause large shifts in the line of action of the load crossing the knee. A small inaccuracy or deformity can then cause abnormally large compression loads on one condyle, coupled to ligament tensions at the other side of the joint (Fig. 31.19). Maquet (1984) has popularized corrective osteotomies for such cases.

Knee replacements

The earliest types of knee replacement have come to be known as 'fully constrained' hinges. This is not an accurate nomenclature, since full constraint prevents any movement, but reflects the fact that these hinge joints constrained all motion apart from rotation about a single flexion axis. These implants were necessarily massive because they prevented secondary tibiofemoral motions into varus–valgus or internal–external ro-

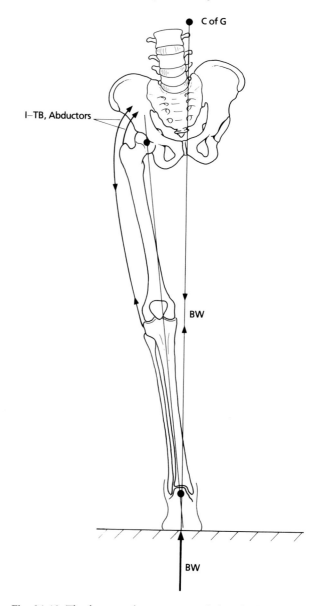

Fig. 31.18 The force resultant passes medial to the knee in the stance phase, leading to the compressive load concentrating on the medial condyle. Tension in the iliotibial band is required to maintain stability.

tation, and hence had to absorb the forces or moments associated with this. Massive fixation means were needed in order to transmit such loads into the bones, and it became normal to have long intramedullary stems plus external patellar flanges. Such implants went out of fashion because their inherently rigid constraint predisposed them to loosening; since the surrounding ligaments and capsule only stabilize the knee after being stretched, they have no chance to participate around a rigidly constrained joint, and so the implant fixation has to transmit all the load. A further point was that limits

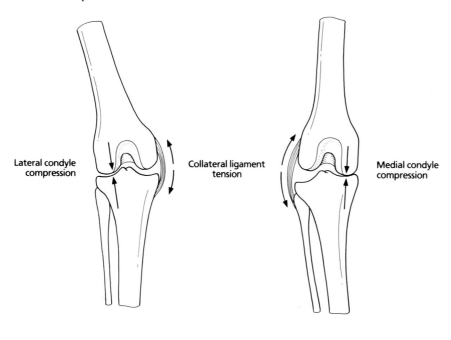

Lateral condyle compression

Collateral ligament tension

Medial condyle compression

(a) Valgus knee

(b) Varus knee

Fig. 31.19 Varus or valgus deformity of the knee leads to collateral ligament tension and the joint force acting on one condyle if the resultant force passes outside the centre of rotation of the femoral condyle.

to motion of these joints, such as full extension, often caused direct metal-to-metal impacts, leading to high-load peaks. These mechanical factors, allied to the inherently poor salvage prospects, led to the relegation of such implants to use in salvage procedures.

Engineers soon realised that prostheses could be designed which would allow the femur to move around on the tibia, leaving the soft-tissue restraints to limit secondary displacements and rotations, thus relieving the implant fixation of all loads except the compressive joint force. Perhaps the ultimate design in this respect was the 'sledge' prosthesis (Stockley *et al.*, 1990), in which the tibial plateaux were completely flat. Consideration of tibiofemoral contact in such a joint, however, shows that there can only be points of contact under load, leading to excessive articular surface pressures, predisposing the surface to damage (Wright and Bartel, 1986). Furthermore, such an implant depends on the ligaments completely, perhaps more than the natural knee. Such considerations led Swanson and Freeman (1974) to design a prosthesis in which the femoral component was primarily a roller of constant radius, which articulated against a matching, but very shallow, trough in the tibial component (Fig. 31.20). The anterior–posterior slopes on the tibial plateau located the femoral component in normal use, since this implant required cruciate excision. If a large shearing force were applied, the roller could glide 'uphill' out of the trough, allowing the capsule and muscles to act and preventing the

transmission of a loosening force to the bone fixation interface. This implant covered the entire bone ends, thus minimizing the compressive stresses arising from the joint force, but also allowed a radical reduction in bone removal. The concept of the femoral component having to 'climb uphill' out of the most stable close-packed configuration was refined further by Walker *et al.* (1974), who used the stability of the natural knee as a guide to the curvatures needed in a prosthesis, if it were to have similar characteristics. This approach still leads to relatively highly-stressed and mobile contact areas. An elegant way around the problem of reconciling motion and conformity is to mimic the natural knee, using menisci. This allows the upper articulation to be spherical and the lower to be flat, so both maintain large contact areas during knee motion (Goodfellow and O'Connor, 1978) (Fig. 31.20). A range of thicknesses of meniscal components allows the soft tissues to be tensed at operation, but meniscal dislocations have been reported (Bert, 1990).

With time, it became apparent that polyethylene tibial plateaux with shallow fixation tended to fail in a varus–valgus 'rocking' mode, reflecting the medial–lateral shifts of the force vector noted above. Subsequent analyses, both experimental (Walker *et al.*, 1981) and theoretical (Lewis *et al.*, 1982) led to the adoption of metal undertrays to limit bending deflections and either 'twin-peg' or 'central post' fixations to limit the rocking motion (Fig. 31.20). The central posts are usually tapered

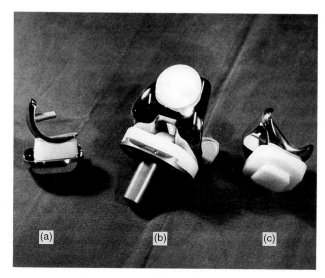

Fig. 31.20 Knee prostheses. (a) Oxford meniscal bearing implant, normally used as a unicondylar replacement; (b) typical recent design (Insall—Burstein), with metallic tray to support tibial plateau and short fixation stems; (c) early Freeman—Swanson type, requiring minimal bone resection.

on the posterior aspect and dimensioned so that loads are transmitted to the adjacent posterior tibial cortex. Implantation of a knee with central fixation means that the cruciates must be removed. Although some implants have been designed to retain these ligaments, smooth function then depends on an accurate relationship between the implant shell and the ligament attachments, otherwise the ligaments may tighten and block motion. Implants which do not preserve the cruciates often have a lug protruding from the tibial component to control anterior—posterior movement of the femur. This could lead to loosening if anterior—posterior forces act on the component at some height above the fixation, but these implants are designed so that the cam action of the lug operates in flexion in normal activities, when the knee will already be supporting a much larger compressive load and hence remain stable (Insall *et al.*, 1982; Insall, 1985).

ANKLE AND FOOT

The foot can be divided anatomically into the hindfoot—the talus and calcaneus, the midfoot—the navicular, cuboid and cuneiform bones, and the forefoot—the metatarsals and phalanges. The bones of these three anatomical units are bound together by interosseous ligaments which allow little mobility, but the units move in relation to each other, via Lisfranc's 'joint' between the forefoot and midfoot, and via Chopart's joint between the midfoot and hindfoot (Heckman, 1984).

Motion

The ankle is essentially a hinge joint, with a transverse axis passing through the tips of the malleoli. The roller-shaped convexity of the superior surface of the talus allows plantarflexion and dorsiflexion as it slides through the tibiofibular mortice joint. The close deformity of the malleoli to the sides of the talus ensures that it cannot deviate from a linear sliding motion in an anterior—posterior direction. Rasmussen and Torborg-Jensen (1982) noted a wide range of ankle mobility reported in earlier literature, with values for dorsiflexion ranging from 10° to 51°, and plantarflexion from 15° to 56°. Using a loading rig to apply 1.5-Nm moment to cadaveric ankles, they reported a mean range of 18° dorsiflexion and 32° plantarflexion. Stauffer (1979) reported that the ankle joint undergoes 6° rotation out of the sagittal plane during flexion—extension, arising from different radii of curvature at the medial and lateral sides of the joint. Ankle motion when walking was measured from high-speed cine films, showing 10° dorsiflexion and 14° plantarflexion. This range of motion increased to 56° when descending stairs.

The subtalar joint, between talus and calcaneus, has an axis slanting from the lateral plantar surface of the calcaneus to the medial dorsal aspect of the navicular. This allows inversion and eversion of the foot, which is vital for correct adaptation to uneven ground when walking. This subtalar adaptation then allows a normal anterior—posterior slide of the ankle joint. The combined actions of tibiotalar and subtalar joints thus approximate to a universal joint.

The normal pattern of ankle motion in walking involves rapid plantarflexion during heel-strike until the foot is flat on the floor, followed by dorsiflexion as the body passes overhead in stance, then plantarflexion to raise the heel and push-off with the toes. During the swing phase the foot is dorsiflexed to a neutral position ready for heel strike (Murray *et al.*, 1964; Stauffer *et al.*, 1977) (Fig. 31.1).

In the latter part of stance phase the metatarsophalangeal joints must all extend simultaneously. These joints have a range of motion of approximately 30° flexion to 90° extension, accommodated by the concave bases of the phalanges sliding over the convex metatarsal heads. The heads of the metatarsals are barrel-shaped, allowing a small arc of lateral motion by slackness in the collateral ligaments. Sammarco (1989) showed that the centre of flexion motion lay inside the metatarsal heads, whereas the abduction/adduction was centred proximally in the metatarsal.

Function during locomotion

During the stance phase between heel-strike and toe-off, the centre of mass of the body progresses forward at walking speed. This is reflected by the foot-to-floor contact—the centre of pressure starting at the heel, then moving towards the toes (Simkin, 1981). The area of the metatarsal heads takes most of the load during the push-off phase, with the second ray taking greatest load (Collis and Jayson, 1972). Finally, the great toe is last to leave the ground.

When viewed laterally, the bony structure of the foot forms a pointed arch, with the talus at its apex. The talus has a superior articulation with the tibia and an accessory articulation with the fibula, and the weight of the body is borne on it. The effect of such loading is to spread out and hence flatten the foot. This tendency is resisted by the plantar fascia, which acts as a tensile tie across the base of the foot (Fig. 31.21). The fascia originates from the calcaneus and dissipates into the plantar aspects of the proximal phalanges, thus crossing

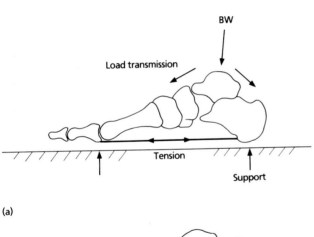

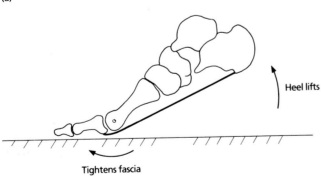

Fig. 31.21 (a) The plantar fascia acts as a tie to prevent collapse of the pointed arch configuration under load. (b) The insertion into the phalanx causes the fascia to be tensed as the heel lifts from the floor, dorsiflexing the metatarsophalangeal joint, thus restoring the arch height.

the metatarsophalangeal joints. The vertical forces are similar to body weight when walking, but can be 2.5 times body weight when running. Foot-flattening reduces the rise and fall of the body mass as it passes overhead with each stride, thus aiding efficiency of locomotion. Since the plantar fascia inserts into the proximal phalanges, it is tensed by the forced dorsiflexion of the metatarsophalangeal joints as the heel is raised from the floor, which helps to restore the normal arch height (Fig. 31.21).

The pelvis swings about a vertical axis when walking, one side then the other being swung forwards in readiness for heel-strike (Murray *et al.*, 1964). At heel-strike, the foot points forward from an internally rotated femur and tibia, which is allowed by eversion of the subtalar joint. This unlocks the transverse tarsal joint, allowing the arch of the foot to flatten as a shock-absorbing mechanism. There is progressive external rotation of the limb as the pelvis moves forwards and externally rotates in relation to the fixed foot. External rotation of the stance leg causes inversion of the subtalar joint and locking of the transverse tarsal joint, which produces a rigid forefoot ready for push-off (Mann, 1980). This mechanism depends on ankle stability to transmit the rotation effect from the tibia to invert the subtalar joint. Inversion of the ankle, however, is a common injury mechanism leading to collateral ligament damage. It is a common misconception to think that these injuries lead to varus instability, which is then checked by an anterior–posterior radiograph for talar tilt. Glasgow *et al.* (1980), showed that the anterior talofibular ligament is damaged most often during inversion, leading to an *anterior* instability. Varus instability only reveals itself if damage spreads to the more vertically oriented calcaneofibular ligament. It is the anterior instability of the lateral side of the talus, effectively an anterolateral rotatory instability (Rasmussen and Torborg-Jensen, 1982) which interferes with the transmission of external rotation from the tibia during the stance phase of walking to invert and stiffen the foot prior to push-off.

Static forces analysis

If a person rises onto the ball of the foot, the ankle moves into plantarflexion due to Achilles' tendon tension. For the ankle to be in equilibrium the dorsiflexion moment, due to the external load, must be equal and opposite to the plantarflexion moment, due to the Achilles' tendon tension (Fig. 31.22). For a typical adult foot size and single leg stance:

$$BW \times 120 = T \times 55$$

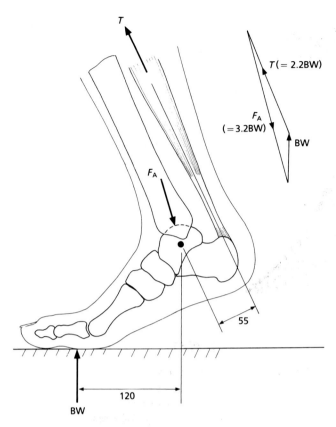

Fig. 31.22 Static analysis of forces when standing with the heel raised. The tendon must impose an equal and opposite plantarflexion moment to the dorsiflexion moment imposed by the floor reaction force, about the axis of the ankle.

so Achilles' tendon tension, $T = 2.2\,BW$. This is normally in a posture which includes knee flexion, so that the knee axis is close to the line of action of the external force, giving a tibial inclination of 20°. The joint force must resist the combined effects of BW and T at the ankle, and may be found by constructing a force vector diagram (Fig. 31.22), leading to ankle joint force = 3.2 BW. Lambert (1971) reported that one-sixth of the load across the ankle is transmitted to the fibula. This arises because of the slope of the talofibular joint away from the sagittal plane.

Dynamic force analysis

The dynamic effects of locomotion increase ankle force above the static load calculated above, partly because the body mass must be accelerated upwards during the push-off phase. Stauffer *et al.* (1977) and Proctor and Paul (1982) used force plates to measure the foot-to-floor reaction forces, and motion analysis of the limb, to predict ankle forces rising to nearly 5 BW during the push-off phase of walking. This coincided with a posterior shear force of 0.7 BW, which causes the compressive joint load to deviate <10° from the tibial axis. Stauffer *et al.* (1977) noted that the force curve was double-peaked, corresponding to heel-strike and toe-off, at a normal cadence.

Ankle-joint prostheses

Protagonists of ankle-joint replacement have noted a significant rate of complications following arthrodesis and have hoped to avoid this by not interfering with the mechanics of the foot. There were several designs on trial in the late 1970s (Kempson *et al.*, 1975; Newton, 1979; Dini and Bassett, 1980; Stauffer and Segal, 1981), but these suffered significant complication rates in the long term and have not gained widespread acceptance. The ankle prostheses were in two groups, depending on the degree of constraint built into their articulations. The more constrained geometry was a cylindrical approximation to the tibiotalar joint, giving a single axis for plantarflexion and dorsiflexion (Fig. 31.23). This geometry gave a large area of contact between the components, thus lowering the contact pressure and, hence, the rate of penetration of the polyethylene component by creep and wear. A side effect of the 'roller-in-trough' geometry is that rotation is prevented until the torque is large enough to make the roller climb 'uphill' out of its trough against the influence of any joint load. This means that rotational torques are transmitted by the implant fixation in normal use, the shear forces leading to loosening. The surrounding ligaments, being compliant, will not transmit loads until they have been stretched to some extent. A less-constrained geometry is more spherical in shape, thus allowing the ankle some freedom for inversion–eversion and rotation, which helps those patients whose subtalar joints have been arthrodesed.

Arthrodesis

Joints of the foot and ankle are still arthrodesed because of the lack of a reliable joint replacement. Unfortunately, this destroys normal gait. In the load-bearing stance phase of the walking cycle, as the body moves forwards over the foot, knee flexion allows the centre of mass of the body to progress forwards with little change in height. A stiff ankle prevents this, because the heel lifts from the ground prematurely—the pivot point having moved from the ankle to the metatarsophalangeal joints. This abnormal gait is not only wasteful of energy—and hence tiring—but it throws abnormal bending loads

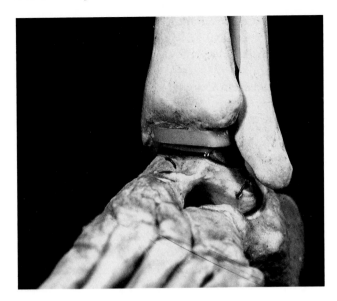

Fig. 31.23 A typical roller-in-trough ankle prosthesis. (Kempson *et al.*, 1975).

onto the tarsometatarsal joints, which are then prone to problems. The prevention of ankle dorsiflexion during the latter part of the stance phase prevents the normal stretching of the calcaneal tendon complex, which stores energy elastically as the body moves forward in stance. The push-off phase of gait is thus deprived of this stored energy as well as the muscular effort as the foot pushes off with a plantarflexion force. Thomas (1969) noted that arthrodesed ankles often led to osteoarthrosis of the subtalar and midtarsal joints, presumably because of the abnormal forces, while Lance *et al.* (1979) reported an increased likelihood of foot pain if ankle arthrodesis is combined with subtalar arthrodesis. This is because the loss of subtalar joint motion prevents the foot adapting to rough ground. Mazur *et al.* (1979) found that patients compensated during normal walking by having shoes with a raised heel that helped movement during the stance phase, combined with larger-than-normal movements in the subtalar and midtarsal joints. This gave nearly normal gait. However, these patients had difficulty in walking barefoot, and could not run. In a similar study of a series of six different types of ankle prosthesis, Demottaz *et al.* (1979) found inferior results for normality of gait and pain relief. Also, at only short-term review (15 months), the majority of implants had progressive radiolucencies around their fixation. Therefore arthrodesis remained the treatment of choice, despite its drawbacks.

Hallux valgus

This deformity results from prolonged loading of the medial aspect of the hallux arising from ill-fitting shoes with a pointed-toe region. The hallux is normally kept straight by soft-tissue balance, especially between abductor and adductor hallucis, but Sammarco (1989) described a mechanism of lateral collateral ligament stretching and medial ligament contraction at the metatarsophalangeal joint. As the phalanx moves laterally, the tendons change their relationship to the metacarpal head, the abductor hallucis slipping laterally under the joint until it acts to flex and pronate the phalanx, rather than abducting it (Mann and Coughlin, 1981). Thus the toe is unbalanced and the adductor hallucis pulls the toe laterally.

THE SHOULDER

Motion

Shoulder motion is usually defined as that of the humerus in relation to the stationary thorax. This encompasses movements within the shoulder girdle as a whole, giving a summation of glenohumeral and scapulothoracic motions. With both shoulder flexion and abduction approaching 180° (Murray *et al.*, 1985), there is greater mobility here than at any other articulation in the human body (Kapandji, 1970). Scapulothoracic mobility does not arise at a true joint, but is controlled by the scapulothoracic muscles and the clavicle. Sternoclavicular motion allows the clavicle to move vertically (elevation) or anteriorly (protraction), combinations of which allow the acromioclavicular joint, and hence the glenoid, to move over a spherical locus centred on the sternoclavicular joint. The orientation of the scapula about a vertical axis then depends on its thin medial border resting on the ribs. The clavicle does not rotate during shoulder motion, but moves in arcs of circumduction, which are accommodated at the sternoclavicular joint by a saddle-like articulation. Scapular motion is normally complementary to that of the humerus, orienting the glenoid towards the direction of the humerus. This action delays impingement of the neck of the humerus against the rim of the glenoid at the extremes of motion. Since the glenohumeral joint accommodates a large range of motion, the glenoid necessarily subtends a small arc and is thus shallow. The shoulder muscles tend to pull the humerus towards the scapula, so this orientation aids stability. Studies of abduction movement have shown that the velocity ratio between glenohumeral and scapulothoracic movements varies through the arc of motion, but is approximately 1.5:1, with 105° gleno-humeral motion in 180° abduction (Inglis, 1982).

The clavicle

The clavicle acts primarily as a strut loaded in compression, its main job being to resist the tensions of the pectoral and trapezium muscles and thus maintain the scapular position against medially-directed loads. These forces must pass through the acromioclavicular joint, where the lateral end of the clavicle meets the upward sloping joint surface on the medial aspect of the acromion (Bateman and Fornasier, 1978). The clavicle is obviously likely to subluxate up the slope if the scapula is forced medially (Fig. 31.24), and it is this tendency which causes rupture of the acromioclavicular ligaments, rather than elevation forces applied by the muscles. Similarly, fractures of the clavicle arise from lengthwise compression forces, which cause buckling failure of a curved strut. The injury mechanism is likely to be a combination of direct impact force on the shoulder and pectoral muscle loading, rather than the tensile load which may at first appear likely during a fall onto the outstretched hand.

Shoulder forces

The spherical glenohumeral joint is only stable as long as the resultant load acting across it passes within the rim of the glenoid, otherwise it will tend to sublux. The resultant load will be largely a reaction force against the muscle tensions crossing the joint, plus any force acting on the hand, and the limb weight. Subluxation could arise during attempts to elevate the arm from a position of 30° abduction, for example, when the deltoid tension tends to pull the humerus superiorly off of the glenoid as in Fig. 31.25(a) (Post, 1988). In most joints, which are constrained more than the shoulder, the ligaments restrain subluxation. This is not practicable at the shoulder because non-contractile tissues can only act at the extremes of motion. The 'rotator cuff' overcomes this problem by forming a contractile hood over the humeral head, composed of the insertions of subscapularis, supraspinatus, infraspinatus and teres minor. Simultaneous and antagonistic actions of these muscles, primarily supraspinatus, pull the humeral head into the glenoid (Basmajian, 1978). This brings the resultant force into the concavity of the articulation, a stable situation (Fig. 31.25b).

Forces acting on the shoulder have not been analysed in detail. Data are available on shoulder strength (Hunsicker, 1955; Murray *et al.*, 1985), but until recently the only force analysis referred to the unloaded limb, with muscle forces opposing limb weight (Poppen and Walker, 1978). Thus prostheses have been 'designed' without knowing what their fixation must withstand, so loosening failures are not surprising. A simplified analysis by Amis (1990) has shown that glenohumeral forces can exceed 3 BW. If the abducted arm supports a load of 80 N at the hand (0.12 BW) the adduction moment created about the humeral head must be resisted by the shoulder abductor muscles (Fig. 31.26), principally the deltoid, which is assumed to act alone. This simplifying assumption will give the lowest joint force, neglecting other cooperating or antagonistic actions. The deltoid moment must be equal and opposite to the moments caused by the external load plus limb weight. Thus F deltoid $\times$ 0.03 m = 0.12 BW $\times$ 0.65 m +

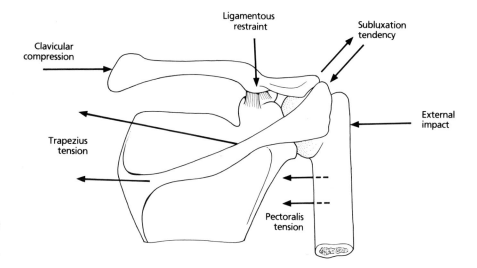

Fig. 31.24 Acromioclavicular joint disruption occurs as a result of forces acting medially on the scapula, when the clavicle subluxes up the sloping endface of the acromion, rupturing the ligaments.

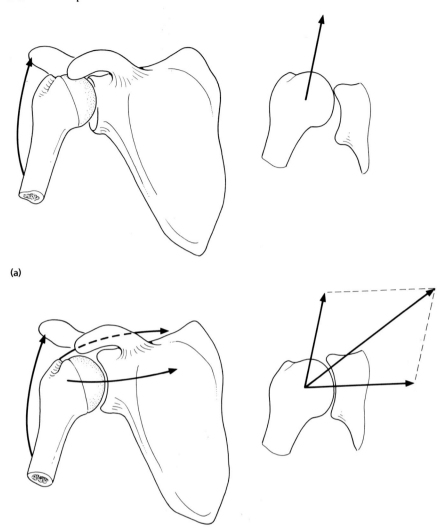

(a)

(b)

Fig. 31.25 (a) Abduction of the shoulder by the deltoid alone will cause superior subluxation of the humerus. (b) The muscles of the rotator cuff pull the head of humerus medially, which swings the resultant force round into the concavity of the glenoid, a stable situation.

0.09 BW × 0.3 m, so F deltoid = 3.5 BW. The joint reaction force closes the force vector triangle, as in Fig. 31.26, and equals 3.45 BW. Since the force vectors are drawn to scale, this shows clearly how muscle forces are the prime cause of joint force.

Shoulder joint prostheses

Various types of shoulder joint replacement have been developed, falling into three types (Fig. 31.27): (i) humeral hemi-arthroplasty; (ii) total replacements

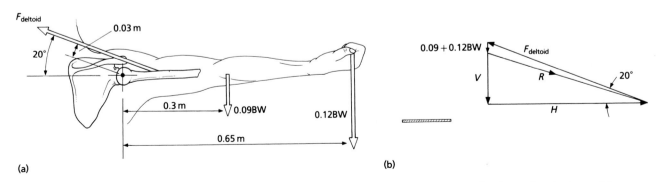

(a)

(b)

Fig. 31.26 Simplified analysis of abduction of the shoulder. The force vector triangle, drawn to scale, shows that the internal forces are much greater than the external load.

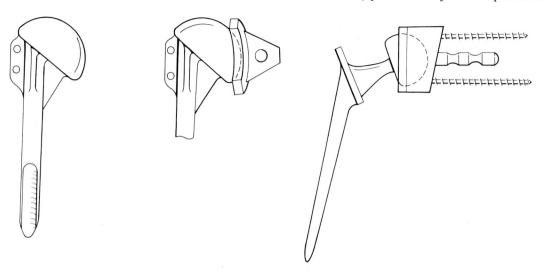

Fig. 31.27 The three main types of shoulder prosthesis: humeral hemi-arthroplasty, surface replacement of the glenoid, captive assembly.

with shallow glenoid geometry; and (iii) total replacements with 'captive' articulations. The main factors deciding which type to use are rotator cuff and glenoid integrity (Bateman and Fornasier, 1978). The lack of bone volume in the scapula is the main problem for shoulder replacement, limiting the possibilities for designing or making a secure fixation for the glenoid component. Thus humeral hemi-arthroplasty is a popular choice, but this requires preservation of the concave glenoid for articulation and a functioning rotator cuff for stability. If the glenoid has been destroyed it must also be replaced, and a shallow onlay component may be chosen as long as the rotator cuff is still functional (Neer *et al.*, 1982). In this case the localized fixation is adequate because the joint is stabilized by the cuff; the humeral head should always be pulled into the shallow glenoid concavity, loading it in compression. Deficiency of the cuff will allow subluxation but without imposing large shearing forces on the glenoid fixation. Subluxation will inevitably occur if the rotator cuff is not restorable, so a deep socket or 'captive' snap-fit assembly is then required for stability. The lack of compressive action from the cuff means that the remaining muscle forces will tend to shear the joint to a greater extent than normal, and the captive geometry causes the shear forces to be transmitted to the prosthesis fixation. This will tend to wobble the glenoid component loose. Various designs have attempted to overcome this by putting fixation stems or screws into the spine or thick lateral border of the scapula (Post *et al.*, 1979), but glenoid component fixation is still a problem. The magnitude of the forces which the fixation must withstand was emphasized by Post (1988), who had a 42% failure

rate in the necks of humeral components with a yield strength of 3.6 kN (5 BW). He found that secure glenoid fixation depended on an intact subchondral bone plate.

THE ELBOW

Motion

Elbow flexion–extension motion takes place around a single fixed axis which passes through the centre of the circular sagittal sections of capitellum and trochlea. The congruence of the joint surfaces means that the relative motion between the humerus and forearm bones is sliding around the fixed axis. This axis is inclined approximately 6° from perpendicular to the humeral shaft, in the coronal plane, sloping superiorly and laterally, so that it bisects the carrying angle in full extension. The carrying angle is approximately 12° in adults, slightly larger in females than males (Amis and Miller, 1982). This geometry causes the forearm to overlay the arm in full flexion, as the carrying angle varies sinusoidally towards zero (Amis *et al.*, 1977). Rotation of the forearm takes place about an axis which passes through the centre of the wrist, so that the hand remains in one place as it is pronated or supinated. Examination of the skeleton suggests that the axis of rotation passes between the centres of the heads of radius and ulna, at elbow and wrist respectively. If this axis were fixed, the hand would rotate about the little finger (approximately in line with the distal ulna) and shift laterally in supination. This does not occur because pronation is accompanied by ulnar abduction at the elbow, a function of anconeus, and supination by adduction. This motion, of 9°, is allowed by collateral ligament laxity (Amis *et al.*, 1977), which is not demonstrable clinically but has been proved by double-exposure radiography (Ray *et al.*, 1951).

Elbow forces

Forces acting on the elbow normally arise from actions of the hand, such as lifting or pulling, and many of the extrinsic hand muscles and wrist stabilizing muscles cross the elbow joint. Thus an elbow force analysis must take account of the flexor digitorum superficialis which acts when grasping an object, then the flexors and extensors carpi radialis and ulnaris which ensure wrist stability by antagonistic contractions. In flexion, biceps, brachialis, brachioradialis and pronator teres cooperate (Basmajian, 1978), with biceps and pronator teres giving antagonistic control of rotation. Allowance for all these muscle actions, sometimes also with triceps antagonism to stabilize the elbow, leads to predictions of forces acting on the end of the distal humerus in extended postures, swinging round to act on the anterior aspect in flexion (Amis *et al.*, 1980) (Fig. 31.28). It can be seen in Fig. 31.28 that the forces are largest in extended postures and reduce with flexion. This is due to the muscles being close to the flexion axis as they lay against the joint near extension—the flexors lift away from the elbow as it is flexed, so act at less of a mechanical disadvantage, while their isometric tension capability will have dropped due to shortening (Elftman, 1966). Similar forces are predicted on radius and ulna during flexion, despite the humeroradial joint being smaller than the humeroulnar.

Analysis of the muscles, though, shows that more act across the joint line from the common extensor origin than from the flexor origin. Thus the elbow normally acts as a bicondylar joint during flexion actions, an equilibrium which is destroyed by radial head excision (Fig. 31.29). This is a controversial procedure, with some studies of post-trauma cases finding significant problems due to wrist and/or medial collateral elbow ligament pain. The procedure appears more innocuous in rheumatoid patients, because of their lower demands. Biomechanically, the force acting on the coronoid is approximately doubled, while a medial ligament tension must resist the valgus action of the muscles inserting into the headless radius. Wrist pain arises from the proximal pull of biceps, brachioradialis and pronator teres, which stretch the interosseous membrane and triangular fibrocartilage as the radius migrates proximally.

In extension activity, the triceps can exert a tension of 2 kN on the olecranon, being the strongest muscle acting on the elbow. It follows that repairs of olecranon fractures are easily disrupted by this tensile action, and that the olecranon should be excavated as little as possible when implanting a joint replacement (Amis *et al.*, 1979).

Elbow-joint prostheses

Elbow-joint replacements were originally of the constrained hinge type, which required excision of the distal humerus and used intramedullary fixation (Souter, 1973). This, unfortunately, predisposed them to loosen-

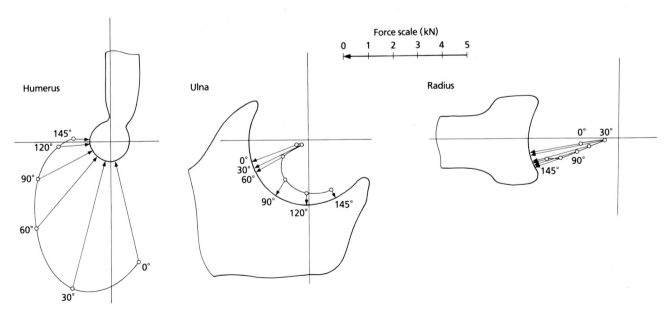

Fig. 31.28 Elbow forces during maximal isometric flexion effort. Radial and ulnar loads are similar and diminish with flexion. The resultant force swings round onto the front of the humerus with flexion.

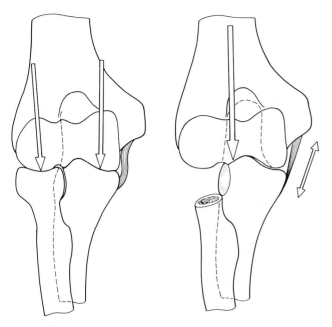

Fig. 31.29 Radial head excision prevents bicondylar load sharing, increasing the coronoid force and requiring ligament tension to prevent valgus deformity.

for the distal humerus have had their fixation reliability improved by adding stems which transmit loads to the adjacent cortical bone (Kudo and Iwano, 1990). Thus, if loosening is the sole criterion, reliability can be obtained by combining a minimally constrained articulation with extensive fixation means (Ewald and Jacobs, 1984).

Elbow replacements incorporating a radial head have been developed (Amis and Miller, 1984; Ewald and Jacobs, 1984), but problems with ensuring correct balance across the articulation have not been matched by significantly better results. Thus the case for radial head replacement in total elbow arthroplasty has not been proven clinically, despite the biomechanical case for their use.

ing. If the hands are pressed together with the elbows flexed 90°, the inward-rotation torque in the humerus is transmitted across the natural elbow by a force couple: tension in the medial collateral ligament and compression of the radial head (Fig. 31.30). The width of the joint provides a moment arm of approximately 55 mm between the forces. If the torque must be resisted by intramedullary fixation alone, with a diameter of only 8 mm, the shear forces between cement and bone are extremely high. Morrey and Bryan (1982) reported that humeral component loosening was reduced by 'semi-constrained' prostheses. These were still hinge-type implants with stem fixation, but they preserved the collateral attachments to the epicondyles and incorporated a small range of lateral motion. This allowed the soft tissues to absorb the torsion loads. These implants still required extensive bone excavation so, following experience at the knee, surface replacements were devised (Kudo *et al.*, 1980; Tuke *et al.*, 1981; Amis and Miller, 1984). These preserve bone stock and utilize soft-tissue stabilization, but they can dislocate if the tissues are not reconstituted meticulously at operation. Knowledge of the forces acting allows the prosthetic articulation to be designed so that it will sublux rather than transmit a damaging force to the bone fixation (Amis and Miller, 1984); there is a general trend for implants with the fewest constraints to be the most successful. As with the knee, however, the most conservative onlay components

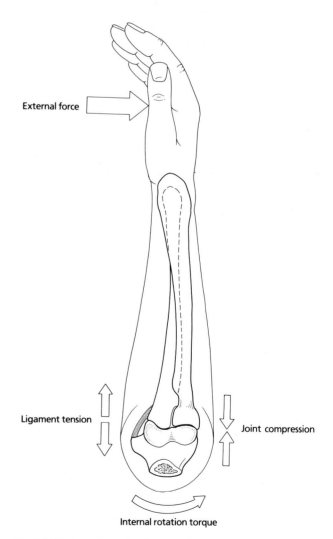

Fig. 31.30 Inward rotation is resisted by a force couple of soft-tissue tension and articular compression, the width of the joint lending stability.

THE WRIST

Wrist motion and stability

The hand has a large range of motion at the wrist, with some 160° of flexion−extension and 50° radial−ulnar deviation. This allows the hand to occupy any position within a wide cone of space, which is accomplished by circumduction motions and not rotation at the wrist (Kapandji, 1970). The radiocarpal articulation has a much smaller radius of curvature in the sagittal than in the coronal plane, so the barrel shape of the proximal face of the carpus is inherently stable in the curved groove of the distal radius in only one position of rotation. Despite the wide range of motion in the normal wrist, Brumfield and Champoux (1984) found that a variety of daily activities were accomplished with only 45° range of flexion−extension motion. This may explain why arthritic patients are usually satisfied after wrist fusion. The carpus is usually divided into proximal and distal rows of bones as functional units for analysis, and different studies have reported various ranges of motion for these. Although the bones in each of the two rows are bound together by a comprehensive system of inter-carpal ligaments that prevent most interosseous move-ment, Taleisnik (1985) has shown that secondary movements occur within the rows, such as scaphoid flexion accompanying radial deviation. Despite this com-plexity, the wrist as a whole behaves in a simple manner kinematically; Youm *et al.* (1978) found that both flexion−extension and radial−ulnar deviation motions

were centred within the proximal part of the capitate (Fig. 31.31). This means that normal movement of the hand in relation to the forearm can be created by a simple prosthetic articulation—a sphere centred at this point. This is the basis of the Meuli (1984) implant, also seen in Fig. 31.31.

Even a casual examination of the wrist suggests that this assembly of carpal bones is inherently unstable and liable to zig-zag collapse. The hand is stabilized on the forearm by antagonistic actions of all the extrinsic muscles during powerful gripping actions (Long *et al.*, 1970; Basmajian, 1978), like the guylines around a marquee. Innervation is strongest in the direction in which force must be applied (Dempster and Finerty, 1947). Actions such as those accompanying prehensile grasping, when the wrist is dorsiflexed in radial deviation by the extensors carpi radialis as a pen is grasped, for example, are virtually automatic. The extrinsic tendons, however, bridge the intercarpal and radiocarpal joints, leaving the buckling tendency undiminished. Stability thus depends on the system of intercarpal ligaments which control bones within the rows, precise packing together of the rows, and on radiocarpal and ulnocarpal ligaments which control the position of the carpus during movements. Sennwald (1987) and Taleisnik (1985) have described V-shaped ligament formations based on the radius and ulna, which converge distally towards the centre of the carpus. By tethering this zone, the hand is forced to rotate about the proximal capitate axis found by Youm *et al.* (1978), so that in radial deviation the proximal carpal row slides ulnarly, yet is

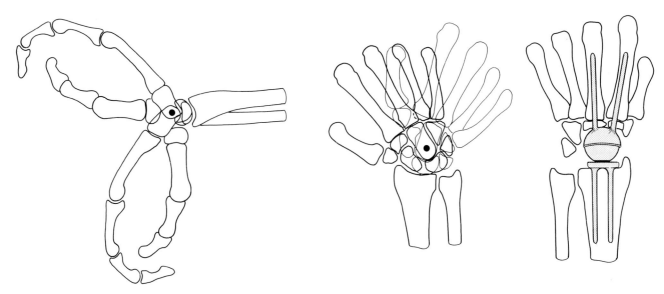

Fig. 31.31 The hand rotates about a point in the proximal capitate, which can be reproduced by a simple spherical prosthesis geometry. The Meuli (1984) prosthesis is shown.

prevented from sliding off of the sloping endface of the radius by the radiolunate and radioscaphocapitate ligaments that form one arm of the V-formation.

Wrist forces

Force transmission through the wrist depends on the hand posture and mode of loading, but it seems likely that force is channelled largely through the capitate–scaphoid–lunate assembly. Since the hand is often positioned so that the thenar region is prominent during falls onto the outstretched hand, it is not surprising that the scaphoid or distal radius are frequently damaged. The muscles can impose forces greater than body weight across the wrist in normal strenuous activity. If the hand supports a load of 200 N, as shown in Fig. 31.32, the wrist flexors must impose an equal and opposite flexion moment to maintain equilibrium. Thus F_{wf} (representing a single notional 'mean wrist flexor' force) $\times 17 \, mm = 200 \, N \times 75 \, mm$, giving $F_{wf} = 882 \, N$.

Wrist-joint prostheses

Wrist-joint replacements have been developed for patients who demand mobility and for whom a fusion would be unsatisfactory. Meuli (1984) found that his spherical design (Fig. 31.31) originally misplaced the centre of the articulation, leading to abnormal hand deviations, so the fixation stems had to be offset. Volz (1984) developed a semi-constrained implant with separate articulations

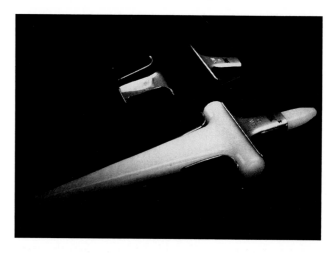

Fig. 31.33 Silastic wrist prosthesis: the silicone rubber stems are not cemented, but slide within the titanium grommets that protect the rubber from abrasion on the edges of the bones.

for flexion–extension and radial–ulnar deviation and no rotational freedom. This, too, required modification of the stem positions in relation to the articulation in order to obtain consistently good hand positions. Volz noted, in particular, that rheumatoid patients often suffered an inhibition of the wrist extensor muscles, so he moved the axis of flexion–extension towards the palm. The enhanced extensor moment arm prevented flexion deformity. Both Meuli and Volz felt that post-operative balancing of the tendons crossing the wrist was the most difficult aspect of total wrist arthroplasty. Use of a flexible silicone rubber implant was reviewed by Swanson *et al.* (1984). As with the Meuli and Volz implants, it was located by intramedullary stems into the radius and third metacarpal. The one-piece moulding was thin in an anterior–posterior direction, to allow hinge bending, but wide, to limit sideways deviation (Fig. 31.33). It produced a mean flexion–extension range of 60°, which Brumfield and Champoux (1984) had shown to be adequate for daily activities. Metallic bone liners protected the rubber against cutting or abrasion on sharp edges, as implant failures had occurred for this reason. However, the reliability and acceptability of arthrodesis have meant that there has been little demand for wrist replacement.

THE FINGERS

Joint motion and stability

When examined in the sagittal plane, both the metacarpophalangeal and interphalangeal joints are found to have circular sections for the heads of the proximal

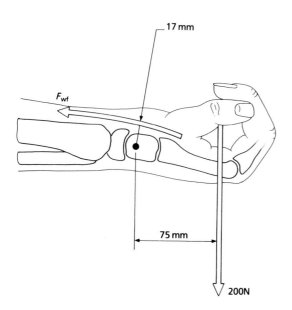

Fig. 31.32 Simplified analysis of wrist flexion, showing that the flexor tendons can impose forces in excess of body weight across the carpus.

bones. This means that all of the finger joints rotate about fixed axes of flexion, with the concave bases of the distal bones sliding, rather than rolling, during movement. Coronal sections also reveal circular contours for the metacarpal heads, which are effectively spherical distally. This geometry obviously allows the proximal phalanx to rotate in flexion−extension, abduction−adduction and pronation−supination. These movements are controlled by the surrounding soft tissues, particularly the collateral structures which fan out distally and in a palmar direction from tubercles on the metacarpal heads. Because the ligaments of the metacarpophalangeal joint originate eccentrically from the flexion axis, they slacken in extension, allowing abduction−adduction, but tighten progressively with flexion to limit this freedom. Rotational effects occur frequently, such as when the side of the index finger tip is loaded in the 'key pinch' posture. This is resisted by the palmar parts of the collateral ligaments, which effectively spiral around the joint to the palmar region of the base of the proximal phalanx and adjacent volar plate, and are thus adapted to resist torsion loads across the joint. Further stability is gained in flexion from a bicondylar shape on the palmar aspect of the more radial metacarpal heads (Hagert, 1981).

The interphalangeal joints are effectively bicondylar articulations—the distal aspects of the proximal phalanges bearing a resemblance to the distal aspect of the femur—and have collateral ligaments originating around the flexion axis. They are thus stable against varus−valgus angulation at all positions of flexion. As with the wrist, the column of bones which make up a finger is intrinsically unstable, and depends on coordinated actions from soft-tissue stabilizers—principally the tendons—to maintain normal controlled postures (Idler, 1985). The sheer bulk of the extrinsic flexor muscles and tendons suggests that the majority of the strength of pinching or gripping actions comes from them, but the interlinking actions of apparently minor intrinsic structures are necessary to control and coordinate joint positions. This is demonstrated by the frequency of boutonnière and swan-neck deformities arising from rheumatoid disease, when synovitic swelling alters the relationships of the intrinsic muscles and lateral bands of the extensor apparatus to the axes of flexion of the joints.

Finger-joint and soft-tissue forces

Large forces can be imposed on the finger joints during daily activities, which may be divided into gripping and pinching actions. A simple two-dimensional analysis of a finger-tip pinching action (Fig. 31.34) shows that the moment arm of the line of action of the applied force increases proximally. This means that a greater flexion moment must be applied by the flexor tendons about the proximal joints to maintain equilibrium. Thus the distal interphalangeal joint is stabilized by the flexor digitorum profundus, while the proximal joint has the added superficialis action. The metacarpophalangeal joint obtains equilibrium because the flexor tendons have larger moment arms about its axis, plus the intrinsic muscle contribution. Tip pinch can include a range of postures, as the interphalangeal joints flex and the metacarpophalangeal joint extends, with a typical maximum force of 70 N in normal adults (Weightman and Amis, 1982; An *et al.*, 1985). In the posture shown in Fig. 31.34, this applies an extension moment of 70 N × 80 mm, or 5.6 Nm to the metacarpophalangeal joint. The flexor tendons have moment arms of approximately 17 mm in the posture shown, so they must have a combined tension of 330 N to oppose the 5.6 Nm caused by the external force. With the finger joints in the flexed posture shown, the flexor tendons follow a curving path into the palm of the hand. This gives the tendon tension the axial and shear components shown, which tend to compress the joint and sublux the phalanx volarly, respectively. A similar situation applies at the interphalangeal joints. Because the concavity at the base of the proximal phalanx is shallow, the articulation of the metacarpophalangeal joint cannot resist the subluxation force, so the slanting

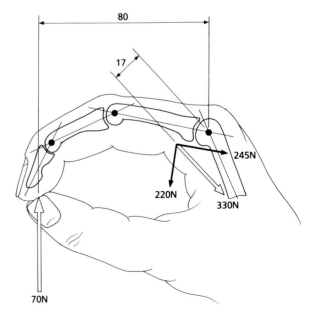

Fig. 31.34 Analysis of finger tip pinch action: the flexor tendons compress the phalanx axially and also apply a palmar shear force, which is resisted by the slanting orientation of the ligament fibres.

fibres of the collateral ligaments must do this, particularly those which insert into the volar plate and hence support the flexor tendon A1 'pulley' (Jones and Amis, 1988) at this joint. In rheumatoid disease, erosion of the base of the phalanx slackens the ligaments, so they cannot then prevent volar subluxation of the metacarpophalangeal joints (Smith *et al.*, 1964).

The flexor tendons pull the phalanges in a volar direction whenever they act on a flexed joint — this is the basis of gripping. The volar action is transmitted to the bones by tension in the 'pulleys' of the fibrous flexor tendon sheath (Fig. 31.35). The tendons would otherwise 'bowstring' towards a straight line, which can occur if the pulleys are damaged by trauma or surgical incisions. Because the finger flexor muscles have limited active excursion, such damage may mean loss of finger flexion. Doyle and Blyth (1975) found that the A2 and A4 pulleys, positioned at the midpoint of the proximal and middle phalanges, were the most important in preventing loss of motion. The annular pulley fibres insert into the margins of the phalanges, giving a structure adapted to

withstand the volar load shown in Fig. 31.35. With a tip pinch tendon tension of 330 N, the pulley shown must support a load of 420 N, so any reconstructive procedure must be strong.

If a force of 70 N is applied to the radial side of the index finger tip as shown in Fig. 31.36, a torque of 2.8 Nm will act on the proximal phalanx and metacarpophalangeal joint. Since the soft tissues here act at a radius of approximately 9 mm from the axis of rotation, a ligament tension of 311 N (nearly 0.5 BW) can be caused. The bicondylar width of the interphalanged joints allows the load to be resisted by radial collateral ligament tension and ulnar joint facet compression (Fig. 31.36).

Finger-joint prostheses

The joint loads have caused failures of finger-joint replacements — the stems of the metallic hinges of Flatt and Ellison (1972) cutting out sideways through the bone cortices, or the silicone rubber implants of Swanson

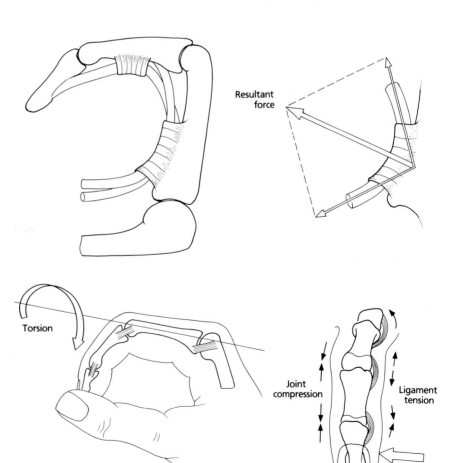

Fig. 31.35 The pulleys transmit tendon forces to the phalanges as the tendons change direction.

Fig. 31.36 Key pinch loading causes large torsion effects on the proximal phalanx and metacarpophalangeal joint. The radial collateral structures of all the joints are tensed, while the ulnar condyles of the interphalangeal joints are compressed.

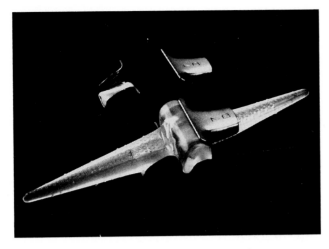

Fig. 31.37 Silastic metacarpophalangeal joint replacement.

(1973) tending to break after bony attrition (Dryer *et al.*, 1984). The silicone rubber implants (Fig. 31.37) have become popular largely because of their simple insertion procedure, but do not act in the same way as a normal joint. The rubber is soft, so the implants deform significantly under physiological loads. This allows forces to transfer to the surrounding soft tissues. The role of the implant is largely to act as a template during the reformation of a fibrous capsule, and such implants are aimed predominantly at rheumatoid patients with low functional demands. Reports that replaced finger joints lose their range of motion with time (Dryer *et al.*, 1984) have been linked to tissue reactions to rubber wear particles. It seems likely, therefore, that a new generation of finger-joint replacements will soon appear, with minimally constrained joint surfaces so that loosening forces should not be transmitted.

CONCLUSIONS

In conclusion, some guiding principles which can be discerned are as follows:
1 The majority of the force acting on a joint arises from the muscles and tendons which cross the joint, and not from the load supported, such as the weight of the body.
2 Because the muscles cross the joints, joints are virtually always compressed during activity, even when carrying a weight in the hand, for example.
3 The degree of constraint between the components of a joint replacement controls the nature of forces which can be transmitted by it. Since excess force transmission leads to loosening, the minimum constraint possible, compatible with the state of the soft-tissue stabilizers, should be chosen.
4 The joints of the upper limb may be 'non-weight-

bearing', but their smaller bones and implant fixations mean that they will be as highly stressed as in the lower limb.

ACKNOWLEDGEMENTS

The author thanks the personnel of the Biomet, Corin, Dow Corning, Howmedica and Zimmer companies for lending the implants illustrated.

REFERENCES

Amis A.A. (1990) Biomechanics: upper limb. Part 1. Upper limb function, shoulder and elbow. *Curr. Orthop.* **4**, 21–26.

Amis A.A. and Miller J.H. (1982) The elbow. Measurement of joint movement. *Clin. Rheum. Dis.* **8**, 571–593.

Amis A.A. and Miller J.H (1984) Design, development and clinical trial of a modular elbow replacement incorporating cement-free fixation. *Engineering and Clinical Aspects of Endoprosthetic Fixation*, Bury St. Edmunds, Mechanical Engineering Press, pp. 121–126.

Amis A.A., Dowson D., Wright V., Miller J.H. and Unsworth A. (1977) An examination of the elbow articulation with particular reference to the variation of the carrying angle. *Eng. Med.* **6**, 76–80.

Amis A.A., Dowson D., Wright V. and Miller J.H. (1979) The derivation of elbow joint forces and their relation to prosthesis design. *J. Med. Eng. Technol.* **3**, 229–234.

Amis A.A., Dowson D. and Wright V. (1980) Elbow joint force predictions for some strenuous isometric actions. *J. Biomech.* **13**, 765–775.

Amis A.A., Bromage J.D. and Larvin M. (1987) Fatigue fracture of a femoral sliding compression screw-plate device after bone union. *Biomaterials* **8**, 153–157.

An K.N., Chao E.Y., Cooney W.P. and Linscheid R.L. (1985) Forces in the normal and abnormal hand. *J. Orthop. Res.* **3**, 202.

Basmajian J.V. (1978) *Muscles Alive — Their Functions Revealed by Electromyography*, 4th edn. Baltimore, Williams & Wilkins.

Bateman J.E. and Fornasier V.L. (1978) *The Shoulder and Neck*, 2nd edn. Philadelphia, W.B. Saunders.

Bert J.M. (1990) Dislocation/subluxation of meniscal bearing elements after New Jersey low contact stress total knee arthroplasty. *Clin. Orthop.* **254**, 211–215.

Berme N. and Paul J.P. (1979) Force actions transmitted by implants. *J. Biomed. Eng.* **1**, 268–272.

Brown T.R.M., Nicol A.C. and Paul J.P. (1984) Comparison of loads transmitted by Charnley and CAD Müller total hip arthroplasties. *Engineering and Clinical Aspects of Endoprosthetic Fixation.* Bury St. Edmunds, Mechanical Engineering Press, pp. 63–68.

Brumfield R.H. and Champoux J.A. (1984) A biomechanical study of normal functional wrist motion. *Clin. Orthop.* **187**, 23–25.

Burstein A.H., Reilly D.T. and Martens M. (1976) Ageing of bone tissue: mechanical properties. *J. Bone Joint Surg.* **58A**, 82–86.

Charnley J. (1967) Total prosthetic replacement of the hip. *Physiotherapy* **53**, 407–409.

Charnley J. (1971) Stainless steel for femoral hip prostheses in combination with a high density polythene socket. *J. Bone Joint Surg.* **53B**, 343.

Charnley J. (1973) Biomechanical considerations in total hip prosthetic design. *The Hip.* St. Louis, C.V. Mosby.

Charnley J. and Kettlewell J. (1965) The elimination of slip between prosthesis and femur. *J. Bone Joint Surg.* **47B**, 56−60.

Collis J.M.F. and Jayson M.I.V. (1972) Measurement of pedal pressures − an illustration of a method. *Ann. Rheum. Dis.* **31**, 215−217.

Crock H.V. (1980) An atlas of the arterial supply of the head and neck of the femur in man. *Clin. Orthop.* **152**, 17−27.

Demottaz J.D., Mazur J.M., Thomas W.H., Sledge C.B. and Simon S.R. (1979) Clinical study of total ankle replacement with gait analysis. *J. Bone Joint Surg.* **61A**, 976−988.

Dempster W.T. and Finerty J.C. (1947) Relative activity of wrist moving muscles in static support of the wrist joint: An electromyographic study. *Am. J. Physiol.* **150**, 596−606.

Denham R.A. and Bishop R.E.D. (1978) Mechanics of the knee and problems in reconstructive surgery. *J. Bone Joint Surg.* **60B**, 345−352.

Dini A.A. and Bassett F.H. (1980) Evaluation of the early result of Smith total ankle replacement. *Clin. Orthop.* **146**, 228−230.

Doyle J.R. and Blythe W. (1975) The finger flexor tendon sheath and pulleys: anatomy and reconstruction. *AAOS Symposium on Tendon Surgery in the Hand.* St. Louis, C.V. Mosby, pp. 81−87.

Dryer F.R., Blair W.F., Shurr D.G. and Buckwalter J.A. (1984) Proximal interphalangeal joint anthroplasty. *Clin. Orthop.* **185**, 187−194.

Elftman H. (1966) Biomechanics of muscle. *J. Bone Joint Surg.* **48A**, 363−377.

Ellis M.I. and Stowe J. (1982) The hip. Measurement of joint movement. *Clin. Rheum. Dis.* **8**, 655−675.

Ewald F.C. and Jacobs M.A. (1984) Total elbow arthroplasty. *Clin. Orthop.* **182**, 137−142.

Flatt A.E. and Ellison M.R. (1972) Restoration of rheumatoid finger joint function. III. A follow-up note after fourteen years of experience with a metallic hinge prosthesis. *J. Bone Joint Surg.* **54A**, 1317−1322.

Fowler J.L., Gie G.A., Lee A.J.C. and Ling R.S.M. (1988) Experience with the Exeter total hip replacement since 1970. *Orthop. Clin. N. Am.* **19**, 477−489.

Glasgow M., Jackson A. and Jamieson A.M. (1980) Instability of the ankle after injury to the lateral ligament. *J. Bone Joint Surg.* **62B**, 196−200.

Goldie I.F., Bunketorp O., Gunterberg B., Hansson T. and Myrhage R. (1979) Resurfacing arthroplasty of the hip − biomechanical, morphological, and clinical aspects based on the results of a preliminary clinical study. *Arch. Orthop. Traumat. Surg.* **95**, 149−157.

Goodfellow J. and O'Connor J. (1978) The mechanics of the knee and prosthesis design. *J. Bone Joint Surg.* **60B**, 358−369.

Hagert C.G. (1981) Anatomical aspects on the design of metacarpophalangeal implants. *Reconstr. Surg. Traumatol.* **18**, 92−110.

Harrington I.J. (1974) The effect of congenital and pathological conditions on the load action transmitted at the knee joint. In *Total Knee Replacement*, London, Institute of Mechanical Engineering Press, pp. 1−7.

Harris W.H. (1984) Advances in total hip arthroplasty − the metal-backed acetabular component. *Clin. Orthop.* **183**, 4−11.

Heckman J.D. (1984) Fractures and dislocations of the foot. In Rockwood C.A. and Green D.P. (eds) *Fractures in Adults*, 2nd edn. Philadelphia, J.B. Lippincott, pp. 1703−1832.

Hunsicker P. (1955) Arm strength at selected degrees of elbow flexion. *W.A.D.C. Tech. Report* 54−548. Wright-Patterson AFB, Ohio.

Idler R.S. (1985) Anatomy and biomechanics of the digital flexor tendons. *Hand Clin.* **1**, 3−11.

Inglis A.E. (ed.) (1982) *American Academy of Orthopaedic Surgeons Symposium on Total Joint Replacement in the Upper Extremity.* St. Louis, C.V. Mosby.

Insall J.N., Lachiewicz P.F. and Burstein A.H. (1982) The posterior stabilised condylar prosthesis: a modification of the total condylar design. Two to four year clinical experience. *J. Bone Joint Surg.* **64A**, 1317−1323.

Insall J.N., Binazzi R, Soudry M. and Mestriner L.A. (1985) Total knee arthroplasty. *Clin. Orthop.* **192**, 13−22.

Jacob H.A.C., Huggler A.H., Dietschi C. and Schreiber A. (1976) Mechanical function of subchondral bone as experimentally determined on the acetabulum of the human pelvis. *J. Biomech.* **9**, 625−627.

Jolley M.N., Salvati E.A. and Brown G.C. (1982) Early results and complications of surface replacement of the hip. *J. Bone Joint Surg.* **64A**, 366−377.

Jones M.M. and Amis A.A. (1988) The fibrous flexor sheaths of the fingers. *J. Anat.* **156**, 185−196.

Judet J. and Judet R. (1950) The use of an artificial femoral head for arthroplasty of the hip joint. *J. Bone Joint Surg.* **32B**, 166−173.

Kapandji I.A. (1970) *The Physiology of the Joints.* Vol. 1. *Upper limb.* Edinburgh, Churchill Livingstone.

Kempson G.E., Freeman M.A.R. and Tuke M.A. (1975) Engineering considerations in the design of an ankle joint. *J. Biomech. Eng.* **16**, 166−171.

Kudo H. and Iwano K. (1990) Total elbow arthroplasty with a non-constrained surface replacement prosthesis in patients who have rheumatoid arthritis − a long-term follow-up study. *J. Bone Joint Surg.* **72A**, 355−362.

Kudo H., Iwano K. and Watanabe S. (1980) Total replacement of the rheumatoid elbow with a hingeless prosthesis. *J. Bone Joint Surg.* **62A**, 277−285.

Kwong K.S.C. (1990) The biomechanical role of the collar of the femoral component of a hip replacement. *J. Bone Joint Surg.* **72B**, 664−665.

Lambert K.L. (1971) The weight-bearing function of the fibula: a strain gauge study. *J. Bone Joint Surg.* **53A**, 507−513.

Lance E.M., Paval A., Fries I., Larsen I. and Patterson R.L. (1979) Arthrodesis of the ankle joint − a follow up study. *Clin. Orthop.* **142**, 146−158.

Levens A.S., Inman V.T. and Blosser J.A. (1948) Transverse rotation of the segments of the lower extremity in locomotion. *J. Bone Joint Surg.* **30A**, 859−872.

Lewis J.L., Askew M.J. and Jaycox D.P. (1982) A comparative evaluation of tibial component designs of total knee prostheses. *J. Bone Joint Surg.* **64A**, 129−135.

Long C., Conrad P.W., Hall E.A. and Furler S.L. (1970) Intrinsic−extrinsic muscle control of the hand in power grip and precision handling. An electromygraphic study. *J. Bone Joint Surg.* **52A**, 853−867.

Lord G.A., Hardy J.R. and Kummer F.J. (1979) An uncemented total hip replacement − experimental study and review of 300

Madreporique arthroplasties. *Clin. Orthop.* **141**, 2−16.

Mann R.A. (1980) Surgical implications of biomechanics of the foot and ankle. *Clin. Orthop.* **146**, 111−118.

Mann R.A. and Coughlin M.J. (1981) Hallux valgus—etiology, anatomy, treatment and surgical considerations. *Clin. Orthop.* **157**, 31−41.

Maquet P.G.J. (1984) *Biomechanics of the knee—with application to the pathogenesis and the surgical treatment of osteoarthritis*, 2nd edn. Berlin, Springer-Verlag.

Maquet P.G.J. (1985) *Biomechanics of the hip as applied to osteoarthritis and related conditions*. Berlin, Springer-Verlag.

Mazur J.M., Schawartz E. and Simon S.R. (1979) Ankle arthrodesis: long term follow-up with gait analysis. *J. Bone Joint Surg.* **61A**, 964−975.

McKee G.K. and Watson-Farrar J. (1966) Replacement of arthritic hips by the McKee−Farrar prosthesis. *J. Bone Joint Surg.* **48B**, 245−259.

Meuli H.C. (1984) Meuli total wrist arthroplasty. *Clin. Orthop.* **187**, 107−111.

Moore A.T. (1952) Metal hip joint: new self-locking vitallium prosthesis. *South. Med. J.* **45**, 1015−1019.

Morrey B.F. and Bryan R.S. (1982) Complications of total elbow arthroplasty. *Clin. Orthop.* **170**, 204−212.

Morrison J.B. (1968) Bioengineering analysis of force actions transmitted by the knee joint. *Bio-Med. Eng.* **3**, 164−170.

Morrison J.B. (1969) Function of the knee joint in various activities. *Bio-Med. Eng.* **4**, 573−580.

Mulroy R.D. and Harris W.H. (1990) The effect of improved cementing techniques on component loosening in total hip replacement—an 11 year radiographic review. *J. Bone Joint Surg.* **72B**, 757−760.

Murray M.P., Drought A.B. and Kory R.C. (1964) Walking patterns in normal men. *J. Bone Joint Surg.* **46A**, 335−360.

Murray M.P., Gore D.R., Gardner G.M. and Mollinger L.A. (1985) Shoulder motion and muscle strength of normal men and women in two age groups. *Clin. Orthop.* **192**, 268−273.

Neer C.S., Watson K.C. and Stanton F.J. (1982) Recent experience in total shoulder replacement. *J. Bone Joint Surg.* **64A**, 319−337.

Newton St. E. (1979) An artificial ankle joint. *Clin. Orthop.* **142**, 141−145.

Nordin M. and Frankel V.H. (eds) (1989) *Basic Biomechanics of the Musculoskeletal System*, 2nd edn. Philadelphia, Lea & Febiger.

Nunn D., Freeman M.A.R., Tanner K.E. and Bonfield W. (1989) Torsional stability of the femoral component of hip arthroplasty. *J. Bone Joint Surg.* **71B**, 452−455.

Oh I., Sander T.W. and Treharne R.W. (1985) Total hip acetabular cup flange design and its effect on cement fixation. *Clin. Orthop.* **195**, 304−309.

Paul J.P. (1967) Forces transmitted by joints in the human body. *Proc. Inst. Mech. Eng.* **181**, 8−15.

Poppen N.K. and Walker P.S. (1978) Forces at the glenohumeral joint in abduction. *Clin. Orthop.* **135**, 165−170.

Post M. (1988) *The Shoulder—Surgical and Nonsurgical Management*, 2nd edn. Philadelphia, Lea & Febiger.

Post M., Jablon M., Miller H. and Singh M. (1979) Constrained total shoulder joint replacement: a critical review. *Clin. Orthop.* **144**, 135−150.

Proctor P. and Paul J.P. (1982) Ankle joint biomechanics. *J. Biomech.* **15**, 627−634.

Rasmussen O. and Torborg-Jensen I. (1982) Mobility of the ankle joint. *Acta Orthop. Scand.* **53**, 155−160.

Ray R.D., Johnson R.J. and Jameson R.M. (1951) Rotation of the forearm: an experimental study of pronation and supination. *J. Bone Joint Surg.* **33A**, 993−996.

Ring P.A. (1968) Complete replacement arthroplasty of the hip by the Ring prosthesis. *J. Bone Joint Surg.* **50B**, 720−731.

Ritter M.A., Keating E.M., Faris P.M. and Brugo G. (1990) Metal-backed acetabular cups in total hip arthroplasty. *J. Bone Joint Surg.* **72A**, 672−677.

Rothman R.H. and Cohn J.C. (1990) Cemented versus cementless total hip arthroplasty—a critical review. *Clin. Orthop.* **254**, 153−169.

Rydell N.W. (1966) Forces acting on the femoral head prosthesis. A study on strain gauge supplied prostheses in living persons. *Acta Orthop. Scand.* (Suppl. 88), 1−132.

Sammarco G.J. (1989) Biomechanics of the foot. In Nordin M. and Frankel V.H. (eds) *Basic Biomechanics of the Musculoskeletal System*, 2nd edn. Philadelphia, Lea & Febiger, pp. 163−181.

Sennwald G. (1987) *The Wrist—Anatomical and Pathophysiological Approach to Diagnosis and Treatment*. Berlin, Springer-Verlag.

Simkin A. (1981) The dynamic vertical force distribution during level walking under normal and rheumatic feet. *Rheum. Rehab.* **20**, 88−97.

Smith E.M., Juvinall R.C. and Bender L.F. (1964) Role of the finger flexors in rheumatoid deformities of the metacarpophalangeal joints. *Arthritis Rheum.* **7**, 467−480.

Souter W.A. (1973) Arthroplasty of the elbow with particular reference to metallic hinge arthroplasty in rheumatoid patients. *Orthop. Clin. N. Am.* **4**, 395−413.

Stauffer R.N. (1979) Total joint arthroplasty—the ankle. *Mayo Clinic Proc.* **54**, 570−575.

Stauffer R.N. and Segal N.M. (1981) Total ankle arthroplasty: four years experience. *Clin. Orthop.* **160**, 217−221.

Stauffer R.N., Chao E.Y.S. and Brewster R.C. (1977) Force and motion analysis of the normal, diseased and prosthetic ankle. *Clin. Orthop.* **127**, 189−196.

Stockley I., Douglas D.L. and Elson R.A. (1990) Bicondylar St. Georg sledge knee arthroplasty. *Clin. Orthop.* **255**, 228−234.

Swanson A.B. (1973) *Flexible Implant Resection Arthroplasty in the Hand and Extremities*. St. Louis, C.V. Mosby.

Swanson A.B., Swanson G.G. and Maupin B.K. (1984) Flexible implant arthroplasty of the radiocarpal joint—surgical technique and long-term study. *Clin. Orthop.* **187**, 94−106.

Swanson S.A.V. and Freeman M.A.R. (1974) The design of a knee joint implant. *Biomed. Eng.* **9**, 348−352.

Taleisnik J. (1985) *The Wrist*. New York, Churchill-Livingstone.

Thomas F.B. (1969) Arthrodesis of the ankle. *J. Bone Joint Surg.* **51B**, 53−59.

Thompson F.R. (1952) Vitallium intramedullary hip prosthesis; preliminary report. *NY State J. Med.* **52**, 3011−3020.

Tuke M.A., Roper B.A., Swanson S.A.V. and O'Riordan S. (1981) The ICLH elbow. *Eng. Med.* **10**, 75−78.

Turner T.M., Sumner D.R., Urban R.M., Rivero D.P. and Galante J.O. (1986) A comparative study of porous coatings in a weight-bearing total hip arthroplasty model. *J. Bone Joint Surg.* **68A**, 1396−1409.

Vasu R., Carter D.R. and Harris W.H. (1982) Stress distribution in the acetabular region—before and after total joint replacement. *J. Biomech.* **15**, 155–164.

Volz R.G. (1984) Total wrist arthroplasty—a clinical review. *Clin. Orthop.* **187**, 112–120.

Walker P.S., Wang C.J. and Masse Y. (1974) Joint laxity as a criterion for the design of condylar knee prostheses. *Total Knee Replacement*. London, Institute of Mechanical Engineering Press, pp. 22–29.

Walker P.S., Reilly D., Thatcher J., Ben Dov M. and Ewald F.C. (1981) Fixation of tibial components of knee prostheses. *J. Bone Joint Surg.* **63A**, 258–267.

Weightman B.O. and Amis A.A. (1982) Finger joint force predic-

tions related to design of joint replacements. *J. Biomed. Eng.* **4**, 197–205.

Williams J.F. and Svensson N.L. (1968) A force analysis of the hip joint. *Bio-Med. Eng.* **3**, 365–370.

Wright T.M. and Bartel D.L. (1986) The problem of surface damage in polyethylene total knee components. *Clin. Orthop.* **205**, 67–74.

Wroblewski B.M. (1979) A method of management of the fractured stem in total hip replacement. *Clin. Orthop.* **141**, 71–73.

Youm Y., McMurthy R.Y., Flatt A.E. and Gillespie T.E. (1978) Kinematics of the wrist. *J. Bone Joint Surg.* **60A**, 423–431.

Chapter 32
Microsurgical Techniques in Orthopaedics

R.W.H. Pho, V.P. Kumar, K. Satku & A.K. Kour

INTRODUCTION

Microsurgery is a technique of magnifying the visual horizon of the surgeon to enable him or her to see better, dissect better and perform micromanipulation with great accuracy. This is to help the surgeon to perform precision surgery that was not possible to achieve in the past. The greatest impact of microsurgery has been in our ability to suture small vessels and to allow us to move tissue readily from one part of the body to other sites.

The applications of microsurgical technique in orthopaedics are as follows.

1 They are an integral part of the training of young orthopaedic surgeons. Surgeons who have been exposed to this technique are often more meticulous in tissue handling, paying more respect to the tissue, anatomy and pathology and are technically more dexterous in fine manipulation in reconstructive orthopaedic surgery.

2 It can be considered as a form of 'spare-part surgery' by using biological tissue consisting of skin, bone, cartilage, muscle, tendon, nerve, toe and digit for reconstruction. This application is widely accepted in limb preservation surgery for trauma, tumour, congenital abnormality and infection. In organ and tissue transplants, musculoskeletal tissue and organs from the patient are now being recognized as important potential sources of biological tissue for replacement of the diseased part.

3 Microsurgical techniques enable the surgeon to augment vascular supply to the ischaemic limb, to avascular bone, to avascular scarred bed and to problematic non-unions.

4 The technique has enabled the surgeon to have a better understanding of micro-anatomy for microvessel and microneural surgery and micromanipulation of tissue. Surgeons are able to develop different new surgical techniques in different parts of the body, e.g.

microdiscectomy for the lumbar disc. This technique has shortened the hopitalization time of patients who are now being rehabilitated faster.

The impact of microsurgery has made development of new diagnostic tools and therapeutic procedures possible.

Although the microsurgical technique in orthopaedics has created a new realm of surgical experience, the complexity of microsurgical procedures that can be undertaken is often said to be limited by the skill and innovative creation of the surgeon. The technique, however, is not intended for use by all surgeons but only for those who have opted to adapt it and have acquired the skill in the laboratory. Wide experience in reconstructive orthopaedic surgery is essential in selecting the correct case, assessing the technical problems and balancing the beneficial result of the technique over conventional methods.

GENERAL PRINCIPLES

It is essential that the surgeon master the technique of micromanipulation, microdissection and microsuture of different types of tissues, i.e. skin and its contents of nerves, vessels, muscles, tendons, bones and joints. A good microsurgical technique can only be performed with good quality fine instruments and the basic technique of microsurgery must be learned and perfected in the laboratory with diligence and practice.

Instruments

The basic microvascular instrument requirements are:
1 loupe and operating microscope;
2 microscissors, dissecting forceps and needle holder;
3 vascular clamps and clips;
4 suture materials;
5 syringes, needles and background materials.

These instruments must be well maintained. It takes only a little carelessness to permanently damage them.

LOUPE MAGNIFICATION

Loupe magnification is easily applied and very practical. It is excellent for semimicro work with magnification varying from ×2 to ×4.5 and allows the working distance to vary from 200 to 400 mm. It has the following disadvantages.
1 The magnification is limited and fixed (Fig. 32.1).
2 The light intensity is not adjustable and an extra light source is required.
3 There is always the initial problem of adjustment. Its greatest disadvantage is that the field of vision is limited and working distance requires the head to be held still all the time. Very often the surgeon gets fatigue and develops neck stiffness.

OPERATING MICROSCOPE

The operating microscope has the following advantages.
1 A variable range of magnification from ×6 to ×40.
2 The light intensity can be increased. The fibre-optic light source is powerful and increases sharpness of image without increase in heat sufficient to produce tissue desiccation.
3 Foot control for focusing and zooming for change of magnification reduces frustration, fatigue and unwanted hand movements.
4 The head and neck can be rested on the eye-piece and thus reduce fatigue.
5 Both the surgeon and the assistant can view the same operative field.
6 One can install a camera for static photographs and for recording on video film.

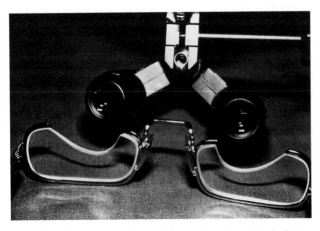

Fig. 32.1 Magnifying glasses used in combination with the loupe.

However, with the operating microscope, the surgeon is restricted in mobility and sometimes has difficulty in adjusting hand movement to compensate for visual magnification. Despite this limitation with the operating microscope one can achieve better control of micromanipulation and microdissection to produce minimal trauma and to achieve precision surgery that is unmatched by other techniques.

Microsurgical techniques are often prolonged and adherence to ergonomic principles to avoid unwanted movement of the hands and fatigue are essential. The surgeon must have good mental control and have a comfortable posture. The seat must be adjustable for height control.

Frustration associated with microsurgery is often due to poor quality of instruments and incorrect accommodation or adjustment of the eye-piece in the operating microscope. In addition, a poor posture predisposes to fatigue and a difficult dissection and handling of the vessel can be very trying. There are also a number of initial problems that one encounters with microsurgical technique such as finding lost needles, breaking sutures and suture pull-through. These can be overcome by constant practice to ensure that finger movement can be reduced to compensate for visual magnification. In free-tissue transplantation, frustration often results from inadequate planning and preparation of the patient and a failure to anticipate the problems of vessel dissection and vessel loss.

MICROSURGICAL TECHNIQUE

Microsuture technique must be practised constantly under the operating microscope so that it can be executed with ease when the need arises. The surgeon must become familiar with the handling of the instruments, the holding of the sutures, the placing of sutures and tying of knots. Inappropriate handling may result in damage to the suture and frequent breakage when tying knots. Microsurgical knots must be tied squarely and the tension adjusted not by sensory control of the hands but by visual observation under the microscope. The initial knot should consist of two loops and should be square. A second and third throw should follow the initial knot. One should evolve a set pattern of handling, placing and of relocating the tiny needle so that the frustration of finding lost needles can be avoided.

Principles of microvascular anastomosis

The vessels to be sutured must be handled gently. The dissection should be performed parallel to the vessel to avoid accidental puncture and to see the lumen of the vessel. Tributaries must be ligated close to the main vessel to avoid turbulence in a potential blind sac. The adventitia from the cut ends of the vessel should be gently teased away and pulled down well over the end of the vessel and then cut and allowed to retract to expose the clear media. This prevents the adventitia from projecting into the lumen and compromising the anastomosis. The vessel lumen should be syringed with heparin solution to clear it of all debris and soft thrombi. The vessel lumen should also be inspected for intimal tears, and cut back to a healthy segment. The antegrade and retrograde blood flow must be tested and be good. Any compromise will result in failure.

The other problems encountered in microvascular anastomosis include discrepancy in the dimensions of the lumen between the recipient and donor vessels, vessel spasm, inadequate length of the donor and recipient vessels and loss of vessels. Discrepancy in vessel size may be overcome by dilatation of the smaller lumen, by an oblique or oblique-and-longitudinal cut of the smaller vessel (Fig. 32.2) or by an end-to-side anastomosis. Vascular spasm can be minimized by ensuring that the patient had adequate fluid replacement, by gentle handling of the vessels and by keeping the vessels moist with warm saline. A 2% lignocaine solution may help to ease spasm or prevent it. Hydrostatic dilatation may occasionally be necessary but must be undertaken with caution. Vessel loss or potential tension at the anastomotic site can be minimized by a bone resection and shortening the limb or digit to be replanted. The interposition of a vein graft to bridge vessel loss is the other common method used to overcome this problem. The best source of vein graft is a cutaneous vein on the dorsum of the foot or the saphenous vein. These vessels tend to have a thick wall with minimal branches and few valves. The large vessel size may pose a problem but the opening of the recipient vessel must be adapted appropriately. It is always important to remember that the vein graft should be positioned so that the valves will not impede the flow of the arterial circulation.

Cobbett's modification of Carroll's principle of triangulation should be used when suturing the vessels.

The first two sutures are placed at an angle of 120° with respect to each other (Fig. 32.3). This causes the posterior wall to fall away from the anterior wall and facilitates suture of the anterior wall. The entry point of the suture from the edge of the vessel should be about the same thickness as the vessel wall in the case of the artery and twice the thickness of the vessel wall in the case of the vein. Once the anterior wall is sutured the first two guide sutures placed at a 120° angle to each other are twisted around 180° to bring the posterior wall anteriorly for suturing.

Principles of microneural suture

Nerve suture should be primary whenever possible. In the presence of adverse factors like gross contamination, however, delayed repair is preferred. In this instance the cut ends must be tagged together to prevent retraction of the nerve ends.

When a decision has been made to repair the nerve, it should be possible to approximate the nerve ends without tension. Should tension be significant, excessive scar-tissue formation at the suture will compromise results. Tension is minimized by mobilization of the nerve ends, flexion of adjacent joints, rerouting of the nerves when possible and most importantly by the use of

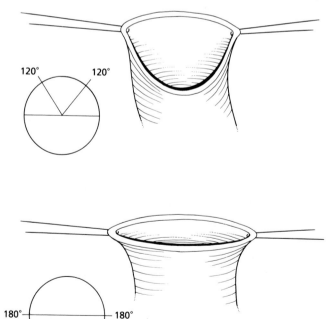

Fig. 32.3 The placement of the first two stay sutures when co-apting vessels. Placing them at an angle of 120° allows the posterior wall to fall away.

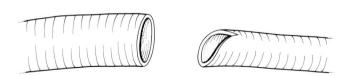

Fig. 32.2 Demonstration of the technique of managing unequal vessel size by oblique and longitudinal cuts on smaller vessel.

autologous nerve graft. Mobilization of the nerve ends must be kept to a minimum as additional nerve injury may occur either by interference with its vascularity or by scar formation in the perineurial gliding tissue. Flexion of the adjacent joint to minimize tension should not be excessive. For instance flexion of the wrist to reduce tension at the anastomotic site of the median or ulnar nerve in the vicinity of the wrist should not exceed 30°. Excessive flexion would be uncomfortable for the patient and when the joint is finally mobilized, damage the already regenerated fibres. Rerouting of the nerve is of use only in certain special circumstances and situations. The anterior transposition of the ulnar nerve when dealing with injury of the ulnar nerve at the elbow is the most appropriate example. Grafting is the best method to avoid tension. The sources of nerve graft include the sural nerve and the medial cutaneous antebrachial nerve. The sural nerve is harvested by series of three to five small transverse or longitudinal incisions along its course. The distal identification of the nerve begins behind the lateral malleolus where the nerve lies in close proximity to the short saphenous vein. Once the nerve has been isolated, by exerting light traction on the nerve, its proximal course can be identified and dissected. The appropriate length of the nerve is then resected to be used as a graft. Once harvested, the graft is laid between the proximal and distal cut ends and sutured. The survival of the graft depends on revascularization from the surrounding bed. A scarred bed would compromise the result.

Unless the nerve ends have been cut cleanly, the ends must be cut back to healthy tissue with a razor blade. The nerve ends are then orientated. The epineurial vascular pattern and the internal fascicular topography could be utilized to achieve the appropriate orientation. The final co-aptation may take the form of epineurial co-aptation, fascicular co-aptation or co-aptation between groups of fascicles. In the latter instances, the fascicles or groups of fascicles must be carefully dissected longitudinally from the cut end to facilitate suture. When the co-aptation of the nerve ends is done by epineurial sutures, the occasional perineurial stitch between corresponding fascicles will enhance co-aptation. In mono- or oligofascicular nerves, fascicular repair is preferred.

The suture materials generally used include 8−0, 10−0 or 11−0 monofilament nylon thread swaged on a tapered flat bodied needle 50−75 μm in diameter.

The repair of a partially transected nerve poses a difficult problem. The epineurium on either side of the transection is incised longitudinally and the fascicles identified. The fascicles are then dissected towards the lesion, taking care not to damage the perineurium. The transected fascicles are then repaired. In chronic injuries, nerve grafts may be necessary to bridge the gap between transected fascicles.

Following repair of the nerve, the limb is immobilized for 3−4 weeks. The regeneration of the nerve is subsequently monitored both clinically and by electrophysiological means. The location of the Tinel sign and its distal progression should be noted regularly. Sensory and motor recovery should be noted clinically and documented. Electromyographic and nerve conduction studies are undertaken to ascertain the level and degree of recovery.

SPECIAL CONSIDERATIONS

Microsurgical procedures have certain inherent characteristics that necessitate special preparation. In microvascular reconstruction vessel anastomosis only forms a very small part of the surgery, yet it is a step done near the end of an operation which will lead to failure if not executed properly. The more complex the case, the longer the operative time and it is likely that the surgeon will tire easily.

Pre-operative planning

Pre-operative preparation must include an angiographic study of the recipient and donor sites to delineate vessels for anastomosis. This is especially so in congenital and post-traumatic conditions where absence or anomalies of vessels and loss or distortion of vessel anatomy are often encountered. This abnormality must be determined pre-operatively. The vascular anatomy of the donor skin and bone should also be similarly studied before surgery. Selection of the right case and anticipation of the problems that one is likely to encounter during surgery is important. An alternative salvage procedure should also be prepared should the original plan fail. Team support should always be readily available.

Intra-operative planning

1 The procedure is long, sometimes taking more than 10 hours. An experienced anaesthetist is necessary to maintain a normal blood volume, normothermia and deep anaesthesia to avoid vessel spasm. The patient should be well hydrated pre- and intra-operatively. The room temperature has to be properly controlled together with patient's body temperature.

The surgeon must avoid operating when fatigued and must be well prepared for the prolonged surgery.

The operative area should be well prepared along

with the possible areas for donor tissue and vein graft.

2 Blood loss is often insidious and occurs from large open wounds and this coupled with long duration of the operation may lead to excessive blood loss with changes in blood pressure and tissue perfusion. The patient may be soaked in a pool of blood or cold solution, thus producing hypothermia. Routine continuous intra-arterial pressure monitoring and monitoring of the urinary output to assess tissue perfusion is helpful. Urinary catheterization prevents bladder distension and reduces autonomic changes that may complicate monitoring.

3 Although in the adult patient, hypothermia is not a problem, in the child the large exposed surface areas coupled with low ambient temperature necessary for the comfort of the surgeons may induce hypothermia and attendant problems.

4 Patients often remain in an awkward position for long periods to facilitate adequate exposure of both the donor and recipient areas and this necessitates satisfactory padding of potential pressure points to prevent pressure sores and nerve palsies.

5 To minimize blood loss, a tourniquet is often necessary, ischaemic time must be carefully monitored, kept to a minimum and when necessary the tourniquet deflated and re-inflated.

6 The prolonged exposure of the tissues to theatre environment and the increased number of personnel in the theatre necessitates strict aseptic principles and the use of prophylactic antibiotics to minimize the risk of infection.

7 To minimize operative time, team approach by simultaneous work at both the donor and recipient sites will have to be planned. A two-team approach is useful to reduce operative time.

8 During harvesting and preparation of the recipient site it is important to mark the arteries and veins from the start. Always choose a large vessel for anastomosis. Any possible damaged segment of vessel must be excised. Attempt to suture only normal vessels of the same size with good forward flow and no tension. Attempt to ensure the vessel pedicle is of sufficient length. If in doubt, a vein graft must be used and this can be facilitated by anastomosing the vein graft as a bench exercise before seating of the composite tissue in the recipient area.

9 Do not compromise the orthopaedic principle of bony fixation. The composite tissue transfer should be placed to facilitate bony fixation and vessel anastomosis. It is therefore important to plan the seating of skin flap, bone and vessel together so that one can fix the bone and close the skin without much tension and at the same time vessel anastomosis can be facilitated. In highly

scarred areas, the recipient vessel should be harvested high up in the virgin field and the donor pedicle is lengthened with a vein graft. On completion of vessel anastomosis, it is important that the area should be drained prior to skin closure.

10 Donor site precautions. Once the transplant tissue has been harvested, the closure of the donor site is often left to junior staff. To minimize donor site morbidity, attention to strict surgical principles is necessary. Complications like compartmental syndrome and infections have been noted and are avoidable.

Post-operative management

1 Anti-coagulation with low dose aspirin 150 mg t.d.s. and Rheomacrodex 500 ml to 1 litre per 24 h are indicated to prevent thrombosis at the vascular anastomotic site. We normally maintain this regimen for 5 days to 1 week after surgery.

2 Close monitoring of circulation to the transplanted tissue is necessary to assess vascular insufficiency and to decide whether re-exploration is necessary. Monitoring would be best done by checking the colour and temperature and if in doubt by use of a needle prick to assess the circulation. When bone is used we normally use an island of skin to monitor circulation and patency of the underlying anastomosed vessels.

3 The limb must be positioned so that external splintage or bandages do not compress against the vessels.

APPLICATION OF MICROSURGICAL TECHNIQUE IN ORTHOPAEDICS

This can be grouped under:
1 re-implantation surgery;
2 reconstruction with skin and soft-tissue transplant;
3 muscle transfer;
4 foot as donor tissue in hand reconstruction;
5 bone joint transfer;
6 epiphyseal transplant.

Re-implantation surgery

The concept of limb transplant was introduced and attempted by Hopfner and Carrel. They attempted to do heterotransplant of dogs' limbs with no knowledge of immunological rejection. Their work was not recognised until Lapchinsky's successful re-implantation of a dog's leg in 1960. The success of Ronald Malt's re-implantation for an amputated right arm in 1962 followed with the Chinese work in 1963 and Tamai's work in 1965 had produced a wide interest in the field of transplantation of the limb and digits and clinical re-implantation of tissues became widely adopted as an acceptable technique in the practice of orthopaedic surgery.

At the present stage, where there is no successful prosthesis that can substitute for the human hand, re-implantation of an amputated part should be attempted whenever feasible. While this may be the case, re-implantation surgery is not without problems. Each case is different with its own different problems.

Re-implantation of limbs can be divided into major upper-limb re-implantation, minor or digital-limb re-implantation and lower-limb re-implantation. Although traumatic amputation is by far the commonest indication for re-implantation, limb replants are occasionally carried out for congenital deformities and following segmental resection of limb for tumour control.

ASSESSMENT OF MAJOR TRAUMATIC AMPUTATION IN RE-IMPLANTATION SURGERY

Experience has indicated that survival of re-implanted limbs cannot be taken for granted. Very often a successful re-implantation with good function acceptable to the patient can only be achieved if one had carried out an accurate assessment and had anticipated the problems and avoided complications at the time of surgery, and if a total primary reconstruction was carried out. Very often the amputation occurs in the area in which re-implantation service is not available. The following management and guidelines are important in the care of amputated cases before transfer to the re-implantation centre.

A patient with a major limb amputation is no different from a patient suffering from multiple injuries. The principle of saving the patient's life should be given priority by keeping the airway clear and controlling haemorrhage through pressure dressing, elevation and fluid replacement. Assessment of other injuries in other parts of the body such as the head, chest and abdomen is mandatory. Medication consisting of analgesics, antibiotics and anti-tetanus should be given. It is very important that during transportation, systemic support of the patient should continuously be given until the patient reaches the re-implantation centre.

The amputated limb should be cleaned and rinsed with sterile saline containing antibiotic solution. It should be wrapped in sterile dry gauze or a towel. This should then be placed in a plastic bag and placed in an ice-box to ensure cooling of the amputated part. The limb should not have direct contact with the ice. In cases where there has been incomplete amputation the cooling may be difficult. Packing of the ice to the incompletely amputated part may be useful but this will make nursing and transportation difficult. Where the skin bridge shows no nerve continuity and the limb is completely devascularized, it is best that the skin bridge be divided to facilitate preservation of the amputated part for transportation.

At the re-implantation centre, further assessment should be carried out.

SUITABILITY OF THE CANDIDATE FOR RE-IMPLANTATION

A detailed medical history of the patient including history of systemic disease or psychiatric illness should be taken. Re-implantation surgery does not follow the 'all-or-none rule'. Even if the re-implanted limb has survived, it may not necessarily be functional. The case must be selected carefully. The patient must be young and well motivated, and suitable for rehabilitation; otherwise the patient may reject the limb or be crippled significantly by the re-attached limb. A self-mutilated amputated limb in the psychologically unstable patient is not suitable for re-implantation. Always try to avoid the tragedy of seeing the initial triumph of the surgical exercise turning to a total failure for the patient and the surgeon.

ASSESSING THE ASSOCIATED INJURIES

Saving the patient's life is more important than saving the patient's limb. The operative risk of the associated conditions in a patient who has peptic ulcer, current infection, diabetes, arteriosclerosis or other injuries should be taken into account as to whether re-implantation is worthwhile. If re-implantation surgery is going to interfere with the surgical management of other vital organs, re-implantation surgery should be abandoned or postponed by cooling the amputated part. Alternatively, a simple procedure could be carried out by attaching it to another part of the body by joining the vessels for simple revascularization as a preservation until further definitive reconstruction can be carried out at a later date.

One must *assess the suitability of the amputated part* for re-implantation. The following factors should be considered.

1 *Ischaemic time.* In major limb amputation the warm ischaemic time is very critical and should not exceed 6 hours. The more proximal the amputation, the more muscle bulk there is and the risk of developing re-implantation toxaemia is higher. The possibility of irreversible Volkmann's ischaemic contracture must also be considered.

2 Soft-tissue injuries. Crushing and degloving injuries indicate extensive damage to the underlying soft tissue including vessels, nerves and skin which may require radical resection. Multiple levels amputation invariably means that the middle segment has been crushed and vessel damage and muscle necrosis are often present. Problems of vessel thrombosis, re-implantation toxaemia and Volkmann's ischaemia are likely.

3 Bone loss. Segmental bone loss and crushing to the bone near the joint make bony fixation difficult. When amputation is near the joints, arthrodesis may be indicated to spare the repair of extensor and flexor tendons, especially around the wrist joint. The tendons can then be used as a motor unit to replace other lost tendons for finger flexion and extension.

In the upper limb, limb shortening is well compensated and has the following advantages:

(a) It will overcome vessel and nerve loss and therefore allows suturing of healthy vessels and nerves without tension or interposition with vessel or nerve graft.

(b) All contused muscles and tendons can be excised radically.

(c) Shortening will facilitate skin closure.

Bone shortening will produce the following problems:

(a) In incomplete amputation, buckling and redundancy of intact structures may be present.

(b) Difficulty will be experienced in adjusting the tension during repair of flexor and extensor tendons.

(c) Cosmetically, this may not be acceptable in a female patient who will not accept a shortened limb.

4 Vessel and nerve loss. In an incomplete amputation the presence of intact nerves means that the patient will almost certainly recover sensation and motor functions distally provided the limb can be revascularized adequately. Nerve loss or failure to regenerate properly is one of the greatest contributing factors for failure in re-implantation surgery. The limitation of proximal re-implantation surgery is principally from unpredictable nerve regeneration, especially in those cases where the nerve has been avulsed. In a degloving or crushing injury, vessel contusion must be assessed adequately and all the damaged vessels should be resected. One should aim at suturing only healthy vessels without tension.

5 Primary reconstruction. Primary reconstruction should be carried out whenever feasible. We should regard an injured limb as one, with regional tissue injury of skin and its contents and should attempt primary reconstruction of bone, vessels, nerves, tendons and skin with detailed planning. Attention should be given to

bony fixation in order to facilitate soft-tissue reconstruction. The time spent in total reconstruction is often worthwhile as this will allow early rehabilitation of the re-implanted limb rather than subjecting the patient to multiple-stage operations where each additional surgery is an additional setback to the rehabilitation of the patient (Fig. 32.4a,b).

One must consider the limb and whether it is worthwhile to do limb preservation or amputation. There are many factors such as age of the patient, site of the long bone which is affected, the viability of the injured limb, the extent of crushing, contamination and possible infection in the injured limb, the extent of regional soft tissue and bone loss and other related general medical conditions that may be equally important in determining whether one should opt for amputation or limb preservation. In assessing factors favouring amputation,

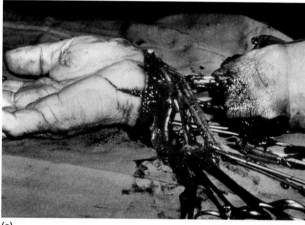

(a)

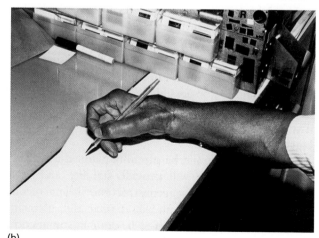

(b)

Fig. 32.4 (a) Traumatic amputation through the right wrist joint. Tendons, vessels and nerves are being identified and tagged. (b) Function 18 months following surgery.

lower-limb amputation is more acceptable because such functional prostheses as the below-knee patellar-tendon-bearing prosthesis are available. In the upper limb destruction of muscle and tendons favours amputation. In the lower limb, the loss of major nerve is a strong indication for amputation. The loss of bone and joint is relatively low on the scoring in the indication for amputation of extremities. We must remember that an injured limb with bone and soft-tissue loss and a limb which is painful and insensitive in the sole is better amputated and a prosthesis fitted.

In limb preservation, shortening is acceptable in the upper limb but in the lower limb we will maintain length. We will expect nerve recovery to be better and perhaps more predictable in the upper limb than in the lower limb. In the upper limb, muscle and tendon reconstructions are indicated to restore functional grip as compared to the lower limb where one can sacrifice one compartment of the muscle without much disability.

OPERATIVE TECHNIQUE

The patient should be catheterized. A two-team approach is recommended, one exploring the recipient proximal stump and the other exploring and debriding the amputated part. Several points are noted.

1 The amputated stump is normally explored and prepared as soon as the theatre can be organized without waiting for general anaesthetic.

2 In an incomplete amputation where there is only skin bridge without any neurovascular bundle connection, the skin bridge is divided to allow a two-team approach and also to facilitate shortening of the bone for bony stabilization.

3 The debridement should be radical with all possibly contaminated and crushed tissue excised. Both nerves and vessels are normally explored under magnification to ensure there is no damage to the endothelium and surrounding structures. All muscle tissues where re-innervation is not possible is excised to ensure that there is no tissue bulk left that will impede skin closure. The neurovascular bundles should be identified and tagged with a marker.

4 Bony fixation should be carefully planned using different methods that will provide stability and least interference to soft-tissue reconstruction. Skeletal reconstruction is very important. Shortening and adequate stabilization of the bone has to be done in conjunction with the total assessment of soft-tissue reconstruction of nerve, tendon and vessels. Bony fixation should be carried out and planned so as to facilitate repair of these soft tissues.

VESSEL ANASTOMOSIS

When a vein graft is indicated it is best that this is sutured to the distal amputated part as a bench exercise before bony fixation. In prolonged ischaemic time, we prefer to do arterial anastomosis first but this invariably results in excessive blood loss. Repair of nerve and tendon should be performed prior to vessel anastomosis where ischaemic time is not critical. This will facilitate surgery in the bloodless field and thus shorten operative time. Following closure of the wound, drainage should be carried out. Fasciotomy is indicated in those cases with prolonged ischaemia.

DIGITAL AMPUTATION

Amputated digits provide a large volume of clinical materials for surgeons to perfect their microsurgical technique of re-implantation. It is now a relatively common emergency operation that is being performed routinely in any medical centre where expertise is available with survival rates reaching 90%. In incomplete amputation revascularization to restore circulation should be carried out. It is important to remember that survival of the digit does not mean success. The ultimate aim is to restore hand function. A digit that is non-functional may interfere with other digits and therefore interfere with the total function of the whole hand. It is the selection of the case that will determine whether the procedure is a triumph and each case must be considered on its own merit. The patient should be selected, based on the case of patient's general health, associated injuries, age and mental state. Whenever it is feasible we recommend re-implantation in all cases in children as nerve regeneration and adaptability will often produce good results. In elderly patients one should be more cautious and selective. For those who are very well motivated and active, re-implantation may be considered. Patients who are psychologically stable and cooperative with post-operative rehabilitation will have better functional results. Although the re-implanted digit may survive, the psychologically ill-prepared patient may feel significantly crippled and end up with a protracted and unrewarding period of rehabilitation.

Types of injury

Clean-cut injuries do far better than crushing injuries, both in survival and restoration of function. In severe crushing, avulsion or degloving type of injury, there is often associated damage to a long segments of the vessels, nerves and tendons (Fig. 32.5). This will often

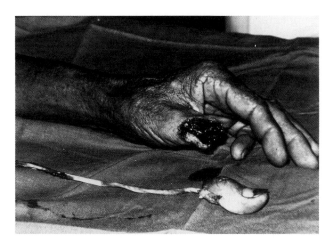

Fig. 32.5 Avulsion injury of left thumb. Note tendon of flexor pollicis longus avulsed from muscle belly in forearm.

require major resection of damaged vessels and surrounding structures. Technically, salvaging the digit is more difficult and the failure rate is higher.

Level of amputation

The more distal the amputation the more difficult it is to identify minute vessels for anastomosis. Very often only small terminal branches of digital artery and vein can be identified for suture. However, despite the practical problems, the ultimate result is better as arthrodesis of the distal interphalangeal joint without tendon reconstruction gives good stability and nerve regeneration is more predictable. In these cases, tendon repair may not be indicated. Similarly, when there is a venous problem, we can do without venous repair and venous return relied solely on external bleeding through the wound. The preservation of the terminal digit will be better than fitting a cosmetic prosthesis. For the more proximal amputations one has to be more selective.

Type and number of digits

For the thumb, we advocate that every attempt must be made to replace an amputated thumb whenever it is feasible as there is no other tissue replacement or prosthesis that can substitute a successful re-implanted thumb both in function and cosmesis.

In single digit amputation, one has to be very selective. Fingers work as a team. If one digit is not functioning it will affect the function of the hand as a whole. By re-implanting one single digit the patient will be off work for at least 3–6 months. This may be more crippling to the patient and his family than the loss of one single digit. Re-implantation of a single digit is recommended for a child at any part and any level. It is recommended in young girls for cosmetic reasons or occupational needs. The index finger of highly skilled technicians and any digit for cosmetic reasons in a model, doctor or musician may be re-implanted. Patient's own wish and social reasons are other indications for re-implantation.

In multiple amputations, one aims to re-implant the digit that will produce the highest success rate both in survival and function. The possibility of salvaging part of a finger that can be used as a 'bank' for future reconstruction should also be entertained.

In the pre-operative assessment, we emphasize on planning to stabilize the patient and perform an accurate assessment on whether the part can be re-implanted and whether it requires special procedures such as skin flap, nerve graft or vein graft. Radiography of extremities is very important to assess the type of bony fixation to be carried out.

The sequence of re-implantation is as follows. First, perform skin debridement and identification of neurovascular bundles. Bony fixation, tendon repair and digital nerve repair follow. Vessel anastomosis is normally done last provided the ischaemic time is not compromised. If there has been adequate planning of skin debridement, identification of neurovascular bundles, shortening of bone with stable bony fixation, vessel approximation should cause no problems. Vessel resection should be carried out such that end-to-end suture of healthy vessels can be achieved with no tension. We prefer to do arterial anastomosis first. This facilitates the identification of suitable, well-drained veins distally for anastomosis. This also ensures that the vein is not twisted and is draining well. In addition, this will also reduce ischaemic time. The main disadvantage is excessive blood loss which can amount to 1 litre per digit, and venous anastomosis is done in a relatively bloody field. We prefer to do one artery and two venous anastomoses for digital re-implantation. Fasciotomy should be done in those cases where there is prolonged ischaemic time from delayed transport, in multiple digit amputations and in those cases with inadequate venous return from poor venous anastomoses.

In avulsion injury, where there is vessel and nerve loss, do not hesitate to use the neighbouring digital artery, dorsal digital vein, digital nerve or vein graft. Skin closure should be carried out with no tension. When indicated, relaxing incisions should be done. The digit should be immobilized in the most comfortable position where optimal tension will occur at the extensor and flexor anastomotic sites. Although we rely on post-operative low-molecular-weight dextran and aspirin, we believe that accurate placing of sutures, minimal handling of vessel wall and anastomosis of healthy vessels with strong forward flow with no tension are important in ensuring patency of anastomosis.

The best functional results of re-implantation of digits are in those cases where total reconstruction is possible at the time of surgery. This is especially seen in the thumb where total reconstruction will provide good results. Attempts at comparing re-implantation against amputation in terms of function showed that there is relatively little difference in terms of hospitalization period. However in thumb re-implantation the result is often superior to amputation.

We have attempted to classify re-implanted digits into three groups:
1 near normal digit;
2 useful digit;
3 useless digit.
This is based on whether the patient regards the re-attached digit as useful, painful or hyperaesthetic with cold intolerance. The findings also include sensibility, both protective as well as two point discrimination, joint stiffness, deformity and atrophy of the digit and pinch strength. About 70% of re-implanted thumbs can be grouped under near normal digit and 30% in the useful digit group. In re-implantation of fingers, approximately 10% can be grouped as near normal digits, 70% as useful digits and 20% as failures. In the last group the re-implanted digit is painful, stiff and useless, and requires amputation.

Our results indicate that re-implantation of the thumb is most rewarding and should always be attempted. As regards other digits it would appear that one has to be very selective. It is important also to amputate a failed re-implanted digit as soon as possible once there is evidence that it is not acceptable to the patient and if it interferes with the overall function of the hand.

LOWER-EXTREMITY RE-IMPLANTATION IN TRAUMA

Indications for lower extremity re-implantation are limited. Traumatic amputations in the lower limb are uncommon. They tend to be severe and often of the avulsion type. Neural recovery is unpredictable and the sole of the foot is left anaesthetic with trophic problems. Limb shortening is less well tolerated. The longest acceptable limb length inequality is 8–10 cm. Effective prostheses for the lower limb make primary amputation acceptable.
1 Bilateral lower limb amputations may be an indication to re-implant one or both limbs.

Pre-operative preparations include correction of haemorrhagic shock and perfusion of the amputated limb with heparinized saline. Perfusion should be possible without resistance and flow from veins, other arteries and medullary cavity of the bones should be equal to the perfusate. Perfusion also clears the limb of all toxic products of prolonged ischaemia and myoglobin, and avoids re-implantation toxaemia. Any resistance to the perfusion or excessive bulging of parts of the limb indicate widespread arterial and or venous injury and contraindicates re-implantation.
2 Warm ischaemia time should not exceed 8 hours.
3 A two-team approach is used.
4 The neurovascular structures are identified and resected back to healthy tissue. The skeleton is stabilized followed by repair of the musculotendinous units and nerves. Venous anastomosis should precede arterial repair to avoid excessive blood loss. Not only are the superficial veins repaired but the deep as well, as deep-tissue necrosis might otherwise ensue. Gaps in vessels and nerves are grafted. Fasciotomy is routine.
5 Post-operative management is along the same lines as for upper-limb re-implantations.
6 Complication of major limb reimplantation include renal failure from myoglobinuria, fat embolism, infection and vascular thrombosis.

Although microsurgical techniques would be more relevant for distal limb, especially digital re-implantations, these techniques are important in major limb re-implantations as well. Proper assessment of arterial and venous injury, especially in relation to intimal tears, allows adequate resection of the unhealthy vessel ends before anastomosis. Extent of nerve injury may also be better assessed under the operating microscope. Vessel and nerve ends are also co-apted accurately with magnification.

RE-IMPLANTATION OF EXTREMITIES AFTER SEGMENTAL RESECTION OF BONE TUMOUR

Limb salvage procedures following segmental tumour resection is increasingly recognized as a valuable method of preserving limb function. It has the following advantages:
1 it avoids phantom pain and stump neuroma by preserving the major nerves;
2 it avoids fitting with cumbersome prostheses;
3 in partial limb preservation, it facilities fitting with a better and lighter prosthesis for better functional results, such as following the Van Ness procedure.
Most of the resection in the lower limb is no different from ablative surgery in the sense that the surgeon's aim

is to preserve the important structures to retain function rather than worry about what is to be resected. The most important structure is the neurovascular bundle. One has to ensure that the local control of tumour is not compromised. In reconstruction for limb function one must consider the following factors.

1 The lower limb is to withstand weight-bearing stress for locomotion. Support should be strong or else fracture is likely. This can be achieved by strong bone-to-bone contact and reinforcement with an internal or external splint.

2 Because of weight-bearing stress, joint reconstruction tends to fail. Arthrodesis may be selected if there is no muscle control for joint function.

3 There should not be too much limb length discrepancy in the newly reconstructed limb. However, in certain circumstances, gross limb length discrepancy is acceptable such as in the Van Ness procedure where resection of the knee joint is followed with derotation of the ankle joint to provide extension and flexion of the ankle joint to replace the knee joint. This will facilitate fitting with a lighter and functional prosthesis.

4 When tumour exists around the shoulder joint, the Tikoff—Linberg procedure can be used. The upper half of the humerus and scapula can be excised and the distal half of the humerus re-attached to the chest wall. This provides a relatively unstable shoulder but excellent elbow and hand function if the neurovascular bundles can be preserved.

Skin and soft-tissue transplant

In the traumatized limb, bone is only one of the tissues injured in the segment. Careful assessment of zone of regional tissue injury around the bone is essential. The surgeon's judgement should not be based only on the interpretation of the shadow on radiography. Adequate skin and soft-tissue cover is essential in promoting early wound healing and bone union. Immediate or late reconstruction of muscle, tendon and nerve facilitates rehabilitation for early return of limb function.

A free skin graft is a safe and reliable method of achieving desired skin cover in a superficial or partial cutaneous loss with a good vascular bed in non-contact or weight-bearing areas. When underlying structures such as bone, joint, tendons or nerves are exposed, a skin flap is indicated. A skin flap can be raised incorporating the muscle, tendon and bone as a composite graft to replace the deficiency in the recipient site. It can be raised as a pedicled or island flap and has been widely used provided the anatomy of the donor tissue is well understood by the surgeon. When a flap is raised close

to the traumatized zone, it is important to avoid creating circumferential skin loss on the injured limb that may impair lymphatic and venous drainage. By division of its pedicle an island flap can be transferred to a distant area as a free flap to facilitate reconstructive surgery.

In replacement of skin and soft tissue loss with a flap, it is important to select the technique that is the simplest, safest and produces consistent and predictable results. A pedicled, regional or island flap should be the first choice. A free flap has the advantages of being a one-stage operation and avoids some of the problems seen in pedicled flaps such as prolonged hospitalization, acrobatic immobilization and occasional psychological disturbance in the patient.

INDICATIONS FOR FLAP TRANSFER

1 Extensive skin loss in a traumatized limb with a bare bone, nerve, tendon or vessel exposed.

2 A composite osteomyocutaneous flap for replacement of bone with skin and soft-tissue loss.

3 A sensory neurovascular flap for restoring sensation and soft-tissue padding in the weight-bearing heel and in the contact areas such as the palmar aspect of the hand and digits.

SELECTION OF DONOR FLAP

Skin flaps can be raised with subcutaneous fat, fascia, nerves, muscles, and bone as neurocutaneous, myocutaneous or osteocutaneous flaps. The donor flap must have the following characteristics.

1 A vascular pedicle of sufficient size and length and predictable course must be available.

2 The area of skin supplied by the vascular pedicle must be known.

3 Skin texture and hair-bearing properties should be similar to the recipient site.

4 The secondary donor defect must be minimal.

In the *upper limb* the following flaps can be used:
- Scapular flap
- Latissimus dorsi flap
- Pectoralis major flap
- Serratus anterior flap
- Deltoid flap
- Medial arm flap
- Lateral arm flap
- Forearm flap either based on posterior or anterior interosseous, ulnar or radial vascular pedicles
- Various digital flaps that can be raised from the hand and fingers

In the *lower limb*, the following flaps can be used:

- Groin flap
- Gracilis flap
- Sartorius flap
- Tensor fascia lata flap
- Saphenous flap
- Gastrocnemius flap
- Anterior tibialis flap
- Peroneal flap
- Insole flap
- Dorsalis pedis flap
- Digital web space flap

The *neurovascular flaps or innervated flaps* can be raised incorporating sensory fibres to the flap:

- Intercostal flap
- Medial arm flap
- Lateral arm flap
- Forearm flap
- Local flap from the arm and digits
- Saphenous flap
- Dorsalis pedis and plantar flaps

The *common myocutaneous flaps* are:

- Latissimus dorsi flap
- Pectoralis major flap
- Gracilis flap
- Tensor fascia lata flap
- Gastrocnemius flap
- Dorsalis pedis flap
- Abductor hallucis flap

The *common osteocutaneous flaps* are:

- Fibular flap
- Anterior tibial flap
- Groin flap incorporating the iliac crest
- Intercostal flap incorporating the rib
- Dorsalis pedis flap incorporating metatarsal bone
- Radial forearm flap incorporating the radius

Groin flap

This is a versatile flap in which the detailed vascular pattern was worked out by McGregor. It provides a large skin flap, exceeding 30×15 cm. The donor site can be closed primarily and the donor scar can be hidden. It is based mainly on the superficial circumflex iliac vessel and superficial epigastric vessel. The use of the deep circumflex iliac vessel allows incorporation of the iliac bone. Its main disadvantages are:

1 the vascular pattern varies greatly;
2 the calibre of the vessels is generally small;
3 the subcutaneous fat is too bulky in obese patients.

Forearm flap

Yang Guo-Fang was the first to report the use of the forearm flap in 1981. The flap is based on the radial artery, its venae commitantes and cephalic vein. The superficial radial nerve and the lateral cutaneous nerve of the forearm can be incorporated to provide sensation. The flap has the following features.

1 The subcutaneous tissue is thin and can be incorporated as a fascial flap. The skin colour and texture are similar to those of the hand.
2 The vessels are very constant and large.
3 The flap can be innervated.
4 A sizeable section of the skin can be incorporated with bone as an osteocutaneous flap or tendons as a tenoneurocutaneous flap. However, in the incorporation of the radius, there is risk of fracture.
5 It can be used as a reversed or antegrade pedicular flap.

The major disadvantage is having to sacrifice one major vessel and cosmetically the donor site is unacceptable. Currently this flap has been extended to incorporate the pedicle based on the ulnar artery, the anterior or posterior interosseous vessels with a different combination of composite tissue.

Scapular flap

This flap was first described by Dos Santos in 1980. The advantages of this flap are:

1 the pedicle runs a constant course;
2 the pedicle consists of one artery and two veins with their calibre measuring $1-1.5$ mm;
3 a very large flap is available and it ranges from 15×15 cm and the donor defect can be closed primarily;
4 the flap is thin for easy moulding to contour the recipient site.

Innervated flaps

Restoration of protective sensation is important in the weight-bearing heel or on the palmar aspect of the hand and in the sacral area of paraplegia patients. An innervated flap raised as a neurovascular island flap, preserving it neurovascular pedicle, is capable of retaining the original sensation in the flap at its new site. Neurovascular island flaps have been widely used in hand surgery since Littler first described the heterofinger neurovascular island flap. The problem of disorientation of sensation of the island flap is well documented. It can be overcome by transection of the nerve and suturing it to the recipient nerve at its new site.

An innervated free flap involves the division of the neurovascular pedicle of an island flap and direct transfer of the flap with anastomosis of its neurovascular pedicle at its new recipient site. The innervated flap will have sensation provided by the recipient nerve with additional contribution from the surrounding skin. This limits the long drawn out and difficult problem of re-educating the patient to correctly orientate sensation in the transferred flap.

The types of neurovascular flaps available are:
1 heterofinger neurovascular island flap;
2 local composite neurovascular island flap;
3 radial transposition island flap;
4 forearm flap;
5 first web space flap;
6 dorsalis pedis flap;
7 abductor hallucis brevis flap;
8 saphenous flap.

A sensate flap with sufficient thickness of the skin for the sole of the foot has so far not been designed although the dorsalis pedis flap with the superficial peroneal nerve incorporated has been used with fairly satisfactory results.

The innervated flap is commonly used in the upper extremity with very good results. Innervated flaps based on the intercostal nerve and vessels can be raised to cover the anaesthesic area of the sacrum in paraplegics. The nerve in the flap can be sutured directly or via nerve transfer to the intercostal nerve just above the level of cord injury. Sacral sores can thereby be treated effectively. The patient's motivation, however, is important in preventing recurrent pressure sores.

Muscle transfer in orthopaedic surgery

The use of muscle and musculocutaneous flaps in orthopaedic surgery is gaining important recognition because of its wide application and a precise understanding of the vascular anatomy of the muscle makes every muscle a potential donor in flap transfer.

The selection of these muscles must be based on the following factors.
1 A precise knowledge of its anatomy and its vascular pedicle.
2 The muscles must be located superficially and must be easily dissected incorporating the surrounding skin, fascia and bone for composite tissue transfer.
3 There should be minimal functional deficit at the donor site.
4 The muscle can be used safely either as a pedicle or as a free-tissue transfer.

TYPES OF MUSCLE TRANSFER

1 Myocutaneous flap incorporating the skin.
2 Myo-osteocutaneous flap incorporating the skin and bone.
3 Fascial flap incorporating mainly the fascia.

Vascularized muscle transfer is indicated in the following conditions:
1 To provide a soft-tissue coverage of vessel, nerve, joint and bone.
2 To provide a vascular bed in traumatized limb for secondary tendon, nerve, bone and joint reconstruction.
3 To introduce new vascular bed to promote wound healing and in management of chronic osteomyelitis.
4 To provide a filling defect to restore contour of a traumatized limb.
5 To provide a voluntary contractile unit for active movement of extremities.

When the muscle is transferred purely to provide soft-tissue coverage and vascular bed it can be transferred without its nerve supply. The muscle, however, will show diffuse atrophy with time.

When the muscle is used as a contractile unit to restore power and active joint movement to the extremities, the neurovascular pedicle must be preserved and the muscle should be innervated. The traumatized limb must have good sensation with passive range of individual joint movement. The choice of donor muscle should adhere to the principles of tendon transfer. The donor muscle should be strong, have good excursion and be expendable. The recipient nerve should provide adequate motor innervation matching the fascicles in the nerves of the donor muscle, i.e. the funicular pattern of the donor and recipient nerves should be matched as closely as possible. It is, therefore, very important that only pure motor nerve is used as a recipient nerve.

Muscle transfer to provide soft-tissue coverage, vascular bed and as space filler

Viable muscle is excellent as a large vascular bed and as a soft-tissue replacement. These procedures are indicated commonly in combined skin loss and soft-tissue defects seen in severely traumatized limb, failed joint replacement and following tumour resection.

In the lower extremities, the knee and the anterior aspect of the leg have little muscle and other soft-tissue cover. The gastrocnemius flap has proved to be valuable in providing soft-tissue and skin cover to these sites. In the upper extremity, the abductor digiti minimi transfer is useful to replace soft-tissue loss in the volar aspect of the wrist or as a contractile unit for thumb abduction in place of a missing abductor pollicis brevis.

In scarred avascular area following injury or radiation, myocutaneous transfer is a useful technique to provide pliable soft tissue and vascular bed before proceeding to secondary tendon, nerve or bone reconstruction.

In orthopaedic surgery, chronic osteomyelitis has proved to be a difficult problem to manage and has very often been resistant to any treatment. With the introduction of muscle transfer and resection of the infected bone, the old statement of 'once osteomyelitis, always osteomyelitis' is no more true. The main problem is defining the extent of infected necrotic bone as sequestrectomy tends to be limited for fear of a pathological fracture. Sequestrectomy is often incomplete invariably leaving behind areas of infected necrotic bone which is the cause of recurrent flare-up of infection and sinus formation.

Muscle flaps have the following advantages.
1 They allow the occlusion of large cavities of dead space after sequestrectomy.
2 They introduce a large vascular bed to facilitate clearance of infection and resorption of infected avascular necrotic bone and introduce neovasculature to the scarred and sequestrated area.
3 When incorporated with bone, the transfer promotes bony union, strengthens the weakened bone and bridges the bony gap in an osteomyelitic non-united bone.
4 In severe trauma, soft-tissue defect with or without bone loss often produces a cosmetically unacceptable appearance. The muscle harvested can be contoured to fill the defect before covering with a skin graft.

Free muscle transfer as a contractile unit

Transplantation of free vascularized skeletal muscle as a contractile unit is now a proven procedure. It involves microvascular anastomosis of vessels and nerves of transplanted muscles in recipient limbs. This technique is indicated where pedicular muscle or tendon transfer is not feasible. This is seen in irreversible, severe brachial plexus injury, Volkmann's ischaemic contracture and following radical resection of bone tumour. The technique has been established as providing useful and predictable results for active elbow and finger flexion during transfer. One must be careful of the ischaemic time and the loss of muscle bulk following transfer as muscle function is related to the muscle tissue of the transplanted muscle and re-innervation of the muscle.

The transplanted muscle must satisfy the following criteria:

1 the dominant vascular pedicle must be of sufficient size and length to allow anastomosis for adequate perfusion of the muscle;
2 the nerve must have fasciculi which match the corresponding nerve at the recipient site;
3 the muscle is dispensable with no functional loss at the donor site;
4 the muscle must demonstrate an adequate dynamic strength and excursion.

The gracilis, pectoralis major and latissimus have been widely used for the transfer. Gracilis is a striped muscle, the fibres are arranged parallel to the pull of the muscle. Its contractile capacity is estimated to be around 12 cm. Pectoralis major has a contractile capacity of 10 cm because of its pennate nature with shorter muscle fibres. However, it has greater cross-sectional area and therefore provides a more powerful contraction. Latissimus dorsi has a long thoracodorsal vascular pedicle measuring 1.5 mm in diameter with a pedicle length of 7–10 cm. The muscle is superficial. It can be raised with ease. It can be incorporated as a myocutaneous transfer. It can be raised as a free contractile unit to restore finger movement or elbow flexion. It is important to select the muscle with greatest range of movement in its normal site that is required in the newly transplanted site as factors such as adhesion and problem of selecting the physiological resting length will reduce the final range of movement.

In clinical practice, the transplanted muscle must have optimal tension and excursion during anchorage at the proximal and distal junctures. If tension is excessive, ischaemia and fibrosis of the muscle will develop. On the other hand, if the transferred muscle is too lax, contraction will be ineffective. It is extremely difficult to estimate the physiological resting length in an ischaemic transplanted muscle.

In order for the transferred muscle to function normally and to maintain normal volume, re-innervation of the motor nerve to the muscle must be complete. This can only be achieved if the funicular patterns of the donor and recipient nerves are matched as closely as possible. It is also desirable that pure motor nerve is used and nerve suture is close to the neuromuscular juncture to minimize the distance for nerve regeneration. In restoring finger flexion, the anterior interosseous nerve is the best choice. It is the nerve responsible for directing finger movement and is often spared from injury because of its deep location.

Gracilis muscle transfer combined with intercostal nerve can be used in restoring elbow flexion. The intercostal nerve, however, is not a pure motor fibre and therefore when used as a recipient nerve the result is unpredictable. In addition the nerve tends to branch out and becomes smaller at its terminal ends, thus making harvesting of the nerve very difficult. It is preferable to harvest the intercostal nerve posteriorly and bridge it with a nerve graft to the nerve of the gracilis muscle. However, one tends to mix the motor and sensory fibres in the donor nerve. Another distinct disadvantage of using intercostal nerve as recipient nerve is that when the patient coughs, the hand and elbow may flex violently and involuntarily hit the patient's face. However, this will phase out after rehabilitation. Muscle transfer as a contractile unit is technically demanding and return of function may take up to 18 months.

Foot as donor tissue in hand reconstruction

The foot is designed to bear weight. It is now playing an increasingly important role as a donor tissue in free-tissue transplant for reconstruction of the hand since the advancement of microsurgical technique and better understanding of micro-anatomy of the foot. The tissues to be removed do not affect the weight-bearing sole and therefore are predominantly harvested from the dorsal aspect based on the dorsalis pedis vascular system.

Nicoladoni in 1898 introduced the concept of using free-tissue transfer of the foot by using the second toe to reconstruct the missing thumb in the hand. The dorsum of the foot provides an excellent variety of donor tissue for free-tissue transfer:

- Dorsalis pedis flap
- First web space flap
- Hemi-pulp
- Second toe
- Combined second and third toe
- Big toe
- Big toe wrap around flap
- Extensor digitorum brevis
- Extensor tendons
- Second metatarsal
- Second metatarsophalangeal joint
- Composite osteocutaneous tendon graft

PROBLEMS IN FREE-TISSUE TRANSFER FROM THE FOOT

Selection of donor toe

Both the big and second toe for reconstructing the thumb are aesthetically acceptable to the patient in terms of length, strength and mobility for prehension and satisfactory sensation. Big toe transfer for replacement of thumb loss has the advantage that the size of the transferred big toe tends to atrophy and thus resembles the thumb both in appearance and size. It has a large pulp for stability and increased pulp pinch and grip strength. However, the transferred big toe tends to have poor range of movement. Sometimes it may be too big and clumsy. There is also significant donor morbidity especially in terms of cosmesis.

Second-toe transfer for replacement of a missing digit or thumb has the advantage that one can incorporate the adjacent dorsalis pedis flap to provide skin cover with relatively minimal donor morbidity (Fig. 32.6a,b). However, second-toe transfer will always look like a second toe and it has a small pulp (Fig. 32.6c). The small toe may not replace the thumb in pulp pinch strength and cosmetically may not be acceptable. The metatarsophalangeal joint is designed for extension and this joint tends to be in a hyperextended position with the interphalangeal joint in flexed position producing a claw deformity (Fig. 32.6c). In thumb reconstruction, excellent function will be obtained provided there is adequate thenar muscle function.

In children, second and third toes have been used for treatment of congenital hand deformities such as constriction bands, congenital amputations and aplasias. The transferred toe has been shown to have reduced active mobility but will grow if the transplanted toe is functional. However, we noticed that in congenital aplasia of the digits, the deficiency of the tendon and nerve at the recipient site makes reconstruction difficult.

Foot anatomy

The anatomy of the foot which requires tedious dissection to identify anatomical variations of the dorsalis pedis artery, first dorsal metatarsal artery and their branches must be known. Vessel spasm is often encountered in these cases.

FREE VASCULARIZED JOINT TRANSFER IN HAND SURGERY

Indications

1 Non-functioning, painful, unstable or stiff arthritic small joints.
2 Congenital deficiency or abnormality of the joints.
3 Traumatic joint loss including the epiphyses in children.

Joint transfer should be done only if there is adequate skin cover and good sensation with intact tendon apparatus for mobility. The joints of choice are the second to fourth toe metatarsophalangeal joints. The

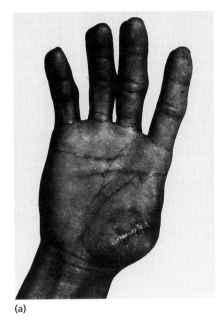
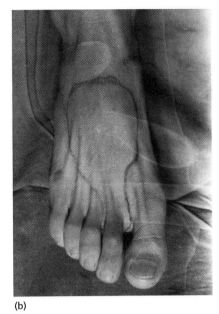
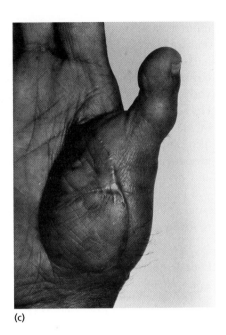

(a)   (b)   (c)

Fig. 32.6 (a) Loss of thumb following trauma. (b) Design of vascularized second-toe transplant based on first dorsal metatarsal artery. (c) Reconstruction of a new 'thumb' using the second toe.

size of the transferred joint must match the healthy finger joint based on radiological appearance.

The metatarsophalangeal joint of the toe has a thick capsule and ligament on the plantar side with strong collateral ligaments. It matches the metacarpophalangeal joint in the hand with the exception of its excessive dorsal extension which is opposite to the dominant palmar flexion of metacarpophalangeal joint. Therefore in the transfer, rotate the metatarsophalangeal joint 180° to reverse extension for flexion.

The blood supply to the second metatarspophalangeal joint is based mainly on the articular branch of the first dorsal metatarsal artery with its accompanying veins for venous drainage. There are often anomalies of this vessel which has to be carefully dissected and preserved.

In digital transfer, sometimes the bone has to be fixed in a relatively flexed position to prevent hyperextension of the metatarsophalangeal joint.

The defect created by harvesting the metatarsophalangeal joint can be replaced with metatarsophalangeal arthrodesis to preserve the toes and to reduce donor morbidity.

Vascularized bone transplant

Vascularized bone grafts were first described by Huntington in 1905. He transposed the fibula with its muscular pedicle to bridge a large defect in the tibia. Taylor Miller and Ham reported on the use of the free vascularized fibula graft in 1975. Since then, large bone defects following trauma, tumour resection and congenital defects have all been reconstructed using free vascularized bone grafts.

Besides the fibula, the rib and iliac crest have also been used as free vascularized transplants to bridge large bone defects. The fibula and iliac crest can also be raised as osteocutaneous transplants when necessary.

Following transplant, the vascularized graft behaves as a segmental fracture and unites with the host bone. However the initial 'immobilization' and disuse results in osteoporosis and weakening of the graft. With optimal stress the vascularized graft rapidly recovers its lost strength and hypertrophies circumferentially. The phenomenon is marked in children where the transplant in time assumes the configuration of the host bone.

During the initial stages stress fractures are not infrequent. It is pertinent to note that stress fractures often present only as a mildly painful swelling, the swelling due to the fracture haematoma and the pain from compression of the surrounding tissue. The vascularized bone graft is aneural and hence insensitive. Radiological assessment reveals the fracture.

DONOR BONE

The *vascularized rib graft* has been used in reconstructing the mandible as the rib is a membraneous bone and conforms to the shape of the mandible. Its blood supply comes from the posterior intercostal, anterior intercostal and the thoracodorsal vessels. The rib may be raised on any one of these pedicles.

The *vascularized iliac crest graft* is supplied by the deep circumflex iliac artery. The origin and course of the vessel is constant. The vessel is large (1.5–2.5 mm in diameter) and suitable for anastomosis.

The overlying skin can be harvested with the bone as an osteocutaneous flap and the donor area can be closed primarily.

The *vascularized fibular graft* has no equal for bridging gaps more than 7.5 cm. It has wide applications.

The advantages are:

1 the fibula is readily available with lengths reaching up to 30 cm;
2 it is a strong cortical bone and designed to withstand weight-bearing stress;
3 its vascular pedicle is constant and large, though short;
4 the proximal fibrocartilaginous head can be harvested as a hemivascularized joint transplant;
5 skin (20 × 10 cm) can be incorporated and the graft raised as an osteocutaneous flap;
6 morbidity from loss of the fibula is minimal.

The rationale for using the free vascularized fibular transplant is that it provides an ideal material for bridging bone defects in most circumstances and introduces the critically needed new vasculature to areas with post-traumatic, post-irradiation and post-infective scarring.

It has been used in the following situations:

1 In management of congenital pseudoarthrosis of tibia, ulna and radius.

2 In management of bone defects following trauma and infective non-union.
3 In reconstruction of large bony defects after tumour resection.

CONGENITAL PSEUDOARTHROSIS OF THE TIBIA (see also Chapter 8.2b)

The primary pathology of this entity is poorly understood. It manifests in young children as a recalcitrant non-union following a pathological fracture. Secondary problems soon ensue and include shortening and atrophy of the affected limb and deformity and stiffness of the adjacent joint. The child is subjected to multiple surgical procedures and not infrequently ends with amputation of the limb.

The treatment for this condition was revolutionized with the use of microsurgical techniques. The pathological tissue adjacent to the non-union was excised radically and the resulting defect bridged with a vascularized fibula graft. The deformity at the non-union and the adjacent joint and shortening of the limb are corrected as a one-stage procedure. Any residual shortening is minimized further by the increased growth of the adjacent epiphysis following the introduction of the new vasculature and weight-bearing stress. The transplanted fibula hypertrophies and becomes tibialized by assuming the character of the host bone for weight-bearing stress.

A problem that gave rise to numerous and varied futile surgical assaults has now been resolved (Fig. 32.7a,b).

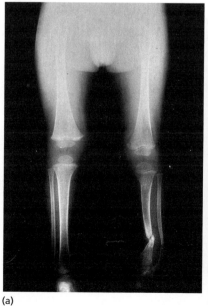 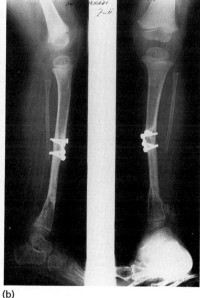

Fig. 32.7 (a) Congenital pseudoarthrosis of left tibia. Note deformity at fracture site and shortening of limb. (b) Following a vascularized fibula graft. Fracture has united. Deformity is corrected and limb growth has taken place.

(a)   (b)

FREE VASCULARIZED BONE TRANSPLANT IN INFECTED NON-UNION WITH LARGE BONE GAPS

Infected non-union in an extensively traumatized limb where the adjacent bed is badly scarred and overlying skin unhealthy is an orthopaedic nightmare. Amputation of the limb has been regularly advised to end the problem.

The advent of the free vascularized bone graft has resolved this problem to a large extent. All dead and doubtfully viable and infected bone and soft tissue are radically excised and the endoskeleton stabilized with an external fixator. Any residual infected sequestra will jeopardise the subsequent procedure.

At the second stage, after the infection has been controlled the free vascularized bone transplant with or without skin is used to bridge the bone defect and provides any necessary skin cover. The neovasculature helps deliver antibiotics in adequate quantities and also facilitates the host to mount a satisfactory immune response in the vicinity in the event of a recrudescence of the infection.

FREE VASCULARIZED BONE IN LIMB SALVAGE FOLLOWING BONE-TUMOUR RESECTION

Limb salvage procedures with wide resection of bone and soft-tissue tumour has now been shown to have similar survival rate as compared to ablative surgery and therefore have gained wide acceptance.

The bony defect following tumour resection may be bridged by custom-made prostheses, allografts, autografts or vascularized autografts. Each of these techniques has its very own inherent advantages and disadvantages. Vascularized bone graft has the advantage of providing soft-tissue coverage and reasonable immediate strength and hypertrophy of bone with time. It may take six months to two years before the graft finally consolidates. Once healed the solution is permanent.

In the lower limb, arthrodesis of the adjacent joint is often indicated as most bone tumours are juxta articular in location and at least one of the joint surfaces must be sacrificed. The small size of the fibula available often necessitates the use of two vascularized fibular grafts to bridge defects in the lower limbs to prevent stress fractures. This is especially so following resection of tumours around the knee.

In the upper limb a single graft is often adequate and following consolidation of the graft rehabilitation is rapid. Following distal radial resection, the proximal fibula including its articular surface may be used as a hemi-vascularized joint transplant to allow preservation of some wrist movement (Fig. 32.8a,b).

Following proximal humeral resection for tumour arthrodesis of the shoulder is preferred with a single graft but stress fractures are not infrequent. Despite these problems, vascularized grafts are still frequently employed as the other alternatives are similarly plagued with complications.

Epiphyseal transplantation

Although free epiphyseal transfer without vascular supply have been partially successful and used by Straub (1929), Wenger (1954), Graham (1954) and others, experimental work has clearly demonstrated viability of the epiphyseal plate for continued longitudinal growth when the epiphysis is vascularized.

The epiphyses selected for transplant should have minimal functional loss at the donor site. Fibular epiphyses and the epiphyses of the toe have been used by the authors.

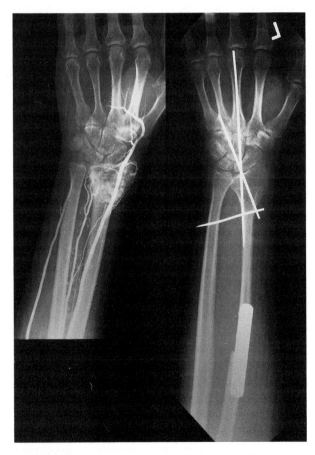

Fig. 32.8 (a) Angiogram in a patient with giant-cell tumour of distal radius. (b) Following wide resection and a vascularized fibula graft. Note reasonable restoration of joint surface by inclusion of fibula head with articular cartilage.

INDICATIONS

Although the procedure is still at an experimental stage, it is a valuable technique and applicable to growing children with: (i) localized epiphyseal growth arrest secondary to surgery, infection or tumour, or with (ii) congenital deficiency of bone and joint especially of the upper extremity.

A careful balance between morbidity of the procedure and benefit to the recipient site should be obtained before this technically demanding microsurgical procedure is undertaken.

CONCLUSION

Microsurgical techniques have opened whole new fields and new possibilities in orthopaedics. Procedures not performed previously are now possible. Microvascular techniques can now even be applied to allografts and experimental work in animals have demonstrated the benefits of microvascular allograft bone transplants. Microvascular procedures are demanding technically and can only be carried out with adequate institutional and personnel support. Careful selection and assessment of patients, skillful execution of the procedure and close post-operative monitoring and careful rehabilitation will keep morbidity both at donor and recipient sites to the minimum and allow the patient to appreciate the results of the reconstruction.

FURTHER READING

Acland R.D. (1979) The free iliac flap. A lateral modification of the free groin flap. *Plastic Reconstruct. Surg.* 64, 30−36.

American Replantation Mission to China (1973) Replantation surgery in China. *Plastic Reconstruct. Surg.* 52, 476−489.

Barwick W.J., Goodking D.J. and Serafin D. (1982) The free scapular flap. *Plastic Reconstruct. Surg.* 69, 779−785.

Barr J.S. (1954) Autogenous epiphyseal transplant. *J. Bone Joint Surg.* 36A, 688.

Bisgard J.D. (1939) Transplantation of epiphyseal cartilage. *Arch. Surg.* 39, 1028.

Bostwick J., Nahal F., Wallace J.C. and Vasconez L.O. (1979) Sixty latissimus dorsi flaps. *Plastic Reconstruct. Surg.* 63, 31−41.

Buncke S.G. and Wearner P.S. (1965) Experimental digital amputation and reimplantation. *Plastic Reconstruct. Surg.* 36, 62−70.

Buncke H.J., Daniller A.I., Schultz W.P. and Chase R.A. (1967) The fate of autogenous whole joints transplanted by microvascular anastomoses. *Plastic Reconstruct. Surg.* 39, 333−341.

Buncke H.J., McLean D.H., George P.T. *et al.* (1973) Thumb replacement: great toe transplantation by microvascular anastomosis. *Br. J. Plastic Surg.* 26, 194−201.

Buncke H.J. and The American Replantation Mission to China (1973) Replantation Surgery in China. Report of the American Replantation Mission to China. *Plastic Reconstruct. Surg.* 52, 476−489.

Buncke S.J., Furnas D.W., Gordon L. and Achauer P. (1977) Free osteocutaneous flap from a rib to the tibia. *J. Plastic Reconstruct. Surg.* 59, 799−805.

Chang T.S. and Wang W. (1981) The use of free forearm flap in hand surgery. *J. Shanghai Med.* 4, 466.

Chen C.W., Chien Y.C. and Poa Y.S. (1963) Salvage of the forearm following complete traumatic amputation. Report of a case. *Chinese Med. J.* 82, 632−638.

Chen Z.W., Chien Y.G., Pao Y.S. and Lin C.T. (1965) Further experiences in the restoration of amputated limbs. *Chinese Med. J.* 84, 225−231.

Chen Z.W. *et al.* (1978) Extremity replantation. *World J. Surg.* 2, 513−524.

Chen Z.W., Yu Z.J. and Wang Y. (1979) A new method of treatment of congenital tibial pseudoarthrosis using free vascularized fibular graft. A preliminary report. *Ann. Acad. Med. Singapore* 8, 465−473.

Chen Z.W., Meyer V.E. and Beasley R.W. (1981) The versatile second toe microvascular transfer. *Orthop. Clin. North Am.* 12, 827−834.

Chen Z.W., Meyer V.E., Kleinert H.E. and Beasley R.W. (1981) Present indications and contraindications for replantation as reflected by long term functional results. *Orthop. Clin. North Am.* 12, 849−870.

Chen Z.W., Quing Q.Y., Jia Y.Z. *et al.* (1982) Free toe transfer. In *Microsurgery.* New York, Springer-Verlag.

Dibbell D.G. (1974) Use of long island flap to bring sensation to the sacral area in young paraplegics. Case report. *Plastic Reconstruct. Surg.* 54, 220−223.

Doi K. (1976) Reimplantation of avulsed thumb with application of neurovascular pedicle. *The Hand* 8, 258−260.

Doi K. (1982) Microsurgical thumb reconstruction—report of six cases with a wrap-around free flap from the big toe and an iliac bone graft. *Ann. Acad. Med.* 11, 225−230.

Donski P.K., Carwell G.R., Scharzer L.A., *et al.* (1979) Growth in revascularized bone grafts in young puppies. *Plastic Reconstruct. Surg.* 64, 239−243.

Dos Santos L.F. (1980) The scapular flap: a new microsurgical free flap. *Boll. Clin. Plastica* 70, 133.

Eiken O., Nabseth D.C. and Deterling R.E. (1964) Limb reimplantation—The pathophysiological effects. *Arch. Surg.* 88, 54−65.

Enneking W.F., Eady J.L. and Burchardt H. (1980) Autogenous cortical bone graft in the reconstruction of segmental skeletal defects. *J. Bone Joint Surg.* 62A, 1039−1058.

Feldman J.J., Cohen B.E. and May J.W. (1978) The medial gastrocnemius myocutaneous flap. *Plastic Reconstruct. Surg.* 60, 531−539.

Freeman B.S. (1959) Growth studies of transplanted epiphyses. *Plastic Reconstruct. Surg.* 23, 584−588.

Gilbert A. and Test L. (1982) The free scapular flap. *Plastic Reconstruct. Surg.* 69, 601−604.

Fitzgerald R.H. Jr. (1980) Experimental osteomyelitis: description of a canine model and the role of depot administration of antibiotics in the prevention and treatment of sepsis. *J. Bone Joint Surg.* 65A, 371−380.

Harii K., Ohmori K., Toru S. *et al.* (1975) Free groin skin flaps. *Br. J. Plastic Surg.* 28, 225−237.

Horn J.S. (1964) Successful reattachment of a completely severed forearm. *Lancet*, **i**, 1152−1154.

Hovnanin A.P. (1956) Latissimus dorsi transfer to restore elbow flexion. *Ann. Surg.* **143**, 493–499.

Ikuta Y., Kubo T. and Tsuge K. (1976) Free muscle transplantation by microsurgical technique to treat severe Volkmann's contracture. *Plastic Reconstruct. Surg.* **58**, 407–441.

Inoue T., Toyoshima Y. and Fukosumi H. (1967) Replantation of severed limbs. *J. Cardiovasc. Surg.* **8**, 31–39.

Jabaley M.E. (1981) Current concepts of nerve repair. *Clin. Plast. Surg.* **8**, 33–44.

Kleinert H.E., Juhala C.A., Tsai T.M. and Van Beek A. (1977) Digital replantation—selection, technique and results. *Orthop. Clin. North Am.* **8**, 309–318.

Kleinert H.E., Jablon M. and Tsai T.M. (1980) An overview of reimplantation and result of 347 reimplants in 245 patients. *J. Trauma* **20**, 390–398.

Komatsu S. and Tamai S. (1968) Successful replantation of completely cut off thumb. *Plastic Reconstruct. Surg.* **42**, 374–377.

Kuo, E.T. *et al.* (1980) Free vascularised small joint transplant — preliminary report of the second metatarsophalangeal joint transfer for reconstruction of damaged metacarpo-phalangeal joint. *Chinese Acad. J. Second Military Med. Coll. Pla.* 1, 2, 12.

Leung P.C. (1981) A new vascular pedicle bone graft for reconstruction of the femoral neck and proximal femur after extensive excision of bone tumour in that region. In *Proceedings of 15th World Congress of SICOT Meeting*.

Leung P.C. (1983) Congenital pseudoarthrosis of the tibia. A report on three cases treated with free vascularised iliac crest graft. *Clin. Orthop. Related Res.* **175**, 45–50.

Leung P.C. (1983) Reconstruction of a large femoral defect using a vascular-pedicled bone graft. *J. Bone Joint Surg.* **65A**, 1179–1180.

Leung P.C. and Kok L.C. (1980) Transplantation of the second toe to the hand. A preliminary report of sixteen cases. *J. Bone Joint Surg.* **62A**, 990–996.

Lichtman D.M., Ahbel D.E., Murphy R.B. and Buncke H.J. (1982) Microvascular double toe transfer for opposable digits — case report and rationale for treatment. *J. Hand Surg.* **7**, 279–283.

Littler J.W. (1960) Neurovascular skin island transfer in reconstructive hand surgery. In *Transactions of the International Society of Plastic Surgeons, Second Congress*. London, Livingstone, pp. 175–178.

Malt R.A. and McKhann C.F (1964) Replantation of severed arm. *J. Am. Med. Ass.* **189**, 716–722.

Manktelow R.T. and McKee N.H. (1978) Free muscle transplantation to provide active finger flexion. *J. Hand Surg.* **3**, 416.

Mathes S.J., Alpert B.S. and Chang N. (1982) Use of the muscle flap in chronic osteomyelitis: experimental and clinical correlation. *Plastic Reconstruct. Surg.* **69**, 815–828.

May J.W. and Daniel R.K. (1978) Great toe to hand tissue transfer. *Clin. Orthop. Related Res.* **133**, 140.

May J.W., Smith R.J. and Peimer C.A. (1981) Toe-to-hand free tissue transfer for thumb construction with multiple digit aplasia. *Plastic Reconstruct. Surg.* **67**, 205.

McCraw J.B., Fishman J.H. and Sharzer L.A. (1978) The versatile gastrocnemius myocutaneous flap. *Plastic Reconstruct. Surg.* **62**, 15–23.

Millesi H. (1979) Microsurgery of peripheral nerves. *World J. Surg.* **3**, 67–69.

Morrison W.A., O'Brien McC. and McLeod A.M. (1978) Digital reimplantation revascularisation — a long term review of 100 cases. *The Hand* **10**, 125–134.

Morrison W.A., O'Brien B.M. and MacLeod A.M. (1980) Thumb reconstruction with a free neurovascular wraparound flap from the big toe. *J. Hand Surg.* **5**, 575–583.

Murray J.F. and Gaveline E. (1967) The neurovascular island pedicle flap. An assessment of late results in sixteen cases. *J. Bone Joint Surg.* **49A**, 1285–1297.

O'Brien B. McC. (1977) *Microvascular Reconstructive Surgery*. London, Churchill Livingstone, pp. 267–289.

O'Brien B.M, Brennen M.D. and MacLeod A.M. (1978) Simultaneous double toe transfer for severely disabled hands. *Hand*, **3**, 232–240.

O'Brien B., MacLeod A.M., Sykes P.J. *et al.* (1978) Microvascular second toe transfer for digital reconstruction. *J. Hand Surg.* **3**, 123–133.

Ohmori K. and Harii K. (1975) Free groin flaps: their vascular basis. *Br. J. Plastic Surg.* **28**, 238–243.

Paletta F.X. (1968) Reimplantation of the amputated extremity. *Ann. Surg.* **168**, 720–726.

Pho R.W.H. (1979) Free vascularized fibular transplant for replacement of lower radius. *J. Bone Joint Surg.* **61B**, 362–365.

Pho R.W.H. (1979) Local composite neurovascular island flap for skin cover in pulp loss of the thumb. *J. Hand Surg.* **4**, 11–15.

Pho R.W.H. (1981) Malignant giant cell tumour of the distal end of the radius treated by free vascularized fibular transplant. *J. Bone Joint Surg.* **63A**, 877–884.

Pho R.W.H. (1983) Free vascularized bone and joint transplant in bone tumour resection. In *The Design and Application of Tumour Prostheses for Bone and Joint Reconstruction*. New York, Thieme-Stratton, pp. 93–97.

Pho R.W.H. and Levack B. (1986) Preliminary observations on epiphyseal growth rate (after free) vascularized fibular graft in congenital pseudoarthrosis of tibia. *Clin. Orthop. Related Res.* **206**, 104–108.

Pho R.W.H., Chacha P.B. and Yeo K.Q. (1979) Rerouting of vessels and nerves from other digits in replanting an avulsed and degloved thumb. *J. Plastic Reconstruct. Surg.* **64**, 330–335.

Pho R.W.H., Chacha P.B., Yeo K.Q. and Daruwalla J.S. (1979) Reimplantation of digits using microvascular technique. *Ann. Acad. Med.* **8**, 398–403.

Pho R.W.H., Vajara R. and Satku K. (1983) Free vascularized bone transplant in problematic non-union of fracture. *J. Trauma* **23**, 341–349.

Pho R.W.H., Levack B., Satku K. and Patradul A. (1985) Free vascularized fibular graft in the treatment of congenital pseudoarthrosis of the tibia. *J. Bone Joint Surg.* **67A**, 64–70.

Ring P.A. (1955) Transplantation of epiphyseal cartilage, an experimental study. *J. Bone Joint Surg.* **37B**, 642–657.

Schenck R. (1977) Free muscle transplantation and composite skin transplantation by microvascular anastomose. *Orthop. Clin. North Am.* **8**, 367–375.

Serafin D., Billarreal-Rios A. and Georgiade N. (1969) A rib containing free flap to reconstruct mandibular defects. *Br J. Plastic Surg.* **30**, 735–745.

Sunderland S. (1978) *Nerves and nerve injuries*, 2nd edn. Edinburgh, Churchill Livingstone.

Sunderland S. (1979) The pros and cons of funicular nerve repair. *J. Hand Surg.* **4**, 201.

Tamai S. (1978) Digits reimplantation. An analysis of 163 replantations in an 11-year old period. *Clin. Plastic Surg.* **5**, 195–209.

Tamai S., Komatsu S., Sakamoto H. *et al.* (1970) Free muscle transplants in dogs with microsurgical neurovascular anastomoses. *Plastic Reconstruct. Surg.* **46**, 219–225.

Tamai S., Micon J., Tupper J. and Flemming J. (1983) Report of subcommittee on reimplantation. *J. Hand Surg.* **8**, 730–732.

Taylor G.I. and Watson N. (1978) One stage repair of compound leg defects with free vascularized flaps of groin skin and iliac bone. *Plastic Reconstruct. Surg.* **61**, 494–506.

Taylor G.I., Miller G.D. and Ham S.J. (1975) The free vascularized bone graft. *J. Plastic Reconstruct. Surg.* **55**, 533–544.

Taylor G.I., Townsend P. and Corlett R. (1979) Superiority of the deep circumflex iliac vessels as the supply for free groin flaps. Clinical work. *Plastic Reconstruct. Surg.* **64**, 745–759.

Terzis J.K. (eds) (1984) Peripheral nerve microsurgery. *Clin. Plastic Surg.* **11**.

Tubiana R. and Duparc J. (1961) Restoration of sensibility in the hand by neurovascular skin island transfer. *J. Bone Joint Surg.* **43B**, 474–480.

Weiland A.J. and Daniel R.K. (1980) Congenital pseudoarthrosis of tibia. Treatment with vascularized autogenesis fibular graft. A preliminary report. *Johns Hopkins Med. J.* **147**, 89–95.

Wenger H.L. (1954) Transplantation of epiphyseal cartilage. *Arch. Surg.* **50**, 148–151.

Wray R.C., Mathes S.M., Young V.L. and Weeks P.M. (1981) Free vascularized whole joint transplants with ununited epiphyses. *Plastic Reconstruct. Surg.* **67**, 519–525.

Yang G.F. (1981) Free forearm flap transfer. A report of 100 cases. In *Proceedings of the Symposium of Free Flap Transfer*, Shenyang, Liaoning, China.

Chapter 33
Management of Spinal Cord Injuries

G. Ravichandran & H.L. Frankel

INTRODUCTION

Traumatic and non-traumatic spinal cord lesions have existed since the early days of the evolution of mankind. For many centuries patients who suffered traumatic spinal cord injury, often as a result of war, died in the battlefield. The Edwin Smith Surgical Papyrus (Bearsted, 1930; Trevor-Hughes, 1988) translated by Dr Breasted not only gives the details of the clinical nature of the patient with paralysis, but also records that this is an ailment that is not to be treated. It is generally believed that surgical intervention on the vertebral column or the spinal cord in patients with traumatic spinal cord injury did not improve the outcome. Lord Nelson, the victor at the Battle of Waterloo, suffered a gunshot injury to his spinal cord and died as a result. The surgeon general, Mr Beatty, is said to have replied to Lord Nelson: 'My Lord, unhappily for our country nothing can be done for you.' Survival following spinal cord injury depended largely on the severity of the neurological lesions. Mortality during the first few months after spinal cord injury for soldiers in the British Army during the First World War was of the order of 50% and the overall mortality rate at 3 years was estimated at 80% (Thompson-Walker, 1937). An interesting account of the history of the management of spinal cord injury in the 20th century has been given by Sir George Bedbrook (Bedbrook, 1987, 1992). The pioneering and uncompromising work of Sir Ludwig Guttman during the latter part of the Second World War formed the foundation of the modern care of paraplegia. He recognized that unlike other forms of injury, a person with spinal cord injury required a team of dedicated doctors, nurses and therapists who have an in-depth understanding on all aspects of care. He pioneered a doctrine of comprehensive care involving not merely the orthopaedic aspects of trauma but the emotional, the psychological and vocational care in addition to a myriad physiological

lesions that are unique to a patient with spinal cord injury. The cost-effectiveness of this comprehensive care has been recognized throughout the world to the extent that even developing countries are now able to offer a high level of care to their patients (Bedbrook, 1992; Young, 1992).

The current model of spinal injury care in the UK is one where an appropriately trained physician or surgeon leads a team of highly trained nurses, physiotherapists, occupational therapists, social workers and others all dedicated to provide a maximum care to the patient with spinal cord injury. This has resulted in a significant increase in the survival of patients with very high cervical cord lesions. There are at least 20 ventilator-dependent tetraplegic patients in this country at present, some of whom have survived for 11 years or more. Such a team, in addition to providing the necessary medical support, liaises with the community and the various social service organizations so that the patient with disability can be treated on an equal footing by employment agencies, housing authorities and in the field of sports.

Sport has assumed an important role in patients with spinal cord injury, most of whom are young men and women in their productive and competitive stages of life. The first Wheelchair Games were held in 1945 and by 1948 the games took on a more official role. The Sports Organization for the disabled throughout the world began to exchange ideas and, in 1952, the first International Games between wheelchair athletes took place at Stoke Mandeville Hospital in the UK. International games for wheelchair athletes have since been held in Rome, Tokyo, Tel Aviv, Heidelburg, Holland, Toronto and Stoke Mandeville.

Along with developments in the field of sport for the disabled, the medical and paramedical fraternity began to share their experiences. This desire to exchange the knowledge between physicians from different parts of the globe resulted in the formation of the International

Medical Society of Paraplegia (IMSOP). The first meeting of IMSOP was held in 1960. Annual meetings of IMSOP are held in different venues throughout the world and its membership now exceeds 1000. The Society also has several associate members and takes a leading and active role in encouraging members from developing countries to participate in international conferences by offering fellowships and scholarships to suitable candidates.

With increasing awareness among a variety of physicians in the care of patients with spinal cord injury, many nations now have their own national or regional spinal cord societies. In addition the paralysed patients have organized their own societies/associations, to represent their views not only to their governments but also to the physicians who treat them. Survival following traumatic spinal cord injury has improved enormously over the years as a result of an integrated approach in the management of the paralysed (Koning *et al.*, 1987). Unfortunately patients who suffer from other conditions, such as demyelinating lesions of the spinal cord or motor neurone disease, do not receive such a comprehensive care by a dedicated team led by a physician and do not survive as well or as long as patients with traumatic/non-traumatic spinal cord injury.

AETIOLOGY

In the Western world, road traffic accidents are by far the commonest cause of acute traumatic spinal cord injury. Motor cars, motor vehicles and pedestrian accidents constitute over 50% of all traumatic admissions to a spinal injuries unit. Each year around 15 per million residents of the UK are likely to suffer from major paralysis as a result of spinal cord injury (Kurtzke, 1975; Krans *et al.*, 1975; Yashon, 1986). Necropsy studies following road traffic accidents put this incidence at 50 per million per year. There is a wide geographical variation in the cause and incidence of spinal cord injury. Gunshot wounds leading to spinal cord injury are not uncommon in California while bicycle-spoke injuries (where a shortened bicycle spoke is thrust under the lamina of the cervical spine to produce paralysis) is one cause of tetraplegia in Southern Africa. A recent epidemiological study concludes that the current rate of traumatic spinal cord injury is of the order of 30–40 new cases per million population (Harvey *et al.*, 1990). Falls at home and industrial accidents are responsible for 10–30% of traumatic spinal cord injury in the Western world. Fall of masonry on workers and fall from a height or a tree are common causes leading to spinal cord injury in South-East Asia. Sporting accidents often due to diving, gymnastics and rugby are not an uncommon cause of traumatic spinal cord injury.

Traumatic spinal cord injury is three to four times more common among men compared to women.

Cervical spine

Injuries to the cervical spine may occur following a fall down a flight of steps or following diving. Motor vehicle accidents, often a rear shunting one, result in a violent extension followed by flexion injury to the neck resulting in tetraplegia. Elderly patients suffer a hyperextension type of cervical spinal cord injury following a minor fall banging their forehead against a hard object.

Thoracic spine

Compression fractures with or without dislocation of the upper thoracic spine are commonly seen following a collision between a motor cycle rider and an automobile. The regulation demanding the use of full-face helmet appears to protect the cervical spine of the motor cyclist by transferring the forces of a collision to the upper thoracic spine. In many cases, radiography following such accidents shows an alarming widening of the superior mediastinum giving a false picture of an aortic injury. Occasionally such cases are associated with injuries to the brachial plexus. Thoracic spine injury is not uncommonly seen in osteoporotic women following minor falls. Injuries to the thoracic spine are less commonly seen among drivers of motor vehicles while it is not uncommon among back seat passengers.

Thoracolumbar junction

This is a relatively mobile part of the vertebral column and injuries between T11 and L2 are frequently seen. In addition to motor vehicle accidents, injuries to the thoracolumbar spine occur as a result of a fall of an object onto the back, typically in the coal-mining industry. Horse-riding accidents can result in injuries to the lower thoracic and upper lumbar spine. Neurological damage to the spinal cord is often incomplete. Surgical stabilization of the vertebral column in certain cases reduces pain and morbidity. Injuries to the bony architecture are often complex as a result of a flexion rotation component at the time of the accident. Soft-tissue bruising may be extensive and sometimes associated with rib injuries, kidney injuries and splenic/liver injury.

Lumbar spine

Injuries to the lumbar spine generally follow a road traffic accident when the restraining lap strap produces acute flexion of the lumbar spine following a head-on collision. Damage to the conus of the spinal cord results in flaccid paraplegia. Damage to the cauda equina results in an incomplete paralysis of the lower extremities. Surgical stabilization where appropriate of these vertebral column injuries results, not only in early mobilization of the victim, but also a significant reduction in pain in the acute and chronic phase.

Non-traumatic spinal lesions

Vascular lesions to the spinal cord are seen usually in the elderly. Anterior spinal artery thrombosis might occur following minor illness such as cold or flu. Spinal cord damage may be associated with pre-existing arteriovenous malformation of the spinal cord. Major cord lesions have been caused during anaesthesia (hypoxic) and during surgical correction of scoliosis either due to distraction or impingement on the cord. Paralysis has occurred as a result of corrective osteotomy of the spine and following dorsal disc surgery. Minor lesions of the cauda equina are not uncommon following disc surgery resulting in some degree of bladder/bowel/sexual dysfunction. Infections to either the vertebral column (tuberculous/pyogenic/parasitic) or the epidural space can lead to paralysis. Spontaneous spinal haematoma has been reported leading to paraplegia. Pre-existing conditions such as rheumatoid arthritis and ankylosing spondylitis can complicate the outcome from spinal cord injury due to minor falls. Paraplegia can be of a slow onset in patients who have had radiation to their vertebral column. Radiation myelitis tends to be slow in onset but progressive in nature. Other unrelated conditions such as Paget's disease of the vertebral column, rapid decompression following deep-sea diving and spinal anaesthesia are but a few of many causes that can and do cause paraplegia (Kurtzke, 1975; Krans *et al.*, 1975; Yashon, 1986; Harvey *et al.*, 1990). Neoplasic conditions of the spine, spinal cord or metastatic deposits from a distant primary causing spinal cord lesions will not be considered in this chapter.

RECOGNITION OF SPINAL CORD INJURY

Injuries to the spine that have the potential to lead to neuraxis trauma are often difficult to assess on clinical grounds alone. In general, spinal injuries should be suspected in patients who are unconscious and who have a head injury following a trauma and in those who have multiple injuries following accidents. Pain and spasm around the spine should arouse suspicion of possible spinal cord injury. In the cervical spine, a rotation of the neck (Cock Robin pose) may be seen not only in dislocations of C1/2 but also unifacet dislocations of the cervical spine (Ravichandran, 1978). Careful palpation of the spinous processes might show either a sudden change in the alignment of the spinous process or a palpable gap (usually seen in bifacet dislocation). A palpable gap can be recognized in patients with dorso-lumbar spinal injury who often have associated extensive soft-tissue bruising surrounding the site of maximum tenderness.

In a conscious patient, neurological assessment often reveals loss of either sensation and/or muscle power in the lower extremities. In an unconscious patient, however, examination is often difficult since precise neurological signs depend on the cooperation of a conscious patient. The seven major causes of failure to recognize vertebral or spinal cord injury are shown in Table 33.1. It is important that every patient arriving at the emergency room after a major accident is thoroughly examined and assessed to exclude spinal cord injury. Many instances of missed injuries of spinal cord have been documented (Ravichandran and Silver, 1982). In addition to causing severe disability to the victim, failure to recognize spinal cord injury leading to mismanagement inevitably ends in medical malpractice litigation

Table 33.1 Conditions contributing to a failure to recognise spinal cord injury

Clinical state	Cause
Unconsciousness due to head injury	Lack of relevant history and difficult neurological assessment
Drug/alcohol intoxication	Misinterpretation of neurological signs as relating exclusively to intoxication
Pre-existing locomotor dysfunction, e.g. ankylosing spondylitis, multiple sclerosis	Failure to interpret pre-existing disability and assumption that present disability is unrelated to the accident
Minimal paralysis	Mistaken and disregarded as post-injury pain inhibition
Ambience of the accident, e.g. stolen-vehicle driver being chased by police before accident presenting with 'paralysis'	Medical officer incorrectly influenced by the circumstances of the accident and assuming 'malingering' by the victim
Radiological problems	Poor-quality radiograph, radiography of the wrong part, too much reliance for radiological demonstration of the fracture
Multiple injury	Attention of the doctor being drawn to life-saving measures

against the health service. The American College of Emergency Physicians recommends that patients with a potential to have spinal cord injury should be examined for pain with radiation, impairment of movements in the lower extremities, presence or absence of neurogenic paradoxical ventilatory movements, and impaired movements of the intrinsics of the hand musculature (Kelley, 1979).

NEUROLOGICAL EVALUATION

This should be done methodically and thoroughly. Even in an unconscious patient certain cardinal signs could be elicited so that the presence of spinal cord injury could be suspected. Clinical examination should include the documentation of blood pressure, pulse, respiratory rate, pupillary reaction and state of consciousness. Any symptoms of root irritation, either in the upper or in the lower extremities, should be documented (Fig. 33.1). Localized tenderness over the spine is an invaluable sign. In an unconscious patient, withdrawal of the extremity from a painful stimulus will be noticed normally above the level of the spinal lesion but will be absent below. Priapism in a male patient can be suggestive of spinal cord injury. Except in a deeply unconscious patient absent tendon reflexes very often indicate spinal shock. On occasions, patients may present with unexplained retention of urine due to a conus lesion.

A low blood pressure, without concomitant tachycardia, is seen in patients with cervical spinal cord injury. As a result of sympathetic paralysis in these patients there is associated peripheral vasodilatation. The extremities are warm. In the absence of obvious blood loss, such as might follow an extremity fracture, these patients do not require rapid transfusion or infusion provided the systolic blood pressure is not significantly below 80 mmHg. The central venous pressure also remains low in these patients. A fluid challenge fails to alter the central venous pressure.

The pulse rate in a complete tetraplegic patient is low and may be in the region of 50−60 beats per minute.

The patient might by hypothermic, particularly if exposed to cold weather prior to transfer to the Accident and Emergency Department. The patient may be confused due to hypothermia which will be difficult to distinguish from an associated head injury. These patients should not be warmed rapidly and the use of hot water bottles is strongly condemned.

Sensory assessment should be done in a methodical and dermatomal fashion (Fig. 33.2). Hypodermic needles should not be used to test pin-prick sensation. Disposable 'neurotips' (blunt pins) are preferable to a common pin.

The practice of using the same sharp pin on a large number of patients is inadvisable. Neurological assessment often commences at the sole of the foot (S1) and progresses along the anterior aspect of the lower extremity to the anterior superior iliac spine (D12/L1). Sensory assessment should then proceed towards the umbilicus (D10) and outwards towards the axilla (D2/3). Because of the overlap of C4 and D2 dermatomes on the anterior aspect of the chest, sensory assessment in tetraplegic patients should extend to the axilla and then towards the medial aspect of the arm and forearm. Evidence for any sacral sensory sparing should be searched in the Accident and Emergency Department because of its great prognostic significance. Minor sacral sensory sparing may subsequently disappear due to cord oedema, only to re-appear several days later. Failure to document these can lead to the erroneous conclusion that a therapeutic manoeuvre such as administration of steroid or an operative intervention has influenced the neurological outcome.

Assessment of motor power of individual muscles is often difficult in the presence of soft-tissue/bony injuries in the lower extremities. Certain specific muscles in the upper and lower extremities together with an assessment of the muscle power of the diaphragm, intercostals and abdominals will often give an overview of the extent of preserved voluntary motor power (Fig. 33.1). Proper documentation of the muscle power will usually help in evaluating any deterioration of spinal cord function while undergoing treatment.

Tendon reflexes in the upper and lower extremities, together with superficial reflexes (abdominal, cremasteric) should be documented. Two further superficial reflexes should be assessed in patients with suspected spinal cord injury. The bulbo cavernosus reflex (S2−S4) is demonstrated by gently squeezing the glans penis or a sharp pin-prick over the clitoris while observing the contraction of the bulbo cavernous muscle. Anal skin reflex (S5) is elicited by stimulating the para-anal skin with a sharp pin which results in the anal muscle contraction. These reflexes may disappear after a few hours due to spinal shock and tend to re-appear a few weeks later. The presence or absence of these reflexes during examination does not by itself give any clue as to the prognosis following spinal cord injury. The presence of these reflexes, however, usually helps clinicians in planning the appropriate bladder and bowel management of the paralysed. Thus, patients with anal reflex often respond to suppositories and their bladders will eventually void reflexly.

2 yr	1 yr	6 mo	3 mo	1 mo	1 wk	init	Date	Left (50)	Muscles		(50) Right	Date	init	1 wk	1 mo	3 mo	6 mo	1 yr	2 yr
									TRAUMA MOTOR INDEX										
								0–5	Biceps	C–5	0–5								
								0–5	Wrist ext	C–6	0–5								
								0–5	Triceps	C–7	0–5								
								0–5	Flex prof	C–8	0–5								
								0–5	Intrinsic	T–1	0–5								
								0–5	Iliopsoas	L–2	0–5								
								0–5	Quadricep	L–3	0–5								
								0–5	Tib anter	L–4	0–5								
								0–5	Ex hallucis	L–5	0–5								
								0–5	Gastroc	S–1	0–5								
									Bilateral total		100								
								0/+	Diaphragm		0/+								
								0/+	Intercost		0/+								
								0/+	Abdominal		0/+								
								0/+	Anal sph		0/+								
									Reflexes										
									Biceps	C5–6									
									Triceps	C–6									
									Supinator	C–7									
									Knee	L3–4									
									Ankle	L5–S1									
									Abdominal	D7–12									
									Cremasteric	L2									
									B–C reflex	S3–4									
									Anal	S5									
									Plantar	S1									

Fig. 33.1 Spinal injury chart. Minimum number of muscles that should be assessed following spinal cord injury. A recommended way of documenting the neurological deficit by the emergency room physician.

CLINICAL SYNDROMES

The various sensory and motor tracts are arranged in a lamellar fashion within the spinal cord. The spinal cord is normally supplied by a large anterior median sulcal artery and two posterior arteries. Radicular feeding arteries arise on either side at different levels often in association with the nutrient artery to the vertebral body from the intercostal artery. Because of the lamellar orientation of the various tracts within the spinal cord,

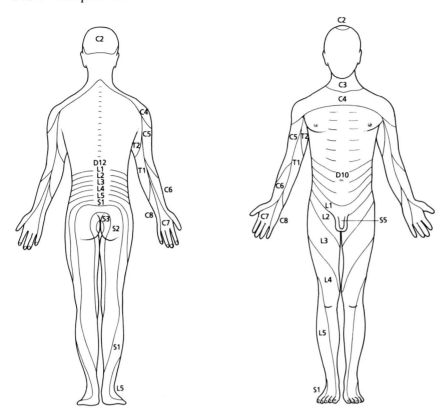

Fig. 33.2 Anterior and posterior view of sensory distribution of various dermatomes. Note overlap of C4 with T2 on the anterior aspect of the chest.

it is possible to clinically divide the lesions into various syndromes.

Complete paralysis is said to exist when there is no sensory or motor sparing below a given neurological level. This is often referred to as Frankel Grade A lesions (Frankel *et al.*, 1969) (Table 33.2). Incomplete spinal cord injury may present with either sensory or motor sparing (Fig. 33.3).

Anterior cord syndrome

When the injury is predominantly confined to the anterior part of the spinal cord, as might happen following a massive disc protrusion or an occlusion of the anterior spinal artery, most of the tracts that are situated anteriorly and supplied by the anterior spinal artery

are damaged resulting in anterior spinal cord syndrome. These patients have varying degrees of motor deficit but will have intact light touch and joint position sense. Pain and temperature sense are usually compromised.

Posterior cord syndrome

This clinical condition arises following neurosurgical procedures, such as removal of an ependymoma through a dorsal myelotomy. The posterior tracts normally responsible for light touch and position sense are compromised. There may be associated damage to the posterior spinal arteries. Most patients with posterior cord syndrome have some degree of motor sparing due to intact anterior cortico-spinal tract and, to some degree, lateral cortico-spinal tract.

Central cord syndrome

This condition is commonly seen in elderly patients, often following a trivial fall when the neck is forcibly extended. The cord is compressed between the thickened ligamentum flavum posteriorly and the osteophytes between the vertebrae anteriorly. A bleed into the spinal cord, usually at the centre of the cord occurs which gradually spreads outwards. Thus, the spinal tracts which are located towards the centre of the spinal

Table 33.2 Frankel grading

Grade	Observation
Grade A	Complete sensory motor loss at a certain level
Grade B	Sensory sparing only below the level of the lesion
Grade C	Functionally useless motor sparing
Grade D	Useful motor sparing below the lesion
Grade E	Neurologically symptom free but abnormal reflexes may be present

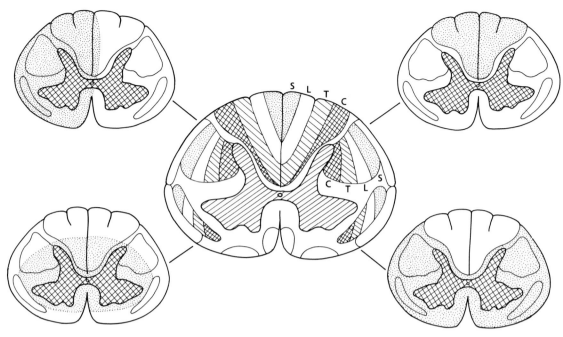

Fig. 33.3 Spinal cord syndromes. Top left, Brown−Sequard's syndrome; top right, posterior cord syndrome; bottom right, anterior cord syndrome; bottom left, central cord syndrome. S = sacral, L = lumbar, T = thoracic, C = cervical.

cord are more frequently damaged than those which are further away from the centre of the spinal cord. Thus the cervical and thoracic tracts which are closer to the centre of the cord tend to be more compromised than the innervation of the lower extremities. These patients have varying degrees of sensory motor preservation in the lower extremities and are often able to walk following rehabilitation. The skeletal damage is often minimal and orthopaedic intervention unnecessary.

Brown−Sequard syndrome

This condition arises when the damage to the spinal cord is localized to one half of the spinal cord as might follow a stab injury. The neurological picture is very distinct. Since pyramidal (cortico-spinal) tracts have already crossed to the appropriate side of the spinal cord, there is often a dense motor paralysis on the side of the lesion with a relative preservation of sensation (spinal thalamic function, pain and temperature). On the unaffected side of the spinal cord there is loss of spinal thalamic function with preserved motor power.

PATHOPHYSIOLOGY OF SPINAL CORD INJURY

Immediately after traumatic spinal cord injury there is seldom a macroscopic change on the spinal cord.

Petecheal haemorrhages usually begin at the centre of the spinal cord, possibly releasing catecholamines. There is gradual loss of electrolytes, such as potassium, from the neural tissue (Lewin *et al.*, 1974). This leads to altered membrane potential and oedema. The extra-cellular fluid which is rich in potassium is thought to be responsible for the clinical phenomenon referred to as 'spinal shock' (Bach-y-Rita and Illis, 1993). There is, however, very seldom a true increase in serum potassium (Fig. 33.4).

A few hours after the spinal cord injury the central bleeding has progressed to central necrosis and there is tissue destruction, chromatolysis and a gradual swelling of the nerve ends. There is fragmentation of intracellular bodies (neurofibrils). Histological changes that are observed in the nerve tracts appear to progress at a substantially slower speed than those observed in the cerebral cortex following trauma. There is temporal discrepancy between the histological damage observed following spinal cord trauma and the clinical picture. Thus, the clinical signs and symptoms lag behind the destructive process progressing at the level of the spinal cord (Ducker *et al.*, 1978).

The extent of central grey matter damage seems to be influenced by the magnitude of initial violence and the systemic blood pressure. In animal experiments, when the trauma is relatively small, causing neuropraxia only; the histological changes show minimal oedema but there

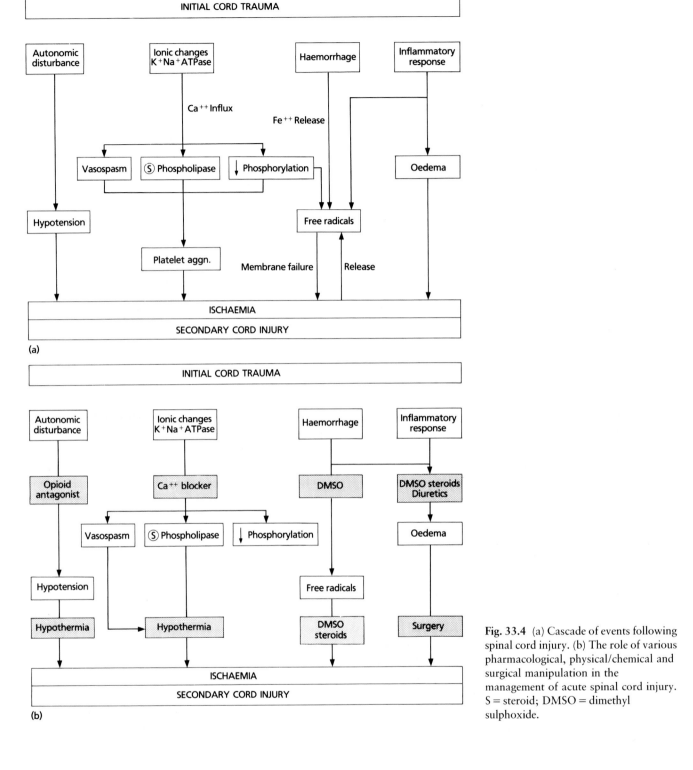

Fig. 33.4 (a) Cascade of events following spinal cord injury. (b) The role of various pharmacological, physical/chemical and surgical manipulation in the management of acute spinal cord injury. S = steroid; DMSO = dimethyl sulphoxide.

is still chromatolysis, vacuolation and alterations in cytoplasmic density. However, when the trauma to the spinal cord is sufficient to produce permanent neurological deficit in these animals there is profound haemorrhage and, at a later stage, there is phagocytosis, vacuolation and formation of a cavity inside the spinal cord. The cavitation is a result of replacement of the destroyed neural tissue with a glial scar.

When central haemorrhage is extensive following acute trauma, the cavities may be extensive. Haematomyelia (bleeding inside the spinal cord) could lead to further neurological deterioration in the acute phase. In the long term these cavities may communicate with subarachnoid space and remain collapsed. In some instances, however, the cavities may distend to produce neurological change due to syringomyelia (Fig. 33.5).

Following spinal cord trauma there is an alteration of spinal cord perfusion. Several chemicals are released at the site of injury which seem to have an adverse effect on the cord perfusion. Experimental studies show that immediately after spinal cord injury there is loss of blood circulation over the central haemorrhagic area. The central grey matter is in a state of haemorrhagic non-profusion for about 2 hours. Angiographic studies show that there is a focal constriction of spinal cord blood vessels and occasional distension of distal arteries inside the spinal cord. There is some evidence to suggest that spinal cord profusion may be influenced by P_{CO_2}. There is experimental evidence to suggest that failure of neurovascular membranes leading to leaking from the capillaries contribute to oedema which further compresses the blood vessels causing ischaemia and neuronal damage (Fig. 33.4).

It has been shown that there is a fall in the level of biogenic amines including dopamine lasting for several days after the spinal cord injury. More recently an impressive array of neuropeptides such as neuropeptide Y, vasopressin, oxytocin, vasoactive intestinal peptides, Substance P and metenkephalins have been seen in the lateral horn of the spinal cord. The evidence, to date, seems to suggest that a complex series of biochemical reactions take place following spinal cord injury. These are influenced by P_{O_2}, P_{CO_2} and arterial blood pressure (Bannister, 1988).

It will be evident from the above brief description that complex biochemical changes follow acute spinal cord injury. Various pharmacological agents have been used by different investigators in order to reduce cord damage. Steroids (Brachen *et al.*, 1990) and gangliosides (Geisler *et al.*, 1992) have been reported in humans to improve recovery of spinal cord function. Early administration of steroids is now considered important in certain states in the USA. An initial improvement in function in patients treated with steroids soon after injury fails to be statistically significant when compared at one year. Ganglioside therapy appears to show some improvement in function even when given a few days after injury. Others have claimed some therapeutic success following surgery and cooling of the cord (Fig. 33.4).

Unfortunately the various therapeutic regimens do not show convincing evidence of producing recovery of function following spinal cord trauma.

TRANSPORT

It is important to question all victims of motor vehicle accidents if they have any pain over the spine. Equally, attempts should be made to elicit voluntary movement of the lower extremities before transporting a victim of a road traffic accident provided there is no obvious extremity fracture. Clearly a conscious patient reporting pain in his lower extremity is unlikely to have suffered major neurological damage. If the patient is trapped under a vehicle, during extraction the use of a Heinz cervical splint or a spinal board will prevent unnecessary movement to the neck and upper thoracic spine. If unconscious and there is a risk of vomiting during transport, the patient will be transferred in a stable lateral position provided the alignment of the neck and the thoracic spine is maintained. A conscious patient with suspected cervical spine injury should be transported with either a soft collar or a stiff neck collar

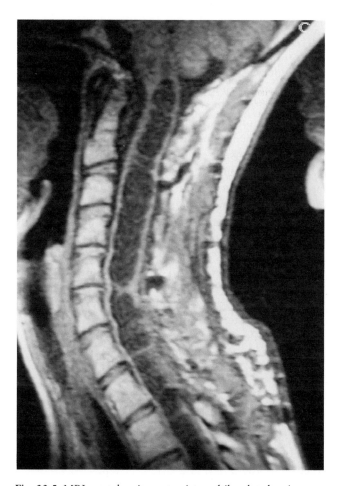

Fig. 33.5 MRI scan showing extensive multiloculated syrinx extending to C1 level in a patient with D3/4 paraplegia 3 months after a road traffic accident.

(Fig. 33.6). The neck may be further immobilized with the use of sandbags on either side of the head. It would be foolish to attribute the victim's inability to move lower extremities or walk to any pre-existing cause such as arthritis, ankylosing spondylitis or drunkeness (Table 33.1). Patients have been transported from the site of an accident with normal lower extremity movement, only to arrive at the Accident and Emergency Department totally paralysed due to unsupported neck movements in transit.

If the patient has to be lifted care should be taken to organize the lift so that the three- or four-person lift does not produce undue shift of the vertebral column. Any sharp objects on the person of the paralysed should be removed before transfer.

The paralysis of the sympathetic nervous system as a result of spinal cord injury may lead to peripheral vasodilatation with consequent loss of body temperature. Care should be taken to warm the patient gradually with appropriate blankets during transit.

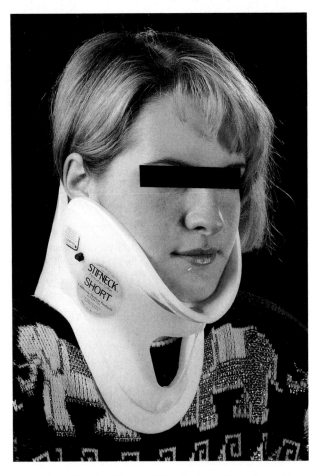

Fig. 33.6 Stiff neck collar, available in three sizes. It provides reasonably rigid fixation to the cervical spine of acutely injured patients.

Apart from victims in inaccessible sites, such as a ravine following fall from a cliff face, in most instances the patient may be transported using an ambulance to the nearest Accident and Emergency Department. Particular attention should be made to prevent the development of hypothermia during transfer of patients in a helicopter.

MANAGEMENT OF ACUTE SPINAL CORD INJURY

Radiological evaluation

If the paralysis is clinically obvious, radiography of the appropriate part of the spinal column should be supervised by a senior medical officer and a team of nurses who are able to supervise the transfer of the patient onto the radiography table. The use of an Easiglide (a transfer aid which is a soft rolling mattress) will reduce unnecessary lifting of the patient.

Attempts should be made to obtain the best possible radiography of the spine in order that the management can be planned. It is often difficult to visualize the cervico-thoracic junction in a patient with lower cervical spinal injury. Associated spasm and a lack of cooperation by the patient could prevent easy radiological demonstration of this area of the neck. Unsupervised and strong pull on the shoulder of paralysed and unco-operative patient could result in the neck being rolled into hyperextension position. This has the potential to cause further neurological damage and should not be attempted without appropriate supervision of the patient by trained medical and nursing staff.

If spinal cord injury is suspected from history of the accident but could not be confirmed on clinical grounds, preliminary radiography should include anterior posterior and lateral views of the suspected part of the vertebral column. Following evaluation of these radiographs, further radiography may be organized.

Anterior posterior radiographs of the cervical spine often give details which may be masked in a poor quality lateral radiograph (Fig. 33.7) (Scher, 1979; Ravichandran and Silver, 1984).

Supine oblique radiography, or 20° oblique views, usually gives details of the entire cervical spine and the apophyseal joints. These radiographs help, not only in initial evaluation, but also to evaluate when the reduction of a cervical dislocation is achieved following traction (Figs 33.8 and 33.9).

Antero-posterior and lateral tomograms may be required to get adequate details of the upper thoracic and mid-thoracic fractures. Such radiography should be

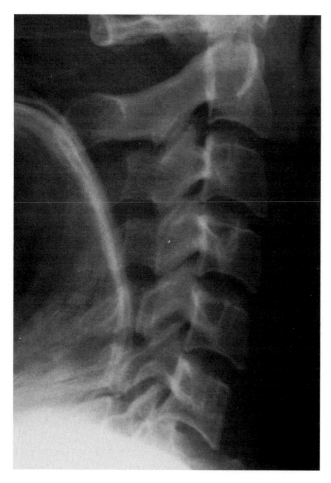

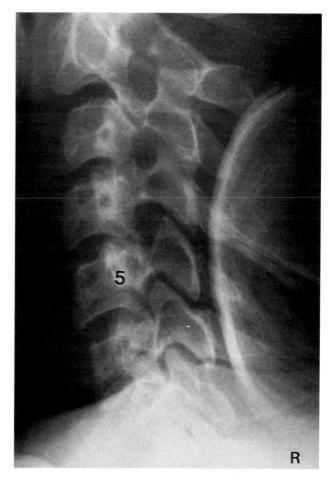

Fig. 33.7 Lateral view of cervical spine showing burst fracture C7 with complete tetraplegia below.

Fig. 33.8 A 20° oblique view (Lodge Moor oblique view) of the same patient in Fig. 33.7 showing details of right apophyseal joint. The radiograph was obtained by elevating the left shoulder on a pillow while the cervical traction is maintained. The radiographic beam passes parallel to the bed.

done after positioning the patient with minimal malalignment of the vertebral column.

Chest radiographs are often required in tetraplegic patients to ascertain any pre-existing pulmonary pathology. Patients with upper thoracic injury may have paravertebral haemotama which might mimic an aortic injury. There may be associated haemopneumothoraces. It must be remembered that, on occasions, there may be more than one vertebral column injury. It is a useful practice to radiograph the entire spinal column.

Fractures to the lower extremities in a paralysed victim may be overlooked as a result of loss of sensation and pain. After careful examination, any suspected soft-tissue bruise in the extremities should be radiologically examined to exclude a bony injury.

Intrathecal contrast examination following spinal cord injury has limited value and the technique of myelography can itself lead to further neurological trauma. Computed tomography of the vertebral column offers a significant advantage in understanding the bony archi-

tecture and the extent of spinal canal compromise following a vertebral fracture (Fig. 33.10). It must be remembered that the presence of a bony fragment causing spinal canal compromise does not constitute an absolute indication for decompressive surgery. Many patients with severe spinal column damage have escaped spinal cord injury (Fig. 33.11).

Magnetic resonance imaging (MRI) offers by far the safest method of evaluating the spinal cord. Even in the acute stage, MRI scans reveal specific changes inside the spinal cord in patients with paralysis. MRI images can be enhanced using gadolinium. Signal suppression reduces various artefacts that are normally seen in MRI scan and it is now possible to generate a three-dimensional image of the spinal cord using volume acquired imaging techniques. It is even possible to study spinal cord blood flow using magnetic resonance and angiography (Perovitch and Wang, 1992).

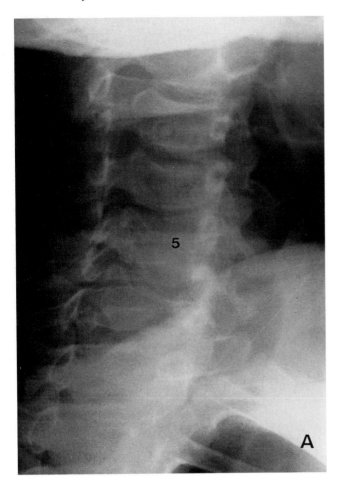

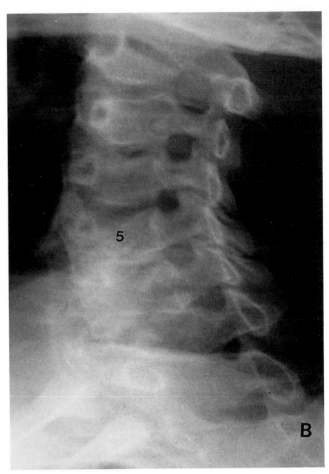

Fig. 33.9 (a,b) Left and right supine oblique views of the cervical spine of the patient shown in Fig. 33.7. The left oblique view is obtained by placing the radiographic plate behind left shoulder and left side of the neck of the patient while the radiographic beam centres at the midpoint of the right sternomastoid muscle inclined at an angle of 45° to coronal plane. Note the separation of C6—C7 apophyseal joints and fracture of left C6 lamina.

General considerations

There is no immediate need to inform either the patient or relatives details of the consequences of spinal cord injury. Insensitive handling of either the patient or the relative by the physician attending in the Accident and Emergency Department often leads to a long-lasting antagonism towards the primary hospital. It also causes unnecessary emotional trauma to the patient. In most cases it is impossible to state, with any degree of certainty, the extent of spinal cord damage soon after admission to the Accident and Emergency Department. Any attempt at counselling the patient or the relative on the prognosis should therefore be recorded.

An intravenous line must be set up using a crystalloid since the paralysed patient is unlikely to be able to take adequate oral fluids for several days. If the patient has no other injury, fluid replacement should be moderate since excessive fluid infusion could lead to pulmonary oedema. Most patients develop paralytic ileus even though bowel sounds may be present for a few hours after the spinal cord injury. Unless there is a risk of vomiting there is no indication for routine nasogastric intubation and aspiration.

In addition to estimation of routine haematological and biochemical parameters, liver function must be assessed. Serum amylase may be raised a few days after spinal cord injury in patients who have had hypothermia.

Acute withdrawal of nicotine and alcohol following spinal cord injury might precipate symptoms not dissimilar to anxiety neurosis and might mimic at times a clinical picture similar to fat embolism. In tetraplegic patients, smoking should be prohibited and the use of alcohol should be discouraged. Prompt supportive

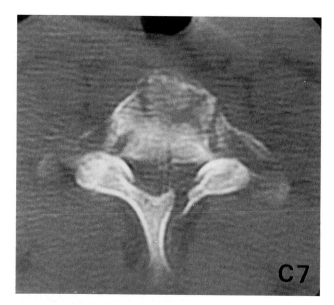

Fig. 33.10 Computed tomography scan. Fracture of C7 showing lamina fracture and destruction of the body.

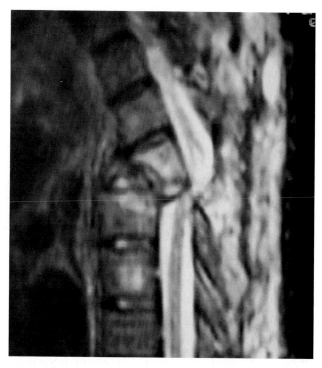

Fig. 33.11 Paraparesis due to tuberculosis of the spine. Neurology deteriorated following decompressive surgery (costotransversectomy). The patient became completely paralysed over a 3-week period. MRI scan showing significant spinal canal compromise. He subsequently made good neurological recovery without further surgical intervention.

therapy for patients who suffer from acute alcohol withdrawal will reduce general distress faced by the patient and their relatives.

Nursing management (Couldwell and Carlisle, 1990)

Nursing care for a paralysed person is a team activity, initially by trained nurses and ancillary staff and subsequently by the patient's carer and the patient himself or herself. The object is most instances is an interaction between a conscious patient and the lead nurse carrying out a particular manoeuvre. Such an interaction provides a willing participation on the part of the patient in care. By this understanding of care, the patient is able to plan future care requirements and instruct carers on the appropriateness of the care given. A variety of mechanized and manual beds are now used in the care of the paralysed. Similarly, there are many mattresses which may be appropriate in a given situation. In this section the authors will aim primarily on the safest and the most convenient way of nursing a patient in an orthopaedic environment.

As mentioned previously, soon after the spinal cord injury there is often vasodilatation and fall in systemic blood pressure in a tetraplegic patient. Before the transfer of the patient from the site of accident to an ambulance, attempts should be made to remove sharp objects that may be on the person of the injured so that pressure sores do not develop during transit. A scoop stretcher is often a convenient way of lifting the patient between surfaces. Once the patient is admitted to the Accident and Emergency Department the clothing should be removed carefully without undue movement of the spine or any injured extremity. Care should be taken to avoid hypothermia during these manoeuvers. Transfer of the patient from the examination couch onto a radiography table could be carried out by the use of an Easiglide. After initial radiological and neurological assessment the patient could be nursed either in a conventional hospital bed or on specialized beds such as an Egerton electric turning bed.

STOKE EGERTON BED

This bed is divided into three longitudinal segments. The central segment can be tilted up or down together with any one of the lateral segments by operating an electric motor. The patient can therefore be turned over a 45° angle to the right or to the left.

STRYKER BED

This consists of two frames which support the front and

back of the patient. The patient can be axially rotated when both frames are applied and locked in position. Cervical traction can also be maintained.

Lifting

Straight lifting of the patient with neck injuries can be carried out by four people, a senior nurse holds the head between his or her forearm while supporting the neck with his or her hand. The nurse will then instruct the other three lifters to insert their arms under the back, pelvis and legs taking care to avoid lateral movements of the spinal column. When the arms of the lifters are in position, the patient is lifted at the instruction of the nurse who supports the head of the patient. After the lift and appropriate adjustment to the bed the patient is repositioned on the bed and the arms are withdrawn without disturbing the spinal alignment.

Dorsal and lumbar lesions: log rolling

Paraplegic patients with either a dorsal or lumbar lesion can be log rolled by three members of staff (Fig. 33.12). The patient is usually positioned with a pillow under his head and a pillow at the dorsolumbar junction (lumbar pillow). To achieve a left lateral position by log roll, the transverse lumbar pillow is used to roll him onto his left. The rolling manoeuvre is carried out in such a way that the spinal alignment is maintained. The shoulder and the lumbar pillow are usually moved during the roll by one member of staff while the right lower extremity is supported by another member of staff. Care should be taken to avoid undue drag on the urinary drainage system. The left lower extremity is positioned with a slight flexion of the knee while the right lower extremity, separated from the left by pillows is kept straight and behind the left knee. The ankles are positioned using pillows to achieve a plantigrade position of the feet. The patient is supported on the left lateral position by the use of an additional pillow under the lumbar pillow (Fig. 33.13). In this technique the patient is rolled from side to side and on to his or her back every 2 hours.

Cervical lesions: pelvic twist

Patients with tetraplegia or cervical spine injury can be turned from side to side using mechanical/electrical turning beds. If such beds are not available they can be turned on an ordinary bed using a technique referred to as 'pelvic twist'. One member of staff will be required to stabilize the neck and shoulder by applying firm downward pressure on either shoulder while supporting the

head with the forearm. To achieve relief of pressure from the left buttock and thigh, a member of staff will then twist the pelvis so that the right trochanter and the right half of the pelvis is towards the centre of the bed. The left buttock is lifted off the bed by a wedge-shaped triangular form inserted under the left loin. The left knee is slightly flexed and supported on two pillows. The feet are maintained in a plantigrade position. Pelvic twist, either to the left or to the right should be carried out every 2 hours and skin over the back and heel inspected during every turn (Fig. 33.12).

It is important to ascertain that the mattress on which the patient is laid is not old, lumpy and sagging in the middle. Pressure sores develop very easily in paralysed patients and are often very difficult to cure.

The frequency of turns can be reduced during the rehabilitation phase. Established paraplegics can be encouraged to sleep prone without any turns during the night. Prone lying, in the long term reduces the incidence of contractures around the hip and knee.

If the paralysed person requires surgical intervention he or she should be nursed on pillows or special mattresses to avoid prolonged pressure over bony prominences during surgery.

Cardio-respiratory management

The systolic blood pressure is often low in the paralysed patient due to associated sympathetic paralysis causing peripheral vasodilatation. The capacitance of the peripheral vasculature is so large that infusion of large quantities of fluids does not often produce a raise in blood pressure (Frankel and Mathias, 1976). In tetraplegic patients, transfusion or infusion of large quantities of fluids is unwise since this can lead to precipitous pulmonary oedema and associated respiratory complications. There is a reduction in circulating catecholamines leading to postural hypotension. Following the acute management when patients are mobilized, most of them suffer severe postural hypotension. The mobilization of a paralysed patient should therefore be a gradual process, increasing the sitting time initially in the bed and subsequently in a wheelchair gradually. This process of training activates the renin–angiotensin system allowing release of vasopressin. Paralysed patients with incomplete spinal cord lesion should not be allowed to suffer severe postural hypotension. It has been shown that such hypotension in incomplete lesions may be associated with neurological compromise (El Asri, 1993).

Deep venous thrombosis and pulmonary embolism are well-known complications of paraplegia. Routine

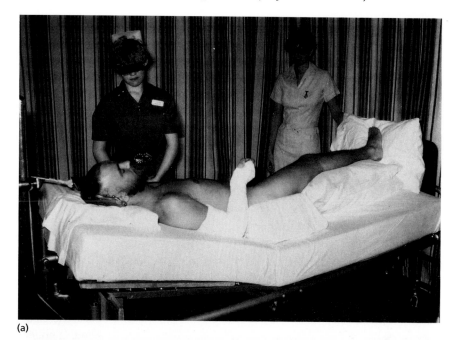

(a)

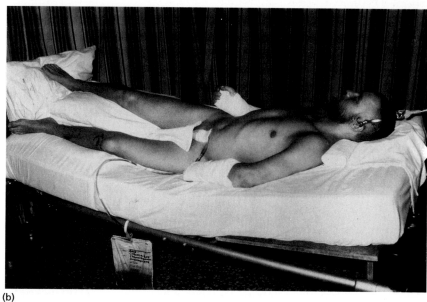

Fig. 33.12 Pelvic twist. The shoulders are held steady by a nurse while the pelvis is twisted by gently rotating one hip over the other and supporting the lifted hemi-pelvis on a triangular piece of foam. Two views of the same patient. Note Gardner–Wells traction, indwelling urethral catheter. Patient has associated orthopaedic injuries to the extremity.

(b)

anti-coagulation therapy using warfarin, often supplemented with heparin during the first few days should be considered in most patients. The majority of fatal pulmonary emboli seem to occur between the end of the first week following spinal cord injury and the third week. Mortality can be significantly reduced with appropriate anti-coagulant therapy (Watson, 1978).

Tetraplegic patients suffer at least 50% reduction in the vital capacity as a result of intercostal paralysis during the acute phase. PaO_2 and oxygen saturation remain low for several weeks due to pulmonary arteriovenous shunting. With the return of tone in the inter-

costal muscles and possibly improved and efficient use of the diaphragm, in the young paraplegic patient the vital capacity gradually improves during the first 6 or 8 weeks.

Tetraplegic patients with a vital capacity of at least 1 litre seldom require ventilatory support provided appropriate chest physiotheapy could be carried out by trained therapists. Turning the patient from side to side, as explained above, will improve drainage and reduce collapse of the lobes.

When the tidal volume is below 400 ml (vital capacity below 1 litre) patients will require elective ventilation.

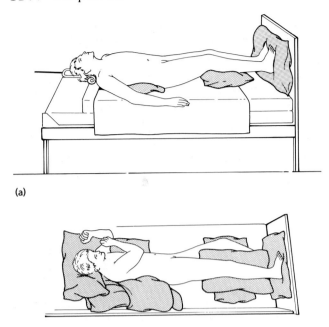

(a)

(b)

Fig. 33.13 (a) Supine nursing for a tetraplegic patient. Note the position of the neck roll and lumbar pillow. Feet are supported on a pillow, the heel is free of pressure and the ankle is dorsiflexed to 90°. An additional pillow to support the head may be useful. (b) Log rolling of a paraplegic patient is usually accompanied by the use of a transverse lumbar pillow positioned at the dorsolumbar junction. The patient is rolled from the supine to lateral position using the pillow to protect the upper part of the torso, while at the same time a helper moves the lower extremities and repositions them on the pillows. The lumbar pillow is then used to support the back and maintain the lateral position with an additional pillow.

Paralysed patients with minor degrees of respiratory insufficiency can benefit from the use of 'mini-tra-cheostomy' and avoid the need for management in the intensive care unit. Inefficient clearance of tracheo-bronchial secretions will lead to atelectasis. Repeated chest physiotherapy by a trained therapist during the acute phase is vital.

When elective ventilation is instituted, either using nasotracheal intubation, or through a tracheostomy, it is important to provide adequate emotional support to these patients. Attempts should be made to wean the patients off the ventilator as soon as is possible.

Respiratory compromise can arise as a result of rib fractures, haemopneumothoraces and collapse of the lung complicating spinal cord injury.

Most paraplegics and all tetraplegics are taught an effective method of coughing during their rehabilitation. The carers of tetraplegic patients are also taught methods of producing assisted cough so that incidence of chest infection could be reduced.

Gastrointestinal tract

Paralysis of the sympathetic and parasympathetic system that follow acute traumatic spinal cord injury usually leads to varying degrees of reduced mobility of the gastrointestinal tract. Even though bowel sounds may be present for a few hours after the injury in most cases there is a significant reduction of bowel sound after about 8 hours. Provided these patients are not rehydrated with oral fluids there is gradual return of bowel motility during the subsequent 24–48 hours. During the first 2 days, oral fluids should be restricted and normal diet withheld. Patients with thoracolumbar fractures often develop paravertebral haematoma and extensive retro-peritoneal haematoma. This is commonly associated with prolonged paralytic ileus. The use of a large lumbar pillow which might hyperextend the thoracolumbar junction aggravates the situation causing, on occasions, paralytic ileus which may persist for several weeks. Some patients develop a condition referred to as 'superior mesenteric artery syndrome'. In these patients, due to hyperextension of the thoracolumbar junction and associated weight loss, there appears to be a partial obstruction to the third part of the duodenum by the superior mesenteric artery leading to gastric dilatation and prolonged paralytic ileus.

Stress ulceration of the gastric mucosa is well known and may be troublesome in young patients with a history of regular alcohol intake. The concurrent use of corticosteroids and full anti-coagulation therapy appears to increase the risk of gastrointestinal bleeding in some patients. Some authors have regularly used prophylactic H_2-receptor blockers during the acute phase. Metoclo-promide may be used in some patients to improve gastric emptying without increasing gastric secretion. This drug also increases small intestinal motility but appears to have very little effect on the large bowel (Epstein *et al.*, 1981).

Because of the paralysis, the oro-caecal transit time has been shown to increase severalfold and it is import-ant that most patients with spinal cord injury take regular aperients. Bowel evacuation should be carried out as appropriate to the patient with rectal stimulants or by manual evacuation. Patients who have intact anal reflex respond to suppositories. Patients with lower motor neuron lesion (with absent anal reflex), can rarely empty their bowels by straining. They usually require gentle persistent digital evacuation in order to avoid 'bowel accidents'.

Bladder management (Thomas, 1982)

Male patients with suprasacral spinal cord injury often exhibit pseudopriapism due to sympathetic loss. This may persist for a few hours and can be intermittent. The bladder of a newly injured patient can be managed with an indwelling urethral catheter. Because of a degree of fluid retention that follows spinal cord injury, the urine output is often variable.

After about 72 hours, provided the fluid intake is satisfactory, it is possible to manage a male patient's bladder by intermittent catheterization. Fluid intake is restricted so that the bladder does not distend to more than 600–800 ml between catheterization. Catheterizations by trained staff are carried out in an aseptic environment initially four times a day. A greater or smaller frequency of catheterization may be required depending on the urine output. In patients with intact sacral reflexes, reflex voiding can occur some 4–6 weeks after injury. When reflex voiding commences and the residual urine after reflex voiding reduces to 200 ml the number of catheterizations can be reduced. When the detrusor activity adequately empties the bladder with residual urine of less than 50–100 ml, intermittent catheterization can be discontinued. In male patients, a condom urinal is applied to the penis to achieve continence.

Intermittent catheterization in female patients confined to bed following vertebral column injury often provides nursing problems. In such patients a fine-bore suprapubic catheter or a small (size 12–14 fr) urethral catheter may be a safe alternative to intermittent catheterization. If a decision is made to manage the bladder with an indwelling catheter, it is advisable to periodically clamp the catheter to maintain bladder volume of between 400 and 600 ml.

Autonomic dysreflexia (hyper-reflexia)

Painful stimuli in the paralysed part of the body, either due to distension of bladder or pathological fractures, often can induce a sudden rapid raise in blood pressure. This is usually associated with bradycardia, profuse sweating and patchy dilatation of blood vessels under the skin producing a blotchy erythema. The blood pressure raise is often very dramatic with systolic and diastolic hypertension. Systolic blood pressure may reach 200 mmHg. Diastolic hypertension of 120–140 is particularly dangerous to the patient and prompt action should be taken to alleviate the cause.

If the autonomic dysreflexia is due to bladder distension, an indwelling urethral catheter usually will reduce the blood pressure. Sublingual glyceryl trinitrate is an effective method of reducing hypertension due to autonomic dysreflexia. Such a treatment should be initiated by the nursing staff, even before medical help could be obtained. On occasions nifedipine may be combined with glyceryl trinitrate to achieve a more sustained reduction of blood pressure. Autonomic dysreflexia may accompany such disparate conditions like toenail infection, parturition, haemorrhoids, anal fissure and pressure sores in addition to conditions already described.

Nutrition

Endogenous fuel reserves are very rapidly depleted following traumatic spinal cord injury. In most patients the carbohydrate reserves are expended within the first 1–2 days. Even though there is a large amount of fat reserve in most patients, the metabolic pathway of fat breakdown is complicated and most glucose-dependent cells do not get adequate quantities of carbohydrate as the energy source. A 70 kg man under unstressed conditions, in bed rest, will usually require 20 kcal/kg body weight in addition to about 0.8 g protein/kg body weight. During the first 24–48 hours, most acute traumatic spinal cord-injured patients are treated with crystalloid. Infusion of 3 litres of 5% dextrose providing no more than 510 kcal/day seldom prevents protein catabolism. It is therefore important to consider food supplement parenterally early on in the management of patients with acute traumatic spinal cord injury. Such patients will initially benefit from 1–2 litres of dextrose/amino acid mixture per day, and where required, supplemented with 10–20% lipid solutions. Long-term parenteral feeding requires the specialist knowledge of a dietician (Visuete, 1989).

Associated injuries

It is not surprising that a significant proportion of patients with acute traumatic spinal cord injury have associated extremity and/or visceral injury. In many patients with spinal cord injury, non-continuous vertebral fractures have been noted. Previous studies tend to indicate that 20–30% of patients with spinal cord injury have associated other injuries (Meinecke, 1968; Calenoff *et al.*, 1978; Silver *et al.*, 1980). On many occasions intra-abdominal injuries have been missed due to lack of classical signs and symptoms. It is important that extremity fractures are immobilized with appropriate surgery as soon as possible. This will enable appropriate nursing of the patient and prevent long-term complications like contractures.

MANAGEMENT OF VERTEBRAL COLUMN INJURIES ASSOCIATED WITH SPINAL CORD INJURY

This section will provide an overview of the role of surgical intervention on the osseous structure surrounding the neuraxis. The techniques of surgical intervention and the superiority of one form of surgery to another is, however, beyond the scope of this chapter. The reader should consult appropriate textbooks on the spine to get greater insight into relative values of different types of fixation.

There is considerable controversy on the effectiveness and efficiency of vertebral column stabilization in paralysed patients. Surgical stabilization with or without decompression of the spinal canal is considered useful in the following conditions:

1 Where there is progression of neurological lesion under observation.

2 Where gross malalignment of the vertebra precludes conservative management.

3 Where reduction of a dislocation is likely to improve function of the nerve root at the level of the dislocation (in the cervical spine).

Presence of foreign body in the spinal canal, compound wounds communicating with the vertebral column and locked facets in the neck are other relative indications for surgical intervention. Decompressive laminectomy, particularly of the dorsal spine, can contribute to further neurological deficit and should be avoided (Lucas and Ducker, 1980). There is inconclusive evidence to suggest neurological improvement following either decompressive surgery or reduction of a fracture followed by stabilization (Bradford and Thompson, 1976; Collins, 1984).

Incomplete spinal cord injuries generally tend to improve even though the extent of neurological recovery remains unpredictable (Frankel *et al.*, 1969; Kinoshita *et al.*, 1993).

Unstable injuries of the spine, however, require prolonged recumbency and a very highly specialized team of nurses. There is always a risk of neurological deterioration during routine nursing management, particularly if the spine is very unstable.

Modern spinal surgical techniques, together with improved anaesthesia and spinal cord monitoring has allowed safe and appropriate surgical intervention in patients with specific spinal cord lesions. The authors believe that surgical stabilization of all vertebral fractures, complicated by spinal cord lesion is inappropriate. Complications following spinal cord injury are significantly higher in the group of patients who had surgical intervention to their vertebral column compared to those treated conservatively (Kinoshita *et al.*, 1993).

Cervical spine injuries

In the upper cervical spine, fracture to the odontoid peg is by far the commonest. Hangman's fracture of C2 and Jefferson fracture of C1 are often associated with minimal neurological deficit. Generally these fractures are treated by skeletal traction and subsequently mobilized in an appropriate halo-jacket fixation. Late instability as a result of subluxation between C1 and C2 is a well-recognized problem and on occasions may require craniocervical fusion. If the patient is managed conservatively during the period of traction it is important to take frequent radiographs of the upper cervical spine to avoid distraction.

Bifacetal dislocation to the cervical spine can often be reduced with sustained traction in a flexed position (Fig. 33.14). A gradual increase in the traction force in most cases will unlock the dislocation. The neck can then be extended followed by a reduction in the traction force. The most commonly used skull caliper is Gardner–Wells' tongs. It is very easy to apply this caliper under local anaesthesia. The pins are usually located just below temperoparietal prominence in the mid-sagittal plane (Fig. 33.15).

Unilateral locked facets are generally more difficult to reduce and will require a greater traction. On occasions, manipulation under general anaesthesia and radiographic control will be required. Manipulation under anaesthesia and muscle relaxation is seldom successful after the first 24–48 hours from the time of injury. During reduction of unilateral facet dislocation, under general anaesthesia, in addition to traction, a lateral flexion away from the dislocated site is required initially. This should be followed after reduction by a rotation towards the site of dislocation. Gentle traction should be maintained throughout the procedure (Evans, 1961). Surgical stabilization of the mid-cervical and lower cervical vertebra can be carried out either anteriorly or posteriorly. Anterior interbody fusion using iliac crest bone graft often produces a satisfactory fixation and the patient can be mobilized within a few weeks after the injury. Interpedicular screw fixation using a hook-plate limits the total damage to the adjacent apophyseal joint (Fig. 33.16). Because of the risk of developing syringomyelia, and the magnetic interference caused by metal plates, one of the authors prefers to stabilize the spine posteriorly using a nylon tape between the spinous process in addition to intravertebral onlay grafting. Such a fixation is often inadequate for early mobilization and patients will require to remain in bed without skull traction for 4–8 weeks.

Tetraplegic patients with either a fracture or dislocations of the cervical spine but treated conservatively,

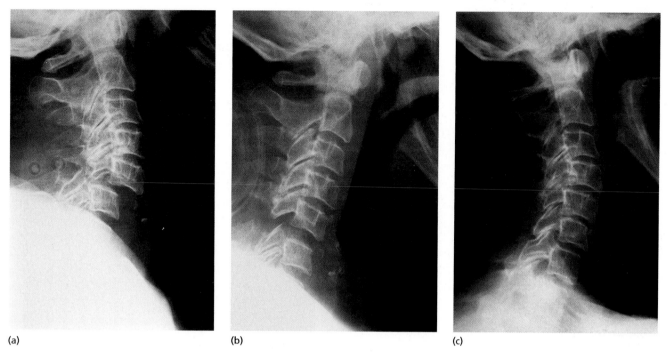

Fig. 33.14 (a) Bifacet dislocation C5−C6. (b) Reduction achieved with traction in flexion. (c) Appearance after reduction of the dislocation, traction weight has been reduced and the neck held in slight extension.

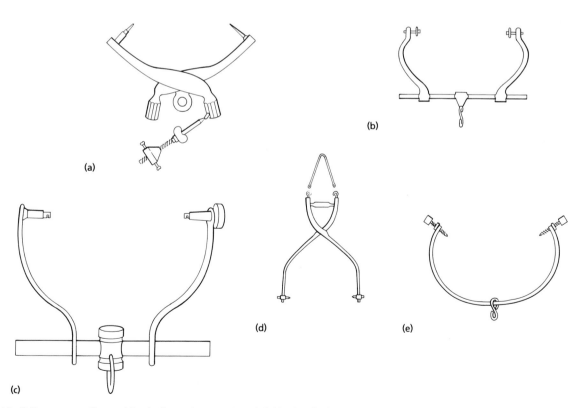

Fig. 33.15 Calipers normally used in skull traction. (a) Crutchfield; (b) Blackburn; (c) Vinke; (d) Cones; (e) Gardner−Wells.

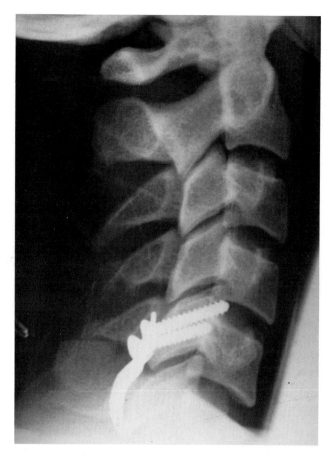

Fig. 33.16 C5—C6 dislocation. Reduced and treated with hook plate fixation.

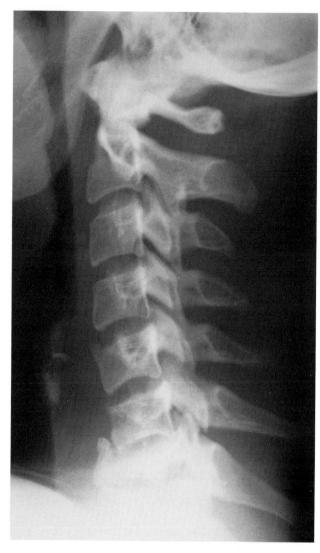

Fig. 33.17 C7 fracture, 14 weeks after injury. Treated with bed rest for 10 weeks. Note development of early kyphotic deformity but satisfactory union. There is an additional fracture of C5 vertebral body which did not cause the paralysis.

remain on traction for between 6 and 8 weeks. They are then mobilized with an appropriate well-fitting collar. Flexion—extension radiographs of the cervical spine are taken at 3 months. Burst fractures of the cervical spine can often be treated conservatively. Even patients with burst fractures who have been treated conservatively by traction and bed rest for 10 weeks show minor late kyphotic deformity of the spine. However such deformities do not cause long-term problems (Fig. 33.17). Paralysed patients who are treated surgically will also require a cervical collar for the same length of time.

If there was radiological evidence of bony compression of one of the cervical nerves an anterior vertebraectomy followed by stabilization will be appropriate. Certain cases of severe hyperextension injury lead to dislocation of the vertebral body in association with fracture to the posterior complex (pars interarticularis, facet and base of the spinous process). These injuries occur as a result of severe violence and are often very unstable. They invariably require stabilization if one should avoid late instability.

Thoracic spine

A large number of injuries to the upper thoracic spine occur in young patients following motor cycle accidents. They may, on occasions be associated with rib fractures and brachial plexus lesion. Most of the vertebral column fractures in this region are treated conservatively in patients with paraplegia. Some degree of correction of vertebral displacement is possible by postural reduction using a firm pillow positioned over the apex of the kyphus. Even in patients with significant displacement of vertebral bodies, the splinting action of the rib cage appears to provide some degree of stability, and conservative management is all that is required for the majority of these patients. Most patients with upper dorsal spinal cord injury remain completely paralysed. Any kyphotic deformity that ensues as a result of displacement is seldom found to be of clinical significance to the patient and does not interfere with normal day-to-day activities.

When surgical intervention is contemplated, attempts should be made to obtain as much detail of the bony architecture as possible using tomography, computed tomography scanning and on occasions MRI scan. The presence of large bony fragments in the neural canal, particularly in the thoracic spine in patients with minimal or no neurological signs, raises a significant risk of late-onset paralysis. Closed reduction (postural) of thoracic spine fracture with a vertebral fragment lying anterior to the spinal cord seldom re-aligns the fragment. Surgical stabilization using long Harrington rods or Hartshill rectangle have been known to compromise physical rehabilitation when the patient is mobilized. On many occasions these rods/plates require to be removed, and this is usually followed by further collapse of the vertebral body. Bony fragments in the spinal canal can be best removed by an anterior or anterolateral approach followed by interbody fusion (Bohlman, 1974; Bedford *et al.*, 1977; McSweeney, 1979; Young *et al.*, 1981; Jelsma *et al.*, 1982).

Thoracolumbar fracture

Fractures of the thoracolumbar spine (T9–L2) are very common and the injuries tend to be complex. A significant proportion of patients with bony injury to the thoracolumbar spine have incomplete neurological lesion. Many authors have attributed neurological recovery to any surgical procedure that was employed. There has never been an adequately controlled randomized study to evaluate any benefit of surgical intervention in patients with thoracolumbar spinal injury complicating paraplegia. This lack of statistical information continues to cause a dilemma in deciding the optimal treatment for patients with spinal cord injury following thoracolumbar trauma. Injuries to the thoracolumbar junction often follow major violence with extensive bruising of the surrounding soft tissue. Pain is very common and is a significant disability during the acute phase. Surgical stabilization can relieve the discomfort and contribute to ease of nursing. The choice of surgical instrumentation would be dictated by the type of fracture and associated injury. It is advisable that the fusion is restricted to one or two segments and any implants used do not cause significant artifacts for future investigation using computed tomography or MRI. In our experience interpedicular screw fixation appears to be the safest and easiest form of immobilizing a single segment in this group of patients (Fig. 33.18).

Several surgical techniques using a variety of screws, plates and wires have been used to achieve varying degrees of spinal stabilization. A concept of stability or instability evolved by Nicol (1949) Watson-Jones (1949) and Holdsworth (1970) was modified by Roy-Camille

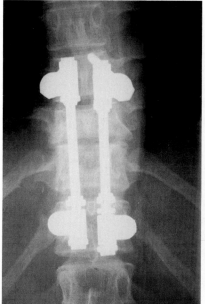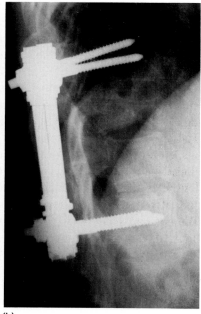

Fig. 33.18 (a, b) Interpedicular screw fixation for fracture of D10 in a patient with minimal neurological deficit. Mobilized with a brace 3 weeks after surgery.

(a)

(b)

et al. (1973) with the introduction of 'middle vertebral segment'. Concepts of stability and instability that evolved from cadaveric spine do not necessarily apply to patients with spinal cord injury. Most of these patients are confined to bed for several weeks for reasons other than the injury to their vertebral column. Bony union most often occurs by conservative management, and rigid fixation at the expense of mobility is seldom an avantage to these patients. Progressive deterioration of neurological level is often considered as an indication for exploration followed by appropriate minimal surgical stabilization. Technically superior surgical stabilization of the thoracolumbar fractures have suffered from serious complications such as sepsis due to inadequate post-operative nursing. The specialized and expert nursing normally available in a spinal injuries centre is often a prerequisite before complex procedures are carried out on the spine of the paralysed.

Fractures of the lumbar spine generally produce damage to the cauda equina. On occasions the artery of Adamkiewicz might be damaged in association with vertebral fracture of L2 or L3 and can produce flaccid paraplegia. On a few occasions, the neurology might ascend several segments due to vascular compromise, unrelated to any bony compression of the cauda equina. When paralysis is incomplete following a fracture of the lumbar vertebra, appropriate stabilization usually offers an efficient way of early mobilization.

CONSERVATIVE MANAGEMENT OF VERTEBRAL COLUMN INJURY

The majority of the patients with spinal cord injury with an associated vertebral injury are treated conservatively. Neurological recovery appears to depend on the severity of initial violence rather than the promptness with which bony re-alignment is achieved with or without surgical intervention. Frankel *et al.* (1969) in a large study showed that 81% of paraplegic patients with dorsal spine injury and 61% with dorsal lumbar injury had incomplete lesions. Bohlman *et al.* (1985) reported no neurological recovery in a group of 149 patients with dorsal spine injury who were admitted with a complete lesion. There was no significant difference in the neurological outcome irrespective of surgical intervention. Wilmot and Hall (1986) and Donovan *et al.* (1984) showed that complications following surgical intervention were significantly greater in patients who underwent internal fixation than those who were treated conservatively. This study also confirmed that there was no significant difference in the neurological outcome between the two groups. The authors believe that con-

servative management of vertebral fractures in patients with neuraxis trauma remains a valid treatment in most instances.

REHABILITATION PROGRAMME

The realization of permanent paralysis has a devastating effect on the psychological state of patients and their families. An initial period of denial of the condition is soon replaced by a realization and a sense of despair. Physical, social, emotional and vocational support that a patient with spinal cord injury receives during his acute treatment and rehabilitation in a spinal injuries centre is crucial to the long-term well-being and health of that individual. The rehabilitation of the paralysed is a team effort and is invariably influenced by the various therapists and support staff. The medical practitioner often takes a limited role but is always guided by specialists such as physiotherapists and occupational therapists.

Physiotherapy

A high tetraplegic often requires considerable assistance from a physiotherapist during the acute phase. Periodic assisted cough to clear the airways is vital. In a spinal injuries unit, every member of staff is aware and proficient in assisting a tetraplegic patient to achieve a satisfactory cough to expectorate and clear the airways of any secretions. All the joints in the upper and lower extremities are normally put through a full range of movements each day to prevent contractures and to maintain optimum range. This ensures greater range of mobility of the extremities when the patient is able to sit in a wheelchair. By appropriately splinting the wrist of C5–C6 tetraplegic patients, an efficient tenodesis grip could be achieved. Thus a C6 tetraplegic with retained function in the extensor carpi radialis longus can achieve a 'grip' if the long flexors to the fingers are allowed to contract to a limited extent. Dorsiflexion achieved by such action will produce flexion of the metacarpophalangeal and interphalangeal joints due to the relative shortening of the long finger flexors. The use of a short opponens splint in these patients will provide a lateral pinch grip (Lamb, 1987). The therapist will also attempt to maintain the muscle bulk and tone by passive movements of the extremities. Partially paralysed muscle can be made stronger by specific exercise even when the patient is confined to bed. The use of springs and weights to improve upper extremity muscle function in paraplegic patients will be of great value during subsequent rehabilitation. More recently the use of functional electrical stimulation has shown some promise of a more rapid strengthening of partially paralysed muscles.

When the patient is able to sit in a wheelchair, he or she learns to manoeuvre the wheelchair. Once adequate sitting balance has been achieved, depending on the level of the patient and his or her overall physical fitness, most paraplegics should be able to transfer between surfaces (Fig. 33.19) thus achieving wheelchair independence. A paraplegic should be able to get into a car without any assistance. They should be able to transfer onto a toilet seat and attend to their own bowel programmes. Modern lightweight wheelchairs allow easy transfer of the wheelchair into a car. The therapist will also advise on the choice of appropriate wheelchair cushions for the paralysed. Certain wheelchairs have the option to stand from a sitting position using levers attached to them. The Levo active wheelchair is suitable to a few paralysed patients in their normal day-to-day activities.

Wheelchair-design concepts have radically changed in the last few years and it is now possible to use different wheelchairs to achieve different functions (Fig. 33.20). There are wheelchairs designed exclusively for track racing and others for use on soft grass. High-spinal tetraplegic patients can now use electric wheelchairs which have integral environment control systems. Thus some of these wheelchairs, far from restricting

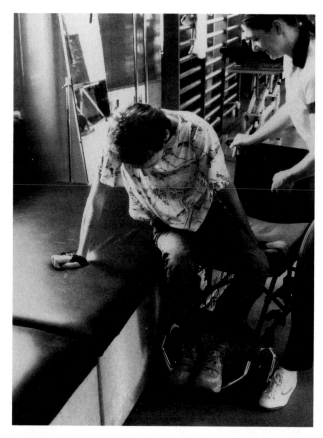

Fig. 33.19 C6 tetraplegic without any triceps function doing wheelchair—bed transfer.

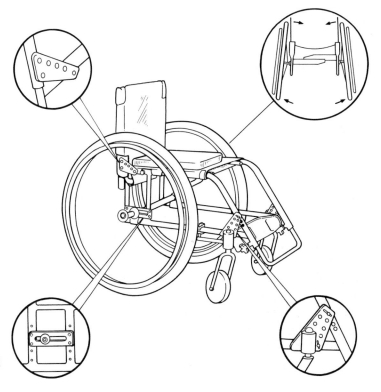

Fig. 33.20 Outline of a modern lightweight wheelchair. Inset showing adjustable back-rest, variable camber, adjustable and changeable castors, variable height, forward rear positioning of the wheel axle.

patients' mobility, enables them to interact with their environment.

Young paraplegic patients with a spinal cord injury below D9 should be able to walk with appropriate long-leg calipers. Modern reciprocating gait orthosis (Fig. 33.21) or hip guidance orthosis enables paraplegic patients to walk on level ground with low energy cost (Bajd *et al.*, 1985; Summers *et al.*, 1988; Isakov *et al.*, 1992). In most spinal injuries centres, physiotherapists often introduce the paralysed to a variety of appropriate sporting activities. Young paraplegic patients derive immense pleasure from these sporting activities. Paraplegic sport has now achieved international standards and the Para-Olympics are held on a regular basis (Fig. 33.22).

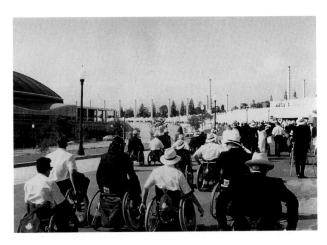

Fig. 33.22 Para-Olympics, Barcelona, 1992.

Occupational therapy

During the acute phase, the occupational therapist assists the physical therapist in obtaining appropriate splints to achieve optimum functional position in the upper extremities of the tetraplegic patient. The occupational therapist, after a long dialogue with the patient and the family, organizes assessment of the home of the paralysed. Traditionally-held views that an occupational therapist provides bed-based entertainment is no longer tenable. Highly-skilled spinal injury occupational therapists set up intricate environmental-controlled systems to enable severely-disabled patients to achieve as much control over the environment as possible while still in bed. Most paraplegic patients easily master personal care. Thus they are able to dress and undress with relative ease. A tetraplegic on the other hand has significant problems in learning to get dressed. Paralysed patients are taught most activities of daily living, such as cooking, toileting, washing and ironing. They also learn about appropriate adaptations that are required to overcome their physical disability to achieve optimum function. A planned home visit is usually made by the occupational therapist who liaises with community-based services so that proper assessment of the home environment and its suitability for use by a wheelchair-dependent patient could be made. Most centres encourage paraplegic patients to undertake driving lessons in an appropriately adapted motor vehicle. Paralysed patients also learn about alternative equipment that they would need to use in their place of employment.

Paraplegic patients and most tetraplegic patients can stand using a standing frame (Fig. 33.23). Standing reduces spasm and contractures. Axial loading of the long bones during standing decreases immobilization osteoporosis and reduces the incidence of pathological fractures. Tetraplegic patients on occasions benefit from surgical procedures in their upper extremities to achieve greater function. Appropriately trained spinal occupational therapists will be able to assess specific needs of

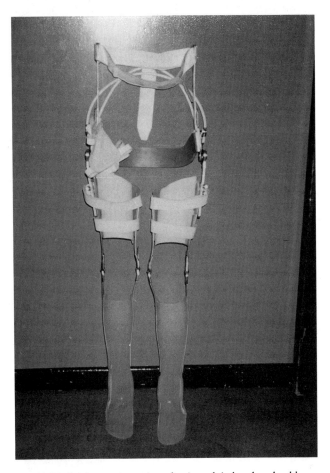

Fig. 33.21 Reciprocating gait orthosis; pelvic band and cable provide a low-energy erect ambulation.

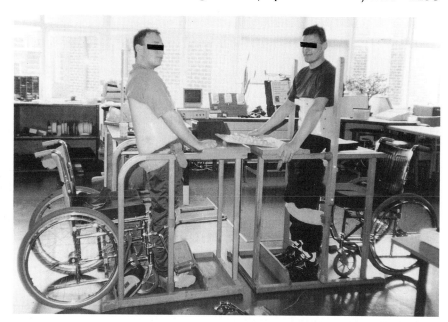

Fig. 33.23 Paraplegic patients standing using Oswestry standing frame. Note three-point fixation—straps behind the heel, in front of the knee and behind the buttocks.

the patient and advise if the planned hand surgery is of value to the patient.

Social support

Social workers attached to the spinal injuries unit are key workers in the rehabilitation of the paralysed. The long, hard struggle to return the paralysed back to the community commences on the day of admission. Paralysis, brings with it financial hardships (Stover and Fine, 1987). Many families have great difficulty in arranging appropriate transport to visit the patient. During the early days of paraplegia, patients feel isolated and these visits from their relatives are of crucial importance in maintaining the morale of the paralysed. The primary role of the social worker is to help the disabled plan the future. The social worker will liaise with the community services and arrange for an assessment of the patient's home to be carried out to ascertain its suitability for the disabled. When required, the social worker negotiates with the local authority to obtain the necessary funding so that the paralysed person can be cared for in an appropriate nursing home. Liaising with the Local Educational Authority so that a paralysed young person can continue with education or training falls within the domain of the social worker. Similarly the social worker negotiates with employers so that the work environment can be adequately adapted to suit the needs of the paralysed person who might still be able to continue with a useful and productive occupation. In the long term, a social worker who has gained the trust of the paralysed is often the first to know the personal

triumphs achieved by the disabled or the tragedy that befell.

Psychological support

The multi-system trauma suffered by the spinal cord injured inevitably leads to significant emotional and psychological effects. Sustained and informed support to the paralysed by trained and experienced staff is important if one is to avoid maladjustment and long-term bitterness. In most cases there is no immediate need for the road traffic accident victim, who might have spinal cord injury, to know the extent of paralysis and its long-term consequences. Blunt and insensitive handling during the acute phase in the Accident and Emergency Department has on many occasions caused deep-seated mistrust of the primary caregivers. The patient and the family need only to have an overview of the injury at that stage. Additional details are often provided after the transfer of the patient to appropriate spinal centres. The staff in these units tend to give a comprehensive and more complete picture of the overall rehabilitation programme, in addition to giving a more realistic prognosis. Both the patient and their family begin to gradually appreciate the complexity of the multi-system damage that follows spinal cord injury, and the present inability to significantly alter the prognosis by any surgical or medical manipulations. In spite of giving adequate, lengthy and compassionate description of the course of treatment in a hospital, most patients choose to deny the injury for several days in the hope that the medical or nursing people could be incorrect. A clinical psychologist, with appropriate training in the field of catastrophic and permanent injuries often is able to alleviate the deep-seated fears and depression that follows spinal cord injury (Trieschmann, 1988, 1992; Ramsay, 1990).

The extent of physical handicap seems to manifest in a more intense way when the patient is mobilized and patients suffer a second spell of temporary depression. However, in an environment, similar to those present in spinal injuries units, where other patients are similarly striving to get independence, patients often adjust very easily. In most cases the 'work' of psychological re-orientation is achieved by the 'patient community'. Specialists in the field generally believe that the depression, anger, denial and periods of reactive depression prevalent in the acute patient with spinal cord injury has to be considered as a normal response to trauma. Patients with minimal neurological deficit or incomplete lesions generally have a greater difficulty in accepting their residual disability and on occasions suffer from post-traumatic stress disorder (Ramsay, 1990).

Psychosexual responses

It is well known that many young male and female paraplegic/tetraplegic patients become very concerned with their sexual role as a result of the injury. This anxiety appears to manifest itself very soon after injury with a series of targeted questions to the nurses and other support staff. During their rehabilitation phase, further emotional trauma becomes manifest by their need to express their sexuality and their difficulties in receiving appropriate responses from their partner. A prolonged hospital stay away from their sexual partner becomes a major hardship to the disabled person. Sexual attractiveness or the lack of it, is generally a major concern to the female rather than the male patient in a wheelchair. The relative preponderance of female members of staff in the caring profession (nurses, physiotherapists, occupational therapists) somehow appears to reassure young male paraplegic patients, while a similar reassurance is lacking in the case of the female paralysed. The relationship between a couple, one of whom is paralysed, suffers a major jolt during the first home visit. The apparent lack of enthusiasm on the part of the non-paralysed partner and the need for reassurance on the part of the paralysed partner generally causes emotional trauma. On the whole, most couples where a partner is disabled and who have had appropriate discussions with the caregivers, manage to re-establish sexual relationships. It takes many months before the long-term survival of this relationship becomes apparent.

Male sexuality

In young patients with suprasacral spinal cord lesion the sacral reflexes are preserved and as a result a reflex erection is possible. To a limited degree this reflex erection could be utilised for intercourse. However, the unreliability of penile tumescence obtained by reflex activity leads to frustration between the partners. After initial rehabilitation, a proportion of patients elect to supplement their reflex erection with the use of constriction therapy (rubber band at the base of the penis) or the vacuum penile tumescence technique (Heller *et al.*, 1992). The use of an intracarporal vasoactive drug such as papaverine has widened the horizon of satisfactory sexual intimacy between a paralysed male and his partner.

Ejaculatory dysfunction can now be controlled in some circumstances with the use of a rectal probe electro-ejaculator (Halstead, 1987; Siosteen *et al.*, 1990). The success of antegrade electro-ejaculation appears to be influenced by the intactness of reflex pathways, any previous bladder outlet surgery, and the presence or absence of recurrent urinary-tract infections. On occasions, a retrograde ejaculate obtained following electric stimulation may be used with appropriate motile spermatozoal concentration techniques. The quality and quantity of sperm vary with chronicity of lesion and on occasion the presence or absence of long-term indwelling urethral catheter. There is some evidence to suggest that repeated periodic electro-ejaculation can improve the quality and quantity of semen (Siosteen *et al.*, 1990). The use of vas aspiration after insertion of artificial spermatocoele and in rare cases testicular aspiration has been known to produce small quantities of motile spermatozoa, thus improving the prospect for parenthood.

Anorgasmia may be seen even in patients with a very minor spinal cord dysfunction. There is, as yet, no satisfactory method of achieving satisfactory orgasm in paralysed men. Stimulation of the autonomic nerve to the bladder and the vas deferens using implanted electrodes, currently under trial has produced in some patients ejaculation, but anorgasmia persists.

It should be remembered that electro-ejaculation in patients with spinal cord lesions at T5 or above carries the risk of inducing severe autonomic dysreflexia.

Female sexuality

Following spinal cord injury, many young female patients suffer a prolonged period of amenorrhoea which may last up to one year. Pregnancy and parturition are options open to the paralysed female patient since, in general, fertility appears to be unaffected by the spinal cord injury after this period of amenorrhoea. Vaginal delivery is still possible and in tetraplegic patients outlet forceps or an elective Caesarean section may be indicated. A proportion of women continue to suffer from lack of confidence, lack of spontaneity and lack of orgasm (Griffith, 1975; Charlifue *et al.*, 1992). Care should be taken by the non-paralysed male partner not to traumatize the paralysed genitalia during intercourse. Female patients with a low-spinal cord injury, have on occasions reported a relative reduction of vaginal lubrication during intercourse, causing discomfort to the partner.

Conception

In general, couples where the male partner has sexual dysfunction due to spinal cord injury suffer great difficulties in achieving conception. The use of gamete intrafallopian transfer with sperm obtained, either by electro-ejaculation or vas aspiration, has on occasions produced satisfactory results (Macourt *et al.*, 1991). *In vitro* fertilization in men with poor-quality ejaculate remain the best option in these conditions.

MANAGEMENT OF LONG-TERM PARAPLEGIA

Pressure sore and its management

Pressure sores are not uncommon among the paralysed. Acute and long-term paralysed patients do suffer from pressure sores. The capillary perfusion pressure of skin and the subcutaneous tissue is of the order of 20–30 mmHg and this pressure is easily exceeded when a person sits or lies on a relatively unyielding mattress. In addition to generating pressure at the points of contact over bony prominences, the tissue between the bone and the skin undergoes deformation (sheer force). The combination of pressure and sheer force when sustained beyond the physiological tolerance leads to progressively irreversible damage to the tissues between the skin and the bone. The extent of tissue damage is also influenced by the general health of the patient and the age of the patient. Thus patients with malnutrition, anaemia, hypoproteinaemia or systemic infection tend to develop pressure sores more easily.

Acute paraplegic patients may develop pressure sores soon after the accident while lying on a roadside following a road traffic accident. The hard unyielding surface of the road together with any sharp objects that a person might carry on his person tend to produce significant tissue damage which might escape the attention of the admitting doctor. Further tissue destruction can be avoided by informed nursing care which includes regular turns of the patient on an appropriate mattress.

During the rehabilitation phase, all patients are taught the best method of relieving pressure from their seat and bony prominences, such as the heel, knee and elbow. The use of appropriate cushions and adjustments to the footplate of a wheelchair reduces the risk of a paraplegic patient developing pressure sores when in a wheelchair. Similarly, the use of an appropriate mattress or an overmattress in addition to regular turning prevents the development of pressure sores. The normal protective reflexes which are present in the non-paralysed, which encourages regular involuntary turns during sleep is clearly absent in the paralysed thus putting him or her at risk. In spite of the paralysis many paraplegics and tetraplegics escape pressure sores for several years. In general, pressure sores in these well rehabilitated occur due to a combination of factors such as urinary infection, contractures, malnutrition, a defective cushion or a pathological fracture. A proportion of patients who have escaped pressure sores at home tend to develop pressure sores as a result of injudicious management in hospitals where they may be admitted for unrelated conditions. Many patients have developed heel and upper-thigh pressure sores as a result of unnecessary rigid immobilization of a lower extremity fracture in a cast. On occasion, the rigid immobilization of one lower extremity reduces the overall mobility of the patient in the home, necessitating prolonged recumbency leading to development of pressure sores.

First evidence of significant tissue damage to the underlying tissue is heralded by the appearance of a fixed erythema over a bony prominence. Patients who recognize the appearance of erythema possibly with underlying induration usually confine themselves to bed, taking care not to add further pressure to that area. It may take several days before the erythema disappears. However, should the soft-tissue destruction be more extensive, irreversible damage occurs, which gradually leads to liquefaction and formation of a sterile abscess. In a proportion of these patients, because of skin necrosis, there is secondary infection, with the formation of a true abscess. The underlying bony prominence undergoes changes in contour and texture, possibly due to hyperaemia and infection, and a chronic sinus eventually results. If the general condition of the patient is poor, there will be associated bacteraemia and septicaemia. Multiple pressure sores in vulnerable patients can lead to death.

A recent study reported that 43 per 10 000 of the population suffer from pressure ulcers (Allman *et al.*, 1986). Some 25% of these were either hospitalized or treated in a nursing home. It is estimated that the cost per patient with pressures sores is of the order of £14 000 with an annual cost for the National Health Service of £350 million. A further £600 million is spent in treating other forms of ulcers in the community (National Pressure Ulcer Advisory Panel, 1989; Cockhill, 1992).

The precise incidence of pressure sores in paraplegic patients is variable and is influenced by many factors. The incidence of pressure sores increases with a chronicity of the condition and most patients who have been paralysed for 10 years or more would have had at least one pressure sore.

If the tissue destruction is minor, and there is no skin necrosis, conservative management is often adequate. If the patient develops a large abscess cavity, in addition to drainage of the abscess, formal secondary closure is often indicated (Figs 33.24 and 33.25). Underlying bone such as the ischeum or trochanter will require to be partially excised leaving a smooth surface. This will reduce recurrence. Paraplegics are likely to get further pressure sores during the course of their life. Attempts should be made to avoid aggressive excision of partially devitalized tissue during the de-sloughing (Fig. 33.25). Similarly, whenever possible attempts should be made to achieve primary closure of the sores without resorting to the use of myocutaneous flaps. Pre- and post-operative nursing is paramount in the management of pressure sores. It is inadvisable to embark on extensive surgical repair, including the use of flaps on paraplegic patients in an environment where 24-hour informed nursing care that is appropriate for the paralysed is not available. Wound sepsis and haematoma formation can devitalize flaps leading to the development of larger sores. The use of low air loss mattress or fluidized bed therapy can complement, in some instances, the need for expert nursing care.

Kyphoscoliosis, fractures, contractures

KYPHOTIC DEFORMITIES

Unlike patients with myelomeningocoele, adult-onset paraplegia does not lead to a rapid and disabling kyphoscoliotic deformity of the vertebral column. Bony injuries to the vertebral column leading to neuraxis trauma in adults are normally treated conservatively with periods of bed rest for up to 10 weeks or more. These patients develop further kyphotic deformity during the period of mobilization and rehabilitation. The increase in kyphotic

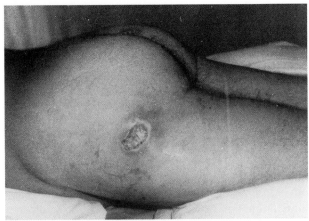
(a)

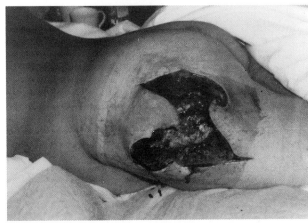
(b)

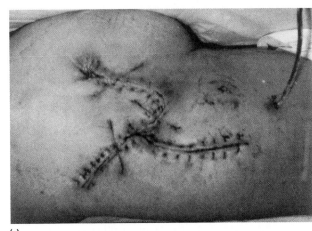
(c)

Fig. 33.24 Left trochanteric pressure sore on a 46-year-old male paraplegic. (a) On admission showing the area of skin destruction. (b) Appearance after de-sloughing, showing extensive soft-tissue destruction. (c) Following repair 3 weeks later.

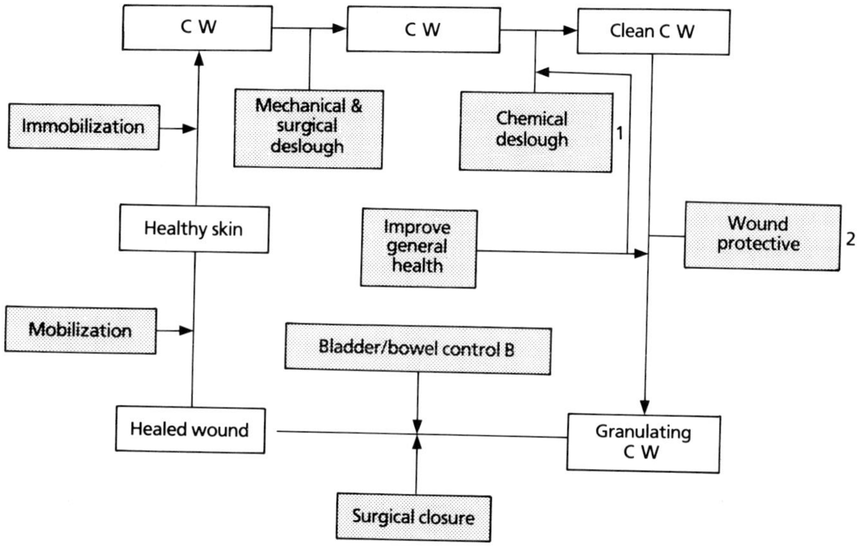

Fig. 33.25 Cycle of decubiti. Pressure sores with full thickness skin loss form a cavity wound (CW) which will require surgical removal of the slough. When the cavity has been adequately treated using chemical de-sloughing agents and wound protective, it granulates. It is then surgically closed. (1) Chemical de-sloughing agents such as hydrogen peroxide, streptokinase/streptodronase, Eusol; (2) Wound protective: hydrogels, hydrocolloids, alginates, polysacroid paste.

angle is seldom functionally disabling and rarely causes cosmetic problems. Patients who have had laminectomy during the initial management for traumatic paraplegia appear to develop a very prominent knuckle just above the site of the laminectomy which will form a bursa and secondarily get infected due to repeated trauma against the canvas of the back rest of a wheelchair. In a series of over 300 patients who have had dorsal and lumbar spine injury associated with paraplegia, the authors found an average kyphotic angle of about 20° at the site of fracture. The deformity was more pronounced in patients with a fracture of the dorsolumbar junction. No further deterioration of the deformity was noticed after the first year of paraplegia.

SCOLIOTIC DEFORMITY

Paralytic scoliosis, of a minor degree can be seen in young adults with paraplegia. Like the kyphotic deformity these do not progress. Children with paraplegia or tetraplegia however, are very vulnerable to the development of severe scoliosis which, if inadequately corrected or contained causes major disability to the patient in adult life. Most specialists dealing with paralysed children routinely brace the thoracolumbar spine until bony maturity is achieved. These patients are encouraged to walk with appropriate orthosis whenever possible and their sitting time in a wheelchair is reduced by alternative methods of ambulation. Some of these patients develop pelvic obliquity causing subluxation or dislocation of the hip joint in addition to the development of pressure sores over bony prominences. Routine and regular follow-up of these children is imperative to avoid these

complications. Most of these children are taught to lie prone at night to prevent hip contractures. Hyperlordosis associated with flexion deformities of hips and knees will compromise their independence in their bladder and bowel care and should be avoided.

Attempts to correct spinal deformity should be carefully planned. Cooperation and support from the local spinal injuries unit is often an added advantage in the pre- and post-operative management of the child. Surgical stabilization should not compromise the mobility of the spine significantly thereby reducing the independence of the young adult. A detailed description of the various surgical techniques and methods of bracing the children are beyond the scope of this chapter.

CONTRACTURES

Bad sitting posture, incorrectly adjusted cushions and foot rest can lead to joint deformities and the development of contractures. Uncontrolled spasticity which causes flexion adduction deformities of the hips will lead to neuropathic changes around the hip joints with disorganization of the femoral head. In extreme cases, the capsule of the hip joint distends with osseous and cartilaginous matter and the hip dislocates. This further increases the spasticity restricting the mobility and independence of the paralysed.

In adults, contractures of the hips and knees can be reduced by prolonged, sustained traction using minimum weight through a tibial pin. Because the traction has to be maintained for three weeks or more, such procedures are best carried out in an environment where the patient can be best nursed. During the period of traction drug manipulation to control spasticity is essential. The use of baclofen, Valium and Dantrium will hasten the correction of the deformities. Fixed deformities caused by isolated muscles such as the sartorious or hamstring can then be released either by closed tenotomy or by open soft-tissue release operations. Closed adductor tenotomy in most patients is a prerequisite to achieve better personal hygiene. Patients must be encouraged to sleep prone with the knees separated by pillows after such corrective procedures.

FRACTURES

There is a continuous loss of bone mass from the paralysed extremities in these patients. The maximum loss of bone measured by the excretion of urinary hydroxyproline occurs between 6 and 12 weeks after injury. However, the levels of urinary hydroxyproline remain high for the rest of their life with transient increases during periods of immobilization due to concurrent infections or disease. Paralysed patients are encouraged to stand using a standing frame or calipers and crutches where appropriate (Figs 33.21 and 33.23). This has the effect of reducing further demineralization of the bone in the lower extremities. However, pathological fractures, usually of the lower end of the femur, are not uncommon in the paralysed and tend to occur in young adults following vigorous sporting activities or in older patients as a result of a defective transfer between two surfaces. Fractures of the lower extremities have occurred during such mundane activities as crossing one's knees to adjust the sock. In general, the fractures to the long bones in the lower extremities are treated conservatively except in the acute phase. Internal fixation using plates and cancellous screws, together with an appropriate well-padded external cast, has the advantage of returning the patient home earlier. It is important to ascertain that adequate home care is available to the disabled prior to discharge from the hospital. Failure to do so will lead to further complications in the form of pressure sores, urinary infections and depression.

Heterotopic bone formation

Heterotopic bone formation, formerly known as 'myositis ossificans' is a well-known complication of spinal cord injury and head injury. Heterotopic bone formation can lead to considerable morbidity due to ankylosis of major joints usually in the lower extremities. The hip joint is by far the commonest site of involvement in this process. The precise conditions that trigger the formation of soft-tissue calcification in the paralysed

patient remain uncertain. Primitive mesenchymal tissue with a potential to form bone appears to respond to minor soft-tissue trauma in paralysed patients. The clinical picture initially is one of inflammation around a joint. There is swelling, induration and on occasion compression of adjacent venous channels leading to a picture roughly similar to that of deep venous thrombosis. Radiological evidence of calcification of soft tissue may take 3−6 weeks from the onset of heterotropic bone formation. However, ultrasound examinations of the soft tissue can prove invaluable not only in excluding deep venous thrombosis, but also in identifying muscle necrosis and the commencement of early calcification before radiological demonstration becomes feasible (Burning, 1975; Cassar-Pallicino *et al.*, 1993).

In the early stages, rest and anti-inflammatory drugs are necessary. Recently, the use of sodium etidronate has been shown to reduce the florid evolution of heterotropic bone formation seen in some patients (Stover, 1976). Untreated patients progress to extensive and diffuse calcification usually around a hip joint which may take many months before maturation of the bone. During the phase of bone formation serum alkaline phosphatase is significantly elevated and remains so for many weeks. The primitive osteoid tissue gradually undergoes a zonal maturation and complete bone maturation may take some 6−18 months. During this period there is a gradual decline in serum alkaline phosphatase.

During the acute phase, once the inflammatory response has subsided, attempts should be made to maintain a reasonable range of movements around the joint. In spite of efforts, on occasions ankylosis will occur and in such cases it is preferable to allow the ankylosis to take place with a hip abducted at 15° and flexed at 45°.

Surgical removal of the mature heterotropic bone formation should not be contemplated until serial radiography over a six-month period fail to shown an increase in the size of the new bone. Levels of serum alkaline phosphatase are unreliable indicators of bone maturation in these patients. Surgical removal of the bone in a patient with ankylosed or severely restricted movements around the hip joint should be complemented with use of sodium etidronate in the peri-operative phase (Stover *et al.*, 1976). Excision of the bone should be just adequate to achieve the range desired. Extensive dissection of the soft tissue to remove the entire ossific mass can (and often does) lead to re-occurrence of calcification in the post-operative phase. Mobilization of the affected joint in the post-operative phase should be gentle and persistent. Careful planning of pre- and post-operative nursing and subsequent mobilization in an appropriate wheelchair is important in the overall management of this condition.

Syringomyelia

Post-traumatic and post-arachnoiditic syringomyelia is not an uncommon complication of long-term paraplegia. Increased use of the magnetic resonance scan following acute traumatic spinal cord injury has shown that intrinsic changes in the spinal cord can be seen very soon after the trauma and large cysts have now been known to occur in a few patients during the phase of acute rehabilitation (less than 12 weeks) (Fig. 33.5). The previously-held view that the condition is of late onset has now been challenged by more recent workers in this field. Until recently, the incidence of post-traumatic syringomyelia leading to further neurological deficit due to enlarging cysts was thought to be 5%. The incidence of asymptomatic (silent) cysts in the spinal cord may be much higher, and some studies put this incidence at 50–60%. The precise reason for the development of post-traumatic syringomyelia remains unknown. However, it is believed that a cavity is formed by the liquefaction of cord tissue damaged at the time of the injury. Haematoma within the spinal cord is considered to be a contributory cause in the development of the cyst which gradually distends. Adhesive arachnoiditis following trauma both above and below the site of bony lesion might cause changes to the CSF flow. CSF flow dynamics may have a role in determining the extent of the cyst (Rossier *et al.*, 1985; William, 1990; Silberstein and Hennessy, 1992).

In severe cases with large cysts, the neurological deterioration and the level of disability could change dramatically. Neurosurgical procedures for such cysts include drainage, syringostomy and insertion of shunt. Periodic follow-up with appropriate radio-diagnostic investigation in these patients is mandatory.

Pain

Pain due to soft-tissue injuries and fractures to the spinal column can be adequately controlled with conventional analgesics. Most patients however, appear to develop 'central pain', which is of a dysaesthetic nature. The perception of pain is commonly influenced by psychological factors. Spinal injury units often reassure these patients and explain the nature of the dysaesthetic pain. Such reasoned explanations, usually by senior members of staff, may reduce the intensity of pain and the need for regular analgesics. Anxiety, uncertain prognosis and pre-existing domestic/vocational problems adversely influence the perception of pain by the patient. The opportunity to share and discuss the nature of their pain with other patients within a spinal injuries unit enables most patients to accept certain levels of discomfort perceived over the paralysed part of the body.

Rarely, surgical procedure may be of value, particularly if the pain is restricted to one or two peripheral nerve distributions. Transcutaneous electrical nerve stimulation has been found to be of value in some of these patients. In patients with a disabling chronic pain, not controlled with analgesics, certain types of anti-epileptics, anxiolytics and sedatives are useful; several destructive procedures may be appropriate. Such procedures include dorsal-root entry zone coagulation, commissurotomy, stereotactic procedures on the thalamus, intraneural injections of caustic agents and cryoprobe destruction of nerves. In a small number of patients, implantation of neuroprostheses which deliver opioid analgesics into the subarachnoid space has been found to be an efficient way of improving the quality of life.

Urological complications

Most male patients with suprasacral spinal cord injury (with intact reflex pathways) usually remain socially continent by the use of a penile sheath. Reflex voiding of urine occurs due to distension of the bladder and a large proportion of these patients have low residual urine after reflex micturition. The ability to satisfactorily empty the bladder is influenced by the chronicity of the disease, associated infection, age in addition to the primary lesion. Regular urological assessment particularly to evaluate the function of the kidneys is important. Most spinal injury units carry out periodic intravenous urograms or ultrasound examinations of the kidneys in patients with spinal cord injury. Clinically asymptomatic patients do not require regular bacteriological assessment of urine. Asymptomatic bacteriuria in patients with low post-micturition residual volume does not require active antimicrobial treatment. However, patients who suffer recurrent urinary-tract infection will benefit from low-dose, long-term antimicrobial treatment.

Elderly patients and female patients with severe disability (tetraplegics) are often managed with an indwelling long-term urethral catheter. In young female patients, periodic clamping of the catheter to maintain bladder volume will reduce long-term problems of bladder contraction, stone formation and catheter blockage. Continuous urinary drainage in female patients often leads to a small contracted bladder which eventually leads to catheter extrusion and urethral erosion causing urinary incontinence. Bladder distension due to a blocked catheter will lead to autonomic dysreflexia (hyper-reflexia). Patients with autonomic dysreflexia complain of violent pounding headache due to severe hypertension which may be associated with sweating and blotchy vasodilatation of the skin. Prompt drainage of the bladder is mandatory.

Both male and female paraplegic patients with supra-sacral spinal cord injury can be managed by self-intermittent catheterization. The uninhibited detrusor activity can be reduced with appropriate medication in most instances and such patients can avoid the need to wear an incontinence device (Table 33.3, Fig. 33.26).

Paraplegic patients with sacral lesion (lower motor neuron bladder) often have minimal detrusor activity and may have sufficient sphincter activity so that their bladders could be managed satisfactorily by intermittent catheterization (Fig. 33.26).

Increased irritability of the bladder in female patients with a long-term indwelling urethral catheter can be reduced by injection of intravesical phenol under the trigone. Other procedures such as Stamey suspension or colpo-suspension can also reduce the incidence of incontinence in female patients. Both male and female patients with irritable bladder can achieve continence by augmentation of the bladder with small bowel (augmentation cystoplasty) and implantation of artificial urethral sphincter. Patients who do not have bladder-neck incompetence, as seen during video urodynamic studies, may benefit by implantation by sacral anterio-stimulator. This procedure involves stimulation of S2–S4 anterior nerve root using implanted electrodes and a receiver unit. The receiver unit is activated using a hand-held external coupling device. In a small proportion of patients, such a stimulation can also achieve erection. More recently, it has been shown that bowel evacuation is hastened with the use of a sacral anterio-stimulator (MacDonagh *et al.*, 1990).

Reconstructive surgery

Reconstructive surgery to the upper extremity by transfer of appropriate muscle to achieve greater function is now well-established practice in certain centres. Transfer of posterior deltoid to the olecranon (deltoid-to-triceps transfers) will provide elbow extension in patients who have reasonable hand function. Similarly, the transfer of one of the extensors of the wrist to the common flexor in patients with active finger extension can result in active finger flexion. C6 tetraplegic patients with intact radial wrist extensors achieve significant benefit by a key-grip (Fig. 33.27) (McDowell *et al.*, 1986) procedure where the flexor pollicis longus tendon is tenodesed to the lower end of radius (Lamb, 1987). Patients selected for tendon surgery must be assessed by an occupational therapist pre-operatively. The value of trained hand physiotherapists and the nursing care that is appropriate for the patient in the post-operative phase cannot be overemphasized.

Spasticity

Uncontrolled spasticity in patients with suprasacral lesion inevitably leads to increased disability. In addition

Table 33.3 The influence of detrusor and sphincter activity on neurogenic bladder management

	D+ S+	D+ S−	D− S+	D− S−	
Reflex voiding	Yes	Yes	No	No	Condom in men, pads in women; voiding may be augmented with carbachol, bethanechol and/or phenoxybenzamine
Intermittent self-catheterization	Yes	Yes	Yes	Yes	Usually with oxybutynin and/or propantheline, sometimes with imipramine
Straining	No	?	Yes	Yes	
Indwelling catheter	Yes	Yes	Yes	Yes	Periodic bladder washouts; propantheline may be needed

D+ = reflex detrusor activity.
S+ = reflex activity of external urethral sphincter.
D− = absent reflex detrusor activity.
S− = absent external urethral sphincter activity.

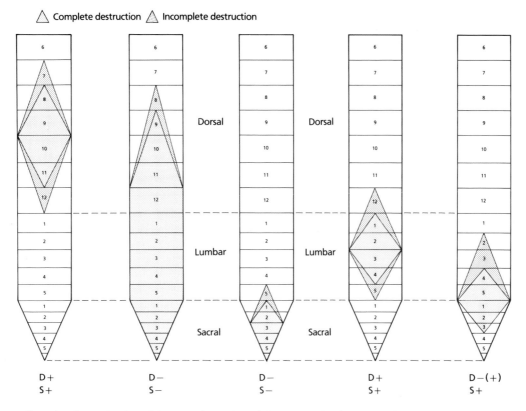

Fig. 33.26 The effect of different levels and degrees of spinal cord damage on the detrusor and external sphincter function. Note the numbers represent the various spinal cord levels and do not correspond to the bony levels. (Redrawn with permission from Mr. D.G. Thomas and Heinemann.)

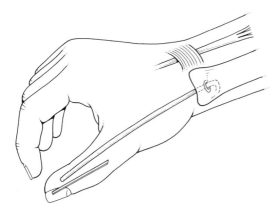

Fig. 33.27 Key grip procedure. In patients with good dorsiflexion, the flexor pollicis longus tendon is divided at the wrist, attached to the volar or lateral aspect of the radius. The interphalangeal joint of the thumb is stabilized. When active wrist extension is attempted, flexor pollicis longus tendon presses the thumb against the side of the index finger providing the key grip. Occasionally, division of the extensor retinaculum may be of value.

to developing contractures, patients with uncontrolled spasticity suffer pathological fractures as a result of fall and pressure sores due to inappropriate seating. Spasm can be reduced by a variety of means. Many patients regularly take anti-spasmodics such as baclofen and dantrolene sodium. Prone lying at night often reduces spasticity and delays the development of contractures around hips and knees. Spasm may be aggravated by minor conditions such as ingrowing toenail, constipation or septic spots in the paralysed part. Spasm has been known to increase during menstruation. Renal calculi, bladder calculi and urinary tract infection generally increase spasticity.

Spasm of the lower extremity can be controlled by a selective block of the spinal nerves. Intrathecal injections of phenol can abolish extremity muscle spasm. Unfortunately, such injections can affect the management of bladder and bowel function. Intrathecal injections can convert a reflex bladder into one that requires indwelling urethral catheterization. Similarly, anal and rectal reflexes can be damaged with the use of intrathecal phenol. Patients who have previously used a rectal stimulant to achieve defaecation will require manual evacuation after instillation of intrathecal phenol.

Phenol can also be used to selectively block peripheral nerves in suitable cases using nerve tracer.

Rarely, intrathecal alcohol has been used to abolish spasticity affecting the lower extremities and the trunk. These are drastic and destructive procedures and should be used only after other methods of containing spasm have failed to improve the quality of life.

More recently, intrathecal administration of baclofen has been shown to control spasticity without adverse central side effects seen in patients who take large amounts of oral baclofen. Various delivery systems are now available. Some of the implanted pumps delivering intrathecal baclofen have a constant infusion rate while others are demand-driven.

Chronic spasticity will inevitably lead to contractures particularly around the hip joint and closed tenotomys or open soft release procedures may be indicated in some patients. Isolated adductor spasticity can often be relieved by obturator neurectomy. The choice of treatment must always be discussed with the patient and the carer, and the complications explained in detail in each case.

Sports and paraplegia

Social re-integration of the paralysed person involves participation in a variety of activities that are available to the able-bodied. Since the disability in most patients precludes their return to a former vocation which involved manual strength and dexterity, disabled sports has become the forum to express the innate competitiveness of human beings. The value of competitive sport was recognized by Sir Ludwig Guttmann early in 1945. A variety of sports are now open to disabled athletes and the Para-Olympics are held on a regular basis (Fig. 33.22). Archery, table tennis and quad ball are sports played predominantly by tetraplegic athletes, while basketball and tennis are more common among paraplegics. There is no doubt that sports play a very important role in the emotional re-integration of the paralysed with the community at large.

Wheelchair/orthosis

Modern lightweight wheelchairs incorporate a variety of advanced design concepts to suit the needs of different patients. Some of these chairs weigh about 8.5 kg without the wheels. Most of these chairs have detachable wheels and folding back-rests. The materials used in the construction of these modern chairs are extremely strong. The design is, in some cases, modular, allowing for variable back-rest height, variable back-rest angle, and adjustment to the rear axle wheel in order to change the centre of gravity and seat height. They also have the ability to alter the camber and come with a choice of casters to suit their requirements. Some of these wheelchairs have mechanical or hydraulic devices which allow the patient to stand. There are specially-designed wheelchairs used by athletes which enable wheelchair athletes participating in marathons to compete with the able-bodied person on an even keel. Appropriate seating, back-rest and foot-rest are vital to achieve maximum independence during rehabilitation (Fig. 33.20).

Hip guidance orthosis is a device which stabilizes the ankle and knee with an articulation for the hip placed anterior to the hip joint. The design features of hip guidance orthosis allows a low-energy erect ambulation of the paralysed patient. The key to a successful functional use of either hip guidance orthosis or reciprocating gait orthosis is motivation. Using a small portable electronic-pulse generator that produces square pulses of 20–50 Hz with a pulse width of 150–300 μs and a potential difference on a 1 kΩ open resistance of 120–200 V, it is possible to stimulate paralysed muscles where there is an intact reflex arc. With appropriate lightweight low-energy orthosis, erect ambulation may become feasible for many paraplegic and tetraplegic patients (Fig. 33.21).

MEDICO-LEGAL ASPECTS

A small proportion of patients with spinal cord injury or a potential for spinal cord injury due to associated vertebral column injury remain unrecognized during the acute management in the Accident and Emergency Department. Four per cent of patients with paraplegia and 8% of patients with tetraplegia appear to have escaped initial detection of their neurological deficit by the admitting team. Many contributory factors have been identified. Minimal, or no, neurological deficit at the time of first admission, head injury and an inability to give appropriate history and multiple injury presenting with life-threatening conditions in the Accident and Emergency Department are not uncommonly seen in the group of patients with missed injuries of the spinal cord (Table 33.1). Other causes such as ambience, where the medical officer's clinical judgement is clouded by historic data (such as the patient being drunk or being in possession of a stolen vehicle) should not lead to an error in the diagnosis of spinal cord injury. Drug and alcohol abuse are not uncommonly seen in patients in whom spinal cord injury is unrecognized. Undue reliance on radiographic demonstration of a vertebral fracture is regrettable. Many patients have had significant neurological deficit without a radiological demonstration of bony injury.

Inevitably, missed injury to the spinal cord leads to mismanagement. In many cases, such missed injuries lead to litigation against the hospital. A careful evaluation of all cardinal signs of spinal cord injury in every patient will inevitably reduce the incidence of missed/ mismanaged/negligently managed injuries to the spinal cord (Reid *et al.*, 1987; Ravichandran, 1989; Silver *et al.*, 1990).

REFERENCES

Allman R.M., Laprade C.A., Noel L.B. and Walker J. (1986) Metal pressure sores among hospitalised patients. *Ann. Intern. Med.* **105**, 337–342.

Bach-y-Rita P. and Illis L.S. (1993) Spinal shock: possible role of receptor plasticity and non-synaptic transmission. *Paraplegia* **31**, 82–87.

Bajd T., Andrews B.J., Kiarlj A. and Katakis J. (1985) Restoration of walking in patients with incomplete spinal cord injury by the use of surface electrical stimulation — preliminary studies. *Prost. Orthot. Int.* **9**, 109–111.

Bannister R. (1988) In *Autonomic Failure*. Oxford, Oxford Medical Publications, pp. 511–521.

Bearsted J.H. (1930) In *The Edwin Smith Surgical Papyrus*, Vol. 1, Chicago, pp. 316–428. See Trevor-Hughes J. (ibid).

Bedbrook G.M. (1987) The development and care of spinal cord paralysis 1918–1986. *Paraplegia* **25**, 172–184.

Bedbrook G.M. (1992) Fifty years on fundamentals in the spinal cord injury are still important. *Paraplegia* **30**, 10–13.

Bedford D.S., Behrooz A., Winter R.B. and Seljeskog E.L. (1977) Surgical stabilisation of fracture and fracture dislocations of the thoracic spine. *Spine* **2**, 185–196.

Bohlman H.H. (1974) Traumatic fractures of the upper thoracic spine with paraplegia. *J. Bone Joint Surg.* **56A**, 1299.

Bollman H.H., Freehafer A. and Dejak J. (1985) The result of treatment of acute injuries of the upper thoracic spine with paralysis. *J. Bone Joint Surg.* **67A**, 360–369.

Brachen M.B., Shephard M.J., Collins W.F. *et al.* (1990) A randomised controlled trial of methyl prednisolone or naloxone in the treatment of acute spinal cord injury. *New Engl. J. Med.* **332**, 1405–1411.

Bradford D.S. and Thompson R.C. (1976) Fracture and dislocations of spine. Indications for surgical intervention. *Minn. Med.* **58**, 711–720.

Burning K. (1975) On the origin of cells in heterotropic bone formation. *Clin. Orthopaed.* **110**, 293–302.

Calenoff L., Chessave, J.W., Rogers L.F. *et al.* (1978) Multiple level spinal injuries — importance of early recognition. *Am. J. Roentg.* **130**, 665–669.

Cassar-Pallicino U.N., McClelland M.R., Badwan D.A.H. *et al.* (1993) Sonographic diagnosis of heterotropic bone formation in spinal injury patients. *Paraplegia* **31**, 40–50.

Charlifue S.W., Gerhart K.A., Menter R.R. *et al.* (1992) Sexual issues in women with spinal cord injury. *Paraplegia* **30**, 192–199.

Cockhill S.M.E. (1992) Wound care problems in the community. In *Proceedings of First European Conference on Advances in Wound Management*. London, Macmillan Magazine Ltd., pp. 3–6.

Collins W.F. (1984) A review of treatment of spinal cord injury. *Br. J. Surg.* **71**, 974–975.

Couldwell D. and Carlisle M. (1990) Nursing care of spinal cord injuries. In Alderson J.D. and Frost E.A. (eds) *Spinal Cord Injuries. Anaesthetic and Associated Care*. London, Butterworth, Vol. 9, pp. 126–138.

Donovan W.H., Carter R.E., Bedbrook G.M. *et al.* (1984) Incidents of medical complications in spinal cord injury: patients in specialised compared with non-specialised centres. *Paraplegia* **22**, 282–290.

Ducker T.M., Salaman M., Perot P.L. and Ballantine D. (1978) Experimental spinal cord trauma. I. Correlation of blood flow, tissue oxygenation and neurologic status in the dog. *Surg. Neurol.* **10**, 60–63.

El Asri W. (1993) Physiological instability of the injuries spinal cord. *Paraplegia* **31** (in press).

Epstein N., Hood D.C. and Ransohoff J. (1981) Gastrointestinal bleeding in patients with spinal cord trauma. *J. Neurosurg.* **54**, 16–20.

Evans D.K. (1961) Reduction of cervical dislocation. *J. Bone Joint Surg.* **43B**, 552–555.

Frankel H.L. and Mathias C.J. (1976) The cardiovascular system in tetraplegia and paraplegia. In Vinken P.J. and Bruyn (eds) *Handbook of Clinical Neurology*. Amsterdam, Vol. 26, pp. 313–333.

Frankel H.L., Hancock D.O., Hyslop G. *et al.* (1969) The value of postural reduction in the initial management of closed injuries of the spine with paraplegia and tetraplegia. *Paraplegia* **7**, 179–192.

Geisler F.H., Dorsey F.C. and Coleman W.P. (1992) Recovery of motor function after a spinal cord injury — a randomised placebo controlled trial with GM-1 ganglioside. *New Engl. J. Med.* **324**, 1829–1838.

Griffith E.R. and Trieschmann R.B. (1975) Sexual function in women with spinal cord injury. *Arch. Phys. Med. Rehabil.* **56**, 18–21.

Halstead L.S. (1987) Rectal probe electrostimulation in the treatment of anejaculatory spinal cord men. *Paraplegia* **25**, 120–129.

Harvey C., Rothschild B.B., Asmann A.J. and Stripling T. (1990) New estimates of traumatic spinal cord injury prevalence: a survey based approach. *Paraplegia* **28**, 537–544.

Heller L., Keren O., Aloni R. and Davidoff G. (1992) An open trial of vacuum penile tumescence: constriction therapy for neurological impotence. *Paraplegia* **30**, 550–553.

Holdsworth F. (1970) Fracture, dislocations and fracture–dislocations of the spine. *J. Bone Joint Surg.* **52A**, 1534–1552.

Isakov E., Douglas R. and Berns P. (1992) Ambulation using the reciprocating gait orthosis and functional electrical stimulation. *Paraplegia* **30**, 246–252.

Jelsma R.K., Kirsch P.T., Jelsma L.F. *et al.* (1982) Surgical treatment of thoracolumbar fractures. *Surg. Neurol.* **18**, 156–166.

Kelley T.A. (1979) Emergency case recognition of spinal cord injury. *J. Am. Coll. Emerg. Physicians* **8**, 493.

Kinoshita H., Nagata Y., Ueda H. and Kisih K. (1993) Conservative management of burst fracture of thoracolumbar and lumbar spine. *Paraplegia* **31**, 58–67.

Koning W., Forwein R.A. and Firsching R. (1987) Epidemiology of spinal cord injury. In Harris (ed.) *Advances in Neurotraumatology*, Vol. 2. Vienna, Springer-Verlag, pp. 1–12.

Krans J.F., Franti C.E., Riggins R.S. *et al.* (1975) Incidents of traumatic spinal cord lesions. *J. Chronic Dis.* **28**, 471–492.

Kurtzke J.F. (1975) Epidemiology of spinal injury. *Exp. Neurol.* **48**, 163–236.

Lamb D.W. (1987) The upper limb and hand in traumatic tetraplegia. In Lamb D.W. (ed.) *The Paralysed Hand*. Edinburgh, Churchill Livingstone, pp. 136–152.

Lewin M.G., Hansbout R.R. and Papius H.M. (1974) Chemical characteristics of traumatic spinal cord oedema. *J. Neurosurg.* **40**, 65–75.

Lucas J.T. and Ducker T.B. (1980) Laminectomy in spinal cord trauma: harmful or helpful? *Neurosurgery* **6**, 688–689.

MacDonagh R.P., Sun W.M., Smallwood R. *et al.* (1990) Control of defaecation in patients with spinal cord injury by stimulation of sacral anterior nerve roots. *Br. Med. J.* **300**, 1494–1497.

McDowell C.L., Moberg E.A. and House J.H. (1986) Proceedings of the Second International Conference on Surgical Rehabilitation of the Upper Limb in Tetraplegia (Quadraplegia). *J. Hand Surg.* **11A**, 604–608.

Macourt D., Engel S., Jones R.F. and Zaki M. (1991) Pregnancy by gamete intrafallopian transfer (GIFT) with sperm aspirated from vasoepididymal junction of spinal injured men: case report. *Paraplegia* **29**, 550–553.

McSweeney T. (1979) Fractures, fracture–dislocations and dislocations of the cervical spine. In Jeffreys E. (ed.) *Disorders of the Cervical Spine*. London, Butterworth.

Meinecke F.W. (1968) Frequency and distribution of associated injuries in traumatic paraplegia and tetraplegia. **5**, 196–211.

National Pressure Ulcer Advisory Panel (1989) Report. West Seneca, New York, NPUAP.

Nicoll E.A. (1949) Fracture of the dorsolumbar spine. *J. Bone Joint Surg.* **31**, 376–394.

Perovitch M. and Wang H. (1992) The evolution of neuroimaging of spinal cord injury patients over the last decade. *Paraplegia* **30**, 39–42.

Ramsay R. (1990) Post-traumatic stress disorder—a new clinical entity. *J. Psychosomatic Res.* **34**, 355–365.

Ravichandran G. (1978) Traumatic single facet subluxation without neurological damage of the cervical spine—a new clinical sign. *Arch. Orthop. Trauma. Surg.* **92**, 221–224.

Ravichandran G. (1989) Errors and omissions in the acute management of spinal cord injury. *J. Med. Defence Union* **5**, 14–16.

Ravichandran G. and Silver J.R. (1982) Missed injuries of the spinal cord. *Br. Med. J.* **284**, 953–956.

Ravichandran G. and Silver J.R. (1984) Recognition of spinal cord injury. *Hosp. Update* 77–86.

Reid D.C., Henderson R., Saboe L. and Miller J.D.R. (1987) Aetiology and clinical course of missed spine fracture. *J. Trauma.* **27**, 980–986.

Rossier A.B., Foo D. and Shillito J. (1985) Post-traumatic syringomyelia. Incidence, clinical presentation, electrophysiological studies, syrinx protein and results of conservative and operative treatment. *Brain* **108**, 439–461.

Roy-Camille R., Demeulenaere C., Saillant G. and Barsat E. (1973) Ostéosynthèse du rachis dorsal et lombaire par voie postérieure. *Nouv. Presse Med.* **2**, 1309–1312.

Scher A.T. (1979) The value of anterio-posterior radiograph in 'hidden' fractures and dislocations of the lower cervical spine. *S. Afr. Med. J.* **55**, 221–224.

Silberstein M. and Hennessy O. (1992) Cystic cord lesions and neurological deterioration in spinal cord injury: operative considerations based on magnetic resonance imaging. *Paraplegia* **30**, 661–668.

Silver J.R. and Frankland L.A. (1990) Traumatic spinal cord injury. In Foy M.A. and Fagg P.S. (eds) *Medico-Legal Reporting in Orthopaedic Trauma*. London, Churchill Livingstone, Vol. 17, pp. 417–430.

Silver J.R., Morris W.R. and Wotfinowski J.S. (1980) Associated injuries in patients with spinal cord injury. *Injury* **12**, 219–224.

Siosteen A., Forssman L., Steen Y. *et al.* (1990) Quality of semen after repeated ejaculation treatment in spinal cord injured men. *Paraplegia* **28**, 96–104.

Stover S.L. and Fine R.R. (1987) The epidemiology and economics of spinal cord injury. *Paraplegia* **25**, 225–228.

Stover S.L., Niemann K.M.W. and Miller J.M. (1976) Disodium etidronate in the prevention of post-operative recurrence of heterotropic ossification in spinal cord injured patients. *J Bone Joint Surg.* **58A**, 683–688.

Summers B.N., McClelland M.R. and El Masri W.S. (1988) A clinical review of adult hip guidance orthosis (para Walker) in traumatic paraplegics. *Paraplegia* **26**, 19–26.

Thomas D.G. (1982) The urinary tract following spinal cord injury. In Chisholm G.D. and Williams (eds) *Urology*. London, Heinemann.

Thompson-Walker, Sir J. (1937) *Proc. R. Soc. Med.* **30**, 1233.

Trevor-Hughes J. (1988) The Edwin Smith surgical papyrus—an analysis of the first case reports of spinal cord injury. *Paraplegia* **26**, 71–82.

Trieschmann R.B. (1988) *Spinal Cord Injuries: Psychological Social and Vocational Rehabilitation*. New York, Demos Publications.

Trieschmann R.B. (1992) Psychological research in spinal cord injury: the state of the art. *Paraplegia* **30**, 58–60.

Vizuete S.F. (1989) Nutritional management in acute spinal cord injury. In Whiteneck (ed.) *The Management of High Quadraplegia—Comprehensive Neurological Rehabilitation*. New York, Demos Publications, pp. 77–93.

Watson N. (1978) Anticoagulant therapy in the prevention of venous thrombosis and pulmonary embolism in spinal cord injury. *Paraplegia* **16**, 265–269.

Watson-Jones R. (1949) Fractures of the spine. *J. Bone Joint Surg.* **31B**, 322–325.

William B. (1990) Post-traumatic syringomyelia, an update. *Paraplegia* **20**, 296–313.

Wilmot C.B. and Hall K. (1986) Evaluation of acute surgical intervention in traumatic paraplegia. *Paraplegia* **24**, 71–76.

Yashon D. (1986) Aetiology and predisposing factors. In Yashon D. (ed.) *Spinal Injury*. Connecticut, Appleton–Century–Crofts, pp. 39–69.

Young B., Brooks W.H. and Tibbs P.A. (1981) Anterior decompression and fusion of thoracolumbar fracture with neurologic deficits. *Acta Neurochir. Vienna* **57**, 287–298.

Young G.S. (1992) The spinal cord injury primary physician—one riot, one ranger. *Paraplegia* **30**, 17–19.

Chapter 34
Orthotics

R.G.S. Platts

INTRODUCTION

The word 'orthotics' has come to mean the science and practice of applying externally worn devices which perform a variety of mechanical functions to the body or body parts to which they are applied. The devices themselves are called 'orthoses' and they are named by the first letter of the joints or body parts that they span. For example, there is the knee−ankle−foot orthosis or **KAFO**, and cervical thoracolumbar orthosis or **CTLO**. This nomenclature is now accepted but the use of eponyms is still fairly general and has some merit as a rapid way of describing a form of orthosis. Here orthoses will be referred to in full.

The professionally trained fitter who measures the patient, writes the manufacturing details, fits the orthosis on the patient and gives instructions in its use is called an 'orthotist'.

The training to become an orthotist has recently become a four-year degree course at one of the two schools in the UK.

The main groups of functions which orthoses may be intended to perform are as follows:

1 *Support.* For example, a thoracolumbar orthosis to support a collapsing paretic spine, or to relieve weight from some of the skeleton of the lower leg with a knee−ankle−foot orthosis.

2 *Limitation of movement.* For example, a knee orthosis to prevent hyperextension.

3 *Correction of deformity.* For example, a thoracolumbar sacral orthosis to correct an idiopathic scoliosis and redirect growth.

4 *Assistance to movement.* For example, a hand orthosis with active springs to assist finger extension.

Many orthoses combine several functions, for instance a knee−ankle−foot orthosis for a leg resulting from a history of poliomyelitis will give support, will limit movement at the knee and perhaps the ankle, it may help to correct a varus ankle and have a spring to assist dorsiflexion. This is not an exhaustive list and examples of other less common functions will emerge during this chapter.

Almost invariably orthoses have to strike a balance between the often conflicting requirements of function, cosmesis and acceptability. The ideal orthosis is, of course, invisible and weightless but nonetheless, performs its desired function. Orthoses need, too, to be provided or replaced quickly, to be hygienic, safe and reliable.

There are all kinds of other factors which need to be considered when recommending orthoses.

1 *Employment.* The level and type of activity at work. Whether the work is mainly sedentary or involves much walking, lifting weights, stairs, etc. The footwear required. The need to wear wellington boots.

2 *Driving.* The type of car, manual or automatic, the need to use both feet, movement at the ankle, hand controls, visibility in regard to neck movements. The room for stiff knees to get in and out, etc.

3 *Dress.* Whether trousers are worn, e.g. in relation to wear from orthotic knee joints, donning and doffing the orthosis.

4 *Hand and other function.* Particularly in relation to donning and doffing. The ability to work buckles, Velcro, stud fasteners; to lace eyelets, pass straps through D-buckles. The ability to reach the necessary parts, e.g. back and hip flexion to reach the foot−with one hand or both. Other pathology with orthotic implications.

5 *Durability required.* Is it to last as long as possible? What is the duration of a treatment period? Or, will it soon be outgrown?

6 *Weight, age and activity level.* A knee orthosis for a frail elderly lady using a walking frame will need to be a very different structure from one performing the same function for a young active person.

7 *Pregnancy.* Apart from the obvious considerations of

girth and weight, pregnancy affects the ability to reach the feet, the balance and spinal posture.

8 *Contralateral limb function.* This will clearly affect the limb under consideration.

9 *Intelligence, motivation and cosmesis.* Judgements need to be made on these factors to determine the likelihood of the orthosis being used.

PRESCRIPTION

The essence of successful orthotic treatment is impeccably careful matching of the patient with the orthosis. The process of prescription should ideally follow the following sequence:

1 Clinical decision that orthotic treatment is desirable.

2 Further clinical examination with a view to the desirable orthotic prescription.

3 Written functional description by the prescriber of the functions expected of the orthosis.

4 Examination, measurement, casting (if necessary) of the patient by the orthotist.

5 Discussion (if required) between the prescriber and the orthotist as to details of the orthosis.

6 Written specification of the orthosis by the orthotist sufficient for the manufacturer to complete the job.

7 Manufacture (if necessary with liaison between the orthotist and the manufacturer, e.g. for cast rectification, trim lines, etc.).

8 (If required) trial fitting by the orthotist of the orthosis in a partly completed state.

9 Fitting and supply of the orthosis by the orthotist.

10 Instruction of the patient by the orthotist on donning, doffing, usage, care, maintenance, cleaning, etc.

11 Inspection by the prescriber.

12 Follow-up by the prescriber.

The need for the prescription to take the form of a functional description of what the orthosis was required to do was recognized by the American Academy of Orthopaedic Surgeons in 1974, who produced elaborate charts. Completion of the chart focussed the mind of the prescriber on the precise biomechanical deficiencies of the patient which were intended to be replaced by the mechanical functions of the orthosis. All identified in great detail. Use of these forms has not gained general acceptance because of the time they take to complete. However, the need to focus attention on the patient's biomechanical deficits and the orthotic substitutes for them has not gone away. The practitioner will be doing his or her job only if he or she thinks in terms of function and provides functional descriptions for the orthotist to translate into hardware. There is currently much waste due to inadequate prescription. Sometimes too much is left to the orthotist so that he or she has

to make decisions on functional requirements which should properly be made by the prescribing doctor. At other times the prescriber stipulates too precisely the form of the orthosis without adequate knowledge of manufacturing techniques and the possibilities for different materials. It then becomes an inappropriate prescription. This is obviously wasteful and is not to the advantage of either the patient or the orthotist.

Effective orthotic supply can only be achieved if the correct relationship exists between prescriber and orthotist. The orthotist should be a highly trained professional with expert knowledge of his craft. The prescriber needs to recognise and rely on this and confine his or her own input to the area in which he or she is trained. Mutual respect of each other's areas of expertise should encourage discussion, and the most appropriate place is the clinic. Too often the visiting orthotist is separated from the prescriber either due to being in different clinic rooms or in time because he/she does not attend on the same day.

To further emphasize this important relationship some examples of what is meant by functional requirement of the orthosis — which is what should be prescribed — are given.

Examples of functional prescribing

EXAMPLE 1

Consider the case of a 50-year-old man who has had several surgical procedures in his early life to deal with his congenital talipes equino-varus. He is left with a 30° varus foot which has 30% range of motion in the ankle on either side of neutral, only slight subtalar movement and relatively normal passive movement in the forefoot. He has Grade 4 plantar and dorsiflexion. He is used to taking weight on the lateral border of his foot and has built up good weight-bearing callous. He comes for the prescription of better surgical footwear, his present boots collapsing laterally and wearing excessively.

Clearly shoes or boots are not going to have any corrective effect. One needs to accommodate the varus deformity leaving what ankle movement there is and make the weight-bearing axis as normal as possible with regard to the knee. The foot would need to be held so that the subtalar joint is minimally varus or else the poor mechanics of the situation are aggravated.

The prescription, following the functional requirements, might be: 'Footwear for everyday use in the office and home to accommodate the minimum of the existing varus and retaining the existing limited ankle movement (for gait and accelerator pedal)'.

EXAMPLE 2

A 43-year-old healthy woman who had poliomyelitis as a child. She was left with residual weakness in the intrinsic muscles of both hands and the right arm is generally weaker than the left, but this is of no great functional significance. The right leg is nearly totally flail. A little abductor power at the hip is used for flexion and hip extension is Grade 2. There is no power of flexion or extension at the knee and it hyperextends to 25°. To passive movements (unloaded) there is appreciable lateral instability. There is no power in the foot or ankle and movement is limited to a few degrees by a previous triple arthrodesis. The range is 10–15° of plantarflexion (i.e. 10° of fixed equinus). The foot is somewhat cavus. On the left the power about the hips is near normal and she has Grade 4 extensors at the knee with a normal range of movement. The ankle and subtalar joints have about 50% of normal range as a result of an arthodesis which has not been fully sustained. There is no power at the ankle and it is therefore unstable laterally with a tendency to valgus. She can plantarflex her toes. The right leg is 2 cm shorter than the left to the malleoli. This shortening is, of course, effectively reduced by the equinus foot when standing barefoot. Both legs are wasted below the knees and the right above the knee as well.

She has always worn a below-knee orthosis on the left and as a child wore a knee–ankle–foot orthosis on the right too. She wears an old fashioned ankle boot on the left with an inside iron and T-strap and a custom made shoe to match on the right. She lives at home with her two teenage children, works in an office and drives an automatic car modified with the accelerator on the left. She is self-conscious of her orthosis and boot and for this reason usually wears slacks.

She comes complaining of increasing pain in the right knee when weight bearing and generally being unable to get about as well as she used to and as she would wish.

If we assume that the pain is coming from the hyperextension, which is likely, it needs controlling. Clearly, too, it is important to retain the movement which she has in the left foot. Cosmesis, is as usual, an important consideration and donning and doffing needs to be easy, especially for a busy person like this.

Control of knee hyperextension can be achieved orthotically by a range of devices from the short lever-arm Swedish knee cage (see p. 1176) through to a full-length knee–ankle–foot orthosis with a gutter down the back of the leg to increase the contact area. The shorter devices are sometimes difficult to maintain in position especially if the leg is basically conical in shape. How long the lever arm should be is a matter of judgement. People used to obtaining stability by means of

hyperextension, as in this lady's case, do not feel safe if the knee is stopped at only just neutral. They will often feel the need for a substantial degree of hyperextension to be built in. This will add mechanical stress and, of course, further load the tissues above and below the knee. The question of whether there needs to be any orthotic contribution to lateral stability will also influence the design. This is the kind of matter which is probable best managed by a discussion with the orthotist.

Whether improvements can be made to the equipment on her left leg is again a matter of judgement. The mechanical requirement is to support the valgus tendency in the ankle, to prevent the foot dropping to the extent that it interferes with gait but to retain some motion at the ankle to enable the knee flexors and extensors to work the foot for driving, pivoting on the heel. It would obviously be cosmetically desirable to use a shoe rather than a boot but her boot probably fulfils both sagittal and coronal-plane mechanical functions. Hinged plastic ankle–foot orthoses which go inside a shoe will do all these things but are not easy to make satisfactorily and may be difficult to don in the presence of weak thumbs. Again, a discussion with the orthotist would be desirable.

A suitable prescription might be: 'Right knee orthosis to control hyperextension to about 10°. Left ankle–foot orthoses to control varus, stop foot drop below 20° (with 3-cm heel) and retain ankle movement above this.'

REGIONAL ORTHOSES

The following sections describe orthoses region by region, emphasizing the functional aspects of each.

Spinal orthoses

CERVICAL

The almost invariable functional requirements of cervical orthoses are to limit spinal movement or to partially unload the weight of the head on to the pectoral girdle. A useful additional effect can be to reduce heat loss.

It is generally not possible to regulate movements at some joints of the cervical spine and not at others. Either the head is fixed (to a variable degree) in relation to the shoulders and trunk or it is not and individual cervical vertebrae will participate differentially in the same way that they move physiologically over the same range. There may, of course, be pathological factors altering movement patterns.

If rotatory movements are to be controlled the chin must be incorporated in a shaped mandibular section.

Orthoses are generally not indicated for chronic torticollis resulting from rheumatic fever or drugs, or for adult spastic torticollis.

Clearly the most effective limitation of movement occurs with the halo-jacket (Fig. 34.1). The next best in terms of immobilization and weight relief is probably a custom-shaped brace with a brow band (Fig. 34.2). There are several forms of modular or pre-fabricated orthoses like the SOMI brace (sterno-mandibular occipital immobilizer) (Fig. 34.3) or those not reaching so far down with alterable struts of various forms (Fig. 34.4). The least demanding, more cosmetic and more heat retentive are the many collars made of materials of varying softness (Fig. 34.5).

THORACIC

There are virtually no orthoses in current use whose function is confined to the thoracic spine. Many orthoses applied to the trunk extend down to the sacrum. Consideration of trunk orthoses will therefore be combined as thoracolumbar sacral orthoses.

Thoracolumbar spinal orthoses fulfil many functions. For simplicity they may be divided as follows but in practice there will be overlapping functions.

Support of collapsing spine and/or weight relief

The spine is an intrinsically unstable mechanical struc-

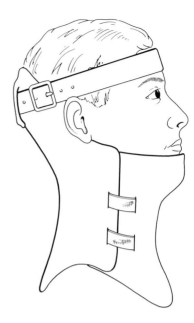

Fig. 34.2 Custom-made cervical brace with brow band.

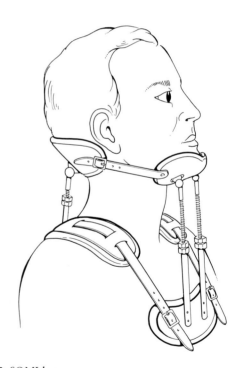

Fig. 34.3 SOMI brace.

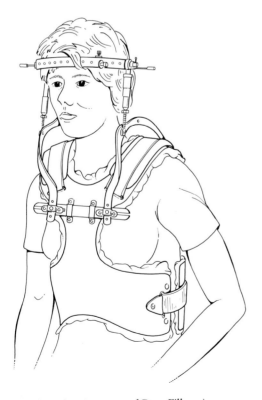

Fig. 34.1 Halo jacket (courtesy of Durr Fillauer).

ture. To maintain its physiological form it needs active muscles and intact bony and ligamentous architecture. Whenever any of these is lacking, for instance in spina bifida, a tuberculous spine or Marfan's syndrome, the requirement is to hold the thorax in relation to the pelvis indirectly to support the spine. In most cases support delivered by roughly horizontal forces will be enough. If

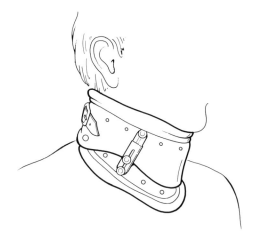

Fig. 34.4 Collar with variable struts.

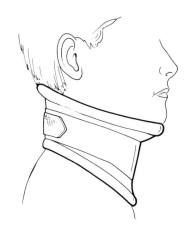

Fig. 34.5 Soft collar.

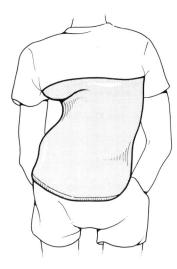

Fig. 34.6 Moulded block leather supportive thoracolumbar spinal orthosis.

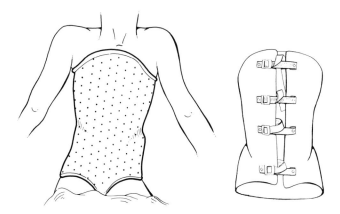

Fig. 34.7 Plastic supportive thoracolumbar spinal orthosis (back opening).

the collapse is severe or there is a particular need to unload the compressive forces, there may need to be an element of distraction taking the vertical load under the axillae or supporting the trunk on a wheelchair frame as in the 'suspension orthosis' (see Fig. 34.8); see also the relief of compressive forces discussed below.

Effective supports can be made in many different forms and in many materials. Some variations are shown in Figs 34.6–34.8. Provided that the structure is strong enough to deliver the required support the relative merits of each style of orthosis and the decision as to which style should be chosen depends more on factors other than purely functional ones. Of particular relevance are:

- Ventilation requirements
- Skin tolerance
- Likelihood of soiling
- Donning and doffing capability
- What the patient is accustomed to

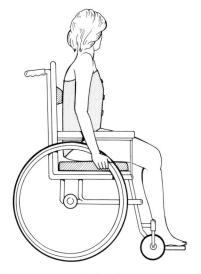

Fig. 34.8 Thoracolumbar spinal orthosis with suspension on to wheelchair back-rest.

Restriction of movement

The usual need for limiting thoracolumbar spinal motion is for pain. Orthoses generally need to be quite rigid and to take firm purchase on the pelvis. Rotational movements (about the vertical axis of the spinal column) are not effectively restricted unless the shoulders and pelvis are contained. Flexion, sideways and backwards and forwards is often limited by impingement of the upper or lower edges of the orthosis on the thorax or pelvis. In this case the mechanism is really autolimitation due to discomfort produced rather than by actually preventing the movement taking place (Fig. 34.9).

Corsets do little to limit spinal movements but obviously if they are deep and well stiffened, with the modern equivalent of whalebones, there will be some restriction.

The traditional style of orthosis for restriction of movement is shown in Fig. 34.10. These can now be made in thermoplastic materials and may need reinforcing with metal or further plastic stiffeners to achieve the required effect. The same kind of considerations on the matter of choice of style apply as in the case of supporting orthoses discussed above.

Correction of deformity

Low back pain. The rationale for the use of fabric corsets or other forms of orthosis for low back pain has been much debated. Studies of their efficacy have been complicated by the difficulties in identifying the precise

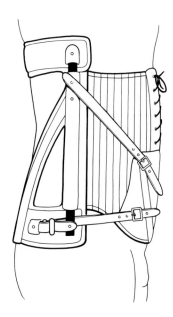

Fig. 34.9 Chair-back brace.

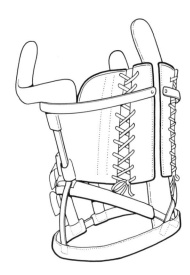

Fig. 34.10 Fischer jacket.

pathology and the cause of the pain and comparing like with like. Other complications arise from the fact of spontaneous recovery and the many other variables involved.

Probably the main mechanical effect of fabric corsets is to re-adjust spinal posture which they do by containing abdominal ptosis and restituting normal lumbar lordosis. (It may be noticed that a corset will seldom be found effective in thin people.) If tight, they will slightly increase intra-abdominal pressure and thereby relieve compressive force on the lumbar spine particularly during extension from forward bending as in lifting. They may also have placebo and warming effects.

Many forms of 'instant' corsets are on the market. Because they are pre-fabricated and not custom-shaped they tend to be short in height. They are frequently prescribed as a form of test to see if a corset will be effective. Because they are not correctly shaped they do not provide an effective test for one that is correctly shaped although they may provide the intra-abdominal, placebo and warming effects.

A recent development for a test device is the Willner Instrument for Spinal Stabilization or WISS device (Fig. 34.11). This is an adjustable frame within which various pads and straps can apply forces to the trunk. It is not something which can be worn for long periods, but providing pain relief can be safely determined fairly promptly, it is useful both for the test and for characterizing the definitive orthosis.

For sagittal plane deformities, kyphosis etc. Three-point fixation devices work well for correction and maintenance of forward flexion deformities. For idiopathic kyphosis, however, the attitude of the pelvis needs to be

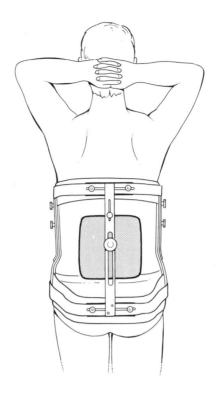
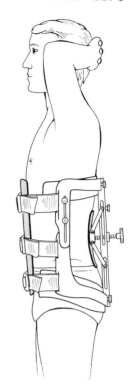

Fig. 34.11 Willner trial brace (courtesy of Camp (UK) Ltd).

controlled as well since the deformity extends, at least functionally if not radiologically, into the lumbar spine.

The traditional three-point fixation orthosis is the Jewett but there are satisfactory modular devices like that shown in Fig. 34.12.

For idiopathic kyphosis a plastic, front opening, thoracolumbar spinal orthoses with clavicle pads (Fig. 34.13) or with shoulder straps provide satisfactory control but there is still some preference for the Milwaukee brace with central pads at the back (Fig. 34.14). This, of

course, suffers cosmetic disadvantages compared with the thoracolumbar spinal orthoses.

For idiopathic scolosis. The condition remains the 'enigma wrapped in a mystery'. As a consequence, orthotic treatment for idiopathic scoliosis is marked by

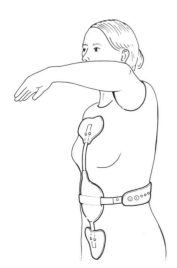

Fig. 34.12 Teufel three-point brace (modular).

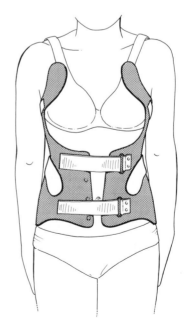

Fig. 34.13 Thoracolumbar spinal orthosis with clavicle pads.

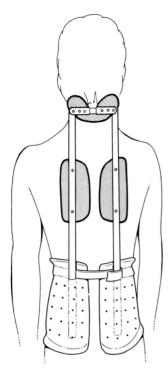

Fig. 34.14 Milwaukee for kyphosis.

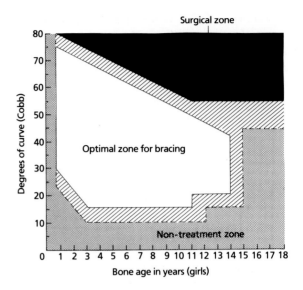

Fig. 34.15 Indications by severity of scoliosis and age (in girls) for orthotic treatment of idiopathic scoliosis (after Blount and Moe, 1973).

a wide variety of styles of orthosis reflecting changing trends in treatment fashions. Although brace treatment has been in and out of fashion in the last decade or two and individual scoliosis specialists will emphasize more aggressive surgery on the one hand or wider use of bracing on the other, the best general description of criteria for brace treatment remains that drawn by Blount (Fig. 34.15).

The essential purpose in any orthotic treatment is to redirect growth. This is achieved by applying approximately horizontally directed forces to the trunk in order to:

1 flatten any excessive lordosis (for which it is necessary to bring the orthosis down well under the buttocks);

2 correct any axial (transverse plane) rotation which may exist between pelvis, trunk and shoulders;

3 apply lateral forces to the sagittal plane deviations (see Fig. 34.16).

The results of orthotic treatments with different forms of orthoses do not differ substantially so that the style of orthosis would not seem to matter provided that it delivers the required forces, and is constructed and applied with care and with due regard to the radiological and clinical findings. The orthoses must, of course, be worn for sufficient time for them to act. We do not know what this is, for how long, in what postures or activities, or at what stages of skeletal maturation.

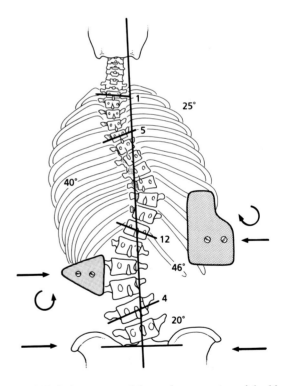

Fig. 34.16 Pad placement and forces for correction of double curve.

There is a pressing need to put some objectivity into these matters with the use of reliable brace compliance monitors.

For lumbar curves, especially in younger children, the three-point devices of the French school (see Fig. 34.17) are satisfactory. Higher curves need higher braces. The Boston modular system (Fig. 34.18) has gained general acceptance for curves with their apex up to T8 or T9. Modular orthoses like these are more suitable for milder curves (e.g. 35° Cobb and under) because they force the body into a symmetrical brace. For larger curves or where the more obtrusive appearance of modular braces becomes a factor, a similar style of thermoplastic orthosis can be custom-shaped (Fig. 34.19). For these, the correction is achieved in three stages; at casting, during modification of the positive mould ('rectification') and by adding foam pads to the interior. For curves with an element above T8 that needs treating the Milwaukee brace (Fig. 34.20) is still favoured. A neck ring with 'throat mould' is used to provide for autocentralization of the head and neck, earlier research having shown that 'distraction' provided by mandibular and occipital pads was unlikely to have any mechanical effect.

Lower extremity orthoses

HIP

Not many orthoses are applied specifically to the hip joint alone. Leaving aside abduction and weight relief orthoses for Legg–Perthes' disease (which seem to have lost favour in recent years) there remain those required to stabilize the hip and occasionally to correct internal rotation. In adults, the requirement for stabilization usually follows removal of the joint for one reason or another.

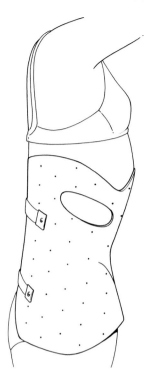

Fig. 34.18 Boston thoracolumbar spinal orthosis.

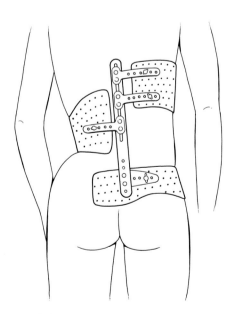

Fig. 34.17 Michel three-point brace for lumbar curves.

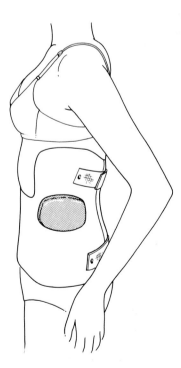

Fig. 34.19 Custom-made thoracolumbar spinal orthosis for a lumbar curve.

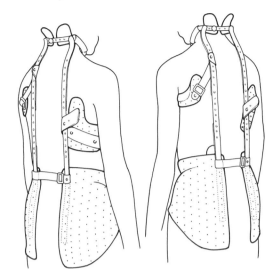

Fig. 34.20 Milwaukee brace.

The functional demand is to hold the femur in relation to the pelvis and prevent it moving upwards or outwards in abduction. It may sometimes be necessary to prevent flexion and extension movements as well.

An effective hip spica may be made in half-shells of thermoplastic (Fig. 34.21). If it is desired to have some flexion and extension movements a satisfactory device is the modular form called Erlanger (see Fig. 34.22).

In infants, congenital dislocation is the main reason for an orthosis. The functional requirements in this case are to maintain the hips flexed at least 90° and abducted at least 40° (each). The ability to perform toiletting without removal of the splint is obviously an advantage.

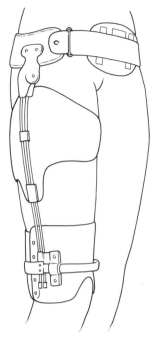

Fig. 34.22 Teufel Erlanger hip control orthosis.

The two most commonly used forms are the van Rosen (Fig. 34.23) which has malleable metal supports suitably covered and the Pavlik harness (Fig. 34.24) which is made of straps only.

In children, where there is an established need to intervene for persistent internal rotation of the hip, orthotic treatment is less favoured nowadays than osteo-

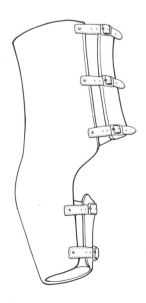

Fig. 34.21 Hip spica.

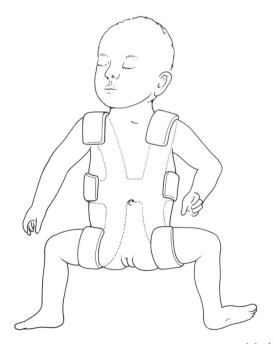

Fig. 34.23 Van Rosen splint for congenital dislocation of the hip.

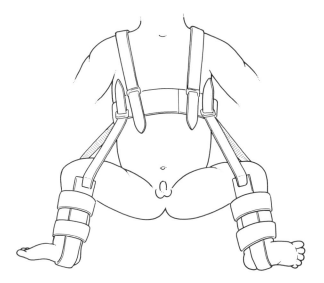

Fig. 34.24 Pavlik harness.

tomies. However a 'twister' orthosis may occasionally be useful on a temporary basis either for training for improved walking or while waiting for surgery or spontaneous recovery in children who persistently trip themselves up. The orthosis consists of a tortional cable which takes purchase from a belt around the pelvis and

is applied to cuffs above and below the knee. A modular form in several sizes is available.

For unloading the hip joint by means of knee–ankle–foot orthoses, see below.

HIP–KNEE–ANKLE–FOOT ORTHOSES

Paralytic conditions which affect some of the trunk and abdominal muscles as well as the legs will need orthoses with connections across the hip, knee and foot. Examples are those required for spina bifida and low spinal cord lesions. New orthotic designs appear very infrequently, but orthoses to enable paraplegics to walk have enjoyed much greater development effort in recent years.

The functional requirement is to hold the pelvis in a roughly neutral position, keep the knees extended, stabilize the feet and ankles, prevent the hips from adducting and assist reciprocal motion of the legs either by gravity or by connection of a reciprocating linkage between the legs.

Two quite well-tried orthoses which meet these demands are the hip guidance orthosis (HGO) which stemmed from work at Oswestry and the reciprocal gait orthosis or RGO which was developed at Louisiana State University (see Fig. 34.25).

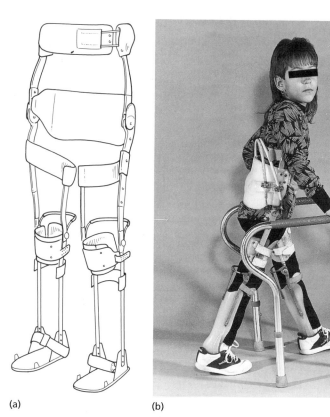

(a)

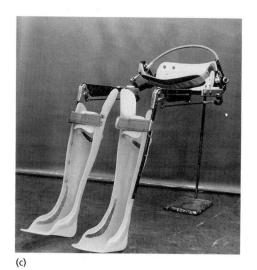

(b)

(c)

Fig. 34.25 Hip guidance orthosis. (b) Reciprocal gait orthosis. (c) Advanced reciprocal gait orthosis.

These orthoses should only be prescribed where there is a closely cooperating team of physician/surgeon, orthotist and physiotherapist. Patients report subjective benefits from the erect posture and the exercise their use entails but there is little objective evidence of physiological benefit. Serious consideration should therefore be given before prescription as both these orthoses require sustained enthusiasm on the part of the user and they are an energy-expensive method of ambulation. They also require strong muscles in the upper trunk, pectoral girdle and arms. The HGO is easier to don and doff and will therefore be preferred for those who will use it only for short periods. The RGO is closer fitting and therefore more cosmetic, but it can tolerate less fixed angular deformity or oedema in the leg than the HGO. The RGO is also rather more expensive. Locking of the hip joint, which may be necessary on account of spasticity, is more easily performed in the HGO. Further details of these two orthoses and their relative merits may be seen in Health Equipment Information No. 192 (1989).

A more recently developed orthosis for the same purpose is the Steeper ARGO or advanced RGO. It has a linkage between hip joint and knee joint which offers assisted standing from sitting. It is rapidly gaining acceptance, especially abroad, and it takes much less time to fabricate than the other orthoses.

Knee orthoses

Orthoses which relieve weight from the knee joint are discussed below. The main requirements of other orthoses for the knee are for stabilization — or preventing unwanted movements. These can be in the three different planes: sagittal, coronal or transverse. Occasionally one may need to assist extension.

Elementary mechanics dictates that the heavier the mechanical demand placed on the orthosis (e.g. a severely valgus knee) the longer is the length of device required for application above and below the knee. Thus short orthoses around the knee joint can only be suitable for relatively undemanding mechanical situations.

ANTERO-POSTERIOR (SAGITTAL PLANE) CONTROL

For hyperextension

The Swedish knee cage (Fig. 34.26) is suitable for mild cases but unless there is reduced girth just above the knee (in contrast to a conical-shaped leg) there is often the problem of the orthosis slipping down. A good modular form of the device is available from Teufel.

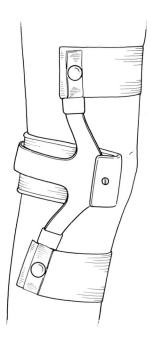

Fig. 34.26 Swedish knee cage.

More demanding situations need to be met with longer devices. Ultimately a full knee−ankle−foot orthosis (see below) is required.

For resistance to flexion

In the presence of flail knee extensors and a plantigrade foot that does not need supporting at the ankle, it is theoretically possible to use a lockable knee orthosis for stiff-legged gait. Normally a full knee−ankle−foot orthosis (see below) is required.

For assistance to extension

It is possible to recruit the ground reaction force to assist knee extension during weight-bearing. It is necessary either to have active plantar flexors or a rigid ankle with the line of force passing in front of the knee (see Fig. 34.27). The ankle may be rigid from an arthrodesis or from a rigid ankle orthosis.

There have been a number of attempts to provide assistance to extension by spring-loaded orthotic knee joints for standing from sitting or during gait, but they have not been attended by much success.

Occasionally an extensor lag may be helped by simple springs or elastic around the joint to help with the last few degrees of extension.

There is considerable scope for the development of flexion control orthotic knee joints on the style of the modern prosthetic joints so as to enable a flaccid knee to flex during the swing phase of gait.

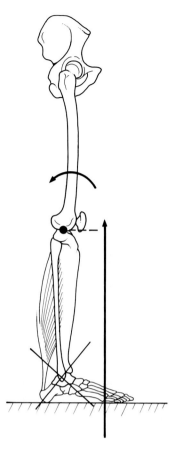

Fig. 34.27 Ground reaction vector in front of knee with stiff ankle assists knee extension.

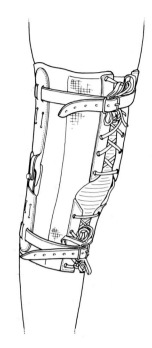

Fig. 34.28 Elasticated knee orthosis.

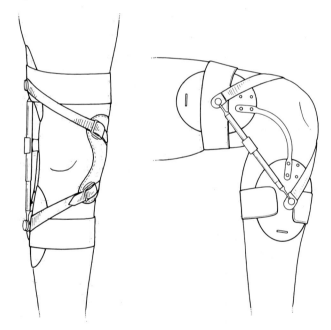

Fig. 34.29 Telescopic varus–valgus splint (TVS).

LATERAL (CORONAL PLANE) CONTROL

It is often surprising how effective a simple elastic knee cap or bandage is for a mildly unstable knee. Whether there is any real mechanical function through proprioceptive or other mechanism, or whether it serves as a reminder to guard the knee has yet to be determined.

There are a number of elasticated knee orthoses with rigid or semi-rigid side stems sewn into them on the market (Fig. 34.28).

The telescopic varus–valgus splint (TVS) in Fig. 34.29 is effective for controlling mild (15° or less) lateral instability though it, too, has problems of retention with conical-shaped knees.

More severely unstable knees need to be controlled with more robust devices with longer lever arms. Ultimately a full knee–ankle–foot orthosis is required to bring the forces to the floor through the shoe (Fig. 34.30).

TRANSVERSE PLANE CONTROL

Torsional instability—most frequently due to anterior cruciate deficiency—has brought a spate of devices to the market. The mechanical requirement is to limit anterior translation and external rotation of the tibia in relation to the femur and at up to 30° of flexion.

Mechanically, the most effective orthosis appears to be the Lennox Hill (Fig. 34.31). It is custom-made from a cast in the USA. There are a number of others for which claims of similar function are made.

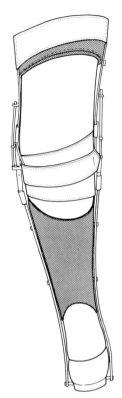

Fig. 34.30 Full-length knee—ankle—foot orthosis for control of severe lateral knee instability (posterior view).

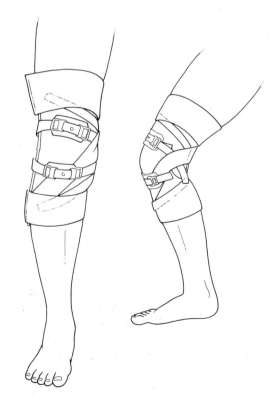

Fig. 34.31 Lennox-Hill knee brace.

Of the 'off-the-shelf' designs there is some evidence that the Don Joy four-point brace is mechanically the most effective. A different style which has appeared recently is an all-plastic orthosis which encloses the whole tibia and rests on the malleoli to prevent it slipping down. It offers some promise but has not yet been widely tested.

Knee—ankle—foot orthoses

These are used to substitute for biomechanical deficiencies at the knee, ankle and foot. The essential components are a thigh attachment or corset, knee joints (or not), a below-knee section and a foot section.

The thigh corset is preferably a complete cylinder of either leather or plastic material. If the foot or knee cannot pass through it, it will have to be an incomplete cylinder and closed with straps. Such orthoses, if made predominantly of plastics and required to take vertical load as well as other stresses should have some keying of one-half with the other so as to avoid shearing movements. Whether the corset is made of plastic or leather will depend on the style of the orthosis, what the user is used to and other factors.

If the orthosis is required to relieve weight from the skeleton of the leg, the thigh corset needs to be moulded with an ischial-bearing fold posteromedially. The fold is better filled externally with a foam-like Plastazote so as to make it easier to sit on hard surfaces (like lavatory seats).

If there is normal (not wasted) musculature, a quadrilateral-shaped corset like those used in prosthetics for stumps provides better purchase.

A number of variations are possible at the orthotic knee joint:

1 No joint, e.g. for arthrodesed knees or as a trial for, perhaps, weight relief.

2 Free joint, e.g. where sufficient knee-extensor power is present or effective substitutes are available at the hip and ankle (see p. 1176).

3 Locking joint (see Fig. 34.32).

(a) Spring-loaded bale locks; either individual or linked with a cord or bar.

(b) Spring-loaded ring lock.

(c) Gravity-loaded ring lock.

(d) Stay-up, stay-down ring lock with spring-loaded ball catch.

(e) One side (b), the other (d) for one-handed operation.

(f) Other designs.

4 Spring-assisted joints. These have been discussed on p. 1176.

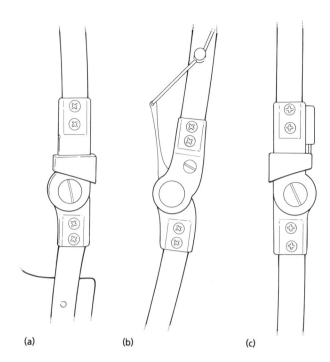

Fig. 34.32 Orthotic knee joints. (a) Ring lock gravity locking; (b) bale lock with cord; (c) ring lock spring loaded.

Several variations are also possible at the ankle joint:
1 Rigid ankle. From a deep plastic ankle—foot orthosis, a high, stiff boot, or spurs or joints with stops.
2 Ankle with limited movement. Spurs or other joint with limited movement built in to the mechanism, or semi-flexible footpiece to 'cosmetic' orthosis which allows dorsiflexion but not plantarflexion.
3 Free ankle joint. Joint on stirrup or spurs or a plastic ankle joint with no stops.

The footpieces to plastic knee—ankle—foot orthoses can often fit inside normal shoes or boots. This is preferable as it gives the patient a wider choice of footwear. It also offers the opportunity for wearing Wellington boots or other special-purpose footwear. For a slightly more cosmetic appearance at the ankle they can also fit into custom-made 'surgical' footwear. If a plastic footpiece is not possible, the metal side stems have to lead to either an ankle joint and a stirrup or to spurs into sockets made up in an adapted heel. Many modern shoes have moulded soles and heels and the heel is hollow. This presents problems in fitting the sockets.

There are thus a number of possible combinations of the component parts which need to be put together to fulfil the function required.

Three examples (below) will indicate some of the possibilities.

For bilateral paraplegia

Spinal cord lesions at T6 and below can achieve a degree of indirect hip stabilization by careful alignment in the sagittal plane (see Fig. 34.33). The centre of gravity has to fall through the pelvis to the middle of the support area on the floor. Lumbar lordosis is exaggerated and the knees are held rigid. The shoes are built with a very rigid base and stirrup connecting to the side stems at an ankle joint with adjustable stops.

An interesting new device from Poland has the same basic components except that, instead of the knee joint, there is a telescoping rod and the thigh section is attached to it and hinged so that when the knee is flexed it is horizontal (Fig. 34.34). It has not gained much general acceptance in the UK but is used more extensively abroad. It is unlikely to be effective for spinal lesions above T6. It may serve as a useful trial orthosis.

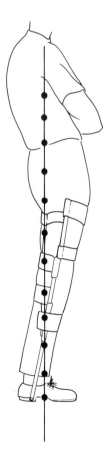

Fig. 34.33 Line of centre of gravity for partial hip stabilization in paraplegics.

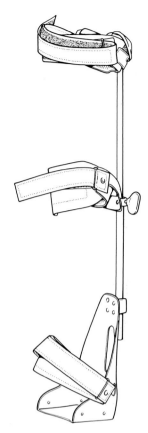

Fig. 34.34 Lower extremity telescopic orthosis (LETOR).

For unilateral flail leg (e.g. a history of poliomyelitis) with lateral instability at the ankle

If there is no serious (more than 15°) angular deformity and there is less than 5 cm shortening, a plastic 'cosmetic' knee–ankle–foot orthosis with an added wing for the ankle and footpiece into the shoe may be considered (Fig. 34.35).

For severe lateral instability at the knee

Plastic thigh and leg sections giving maximum contact area are connected with side stems which become sockets engaging in the heel of the shoe (Fig. 34.30).

Ankle–foot orthoses

The usual mechanical demands on ankle–foot orthoses are to:
1 control lateral instability at the ankle, subtalar or midtarsal joints;
2 limit plantar- and dorsiflexion;
3 take some weight under the knee and transfer it to below the foot;

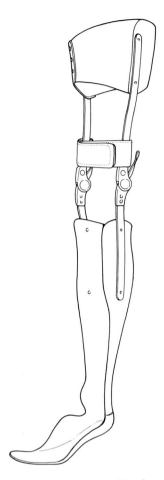

Fig. 34.35 Plastic cosmetic knee–ankle–foot orthosis with wings for valgus foot.

4 provide a shoe-shaped lower part to accommodate small or deformed feet in normal, shop-bought shoes.

The design of any orthosis for controlling lateral instability will depend on the need for ankle movement and the style of footwear to be used. A completely enclosing ankle–foot orthosis made in block leather or plastic (Fig. 34.36) will, of course, prevent such movement altogether.

Lateral support with free movement at the ankle can be provided by a plastic hinged orthosis (Fig. 34.37). The conventional device allowing some ankle movement is the single 'iron' on the appropriate side with a T-strap. The strap should come from a loop or lug on the iron to improve the direction of support (Fig. 34.38). The iron engages in sockets built into the heel of the shoe and stops can be added to control the amount of ankle movement. Off the shelf devices with pads of gel or air or both are available for supporting sprained ankles.

The below-knee iron without a T-strap becomes an

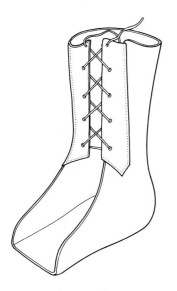

Fig. 34.36 Moulded block leather anklet.

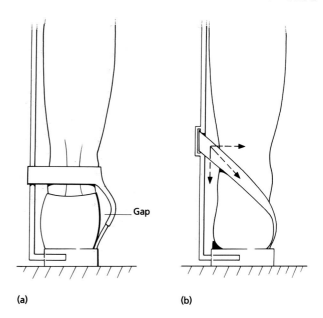

(a)   **(b)**

Fig. 34.38 Ankle—foot orthosis for lateral support. Strap retainer in (b) improves the direction of pull.

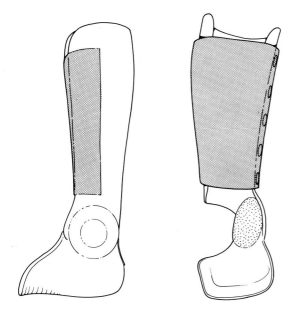

Fig. 34.37 Hinged plastic ankle—foot orthosis for lateral instability.

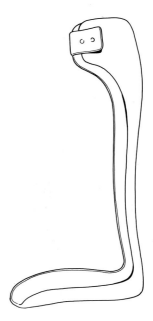

Fig. 34.39 Ortholen foot drop splint.

orthosis fulfilling the second functional category. A simple orthosis for the prevention of foot drop is the Ortholene 'leaf spring' (Fig. 34.39). It allows dorsiflexion but not plantarflexion from a datum—for different heel heights—which is determined at the initial casting. The material is partly ductile and can be hammered to alter the amount of dorsiflexion.

There is a variety of pre-fabricated devices for foot drop such as that in Fig. 34.40.

Taking weight under the knee borrows technology from below-knee prosthetics. The orthosis is very close

fitting all around below the knee and emphasizes the patella tendon bar (Fig. 34.41).

It is possible for some small or deformed and small feet to be accommodated in normal shop-bought footwear. At times there is also the requirement to provide either lateral stability or some means of retention of the footwear on a foot with absent foreparts. In these cases an ankle—foot orthosis can be made to accommodate the foot with a suitably shaped foam filler (Fig. 34.42).

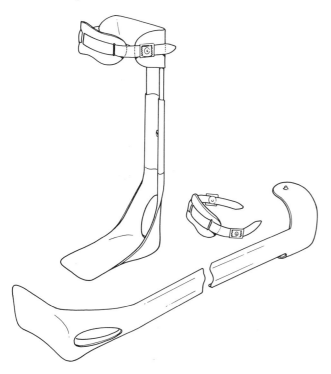

Fig. 34.40 Modular foot drop splint (courtesy of VM Marketing).

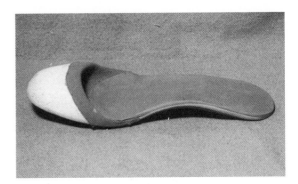

Fig. 34.42 Foam inlay filler for short foot into standard shoe.

It should be noted that any leg orthosis (hip, knee or below-knee) passing down into the *inside* of footwear should have that part of its external shape a congruent fit with the internal shape of the shoe (i.e. the last shape) This is to ensure maximum stability between orthosis and shoe, for the shoe is only held in place by friction, laces and buckles, etc. If the relatively rigid plastic footpiece is made the shape of the anatomical foot, it will not fit the shoe properly. Any mouldings, metartarsal pads, arch supports, etc., can be placed in the inside of the footpiece.

Footwear and foot orthoses

Of all the different orthoses which may be provided, footwear seems to be the most frequent cause of dissatisfaction on the part of both patients and prescribers. Part of this problem is almost certainly because painful feet is a common symptom (the majority of cases with rheumatoid arthritis will have affected feet at some time) and patients tend to look to their footwear for relief of the pain. In a number of cases no design of shoe or orthosis can relieve this pain and it is important that prescribers warn such patients so that unrealizable expectations are not raised. That said, there are undoubtedly many poorly prescribed or poorly made and poorly fitting shoes which are justifiable reasons for complaint. Delays in provision also feature prominently as complaints.

The essential purpose of footwear in temperate climates is to clothe the foot. Sometimes this is the only purpose for which special footwear is prescribed. In addition to this there is a whole range of devices either placed separately within the footwear or incorporated within the construction of it. The chief functional purposes are:

1 to correct or support deformities or potential deformities;

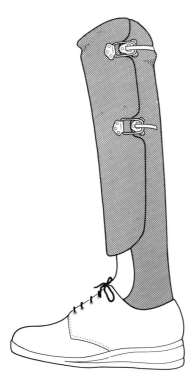

Fig. 34.41 Patellar tendon-bearing plastic ankle–foot orthosis.

2 to redistribute plantar surface load for relief of pain, ulceration or danger of it, etc.;

3 to substitute for absent parts of the foot;

4 to provide a means for compensation of leg length inequalities.

Lateral instability can be supported or corrected outside the shoe with wedging or float-outs (Fig. 34.43), inside the shoe with wedged inlays or by recruiting body weight and converting the force with a heel cup (Fig. 34.44).

There are some modular heel cups available for children but for adults they are best made from an individual cast. This should be taken weight-bearing so that it fits the compressed heel and is nearer the shape of the last.

The redistribution of plantar loading often entails the need for increased depth in the shoe in order to accommodate inlays with thickness sufficient to provide the mechanical effect. A range of ready-made shoes is now available, generally called 'extra-depth shoes'. Many are quite reasonable in appearance and cost about one-fifth of a custom-made shoe (Fig. 34.45).

One of the most common reasons for needing to alter the weight distribution is for neuropathic ulceration in, for example, leprosy, diabetes and spina bifida. In these cases it is not simply a matter of altering the static weight distribution but also of reducing pathological subcutaneous shearing. The normal metatarsal head rolls within the more superficial tissues during the stance phase of gait. The neuropathic subcutaneous tissue is scarred and thinned and cannot sustain normal rolling. The consequent shearing is a major factor in the development of ulceration. The orthotic solution to reduce this shearing is to transfer the rolling elsewhere and keep the forces on the plantar surface as near as possible at right angles to the skin. As indicated in Fig. 34.46, the heel is cut away and perhaps made softer with foam, the base of the shoe is made rigid and the tread and toe area is tapered to provide for the rocking motion between foot flat and toe-off. Shoes modified in this way are not attractive in appearance and patients need to be warned and well motivated.

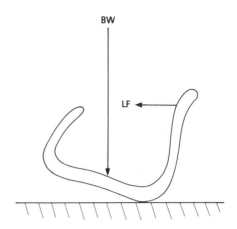

Fig. 34.44 Action of the heel cup. Body weight (BW) converts to lateral force (LF).

As yet, there is no completely objective method of arriving at the optimum shape for an even distribution of plantar surface load at all phases of the gait cycle. It is not always clear that an even distribution is desired since some areas of the foot are better designed to bear weight than others. There are many devices which indicate pressure distribution when standing or walking on flat surfaces. There are also devices which provide pressure readings on discrete areas of the foot over contoured surfaces. But these do not have the spatial discrimination for determining optimal shape over the whole surface. Also the deformation characteristics of different areas of the foot cannot be known until they are actually deformed. Thus, although some useful information may be had from pressure mapping devices, particularly in recording changes over periods of time, there still remains an element of art and experience in making inlays with the optimum combination of different materials and their shape.

Another frequent reason for the need to redistribute the loading on the foot is for metatarsalgia. The effects of maldistribution of load on the metatarsal heads can be alleviated by use of metatarsal domes. These move the loading further behind the head and help to reduce

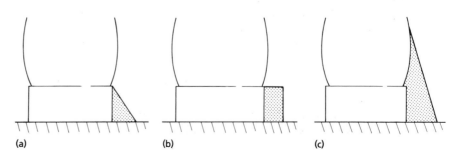

Fig. 34.43 Various ways of floating out the heel for increased lateral stability.

(a)   **(b)**   **(c)**

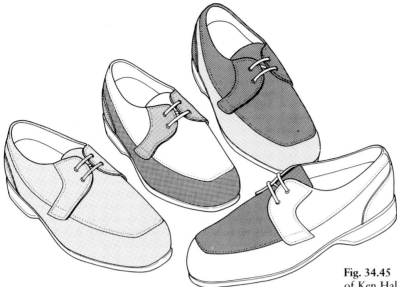

Fig. 34.45 Various forms of standard extra-depth shoes (courtesy of Ken Hall Ltd.).

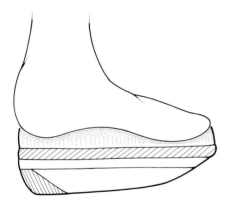

Fig. 34.46 Layered rocker base for diabetic neuropathy.

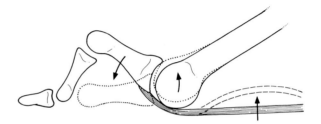

Fig. 34.47 Action of metatarsal dome.

hyperextension at the proximal interphalangeal joint (Fig. 34.47).

For absent parts of the foot it is often possible merely to add fillers to ordinary shop-bought shoes. In the case of absent toes or a short foot the filler may only be required for the sake of the shoe's appearance — to avoid it collapsing and (Fig. 34.42) creasing — rather than for any functional relationship with the foot. It is uncomfortable for toes or the distal end of the foot with amputated toes to touch the end of the shoe. The lacing or other fastening of the shoe should hold the foot back into the heel.

Midfoot amputations, congenital or acquired, can frequently be accommodated in ordinary shoes provided they are high enough in the front and have a good grip of the heel in order to provide adequate retention during the swing phase of gait. If retention is a problem, one

may have to resort to an ankle—foot orthosis as described above. Sometimes, just a plastic clip above the ankle is required only for the purpose of heel retention (Fig. 34.48).

Where the functional amputation is around the midfoot and the sole of the shoe is flexible it may be necessary to artificially stiffen it in order to bring the flexion movement of the shoe further distally. This will, of course, exacerbate the problem of retention at the heel due to extending the lever arm (Fig. 34.49) and a biomechanical compromise has to be reached in each case.

Lateral deficiencies, as in absent rays, can also often be dealt with by inlays in normal shoes.

Shoe raises for leg-length discrepancies may be inside or outside the shoe (Fig. 34.50). Lateral instabilities at the ankle and knee are enhanced by high raises. It is common practice to increase the equinus as the heel height is increased. For example, a 3 cm raise on a 2 cm heel will usually have the tread raised about 2 cm and the toe tapered to 1 cm. If the raise is used in conjunction

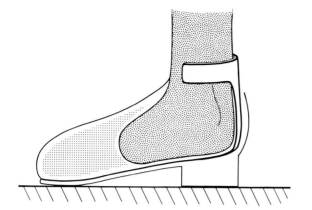

Fig. 34.48 Ankle–foot orthosis clip for heel retention.

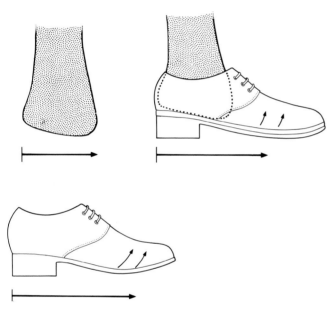

Fig. 34.49 Biomechanical compromise with shoe stiffener.

with an orthosis, as is often the case, it is important to determine the effect of the increased plantarflexion on the orthosis. Naturally if the ankle is rigid or if there are stops to control its movement the raise will need to be uniform throughout the length of the shoe.

The discussion on footwear so far has involved the use of shop-bought shoes, pre-fabricated deep shoes and custom-made 'surgical' shoes. It is in the interest of both the patient and the economy that the selection of appropriate footwear for particular foot problems should consider these three different classes in that same sequence. It should be possible to use shop-bought shoes if the foot dimensions do not exceed those of the shoe in any direction. Likewise, extra-depth shoes should be considered next taking account of the dimensions of inlays or orthoses as well. Use of custom-made shoes should be considered only after the other two types have been excluded.

Upper-extremity orthoses

SHOULDER AND SCAPULO-HUMERAL COMPLEX

The generalization that the more complicated a joint is, the more difficult it is to provide satisfactory orthoses around it, is exemplified at the shoulder and scapulo-humeral complex. There are comparatively few successful orthoses and many occasions when there is an unmet functional demand.

Retention of scapula — prevention of winging

Mechanically this is a demanding situation. Considerable force needs to be applied, anteriorly directed, to prevent winging. This can only be provided by either a cantilever from further down the back (which effectively stiffens the back) or by a counter force from the front from a thoracic 'bodice'. Such a bodice must be custom built and to provide the necessary forces will inevitably restrict

Fig. 34.50 Shoe raises: (a) outside; (b) inside.

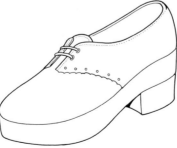

(a)

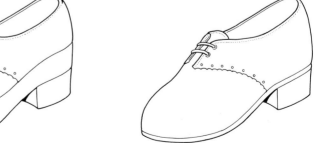

(b)

full respiratory excursion. In order not to be uncomfortably tight during shallow respiration, users learn to increase thoracic volume and tighten the bodice at moments when the scapula is in need of support.

Arm abduction

There is a not-infrequent need to hold the arm abducted following surgery or trauma. The elbow is usually at 90°. It is a purely static requirement though in some cases there would be an advantage in being able to bring the abducted arm across the front of the body.

Many practitioners prefer to use plaster of Paris but there are several forms of modular Airplane splint on the market, for example as in Fig. 34.51.

Prevention of subluxation

Flail arms have a tendency to subluxate, e.g. in brachial plexus lesions or hemiplegia. The functional requirement is to support the weight of the arm and hold the upper end of the humerus in position.

The use of a conventional sling is limited by the load that can be taken on the contralateral neck and shoulder. Substantial support for sports players can be had from a moulded plastic brace (Fig. 34.52) and lesser degrees of support can be provided by various modular slings and fabric supports as in Fig. 34.53 which probably help more as a reminder than in any strictly mechanical sense.

FLAIL ARMS AND THEIR SUPPORT

Orthotics for brachial plexus lesions have not advanced much in recent years although there are great opportunities to bring technology to bear on upper-extremity substitution systems with a combination of prosthetics, orthotics and robotics.

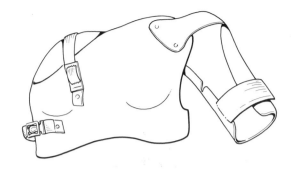

Fig. 34.52 Moulded plastic shoulder subluxation inhibitor.

Functional flail arm splints

For the ambulant case, the objectives to be persued are the provision of a tool — clamp or mobile mini vice — in the appropriate working area in front of the body for the other hand to work against. There thus needs to be effective retention and stabilization around the shoulder and thorax to take the weight of the arm flexed at the elbow and a tool, split hook, clamp, etc., at a position equating to the hand but clear of it so that it does not get in the way (see Fig. 34.54). The tool is normally body powered with a shoulder harness but can be provided with external power.

The Stanmore Steeper flail arm splint (Fig. 34.54 and 34.55) is the most widely used orthosis although it has a number of deficiencies.

For incomplete lesions, the French helicoidal splint from Nancy (Fig. 34.56) offers much easier donning and doffing.

Another development from France for chair-bound people is a remarkably free running arm support called the MAG (mouvements assistes par glissieres). It is a forearm gutter-and-hand support mounted on a pivot on the travelling gear. It can be mounted sloping in the direction that needs assistance and it successfully

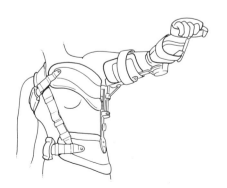

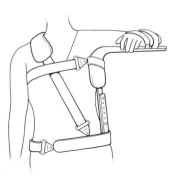

Fig. 34.51 Modular Airplane splint.

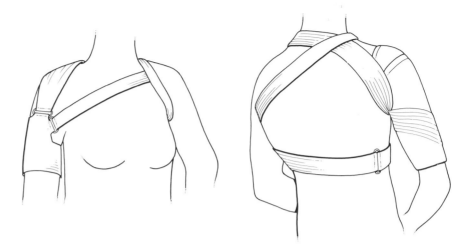

Fig. 34.53 Modular slings rewind the wearer.

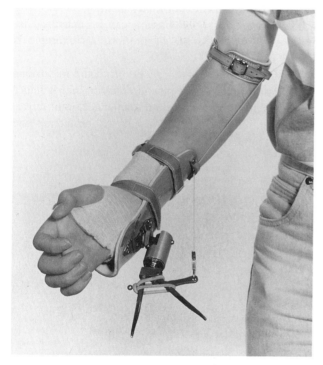

Fig. 34.54 Tool on flail arm splint. Level with the hand but clear of it.

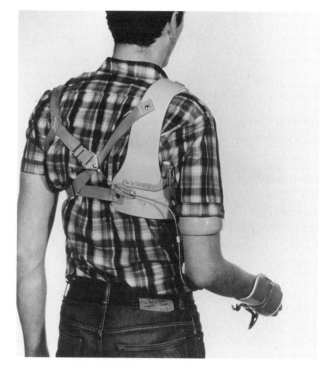

Fig. 34.55 The Stanmore Steeper flail arm splint.

converts weak shoulder power, as in C5 spinal quadriplegia, to work a normal joystick attached to the orthotic element or to use a computer or typewriter keyboard with a stick. Vertical movements to lift the stick to new positions are achieved by depressing the shoulder which pivots the orthosis and lifts the distal end.

ELBOW ORTHOSES

The need for orthotic treatment at the elbow usually stems from the need to stabilize a disrupted joint or to substitute for lost biceps and brachioradialis function. Occasionally a resting splint is required.

Stabilization of the elbow joint

Clearly, retaining upper- and lower-arm long bones in relative position to each other requires cuffs around each and a connecting, stiff linkage between. The two main difficulties are that the upper cuff often tends to slip down and the lower cuff, if it is long enough and tight enough to provide adequate purchase, will prevent

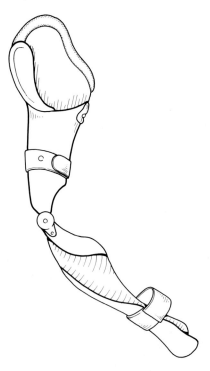

Fig. 34.56 The Nancy helicoidal splint for incomplete lesions provides easier donning and doffing.

full rotation of the wrist. For the former, consideration should be given to suspension straps over the shoulder and around the thorax. The latter problem is solved mainly by realising its existence. Of course the wrist can be held in neutral pronation–supination to improve function.

The linkage and orthotic joint can take different forms according to the requirement for rigidity or mobility. The range would include:

1 no joint;
2 Hinged
   (a) free,
   (b) with stops to limit range,
   (c) with ratchet,
   (d) with spring assist, etc.

HAND AND WRIST ORTHOSES

Orthotics for the hand and wrist are also difficult, but for different reasons. The hand, being a highly sensitive and multi-jointed structure is difficult to follow externally. Devices tend to be complicated in construction and highly visible. Even if they enable a function otherwise impossible, there will almost certainly be some negative effects. There is always a compromise and prescribers, orthotists and, particularly patients, need to be aware of all the factors to avoid rejection. Lack of

such recognition is the predominant cause of the high failure rate often experienced.

The biomechanical requirements demanding the use of wrist and hand orthoses may be divided into the following categories:

1 limiting the movements of joints, either preventing any movement or limiting the range;
2 correcting a deformity;
3 assisting joint movement, either with springs or with body power transferred from elsewhere, or with external power.

Movement-limiting orthoses

If immobilization of the wrist is required, plaster of Paris, Hexcellite, Scotchplast, etc., splintage is normally needed first. Later rehabilitation can be enhanced by orthoses limiting the arc of motion. An example is shown in Fig. 34.57.

The fingers and thumb can be protected in various ways. An example is the plastic or metal mallet finger splint which prevents distal interphalangeal joint movement (Fig. 34.58) or a thumb spica protecting the proximal joint.

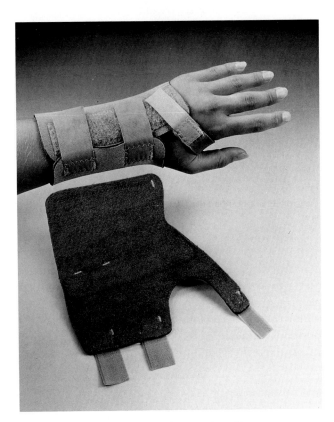

Fig. 34.57 Movement-limiting elastic wrist splint.

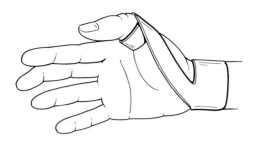

Fig. 34.58 Elastic applies corrective effect to pull thumb to opponens position.

Correcting deformities

Ulnar deviation in rheumatoid arthritis could probably be largely prevented by timely corrective splinting. But so far there is little evidence that anyone has succeeded because of a general reluctance to be involved with any form of splinting unless the need for it is obvious. The time to do it in rheumatoid arthritis is well before it is obvious.

Contractures can have a progressive application of force, either with a spring mechanism using spring wire or elastic or with a turnbuckle type of arrangement. Examples are shown in Figs 34.59 and 60.

Assisting joint movement

A modular set of hand orthoses has recently become available (see Fig. 34.60). With the Steeper Tayside system it is possible to build a variety of different functionalities from the off-the-shelf modules.

Where wrist extension power is preserved but there is no prehension the so-called flexor hinge orthosis can be effective (Fig. 34.61). The power of wrist extension is converted to a movement which approximates the first two digits to the thumb which is held fixed.

A similar device using a small battery powered electric motor is available from the USA for when there is no extensor power (Fig. 34.62).

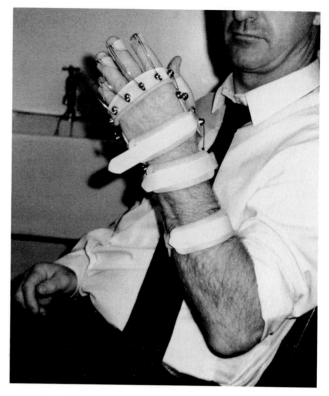

Fig. 34.60 The Steeper Tayside modular system.

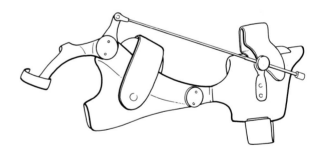

Fig. 34.61 Wrist extension powered prehension orthosis.

Fig. 34.59 (a) Turnbuckle applies successively adjusted corrective effect. (b) Elastic applies corrective forces to flexion contracture of the proximal interphalangeal joint.

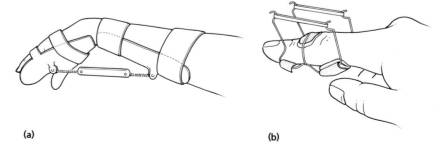

(a)   (b)

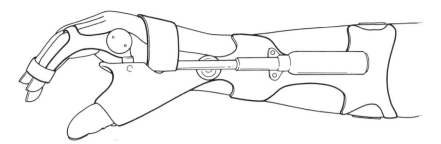

Fig. 34.62 Electrically powered prehension orthosis.

For hand splinting, specialized texts should be consulted. The *Atlas of Orthotics* (American Academy of Orthopaedic Surgeons, 1975) and *A Manual of Static Hand Splinting* (Malick) are starting points.

REFERENCES

American Academy of Orthopaedic Surgeons (1975) *Atlas of Orthotics*. Philadelphia, C.V. Mosby Co.

Blount W.P. and Moe J.H. (1973) *The Milwaukee Brace*. Baltimore, Williams and Wilkins.

Health Equipment Information No. 192 (1989). *A Comparative Evaluation of the Hip Guidance Orthosis (HGO) and the Reciprocating Giant Orthosis (RGO)*. London, NHS Procurement Directorate.

Malick M.H. *Manual of Static Handsplinting*. Pittsburg, Harmaville Rehabilitation Centre.

Chapter 35
Amputations

B.G. Andrews & S. Sooriakumaran

LOWER-LIMB AMPUTATIONS

> One of the meanest and yet one of the greatest operations in surgery mean, when resorted to where better may be done great as the only step to give comfort and prolonged life.
>
> Ferguson (1865)

Amputation is as old as surgery itself. There is a reference in the Rig Veda stories, written in Sanskrit in about 1800 BC, of a Queen Vishpla being fitted with an iron leg following the loss of a leg in battle, but the earliest reference to amputation itself is usually considered to be Herodotus (424 BC) who tells of Hegistratus, a seer, who is condemned to death by the Spartans. He was tethered by a leg to await execution, but escaped by amputating his foot himself, and travelling 30 miles to Tradgia. He was later captured by the Spartans, who this time put him to death, but recorded that he had been provided with a wooden foot. Trauma associated with infection was the overwhelmingly commonest reason for amputation until the First World War.

Larrey, who was Napoleon's personal surgeon, during one of the battles, was said to have performed 200 amputations in 24 hours: a performance indicator that is not likely to be improved upon!

The First World War produced an awesome number of amputees, perhaps more than 100 000 in Europe; 40 000 were British and 26 000 of them were treated at Roehampton. Since that time, more conservative surgery, modern techniques, and antibiotics have reduced the need for amputation following injury and infection. At the same time, there has been a substantial increase in the average age of the population, and with it an increasing incidence of arteriovascular disease and diabetes mellitus, so that by 1982, 75% of the patients in the UK referred to limb fitting centres were suffering from peripheral vascular disease. The other 25% were due to trauma or tumour, occasionally infection or congenital anomalies, and sometimes neurological disorders.

Vascular disease

A detailed discussion of the place of amputation in the management of peripheral vascular disease would be inappropriate in this text, but a few comments may be helpful. Ischaemic disease is now responsible for nearly 80% of all lower-limb amputations, and, with the exception of a small group of younger patients with thrombo-angiitis obliterans, these are all elderly patients who pose serious problems in management and rehabilitation. Many will develop ischaemic lesions elsewhere, particularly myocardial and cerebral infarctions. In addition, approximately 30% of single-leg amputees, suffering from peripheral vascular disease, will become bilateral amputees within 3 years. In dysvascular patients, over 80% of those who have a single below-knee amputation will be able to walk, whereas only 50% of those with above-knee amputations will be able to do so. With bilateral below-knee amputations, walking can still be achieved by a proportion of dysvascular patients, but bilateral above-knee amputation inevitably means a wheelchair existence.

The preservation of the knee joint, therefore, is of great importance in dysvascular individuals, as it is in all other leg amputations.

In 1961, there were three above-knee amputations performed for every below-knee amputation in vascular disease. By the early 1980s, these figures had been reversed so that almost 80% of patients with peripheral vascular disease and diabetes mellitus requiring amputation have done so below the knee. This dramatic change, which marks the most significant progress achieved in amputation surgery in the past 50 years, followed the introduction of long posterior flap including the calf musculature. The operation was first performed by Verduyn in 1695. It was subsequently revived by Kendrick in the UK in 1954 and popularized by Burgess in Seattle in the 1960s.

Tumours

Primary malignant tumours of bone or the soft tissues of the leg may require amputation, and in exceptional circumstances metastatic bone disease in the limb may also be treated by amputation as a palliative and pain-relieving measure. However, increasing improvement and sophistication of prosthetic joint replacement and adjuvant chemotherapy have diminished the role of amputation in the treatment of primary disease. It can be considered usefully in an overall view of the management of limb tumours, which is featured in Chapter 28. Suffice it to say here that the old view that amputation for malignant disease of bone must always take place at or above the level of the proximal joint no longer holds sway. Prosthetic replacement of malignant tumours has clearly shown that the risks of intramedullary spread of tumours were exaggerated and the risk of stump recurrence, stressed so much in the past, was clearly an overstatement.

Trauma

It is in the field of trauma that the place of amputation is most controversial. The basic question that must be asked is whether the limb preserved will be functionally and cosmetically better than a prosthesis. A knowledge, therefore, of what can and cannot be achieved with a prosthesis is mandatory before any decision can rationally be taken about the desirability of amputation. In the arm, the indications for amputation following trauma are few. The arm is not only an extraordinary complex and subtle mechanical instrument, but its value is also very dependent upon its tactile and sensory nature. The movements that can be reproduced by a prosthesis are crude, limited and clumsy. What is more important, however, is that the prosthesis has no sensation and without this sensory input, the need or desire to use a prosthesis is greatly reduced. The attempts so far to produce a cosmetic arm with even minimal function have been disappointing. The prostheses are clearly inanimate and unsightly, and for many amputees and their friends and family, less acceptable than an empty sleeve.

Preservation of a severely mutilated arm may therefore be preferable to amputation provided that some sensation in a part of a hand is retained, and that there is a little movement. While not necessarily associated with upper-limb injury, damage to the brachial plexus may result in severe or total loss of movement and sensation in the arm. Seddon and Yeoman advised relatively early amputation of the limb in the absence of any neurological recovery. They advocated that early amputation and prosthetic replacement would encourage and facilitate the use of a prosthesis and hasten the return of the patient to a useful role in society. Their early enthusiasm has not been justified by the passage of time. Very few patients, with amputations following brachial plexus injuries, make regular use of their prosthesis. Occasionally, patients feel that the simple grasping function of a prosthesis might help them functionally in terms of gaining employment, and, providing they have a clear understanding of the limitations of a prosthesis and a well-defined objective in terms of rehabilitation, then amputation may be justifiable. A few patients also may find the useless totally paralysed arm such an encumbrance and social embarrassment that they may prefer amputation and an empty sleeve. Causalgic pain may be a feature of brachial plexus injuries. Its cause and nature are not clearly understood. It can be very distressing for the patient and amputation is sometimes sought in the mistaken belief that that will rid them of the pain; nothing could be further from the truth. They will develop a painful phantom and are likely to be even more distressed by their symptoms.

In comparison with the arm, replacement of the leg presents less of a problem. The leg is primarily an organ of locomotion and this can be more adequately replaced by a prosthesis. The physical achievement of leg amputees can sometimes be quite remarkable. Providing the knee joint has been preserved and there is a sufficient below-knee stump, a virtually normal existence can be expected. Many can walk without any trace of a limp, and they can hurry if not actually run. Tennis, squash, skiing on two skis, and swimming are all within their capabilities, and a few exceptional individuals can even achieve more. One double below knee amputee achieved a very good standard of cricket at a County Second XI level as a medium-pace left-arm bowler, and another well-known climbing amputee with bilateral below-knee amputations has scaled Aconcagua at 23 000 feet, the highest mountain in the Andes and is a well-known and well-established rock climber. The absence of sensation in a below-knee prosthesis does not present the same disadvantages as it does in arm prostheses. Marginally better levels of function can be anticipated in those few individuals who suffer an amputation at the level of the ankle joint or through the anterior part of the foot. The loss of the leg through the thigh resulting in the loss of the knee joint, however, results in a very much reduced level of performance. All above-knee amputees walk with a detectable limp. They can stand and walk for long periods, but find it difficult to hurry, partly because this is very tiring and also because of the mechanics of the knee mechanism itself, which functions less well and less smoothly if an attempt is made to speed up the gait. Walking with an above-knee prosthesis puts considerable stress upon the back, and substantially more strain on the remaining limb. Bilateral above-knee amputees have considerable difficulty in walking. Fortunately, the number of young people with bilateral above-knee amputations are few. They can generally stand and walk with very considered effort over short distances, many often requiring the support of a stick. The majority of people with bilateral above-knee amputations are dysvascular patients and these are almost invariably confined to a wheelchair existence. The combination of one above- and one-below knee amputation is less seriously disabling, but still puts substantial demands upon both the individual's physical and mental capabilities. Yet, achievements can sometimes still be remarkable.

In the severely injured leg, it is reasonable to consider the place of amputation at three different stages: firstly, at a stage within a few hours of the injury; then at a second stage extending for up to a period of 4 weeks; finally, extending from thereon through months and occasionally into years. As a result of trauma, an amputation of the leg may have already taken place. Success can now frequently be claimed for re-implantation of a detached arm and indeed if survival of the re-attached limb is accompanied by the return of useful sensation, then undoubtedly that could be rated a success. In the leg, however, the chances of sensation returning are remote, and it is very doubtful indeed whether any re-attached legs function as well as a prosthesis. Improved techniques of anastomosis and bone stabilization and nerve repair may change that, but the authors suspect, only marginally, and the indications for re-attachment of the leg will remain for the foreseeable future virtually nil. In the acutely injured leg, the only overriding case for immediate amputation is the ischaemic leg in which the vascular injury cannot be repaired; or when overwhelming sepsis develops in the ischaemic leg (gas gangrene). The degree of ischaemia can initially be very difficult to assess and it is surprising and sometimes gratifying to see how white, apparently avascular legs, will recover. The restoration of the blood pressure, adequate oxygenation, and, in particular, the reduction and temporary stabilization of severely displaced fractures may have a dramatic effect upon the circulation in the periphery of the injured limb. Should the part distal

to the injury remain ischaemic and not be amenable to vascular reconstruction, then an amputation of those parts compatible with the removing of all dead tissue should be undertaken. At this stage, however, it is generally wise to preserve all viable tissue and not undertake a definitive amputation. In a similar manner, if a patient presents already having sustained a traumatic amputation, debridement compatible with removing remaining dead tissue and contaminated tissue should be undertaken, and definitive amputation surgery should not be performed until the true extent of the damage can be properly assessed. This may take several days; in particular, skin that has a compromised blood supply may be compromised further by definitive surgery or definitive surgery may subsequently prove to be inadequate and have to be revised.

During the first few days following the injury, the patient's physical state will become stabilized and a more rational assessment of the extent of the injury can be undertaken. A number of factors will have to be taken into account in deciding whether or not the limb is worth preserving. These factors include: (i) partial or total loss of the nerve supply; (ii) the adequacy of the circulation; (iii) the loss of tissue, be it skin, bone or muscle; or (iv) a combination of all three. The loss of bone, muscle and skin, particularly below the knee, is not an uncommon situation in road traffic accidents, and it is essential that a rational, and not overoptimistic, view is taken of the prospects of recovery even following extensive surgery. Too often a prolonged series of operations is undertaken with the object of producing good skin cover and bone union without a clear understanding of what the likely functional outcome is to be or what period will be involved and whether the end result, after a year or two of surgery, will produce a leg that functions better than a prosthesis. Pozo *et al.* have shown that substantial loss of bone, soft tissue and skin carries a very poor prognosis, and they showed that the end result, often after many years of surgery, still resulted in amputation. Many of the patients that they examined were young and had had twenty or more operations, extending over periods up to seven years. It is evident that both for the patient and the doctor the decision to undertake an amputation, when so much time and effort has been involved in the surgical treatment, is very difficult. It is in this situation that a second opinion may be of enormous value, and should be sought sooner rather than later. It is sometimes easier for an independent orthopaedic surgeon to take a more rational view of such a clinical problem. Equally, a clear understanding from both the doctor's and the patient's point of view of what an amputation entails and what can be achieved with a prosthesis makes that decision to 'cut one's losses' easier to take. This leads on to the third stage of decision-making about amputation, where a relatively stable clinical state has been achieved. The persistence of neurological loss and of claudication-like pain associated with ischaemia, loss of movement in joints, muscle weakness, non-union or malunion of fractures, contractures, the patient's age and general health and ambitions will all influence the decision about amputation. Patients are often helped by talking to other people who have lost their legs in similar circumstances and the advantages and disadvantages of amputation being clearly explained to them by a prosthetic expert. With the benefit of hindsight, it may be obvious that the limb was never worth preserving, and it is important that the surgeon considers that question at an early rather than a late stage. With increasing surgical skills and medical advances, the successful preservation of limbs will continue to advance, but there will always be a group in which excessive optimism on the part of the doctor may still commit a patient to years of surgery and increasing frustration and bitterness at the disappointing outcome, and so often in these generally young people they will have lost some of the most fruitful and formative years of their lives.

A number of other orthopaedic conditions may occasionally best be treated by amputation. Persistent bony infection, uncontrollable ulceration, painful joints, particularly those in which arthroplasty or arthrodesis have failed, may all result in a clinical situation in which amputation is to be preferred. One must sound a word of warning, however. A few patients following injury or surgery may find it very difficult to come to terms with their physical disability, and complain bitterly of pain in the affected part. They may plead for a radical solution to their problem, even amounting to an amputation. Unless there is clear, unequivocal evidence for a cause for their complaint then their desire to have an amputation should be treated with great caution and scepticism. Patients are occasionally seen who present with 'severe pain' in a soundly fused ankle or fused knee, demanding that this problem be resolved by an amputation. Occasionally, their wishes have been granted, and, in the author's (B.A.) experience they have always complained even more bitterly about pain in their amputation stump and an inability to use an artificial limb. These patients are particularly difficult to deal with for they visit numerous orthopaedic surgeons, hoping to persuade one of them to remove the limb. While there is no easy answer to the problem, amputation will certainly not solve it. Many of these patients are severely depressed and a number have a compensation neurosis which may be helped by psychiatric treatment and psychotropic agents. They may be persuaded to take such advice, but that, regrettably, is not very often.

Neurological problems

The commonest neurological disorder that may result in amputation is spina bifida. Most frequently these are patients with low lesions affecting the IVth and Vth lumbar and sacral nerve roots; in other words, the least obviously disabled. Reconstructive surgery and ankle foot orthoses generally allow patients in this category to walk, often with a relatively normal gait. The sensory loss in these patients is patchy, but frequently the sole of the foot is anaesthetic. There is often some deformity of the foot and loss of movement, and with increasing age the uneven pressures and anaesthesia eventually result in ulceration of a trophic nature. This may prove resistant to treatment or impossible to heal, and may often be associated with underlying osteomyelitis. Sometimes, this presents as an intractable problem in children of the age of 10 years upwards, but, most frequently, it is seen in patients over 20 years and may often be a bilateral problem. Most patients with this level of neurological disability cope well with below knee amputations and patellar tendon bearing prostheses. They usually have adequate sensation over the area of the patellar tendon and the tibial flare, where the pressures are directed in the amputation stump, and so the risk of skin breakdown is small. They have a good quadriceps mechanism which allows them to walk well, even if the hamstring musculature is less than normal. Spina bifida patients with a higher level of neurological involvement are commonly wheelchair bound or can only walk and stand for very limited distances with the aid of long-leg orthoses and are therefore much less likely to develop trophic ulceration in the foot. The only other neurological problem worth discussing that may occasionally be helped by amputation is anterior poliomyelitis. This now uncommon condition in the Western world still appears quite frequently in underdeveloped countries. The only situation in which amputation is worth considering is in those patients who have a flail limb, and, in addition, have some painful problem either with the knee or ankle often after previous fracture or injury. The functional difference between the patient with a flail leg controlled by a long-leg caliper and a patient with an above-knee amputation wearing a prosthesis is marginal, as the muscles that stabilize the hip are almost invariably paralysed. A stabilizing pelvic band has to be worn on the prosthesis, and the gait is invariably cumbersome.

Amputation is therefore only worthwhile if it eradicates some other problem, such as a painful joint or ulceration occasionally seen as a result of a poor skin circulation.

Other locomotor problems requiring or benefiting from amputation are rare. Chronic infection has already been alluded to, and the commonest cause of this is past injury to the tibia, generally complicated by failed internal fixation. Below-knee amputation does not generally result in any problems, providing the skin is healthy, even if there appears to be infection throughout much of the medullary shaft at the time. This may be because amputation converts the tibia into an open-ended structure, which is less likely to be infected further. Intractable venous ulceration may occasionally be an indication for amputation. Such ulceration, however, is often associated with previous deep-vein thrombosis, and this may result in greater than normal changes in the daily size of the amputation stump. This, in turn, may present fitting problems with a prosthesis. In a similar and more striking way, those patients with gross lymphatic disorders of the legs, in particular Milroy's disease and lymphatic hypoplasia, are likely to develop gross swelling of an amputation stump, rendering the use of a prosthesis almost impossible.

Congenital problems

The prosthetic and surgical management of congenital limb deficiency is discussed in Chapter 9. It is therefore appropriate only to make some comments about the role of amputation in the management of these problems. In only a small proportion of children with congenital limb deficiency is amputation the best form of treatment. If considered, then timing is of great importance. Some children with congenital absence of the fibula, almost all children with congenital absence of the tibia and children with gross proximal femoral deficiency, cannot be treated successfully by reconstructive surgery. They can only be made ambulant by an extension prosthesis, and with severe deformities these may be heavy, cumbersome and unsightly. Most severe deformities associated with congenital absence of the fibula and congenital absence of the tibia are best treated by amputation at an early stage. This may involve a simple ankle disarticulation in a child with congenital absence of the fibula. In the much rarer, congenital absence of the tibia, a tibial remnant with an extensor mechanism is sometimes present and allows a below-knee amputation. These operations should be undertaken at about the age of one year, so that the child can be fitted with a prosthesis at that stage, and grow up as an amputee. Parents, understandably, find that decision a very difficult one to make, and a second opinion from someone experienced in the field is generally necessary. All too often the decision is not taken at that stage, and the child is then subjected to reconstructive operations that are doomed to failure and the need to wear an often ugly orthosis. It is not uncommon, at about the time the child goes to school, for the parents, grandparents or schoolteacher to begin to question whether or not an amputation would be preferable, but to a child that has got used to its body image and has no pain that decision may be extremely hard for them to take, and there is a danger of producing serious psychological disturbances. Unless there are overwhelming reasons to the contrary, it is better to let the children grow up to an age and level of maturity where they can take part in the decision-making, can understand the physical loss that is entailed, and the prosthetic, cosmetic and functional gains that can be made. If amputation is undertaken at an early stage in childhood, then it is important to warn the parents of the inevitable overgrowth of the stump that occurs. This is most commonly seen in the fibula, which may require trimming two or three times during the growing phase. It ceases at skeletal maturity and cannot be prevented. It can also occur in congenital amputations of a true congenital nature, although it is less common.

Pre-operative assessment

Since amputation is such an irrevocable step, it is wise to advise and even encourage the patient to seek a second opinion. It is essential that the patient understands what problems may arise as a result of an amputation, and even more essential that the individual has a clear understanding of what a prosthesis consists of, and what can and cannot be achieved with its use. Optimal care of a potential amputee is best conducted by a team of specialists, not only the surgeon but the prosthetist, physiotherapist, and occupational therapist all have an important and different role to play, and time needs to be spent with each of these individuals before the amputation, so that the patient has a chance to discuss all of the intimate details involved in wearing a limb and has a clear view of the rehabilitation programme. The physical and psychological trauma of an amputation cannot be overstated, and it will have repercussions on family and friends. The approach of the team has to be optimistic and enthusiastic. The idea has to be firmly implanted in the patient's mind that the amputation presents them with new opportunities, that they are shedding an organ that has become an encumbrance and a nuisance, they are getting something new with which they can lead a fuller and happier existence. This physical and emotional support must continue through the post-operative rehabilitative programme and may need to continue for many weeks until the patient is thoroughly adjusted and satisfied with the outcome. Many patients find it immensely difficult to come to terms with life as an amputee. Continuing vigorous and enthusiastic support designed to integrate them back in to their social and working environment helps the great majority to lead a happy existence.

In general surgical terms, pre-operative assessment does not differ significantly from other surgical procedures. The level of the amputation will generally have been determined by the nature of the pathology. The presence of other joint abnormalities in the legs and, in particular, evidence of ankylosis or fixed deformity in the limb that is to be amputated may affect the optimal level of amputation, and needs to be thoroughly discussed with the prosthetist.

Surgery

Precise details of the operative techniques are inappropriate in this text. Some comments, however, on the advantages and disadvantages of amputation at various levels and upon special aspects of the technique are worth making. The most frequent levels of amputation are below and above the knee. Less commonly performed are amputations just above the ankle joint, amputations through or round the knee joint, and amputations at the level of the hip joint or through the pelvis.

AMPUTATIONS THROUGH THE MIDFOOT

The operation of disarticulation at the tarso-metatarsal joint attributed to Lisfranc, and the amputation of the foot through the midtarsal joint attributed to Chopart are only of historical interest. Patients with Chopart amputations are still occasionally seen. Few if any, however, have satisfactory stumps because the uneven balance of muscles on the foot remnant pulls the stump into an equino-varus position. Excessive weight is then borne on the antero-lateral aspect of the stump, which becomes painful and ulcerates over the end of the stump and a terminal scar does not compromise this.

Digital or single-ray amputations scarcely interfere with foot function. A transmetatarsal amputation removes the anterior pillar of the arch and necessitates a forefoot filler with longitudional arch support and plantar stiffener. The Lisfranc and Chopart disarticulations through the midfoot require more proximal sockets, which limit subtalar movement.

Recent applications of more flexible material such as Eurothane elastomer and reinforced silicone have resulted in more flexible and cosmetically appealing replacements.

SYMES AMPUTATION

The indications and opportunities for using this type of amputation are now very uncommon. Nevertheless it still has a place in the field of amputation surgery. The benefit that Symes' amputation confers upon the amputee is that the stump is end-bearing, and in fact a patient can bear their full weight on the end of the stump, providing that the heel flap is stable. Therefore, on those rare occasions when the trauma is limited to the forepart of the foot and the heel skin is not compromised, a Symes' amputation may confer upon the individual a degree of stability and an ability to walk without the need for a prosthesis that would be denied with a below-knee amputation. Symes' amputation, though surgically demanding, has the advantages in retaining the growth plate in children and the production of an end-bearing stump enables the amputee to walk short distances without the need of a prosthesis. However, the retention of maleolli though enabling self-suspension tends to make the prosthesis rather bulky at ankle level. Limited space between the distal end of stump and ground limits choice of prosthetic feet. Another disadvantage of the Symes' prosthesis is that is it cosmetically less satisfactory than a patellar tendon-bearing prosthesis, and, as such, is unacceptable to women.

Harris' description of Symes' amputation is still the method of choice. Attempts to modify Symes' amputation by sectioning the tibia and fibula at a slightly higher level or removing the malleoli, designed initially to improve the cosmesis, do in fact reduce the weight-bearing area of the stump significantly and thus reduce considerably the end-bearing potential of the stump. The important surgical factors to be stressed in the operation are that the cut surface of the bone must be absolutely parallel to the ground surface when the individual is standing, and a good deal of effort may have to be devoted to stabilizing the heel flap beneath the stump. Should it not come to stabilize in a satisfactory position, then the end-bearing quality of the stump is lost, and the virtue of Symes' amputation then disappears.

AMPUTATION AT BELOW-KNEE LEVEL

This is the next level of choice after the transmetatarsal in a dysvascular limb. Since the introduction of patellar tendon-bearing prostheses by Radcliffe and Foort (1961) this is perhaps the most favoured and succesful level of amputation. A motivated patient with a myoplastic stump suitably fitted with a patellar tendon-bearing prosthesis should achieve rehabilitation to pre-morbid level.

Some variation in the level of bone section below the knee joint is now permissible and in fact, is encouraged. The old concept of a site of election is outmoded and the level of bone section should be determined by the quality of the skin and by the height of the individual. In general terms, the longer the stump, the better the function, and certainly the better the power. Factors that limit the length of the stump are that firstly, if the stump is too long, then it will have poor skin cover with a lack of muscle underneath and a tendency therefore to be poorly nourished and a tendency to break down. Similarly, if the stump is too long, then, when it is contained within its prosthesis, its bulk will mean that the prosthesis is substantially bulkier than the normal leg.

Taking these two factors into consideration, however, means that the stump can often be several centimetres longer than the accepted site of election.

Details of techniques of below-knee amputation are well described in the book literature. The two common methods used are either the conventional amputation using equal anterior and posterior flaps with a terminal scar or, as an alternative, the long posterior flap operation, in which the scar comes to lie anteriorly. Most surgeons now favour the long posterior flap operation, at least in part, because their training has often been on dysvascular patients in which this operation is undoubtedly preferable. In the otherwise fit individual, however, who is having an amputation possibly because of trauma or tumour, the operation involving equal anterior and posterior flaps is to be preferred for two reasons. Firstly, the flaps are less bulky and so the stump reaches a state of maturity in which a well-fitting prosthesis can be worn at a very much earlier stage. Secondly, the scar is terminal and is not subjected to pressure when a patellar tendon-bearing prosthesis is actively used. In a vigorous walker, the force driving the prosthesis is transmitted through the anterior/inferior aspect of the stump, and it is therefore a particularly unfortunate place to have a scar, especially in a young vigorous walker.

The operation using equal anterior and posterior flaps is designed to produce a blunt stump rather than the tapered stump that was favoured in the prosthetists in the past. This means that the fibula should be only cut marginally shorter than the tibia and it is important that the bone is well enclosed by a snug envelope of anterior and postero-tibial musculature with periosteum being used anteriorly to support the limited antero-tibial muscles. Considerable attention must be paid to the tibial crest, which must be properly trimmed and chamfered, so that it does not have any rough or sharp edges. If it does, it would certainly cause pain and may well break down and necessitate revision of the stump.

The long posterior flap operation, and the variation of it, the skew flap operation, have both been widely described in the literature.

For the prosthesis, a plaster cast of the stump is used to make a positive model which is then rectified to make the socket so that the main load is on the patella tendon and paratibial area, the popliteal area giving the counter-pressure. Pressure sensitive areas such as the head of fibula, crest of tibia and end of stump are given clearance. Patellar tending-bearing prostheses are designed to retain the full function of the knee joint. Patients with instability of knee or short stump require a thigh corset. The socket is connected to the ankle by a shin tube through an alignment device. The ankle can be uniaxial or polyaxial. The uniaxial ankle has a plantar/dorsiflexion rubber bumper and toe break in a wood/plastic foot. A polyaxial foot has a rubber ball in a snubber ring in the ankle to simulate dorsi/plantar flexion and supination/pronation. The solid ankle cushion heel (SACH) system does not have any moving parts. The ridge of cushion in the heel and an internal keel replacing the normal movements. Research and development into more energy storing ankle−foot mechanisms such as the flex foot based on carbon fibre construction has enabled athletically active amputees to improve their sprinting performances.

AMPUTATIONS AT THE KNEE-JOINT LEVEL

The indications for amputation at this level are now few and far between. The success of below-knee amputations in dysvascular patients has reduced substantially the need for amputation at the knee-joint level for patients in this group. There has been some controversy for many years as to which of the operations at the knee-joint level is best. There are three options. First there is true disarticulation at the knee joint with preservation of the patella, anchoring the patellar tendon to the cruciate ligaments and utilizing more or less equal medial and lateral skin flaps, so that the skin scar sits in the intercondylar region of the femur. This operation used to be known in Continental Europe as the English amputation.

The second option is to perform the operation described at the end of the last century by Gritti and Stokes. This is still practised, but fortunately not widely. The principle of the operation is to section the femur just at the level of the beginning of the condylar flares and fix the patella onto the lower end of the femur in the misconceived hope that the stump will then be end-bearing.

The third option is simply to section the femur at trans- or just supra-femoral condylar level. The advantages of the true through-knee disarticulation are that the stump is end-bearing and the operation is quick and easy to do, and virtually bloodless. Its disadvantage is that, although it is end-bearing and because of its shape, the prosthesis can be, to a degree, self-supporting over the flare of the condyles, but it does not allow any space in the prosthesis for a sophisticated knee mechanism. The knee mechanism has to be either external to the prosthesis in some hinge form or concealed within the shank of the tibial part of the prosthesis, and these do represent substantial prosthetic disadvantages. Occasionally, a heavy middle-aged man, who needs a robust end-bearing stump rather than an above-knee amputation, will find that the stability of the stump outweighs the prosthetic disadvantages. The claims made on behalf of the Gritti–Stokes amputation are that it heals better than the through-knee amputation, that it is easier to fit into a prosthesis and that it is end-bearing. It is probably true to say that skin healing is somewhat better, but it is incorrect to say that it is end-bearing, for it is seldom that the patella ever attaches itself firmly to the lower end of the femur. Therefore it has all the disadvantages, from a prosthetic point of view, that the through-knee amputation has, and it should not be practised. Similarly, a trans-condylar amputation, while not claiming any merits in terms of end-bearing, still involves prosthetic modifications and loss of the normal mechanical knee joint in the prosthesis, and it therefore has no advantages over an above-knee amputation. With the occasional exception of through-knee amputation, these operations should be abandoned.

ABOVE-KNEE AMPUTATION

The same principle enunciated with choice of level below the knee applies equally well above the knee. There is no absolute site of election. The length of the stump should be tailored to the needs of the individual, taking into account the demands made upon it by the type of prosthesis available. The longer the amputation stump, the easier it is to fit, and it confers a greater sense of stability. Enough bone, however, must be removed to allow for the knee mechanism to be contained within the lower part of the thigh component of the prosthesis. Most sophisticated mechanisms currently occupy 11 cm. A further 3–4 cm needs to be allowed for the soft-tissue covering of the bone, which means the level of bone section should be measured up from the knee joint line, a distance of approximately 14 cm. The technique is well document in the literature.

There are one or two points of technique, however, that are worth stressing. It is essential that the femoral shaft is securely contained within an enveloping sheath of muscle. Should it not be so, it will come to rest under the skin, most frequently on the lateral side of the stump. Where the skin is subjected to excessive pressure, it will be uncomfortable and painful with prolonged use. With good musculature, the easiest way to produce a secure myoplasty is to section the hamstrings and the adductors and the ilio-tibial tract at the level of bone section, and fashion a long anterior flap from the quadriceps mechanism that can then be sutured to the other sectioned muscles, neatly encapsulating the end of the femur. Alternatively, if the muscles are thin and providing the stump is not too short, the adductors can first be sutured to the ilio-tibial tract, and the quadriceps sutured to the hamstrings on top. Neuromata always form after nerves have been sectioned, and the neuroma that forms after cutting the sciatic nerve can be quite large. It is therefore essential that the nerve is sectioned at high level so that this neuroma is not subjected to pressure within the prosthesis, particularly when the patient is sitting. The sciatic nerve bleeds quite profusely and can safely be ligatured with an absorbable material at a higher level. Antibiotics should always be used with above-knee amputations because of the risk of contamination from the perineum. There is no need to use antibiotics at the lower levels of amputation unless there is obvious evidence of infection.

In a suitably performed myoplastic stump of adequate length, a total contact self-suspending socket made of semi-flexible material gives greater freedom of muscle activity during ambulation with more tactile feedback. Weight is mainly transmitted through an ischial seat built on the socket brim. Patients with non-myoplastic stump unable to use suction sockets use a pelvic belt with or without shoulder suspension. Sockets may be made of wood, metal, or the more commoner thermoplastic (polypropylene, polyethylene and surlyn).

Knee joints may be uni- or polyaxial using four-bar linkage. The knee joint can be locked by extension of the knee to provide a stiff knee gait or a optional locking device to enable free knee gait option. In more active amputees, free knee-stabilized mechanisms are used. Pneumatic and hydraulic devices are used to assist swing phase. The alignment of the socket, the knee joint and the foot are important to achieve the best possible prosthetic gait.

HIP DISARTICULATION AND HINDQUARTER AMPUTATIONS

Mercifully, neither of these operations is frequently required. Occasionally, a choice may have to be made as to whether or not to perform a high above-knee amputation or a hip disarticulation. Providing there is 3 cm of length below the adductor tendon, an above-knee prosthesis can be fitted adequately. Anything shorter than this presents considerable prosthetic difficulties and a better fit and greater comfort can be obtained with through-hip amputation. Disarticulation of the hip is a perfectly straightforward operation. It is simply an anatomical exercise, most easily performed with anterior and posterior flaps, the posterior flap being much longer and containing the bulk of the gluteal musculature. This allows early control of the main vessels and minimizes haemorrhage. Hindquarter amputation is rarely performed. It can be quite difficult, particularly in controlling bleeding from the ilio-lumbar veins, and those few patients that require such an operation are best referred to an expert.

With prostheses at these levels, the socket embraces the pelvis. In disarticulation the weight is transmitted through the ipsilateral ischium, and in the hindquarter through the contralateral ischium and abdominal wall. In the Canadian design of prosthesis, the hip joint is built anterior to the socket and the movement of the hip is controlled by a limiter. The alignment requires the knee joint to be aligned in hyperextension to achieve stability.

Post-operative care and rehabilitation

The vogue for rigid post-operative plaster dressing and immediate post-operative fitting have largely fallen into disuse. Crêpe bandages, fairly loosely applied, make an adequate post-operative dressing. If attempts are made to apply them tightly, the bandages will have a tourniquet effect and produce stump swelling. Sutures should be left for 2 weeks and 3 weeks in patients with dysvascular disease or diabetes. Early mobilization is beneficial both from the patient's point of view as well as the health of the stump. Use is now widely made of the Pam aid which consists of a simple pneumatic pylon enabling the patient to bear some weight through the amputation stump 5–6 days after the amputation. This does not compromise stump healing. In ideal circumstances, a patellar tendon-bearing pylon with a shin and foot can be fitted within 2 weeks of the amputation, and fit young people can be expected to walk tolerably well on such a device 2 weeks from the time of the operation with the aid of two sticks.

Rehabilitation requires a team approach, and its early effective use is crucial. Delays in the provision of a prosthesis and a lack of urgency in learning to use it will reduce substantially the chances of a successful outcome. An early return to a normal social and working environment should be the objective. The artificial limb is made of a socket, articulations, suspension mechanisms, alignment devices and cosmetic cover. Most modern prostheses are built of modular components in an endoskeletal system with an axial tube made of either carbon fibre or titanium.

POST-AMPUTATION PROBLEMS

There is a widely held belief that amputation stumps are particularly painful, and that this pain may continue for weeks post-operatively, and be associated with a reputedly intractable problem of a painful phantom. Amputation stumps are probably no more painful than other orthopaedic operations involving bone section of a comparable magnitude. Adequate control with analgesia in the first 3–4 days, however, will do much to allay the patient's anxiety about the problems of a painful stump. The patient always perceives a phantom limb. This needs to be clearly explained to them before the operation. Many amputees continue to experience this phantom limb for the rest of their lives, and will often describe how they can still feel their toes or fingers at the end of the stump, but cannot feel the intermediate missing part. Children also experience this phantom sensation following amputation, but it generally disappears completely within a short period. Phantoms are not painful, and this also needs to be stressed to the patient pre-operatively. Painful phantoms and causalgia were first described by Weir Mitchell after the American Civil War. Painful phantoms have added such colour and drama to many plays and books so that they have now become an accepted part of life for an amputee. No rational explanation has ever been provided as to why a phantom should be painful, and no successful treatment has yet been described. Nerve blocks, division of nerves, division of spinal roots and spinal columns have all been attempted and have been unsuccessful. Patients can be very persistent in their complaint. They sometimes persuade the surgeon to amputate the limb at a higher level; this never works. The patient must be persuaded that further surgery will not ease their problem. The patient with a painful phantom is usually depressed and may have insoluble domestic and employment problems. In a neurotic patient, there is no easier place for their neurosis to repose than in an amputation stump. Occasionally, psychiatric treatment is of value, particularly if there is an obvious element of depression when psychotropic agents may also be of assistance. Every possible help must be given, from a social point of view, to facilitate the patient's return to a normal environment. This is the most useful, positive approach, but will not always be successful. Some patients will persist with their painful phantom, and this cannot be treated. What must be avoided is further surgery, which will not only fail to relieve the patient's pain, but subject them to further physical and psychological trauma, making a satisfactory resolution of the problem even more unlikely.

Neuromata always form in amputation stumps, and there is no method of preventing their occurrence. They do not cause spontaneous pain, and are not the cause of painful phantoms. If they occur, however, in places where they are subjected to pressure in the prosthesis or if they are subjected to traction because of attachment to ill-placed scars, then they will cause pain, and need to be excised adequately, so that when a further neuroma forms it is not in a vulnerable position. Most of the other problems that arise in an amputation stump are due to its potentially unhealthy environment within a prosthesis. Inevitably, the skin within the prosthesis will get moist, and with inadequate hygiene, infection and stump breakdown can occur. Abnormal pressures due to an ill-fitting prosthesis can produce ulceration, and some individuals, particularly those with a lot of hair, are prone to develop sebaceous cysts and infected implantation dermoids in the skin in contact with the socket rim. Bone spurs sometimes occur and these can be seen if the stump is radiographed, but they do not cause symptoms. Below-knee amputees are not more prone to develop osteoarthritic changes in other joints, although clearly these joints are subjected to rather greater stress than in a two-legged individual. This is probably because the amputee generally leads a less vigorous life. With an above-knee amputee, there is considerable stress involved in walking, particularly upon the lumbar spine, and some long-term degenerative changes in the lumbosacral spine are to be expected in an above-knee amputee of long-standing.

UPPER LIMB

Replacement of upper-limb function compared to lower limb is a major prosthetic and bioengineering challenge. The agile, dexterous and coordinated actions of the hand require good sensation. Though a great deal of upper-limb function is bimanual, loss of one hand does not preclude regaining independence with the remaining normal hand. The complexity of upper-limb prostheses and the ability of patient to function quite effectively with the remaining arm, decrease motivation in unilateral amputees, more so in proximal levels. Motivation varies, between patients born with congenital absence of an upper limb, who have learned to carry out all activities one-handed and have grown with that body image, and active adults who suddenly face the loss of an arm, especially if it is the dominant side. The relevance of the prosthesis and the type of terminal device would also depend on the aesthetic requirements, vocation and social activities of the patient. In fact, careful consideration of all these factors should be considered, functional requirements assessed, and realistic potentials set prior to embarking on prosthetic prescription and training. This is best carried out by teamwork, consisting of all the professionals involved, such as rehabilitation clinician, prosthetists and therapists. The surgeon performing the amputation must know of the types of prostheses and the optimal stump features for different levels to improve prospects of outcome. Generally, in upper-limb ablation maximum conservation of length is advocated, but certain sites, such as disarticulation through wrist or elbow, present difficulties and are not favoured by prosthetists. Prosthetic substitution and management of congenital upper-limb deficiencies differ quite markedly and they are dealt with in Chapter 9.

The prosthesis is designed for cosmesis, function or both. Purely cosmetic replacement is achieved by a hand made of foam with digits strengthened with wires permitting passive position of fingers and covered with a glove. Recently, the cosmetic results of the glove have been improved by giving a wider choice of skin colours and paying more attention to features such as skin creases, nail and venous markings.

Prostheses for function are still unsightly, heavy, cumbersome and limited. There is a variety of optional terminal devices available but none of them matches the prehensile and non-prehensile function of the normal hand. The conventional split hook which is available in a range of different sizes and shapes achieves a grip with variable power and precision. The commonest type of mechanical hand supplied provides a lateral pinch between the pad of the thumb which is mobile against the immobile index finger. A range of interchangeable devices can be fitted to the wrist component. These are mobile or static. Examples include pliers, universal grips and aids for typing, feeding, sports and musical instruments.

The split hook is voluntarily opened against the variable tension provided by rubber bands placed at the stem of the hook. The power needed to open the hook is transmitted by a cable attached to the harnessing system and the basic motion required is forward flexion of the humerus with some assistance from bi-scapular abduction. The myoelastic limb is the most common example of an externally powered functional prosthesis. Electrodes implanted in the socket pick up myoelectric potentials from contractions of muscle groups and operate the electric motor housed in the hand. The external power source is from rechargeable batteries. The type of hand movement is limited to a three-point chuck grip between the thumb, index and midfinger, the last two fingers being cosmetic. The appliance is heavy. It combines a degree of function with a more cosmetically acceptable device than a split hook and is also free of the harnessing system, relying on a self-suspending socket.

Amputations in the hand can leave a wide variety of residual hand deformities and functional limitations and prosthetic replacements are meant to complement this. Isolated digit losses can be replaced with thimble-fitting cosmetic fingers without interfering with the residual digit function. The prostheses act as a post to provide opposition as in a hand with a mobile sensate thumb but with no other digits. The wrist gauntlet made of leather to house feeding or writing aids can be appropriate in certain patients.

In wrist disarticulation and long below-elbow (more than 80° of the length) ablation, the patient has ability to supinate and pronate, and the split sockets are used to house the terminal device to retain this movement. Below-elbow amputation is performed through the junction of the proximal two-thirds and distal one-third leaving adequate clearance to fit the wrist rotary to simulate supination and pronation. Disarticulation of the elbow is generally not favoured as the prosthesis tends to be bulky and cosmetically unacceptable. Although retention of the condyles improves suspension and rotatory stability, the joints have to be set outside the socket.

In above-elbow amputation, the lowest-level surgically compatible should be sought. A very short above-elbow amputation is much preferred to shoulder disarticulation. The surface contour provided by the retained head improves both cosmesis and prosthetic restoration. However, stumps shorter than the deltoid insertion do not allow effective control of shoulder joints. The elbow mechanism is a simple uniaxial joint allowing 60° of flexion and 180° of extension. Flexion is obtained passively, or actively using the flexion cord. When tensed by rounding the shoulder or by humeral flexion, or both, the cord will first flex the forearm and when locked will actuate the terminal device. The elbow can be locked at variable degrees of flexion to carry or push any load. A ring device is fitted above the elbow joint to allow rotation about the long axis and the desired position maintained either by friction or by a bolt locking into holes on the turntable. These prostheses are suspend by three webbing straps which meet above the shoulder and are attached to a webbing loop passing around the opposite axilla.

A true shoulder disarticulation empties the glenoid fossa and leaves the acromion and clavicle projecting laterally to present a sharp angle, whereas retaining the head of humerus maintains a round contour and enables provision of a more comfortable prosthesis. The socket is made of block leather from a plaster cast incorporating the chest wall for weight distribution and stability. The rest of the components are based along the lines of above-elbow prosthesis but the operation involves the opposite hand due to lack of shoulder control.

At forequarter level, the immediate need is for reduction of deformity and this is provided by a light shoulder cap to fill up the shoulder of the clothing to give a normal outline and to carry the shoulder straps of underclothing. These are made of foam plastic materials which are light and semi-flexible and covered with a washable nylon cover held with a zipper. Full prostheses at this level become cumbersome and heavy and necessitate extension of socket to encircle the neck. They are scarcely used.

Prosthetic training

It is important to ensure that the amputee begins training with the equipment at its maximum efficiency. The prosthesis should conform to the prescription in regards to length, socket fit, range of motion, efficiency of terminal device, suspension, stability, workmanship and cosmesis. During the training stage the amputee should gain adequate orientation of the prosthesis to detect any mechanical faults. Donning and doffing methods are also taught. Amputees are trained to pre-position the terminal device and approach the object correctly without unnecessary and awkward body movements.

Prehension training involves drills in approach, grasp and release of various sizes of objects and different types of materials. The objects include a sponge rubber cube, a wooden block, a cotton ball, a paper cup and even an ice-cream cone. Amputees learn harness feedback to adjust the necessary tension on the object. Once these basic operations are learned they are then applied to practise activities of daily living. The amputee, however, relies on vision and hearing.

Once the prime activities, such as feeding, dressing and grooming are completed, more specialized tasks such as communication skills involving the use of telephone or typewriter are attempted. Vocational and recreational interests are encouraged. Once a good foundation for basic independence has been established the initial prosthetic training can be considered complete. Amputees will improve on this, and difficulties addressed in review clinics. The prosthesis is modified as needed.

It is now standard practice to commence stump exercises and use of walking aids such as PPAM Aid and Tulip limbs as early as 5 days' post-amputation. At 2—4 weeks after amputation, the stump measurements or plaster cast is taken to begin fabrication. Patients then progress to various stages of training in the physiotherapy department. Long term, the patient attends for monitoring of stump problems, hardware maintenance, and updating to incorporate new prosthetic advances. Sockets are replaced as the stump matures. The patient continues attending for review of stump problems, prosthetic maintenance and modification.

Chapter 36
Orthopaedic Malpractice

N.H. Harris

INTRODUCTION

It is not the purpose of this chapter to indicate how a surgeon may reduce the chances of being sued for malpractice. Rather it is to discuss standards of practice and how some of the more common errors might be avoided.

In 1978, settled cases of malpractice in the UK amounted to 1 in 1000, and in 1988 it was 13 per 1000, and although figures are not available for the current position—mainly due to the fact that these cases have been dealt with by health authorities under the Crown Indemnity Scheme since January 1990—the incidence is undoubtedly much higher.

For the most part these cases are obstetric, anaesthetic and orthopaedic, including trauma. It has been estimated that an orthopaedic surgeon is 2.5 times more likely to be sued than the average doctor. Glyn Thomas (1986) made the interesting observation that during 25 years of consultant orthopaedic practice, and taking into account ward rounds, operating sessions and out-patient clinics, there are 402 500 opportunities to make a fool of yourself!

Other recent reports have also indicated concern about the explosion in orthopaedic malpractice actions; Lacombe and O'Keefe (1989), Woodyard (1990), Vickers (1991) and Harris (1990).

CAUSES OF INCREASED LITIGATION IN ORTHOPAEDIC PRACTICE

There are a number of possible explanations for increasing litigation. Patient expectations have significantly increased in recent years and during a period of rapid growth in medical technology, the profession has had the ability to palliate and sometimes cure conditions hitherto considered untreatable. None of this is surprising and applies to all branches of medicine.

As far as orthopaedic practice is concerned, the steadily rising number of trauma victims, including some multiple injuries of great complexity, continue to dominate the workload of most Accident and Emergency and orthopaedic departments. It is not always the case that these departments are staffed by adequate numbers and quality of medical, nursing and ancillary staff. Inevitably, this brings into question the urgent need for major accident centres, and the closure of small poorly staffed and equipped units.

Inadequate staffing and facilities are not put forward as an excuse for inferior standards of practice; it is, in fact, not a defence in law because it is a doctor's duty to inform management in writing if he or she considers that lack of facilities are dangerous for patients. If the doctor fails to do so and a medical accident occurs, he or she may be liable (Medical Defence Union, 1986).

Fractures are now very commonly treated by internal fixation which increases the hazards. Joint replacement has been so successful over the last 20 years that some patients expect a guarantee of success and no complications. Some recent advances such as arthroscopic surgery have brought with it complications and errors which have prompted litigation.

In the course of investigating possible negligence in over 400 orthopaedic patients in the last 15 years, it has become apparent to the author that avoidable errors have occurred because responsibility for decision-making and treatment, including surgery, has been inappropriately delegated to junior and inexperienced doctors. In John Woodyard's survey (1990), 81 of 236 accidents could be attributed to inappropriate delegation of responsibility.

The author's own concern on this aspect of the problem, and Woodyard's survey, was confirmed by the confidential inquiry into peri-operative deaths (1987, 1992), and as a consequence, the advice was that all new patients in out-patient clinics, and all patients before surgery, should be seen by senior medical staff; and major and complex conditions should be operated on, or closely supervised by them. It should be emphasized that these reports are concerned only with perioperative deaths; they do not reflect the much larger number of patients who sustain injury and disability as a result of errors in medical practice.

A most important and revealing report on the management of skeletal trauma in the UK has recently been published by the British Orthopaedic Association (1992). Serious deficiencies in staffing and workload are widespread, leading to unavailability of consultant supervision and inappropriate delegation of work to junior doctors; deficiencies in facilities such as intensive care and specialized equipment and poor organization (such as a low level of referral to surgery with special expertise) are also discussed.

It is arguable that in some of the matters discussed, a doctor has been negligent and that blame cannot necessarily always be attributed to poor staffing or lack of facilities, for example because surgeons should not be knowingly offering a second-rate service. This is not a defence in law.

What is not in doubt from the survey, is that 12% of patients were judged to have significant preventable disability. The estimate is that 108 000 patients per year had a serious disability which could have been prevented by the elimination of the deficiencies to which the report courageously draws attention.

NEGLIGENCE

Negligence is a legal term and is not synonymous with carelessness, though the two may coexist. In the UK, the law imposes on a doctor a duty of care to a standard that would be acceptable to a reasonable body of their peers, and at the time the incident occurred. In other words, the standard of medical practice, including consent, diagnosis and treatment, is determined by the medical profession, not the courts. The test is an objective one and is referred to as the Bolam test; it may be summarized as follows: It is the standard of the ordinary skilled man exercising and professing to have a special skill; a man need not profess to the highest expert's skill; it is well established in law that it is sufficient if he exercises the ordinary skill of a competent man exercising that particular art. The art is judged in the light of the practitioner's specialty and the post that he holds.

Lest the orthopaedic surgeon thinks that the increasing risk of being sued and the law is interfering with his or her clinical practice, it is appropriate to bear in mind the following judgements. Lord Clyde (1985) said:

> In the realm of diagnosis and treatment there is ample scope for differences of opinion, and one man [*sic*] is clearly not negligent because his conclusions differ from that of another professional man, nor because he had displayed less skill or knowledge that others would have shown.
>
> The true test for establishing negligence in diagnosis or treatment on the part of a doctor, is whether he has proved to be guilty of such failure that no doctor of ordinary skill would be guilty of it, acting with ordinary care.

Lord Scarman (1983) said in the House of Lords' judgement:

> Differences of opinion in practice exist, and will always exist, in medical and other professions. There is seldom any one answer exclusive to all others, to problems of professional judgement, but that is no basis for a conclusion of negligence.

In the light of the above the author suggests there really is no valid excuse for an orthopaedic surgeon to engage in the practice of defensive medicine.

The profession, including orthopaedic surgeons, has the ability to influence the standard of practice. Under the present adversarial system, the courts have to distinguish the reasonably held difference of expert medical opinion from unacceptable medical practice. For the first time in the UK there are published guidelines provided by all disciplines which form a basis for setting objective standards of practice (Powers and Harris, 1994).

CONSENT

Obtaining the consent of the patient after explaining the nature of the procedure, and mentioning risks and possible complications, is one of the components of the general duty held by a doctor to his or her patient. The problems which arise are not unique to orthopaedic surgery and it is not therefore appropriate to discuss the matter here. However, one general point needs to be made. With regard to elective orthopaedic practice, the vast majority are not done for life-threatening conditions. It is important, therefore, that the nature of the procedure is discussed and also possible risks and complications and alternative treatments, and what is likely to happen if surgery is not done. The standard consent forms do not include this information. The patient never remembers what they have been told and therefore it is a sensible precaution to write in the notes a short summary of the information given to the patient.

COMMON ERRORS IN ORTHOPAEDIC PRACTICE

The areas which regularly come to litigation include misdiagnosis or late diagnosis, nerve damage, circulatory impairment, errors of operative technique and wound infection.

Diagnostic errors

Failure to make a correct diagnosis is not necessarily an indication of a poor standard of care. However, a doctor will be held liable if it can be shown that there was failure to exercise reasonable skill and care. In his review of 100 allegations of negligence, Vickers lists 14 failed in which diagnosis was delayed and 28 failures to X-ray, or incorrect interpretation of radiographs, which usually leads to delay in diagnosis—a total of 42. In other words, very nearly half the cases were concerned with diagnostic errors. This is in accordance with the authors own experience. Many of these errors occur in Accident and Emergency departments which fail to take a radiograph following trauma. If one is taken, the fracture may not be seen, and the patient is sent away— often without any specific instructions. In most cases the error is picked up early (within 48 hours) if the hospital has a reliable mechanism for recalling patients after inspection of the radiograph by a radiologist. Sadly, such an arrangement does not always exist. It is the duty of the orthopaedic surgeon to make certain that a mechanism exists for the prompt recall of patients following the correct radioraphic diagnosis.

The consequences of late diagnosis may be serious— congenital dislocation of the hip, adolescent coxa vara, a deep-wound infection after total hip replacement, femoral neck and scaphoid fractures leading to increased risk of avascular necrosis and non-union and posterior dislocation of the shoulder—are a few examples, all of which repeatedly give rise to litigation.

In other instances, late diagnosis has no material effect on the eventual outcome. Thus an undisplaced fracture of a metacarpal, distal radius or fibula will heal without disability even if no treatment is given. Occasionally an accident causes damage which will lead to complications and permanent disability even if prompt diagnosis and treatment is given; an example is femoral neck fracture with displacement in a child.

The basis for a diagnostic error is inadequate history-taking which leads to deficiencies in the examination. It is undoubtedly true that a doctor who cannot take a good history and a patient who cannot give one, are in danger of giving and receiving poor treatment. A good history indicates the likely site of the disease and the probable diagnosis, and then the appropriate radiograph can be requested. Fractures and dislocations which are complicated by nerve and vascular damage require particularly careful and prompt assessment by an experienced orthopaedic surgeon, if serious and disabling consequences are to be avoided. The following case histories illustrate the foregoing points.

CASE REPORTS

Case 1

A middle-aged woman complained of increasingly severe lumbodorsal back pain over a period of 3 months, by which time she had night sweats, difficulty with walking (due to paraplegia) and retention of urine. At no time was she examined by her doctor during four consultations. After 2 months, having assumed the pain was in the lumbar region, a lumbar spine radiograph was done and reported as normal. A week or two later she was admitted to hospital when advanced tuberculosis of the lower dorsal spine was diagnosed; it was associated with a large abscess and paraplegia. Emergency surgery failed to prevent permanent neurological damage or relieve the bladder paralysis.

More careful history-taking and a clinical examination would have revealed the source of pain at an early stage leading to a request for the appropriate radiography. This case was indefensible.

Case 2

An infant's hips were routinely checked at birth and at 6 weeks by the general practitioner; a further check at the health centre at the age of 7 months reported normal hips. At 15 months, the mother was concerned the child was not walking. When walking had started between 16 and 18 months, the mother noticed a limp. Despite the history of late walking and a limp, the general practitioner did not examine the hips.

At 24 months, the health visitor confirmed the mother's continued concern about an awkward gait, and the left leg looked different to the right. This was reported to the general practitioner who did not find an abnormality. No radiograph was requested. At 30 months, a radiograph was requested and a diagnosis of left congenital hip dislocation was confirmed. Subsequently, after closed reduction, a Salter innominate osteotomy was performed. At the age of 9 years, a significant defect of the acetabulum persists.

This case illustrates how important it is to listen to what a mother is saying about her child and to act accordingly; it also illustrates the importance of a careful clinical examination of a child's hips by an experienced doctor who has been trained in the appropriate techniques. This is the orthopaedic surgeon's responsibility with the health authority to ensure that satisfactory arrangements exist for the routine screening of children's hips.

Case 3

A 15-year-old boy represented to his general practitioner with a 2 months' history of knee pain; there was no history of trauma and the general health was good. He was promptly referred to hospital as a possible hip problem. The hospital doctor thought he may have Still's disease; no radiographs were taken and 1 month after first presenting, he was referred to a rheumatologist. A total of 19 blood investigations were done and all major joints were radiographed; the hip had an antero-posterior projection only, and these films were reported as normal. Aspirin was prescribed and he was told to return in 6 months. He was seen again 4 months later, still complaining of knee pain but no examination of the hips took place. At 6 months after presenting, the hips were examined by the rheumatologist and radiographs revealed a very severe chronic epiphyseal displacement with fusion of the growth plate.

This case illustrates a failure to understand the significance of the history leading to failure to examine the hips and request lateral hip radiography. The general practitioner and the doctor in the Accident and Emergency department are usually the first to see children who complain of knee pain. Regrettably, it is usual to examine and radiograph the knee and ignore the hip.

The radiologist made his report on the basis of an antero-posterior projection only and failed to notice the metaphyseal changes, widening of the epiphyseal plate and a positive Trethowen's sign, and a break in Shenton's line. The consultant rheumatologist accepted the radiological report and did not inspect the radiograph.

It should, of course, be routine to take two projections for the study of joint pathology. Another all-too-common example is a failure to diagnose posterior dislocation of the shoulder because an axial projection is not taken (see Chapter 23). This case also illustrates the common discrepancy between generalist radiologist opinion on bone and joint pathology and that of an orthopaedic surgeon who will always interpret the radiographs and ensure the appropriate projections have been done.

Case 4

A 40-year-old man who played sport regularly suddenly felt pain at the back of his ankle when playing squash. He told the doctor in the Accident and Emergency department, 'It feels as if a brick has been thrown at me, and I fell to the ground'. Despite the typical history of a ruptured Achilles' tendon, the diagnosis was missed. After 2 days he told the general practitioner that he was not improving, and physiotherapy was ordered without a clinical examination. After 2 months he reported no improvement and was referred to an orthopaedic surgeon who confirmed the diagnosis. Complex reconstructive surgery and inevitable permanent disability could have been prevented by correctly interpreting the history and a more careful examination. The case was indefensible.

Case 5

A 42-year-old man sustained a head injury in a road traffic accident and was knocked unconscious but recovered on arrival at hospital, when he complained of neck pain. A radiograph of the cervical spine was considered to be normal (and subsequently reported as such by the radiologist).

During the course of the next few days, the patient complained increasingly of weakness in the arms and hands with paraesthesia, weakness of the legs and inability to stand, and interference with bladder function. At first these symptoms were ignored by medical staff; no record was made and no clinical examination was carried out (which would have revealed gross neurological signs in the limbs). It was not until 2 weeks after injury that repeat radiography of the cervical spine confirmed a fracture–dislocation of the cervical spine at the C5–C6 level. Serious permanent disability resulted. The error was that the first radiograph was totally inadequate because C6 and C7 vertebrae were obscured by the shadow of the shoulder joint. The clinician and radiologist failed to appreciate the inadequacies of the radiograph. The error may not have had serious consequences if the patient repeated complaints had been taken seriously and a clinical examination carried out.

This case emphasizes the importance of routine cervical spine radiography in head injury patients and illustrates the importance of checking that the full length of the cervical spine is visible.

Nerve damage

There are two groups of patients which may lead to malpractice litigation: nerve injuries following trauma diagnosed late and iatrogenic nerve injuries.

POST-TRAUMATIC NERVE INJURY

The only way that the incidence of misdiagnosis can be reduced is for the examining doctor in the Accident and Emergency department and fracture clinics to have a high index of suspicion that nerve damage is a possibility after certain injuries. The common examples are laceration on the flexor aspect of the wrist and fingers, supracondylar fractures of the humerus in a child, shoulder dislocations and fractures leading to a compartment syndrome. Routine testing of nerve function by a reasonably experienced clinician and detailed recording of the results is of critical importance.

IATROGENIC NERVE INJURY

This is discussed in more detail in Chapter 27, and was reviewed by Bonney in 1987 and Birch *et al.* in 1991.

Birch has more recently pointed out (1992) that since 1990, the peripheral nerve injury unit at the Royal National Orthopaedic Hospital has treated 44 patients with iatrogenic peripheral nerve injuries, 22 of which occurred during day-case operation procedures; 11 of these resulted from operations on the posterior triangle of the neck, nine from operations on the upper limb, and two following operations for varicose veins. It was exceptional to make an early diagnosis, and in only four patients was the diagnosis made by the operating surgeon who rarely saw the patient again.

The message is clear—day-case surgery is not necessarily a minor procedure; operations should not be done by minor surgeons! Consultants or senior registrar surgeons and anaesthetists who should do this work, must not give in to pressure from management to do more day-case surgery unless they are satisfied with the arrangements for the patient's safety and that the general organization is of an appropriate standard.

Direct damage occurs in the field of operation—usually by cutting, encircling with a ligature, pressure or traction. Traction or pressure may also damage nerves not in the field of operation. Nerve damage is inexcusable and is usually the result of carelessness or the operation has been delegated inappropriately to a junior doctor with inadequate experience. Direct damage may occur from the application of a tourniquet—particularly in susceptible patients (muscle atrophy and lack of subcutaneous fat as seen in some cases of rheumatoid arthritis). Tourniquet damage ought to be preventable if the equipment is regularly serviced, protective padding is applied to the limb and pressure in the upper limb of the adult does not exceed 250 mmHg (200 mmHg for children) and in the lower limb 300 mmHg.

Examples which regularly lead to litigation are damage to the musculocutaneous nerve in the arm, during the anterior approach to the shoulder, the posterior interosseus when exposing the radial head, digital nerves during operations for Dupuytren's contracture, the radial nerve in exposure of the humeral shaft, the sciatic nerve during hip-replacement operations and the accessory nerve during removal of a lymph gland from the posterior triangle of the neck.

It is surprising how often a post-operative nerve injury is treated by a 'wait-and-see' policy. The rule should be that loss of nerve function in the presence of an open wound (traumatic or operative) must be presumed to result from nerve division and early exploration is therefore obligatory. If the affected nerve is not in the field of operation, it may be reasonable to adopt a 'wait-and-see' policy in anticipation that the nerve has been damaged by pressure or traction and that spontaneous recovery will occur; in such cases electromyography after about two weeks may be helpful. Not all orthopaedic surgeons are experienced in treating peripheral nerve injuries. Patients will benefit and litigation will be reduced if these patients are promptly referred to centres with the appropriate expertise.

In operations to remove a malignant tumour, nerves may have to be sacrificed if excision is to be effective; in such cases, the risk must be explained to the patient. It is inexcusable to damage nerves during excision of a benign tumour; a good example is excision of a schwannoma with a portion of nerve trunk on the assumption that it is a ganglion.

Special problems arise with regard to lumbar disc surgery because nerve roots have to be exposed and retracted. Excessive traction can be applied without the surgeon being aware of it. Operative difficulties arise sometimes—excessive bleeding, difficulty with exposure and cerebral spinal fluid leakage are some examples. The disability from nerve damage may be significant and is often permanent. The risk can be reduced to a minimum if a pre-operative myelogram or scan is done, the surgeon is experienced, the patient is properly positioned and given hypotensive anaesthesia, and there must be adequate exposure and gentle handling of nerve roots.

In conclusion, it is worth emphasizing that only a few years ago, if a case of nerve injury came to litigation, the statement of claim would indicate the surgeon failed to explore the nerve at the optimum time, or alternatively no exploration was carried out. The defence would have been that nerve repair would be too difficult or likely to fail. Nowadays such a defence is invalid because of greatly improved nerve repair techniques, including grafting.

CASE REPORTS

These illustrate some of the points made above.

Case 1

A 24-year-old dentist had a Putti–Patt operation for recurrent dislocation of the shoulder, following which he manifested signs of damage to the musculocutaneous nerve. A 'wait-and-see' policy was adopted. The clinical picture of a deep motor paralysis and sensory loss persisted, and even at 8 months no thought was given to the possibility that the nerve might have been divided. No exploration was carried out and it was not until 30 months after the event that he was referred to the orthopaedic expert, when it was clearly too late to produce benefits from surgery.

Case 2

A 60-year-old man had a Charnley total hip replacement for osteoarthritis with moderate protrusio of the acetabulum, performed through a postero-lateral incision. Following the operation he had a sciatic nerve palsy. Two days later, the surgeon explored the nerve and found the medial division had been cut, the proximal end of which was retracted under the gluteus maximus. The surgeon also noted unconstrained cement from the acetabulum, and attributed the nerve injury to a burn from this material. Nothing was done about the nerve injury and an opinion from an expert was not obtained. All the evidence was in favour of surgical division of the nerve but even if cement was responsible it certainly should have been preventable.

Case 3

A 49-year-old man presented with a 3-year history of a lump on the flexor aspect of the wrist, and it was diagnosed as a probable ganglion. An inexperienced junior doctor excised the lump which was described as neuroma arising from a branch of ulnar nerve.

In fact, the tumour was excised with a portion of the motor branch of the ulnar nerve, and histologically proved to be a neurilemmoma. Surprisingly a second opinion was obtained from a plastic surgeon who advised nerve grafting would be required but was likely to fail, so he was never given the chance to obtain the opinion of a nerve repair expert. This sequence of events is not uncommon. It illustrates the fact that minor operations require the skill of a qualified surgeon; an inappropriate delegation, as in this case, is to be deplored.

Vascular damage

Almost all cases that come to litigation are the result of trauma leading to vascular deficiency, which is not recognized until irreversible changes have occurred.

As with peripheral nerve injuries, prompt diagnosis and a high index of suspicion by the examining doctor, and routine assessment of the peripheral circulation in all cases of limb trauma; in the upper limb, a supra-condylar fracture in a child and tibial fracture in adults are the two common sites of vascular trauma.

A compartment syndrome of variable severity is very common after a tibial fracture, and warning symptoms are frequently ignored and the signs of ischaemia are missed, leading to permanent disability from ischaemic changes in the foot and toes. The following case is a good example.

Case history

A 13-year-old boy sustained a displaced and angulated distal tibial fracture which was manipulated into a satisfactory position, and a complete plaster cast was applied; it was not split.

A few hours later he complained of much pain accompanied by a burning sensation in the foot and toes which were swollen. At 48 hours there was evidence of reduced sensation in the toes. He went home on day 5. The plaster was removed at 2 months and since then he has noticed an increasing foot deformity. At 10 years after the fracture (when aged 23) he complained of a burning pain in the ankle, which had persisted since the injury, and inability to put the foot to the ground. He was noticed to have a 45° plantaris deformity, and considerable calf atrophy, claw toes and absent intrinsic muscle function; the skin on the sole of the foot was hypersensitive.

The history and clinical findings are consistent with an ischaemic episode which occurred soon after the application of the plaster.

Even if the diagnosis of compartment syndrome was suspected, a 'wait-and-see' policy is not justified. If splitting the plaster and underlying padding does not rapidly relieve the symptoms and unequivocally restore the circulation, then urgent exploration and decompression is obligatory.

Errors of operative technique

It is clearly impossible to give an account of every possible error. Some of those which occur most often, and following standard procedures, will be discussed.

THE TOURNIQUET

The risks of tourniquet are injury to peripheral nerves which are susceptible to damage by the tourniquet cuff. Certain patients are more susceptible to accepted pressure levels, namely rheumatoid arthritics whose limbs are thin and devoid of subcutaneous fat, some patients with carcinoma, alcoholics and diabetics. With these cases, either special precautions should be taken and protective padding applied, or a tourniquet is avoided. In other patients, it may be that the cuff pressure has been too high. The other principal risk is ischaemia from prolonged use. The operating surgeon is clearly responsible for the application and removal of the tourniquet. To summarize, a generally accepted protocol is as follows: only use a pneumatic-type tourniquet and check the apparatus at regular intervals. It should only be applied under the direct supervision of a surgeon. Record the time of application and removal. Direct damage of normal nerves can be avoided by protecting them with a soft layer of material, and avoiding pressure above 250 mmHg in the adult upper limb (200 mmHg in children) with susceptible nerves and in patients when there is evidence of peripheral vascular disease. A safer approach is to avoid using a tourniquet in such cases.

Most orthopaedic surgeons would accept 1 hour as a safe upper limit for time of application.

OPERATING ON THE WRONG LIMB

This indefensible disaster still occurs occasionally; it is entirely preventable if normal procedures for the preparation of patients for operations are followed.

IATROGENIC NERVE INJURIES

Iatrogenic nerve injuries are discussed in Chapter 27.

Other common intra-operative errors

INTERNAL FIXATION OF FRACTURES

The following examples of internal fixation of fractures illustrate avoidable errors, all of which at one time or another have been subject to litigation and are difficult to defend.

The principal errors here are the use of an inappropriate form of fixation and inadequate technique. This type of operation is frequently delegated to a junior doctor and it needs to be emphasized, therefore, that errors will be avoided if these operations are performed by an experienced and adequately trained surgeon.

Case reports

Case 1. A 36-year-old woman sustained a minimally displaced fracture of the proximal third of the ulna; 6 days later internal fixation with six-hole plate was performed by a senior house officer. At 3 days later the plaster was removed because of hand swelling and she had a sling for the next 11 days. A comment was made from the post-operative radiograph about the poor quality of fixation; four screws passed into the proximal fragment, one through the fracture and one into the distal fragment. A further radiograph was not taken and a plaster-back splint was applied. The next radiograph at 6 weeks showed a loss of fixation and significant angulation of the fracture. It was allowed to unite without correction of the deformity. She was left with an unsightly deformity, 40° loss of supination and 30° loss of pronation.

Due to a technical error, the internal fixation was wholly inadequate, and it is likely that angulation would have occurred, even in a cast.

Case 2. A 25-year-old sustained a compound fracture of the tibia and fibula without complication. He had conservative treatment for a month followed by internal fixation with a plate; the surgeon was an inexperienced junior doctor. Post-operative radiographs showed a 20–25° angulation and 45° of external rotation deformity. As a consequence, he has a clumsy gait with an abnormal foot strike. This relatively common error of operative technique is preventable.

ARTHRODESIS

It is a long-established principle that the joint must be placed in a functional position which will vary accordingly to the joint affected, the patient's occupation, and sex, if footwear is effected.

The usual error is failure to achieve a position of function. The shoulder, hip and knee are not now so commonly fused as hitherto, but the metatarsophalangeal joint of the hallux remains a common site for operation; malposition of the hallux is a frequent occurrence, usually in women.

OSTEOTOMY

Internal fixation is the usual practice for most of these standard and very common orthopaedic procedures. The errors are generally due to poor operative technique; the deformity is not fully corrected and the quality of fixation may be poor, leading to loss of position.

TOTAL HIP REPLACEMENT

Leaving aside the known complications which rarely give rise to litigation, nerve injury — usually the sciatic — and intraoperative fracture of the femoral shaft are the two most common. The fracture results from carelessness during manipulation to dislocate the joint; the joint may be very stiff with protrusio of the acetabulum, and excessive force is used to attempt dislocation of the joint. In other cases the quality of the bone may be poor and it is not recognised by the surgeon. Occasionally fractures occur during insertion of the femoral component and this is inexcusable. If it occurs during revision surgery, it may well be unavoidable and the patient should be warned accordingly.

LUMBAR DISC SURGERY

Failure to relieve symptoms following surgery for a clinically and radiological demonstrable prolapse is likely to be due to operation at the wrong level. It should not occur; negative exploration at the expected level does no harm, but should be followed by exploration above or below as may be appropriate. Nerve root damage has been discussed earlier (p. 1207).

Post-operative deep wound infection

Although it is difficult to generalize, and perhaps unwise to do so, in orthopaedic practice under ideal conditions the overall infection rate should not be higher than 1%. In many centres it is likely to be 0.5% or less. If it is 2%, or higher, then this would not be acceptable to most orthopaedic surgeons.

Infection is recognized as a natural hazard of all surgical procedures; if implants are used, the surgery is complex and lasts several hours, and the patient has poor resistance for some reason, infection is **more** likely to occur. Notwithstanding the natural hazard, the surgeon has a duty to take all reasonable steps to reduce the chance of infection. Some of the more obvious measures under the control of the surgeon are to avoid surgery in the presence of a focus of infection, to avoid too long an exposure of the wound, to handle tissues with care and avoid haematomas and to use suction drainage and prophylactic antibiotics where appropriate. With regard to the last, there is strong evidence that antibiotic-loaded cement significantly reduces the incidence of deep infection, and it is reasonable to suggest that its use is obligatory (see Chapter 15).

Some precautions are relative such as using surgical implants in the presence of a compound wound, and it would be unwise to condemn such a procedure, when clearly in some instances, the practice would be the method of choice.

The consequences of deep infection may vary from delayed discharge from hospital to serious permanent disability. Nevertheless, in the UK the occurrence of deep infection is not usually a reason for litigation. As the following two cases illustrate, patients seek redress in the courts because of failure to diagnose and treat the complication at an early stage.

CASE REPORTS

Case 1

A young woman entered hospital for a meniscectomy, following which her knee remained painful and swollen. A subacute septic arthritis was not diagnosed (and therefore not treated) for several weeks. At diagnosis the articular surface of the joint had been destroyed. After 2 years or so a joint replacement was performed.

Case 2

A young man sustained an Achilles' tendon rupture which was surgically treated. Following deep-wound infection it broke down and the tendon was exposed. Definitive treatment was delayed because the wound infection was thought to be superficial. After a short time, a 5-cm length of tendon had been destroyed leading to permanent and severe loss of calf function.

In both cases, the patient claimed compensation — not for the occurrence of deep infection — but because it was not recognized and treated in the early stages. These two cases illustrate that an error of clinical judgement may be of such a degree that it amounts to negligence (Lord Edmund-Davis, 1981).

CONCLUSIONS

Some of the avoidable injuries to patients that occur in current orthopaedic practice have been outlined. The incidence can be reduced, but probably never eliminated. In conclusion, the following eight points summarize the prerequisites for so doing. No apology is made for stressing these measures, which amount simply to the application of common sense.

1 Improve the supervision of junior doctors by experienced orthopaedic surgeons and Accident and Emergency department consultants.

2 Poor-quality staffed Accident and Emergency departments without expert supervision continue to receive emergencies, including trauma, in some parts of the UK; the number of attending patients whose litigation has been successful, is quite striking. These departments should be closed.

3 History-taking is a neglected art. Inspection of clinical records of many hundreds of patients from a variety of hospitals indicates that the recording of clinical details including the examination, probable diagnosis and suggested treatment, and post-operative day-to-day recording of the patients condition, are not only deficient but frequently illegible and unsigned. The nursing records generally set a standard which highlights these deficiencies.

4 Only orthopaedic surgeons — some of whom will have special experience — should treat patients after trauma to bones, joints, nerves, muscles and tendons.

5 All patients after trauma, and those referred by general practitioners for an opinion, should be seen by a senior registrar or consultant.

6 No patient should have elective surgery unless first seen by a consultant or senior registrar.

7 Operations must be undertaken only by surgeons

with the appropriate qualifications and experience — usually a consultant, senior registrar or registrar. The same applies to the discharge of patients from the ward.

8 Finally, and perhaps most important of all, more time must be spent talking to patients and listening to their complaints. If something untoward occurs, it is especially important to explain matters, and answer questions truthfully and give appropriate reassurance.

Litigation will not arise if the normal accepted standards of practice are maintained. The amount of litigation that may follow from a medical accident is for the most part inversely proportional to the quality of communication with the patient.

REFERENCES

Birch R. (1992) Letter. *J. Med. Def. Union* 8(3), p. 71.

Birch R., Bonney G., Dowell J. and Hollingdale J. (1991) Iatrogenic injuries of peripheral nerves. *J. Bone Joint Surg.* **73B**, 280.

Bonney G. (1987) Iatrogenic injuries of nerves. *J. Med. Def. Union* no. 3, p. 4 and no. 3, p. 2.

British Orthopaedic Association (1992) *The Management of Skeletal Trauma in the UK.* London, BOA.

Buck N., Devlin H.B. and Lunn J.N. (1987) *The Confidential Enquiry into Perioperative Deaths.* London, Nuffield Provincial Hospital Trust, King's Fund.

Campling E.A., Devlin H.B., Hoile R.W. and Lunn J.N. (1992) *The Report of the National Confidential Inquiry into Perioperative Deaths, 1990,* London, Nuffield Provincial Hospital Trust, King's Fund.

Clyde Lord, Hunter N. and Hanley V. (1985) SGT, 213.

Edmund-Davis Lord (1981) *Whitehouse* v. *Jordan* 1, Aller 26.

Glyn T.T. (1986) Orthopaedic manholes and rabbit holes: some thoughts on medical negligence. *J. Law Soc. Med.* 79, 701.

Harris N.H. (1990) *Medical Negligence.* London, Butterworth Law, p. 659.

Medical Defence Union (1986) Economics and the National Health Service; are doctors liable? *J. Med. Def. Union*, 1, 1.

Lacombe D.C. and O'Keefe T.J. (1989) Legal aspects of medical practice for the orthopaedic surgeon. *Curr. Orthop.* 3, p. 115.

Powers M.J. and Harris N.H. (1994) *Medical Negligence.* London, Butterworths.

Scarman Lord (1983) *Maynard* v. *West Midlands Health Authority,* 1WLR.

Vickers R. (1991) Risk management in trauma and orthopaedics. *J. Med. Def. Union* 7(3), 72.

Woodyard J. (1990) Orthopaedic negligence: the tip of the iceberg? *J. Hosp. Med.* 44, 163.

Index

Page numbers in *italic* refer to figures and/or tables